RANG & DALE'S

Pharmacology

Image on the cover shows an siRNA-loaded RISC (RNAi-induced silencing complex) cleaving and degrading a target mRNA.
Image credit: Alnylam Pharmaceuticals.

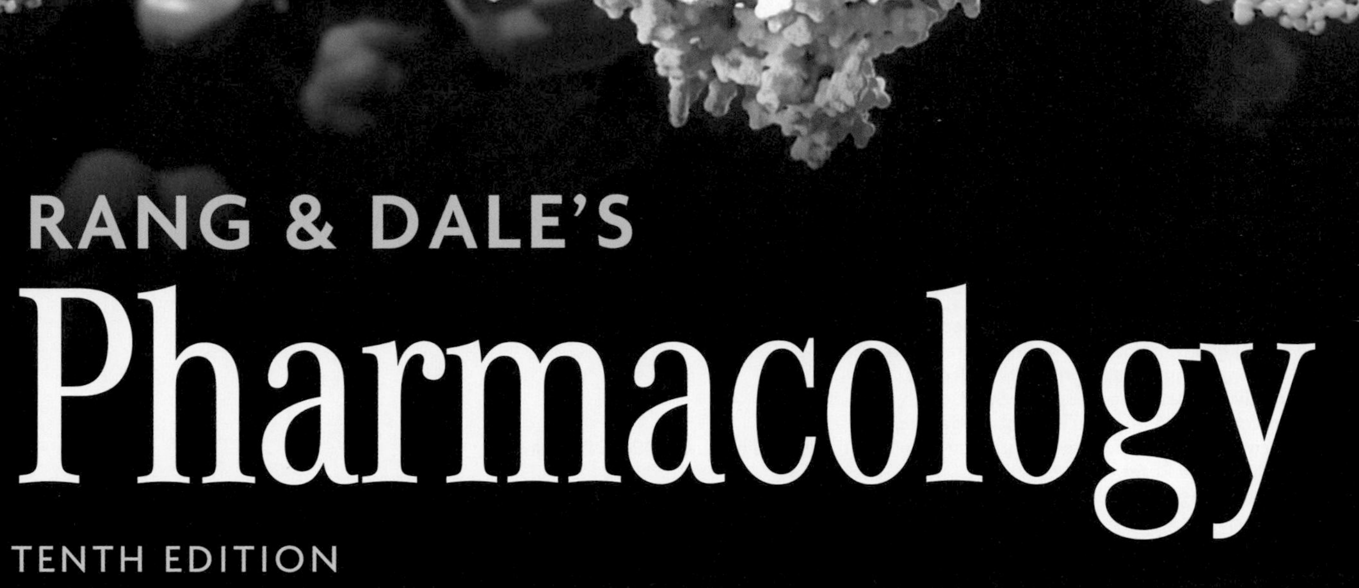

RANG & DALE'S

Pharmacology

TENTH EDITION

JAMES M. RITTER
DPhil FRCP HonFBPhS FMedSci
Emeritus Professor of Clinical Pharmacology
King's College London
London, United Kingdom

ROD FLOWER
PhD LLD DSc HonFBPhS FMedSci FRS
Emeritus Professor of Pharmacology
Bart's and the London School of Medicine
Queen Mary, University of London
London, United Kingdom

GRAEME HENDERSON
PhD, FRSB, HonFBPhS
Professor of Pharmacology
University of Bristol
Bristol, United Kingdom

YOON KONG LOKE
MBBS MD FRCP FBPhS
Professor of Medicine and Pharmacology
Norwich Medical School, University of East Anglia
Norwich, United Kingdom

DAVID MacEWAN
PhD FRSB FBPhS SFHEA
Professor of Molecular Pharmacology/Toxicology
Deputy Executive Dean
University of Liverpool
Liverpool, United Kingdom

EMMA ROBINSON
PhD FBPhS
Professor of Psychopharmacology
University of Bristol
Bristol, United Kingdom

JAMES FULLERTON
MA MBChB MRCP PhD FHEA
Associate Professor of Clinical Therapeutics
University of Oxford
Consultant in Acute General Medicine and Clinical Pharmacology
Oxford University Hospitals NHS Foundation Trust
Oxford, United Kingdom

Visit Elsevier eBooks+ (eBooks.Health.Elsevier.com) for additional online content

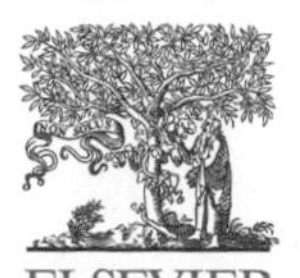

London New York Oxford Philadelphia St Louis Sydney 2024

Potential Competing Financial Interests Statements for Rang & Dale 10E (2018–2022)
JMR: has no competing financial interest to declare.
RJF: serves as a board member for Antibe Therapeutics.
GH: has no competing financial interests to declare.
YKL: has received consultancy fees from Syri Ltd.
DJM: has no competing financial interests to declare.
ER: has received collaborative research funding from Boehringer Ingelheim, COMPASS Pathways, Eli Lilly, MSD and Pfizer.
JF: has no competing financial interests to declare.

Notice

Practitioners and researchers must always rely on their own experience and knowledge in evaluating and using any information, methods, compounds or experiments described herein. Because of rapid advances in the medical sciences, in particular, independent verification of diagnoses and drug dosages should be made. To the fullest extent of the law, no responsibility is assumed by Elsevier, authors, editors or contributors for any injury and/or damage to persons or property as a matter of products liability, negligence or otherwise, or from any use or operation of any methods, products, instructions, or ideas contained in the material herein.

ISBN: 978-0-323-87395-6
IE ISBN: 978-0-323-87396-3

Senior Content Strategist: Alexandra Mortimer
Content Development Specialist: Nicholas Henderson
Project Manager: Joanna Souch
Design: Renee Duenow
Marketing Manager: Deborah Watkins

Printed in the UK

Last digit is the print number: 9 8 7 6 5 4 3 2 1

Contents

SECTION 1 General principles

SECTION 2 Chemical mediators

SECTION 5 Drugs used for the treatment of infections and cancer

Self-assessment questions compiled by Dr. Christine Edmead, University of Bath, are available through eBooks.Health.Elsevier.com

Video and Case Study Contents

 Online content accessible via https://ebooks.health.elsevier.com using the pin in the front of the book.

VIDEOS

In conversation with Humphrey Rang
Interview with Humphrey Rang of *Rang & Dale's Pharmacology* textbook. In discussion with David MacEwan, Humphrey recalls the history and development of the textbook and reflects on his distinguished career.

In conversation with Jim Ritter
Interview with Jim Ritter, author of *Rang & Dale's Pharmacology* textbook. In discussion with David MacEwan, Jim reflects on how the textbook has developed during his time as one of the longest-serving authors.

In conversation with Rod Flower
Interview with Rod Flower, one of the earliest authors of *Rang & Dale's Pharmacology* textbook. In conversation, Rod reflects on changes during his time working on the popular textbook.

In conversation with Graeme Henderson
Interview with Graeme Henderson, author of *Rang & Dale's Pharmacology* textbook. Here, Graeme reflects on how the textbook has developed during his time as its Editor and how *Rang & Dale's Pharmacology* has impacted the teaching of pharmacology and drug use over the years.

In conversation with Yoon Loke
Interview with Yoon Loke, author of *Rang & Dale's Pharmacology* textbook. In dialogue with David MacEwan, Yoon discusses his experiences co-authoring the successful textbook and how it has influenced teaching of pharmacology to medical students.

In conversation with Emma Robinson
Interview with Emma Robinson, one of the most recent co-authors of *Rang & Dale's Pharmacology* textbook. In discussion, Emma discusses her early impressions as co-author of the successful book, and how she tries to incorporate her own teaching method into the textbook.

In conversation with James Fullerton
Interview with James Fullerton, co-author of *Rang & Dale's Pharmacology* textbook. In discussion with David MacEwan, James discusses his impressions of the textbook and how it influences how medical school students learn about drugs, applying that knowledge in the clinic.

Pharmacology in practice: clinical overdose
Topic video with Adam Danashmend, clinical registrar in London. Adam gives his advice on the importance of pharmacology to doctors, and opioid overdose cases in the clinic.

Pharmacology in practice: role of pharmacology in undergraduate medical education
Dr Mohammad Sarwar describes the clinical use of anaesthetics and pain relief in preoperative, operative and postoperative clinical settings, to inform students of the most appropriate drug combinations used by anaesthesiologists.

Pharmacology in practice: importance of chemistry, drug-receptor interactions and pharmacokinetics to people who use opioids
Rang & Dale author Graeme Henderson describes opioid use and misuse, outlining how agonists and antagonists are used on the street and the pharmacological knowledge underlying their use.

Pharmacology in practice: investigation of the frequency of narcotic misuse
Pharmacology graduate Meurig Shotton describes his project analysing the purity of narcotics and use of cutting-agents in social nonclinical settings, such as music festivals.

Topic: what are drugs and how do they work? Understanding receptor theory better
Rang & Dale author David MacEwan describes drugs, receptors and receptor theory in more depth to help students understand these pharmacology basics.

Topic: enzyme inducers and inhibitor – the logical approach
Rang & Dale author Yoon Loke describes how enzyme inducers and inhibitors have the ability to modify the actions of other drugs taken concurrently.

CASE STUDIES

Rang & Dale's Pharmacology Tenth Edition Preface

'Things will have to change in order that they remain the same.' (Prince Don Fabrizio Salina, in Il Gattopardo*)*

'Pharmacology', first published by Churchill Livingstone in 1987 and dedicated to the memory of Professor HO Schild, was the brainchild of Humphrey Rang. Its predecessor, Schild's *'Applied Pharmacology'*, set a standard that the authors tried to maintain. *'Rang & Dale's Pharmacology'*, as it is now known, has gone through nine editions and been published in 11 languages since the fifth edition. This present (tenth) edition is the first that has not benefitted from Humphrey's hands-on leadership and, while he remains very much alive and kicking, we have tried in a similar spirit to maintain the standards that he has set over the past 35 years. In this spirit, and in line with the sentiment expressed by Prince Don Fabrizio and quoted above, we have welcomed two younger colleagues Professor Emma Robinson (Bristol) and Dr James Fullerton (Oxford) who have ably assisted us in writing this present edition.

In this edition, as in its predecessors, we set out not just to describe what drugs do but to explain the mechanisms by which they act. This entails analysis of physiological mechanisms and pathological disturbances at the cellular and molecular level. Pharmacology has its roots in therapeutics as well as in organic chemistry and biotechnology, so we have attempted to make the link between effects at the molecular and cellular level and the range of beneficial and harmful effects that humans experience when drugs are used for therapeutic or other reasons. Many psychoactive drugs are not prescribed as medicines or sold over the counter. Some of these are widely used for pleasure, especially by young people, sometimes with harmful consequences. While our main emphasis is on therapeutic use, psychoactive drugs, drug addiction and tolerance are also covered. Similarly, there is a chapter on drugs used (or abused) in sport and for other lifestyle purposes.

Pharmacology remains a fast-moving field. In 2021 the European Medicines Agency approved 54 new active substances. Of these, seven related to COVID-19 but other indications were also widely represented: other infections (two), cardiovascular (three), metabolic (two), reproduction (three), gastro-intestinal (one), neurological (five), endocrine (four), skin (three), eyes (two), rheumatology (three), haematology (five), cancer (12) and vaccines other than those directed against SARS-CoV2 (two). In previous editions we have not covered vaccines, whether live attenuated organisms or nonliving material derived from pathogenic organisms, opting to concentrate on molecular entities of defined chemical structure. The current wave of vaccines do have defined chemical structures that act as specific targets for the immune cells of the recipient, and we mention these in relevant sections such as that on COVID-19 in the chapter on antiviral drugs, but without going into detail. Macromolecular drugs (including monoclonal antibody and RNA drugs) that act specifically to cause effects in the host via high affinity binding to targets such as surface membrane receptors represent a new frontier in pharmacology. They contrast in pharmacokinetics, specificity, therapeutic efficacy and range of harmful effects from the small molecule chemical entities that still constitute the main armamentarium of therapeutic drugs. They are covered in greater depth than the novel vaccines in the relevant organ-specific chapters, and the chapter on biopharmaceuticals has been completely revised and updated and now includes a much larger section on RNA drugs. We also, as in previous editions, cover drugs such as anaesthetics and immunosuppressants that enable other therapeutic modalities such as surgery and transplantation. The surprisingly tricky question of 'what is a drug?' raised by such distinctions is addressed in more detail in Chapter 1.

Pharmacology is a lively scientific discipline in its own right, with an importance beyond that of providing a basis for the use of drugs in therapy or for other purposes, and we aim to provide a firm background, not only for future doctors but also for scientists and practitioners of other disciplines such as pharmacy and other professions allied to medicine, especially those who contemplate the possibility of a career in drug discovery and development, which are covered in a separate chapter. We have therefore, where appropriate, described how drugs are used as probes for elucidating cellular and physiological functions, even when they have no clinical use.

Nomenclature. Names of drugs and related chemicals are established through usage and sometimes there is more than one name in common use. For prescribing purposes, it is important to use standard names, and we follow as far as possible the World Health Organization's list of recommended international non-proprietary names (rINNs). Sometimes these conflict with the familiar names, e.g. amphetamine becomes amfetamine in the rINN list, and the endogenous mediator prostaglandin I_2, the standard name in the scientific literature, becomes 'epoprostenol'– a name unfamiliar to most scientists – in the rINN list. Some trade names have become so familiar as to be widely used outside their original remit. UK consumers once talked of 'hoovering the carpet', and among consumers (patients, doctors and others) 'Heroin', the Bayer trade mark for diamorphine, was similarly colloquialized and extended from the synthetic product to various resins and mixtures obtained by acetylating opium extract; diamorphine (the rINN) is preferred. The same goes for more recent instances (e.g. Herceptin/trastuzumab and Viagra/sildenafil), but with the caveat for prescribers and pharmacists that there are cases where prescribing by trade name is recommended by the British National Formulary because of clinically important pharmacokinetic differences between products. In general, we use rINN names as far as possible in the context of therapeutic use, but often use the common name in describing mediators and familiar drugs. Sometimes English and American usage varies (as with adrenaline/epinephrine and noradrenaline/

norepinephrine). Adrenaline and noradrenaline are the official names in EU member states and relate clearly to terms such as 'noradrenergic', 'adrenoceptor' and 'adrenal gland' and we prefer them for these reasons.

Organization. Drug action can be understood only in the context of what else is happening in the body. So, at the beginning of most chapters, we briefly discuss the physiological and biochemical processes relevant to the action of the drugs described in that chapter. As regards the chemical structures of drugs, we have included these only where this helps in understanding how those drugs act or are handled by the body, since chemical structures are readily available for reference online.

The overall organisation of the book has been retained, with sections covering: (1) the general principles of drug action; (2) the chemical mediators and cellular mechanisms with which drugs interact in producing their therapeutic or other effects; (3) the action of drugs on specific organ systems; (4) the action of drugs on the nervous system; (5) the action of drugs used to treat infectious diseases and cancer; (6) a range of special topics comprising harmful effects of drugs, lifestyle drugs and drugs in sport and drug discovery and development. This organization reflects our belief that drug action needs to be understood, not as mere description of the effects of individual drugs and their uses, but as a chemical intervention that perturbs the complex network of chemical and cellular signalling that underlies the function of any living organism. In addition to updating all of the chapters, we have, within this general plan, reorganised the text in various ways, to keep abreast of modern developments:

- A completely revised 'biopharmaceuticals' chapter (Ch. 5) updated and now including a much larger section on RNA drugs.
- Chapter 24 *Haemopoietic system and treatment of anaemia*: updated to incorporate recent advances in oxygen sensing and response to reduced oxygen tension, with a new figure, and safe and effective drugs stemming from this (e.g. daprodustat)
- A new chapter on drugs and the eye (Ch. 27) has been included.
- Chapter 40 *Neurodegenerative diseases,* has been rewritten to broaden its focus on Alzheimer's disease to include other forms of dementia (dementia associated with Lewy bodies and vascular dementia) and their treatment.
- A new chapter (Ch. 42) on the pharmacological management of headache (includes the new CGRP antagonists for migraine prophylaxis)
- Chapter 43 *Analgesic drugs*: a new section on drug treatment of chronic pain.
- A revised chapter (Ch.51) on 'Basic principles of antimicrobial therapy' featuring new diagrams illustrating sites of action of antibiotics at ribosomes.
- A completely revised chapter (Ch. 53) on antivirals incorporating more information on their mode of replication and a section on COVID-19.
- A significantly updated chapter on Anticancer drugs (Ch. 57) which incorporates the great expansion in different types of new anticancer agents that have exploded into the clinic setting in recent years.
- A new section on the background to drug discovery highlighting the current successes and future potential of small interfering RNA drugs in structure-based drug design which appear set to access many new drug targets and revolutionise medicine.

In selecting new material for inclusion, we have taken into account not only new agents but also recent extensions of basic knowledge that presage further drug development. And where possible, we have given a brief outline of new treatments in the pipeline. We have cut out drugs that have become obsolete, and theories that have had their day.

References and further reading lists are largely restricted to guidance on further reading and review articles that list key original papers.

ACKNOWLEDGEMENTS

We would like to thank the following for their help and advice in writing this edition: Dr Peggy Frith, Professor Eamonn Kelly, Dr Jan Melichar, Dr Katy Sutcliffe, Professor Andrew Owen and Dr William Brown.

We would also like to thank Dr Christine Edmead for her work on the self-assessment questions which are available as additional material in the online edition of this book.

We would like to put on record our appreciation of the team at Elsevier who worked on this edition: Alexandra Mortimer (content strategist), Nicholas Henderson (content development specialist) and Joanna Souch (project manager).

We are also very grateful to readers who have taken the trouble to write to us with constructive comments and suggestions. We have done our best to incorporate these. Comments on the new edition will be welcome.

James M. Ritter
Rod Flower
Graeme Henderson
Yoon Kong Loke
David MacEwan
Emma Robinson
James Fullerton

1 What is pharmacology?

OVERVIEW

In this introductory chapter we explain how pharmacology came into being and evolved as a scientific discipline and describe the present-day structure of the subject, how it continues to develop and its links to other biomedical sciences. The structure that has emerged forms the basis of the organisation of the rest of the book. Readers in a hurry to get to the here-and-now of pharmacology can safely skip this chapter.

WHAT IS A DRUG?

For the purposes of this book, a drug can be defined as *a chemical substance of known structure, other than a nutrient or an essential dietary ingredient,*[1] *which, when administered to a living organism, produces a biological effect.*

A few points are worth noting. Drugs may be synthetic chemicals, chemicals obtained from plants or animals or products of biotechnology (biopharmaceuticals). A *medicine* is a chemical preparation, which usually, but not necessarily, contains one or more drugs, administered with the intention of producing a therapeutic effect. Medicines usually contain other substances (excipients, stabilisers, solvents, etc.) besides the active drug, to make them more convenient to use. To count as a drug, the substance must be administered as such, rather than released by physiological mechanisms. Many substances, such as insulin or thyroxine, are endogenous hormones but are also drugs when they are administered intentionally. Many drugs are not used commonly in medicine but are nevertheless useful research tools. The definition of a drug also covers toxins, one or two of which are administered in the clinic whilst many are critical pharmacological tools. In everyday parlance, the word *drug* is often associated with psychoactive substances and addiction – unfortunate negative connotations that tend to bias uninformed opinion against any form of chemical therapy. In this book we focus mainly on drugs used for therapeutic purposes but also describe psychoactive drugs, lifestyle drugs as well as drugs used in sport to enhance performance and provide important examples of drugs used as experimental tools. Poisons fall strictly within the definition of drugs, and indeed 'all drugs are poisons… it is only the dose which makes a thing poison' (an aphorism credited to Paracelsus, a 16th century Swiss physician); conversely, poisons may be effective therapeutic agents when administered in sub-toxic doses. Botulinum toxin ('Botox', see Ch. 14) provides a striking example: it is the most potent poison known in terms of its lethal dose but is widely used both medically and cosmetically. General aspects of harmful effects of drugs are considered in Chapter 58. Toxicology is the study of toxic effects of chemical substances (including drugs), and toxicological testing is undertaken on new chemical entities during their development as potential medicinal products (see Ch. 60), but the subject is not otherwise covered in this book.

Historically the definition of a drug – a chemical substance of known structure – precluded vaccines being included as drugs given that typically they were preparations of antigens made from weakened or killed forms of microbes or viruses, their toxins or their surface proteins. Modern vaccine technology now uses sequences of DNA or RNA of known structure, allowing them to come under our definition of a drug.

ORIGINS AND ANTECEDENTS

Pharmacology can be defined as the study of the effects of drugs on the function of living systems. As a science, it was born in the mid-19th century, one of a host of new biomedical sciences based on principles of experimentation rather than dogma or intuition that came into being in that remarkable period. Long before that – indeed from the dawn of civilisation – herbal remedies were widely used, pharmacopoeias were written, and the apothecaries' trade flourished. However, nothing resembling scientific principles was applied to therapeutics, which was known at that time as *materia medica.*[2] Even Robert Boyle, who laid the scientific foundations of chemistry in the middle of the 17th century, was content, when dealing with therapeutics (*A Collection of Choice Remedies*, 1692), to recommend concoctions of worms, dung, urine and the moss from a dead man's skull. The impetus for pharmacology came from the need to improve the outcome of therapeutic intervention by doctors, who were at that time skilled at clinical observation and diagnosis but broadly ineffectual when it came to treatment.[3] Until the late 19th century, knowledge of the normal and abnormal functioning of the body was too rudimentary to provide even a rough basis for understanding drug effects; at the same time, disease and death were regarded as semi-sacred subjects, appropriately dealt with by authoritarian inclinations, rather than scientific doctrines. Clinical practice often displayed an

[1]Like most definitions, this one has its limits. For example, there are a number of essential dietary constituents, such as iron and various vitamins, which are used as medicines. Furthermore, some biological products (e.g. **epoietin**) show batch-to-batch variation in their chemical constitution that significantly affects their properties. There is also the study of pharmaceutical-grade nutrients or 'nutraceuticals'.

[2]The name persists today in some ancient universities, being attached to chairs of what we would call clinical pharmacology.

[3]Oliver Wendell Holmes, an eminent physician, wrote in 1860: '[I] firmly believe that if the whole materia medica, as now used, could be sunk to the bottom of the sea, it would be all the better for mankind and the worse for the fishes' (see Porter, 1997).

obedience to authority and ignored what appeared to be easily ascertainable facts. For example, cinchona bark was recognised as a specific and effective treatment for malaria, and a sound protocol for its use was laid down by Lind in 1765. In 1804, however, Johnson declared it to be unsafe until the fever had subsided, and he recommended instead the use of large doses of calomel (mercurous chloride) in the early stages – a murderous piece of advice that was slavishly followed for the next 40 years.

The motivation for understanding what drugs can and cannot do came from clinical practice, but the science could be built only on the basis of secure foundations in physiology, pathology and chemistry. It was not until 1858 that Virchow proposed the cell theory. The first use of a structural formula to describe a chemical compound was in 1868. Bacteria as a cause of disease were discovered by Pasteur in 1878. Previously, pharmacology hardly had the legs to stand on, and we may wonder at the bold vision of Rudolf Buchheim, who created the first pharmacology institute (in his own house) in Estonia in 1847.

In its beginnings, before the advent of synthetic organic chemistry, pharmacology concerned itself exclusively with understanding the effects of natural substances, mainly plant extracts – and a few (mainly toxic) chemicals such as mercury and arsenic. An early development in chemistry was the purification of active compounds from plants. Friedrich Sertürner, a young German apothecary, purified morphine from opium in 1805. Other substances quickly followed, and, even though their structures were unknown, these compounds showed that chemicals, not magic or vital forces, were responsible for the effects that plant extracts produced on living organisms. Early pharmacologists focused most of their attention on such plant-derived drugs as quinine, digitalis, atropine, ephedrine, strychnine and others (many of which are still used today and will have become old friends by the time you have finished reading this book).[4]

PHARMACOLOGY IN THE 20TH AND 21ST CENTURIES

Beginning in the 20th century, the fresh wind of synthetic chemistry began to revolutionise the pharmaceutical industry, and with it the science of pharmacology. New synthetic drugs, such as barbiturates and local anaesthetics, began to appear, and the era of antimicrobial chemotherapy began with the discovery by Paul Ehrlich in 1909 of arsenical compounds for treating syphilis. Around the same time, William Blair-Bell was world renowned for his pioneering work at Liverpool in the treatment of breast cancers with another relatively poisonous agent, lead colloid mixtures. The thinking was that, yes, drugs were toxic, but they were slightly more toxic to a microbe or cancer cell. This early chemotherapy has laid the foundations for much of the antimicrobial and anticancer therapies still used today. Further breakthroughs came when the sulfonamides, the first antibacterial drugs, were discovered by Gerhard Domagk in 1935 and with the development of penicillin by Chain and Florey during the Second World War, based on the earlier work of Fleming.

These few well-known examples show how the growth of synthetic chemistry, and the resurgence of natural product chemistry, caused a dramatic revitalisation of therapeutics in the first half of the 20th century. Each new drug class that emerged gave pharmacologists a new challenge, and it was then that pharmacology really established its identity and its status among the biomedical sciences.

In parallel with the exuberant proliferation of therapeutic molecules – driven mainly by chemistry – which gave pharmacologists so much to think about, physiology was also making rapid progress, particularly in relation to chemical mediators, which are discussed in depth throughout this book. Many hormones, neurotransmitters and inflammatory mediators were discovered in this period, and the realisation that chemical communication plays a central role in almost every regulatory mechanism that our bodies possess immediately established a large area of common ground between physiology and pharmacology, for interactions between chemical substances and living systems were exactly what pharmacologists had been preoccupied with from the outset. Indeed, these fields have developed hand-in-hand as wherever there is either a physiological or pathological mechanism, pharmacology could be there to exploit it with a drug. The concept of 'receptors' for chemical mediators, first proposed by Langley in 1905, was quickly taken up by pharmacologists such as Clark, Gaddum, Schild and others and is a constant theme in present-day pharmacology (as you will soon discover as you plough through the next two chapters). The receptor concept, and the technologies developed from it, have had a massive impact on drug discovery and therapeutics. Biochemistry also emerged as a distinct science early in the 20th century, and the discovery of enzymes and the delineation of biochemical pathways provided yet another framework for understanding drug effects. The picture of pharmacology that emerges from this brief glance at history (Fig. 1.1) is of a subject evolved from ancient prescientific therapeutics, involved in commerce from the 17th century onwards, and which gained respectability by donning the trappings of science as soon as this became possible in the mid-19th century. Pharmacology grew rapidly in partnership with the evolution of organic chemistry and other biomedical sciences, and was quick to assimilate the dramatic advances in molecular and cell biology in the late 20th century. Now, in the 21st century, we are in the exciting new era of molecular modelling. The elucidation of protein structures at the atomistic level, especially of receptor proteins, allows the use of high-powered in silico modelling and mathematical simulation approaches to reveal how drugs interact with receptors and ion channels. As well as telling us more about how current drugs work, such approaches are revolutionising the design of new drugs.

[4]A handful of synthetic substances achieved pharmacological prominence long before the era of synthetic chemistry began. Diethyl ether, first prepared as 'sweet oil of vitriol' in the 16th century, and nitrous oxide, prepared by Humphrey Davy in 1799, were used to liven up parties before being introduced as anaesthetic agents in the mid-19th century (see Ch. 41). Amyl nitrite (see Ch. 19) was made in 1859 and can claim to be the first 'rational' therapeutic drug; its therapeutic effect in angina was predicted on the basis of its physiological effects – a true 'pharmacologist's drug' and the smelly forerunner of the nitrovasodilators that are widely used today. Aspirin (Ch. 25), the most widely used therapeutic drug in history, was first synthesised in 1853, with no therapeutic application in mind. It was rediscovered in 1897 in the laboratories of the German company Bayer, who were seeking a less toxic derivative of salicylic acid. Bayer commercialised aspirin in 1899 and made a fortune.

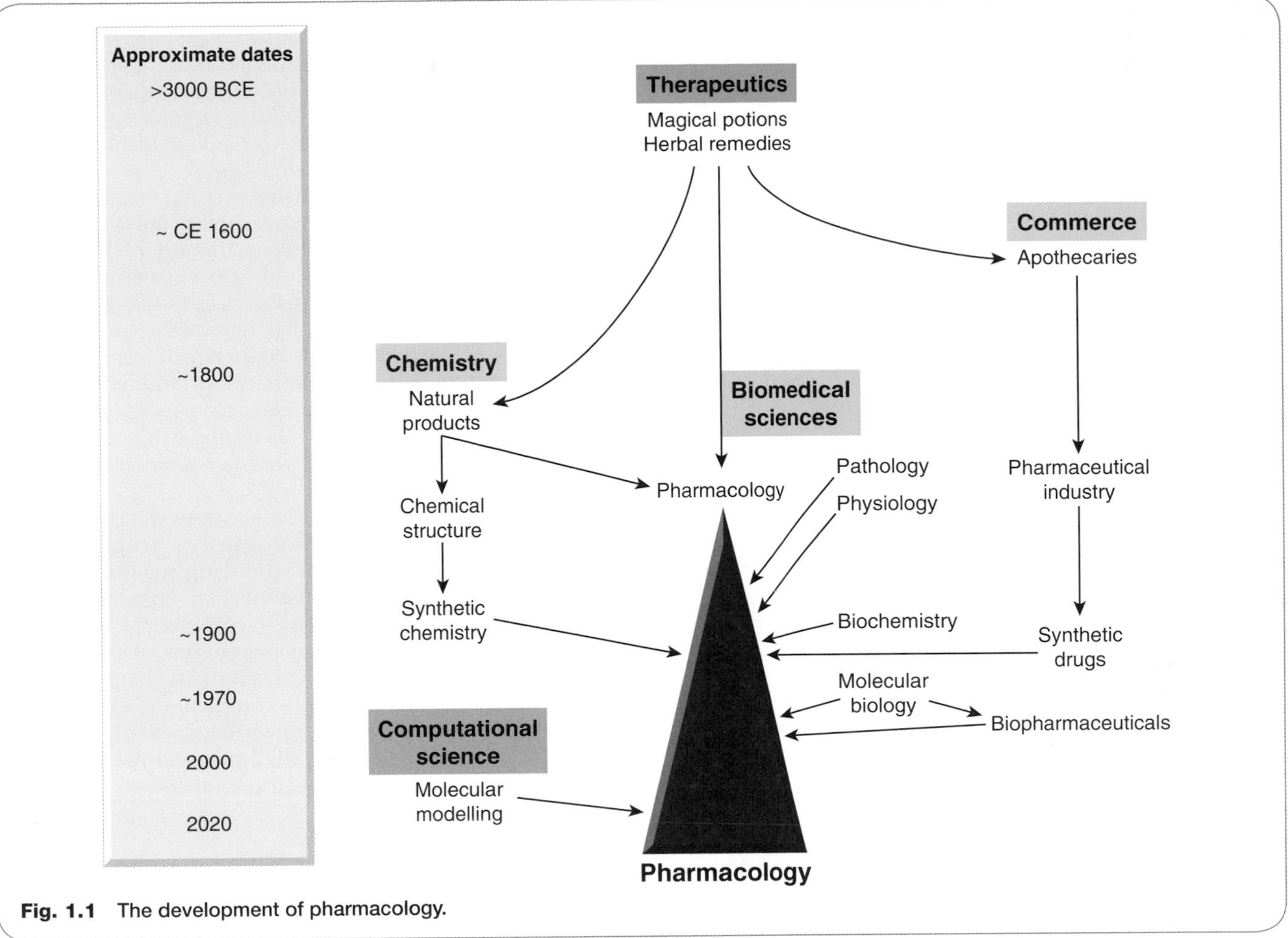

Fig. 1.1 The development of pharmacology.

ALTERNATIVE THERAPEUTIC PRINCIPLES

Modern medicine relies heavily on drugs as the main tool of therapeutics. Other therapeutic procedures, such as surgery, vaccination, diet, exercise, psychological treatments, radiotherapy, etc., are also important, of course, as is deliberate non-intervention, but none is so widely applied as drug-based therapeutics.

Before the advent of science-based approaches, repeated attempts were made to construct systems of therapeutics, many of which produced even worse results than pure empiricism. One of these was *allopathy*, espoused by James Gregory (1735–1821). The favoured remedies included bloodletting, emetics and purgatives, which were used until the dominant symptoms of the disease were suppressed. Many patients died from such treatment, and it was in reaction against it that Hahnemann introduced the practice of *homeopathy* in the early 19th century. The implausible guiding principles of homeopathy are:

- like cures like
- activity can be enhanced by dilution

The system rapidly drifted into absurdity: for example, Hahnemann recommended the use of drugs at dilutions of $1{:}10^{60}$, equivalent to one molecule in a sphere the size of the orbit of Neptune.

Many other systems of therapeutics have come and gone, and the variety of dogmatic principles that they embodied have tended to hinder rather than advance scientific progress. Currently, therapeutic systems that have a basis that lies outside the domain of science remain popular under the general banner of 'alternative' or 'complementary' medicine. Mostly, they reject the 'medical model', which attributes disease to an underlying derangement of normal function that can be defined in physiological or structural terms, scientifically detected by objective means, and influenced beneficially by appropriate chemical or physical interventions. They focus instead mainly on subjective malaise, which may be disease associated or not. Abandoning objectivity in defining and measuring disease goes along with a similar departure from scientific principles in assessing therapeutic efficacy and risk, with the result that principles and practices can gain acceptance without satisfying any of the criteria of validity that would convince a critical scientist, and that are required by law to be satisfied before a new drug can be introduced into therapy. Demand for 'alternative' therapies by the general public, alas, has little to do with demonstrable efficacy.[6]

[6]The UK Medicines and Healthcare Regulatory Agency (MHRA) requires detailed evidence of therapeutic efficacy based on controlled clinical trials before a new drug is registered, but no clinical trials data for homeopathic products or for the many herbal remedies that were on sale before the Medicines Act of 1968.

THE EMERGENCE OF BIOTECHNOLOGY

Since the 1980s, biotechnology has emerged as a major source of new therapeutic agents in the form of antibodies, enzymes, various regulatory proteins, oligonucleotides and DNA/RNA vaccines (Clark and Pazderink, 2015; Theobold, 2020). Although such products (known as *biopharmaceuticals*) are generally produced by genetic engineering rather than by synthetic chemistry, the pharmacological principles are essentially the same as for conventional drugs, although the details of absorption, distribution and elimination, specificity, harmful effects and clinical effectiveness all differ markedly between high-molecular-weight biopharmaceuticals and low-molecular-weight drugs – as does their cost! In recent years the development of gene- and cell-based therapies has gathered pace, taking therapeutics into a new domain (see Ch. 5). The principles governing gene suppression, gene editing to repair faulty genes (notably through advances in CRISPR-Cas9 gene-editing technologies) and the design, delivery and control of functioning artificial genes introduced into cells, or of engineered cells introduced into the body, are very different from those of drug-based therapeutics and require a different conceptual framework.

PHARMACOLOGY TODAY

As with other biomedical disciplines, the boundaries of pharmacology are not sharply defined, nor are they constant. Its exponents are, as befits pragmatists, ever ready to poach on the territory and techniques of other disciplines. If it ever had a conceptual and technical core that it could really call its own, this has now dwindled almost to the point of extinction, and the subject is defined by its purpose – to understand what drugs do to living organisms, and more particularly how their effects can be applied to therapeutics – rather than by its scientific coherence.

Fig. 1.2 shows the structure of pharmacology as it appears today. Within the main subject fall a number of compartments (neuropharmacology, immunopharmacology, pharmacokinetics, etc.), which are convenient, if not watertight, subdivisions. These topics form the main subject matter of this book. Around the edges are several interface disciplines, not covered in this book, which form important two-way bridges between pharmacology and other fields of biomedicine. Pharmacology tends to have more of these than other disciplines. Recent arrivals on the fringe are subjects such as pharmacogenomics, pharmacoepidemiology and pharmacoeconomics.

Pharmacogenomics. Pharmacogenetics, the study of genetic influences on responses to drugs, initially focused on familial idiosyncratic drug reactions, where affected individuals show an abnormal – usually adverse – response to a class of drug (see Nebert and Weber, 1990). Rebranded as pharmacogenomics, it now covers broader genetically based variations in drug response, where the genetic basis is more complex, the aim being to use genetic information to guide the choice of drug therapy on an individual basis – so-called personalised medicine

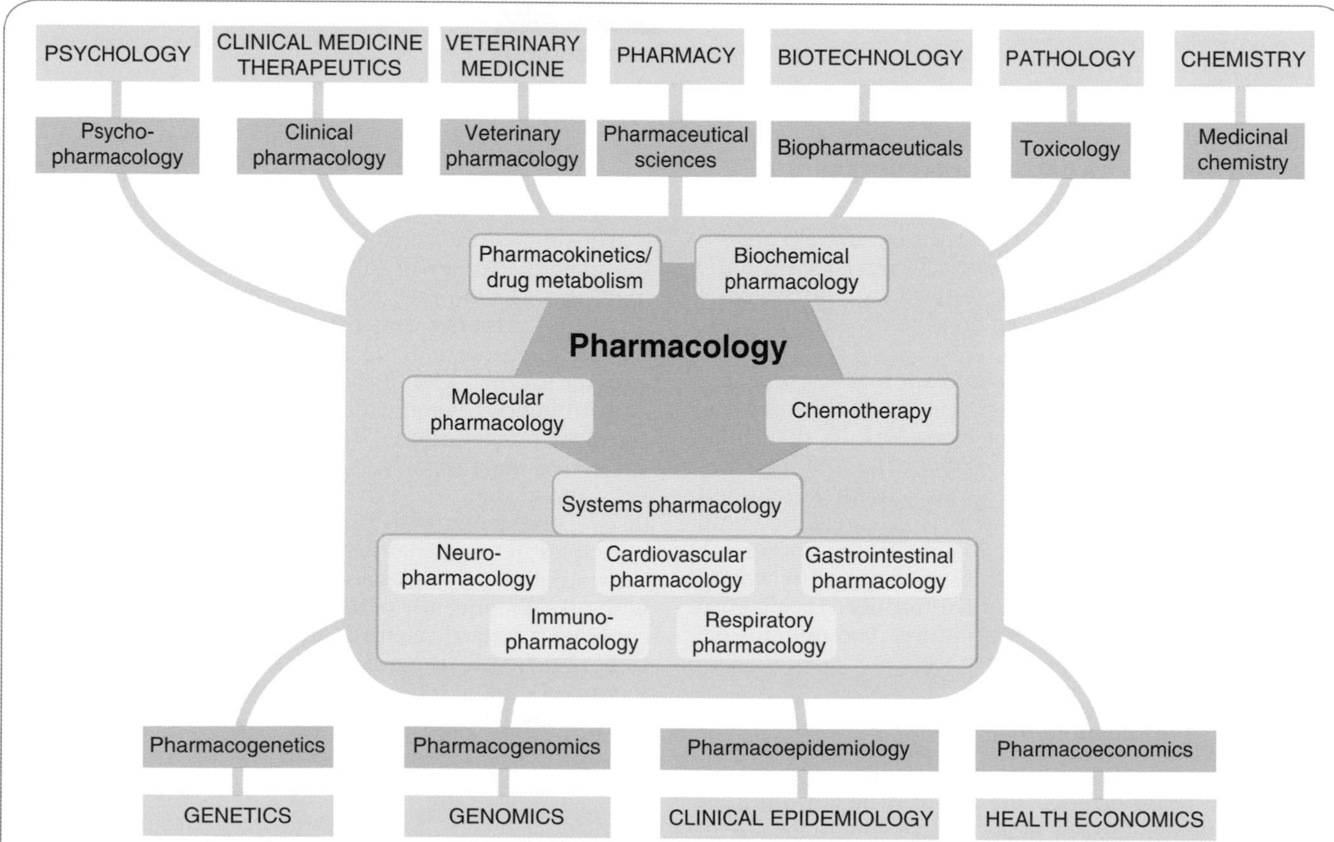

Fig. 1.2 Pharmacology today with its various subdivisions. The *grey box* contains the general areas of pharmacology covered in this book. Interface disciplines *(brown boxes)* link pharmacology to other mainstream biomedical disciplines *(green boxes)*.

(see Ch. 12). The underlying principle is that differences between individuals in their response to therapeutic drugs can be predicted from their genetic make-up. Examples that confirm this are steadily accumulating (see Ch. 12). So far, they mainly involve genetic polymorphism of drug-metabolising enzymes or receptors. Ultimately, linking specific gene variations with variations in therapeutic or unwanted effects of a particular drug should enable the tailoring of therapeutic choices on the basis of an individual's genotype. Steady improvements in the cost and feasibility of individual genotyping will increase its applicability potentially with far-reaching consequences for therapeutics (see Ch. 12).[7]

Pharmacoepidemiology. This is the study of drug effects at the population level (see Caparrotta et al., 2019). It is concerned with the variability of drug effects between individuals in a population, and between populations. It is an increasingly important topic in the eyes of the regulatory authorities who decide whether or not new drugs can be licensed for therapeutic use. Variability between individuals or populations detracts from the utility of a drug, even though its overall effect level may be satisfactory. Pharmacoepidemiological studies meta-analyse randomised controlled clinical trials, and also take into account patient compliance and other factors that apply when the drug is used under real-world settings.

Pharmacoeconomics. This branch of health economics aims to quantify in economic terms the cost and benefit of drugs used therapeutically. It arose from the concern of many governments to provide for healthcare from tax revenues, raising questions of what therapeutic procedures represent the best value for money. This, of course, raises fierce controversy, because it ultimately comes down to putting monetary value on health and longevity, often using a measure of quality-adjusted life year (QALY) to measure the impact of new therapeutic interventions to judge whether society *should* fund a new drug and for what societal gains. As with pharmacoepidemiology, regulatory authorities are increasingly requiring economic analysis, as well as evidence of individual benefit, when making decisions on licensing. For more information on this complex subject, see Franklin et al. (2019).

[7]Whole genome sequencing is now offered directly to the public and costs as little as £50.

REFERENCES AND FURTHER READING

Caparrotta, T.M., Dear, J.W., Colhoun, H.M., Webb, D.J., 2019. Pharmacoepidemiology: using randomised control trials and observational studies in clinical decision-making. Br. J. Clin. Pharmacol. 85, 1907–1924.

Clark, D.P., Pazderink, N.J., 2015. Biotechnology. Elsevier, New York.

Franklin, M., Lomas, J., Walker, S., Young, T., 2019. An educational review about using cost data for the purpose of cost-effectiveness analysis. Pharmacoeconomics 37, 631–643.

Nebert, D.W., Weber, W.W., 1990. Pharmacogenetics. In: Pratt, W.B., Taylor, P. (Eds.), Principles of Drug Action, third ed. Churchill Livingstone, New York.

Porter, R., 1997. The Greatest Benefit to Mankind. Harper-Collins, London.

Theobold, N., 2020. Emerging vaccine delivery systems for COVID-19. Drug Discov. Today 25, 1556–1558.

2 How drugs act: general principles

OVERVIEW

The emergence of pharmacology as a science came when the emphasis shifted from describing what drugs do to explaining how they work. In this chapter we set out some general principles underlying the interaction of drugs with living systems (Ch. 3 goes into some of the more molecular aspects in detail). The interaction between drugs and cells is described, followed by a more detailed examination of different types of drug–receptor interaction. The receptor concept has been described as the 'big idea' of pharmacology (Rang, 2006) and will be a recurring theme throughout this book.

INTRODUCTION

To begin with, we should gratefully acknowledge Paul Ehrlich for insisting that drug action must be explicable in terms of conventional chemical interactions between drugs and tissues, and for dispelling the idea that the remarkable potency and specificity of action of some drugs put them somehow out of reach of chemistry and physics and required the intervention of magical 'vital forces'. Although many drugs produce effects in extraordinarily low doses and concentrations, low concentrations still involve very large numbers of molecules. One drop of a solution of a drug at only 10^{-10} mol/L still contains about 3×10^9 drug molecules, so there is no mystery in the fact that it may produce an obvious pharmacological response. Some bacterial toxins (e.g. diphtheria toxin) act with such precision that a single molecule taken up by a target cell is sufficient to kill it.

One of the basic tenets of pharmacology is that drug molecules must exert some chemical influence on one or more cell constituents in order to produce a pharmacological response. In other words, drug molecules must get so close to these constituent cellular molecules that the two interact chemically in such a way that the function of the latter is altered. Of course, the molecules in the organism vastly outnumber the drug molecules, and if the drug molecules were merely distributed at random, the chance of interaction with any particular class of cellular molecule would be negligible. Therefore pharmacological effects require, in general, the non-uniform distribution of the drug molecule within the body or tissue, which is the same as saying that drug molecules must be 'bound' to particular constituents of cells and tissues in order to produce an effect. Ehrlich summed it up thus: '*Corpora non agunt nisi fixata*' (in this context, 'A drug will not work unless it is bound').[1]

These critical binding sites are often referred to as 'drug targets' (an obvious allusion to Ehrlich's famous phrase 'magic bullets', describing the potential of antimicrobial drugs). The mechanisms by which the association of a drug molecule with its target leads to a physiological response constitute the major thrust of pharmacological research. Most drug targets are protein molecules. Even general anaesthetics (see Ch. 41), which were long thought to produce their effects by an interaction with membrane lipid only, now appear to interact mainly with membrane proteins (see Franks, 2008).

All rules need exceptions, and many antimicrobial and antitumour drugs (see Chs 51 and 57), as well as mutagenic and carcinogenic agents (see Ch. 58), interact directly with DNA rather than protein; bisphosphonates, used to treat osteoporosis (see Ch. 36), bind to calcium salts in the bone matrix, rendering them toxic to osteoclasts. There are also exceptions among the new generation of *biopharmaceutical drugs* that include nucleic acids, proteins and antibodies (see Ch. 5), although these do interact with cellular components to produce their effects.

PROTEIN TARGETS FOR DRUG BINDING

Four main kinds of regulatory protein are commonly involved as primary drug targets, namely:

- receptors
- enzymes
- carrier molecules (transporters)
- ion channels

Furthermore, many drugs bind (in addition to their primary targets) to plasma proteins (see Ch. 9) and other tissue proteins, without producing any obvious physiological effect. Nevertheless, the generalisation that most drugs act on one or other of the four types of protein listed earlier serves as a good starting point.

Further discussion of the mechanisms by which such binding leads to cellular responses is given in Chapters 3 and 4.

DRUG RECEPTORS

WHAT DO WE MEAN BY RECEPTORS?

As emphasised in Chapter 1, the concept of receptors is central to pharmacology, and the term is most often used to describe the target molecules through which soluble physiological mediators – hormones, neurotransmitters, inflammatory mediators, etc. – produce their effects. Examples such as acetylcholine receptors, cytokine receptors, steroid receptors and growth hormone receptors abound in this book, and generally the term *receptor* indicates a recognition molecule for a chemical mediator through which a response is transduced. Receptor molecules have evolved to allow fine-tuning of the homeostatic control of

---

[1]There are, if one looks hard enough, exceptions to Ehrlich's dictum – drugs that act without being bound to any tissue constituent (e.g. osmotic diuretics, osmotic purgatives, antacids and heavy metal chelating agents). Nonetheless, the principle remains true for the great majority.

Targets for drug action

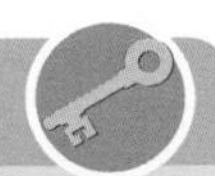

- A drug is a chemical applied to a physiological system that affects its function in a specific way.
- With some exceptions, drugs act on target proteins, namely:
  - receptors
  - enzymes
  - carriers
  - ion channels.
- The term *receptor* is used in different ways. In pharmacology, it describes protein molecules whose function is to recognise and respond to endogenous chemical signals. Other macromolecules with which drugs interact to produce their effects are known as *drug targets.*
- Specificity is reciprocal: individual classes of drug bind only to certain targets, and individual targets recognise only certain classes of drug.
- No drugs are completely specific in their actions. In many cases, increasing the dose of a drug will cause it to affect targets other than the principal one (so called 'off-target' effects), and this can lead to side effects.

cells and physiological functions – pharmacology often hijacks these innate control steps.

'Receptor' is sometimes used to denote *any* target molecule with which a drug molecule (i.e. a foreign compound rather than an endogenous mediator) has to combine in order to elicit its specific effect. For example, the voltage-sensitive sodium channel is sometimes referred to as the 'receptor' for **local anaesthetics** (see Ch. 44), or the enzyme dihydrofolate reductase as the 'receptor' for **methotrexate** (see Chs 51 and 57). The term *drug target*, of which receptors are one type, is preferable in this context.

In the more general context of cell biology, the term receptor is used to describe various cell surface molecules (such as *T-cell receptors, integrins, Toll receptors*, etc.; see Ch. 7) involved in the cell-to-cell interactions that are important in immunology, cell growth, migration and differentiation, some of which are also emerging as drug targets. These receptors differ from conventional pharmacological receptors in that they respond to proteins attached to cell surfaces or extracellular structures, rather than to soluble mediators.

Enzymes exist to mediate the biochemical signals within cells or tissues. Some drugs can modulate the activities of these enzymes for our benefit. For example, common anti-inflammatory drugs (NSAIDs; see Ch. 25) are used to relieve pain and inflammation – they achieve their effects through inhibiting cyclooxygenase enzymes.

Various carrier proteins are often referred to as receptors, such as the *low-density lipoprotein receptor* that plays a key role in lipid metabolism (see Ch. 22) and the *transferrin receptor* involved in iron absorption (see Ch. 24). These entities have little in common with pharmacological receptors. Although quite distinct from pharmacological receptors, these proteins play an important role in the action of drugs such as statins (see Ch. 22).

RECEPTORS IN PHYSIOLOGICAL SYSTEMS

Receptors form a key part of the system of chemical communication that all multicellular organisms use to coordinate the activities of their cells and organs. Without them, we would be unable to function.

Some fundamental properties of receptors are illustrated by the action of **adrenaline** (epinephrine) on the heart. Adrenaline first binds to a receptor protein (the β_1 *adrenoceptor*, see Ch. 15) that serves as a recognition site for adrenaline and other catecholamines. When it binds to the receptor, a train of reactions is initiated (see Ch. 3), leading to an increase in force and rate of the heartbeat. In the absence of adrenaline, the receptor is normally functionally silent. This is true of most receptors for endogenous mediators (hormones, neurotransmitters, cytokines, etc.), although there are examples (see Ch. 3) of receptors that are 'constitutively active' – that is, they exert a controlling influence even when no chemical mediator is present.

There is an important distinction between *agonists*, which 'activate' the receptors, and *antagonists*, which combine at the same site without causing activation, and block the effect of agonists on that receptor. The distinction between agonists and antagonists exists only for pharmacological receptors; we cannot usefully speak of 'agonists' for the other classes of drug target described earlier.

The characteristics and accepted nomenclature of pharmacological receptors and other drug targets are detailed in the Guide to Pharmacology, an extensive online database as well as in a regularly updated summary (Alexander et al., 2019). The origins of the receptor concept and its pharmacological significance are discussed by Rang (2006).

DRUG SPECIFICITY

For a drug to be useful as either a therapeutic or a scientific tool, it must act selectively on particular cells and tissues. In other words, it must show a high degree of binding site specificity. Conversely, proteins that function as drug targets generally show a high degree of ligand specificity; they bind only molecules of a certain precise type.

These principles of binding site and ligand specificity can be clearly recognised in the actions of a mediator such as **angiotensin** (see Ch. 21). This peptide acts strongly on vascular smooth muscle, and on the kidney tubule, but has very little effect on other kinds of smooth muscle or on the intestinal epithelium. Other mediators affect a quite different spectrum of cells and tissues, the pattern in each case reflecting the specific pattern of expression of the protein receptors for the various mediators. A small chemical change, such as conversion of one of the amino acids in angiotensin from L to D form, or removal of one amino acid from the chain, can inactivate the molecule altogether, because the receptor fails to bind the altered form. The complementary specificity of ligands and binding sites, which gives rise to the very exact molecular recognition properties of proteins, is central to explaining many of the phenomena of pharmacology. It is no exaggeration to say that the ability of proteins to interact in a highly selective way with other molecules – including other proteins – is the basis of living machines. Its relevance to the understanding of drug action will be a recurring theme in this book.

Finally, it must be emphasised that no drug acts with complete specificity. Thus tricyclic antidepressant drugs (see Ch. 48) act by blocking monoamine transporters but are notorious for producing side effects (e.g. dry mouth) related to their ability to block various other receptors. In general, the lower the potency of a drug and the higher the dose needed, the more likely it is that sites of action other than the primary one will assume significance. In clinical terms, this is often associated with the appearance of unwanted 'off-target' side effects[2] of which no drug is free.

Since the 1970s, pharmacological research has succeeded in identifying the protein targets of many different types of drug. Drugs such as opioid analgesics (see Ch. 43), cannabinoids (see Ch. 18) and benzodiazepines (see Ch. 45), whose actions have been described in exhaustive detail for many years, are now known to target well-defined receptors, many of which have been fully characterised by gene-cloning and protein crystallography techniques (see Ch. 3).

RECEPTOR CLASSIFICATION

Where the action of a drug can be associated with a particular receptor, this provides a valuable means for classification and refinement in drug design. For example, pharmacological analysis of the actions of histamine (see Ch. 17) showed that some of its effects (the H_1 effects, such as smooth muscle contraction) were strongly antagonised by the competitive histamine antagonists then known. Black and his colleagues suggested in 1970 that the remaining actions of histamine, which included its stimulant effect on gastric secretion, might represent a second class of histamine receptor (H_2). Testing a number of histamine analogues, they found that some were selective in producing H_2 effects, with little H_1 activity. By analysing which parts of the histamine molecule conferred this type of specificity, they were able to develop selective H_2 antagonists, which proved to be potent in blocking gastric acid secretion, a development of major therapeutic significance (see Ch. 30).[3] Two further types of histamine receptor (H_3 and H_4) were recognised later.

Receptor classification based on pharmacological responses continues to be a valuable and widely used approach. Subsequently, newer experimental approaches produced other criteria on which to base receptor classification. The direct measurement of ligand binding to receptors (see later) allowed many new receptor subtypes to be defined that could not easily be distinguished by studies of drug effects. Molecular sequencing of the amino acid structure (see Ch. 3) provided a completely new basis for classification at a much finer level of detail than can be reached through pharmacological analysis. Finally, analysis of the biochemical pathways that are linked to receptor activation (see Ch. 3) provides yet another basis for classification.

The result of this data explosion was that receptor classification suddenly became much more detailed, with a proliferation of receptor subtypes for all the main types of ligand. As alternative molecular and biochemical classifications began to spring up that were incompatible with the accepted pharmacologically defined receptor classes, the International Union of Basic and Clinical Pharmacology (IUPHAR) convened expert working groups to produce agreed receptor classifications for the major types, taking into account the pharmacological, molecular and biochemical information available. These wise people have a hard task; their conclusions will be neither perfect nor final but are essential to ensure a consistent terminology. To the student, this may seem an arcane exercise in taxonomy, generating much detail but little illumination. There is a danger that the tedious lists of drug names, actions and side effects that used to burden the subject will be replaced by exhaustive tables of receptors, ligands and transduction pathways. In this book, we have tried to avoid detail for its own sake and include only such information on receptor classification as seems interesting in its own right or is helpful in explaining the actions of important classes of drugs.

DRUG–RECEPTOR INTERACTIONS

Occupation of a receptor by a drug molecule may or may not result in *activation* of the receptor. By activation, we mean that the receptor is affected by the bound molecule in such a way as to alter the function of the cell and elicit a tissue response. The molecular mechanisms associated with receptor activation are discussed in Chapter 3. Binding and activation represent two distinct steps in the generation of the receptor-mediated response by an agonist (Fig. 2.1). If a drug binds to the receptor without causing activation and thereby prevents the agonist from binding, it is termed a *receptor antagonist*. The tendency of a drug to bind to the receptors is governed by its *affinity*, whereas the tendency for it, once bound, to switch the receptor into its active conformation is denoted by its *efficacy*. These terms are defined more precisely later. Drugs of high potency generally have a high affinity for the receptors and thus occupy a significant proportion of the receptors even at low concentrations. Agonists also possess significant *efficacy*,

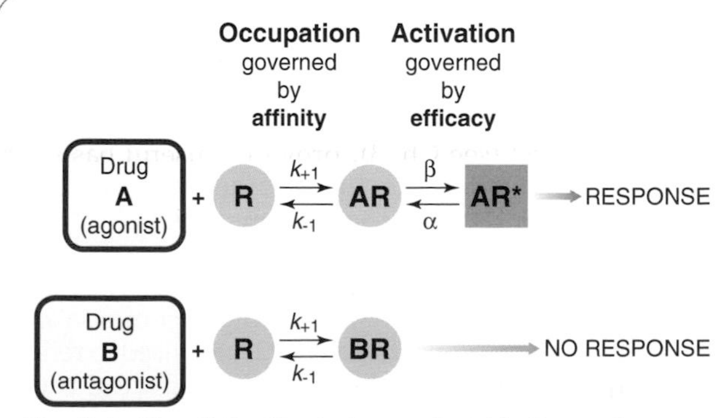

Fig. 2.1 The distinction between drug binding and receptor activation. Ligand *A* is an agonist, because when it is bound, the receptor *(R)* tends to become activated, whereas ligand *B* is an antagonist, because binding does not lead to activation. It is important to realise that for most drugs, binding and activation are reversible, dynamic processes. The rate constants k_{+1}, k_{-1}, α and β for the binding, unbinding and activation steps vary between drugs. For an antagonist, which does not activate the receptor, β = 0.

[2]'On-target' side effects are unwanted effects mediated through the same receptor as the clinically desired effect, for example constipation and respiratory depression by opioid analgesic drugs (see Ch. 43), whereas 'off-target' side effects are mediated by a different mechanism.

[3]For this work, and the development of β-adrenoceptor antagonists by a similar experimental approach, Sir James Black was awarded the 1984 Nobel Prize in Physiology or Medicine.

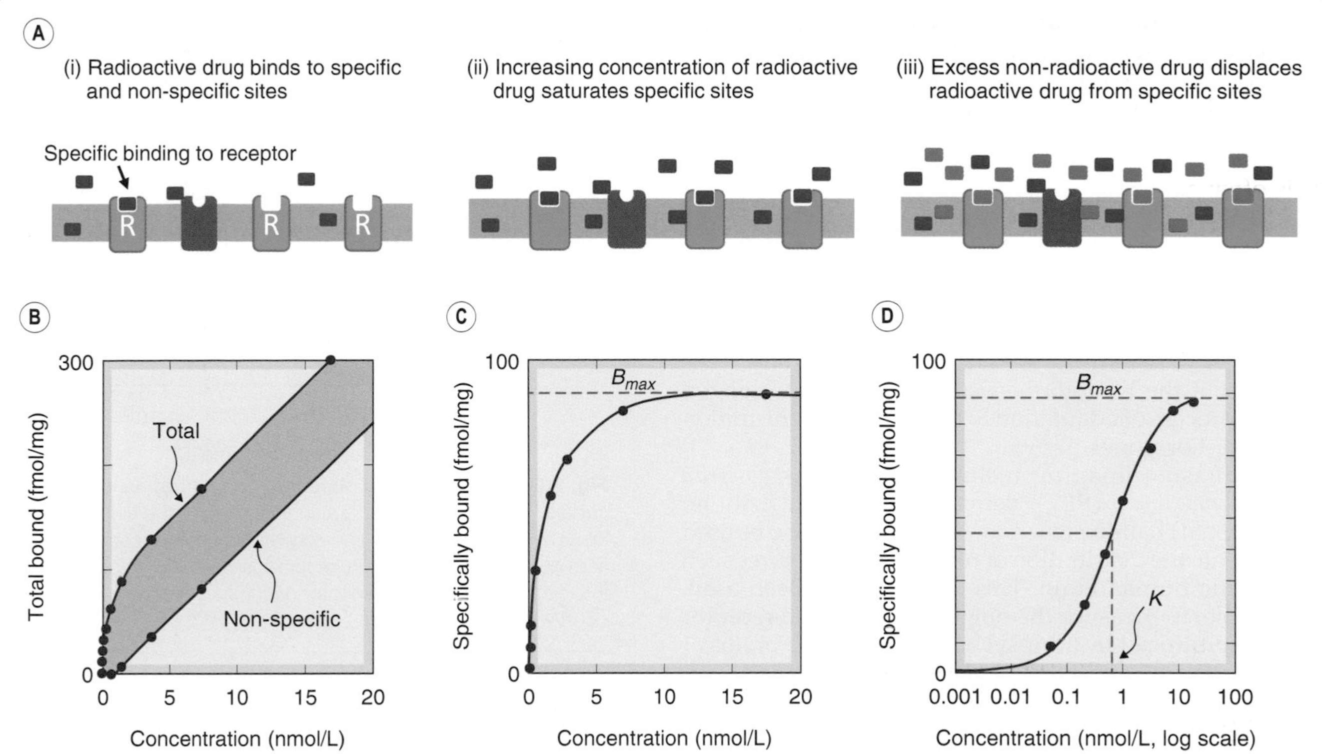

Fig. 2.2 Measurement of receptor binding. (A) (i) Cartoon depicting radioligand (shown in red) binding to its receptor *(R)* in the membrane as well as to non-specific sites on other proteins and lipid. In (ii) when the concentration of radioligand is increased all the specific sites become saturated but non-specific binding continues to increase. In (iii) the addition of a high concentration of a non-radioactive drug *(shown in green)* that also binds to R displaces the radioactive drug from its receptors but not from the non-specific sites. (B–D) Illustrate actual experimental results for radioligand binding to β-adrenoceptors in cardiac cell membranes. The ligand was [^{3}H]-cyanopindolol, a derivative of pindolol (see Ch. 15). (B) Measurements of total and non-specific binding at equilibrium. Non-specific binding is measured in the presence of a saturating concentration of a non-radioactive β-adrenoceptor agonist, which prevents the radioactive ligand from binding to β-adrenoceptors. The difference between the two lines represents specific binding. (C) Specific binding plotted against concentration. The curve is a rectangular hyperbola (Eq. 2.5). (D) Specific binding as in (C) plotted against the concentration on a log scale. The sigmoid curve is a *logistic curve* representing the logarithmic scaling of the rectangular hyperbola plotted in panel (C) from which the binding parameters *K* (the equilibrium dissociation constant) and B_{max} (the binding capacity) can be determined.

whereas antagonists, in the simplest case, have zero efficacy. Drugs with intermediate levels of efficacy, such that even when 100% of the receptors are occupied the tissue response is submaximal, are known as *partial agonists*, to distinguish them from *full agonists*, the efficacy of which is sufficient that they can elicit a maximal tissue response. These concepts, although clearly an oversimplified description of events at the molecular level (see Ch. 3), provide a useful basis for characterising drug effects.

We now discuss certain aspects in more detail, namely drug binding, agonist concentration–effect curves, competitive antagonism, partial agonists and the nature of efficacy. Understanding these concepts at a qualitative level is sufficient for many purposes, but for more detailed analysis a quantitative formulation is needed (see later in the chapter).

THE BINDING OF DRUGS TO RECEPTORS

The binding of drugs to receptors can often be measured directly by the use of drug molecules (agonists or antagonists) labelled with one or more radioactive atoms (usually ^{3}H, ^{14}C or ^{125}I). The usual procedure is to incubate samples of the tissue (or membrane fragments) with various concentrations of radioactive drug until equilibrium conditions are reached (i.e. when the rates of association [binding] and dissociation [unbinding] of the radioactive drug are equal). The bound radioactivity is measured after removal of the supernatant and any unbound labelled drug.

In such experiments, the radiolabelled drug will exhibit both specific binding (i.e. binding to receptors, which is saturable as there are a finite number of receptors in the tissue) and a certain amount of 'non-specific binding' (i.e. drug taken up by structures other than receptors, which, at the concentrations used in such studies, is normally non-saturable), which obscures the specific component and needs to be kept to a minimum (Fig. 2.2A,B). The amount of non-specific binding is estimated by measuring the radioactivity taken up in the presence of a saturating concentration of a (non-radioactive) ligand that inhibits completely the binding of the radioactive drug to the receptors, leaving behind the non-specific component. This is then subtracted from the total binding to give an estimate of specific binding (Fig. 2.2C). The *binding curve* (Fig. 2.2C,D) defines the relationship between concentration and the amount of drug bound (B), and in most cases it fits well to the relationship predicted theoretically (see Fig. 2.14), allowing the affinity of the drug for the receptors to be estimated, as well as the maximal *binding capacity* (B_{max}), representing the density of receptors in the tissue. When combined with functional studies, binding measurements have proved very valuable. It has, for example, been confirmed that the *spare receptor hypothesis* for muscarinic receptors in smooth muscle is correct; agonists are found to bind, in general, with rather low affinity, and a maximal biological effect occurs at low receptor occupancy. It has also been shown, in skeletal muscle and other tissues, that denervation leads to an increase in the number of receptors in the target cell, a finding that accounts, at least in part, for the phenomenon of *denervation supersensitivity*. More generally, it appears that receptors tend to increase in number, usually over the course of a few days, if the relevant hormone or transmitter is absent or scarce, or to decrease in number if the receptors are activated for a prolonged period, a process of adaptation to continued administration of drugs or hormones.

Non-invasive imaging techniques, such as *positron emission tomography* (PET), using drugs labelled with an isotope of short half-life (such as ^{11}C or ^{18}Fl), can also be used to investigate the distribution of receptors in structures such as the living human brain. This technique has been used, for example, to measure the degree of dopamine-receptor blockade produced by antipsychotic drugs in the brains of patients with schizophrenia (see Ch. 47).

Binding curves with agonists often reveal an apparent heterogeneity among receptors. For example, agonist binding to muscarinic receptors (see Ch. 14) and also to β-adrenoceptors (see Ch. 15) suggests at least two populations of binding sites with different affinities. This may be because the receptors can exist either unattached or coupled within the membrane to another macromolecule, the G protein (see Ch. 3), which constitutes part of the transduction system through which the receptor exerts its regulatory effect. Antagonist binding does not show this complexity, probably because antagonists, by their nature, do not lead to the secondary event of G protein coupling. Because agonist binding results in activation, agonist affinity has proved to be a surprisingly elusive concept, about which aficionados love to argue.

THE RELATION BETWEEN AGONIST CONCENTRATION AND EFFECT

Although binding can be measured directly, it is usually a biological response, such as a rise in blood pressure, contraction or relaxation of a strip of smooth muscle in an organ bath, the activation of an enzyme, or a behavioural response, that we are interested in, and this is often plotted as a *concentration–effect curve* (in vitro) or *dose–response curve* (in vivo), as in Fig. 2.3. This allows us to estimate the *maximal response/effect* that the drug can produce (E_{max}) and the concentration or dose needed to produce a 50% maximal response (EC_{50} or ED_{50}). A logarithmic concentration or dose scale is often used. This transforms the curve from a rectangular hyperbola to a sigmoidal curve in which the mid portion is essentially linear (the importance of the slope of the linear portion will become apparent later in this chapter when we consider antagonism and partial agonists). The E_{max}, EC_{50} and slope parameters are useful for comparing different drugs that produce qualitatively similar effects (see Fig. 2.7 and Ch. 8). Although they look similar to the binding curve in Fig. 2.2D, concentration–effect curves cannot be used to measure the affinity of agonist drugs for their receptors, because the response produced is not, as a rule, directly proportional to receptor occupancy. This often arises because the maximum response of a tissue may be produced by agonists when they occupy less than 100% of the receptors. Under these circumstances the tissue is said to possess spare receptors (see later).

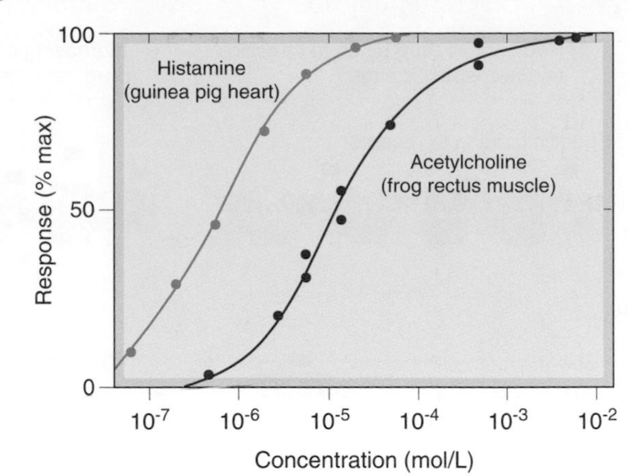

Fig. 2.3 Experimentally observed concentration–effect curves. Although the lines, drawn according to the binding Eq. 2.5, fit the points well, such curves do not give correct estimates of the affinity of drugs for receptors. This is because the relationship between receptor occupancy and response is usually non-linear.

In interpreting concentration–effect curves, it must be remembered that the concentration of the drug at the receptors may differ from the known concentration in the bathing solution. Agonists may be subject to rapid enzymic degradation or uptake by cells as they diffuse from the surface towards their site of action, and a steady state can be reached in which the agonist concentration at the receptors is very much less than the concentration in the bath. In the case of acetylcholine, for example, which is hydrolysed by cholinesterase present in most tissues (see Ch. 14), the concentration reaching the receptors can be less than 1% of that in the bath, and an even bigger difference has been found with noradrenaline (norepinephrine), which is avidly taken up by sympathetic nerve terminals in many tissues (see Ch. 15). The problem is reduced but not entirely eradicated by the use of recombinant receptors expressed in cells in culture. Thus, even if the concentration–effect curve, as in Fig. 2.3, looks just like a facsimile of the binding curve (see Fig. 2.2D), it cannot be used directly to determine the affinity of the agonist for the receptors.

SPARE RECEPTORS

Stephenson (1956), studying the actions of acetylcholine analogues in isolated tissues, found that many full agonists were capable of eliciting maximal responses at very low occupancies, often less than 1%. This means that the mechanism linking the response to receptor occupancy has a substantial reserve capacity. Such systems may be said to possess *spare receptors*, or a receptor reserve. The existence of spare receptors does not imply any functional subdivision of the receptor pool, but merely that the pool is larger than the number needed to evoke a full response. This surplus of receptors over the number actually needed might seem a wasteful biological arrangement. But in fact it is highly efficient in that a given number of agonist–receptor complexes, corresponding to a given level of biological response, can be reached with a lower concentration of hormone or neurotransmitter than would be the case if fewer receptors were provided. Economy of hormone or transmitter secretion is thus achieved at the expense of providing more receptors.

COMPETITIVE ANTAGONISM

Although one drug can inhibit the response to another in several ways, competition at the receptor level is particularly important, both in the laboratory and in the clinic, because of the high potency and specificity that can be achieved.

In the presence of a competitive antagonist, the agonist occupancy (i.e. proportion of receptors to which the agonist is bound) at a given agonist concentration is reduced, because the receptor can usually accommodate only one molecule at a time. However, because the two are in competition, raising the agonist concentration can restore the agonist occupancy (and hence the tissue response). The antagonism is therefore said to be *surmountable*, in contrast to other types of antagonism (see later) where increasing the agonist concentration fails to overcome the blocking effect. A simple theoretical analysis (see Quantitative Aspects of Drug–Receptor Interactions later) predicts that in the presence of a fixed concentration of the antagonist, the log concentration–effect curve for the agonist will be shifted to the right, without any change in slope or maximum – the hallmark of competitive antagonism (Fig. 2.4A). The shift is expressed as a *dose ratio*, *r* (the ratio by which the agonist concentration has to be increased in the presence of the antagonist in order to restore a given level of response). Theory predicts that the dose ratio increases linearly with the concentration of the antagonist. These predictions are often borne out in practice (Fig. 2.5A), providing a relatively simple method for determining the equilibrium dissociation constant of the antagonist (K_B; Fig. 2.5B). Examples of competitive antagonism are very common in pharmacology. The surmountability of the block by the antagonist may be important in practice, because it allows the functional effect of the agonist to be restored by an increase in concentration. With other types of antagonism (as detailed later), the block is usually insurmountable.

The salient features of competitive antagonism are:

- a shift of the agonist log concentration–effect curve to the right, without change of slope or maximum (i.e. antagonism can be overcome by increasing the concentration of the agonist)
- linear relationship between agonist dose ratio and antagonist concentration
- evidence of competition from binding studies

Competitive antagonism is the most direct mechanism by which one drug can reduce the effect of another (or of an endogenous mediator).

The characteristics of *reversible competitive antagonism* described previously reflect the fact that agonist and competitive antagonist molecules do not stay bound to the receptor but dissociate and rebind continuously. The rate of dissociation of the antagonist molecules is sufficiently high that a new equilibrium is rapidly established on addition of the agonist. In effect, agonist molecules are able to replace the antagonist molecules on the receptors when the antagonist unbinds, although they cannot, of course, evict bound antagonist molecules. Displacement occurs

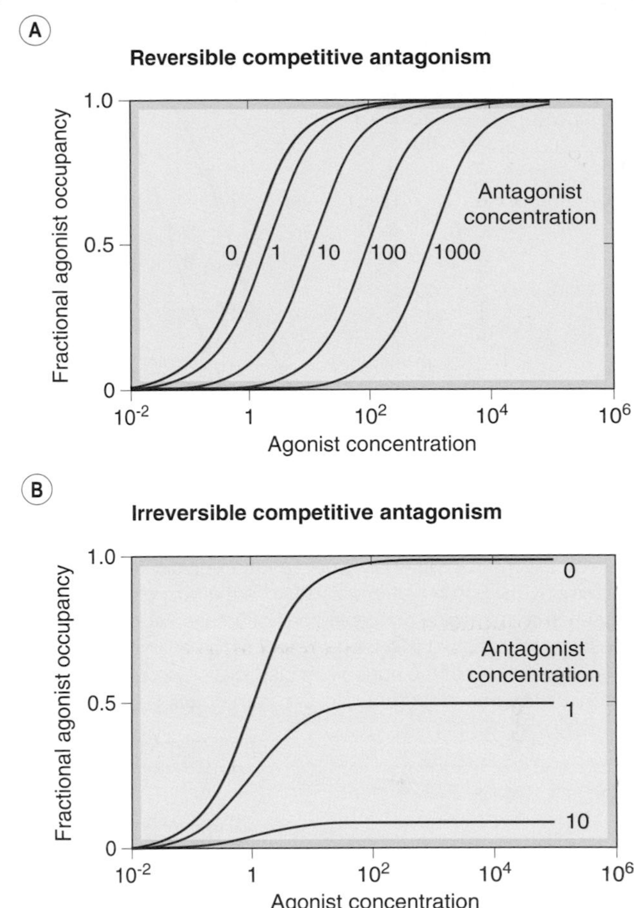

Fig. 2.4 Hypothetical agonist concentration–occupancy curves in the presence of reversible (A) and irreversible (B) competitive antagonists. The concentrations are normalised with respect to the equilibrium dissociation constants, *K* (i.e. 1.0 corresponds to a concentration equal to *K* and results in 50% occupancy). Note that in (A) increasing the agonist concentration overcomes the effect of a reversible antagonist (i.e. the block is surmountable), so that the maximal response is unchanged, whereas in (B) the effect of an irreversible antagonist is insurmountable and full agonist occupancy cannot be achieved.

Competitive antagonism

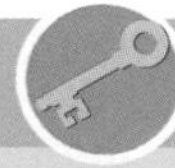

- Reversible competitive antagonism is the commonest and most important type of antagonism; it has two main characteristics.
  - In the presence of the antagonist, the agonist log concentration–effect curve is shifted to the right without change in slope or maximum, the extent of the shift being a measure of the *dose ratio.*
  - The dose ratio increases linearly with antagonist concentration.
- Antagonist affinity, measured in this way, has been widely used as a basis for receptor classification.

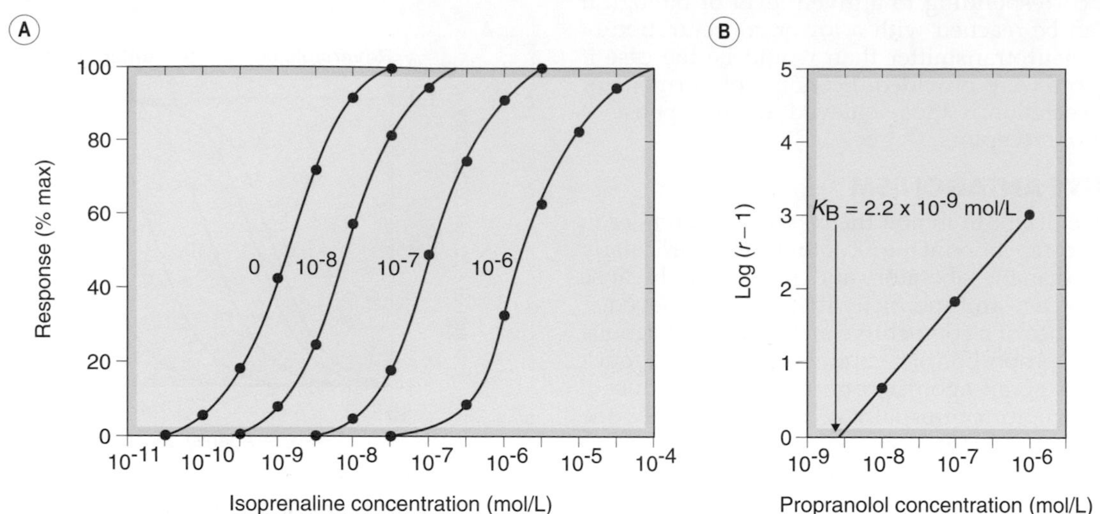

Fig. 2.5 Competitive antagonism of isoprenaline by propranolol measured on isolated guinea pig atria. (A) Concentration–effect curves at various propranolol concentrations (indicated on the curves). Note the progressive shift to the right without a change of slope or maximum. (B) Schild plot (Eq. 2.10). '*r*' is the ratio of the concentration of agonist that produces a given level of response in the presence and absence of increasing concentrations of antagonist (discussed later in Quantitative Aspects of Drug Receptor Interactions). The equilibrium dissociation constant (K_B) for propranolol is given by the abscissal intercept, 2.2 × 10^{-9} mol/L. Note that the subscript 'B' is now used in 'K_B' to indicate that the equilibrium dissociation constant is that of the antagonist (designated drug B) measured in the presence of the agonist (designated drug A). (Results from Potter, L.T., 1967. Uptake of propranolol by isolated guinea pig atria. J. Pharmacol. Exp. Ther. 55, 91–100.)

because, by occupying a proportion of the vacant receptors, the agonist effectively reduces the rate of association of the antagonist molecules; consequently, the rate of dissociation temporarily exceeds that of association, and the overall antagonist occupancy falls.

IRREVERSIBLE COMPETITIVE ANTAGONISM

Irreversible competitive (or *non-equilibrium*) *antagonism* occurs when the antagonist binds to the same site on the receptor as the agonist but dissociates very slowly, or not at all, from the receptors, with the result that no change in the antagonist occupancy takes place when the agonist is applied.[4]

The predicted effects of reversible and irreversible antagonists are compared in Fig. 2.4.

In some cases (Fig. 2.6A), the theoretical effect is accurately reproduced with the antagonist reducing the maximum response. However, the distinction between reversible and irreversible competitive antagonism (or even non-competitive antagonism) is not always so clear. This is because of the phenomenon of spare receptors; if the agonist occupancy required to produce a maximal biological response is very small (say 1% of the total receptor pool), then it is possible to block irreversibly nearly 99% of the receptors without reducing the maximal response. The effect of a lesser degree of antagonist occupancy will be to produce a parallel shift of the log concentration–effect curve that is indistinguishable from reversible competitive antagonism (Fig. 2.6B). Only when the antagonist occupancy exceeds 99% will the maximum response be reduced.

Irreversible competitive antagonism occurs with drugs that possess reactive groups that form covalent bonds with the receptor. These are mainly used as experimental tools for investigating receptor function, and few are used clinically. Irreversible enzyme inhibitors that act similarly are clinically used, however, and include drugs such as **aspirin** (see Ch. 25), **omeprazole** (see Ch. 30), monoamine oxidase inhibitors (see Ch. 48) and **ibrutinib** (see Ch. 57).

PARTIAL AGONISTS AND THE CONCEPT OF EFFICACY

So far, we have considered drugs either as agonists, which in some way activate the receptor when they occupy it, or as antagonists, which cause no activation. However, the ability of a drug molecule to activate the receptor – namely its efficacy – is actually a graded, rather than an all-or-nothing, property. If a series of chemically related agonist drugs acting on the same receptors is tested on a given biological system, it is often found that the largest response that can be produced differs from one drug to another. Some compounds (known as *full agonists*) can produce a maximal response (the largest response that the tissue is capable of giving), whereas others (*partial agonists*) can produce only a submaximal response. Fig. 2.7A shows concentration–effect curves for several α-adrenoceptor agonists (see Ch. 15), which cause contraction of isolated strips of rabbit aorta. The full agonist **phenylephrine** produced the maximal response of which the tissue was capable; the other compounds could produce only submaximal responses and are partial agonists. The difference between full

---

[4]This type of antagonism is sometimes called non-competitive, but that term is ambiguous and best avoided in this context.

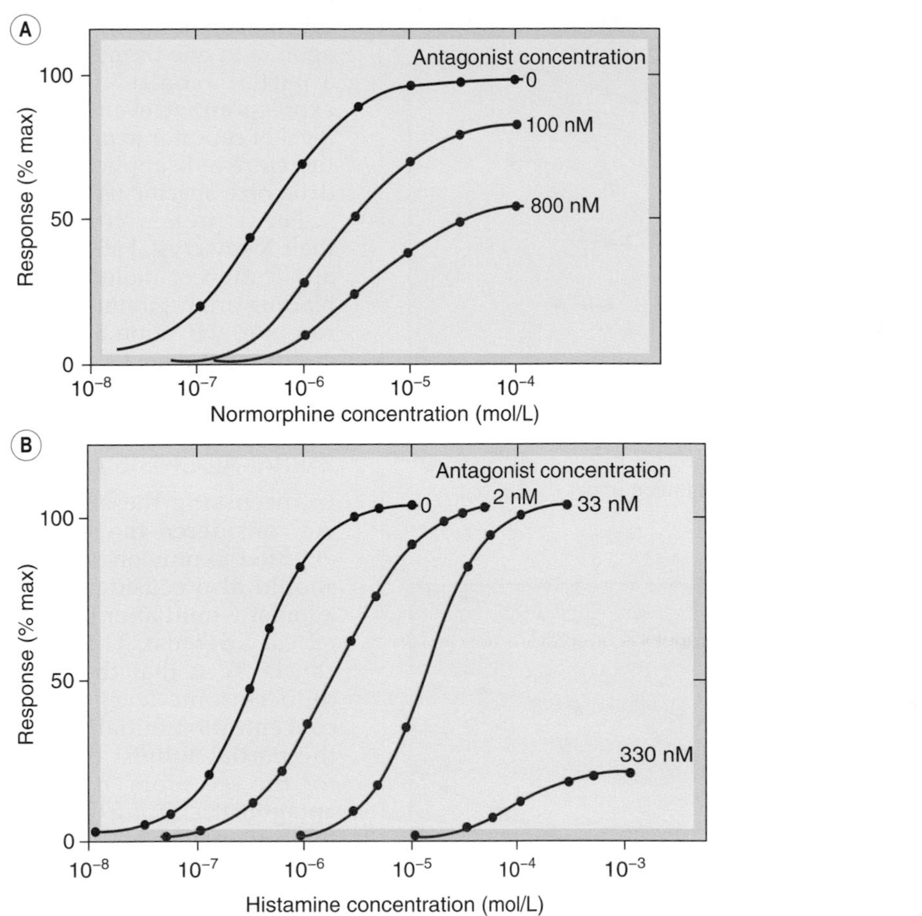

Fig. 2.6 Effects of irreversible competitive antagonists on agonist concentration–effect curves. (A) Rat brain neurons responding to the opioid agonist normorphine before and after being exposed to the irreversible competitive antagonist β-funaltrexamine for 30 minutes and then washed to remove the antagonist. Note the depression of the maximum response. (B) Responses of the guinea pig ileum to histamine before and after treatment with increasing concentrations of a receptor alkylating agent (GD121) for 5 minutes and then washed to remove the antagonist. Note the concentration–response curve is initially shifted to the right with no depression of the maximum response. (Panel [A] after Williams, J.T., North, R.A., 1984. Mol. Pharmacol. 26, 489–497; panel [B] after Nickerson, M., 1955. Nature 178, 696–697.)

and partial agonists lies in the relationship between receptor occupancy and response. In the experiment shown in Fig. 2.7 it was possible to estimate the affinity of the various drugs for the receptor, and hence (based on the theoretical model described later) to calculate the fraction of receptors occupied (known as *occupancy*) as a function of drug concentration. Plots of response as a function of occupancy for the different compounds are shown in Fig. 2.7B, showing that for partial agonists the response at a given level of occupancy is less than for full agonists. The weakest partial agonist, **tolazoline**, produces a barely detectable response even at 100% occupancy, and is usually classified as a *competitive antagonist* (see Ch. 15).

These differences can be expressed quantitatively in terms of *efficacy* (e), a parameter originally defined by Stephenson (1956) that describes the 'strength' of the agonist–receptor complex in evoking a response of the tissue. In the simple scheme shown in Fig. 2.1, efficacy describes the tendency of the drug–receptor complex to adopt the active (AR*), rather than the resting (AR), state. A drug with zero efficacy (e = 0) has no tendency to cause receptor activation, and causes no tissue response. A full agonist is a drug who efficacy[5] is sufficient that it produces a maximal response when less than 100% of receptors are occupied. A partial agonist has lower efficacy, such that 100% occupancy elicits only a submaximal response.

Subsequently it was appreciated that efficacy is composed of drug-dependent and tissue-dependent components. The drug-dependent component is referred to as the *intrinsic efficacy*, which is the ability of the agonist drug molecule, once bound, to activate the receptor protein (see Kelly, 2013). The tissue-dependent components of efficacy include the number of receptors that it expresses and the efficiency of coupling of receptor activation to the measured tissue response. The number of receptors expressed is especially relevant to the study of receptors in

[5]In Stephenson's formulation, efficacy is the reciprocal of the occupancy needed to produce a 50% maximal response, thus e = 25 implies that a 50% maximal response occurs at 4% occupancy. There is no theoretical upper limit to efficacy; indeed, some agonists are termed *super agonists* because they possess greater efficacy than the receptor's own endogenous agonist (e.g. dexmedetomidine, an α_2 adrenoceptor agonist with greater efficacy than that of either adrenaline or noradrenaline).

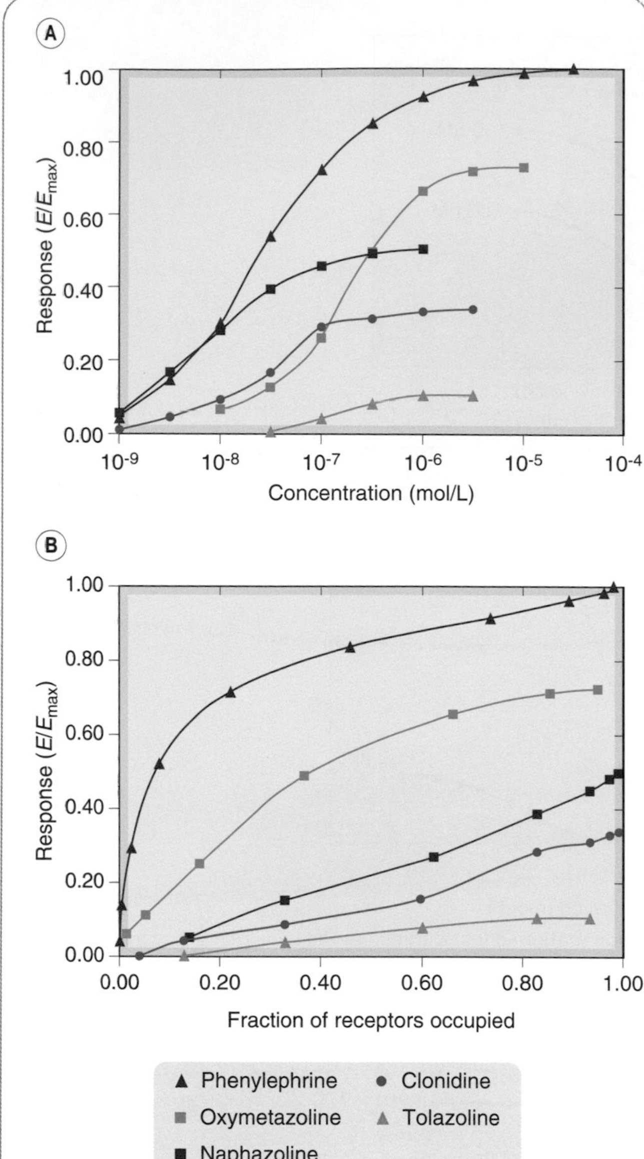

Fig. 2.7 Partial agonists. (A) Log concentration–effect curves for a series of α-adrenoceptor agonists causing contraction of an isolated strip of rabbit aorta. Phenylephrine is a full agonist. The others are partial agonists with different efficacies. The lower the efficacy of the drug the lower the maximum response and slope of the log concentration–response curve. (B) The relationship between response and receptor occupancy for the series. Note that the full agonist, phenylephrine, produces a near-maximal response when only about half the receptors are occupied, whereas partial agonists produce submaximal responses even when occupying all of the receptors. The efficacy of tolazoline is so low that it is classified as an α-adrenoceptor antagonist (see Ch. 15). In these experiments, receptor occupancy was not measured directly, but was calculated from pharmacological estimates of the equilibrium constants of the drugs. (Data from Ruffolo, R.R. Jr, et al., 1979. J. Pharmacol. Exp. Ther. 209, 429–436.)

recombinant expression systems when receptors are often very highly expressed and intermediate efficacy agonists then appear as full agonists. Across different cell types expressing the same receptor but at different densities, a given drug of intermediate efficacy may appear as a full agonist in one tissue (high level of receptor expression), a partial agonist in another (lower level of receptor expression) and even as an antagonist in another (very low level of receptor expression). The term 'partial agonist' is therefore only applicable when describing the action of a drug on a specific tissue or cell type.

For G protein–coupled receptors the elucidation of their X-ray crystal structures (described in Ch. 3) and the application of molecular dynamic simulations of drug binding are beginning to tease out the molecular basis of receptor activation and why some ligands are agonists and some are antagonists. For students starting to study pharmacology the simple theoretical two-state model described later provides a useful starting point.

PARTIAL AGONISTS AS ANTAGONISTS

In discussing the efficacy of partial agonists earlier, we considered the situation in which the tissue was exposed to only one drug, the partial agonist. What we should also consider is how the presence of a partial agonist would alter the response of a tissue to a higher efficacy agonist. This is depicted in Fig. 2.8 where it can be seen that the presence of the partial agonist induces some level of response dependent upon the concentration initially applied, but in addition because the partial agonist is competing with the full agonist for the receptors, it effectively acts as a competitive antagonist, shifting the concentration–response curve of the full agonist to the right. This is not just an obscure theoretical point but something which occurs in clinical practice. In the treatment of heroin users, buprenorphine, a weak partial agonist, not only acts as a weak opioid substitute but also acts as an antagonist and reduces the likelihood of overdose when users relapse and take heroin again (see Ch. 50).

CONSTITUTIVE RECEPTOR ACTIVATION AND INVERSE AGONISTS

Although we are accustomed to thinking that receptors are activated only when an agonist molecule is bound, there are examples (see De Ligt et al., 2000) where an appreciable level of activation (*constitutive activation*) may exist even when no ligand is present. These include receptors for benzodiazepines (see Ch. 45), cannabinoids (see Ch. 18), 5-hydroxytryptamine (see Ch. 16) and several other mediators. Furthermore, receptor mutations occur – either spontaneously, in some disease states (see Bond and Ijzerman, 2006), or experimentally created (see Ch. 4) – that result in appreciable constitutive activation. If a ligand reduces activity below the basal level of constitutive activation such drugs are known as *inverse agonists* (Fig. 2.9; see De Ligt et al., 2000) to distinguish them from *neutral antagonists*, which do not by themselves affect the level of activation. Inverse agonists can be regarded as drugs with negative efficacy, to distinguish them from agonists (positive efficacy) and neutral antagonists (zero efficacy). Neutral antagonists, by binding to the agonist binding site, will antagonise both agonists and inverse agonists. Inverse agonism was first observed at the benzodiazepine receptor (see Ch. 45) but such drugs are proconvulsive and thus not therapeutically useful! New examples of constitutively active receptors and inverse agonists are emerging with

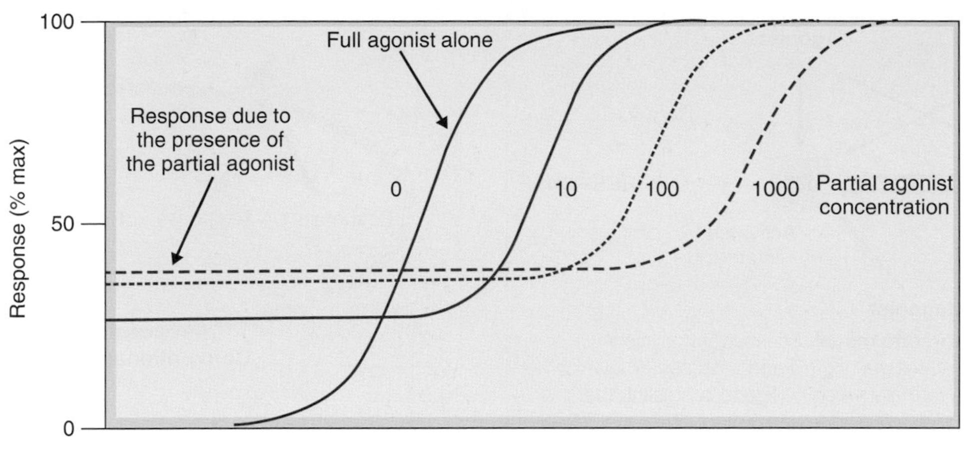

Fig. 2.8 Hypothetical concentration–response curves for a full agonist in the absence and presence of increasing concentrations of a partial agonist. The partial agonist will have agonist action and hence the initial response increases as the partial agonist concentration increases, reaching a maximum equal to the maximum response of the partial agonist. However, when the full agonist is added in the presence of the partial agonist its concentration–response curve is shifted to the right.

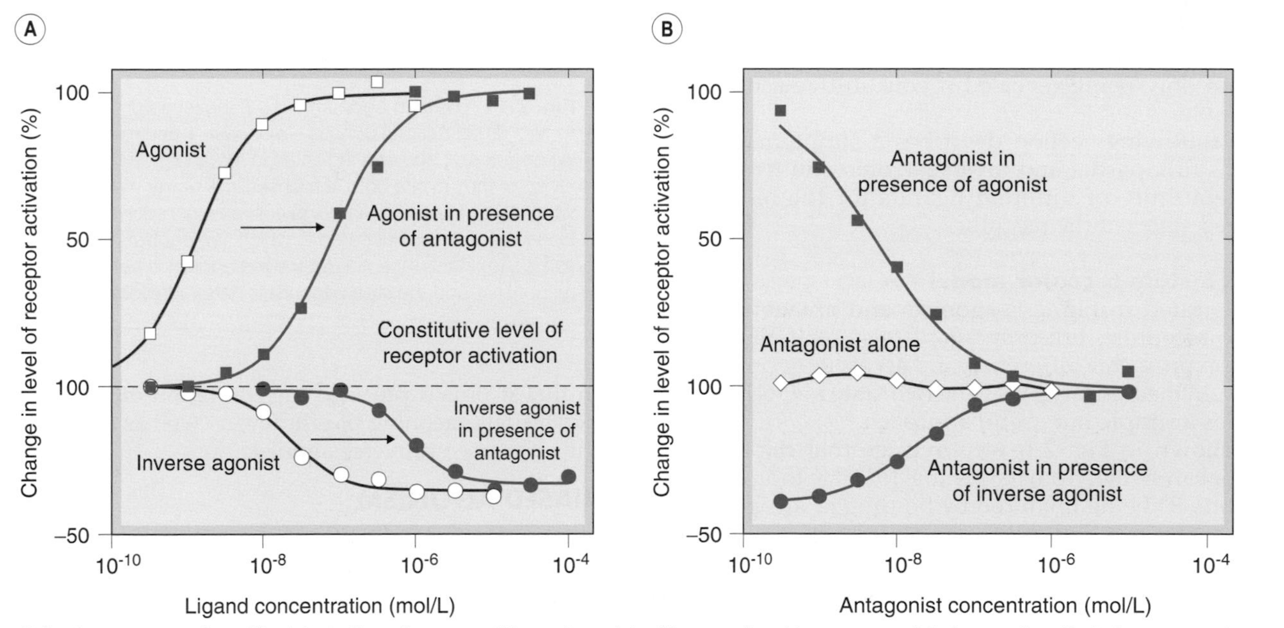

Fig. 2.9 Inverse agonism. The interaction of a competitive antagonist with normal and inverse agonists in a system that shows receptor activation in the absence of any added ligands (constitutive activation). (A) The degree of receptor activation (vertical scale) increases in the presence of an agonist *(open squares)* and decreases in the presence of an inverse agonist *(open circles)*. The addition of a competitive antagonist shifts both curves to the right *(closed symbols)*. (B) The antagonist on its own does not alter the level of constitutive activity *(open symbols)*, because it has equal affinity for the active and inactive states of the receptor. In the presence of an agonist *(closed squares)* or an inverse agonist *(closed circles)*, the antagonist restores the system towards the constitutive level of activity. These data were obtained with cloned human 5-hydroxytryptamine (5-HT) receptors expressed in a cell line. (Agonist, 5-carboxamidotryptamine; inverse agonist, spiperone; antagonist, WAY 100635; see Ch. 16 for information on 5-HT receptor pharmacology.) (Reproduced with permission from Newman-Tancredi, A., et al., 1997. Br. J. Pharmacol. 120, 737–739.)

increasing frequency (mainly among G protein–coupled receptors). **Pimavanserin**, an inverse agonist at the 5-HT_{2A} receptor, has recently been developed for the treatment of psychosis associated with Parkinson's disease (see Chs 40 and 47). It turns out that most of the receptor antagonists in clinical use are actually inverse agonists when tested in systems showing constitutive receptor activation. However, most receptors – like cats – show a preference for the inactive state, and for these there is no practical difference between a competitive antagonist and an inverse agonist, inverse

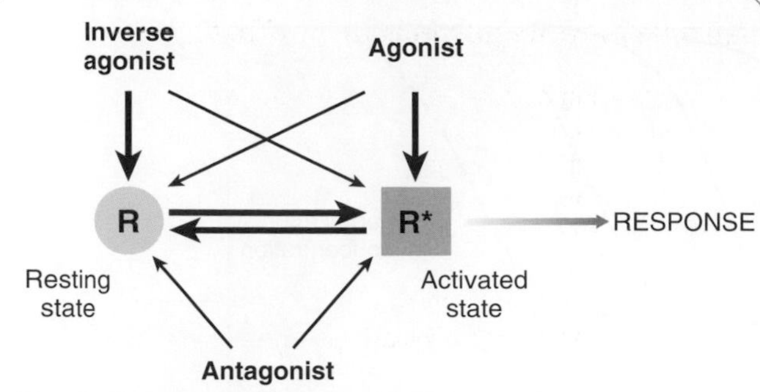

Fig. 2.10 The two-state model. The receptor is shown in two conformational states, *resting (R)* and *activated (R*)*, which exist in equilibrium. Normally, when no ligand is present, the equilibrium lies far to the left, and few receptors are found in the R* state. For constitutively active receptors, an appreciable proportion of receptors adopt the R* conformation in the absence of any ligand. Agonists have higher affinity for R* than for R, so shift the equilibrium towards R*. The greater the relative affinity for R* with respect to R, the greater the efficacy of the agonist. An inverse agonist has higher affinity for R than for R* and so shifts the equilibrium to the left. A *neutral* antagonist has equal affinity for R and R* so does not by itself affect the conformational equilibrium but reduces by competition the binding of other ligands.

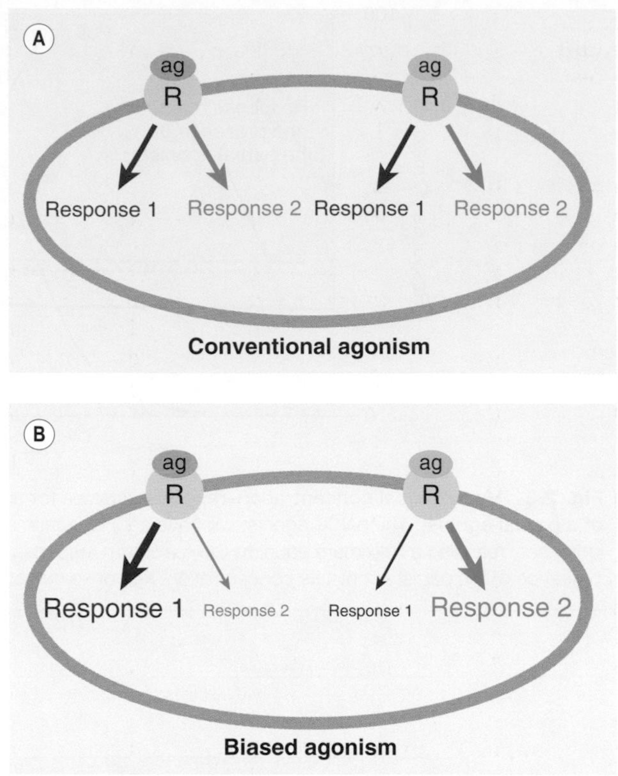

Fig. 2.11 Biased agonism. In (A), the receptor *(R)* is coupled to two intracellular responses – *response 1* and *response 2*. When different agonists indicated in *red* and *green* activate the receptor they evoke both responses in a similar manner. This is what we can consider as being conventional agonism. In (B), biased agonism is illustrated in which two agonists bind at the same site on the receptor yet the *red* agonist is better at evoking response 1 and the *green* agonist is better at evoking response 2.

agonism only being revealed if constitutive activation is observable.

The following section describes a simple model that explains full, partial and inverse agonism in terms of the relative affinity of different ligands for the resting and activated states of the receptor.

The two-state receptor model

As illustrated in Fig. 2.1, agonists and antagonists both bind to receptors, but only agonists activate them. How can we express this difference, and account for constitutive activity, in theoretical terms? The two-state model (Fig. 2.10) provides a simple but useful approach.

As shown in Fig. 2.1, we envisage that the occupied receptor can switch from its 'resting' (R) state to an activated (R*) state, R* being favoured by binding of an agonist but not an antagonist molecule.

As described earlier, receptors may show constitutive activation (i.e. the R* conformation can exist without any ligand being bound), so the added drug encounters an equilibrium mixture of R and R* (see Fig. 2.10). If it has a higher affinity for R* than for R, the drug will cause a shift of the equilibrium towards R* (i.e. it will promote activation and be classed as an agonist). If its preference for R* is very large, nearly all the occupied receptors will adopt the R* conformation and the drug will be a full agonist; if it shows only a modest degree of selectivity for R* (say 5- to 10-fold), a smaller proportion of occupied receptors will adopt the R* conformation and it will be a partial agonist; if it shows no preference, the prevailing R : R* equilibrium will not be disturbed and the drug will be a neutral antagonist (zero efficacy), whereas if it shows selectivity for R it will shift the equilibrium towards R and be an inverse agonist (negative efficacy). We can therefore think of efficacy as a property determined by the relative affinity of a ligand for R and R*, a formulation known as the *two-state model*, which is useful in that it puts a physical interpretation on the otherwise mysterious meaning of efficacy, as well as accounting for the existence of inverse agonists.

BIASED AGONISM

A major problem with the two-state model is that, as we now know, receptors are not actually restricted to two distinct states but have much greater conformational flexibility, so that there is more than one inactive and active conformation. The different conformations that they can adopt may be preferentially stabilised by different ligands, and may produce different functional effects by activating different signal transduction pathways (see Ch. 3).

Receptors that couple to second messenger systems (see Ch. 3) can couple to more than one intracellular effector pathway, giving rise to two or more simultaneous responses. One might expect that all agonists that activate the same receptor type would evoke the same array of responses (Fig. 2.11A). However, it has become apparent that different agonists can exhibit bias for the generation of one response over another even though they are acting through the same receptor (Fig. 2.11B), probably because they stabilise different activated states of the receptor (see Kelly, 2013). Agonist bias has become an important concept in pharmacology.

Redefining and attempting to measure agonist efficacy for such a multistate model is problematic, however, and requires a more complicated state transition model than the two-state model described previously. The errors, pitfalls and a possible way forward have been outlined by Kenakin and Christopoulos (2013).

ALLOSTERIC MODULATION

In addition to the agonist binding site (now referred to as the *orthosteric* binding site), to which competitive antagonists also bind, receptor proteins possess many other *(allosteric)* binding sites (see Ch. 3) through which drugs can influence receptor function in various ways, by increasing or decreasing the affinity of agonists for the agonist binding site, by modifying efficacy or by producing a response themselves (Fig. 2.12). Depending on the direction of the effect, the ligands may be allosteric antagonists or allosteric facilitators of the agonist effect, and the effect may be to alter the slope and maximum of the agonist log concentration–effect curve (see Fig. 2.12). This type of allosteric modulation of receptor function has attracted much attention recently and occurs at different types of receptors (see review by Changeux and Christopoulos, 2016). Well-known examples of allosteric facilitation include glycine at *N*-methyl-D-aspartate (NMDA) receptors (see Ch. 38), benzodiazepines at $GABA_A$ receptors (see Ch. 45) and **cinacalcet** at the Ca^{2+} receptor (see Ch. 36). One reason why allosteric modulation may be important to the pharmacologist and future drug development is that across families of receptors such as the muscarinic receptors (see Ch. 14) the orthosteric binding sites are very similar and it has proven difficult to develop selective agonists and antagonists for individual subtypes. The hope is that there will be greater variation in the allosteric sites and that receptor-selective allosteric ligands can be developed. Furthermore, positive allosteric modulators (PAMs) will exert their effects only on receptors that are being activated by endogenous ligands and have no effect on those that are not activated. This might provide a degree of selectivity (e.g. in potentiating spinal inhibition mediated by endogenous opioids, see Ch. 43) and a reduction in side effect profile.

BITOPIC AGONISTS

To further complicate the issue of drug–receptor interactions, some agonists may display a combination of orthosteric and allosteric actions at the same receptor, providing direct agonist and modulatory functions (see Volpato et al., 2020). These are termed bitopic agonists and we are likely to hear more about such drugs in the future.

OTHER FORMS OF DRUG ANTAGONISM

Other mechanisms can also account for inhibitory interactions between drugs.

The most important ones are:

- chemical antagonism
- pharmacokinetic antagonism
- block of receptor–response linkage
- physiological antagonism

CHEMICAL ANTAGONISM

Chemical antagonism refers to the uncommon situation where the two substances combine in solution; as a result, the effect of the active drug is lost. Examples include the use of chelating agents (e.g. **dimercaprol**) that bind to heavy metals and thus reduce their toxicity, and the use of the neutralising antibody **infliximab**, which has an anti-inflammatory action due to its ability to sequester the inflammatory cytokine tumour necrosis factor (TNF; see Ch. 17).

Agonists, antagonists and efficacy

- Drugs acting on receptors may be *agonists* or *antagonists.*
- Agonists initiate changes in cell function, producing effects of various types; antagonists bind to receptors without initiating such changes.
- Agonist potency depends on two parameters: *affinity* (i.e. tendency to bind to receptors) and *efficacy* (i.e. ability, once bound, to initiate changes that lead to effects).
- For antagonists, efficacy is zero.
- *Full agonists* (which can produce maximal effects) have high efficacy; *partial agonists* (which can produce only submaximal effects) have intermediate efficacy.
- According to the two-state model, efficacy reflects the relative affinity of the compound for the resting and activated states of the receptor. Agonists show selectivity for the activated state; antagonists show no selectivity. This model, although helpful, fails to account for the complexity of agonist action.
- *Inverse agonists* show selectivity for the resting state of the receptor, this being of significance only in situations where the receptors show *constitutive activity.*
- *Allosteric modulators* bind to sites on the receptor other than the agonist binding site and can modify agonist activity.

PHARMACOKINETIC ANTAGONISM

Pharmacokinetic antagonism describes the situation in which the 'antagonist' effectively reduces the concentration of the active drug at its site of action. This can happen in various ways. The rate of metabolic degradation of the active drug may be increased (e.g. the reduction of the anticoagulant effect of **warfarin** when an agent that accelerates its hepatic metabolism, such as **phenytoin**, is given; see Chs 10 and 58). Alternatively, the rate of absorption of the active drug from the gastrointestinal tract may be reduced, or the rate of renal excretion may be increased. Interactions of this sort, discussed in more detail in Chapter 58, are common and can be important in clinical practice.

BLOCK OF RECEPTOR–RESPONSE LINKAGE

Non-competitive antagonism describes the situation where the antagonist blocks at some point downstream from the agonist binding site on the receptor, and interrupts the chain of events that leads to the production of a response by the agonist. For example, **ketamine** enters the ion channel pore of the NMDA receptor (see Ch. 38) blocking it, thus preventing ion flux through the channels. Drugs such as **verapamil** and **nifedipine** prevent the influx of Ca^{2+} through the cell membrane (see Ch. 21) and thus non-selectively block the contraction of smooth muscle produced

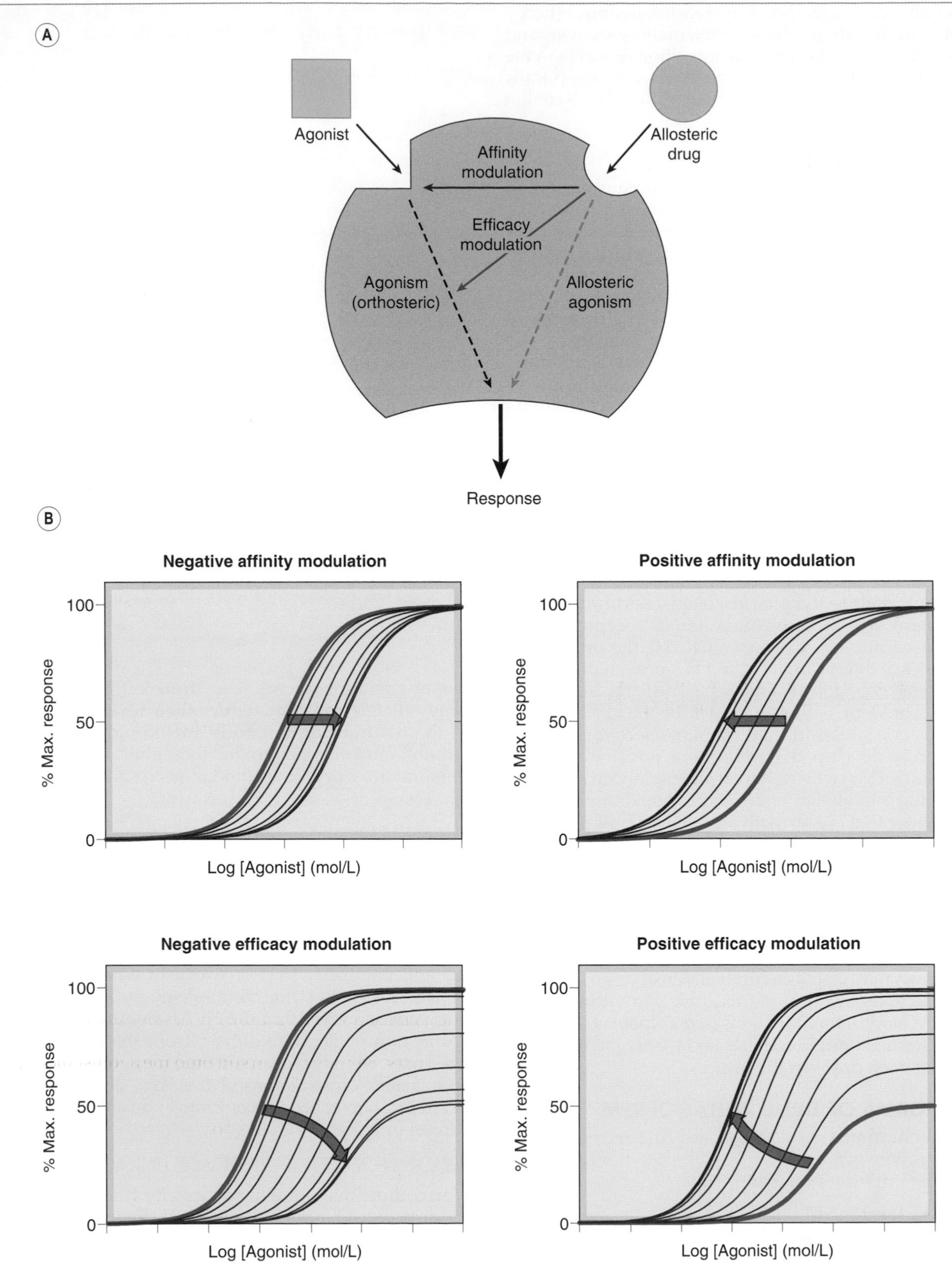

Fig. 2.12 Allosteric modulation. (A) Allosteric drugs bind at a separate site on the receptor to 'traditional' agonists (now often referred to as 'orthosteric' agonists). They can modify the activity of the receptor by (i) altering agonist affinity, (ii) altering agonist efficacy or (iii) directly evoking a response themselves. (B) Effects of affinity- and efficacy-modifying allosteric modulators on the concentration–effect curve of an agonist *(blue line)*. In the presence of the allosteric modulator the agonist concentration–effect curve *(now illustrated in red)* is shifted in a manner determined by the type of allosteric modulator until a maximum effect of the modulator is reached. (Panel [A] adapted with permission from Conn et al., 2009. Nat. Rev. Drug Discov. 8, 41–54; panel [B] courtesy Christopoulos, A.)

by drugs acting at any receptor that couples to these calcium channels. As a rule, the effect will be to reduce the slope and maximum of the agonist log concentration–response curve, although it is quite possible for some degree of rightward shift to occur as well.

PHYSIOLOGICAL ANTAGONISM

Physiological antagonism is a term used loosely to describe the interaction of two drugs whose opposing actions in the body tend to cancel each other. For example, **histamine** acts on receptors of the parietal cells of the gastric mucosa to stimulate acid secretion, while **omeprazole** blocks this effect by inhibiting the proton pump; the two drugs can be said to act as physiological antagonists.

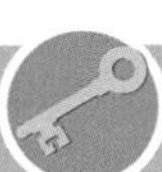

Types of drug antagonism

Drug antagonism occurs by various mechanisms:

- chemical antagonism (interaction in solution)
- pharmacokinetic antagonism (one drug affecting the absorption, metabolism or excretion of the other)
- competitive antagonism (both drugs binding to the same receptors); the antagonism may be reversible or irreversible
- interruption of receptor–response linkage
- physiological antagonism (two agents producing opposing physiological effects)

DESENSITISATION AND TOLERANCE

Often, the effect of a drug gradually diminishes when it is given continuously or repeatedly. *Desensitisation* and *tachyphylaxis* are synonymous terms used to describe this phenomenon, which often develops in the course of a few minutes. The term *tolerance* is conventionally used to describe a more gradual decrease in responsiveness to a drug, taking hours, days or weeks to develop, but the distinction is not a sharp one. The term *refractoriness* is also sometimes used, mainly in relation to a loss of therapeutic efficacy. *Drug resistance* is a term used to describe the loss of effectiveness of antimicrobial or antitumour drugs (see Chs 51 and 57). Many different mechanisms can give rise to these phenomena. They include:

- change in receptors
- translocation of receptors
- exhaustion of mediators
- increased metabolic degradation of the drug
- physiological adaptation
- active extrusion of drug from cells (mainly relevant in cancer chemotherapy; see Ch. 57)

CHANGE IN RECEPTORS

Among receptors directly coupled to ion channels (see Ch. 3), desensitisation is often rapid and pronounced. At the neuromuscular junction (Fig. 2.13A), the desensitised state is caused by a conformational change in the receptor, resulting in tight binding of the agonist molecule without the opening of the ionic channel. Phosphorylation of intracellular regions of the receptor protein is a second, slower mechanism by which ion channels become desensitised.

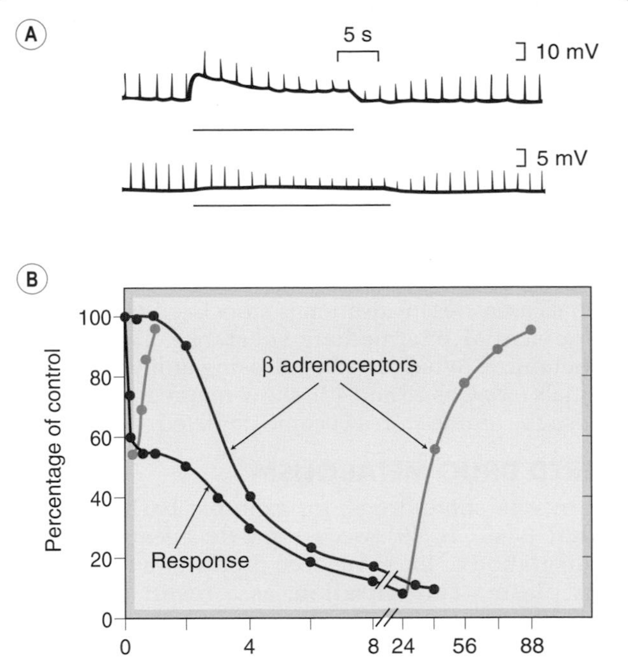

Fig. 2.13 Two kinds of receptor desensitisation. (A) Acetylcholine (ACh) at the frog motor endplate. Brief depolarisations *(upward deflections)* are produced by short pulses of ACh delivered from a micropipette. A long pulse *(horizontal line)* causes the response to decline with a time course of about 20 seconds, owing to desensitisation, and it recovers with a similar time course. (B) β-Adrenoceptors of rat glioma cells in tissue culture. Isoproterenol (1 μmol/L) was added at time zero, and the adenylyl cyclase response and β-adrenoceptor density measured at intervals. During the early uncoupling phase, the response *(blue line)* declines with no change in receptor density *(red line)*. Later, the response declines further concomitantly with disappearance of receptors from the membrane by internalisation. The *green* and *orange lines* show the recovery of the response and receptor density after the isoproterenol is washed out during the early or late phase. (Panel [A] from Katz B., Thesleff S., 1957. J. Physiol. 138, 63; panel [B] from Perkins, J.P., 1981. Trends Pharmacol. Sci. 2, 326.)

Most G protein–coupled receptors (see Ch. 3) also show desensitisation (Fig. 2.13B). Phosphorylation of the receptor interferes with its ability to activate second messenger cascades, although it can still bind the agonist molecule. The molecular mechanisms of this 'uncoupling' are considered further in Chapter 3. This type of desensitisation usually takes seconds to minutes to develop, and recovers when the agonist is removed.

It will be realised that the two-state model in its simple form, discussed earlier, needs to be further elaborated to incorporate additional desensitised states of the receptor.

TRANSLOCATION OF RECEPTORS

Prolonged exposure to agonists often results in a gradual decrease in the number of receptors expressed on the cell surface, as a result of *internalisation* of the receptors. This is shown for β adrenoceptors in Fig. 2.13B and is a slower process than the uncoupling described earlier. Similar changes have been described for other types of receptor, including those for various peptides. The internalised receptors are taken into the cell by endocytosis of patches of the membrane, a process that normally depends on receptor phosphorylation and the subsequent binding of *arrestin* proteins to the phosphorylated receptor (see Ch. 3, Fig. 3.16). This type of adaptation is common for hormone receptors and has obvious relevance to the effects produced when drugs are given for extended periods. It is generally an unwanted complication when agonist drugs are used clinically.

EXHAUSTION OF MEDIATORS

In some cases, desensitisation is associated with depletion of an essential intermediate substance. Drugs such as **amphetamine**, which acts by releasing amines from nerve terminals (see Chs 15 and 49), show marked tachyphylaxis because the amine stores become depleted.

ALTERED DRUG METABOLISM

Tolerance to some drugs, for example **barbiturates** and **ethanol** (see Ch. 49), occurs partly because repeated administration of the same dose produces a progressively lower plasma concentration, as a result of increased metabolic degradation. The degree of tolerance that results is generally modest, and in both of these examples other mechanisms contribute to the substantial tolerance that actually occurs. However, the pronounced tolerance to **nitrovasodilators** (see Chs 19 and 21) results mainly from decreased metabolism, which reduces the release of the active mediator, nitric oxide.

PHYSIOLOGICAL ADAPTATION

Diminution of a drug's effect may occur because it is nullified by a homeostatic response. For example, the blood pressure-lowering effect of **thiazide diuretics** is limited because of a gradual activation of the renin–angiotensin system (see Ch. 21). Such homeostatic mechanisms are very common, and if they occur slowly the result will be a gradually developing tolerance. It is a common experience that many side effects of drugs, such as nausea or sleepiness, tend to subside even though drug administration is continued. We may assume that some kind of physiological adaptation is occurring, presumably associated with altered gene expression resulting in changes in the levels of various regulatory molecules, but little is known about the mechanisms involved.

QUANTITATIVE ASPECTS OF DRUG–RECEPTOR INTERACTIONS

Here we present some aspects of so-called receptor theory, which is based on applying the Law of Mass Action to the drug–receptor interaction and which has served well as a framework for interpreting a large body of quantitative experimental data (see Colquhoun, 2006).

THE BINDING REACTION

The first step in drug action on specific receptors is the formation of a reversible drug–receptor complex, the reactions being governed by the Law of Mass Action. Suppose that a piece of tissue, such as heart muscle or smooth muscle, contains a total number of receptors, N_{tot}, for an agonist such as adrenaline. When the tissue is exposed to adrenaline at concentration x_A and allowed to come to equilibrium, a certain number, N_A, of the receptors will become occupied, and the number of vacant receptors will be reduced to $N_{tot} - N_A$. Normally, the number of adrenaline molecules applied to the tissue in solution greatly exceeds N_{tot}, so that the binding reaction does not appreciably reduce x_A. The magnitude of the response produced by the adrenaline will be related (even if we do not know exactly how) to the number of receptors occupied, so it is useful to consider what quantitative relationship is predicted between N_A and x_A. The reaction can be represented by:

$$\begin{array}{ccccc} A & + & R & \underset{k_{-1}}{\overset{k_{+1}}{\rightleftharpoons}} & AR \\ \text{drug} & + & \text{free receptor} & & \text{complex} \\ (x_A) & & (N_{tot} - N_A) & & (N_A) \end{array}$$

The Law of Mass Action (which states that the rate of a chemical reaction is proportional to the product of the concentrations of reactants) can be applied to this reaction.

$$\text{Rate of forward reaction} = k_{+1} x_A (N_{tot} - N_A) \quad \textbf{(2.1)}$$

$$\text{Rate of backward reaction} = k_{-1} N_A \quad \textbf{(2.2)}$$

At equilibrium, the two rates are equal:

$$k_{+1} x_A (N_{tot} - N_A) = k_{-1} N_A \quad \textbf{(2.3)}$$

The *affinity constant* of binding is given by k_{+1}/k_{-1} and from Eq. 2.3 equals $N_A / x_A(N_{tot} - N_A)$. Unfortunately, this has units of reciprocal concentration (L/mol) which for some of us is a little hard to get our heads around. Pharmacologists therefore tend to use the reciprocal of the affinity constant, the equilibrium dissociation constant *(K)*, which has units of concentration (mol/L).

For drug A its equilibrium dissociation constant (K_A)[6] can be represented as

$$K_A = k_{-1} / k_{+1} = x_A (N_{tot} - N_A) / N_A \quad \textbf{(2.4)}$$

The proportion of receptors occupied, or occupancy (P_A), is N_A/N_{tot}. If we manipulate Eq. 2.4 then

$$P_A = \frac{x_A}{x_A + k_{-1}/k_{+1}} = \frac{x_A}{x_A + K_A} \quad \textbf{(2.5)}$$

Thus if the equilibrium dissociation constant of a drug is known we can calculate the proportion of receptors it will occupy at any concentration as it is independent of N_{tot}.

Eq. 2.5 can be written as:

$$P_A = \frac{x_A / K_A}{x_A / K_A + 1} \quad \textbf{(2.6)}$$

This important result is known as the Hill-Langmuir equation.[7]

The *equilibrium dissociation constant*, K_A, is a characteristic of the drug and of the receptor; it has the dimensions of

[6]Here we now use 'K_A' rather than just 'K' because we will in the next section be going on to consider the situation when two drugs, A and B, are present and there we will use 'K_A' and 'K_B' to denote the equilibrium dissociation constants of the two drugs.

[7]A.V. Hill first published it in 1909, when he was still a medical student. Langmuir, a physical chemist working on gas adsorption, derived it independently in 1916. Both subsequently won Nobel Prizes. Until recently, it was known to pharmacologists as the Langmuir equation, even though Hill deserves the credit.

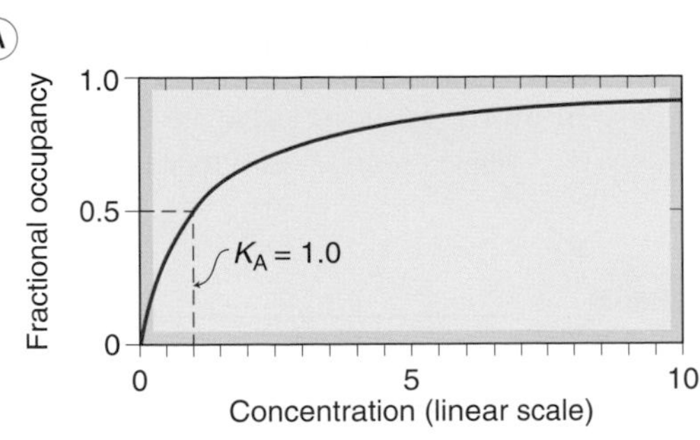

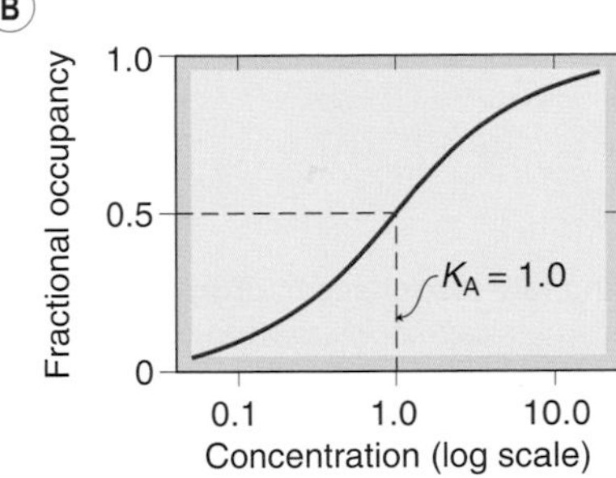

Fig. 2.14 Theoretical relationship between occupancy and ligand concentration. The relationship is plotted according to Eq. 2.5. (A) Plotted with a linear concentration scale, this curve is a rectangular hyperbola. (B) Plotted with a log concentration scale, it is a symmetrical sigmoid curve. K_A is defined in the text and footnote 6.

concentration and is numerically equal to the concentration of drug required to occupy 50% of the sites at equilibrium. (Verify from Eq. 2.5 that when $x_A = K_A$ then $P_A = 0.5$.) The higher the affinity of the drug for the receptors, the lower will be the value of K_A. Eq. 2.6 describes the relationship between occupancy and drug concentration, and it generates a characteristic curve known as a *rectangular hyperbola*, as shown in Fig. 2.14A. It is common in pharmacological work to use a logarithmic scale of concentration; this converts the hyperbola to a symmetrical sigmoid curve (Fig. 2.14B).

The same approach is used to analyse data from experiments in which drug binding is measured directly (see Fig. 2.2). In this case, the relationship between the amount bound (B) and ligand concentration (x_A) should be:

$$B = B_{\max} x_A / (x_A + K_A) \tag{2.7}$$

where B_{max} is the total number of binding sites in the preparation (often expressed as pmol/mg of protein). To display the results in linear form, Eq. 2.6 may be rearranged to:

$$B / x_A = B_{\max} / K_A - B / K_A \tag{2.8}$$

A plot of B/x_A against B (known as a *Scatchard plot*, named after the American physicochemist George Scatchard) gives a straight line from which both B_{max} and K_A can be estimated. Statistically, this procedure is not without problems, and it is now usual to estimate these parameters from the untransformed binding values by an iterative non-linear curve-fitting procedure.[8]

To this point, our analysis has considered the binding of one ligand to a homogeneous population of receptors. To get closer to real-life pharmacology, we must consider (a) what happens when more than one ligand is present, and (b) how the tissue response is related to receptor occupancy.

BINDING WHEN MORE THAN ONE DRUG IS PRESENT

Suppose that two drugs, A and B, which bind to the same receptor with equilibrium dissociation constants K_A and K_B, respectively, are present at concentrations x_A and x_B. If the two drugs compete (i.e. the receptor can accommodate only one at a time), then, by application of the same reasoning as for the one-drug situation described earlier, the occupancy by drug A is given by:

$$P_A = \frac{x_A / K_A}{x_A / K_A + x_B / K_B + 1} \tag{2.9}$$

Comparing this result with Eq. 2.5 shows that adding drug B, as expected, reduces the occupancy by drug A. Fig. 2.4A shows the predicted binding curves for A in the presence of increasing concentrations of B, demonstrating the shift without any change of slope or maximum that characterises the pharmacological effect of a competitive antagonist (see Fig. 2.5). The extent of the rightward shift, on a logarithmic scale, represents the ratio (r_A, given by x_A'/x_A where x_A' is the increased concentration of A) by which the concentration of A must be increased to overcome the competition by B. Rearranging Eq. 2.9 shows that

$$r_A = (x_B / K_B) + 1 \tag{2.10}$$

Thus r_A depends only on the concentration and equilibrium dissociation constant of the competing drug B, not on the concentration or equilibrium dissociation constant of A.

If A is an agonist, and B is a competitive antagonist, and we assume that the response of the tissue will be an unknown function of P_A, then the value of r_A determined from the shift of the agonist concentration–effect curve at different antagonist concentrations can be used to estimate the equilibrium dissociation constant K_B for the antagonist. Such pharmacological estimates of r_A are commonly termed *agonist dose ratios* (more properly concentration ratios, although most pharmacologists use the older term). This simple and very useful Eq. 2.10 is known as the *Schild equation*, after the pharmacologist who first used it to analyse drug antagonism.

Eq. 2.10 can be expressed logarithmically in the form:

$$\log (r_A - 1) = \log x_B - \log K_B \tag{2.11}$$

Thus a plot of log (r_A−1) against log x_B, usually called a Schild plot (as in Fig. 2.5, earlier), should give a straight line with unit slope (i.e. its gradient is equal to 1) and an abscissal intercept equal to log K_B. Following the pH and pK notation, antagonist potency can be expressed as a pA_2 value; under conditions of competitive antagonism, $pA_2 = -\log K_B$. Numerically, pA_2 is defined as the negative logarithm of the molar concentration of antagonist required to produce an agonist dose ratio equal to 2. As with pH notation, its principal advantage is that it produces simple numbers, a pA_2 of 6.5 being equivalent to a K_B of 3.2×10^{-7} mol/L.

[8]Such iterative non-linear curve-fitting computer programmes were not available to our pharmacological forebears.

For competitive antagonism, r shows the following characteristics:

- It depends only on the concentration and equilibrium dissociation constant of the antagonist, and not on the size of response that is chosen as a reference point for the measurements (so long as it is submaximal).
- It does not depend on the equilibrium dissociation constant of the agonist.
- It increases linearly with x_B, and the slope of a plot of $(r_A - 1)$ against x_B is equal to $1/K_B$; this relationship, being independent of the characteristics of the agonist, should be the same for an antagonist against all agonists that act on the same population of receptors.

These predictions have been verified for many examples of competitive antagonism (see Fig. 2.5).

In this section, we have avoided going into great detail and have oversimplified the theory considerably. As we learn more about the actual molecular details of how receptors work to produce their biological effects (see Ch. 3), the shortcomings of this theoretical treatment will become more obvious. The two-state model can be incorporated without difficulty, but complications arise when we include the involvement of G proteins (see Ch. 3) in the reaction scheme (as they shift the equilibrium between R and R*), and when we allow for the fact that receptor activation is not a simple on–off switch, as the two-state model assumes, but may take different forms. Despite strenuous efforts by theoreticians to allow for such possibilities, the molecules always seem to remain one step ahead. Nevertheless, this type of basic theory applied to the two-state model remains a useful basis for developing quantitative models of drug action. The book by Kenakin (1997) is recommended as an introduction, and the later review (Kenakin and Christopoulos, 2011) presents a detailed account of the value of quantification in the study of drug action.

Binding of drugs to receptors

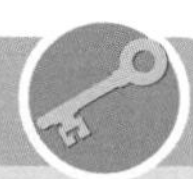

- Binding of drugs to receptors necessarily obeys the *Law of Mass Action.*
- At equilibrium, receptor occupancy is related to drug concentration by the *Hill–Langmuir equation* (Eq. 2.6).
- The higher the affinity of the drug for the receptor, the lower the concentration at which it produces a given level of occupancy.
- The same principles apply when two or more drugs compete for the same receptors; each has the effect of reducing the apparent affinity for the other.

THE NATURE OF DRUG EFFECTS

In discussing how drugs act in this chapter, we have focused mainly on the rapid consequences of receptor activation. Details of the receptors and their linkage to effects at the cellular level are described in Chapter 3. We now have a fairly good understanding at this level. It is important, however, particularly when considering drugs in a therapeutic context, that their direct effects on cellular function generally lead to secondary, delayed effects, which are often highly relevant in a clinical situation in relation to both therapeutic efficacy and harmful effects (Fig. 2.15). For example, activation of cardiac β-adrenoceptors (see Chs 3 and 20) causes rapid changes in the functioning of the heart muscle, but also slower (minutes to hours) changes in the functional state of the receptors (e.g. desensitisation), and even slower (hours to days) changes in gene expression that produce long-term changes (e.g. hypertrophy) in cardiac structure and function. Opioids (see Ch. 43) produce an immediate analgesic effect, but after a time, tolerance and dependence ensue. In these and many other examples, the nature of the intervening mechanism is unclear, although as a general rule any long-term phenotypic change necessarily involves alterations of gene expression. Drugs are often used to treat chronic conditions, and understanding long-term as well as acute drug effects is very important. Pharmacologists have traditionally tended to focus on short-term physiological responses, which are much easier to study, rather than on delayed effects. The focus is now clearly shifting.

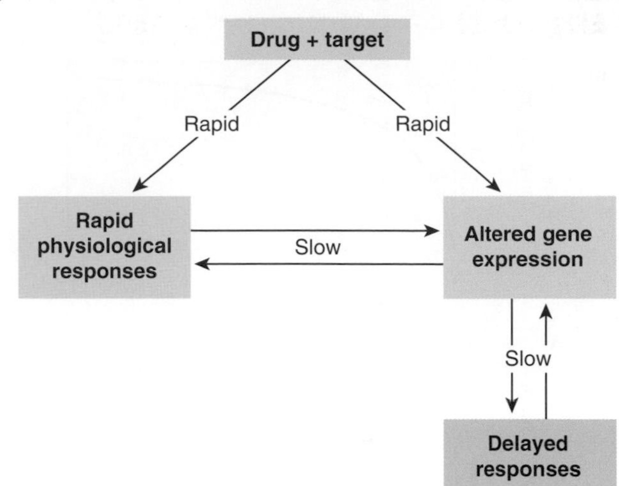

Fig. 2.15 Early and late responses to drugs. Many drugs act directly on their targets *(left-hand arrow)* to produce a rapid physiological response. If this is maintained, it is likely to cause changes in gene expression that give rise to delayed effects. Some drugs *(right-hand arrow)* have their primary action on gene expression, producing delayed physiological responses. Drugs can also work by both pathways. Note the bidirectional interaction between gene expression and response.

Drug effects

- Drugs act mainly on cellular targets, producing effects at different functional levels (e.g. biochemical, cellular, physiological and structural).
- The direct effect of the drug on its target produces acute responses at the biochemical, cellular or physiological levels.
- Prolonged receptor activation generally leads to *delayed long-term effects*, such as desensitisation or down-regulation of receptors, hypertrophy, atrophy or remodelling of tissues, tolerance and dependence.
- Long-term delayed responses result from changes in gene expression, although the mechanisms by which the acute effects bring this about are often uncertain.
- Therapeutic effects may be based on acute responses (e.g. the use of bronchodilator drugs to treat asthma; Ch. 28) or delayed responses (e.g. antidepressants; Ch. 48).

REFERENCES AND FURTHER READING

General

Alexander, S.P.H., Kelly, E., Mathie, A., et al., 2019. The concise guide to pharmacology. Br. J. Pharmacol. 176 (S1), S1–S493.

Colquhoun, D., 2006. The quantitative analysis of drug–receptor interactions: a short history. Trends Pharmacol. Sci. 27, 149–157.

Franks, N.P., 2008. General anaesthesia: from molecular targets to neuronal pathways of sleep and arousal. Nat. Rev. Neurosci. 9, 370–386.

Guide to Pharmacology. Available at: https://www.guidetopharmacology.org/.

Kenakin, T., 1997. Pharmacologic Analysis of Drug–Receptor Interactions, third ed. Lippincott-Raven, New York.

Kenakin, T., Christopoulos, A., 2013. Signalling bias in new drug discovery: detection, quantification and therapeutic impact. Nat. Rev. Drug Discov. 12, 205–216.

Rang, H.P., 2006. The receptor concept: pharmacology's big idea. Br. J. Pharmacol. 147 (Suppl. 1), 9–16.

Stephenson, R.P., 1956. A modification of receptor theory. Br. J. Pharmacol. 11, 379–393.

Receptor mechanisms: agonists and efficacy

Bond, R.A., Ijzerman, A.P., 2006. Recent developments in constitutive receptor activity and inverse agonism, and their potential for GPCR drug discovery. Trends Pharmacol. Sci. 27, 92–96.

Changeux, J.P., Christopoulos, A., 2016. Allosteric modulation as a unifying mechanism for receptor function and regulation. Cell 166, 1084–1102.

De Ligt, R.A.F., Kourounakis, A.P., Ijzerman, A.P., 2000. Inverse agonism at G protein-coupled receptors: (patho)physiological relevance and implications for drug discovery. Br. J. Pharmacol. 130, 1–12.

Kelly, E., 2013. Efficacy and ligand bias at the μ-opioid receptor. Br. J. Pharmacol. 169, 1430–1446.

Kenakin, T., Christopoulos, A., 2011. Analytical pharmacology: the impact of numbers on pharmacology. Trends Pharmacol. Sci. 32, 189–196.

May, L.T., Leach, K., Sexton, P.M., Christopoulos, A., 2007. Allosteric modulation of G protein-coupled receptors. Annu. Rev. Pharmacol. Toxicol. 47, 1–51.

Volpato, D., Kauk, M., Messerer, R., et al., 2020. The role of orthosteric building blocks of bitopic ligands for muscarinic M1 receptors. ACS Omega 5, 31706–31715.

3 How drugs act: molecular aspects

OVERVIEW

In this chapter, we move from the general principles of drug action outlined in Chapter 2 to the molecules that are involved in recognising chemical signals and translating them into cellular responses. Molecular pharmacology is advancing rapidly, and the new knowledge is changing our understanding of drug action and opening up many new therapeutic possibilities, further discussed in other chapters.

First, we consider the types of target proteins on which drugs act. Next, we describe the main families of receptors and ion channels. Finally, we discuss the various forms of receptor–effector linkage (signal transduction mechanisms) through which receptors are coupled to the regulation of cell function. The relationship between the molecular structure of a receptor and its functional linkage to a particular type of effector system is a principal theme. In the next two chapters, we see how these molecular events alter important aspects of cell function – a useful basis for understanding the effects of drugs on intact living organisms. We are confident that tomorrow's pharmacology will rest solidly on the advances in cellular and molecular biology that are discussed here.

PROTEIN TARGETS FOR DRUG ACTION

The protein targets for drug action on mammalian cells (Fig. 3.1) that are described in this chapter can be broadly divided into:

- receptors
- ion channels
- enzymes
- transporters (carrier molecules)

The great majority of important drugs act on one or other of these types of protein, but there are exceptions. For example, **colchicine**, used to treat arthritic gout attacks (see Ch. 25), interacts with the structural protein tubulin, while several immunosuppressive drugs (e.g. **ciclosporin**; see Ch. 25) bind to cytosolic proteins known as immunophilins. Therapeutic antibodies act by sequestering mediators of inflammation (see Chs 5, 25 and 40) and oligonucleotide sequences act as antisense or transgenes to alter protein expression (see Ch. 40). Targets for chemotherapeutic drugs (see Chs 51–57), where the aim is to suppress invading microorganisms or cancer cells, include DNA and cell wall constituents as well as other proteins.

RECEPTORS

Receptors (see Fig. 3.1A) are the sensing elements in the system of chemical communications that coordinate the function and responses of all the different cells in the body, the chemical messengers being the various hormones, transmitters and other mediators discussed in Section 2 of this book. Many therapeutically useful drugs act, either as agonists or antagonists, on receptors for known endogenous mediators. In most cases, the endogenous mediator was discovered before – often many years before – the receptor was characterised pharmacologically and biochemically. In some cases, such as the cannabinoid and opioid receptors (see Chs 18 and 43), the endogenous mediators were identified later; in others, known as *orphan receptors* (see later) the mediator, if it exists, still remains unknown. The host defence system also utilises a set of receptors (e.g. the 'Toll' receptors) that are adept at recognising fragments of 'foreign' bacterial and other invading organisms. These are considered separately in Chapter 7.

ION CHANNELS

Ion channels[1] are essentially gateways in cell membranes that selectively allow the passage of particular ions, and that are induced to open or close by a variety of mechanisms. Two important types are *ligand-gated channels* and *voltage-gated channels*. The former open only when one or more agonist molecules are bound, and are properly classified as receptors, since agonist binding is needed to activate them. Voltage-gated channels are gated by changes in the transmembrane potential rather than by agonist binding.

In general, drugs can affect ion channel function in several ways:

1. By binding to the channel protein itself, either to the ligand-binding (*orthosteric*) site of ligand-gated channels or to other (*allosteric*) sites, or, in the simplest case, exemplified by the action of local anaesthetics on the voltage-gated sodium channel (see Ch. 44), the drug molecule plugs the channel physically (see Fig. 3.1B), blocking ion permeation. Examples of drugs that bind to allosteric sites on the channel protein and thereby affect channel gating include:
   - **benzodiazepines** (see Ch. 45). These drugs bind to a region of the $GABA_A$ receptor–chloride channel complex (a ligand-gated channel) that is distinct from the GABA binding site and facilitate the opening of the channel by the inhibitory neurotransmitter GABA (see Ch. 38)
   - vasodilator drugs of the **dihydropyridine** type (see Ch. 21), which inhibit the opening of L-type calcium channels (see Ch. 4).

[1]'Ion channels and the electrical properties they confer on cells are involved in every human characteristic that distinguishes us from the stones in a field' (Armstrong, C.M., 2003. Voltage-gated K channels. Sci. STKE 188, re10).

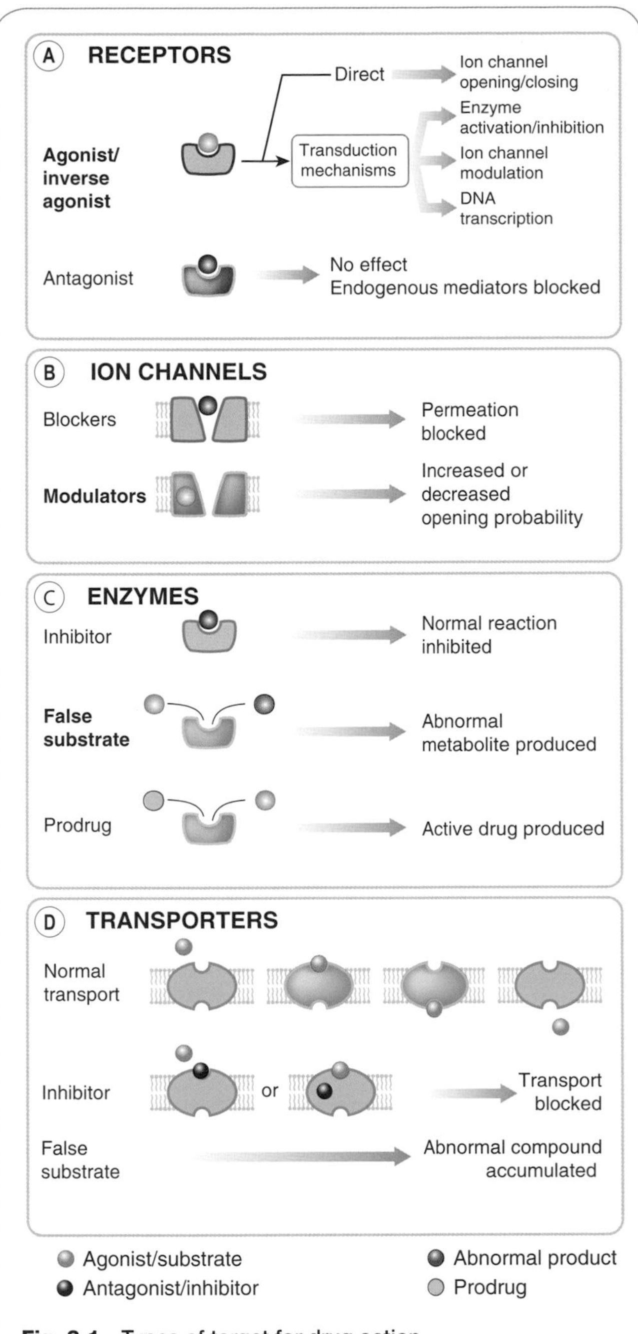

Fig. 3.1 Types of target for drug action.

2. By an indirect interaction, involving an activated G protein subunit or other intermediary.
3. By altering the level of expression of ion channels on the cell surface. For example, **gabapentin** reduces the insertion of neuronal calcium channels into the plasma membrane (see Ch. 46).

A summary of the different ion channel families and their functions is given later.

ENZYMES

Many drugs target enzymes (see Fig. 3.1C). Often, the drug molecule is a substrate analogue that acts as a competitive inhibitor of the enzyme (e.g. **captopril**, acting on angiotensin-converting enzyme; see Ch. 21); in other cases, the binding is irreversible and non-competitive (e.g. **aspirin**, acting on cyclo-oxygenase; see Ch. 25). Drugs may also act as false substrates, where the drug molecule undergoes chemical transformation to form an abnormal product that subverts the normal metabolic pathway. An example is the anticancer drug **fluorouracil**, which replaces uracil as an intermediate in purine biosynthesis but cannot be converted into thymidylate, thus blocking DNA synthesis and preventing cell division (see Ch. 57).

It should also be mentioned that drugs may require enzymic degradation to convert them from an inactive form, the prodrug (see Ch. 10), to an active form (e.g. **enalapril** is converted by esterases to enalaprilat, which inhibits angiotensin-converting enzyme). Furthermore, as discussed in Chapter 58, drug toxicity often results from the enzymic conversion of the drug molecule to a reactive metabolite. **Paracetamol** (see Ch. 25) causes liver damage in this way. As far as the primary action of the drug is concerned, this is an unwanted side reaction, but it is of major practical importance.

TRANSPORTERS

The movement of ions and small polar organic molecules across cell membranes generally occurs either through channels or through the agency of a transport protein (see Fig. 3.1D), because the permeating molecules are often insufficiently lipid-soluble to penetrate lipid membranes on their own. Many such transporters are known; examples of particular pharmacological importance include those responsible for the transport of ions and many organic molecules across the renal tubule, the intestinal epithelium and the blood–brain barrier; the transport of Na^+ and Ca^{2+} out of cells; the uptake of neurotransmitter precursors (such as choline) or of neurotransmitters themselves (such as amines and amino acids) by nerve terminals; and the transport of drug molecules and their metabolites across cell membranes and epithelial barriers. We shall encounter transporters frequently in later chapters.

In many cases, hydrolysis of ATP provides the energy for transport of substances against their electrochemical gradient. Such transport proteins include a distinct ATP-binding site and are termed *ABC* (ATP-Binding Cassette) transporters. Important examples include the sodium pump (Na^+-K^+-ATPase; see Ch. 4) and *multidrug resistance* (MDR) transporters that eject cytotoxic drugs from cancer and microbial cells, often conferring resistance to these therapeutic agents (see Ch. 57). In other cases, including the neurotransmitter transporters, the transport of organic molecules is coupled to the transport of ions (usually Na^+), either in the same direction (*symport*) or in the opposite direction (*antiport*), and therefore relies on the electrochemical gradient for Na^+ generated by the ATP-driven sodium pump. The carrier proteins embody a recognition site that makes them specific for a particular permeating species, and these recognition sites can also be targets for drugs whose effect is to block the transport system (e.g. cocaine blocks monoamine neurotransmitter uptake into nerve terminals; see Ch. 49).

The importance of transporters as a source of individual variation in the pharmacokinetic characteristics of various drugs is increasingly recognised (see Ch. 11).

RECEPTOR PROTEINS

In the 1970s, pharmacology entered a new phase when receptors, which had until then been theoretical entities, began to emerge as biochemical realities. Over the following five decades enormous advances have been made.[2]

A major step forward was in determining the amino acid sequence of receptor proteins first by cloning individual receptors and then thereafter by genome sequencing. Sequence data have revealed many molecular variants (subtypes) of known receptors that had not been evident from pharmacological studies (see IUPHAR/BPS, *Guide to Pharmacology*). Much remains to be discovered about the pharmacological, functional and clinical significance of this abundant molecular polymorphism. It is expected, however, that such variations will account for part of the variability between individuals in response to therapeutic agents (see Ch. 12)

Although we already knew many of the endogenous ligands that activated well-characterised receptors it became apparent from the genome sequencing that there were novel receptors for which the endogenous ligands were so far unknown, and they are described as 'orphan receptors'.[3] Identifying ligands for these presumed receptors was and in some cases still is difficult. Increasingly, there are examples (e.g. free fatty acid receptors) where important endogenous ligands have been linked to hitherto orphan receptors and there is optimism that novel therapeutic agents will emerge by targeting this pool of unclaimed receptors.

Much information has been gained by introducing the cDNA encoding individual receptors into cell lines, producing cells that express the foreign (recombinant) receptors in a functional form. Such engineered cells allow much more precise control of the expressed receptors than is possible with natural cells or intact tissues (e.g. specific mutations can be introduced in the receptor sequence and the resulting changes in receptor function characterised), and recombinant receptor expression is widely used to study the functional and pharmacological characteristics of receptors. Expressed human receptors, which often differ in their sequence and pharmacological properties from their animal counterparts, can be studied in this way.

Many of the difficulties of obtaining crystals of membrane embedded proteins have been overcome. Obtaining crystals of a receptor protein allows its structure to be analysed at very high resolution by X-ray diffraction techniques. X-ray crystallography and more recently cryo-electron microscopy are being used to elucidate the three-dimensional molecular structure of receptors in detail. This then allows the use of sophisticated computational molecular docking and molecular dynamics simulations to study ligand binding to the receptor and subsequent protein conformational changes associated with activation of the receptor.

TYPES OF RECEPTOR

Receptors elicit many different types of cellular effect. Some of them are very rapid, such as those involved in fast synaptic transmission, operating within milliseconds, whereas other receptor-mediated effects, such as many of those produced by thyroid hormone or various steroid hormones, occur over hours or days. There are many examples of intermediate timescales - catecholamines, for example, usually act in a matter of seconds, whereas many peptides take rather longer to produce their effects. Not surprisingly, very different types of linkage between receptor occupation and the ensuing response are involved. Based on molecular structure and the nature of this linkage (the transduction mechanism), we can distinguish four receptor types, or superfamilies (Figs 3.2 and 3.3; Table 3.1).

- Type 1: **ligand-gated ion channels** (also known as **ionotropic** receptors[4]). These are the receptors which mediate fast synaptic transmission in the nervous system (see Table 3.1).
- Type 2: **G protein–coupled receptors** (GPCRs). These are also known as **metabotropic receptors** or **7-transmembrane** (7-TM, serpentine or heptahelical) **receptors.** They are membrane receptors that are coupled to intracellular effector systems primarily via a G protein. They constitute the largest family[5] and include receptors for many hormones and slow transmitters (Table 3.1).
- Type 3: **kinase-linked and related receptors.** This is a large and heterogeneous group of membrane receptors responding mainly to protein mediators. They comprise an extracellular ligand-binding domain linked to an intracellular domain by a single transmembrane helix. In many cases, the intracellular domain is enzymic in nature (with protein kinase or guanylyl cyclase activity). Some lack enzymic activity themselves but link to intracellular effector enzymes through their binding of adaptor proteins.
- Type 4: **nuclear receptors (NRs).** These are receptors that regulate gene transcription.[6] Receptors of this type also recognise many foreign molecules, inducing the expression of enzymes that metabolise them.

MOLECULAR STRUCTURE OF RECEPTORS

The molecular organisation of typical members of each of these four receptor superfamilies is shown in Fig. 3.3. Although individual receptors show considerable sequence variation in particular regions, and the lengths of the main intracellular and extracellular domains also vary from one to another within the same family, the overall structural

[2]Including the awarding of the 2021 Nobel Prize for Physiology and Medicine to David Julius and Ardem Patapoutian, for their discovery of mechano-sensitive and ligand-operated ion channel receptors used in temperature, touch and pain sensation.

[3]An oddly Dickensian term that seems inappropriately condescending. Because we can assume that these receptors play defined roles in physiological signalling, their 'orphanhood' reflects our ignorance, not their status. More information on orphan receptors can be found at www.guidetopharmacology.org/GRAC/FamilyDisplayForward?familyId=115#16.

[4]Here, focusing on receptors, we include ligand-gated ion channels as an example of a receptor family. Other types of ion channels are described later; many are also drug targets, although not receptors in the strict sense.

[5]There are 865 human GPCRs comprising 1.6% of the genome (Fredriksson and Schiöth, 2005). Nearly 500 of these are believed to be odorant receptors involved in smell and taste sensations, the remainder being receptors for known or unknown endogenous mediators - enough to keep pharmacologists busy for some time yet.

[6]The term *nuclear receptor* is something of a misnomer, because some are actually located in the cytosol and migrate to the nuclear compartment when a ligand is present.

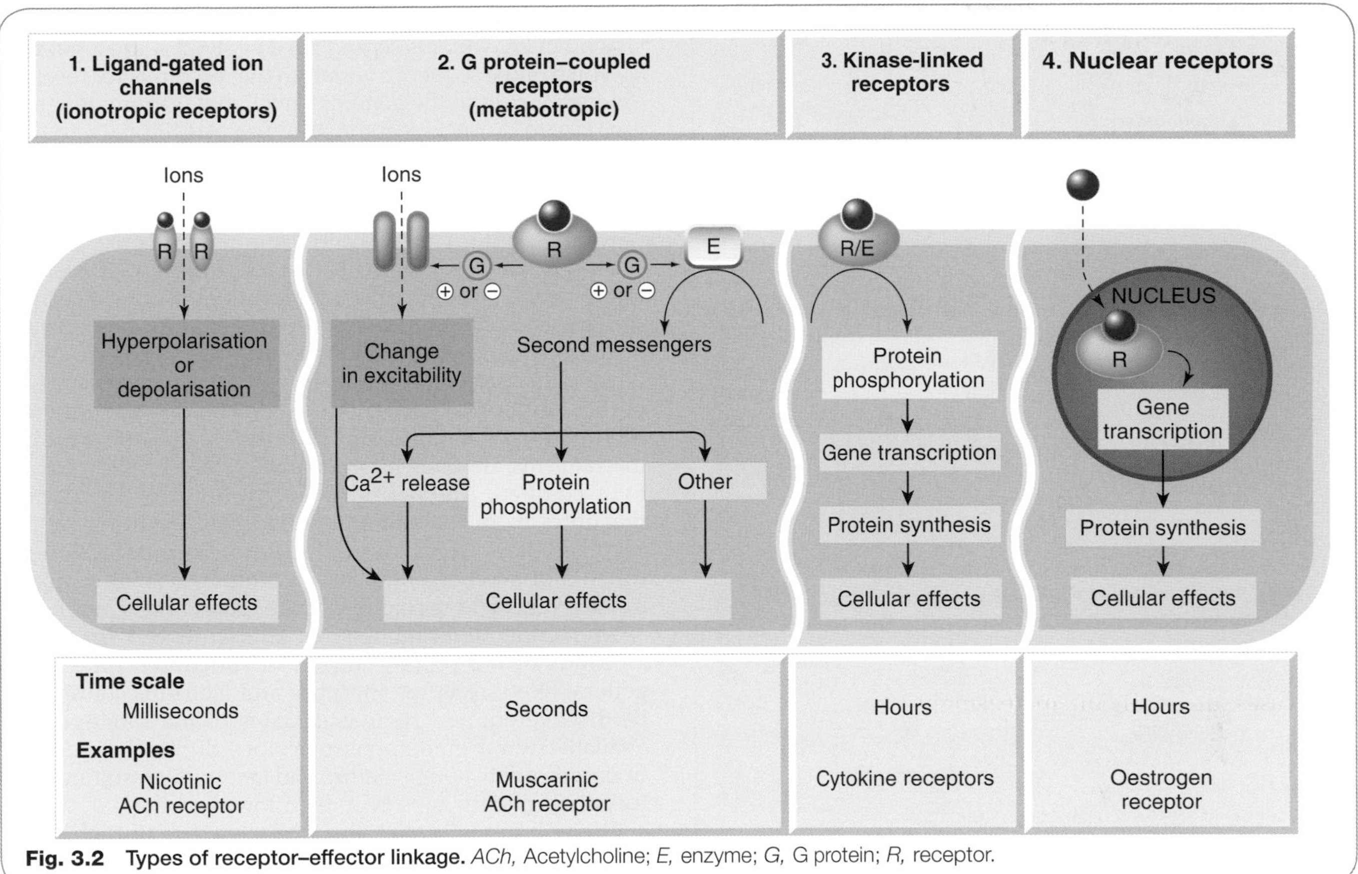

Fig. 3.2 Types of receptor–effector linkage. *ACh,* Acetylcholine; *E,* enzyme; *G,* G protein; *R,* receptor.

Table 3.1 The four main types of receptor

	Type 1: Ligand-gated ion channels	Type 2: G protein–coupled receptors	Type 3: Receptor kinases	Type 4: Nuclear receptors
Location	Membrane	Membrane	Membrane	Intracellular
Effector	Ion channel	Channel or enzyme	Protein kinases	Gene transcription
Coupling	Direct	G protein or arrestin	Direct	Via DNA
Examples	Nicotinic acetylcholine receptor, $GABA_A$ receptor	Muscarinic acetylcholine receptor, adrenoceptors	Insulin, growth factors, cytokine receptors	Steroid receptors
Structure	Oligomeric assembly of subunits surrounding central pore	Monomeric or oligomeric assembly of subunits comprising seven transmembrane helices with intracellular G protein–coupling domain	Single transmembrane helix linking extracellular receptor domain to intracellular kinase domain or kinase-binding ability	Monomeric structure with receptor- and DNA-binding domains

patterns and associated signal transduction pathways are very consistent. The realisation that just four main receptor superfamilies provide a solid framework for interpreting the complex welter of information about the effects of a large proportion of the drugs that have been studied has been one of the most refreshing developments in modern pharmacology.

RECEPTOR HETEROGENEITY AND SUBTYPES

Receptors within a given family generally occur in several molecular varieties, or subtypes, with similar architecture but significant differences in their sequences, and often in their pharmacological properties.[7] Nicotinic acetylcholine receptors are typical in this respect; distinct subtypes occur in different brain regions (see Table 39.2), and these differ from the muscle receptor. Some of the known pharmacological differences (e.g. sensitivity to blocking agents) between muscle and brain acetylcholine receptors correlate with specific sequence differences; however, as far as we know, all nicotinic acetylcholine receptors respond to the same physiological

[7]Receptors for 5-hydroxytryptamine (see Ch. 16) are currently the champions with respect to diversity, with 13 subtypes of GPCR and 1 ligand-gated ion channel all responding to the same endogenous ligand.

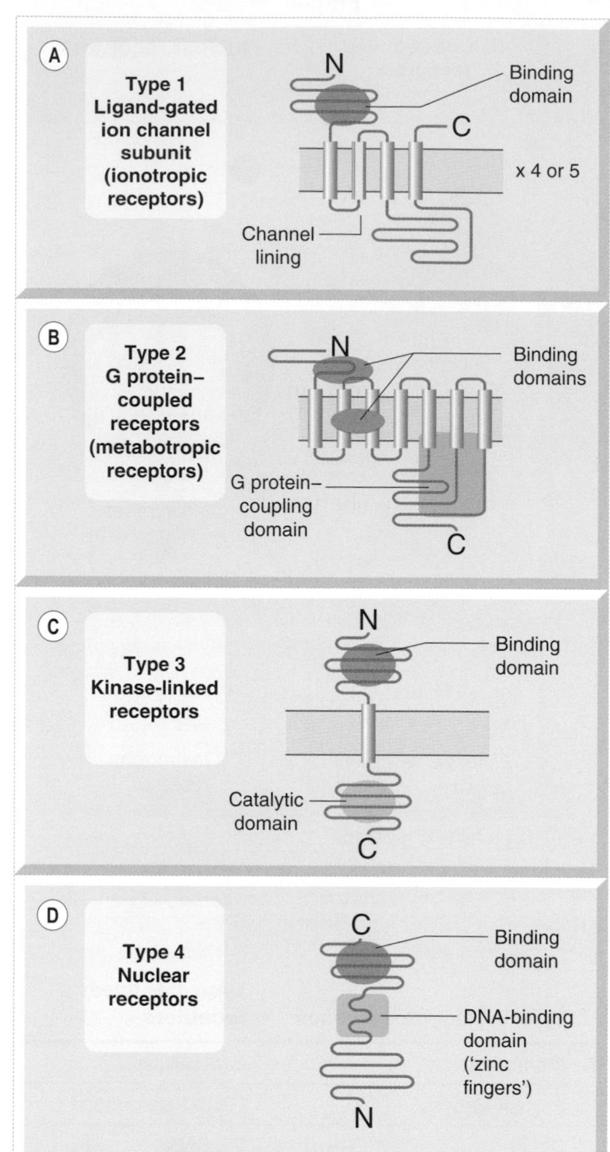

Fig. 3.3 General structure of four receptor families. The rectangular segments represent hydrophobic α-helical regions of the protein comprising approximately 20 amino acids, which form the membrane-spanning domains of the receptors. The *pink shaded areas* illustrate the region of the orthosteric ligand-binding domains. (A) Type 1: ligand-gated ion channel subunit. The example illustrated here shows the subunit structure of the nicotinic acetylcholine receptor. The subunit structure of other ligand-gated ion channels is shown in Fig. 3.5. Many ligand-gated ion channels comprise four or five subunits of the type shown, the whole complex containing 16–20 membrane-spanning segments surrounding a central ion channel. (B) Type 2: G protein–coupled receptors (GPCRs). The two ligand-binding domains shown illustrate the position of the orthosteric ligand-binding domains on different types of GPCRs, there would be only one on each GPCR. (C) Type 3: kinase-linked receptors. Most growth factor receptors incorporate the ligand-binding and enzymatic (kinase) domains in the same molecule, *as shown*, whereas cytokine receptors lack an intracellular kinase domain but link to cytosolic kinase molecules. Other structural variants also exist. (D) Type 4: nuclear receptors that control gene transcription.

mediator and produce the same kind of synaptic response, so why many variants should have evolved is still a puzzle.

Much of the sequence variation that accounts for receptor diversity arises at the genomic level; that is, different genes give rise to distinct receptor subtypes. Additional variation arises from alternative mRNA splicing, which means that a single gene can give rise to more than one receptor isoform. After translation from genomic DNA, the mRNA normally contains non-coding regions (introns) that are excised by mRNA splicing before the message is translated into protein. Depending on the location of the splice sites, splicing can result in inclusion or deletion of one or more of the mRNA coding regions giving rise to long or short forms of the protein. This is an important source of variation, particularly for GPCRs, producing receptors with different binding characteristics and different signal transduction mechanisms, although its pharmacological relevance remains to be clarified. Another process that can produce different receptors from the same gene is mRNA editing, which involves the mischievous substitution of one base in the mRNA for another, and hence potentially a small variation in the amino acid sequence of the expressed receptor.

Molecular heterogeneity of this kind is a feature of all kinds of receptors – indeed of functional proteins in general. New receptor subtypes and isoforms continue to be discovered, and regular updates of the catalogue are available (www.guidetopharmacology.org/). The problems of classification, nomenclature and taxonomy resulting from this flood of data have been mentioned earlier.

We will now describe the characteristics of each of the four receptor superfamilies.

TYPE 1: LIGAND-GATED ION CHANNELS

The nicotinic acetylcholine receptor, which we find at the skeletal neuromuscular junction (see Ch. 14), in autonomic ganglia (see Ch. 14) and in the brain (see Ch. 39), is a typical example of a ligand-gated ion channel, known as the cys-loop receptors (so called because they have in their structure a large intracellular domain between transmembrane domains 3 and 4 containing multiple cysteine residues [see Fig. 3.3A]). Others of this type include the $GABA_A$ and glycine receptors (see Ch. 38) as well as the 5-hydroxytryptamine type 3 ($5\text{-}HT_3$; see Chs 16 and 39) receptor. Other types of ligand-gated ion channel exist – namely ionotropic glutamate receptors (see Ch. 38) and purinergic P2X receptors (see Chs 17 and 39) that differ in several respects from the nicotinic acetylcholine receptor (see Fig. 3.5). In addition to the ligand-gated ion channels found on the cell membrane that mediate fast synaptic transmission, there are also intracellular ligand-gated ion channels – namely the inositol trisphosphate (IP_3) and ryanodine receptors (see Ch. 4) that release Ca^{2+} from intracellular stores.

MOLECULAR STRUCTURE

Ligand-gated ion channels have structural features in common with other ion channels, described later in this chapter. The nicotinic acetylcholine receptor first cloned from the Torpedo electric ray (Fig. 3.4)[8] consists of a pentameric

[8]In early studies, the Torpedo electric ray was used to isolate and purify the nicotinic receptor as it expresses a very high density of nicotinic receptors on its electroplaques. We now realise that the subunit compositions of the mammalian neuromuscular (Ch. 14) and neuronal (Chs 14 and 39) nicotinic receptors are different from that of the Torpedo but here we focus on the Torpedo receptor to keep it simple.

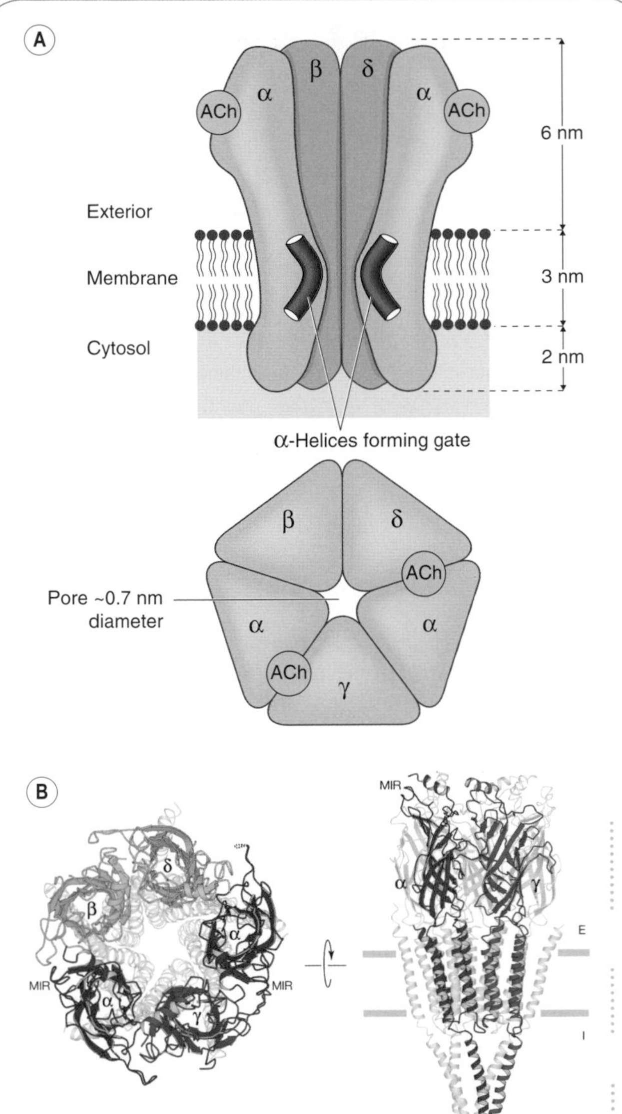

Fig. 3.4 Structure of the nicotinic acetylcholine receptor (a typical ligand-gated ion channel). (A) Schematic diagram in side view *(upper)* and plan view *(lower)*. The five receptor subunits (α_2, β, γ, δ) form a cluster surrounding a central transmembrane pore, the lining of which is formed by the M_2 helical segments of each subunit. These contain a preponderance of negatively charged amino acids, which makes the pore cation selective. There are two acetylcholine binding sites in the extracellular portion of the receptor, at the interface between the α and the adjoining subunits. When acetylcholine binds, the kinked α-helices either straighten out or swing out of the way, thus opening the channel pore. (B) High-resolution image showing revised arrangement of intracellular domains. (Panel [A] based on Unwin, N., 1993. Nicotinic acetylcholine receptor at 9Å resolution. J. Mol. Biol. 229, 1101–1124, and Unwin, N., 1995. Acetylcholine receptor channel imaged in the open state. Nature 373, 37–43; panel [B] reproduced with permission from Unwin, N., 2005. Refined structure of the nicotinic acetylcholine receptor at 4Å resolution. J. Mol. Biol. 346(4), 967–989.)

assembly of different subunits, of which there are four types, termed α, β, γ and δ, each of molecular weight (M_r) 40–58 kDa. The subunits show marked sequence homology, and each contains four membrane-spanning α-helices, inserted into the membrane as shown in Fig. 3.4B. The pentameric structure (α_2, β, γ, δ) possesses two acetylcholine binding sites, each lying at the interface between one of the two α subunits and its neighbour. Both must bind acetylcholine molecules for the receptor to be activated. Fig. 3.4B shows the receptor structure. Each subunit spans the membrane four times, so the channel comprises no fewer than 20 membrane-spanning helices surrounding a central pore.

One of the transmembrane helices (M_2) from each of the five subunits forms the lining of the ion channel (see Fig. 3.4). The five M_2 helices that form the pore are sharply kinked inwards halfway through the membrane, forming a constriction. When acetylcholine molecules bind, a conformation change occurs in the extracellular part of the receptor, which twists the α subunits, causing the kinked M_2 segments to swivel out of the way, thus opening the channel. The channel lining contains a series of anionic residues, making the channel selectively permeable to cations (primarily Na^+ and K^+, although some types of nicotinic receptor are permeable to Ca^{2+} as well).

The use of site-directed mutagenesis, which enables short regions, or single residues, of the amino acid sequence to be altered, has shown that a mutation of a critical residue in the M_2 helix changes the channel from being cation permeable (hence excitatory in the context of synaptic function) to being anion permeable (typical of receptors for inhibitory transmitters such as GABA and glycine). Other mutations affect properties such as gating and desensitisation of ligand-gated channels.

Other ligand-gated ion channels, such as glutamate receptors (see Ch. 38) and P2X receptors (see Chs 16 and 39), whose subunit structures are shown in Fig. 3.5, have a different architecture. Ionotropic glutamate receptors are tetrameric and the pore is built from loops rather than transmembrane helices, in common with many other (non-ligand-gated) ion channels (see Fig. 3.20). P2X receptors are trimeric and each subunit has only two transmembrane domains (North, 2002). The nicotinic receptor and other cys-loop receptors are pentamers with two agonist binding sites on each receptor. Binding of one agonist molecule to one site increases the affinity of binding at the other site (positive cooperativity) and both sites need to be occupied for the receptor to be activated and the channel to open. Some ionotropic glutamate receptors have as many as four agonist binding sites and P2X receptors have three, but they appear to open when two agonist molecules are bound. Once again we realise that the simple model of receptor activation shown in Fig. 2.1 is an oversimplification as it only considered one agonist molecule binding to produce a response. For two or more agonist molecules binding, more complex mathematical models are needed (see Colquhoun, 2006).

THE GATING MECHANISM

Receptors of this type control the fastest synaptic events in the nervous system, in which a neurotransmitter acts on the postsynaptic membrane of a nerve or muscle cell and transiently increases its permeability to particular ions. Most excitatory neurotransmitters, such as acetylcholine at the neuromuscular junction (see Ch. 14) or glutamate in the central nervous system (see Ch. 38), cause an increase in Na^+ and K^+ permeability and in some instances Ca^{2+} permeability. At negative membrane potentials this results in a net inward current carried mainly by Na^+, which

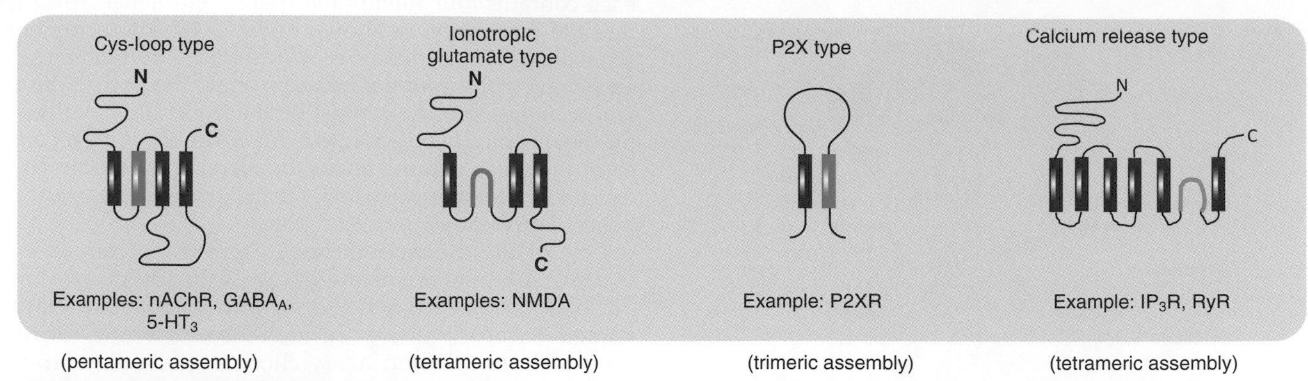

(pentameric assembly) (tetrameric assembly) (trimeric assembly) (tetrameric assembly)

Fig. 3.5 Molecular architecture of ligand-gated ion channels. *Red* and *blue rectangles* represent membrane-spanning α-helices and *blue hairpins* represent the P loop pore-forming regions. *5-HT$_3$*, 5-Hydroxytryptamine type 3 receptor; *GABA$_A$*, GABA type A receptor; *IP$_3$R*, inositol trisphosphate receptor; *nAChR*, nicotinic acetylcholine receptor; *NMDA*, *N*-methyl-D-aspartatic acid receptor; *P2XR*, purine P2X receptor; *RyR*, ryanodine receptor.

depolarises the cell and increases the probability that it will generate an action potential. The action of the transmitter reaches a peak in a fraction of a millisecond, and usually decays within a few milliseconds. The sheer speed of this response implies that the coupling between the receptor and the ion channel is a direct one, and the molecular structure of the receptor–channel complex (see earlier) agrees with this. In contrast to other receptor families, no intermediate biochemical steps are involved in the transduction process.

The *patch clamp recording technique*, devised by Neher and Sakmann, allows the very small current flowing through a single ion channel to be measured directly (Fig. 3.6). The patch clamp technique provides a view, rare in biology, of the physiological behaviour of individual protein molecules in real time, and has given many new insights into the gating reactions and permeability characteristics of both ligand-gated channels and voltage-gated channels. The magnitude of the single channel conductance confirms that permeation occurs through a physical pore through the membrane, because the ion flow is too large (about 10^7 ions per second) to be compatible with a carrier mechanism. The channel conductance produced by different agonists is the same, whereas the mean channel lifetime varies. The ligand–receptor interaction scheme shown in Chapter 2 is a useful model for ion-channel gating. The conformation R*, representing the open state of the ion channel, is thought to be the same for all agonists, accounting for the finding that the channel conductance does not vary. Kinetically, the mean open time is determined mainly by the closing rate constant, α, and this varies from one drug to another. As explained in Chapter 2 (see Fig. 2.1), an agonist of high efficacy that activates a large proportion of the receptors that it occupies will be characterised by $\beta/\alpha \gg 1$, whereas for a drug of low efficacy β/α has a lower value.

At some ligand-gated ion channels, the situation is more complicated because different agonists may cause individual channels to open to one or more of several distinct conductance levels (see Fig. 3.6B). This implies that there is more than one R* conformation. Furthermore, desensitisation of ligand-gated ion channels (see Ch. 2) also involves one or more additional agonist-induced conformational states. These findings necessitate some elaboration of the simple scheme in which only a single open state, R*, is represented and are an example of the way in which the actual behaviour of receptors makes our theoretical models look a little threadbare.

Ligand-gated ion channels

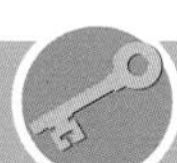

- These are sometimes called ionotropic receptors.
- They are involved mainly in fast synaptic transmission.
- There are several structural families, the commonest being heteromeric assemblies of four or five subunits, with transmembrane helices arranged around a central aqueous channel.
- Ligand binding and channel opening occur on a millisecond timescale.
- Examples include the nicotinic acetylcholine, GABA type A (GABA$_A$), glutamate (e.g. *N*-methyl-D-aspartatic acid receptor [NMDA]) and ATP (P2X) receptors.

TYPE 2: G PROTEIN–COUPLED RECEPTORS

GPCRs constitute the commonest single class of targets for therapeutic drugs. The GPCR family comprises many of the receptors that are familiar to pharmacologists, such as muscarinic AChRs, adrenoceptors, dopamine receptors, 5-HT (serotonin) receptors, receptors for many peptides, purine receptors and many others, including the chemoreceptors involved in olfaction and pheromone detection, and also many 'orphans'. For most of these, pharmacological and molecular studies have revealed a variety of subtypes. All have the characteristic heptahelical structure (see Fig. 3.3B).

Many neurotransmitters, apart from peptides, can interact with both GPCRs and ligand-gated channels, allowing the same molecule to produce fast (through ligand-gated ion channels) and relatively slow (through GPCRs) effects. Individual peptide hormones, however, generally act either on GPCRs or on kinase-linked receptors (see later), but rarely on both, and a similar choosiness applies to the many ligands that act on NRs.[9]

[9]Examples of promiscuity are increasing, however. Steroid hormones, normally faithful to nuclear receptors, make the occasional pass at ion channels and GPCRs, and some eicosanoids act on nuclear receptors as well as GPCRs. Nature is quite open minded, although such examples are liable to make pharmacologists frown and students despair.

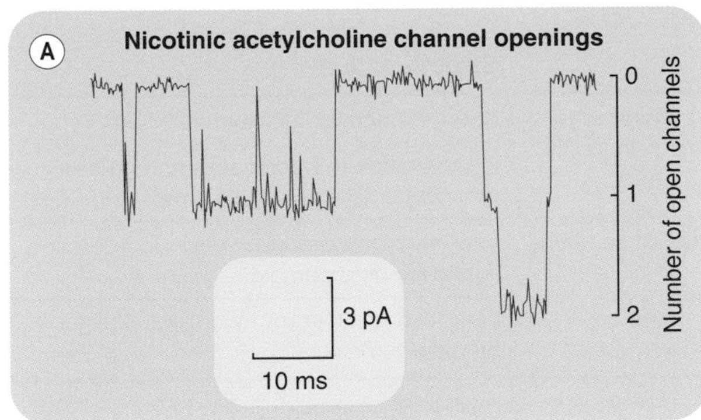

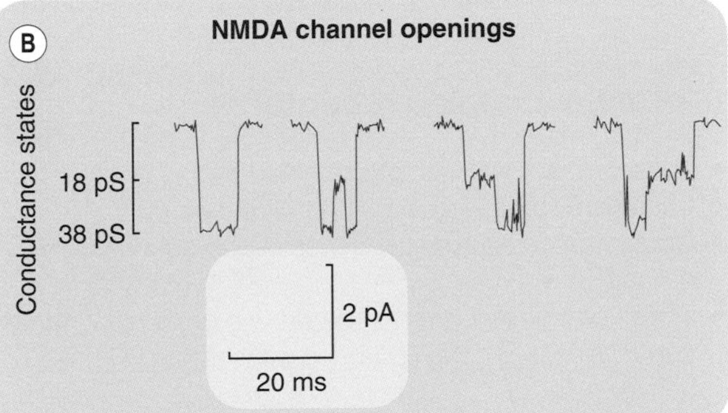

Fig. 3.6 Single channel openings recorded by the patch clamp technique. (A) Acetylcholine-operated ion channels at the frog motor endplate. The pipette, which was applied tightly to the surface of the membrane, contained 10 μmol/L ACh. The downward deflections show the currents flowing through single ion channels in the small patch of membrane under the pipette tip. Towards the end of the record, two channels can be seen to open with a discrete step from the first to the second. (B) Single-channel *N*-methyl-D-aspartic acid receptor (NMDA) receptor currents recorded from cerebellar neurons in the outside-out patch conformation. NMDA was added to the outside of the patch to activate the channel. The channel opens to multiple conductance levels. In (B) the openings to the higher conductance level and the subsequent closings are smooth, indicating that one channel is opening (two channels would not be expected to open and close simultaneously) whereas in (A) there are discrete steps indicating two channels. (Panel [A] courtesy D. Colquhoun and D.C. Ogden; panel [B] reproduced with permission from Cull-Candy, S.G., and Usowicz, M.M., 1987. Multiple-conductance channels activated by excitatory amino acids in cerebellar neurons. Nature 325, 525–528.)

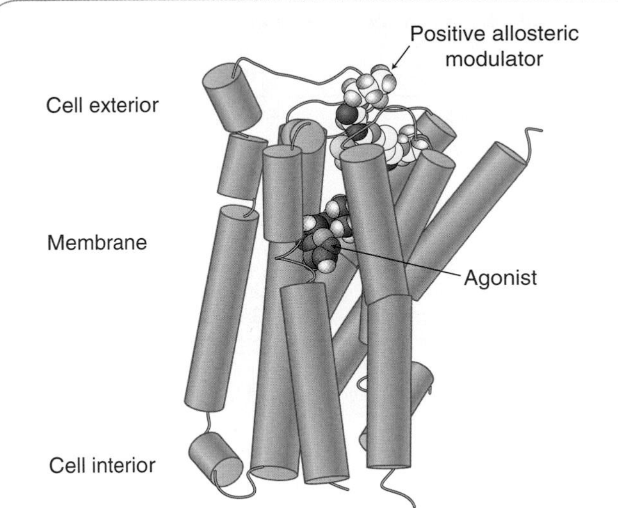

Fig. 3.7 Structure of the M_2 muscarinic receptor. High-resolution image showing the conformation of the M_2 muscarinic receptor bound with both an agonist (orthosteric) and a positive allosteric modulator. The brown cylinders represent the transmembrane domains. The full extent of the N- and C-terminal domains and the third intracellular loop are not shown. (Courtesy A. Christopoulos.)

MOLECULAR STRUCTURE

In 1986 the first pharmacologically relevant GPCR, the β_2 adrenoceptor (see Ch. 15), was cloned. Thereafter molecular biology caught up very rapidly with pharmacology, and with the sequencing of the human genome the amino acid sequence of all the GPCRs hitherto identified by their pharmacological properties was revealed, as was the structure of many novel GPCRs. More recently X-ray crystallography and cryo-electron microscopy have been used to study the three-dimensional molecular structure of these receptors in detail (Fig. 3.7) (Garcia-Nafria and Tate, 2019; Zhang et al., 2015). Also, computational molecular docking, molecular dynamics simulation and nuclear magnetic resonance (NMR) methods have been developed to study ligand binding and subsequent conformational changes associated with activation (see Sounier et al., 2015). This has provided important information on agonist- and antagonist-bound receptor conformations as well as receptor–G protein interactions. From such studies we are gaining a clearer picture of the mechanism of activation of GPCRs and the factors determining agonist efficacy, as well as having a better basis for designing new GPCR ligands.

GPCRs consist of a single polypeptide chain, usually of 350–400 amino acid residues, but in some cases up to 1100 residues. The general anatomy is shown in Fig. 3.3B. Their characteristic structure comprises seven transmembrane α-helices, similar to those of the ion channels discussed previously, with an extracellular N-terminal domain of varying length, and an intracellular C-terminal domain.

GPCRs are divided into three main classes – A, B and C (Table 3.2). There is considerable sequence homology between the members of one class, but little between different classes. They share the same seven transmembrane helix (heptahelical) structures, but differ in other respects, principally in the length of the extracellular N-terminus and the location of the agonist binding domain. Class A is by far the largest, comprising most monoamine, neuropeptide and chemokine receptors. Class B includes receptors for some other peptides, such as calcitonin and glucagon. Class C is the smallest, its main members being the metabotropic glutamate and GABA receptors and the Ca^{2+}-sensing receptors.[10]

[10]The Ca^{2+}-sensing receptor (see Conigrave et al., 2000) is an unusual GPCR that is activated not by conventional mediators but by extracellular Ca^{2+} in the range of 1–10 mmol/L – an extremely low affinity in comparison with other GPCR agonists. It is expressed by cells of the parathyroid gland, and serves to regulate the extracellular Ca^{2+} concentration by controlling parathyroid hormone secretion (Ch. 36). This homeostatic mechanism is quite distinct from the mechanisms for regulating intracellular Ca^{2+}, discussed in Chapter 4.

Table 3.2 Main G protein–coupled receptor classes[a,b]

Class	Receptors[b]	Structural features
A: rhodopsin family	The largest group. Receptors for most amine neurotransmitters, many neuropeptides, purines, prostanoids, cannabinoids, etc.	Short extracellular (N-terminal) tail. Ligand binds to transmembrane helices (amines) or to extracellular loops (peptides)
B: secretin/glucagon receptor family	Receptors for peptide hormones, including secretin, glucagon, calcitonin	Intermediate extracellular tail incorporating ligand-binding domain
C: metabotropic glutamate receptor/calcium sensor family	Small group. Metabotropic glutamate receptors, $GABA_B$ receptors, Ca^{2+}-sensing receptors	Long extracellular tail incorporating ligand-binding domain

[a]Other classes include frizzled G protein–coupled receptors (GPCRs), adhesion GPCRs and receptors for pheromones.
[b]For full lists, see www.guidetopharmacology.org.

For small molecules, such as noradrenaline (norepinephrine) and acetylcholine, the ligand-binding domain of class A receptors is buried in the cleft between the α-helical segments within the membrane (see Figs 3.3B and 3.7), similar to the slot occupied by *retinal* in the *rhodopsin* molecule.[11] Peptide ligands, such as substance P (see Ch. 17), bind more superficially to the extracellular loops, as shown in Fig. 3.3B. From crystal structures and single-site mutagenesis experiments, it is possible to map the ligand-binding domain of these receptors. Recent advances in computational molecular docking of ligands into the ligand–receptor-binding domain have made it possible to design novel synthetic ligands based primarily on knowledge of the receptor structure (see Manglik et al., 2016) – an important milestone in drug development, which has relied up to now mainly on the structure of endogenous mediators (such as histamine) or plant alkaloids (such as morphine) for its chemical inspiration.[12]

PROTEINASE-ACTIVATED RECEPTORS[13]

Although activation of GPCRs is normally the consequence of a diffusible agonist, it can be the result of proteinase activation. Four types of proteinase-activated receptors (PARs) have been identified (see review by Chandrabalan and Ramachandran, 2021). Many proteinases, such as thrombin (a proteinase involved in the blood-clotting cascade; see Ch. 24), activate PARs by snipping off the end of the extracellular N-terminal tail of the receptor (Fig. 3.8) to expose five or six N-terminal residues that bind to receptor domains in the extracellular loops, functioning as a 'tethered agonist'. Receptors of this type occur in many tissues and they appear to play a role in inflammation and other responses to tissue damage where tissue proteinases are released. A PAR can be activated only once, because the cleavage cannot be reversed, and thus continuous resynthesis of the receptor protein is necessary. Inactivation occurs by a further proteolytic cleavage that frees the tethered ligand, or by desensitisation, involving phosphorylation (see Fig. 3.8), after which the receptor is internalised and degraded, to be replaced by newly synthesised protein.

[11]Hydrophilic small molecules access their ligand-binding domain from the extracellular space down the water-filled cleft, however for highly lipophilic molecules, such as those activating the cannabinoid CB_1 and lysophospholipid $S1P_1$ receptors, access appears to be through a membrane-embedded access fenestration in the side of the receptor.
[12]In the past many lead compounds have come from screening huge chemical libraries (see Ch. 60). No inspiration was required, just robust assays, large computers and efficient robotics. Now with the generation of crystal structures we have moved to a more sophisticated age in drug discovery.
[13]These receptors were formerly called protease-activated receptors.

G protein–coupled receptors

- These are sometimes called metabotropic or seven-transmembrane-domain (7-TDM) receptors.
- Structures comprise seven membrane-spanning α-helices.
- The G protein is a membrane protein comprising three subunits (α, β, γ), the α subunit possessing GTPase activity.
- The G protein interacts with a binding pocket on the intracellular surface of the receptor.
- When the G protein binds to an agonist-occupied receptor, the α subunit binds GTP, dissociates and is then free to activate an effector (e.g. a membrane enzyme). In some cases, the βγ subunit is the activator species.
- Activation of the effector is terminated when the bound GTP molecule is hydrolysed, which allows the α subunit to recombine with βγ.
- There are several types of G protein, which interact with different receptors and control different effectors.
- Examples include muscarinic acetylcholine receptors, adrenoceptors, neuropeptide and chemokine receptors, and proteinase-activated receptors.

G PROTEINS AND THEIR ROLE

G proteins comprise a family of membrane-resident proteins whose function is to respond to GPCR activation and pass on the message inside the cell to the effector systems that generate a cellular response. They represent the level of middle management in the organisational hierarchy, intervening between the receptors – choosy mandarins, alert to the faintest whiff of their preferred chemical – and the effector enzymes or ion channels – the blue-collar brigade that gets the job done without needing to know which hormone authorised the process. They are the go-between proteins but were actually called G proteins because of their interaction with the guanine nucleotides, GTP and GDP. For more detailed information on the structure and functions of G proteins, see the review by Li et al. (2020). G proteins

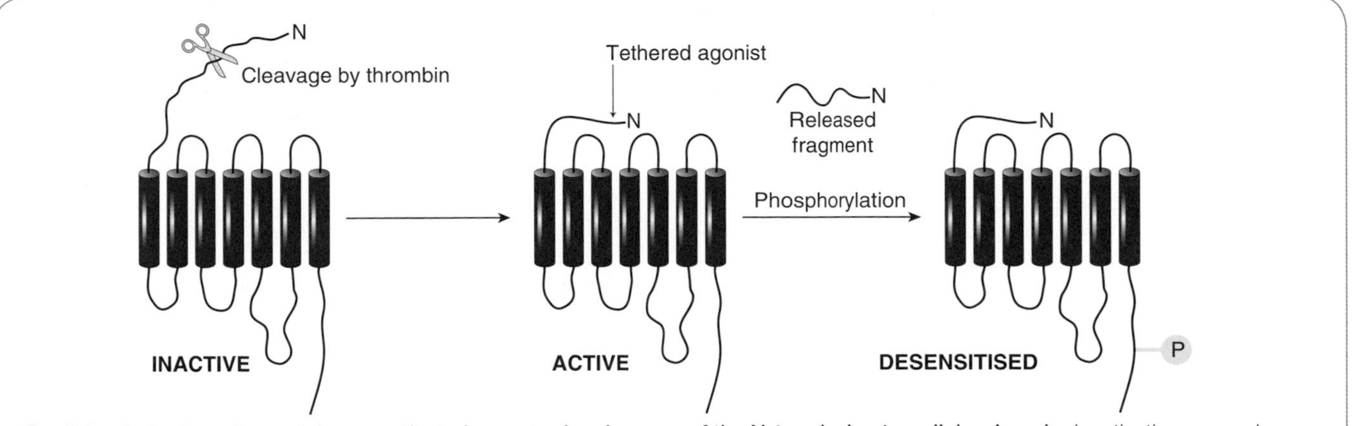

Fig. 3.8 Activation of a proteinase-activated receptor by cleavage of the N-terminal extracellular domain. Inactivation occurs by phosphorylation. Recovery requires resynthesis of the receptor.

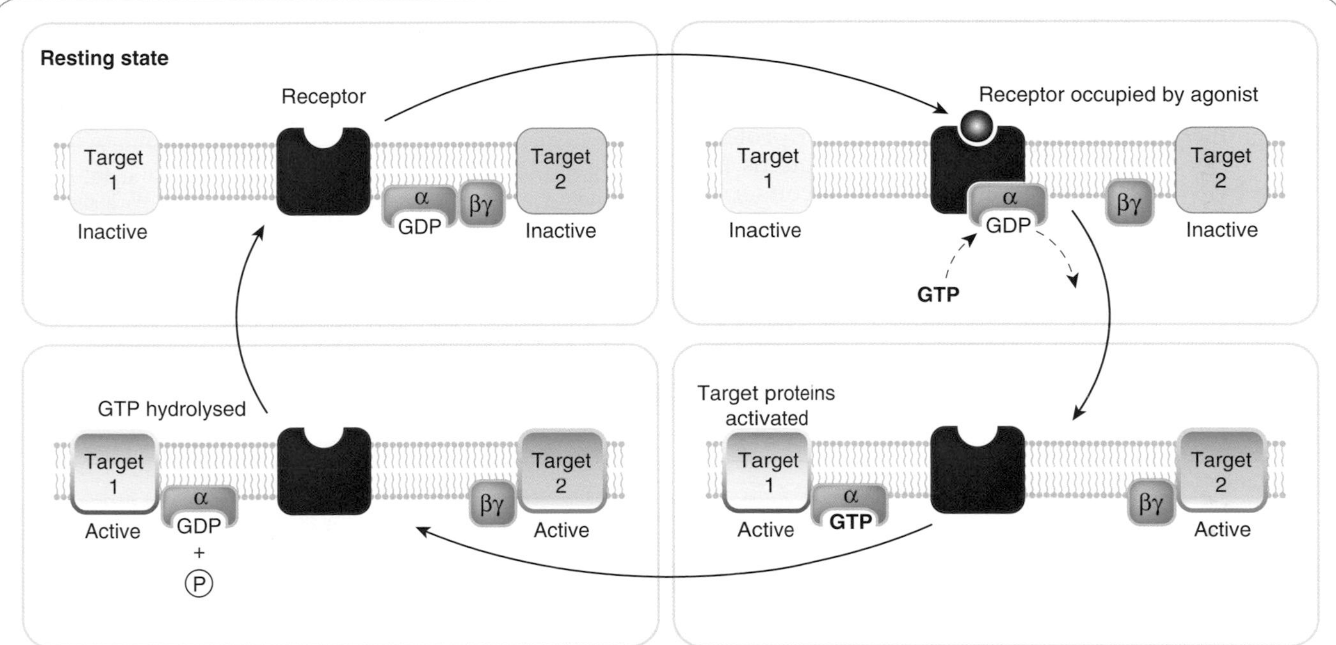

Fig. 3.9 Function of the G protein. The G protein consists of three subunits (α, β, γ), which are anchored to the membrane through attached lipid residues. Coupling of the α subunit to an agonist-occupied receptor causes the bound GDP to exchange with intracellular GTP; the α–GTP complex then dissociates from the receptor and from the βγ complex, and interacts with a target protein (target 1, which may be an enzyme, such as adenylyl cyclase or phospholipase C). The βγ complex also activates a target protein (target 2, which may be an ion channel or a kinase). The GTPase activity of the α subunit is increased when the target protein is bound, leading to hydrolysis of the bound GTP to GDP, whereupon the α subunit reunites with βγ.

consist of three subunits: α, β and γ (Fig. 3.9). Guanine nucleotides bind to the α subunit, which has enzymic (GTPase) activity, catalysing the conversion of GTP to GDP. The β and γ subunits remain together as a βγ complex. The 'γ' subunit is anchored to the membrane through a fatty acid chain, coupled to the G protein through a reaction known as *prenylation*. In the 'resting' state (see Fig. 3.9), the G protein exists as an αβγ trimer, which may or may not be precoupled to the receptor, with GDP occupying the site on the α subunit. When a GPCR is activated by an agonist this induces small changes in residues around the ligand-binding pocket that translate to larger rearrangements of the intracellular regions of the receptor that open a cavity on the intracellular side of the receptor into which the G protein can bind, resulting in a high-affinity interaction of αβγ and the receptor. This agonist-induced interaction of αβγ with the receptor occurs within about 50 ms, causing the bound GDP to dissociate and to be replaced with GTP (GDP–GTP exchange), which in turn causes dissociation of the G protein trimer, releasing α–GTP from the βγ subunits; these are the 'active' forms of the G protein, which diffuse in the membrane and can associate with various enzymes and ion channels, causing activation of the target (see Fig. 3.9). It was originally thought that only the α subunit had a signalling function, the βγ complex serving merely as a chaperone to keep the flighty α subunits out of range of the various effector proteins that they might otherwise excite. However, the βγ complexes actually make assignations of their own, and control effectors in much the same way as the α subunits. The association of α or βγ subunits with target enzymes or channels can cause either activation or inhibition, depending on which G protein is involved (see Table 3.3). G protein activation results in amplification, because a single agonist–receptor complex can activate several G protein molecules in turn, and each of these can remain associated with their effector enzyme for long enough to produce many molecules of product. The product (see later) is often a 'second messenger', and further amplification occurs before the final cellular response is produced. Signalling is terminated when the hydrolysis of GTP to GDP occurs through the inherent GTPase activity of the α subunit. The resulting α–GDP then dissociates from the effector, and reunites with βγ, completing the cycle.

Attachment of the α subunit to an effector molecule actually increases its GTPase activity, the magnitude of this increase being different for different types of effector. Because GTP hydrolysis is the step that terminates the ability of the α subunit to produce its effect, regulation of its GTPase activity by the effector protein means that the activation of the effector tends to be self-limiting. In addition, there is a family of about 20 cellular proteins, regulators of G protein signalling (RGS) proteins (see review by Sjögren, 2017), that possess a conserved sequence that binds specifically to α subunits to increase greatly their GTPase activity, so hastening the hydrolysis of GTP and inactivating the complex. RGS proteins thus exert an inhibitory effect on G protein signalling, a mechanism that is thought to have a regulatory function in many situations.

Different GPCRs couple to different G proteins and thus produce distinct cellular responses. For example, M_2 muscarinic acetylcholine receptors (mAChRs) and β_1 adrenoceptors, both of which occur in cardiac muscle cells, produce opposite functional effects (see Chs 14 and 15). Four main classes of G protein (G_s, G_i, G_o and G_q) are of pharmacological importance (Table 3.3). These differ primarily in the α subunit they contain.[14] G proteins show selectivity with respect to both the receptors and the effectors with which they couple, having specific recognition domains in their structure complementary to specific G protein-binding domains in the receptor and effector molecules. For example, G_s and G_i produce, respectively, stimulation and inhibition of the enzyme *adenylyl cyclase* (Fig. 3.10).

One functional difference that has been useful as an experimental tool to distinguish which type of G protein is involved in different situations concerns the action of two bacterial toxins, *cholera toxin* and *pertussis toxin* (see Table 3.3). These toxins, which are enzymes, catalyse a conjugation reaction (ADP ribosylation) on

[14]In humans there are 21 known subtypes of Gα, 6 of Gβ and 12 of Gγ, providing, in theory, about 1500 variants of the trimer. We know little about the role of different α, β and γ subtypes, but it would be rash to assume that the variations are functionally irrelevant. By now, you will be unsurprised (even if somewhat bemused) by such a display of molecular heterogeneity, for it is the way of evolution.

Table 3.3 The main G protein subtypes and their functions[a]

Subtypes	Main effectors	Notes
Gα subunits[b]		
$G\alpha_s$	Stimulates adenylyl cyclase, causing increased cAMP formation	Activated by cholera toxin, which blocks GTPase activity, thus preventing inactivation
$G\alpha_i$	Inhibits adenylyl cyclase, decreasing cAMP formation	Blocked by pertussis toxin, which prevents dissociation of αβγ complex
$G\alpha_o$	Limited effects of α subunit (effects mainly due to βγ subunits)	Blocked by pertussis toxin. Occurs mainly in nervous system
$G\alpha_q$	Activates phospholipase C, increasing production of second messengers inositol trisphosphate and diacylglycerol thus releasing Ca^{2++} from intracellular stores and activating protein kinase C (PKC)	
$G\alpha_{12/13}$	Activates Rho and thus Rho kinase	
Gβγ subunits		
	Activate potassium channels Inhibit voltage-gated calcium channels Activate GPCR kinases (GRKs) Activate mitogen-activated protein kinase cascade Interact with some forms of adenylyl cyclase and with phospholipase Cβ	Many βγ isoforms identified, but specific functions are not yet known

[a]This table lists only those isoforms of major pharmacological significance. Many more have been identified, some of which play roles in olfaction, taste, visual transduction and other physiological functions.
[b]Initially the subscripts 's' and 'i' were used to denote stimulatory and inhibitory actions on adenylyl cyclase but, subsequently, the terms used, 'q' and '12/13', have little logic behind their use.
GPCR, G protein–coupled receptor.

the α subunit of G proteins. Cholera toxin acts only on G_s, and it causes persistent activation. Many of the symptoms of cholera, such as the excessive secretion of fluid from the gastrointestinal epithelium (leading to 'rice-water stools'), are due to the uncontrolled activation of adenylyl cyclase that occurs. Pertussis toxin specifically blocks G_i and G_o by preventing dissociation of the G protein trimer. Pertussis toxin is released from *Bordetella pertussis* bacteria, which cause whooping cough. As with cholera toxin, the symptoms caused by pertussis toxin are related to its effects on G proteins, but in this case by inhibiting G_i and G_o rather than activating G_s and leading to changes in respiratory tract secretion and a distinctive cough rather than the copious diarrhoea of cholera.

TARGETS FOR G PROTEINS

The main targets for G proteins, through which GPCRs control different aspects of cell function (see Table 3.3), are:

- *adenylyl cyclase*, the enzyme responsible for cAMP formation;
- *phospholipase C*, the enzyme responsible for inositol phosphate and diacylglycerol (DAG) formation;
- *ion channels*, particularly calcium and potassium channels;
- *Rho A/Rho kinase*, a system that regulates the activity of many signalling pathways controlling cell growth, proliferation and motility, smooth muscle contraction, etc.;
- *mitogen-activated protein (MAP) kinase*, a system that controls many cell functions, including cell division and is also a target of several kinase-linked receptors.

The adenylyl cyclase/cAMP system

The discovery by Sutherland and his colleagues of the role of cAMP (cyclic 3′,5′-adenosine monophosphate) as an intracellular mediator demolished at a stroke the barriers that existed between biochemistry and pharmacology, and introduced the concept of second messengers in signal transduction. cAMP is a nucleotide synthesised within the cell from ATP by the action of a membrane-bound enzyme, adenylyl cyclase. It is produced continuously and inactivated by hydrolysis to 5′-adenosine monophosphate (AMP) by the action of a family of enzymes known as phosphodiesterases (PDEs). Many different drugs, hormones and neurotransmitters act on GPCRs and increase or decrease the catalytic activity of adenylyl cyclase (see Fig. 3.10), thus raising or lowering the concentration of cAMP within the cell. In mammalian cells there are 10 different molecular isoforms of the enzyme, some of which respond selectively to $G\alpha_s$ or $G\alpha_i$.

cAMP regulates many aspects of cellular function including, for example, enzymes involved in energy metabolism, cell division and cell differentiation, ion transport, ion channels and the contractile proteins in smooth muscle. These varied effects are, however, all brought about by a common mechanism, namely the activation of protein kinases by cAMP (known as cAMP-dependent protein kinases) in eukaryotic cells. One important cAMP-dependent protein kinase is *protein kinase A* (PKA). Protein kinases regulate the function of many different cellular proteins by controlling protein phosphorylation. Fig. 3.11 shows how increased cAMP production in response to β-adrenoceptor activation affects enzymes involved in glycogen and fat metabolism in liver, fat and muscle cells. The result is a coordinated response in which stored energy in the form of glycogen and fat is made available as glucose to fuel muscle contraction.

Other examples of regulation by PKA include the increased activity of voltage-gated calcium channels in heart muscle cells (see Ch. 20). Phosphorylation of these channels increases the amount of Ca^{2+} entering the cell during the action potential, and thus increases the force of contraction of the heart.

In smooth muscle, PKA phosphorylates (thereby inactivating) another enzyme, *myosin light-chain kinase*, which is required for contraction. This accounts for the smooth muscle relaxation produced by many drugs that increase cAMP production in smooth muscle (see Ch. 4).

As mentioned earlier, receptors linked to G_i rather than G_s inhibit adenylyl cyclase, and thus reduce cAMP formation to elicit opposing responses to those receptors which activate G_s. Examples include certain types of mAChR (e.g. the M_2 receptor of cardiac muscle; see Ch. 14), α_2 adrenoceptors in smooth muscle (see Ch. 15) and opioid receptors (see Ch. 43). Adenylyl cyclase can be activated directly by drugs such as **forskolin**, which is used experimentally to study the role of the cAMP system.

cAMP is hydrolysed within cells by *PDEs*, an important and ubiquitous family of enzymes. Twenty-four PDE subtypes exist, of which some are more selective for cAMP, while others are more selective for cGMP. Most are weakly inhibited by drugs such as methylxanthines (e.g. **theophylline** and **caffeine**; see Chs 28 and 49). **Roflumilast** (used to treat chronic obstructive pulmonary disease [COPD]; see Ch. 28) is selective for PDE_{4B}, expressed in inflammatory cells; **milrinone** (a positive

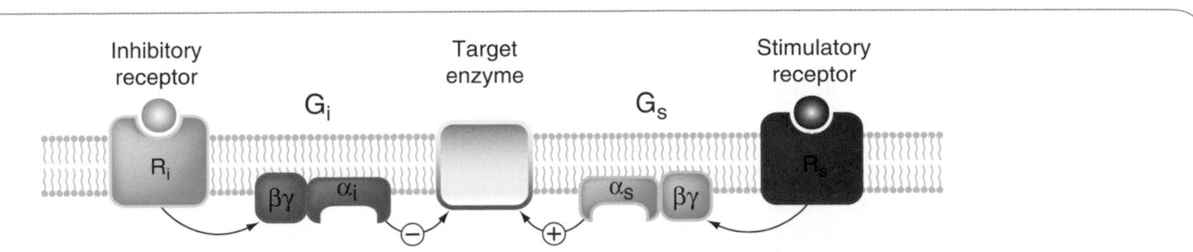

Fig. 3.10 Bidirectional control of a target enzyme, such as adenylyl cyclase by G_s and G_i. Heterogeneity of G proteins allows different receptors to exert opposite effects on a target enzyme.

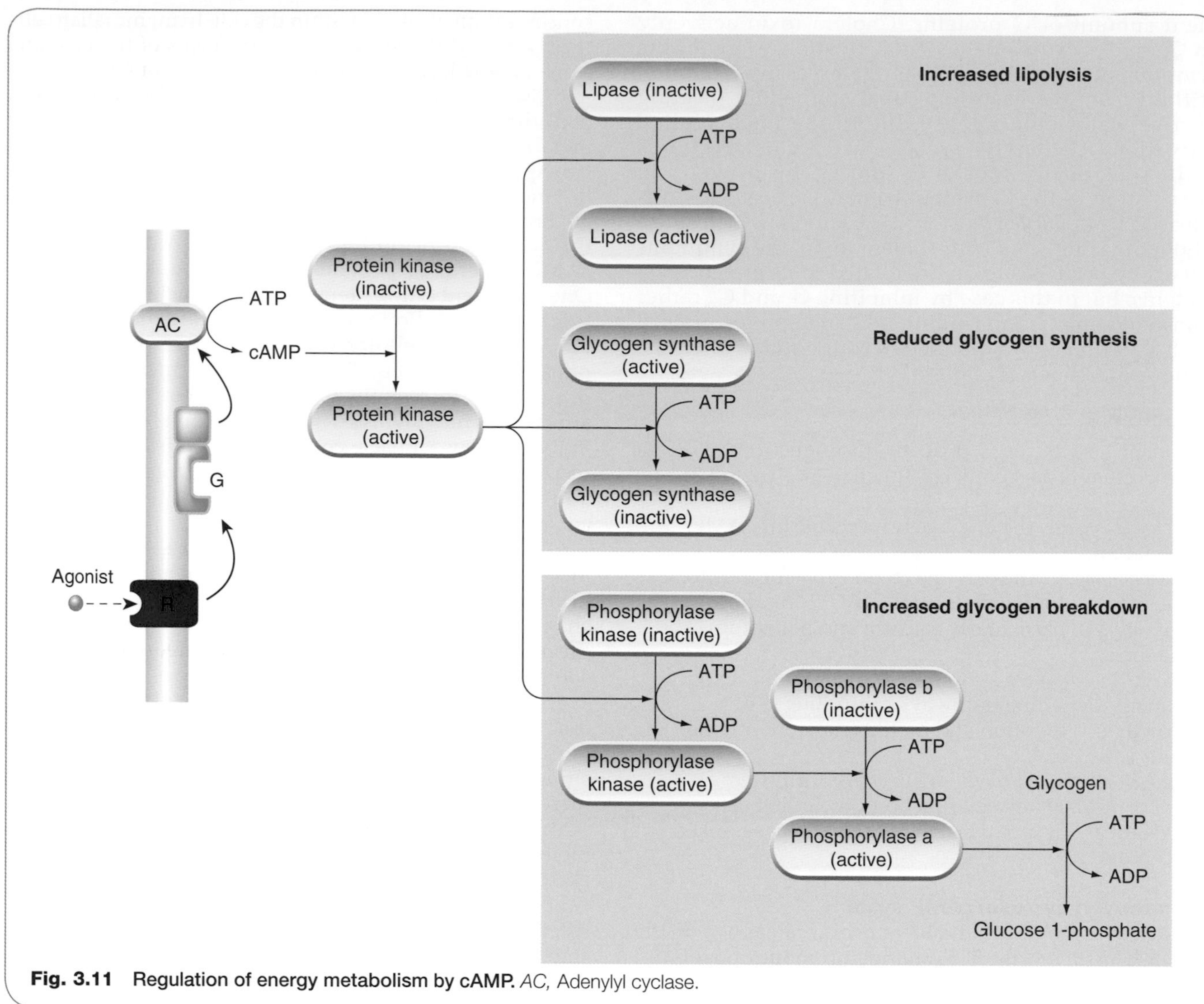

Fig. 3.11 Regulation of energy metabolism by cAMP. *AC,* Adenylyl cyclase.

inotrope that makes the heart beat harder and is sometimes used for symptoms in patients awaiting heart transplantation; see Ch. 20) is selective for PDE_{2A}, which is expressed in heart muscle; **sildenafil** (better known as Viagra; see Ch. 35) is selective for PDE_{5A}, and consequently enhances the vasodilator effects of nitric oxide (NO) and drugs that release NO, whose effects are mediated by cGMP (see Ch. 19). The similarity of some of the actions of these drugs to those of sympathomimetic amines (see Ch. 15) probably reflects their common property of increasing the intracellular concentration of cAMP.

The phospholipase C/inositol phosphate system

The *phosphoinositide* system, an important intracellular second messenger system, was first discovered in the 1950s by Hokin and Hokin, whose recondite interests centred on the mechanism of salt secretion by the nasal glands of seabirds. They found that secretion was accompanied by increased turnover of a minor class of membrane phospholipids known as phosphoinositides (collectively known as PIs; Fig. 3.12). Subsequently, Michell and Berridge found that many hormones that produce an increase in free intracellular Ca^{2+} concentration (which include, for example, muscarinic agonists and α-adrenoceptor agonists acting on smooth muscle and salivary glands) also increase PI turnover. It was later found that one particular member of the PI family, namely phosphatidylinositol (4,5) bisphosphate (PIP_2), which has additional phosphate groups attached to the inositol ring, plays a key role. PIP_2 is the substrate for a membrane-bound enzyme, phospholipase Cβ (PLCβ), which splits it into *DAG* and *inositol (1,4,5) trisphosphate* (IP_3; Fig. 3.13), both of which function as second messengers. The activation of PLCβ by various agonists is mediated through a G protein (G_q, see Table 3.3). After cleavage of PIP_2, the status quo is restored, as shown in Fig. 3.13, DAG being phosphorylated to form phosphatidic acid (PA), while the IP_3 is dephosphorylated and then recoupled with PA to form PIP_2 once again.[15]

[15]Alternative abbreviations for these mediators are PtdIns (PI), PtdIns (4,5)-P_2 (PIP_2), Ins (1,4,5)-P_3 (IP_3).

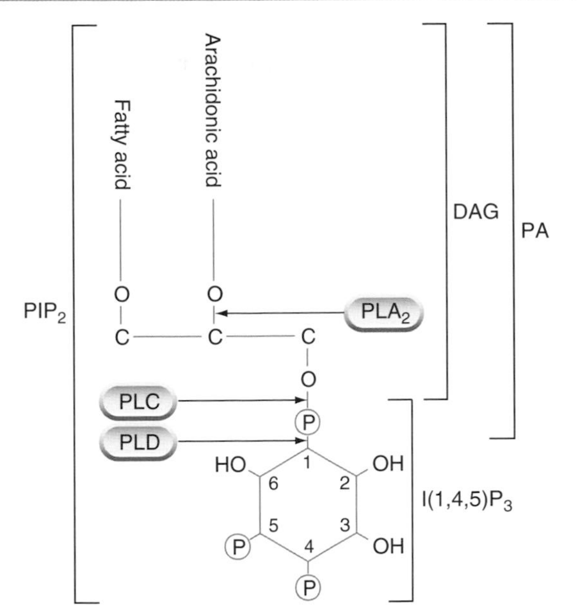

Fig. 3.12 Structure of phosphatidylinositol bisphosphate (PIP_2), showing sites of cleavage by different phospholipases to produce active mediators. Cleavage by phospholipase A2 (PLA_2) yields arachidonic acid. Cleavage by phospholipase C (PLC) yields inositol trisphosphate ($I(1,4,5)P_3$) and diacylglycerol (DAG). *PA*, Phosphatidic acid; *PLD*, phospholipase D.

Lithium, an agent used in psychiatry (see Ch. 48), blocks this recycling pathway (see Fig. 3.13).

Inositol phosphates and intracellular calcium

Inositol (1,4,5) trisphosphate (IP_3) is a water-soluble mediator that is released into the cytosol and acts on a specific receptor – the IP_3 receptor – which is a ligand-gated calcium channel present on the membrane of the endoplasmic reticulum (see Figs 3.5 and 4.1). The main role of IP_3, described in more detail in Chapter 4, is to control the release of Ca^{2+} from intracellular stores. Because many drug and hormone effects involve intracellular Ca^{2+}, this pathway is particularly important.

DAG and protein kinase C

DAG is produced, as well as IP_3, whenever receptor-induced PI hydrolysis occurs. The main effect of DAG is to activate a protein kinase, *protein kinase C* (PKC), which catalyses the phosphorylation of several intracellular proteins. DAG, unlike the inositol phosphates, is highly lipophilic and remains within the membrane. It binds to a specific site on the PKC molecule, causing the enzyme to migrate from the cytosol to the cell membrane, thereby becoming activated. There are at least 10 different mammalian PKC subtypes, which have distinct cellular distributions and phosphorylate different proteins. Several are activated by DAG and raised intracellular Ca^{2+}, both of which are produced by activation of GPCRs.[16] PKCs are also activated by *phorbol esters* (highly irritant, tumour-promoting compounds produced by certain plants), which have been extremely useful in studying the functions of PKC. One of the subtypes is activated by the lipid mediator *arachidonic acid* (see Ch. 17) generated by the action of phospholipase A_2 on membrane phospholipids, so PKC activation can also occur with agonists that activate this enzyme. The various PKC isoforms, like the tyrosine kinases discussed later, act on many different functional proteins, such as ion channels, receptors, enzymes (including other kinases), transcription factors and cytoskeletal proteins. Protein phosphorylation by kinases plays a central role in signal transduction and controls many different aspects of cell function. The DAG–PKC link provides a mechanism whereby GPCRs can mobilise this army of control freaks.

[16]PKCs were originally named as Ca^{2+}-dependent protein kinases (PKC), as opposed to cAMP-dependent PKA. Although later subtypes were found not to be Ca^{2+}-dependent, the PKC name has stuck.

Ion channels as targets for G proteins

Another major function of GPCRs is to control ion channel function directly by mechanisms that do not involve second messengers such as cAMP or inositol phosphates. Direct G protein–channel interaction, through the $\beta\gamma$ subunits of G_i and G_o proteins, appears to be a general mechanism for controlling K^+ and Ca^{2+} channels. In cardiac muscle, for example, mAChRs enhance K^+ permeability in this way (thus hyperpolarising the cells and inhibiting electrical activity; see Ch. 20). Similar mechanisms operate in neurons, where many inhibitory drugs, such as opioid analgesics, reduce excitability by opening certain K^+ channels – known as G protein-activated inwardly rectifying K^+ channels (GIRK) – or by inhibiting voltage-activated N and P/Q type Ca^{2+} channels, thus reducing neurotransmitter release (see Chs 4 and 43).

The Rho/Rho kinase system

The Rho/Rho kinase signalling pathway consists of three small GTPases – Rho A, B and C – that can activate downstream kinases, Rho kinase 1 and 2 (sometimes referred to as ROCK 1 and ROCK 2 – ROCK being an acronym for *Rho-associated coiled-coil containing protein kinase*) (see Porazinski et al., 2020). Rho A can be activated by certain GPCRs (and also by non-GPCR mechanisms), which couple to G proteins of the $G_{12/13}$ type. The free G protein α subunit interacts with a *guanosine nucleotide exchange factor*, which facilitates GDP–GTP exchange at another GTPase, Rho. Rho–GDP, the resting form, is inactive, but when GDP–GTP exchange occurs, Rho are activated, and in turn activate Rho kinases. Rho kinases phosphorylate many substrate proteins and control a wide variety of cellular functions, including smooth muscle contraction and proliferation, cell movement and migration, angiogenesis and synaptic remodelling. They have been implicated in numerous disease states including glaucoma (see Ch. 27), cardiovascular disease (see Chs 20 and 21), neurodegenerative disorders (see Ch. 40) and cancer (see Ch. 57). Rho kinase inhibitors (e.g. **fasudil**, **netarsudil**) have been developed and are used clinically in some countries for the treatment of glaucoma and cognitive decline following stroke. Their progress in clinical trials to determine their efficacy in the treatment of pulmonary hypertension seems to have stalled.

The MAP kinase system

The MAP kinase system involves several signal transduction pathways (Fig. 3.15) that are activated not only by various cytokines and growth factors acting on kinase-linked receptors (Fig. 3.17), but also by ligands activating GPCRs. The coupling of GPCRs to different families of MAP kinases can involve G protein α and $\beta\gamma$ subunits as well as *Src* and *arrestins* – proteins also involved in GPCR desensitisation. The MAP kinase system controls many processes involved

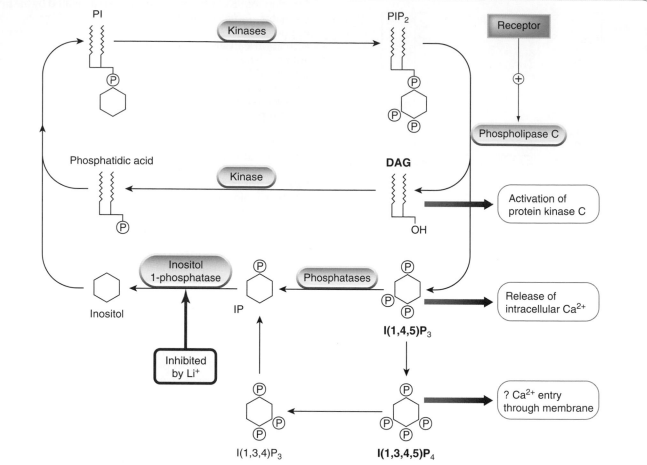

Fig. 3.13 The phosphatidylinositol (PI) cycle. Receptor-mediated activation of phospholipase C results in the cleavage of phosphatidylinositol bisphosphate (PIP_2), forming diacylglycerol (DAG) (which activates protein kinase C) and inositol trisphosphate (IP_3) (which releases intracellular Ca^{2+}). The role of inositol tetraphosphate (IP_4), which is formed from IP_3 and other inositol phosphates, is unclear, but it may facilitate Ca^{2+} entry through the plasma membrane. IP_3 is inactivated by dephosphorylation to inositol. DAG is converted to phosphatidic acid, and these two products are used to regenerate PI and PIP_2.

Effectors controlled by G proteins

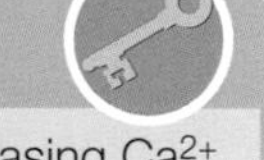

GPCRs couple through G proteins to second messenger pathways and ion channels:

- Adenylyl cyclase/cAMP:
  - can be activated or inhibited by pharmacological ligands, depending on the nature of the receptor and G protein;
  - adenylyl cyclase catalyses formation of the intracellular messenger cAMP;
  - cAMP activates protein kinases such as PKA that control cell function in many different ways by causing phosphorylation of various enzymes, carriers and other proteins.
- Phospholipase C/inositol trisphosphate (IP_3)/DAG:
  - catalyses the formation of two intracellular messengers, IP_3 and DAG, from membrane phospholipid;
  - IP_3 acts to increase free cytosolic Ca^{2+} by releasing Ca^{2+} from intracellular compartments
  - increased free Ca^{2+} initiates many events, including contraction, secretion, enzyme activation and membrane hyperpolarisation;
  - DAG activates various PKC isoforms, which control many cellular functions by phosphorylating a variety of proteins.
- Ion channels:
  - opening potassium channels (GIRKs), resulting in membrane hyperpolarisation;
  - inhibiting voltage-activated calcium channels, thus reducing neurotransmitter release.
- Phospholipase A_2 (and thus the formation of arachidonic acid and eicosanoids).

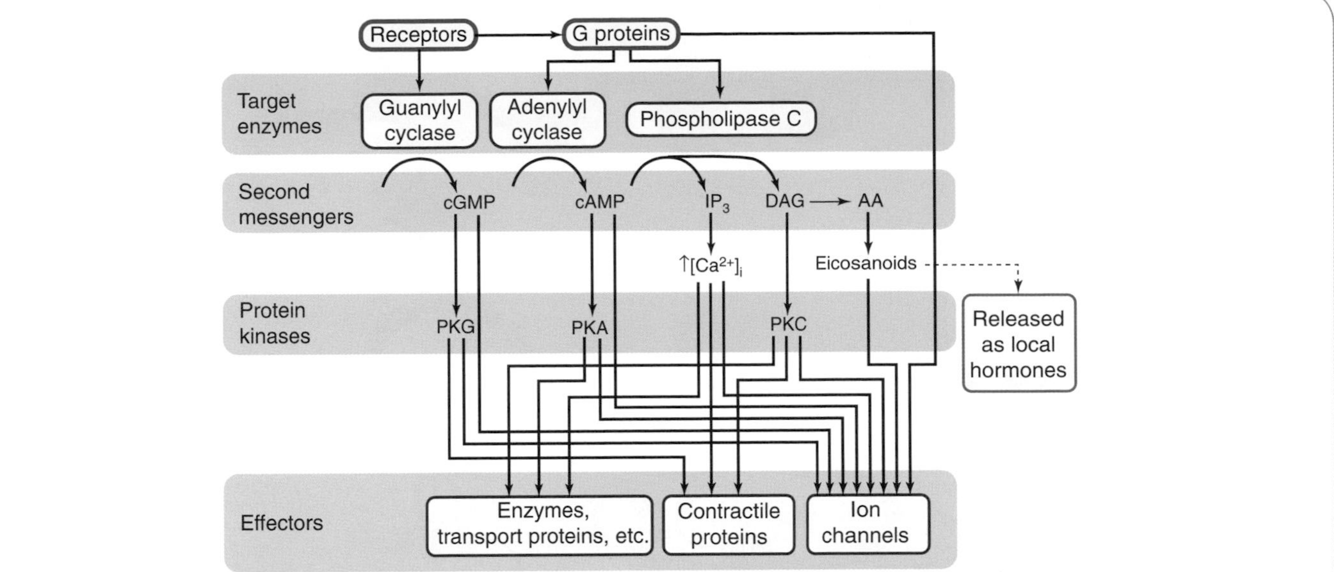

Fig. 3.14 G protein and second messenger control of cellular effector systems. Not shown in this diagram are signalling pathways where arrestins, rather than G proteins, link G protein–coupled receptors to downstream events (see text and Fig. 3.15). *AA,* Arachidonic acid; *DAG,* diacylglycerol; *IP_3,* inositol trisphosphate; *PKA,* protein kinase A; *PKC,* protein kinase C; *PKG,* cGMP-dependent protein kinase.

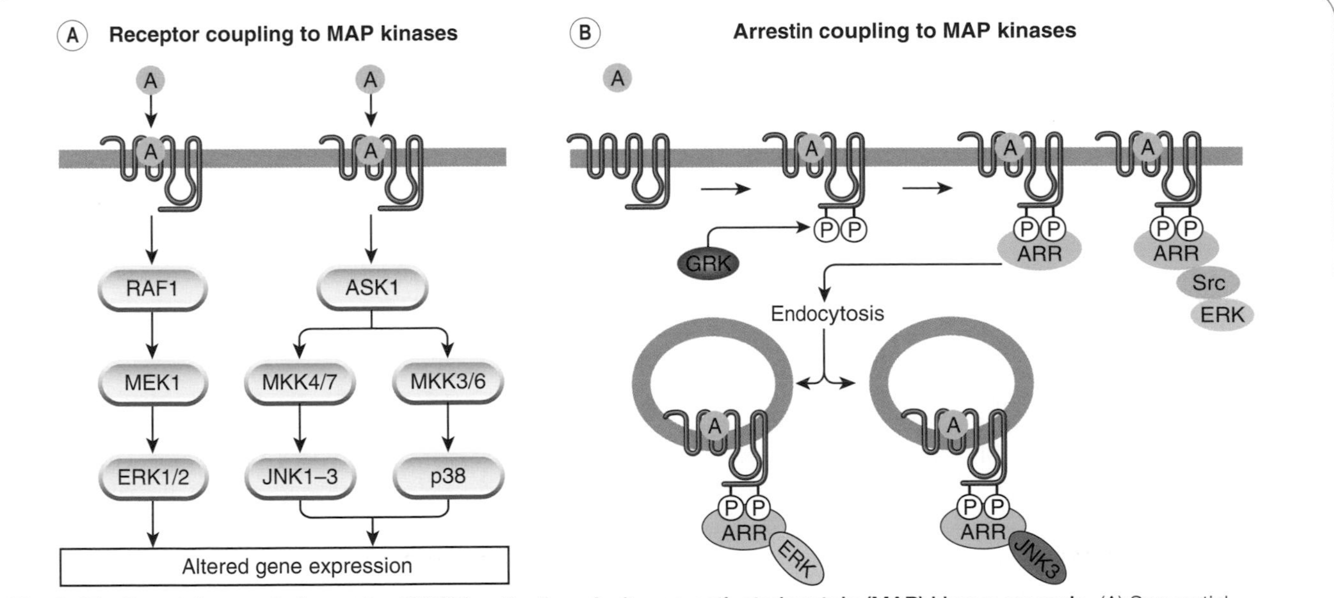

Fig. 3.15 G protein–coupled receptor (GPCR) activation of mitogen-activated protein (MAP) kinase cascade. (A) Sequential activation of the multiple components of the MAP kinase cascade. GPCR activation of MAP kinases can involve Gα and βγ subunits (not shown). (B) Activation of ERK and JNK3 through interaction with arrestins (βARR). Activation of ERK can occur either at the plasma membrane involving Src or by direct activation after internalisation of the receptor/arrestin complex. *ARR,* Arrestin; *GRK,* G protein–coupled receptor kinase.

in gene expression, cell division, apoptosis and tissue regeneration.

The main postulated roles of GPCRs in controlling enzymes and ion channels are summarised in Fig. 3.14.

FURTHER DEVELOPMENTS IN GPCR BIOLOGY

By the early 1990s, we thought we had more or less got the measure of GPCR function, as described previously. Since then, the plot has thickened, and further developments have necessitated a substantial overhaul of the basic model.

GPCR desensitisation

As described in Chapter 2, desensitisation is a feature of most GPCRs, and the mechanisms underlying it have been extensively studied. *Homologous desensitisation* is restricted to the receptors activated by the desensitising agonist, while *heterologous desensitisation* affects other GPCRs in

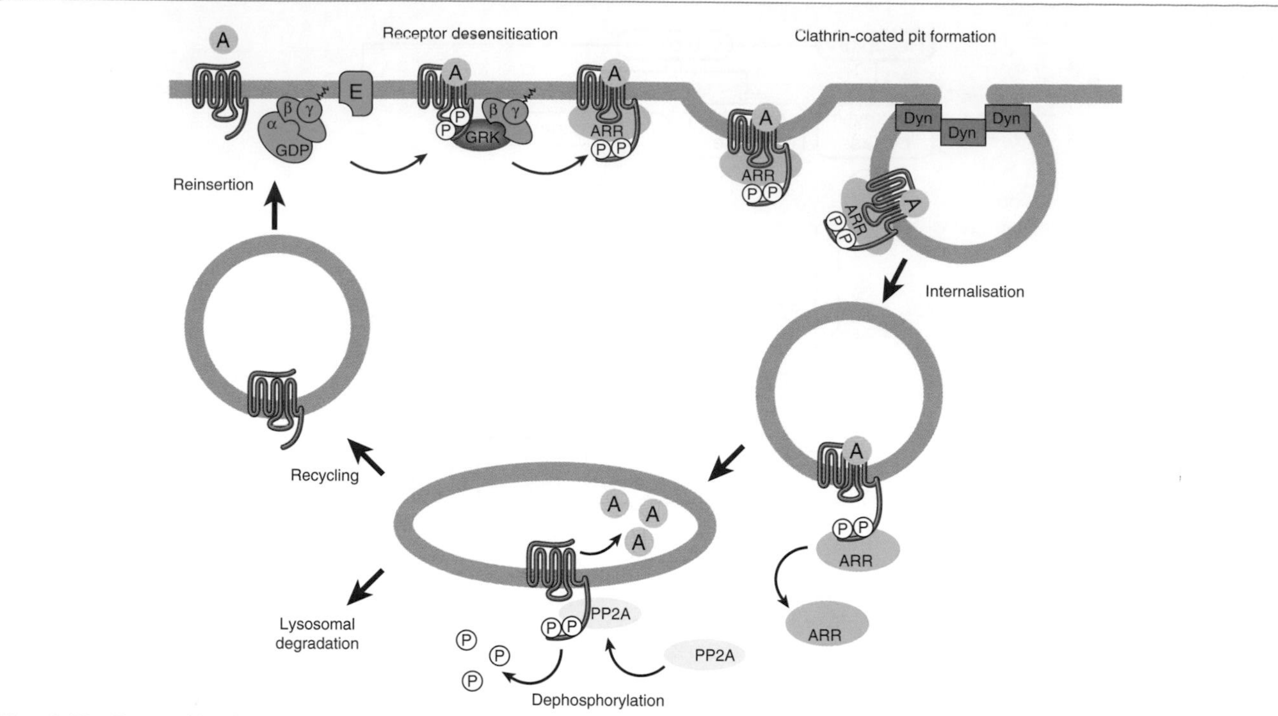

Fig. 3.16 Desensitisation and trafficking of G protein–coupled receptors (GPCRs). On prolonged agonist activation of the GPCR, selective GPCR kinases (GRKs) are recruited to the plasma membrane and phosphorylate the receptor. Arrestin (ARR) then binds and traffics the GPCR to clathrin-coated pits for subsequent internalisation into endosomes in a dynamin-dependent process. The GPCR is then dephosphorylated by a phosphatase (PP2A) and either recycled back to the plasma membrane or trafficked to lysosomes for degradation. *Dyn*, Dynamin; *GRK*, G protein–coupled receptor kinase; *PP2A*, phosphatase 2A.

addition. Two main processes are involved (see Kelly et al., 2008):

- receptor phosphorylation
- receptor internalisation (endocytosis)

The sequence of GPCRs includes certain residues (serine and threonine), mainly in the C-terminal cytoplasmic tail, which can be phosphorylated by specific GPCR kinases (GRKs) and by kinases such as PKA and PKC.

On receptor activation GRK2 and GRK3 are recruited to the plasma membrane by binding to free G protein βγ subunits. GRKs then phosphorylate the receptors in their activated (i.e. agonist-bound) state. The phosphorylated receptor serves as a binding site for arrestins, intracellular proteins that block the interaction between the receptor and the G proteins producing a selective *homologous desensitisation*. Arrestin binding also targets the receptor for endocytosis in clathrin-coated pits (Fig. 3.16). The internalised receptor can then either be dephosphorylated and reinserted into the plasma membrane (*resensitisation*) or trafficked to lysosomes for degradation (*inactivation*). This type of desensitisation seems to occur with most GPCRs but with subtle differences that fascinate the aficionados.

Phosphorylation by PKA and PKC at residues different from those targeted by GRKs generally leads to impaired coupling between the activated receptor and the G protein, so the agonist effect is reduced. This can give rise to either homologous or heterologous desensitisation, depending on whether or not receptors other than that for the desensitising agonist are simultaneously phosphorylated by the kinases, some of which are not very selective. Receptors phosphorylated by second messenger kinases are probably not internalised and are reactivated by dephosphorylation by phosphatases when the agonist is removed.

GPCR oligomerisation

The earlier view that GPCRs exist and function as monomeric proteins (in contrast to ion channels, which generally comprise multimeric complexes) was first overturned by work on the $GABA_B$ receptor. Two subtypes of this GPCR exist, encoded by different genes, and the functional receptor consists of a heterodimer of the two (see Ch. 38). A similar situation arises with G protein–coupled glutamate receptors. Oddly, although the $GABA_B$ dimer has two potential agonist binding sites, one on each subunit, only one is functional and signalling is transmitted through the dimer to the other receptor in the dimer which couples to the G protein (see Fig. 39.9).

Other GPCRs are functional as monomers but it now seems likely that most, if not all, GPCRs can exist as either homomeric or heteromeric oligomers (i.e. dimers or larger oligomers) (Ferré et al., 2015). Within the opioid receptor family (see Ch. 43), the μ receptor was crystallised as a dimer, and stable and functional heterodimers of κ and δ receptors, whose pharmacological properties differ from those of either parent, have been created in cell lines. More diverse GPCR combinations have also been found, such as that between dopamine (D_2) and somatostatin receptors, on which both ligands act with increased potency. Roaming even further afield in search of functional assignations, the

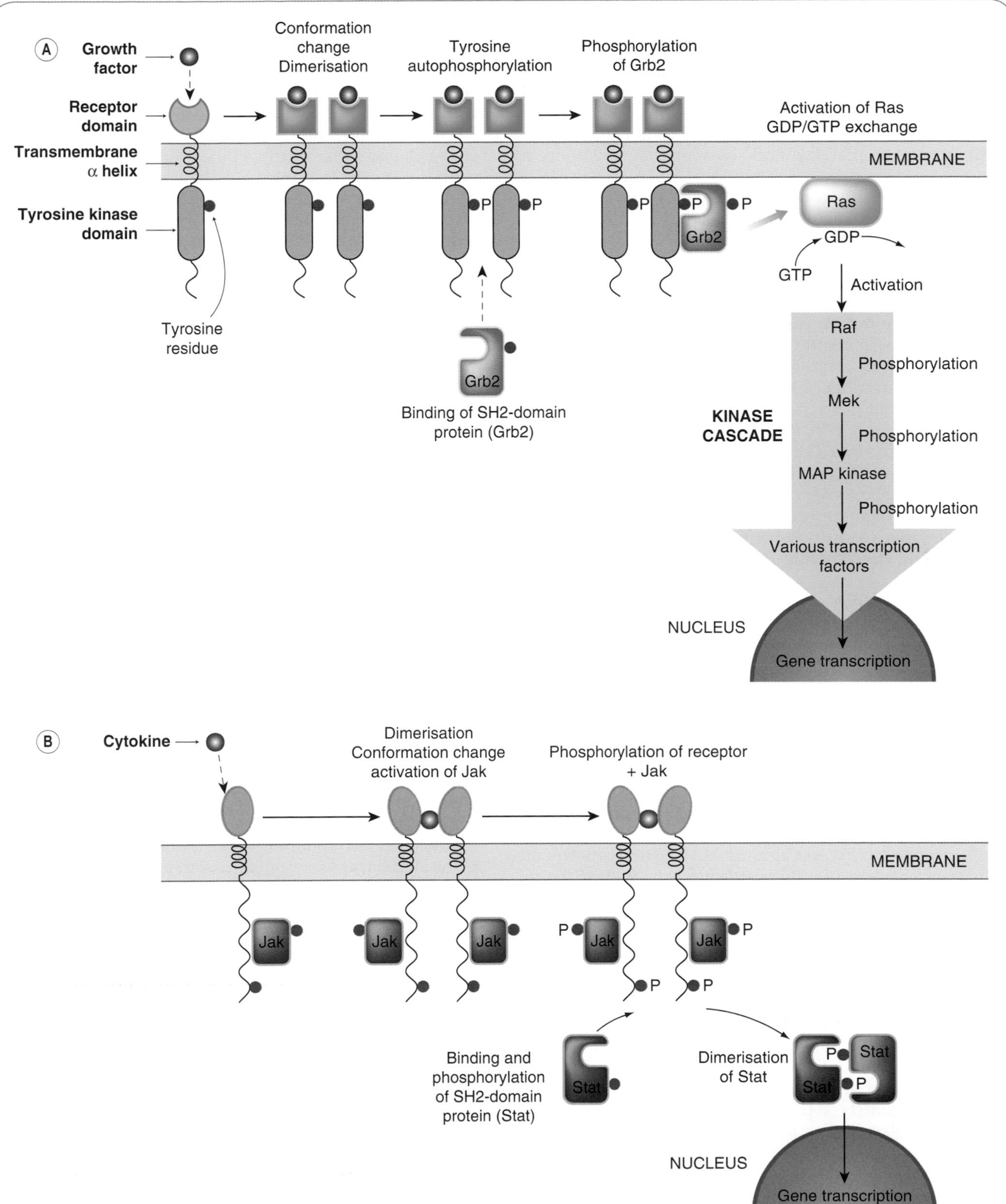

Fig. 3.17 Transduction mechanisms of kinase-linked receptors. The first step following agonist binding is dimerisation, which leads to autophosphorylation of the intracellular domain of each receptor. SH2-domain proteins then bind to the phosphorylated receptor and are themselves phosphorylated. Two well-characterised pathways are shown: (A) the growth factor (Ras/Raf/mitogen-activated protein [MAP] kinase) pathway (see also Ch. 6). Grb2 can also be phosphorylated but this negatively regulates its signalling. (B) Simplified scheme of the cytokine (Jak/Stat) pathway (see also Ch. 57). Some cytokine receptors may pre-exist as dimers rather than dimerise on cytokine binding. Several other pathways exist, and these phosphorylation cascades interact with components of G protein systems.

dopamine receptor D_5 can couple directly with a ligand-gated ion channel, the $GABA_A$ receptor, inhibiting the function of the latter without the intervention of any G protein (Liu et al., 2000). These interactions have so far been studied mainly in engineered cell lines, but they also occur in native cells. Functional dimeric complexes between angiotensin (AT_1) and bradykinin (B_2) receptors occur in human platelets and show greater sensitivity to angiotensin than 'pure' AT_1 receptors (AbdAlla et al., 2001). In women suffering from pregnancy-related hypertension (pre-eclamptic toxaemia), the number of these dimers increases due to increased expression of B_2 receptors, resulting – paradoxically – in increased sensitivity to the vasoconstrictor action of angiotensin.

Constitutively active receptors

GPCRs may be constitutively (i.e. spontaneously) active in the absence of any agonist (see Ch. 2 and review by Costa and Cotecchia, 2005). This was first shown for δ opioid receptors (see Ch. 43). There are now many other examples of native GPCRs that show constitutive activity when studied in vitro. The histamine H_3 receptor also shows constitutive activity in vivo, and this may prove to be a quite general phenomenon. It means that inverse agonists (see Ch. 2), which suppress this basal activity, may exert effects distinct from those of neutral antagonists, which block agonist effects without affecting basal activity.

Agonist specificity

It was thought that the linkage of a particular GPCR to a particular signal transduction pathway depends mainly on the structure of the receptor, which confers specificity for a particular G protein, from which the rest of the signal transduction pathway follows. This would imply, in line with the two-state model discussed in Chapter 2, that all agonists acting on a particular receptor stabilise the same activated (R*) state and should activate the same signal transduction pathway, and produce the same type of cellular response. It is now clear that this is an oversimplification. In many cases, for example, with agonists acting on angiotensin receptors, or with inverse agonists on β adrenoceptors, the cellular effects are qualitatively different with different ligands, implying the existence of more than one – probably many – R* states (sometimes referred to as *biased agonism*; see Ch. 2). Binding of arrestins to GPCRs initiates MAP kinase signalling, such that agonists that induce GRK/arrestin 'desensitisation' will terminate some GPCR signalling but may also activate signalling through arrestins that may continue even after the receptor/arrestin complex has been internalised (see Fig. 3.15).

Biased agonism has profound implications – indeed heretical to many pharmacologists, who are accustomed to thinking of agonists in terms of their affinity and efficacy, and nothing else; it has added a new dimension to the way in which we think about drug efficacy and specificity (see Kenakin and Christopoulos, 2013).

Receptor activity-modifying proteins

Receptor activity-modifying proteins (RAMPs) are a family of membrane proteins that associate with some GPCRs and alter their functional characteristics. They were discovered in 1998 when it was found that the functionally active receptor for the neuropeptide *calcitonin gene-related peptide* (CGRP) (see Chs 16 and 19) consisted of a complex of a GPCR – called calcitonin receptor-like receptor (CRLR) – that by itself lacked activity, with another membrane protein (RAMP1). More surprisingly, CRLR when coupled with another RAMP (RAMP2) showed a quite different pharmacology, being activated by an unrelated peptide, *adrenomedulin*. In other words, the agonist specificity is conferred by the associated RAMP as well as by the GPCR itself. More RAMPs have emerged, and so far nearly all the examples involve Class B peptide receptors (see Table 3.2), the calcium-sensing receptor being an exception. RAMPs are an example of how protein–protein interactions influence the pharmacological behaviour of the receptors in a highly selective way and may be novel targets for drug development (Hay and Pioszak, 2015).

G protein–independent signalling

In using the term *G protein–coupled receptor* to describe the class of receptors characterised by their heptahelical structure, we are following conventional textbook dogma but neglecting the fact that G proteins are not the only link between GPCRs and the various effector systems that they regulate. In this context, signalling mediated through arrestins bound to the receptor, rather than through G proteins, is important (see review by Lefkowitz, 2013). Arrestins can act as an intermediary for GPCR activation of the MAP kinase cascade (see Fig. 3.15B).

There are many examples where the various 'adapter proteins' that link receptors of the tyrosine kinase type to their effectors can also interact with GPCRs (see Brzostowski and Kimmel, 2001), allowing the same effector systems to be regulated by receptors of either type.

In summary, the simple dogma that has underpinned much of our understanding of GPCRs, namely, one GPCR gene – one GPCR protein – one functional GPCR – one G protein – one response, is showing distinct signs of wear. In particular:

- one gene, through alternative splicing, RNA editing, etc., can give rise to more than one receptor protein;
- one GPCR protein can associate with others, or with other proteins such as RAMPs, to produce more than one type of functional receptor;
- different agonists may affect a receptor in different ways and elicit qualitatively different responses;
- the signal transduction pathway from 'GPCR' does not invariably require G proteins, and there can be cross-talk with tyrosine kinase-linked receptors.

GPCRs are evidently versatile and adventurous molecules around which much modern pharmacology revolves, and nobody imagines that we have reached the end of the story.

TYPE 3: KINASE-LINKED AND RELATED RECEPTORS

These membrane receptors are quite different in structure and function from ligand-gated channels and GPCRs. They are activated by a wide variety of protein mediators, including growth factors and cytokines (see Ch. 19), and hormones such as insulin (see Ch. 31) and leptin (see Ch. 32), whose effects are exerted mainly at the level of gene transcription. Most of these receptors are large proteins consisting of a single chain of up to 1000 residues, with a single membrane-spanning helical region, linking a large extracellular ligand-binding domain to an intracellular domain of variable size and function. The basic structure is shown in Fig. 3.3C, but many variants exist (see later). Over 100 such receptors have been cloned, and many structural variations exist. For more detail, see the review by Hubbard and Miller (2007). Examples of the related (indirect) kinase-linked receptor types include cytokine receptors (e.g. tumour necrosis factor [TNF] receptors) and pattern recognition receptors (PRRs) that recognise pathogen-associated molecular patterns (PAMPs) or danger-associated molecular patterns (DAMPs) found in pathogens, which stimulate the innate immune system host defence network (see Ch. 7). PRR receptors include the cell surface Toll-like receptors (TLRs), and the cytoplasmic receptors such as RIG-I-like receptors (RLRs) and NOD-like receptors (NLRs). All these immune receptors signal their intracellular effects through adaptor proteins and kinases to alter the cell's transcription to elicit the correct immune response needed to fight against any pathogenic invaders. All these receptors play a major role in controlling cell division, intermediary metabolism, growth, differentiation, inflammation, tissue repair, apoptosis and immune responses, discussed further in Chapters 6 and 19.

The main types are as follows:

Receptor tyrosine kinases (RTKs). These receptors have the basic structure shown in Fig. 3.17A, incorporating a tyrosine kinase moiety in the intracellular region. They include receptors for many growth factors, such as **epidermal growth factor** and **nerve growth factor**, and also the group of *TLRs* that recognise bacterial lipopolysaccharides and play an important role in the body's reaction to infection (see Ch. 7). The insulin receptor (see Ch. 31) also belongs to the RTK class, although it has a more complex dimeric structure, and links indirectly to intracellular tyrosine kinases.

Receptor serine/threonine kinases. This smaller class is similar in structure to RTKs but they phosphorylate serine and/or threonine residues rather than tyrosine. The main example is the receptor for **transforming growth factor** (TGF).

Cytokine receptors. These receptors (Fig. 3.17B) lack intrinsic enzyme activity. When occupied, they activate various tyrosine kinases, such as Jak (the Janus kinase). Ligands for these receptors include cytokines such as **interferons** and **colony-stimulating factors** involved in immunological responses as well as cell growth and differentiation.

PROTEIN PHOSPHORYLATION AND KINASE CASCADE MECHANISMS

Protein phosphorylation (see Cohen, 2002) is a key mechanism for controlling the function of proteins (e.g. enzymes, ion channels, receptors, transport proteins) involved in regulating cellular processes. Phosphorylation and dephosphorylation are accomplished by *kinases* and *phosphatases*, respectively - enzymes, of which several hundred subtypes are represented in the human genome - which are themselves subject to regulation dependent on their phosphorylation status. Much effort is currently being invested in mapping the complex interactions between signalling molecules that are involved in drug effects and pathophysiological processes such as oncogenesis, neurodegeneration, inflammation and much else. Here we can present only a few pharmacologically relevant aspects of what has become an enormous subject.

In many cases, ligand binding to the receptor leads to dimerisation. The association of the two intracellular kinase domains allows a mutual autophosphorylation of intracellular tyrosine residues to occur. The phosphorylated tyrosine residues then serve as high-affinity docking sites for other intracellular proteins that form the next stage in the signal transduction cascade. One important group of such proteins is known as the *SH2 domain proteins* (standing for *Src* homology, because they were first identified in the *Src* oncogene product).[17] These possess a highly conserved sequence of about 100 amino acids, forming a recognition site for the phosphotyrosine residues of the receptor. Individual SH2 domain proteins, of which many are now known, bind selectively to particular receptors, so the pattern of events triggered by particular growth factors is highly specific. The mechanism is summarised in Fig. 3.17.

What happens when the SH2 domain protein binds to the phosphorylated receptor varies greatly according to the receptor that is involved; many SH2 domain proteins are enzymes, such as protein kinases or phospholipases. Some growth factors activate a specific subtype of phospholipase C (PLCγ), thereby causing phospholipid breakdown, IP_3 formation and Ca^{2+} release. Other SH2-containing proteins couple phosphotyrosine-containing proteins with a variety of other functional proteins, including many that are involved in the control of cell division and differentiation. The end result is to activate or inhibit, by phosphorylation, a variety of transcription factors that migrate to the nucleus and suppress or induce the expression of particular genes. For more

Kinase-linked receptors

- Receptors for various growth factors incorporate tyrosine kinase in their intracellular domain.
- Cytokine receptors have an intracellular domain that binds and activates cytosolic kinases when the receptor is occupied.
- The receptors all share a common architecture, with a large extracellular ligand-binding domain connected via a single membrane-spanning helix to the intracellular domain.
- Signal transduction generally involves dimerisation of receptors, followed by autophosphorylation of tyrosine residues. The phosphotyrosine residues act as acceptors for the SH2 domains of a variety of intracellular proteins, thereby allowing control of many cell functions.
- They are involved mainly in events controlling cell growth and differentiation, and act indirectly by regulating gene transcription.
- Two important pathways are:
  - the Ras/Raf/MAP kinase pathway, which is important in cell division, growth and differentiation;
  - the Jak/Stat pathway activated by many cytokines, which controls the synthesis and release of many inflammatory mediators.

[17] ***v-Src*** is a gene found in Rous sarcoma virus that encodes a tyrosine kinase which causes sarcoma (a malignant tumour) in chickens – it was found to have a closely related sequence to the chicken's own gene termed c-Src (for cellular rather than viral Src). This was the first oncogene to be discovered, in 1979.

detail, see Jin and Pawson (2012). *Nuclear factor kappa B* (NF-κB) is a transcription factor that plays a key role in multiple disorders including inflammation and cancer (see Chs 18 and 57; Karin et al., 2004). It is normally present in the cytosol, complexed with an inhibitor (I-κB). Phosphorylation of I-κB occurs when a specific kinase (IKK) is activated in response to various inflammatory cytokines and GPCR agonists. This results in dissociation of I-κB from NF-κB and migration of NF-κB to the nucleus, where it switches on various proinflammatory and anti-apoptotic genes.

Two well-defined signal transduction pathways are summarised in Fig. 3.17. The Ras/Raf pathway mediates the effect of many growth factors and mitogens. Ras, which is a proto-oncogene product, functions like a G protein, and conveys the signal (by GDP/GTP exchange) from the SH2-domain protein, Grb. Activation of Ras in turn activates Raf, which is the first of a sequence of three serine/threonine kinases, each of which phosphorylates, and activates, the next in line. The last of these, MAP kinase (which is also activated by GPCRs, see earlier), phosphorylates one or more transcription factors that initiate gene expression, resulting in a variety of cellular responses, including cell division. This three-tiered MAP kinase cascade forms part of many intracellular signalling pathways involved in a wide variety of disease processes, including malignancy, inflammation, neurodegeneration, atherosclerosis and much else. The kinases form a large family, with different subtypes serving specific roles. They are thought to represent an important target for future therapeutic drugs. Many cancers are associated with mutations in the genes coding for proteins involved in this cascade, leading to activation of the cascade in the absence of the growth factor signal (see Chs 6 and 57). For more details, see the review by Avruch (2007).

A second pathway, the Jak/Stat pathway (see Fig. 3.17B), is involved in responses to many cytokines. Dimerisation of these receptors occurs when the cytokine binds, and this attracts a cytosolic tyrosine kinase unit (Jak) to associate with, and phosphorylate, the receptor dimer. Jaks belong to a family of proteins, different members having specificity for different cytokine receptors. Among the targets for phosphorylation by Jak are a family of transcription factors (Stats). These are SH2-domain proteins that bind to the phosphotyrosine groups on the receptor–Jak complex, and are themselves phosphorylated. Thus activated, Stat migrates to the nucleus and activates gene expression.

Other important mechanisms centre on *phosphatidylinositol-3 kinase* (PI_3 kinases; see Vanhaesebroeck et al., 1997), a ubiquitous enzyme family that is activated both by GPCRs and RTKs and attaches a phosphate group to position 3 of PIP_2 to form PIP_3. Other protein kinases, particularly protein kinase B (PKB,[18] also known as Akt), have recognition sites for PIP_3 and are thus activated, controlling a wide variety of cellular functions, including apoptosis, differentiation, proliferation and trafficking. Akt also causes NO synthase activation in the vascular endothelium (see Ch. 21).

Recent work on signal transduction pathways has produced a bewildering profusion of molecular detail, often couched in a jargon that is apt to deter the faint-hearted. Perseverance will be rewarded, however, for there is no doubt that important new drugs, particularly in the areas of inflammation, immunology and cancer, will come from the targeting of these proteins (Wilson et al., 2018). A breakthrough in the treatment of chronic myeloid leukaemia was achieved with the introduction of the first explicitly designed kinase inhibitor, **imatinib**, a drug that inhibits a specific tyrosine kinase involved in the pathogenesis of the disease (see Ch. 57).

Fig. 3.18 illustrates the central role of protein kinases in signal transduction pathways in a highly simplified and schematic way. Many, if not all, of the proteins involved, including the receptors and the kinases themselves, are substrates for kinases, so there are many mechanisms for feedback and cross-talk between the various signalling pathways. Given that there are over 500 protein kinases, and similarly large numbers of receptors and other signalling molecules, the network of interactions can look bewilderingly complex. Dissecting out the details has become a major theme in cell biology. For pharmacologists, the idea of a simple connection between receptor and response, which guided thinking throughout the 20th century, is undoubtedly crumbling, although it will take some time before the complexities of signalling pathways are assimilated into a new way of thinking about drug action.

Protein phosphorylation in signal transduction

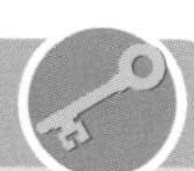

- Many receptor-mediated events involve protein phosphorylation, which controls the functional and binding properties of intracellular proteins.
- Receptor-linked tyrosine kinases, cyclic nucleotide-activated tyrosine kinases and intracellular serine/threonine kinases comprise a 'kinase cascade' mechanism that leads to amplification of receptor-mediated events.
- There are many kinases, with differing substrate specificities, allowing specificity in the pathways activated by different hormones.
- Desensitisation of GPCRs occurs as a result of phosphorylation by specific receptor kinases, causing the receptor to become non-functional and to be internalised.
- There is a large family of phosphatases that act to dephosphorylate proteins and thus reverse the effects of kinases.

TYPE 4: NUCLEAR RECEPTORS

By the 1970s, it was clear from experiments with radiolabelled tracers that receptors for steroid hormones such as oestrogen and the glucocorticoids (Chs 33 and 35) were present in the cytoplasm of cells and translocated into the nucleus after binding with their steroid partner. Other hormones, such as the thyroid hormone T_3 (see Ch. 34) and the fat-soluble vitamins D and A (retinoic acid),

[18]Protein kinase B was named to fill in the gap between protein kinase A (cAMP-dependent) and protein kinase C (Ca^{2+}-dependent). As you can see, nomenclature is highly imaginative!

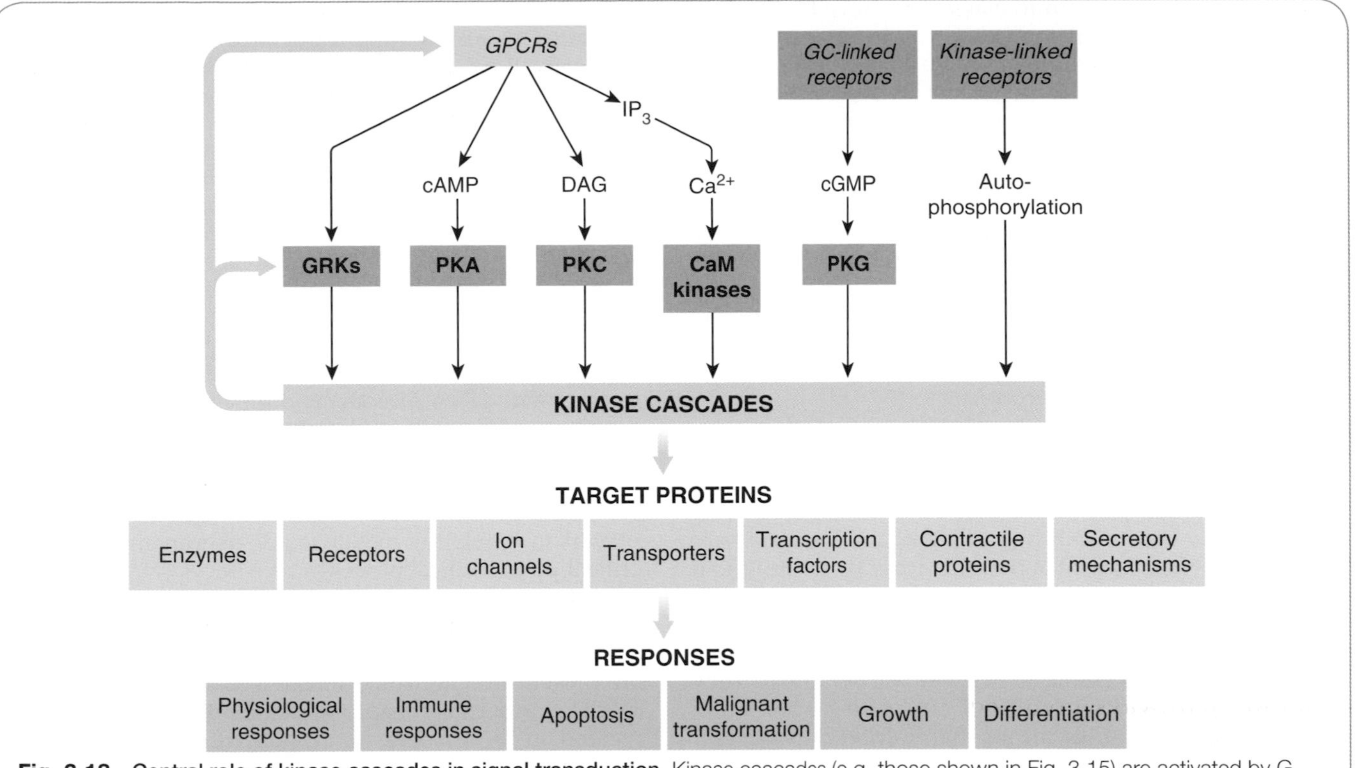

Fig. 3.18 Central role of kinase cascades in signal transduction. Kinase cascades (e.g. those shown in Fig. 3.15) are activated by G protein–coupled receptors (GPCRs), either directly or via different second messengers, by receptors that generate cGMP, or by kinase-linked receptors. The kinase cascades regulate various target proteins, which in turn produce a wide variety of short- and long-term effects. *CaM kinase,* Ca^{2+}/calmodulin-dependent kinase; *DAG,* diacylglycerol; *GC,* guanylyl cyclase; *GRK,* GPCR kinase; *IP_3,* inositol trisphosphate; *PKA,* cAMP-dependent protein kinase; *PKC,* protein kinase C; *PKG,* cGMP-dependent protein kinase.

were found to act in a similar fashion. In the mid-1980s, the genes for oestrogen and glucocorticoid receptors were identified using the (then) relatively new molecular cloning techniques. Comparisons of gene and protein sequence data led to the recognition that these receptors were similar and in fact were members of a much larger family of some 50 related proteins. We now know these as the *nuclear receptor (NR) family*.

The ligands for most endocrine receptors were, of course, already known but the NR family also comprised many (some 36) other *orphan receptors* – receptors with no known well-defined endogenous ligands. The first of these to be described, in the 1990s, was the *retinoid X receptor* (RXR), which was cloned on the basis of its similarity with the vitamin A receptor and which was subsequently found to bind the vitamin A derivative 9-*cis*-retinoic acid (Evans et al., 2014). This event triggered intense interest in the NR field and, during the intervening years, specific binding partners have been characterised for at least 11 further NRs ('adopted orphans', e.g. RXR) were discovered, but the ligands for the remaining 25 'true orphans' have yet to be identified – or perhaps do not exist as such, as one possible function of these receptors is their 'promiscuous' ability to bind to many related compounds (such as dietary factors) with low affinity.

Whilst there are 48 known NRs in man, more proteins may arise through alternative splicing events. While this represents a rather small proportion of all receptors (less than 10% of the total number of GPCRs for example), the NRs are very important drug targets (Burris et al., 2013), being responsible for the biological effects of approximately 10%–15% of all prescription drugs. They can recognise an extraordinarily diverse group of substances (mostly small hydrophobic molecules), which may exhibit full or partial agonist, antagonist or inverse agonist activity. Many NRs which bind their ligands with high affinity (e.g. oestrogen receptor [ER] and glucocorticoid receptor [GR]) are involved predominantly in endocrine signalling, but many bind their ligands with low affinity and probably act as metabolic (e.g. lipid) sensors. They are thus crucial links between our dietary and metabolic status and the expression of genes that regulate the metabolism and disposition of lipids (Goto, 2019). NRs also regulate the expression of many drug-metabolising enzymes and transporters. Pregnane X (PXR) and *constitutive androstane receptor (CAR),* for example, are akin to airport security guards who alert the bomb disposal squad when suspicious luggage is found. When they sense foreign molecules (xenobiotics), they induce drug-metabolising enzymes such as CYP3A (which is responsible for metabolising about 60% of all prescription drugs; see Ch. 10 and di Masi et al., 2009). They also bind some prostaglandins and non-steroidal drugs, as well as the antidiabetic thiazolidinediones (see Ch. 31) and fibrates (see Ch. 22).

CLASSIFICATION OF NRs

NRs are usually classified into subfamilies according to their phylogeny (see Germain et al., 2006). For our purposes, however, it is more useful to classify them on the basis of their molecular mechanism into two main classes (I and II) and two other minor groups of receptors (III, IV).

Class I consists largely of endocrine steroid receptors which normally act as homodimers. These include the GR (2 subtypes) and mineralocorticoid receptors (MRs), as well as the ERs (two subtypes), progesterone and androgen receptors (PR and AR, respectively). The hormones recognised by these receptors generally act in a negative feedback fashion to control biological events (see Ch. 33 for more details). In the absence of their ligand, these NRs are predominantly located in the cytoplasm (although possibly reversibly attached to the cytoskeleton or other intracellular structures) complexed with 'chaperone' heat shock proteins (HSPs) and other 'co-chaperone' factors.

Unlike the receptors in class I, NRs in Class II almost always operate as heterodimers together with RXR, the retinoid X receptor. Two types of heterodimer may then be formed: a *non-permissive heterodimer*, which can be activated only by the RXR ligand itself, and the *permissive heterodimer*, which can be activated either by retinoic acid itself or by its partner's ligand. Class II NRs are generally bound to co-repressor proteins. These dissociate when the ligand binds and allows recruitment of co-activator proteins and hence changes in gene transcription. They tend to mediate positive feedback effects (e.g. occupation of the receptor amplifies rather than inhibits a particular biological event).

Class III NRs are very similar to Class I in the sense that they form homodimers, whereas Class IV NRs may function as monomers or dimers. Many of the remaining orphan receptors belong to these latter classes.

STRUCTURE OF NRs

The NR superfamily probably evolved from a single distant evolutionary ancestral gene by duplication and other events. All NRs are monomeric proteins of 50–100 kDa, which share a broadly similar structural configuration as revealed by X-ray crystallography (see Fig. 3.19 and Bourguet et al., 2000, for further details). Alternative splicing of genes may yield several receptor isoforms, each with slightly different N-terminal regions although in the case of the ER, each of the two subtypes is encoded by a different gene.

The *N-terminal domain* of the receptor family displays the most heterogeneity. It harbours a crucial *activation function 1 (AF1)* site which binds to other cell-specific transcription factors in a ligand-independent way and modifies the binding or regulatory capacity of the receptor itself. In the presence of the ligand, it synergises with a further activation sequence, *AF2,* to produce a fully active complex. The AF2 region is important in ligand-dependent activation and is generally highly conserved, although it is absent in *Rev-erbAα* and *Rev-erbAβ*, NRs that regulate metabolism (and also function as part of a circadian molecular clock mechanism).

The *core domain* of the receptor is highly conserved and consists of the structure responsible for DNA recognition and binding. At the molecular level, this comprises two *zinc fingers* – cysteine- (or cystine-/histidine-) rich loops in the amino acid chain that are held in a particular conformation by zinc ions. The main function of this portion of the molecule is to bind to recognition elements located in the genes that are regulated by this family of receptors, but it also regulates NR receptor dimerisation. The highly flexible *hinge region* is crucial to this latter function of NRs but also regulates the intracellular trafficking of the receptor.

Finally, the *C-terminal domain* contains the *ligand-binding module*. This region is not well conserved amongst NRs (although it is structurally similar) and is specific to each class of receptor, thereby enabling it to recognise its cognate ligands. It is also important in dimerisation and binding co-activator and co-repressor proteins. Also located near the C-terminal are motifs that contain *nuclear localisation signals* and others that may, in the case of some receptors, bind *accessory heat shock* and other proteins.

CONTROL OF GENE TRANSCRIPTION BY NRs

Unlike the other receptors described in this chapter, NRs can interact with DNA directly, and may thus be regarded as *ligand-activated transcription factors* that produce their effects by modifying gene transcription. Through this mechanism they can control the transcription and expression of many genes and proteins so, as might be imagined, they are key players in regulating metabolic, developmental and other critical physiological processes.

Another characteristic property is that NRs are not generally embedded in membranes like GPCRs or ion channels (although there are important exceptions) but are present in other compartments of the cell. Some, such as the endocrine receptors, which are predominately located in the cytoplasm, are activated by their ligand and translocate from the cytoplasm to the nucleus, while others, such as the RXR, probably dwell mainly within the nuclear compartment. Having said this, there is increasing evidence for the existence of small pools of some NRs, such as ERs and GRs associated with the plasma membrane, in organelles such as the mitochondria (Levin and Hammes, 2016) and even in cells without nuclei such as platelets, where they can apparently regulate other targets such as protein kinases to bring about immediate biological actions (Shaqura et al., 2016).

To bring about changes in gene transcription, activated NRs bind to *hormone response elements* (HREs) in the genome. HREs are short (usually 4–6 base pairs) sequences of DNA which are generally present symmetrically in pairs or *half-sites* with one half on each DNA strand. These typically comprise *inverted repeats* separated by three nucleotide bases, although there may different arrangements (e.g. *simple,* rather than inverted repeats). Each NR exhibits a preference for a particular *consensus sequence* and the nucleotide spacing between them, but because of the family homology, they all share a close similarity. Some NRs, particularly those in Class III, function as homodimers but they can bind to HREs, which do not have an inverted repeat sequence, whereas Class IV NRs may function as monomers or dimers but only bind to one HRE half site.

In the nucleus, the AF1 and AF2 domains of the ligand-bound receptor recruit large complexes of other proteins including *co-activators* or *co-repressors* to modify gene expression. Some of these co-activators are enzymes involved in chromatin remodelling, such as histone acetylase/deacetylase which, together with other enzymes, regulate the unravelling of the DNA to facilitate access by polymerase enzymes and hence gene transcription. Co-repressor complexes are recruited by some receptors and comprise histone deacetylase and other factors that cause the chromatin to become tightly packed, preventing further transcriptional activation. The case of the *CAR* (see later)

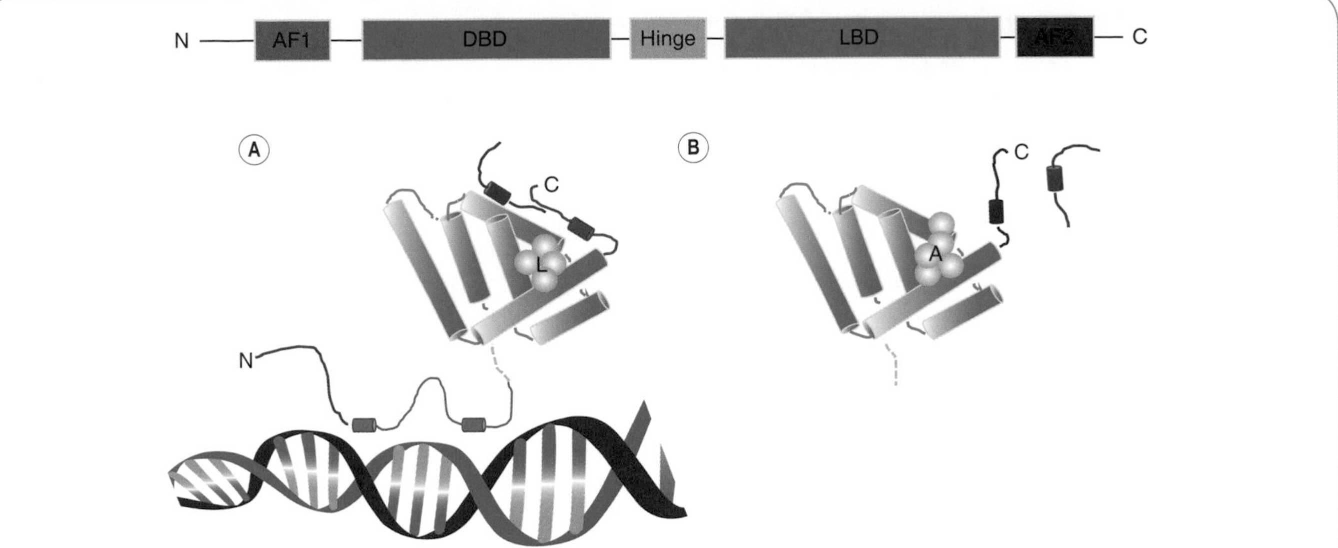

Fig. 3.19 Schematic diagram of a nuclear receptor. A greatly simplified diagram of the functional topology of a nuclear receptor (the oestrogen receptor is picked as an example). A schematic diagram shows the various regions of the receptor including the DNA-binding domain (DBD). *Below* is a diagram illustrating, in the corresponding colours, the configuration of the liganded receptor showing its binding to hormone response elements (HREs) on DNA. In panel A, the ligand (L) is bound in the ligand-binding domain (LBD) and this enables the C-terminal AF2 region to bind to the LBD. In turn, this allows the binding of a co-activator protein at the LBD (only a partial structure shown), which allows gene transcription to proceed. In panel B, an antagonist (A) is bound to the LBD. This sterically inhibits the binding of AF2 and thus the attachment of the co-activator protein. Most nuclear receptors operate as dimers but only a monomer is shown here for clarity. Cylindrical structures represent regions of α-helical protein structure. (Based largely upon Shiau, A.K., Barstad, D., Loria, P.M., et al., 1998. The structural basis of estrogen receptor/coactivator recognition and the antagonism of this interaction by tamoxifen. Cell 95, 927–937.)

is particularly interesting: like some G proteins described earlier in this chapter, CAR can adopt a constitutively active complex that is terminated when it binds its ligand. The mechanisms of negative gene regulation by NRs are particularly complex (see Santos et al., 2011, for a good account).

In addition to agonists, NRs can also be targeted by competitive antagonists, which prevent occupation of the binding site by the endogenous ligand or by inverse agonists (or antagonists), which sterically prevent the binding of co-activator factors, thus reducing the constitutive activity of these receptors. A very interesting development is the identification of selective receptor modulators (e.g. selective ER modulators - SERMs such as **tamoxifen**) which, by altering the binding of co-activator and co-repressor proteins, have agonist activity in some tissues and antagonist activities in others.

REGULATION OF NR ACTIVITY

Many NRs are subject to exquisite post-transcriptional and other regulation. The HSPs play a particularly important part in the functioning of the receptor with HSP90 being essential for GR function (for example) while HSP70 is inhibitory. The dynamic interplay between these HSPs is crucial for the cycling of GR between its active and inactive states (Noddings et al., 2022). Differential phosphorylation of GR also plays an important part in behaviour of the receptor with sites such as *Ser*^{211}, *Ser*^{203} and others being especially significant. For example, phosphorylation of the former residue is associated with receptor activation and nuclear localisation while phosphorylation of the latter has a down-regulatory influence (Wang et al., 2002). Receptor methylation may also be important (Malbeteau et al., 2022).

THE NR FAMILY IN HEALTH AND DISEASE

Given the fact that the NR family of receptors plays a key part in the regulation and coordination of growth, development and organogenesis, reproduction, the immune system and many other fundamental biological processes, it is not surprising that many illnesses are associated with malfunctioning of the NR system. Such conditions include inflammation, cancer, diabetes, cardiovascular disease, obesity and reproductive disorders (see Kersten et al., 2000; Murphy and Holder, 2000).

The discussion here must be taken only as a broad guide to the action of NRs, as many other types of interaction have also been discovered. For example, some of these receptors may bring about non-genomic - or even genomic - actions by directly interacting with factors in the cytosol, or they may be covalently modified by phosphorylation or by protein–protein interactions with other transcription factors such that their function is altered (see Falkenstein et al., 2000).

Table 3.4 summarises the properties of some common NRs of importance to pharmacologists.

ION CHANNELS AS DRUG TARGETS

We have discussed ligand-gated ion channels as one of the four main types of drug receptor. There are many other types of ion channel that represent important drug targets, even though they are not generally classified as

Table 3.4 Some common pharmacologically significant nuclear receptors

Receptor name	Abbreviation	Ligand	Drugs	Location	Ligand binding	Mechanism of action
Type I						
Androgen	AR	Testosterone	All natural and synthetic glucocorticoids (see Ch. 33), mineralocorticoids (see Ch. 29) and sex steroids (see Ch. 35) together with their antagonists (e.g. raloxifene, 4-hydroxy-tamoxifen and mifepristone)	Cytosolic	Homodimers	Translocation to nucleus. Binding to HREs with two half-sites with an inverted sequence. Recruitment of co-activators, transcription factors and other proteins
Oestrogen	ERα, β	17β-oestradiol				
Glucocorticoid	GRα	Cortisol, corticosterone				
Progesterone	PR	Progesterone				
Mineralocorticoid	MR	Aldosterone				
Type II						
Retinoid X	RXR α,β,γ	9-*cis*-retinoic acid	Retinoid drugs (see Ch. 27)	Nuclear	Heterodimers often with RXR	Binding to HREs with two half-sites with an inverted or simple repeat sequence. Complexed with co-repressors, which are displaced following ligand binding, allowing the binding of co-activators
Retinoic acid	RAR α,β,γ	Vitamin A				
Thyroid hormone	TR α,β	T3, T4	Thyroid hormone drugs (see Ch. 34)			
Peroxisome proliferator	PPAR α,β,γ,δ	Fatty acids, prostaglandins	Rosiglitazone, pioglitazone (see Ch. 31)			
Constitutive androstane	CAR	Androstane	Stimulation of CYP synthesis and alteration of drug metabolism (see Ch. 10)			
Pregnane X	PXR	Xenobiotics				

Only examples from Classes I and II are included.
HRE, Hormone response element.

Nuclear receptors

- In humans this protein family comprises 48 soluble intracellular receptors that sense lipid and hormonal signals and modulate gene transcription.
- Their ligands are many and varied, including steroid hormones and drugs, thyroid hormones, vitamins A and D, various lipids and xenobiotics.
- There are two main categories:
  - **Class I** NRs are present in the cytoplasm, form homodimers in the presence of their ligand and migrate to the nucleus. Their ligands are mainly endocrine in nature (e.g. steroid hormones);
  - **Class II** NRs are generally constitutively present in the nucleus and form heterodimers with the RXR. Their ligands are usually lipids (e.g. the fatty acids).
- The liganded receptor complexes initiate changes in gene transcription by binding to HREs in gene promoters and recruiting co-activator or co-repressor factors.
- The receptor family is the target of approximately 10% of prescription drugs, and the enzymes that it regulates affect the pharmacokinetics of some 60% of all prescription drugs.

'receptors' because they are not the immediate targets of fast neurotransmitters, but drugs can act upon them to alter their ability to open and close.[19]

Here we discuss the structure and function of ion channels at the molecular level; their role as regulators of cell function is described in Chapter 4.

Ions are unable to penetrate the lipid bilayer of the cell membrane and can get across only with the help of membrane-spanning proteins in the form of channels or transporters. The concept of ion channels was developed in the 1950s on the basis of electrophysiological studies on the mechanism of membrane excitation (see Ch. 4). Electrophysiology, particularly the *voltage clamp technique*, remains an essential tool for studying the physiological and pharmacological properties of ion channels. Since the mid-1980s, when the first ion channels were cloned by Numa in Japan, much has been learned about the structure and function of these complex molecules. The

[19]In truth, the distinction between ligand-gated channels and other ion channels is an arbitrary one. In grouping ligand-gated channels with other types of receptor in this book, we are respecting the historical tradition established by Langley and others, who first defined receptors in the context of the action of acetylcholine at the neuromuscular junction. The advance of molecular biology may force us to reconsider this semantic issue in the future, but for now we make no apology for upholding the pharmacological tradition.

use of patch clamp recording, which allows the behaviour of individual channels to be studied in real time, has been particularly valuable in distinguishing channels on the basis of their conductance and gating characteristics. Accounts by Ashcroft (2000), Catterall (2000) and Hille (2001) give background information.

Ion channels consist of protein molecules designed to form water-filled pores that span the membrane and can switch between open and closed states. The rate and direction of ion movement through the pore are governed by the electrochemical gradient for the ion in question, which is a function of its concentration on either side of the membrane and of the membrane potential. Ion channels are characterised by:

- their selectivity for particular ion species, determined by the size of the pore and the nature of its lining;
- their gating properties (i.e. the nature of the stimulus that controls the transition between open and closed states of the channel);
- their molecular architecture.

ION SELECTIVITY

Channels are generally either cation selective or anion selective. The main cation-selective channels are selective for Na^+, Ca^{2+} or K^+, or non-selective and permeable to all three. Anion channels are mainly permeable to Cl^-, although other types also occur. The effect of modulation of ion channels on cell function is discussed in Chapter 4.

GATING

VOLTAGE-GATED CHANNELS

In the main, these channels open when the cell membrane is depolarised.[20] They form a very important group because they underlie the mechanism of membrane excitability (see Ch. 4). The most important channels in this group are selective sodium, potassium or calcium channels.

Commonly, the channel opening (activation) induced by membrane depolarisation is short lasting, even if the depolarisation is maintained. This is because, with some channels, the initial activation of the channels is followed by a slower process of inactivation.

The role of voltage-gated channels in the generation of action potentials and in controlling other cell functions is described in Chapter 4.

LIGAND-GATED CHANNELS

These (see Fig. 3.5) are activated by binding of a chemical ligand to sites on the channel molecule. Fast neurotransmitters, such as glutamate, acetylcholine, GABA, 5-HT and ATP (see Chs 14, 16 and 38), act in this way, binding to sites on the outside of the membrane. In addition, there are also ligand-gated ion channels that do not respond to neurotransmitters but to changes in their local environment. For example, the TRPV1 channel on sensory nerves that mediates the pain-producing effect of the chilli pepper ingredient capsaicin responds to extracellular protons when tissue pH falls, as occurs in inflamed tissue, as well as to the physical stimulus, heat (see Ch. 43).

Some ligand-gated channels in the plasma membrane respond to intracellular rather than extracellular signals, the most important being the following:

- Calcium-activated potassium channels, which occur in most cells and open, thus hyperpolarising the cell, when $[Ca^{2+}]_i$ increases.
- Calcium-activated chloride channels, widely expressed in excitable and non-excitable cells where they are involved in diverse functions such as epithelial secretion of electrolytes and water, sensory transduction, regulation of neuronal and cardiac excitability and regulation of vascular tone.
- ATP-sensitive potassium channels, which open when the intracellular ATP concentration falls because the cell is short of energy. These channels, which are quite distinct from those mediating the excitatory effects of extracellular ATP, occur in many nerve and muscle cells, and also in insulin-secreting cells (see Ch. 31), where they are part of the mechanism linking insulin secretion to blood glucose concentration.

Other examples of cell membrane channels that respond to intracellular ligands include arachidonic acid-sensitive potassium channels and DAG-sensitive calcium channels, whose functions are not well understood.

CALCIUM RELEASE CHANNELS

The main ones, IP_3 and **ryanodine** receptors (see Ch. 4), are a special class of ligand-gated calcium channels that are present on the endoplasmic or sarcoplasmic reticulum rather than the plasma membrane and control the release of Ca^{2+} from intracellular stores. Ca^{2+} can also be released from lysosomal stores by nicotinic acid adenine dinucleotide phosphate, which activates two-pore domain calcium channels.

STORE-OPERATED CALCIUM CHANNELS

When the intracellular Ca^{2+} stores are depleted, 'store-operated' channels (SOCs) in the plasma membrane open to allow Ca^{2+} entry. The mechanism by which this linkage occurs involves interaction of a Ca^{2+}-sensor protein in the endoplasmic reticulum membrane with a dedicated Ca^{2+} channel in the plasma membrane (see Stathopulos and Ikura, 2017). In response to GPCRs that elicit Ca^{2+} release, the opening of these channels allows the cytosolic free Ca^{2+} concentration, $[Ca^{2+}]_i$, to remain elevated even when the intracellular stores are running low, and also provides a route through which the stores can be replenished (see Ch. 4).

MOLECULAR ARCHITECTURE OF ION CHANNELS

Ion channels are large and elaborate molecules. Their characteristic structural motifs have been revealed as knowledge of their sequence and structure has accumulated since the mid-1980s, when the first voltage-gated sodium channel was cloned. The main structural subtypes are shown in Fig. 3.20. All consist of several (often four) domains, which are similar or identical to each other, organised either as an oligomeric array of separate subunits or as one large protein. Each subunit or domain contains a bundle of two to six membrane-spanning helices.

Voltage-gated channels generally include one transmembrane helix that contains an abundance of basic (i.e. positively charged) amino acids. When the membrane

[20]There is always an exception to the rule! The members of the HCN family of potassium channels found in neurons and cardiac muscle cells are activated by hyperpolarisation.

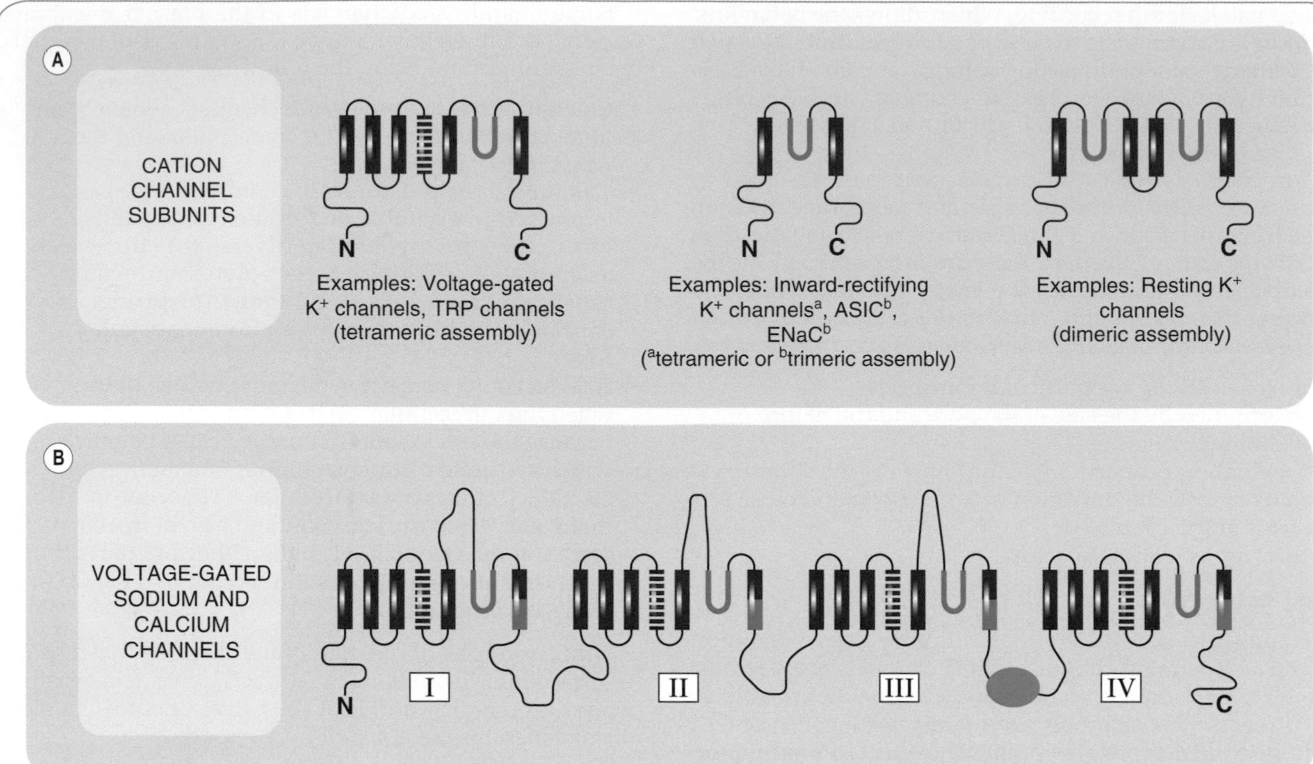

Fig. 3.20 Molecular architecture of ion channels. *Red and blue rectangles* represent membrane-spanning α-helices. *Blue hairpins* are pore loop (P) domains, present in many channels; *blue rectangles* are the pore-forming regions of the membrane-spanning α-helices. *Cross-shaded rectangles* represent the voltage-sensing regions of voltage-gated channels. The *green symbol* represents the inactivating particle of voltage-gated sodium channels. Further information on ion channels is given in Chapter 4. *ASIC*, Acid-sensing ion channel; *ENaC*, epithelial sodium channel; *TRP*, transient receptor potential channel.

is depolarised, so that the interior of the cell becomes less negative, this region – the voltage sensor – moves slightly towards the outer surface of the membrane, which has the effect of opening the channel (see Bezanilla, 2008). Many voltage-activated channels also show *inactivation*, which happens when an intracellular appendage of the channel protein moves to plug the channel from the inside. Voltage-gated sodium and calcium channels are remarkable in that the whole structure with four six-helix domains consists of a single huge protein molecule, the domains being linked together by intracellular loops of varying length (see Fig. 3.20B). Potassium channels comprise the most numerous and heterogeneous class.[21] Voltage-gated potassium channels resemble sodium channels, except that they are made up of four subunits rather than a single long chain. The class of potassium channels known as 'inward rectifier channels' because of their biophysical properties has the two-helix structure shown in Fig. 3.20A, whereas others are classed as 'two-pore domain' channels, because each subunit contains two P loops.

The various architectural motifs shown in Fig. 3.20 only scrape the surface of the molecular diversity of ion channels. In all cases, the individual subunits come in several molecular varieties, and these can unite in different combinations to form functional channels as *hetero-oligomers* (as distinct from *homo-oligomers* built from identical subunits). Furthermore, the channel-forming structures described are usually associated with other membrane proteins, which significantly affect their functional properties. For example, the ATP-gated potassium channel exists in association with the *sulfonylurea receptor* (SUR), and it is through this linkage that various drugs (including antidiabetic drugs of the sulfonylurea class; see Ch. 31) regulate the channel. Good progress is being made in understanding the relation between molecular structure and ion channel function, but we still have only a fragmentary understanding of the physiological role of many of these channels. Many important drugs exert their effects by influencing channel function, either directly or indirectly.

[21]The human genome encodes more than 70 distinct potassium channel subtypes – either a nightmare or a golden opportunity for the pharmacologist, depending on one's perspective.

PHARMACOLOGY OF ION CHANNELS

Many drugs and physiological mediators described in this book exert their effects by altering the behaviour of ion channels.

The gating and permeation of both voltage-gated and ligand-gated ion channels are modulated by many factors, including the following.

- *Ligands that bind directly to various sites on the channel protein.* These include a variety of drugs and toxins that act in different ways, for example by blocking the channel or by affecting the gating process, thereby either facilitating or inhibiting the opening of the channel.

- *Mediators and drugs that act indirectly, mainly by activation of GPCRs.* The latter produce their effects mainly by affecting the state of phosphorylation of individual amino acids located on the intracellular region of the channel protein. As described earlier, this modulation involves the production of second messengers that activate protein kinases. The opening of the channel may be facilitated or inhibited, depending on which residues are phosphorylated. Drugs such as β-adrenoceptor agonists (see Ch. 15) affect calcium and potassium channel function in this way, producing a wide variety of cellular effects.
- *Intracellular signals, particularly Ca^{2+} and nucleotides such as ATP and GTP* (see Ch. 4). Many ion channels possess binding sites for these intracellular mediators. Increased $[Ca^{2+}]_i$ opens certain types of potassium and chloride channels, and inactivates voltage-gated calcium channels. As described in Chapter 4, $[Ca^{2+}]_i$ is itself affected by the function of ion channels and GPCRs. Intracellular ATP binds to and closes a family of potassium channels known as the ATP-gated potassium channels (see Ch. 31) that are also sensitive to sulfonylurea drugs. Intracellular cyclic nucleotides, cAMP and cGMP, activate channels permeable to either calcium and sodium ions or potassium ions.

Fig. 3.21 summarises the main sites and mechanisms by which drugs affect voltage-gated sodium channels, a typical example of this type of drug target.

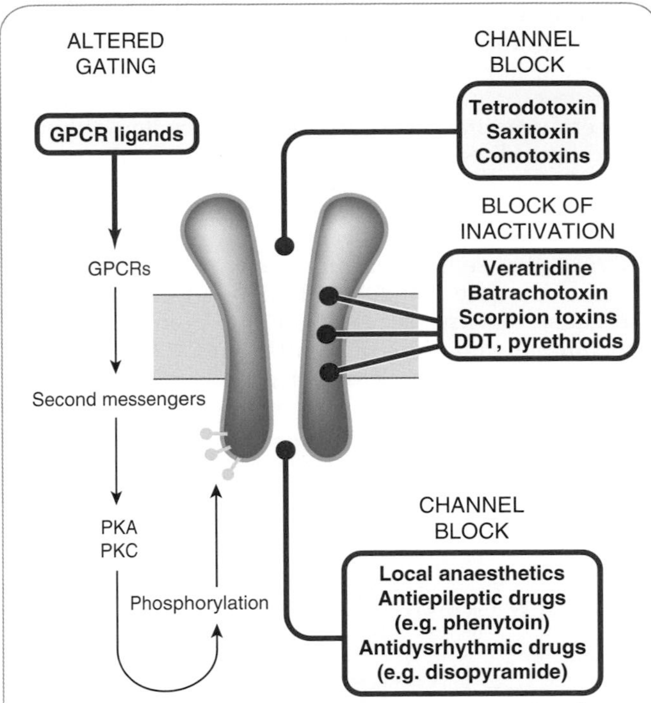

Fig. 3.21 Drug-binding domains of voltage-gated sodium channels (see Ch. 44). The multiplicity of different binding sites and effects appears to be typical of many ion channels. *DDT,* Dichlorodiphenyltrichloroethane (dicophane, a well-known insecticide); *GPCR,* G protein–coupled receptor; *PKA,* protein kinase A; *PKC,* protein kinase C.

CONTROL OF RECEPTOR EXPRESSION

Receptor proteins are synthesised by the cells that express them, and the level of expression is itself controlled, via the pathways discussed previously, by receptor-mediated events. We can no longer think of the receptors as the fixed elements in cellular control systems, responding to changes in the concentration of ligands, and initiating effects through the signal transduction pathway – they are themselves subject to regulation. Short-term regulation of receptor function generally occurs through *desensitisation*, as discussed earlier. Long-term regulation occurs through *an increase or decrease of receptor expression*. Examples of this type of control include the proliferation of various postsynaptic receptors after denervation (see Ch. 13), the up-regulation of various G protein–coupled and cytokine receptors in response to inflammation (see Ch. 17) and the induction of growth factor receptors by certain tumour viruses (see Ch. 6). Long-term drug treatment invariably induces adaptive responses, which, particularly with drugs that act on the central nervous system, can limit their effectiveness as in opioid tolerance (see Ch. 43) or can be the basis for therapeutic efficacy. In the latter instance this may take the form of a very slow onset of the therapeutic effect (e.g. with antidepressant drugs; see Ch. 48). It is likely that changes in receptor expression, secondary to the immediate action of the drug, are involved in delayed effects of this sort – a kind of 'secondary pharmacology', the importance of which is only now becoming clearer. The same principles apply to drug targets other than receptors (ion channels, enzymes, transporters, etc.) where adaptive changes in expression and function follow long-term drug administration, resulting, for example, in resistance to certain anticancer drugs (see Ch. 57).

RECEPTORS AND DISEASE

Increasing understanding of receptor function in molecular terms has revealed a number of disease states directly linked to receptor malfunction. The principal mechanisms involved are:

- autoantibodies directed against receptor proteins;
- mutations in genes encoding receptors, ion channels and proteins involved in signal transduction.

An example of the former is *myasthenia gravis* (see Ch. 14), a disease of the neuromuscular junction due to autoantibodies that inactivate nicotinic acetylcholine receptors. Autoantibodies can also mimic the effects of agonists, as in many cases of thyroid hypersecretion, caused by activation of **thyrotropin** receptors (see Ch. 34).

Inherited mutations of genes encoding GPCRs account for various disease states (see Stoy and Gurevich, 2015). Mutated **vasopressin** and **adrenocorticotrophic hormone** receptors (see Chs 29 and 33) can result in resistance to these hormones. Receptor mutations can result in activation of effector mechanisms in the absence of agonists. One of these involves the receptor for thyrotropin, producing continuous oversecretion of thyroid hormone; another involves the receptor for luteinising hormone and results in precocious puberty. Adrenoceptor polymorphisms are common in humans, and certain mutations of the β_2 adrenoceptor, although they do not directly cause disease, are associated with a reduced efficacy of β-adrenoceptor agonists in treating asthma (see Ch. 28) and a poor prognosis in patients with cardiac failure, potentially through *constitutively active mutations* that render receptors active in the absence of any agonists (see Ch. 20). Mutations in G proteins can also cause disease (see Spiegel and Weinstein, 2004). For example, mutations of a particular Gα subunit cause one form of *hypoparathyroidism*, while mutations of a Gβ subunit result in hypertension. Many cancers are associated with mutations of the genes encoding growth factor receptors, kinases and other proteins involved in signal transduction and cell survival (see Ch. 6).

Mutations in ligand-gated ion channels ($GABA_A$ and nicotinic) and other ion channels (Na^+ and K^+) that alter their function give rise to some forms of idiopathic epilepsy (see Ch. 46 and Thakran et al., 2020).

Research on genetic polymorphisms affecting receptors, signalling molecules, ion channels and effector enzymes is continuing apace, and it is expected that a clearer understanding of the variability between individuals in their disease susceptibility and response to therapeutic drugs (see Ch. 12) will result, in the foreseeable future.

REFERENCES AND FURTHER READING

General

IUPHAR/BPS. Guide to Pharmacology. Avilable at: www.guidetopharmacology.org/.

Nelson, N., 1998. The family of Na^+/Cl^- neurotransmitter transporters. J. Neurochem. 71, 1785–1803.

Ion channels

Ashcroft, F.M., 2000. Ion Channels and Disease. Academic Press, London.

Bezanilla, F., 2008. How membrane proteins sense voltage. Nat. Rev. Mol. Cell Biol. 9, 323–332.

Catterall, W.A., 2000. From ionic currents to molecular mechanisms: the structure and function of voltage-gated sodium channels. Neuron 26, 13–25.

Colquhoun, D., 2006. Agonist-activated ion channels. Br. J. Pharmacol. 147, S17–S26.

Hille, B., 2001. Ionic Channels of Excitable Membranes. Sinauer Associates, Sunderland.

North, R.A., 2002. Molecular physiology of P2X receptors. Physiol. Rev. 82, 1013–1067.

Stathopulos, P.B., Ikura, M., 2017. Store operated calcium entry: from concept to structural mechanisms. Cell Calcium 63, 3–7.

Thakran, S., Guin, D., Singh, P., et al., 2020. Genetic landscape of common epilepsies: advancing towards precision in treatment. Int. J. Mol. Sci. 21, 7784.

G protein-coupled receptors

AbdAlla, S., Lother, H., El Massiery, A., Quitterer, U., 2001. Increased AT_1 receptor heterodimers in preeclampsia mediate enhanced angiotensin II responsiveness. Nat. Med. 7, 1003–1009.

Adams, M.N., Ramachandran, R., Yau, M.K., et al., 2011. Structure, function and pathophysiology of protease activated receptors. Pharmacol. Ther. 130, 248–282.

Audet, M., Bouvier, M., 2012. Restructuring G protein-coupled receptor activation. Cell 151, 14–23.

Chandrabalan, A., Ramachandran, R., 2021. Molecular mechanisms regulating proteinase-activated receptors (PARs). FEBS J. 288, 2697–2726.

Conigrave, A.D., Quinn, S.J., Brown, E.M., 2000. Cooperative multi-modal sensing and therapeutic implications of the extracellular Ca^{2+}-sensing receptor. Trends Pharmacol. Sci. 21, 401–407.

Costa, T., Cotecchia, S., 2005. Historical review: negative efficacy and the constitutive activity of G protein-coupled receptors. Trends Pharmacol. Sci. 26, 618–624.

Ferré, S., Casadó, V., Devi, L.A., et al., 2015. G protein-coupled receptor oligomerization revisited: functional and pharmacological perspectives. Pharmacol. Rev. 66, 413–434.

Fredriksson, R., Schiöth, H.B., 2005. The repertoire of G protein-coupled receptors in fully sequenced genomes. Mol. Pharmacol. 67, 1414–1425.

Garcia-Nafria, J., Tate, C.G., 2019. Cryo-EM structures of GPCRs coupled to G_s, G_i and G_o. Mol. Cell. Endocrinol. 488, 1–13.

Hay, D.L., Pioszak, A.A., 2015. Receptor activity-modifying proteins (RAMPs): new insights and roles. Ann. Rev. Pharmacol. Toxicol. 56, 469–487.

Kelly, E., Bailey, C.P., Henderson, G., 2008. Agonist-selective mechanisms of GPCR desensitization. Br. J. Pharmacol. 153 (Suppl. 1), S379–S388.

Kenakin, T., Christopoulos, A., 2013. Signalling bias in new drug discovery: detection, quantification and therapeutic impact. Nat. Rev. Drug Discov. 12, 205–216.

Lefkowitz, R.J., 2013. A brief history of G-protein coupled receptors. Angew. Chem. Int. Ed. 52, 6366–6378.

Li, J., Ge, Y., Huang, J.X., Strømgaard, K., Zhang, X., Xiong, X.F., 2020. Heterotrimeric G proteins as therapeutic targets in drug discovery. J. Med. Chem. 63, 5013–5030.

Liu, F., Wan, Q., Pristupa, Z., et al., 2000. Direct protein–protein coupling enables cross-talk between dopamine D_5 and γ-aminobutyric acid A receptors. Nature 403, 274–280.

Manglik, A., Lin, H., Aryal, D.K., et al., 2016. Structure-based discovery of opioid analgesics with reduced side effects. Nature 537, 185–190.

Simonds, W.F., 1999. G protein regulation of adenylate cyclase. Trends Pharmacol. Sci. 20, 66–72.

Sjögren, B., 2017. The evolution of regulators of G protein signalling proteins as drug targets – 20 years in the making: IUPHAR Review 21. Br. J. Pharmacol. 174, 427–437.

Sounier, R., Mas, C., Steyaert, J., et al., 2015. Propagation of conformational changes during μ-opioid receptor activation. Nature 524, 375–378.

Spiegel, A.M., Weinstein, L.S., 2004. Inherited diseases involving G proteins and G protein-coupled receptors. Annu. Rev. Med. 55, 27–39.

Stoy, H., Gurevich, V.V., 2015. How genetic errors in GPCRs affect their function: possible therapeutic strategies. Genes Dis. 2, 108–132.

Xie, G.X., Palmer, P.P., 2007. How regulators of G protein signalling achieve selective regulation. J. Mol. Biol. 366, 349–365.

Zhang, D., Zhao, Q., Wu, B., 2015. Structural studies of G protein-coupled receptors. Mol. Cells 38, 836–842.

Signal transduction

Avruch, J., 2007. MAP kinase pathways: the first twenty years. Biochim. Biophys. Acta 1773, 1150–1160.

Brzostowski, J.A., Kimmel, A.R., 2001. Signaling at zero G: G protein-independent functions for 7TM receptors. Trends Biochem. Sci. 26, 291–297.

Porazinski, S., Parkin, A., Pajic, M., 2020. Rho-ROCK signaling in normal physiology and as a key player in shaping the tumor microenvironment. Adv. Exp. Med. Biol. 1223, 99–127.

Vanhaesebroeck, B., Leevers, S.J., Panayotou, G., Waterfield, M.D., 1997. Phosphoinositide 3-kinases: a conserved family of signal transducers. Trends Biochem. Sci. 22, 267–272.

Kinase-linked receptors

Cohen, P., 2002. Protein kinases – the major drug targets of the twenty-first century. Nat. Rev. Drug Discov. 1, 309–315.

Cook, D.N., Pisetsky, D.S., Schwartz, D.A., 2004. Toll-like receptors in the pathogenesis of human disease. Nat. Immunol. 5, 975–979.

Hubbard, S.R., Miller, W.T., 2007. Receptor tyrosine kinases: mechanisms of activation and signaling. Curr. Opin. Cell Biol. 19, 117–123.

Ihle, J.N., 1995. Cytokine receptor signalling. Nature 377, 591–594.

Jin, J., Pawson, T., 2012. Modular evolution of phosphorylation-based signalling systems. Philos. Trans. R. Soc. Lond. B. Biol. Sci. 367, 2540–2555.

Karin, M., Yamamoto, Y., Wang, M., 2004. The IKK-NFκB system: a treasure trove for drug development. Nat. Rev. Drug Discov. 3, 17–26.

Wilson, L.J., Linley, A., Hammond, D.E., et al., 2018. New perspectives, opportunities, and challenges in exploring the human protein kinome. Cancer Res. 78, 15–29.

Nuclear receptors

Bourguet, W., Germain, P., Gronemeyer, H., 2000. Nuclear receptor ligand-binding domains: three-dimensional structures, molecular interactions and pharmacological implications. Trends Pharmacol. Sci. 21, 381–388.
Burris, T.P., Solt, L.A., Wang, Y., et al., 2013. Nuclear receptors and their selective pharmacologic modulators. Pharmacol. Rev. 65, 710–778.
di Masi, A., De Marinis, E., Ascenzi, P., Marino, M., 2009. Nuclear receptors CAR and PXR: molecular, functional, and biomedical aspects. Mol. Aspects Med. 30, 297–343.
Evans, R.M., Mangelsdorf, D.J., 2014. Nuclear receptors, RXR, and the big bang. Cell 157, 255–266.
Falkenstein, E., Tillmann, H.C., Christ, M., Feuring, M., Wehling, M., 2000. Multiple actions of steroid hormones – a focus on rapid non-genomic effects. Pharm. Rev. 52, 513–553.
Germain, P., Staels, B., Dacquet, C., Spedding, M., Laudet, V., 2006. Overview of nomenclature of nuclear receptors. Pharmacol. Rev. 58, 685–704.
Goto, T., 2019. A review of the studies on food-derived factors which regulate energy metabolism via the modulation of lipid-sensing nuclear receptors. Biosci. Biotechnol. Biochem. 83, 579–588.
Kersten, S., Desvergne, B., Wahli, W., 2000. Roles of PPARs in health and disease. Nature 405, 421–424.
Levin, E.R., Hammes, S.R., 2016. Nuclear receptors outside the nucleus: extranuclear signalling by steroid receptors. Nat. Rev. Mol. Cell Biol. 17, 783–797.
Malbeteau, L., Pham, H.T., Eve, L., Stallcup, M.R., Poulard, C., Le Romancer, M., 2022. How protein methylation regulates steroid receptor function. Endocr. Rev. 43, 160–197.
Murphy, G.J., Holder, J.C., 2000. PPAR-γ agonists: therapeutic role in diabetes, inflammation and cancer. Trends Pharmacol. Sci. 21, 469–474.
Noddings, C.M., Wang, R.Y., Johnson, J.L., Agard, D.A., 2022. Structure of Hsp90-p23-GR reveals the Hsp90 client-remodelling mechanism. Nature 601, 465–469.
Santos, G.M., Fairall, L., Schwabe, J.W.R., 2011. Negative regulation by nuclear receptors: a plethora of mechanisms. Trends Endocrinol. Metab. 22, 87–93.
Shaqura, M., Li, X., Al-Khrasani, M., et al., 2016. Membrane-bound glucocorticoid receptors on distinct nociceptive neurons as potential targets for pain control through rapid non-genomic effects. Neuropharmacology 111, 1–13.
Shiau, A.K., Barstad, D., Loria, P.M., et al., 1998. The structural basis of estrogen receptor/coactivator recognition and the antagonism of this interaction by tamoxifen. Cell 95, 927–937.
Wang, Z., Frederick, J., Garabedian, M.J., 2002. Deciphering the phosphorylation "code" of the glucocorticoid receptor in vivo. J. Biol. Chem. 277, 26573–26580.

4 How drugs act: cellular aspects – excitation, contraction and secretion

OVERVIEW

The link between a drug interacting with a molecular target and its effect at the pathophysiological level, such as a change in blood glucose concentration or the shrinkage of a tumour, involves events at the cellular level. Whatever their specialised physiological function, cells generally share much the same repertoire of signalling mechanisms. In this chapter, we describe excitation, contraction and secretion signalling mechanisms that operate mainly over a short timescale (milliseconds to hours), which account for many physiological responses;

The short-term regulation of cell function depends mainly on the following components and mechanisms, which regulate, or are regulated by, the free concentration of Ca^{2+} in the cytosol, $[Ca^{2+}]_i$:

- **ion channels and transporters in the plasma membrane**
- **the storage and release of Ca^{2+} by intracellular organelles**
- **Ca^{2+}-dependent regulation of a variety of functional proteins, including enzymes, contractile proteins and vesicle proteins**

Because $[Ca^{2+}]_i$ plays such a key role in cell function, a wide variety of drug effects result from interference with one or more of these Ca^{2+}-dependent mechanisms. Knowledge of the molecular and cellular details is extensive, and here we focus on the aspects that help to explain drug effects. More detailed coverage of the topics presented in this chapter can be found in Berridge (2014) and Kandel et al. (2021).

REGULATION OF INTRACELLULAR CALCIUM

Ever since the famous accident in 1882 by Sidney Ringer's technician, which showed that using tap water rather than distilled water to make up the bathing solution for isolated frog hearts would allow them to carry on contracting, the role of Ca^{2+} as a major regulator of cell function has never been in question. Many drugs and physiological mechanisms operate, directly or indirectly, by influencing $[Ca^{2+}]_i$. Here we consider the main ways in which it is regulated. Details of the molecular components and drug targets are presented in Chapter 3, and descriptions of drug effects on integrated physiological function are given in later chapters.

The study of Ca^{2+} regulation was greatly facilitated by the development of optical techniques based on the Ca^{2+}-sensitive photoprotein *aequorin*, and fluorescent dyes such as *Fura-2*, which allow free $[Ca^{2+}]_i$ to be continuously monitored in living cells with a high level of temporal and spatial resolution. Addition of an acetoxymethyl ester (AM) moiety to the dye molecule allows them to diffuse into cells and become 'trapped' inside living cells once intracellular esterases cleave the AM group from the dye. Some (e.g. Fura-2) are ratiometric by nature, allowing greater accuracy of $[Ca^{2+}]_i$ quantitation.

Most of the Ca^{2+} in a resting cell is sequestered in organelles, particularly the *endoplasmic* or *sarcoplasmic reticulum* (ER or SR) and the mitochondria, and the free $[Ca^{2+}]_i$ is kept to a low level, about 100 nmol/L. The Ca^{2+} concentration in extracellular fluid, $[Ca^{2+}]_o$, is about 2.4 mmol/L, so there is a large concentration gradient favouring Ca^{2+} entry. Free $[Ca^{2+}]_i$ is kept low (1) by the operation of active transport mechanisms that eject cytosolic Ca^{2+} through the plasma membrane and pump it into the ER and (2) by the normally low Ca^{2+} permeability of the plasma and ER membranes. Regulation of $[Ca^{2+}]_i$ involves three main mechanisms:

- control of Ca^{2+} entry
- control of Ca^{2+} extrusion
- exchange of Ca^{2+} between the cytosol and the intracellular stores

These mechanisms are described in more detail later and are summarised in Fig. 4.1.

CALCIUM ENTRY MECHANISMS

There are four main routes by which Ca^{2+} enters cells across the plasma membrane:

- voltage-gated calcium channels
- ligand-gated and physically-activated calcium channels
- store-operated calcium entry
- Na^+–Ca^{2+} exchange (which can operate in either direction)

VOLTAGE-GATED CALCIUM CHANNELS

The pioneering work of Hodgkin and Huxley on the ionic basis of the nerve action potential identified voltage-dependent Na^+ and K^+ conductances as the main participants. It was later found that some invertebrate nerve and muscle cells could produce action potentials that depended on Ca^{2+} rather than Na^+, and it was then found that vertebrate cells also possess voltage-activated calcium channels capable of allowing substantial amounts of Ca^{2+} to enter the cell when the membrane is depolarised. These voltage-gated channels are highly selective for Ca^{2+} and are not permeable to Na^+ or K^+; they are ubiquitous in excitable cells and cause Ca^{2+} to enter the cell whenever the membrane is depolarised, for example by a conducted action potential.

A combination of electrophysiological and pharmacological criteria has revealed five distinct types

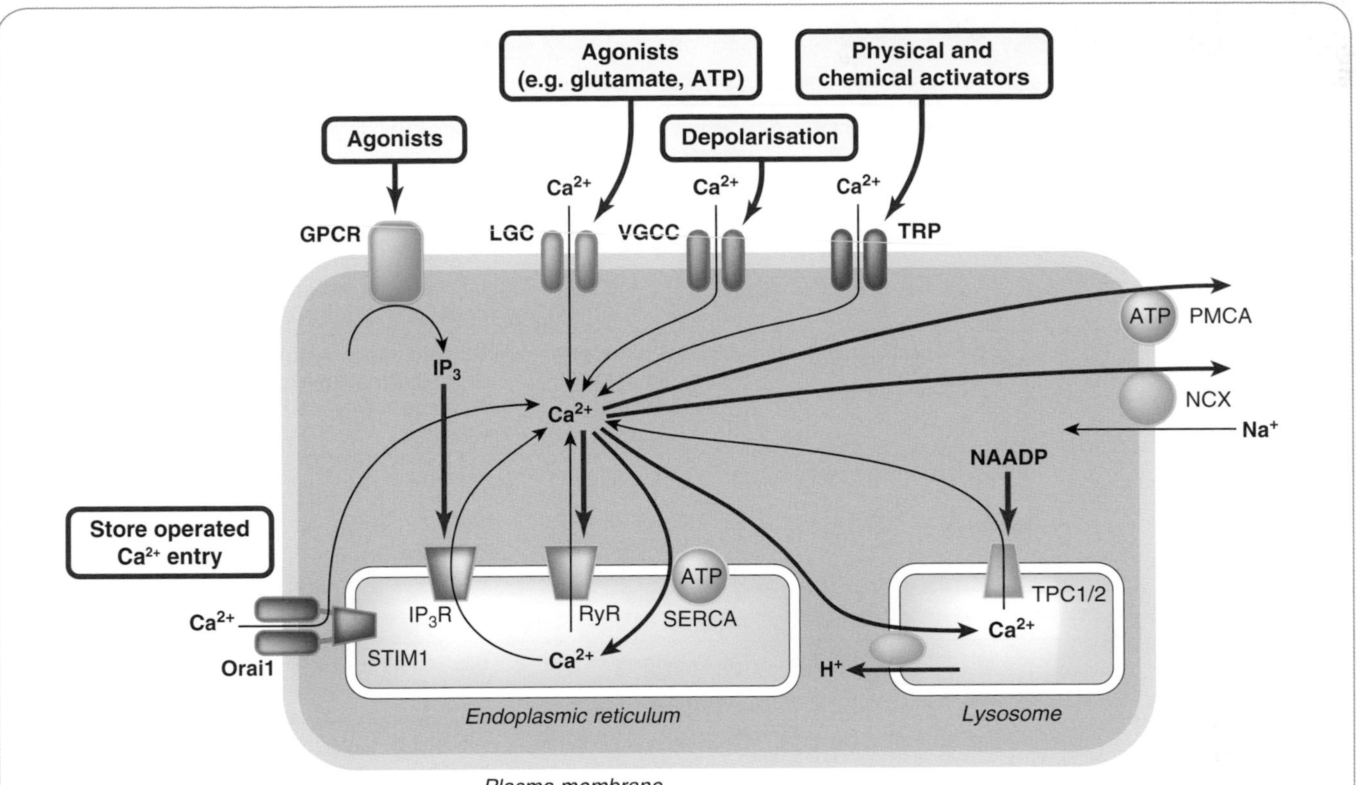

Fig. 4.1 Regulation of intracellular calcium. The main routes of transfer of Ca^{2+} into, and out of, the cytosol, endoplasmic reticulum (ER) and lysosomal structures are shown for a typical cell (see text for details). *Black arrows:* routes into the cytosol. *Blue arrows*: routes out of the cytosol. *Red arrows*: regulatory mechanisms. Ca^{2+} release from the ER activates the sensor protein Stim1, which then interacts directly with Orai1 to promote Ca^{2+} entry when the ER store is depleted. Normally, $[Ca^{2+}]_i$ is regulated to about 10^{-7} mol/L in a 'resting' cell. Mitochondria (not shown) also function as Ca^{2+} storage organelles but release Ca^{2+} only under pathological conditions, such as ischaemia. There is evidence for a lysosomal store of Ca^{2+}, activated by the second messenger nicotinic acid adenine dinucleotide phosphate (NAADP) through a two-pore domain calcium channel (TPC). *GPCR,* G protein–coupled receptor; *IP_3,* inositol trisphosphate; *IP_3R,* inositol trisphosphate receptor; *LGC,* ligand-gated cation channel; *NCX,* Na^+–Ca^{2+} exchange transporter; *PMCA,* plasma membrane Ca^{2+}-ATPase; *RyR,* ryanodine receptor; *SERCA,* sarcoplasmic/endoplasmic reticulum ATPase; *VGCC,* voltage-gated calcium channel.

of voltage-gated calcium channel current: L, T, N, P/Q and R.[1] They vary with respect to their voltage threshold for activation, their activation and inactivation kinetics, their conductance and their sensitivity to blocking agents, as summarised in Table 4.1. The molecular basis for this heterogeneity has been worked out in some detail. The main pore-forming subunit (termed α_1, see Fig. 3.20) occurs in at least 10 molecular subtypes, and associates with other subunits (β, γ and two subunits from the same gene, $\alpha_2\delta$, linked by a disulfide bond) that also exist in different subtypes to form the functional channel. Different combinations of these subunits give rise to the different physiological subtypes.[2] In general, L channel currents are particularly important in regulating contraction of cardiac and smooth muscle, and N channel currents (and also P/Q) are involved in neurotransmitter and hormone release, while T channel currents mediate Ca^{2+} entry into neurons around the resting membrane potential and can control the rate of repolarisation of neurons and cardiac cells, as well as various Ca^{2+}-dependent functions such as regulation of other ion channels, enzymes, etc. Clinically used drugs that act directly on some forms of calcium channel include the group of 'Ca^{2+} antagonists' consisting of *dihydropyridines* (e.g. **nifedipine**), **verapamil** and **diltiazem** (used for their cardiovascular effects; see Chs 20 and 21). Many drugs affect calcium channels indirectly by acting on G protein–coupled receptors (see Ch. 3). A number of toxins act selectively on one or other type of calcium channel (see Table 4.1), and these are used as experimental tools.

LIGAND-GATED AND PHYSICALLY ACTIVATED CHANNELS

Most ligand-gated cation channels (see Ch. 3) that are activated by excitatory neurotransmitters are relatively non-selective, and conduct Ca^{2+} ions as well as other cations. Most important in this respect is the glutamate receptor of the *N*-methyl-D-aspartate (NMDA) type (see Ch. 38), which has a particularly high permeability to Ca^{2+} and is a major contributor to Ca^{2+} uptake by postsynaptic neurons (and also glial cells) in the central nervous system. Activation

[1]P and Q are so similar that they usually get lumped together. The terminology is less than poetic: L stands for *long-lasting;* T stands for *transient;* N stands for *neither long-lasting nor transient*. Although P stands for *Purkinje* – this type of channel current was first observed in cerebellar Purkinje cells – it continued the alphabetical sequence (missing out O of course) and so the next discovered were termed Q and R.

[2]Readers interested in knowing more about the subunit composition of different voltage-gated calcium channels should consult the Guide to Pharmacology at http://www.guidetopharmacology.org/GRAC/FamilyDisplayForward?familyId=80.

Table 4.1 Types and functions of Ca^{2+} channels

Gated by	Main types	Characteristics	Location and function	Drug effects
Voltage	L	High activation threshold Slow inactivation	Plasma membrane of many cells Main Ca^{2+} source for contraction in smooth and cardiac muscle	Blocked by dihydropyridines, verapamil, diltiazem and calciseptine (peptide from snake venom) Activated by BayK 8644 Phosphorylation by PKA (e.g. following β_1 adrenoceptor activation) increases channel opening
	N	High activation threshold Slow inactivation	Main Ca^{2+} source for transmitter release by nerve terminals	Blocked by ω-conotoxin GV1A (component of *Conus* snail venom) and ziconotide (marketed preparation of ω-conotoxin used to control pain) (Ch. 43)
	T	Low activation threshold Fast inactivation	Widely distributed Important in cardiac pacemaker and atria (role in dysrhythmias), also neuronal firing patterns	Blocked by mibefradil
	P/Q	High activation threshold Slow inactivation	Nerve terminals Transmitter release	Blocked by ω-agatoxin-4A (component of funnel-web spider venom)
	R	High activation threshold Fast inactivation	Neurons and dendrites Control of firing patterns	Blocked by low concentrations of SNX-482 (a toxin from a member of the tarantula family)
IP_3	IP_3 receptor	Activated by binding of IP_3 and Ca^{2+}	Located in endoplasmic/ sarcoplasmic reticulum Mediates Ca^{2+} release produced by GPCR activation	Not directly targeted by drugs Some experimental blocking agents known Responds to GPCR agonists and antagonists in many cells
Ca^{2+}	Ryanodine receptor	Directly activated in skeletal muscle via dihydropyridine receptor of T-tubules. Activated by Ca^{2+} in cardiac muscle	Located in endoplasmic/ sarcoplasmic reticulum. Pathway for Ca^{2+} release in striated muscle	Activated by caffeine and ATP in the presence of Ca^{2+} Ryanodine both activates (low concentrations) and closes (high concentrations) the channel. Also closed by Mg^{2+}, K^+ channel blockers and dantrolene Mutations may lead to drug-induced malignant hypothermia, sudden cardiac death and central core disease
Store depletion	Store-operated channels	Activated by sensor protein that monitors level of ER Ca^{2+} stores	Located in plasma membrane	Activated indirectly by agents that deplete intracellular stores (e.g. GPCR agonists, thapsigargin) Not directly targeted by drugs

ER, Endoplasmic reticulum; *GPCR*, G protein–coupled receptor; *IP_3*, inositol trisphosphate; *PKA*, protein kinase A.

of this receptor can readily cause so much Ca^{2+} entry that the cell dies, mainly through activation of Ca^{2+}-dependent proteases but also by triggering *apoptosis* (see Ch. 6). This mechanism, termed *excitotoxicity*, probably plays a part in various neurodegenerative disorders (see Ch. 40).

For many years, there was dispute about the existence of 'receptor-operated channels' in smooth muscle, responding directly to mediators such as adrenaline (epinephrine), acetylcholine and histamine. Now it seems that the P2X receptor (see Ch. 3), activated by ATP, is the only example of a true ligand-gated channel in smooth muscle, and this constitutes an important route for Ca^{2+} entry. As mentioned earlier, many mediators acting on G protein–coupled receptors affect Ca^{2+} entry indirectly, mainly by regulating voltage-gated calcium channels or potassium channels.

The TRP channel superfamily[3] comprises six families of ion channels – TRPC, TRPM, TRPV, TRPA, TRPP and TRPML – that exhibit structural homology. They are permeable to Ca^{2+} as well as Na^+ and K^+. Different TRP channels respond to different stimuli and can be chemically activated (e.g. by extracellular protons or by intracellular second messengers such as diacylglycerol) or physically activated (e.g. by cooling or heating and by stretch). Given their widespread distribution in the body in a variety of tissues and their responses to different stimuli it will come as no surprise therefore that these channels are involved in a myriad of physiological and pathological situations (Blair et al., 2019). For now all we need to be aware of is their role in allowing Ca^{2+} to enter cells in response to different stimuli.

STORE-OPERATED CALCIUM ENTRY

Store-operated calcium entry is through very-low-conductance channels that occur in the plasma membrane and open to allow entry when the ER stores are depleted, but are not sensitive to cytosolic $[Ca^{2+}]_i$. The linkage between the ER and the plasma membrane involves a Ca^{2+}-sensor protein (*Stim1*) in the ER membrane, which connects directly to the channel protein (*Orai1*) in the adjacent plasma membrane (Fig 4.1). Ca^{2+} loss from the ER causes Stim1 to accumulate at junctions between the ER and the plasma membrane where it traps and activates Orai1 resulting in Ca^{2+} entry across the plasma membrane (see Lewis, 2020).

Like the ER and SR channels, these channels can serve to amplify the rise in $[Ca^{2+}]_i$ resulting from Ca^{2+} release from the stores. So far, only experimental compounds are known to block these channels, but efforts are being made to develop specific blocking agents for therapeutic use as relaxants of smooth muscle.

CALCIUM EXTRUSION MECHANISMS

Active transport of Ca^{2+} outwards across the plasma membrane, and inwards across the membranes of the ER or SR, depends on the activity of distinct Ca^{2+}-dependent ATPases,[4] similar to the Na^+/K^+-dependent ATPase that pumps Na^+ out of the cell in exchange for K^+. **Thapsigargin** (derived from a Mediterranean plant, *Thapsia garganica*) specifically blocks the ER pump, causing loss of Ca^{2+} from the ER. It is a useful experimental tool but has no therapeutic significance.

Calcium is also extruded from cells in exchange for Na^+, by Na^+–Ca^{2+} exchange. The exchanger transfers three Na^+ ions for one Ca^{2+}, and therefore produces a net depolarising current when it is extruding Ca^{2+}. The energy for Ca^{2+} extrusion comes from the electrochemical gradient for Na^+, not directly from ATP hydrolysis. This means that a reduction in the Na^+ concentration gradient resulting from Na^+ entry will reduce Ca^{2+} extrusion by the exchanger, causing a secondary rise in $[Ca^{2+}]_i$, a mechanism that is particularly important in cardiac muscle (see Ch. 20).

[1]'TRP' is an abbreviation of 'Transient Receptor Potential' which was the term applied to the first such channel observed in the drosophila retina. Although channels in the TRP superfamily have vastly different biophysical and pharmacological characteristics the term has stuck despite its relevance being questionable. In 2021 David Julius and Ardem Patapoutian were awarded the Nobel Prize in Physiology or Medicine for their work on TRP channels.

[3]These pumps have been likened to Sisyphus, condemned endlessly to push a stone up a hill (also consuming ATP, no doubt), only for it to roll downhill again.

Digoxin (derived from the *Digitalis* or 'Foxglove' plant), which inhibits Na^+ extrusion, acts on cardiac muscle in this way (see Ch. 20), causing $[Ca^{2+}]_i$ to increase.

CALCIUM RELEASE MECHANISMS

There are two main types of calcium channel in the ER and SR membrane, which play an important part in controlling the release of Ca^{2+} from these stores.

- The *inositol trisphosphate receptor* (IP_3R) is activated by inositol trisphosphate (IP_3), a second messenger produced by the action of many ligands on G protein–coupled receptors (see Ch. 3). IP_3R is a ligand-gated ion channel, although its molecular structure differs from that of ligand-gated channels in the plasma membrane (see Berridge, 2016). This is the main mechanism by which activation of Gq-coupled receptors causes an increase in $[Ca^{2+}]_i$.
- *Ryanodine receptors* (RyRs) are so called because they were first identified through the specific blocking action of the plant alkaloid **ryanodine.** There are three isoforms – RyR1–3 (Van Petegem, 2012), which are expressed in many different cell types. RyR1 is highly expressed in skeletal muscle, RyR2 in the heart and RyR3 in brain neurons. In skeletal muscle, RyRs on the SR are physically coupled to *dihydropyridine receptors (DHPRs)* on the T-tubules (see Fig. 4.9); this coupling results in rapid Ca^{2+} release following the action potential in the muscle fibre. In other muscle types, RyRs respond to Ca^{2+} that enters the cell through membrane calcium channels by a mechanism known as *calcium-induced calcium release* (CICR).

The functions of IP_3Rs and RyRs are modulated by a variety of other intracellular signals (see Berridge, 2016; Van Petegem, 2012), which affect the magnitude and spatiotemporal patterning of Ca^{2+} signals. Fluorescence imaging techniques have revealed a remarkable level of complexity of Ca^{2+} signals, and much remains to be discovered about the importance of this patterning in relation to physiological and pharmacological mechanisms. The Ca^{2+} sensitivity of RyRs is increased by **caffeine**, causing Ca^{2+} release from the SR even at resting levels of $[Ca^{2+}]_i$. This is used experimentally but rarely happens in humans, because the other pharmacological effects of caffeine (see Ch. 49) occur at much lower doses. The blocking effect of **dantrolene**, a compound related to ryanodine, is used therapeutically to relieve muscle spasm in the rare condition of *malignant hyperthermia* (see Ch. 41), which is associated with inherited abnormalities in the RyR protein.

A typical $[Ca^{2+}]_i$ signal resulting from activation of a Gq-coupled receptor is shown in Fig. 4.2A. The response produced in the absence of extracellular Ca^{2+} represents release from intracellular stores. The larger and more prolonged response when extracellular Ca^{2+} is present shows the contribution of store-operated calcium entry. The various positive and negative feedback mechanisms that regulate $[Ca^{2+}]_i$ give rise to a variety of temporal and spatial oscillatory patterns (Fig. 4.2B) that are responsible for spontaneous rhythmic activity in smooth muscle and nerve cells (see Berridge, 2008).

OTHER SECOND MESSENGERS

Two intracellular metabolites, cyclic ADP-ribose (cADPR) and nicotinic acid adenine dinucleotide phosphate (NAADP) formed from the ubiquitous coenzymes

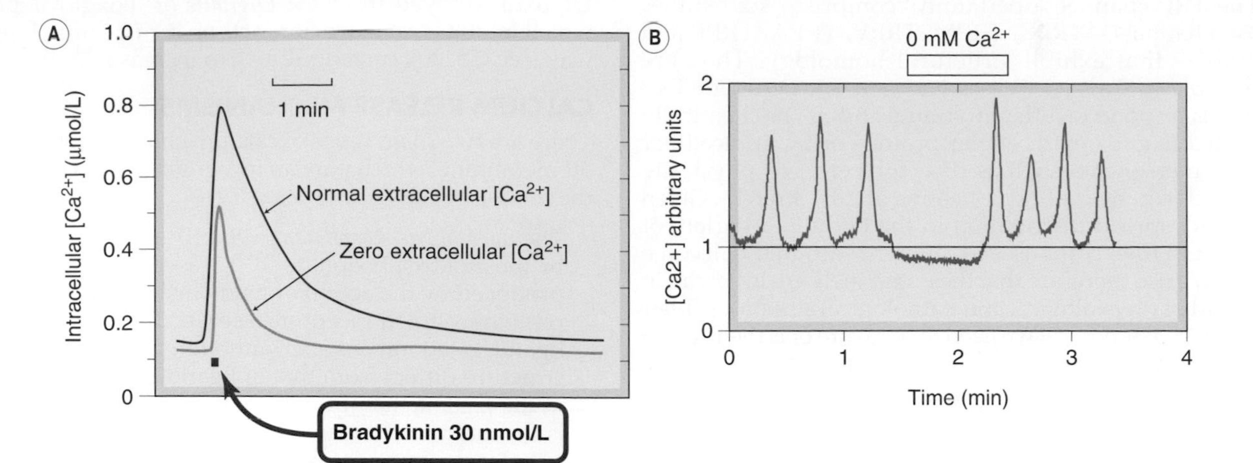

Fig. 4.2 (A) Increase in intracellular free calcium concentration in response to receptor activation. The records were obtained from a single rat sensory neuron grown in tissue culture. The cells were loaded with the fluorescent Ca^{2+} indicator Fura-2, and the signal from a single cell monitored with a fluorescence microscope. A brief exposure to the peptide bradykinin, which causes excitation of sensory neurons (see Ch. 43), causes a transient increase in $[Ca^{2+}]_i$ from the resting value of about 150 nmol/L. When Ca^{2+} is removed from the extracellular solution, the bradykinin-induced increase in $[Ca^{2+}]_i$ is still present but is smaller and briefer. The response in the absence of extracellular Ca^{2+} represents the release of stored intracellular Ca^{2+} resulting from the intracellular production of inositol trisphosphate. The difference between this and the larger response when Ca^{2+} is present extracellularly is believed to represent Ca^{2+} entry through store-operated ion channels in the cell membrane. (B) Spontaneous intracellular calcium oscillations in pacemaker cells from the rabbit urethra that regulate the rhythmic contractions of the smooth muscle. The signals cease when external Ca^{2+} is removed, showing that activation of membrane Ca^{2+} channels is involved in the mechanism. (A, Figure kindly provided by G. M. Burgess and A. Forbes, Novartis Institute for Medical Research. B, From McHale, N., Hollywood, M., Sergeant, G., Thornbury, K., 2006. Origin of spontaneous rhythmicity in smooth muscle. J. Physiol. 570, 23–28.)

nicotinamide adenine dinucleotide (NAD) and NAD phosphate, also affect Ca^{2+} signalling (see Morgan et al., 2015; Parrington et al., 2015). cADPR acts by increasing the sensitivity of RyRs to Ca^{2+}, thus increasing the 'gain' of the CICR effect, whereas NAADP has been proposed to release Ca^{2+} from lysosomes by activating two-pore domain calcium channels (Fig. 4.1).

The levels of these messengers in mammalian cells may be regulated mainly in response to changes in the metabolic status of the cell, although the details are still not clear. Abnormal Ca^{2+} signalling is involved in many pathophysiological conditions, such as ischaemic cell death, endocrine disorders and cardiac dysrhythmias, where cADPR and NAADP, and their interaction with other mechanisms that regulate $[Ca^{2+}]_i$, may be important.

THE ROLE OF MITOCHONDRIA

Under normal conditions, mitochondria accumulate Ca^{2+} passively as a result of the intramitochondrial potential, which is strongly negative with respect to the cytosol. This negativity is maintained by active extrusion of protons, and is lost - thus releasing Ca^{2+} into the cytosol - if the cell runs short of ATP, for example under conditions of hypoxia. This only happens *in extremis*, and the resulting Ca^{2+} release contributes to the cytotoxicity associated with severe metabolic disturbance. Cell death resulting from brain ischaemia or coronary ischaemia (see Chs 20 and 40) involves this mechanism, along with others that contribute to an excessive rise in $[Ca^{2+}]_i$.

CALMODULIN

Calcium exerts its control over cell functions by virtue of its ability to regulate the activity of many different proteins, including enzymes (particularly kinases and phosphatases), channels, transporters, transcription factors, synaptic vesicle proteins and many others either by binding directly to these proteins or through a Ca^{2+}-binding protein that serves as an intermediate between Ca^{2+} and the regulated functional protein, the best known such binding protein being the ubiquitous *calmodulin*. This regulates at least 40 different functional proteins - indeed a powerful fixer. Calmodulin (short for calcium-modulated protein, often abbreviated further to CaM) is a dumbbell-shaped protein with a globular domain at either end, each with two Ca^{2+} binding sites. When all are occupied, the protein undergoes a conformational change, exposing a 'sticky' hydrophobic domain that lures many proteins into association, thereby affecting their functional properties.

EXCITATION

Excitability describes the ability of a cell to show a regenerative all-or-nothing electrical response to depolarisation of its membrane, this membrane response being known as an *action potential*. It is a characteristic of most neurons and muscle cells (including skeletal, cardiac and smooth muscle) and of many endocrine gland cells. In neurons and muscle cells, the ability of the action potential, once initiated, to propagate to all parts of the cell membrane, and often to spread to neighbouring cells, explains the importance of membrane excitation in intra- and intercellular signalling. In the nervous system and in skeletal muscle, action potential propagation is the mechanism responsible for communication over long distances at high speed, indispensable for large, fast-moving creatures. In cardiac and smooth muscle, as well as in some central neurons, spontaneous rhythmic activity occurs. In

Calcium regulation

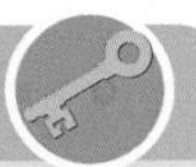

Intracellular Ca^{2+} concentration, $[Ca^{2+}]_i$, is critically important as a regulator of cell function.

- Intracellular Ca^{2+} is determined by (a) Ca^{2+} entry; (b) Ca^{2+} extrusion; and (c) Ca^{2+} exchange between the cytosol, endoplasmic or sarcoplasmic reticulum (ER, SR), lysosomes and mitochondria.
- Calcium entry occurs by various routes, including voltage- and ligand-gated calcium channels and Na^+–Ca^{2+} exchange.
- Calcium extrusion depends mainly on an ATP-driven Ca^{2+} pump.
- Calcium ions are actively taken up and stored by the ER/SR, from which they are released in response to various stimuli.
- Calcium ions are released from ER/SR stores by (1) the second messenger inositol trisphosphate (IP_3) acting on IP_3receptors; or (2) increased $[Ca^{2+}]_i$ itself acting on ryanodine receptors, a mechanism known as Ca^{2+}-induced Ca^{2+} release.
- Other second messengers, cyclic ADP-ribose and nicotinic acid dinucleotide phosphate, also promote the release of Ca^{2+} from Ca^{2+} stores.
- Depletion of ER/SR Ca^{2+} stores promotes Ca^{2+} entry through the plasma membrane, via store-operated channels.
- Calcium ions affect many aspects of cell function by binding to proteins such as calmodulin, which in turn bind other proteins and regulate their function.

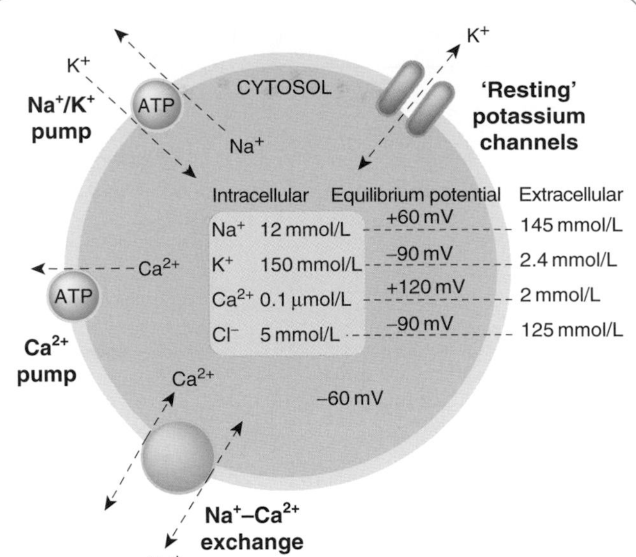

Fig. 4.3 Simplified diagram showing the ionic balance of a typical 'resting' cell. The main transport mechanisms that maintain the ionic gradients across the plasma membrane are the ATP-driven Na^+–K^+ and Ca^{2+} pumps and the Na^+–Ca^{2+} exchange transporter. The membrane is relatively permeable to K^+, because some types of potassium channel are open at rest, but impermeable to other cations. The unequal ion concentrations on either side of the membrane give rise to the 'equilibrium potentials' shown. The resting membrane potential, typically about −60 mV but differing between different cell types, is determined by the equilibrium potentials and the permeabilities of the various ions involved and by the 'electrogenic' effect of the transporters. For simplicity, anions and other ions, such as protons, are not shown, although these play an important role in many cell types.

gland cells, the action potential, where it occurs, serves to amplify the signal that causes the cell to secrete. In each type of tissue, the properties of the excitation process reflect the special characteristics of the ion channels that underlie the process. The molecular nature of ion channels, and their importance as drug targets, is considered in Chapter 3; here we discuss the cellular processes that depend primarily on ion channel function. For more detail, see Hille (2001).

THE 'RESTING' CELL

The resting cell is not resting at all but very busy controlling the state of its interior, and it requires a continuous supply of energy to do so. In relation to the topics discussed in this chapter, the following characteristics are especially important:

- membrane potential
- permeability of the plasma membrane to different ions
- intracellular ion concentrations, especially $[Ca^{2+}]_i$

Under resting conditions, all cells maintain a negative internal potential between about −30 and −80 mV, depending on the cell type. This arises because (1) the membrane is relatively impermeable to Na^+ and (2) Na^+ ions are actively extruded from the cell in exchange for K^+ ions by an energy-dependent transporter, the Na^+ pump (or Na^+-K^+-ATPase). The result is that the intracellular K^+ concentration, $[K^+]_i$, is higher, and $[Na^+]_i$ is lower, than the respective extracellular concentrations (Fig. 4.3). In many cells, other ions, particularly Cl^-, are also actively transported and unequally distributed across the membrane. In many cases (e.g. in neurons), the membrane permeability to K^+ is relatively high, and the membrane potential settles at a value of −60 to −80 mV, close to the equilibrium potential for K^+ (Fig. 4.3). In other cells (e.g. smooth muscle), anions play a larger part, and the membrane potential is generally lower (−30 to −50 mV) and less dependent on K^+.

ELECTRICAL AND IONIC EVENTS UNDERLYING THE ACTION POTENTIAL

Our present understanding of electrical excitability rests firmly on the work of Hodgkin, Huxley and Katz on squid axons, published in 1949–1952. Their experiments (see Katz, 1966) revealed the existence of voltage-gated ion channels and showed that the action potential is generated by the interplay of two processes:

1. A rapid, transient increase in Na^+ permeability that occurs when the membrane is depolarised beyond about −50 mV.
2. A slower, sustained increase in K^+ permeability.

Because of the inequality of Na^+ and K^+ concentrations on the two sides of the membrane, an increase in Na^+ permeability causes an inward (depolarising) current of Na^+ ions, whereas an increase in K^+ permeability causes an

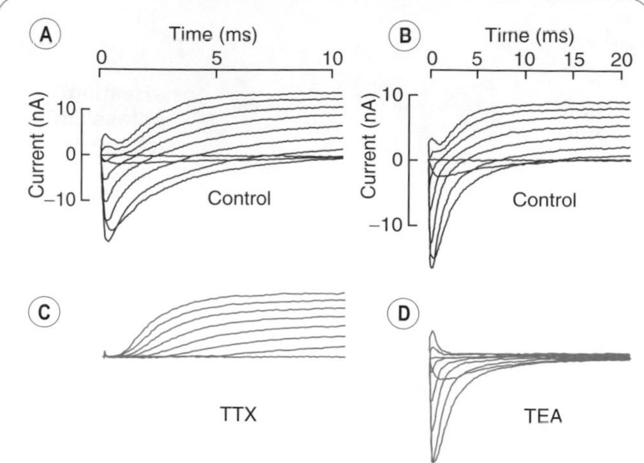

Fig. 4.4 Separation of sodium and potassium currents in the nerve membrane. Voltage clamp records from the node of Ranvier of a single frog nerve fibre. At time 0, the membrane potential was stepped to a depolarised level, ranging from −60 mV (lower trace in each series) to +60 mV (upper trace in each series) in 15-mV steps. (A and B) Control records from two fibres. (C) Effect of tetrodotoxin (TTX), which abolishes Na^+ currents. (D) Effect of tetraethylammonium (TEA), which abolishes K^+ currents. (From Hille, B., 1970. Ionic channels in nerve membranes. Prog. Biophys. Mol. Biol. 21, 1–32.)

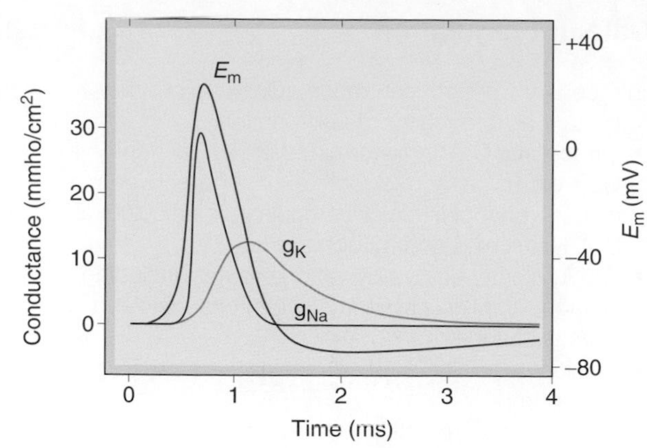

Fig. 4.5 Behaviour of sodium and potassium channels during a conducted action potential. Rapid opening of sodium channels occurs during the action potential upstroke. Delayed opening of potassium channels, and inactivation of sodium channels, causes repolarisation. E_m, Membrane potential; g_K, membrane conductance to K^+; g_{Na}, membrane conductance to Na^+.

outward (repolarising) current. The separability of these two currents can be most clearly demonstrated by the use of drugs blocking sodium and potassium channels, as shown in Fig. 4.4. During the physiological initiation or propagation of a nerve impulse, the first event is a small depolarisation of the membrane, produced either by transmitter action or by the approach of an action potential passing along the axon. This opens sodium channels, allowing an inward current of Na^+ ions to flow, which depolarises the membrane still further. The process is thus a regenerative one, and the increase in Na^+ permeability is enough to bring the membrane potential towards E_{Na}. The increased Na^+ conductance is transient, because the channels inactivate rapidly and the membrane returns to its resting state.

In many types of cell, including most nerve cells, repolarisation is assisted by the opening of voltage-dependent K^+ channels. These function in much the same way as sodium channels, but their activation kinetics are about 10 times slower and they do not inactivate appreciably. This means that the potassium channels open later than the sodium channels, contributing to the rapid termination of the action potential and to the slower after-hyperpolarisation that follows the depolarising phase. The behaviour of the sodium and potassium channels during an action potential is shown in Fig. 4.5.

The foregoing account, based on Hodgkin and Huxley's work 70 years ago, involves only Na^+ and K^+ channels. Subsequently, voltage-gated calcium channels (see Fig. 4.1) were discovered. These function in basically the same way as sodium channels, if on a slightly slower timescale; they contribute to action potential generation in many cells, particularly cardiac and smooth muscle cells, but also in neurons and secretory cells. Ca^{2+} entry through voltage-gated calcium channels plays a key role in intracellular signalling.

CHANNEL FUNCTION

The discharge patterns of excitable cells vary greatly. Skeletal muscle fibres are quiescent unless stimulated by the arrival of a nerve impulse at the neuromuscular junction (see Ch. 14). Cardiac muscle fibres discharge spontaneously at a regular rate (see Ch. 20). Neurons may be normally silent, or they may discharge spontaneously, either regularly or in bursts; smooth muscle cells show a similar variety of firing patterns. The frequency at which different cells normally discharge action potentials also varies greatly, from 100 Hz or more for fast-conducting neurons, down to about 1 Hz for cardiac muscle cells. These very pronounced functional variations reflect the different characteristics of the ion channels expressed in different cell types. Rhythmic fluctuations of $[Ca^{2+}]_i$ underlie the distinct firing patterns that occur in different types of cell (see Berridge, 2016).

Drugs that alter channel characteristics, either by interacting directly with the channel itself or indirectly through second messengers, affect the function of many organ systems, including the nervous, cardiovascular, endocrine, respiratory and reproductive systems, and are a frequent theme in this book. Here we describe some of the key mechanisms involved in the regulation of excitable cells.

In general, action potentials are initiated by membrane currents that cause depolarisation of the cell. These currents may be produced by synaptic activity, by an action potential approaching from another part of the cell, by a sensory stimulus or by spontaneous *pacemaker* activity. The tendency of such currents to initiate an action potential is governed by the *excitability* of the cell, which depends mainly on the state of (1) the voltage-gated sodium and/or calcium channels and (2) the potassium channels of the resting membrane. Anything that increases the number of available sodium or calcium channels, or reduces their activation threshold, will tend to increase excitability, whereas increasing the resting K^+ conductance reduces it. Agents that do the reverse, by blocking channels or interfering with their opening, will

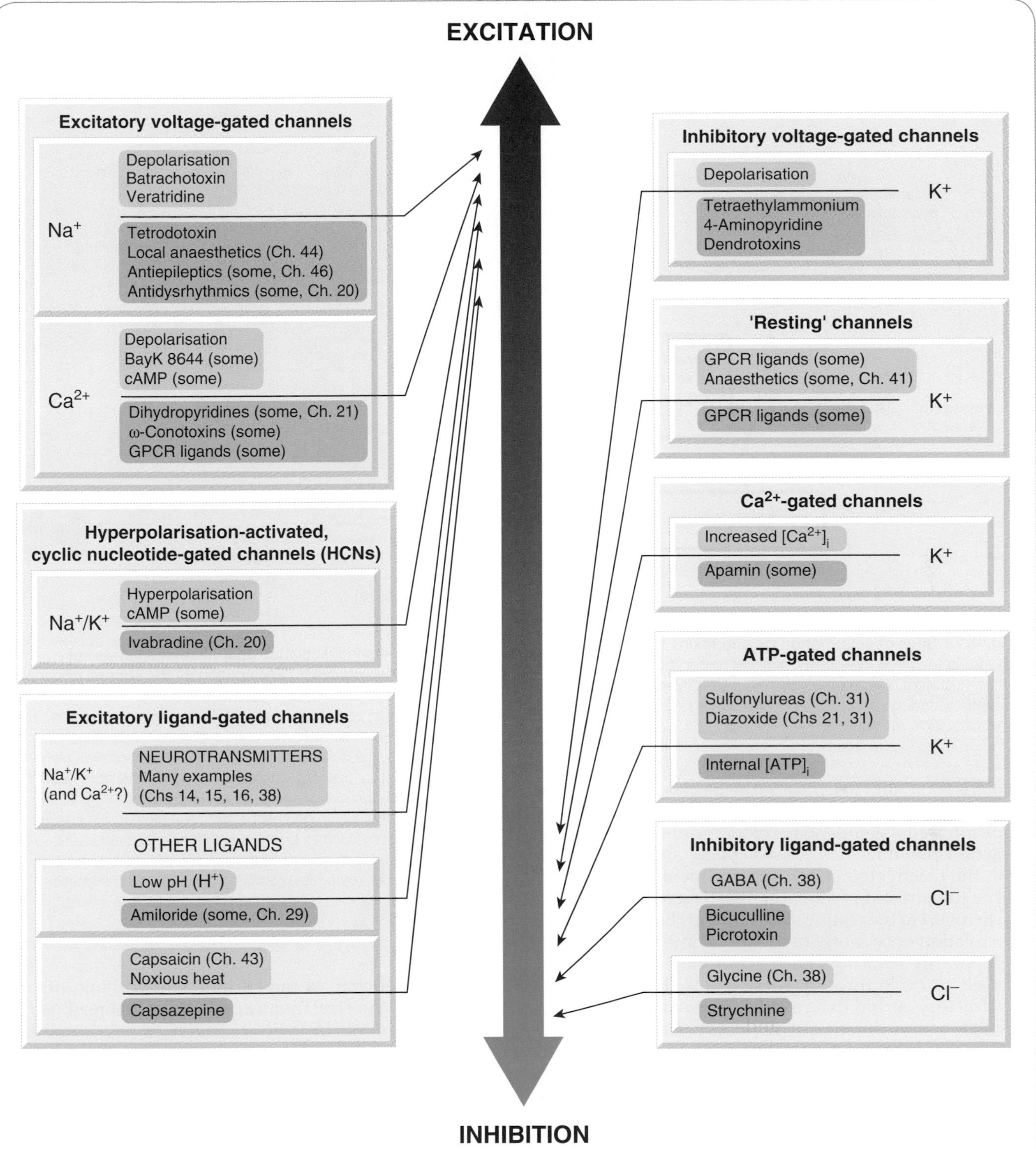

Fig. 4.6 Ion channels associated with excitatory and inhibitory membrane effects, and some of the drugs and other ligands that affect them. Channel openers are shown in *green boxes*, and blocking agents and inhibitors, in *pink boxes*. Hyperpolarisation-activated Na^+/K^+ channels are known as hyperpolarisation-activated, cyclic nucleotide-gated channels (HCNs); H^+ activated channels are known as acid-sensing ion channels (ASICs). *GPCR,* G protein–coupled receptor.

have the opposite effect. Some examples are shown inFigs 4.6 and 4.7. Inherited mutations of channel proteins are responsible for a wide variety of neurological and other genetic disorders (see Imbrici et al., 2016).

USE DEPENDENCE AND VOLTAGE DEPENDENCE

Voltage-gated channels can exist in three functional states (Fig. 4.8): *resting* (the closed state that prevails at the normal resting potential), *activated* (the open state favoured by brief

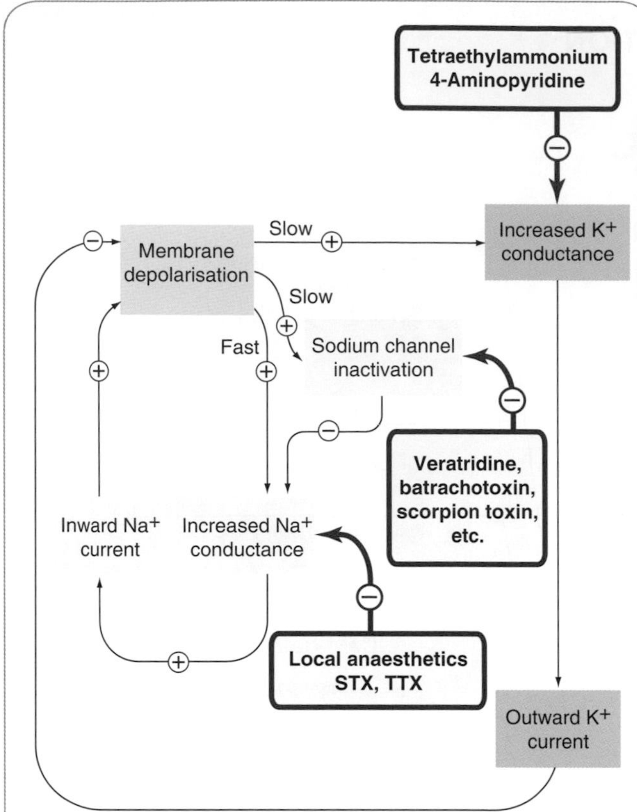

Fig. 4.7 Sites of action of drugs and toxins that affect channels involved in action potential generation. Many other mediators affect these channels indirectly via membrane receptors, through phosphorylation or altered expression. *STX*, Saxitoxin; *TTX*, tetrodotoxin.

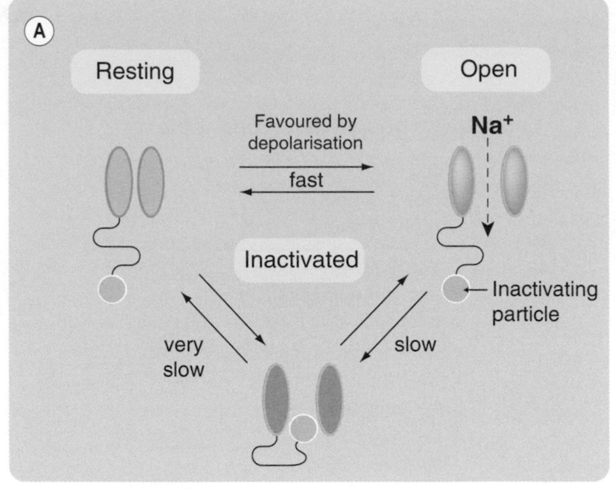

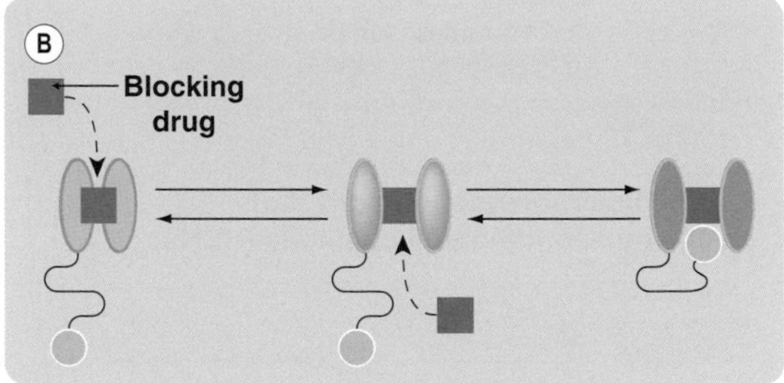

Fig. 4.8 Resting, activated and inactivated states of voltage-gated channels, exemplified by the sodium channel. (A) Membrane depolarisation causes a rapid transition from the resting (closed) state to the open state. The inactivating particle (part of the intracellular domain of the channel protein) is then able to block the channel. With prolonged depolarisation below the threshold for opening, channels can go directly from resting to inactivated without opening. (B) Some blocking drugs (such as tetrodotoxin) block the channel from the outside like a plug, whereas others (such as local anaesthetics and antiepileptic drugs) enter from the inside of the cell and often show preference for the open or inactivated states, and thus affect the kinetic behaviour of the channels, with implications for their clinical application.

depolarisation) and *inactivated* (the blocked state resulting from a trapdoor-like occlusion of the open channel by a floppy intracellular appendage of the channel protein). After the action potential has passed, many sodium channels are in the inactivated state; after the membrane potential returns to its resting value, the inactivated channels take time to revert to the resting state and thus become available for activation once more. In the meantime, the membrane is temporarily *refractory*. Each action potential causes the channels to cycle through these states. The duration of the refractory period determines the maximum frequency at which action potentials can occur. Drugs that block sodium channels, such as local anaesthetics (see Ch. 44), antidysrhythmic drugs (see Ch. 20) and antiepileptic drugs (see Ch. 46), commonly show a selective affinity for one or other of these functional states of the channel, and in their presence the proportion of channels in the high-affinity state is increased. Of particular importance are drugs that bind most strongly to the inactivated state of the channel and thus favour the adoption of this state, prolonging the refractory period and reducing the maximum frequency at which action potentials can be generated. This type of block is called *use dependent*, because the binding of such drugs increases as a function of the rate of action potential discharge, which governs the rate at which inactivated – and therefore drug-sensitive – channels are generated. This is important for some antidysrhythmic drugs (see Ch. 20) and for antiepileptic drugs (see Ch. 46), because high-frequency discharges can be inhibited without affecting excitability at normal frequencies. Drugs that readily block sodium channels in their resting state (e.g. some local anaesthetics, see Ch. 44) prevent excitation at low as well as high frequencies.

Most sodium channel-blocking drugs are cationic at physiological pH and are therefore affected by the voltage gradient across the cell membrane. Some drugs block the channel from the inside, so that their blocking action is favoured by depolarisation. This phenomenon, known as *voltage dependence*, is also of relevance to the action of antidysrhythmic and antiepileptic drugs, because the cells that are the seat of dysrhythmias or seizure activity are generally somewhat depolarised and therefore more strongly blocked than healthy cells. Similar considerations apply also to drugs that block potassium or calcium channels, but we know less about the importance of use and voltage dependence for these than we do for sodium channels.

SODIUM CHANNELS

In most excitable cells, the regenerative inward current that initiates the action potential results from activation of voltage-gated sodium channels. The early voltage clamp studies by Hodgkin and Huxley on the squid giant axon revealed the essential functional properties of these channels. Later, advantage was taken of the potent and highly selective blocking action of **tetrodotoxin** (TTX, see Ch. 44) to label and purify the channel proteins, and subsequently to clone them. Sodium channels consist of a central, pore-forming α subunit (shown in Fig. 3.20) and two auxiliary β subunits. Nine α-subunits ($Na_v1.1$ through $Na_v1.9$) and four β subunits have been identified in mammals. The α subunits contain four similar domains, each comprising six membrane-spanning helices (see Catterall et al., 2020). One of these helices, S4, which contains several basic amino acids and forms the voltage sensor, moves outwards, thus opening the channel, when the membrane is depolarised. One of the intracellular loops is designed to swing across and block the channel when S4 is displaced, thus inactivating the channel.

It was known from physiological studies that the sodium channels of heart and skeletal muscle differ in various ways from those of neurons. In particular, cardiac sodium channels (and those of some sensory neurons) are relatively insensitive to TTX and slower in their kinetics, compared with most neuronal sodium channels. This is explained by the relative insensitivity of some α subunits ($Na_v1.5$, $Na_v1.8$ and $Na_v1.9$) to TTX. Changes in the level of expression of some sodium channel subunits is thought to underlie the hyperexcitability of sensory neurons in different types of neuropathic pain (see Ch. 43).

In addition to channel-blocking compounds such as TTX, other compounds affect sodium channel gating. For example, the plant alkaloid **veratridine** and the frog skin poison **batrachotoxin** cause persistent activation, while various scorpion toxins prevent inactivation, mechanisms resulting in enhanced neuronal excitability.

POTASSIUM CHANNELS

In a typical resting cell (Fig. 4.3), the membrane is selectively permeable to K^+ and the membrane potential (about −60 mV) is somewhat positive to the K^+ equilibrium (about −90 mV). This resting permeability comes about because some potassium channels are open. If more potassium channels open, the membrane hyperpolarises and the cell is inhibited, whereas the opposite happens if potassium channels close. As well as affecting excitability in this way, potassium channels also play an important role in regulating the duration of the action potential and the temporal patterning of action potential discharges; altogether, these channels play a central role in regulating cell function. As mentioned in Chapter 3, the number and variety of potassium channel subtypes are extraordinary, implying that evolution has been driven by the scope for biological advantage to be gained from subtle variations in the functional properties of these channels. There are over 60 different pore-forming subunits, plus another 20 or so auxiliary subunits. An impressive evolutionary display, maybe, but hard going for most of us.

Potassium channels fall into three main classes (Table 4.2),[5] of which the structures are shown in Fig. 3.20.

- *Voltage-gated potassium channels*, which possess six membrane-spanning helices, one of which serves as the voltage sensor, causing the channel to open when the membrane is depolarised. Included in this group are channels responsible for most of the voltage-gated K^+ currents familiar to electrophysiologists, and others such as Ca^{2+}-activated potassium channels, and HERG channels important in the heart. Many of these channels are blocked by drugs such as **tetraethylammonium** and **4-aminopyridine.**
- *Inwardly rectifying potassium channels*, so called because they allow K^+ to pass inwards much more readily than outwards. These have two membrane-spanning helices and a single pore-forming loop (P loop). These channels are regulated by interaction with G proteins (see Ch. 3) and mediate the inhibitory effects of many agonists acting on G protein–coupled receptors. Certain types are important in the heart, particularly in regulating the duration of the cardiac action potential (see Ch. 20); others are the target for the action of **sulfonylureas** (antidiabetic drugs that stimulate insulin secretion by blocking them; see Ch. 31) and smooth muscle relaxant drugs, such as **minoxidil** and **diazoxide**, which open them (see Ch. 21).
- *Two-pore domain potassium channels*, with four helices and two P loops. These show outward rectification and therefore exert a strong repolarising influence, opposing any tendency to excitation. They may contribute to the resting K^+ conductance in many cells and are susceptible to regulation via G proteins; certain subtypes have been implicated in the action of volatile anaesthetics such as **isoflurane** (see Ch. 41).

For more details, and information on potassium channels and the various drugs and toxins that affect them, see Jenkinson (2006) and Alexander et al. (2021).

Inherited abnormalities of potassium channels (channelopathies) contribute to a rapidly growing number of cardiac, neurological and other diseases. These include the *long QT syndrome* associated with mutations in cardiac voltage-gated potassium channels, causing episodes of ventricular arrest that can result in sudden death. Drug-induced prolongation of the *QT* interval is an unwanted side effect of several drugs (see Chs 20 and 58), including **methadone** and various antipsychotic agents. Nowadays, new drugs are screened for this property at an early stage in the development process (see Ch. 60). Certain familial types of deafness and epilepsy are associated with mutations in voltage-gated potassium channels (Imbrici et al., 2016).

[4]Potassium channel terminology is confusing, to put it mildly. Electrophysiologists have named K^+ currents prosaically on the basis of their functional properties (I_{KV}, I_{KCa}, I_{KATP}, I_{KIR}, etc.); geneticists have named genes somewhat fancifully according to the phenotypes associated with mutations ('shaker', 'ether-a-go-go', etc.), while molecular biologists have introduced a rational but unmemorable nomenclature on the basis of sequence data (KCNK, KCNQ, etc., with numerical suffixes). The rest of us must make what we can of the unpoetic jargon of labels such as HERG (which – don't blink – stands for 'Human Ether-a-go-go Related Gene'), TWIK, TREK and TASK.

Table 4.2 Types and functions of K^+ channels

Structural class[a]	Functional subtypes[b]	Functions	Drug effects	Notes
Voltage-gated (6T, 1P)	Voltage-gated K^+ channels	Action potential repolarisation	Blocked by tetraethylammonium, 4-aminopyridine	Subtypes in the heart include HERG and LQT channels, which are involved in congenital and drug-induced dysrhythmias Other subtypes may be involved in inherited forms of epilepsy
		Limits maximum firing frequency	Certain subtypes blocked by dendrotoxins (from mamba snake venom)	
	Ca^{2+}-activated K^+ channels	Inhibition following stimuli which increase $[Ca^{2+}]_i$	Certain subtypes blocked by apamin (from bee venom), and charybdotoxin (from scorpion venom)	Important in many excitable tissues to limit repetitive discharges, also in secretory cells
Inward rectifying (2T, 1P)	G protein-activated	Mediate effects of Gi/Go-coupled GPCRs which cause inhibition by increasing K^+ conductance	GPCR agonists and antagonists Some are blocked by tertiapin-Q (from honey bee venom)	Other inward rectifying K^+ channels important in kidney
	ATP-sensitive	Found in many cells Channels open when [ATP] is low, causing inhibition Important in control of insulin secretion in the pancreas	Association of one subtype with the sulfonylurea receptor (SUR) results in modulation by sulfonylureas (e.g. **glibenclamide**) which close channel, and by K^+ channel openers (e.g. **diazoxide, minoxidil**) which relax smooth muscle	
Two-pore domain (4T, 2P)	Several subtypes identified (TWIK, TRAAK, TREK, TASK, etc.)	Most are voltage-insensitive; some are normally open and contribute to the 'resting' K^+ conductance Modulated by GPCRs	Certain subtypes are activated by volatile anaesthetics (e.g. isoflurane) No selective blocking agents	The nomenclature is misleading, especially when they are incorrectly referred to as two-pore channels

[a]K^+ channel structures (see Fig. 3.20) are defined according to the number of transmembrane helices (T) and the number of pore-forming loops (P) in each α subunit. Functional channels contain several subunits (often four) which may be identical or different, and they are often associated with accessory (β) subunits.
[b]Within each functional subtype, several molecular variants have been identified, often restricted to particular cells and tissues. The physiological and pharmacological significance of this heterogeneity is not yet understood.
GPCR, G protein–coupled receptor; HERG, human ether-a-go-go related gene; *LQT,* longQT syndrome.

Ion channels and electrical excitability

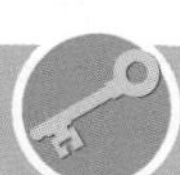

- Excitable cells generate an all-or-nothing action potential in response to membrane depolarisation. This occurs in most neurons and muscle cells, and in some gland cells. The ionic basis and time course of the response varies between tissues.
- The regenerative response results from the depolarising current associated with opening of voltage-gated cation channels (mainly Na^+ and Ca^{2+}). It is terminated by inactivation of these channels accompanied by opening of K^+ channels.
- These voltage-gated channels exist in many molecular varieties, with specific functions in different types of cell.
- The membrane of the 'resting' cell is relatively permeable to K^+ but impermeable to Na^+ and Ca^{2+}. Drugs or mediators that open K^+ channels reduce membrane excitability, as do inhibitors of Na^+ or Ca^{2+} channel function. Blocking K^+ channels or activating Na^+ or Ca^{2+} channels increases excitability.
- Cardiac muscle cells, some neurons and some smooth muscle cells generate spontaneous action potentials whose amplitude, rate and rhythm are affected by drugs that affect ion channel function.

MUSCLE CONTRACTION

The effects of drugs on the contractile machinery of smooth muscle are the basis of many therapeutic applications, for smooth muscle is an important component of most physiological systems, including blood vessels and the gastrointestinal, respiratory and urinary tracts. For many decades, smooth muscle pharmacology with its trademark technology – the isolated organ bath – held the centre of the pharmacological stage, and neither the subject nor the technology shows any sign of flagging, even though the stage has become much more crowded. Cardiac and skeletal muscle contractility is also the target of important drug effects.

Although in each case the basic molecular basis of contraction is similar, namely an interaction between actin and myosin, fuelled by ATP and initiated by an increase in $[Ca^{2+}]_i$, there are differences among these three kinds of muscle that account for their different responsiveness to drugs and chemical mediators.

These differences (Fig. 4.9) involve (1) the linkage between membrane events and increase in $[Ca^{2+}]_i$ and (2) the mechanism by which $[Ca^{2+}]_i$ regulates contraction.

SKELETAL MUSCLE

Skeletal muscle possesses an array of transverse T-tubules extending into the cell from the plasma membrane. The action potential of the plasma membrane depends on voltage-gated sodium channels, as in most nerve cells, and propagates rapidly from its site of origin, the motor endplate (see Ch. 14), to the rest of the fibre. The T-tubule membrane contains voltage-gated calcium channels termed *dihydropyridine receptors* (DHPRs),[6] that respond to membrane depolarisation conducted passively along the T-tubule when the plasma membrane is invaded by an action potential. DHPRs are located extremely close to *RyRs* (see Ch. 3) in the adjacent SR membrane and activation of these RyRs causes release of Ca^{2+} from the SR. Direct coupling between the DHPRs of the T-tubule and the RyRs of the SR (as shown in Fig. 4.9) causes the opening of the RyRs on membrane depolarisation. Through this link, depolarisation rapidly activates the RyRs, releasing a short puff of Ca^{2+} from the SR into the sarcoplasm. The Ca^{2+} binds to troponin, a protein that normally blocks the interaction between actin and myosin. When Ca^{2+} binds, troponin moves out of the way and allows the contractile machinery to operate. Ca^{2+} release is rapid and brief, and the muscle responds with a short-lasting 'twitch' response. This is a relatively fast and direct mechanism compared with the arrangement in cardiac and smooth muscle (see later), and consequently less susceptible to pharmacological modulation.

CARDIAC MUSCLE

Cardiac muscle differs from skeletal muscle in several important respects. The nature of the cardiac action potential, the ionic mechanisms underlying its inherent rhythmicity and the effects of drugs on the rate and rhythm of the heart are described in Chapter 20. The cardiac action potential varies in its configuration in different parts of the heart, but commonly shows a plateau lasting several hundred milliseconds following the initial rapid depolarisation. T-tubules in cardiac muscle contain L-type calcium channels, which open during this plateau and allow Ca^{2+} to enter. This Ca^{2+} entry acts on RyRs (a different molecular type from those of skeletal muscle) to release Ca^{2+} from the SR (see Fig. 4.9). With minor differences, the subsequent mechanism by which Ca^{2+} activates the contractile machinery is the same as in skeletal muscle. Ca^{2+}-induced Ca^{2+} release via RyRs may play a role in some forms of cardiac arrhythmia. Mutations of RyRs are implicated in various disorders of skeletal and cardiac muscle function (see Priori and Napolitano, 2005).

SMOOTH MUSCLE

The properties of smooth muscle vary considerably in different organs, and the mechanisms linking membrane events and contraction are correspondingly variable and more complex than in other kinds of muscle. Spontaneous rhythmic activity occurs in many organs, by mechanisms producing oscillations of $[Ca^{2+}]_i$ (see Fig. 4.2B). The action potential of smooth muscle is generally a rather lazy and vague affair compared with the more military behaviour of skeletal and cardiac muscle, and it propagates through the tissue much more slowly and uncertainly. The action potential is, in most cases, generated by L-type calcium channels rather than by voltage-gated sodium channels, and this is one important route of Ca^{2+} entry. In addition, many smooth muscle cells possess P2X receptors, ligand-gated cation channels, which allow Ca^{2+} entry when activated by ATP released from autonomic nerves (see Ch. 13). Smooth muscle cells also store Ca^{2+} in the ER, from which it can be released when the IP_3R is activated (see Ch. 3). IP_3 is generated by activation of many types of G protein–coupled receptor. Thus in contrast to skeletal and cardiac muscle, Ca^{2+} release and contraction can occur in smooth muscle when such receptors are activated without necessarily involving depolarisation and Ca^{2+} entry through the plasma membrane. RyRs are also present in many smooth muscle cells, and calcium-induced Ca^{2+} release via these channels may play a role in generating muscle contraction (see Fig. 4.9) or couple to plasma membrane calcium-activated K^+ channels resulting in cell hyperpolarisation, thereby reducing Ca^{2+} entry through voltage-gated calcium channels (Fig. 4.10).

The contractile machinery of smooth muscle is activated when the *myosin light chain* undergoes phosphorylation, causing it to become detached from the actin filaments. This phosphorylation is catalysed by a kinase, *myosin light-chain kinase* (MLCK), which is activated when it binds to Ca^{2+}–calmodulin (Fig. 4.9). A second enzyme, *myosin phosphatase*, reverses the phosphorylation and causes relaxation. The activity of MLCK and myosin phosphatase thus exerts a balanced effect, promoting contraction and relaxation, respectively. Both enzymes are regulated by cyclic nucleotides (cAMP and cGMP; see Ch. 3), and many drugs that cause smooth muscle contraction or relaxation mediated through G protein–coupled receptors or through guanylyl cyclase-linked

[5]Although these are, to all intents and purposes, just a form of L-type calcium channel the term *dihydropyridine receptor* (DHPR) is used to reflect that they are not identical to the L-type channels in neurons and cardiac muscle.

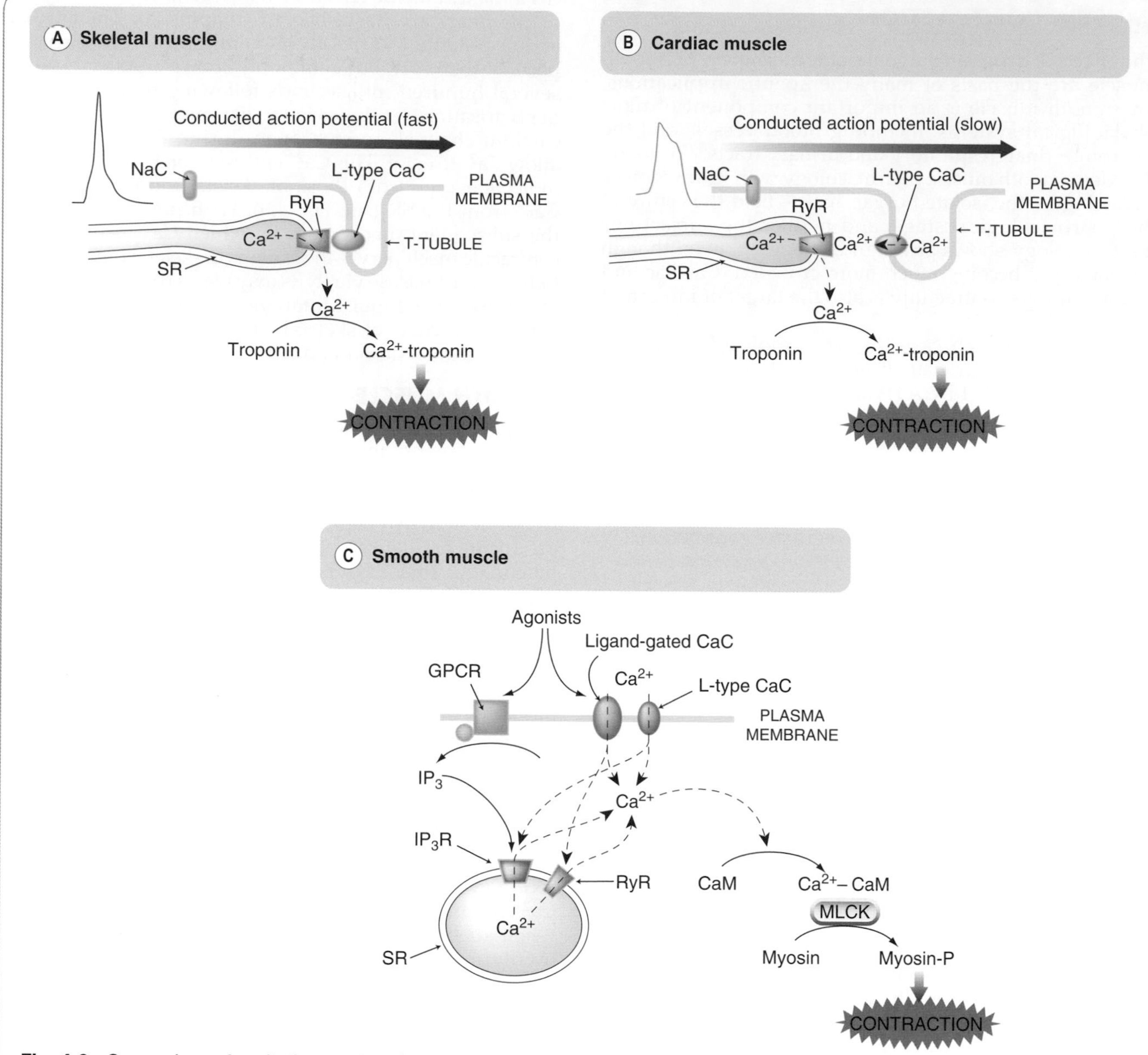

Fig. 4.9 Comparison of excitation–contraction coupling in (A) skeletal muscle, (B) cardiac muscle and (C) smooth muscle. Skeletal and cardiac muscle differ mainly in the mechanism by which membrane depolarisation is coupled to Ca^{2+} release. The calcium channel (CaC) and ryanodine receptor (RyR) are very closely positioned in both types of muscle. In cardiac muscle, Ca^{2+} entry via voltage-gated calcium channels initiates Ca^{2+} release through activation of the Ca^{2+}-sensitive RyRs, whereas in skeletal muscle the sarcolemmal calcium channels activate the RyRs through a voltage-dependent physical interaction. The control of intracellular Ca^{2+} in smooth muscle cells may vary depending upon the type of smooth muscle. In general terms, smooth muscle contraction is largely dependent upon inositol trisphosphate (IP_3)-induced Ca^{2+} release from SR stores through IP_3 receptors (IP_3R). Smooth muscle contraction can also be produced either by Ca^{2+} entry through voltage- or ligand-gated calcium channels. The mechanism by which Ca^{2+} activates contraction is different, and operates more slowly, in smooth muscle compared with in skeletal or cardiac muscle. *CaM,* Calmodulin; *GPCR,* G protein–coupled receptor; *MLCK,* myosin light-chain kinase; *NaC,* voltage-gated sodium channel; *SR,* sarcoplasmic reticulum.

receptors act in this way. Fig. 4.10 summarises the main mechanisms by which drugs control smooth muscle contraction. The complexity of these control mechanisms and interactions explains why pharmacologists have been entranced for so long by smooth muscle. Many therapeutic drugs work by contracting or relaxing smooth muscle, particularly those affecting the cardiovascular, respiratory and gastrointestinal systems, as discussed in later chapters, where details of specific drugs and their physiological effects are given.

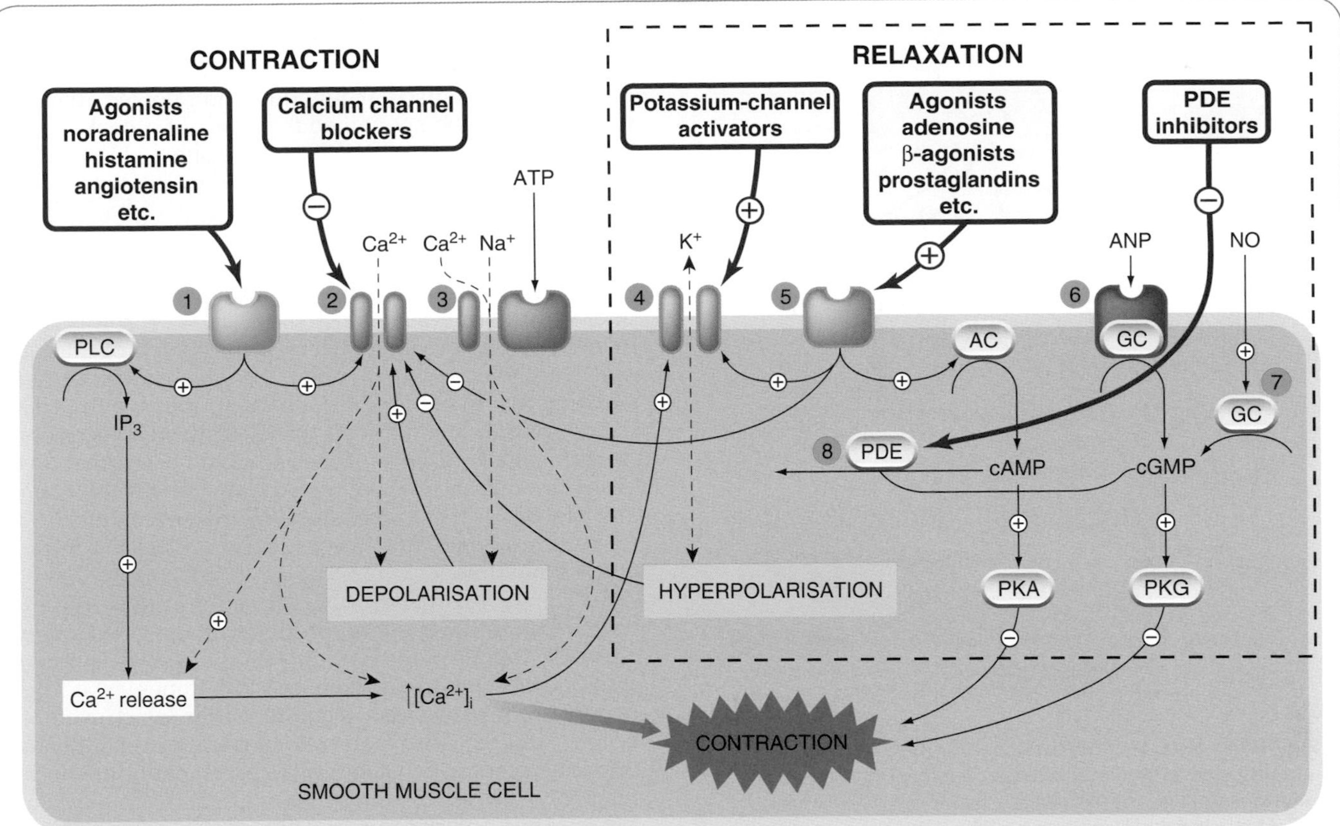

Fig. 4.10 Mechanisms controlling smooth muscle contraction and relaxation. *1.* G protein–coupled receptors for excitatory agonists, mainly regulating inositol trisphosphate formation and calcium channel function. *2.* Voltage-gated calcium channels. *3.* P2X receptor for ATP (ligand-gated cation channel). *4.* Potassium channels. *5.* G protein–coupled receptors for inhibitory agonists, mainly regulating cAMP formation and potassium and calcium channel function. *6.* Receptor for atrial natriuretic peptide (ANP), coupled directly to guanylyl cyclase (GC). *7.* Soluble GC, activated by nitric oxide (NO). *8.* Phosphodiesterase (PDE), the main route of inactivation of cAMP and cGMP. *AC,* Adenylyl cyclase; *PKA,* protein kinase A; *PKG,* protein kinase G; *PLC,* phospholipase C.

Muscle contraction

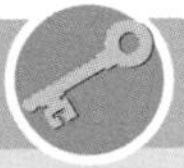

- Muscle contraction occurs in response to a rise in $[Ca^{2+}]_i$.
- In skeletal muscle, depolarisation causes rapid Ca^{2+} release from the sarcoplasmic reticulum (SR); in cardiac muscle, Ca^{2+} enters through voltage-gated channels, and this initial entry triggers further release from the SR; in smooth muscle, the Ca^{2+} signal is due partly to Ca^{2+} entry and partly to inositol trisphosphate (IP_3)-mediated release from the SR.
- In smooth muscle, contraction can occur without action potentials, for example, when agonists at G protein–coupled receptors lead to IP_3 formation.
- Activation of the contractile machinery in smooth muscle involves phosphorylation of the myosin light chain, a mechanism that is regulated by a variety of second messenger systems.

RELEASE OF CHEMICAL MEDIATORS

Much of pharmacology is based on interference with the body's own chemical mediators, particularly neurotransmitters, hormones and inflammatory mediators. Here we discuss some of the common mechanisms involved in the release of such mediators, and it will come as no surprise that Ca^{2+} plays a central role. Drugs and other agents that affect the various control mechanisms that regulate $[Ca^{2+}]_i$ will therefore also affect mediator release, and this accounts for many of the physiological effects that they produce.

Chemical mediators that are released from cells fall into two main groups (Fig. 4.11):

- Mediators that are preformed and packaged in storage vesicles – sometimes called storage granules – from which they are released by *exocytosis*. This large group comprises all the conventional neurotransmitters and neuromodulators (see Chs 13 and 37), and many hormones. It also includes secreted proteins such as cytokines and various growth factors (see Ch. 17).
- Mediators that are produced on demand and are released by diffusion or by membrane carriers.[7] This group includes nitric oxide (see Ch. 19) and many lipid mediators (e.g. prostanoids, see Ch. 17) and endocannabinoids (see Ch. 18), which are released

[7]Carrier-mediated release can also occur with neurotransmitters that are stored in vesicles but is quantitatively less significant than exocytosis.

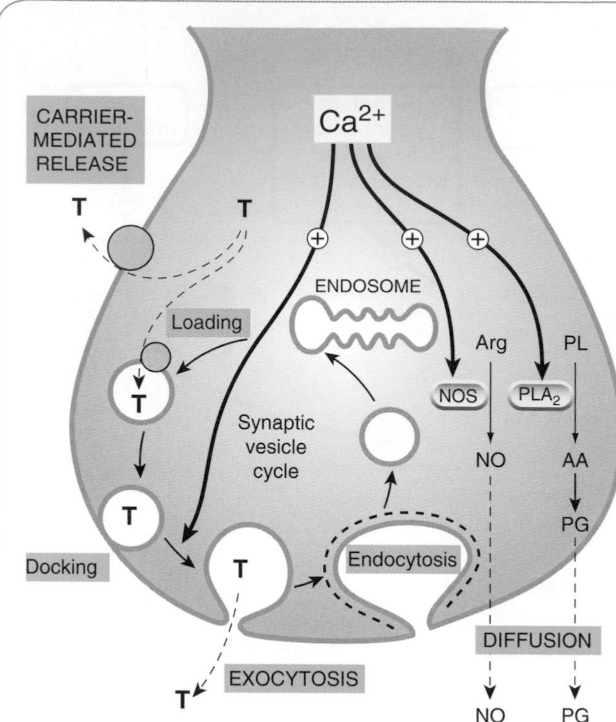

Fig. 4.11 Role of exocytosis, carrier-mediated transport and diffusion in mediator release. The main mechanism of release of monoamine and peptide mediators is Ca^{2+}-mediated exocytosis, but carrier-mediated release from the cytosol also occurs. T represents a typical amine transmitter, such as noradrenaline (norepinephrine) or 5-hydroxytryptamine. Nitric oxide (NO) and prostaglandins (PGs) are released by diffusion as soon as they are formed, from arginine (Arg) and arachidonic acid (AA), respectively, through the action of Ca^{2+}-activated enzymes, nitric oxide synthase (NOS) and phospholipase A_2 (PLA_2) (see Chs 17 and 19 for more details).

from the postsynaptic cell to act on nerve terminals in a retrograde manner.

Calcium ions play a key role in both cases, because a rise in $[Ca^{2+}]_i$ initiates exocytosis and is also the main activator of the enzymes responsible for the synthesis of diffusible mediators.

In addition to mediators that are released from cells, some are formed from precursors in the plasma, two important examples being *kinins* (see Ch. 17) and *angiotensin* (see Ch. 21), which are peptides produced by protease-mediated cleavage of circulating proteins.

EXOCYTOSIS

Exocytosis, occurring in response to an increase of $[Ca^{2+}]_i$, is the principal mechanism of transmitter release (see Fig. 4.11) in the peripheral and central nervous systems, as well as in endocrine cells and mast cells. The secretion of enzymes and other proteins by gastrointestinal and exocrine glands and by vascular endothelial cells is also basically similar. Exocytosis (see Thorn et al., 2016) involves fusion between the membrane of synaptic vesicles and the inner surface of the plasma membrane. The vesicles are preloaded with stored transmitter, and release occurs in discrete packets, or quanta, each representing release from a single vesicle. The first evidence for this came from the work of Katz and his colleagues in the 1950s, who recorded spontaneous 'miniature endplate potentials' at the frog neuromuscular junction and showed that each resulted from the spontaneous release of a packet of the transmitter, acetylcholine.[8] They also showed that release evoked by nerve stimulation occurred by the synchronous release of several hundred such quanta and was highly dependent on the presence of Ca^{2+} in the bathing solution. Unequivocal evidence that the quanta represented vesicles releasing their contents by exocytosis came from electron microscopic studies, in which the tissue was rapidly frozen in mid-release, revealing vesicles in the process of extrusion, and from elegant electrophysiological measurements showing that membrane capacitance (reflecting the area of the presynaptic membrane) increased in a stepwise manner as each vesicle fused and then gradually returned as the vesicle membrane was recovered from the surface. There is also biochemical evidence showing that, in addition to the transmitter, other constituents of the vesicles are released at the same time.

In nerve terminals specialised for fast synaptic transmission, Ca^{2+} enters through voltage-gated calcium channels, mainly of the N and P/Q type (Table 4.1), and the synaptic vesicles are 'docked' at active zones – specialised regions of the presynaptic membrane from which exocytosis occurs, situated close to the relevant calcium channels and opposite receptor-rich zones of the postsynaptic membrane. Elsewhere, where speed is less critical, Ca^{2+} may come from intracellular stores and the spatial organisation of active zones is less clear. It is common for secretory cells, including neurons, to release more than one mediator (for example, a 'fast' transmitter such as glutamate and a 'slow' transmitter such as a neuropeptide) from different vesicle pools (see Ch. 13). The fast transmitter vesicles are located close to active zones, while the slow transmitter vesicles are further away. Release of the fast transmitter, because of the tight spatial organisation, occurs as soon as the neighbouring calcium channels open, before the Ca^{2+} has a chance to diffuse throughout the terminal, whereas release of the slow transmitter requires the Ca^{2+} to diffuse more widely. As a result, release of fast transmitters occurs impulse by impulse, even at low stimulation frequencies, whereas release of slow transmitters builds up only at higher stimulation frequencies. The release rates of the two therefore depend critically on the frequency and patterning of firing of the presynaptic neuron (Fig. 4.12). In non-excitable cells (e.g. most exocrine and endocrine glands), the slow mechanism predominates and is activated mainly by Ca^{2+} release from intracellular stores.

Calcium causes exocytosis by binding to the vesicle-bound protein synaptotagmin, and this favours association between a second vesicle-bound protein, *synaptobrevin*, and a related protein, *syntaxin*, on the inner surface of the plasma membrane. This association brings the vesicle membrane into close apposition with the plasma membrane, causing membrane fusion. This group of proteins, known collectively as SNAREs, plays a key role in exocytosis.

[8]For this work Sir Bernard Katz was awarded the Nobel Prize in Physiology or Medicine in 1970. He shared the prize with Ulf Von Euler and Julius Axelrod, who worked on aspects of noradrenergic transmission.

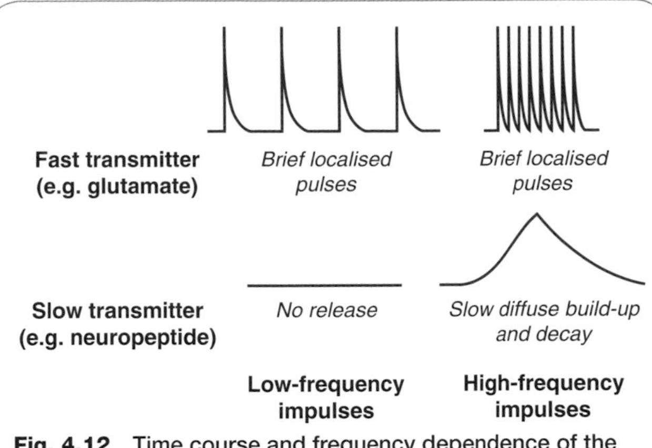

Fig. 4.12 Time course and frequency dependence of the release of 'fast' and 'slow' transmitters. Fast transmitters (e.g. glutamate) are stored in synaptic vesicles that are 'docked' close to voltage-gated calcium channels in the membrane of the nerve terminal and are released in a short burst when the membrane is depolarised (e.g. by an action potential). Slow transmitters (e.g. neuropeptides) are stored in separate vesicles further from the membrane. Release is slower, because they must first migrate to the membrane, and occurs only when $[Ca^{2+}]_i$ builds up sufficiently.

Having undergone exocytosis, the empty vesicle[9] is recaptured by endocytosis and returns to the interior of the terminal, where it fuses with the larger endosomal membrane. The endosome buds off new vesicles, which take up transmitter from the cytosol by means of specific transport proteins and are again docked on the presynaptic membrane. This sequence, which typically takes several minutes, is controlled by various trafficking proteins associated with the plasma membrane and the vesicles, as well as cytosolic proteins. So far, there are few examples of drugs that affect transmitter release by interacting with synaptic proteins, although the botulinum neurotoxins (see Ch. 14) produce their effects by proteolytic cleavage of SNARE proteins.

NON-VESICULAR RELEASE MECHANISMS

If this neat and tidy picture of transmitter packets ready and waiting to pop obediently out of the cell in response to a puff of Ca^{2+} seems a little too good to be true, rest assured that the picture is not quite so simple. Acetylcholine, noradrenaline (norepinephrine) and other mediators can leak out of nerve endings from the cytosolic compartment, independently of vesicle fusion, by utilising carriers in the plasma membrane (see Fig. 4.11). Drugs such as **amphetamines**, which release amines from central and peripheral nerve terminals (see Chs 15 and 39), do so by displacing the endogenous amine from storage vesicles into the cytosol, whence it escapes via the monoamine transporter in the plasma membrane, a mechanism that does not depend on Ca^{2+}.[10]

Nitric oxide (see Ch. 19), arachidonic acid metabolites (e.g. prostaglandins; see Ch. 17) and endocannabinoids (see Ch. 18) are important examples of mediators that are released from the cytosol by diffusion across the membrane or by carrier-mediated extrusion, rather than by exocytosis. The mediators are not stored but escape from the cell as soon as they are synthesised. In each case, the synthetic enzyme(s) is activated by Ca^{2+}, and the moment-to-moment control of the rate of synthesis depends on $[Ca^{2+}]_i$. This kind of release is necessarily slower than the classic exocytotic mechanism, but in the case of nitric oxide is fast enough for it to function as a true transmitter (see Fig. 13.5 and Ch. 19).

Mediator release

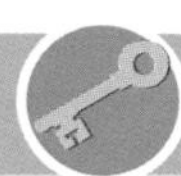

- Most chemical mediators are packaged into storage vesicles and released by exocytosis. Some are not stored but synthesised on demand and released by diffusion or the operation of membrane carriers.
- Exocytosis occurs in response to increased $[Ca^{2+}]_i$ as a result of a Ca^{2+}-mediated interaction between proteins of the synaptic vesicle and the plasma membrane, causing the membranes to fuse.
- After releasing their contents, vesicles are recycled and reloaded with transmitter.
- Many secretory cells contain more than one type of vesicle, loaded with different mediators and secreted independently.
- Stored mediators (e.g. neurotransmitters) may be released directly from the cytosol independently of Ca^{2+} and exocytosis, by drugs that interact with membrane transport mechanisms.
- Non-stored mediators, such as prostanoids, nitric oxide and endocannabinoids, are released by increased $[Ca^{2+}]_i$, which activates the enzymes responsible for their synthesis.

EPITHELIAL ION TRANSPORT

Fluid-secreting epithelia include the renal tubule, salivary glands, gastrointestinal tract and airways epithelia. In each case, epithelial cells are arranged in sheets separating the interior (blood-perfused) compartment from the exterior lumen compartment, into which, or from which, secretion takes place. Fluid secretion involves two main mechanisms, which often co-exist in the same cell and indeed interact with each other. The two mechanisms (Fig. 4.13) are concerned, respectively, with Na^+ transport and Cl^- transport.

In the case of Na^+ transport, secretion occurs because Na^+ enters the cell passively at one end and is pumped out actively at the other, with water following passively. Critical to this mechanism is a class of highly regulated epithelial sodium channels (ENaCs) that allow Na^+ entry.

ENaCs (see Hanukoglu, 2021) are widely expressed, not only in epithelial cells but also in neurons and other excitable cells, where their function is largely unknown. They are regulated mainly by aldosterone, a hormone produced by the adrenal cortex that enhances Na^+ reabsorption by the kidney (see Ch. 29). Aldosterone, like other steroid

[9]The vesicle contents may not always discharge completely. Instead, vesicles may fuse transiently with the cell membrane and release only part of their contents before becoming disconnected (termed *kiss-and-run exocytosis*).

[10]Some cheeses may have high levels of the trace amino acid tyramine, which can act akin to amphetamines and release noradrenaline (particularly in those being treated with monoamine oxidase (MAO) inhibitors, see Ch. 48), giving a dramatic sympathomimetic episode known as a 'cheese effect'.

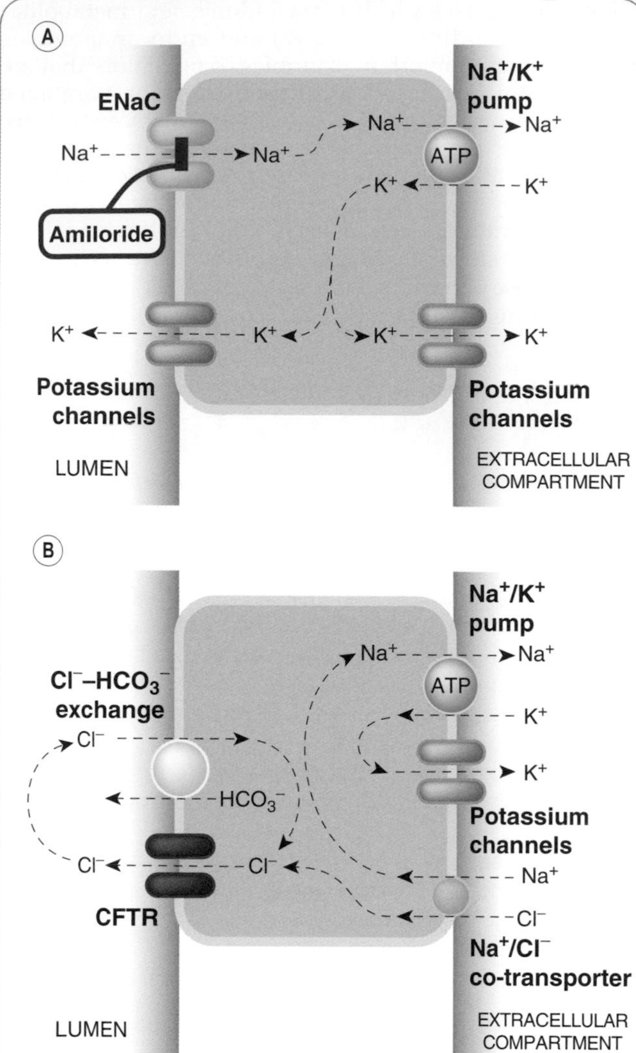

Fig. 4.13 Generalised mechanisms of epithelial ion transport. Such mechanisms are important in renal tubules (see Ch. 29 for more details) and in many other situations, such as the gastrointestinal and respiratory tracts. The exact mechanism may vary from tissue to tissue depending upon channel and pump expression and location. (A) Sodium transport. A special type of epithelial sodium channel (ENaC) controls entry of Na^+ into the cell from the lumenal surface, the Na^+ being actively pumped out at the apical surface by the Na^+–K^+ exchange pump. K^+ moves passively via potassium channels. (B) Chloride transport. Cl^- leaves the cell via a special membrane channel, the cystic fibrosis transmembrane conductance regulator (CFTR), after entering the cell either from the apical surface via the Na^+/Cl^- co-transporter, or at the lumenal surface via the Cl^-/HCO_3^- co-transporter.

hormones, exerts its effects by regulating gene expression (see Ch. 3), and causes an increase in ENaC expression, thereby increasing the rate of Na^+ and fluid transport. ENaCs are selectively blocked by certain diuretic drugs, notably **amiloride** (see Ch. 29), a compound that is widely used to study the functioning of ENaCs in other situations.

Chloride transport is particularly important in the airways and gastrointestinal tract. In the airways it is essential for fluid secretion, whereas in the colon it mediates fluid reabsorption, the difference being due to the different arrangement of various transporters and channels with respect to the polarity of the cells. The simplified diagram in Fig. 4.13B represents the situation in the pancreas, where secretion depends on Cl^- transport. The key molecule in Cl^- transport is the *cystic fibrosis transmembrane conductance regulator* (CFTR), so named because early studies on the inherited disorder cystic fibrosis showed it to be associated with impaired Cl^- conductance in the membrane of secretory epithelial cells, and the CFTR gene, identified through painstaking genetic linkage studies and isolated in 1989, was found to encode a Cl^--conducting ion channel. Severe physiological consequences follow from CFTR mutations and the resulting impairment of secretion, particularly in the airways but also in many other systems, such as sweat glands and pancreas. Studies on the disease-associated mutations of the CFTR gene (see Ch. 28) have revealed much about the molecular mechanisms involved in Cl^- transport (Wang et al., 2014).

Both Na^+ and Cl^- transport is regulated by intracellular messengers, notably by Ca^{2+} and cAMP, the latter exerting its effects by activating protein kinases and thereby causing phosphorylation of channels and transporters. CFTR itself is activated by cAMP. In the gastrointestinal tract, increased cAMP formation causes a large increase in the rate of fluid secretion, an effect that leads to the copious diarrhoea produced by cholera infection (see Ch. 3) and by inflammatory conditions in which prostaglandin formation is increased (see Ch. 17). Activation of G protein–coupled receptors, which causes release of Ca^{2+}, also stimulates secretion, possibly also by activating CFTR. Many examples of therapeutic drugs that affect epithelial secretion by activating or blocking G protein–coupled receptors appear in later chapters.

Epithelial ion transport

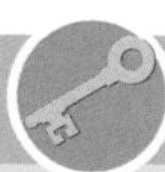

- Many epithelia (e.g. renal tubules, exocrine glands and airways) are specialised to transport specific ions.
- This type of transport depends on a special class of ENaCs which allow Na^+ entry into the cell at one surface, coupled to active extrusion of Na^+, or exchange for another ion, from the opposite surface.
- Anion transport depends on a specific chloride channel (the CFTR), mutations of which result in cystic fibrosis.
- The activity of channels, pumps and exchange transporters is regulated by various second messengers and nuclear receptors, which control the transport of ions in specific ways.

REFERENCES AND FURTHER READING

General references

Alexander, S.P.H., Mathie, A., Peters, J.A., et al., 2021. The concise guide to pharmacology 2020/21: ion channels. Br. J. Pharmacol. 178, S157–S245.

Berridge, M.J., 2014. Cell Signalling Biology. Portland Press, London. Available at: https://doi.org/10.2218/gtopdb/F78/2021.3. www.cellsignallingbiology.org.

Berridge, M.J., 2016. The inositol trisphosphate/calcium signaling pathway in health and disease. Physiol. Rev. 96, 1261–1296.

Blair, N.T., Carvacho, I., Chaudhuri, D., et al., 2019. Transient Receptor Potential Channels (TRP) (Version 2019.3) in the IUPHAR/BPS Guide to Pharmacology Database. IUPHAR/BPS Guide to Pharmacology. Available at: https://doi.org/10.2218/gtopdb/F78/2021.3.

Kandel, E.R., Koester, J.D., Mack, S.H., Siegelbaum, S.A., 2021. Principles of Neural Science, sixth ed. McGraw-Hill, New York.

Katz, B., 1966. Nerve, Muscle and Synapse. McGraw-Hill, New York.

Lewis, R.S., 2020. Store-operated calcium channels: from function to structure and back again. Cold Spring Harb. Perspec. Biol. 12, a035055.

Morgan, A.J., Davis, L.C., Ruas, M., Galione, A., 2015. TPC: the NAADP discovery channel? Biochem. Soc. Trans. 43, 384–389.

Parrington, J., Lear, P., Hachem, A., 2015. Calcium signals regulated by NAADP and two-pore channels–their role in development, differentiation and cancer. Int. J. Dev. Biol. 59, 341–355.

Excitation and ion channels

Catterall, W.A., Lenaeus, M.J., Gamal El-Din, T.M., 2020. Structure and pharmacology of voltage-gated sodium and calcium channels. Ann Rev. Pharmacol. Toxicol. 60, 133–154.

Hille, B., 2001. Ionic Channels of Excitable Membranes. Sinauer Associates, Sunderland.

Imbrici, P., Liantonio, A., Camerino, G.M., et al., 2016. Therapeutic approaches to genetic ion channelopathies and perspectives in drug discovery. Front. Pharmacol. 7, 121.

Jenkinson, D.H., 2006. Potassium channels - multiplicity and challenges. Br. J. Pharmacol. 147 (Suppl. 1), 63–71.

Muscle contraction

Berridge, M.J., 2008. Smooth muscle cell calcium activation mechanisms. J. Physiol. 586, 5047–5061.

Priori, S.G., Napolitano, C., 2005. Cardiac and skeletal muscle disorders caused by mutations in the intracellular Ca^{2+} release channels. J. Clin. Invest. 115, 2033–2038.

Van Petegem, F., 2012. Ryanodine receptors: structure and function. J. Biol. Chem. 287 (31), 31624–31632.

Secretion and exocytosis

Hanukoglu, I., 2021. Epithelial sodium channel (ENaC). IUPHAR/BPS guide to pharmacology. CITE 2021 (2). Available at: https://doi.org/10.2218/gtopdb/F122/2021.2.

Thorn, P., Zorec, R., Rettig, J., Keating, D.J., 2016. Exocytosis in non-neuronal cells. J. Neurochem. 137, 849–859.

Wang, Y., Wrennall, J.A., Cai, Z., Li, H., Sheppard, D.N., 2014. Understanding how cystic fibrosis mutations disrupt CFTR function: from single molecules to animal models. Int. J. Biochem. Cell Biol. 52, 47–57.

5 How drugs act: biopharmaceuticals and gene therapy

OVERVIEW

In this chapter, we discuss the properties of a group of therapeutic agents known collectively as *biopharmaceuticals*. These are relatively recent additions to our therapeutic armoury, but they have already made a major impact on the treatment of rare genetic conditions as well as chronic diseases such as rheumatoid arthritis. The number of biopharmaceuticals approved for clinical use is growing rapidly and the sector will assume even more significance in the future. We first introduce protein- and oligonucleotide-based (largely RNA derived) biopharmaceuticals, highlight the major differences with 'conventional' small molecule drugs and explain how they are manufactured, how they work and how they are metabolised. We then introduce the central concepts of *gene therapy*, discuss the promise and problems associated with this therapeutic modality and highlight some recent successes.

INTRODUCTION

This chapter deals with the general pharmacological characteristics of protein and nucleic acid-based drugs produced using either 'genetic engineering' techniques or synthetic chemistry. Many of these drugs have filled therapeutic niches which other more conventional 'small molecule' drugs have been unable to occupy. Some idea of the vigour of the biopharmaceutical sector may be gained from the total market size which is estimated to be worth over US$320 billion by 2026.

The drugs described in this chapter are termed biopharmaceuticals but, annoyingly for authors of textbooks and their readers, there is no consensus on what actually constitutes a 'biopharmaceutical' as opposed to a conventional drug. An apparently obvious distinguishing feature is whether the drug is predominately 'chemical' in nature (like almost all the small molecule drugs in this book) or of 'biological' origin or manufacture (like insulin or growth hormone, for example). Unfortunately, this simplistic distinction breaks down rather quickly when we consider that 'small molecule' drugs (such as **morphine** or **penicillin**) are plant or fungal products whilst other 'biological molecules' such as short peptides or antisense oligonucleotides (ASOs) can be synthesised using organic chemistry techniques.

A further problem is the stance adopted by the main drug regulatory agencies. Historically, the US Food and Drug Administration (FDA) and their European counterparts have used slightly different definitions when classifying 'biopharmaceuticals' and this has profound effects on the companies that manufacture them, affecting their regulatory obligations, business models, patent filings, investment funding and even public relations. As one commentator (Rader, 2008) put it, 'The result is a Babel-like situation with terminological chaos and anarchy confounding communication, comparative and industry analyses, understanding and regulation'.

There is also another tiresome semantic issue here which should be noted: such drugs are often referred to by the diminutive 'biologics' in academic discussions and papers for the sake of convenience, but this term is also used to refer to *any* biological reagents (e.g. antibody-based laboratory tests, blood products and so on). For reasons of clarity therefore, we will adhere to the term *biopharmaceutical* in this chapter. We will begin with a discussion of protein and oligonucleotide biopharmaceuticals.

PROTEIN AND PEPTIDE BIOPHARMACEUTICALS

The use of proteins as therapeutic agents is not a novel idea; insulin, extracted from animal pancreas tissue (see Ch. 31), and human growth hormone (extracted at one time from human cadaver pituitary glands; see Ch. 33) were among the first therapeutic proteins to be used and, for many years, such purified extracts provided the only option for treating protein hormone deficiency disorders. However, there were problems. Technical difficulties in extraction of the hormone from tissue often led to disappointing yields. Administration of animal hormones (e.g. pig insulin) to humans did not offer an easy solution. These could evoke an immune response and there was also another insidious danger – transmission of infectious agents across species or between people. This was highlighted in the 1970s, when cases of the neurodegenerative *Creutzfeldt–Jakob disease* (see Ch. 40) were seen in patients who had been treated, sometimes decades earlier, with human growth hormone obtained from cadavers,. This serious, and sometimes life-threatening, problem was traced to contamination of the donor pituitary glands with infectious *prions* (see Ch. 40). Fortunately, the advent of 'genetic engineering' techniques offered a new way to deal with these troublesome issues.

The protein biopharmaceuticals in use today are sometimes classified as first- or second-generation agents. *First-generation* biopharmaceuticals are usually straightforward copies of human hormones or other proteins, prepared by *transfecting* the human gene into a suitable *expression system* (a cell line that produces the protein in good yield), then harvesting and purifying the *recombinant protein* for use as a drug. The first agent to be produced in this way was recombinant human insulin in 1982. *Second-generation* biopharmaceuticals are those that have been *engineered* in some way; that is to say, either the gene has been deliberately altered prior to transfection such that the structure of the recombinant protein is changed, or

Table 5.1 Some examples of protein biopharmaceuticals

Class	Biopharmaceutical	Change	Target	Indication	Reason for change
First generation	Human insulin	None	Insulin receptor	Diabetes	N/A
	Human growth hormone	None	Growth hormone receptor (agonist)	Pituitary dwarfism; Turner's syndrome	N/A
Second generation	Insulin	AA sequence	Insulin receptor	Diabetes	Faster acting hormone
	Interferon analogue	AA sequence	Viral replication	Viral infection	Superior antiviral activity
	Glucocerebrosidase	Carbohydrate residue	Glucocerebrosides	Gaucher's disease	Promotes phagocytic uptake
	Erythropoietin analogue	Carbohydrate residue	Erythropoietin receptor	Anaemia	Prolongs half-life
	Human growth hormone	AA sequence; prosthetic group	Growth hormone receptor (antagonist)	Acromegaly	Converts agonist into antagonist with long duration of action

AA, Amino acid.

some alteration is made to the purified end product. Such changes are generally made to improve some aspect of the protein's activity profile. Human recombinant insulins designed to act faster or last longer were among the first in this class to be marketed; Table 5.1 contains other examples.

Production methods

There are several technical and other challenges associated with the manufacture of any type of recombinant protein, and one of the most pressing is the choice of expression system. Recombinant proteins can be conveniently expressed in bacterial systems (*Escherichia coli*, for example), which grow quickly and are generally easy to manipulate. Disadvantages of this approach include the fact that the final product may contain bacterial endotoxins, which must be removed before administration to patients, and also that bacterial cells differ from mammalian cells in patterns of *post-translational processing* (e.g. glycosylation) of proteins, which may affect their biological action. To circumvent these problems, mammalian (e.g. Chinese hamster ovary (CHO)) cells can also be used as expression systems, although such cells require more careful culture, grow more slowly than bacteria and produce less product, all of which contributes to the cost of the final medicine.

A number of emergent technologies are set to transform the production process in the future. The use of plants (see Huebbers and Buyel, 2021; Moon et al., 2019) or algae (see Rosales-Mendoza et al., 2020; Taunt et al., 2018) to produce recombinant proteins obviously has considerable potential. The associated concept of 'therapeutic food' in which biopharmaceuticals or vaccines are incorporated within the plant such that the foodstuff itself becomes the therapeutic agent (see Cebadera Miranda et al., 2020) is one which would have obvious advantages in the treatment of large populations particularly in developing countries if the legislative and ethical challenges, as well as the pharmaceutical problems of delivering such drugs by an oral route, can be surmounted (see Homayun et al., 2019). Looking forward, some biopharmaceutical drugs could be produced in the future using 3D printing technology (Evans et al., 2021) streamlining production considerably.

Engineered proteins

There are several ways in which proteins can be altered prior to expression. Changing the nucleotide sequence of the coding gene can be used to alter single amino acids or, indeed, entire segments of the polypeptide chain. Reasons for modifying proteins in this way include:

- improving pharmacokinetic properties
- creation of novel *fusion* or other proteins
- reducing immunogenicity, for example, by *humanising* the protein

It is often useful to modify the pharmacokinetic properties of recombinant proteins. Changes in the structure of human insulin, for example, provided a form of the hormone that does not self-associate (i.e. 'clump' together) during storage and is therefore faster acting and easier to manage. The half-life of proteins in the blood can often be extended by *PEGylation* (see Ch. 11), that is, the addition of polyethylene glycol (PEG) to the molecule. This *post-translational engineering* approach has been applied to human hormones, such as recombinant growth hormone, interferons and others. This is not merely a convenience to patients; it also reduces the overall cost of the treatment, which is an important factor in the adoption of any type of therapy.

Fusion proteins comprise two or more proteins engineered (by modification of their genes) so as to be expressed as one single polypeptide chain, sometimes joined by a short linker. An example is **etanercept**, an anti-inflammatory drug used in the treatment of rheumatoid arthritis and other conditions (see Ch. 25). Etanercept consists of the ligand-binding domain taken from the tumour necrosis factor (TNF) receptor, joined to the *constant* (Fc) domain of a human immunoglobulin G antibody. The receptor moiety sequesters endogenous TNF, complexing it in an inactive form, while the immunoglobulin fragment increases persistence of the drug in the blood. Reduction of immunogenicity through bioengineering is discussed later.

Perhaps the most exciting idea in protein engineering is the notion that use of a 'modified' genetic code will permit the inclusion of noncanonical amino acids into biopharmaceuticals. This would provide multiple opportunities for novel drug discovery (Kang et al., 2018). Such an approach has already yielded at least one approved veterinary drug (***Pegbovigrastim***, a modified form of granulocyte colony stimulating factor (G-CSF) used to treat mastitis in cattle) and several other agents are already in the developmental pipeline.

MONOCLONAL ANTIBODIES

As with early hormones, the initial use of monoclonal antibodies (mAbs) as therapeutics was achieved via their transfer from humans or animals to patients as 'antisera'. Conventionally, antisera are produced from the blood of humans or animals who have recovered from an infection or have been immunised. Antiserum containing high levels of specific antibodies (e.g. to tetanus toxin, snake venom or, more recently, spike proteins of SARS-CoV-2) is prepared from this serum and this can then be used therapeutically to neutralise pathogens or other dangerous substances in the blood of the recipient patient. While preparations can thus confer *passive immunity*, they suffer from a number of inherent disadvantages that limit their utility.

The endogenous immune response produces a mixture of *polyclonal antibodies* – that is, a *polyvalent* mixture of antibodies from all the plasma cell clones that reacted to that particular antigen. The actual composition and efficacy of this vary over time, and obviously there is a limit to how much immune plasma can be collected on any one occasion. However, in 1975, Milstein and Köhler[1] discovered a method of producing from immunised mice an immortalised *hybridoma*, a fusion of one selected lymphocytic clone with an immortalised tumour cell. The hybridoma cell line could be retained and expanded indefinitely while preserving the integrity of its product. This consequently provided a versatile method of producing *mAbs* – a single species of *monovalent* antibody – at high abundance in vitro against virtually any antigen.

Therapeutic mAbs can be classified into first- or second-generation reagents along similar lines to the other therapeutic proteins discussed earlier. First-generation mAbs were simply murine monoclonals (or fragments thereof) but these encountered several problems in the clinic. As mouse proteins, they provoked an immune response in 50%–75% of all human recipients, had a short half-life in the human circulation and were unable to activate human complement.

Most of these problems have been surmounted by using either *chimeric* or *humanised* mAbs. These two terms refer to the degree to which the immunoglobulin has been modified (see Fig. 5.1); the IgG molecule consists of an Fc domain and the antibody-binding domain (Fab), with *hypervariable* regions that recognise and bind to the antigen in question. The genes for chimeric mAbs are engineered to contain the cDNA of the *murine* Fab domain coupled with

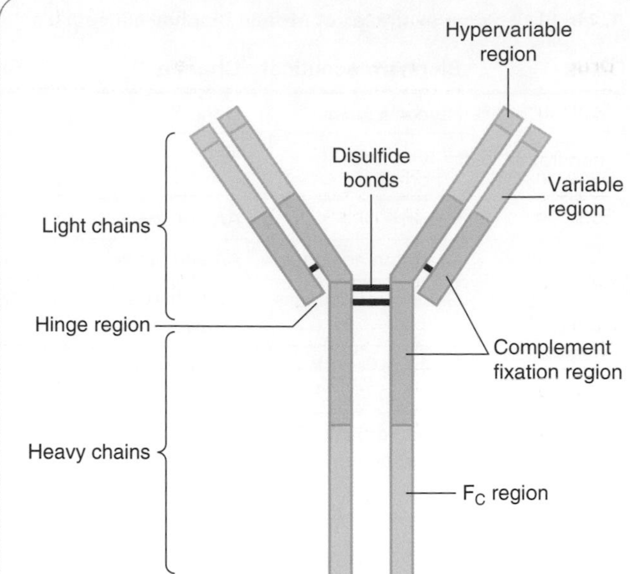

Fig. 5.1 Production of engineered 'chimeric' and 'humanised' monoclonal antibodies. The Y-shaped antibody molecule consists of two main domains: the Fc (constant) domain and the Fab (antigen-binding) domain. At the tip of the Fab regions (on the arms of the 'Y') are the hypervariable regions that actually bind the antigen. Chimeric antibodies are produced by replacing the murine Fc region with its human equivalent by altering and splicing the gene. For humanised antibodies, only the murine hypervariable regions are retained, the remainder of the molecule being human in origin. (After Walsh, G., 2004. Second-generation biopharmaceuticals. Eur. J. Pharm. Biopharm. 58, 185–196.)

the *human* Fc domain sequences. This greatly (around five-fold) extends the plasma half-life because whilst most plasma proteins turn over quite rapidly, immunoglobulins are an exception (it is easy to see why this provides a selective advantage to the host). Incorporation of human Fc sequences also improves the functionality of the antibody in human medicine. A further development (and now the preferred approach) is to replace the *entire* Fc and Fab region with the human equivalent with the exception of the hypervariable regions, giving a molecule which, while essentially human in nature, contains just the minimal segment of murine antibody-binding sites. The anticancer monoclonal **trastuzumab (Herceptin**; see Ch. 57) is an example of such an antibody.

It is now also possible to produce a *wholly human* mAb. The techniques for doing this include using genetically modified (GM) 'humanised' mice which bear human immunoglobulin genes or by using antibody engineering techniques. Such proteins are usually referred to as 'human' mAbs, but it is important to realise that they may still be immunogenic despite being predominantly human proteins (see Harding et al., 2010).

mAb preparations now form by far the largest sector of the biopharmaceutical market and represent the majority of the highest grossing drugs in recent years (quoted in Evans et al., 2021). At the time of writing there are some 80 such preparations on the market (Lu et al., 2020). Table 5.2 contains some examples of these together with an

[1]They won the 1984 Nobel Prize for Physiology or Medicine for this work.

Table 5.2 Some current licensed monoclonal antibody therapies

Drug	Type	Target	Disease
Adalimumab	Fully human mAb	TNF-α	Rheumatoid arthritis and other arthritic diseases; Crohn's disease, ulcerative colitis; uveitis
Bevacizumab	Humanised mAb	VEGF-A	Colorectal cancer; non–small cell lung cancer; some other cancers
Eculizumab	Humanised mAb	Complement protein C5	Paroxysmal nocturnal haemoglobinuria; atypical haemolytic uraemic syndrome; myasthenia gravis; others
Infliximab	Chimeric mAb	TNF-α	Crohn's disease; ulcerative colitis; rheumatoid arthritis and other arthritic diseases
Nivolumab	Fully human mAb	PD-1 'death' receptor	Melanoma; non–small cell lung cancer; some other cancers
Omalizumab	Humanised mAb	Fc region of IgE	Asthma; chronic idiopathic urticaria
Pembrolizumab	Humanised mAb	PD-1 'death' receptor	Melanoma; non–small cell lung cancer; head and neck cancer; lymphoma; some other cancers
Rituximab	Chimeric mAb	CD20 (B cells)	Non-Hodgkin's lymphoma; chronic lymphocytic leukaemia; rheumatoid arthritis; others
Trastuzumab	Humanised mAb	HER2 receptor	Breast cancer; gastric cancer
Ustekinumab	Fully human mAb	IL-12; IL-23	Psoriasis, psoriatic arthritis; Crohn's disease

Therapeutic monoclonal antibody names all end in '-mab', prefixed by an indication of their species nature: *-umab* (human), *-omab* (mouse), *-ximab* (chimera), *-zumab* (humanised).
HER2, Human epidermal growth factor receptor 2; *IgE*, immunoglobulin E; *IL*, interleukin; *mAb*, monoclonal antibody; *PD-1*, programmed cell death protein-1; *TNF-α*, tumour necrosis factor α; *VEGF-A*, vascular endothelial growth factor A.

explanation of the tongue-twisting nomenclature system by which they are known.

In the future, antibodies from other animals may be a useful addition to our armoury. Those from *Camelids* (camels, lamas, etc.) have a simpler molecular structure than human antibodies and are thus easier to manufacture and 'engineer' (see Wrapp et al., 2020).

PHARMACOLOGY OF PROTEIN BIOPHARMACEUTICALS

There are important differences between the pharmacological properties of protein (and oligonucleotide biopharmaceuticals) and those of conventional small molecule drugs (Tables 5.3 and 5.4), which are in part attributable to their difference in molecular mass. Most conventional drugs have molecular masses of less than 1000 and are usually less than 500 – in fact, it is thought that this factor is important in achieving optimal distribution in the body and the biological activity of the drug. In contrast, even the smallest protein biopharmaceutical, insulin, has a molecular mass of almost 6 kDa, while antibodies usually weigh in at about 150 kDa. Roughly, 1 kDa equates to 1000 g/mole. Their size obviously affects the absorption and bioavailability of biopharmaceuticals.

Another distinguishing factor between the two types of drugs is a consequence of their production. 'Conventional' drugs (and short peptides and oligonucleotides) are produced by total (occasionally partial) chemical synthesis, with identical characteristics wherever the compound is made. However, this is not the case with many protein-based biopharmaceuticals. The gene expression system used to produce therapeutically active proteins differs from one company or laboratory to another – deliberately so in most cases because, unlike genes themselves, proprietary constructs and expression systems can be patented, enabling pharma to protect its intellectual property. Each expression system produces a slightly different product in terms of its purity, post-translational modifications and protein 'fingerprint'.[2] This has important consequences for drug regulation, because unlike synthetic small molecule drugs, each biopharmaceutical is unique and a common saying in the biotech industry is that 'the product is the process'. Compared to the first-in-the-field drug, *subsequent entry biologics* (SEBs) or *follow-on biologics* (FOBs) may be *bioequivalents* (i.e. drugs that are interchangeable with, and therapeutically equivalent to, the original preparation); but more often, while still therapeutically effective, they have different clinical properties.[3] However, each preparation requires separate regulatory approval.

Another manufacturing issue concerns the number of steps required to prepare biopharmaceuticals. With chemical synthesis, one can easily assess the exact purity of the final product, but preparations of biopharmaceuticals may not be homogenous and could contain mixtures of different glycoforms of the protein or possibly traces of bacterial proteins or endotoxins. This means that there is a

[2]The 'biological variation' encountered when using living cells to produce a drug is obviously not present in the more precise medicinal chemistry processes. The activity of conventional 'chemical' drugs relates directly to their physicochemical properties such as weight and purity, whereas the activity of biopharmaceuticals can only be measured in activity 'units'.

[3]More bewildering terminology: *biosimilars* are generic drugs with a similar function to the original but with different pharmacology or toxicology; *biobetters* are generic drugs with a similar function to the original but with superior pharmacology or toxicology.

Table 5.3 Differences between biopharmaceuticals and conventional small molecule drugs

Property	Conventional drug	Protein biopharmaceutical	Oligonucleotide biopharmaceutical
Size	Generally <500 kDa	Generally >5000 kDa Small proteins 10^3–10^4 kDa mAbs 10^5 kDa	Generally ~10^3 kDa
Synthesis	Easy to synthesise in identical batches	Most are unique agents requiring complex synthesis and purification.	Generally easy to synthesise in identical batches
Dose-response relationship	Usually a predictable effect relationship between dose and effect	Complex mechanism of action, usually high affinity binding, slow on/off rates, unusual D/R curves	Complex mechanism of action. Unusual D/R relationship
Pharmacokinetics	Often oral administration, variable absorption and bioavailability, phase I and 2 metabolism, excretion of drug in urine or faeces	Usually parenteral administration; bioavailability high, long half-life, atypical distribution and elimination mechanisms	Usually ex vivo or topical administration. Metabolism by nucleases, and clearance by elimination by kidneys
Toxicology and adverse effects	Variable, possible drug interactions. Off-target effects common	Immunogenicity, few drug interactions, generally fewer adverse off-target effects	Immune reactions can be problematic

mAb, Monoclonal antibody.

Table 5.4 A comparison of pharmacokinetics between two conventional small molecule drugs and some biopharmaceuticals

Type	Drug	Route[a]	Dosing frequency	T_{max}	$T_{1/2}$	Bioavailability	*V*
Conventional drug	20 mg simvastatin	p.o.	1 per day	0.7 h	1.5 h	<5%	215 L/kg
	75 mg indometacin	p.o.	1–2 per day	2–3 h	2–3 h	>90%	1.0 L/kg
Biopharmaceutical	25 mg etanercept	i.m.	1–2 per week	69 h	102 h	58%	6–11 L/kg
	40 mg adalimumab	i.m.	1 per 2 weeks	131 h	10–20 days	64%	4.7–6.0 L/kg
	75 mg omalizumab	i.m.	1 per month	7–8 days	26 days	62%	5.5 L/kg

[a]Route of administration: *i.m.*, intramuscular; *p.o.*, by mouth. All data approximated from manufacturer's information.
T_{max}, Time to maximum plasma concentration; $t_{1/2}$, half-life; *V*, volume of distribution.

requirement for greatly enhanced quality control which obviously has profound implications for ease of manufacture and final unit cost (Revers and Furczon, 2010).

Some actions of biopharmaceuticals resemble those of conventional drugs: for example, insulin or growth hormone has identical actions to the native hormone. But others are different. Some mAbs immunoneutralise unwanted substances: for example, **infliximab** directly neutralises the cytokine TNF to produce its therapeutic effect. However, another mAb, **rituximab**, binds to CD20 on lymphocytes, causing actual destruction of the cells to diminish an unwanted immune response. **Ibritumomab tiuxetan** also binds CD20 but delivers ^{90}Y to kill the cells.

Because of these different modes of action, the relationship between dose and effect, so beloved of pharmacologists, is much less clear cut. Agoram (2009) highlights some of the problems. In the case of mAbs for example, high-affinity binding is usual (sometimes a mixture of specific and non-specific binding), slow on- and off-rates are common and the mAb may be internalised, thus modifying the properties of its target cell. Dose–response relationships are sometimes bell shaped or U shaped. Human recombinant erythropoietin has a bell-shaped dose–response and, in the case of many mAbs, there is a single optimal dose at which effective immunoneutralisation occurs, instead of the proportional effects that we are more accustomed to when dealing with small molecule drugs.

The differences in the nature and size of most biopharmaceuticals when compared with conventional drugs also have implications for their pharmacokinetic properties. Because proteins do not usually survive oral administration, most must be administered parenterally and so bioavailability is typically high compared with many small molecule drugs – often in the region of 80%–100%. However, except in the case of intravenous administration, absorption from the injection site is usually slow and the time to attain C_{max} (i.e. the T_{max}) reflects this. Once in the circulation, however, the half-life is typically long. Because antibodies bind to their target with high affinity, the volume of distribution is often small, but transcellular and unusual trafficking may redistribute the drug to other tissues (Zhao et al., 2012). A comparison of the pharmacokinetics of conventional small molecule drugs with several biopharmaceuticals is shown in Table 5.4.

Protein biopharmaceuticals are not removed from the body following metabolic transformation and excretion of the type described for conventional drugs in Chapter 10 and some antibodies can persist in the circulation for weeks. Instead, uptake of large biopharmaceuticals by the lymphatic system is the usual first step, followed by lysosomal degradation. However, some 'small' (<69 kDa) mAbs may be eliminated directly by the kidney. Immunogenicity is an issue that plagued early development of proteins as drugs, and whilst this has been largely overcome by 'humanisation' of antibodies and proteins, it is still important because it may alter the pharmacokinetic properties of the drug (Richter et al., 1999) by increasing its clearance from the circulation.

Drug interactions are less of an issue with protein biopharmaceuticals, as are general toxicity problems and adverse effects (although unwanted biological side effects can be severe), an advantage that is reflected in their relatively rapid approval by regulatory agencies. In part, this is due to their extraordinary specificity. In fact, few drugs currently come closer to the idea of a 'magic bullet'[4] than mAbs which, because of the specificity of the immune system, can inactivate single targets with an extraordinary degree of precision.

Ironically, this latter property can cause major problems when testing these drugs. In 2006, for example, a UK 'first-in-man' phase 1 clinical trial of a new mAb (TGN 1412) designed to activate T cells (see Ch. 7) and thus treat B-cell lymphocytic leukaemia went badly wrong. All six participants became severely ill following a 'cytokine storm' and suffered lasting damage. The incident provoked wide media publicity[5] and, while the subsequent investigation blamed an 'unpredictable' biological reaction for the disaster, it caused many to think hard about how such trials should be conducted in the future (see Muller and Brennan, 2009). Highly specific reagents, such as monoclonals intended for human use, pose particular problems as they may not cross-react with the corresponding proteins of other species, thus evading detection in the usual preclinical animal safety screens. It may be the case that 'surrogate' mAbs which are species specific will have to be developed to test in animal models of the disease prior to testing in humans.

OLIGONUCLEOTIDES

At the time of writing, the most notable advances in this category are the RNA-based biopharmaceuticals. While RNA was discovered just a few years after the ground-breaking publication of the structure of DNA, it was, until the early 1990s, regarded solely as a sort of molecular shuttle which moved genetic information from the genome to the ribosomes where it could be translated into the appropriate protein. The discovery in 1990 that injection of mRNA into muscle tissue could produce an increased synthesis of the corresponding protein was a major conceptual breakthrough in the field and ignited an interest in using RNA therapeutically.

Some 30 years on, we are reaping the harvest of this insight. The use of RNA-based drugs is set to have an enormous impact on pharmacology, greatly enlarging its reach and scope (see Yu et al., 2020). Part of the reason is that RNA molecules are hugely versatile and can be used to target not just other RNA species but also proteins and even DNA itself, in other words, not just the *proteome* but also the *transcriptome* and the *genome* of the cell. Only some 2% of the genome codes for functional proteins; the remainder (previously known arrogantly as 'junk DNA') comprises *pseudogenes*, the molecular remains of ancient viral infections, some (presumably) non-functional or redundant genetic information but significantly, it also includes a huge amount of *long non-coding RNA*. The function of which is only just emerging. The prospect of deploying RNA drugs (or more usually modified analogues) in this part of the transcriptome vastly increases the number of potential drug targets, many of which can now be addressed for the first time. In addition, when used in conjunction with other molecular techniques such as the clustered regulatory interspersed short palindromic repeats (CRISPR)-Cas gene editing system (discussed later), RNA can extend the reach of pharmacology directly into the genome to edit particular genes. It is an astonishing prospect.

In practice we can conveniently divide RNA drugs into four general categories:

- RNA drugs that target proteins
- RNA drugs that target other nucleotides (either RNA or DNA)
- RNA drugs that are actually used to encode proteins
- Miscellaneous other RNA species with pharmacological potential.

The main properties of these species are listed in Table 5.5. We will consider each category separately.

RNA DRUGS THAT TARGET PROTEINS

Aptamers are single-stranded structures of RNA (or DNA). These probably exist naturally in some organisms (e.g. viruses and bacteria) where they fulfil various cellular functions. Because of the ease by which they can be (chemically) synthesised and their ability to adopt many different structures through intramolecular bonding between their constituent nucleotide bases, aptamers can be used to target proteins (and other structures) in much the same way as conventional small molecule drugs, and thus can act at cell surface receptors and other 'pharmacological' targets.

In 2004, the first RNA aptamer approved for clinical use was licensed by the FDA. **Pegaptanid** is a 28-nucleotide structure with an added PEG group. The therapeutic target was age-related macular degeneration (see Ch. 27) and the drug specifically binds to and inhibits the action of an isoform of vascular endothelial growth factor (VEGF)

[4]It was Weber's opera, *Der Freischütz* (The Sharpshooter, 1821), that introduced the idea of a 'magic bullet' which, once fired, always found its mark. Ehrlich liked the idea and thought that it was a good description of a highly specific drug. The term, and the associated aspirational concept, has haunted our discipline ever since.

[5]One tabloid headline read: 'We saw human guinea pigs explode' (quoted by Stobbart et al., 2007).

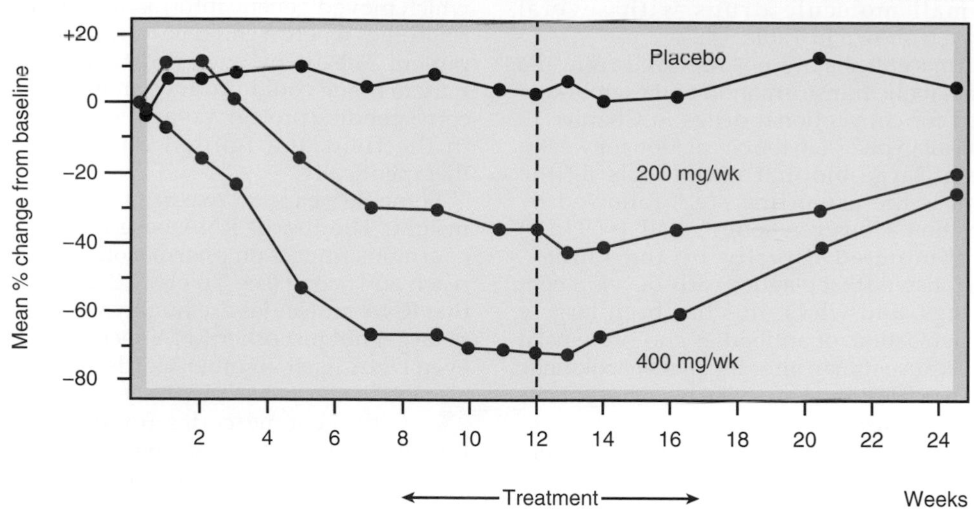

Fig. 5.2 Using antisense oligonucleotides to correct mild-moderate hyperlipidaemia. The antisense oligonucleotide **mipomersen** was administered to 50 patients for 13 weeks. The data show the mean reduction in low-density lipoprotein (LDL) cholesterol expressed in percentage terms from the baseline readings at day 1 with doses of 200 mg/week *(red)* and 400 mg/week *(blue)* compared with a placebo *(black)*. The reduction in expression of apolipoprotein B caused by the drug exactly paralleled the LDL cholesterol data. After discontinuation of the treatment (indicated by *dotted line*) the blood levels showed signs of returning to baseline values but were still depressed by 20%–30% at the conclusion of the study at these doses (Redrawn from Geary, R.S., Baker, B.F., Crooke, S.T., 2015. Clinical and preclinical pharmacokinetics and pharmacodynamics of mipomersen (Kynamro[R]): a second-generation antisense oligonucleotide inhibitor of apolipoprotein B. Clin. Pharmacokinet. 54, 133–146.)

Table 5.5 Types of RNA-based drugs

Type	RNA structure	Mechanism	Comments
Aptamers	Single stranded	Direct action on protein and other targets	Similar to small molecule drugs. Can be modelled and designed to bind to different sites
Antisense oligonucleotides (ASOs)	Single stranded	Binds to specific mRNA by base pairing inactivating it or causing degradation through RNA interference mechanism	Can also be oligo-DNA Works better in nuclear compartment Usually 15–30 base pairs
Small interfering RNAs (siRNAs)	Double stranded	Complex mechanism. Binds to specific mRNA forming a 'RNA-induced silencing' complex, thus inactivating it	Works better for cytoplasmic targets. Larger (20–24 base pairs) than other RNA species
Micro RNAs (miRNAs)	Single stranded	Binds to specific mRNA by base pairing, causing degradation or instability of RNA or less efficient translation by ribosomes	Endogenous non-coding RNA species that regulates gene expression. Synthetic miRNAs can be designed to act in the same way. Can silence multiple targets
Messenger RNA (mRNA)	Single stranded	Acts in a similar way to endogenous mRNA to increase synthesis of specific proteins	Larger than most other RNA drugs. Must contain appropriate structure and an open reading frame to allow for translation to occur
Guide RNA (gRNA)	Single stranded	Binds to a specific target region of DNA	Smaller than other RNA species. Can be used in conjunction with the CRISPR-Cas gene editing system

CRISPR, Clustered regulatory interspersed short palindromic repeats.
From Yu, A.M., Choi, Y.H., Tu, M.J., 2020. RNA drugs and RNA targets for small molecules: principles, progress, and challenges. Pharmacol. Rev. 72, 862–898.

blocking the VEGF receptor thus preventing it from stimulating the growth of new blood vessels.

RNA DRUGS THAT TARGET OTHER NUCLEOTIDES

ANTISENSE OLIGONUCLEOTIDES

Discovered in 1978 and long a staple of laboratory research where they were used with great success to 'knock down' the expression of genes of interest, 'ASOs' have now found their place in the clinic. They are generally chemically modified single-strand oligonucleotides which hybridise to the complementary mRNA (which itself needs to be single stranded to partcipate in translation) for particular proteins and prevent transcription or translation either directly (as the two strands are now duplexed) or because the target mRNA is then degraded by RNAses. They typically have molecular masses in the region of 7–15 kDa.

ASOs can act in several ways: for example, the anti-cytomegalovirus drug **fomiversin** (the first such agent to be introduced but now withdrawn because of lack of demand) halts the progress of cytomegalovirus retinitis by blocking transcription of a key viral protein. **Mipomersin** reduces the expression of apolipoprotein B and has been used for treating hypercholesteraemia (Fig. 5.2), whereas drugs such as **eteplirsen** and **golodirsen** act to mitigate the progress of Duchenne muscular dystrophy in a more complex fashion. The problem here is a mutation (a premature stop codon) in the dystrophin gene which leads to the synthesis of a non-functional protein; this results in gradual atrophy of muscle mass with progressive weakness and eventually paralysis and death. Since it is an X-linked gene, the victims are young boys. **Eteplirsen** and **golodirsen** can interfere with the transcription of the defective gene and reintroduce a new open reading frame resulting in the transcription of a truncated but still functional protein. There are several common mutations (and thus variants of this disease) with different regions of the dystrophin gene being affected. Thus several drugs have been developed which target different exons of the dystrophin gene. **Eteplirsen** targets exon 51, **golodirsen** and **vitolarsen** target exon 53 and a further antisense drug **casimersin** targets exon 45.

SMALL INTERFERING RNAs

Discovered in 1998,[6] and similarly to antisense agents, small interfering RNAs (siRNAs) also target mRNA but through a more complex process. These are double-stranded RNA molecules which comprise a *guide strand* and a *passenger strand*. Following rather complex enzymatic processing, the passenger strand is removed, and the guide strand complexes with the target mRNA to form an *siRNA-induced silencing complex* (RISC). This enhances breakdown of mRNA coding for one specific protein, potentially for long periods (several months). Generally speaking, siRNAs are more effective in silencing cytoplasmic mRNA targets whereas antisense RNAs are more effective in the nuclear compartment. They are highly unstable in plasma, and their use as therapeutic agents depends on chemical modification of the 2′ position of the ribose ring which greatly improves their stability (see Ch. 60). A further hurdle is access to their site of action in the cytoplasm. One method of achieving this is formulation in lipid nanoparticles (see Ch. 9). More recently, for drugs acting on hepatocytes this problem has been addressed by conjugating the chemically modified siRNA with tris-*N*-acetylgalactosamine (Gal-Nac). This binds to asialoglycoprotein (ASGP) receptors expressed by hepatocytes. Binding to ASGP leads rapidly to endocytosis and efficient delivery to a hepatic site of action.

One approved siRNA drug formulated in lipid nanoparticles, **patisiran**, is used to treat the neuropathy caused by the misfolded copies of transthyretin in patients with hereditary transthyretin-mediated amyloidosis. Two other, more recently licensed siRNA drugs are Gal-Nac conjugates, namely **givosiran** (illustrated on our front cover in combination in its RISC complex) and **inclisiran**. **Givosiran** is used to treat patients with hepatic porphyria caused by a disruption of heme biosynthesis in the liver. It works by causing breakdown of mRNA coding for aminolevulinic acid synthase 1 thereby suppressing synthesis of this inducible hepatic enzyme toward normal. **Inclisiran** (see Ch. 22) reduces low-density lipoprotein (LDL)-cholesterol by destabilising mRNA coding for PCSK9 and hence suppressing the synthesis of PSCK9 in hepatocytes. It is administered subcutaneously twice a year, so is potentially useful in primary care. The therapeutic potential of this extraordinarily versatile class of agent for treatment of both rare and common disorders is further discussed in Chapter 60.

MICRO-RNAs

Micro-RNAs (miRNAs) are single-stranded structures with a molecular weight of about 10–12 kDa. They are derived from non-coding RNA involved in post-transcriptional gene regulation. Their mechanism of action is complex but, like the siRNAs, they can form a 'silencing complex' with their target mRNA. Unlike siRNAs, however, they can simultaneously alter the expression of multiple transcripts, making them a versatile experimental (and possibly therapeutic) drug. At the time of writing, there are no miRNA drugs in the clinic but there are several being trialled for, for example, Huntingdon's disease. They also hold out especial promise as possible replacements for tumour suppressing miRNAs (as opposed to pro-tumoural 'oncomiRs') which are lost in some types of cancer.

RNA DRUGS THAT ARE USED TO ENCODE PROTEINS

Since the transcription of (single-stranded) mRNA copies of genes is the usual way in which cells generate proteins, it is obvious that this species could have great therapeutic potential as a form of 'replacement therapy'. If a particular protein is not produced, or at least not in sufficient quantities, administration of the appropriate mRNA to the target cell could provide a very attractive way forward, certainly easier than using DNA or plasmid constructs to do the same job.

One particular application which has achieved recent success (as well as grabbing the headlines) has been its use in vaccines. In the widely used Pfizer-BioNTech COVID-19 vaccine used to prevent infection with SARS-CoV-2 for example, the mRNA for a version of the full-length 'spike' protein of the virus is delivered intramuscularly in

[6]Discovered initially when plant scientists found, to their surprise, that introducing RNA which encoded the colour-producing enzyme in petunias made the flowers *less* colourful, not more so – a process they termed 'gene quelling'. Subsequently siRNA has emerged as an important physiological mechanism for controlling gene expression and was recognised by the award in 2006 of the Nobel Prize to Craig Mello and Andrew Fire for their seminal discoveries in *Caenorhabditis elegans*.

Table 5.6 Some RNA-based drugs in clinical use

Drug	Type	Disease	Target	Mechanism	Dosage form
Pegaptanid[a]	Aptamer	Neovascular age-related macular degeneration	VEGF isoform receptor	Direct antagonist	Intravitreal injection (6-week intervals)
Eteplirsen[a]	Antisense oligonucleotide	Duchenne muscular dystrophy	Exon 51 of dystrophin pre-RNA	Alters splicing of incorrect version of the protein allowing functional protein transcription	Intravenous infusion (weekly)
Golodirsen[a]	Antisense oligonucleotide	Duchenne muscular dystrophy	Exon 53 of dystrophin pre-RNA	Prevents splicing of incorrect version of the protein allowing functional protein transcription	Intravenous infusion (weekly)
Nusinersen	Antisense oligonucleotide	Spinal muscular atrophy	Survival motor neuron (SMN) mRNA	Alters splicing of SMN mRNA to produce correct version of protein	Intrathecal (variable schedule)
Patisiran	Small interfering RNA	Hereditary transthyretin mediated amyloidosis	Transthyretin mRNA	Binds to mRNA to prevent production of protein	Intravenous infusion (every 3 weeks)
Givosiran	Small interfering RNA	Acute hepatic porphyria	d-Aminolevulinic acid synthase 1 mRNA	Binds to mRNA causing degradation of mRNA through RNA interference	Subcutaneous injection (monthly)
Pfizer-BioNtech COVID-19 vaccine	'Spike' protein mRNA	COVID-19 infection (prophylactic protection)	COVID-19 external 'spike' protein	mRNA in muscle cells produces copies of the spike protein which are recognised as immunogenic targets by the host immune system.	Intramuscular injection (two doses at 21-day interval)

[a]Not yet available in the UK.
Data chiefly from Yu, A.M., Choi, Y.H., Tu, M.J., 2020. RNA drugs and RNA targets for small molecules: principles, progress, and challenges. Pharmacol. Rev. 72, 862–898.

nanolipid particles. This mRNA is then translated in the host's muscle to produce copies of the coronavirus spike protein which is then recognised by the immune system which responds with an appropriate antibody and T-cell response. The Moderna COVID-19 vaccine relies on a similar mechanism.[7]

In order to function as mRNA in the cell, the synthetic construct must contain the requisite molecular signals enabling it to be recognised by the protein synthesising machinery. These include the presence of an open reading frame as well as appropriate 5′- and 3′-untranslated groups and a poly(A) tail. Because of this, mRNA constructs tend to be larger than the other RNA-derived drugs in this section. In addition, and like almost all the other species, they must be modified in some way to prevent destruction by RNAses.

MISCELLANEOUS OTHER RNA SPECIES WITH PHARMACOLOGICAL POTENTIAL

This group comprises several other types of RNA species which hold out promise for future use, but which whose current state of development are not yet sufficiently mature to have realised this potential. The group includes *guide RNAs* (gRNAs), small fragments of complementary RNA which can be used in conjunction with the CRISPR-Cas gene editing technique, as well as *ribozymes*, catalytically active RNA.

Table 5.6 shows some examples of RNA-based drugs already in the clinic.

PROBLEMS WITH RNA BIOPHARMACEUTICALS

There are a number of constitutive problems with all types of RNA biopharmaceuticals. One especially troublesome feature of RNA drugs is the fact that the immune system recognises RNA through Toll receptors (particularly TLR 7; see Ch. 7) as being an indicator of the presence of a pathogenic virus and this may trigger an aberrant immune reaction and possibly a cytokine storm.

As is the case with proteins, RNA drugs cannot be administered orally and so must be given by other routes such as intramuscular injection or infusion. Some can be administered topically (see Table 5.6). Polynucleotides have a negative charge and are hydrophilic in nature, making it difficult for them to cross cell membranes, so the development of suitable delivery systems is another hurdle which must be surmounted before any type of RNA is useful in the clinic. Lipid carriers of various compositions have

[7]At the start of 2022, Pfizer and Moderna combined are reportedly making ~$100 million profit per day from these two vaccines alone.

Table 5.7 Some current licensed gene therapies

Gene therapy	Therapeutic indication	Gene	Comments
Yescarta (Axicabtagene ciloleucel)	Large B-cell lymphoma	Chimeric antigen receptor (CAR-T)	Ex vivo use T cells transfected with CAR receptor gene for reinfusion
Strimvelis	Combined immunodeficiency	New copy of adenosine deaminase protein	Ex vivo use CD34 cells transfection with gene for reinfusion
Zynteglo (Betibeglogene autotemcel)	β-thalassaemia	Haemoglobin	Ex vivo use Stem cells transfected with gene for reinfusion
Luxturna (Voretigene neparvovec)	Leber's congenital amaurosis; retinitis pigmentosa	Retinoid isomerohydrolase	In vivo use; subretinal injection Adenovirus delivery system
Zolgensma (Onasemnogene abeparvovec)	Spinal muscular atrophy	New copy of survival motor neuron (SMN1) protein	In vivo use; single IV infusion Adeno-associated virus delivery system
Roctavian (Valoctogene roxaparvovec)	Haemophilia A	Factor VIII	In vivo; IV delivery Adeno-associated virus delivery system (under review)
Imlygic (Talimogene laherparepvec)	Melanoma	GM-CSF	In vivo: direct injection into tumour Herpes simplex virus delivery system

GM-CSF, Granulocyte-macrophage colony stimulating factor; *IV*, intravenous.

been trialled as delivery systems often with some success, but other possibilities include the construction of hybrid molecules in which the RNA is conjugated to other ligands to achieve a more targeted approach. In the case of **givosiran** for example, a conjugated *N*-acetylgalactosamine residue promotes uptake by the target organ, the liver.

As one might also anticipate, as well as cold-storage requirements of RNA therapeutics, the stability of the RNA is itself a major issue. Cells and tissues contain abundant RNAses which could rapidly destroy any administered RNA. RNAses are found in fingerprints, on every surface and even in the air we breathe. To circumvent this, various strategies have been devised by which chemical modification of the nucleotide structure, often using *methylphosphonate* or *phosphorothioate* derivatives, can offer protection against these enzymes. Such modifications may also improve the pharmacokinetic properties of these drugs too although there is the risk of enhanced immunogenicity and possibly toxicity also. The eventual clearance of RNA drugs (or metabolic fragments) from the body is mainly through renal excretion.

GENE THERAPY

Astonishingly, the first study to demonstrate the theoretical feasibility of gene transfer took place in 1944 when Avery and his colleagues showed that a virulence factor could be transferred between two strains of pneumococcus and identified the factor as (what we now call) DNA, which was not even recognised at that time as the genetic material. Following the molecular biology revolution in the 1980s, however, the significance of this experiment became clear and the notion that one could replace faulty or missing genes became a distant – if thrilling – prospect. It is easy to see why; first, it is a (deceptively) simple approach to a radical cure of the literally thousands of rare genetic and other monogenic diseases such as *cystic fibrosis* and the *haemoglobinopathies*, which are collectively responsible for much misery throughout the world. Second, many other more common conditions, including malignant, neurodegenerative and infectious diseases, have a large genetic component. Conventional treatment of such disorders is (as readers of later chapters will appreciate) far from ideal, so the promise of a completely new approach had enormous allure. The field, which had a rather shaky beginning, has now achieved some notable success (see Table 5.7) and despite the fact that only a few gene therapies have so far been approved for clinical use, some experts estimate the sector will be worth US$10–20 billion by 2028.

There are two main gene therapy strategies. Using the *in vivo technique*, the vector containing the therapeutic gene is injected into the patient, either intravenously (in which case some form of organ or tissue targeting is required) or directly into the target tissue (e.g. the retina). When using the *ex vivo strategy* (Figs. 5.3 and 5.4), cells are removed from the patient (e.g. stem cells from bone marrow, cells from the circulating blood or myoblasts from a biopsy of striated muscle) and treated with the vector in the laboratory. The genetically altered autologous cells are injected back into the patient they came from (usually sometime later), thus avoiding any immune rejection.

While many difficulties have been overcome, the technology is still rife with technical and other problems. These include:

- *pharmacokinetics*: delivery of the gene to the interior of appropriate target cells either in vivo (especially those in the central nervous system (CNS)) or in vitro;

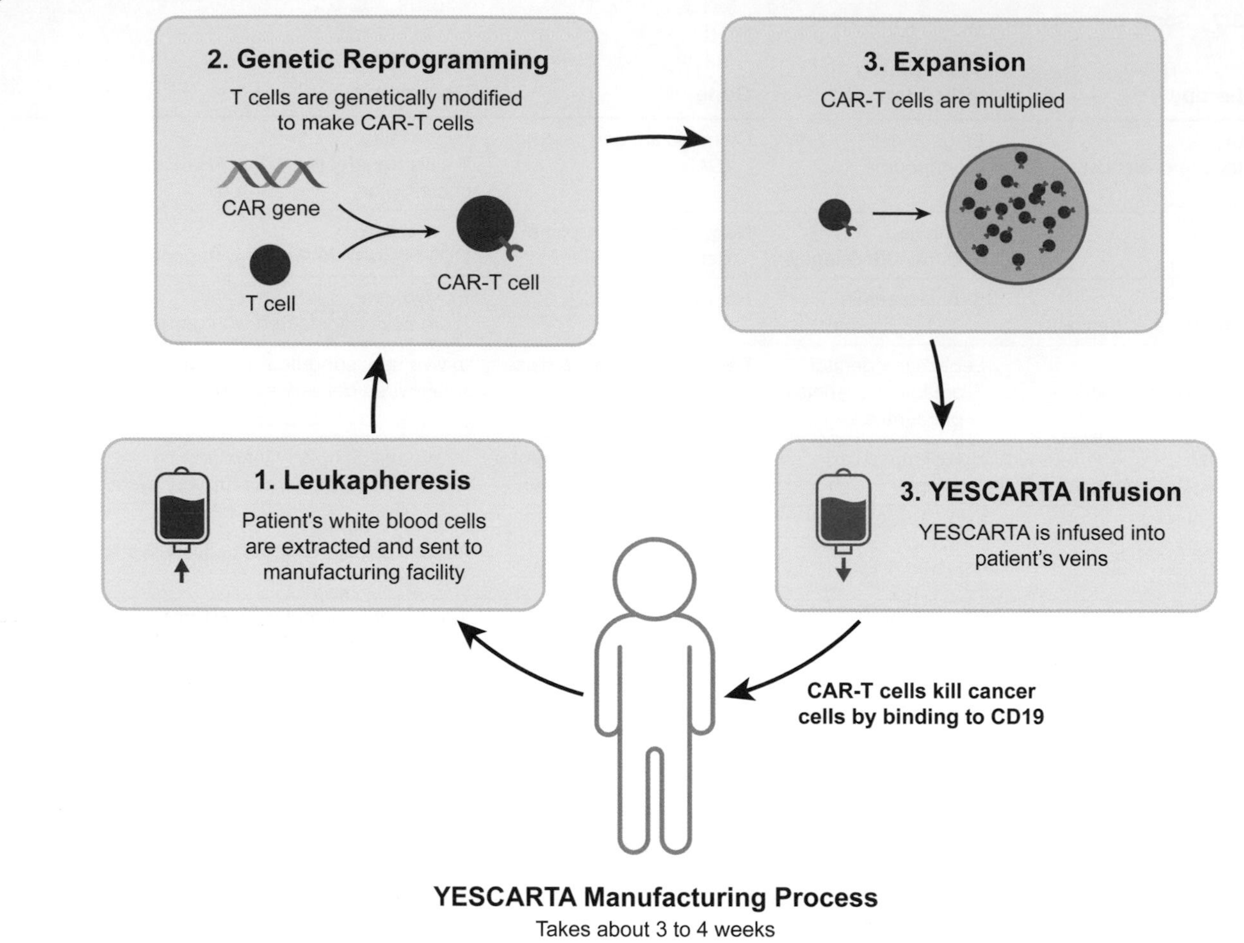

Fig. 5.3 **An example of ex vivo gene therapy. Yescarta** (Axicabtagene ciloleucel) is a gene therapy for treating large B-cell lymphoma. T cells are removed for the patient and, in the laboratory, transfected with the gene for a specific T-cell (chimeric antigen) receptor (CAR-T). After expanding the population, the preparation of autologous T cells is reinfused into the patient who has been prepared with a suitable chemotherapy regime. The modified T cells bind to the CD19 receptor on lymphoma cells and kill the cell. Note that the preparation procedure takes 3–4 weeks to accomplish.

- *pharmacodynamics*: the controlled expression of the gene in question;
- *safety;*
- *clinical efficacy* and *long-term practicability.*

GENE DELIVERY

The transfer of large stretches of recombinant nucleic acid into target cells is critical to the success of gene therapy. In the words of one commentator (Galun, quoted in Bender, 2016), 'Gene therapy is actually three things: delivery, delivery and delivery'. To achieve their therapeutic effects, the constructs must pass from the extracellular space across the plasma and nuclear membranes and be incorporated into the chromosomes. Because DNA is negatively charged and single genes have molecular weights around 10^4 times greater than conventional drugs, the problem is of a different order from the equivalent stage of routine drug development.

There are several important considerations in choosing a gene delivery system; these include:

- the *capacity* of the system (e.g. how much DNA it can carry);
- the *transfection efficiency* (its ability to enter and become utilised by the cell's own machinery);
- the *lifespan* of the transfected material (usually determined by the lifetime of the targeted cells);
- the *safety issue*, especially important in the case of viral delivery systems.

An ideal vector should be safe, highly efficient (i.e. insert the therapeutic gene into a high proportion of target cells and under control of the appropriate promoter) and selective in that it should lead to expression of the therapeutic protein in the target cells but not to the expression of other (e.g. viral proteins). Ideally, and provided that the cell into which it is inserted is itself long lived, the vector should cause persistent expression, avoiding the need for repeated treatment. The latter consideration can be a problem in some tissues. In the autosomal recessive disorder cystic fibrosis, for example, the airway epithelium malfunctions because it lacks a membrane Cl− transporter known as the cystic fibrosis transport regulator (CFTR). Epithelial cells in the airways are continuously dying and being replaced, so even if the unmutated CFTR gene could be stably transfected into the epithelium, there would still be a periodic need for further treatment unless the gene could be inserted into the progenitor (stem) cells. Similar problems are anticipated in other cells that turn over continuously, such as gastrointestinal epithelium and skin.

VIRAL VECTORS

To overcome this first and most fundamental hurdle of gene delivery, techniques borrowed from viruses, which are masters of the sort of molecular hijacking that is required to introduce functional genes into mammalian cells, are often used in gene therapy research.

While seemingly straightforward, there remain substantial practical problems with this *viral vector* approach. As viruses have evolved the means to invade human cells, so humans have evolved immune responses and other protective countermeasures. Although limiting in some respects, this is not all bad news from the point of view of safety. As many of the viruses used for vectors are pathogenic, they are usually modified such that they are 'replication defective' to avoid toxicity.

Retroviruses

If introduced into stem cells, most *retroviral vectors* have long-lasting effects because they are incorporated into, and replicate along with, host genomic DNA, and so the 'therapeutic' gene is passed down to each daughter cell during division. Against this, the *retroviral integrase* inserts the construct into chromosomes randomly, so it may also cause damage. Also, retroviruses could infect germ or non-target cells and produce undesired effects if administered in vivo. For this reason, they have been used mainly for ex vivo gene therapy.

Many viruses are equipped to infect specific cell types, but these are not necessarily the target cell of interest. It is however possible to change the retroviral envelope to alter specificity, such that the vector could be administered systemically but would target only the desired cell population. An example of this approach with a *lentivirus* (a type of retrovirus) is the substitution of the envelope protein of a non-pathogenic vector (e.g. mouse leukaemia virus) with the envelope protein of human vesicular stomatitis virus, to specifically target human epithelial cells.

Most retrovirus vectors are unable to penetrate the nuclear envelope, and because this dissolves during cell division, they only infect dividing cells rather than non-dividing cells (such as adult neurons).

Adenovirus vectors

Adenovirus vectors are popular because of the high transgene expression that can be achieved. They transfer genes to the nucleus of the host cell, but (unlike retroviruses) these are not inserted into the host genome and so do not produce effects that outlast the lifetime of the transfected cell. This property also obviates the risk of disturbing the function of other cellular genes and the theoretical risks of carcinogenicity and germ cell transfection. Because of these favourable properties, adenovirus vectors have been used extensively for in vivo gene therapy. Engineered deletions in the viral genome render it unable to replicate or cause widespread infection in the host while at the same time creating space in the viral genome for the therapeutic transgene to be inserted.

One of the first adenoviral vectors lacked part of a growth-controlling region called E_1, while incorporating the desired transgene. This vector gave excellent results, demonstrating gene transfer to cell lines and animal models of disease, but it proved disappointing as a treatment for cystic fibrosis in human trials. Low doses (administered by aerosol to patients with this disease) produced only a very low-efficiency transfer, whereas higher doses caused inflammation, a host immune response and short-lived gene expression. Furthermore, treatment could not be repeated because of the appearance, in the circulation, of neutralising antibodies. This led to attempts to manipulate adenoviral vectors to mutate or remove the genes that are most strongly immunogenic.

Other viral vectors

Other potential viral vectors used in gene therapy preparations include *adeno-associated virus*, *herpes virus* and disabled versions of *human immunodeficiency virus* (HIV). Adeno-associated virus associates with host DNA but is not activated unless the cell is infected with an adenovirus. It is less immunogenic than other vectors but is difficult to mass produce and cannot be used to carry large transgenes. Herpes virus does not associate with host DNA but is very long lived in nervous tissue (so might have a specific application in treating neurological disease). HIV, unlike most other retroviruses, can infect non-dividing cells such as neurons. It is possible to remove the genes that control replication from HIV and substitute other genes. Alternatively, it may prove possible to transfer to other non-pathogenic retroviruses those genes that permit HIV to penetrate the nuclear envelope.

NON-VIRAL VECTORS

To reduce the potential problems associated with viral vectors, a variety of other substances have been used to deliver genes and other material. These are often collectively known as *nanocarriers*. The list includes the following (but see also Xu et al., 2014).

Liposomes

Non-viral vectors include a variant of liposomes (see Ch. 9). Plasmids (diameter up to approximately 2 μm) are too big to package in regular liposomes (diameter 0.025–0.1 μm), but larger particles can be made from positively charged lipids ('lipoplexes'), which interact with both negatively charged cell membranes and DNA, improving delivery into the cell nucleus and incorporation into the host chromosome. Such particles have been used to deliver the genes for HLA-B7, interleukin-2 and CFTR (as well as COVID-19 vaccines) to cells. They are much less efficient than viruses, and attempts are currently under way to improve this by incorporating various viral signal proteins (membrane fusion proteins, for example) in their outer coat. Direct injection of these complexes into solid tumours (e.g. melanoma, breast, kidney and colon cancers) can, however, achieve high local concentrations within the tumour.

Microspheres

Biodegradable microspheres made from polyanhydride co-polymers of fumaric and sebacic acids can be loaded with plasmid DNA. A plasmid with bacterial β-galactosidase

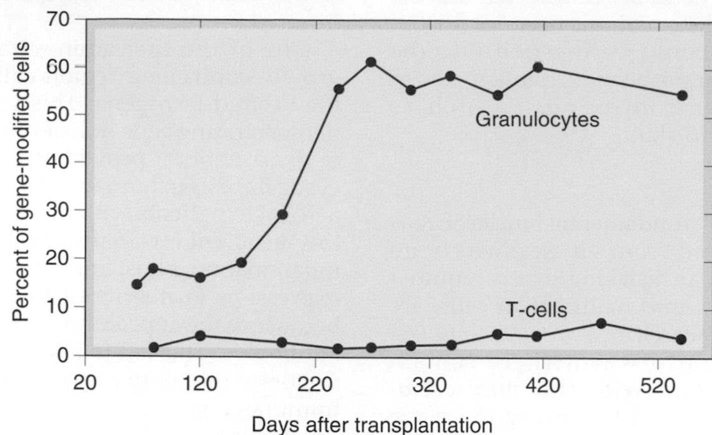

Fig. 5.4 Correcting an inherited defect using gene therapy. In this clinical trial, two patients with X-linked chronic granulomatous disease were transfused with GM-CSF (granulocyte-macrophage colony stimulating factor)-treated peripheral blood cells that had been genetically modified with a retroviral vector bearing the intact *gp91phox* gene ('in vitro protocol' – see text). The graph shows that the number of gene-modified peripheral blood leukocytes remained high for well over a year and this was accompanied by good levels of superoxide production in these cells – a clinical 'cure'. (Data redrawn from Ott, M.G., Schmidt, M., Schwarzwaelder, K., et al., 2006. Correction of X-linked chronic granulomatous disease by gene therapy, augmented by insertional activation of MDS1-EVI1, PRDM16 or SETBP1. Nat. Med. 12, 401–409.)

activity formulated in this way and given by mouth to rats has resulted, surprisingly, in systemic absorption and expression of the bacterial enzyme in the rat liver, raising the eventual possibility of oral gene therapy (Kutzler and Weiner, 2008).

Plasmid DNA

Surprisingly, plasmid DNA itself ('naked DNA', obtained from bacterial cultures) enters the nucleus of some cells and is expressed, albeit much less efficiently than when it is packaged in a vector. Such DNA carries no risk of viral replication and is not usually immunogenic, but it cannot be targeted precisely. Nevertheless, there is considerable interest in the use of naked DNA in vaccines, as the technique has several theoretical advantages (Kutzler and Weiner, 2008; Liu, 2011). At the time of writing the first DNA vaccine, **ZyCoV-D** (for prophylactic treatment of COVID-19 infection), developed by the Indian pharmaceutical company Zydus Cadilla, has been approved for global usage. Many others are in development.

CONTROLLING GENE EXPRESSION

To realise the full potential of gene therapy, it is not enough to transfer the gene selectively to the desired target cells and maintain acceptable expression of its product - difficult though these goals are. It is also essential that the activity of the gene can be controlled. Historically, it was the realisation of the magnitude of this task that diverted attention from the haemoglobinopathies (which were among the first projected targets of gene therapy). Correction of these disorders demands an appropriate balance of normal α- and β-globin chain synthesis to be effective, and for this, and many other potential applications, precisely controlled gene expression, are essential.

It has not yet proved routinely possible to control transgenes precisely in human recipients, but there are techniques that may eventually enable us to achieve this goal. One hinges upon the use of an *inducible expression system*. This is a fairly standard laboratory technique whereby the inserted gene also includes, for example, a **doxycycline**-inducible promoter such that expression of the gene can be switched on or off by treatment with, or withdrawal of, the antibiotic.

The control of transfected genes is important in gene targeting as well. By splicing the gene of interest with a tissue-specific promoter, it should be possible to restrict expression of the gene to the target tissue. Such an approach has been used in the design of gene therapy constructs for use in ovarian cancer, the cells of which express several proteins at high abundance, including the proteinase inhibitor SLP1. In combination with the SLP1 promoter, plasmids carrying various genes were successfully and selectively expressed in ovarian cancer cell lines (Wolf and Jenkins, 2002).

SAFETY AND SOCIETAL ISSUES

Experiments or protocols involving the transfer of genetic material tend to provoke deep unease in some sectors of society - witness the GM crop debate (see Freire et al., 2014), the 'vaccine hesitancy' that we have seen during the recent COVID-19 pandemic as well as the controversy surrounding the MMR vaccine and autism. While this may be traced partly to ignorance or prejudice (not helped by society's politicisation of science and health matters), it is nevertheless a problem that can hinder the introduction of new agents. There is a broad consensus that the *Weismann barrier*[8] should not be breached and so a moratorium has been agreed on making alterations to the DNA of germ cells (which could influence future generations) and gene therapy trials have focused on somatic cells only.

[8]Named after August Weismann (1834–1914), who formulated the concept that inheritance utilises only germ, and not somatic, cells.

Societal issues aside, the technique does raise a number of specific concerns that generally relate to the use of viral vectors. These are usually selected because they are non-pathogenic, or modified to render them innocuous, but there is a concern that such agents might still acquire virulence during use. Retroviruses, which insert randomly into host DNA, may damage the genome and interfere with the protective mechanisms that normally regulate the cell cycle (see Ch. 6), and if they happen to disrupt essential cellular functions, this could increase the risk of malignancy.[9]

Another problem is that immunogenic viral proteins may elicit an inflammatory response. Initial clinical experience was reassuring, but the death of Jesse Gelsinger, an 18-year-old volunteer in a gene therapy trial for the non-fatal disease *ornithine decarboxylase deficiency* (which can be controlled, albeit tediously, by diet and drugs anyway), led to the appreciation that such safety concerns are very real (see Marshall, 1999).

THERAPEUTIC APPLICATIONS

Despite the plethora of technical problems and safety concerns, there have been some encouraging successes and continuing interest in the sector as evidenced by the huge number of papers describing, or proposing, gene therapy solutions for a variety of clinical conditions, ranging from overactive bladder and defective colour vision to life-threatening cancers and neurological conditions. Even so, there are at present only a handful of gene therapies actually approved. Some of these are listed in Table 5.7.

The first to be approved was **Gendicine**, a treatment which aimed to replace the faulty p53 protein that caused head and neck cancer, which was licensed in China in 2003. The European Medicines Agency granted its first license for a gene therapy product, **Alipogene tiparvovec (Glybera),** in 2012.[10] This is an adeno-associated virus construct that delivers a correct copy of lipoprotein lipase to patients lacking this enzyme (a very rare disorder that causes severe pancreatitis), and in 2016, **Strimvelis** was also approved in Europe. This is an ex vivo gene therapy approach to replace adenosine deaminase which is absent from children with a rare (~15 patients per year in Europe) type of severe compromised immunodeficiency (SCID). In the United States, the first gene therapy was approved in 2017: **Kymriah (tisagenlecleucel)**, a treatment for acute lymphoblastic leukaemia. This is also based upon an ex vivo technique whereby T cells from the patient are genetically modified to contain a chimeric antigen receptor (CAR-T) cell, which, when reinfused into the patient, destroys leukaemia cells. Currently, gene therapies for spinal muscular atrophy (one of the common fatal inherited diseases of infancy) and large B-cell lymphoma command the highest market share of this sector.

[9]This risk is more than a theoretical possibility; several children treated for *severe combined immunodeficiency* (SCID) with a retrovirus vector developed a leukaemia-like illness (Woods et al., 2006). The retroviral vector was shown to have inserted itself into a gene called *LMO-2*, mutations of which are associated with childhood cancers.

[10]With an annual cost of at least US$1 million per treatment, Glybera was at that time dubbed 'the most expensive medicine in the world'. This dubious honour has now passed to Zolgensma at £1.79 million per treatment.

FUTURE DIRECTIONS

This biopharmaceutical sector of the market is growing rapidly and major advances appear with bewildering speed.

One field which is especially promising is *gene editing*. Rather than replacing a gene in its entirety, this technique, which is similar in scope to the RNA pharmaceuticals, actually aims to 'edit' the faulty gene in the cell. The mechanism for accomplishing this is a system of gene editing originally discovered in bacteria. Bearing the rather daunting name *clustered regulatory interspersed short palindromic repeats (CRISPR)* it can selectively target nucleases (notably *Cas9*) to precisely edit genes of interest.[11] Viruses can deliver the CRISPR-Cas9 components, thereby acting as delivery vehicles for the biochemical machinery required to repair faulty genes in humans (see for example, Gori et al., 2015; Gee et al., 2017). gRNAs can be used in conjunction with this technique to provide selectivity and specificity. At the time of writing, several studies are underway around the world to use this technique for the treatment of haemoglobinopathies. This new field, together with an assessment of the likely problems and hurdles to overcome, is reviewed by Cornel et al. (2019).

Also worth mentioning is the fact that some small molecule drugs have, rather surprisingly, been discovered to produce their effects through an action on RNA or DNA targets. These include the naturally occurring antibiotics which act on the ribozymes which catalyse the synthesis of growing protein chains at the ribosomes (see Ch. 52) and **ataluren**, a drug which despite being undoubtedly in the small molecule class (m.w. 284.25 kDa) can actually reduce the probability of premature 'stop codons' (such as occur in dystrophin) by interfering with the synthesis of full-length proteins at the ribosomes. Because of this action, it can be used to treat Duchenne muscular dystrophy. Even more extraordinary was the discovery (Jones and Taylor, 1980) that the drug **5′-azacytidine** (see Ch. 57), used for years as an anticancer drug, actually inhibits DNA methylation, in other words it can influence the *epigenetic modification* of genes (see Ghasemi, 2020, for a comprehensive overview of drugs that act through various epigenetic mechanisms). The idea that drugs can work – or can even be designed to work through epigenetic mechanisms – is revolutionary and could open the way to all sorts of useful pharmacology. It would be possible for example to cause fully differentiated cells to revert to stem cells. While this is possible now, this is a technically difficult procedure.

While oligonucleotide and even protein biopharmaceuticals share some of the characteristics of other drugs described in this book, the same cannot be said for gene therapy and this raises some important questions. Is a gene a 'drug'? Is a virus a 'drug'? Is a GM stem cell a 'drug'? You could argue that they satisfy the broad definition that we posited at the start of this book in that 'administration to a living organism produces a biological effect', but it does not seem sensible to discuss the 'pharmacology' of gene therapy as such and most would consider it beyond the scope of our subject at present. They are therapies nonetheless. A gene has no inherent pharmacodynamic or pharmacokinetic properties; most of the toxicity and adverse effects mentioned here are due to the vector or carrier and not the gene itself.

[11]Emmanuelle Charpentier and Jennifer Doudna won the 2020 Nobel Prize for Chemistry for this extraordinary discovery.

And how do you assess the optimal dose of a 'drug' that is self-replicating? Having said that, we make no apologies for including gene therapy in this section. It is becoming a major therapeutic modality and physicians and pharmacologists alike will be called on to assess and comment on the biological effects it produces.

REFERENCES AND FURTHER READING

General reviews on biopharmaceuticals and gene therapy

Agoram, B.M., 2009. Use of pharmacokinetic/pharmacodynamic modelling for starting dose selection in first-in-human trials of high-risk biologics. Br. J. Clin. Pharmacol. 67, 153–160.

Bender, E., 2016. Gene therapy: industrial strength. Nature 537, S57–S59.

Cebadera Miranda, E., Castillo Ruiz-Cabello, M.V., Camara Hurtado, M., 2020. Food biopharmaceuticals as part of a sustainable bioeconomy: edible vaccines case study. Nat. Biotechnol. 59, 74–79.

Evans, S.E., Harrington, T., Rodriguez Rivero, M.C., Rognin, E., Tuladhar, T., Daly, R., 2021. 2D and 3D inkjet printing of biopharmaceuticals – a review of trends and future perspectives in research and manufacturing. Int. J. Pharm. 599, 120443.

Harding, F.A., Stickler, M.M., Razo, J., DuBridge, R.B., 2010. The immunogenicity of humanized and fully human antibodies: residual immunogenicity resides in the CDR regions. MAbs 2, 256–265.

Homayun, B., Lin, X., Choi, H.J., 2019. Challenges and recent progress in oral drug delivery systems for biopharmaceuticals. Pharmaceutics 11, 1–29.

Huebbers, J.W., Buyel, J.F., 2021. On the verge of the market – plant factories for the automated and standardized production of biopharmaceuticals. Biotechnol. Adv. 46, 107681.

Jones, P.A., Taylor, S.M., 1980. Cellular differentiation, cytidine analogs and DNA methylation. Cell 20, 85–93.

Kang, M., Lu, Y., Chen, S., Tian, F., 2018. Harnessing the power of an expanded genetic code toward next-generation biopharmaceuticals. Curr. Opin. Chem. Biol. 46, 123–129.

Kaplon, H., Reichert, J.M., 2021. Antibodies to watch in 2021. mAbs 13, 1860476.

Kutzler, M.A., Weiner, D.B., 2008. DNA vaccines: ready for prime time? Nat. Rev. Genet. 9, 776–788.

Liu, M.A., 2011. DNA vaccines: an historical perspective and view to the future. Immunol. Rev. 239, 62–84.

Lu, R.M., Hwang, Y.C., Liu, I.J., et al. 2020. Development of therapeutic antibodies for the treatment of diseases. J. Biomed. Sci. 27, 1.

Moon, K.B., Park, J.S., Park, Y.I., et al. 2019. Development of systems for the production of plant-derived biopharmaceuticals. Plants (Basel) 9, 1–21.

Rader, R.A., 2008. (Re)defining biopharmaceutical. Nat. Biotechnol. 26, 743–751.

Regolado, A., 2016. The world's most expensive medicine is a bust. MIT Technology Review. May issue. Available at: https://www.technologyreview.com/2016/05/04/245988/the-worlds-most-expensive-medicine-is-a-bust/.

Revers, L., Furczon, E., 2010. An introduction to biologics and biosimilars. Part II: subsequent entry biologics: biosame or biodifferent? Can. Pharm. J. 143, 184–191.

Rosales-Mendoza, S., Solis-Andrade, K.I., Marquez-Escobar, V.A., Gonzalez-Ortega, O., Banuelos-Hernandez, B., 2020. Current advances in the algae-made biopharmaceuticals field. Expert. Opin. Biol. Ther. 20, 751–766.

Taunt, H.N., Stoffels, L., Purton, S., 2018. Green biologics: the algal chloroplast as a platform for making biopharmaceuticals. Bioengineered 9, 48–54.

Verma, I.M., Somia, N., 1997. Gene therapy – promises, problems and prospects. Nature 389, 239–242.

Wrapp, D., De Vlieger, D., Corbett, K.S., et al., 2020. Structural basis for potent neutralization of betacoronaviruses by single-domain camelid antibodies. Cell 181, 1004–1015.e15.

Walker, R.S.K., Pretorius, I.S., 2018. Applications of yeast synthetic biology geared towards the production of biopharmaceuticals. Genes (Basel) 9, 340.

Walsh, G., 2004. Second-generation biopharmaceuticals. Eur. J. Pharm. Biopharm. 58, 185–196.

Wirth, T., Parker, N., Yla-Herttuala, S., 2013. History of gene therapy. Gene 525, 162–169.

Xu, H., Li, Z., Si, J., 2014. Nanocarriers in gene therapy: a review. J. Biomed. Nanotechnol. 10, 3483–3507.

Yu, A.M., Choi, Y.H., Tu, M.J., 2020. RNA drugs and RNA targets for small molecules: principles, progress, and challenges. Pharmacol. Rev. 72, 862–898.

Zhao, L., Ren, T.H., Wang, D.D., 2012. Clinical pharmacology considerations in biologics development. Acta Pharmacol. Sin. 33, 1339–1347.

Problems

Ahmed, B., Zafar, M., Qadir, M.I., 2019. Review: oncogenic insertional mutagenesis as a consequence of retroviral gene therapy for X-linked severe combined immunodeficiency disease. Crit. Rev. Eukaryot. Gene Expr. 29, 511–520.

Check, E., 2002. A tragic setback. Nature 420, 116–118.

Delhove, J., Osenk, I., Prichard, I., Donnelley, M., 2020. Public acceptability of gene therapy and gene editing for human use: a systematic review. Hum. Gene Ther. 31, 20–46.

Freire, J.E., Medeiros, S.C., Lopes Neto, A.V., et al., 2014. Bioethical conflicts of gene therapy: a brief critical review. Rev. Assoc. Med. Bras. (1992) 60, 520–524.

Marshall, E., 1999. Gene therapy death prompts review of adenovirus vector. Science 286, 2244–2245.

Muller, P.Y., Brennan, F.R., 2009. Safety assessment and dose selection for first-in-human clinical trials with immunomodulatory monoclonal antibodies. Clin. Pharmacol. Ther. 85, 247–258.

Reijers, J.A.A., Malone, K.E., Bajramovic, J.J., Verbeek, R., Burggraaf, J., Moerland, M., 2019. Adverse immunostimulation caused by impurities: the dark side of biopharmaceuticals. Br. J. Clin. Pharmacol. 85, 1418–1426.

Richter, W.F., Gallati, H., Schiller, C.D., 1999. Animal pharmacokinetics of the tumor necrosis factor receptor-immunoglobulin fusion protein lenercept and their extrapolation to humans. Drug Metab. Dispos. 27, 21–25.

Stobbart, L., Murtagh, M.J., Rapley, T., et al., 2007. We saw human Guinea pigs explode. BMJ 334, 566–567.

Woods, N.B., Bottero, V., Schmidt, M., von Kalle, C., Verma, I.M., 2006. Gene therapy: therapeutic gene causing lymphoma. Nature 440, 1123.

Therapeutic uses

Ahangarzadeh, S., Payandeh, Z., Arezumand, R., Shahzamani, K., Yarian, F., Alibakhshi, A., 2020. An update on antiviral antibody-based biopharmaceuticals. Int. Immunopharmacol. 86, 106760.

Alnasser, S.M., 2021. Review on mechanistic strategy of gene therapy in the treatment of disease. Gene 769, 145246.

Cornel, M.C., Howard, H.C., Lim, D., Bonham, V.L., Wartiovaara, K., 2019. Moving towards a cure in genetics: what is needed to bring somatic gene therapy to the clinic? Eur. J. Hum. Genet. 27, 484–487.

Gee, P., Xu, H., Hotta, A., 2017. Cellular reprogramming, genome editing, and alternative CRISPR Cas9 technologies for precise gene therapy of Duchenne muscular dystrophy. Stem Cells Int. 2017, 8765154.

Geary, R.S., Baker, B.F., Crooke, S.T., 2015. Clinical and preclinical pharmacokinetics and pharmacodynamics of mipomersen (Kynamro^R): a second-generation antisense oligonucleotide inhibitor of apolipoprotein B. Clin. Pharmacokinet. 54, 133–146.

Ghasemi, S., 2020. Cancer's epigenetic drugs: where are they in the cancer medicines? Pharmacogenomics J. 20, 367–379.

Gori, J.L., Hsu, P.D., Maeder, M.L., Shen, S., Welstead, G.G., Bumcrot, D., 2015. Delivery and specificity of CRISPR-Cas9 genome editing technologies for human gene therapy. Hum. Gene Ther. 26, 443–451.

Hutmacher, C., Neri, D., 2019. Antibody-cytokine fusion proteins: biopharmaceuticals with immunomodulatory properties for cancer therapy. Adv. Drug Deliv. Rev. 141, 67–91.

Murer, P., Neri, D., 2019. Antibody-cytokine fusion proteins: a novel class of biopharmaceuticals for the therapy of cancer and of chronic inflammation. Nat. Biotechnol. 52, 42–53.

Ott, M.G., Schmidt, M., Schwarzwaelder, K., et al., 2006. Correction of X-linked chronic granulomatous disease by gene therapy, augmented by insertional activation of MDS1-EVI1, PRDM16 or SETBP1. Nat. Med. 12, 401–409.

Wolf, J.K., Jenkins, A.D., 2002. Gene therapy for ovarian cancer (review). Int. J. Oncol. 21, 461–468.

Cell proliferation, apoptosis, repair and regeneration

6

OVERVIEW

About 10 billion new cells are created daily in us through cell division and this must be counterbalanced by the elimination of a similar number from the body in an ordered manner. This chapter explains how this homeostasis is managed. We deal with the life and death of the cell – the processes of replication, proliferation, apoptosis, repair and regeneration and how these relate to the actions of drugs. We begin with cell replication. We explain how stimulation by growth factors causes cells to divide and then consider the interaction of how these cells may interact with the extracellular matrix (ECM) which regulates further cell proliferation and development. We describe the crucial phenomenon of apoptosis (the programmed series of events that lead to cell's controlled death), outlining the changes that occur in a cell that is preparing to die and the intracellular pathways that culminate in its demise. We explain how these processes relate to the repair of damaged tissue, to the possibility of its regeneration and whether there is scope for modulating this using novel drugs.

CELL PROLIFERATION

Cell proliferation is, of course, a fundamental biological event. It is integral to many physiological and pathological processes including growth, healing, repair, hypertrophy, hyperplasia and the development of tumours. Because cells need oxygen and nutrients to survive, *angiogenesis* (the development of new blood vessels) is necessary before many of these processes can occur.

Proliferating cells go through what is termed *the cell cycle*, during which they replicate all their components and then divide into two identical daughter cells.[1] The process is tightly regulated by signalling pathways, including receptor tyrosine kinases or receptor-linked kinases and the mitogen-activated protein kinase (MAP kinase) cascade (see Ch. 3). In all cases, the pathways eventually lead to transcription of the genes that control the cell cycle.

THE CELL CYCLE

In the adult, few cells divide repeatedly and most remain in a quiescent phase outside the cycle in the phase termed G_0 (Fig. 6.1). Some cells such as neurons and skeletal muscle cells (considered to be 'terminally differentiated') spend all their lifetime in G_0, whereas others being more stem cell–like in phenotype, including bone marrow cells and the epithelium of the gastrointestinal tract, divide daily.

The cell cycle is an ordered sequential series of phases (see Fig. 6.1). These are known as S (Synthesis), M (Mitosis) and G (Gap between S or M phases), and they always occur in this order:

- G_1: (Gap1) preparation for DNA synthesis
- S: (Synthesis) DNA synthesis and chromosome duplication of the parental cell
- G_2: (Gap2) preparation for division
- M: (Mitosis) division into two identical daughter cells.

In cells that are dividing continuously, G_1, S and G_2 comprise the *interphase* – the phase between one mitosis and the next.

Cell division requires the controlled timing of the critical S phase and M phases. Entry into each of these phases is tightly regulated at *check points* (restriction points) at the start of the S and M phases. Any DNA damage stops the cycle at one or other of these check points to allow repair and thus maintain the integrity of our DNA sequence in each subsequent cell. This process is critical for the maintenance of genetic stability. Failure of the check points to stop the cycle when it is appropriate to do so leads to genetic instability, which is a hallmark of cancer.[2]

Quiescent (G_0) cells enter G_1 after exposure to chemical mediators, some of which are associated with damage. For example, a wound can stimulate a quiescent skin cell to divide, thus repairing the lesion. The impetus for a cell to enter the cycle (i.e. to move from G_0 into G_1) may be *growth factors* acting on *growth factor receptors*, although the action of other types of ligands on G protein–coupled receptors (see Ch. 3) can also initiate this process.

Growth factors stimulate the synthesis of both positive regulators of the cell cycle that control the changes necessary for cell division and negative regulators that counterbalance the positive regulators. The maintenance of normal cell numbers in tissues and organs requires a balance between the positive and the negative regulatory signals. *Apoptosis*[3] also controls cell numbers.

POSITIVE REGULATORS OF THE CELL CYCLE

The cycle begins when a growth factor acts on a quiescent cell, provoking it to divide. Growth factors stimulate production of two families of proteins, namely *cyclins* and serine/threonine protein kinases called *cyclin-dependent*

[1]Not strictly identical in the case of stem cells, as one differentiates and the other remains stem.

[2]The main daily job of our immune system is to detect and destroy cells which have genetic instability, which may become cancerous if missed. This immuno-surveillance removes thousands of incorrectly divided or dangerously damaged cells each day. Occasionally, our immune system will encounter a foreign body such as a virus or bacteria and will then 'moonlight' on that job for a while too.

[3]The term is originally a Greek word that describes the falling of leaves or petals from plants. Termed in 1972 by Professor James Cormack of Aberdeen University's Greek Department, the second 'p' is silent – APE oh TOE sis.

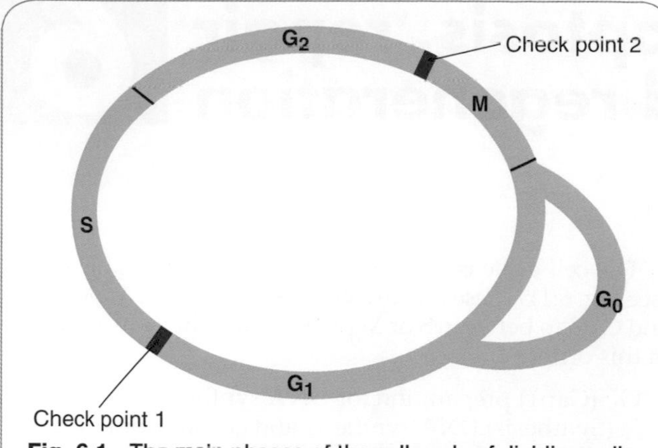

Fig. 6.1 The main phases of the cell cycle of dividing cells.

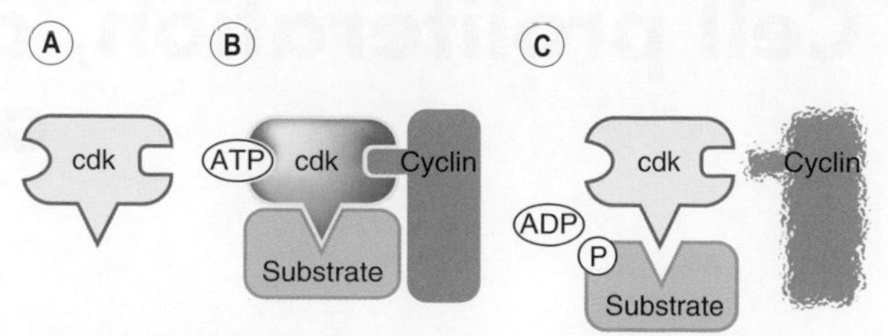

Fig. 6.2 Schematic representation of the activation of a cyclin-dependent kinase (cdk). (A) An inactive cdk. (B) The inactive cdk binds to a cyclin and is activated; it can now phosphorylate a specific protein substrate (e.g. an enzyme). (C) After the phosphorylating event, the cyclin is degraded.

kinases (cdks), coded for by the *delayed response* genes. The cdks sequentially phosphorylate various enzymes – activating some and inhibiting others – to coordinate the progression of the cell through the cycle.

Each cdk is inactive and must bind to a cyclin partner before it can phosphorylate its target protein(s). After such a phosphorylation event the cyclin is degraded (Fig. 6.2) by the *ubiquitin/protease system*. Here, several enzymes sequentially add small molecules of ubiquitin to the cyclin. The resulting ubiquitin polymer acts as an 'address label' that directs the cyclin to the *proteasome* where the polyubiquinated cyclin is readily degraded.

There are eight main groups of cyclins. According to the 'classical model' of the cell cycle (see Satyanarayana and Kaldis, 2009), those of principal importance in the control of the cycle are cyclins A, B, D and E. Each cyclin is associated with, and activates, a particular cdk. Cyclin A activates cdks 1 and 2; cyclin B, cdk 1; cyclin D, cdks 4 and 6; and cyclin E, cdk 2. Precise timing of each step is essential and many cycle proteins are degraded after they have carried out their functions.[4] The actions of the cyclin/cdk complexes throughout the cell cycle are depicted in Fig. 6.3.

The activity of these cyclin/cdk complexes is negatively modulated at one or other of the two check points, holding the cell before embarking onto its next stage. In quiescent G_0 cells, cyclin D is present in low concentration, and an important regulatory protein – the *Rb protein*[5] is hypophosphorylated (i.e. phosphorylated but not in a hyperphosphorylated state). This restrains the cell cycle at check point 1 by inhibiting the expression of several proteins critical for further cycle progression. The Rb protein accomplishes this by binding to transcription factors and preventing them from promoting expression of the genes that code for proteins (such as cyclins E and A, DNA polymerase, thymidine kinase and dihydrofolate reductase) needed for DNA replication during S phase. This configuration is maintained until a cell is instructed to divide thus:

- Growth factor action on a cell in G_0 propels it into G_1, which prepares the cell for S phase. The concentration of cyclin D increases and the cyclin D/cdk complex phosphorylates and activates the proteins required for DNA replication.
- In mid-G_1, the cyclin D/cdk complex phosphorylates the Rb protein, releasing a transcription factor that activates the genes for the components essential for the next phase – DNA synthesis. The action of the cyclin E/cdk complex is necessary for transition from G_1, past check point 1, into S phase.
- Once into S phase, the processes that have been set in motion cannot be reversed and the cell is committed to DNA replication and mitosis. Cyclin E/cdk and cyclin A/cdk regulate progress through the S phase, phosphorylating and thus activating the proteins/enzymes involved in DNA synthesis.
- In G_2 phase, the cell, which now has double the number of chromosomes, produces the messenger RNAs and proteins needed to duplicate all other cellular components for allocation to the two daughter cells.
- Cyclin A/cdk and cyclin B/cdk complexes are active during G_2 phase and are necessary for entry into M phase, i.e. for passing check point 2. The presence of cyclin B/cdk complexes in the nucleus is required for mitosis to commence.

Mitosis occurs in four stages:

- *Prophase.* The duplicated chromosomes (which are at this point a tangled mass in the nucleus) condense, each now consisting of two *daughter chromatids* (the original chromosome and an identical copy). These are released into the cytoplasm as the nuclear membrane disintegrates.
- *Metaphase.* The chromosomes are aligned at the equator of the cell (see Fig. 6.3).
- *Anaphase.* A specialised cytoskeletal device, the mitotic apparatus, captures the chromosomes and draws them to opposite poles of the dividing cell (see Fig. 6.3).
- *Telophase.* A nuclear membrane forms round each set of chromosomes. Finally, the cytoplasm divides between the two forming daughter cells. The last step in mitosis is *cytokinesis*, where the plasma membrane between each daughter cell is pinched-

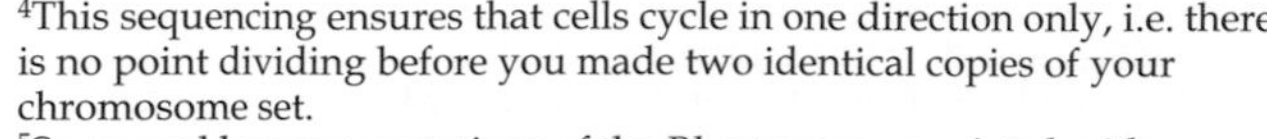

[4]This sequencing ensures that cells cycle in one direction only, i.e. there is no point dividing before you made two identical copies of your chromosome set.

[5]So named because mutations of the *Rb* gene are associated with retinoblastoma tumours.

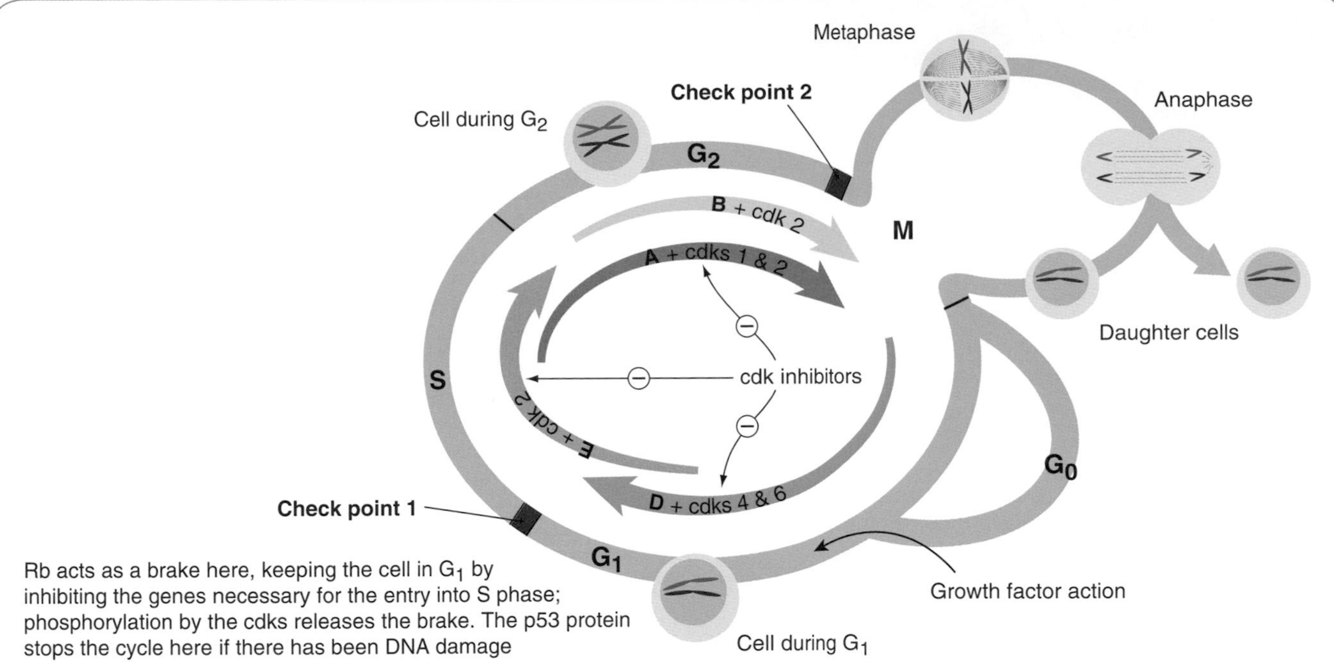

Fig. 6.3 Schematic diagram of the cell cycle, showing the role of the cyclin/cyclin-dependent kinase (cdk) complexes. The processes outlined in the cycle occur inside a cell such as the one shown in Fig. 6.4. A quiescent cell (in G_0 phase), when stimulated to divide by growth factors, is propelled into G_1 phase and prepares for DNA synthesis. Progress through the cycle is determined by sequential action of the cyclin/cdk complexes – depicted here by *coloured arrows*, the arrows being given the names of the relevant cyclins: D, E, A and B. The cdks are given next to the relevant cyclins. The thickness of each arrow represents the intensity of the cdk action at that point in the cycle. The activity of the cdks is regulated by cdk inhibitors. If there is DNA damage, the products of the tumour suppressor gene *p53* arrest the cycle at check point 1, allowing for repair. If repair fails, apoptosis (see Fig. 6.5) is initiated. The state of the chromosomes is shown schematically in each G phase – as a single pair in G_1, and each duplicated and forming two daughter chromatids in G_2. Some changes that occur during mitosis (metaphase, anaphase) are shown in a subsidiary circle. After the mitotic division, the daughter cells may enter G_1 or G_0 phase. *Rb*, Retinoblastoma gene.

off and split.[6] Each daughter cell will be in G_0 phase and will remain there unless stimulated into G_1 phase once more, as described earlier.

During metaphase, the cyclin A and B complexes phosphorylate cytoskeletal proteins, nuclear histones and possibly components of the *mitotic spindle* (the microtubules along which the chromatids are pulled during metaphase).

NEGATIVE REGULATORS OF THE CELL CYCLE

One of the main negative regulators is the Rb protein, which restrains the cell cycle when it is hypophosphorylated.

Inhibitors of the cdks also serve as negative regulators, their main action being at check points. There are two known families of inhibitors: the *CIP family* (cdk inhibitory proteins, also termed KIP or kinase inhibitory proteins) – proteins p21, p27 and p57; and the *Ink family* (inhibitors of kinases) – proteins p16, p19 and p15.

Protein p21 is a good example of the role of a cyclin/cdk inhibitor. It is under the control of the *p53* gene – a particularly important negative regulator which is relevant in carcinogenesis – that operates at check point 1.

[6]The entire cell cycle process, in order, is summed up in the acronym IPMATC: interphase, prophase, metaphase, anaphase, telophase and cytokinesis.

Inhibition of the cycle at check point 1

The *p53* gene has been called the 'guardian of the genome'. It codes for the p53 protein, a transcription factor found in only low concentrations in normal healthy cells. However, following DNA damage, the protein accumulates and activates the transcription of several genes, one of which codes for p21. Protein p21 inactivates cyclin/cdk complexes, thus Rb phosphorylation is prevented, and it becomes hypophosphorylated. This causes arrest of the cycle at check point 1, allowing DNA repair to take place. If the repair is successful, the cycle proceeds past check point 1 into S phase. If the repair is unsuccessful, the *p53* gene triggers apoptosis or cell suicide.[7]

Inhibition of the cycle at check point 2

DNA damage can arrest the cycle at check point 2, but the mechanisms involved are poorly understood. Inhibition of the accumulation of cyclin B/cdk complex in the nucleus seems to be a factor. For more detail on the control of the cell cycle, see section on microRNAs later in this chapter and Swanton (2004).

[7]Thus p53 is 'the guardian of the genome', preventing any unrepairable errors or genomic instability that occur in a cell from passing on to daughter cells by killing the cell and another healthy cell will replace the p53-destroyed cell. It is better for an organism to kill off less than perfect cells than to have any error whatsoever kept for future generations – 'the needs of the many outweigh the needs of the few' as Spock would say.

The cell cycle

- The term *cell cycle* refers to the sequence of events that take place within a cell as it prepares for division. The quiescent or resting state is called G_0.
- Growth factor action stimulates a cell in G_0 to enter the cycle.
- The phases of the cell cycle are:
  - G_1: preparation for DNA synthesis
  - S: DNA synthesis
  - G_2: preparation for division
  - M, mitosis: division into two daughter cells
- In G_0 phase, a hypophosphorylated protein, coded for by the *Rb* gene, arrests the cycle by inhibiting expression of critical factors necessary for DNA replication.
- Progress through the cycle is controlled by specific kinases (cdks) that are activated by binding to specific proteins termed cyclins.
- Four main cyclins D, E, A and B, together with their cdk complexes, drive the cycle; cyclin D/cdk also releases the Rb protein-mediated inhibition.

There are protein inhibitors of cdks in the cell. Protein p21 is particularly important; it is expressed when DNA damage triggers transcription of gene *p53* and arrests the cycle at check point 1.

INTERACTIONS BETWEEN CELLS, GROWTH FACTORS AND THE EXTRACELLULAR MATRIX

Cell proliferation is regulated by the integrated interplay between growth factors, cells themselves, the ECM and the matrix metalloproteinases (MMPs). The ECM is secreted by the cells and provides a supportive framework. It also profoundly influences cell behaviour by signalling through the cell's integrins (proteins on a cell's extracellular surface that sense the ECM and signal to the cell what environment it is in or which cell neighbours it has). Matrix expression by cells is regulated by growth factors and cytokines (see Järveläinen et al., 2009; Verrecchia and Mauviel, 2007). The activity of some growth factors is, in turn, determined by the matrix, because they are sequestered by matrix components and released by proteinases (e.g. MMPs) secreted by the cells.

The action of growth factors acting through receptor tyrosine kinases or receptor-coupled kinases (see Ch. 3) is a fundamental part of these processes. Important examples include *fibroblast growth factor* (FGF), *epidermal growth factor* (EGF), *platelet-dependent growth factor* (PDGF), *vascular endothelial growth factor* (VEGF) and *transforming growth factor* (TGF)-β.

The main components of the ECM are:

- Fibre-forming elements, e.g. *collagen species* (the main proteins of the matrix) and *elastin.*
- Non-fibre-forming elements, e.g. proteoglycans, glycoproteins and adhesive proteins such as *fibronectin.* Proteoglycans have a growth-regulating role, in part by functioning as a reservoir of sequestered growth factors. Other elements are associated with the cell surface, where they bind cells to the matrix. Adhesive proteins link the various elements of the matrix together and also form links between the cells and the matrix through cell surface integrins.

Other proteins in the ECM are *thrombospondin* and *osteopontin*, which are not structural elements but modulate cell–matrix interactions and repair processes. The production of the ECM components is regulated by growth factors, particularly TGF-β.

The ECM is a target for drug action. Both beneficial and adverse effects have been reported. Thus, glucocorticoids decrease collagen synthesis in chronic inflammation and cyclo-oxygenase (COX)-2 inhibitors can modify fibrotic processes apparently through an action on TGF-β. Statins can decrease fibrosis by inhibiting angiotensin-induced connective tissue growth factor production (Rupérez et al., 2007) and reducing MMP expression. This may contribute to their effects in cardiovascular diseases (Tousoulis et al., 2010). The adverse actions of some drugs attributable to an effect on the ECM include the osteoporosis and skin thinning caused by glucocorticoids (discussed in Järveläinen et al., 2009). The ECM is also an important target in the search for new drugs that regulate tissue repair.

THE ROLE OF INTEGRINS

Integrins are transmembrane kinase-linked receptors (see Ch. 3) comprising α and β subunits. Interaction with the ECM elements (e.g. fibronectin) triggers various cell responses, such as cytoskeletal rearrangement (not considered here) and co-regulation of growth factor function.

Intracellular signalling by both growth factor receptors and integrins is important for optimal cell proliferation (Fig. 6.4). Following integrin stimulation an adapter protein and an enzyme *(focal adhesion kinase [FAK])* activate the kinase cascade initiating growth factor signalling. There is extensive cross-talk between the integrin and growth factor pathways (Streuli and Akhtar, 2009). Autophosphorylation of growth factor receptors (see Ch. 3) is enhanced by integrin activation, and integrin-mediated adhesion to the ECM (see Fig. 6.4) not only suppresses the concentrations of cdk inhibitors but also is required for the expression of cyclins A and D, and therefore for the progression of the cell cycle. Furthermore, integrin activation inhibits apoptosis (see later), further facilitating growth factor action (see reviews by Barczyk et al., 2010 and Gahmberg et al., 2009).

Several therapeutic monoclonal antibodies, including **natalizumab** (used to treat multiple sclerosis) and **abciximab** (an antithrombotic; see Ch. 23), target integrins.

THE ROLE OF MATRIX METALLOPROTEINASES

Degradation of the ECM by MMPs is necessary for tissue growth, repair and remodelling. When growth factors stimulate a cell to enter the cell cycle, they also stimulate the secretion of MMPs (as inactive precursors), which then sculpt the matrix, producing the local changes necessary to accommodate the increased cell numbers. Metalloproteinases in turn release growth factors from the ECM and, in some cases (e.g. interleukin [IL]-1β), process them from precursor to their active form. The action of these enzymes is regulated by tissue inhibitors

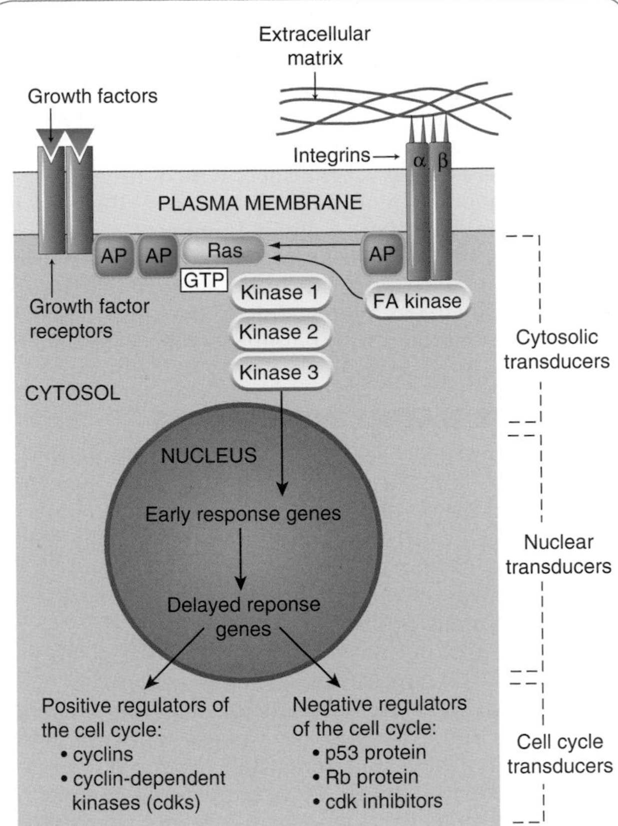

Fig. 6.4 Simplified diagram of the effect of growth factors on a cell in G_0. The overall effect of growth factor action is the generation of the cell cycle transducers. A cell such as the one depicted will then embark on G_1 phase of the cell cycle. Most growth factor receptors have integral tyrosine kinase (see Fig. 3.17). These receptors dimerise, then cross-phosphorylate their tyrosine residues. The early cytosolic transducers include proteins that bind to the phosphorylated tyrosine residues. Optimum effect requires cooperation with integrin action. Integrins (which have α and β subunits) connect the extracellular matrix with intracellular signalling pathways and also with the cell cytoskeleton (not shown here). G protein–coupled receptors can also stimulate cell proliferation, because their intracellular pathways can connect with the Ras/kinase cascade (not shown). *AP*, Adapter protein; *cdk*, cyclin-dependent kinase; *FA kinase*, focal adhesion kinase; *Rb*, retinoblastoma protein.

of metalloproteinases (TIMPs), which are also secreted by local cells.

In addition to their physiological function, metalloproteinases are involved in the tissue destruction that accompanies various diseases, such as rheumatoid arthritis, osteoarthritis, periodontitis, macular degeneration and myocardial restenosis. They also have a critical role in the growth, invasion and metastasis of tumours (Clark et al., 2008; Jackson et al., 2017; Marastoni et al., 2008). Because of this, much effort has gone into developing synthetic MMP inhibitors for treating cancers and inflammatory disorders, although clinical trials so far have shown limited efficacy and significant adverse effects (see Gialeli et al., 2011). **Doxycycline**, an antibiotic, also inhibits MMPs, and is used experimentally for this purpose.

Interactions between cells, growth factors and the matrix

- Cells secrete the components of the ECM and become embedded in this tissue.
- The ECM influences the growth and behaviour of the cells. It also acts as a reservoir of growth factors.
- Integrins are transmembrane cellular receptors that can interact with elements of the ECM. They modulate growth factor signalling pathways and also mediate cytoskeletal adjustments within the cell.
- Growth factors cause cells to release metalloproteinases that degrade the local matrix so that it can accommodate the increase in cell numbers.
- In turn, metalloproteinases release growth factors from the ECM and can activate some that are present in precursor form.

ANGIOGENESIS

Angiogenesis, which normally accompanies cell proliferation, entails the formation of new capillaries from existing small blood vessels. Without this, new tissues (including tumours) cannot feed and grow. Angiogenic stimuli include cytokines and various growth factors, in particular *VEGF*. The sequence of events in angiogenesis is as follows:

1. The basement membrane is degraded locally by proteinases.
2. Endothelial cells migrate out, forming a 'sprout'.
3. Following these leading cells, other endothelial cells proliferate under the influence of VEGF.
4. Matrix material is laid down around the new capillary.

A monoclonal antibody, **bevacizumab**, which neutralises VEGF, is used as adjunct treatment for various cancers (see Ch. 57), and following injection into the eye, to treat age-related macular degeneration, a condition in which retinal blood vessels over-proliferate, causing blindness (see Ch. 27).

APOPTOSIS AND CELL REMOVAL

Apoptosis is cell 'suicide' in a controlled and orderly manner. It is regulated by a built-in genetically programmed self-destruct mechanism consisting of a specific sequence of biochemical events. It is thus unlike *necrosis*, which is a wholly disorganised disintegration of damaged cells that releases substances which trigger the inflammatory response.[8]

Apoptosis plays an essential role in embryogenesis, shaping organs during development by eliminating cells that have become redundant. It is the mechanism that each day unobtrusively removes some 10 billion cells from the

[8]There are other several other forms of programmed cell death (PCD) including *autophagy* and (confusingly) *programmed necrosis* or *necroptosis* (see Galluzzi et al., 2018). Here we will focus on apoptosis, also known as 'Type I PCD'.

human body. It is involved in numerous physiological events, including the shedding of the intestinal lining, the death of time-expired neutrophils and the turnover of tissues as the newborn infant grows to maturity. It is the basis for the development of self-tolerance in the immune system (see Ch. 7) and acts as a first-line defence against carcinogenic mutations by purging cells that could become malignant.

Disorders of apoptosis are also implicated in the pathophysiology of many conditions, including:

- chronic neurodegenerative diseases such as Alzheimer's and Parkinson's disease and multiple sclerosis (see Ch. 40);
- conditions with acute tissue damage or cell loss, such as myocardial infarction (see Ch. 22), stroke and spinal cord injury (see Ch. 40);
- depletion of T cells in HIV infection (see Ch. 53);
- osteoarthritis (see Ch. 36);
- haematological diseases, such as aplastic anaemia (see Ch. 24);
- evasion of the immune response by cancer cells and resistance to cancer chemotherapy (see Ch. 57);
- autoimmune/inflammatory diseases such as myasthenia gravis (see Ch. 14), rheumatoid arthritis (see Ch. 25), and bronchial asthma (see Ch. 28);
- viral infections with ineffective eradication of virus-infected cells (see Ch. 53).

Apoptosis is particularly important in the regulation of the immune response and in the many conditions in which it is an underlying component. There is evidence that T cells have a negative regulatory pathway controlled by surface *PCD receptors* (e.g. the PD-1 receptor), and that there is normally a balance between the stimulatory pathways triggered by antigens and this negative regulatory apoptosis-inducing pathway. The balance is important in the maintenance of peripheral tolerance. A disturbance of this balance is seen in autoimmune disease, in the 'exhaustion' of T cells in chronic viral diseases such as HIV, and possibly in tumour escape from immune destruction (Zha et al., 2004). Indeed PD-1 generally acts to inhibit T-cell receptor signalling, and PD-1 inhibitors (check point inhibitors) cause activation of T cells, allowing them to once more recognise and attack the tumour (see also Ch. 57).

Apoptosis is a *default response*; i.e. continuous active signalling by tissue-specific trophic factors, cytokines and hormones and cell-to-cell contact factors (adhesion molecules, integrins, etc.) are required for cell survival and viability. The self-destruct mechanism is automatically triggered unless it is actively and continuously inhibited by these anti-apoptotic factors. Different cell types require differing sets of *survival factors*, which function only locally. If a cell strays or is dislodged from the area protected by its paracrine survival signals, it will die.

Withdrawal of these survival factors – which has been termed *death by neglect* – is not the only pathway to apoptosis (Fig. 6.5). The death machinery can be activated by ligands that stimulate *death receptors* and by DNA damage. But it is generally accepted that cell proliferation processes and apoptosis are tightly integrated.

MORPHOLOGICAL CHANGES IN APOPTOSIS

As the cell dies it 'rounds up', the chromatin condenses into dense masses, nucleases chop up the genome into unusable different sized fragments (seen on an electrophoretic gel as DNA 'laddering'), the cytoplasm shrinks and there is blebbing of the plasma membrane. Finally, mediated by a family of proteolytic enzymes known as caspases, the cell is transformed into a cluster of membrane-bound entities. This cellular 'corpse' displays 'eat me' signals, such as phosphatidylserine on its surface, which are recognised by macrophages, which then phagocytose the remains. It is important that these cellular fragments are enclosed by a membrane because otherwise the release of cell constituents could trigger an inflammatory reaction. An additional safeguard against this is that phagocytosing macrophages release anti-inflammatory mediators such as TGF-β, annexin-1 and IL-10.

THE MAJOR PLAYERS IN APOPTOSIS

The repertoire of reactions in apoptosis is extremely complex and varies between species and cell types. Yet it could be that the pivotal reaction(s) that lead to either cell survival or cell death, reaching this tipping point can be controlled by either a single gene or a combination of key genes. Either way, these genes are desirable targets for drugs used to treat many proliferative diseases.

Only a simple outline of apoptosis can be given here. Portt et al. (2011) have reviewed the whole area in detail. The major players are a family of cysteine aspartate-directed proteinases (*caspases*) present in the cell in inactive form. These undertake delicate protein surgery, selectively cleaving specific sets of target proteins (enzymes, structural components, all of which contain a characteristic motif recognised by the caspases), inactivating some and activating others. A cascade of about nine different caspases is required, some functioning as initiators that transmit the initial apoptotic signals, and others being responsible for the final phase of cell death (see Fig. 6.5).

The 'executioner' caspases (e.g. caspase 3) directly cleave and inactivate cell constituents such as the DNA repair enzymes, protein kinase C and cytoskeletal components. Activation of a DNAase cuts genomic DNA between the nucleosomes, generating DNA fragments of approximately 180 base pairs.

However, not all caspases are death-mediating enzymes; some have a role in the processing and activating of cytokines (e.g. caspase 8 is active in processing the inflammatory cytokines IL-1 and IL-18).

Besides the caspases, another pathway can be triggered by *apoptotic initiating factor* (AIF), a protein released from mitochondria that enters the nucleus and triggers cell suicide.

PATHWAYS TO APOPTOSIS

There are two main routes to cell death: stimulation of death receptors by external ligands (the *extrinsic pathway*) and an internal *mitochondrial pathway*. Both routes activate initiator caspases and converge on a final common effector caspase pathway.

THE EXTRINSIC PATHWAY

Lurking in the plasma membrane of most cell types are members of the tumour necrosis factor receptor (TNFR) superfamily (also known as Fas receptors), which function as 'death receptors' (see Fig. 6.5). Important family members include TNFR-1 and CD95 (also known as Fas ligands or Apo-1), but there are many others (e.g. PD-1, a death receptor that can be induced on activated T cells, as discussed previously).

Each receptor has a 'death domain' in its cytoplasmic tail. Stimulation of the receptors by a ligand such as tumour necrosis factor (TNF[9]) itself or TRAIL[10] causes them to trimerise and recruit an adapter protein that binds to their death domains. The resulting complex activates caspase 8 (and probably caspase 10), which in turn activates the downstream effector caspases (see Fig. 6.5).

The mitochondrial pathway

This pathway can be triggered by DNA damage, by withdrawal of cell survival factors or other causes. In some way, the cell can 'audit' such damage and decide whether to initiate the apoptotic pathway. It is possible that *promyelocytic leukaemia bodies*, large complexes of proteins in the nucleus, participate in this task (Wyllie, 2010), although how they do so is not clear.

Regulating the apoptotic event are the members of the Bcl-2 protein family, a group of proteins with homologous domains allowing interactions between individual members. If the cell selects the apoptotic route, the p53 protein activates p21 and proapoptotic members of the Bcl-2 family – Bid, Bax and Bak. In addition to these proapoptotic species, this family has antiapoptotic members (e.g. Bcl-2 itself[11]). These factors compete with each other at sites on the surface of the mitochondria and the outcome depends upon the relative competing concentrations of these molecular players. In the case of a proapoptotic signal, oligomers of Bax and or Bak form pores in the mitochondrial membrane through which proteins such as cytochrome C can leak.

When released, cytochrome C complexes with a protein termed Apaf-1 (apoptotic protease-activating factor-1), the pair then combining with procaspase 9 to activate it. This latter enzyme orchestrates the effector caspase pathway. The triumvirate of cytochrome C, Apaf-1 and procaspase 9 is termed the *apoptosome* (see Fig. 6.5 and see Riedl and Salvesen, 2007). Nitric oxide (see Ch. 21) is another mediator that can have proapoptotic or antiapoptotic actions.

In normal cells, survival factors (specified earlier) continuously activate antiapoptotic mechanisms. The withdrawal of survival factors can cause death in several different ways depending on the cell type. A common mechanism is tipping the balance between Bcl-2 family members leading to loss of the antiapoptotic protein action, with the resultant unopposed action of the proapoptotic members of the Bcl-2 family of proteins (see Fig. 6.5).

The two main cell death pathways are connected to each other, in that caspase 8 in the death receptor pathway can activate the proapoptotic Bcl-2 family proteins and thus activate the mitochondrial pathway.

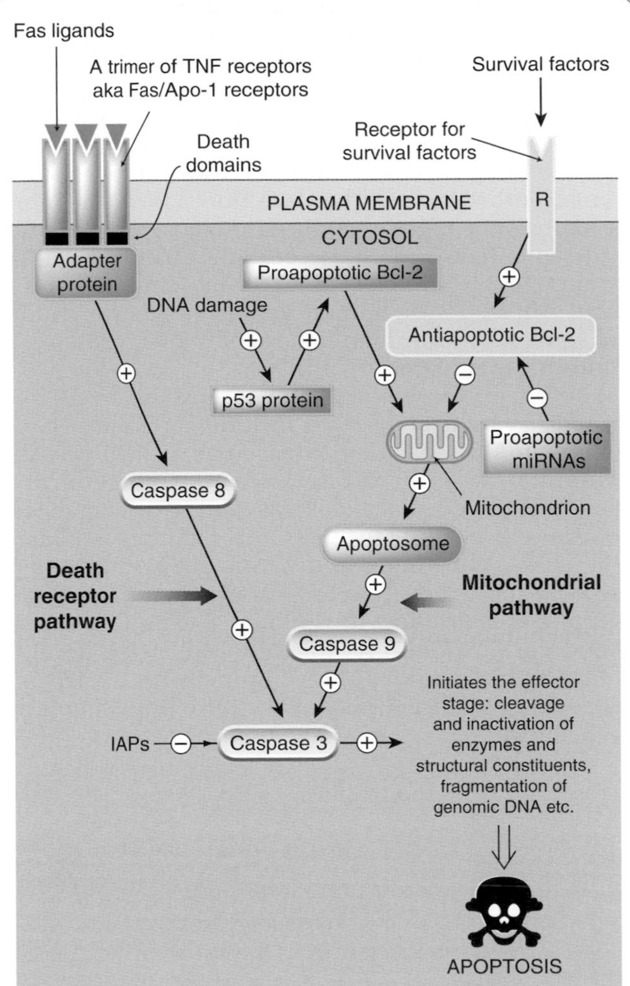

Fig. 6.5 A simplified diagram of the two main signalling pathways in apoptosis. The 'death receptor' pathway is activated when death receptors such as members of the tumour necrosis factor (TNF) family are stimulated by specific death ligands. This recruits adapter proteins that activate initiator caspases (e.g. caspase 8), which in turn activate effector caspases such as caspase 3. The mitochondrial pathway is activated by diverse signals, one being DNA damage. In the presence of DNA damage that cannot be repaired, the p53 protein (see text and Figs 6.3 and 6.4) activates a subpathway that releases cytochrome C from the mitochondrion, with subsequent involvement of the *apoptosome* and activation of an initiator caspase, caspase 9. The apoptosome is a complex of procaspase 9, cytochrome C and apoptotic-activating protease factor-1 (Apaf-1). Both these pathways converge on the effector caspase (e.g. caspase 3), which brings about the demise of the cell. The survival factor sub-pathway normally restrains apoptosis by inhibiting the mitochondrial pathway through activation of the antiapoptotic factor Bcl-2. The receptor labelled *'R'* represents the respective receptors for trophic factors, growth factors, cell-to-cell contact factors (adhesion molecules, integrins), etc. Continuous stimulation of these receptors is necessary for cell survival/proliferation. If this pathway is non-functional *(shown in grey)*, this antiapoptotic drive is withdrawn. *IAP,* Inhibitor of apoptosis.

[9]TNF was first thought to be secreted by bacteria, since it was known that infected tumours would sometimes recede and be cured. This 'bacterial-secreted' *tumour killing factor* was discovered to be TNF, released instead from our macrophages responding to the bacterial infection. A side effect of the TNF was tumour death, hence its name. TNF is also known as *cachexin*, the agent responsible for muscle apoptosis and wastage in cancer patients.

[10]TRAIL is tumour necrosis factor-α–related apoptosis-inducing ligand, of course; what else? See Janssen et al. (2005) for discussion of a role of TRAIL. PD-L1, a ligand for the PD-1 receptor, is found on all haemopoietic cells and many other tissues.

[11]Another brake on cell death is a family of caspase-inhibiting proteins called IAPs (inhibitors of apoptosis proteins).

MicroRNAs, the cell cycle and apoptosis

MicroRNAs (miRNAs), discovered only around the turn of the millennium, are a family of small 'non-protein coding' RNAs present within plants and animals. Coded by sections of the genome found outside the normal protein coding sequences of genes, miRNAs negatively regulate the ribosomal translation processes of many other genes. They are now known to inhibit the expression of genes coding for cell cycle regulation, apoptosis (see Fig. 6.5), cell differentiation and development (Carleton et al., 2007; Lynam-Lennon et al., 2009). About 3% of human genes encode for miRNA and some 30% of human genes coding for proteins are themselves regulated by miRNAs.

Altered miRNA expression is now believed to be linked to a variety of diseases, including diabetes, obesity, Alzheimer's disease, cardiovascular system diseases, inflammatory conditions and neurodegenerative diseases (Barbato et al., 2009), as well as carcinogenesis, metastasis and resistance to cancer therapies (Garzon et al., 2009; Wurdinger and Costa, 2007). miRNAs are also believed to function as oncogenes and/or tumour suppressor genes and to regulate T cells (Zhou et al., 2009). Not surprisingly, miRNAs are being heralded as targets for new drug development for a variety of disease states (Christopher et al., 2016; Rupaimoole and Slack, 2017).

Apoptosis

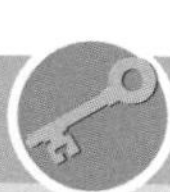

- Apoptosis is PCD. It is an essential biological process and critical, for example, for embryogenesis and tissue homeostasis.
- Apoptosis depends upon a cascade of proteinases called caspases. Two sets of initiator caspases converge on a set of effector caspases, bringing about the apoptotic event.
- Two main pathways activate the effector caspases: the death receptor pathway and the mitochondrial pathway.
  - Stimulation of the TNFR family initiates the death receptor pathway. The main initiator is caspase 8.
  - The mitochondrial pathway is activated by internal factors such as DNA damage, which results in transcription of gene *p53.* The p53 protein activates a sub-pathway that releases cytochrome C from the mitochondrion. This, in turn, complexes with protein Apaf-1 and together they activate initiator caspase 9.
- In undamaged cells, survival factors (cytokines, hormones, cell-to-cell contact factors) continuously activate antiapoptotic mechanisms. Withdrawal of survival factors causes cell death through the mitochondrial pathway.
- The effector caspases (e.g. caspase 3) initiate a cascade of proteases that cleave cell constituents, DNA, cytoskeletal components, enzymes, etc. This reduces the cell to a cluster of membrane-bound entities that are eventually phagocytosed by macrophages.

PATHOPHYSIOLOGICAL IMPLICATIONS

As mentioned before, cell proliferation and apoptosis are involved in many physiological and pathological processes. These are:

- the growth of tissues and organs in the embryo and later during development;
- the replenishment of lost or 'time-expired' cells such as leukocytes, gut epithelium and uterine endometrium;
- immunological responses, including development of immunological tolerance to host proteins;
- repair and healing after injury or inflammation;
- the hyperplasia (increase in cell number and in connective tissue) associated with chronic inflammatory, hypersensitivity and autoimmune diseases (see Ch. 7);
- the growth, invasion and metastasis of tumours (see Ch. 57);
- regeneration of tissues.

The role of cell proliferation and apoptosis in the first two processes listed is self-evident and needs no further comment. Their involvement in immune tolerance is discussed briefly previously but the other processes require further discussion.

REPAIR AND HEALING

Repair occurs when tissues are damaged or lost. It is also implicated in the resolution of the local inflammatory reaction to a pathogen or chemical irritant. In some instances, damage or tissue loss can lead to *regeneration*, which is different from repair and is considered later.

There is considerable overlap between the mechanisms activated in inflammation and repair. Both entail an ordered series of events including cell migration, angiogenesis, proliferation of connective tissue cells, synthesis of ECM and finally remodelling – all coordinated by the growth factors and cytokines that are appropriate for the particular tissue involved. TGF-β is a key regulator of several of these processes.[12]

[12]Next time you cut yourself, have a look at the scar exactly a week later. It may be that almost the scar has nearly vanished. This impressive biological process (bleeding, scabbing, scarring, wound healing) in a week is dependent upon growth factors from the scab stimulating epithelial and endothelial stem cells to remodel and match what was damaged – even down to replicating a fingerprint.

Repair, healing and regeneration

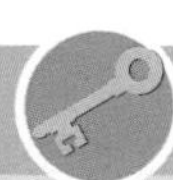

- Repair and healing occur when tissues are damaged. It is a common sequel to inflammation. Connective tissue cells, white blood cells and blood vessels are commonly involved.
- Regeneration is the replacement of the tissue or organ that has been damaged or lost. It depends upon the presence of a pool of primitive stem cells that have the potential to develop into any cell in the body. Complete regeneration of a tissue or organ is rare in mammals. The more rapid repair processes – often accompanied by scarring – usually make good the damage. This may be an evolutionary trade-off in mammals for the lost power of regeneration.
- However, it might be possible eventually to activate regenerative pathways in mammals – at least to some extent and in some organs.

HYPERPLASIA

Hyperplasia (cell proliferation and matrix expansion) is a hallmark of chronic inflammatory and autoimmune diseases such as rheumatoid arthritis (see Chs 7 and 25), psoriasis, chronic ulcers and chronic obstructive lung disease. It also underlies the bronchial hyper-reactivity of chronic asthma (see Ch. 28) and glomerular nephritis.

Cell proliferation and apoptotic events are also implicated in atherosclerosis, restenosis and myocardial repair after infarction (see Ch. 22).

THE GROWTH, INVASION AND METASTASIS OF TUMOURS

Growth factor signalling systems, antiapoptotic pathways and cell cycle controllers are of increasing interest as targets for novel approaches to the treatment of cancer (see Ch. 57).

STEM CELLS AND REGENERATION

Regeneration of tissue replaces that lost following damage or disease and allows restoration of function. Many animals (e.g. amphibians) have impressive regenerative powers and can even regrow an entire organ such as a limb or a tail. The essential process is the activation of *stem cells* – a pool of undifferentiated cells that have the potential to develop into any of the more specialised cells in the body – 'totipotent' or 'pluripotent' cells (Burgess, 2016; Slack, 2014). Not only do amphibians have a plentiful supply of these primitive cells but many of their more specialised cells can de-differentiate, becoming stem cells again. These can then multiply and retrace the foetal developmental pathways that generated the organ, by differentiating into the various cell types needed to replace the missing structure.

However, during evolution, mammals have lost this ability in all but a few tissues. Blood cells, intestinal epithelium and the outer layers of the skin are replaced continuously throughout life but there is a low turnover and replacement of cells in organs such as liver, kidney and bone. This 'physiological renewal' is affected by local tissue-specific stem cells.

Almost alone among mammalian organs, the liver has significant ability to replace itself. It can regenerate to its original size in a remarkably short time, provided that at least 25% has been left intact.[13] The mature parenchymal liver cells participate in this process as well as all the other cellular components of the liver.

It is necessary to distinguish *embryonic stem cells* (ES cells) from *adult stem cells* (AS cells) and *progenitor cells*. ES cells are the true pluripotent cells of the embryo that can differentiate into any other cell type. AS cells have a more restricted capability, whereas progenitor cells are able to differentiate only into a single cell type. ES cells are absent in the adult mammal, but AS cells are present, although they are few in number. In mammals, tissue or organ damage (with the exception of the liver, mentioned previously) normally leads to repair, rather than regeneration.

Until recently, it was assumed (with a few exceptions) that this was an unalterable situation, but recent work has suggested that it might be possible to activate the regenerative pathways in mammals – at least to some extent and in some organs. For this to happen, it is necessary to encourage some stem cells to proliferate, develop and differentiate at the relevant sites; or – and this is a rather more remote prospect in humans – to persuade some local specialised cells to de-differentiate. This can occur in some mammals under special circumstances. However, it may be that repair is the Janus face of regeneration, being an evolutionary trade-off in mammals for the lost power of regeneration.[14]

Where are the relevant stem cells that could be coaxed into regenerative service? Various possibilities are being vigorously investigated and, in some cases, tested clinically. These include:

- ES cells (limited availability and serious ethical issues)
- bone marrow-derived mesenchymal stem cells (Zhang et al., 2017)
- muscle-derived stem cells (Kelc et al., 2013)
- human-induced pluripotent stem cells (Nishikawa et al., 2008)
- tissue-resident progenitor cells.

For a tissue such as the liver to regenerate, local tissue-specific stem cells must be stimulated by growth factors to enter the cell cycle and to proliferate. Other essential processes (already discussed) include angiogenesis, activation of MMPs and the interaction between the matrix and fibronectin to link all the new elements together. The concomitant replacement of components of the lost connective tissue (fibroblasts, macrophages, etc.) is also necessary.

Because most tissues do not regenerate spontaneously, mechanisms that could restore regenerative ability could be of immense therapeutic value. Stem cell therapy has become an attractive prospect for treating all manner of diseases, ranging from erectile dysfunction and urinary incontinence to heart disease and neurodegeneration. Animal studies have confirmed that this is a potentially rewarding area although routine stem cell therapy in humans is still a distant prospect. The literature is daunting, but the following examples provide an insight into the obstacles and aspirations of the field: repair of damaged heart muscle (see Ch. 21; see Lovell and Mathur, 2011), repair of retinal degeneration (Ong and da Cruz, 2012), stroke (Banerjee et al., 2011) and replacement of insulin-secreting cells to treat type 1 diabetes mellitus (see Ch. 32; Voltarelli et al., 2007).

THERAPEUTIC PROSPECTS

Theoretically, all the processes described in this chapter could constitute useful targets for new drug development. In the following, we list those approaches that are proving or are likely to prove fruitful.

[13]There is an account of liver regeneration in Greek mythology. Prometheus stole the secret of fire from Zeus and gave it to mankind. To punish him, Zeus had him shackled to a crag in the Caucasus and every day an eagle tore at his flesh and devoured much of his liver. During the night, however, it regenerated and in the morning was whole again. The legend doesn't say whether the requisite 25% was left after the eagle had had its fill, and the regeneration described seems unrealistically fast – rat liver takes 2 weeks or more to get back to the original size after 66% hepatectomy.

[14]Bovine myosatellite stem cells have been used to grow beefburgers in the lab (so-called 'no-kill' alternatives). The fact that one burger can cost up to £250,000 to make may mean that only professional footballers can afford them for now.

APOPTOTIC MECHANISMS

Compounds that could modify apoptosis are being intensively investigated (MacFarlane, 2009; Melnikova and Golden, 2004). Here we can only outline some of the more important approaches.

Drugs that promote apoptosis by various mechanisms were heralded as a potential new approach to cancer treatment, and are actively being studied, although none has yet been approved for clinical use. Potential proapoptotic therapeutic approaches need to be targeted precisely to the diseased tissue to avoid the obvious risks of damaging other tissues. Examples include the following:

- An antisense compound against Bcl-2 (**oblimersen**) is being tested for chronic lymphocytic leukaemia.
- **Obatoclax** and **navitoclax** are small molecule inhibitors of Bcl-2 action, being tested for treating haematological malignancies. For details see MacFarlane (2009).
- MicroRNA technology could also be used to promote apoptosis (see Fig. 6.5).
- Monoclonal agonist antibodies to the death receptor ligand TRAIL (e.g. **lexatumumab**) are undergoing clinical trials for treatment of solid tumours and lymphomas (MacFarlane, 2009).
- **Bortezomib**, which inhibits the proteasome, is available for the treatment of selected cancers. It causes the build-up of Bax, an apoptotic promoter protein of the Bcl-2 family that acts by inhibiting antiapoptotic Bcl-2. Bortezomib acts partly by inhibiting nuclear factor κB (NF-κB) action (see Ch. 3).
- One of the most cancer-specific genes codes for an endogenous caspase inhibitor, *survivin*. This occurs in high concentrations in certain tumours and a small molecule suppressor of survivin is in clinical trial (Giaccone and Rajan, 2009), the objective being to induce cancer cell suicide.

Inhibiting apoptosis might prevent or treat a wide range of common degenerative disorders. Unfortunately, success in developing such inhibitors for clinical use has so far proved elusive and a number have been found to lack efficacy in clinical trials. Current areas of interest include the following:

- Blocking the PD-1 death receptor with a targeted antibody (such as **nivolumab**) is a potentially fruitful new avenue to explore for the treatment of HIV, hepatitis B and hepatitis C infections, as well as other chronic infections and some cancers that express the ligand for PD-1 (Trivedi et al., 2015).
- Several caspase inhibitors are under investigation for treating myocardial infarction, stroke, liver disease, organ transplantation and sepsis. **Emricasan** is one such candidate undergoing trials in patients requiring liver transplants.

ANGIOGENESIS AND METALLOPROTEINASES

The search for clinically useful anti-angiogenic drugs and MMP inhibitors is continuing but has not so far been successful. At present, only one new drug has been approved for use in cancer treatment: **bevacizumab**, a monoclonal antibody that neutralises VEGF, and which is also used to treat age-related macular degeneration, a disease also associated with excessive proliferation of retinal blood vessels.

CELL CYCLE REGULATION

The main endogenous positive regulators of the cell cycle are the cdks. Several small molecules that inhibit cdks by targeting the ATP-binding sites of these kinases have been developed; an example is **flavopiridol**, which inhibits all the cdks, causing arrest of the cell cycle, and is currently in clinical trials for the treatment of acute myeloid leukaemia; it also promotes apoptosis, has anti-angiogenic properties and can induce differentiation (Dickson and Schwartz, 2009).

Some compounds affect upstream pathways for cdk activation and may find a use in cancer treatment. Examples are **perifosine** (although its future is uncertain at the moment) and **lovastatin** (a cholesterol-lowering drug, see Ch. 22, which may also have anticancer properties).

Bortezomib, a boronate compound, covalently binds the proteasome, inhibiting the degradation of proapoptotic proteins. It is used in treating multiple myeloma (see Ch. 57).

Of the various components of the growth factor signalling pathway, receptor tyrosine kinases, the Ras protein and cytoplasmic kinases have been the subjects of most interest. Kinase inhibitors recently introduced for cancer treatment include **imatinib**, **gefitinib lapatinib**, **sunitinib** and **erlotinib** (see Ch. 57).

REFERENCES AND FURTHER READING

Cell cycle and apoptosis (general)

Ashkenasi, A., 2002. Targeting death and decoy receptors of the tumour necrosis receptor superfamily. Nat. Rev. Cancer 2, 420–429.

Aslan, J.E., Thomas, G., 2009. Death by committee: organellar trafficking and communication in apoptosis. Traffic 10, 1390–1404.

Barbato, C., Ruberti, F., Cogoni, C., 2009. Searching for MIND: microRNAs in neurodegenerative diseases. J. Biomed. Biotechnol. 2009, 871313.

Carleton, M., Cleary, M.C., Linsley, P.S., 2007. MicroRNAs and cell cycle regulation. Cell Cycle 6, 2127–2132.

Christopher, A.F., Kaur, R.P., Kaur, G., Kaur, A., Gupta, V., Bansal, P., 2016. MicroRNA therapeutics: discovering novel targets and developing specific therapy. Perspect. Clin. Res. 7, 68–74.

Cummings, J., Ward, T., Ranson, M., Dive, C., 2004. Apoptosis pathway-targeted drugs – from the bench to the clinic. Biochim. Biophys. Acta 1705, 53–66.

Danial, N.N., Korsmeyer, S.J., 2004. Cell death: critical control points. Cell 116, 205–219.

Dickson, M.A., Schwartz, G.K., 2009. Development of cell-cycle inhibitors for cancer therapy. Curr. Oncol. 16, 36–43.

Elmore, S., 2007. Apoptosis: a review of programmed cell death. Toxicol. Pathol. 35, 495–516.

Galluzzi, L., Vitale, I., Aaronson, S.A., et al., 2018. Molecular mechanisms of cell death: recommendations of the nomenclature committee on cell death 2018. Cell. Death Differ. 25, 486–541.

Garzon, R., Calin, G.A., Croce, C.M., 2009. MicroRNAs in cancer. Annu. Rev. Med. 60, 167–179.

Giaccone, G., Rajan, A., 2009. Met amplification and HSP90 inhibitors. Cell Cycle 8, 2682.

Janssen, E.M., Droin, N.M., Lemmens, E.E., 2005. CD4⁺ T-cell-help controls CD4⁺ T cell memory via TRAIL-mediated activation-induced cell death. Nature 434, 88–92.

Lynam-Lennon, N., Maher, S.M., Reynolds, J.V., 2009. The roles of microRNAs in cancer and apoptosis. Biol. Rev. 84, 55–71.

MacFarlane, M., 2009. Cell death pathways – potential therapeutic targets. Xenobiotica 39, 616–624.

Melnikova, A., Golden, J., 2004. Apoptosis-targeting therapies. Nat. Rev. Drug Discov. 3, 905–906.
Ouyang, L., Shi, Z., Zhao, S., et al., 2012. Programmed cell death pathways in cancer: a review of apoptosis, autophagy and programmed necrosis. Cell Prolif. 45, 487–498.
Portt, L., Norman, G., Clapp, C., Greenwood, M., Greenwood, M.T., 2011. Anti-apoptosis and cell survival: a review. Biochim. Biophys. Acta 1813, 238–259.
Riedl, S.J., Salvesen, G.S., 2007. The apoptosome: signalling platform of cell death. Nat. Rev. Mol. Cell Biol. 8, 405–413.
Riedl, S.J., Shi, Y., 2004. Molecular mechanisms of caspase regulation during apoptosis. Nat. Rev. Mol. Cell Biol. 5, 897–905.
Rupaimoole, R., Slack, F.J., 2017. MicroRNA therapeutics: towards a new era for the management of cancer and other diseases. Nat. Rev. Drug Discov. 16, 203–222.
Satyanarayana, A., Kaldis, P., 2009. Mammalian cell-cycle regulation: several Cdks, numerous cyclins and diverse compensatory mechanisms. Oncogene 28, 2925–2939.
Swanton, C., 2004. Cell-cycle targeted therapies. Lancet 5, 27–36.
Tousoulis, D., Andreou, I., Tentolouris, C., et al., 2010. Comparative effects of rosuvastatin and allopurinol on circulating levels of matrix metalloproteinases in patients with chronic heart failure. Int. J. Cardiol. 145, 438–443.
Trivedi, M.S., Hoffner, B., Winkelmann, J.L., Abbott, M.E., Hamid, O., Carvajal, R.D., 2015. Programmed death 1 immune checkpoint inhibitors. Clin. Adv. Hematol. Oncol. 13, 858–868.
Wurdinger, T., Costa, F.F., 2007. Molecular therapy in the microRNA era. Pharmacogenomics J. 7, 297–304.
Wyllie, A.H., 2010. 'Where, O death, is thy sting?' A brief review of apoptosis biology. Mol. Neurobiol. 42, 4–9.
Yang, B.F., Lu, Y.J., Wang, Z.G., 2009. MicroRNAs and apoptosis: implications in molecular therapy of human disease. Clin. Exp. Pharmacol. Physiol. 36, 951–960.
Zha, Y., Blank, C., Gajewski, T.F., 2004. Negative regulation of T-cell function by PD-1. Crit. Rev. Immunol. 24, 229–237.
Zhou, L., Seo, K.H., Wong, H.K., Mi, Q.S., 2009. MicroRNAs and immune regulatory T cells. Int. Immunopharmacol. 9, 524–527.

Integrins, extracellular matrix, metalloproteinases and angiogenesis

Barczyk, M., Carracedo, S., Gullberg, D., 2010. Integrins. Cell Tissue Res. 339, 269–280.
Clark, I.M., Swingler, T.E., Sampieri, C.L., Edwards, D.R., 2008. The regulation of matrix metalloproteinases and their inhibitors. Int. J. Biochem. Cell Biol. 40, 1362–1378.
Gahmberg, C.G., Fagerholm, S.C., Nurmi, S.M., et al., 2009. Regulation of integrin activity and signalling. Biochim. Biophys. Acta 1790, 431–444.
Gialeli, C., Theocharis, A.D., Karamanos, N.K., 2011. Roles of matrix metalloproteinases in cancer progression and their pharmacological targeting. FEBS. J. 278, 16–27.
Jackson, H.W., Defamie, V., Waterhouse, P., Khokha, R., 2017. TIMPs: versatile extracellular regulators in cancer. Nat. Rev. Cancer 17, 38–53.
Järveläinen, H., Sainio, A., Koulu, M., Wight, T.N., Penttinen, R., 2009. Extracellular matrix molecules: potential targets in pharmacotherapy. Pharmacol. Rev. 61, 198–223.
Marastoni, S., Ligresti, G., Lorenzon, E., Colombatti, A., Mongiat, M., 2008. Extracellular matrix: a matter of life and death. Connect. Tissue Res. 49, 203–206.
Rupérez, M., Rodrigues-Diez, R., Blanco-Colio, L.M., et al., 2007. HMG-CoA reductase inhibitors decrease angiotensin II-induced vascular fibrosis: role of RhoA/ROCK and MAPK pathways. Hypertension 50, 377–383.
Streuli, C.H., Akhtar, N., 2009. Signal co-operation between integrins and other receptor systems. Biochem. J. 418, 491–506.
Verrecchia, F., Mauviel, A., 2007. Transforming growth factor-beta and fibrosis. World J. Gastroenterol. 13, 3056–3062.

Stem cells, regeneration and repair

Aldhous, P., 2008. How stem cell advances will transform medicine. New Scientist 2654, 40–43.
Banerjee, S., Williamson, D., Habib, N., Gordon, M., Chataway, J., 2011. Human stem cell therapy in ischaemic stroke: a review. Age Ageing 40, 7–13.
Burgess, R., 2016. Stem Cells: A Short Course. Wiley-Blackwell. ISBN: 978-1-118-43919-7.
Gaetani, R., Barile, L., Forte, E., et al., 2009. New perspectives to repair a broken heart. Cardiovasc. Hematol. Agents Med. Chem. 7, 91–107.
Kelc, R., Trapecar, M., Vogrin, M., Cencic, A., 2013. Skeletal muscle-derived cell cultures as potent models in regenerative medicine research. Muscle Nerve 47, 477–482.
Lovell, M.J., Mathur, A., 2011. Republished review: cardiac stem cell therapy: progress from the bench to bedside. Postgrad. Med. J. 87, 558–564.
Nature Reviews Neuroscience, 2006. Vol. 7 (August) has a series of articles on nerve regeneration.
Nishikawa, S., Goldstein, R.A., Nierras, C.R., 2008. The promise of human induced pluripotent stem cells for research and therapy. Nat. Rev. Mol. Cell Biol. 9, 725–729.
Ong, J.M., da Cruz, L., 2012. A review and update on the current status of stem cell therapy and the retina. Br. Med. Bull. 102, 133–146.
Rosenthal, N., 2003. Prometheus's vulture and the stem-cell promise. N. Engl. J. Med. 349, 267–286.
Slack, J.M.W., 2014. Genes. A Very Short Introduction. Oxford University Press. ISBN: 9780199603381.
Voltarelli, J.C., Couri, C.E., Stracieri, A.B., et al., 2007. Autologous nonmyeloablative hematopoietic stem cell transplantation in newly diagnosed type 1 diabetes mellitus. JAMA 297, 1568–1576.
Zhang, X., Bendeck, M.P., Simmons, C.A., Santerre, J.P., 2017. Deriving vascular smooth muscle cells from mesenchymal stromal cells: evolving differentiation strategies and current understanding of their mechanisms. Biomaterials 145, 9–22.
Wilson, C., 2003. The regeneration game. New Scientist 179, 2414–2427.

7 Cellular mechanisms: host defence

OVERVIEW

Everyone has experienced an inflammatory episode at some time or other and will be familiar with the typical symptoms which include redness, swelling, heat, pain and loss of function at the site of injury or infection, sometimes accompanied by fever and malaise. Inflammatory mediators are considered separately in Chapter 17; here we focus on the cellular players involved in the host defence response and explain the bare bones of this sophisticated and crucial mechanism. An appreciation of these responses and their functions is key to understanding the actions of anti-inflammatory and immunosuppressant drugs – a major class of therapeutic agents with multiple clinical applications (see Ch. 25).

INTRODUCTION

All living creatures are born into a world that poses a constant challenge to their physical well-being and survival. Evolution, which has equipped us with homeostatic systems that maintain a stable internal environment in the face of changing external temperatures and fluctuating supplies of food and water, has also provided us with mechanisms for combating the ever-present threat of infection and for promoting healing and restoration of normal function in the event of injury. In mammals, this function is subserved by the *innate* (or non-adaptive or non-specific) and *adaptive* (alternatively *acquired or specific*) immune systems. These work together through a variety of mediators and mechanisms to mount the *inflammatory response*. Whilst predominantly protective, dysregulation of the initiation, magnitude, duration, location or resolution of inflammation contributes to a wide spectrum of diseases where drug therapy may help restore order.

The main functions of this host inflammatory response then are *defence, repair* and the restoration of function – in other words, nothing less than the ongoing biosecurity and survival of the organism. Immunodeficiency due to genetic causes (e.g. *leukocyte adhesion deficiency*), untreated infection with organisms such as HIV, radiation overexposure or immunosuppressant drugs is consequently a life-threatening state.

Like airport security systems in the mundane world, the body has the cellular and molecular equivalents of guards, identity checks, alarm systems and a communication network with which to summon back-up when required. It also has access to an astonishing data bank that stores precise molecular details of previous unwanted intruders and prevents them from returning. This host response has two main arms, which work together hand-in-hand. These are:

- *The innate response.* This developed early in evolution and is present in virtually all organisms. In fact, some of the key mammalian gene families and other components were first identified in plants and insects. This is the first line of defence.
- *The adaptive immune response.* This appeared much later in evolutionary terms and is found almost exclusively in vertebrates. It provides the physical basis for our immunological 'memory' and is the second, and supremely effective, line of defence.

While we consider these separately it must be appreciated that their functions and actions are closely intertwined.

The inflammatory response

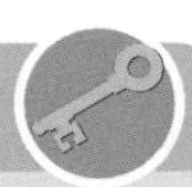

- The inflammatory response occurs in tissues following injury or exposure to a pathogen or other noxious substance.
- It comprises two components: an *innate* non-adaptive response and an *adaptive* (acquired or specific) immunological response.
- These reactions are generally protective, but if inappropriately deployed they are deleterious.
- The normal outcome of the response is healing with or without scarring; alternatively, if the underlying cause persists or the response fails to resolve, chronic inflammation results.
- Many diseases that require drug treatment involve inflammation. Understanding the action and use of anti-inflammatory and immunosuppressive drugs therefore necessitates an understanding of the underlying biology.

THE INNATE IMMUNE RESPONSE

Mucosal epithelial tissues, which are exposed to the external environment, constantly secrete antibacterial proteins such as *defensins* together with a type of 'all-purpose' immunoglobulin known as immunoglobulin A (IgA) as a sort of pre-emptive defensive strategy. Elsewhere the innate response is activated immediately following infection or injury.[1]

[1]One immunologist described the innate immune response as the organism's 'knee jerk' response to infection; it is an excellent description.

The innate immune response

- The innate response occurs immediately on injury or infection. It comprises vascular and cellular elements. Mediators generated by cells or from plasma modify and regulate the magnitude of the response.
- Utilising Toll and other recognition receptors, sentinel cells in body tissues, such as macrophages, mast and dendritic cells detect specific pathogen or damage-associated molecular patterns. This triggers the release of cytokines, particularly interleukin (IL)-1 and tumour necrosis factor (TNF)-α, as well as various chemokines.
- IL-1 and TNF-α act on local postcapillary venular endothelial cells, causing:
  - vasodilatation and fluid exudation
  - expression of adhesion molecules on the cell surfaces
- Exudate contains enzyme cascades that generate bradykinin (from kininogen), and C5a and C3a (from complement). Complement activation lyses bacteria.
- C5a and C3a stimulate mast cells to release histamine, which dilates local arterioles.
- Tissue damage and cytokines release prostaglandins PGI_2 and PGE_2 (vasodilators) and leukotriene (LT) B_4 (a chemokine).
- Cytokines stimulate synthesis of vasodilator nitric oxide, which increases vascular permeability.
- Using adhesion molecules, leukocytes roll on, adhere to and finally migrate through activated vascular endothelium towards the pathogen (attracted by chemokines, IL-8, C5a and LTB_4), where phagocytosis and bacterial killing take place.

PATTERN RECOGNITION

One of the most important functions of any security system is the ability to establish identity. How does an organism decide whether a cell or stray molecule is a bona fide citizen or an unwanted and potentially dangerous intruder? In the case of the innate response this is achieved through a network of *pattern recognition receptors* (PRRs). They recognise *pathogen-associated molecular patterns* (PAMPs) – common products produced by bacteria, fungi, parasites and viruses, which they cannot readily change to evade detection.

PRRs consist of multiple families that may be classified by protein domain homology (see Li and Wu, 2021, for a recent review). These include membrane-bound receptors such as the G protein–coupled FPR (formyl peptide receptor) family which recognise *N*-formylated peptides characteristic of bacterial protein synthesis (and liberated from damaged mitochondria too); *C-type lectin receptors* (CLRs) which predominantly detect fungal beta-glucan and mannose; and cytoplasmic receptors such as the *NOD-like receptors* (nucleotide-binding oligomerisation domain-like receptors), a large family of intracellular proteins that can recognise fragments of bacterial proteoglycan – as well as several other families including *retinoic acid-inducible gene-1* (RIG-1) like receptors and *absent in melanoma-2-like receptors* (ALRs) which detect intracellular pathogen-originated RNA and DNA, respectively. It also includes what is probably the best-studied of these PRRs, the *Toll-like receptors* (TLRs; see Fitzgerald and Kagan 2020, for a recent review).

The Toll[2] gene was first identified in *Drosophila* in the mid-1990s but analogous genes were soon found in vertebrates. It was quickly established that the main function of this family of proteins was to detect highly conserved components in pathogens and to signal their presence to both arms of the immune system.

Humans have a repertoire of 10 TLRs but some other animals have more. Structurally, they are transmembrane glycoproteins belonging to the *receptor tyrosine kinase* family (see Ch. 3). Phylogenetically they are highly conserved. Unlike the antigen receptors on T and B cells that develop and change through life, endowing each lymphocyte clone with a structurally unique receptor (see later), TLRs are encoded for by discrete genes in the host DNA. Table 7.1 lists these receptors and the chief pathogenic products they recognise, where these are known. There are two main types of TLR, located respectively on the cell surface and in endosomes. The latter type generally recognises pathogen RNA/DNA (presumably because they appear in phagosomes), while the former recognises other pathogen components such as cell wall material, endotoxin, etc. Some TLRs also recognise *damage associated molecular patterns* (DAMPs), molecules or motifs released either actively or passively when host cells are damaged (e.g. heat shock proteins). This provides an additional way of detecting internal damage and 'raising the alarm' (indeed, DAMPs are often referred to as *alarmins*).

How a single family of receptors can recognise such a wide spectrum of different chemicals is a molecular mystery. Some solve this problem by acting in concert. TLR 1, 2 and 6 act in this way whereas others recruit additional 'accessory' proteins that modulate their binding properties to achieve the same goal (e.g. TLR 4 with MD-2 and CD14). When activated, Toll receptors dimerise and initiate complex signalling pathways that activate genes coding for proteins and factors crucial to the deployment or modulation of the inflammatory response, many of which we will discuss further. Interestingly, from the pharmacological viewpoint, TLR 7 also recognises some synthetic antiviral compounds such as *imidazoquinolones*. The ability of these drugs to provoke TLR activation probably underlies their clinical effectiveness (see Ch. 53). Conversely, given their role in the initiation of inflammation and the near ubiquity of this process in pathology, TLRs are themselves now the subject of therapeutic targeting in multiple disease states (see Anwar et al., 2019, for a recent review)

TLRs are strategically located on 'sentinel' cells – those likely to come into early contact with invaders. These include *macrophages* as well as *mast cells* and (crucially) the *dendritic cells*, which are especially abundant in skin and other inside–outside interfaces and *intestinal epithelial cells,* which are exposed to pathogens in the food that we eat. Genetic defects in the TLR system have been discovered. These can lead to an inability to mount an effective host defence response or sometimes to a constitutively active inflammatory response.

[2]The name, which loosely translates from German as 'Great!' or 'Eureka!', has remained firmly attached to the family. Discovered in fruit fly experiments, Christiane Nüsslein-Volhard exclaimed 'Das ist ja *toll!*' The name has stuck since then.

Table 7.1 The human Toll-like receptor (TLR) family of pattern recognition receptors (PRRs)

PRR	Pathogen or endogenous product recognised	Ligand	Sites of expression	Location
TLR 2 (usually acting together with **TLR 1**, **TLR 6** and possibly **TLR 10**)	Bacteria (Gm pos) *Mycoplasma* Parasites Yeast Damaged host cells	Lipoproteins Lipoteichoic acid GPI anchors Cell wall carbohydrates Heat shock proteins	Monocyte/macrophages Some dendritic cells B lymphocytes Mast cells	Cell surface
TLR 4[a]	Bacteria (Gm neg) Virus Damaged host cells	Lipopolysaccharide Some viral proteins Heat shock proteins Fibrinogen Hyaluronic acid	Monocyte/macrophages Some dendritic cells Mast cells Intestinal epithelium	
TLR 5	Bacteria	Flagellin	Monocyte/macrophages Some dendritic cells Intestinal epithelium	
TLR 3	Virus	Viral dsRNA	Dendritic cells B lymphocytes	Intracellular (endosomal)
TLR 7	Virus	Viral ssRNA Some synthetic drugs	Monocyte/macrophages	
TLR 8	Virus	Viral ssRNA	Mast cells	
TLR 9	Bacteria	Bacterial CpG containing Bacterial DNA Self DNA	B lymphocytes	

[a]Operates in conjunction with MD-2 (lymphocyte antigen 96, a lipopolysaccharide binding protein) and CD14.
CpG DNA, Unmethylated CG dinucleotide; *dsRNA*, double-stranded RNA; *Gm neg/pos*, Gram-negative/positive (bacteria); *GPI*, glycosylphosphatidylinositol anchoring proteins; *ssRNA*, single-stranded RNA.

Having outlined how 'non-self' pathogens are detected by the innate immune system, we can now describe the events that follow.

RESPONSES TO PATTERN RECOGNITION

Vascular events

The interaction of a PAMP with TLRs triggers the sentinel cells to produce a range of pro-inflammatory polypeptides called *cytokines*, including *tumour necrosis factor* (*TNF*)-*α* and *interleukin* (*IL*)-*1*. The intracellular maturation and processing of IL-1 (and some other cytokines) is managed by *inflammasomes*, multiprotein complexes that vary according to the type of inflammatory stimulus. The inflammasome thus initiates a precisely tailored inflammatory response appropriate to the situation (see Zheng et al., 2020, for a recent overview).

Also released, either as a direct consequence of tissue damage or following cytokine stimulation, are lower-molecular-weight inflammatory mediators including the prostaglandins (PGs), such as PGE_2 and PGI_2 (prostacyclin), and histamine (both being further discussed in Ch. 17). These act on the vascular endothelial cells of the postcapillary venules along with cytokines, to trigger the expression of *adhesion molecules* on the intimal surface and an increase in vascular permeability (allowing immune cells to pass from the blood to the affected tissue). Simultaneously they modulate perfusion, dilatating small arterioles to increase blood flow whilst there is a slowing (and sometimes a cessation) of blood flow in the postcapillary venules promoting exudation of fluid (seen as swelling or oedema).

Leukocytes adhere to the endothelial cells through interactions between their cell surface *integrins* and adhesion molecules on endothelial cells, halting their flow through the microcirculation. They are then able to migrate out of the vessels, attracted by *chemokines* (a subtype of cytokine) generated by the microorganisms themselves or as a result of their interaction with the tissues. Polypeptide chemokines released during TLR activation play an important part in this. (Cytokines and chemokines are considered separately in Ch. 17.)

The resulting fluid exudate contains the components for four proteolytic enzyme cascades: the *complement system*, the *coagulation system*, the *fibrinolytic system* and the *kinin system* (Fig. 7.1). The components of these cascades are inactive proteases that are activated by cleavage, each activated component then activating the next in sequence.

The *complement system* comprises nine major protein components, designated C1 to C9. Activation of the cascade may be initiated by substances derived from microorganisms, such as yeast cell walls or endotoxins.

This pathway of activation is termed the *alternative pathway*, as opposed to the *classic pathway*, which is dealt with later. One of the main events is the enzymatic splitting of C3, giving rise to various peptides, one of which, *C3a* (termed an *anaphylatoxin*), stimulates mast cells to secrete further chemical mediators and can also directly stimulate smooth muscle, while *C3b* (termed an *opsonin*) attaches to the surface of a microorganism, facilitating ingestion by phagocytes. *C5a*, generated enzymatically from C5, also releases mediators from mast cells and is a powerful chemotactic attractant and activator of leukocytes.

The final components in the sequence, complement-derived mediators C5 to C9, coalesce to form a *membrane attack complex* that can attach to, and lyse, some bacterial membranes. Complement can therefore mediate the destruction of invading bacteria and damage multicellular parasites; however, it may sometimes cause injury to the host. The principal enzymes of the coagulation and fibrinolytic cascades, thrombin and plasmin, can also activate the cascade by hydrolysing C3, as can enzymes released from leukocytes.

The *coagulation system* and the *fibrinolytic system* are described in Chapter 23. Factor XII is activated to XIIa (e.g. by collagen), and the end product, fibrin, laid down during a host–pathogen interaction, may also serve to limit the extent of the infection. Thrombin is additionally involved in the activation of the kinin and, indirectly, the fibrinolytic systems (see Ch. 23). The *kinin system* is another enzyme cascade activated in inflammation. It yields several pro-inflammatory and pain-producing mediators, in particular bradykinin.

Eventually, the inflammatory exudate drains through the lymphatics to local lymph nodes or lymphoid tissue. Here, specialised leukocytes recognise the products of the invading microorganism and trigger the adaptive phase of the response.

Cellular events

Of the cells involved in inflammation, some (e.g. vascular endothelial cells, mast cells, dendritic cells and tissue macrophages) are normally present in tissues, while other actively motile cells (e.g. neutrophils) gain access from the circulating blood.

Polymorphonuclear leukocytes

Neutrophil polymorphs – the 'shock troops' of inflammation – are the first blood leukocytes to enter an infected or damaged tissue (Fig. 7.2). The whole process is cleverly choreographed: under direct observation, the neutrophils may be seen first to *roll* along the activated endothelium, then to *adhere* and finally

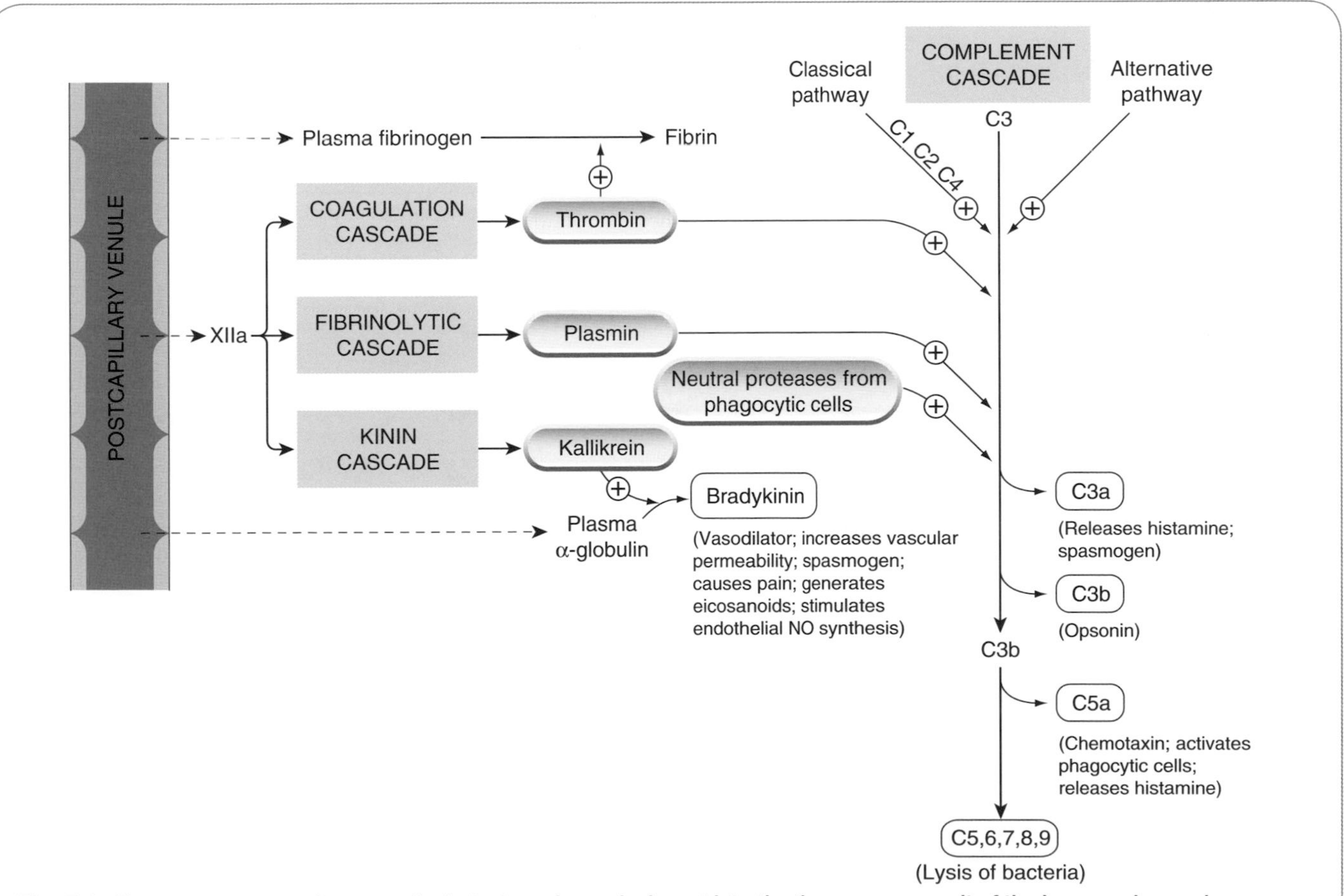

Fig. 7.1 Four enzyme cascades are activated when plasma leaks out into the tissues as a result of the increased vascular permeability of inflammation. Factors causing cellular migration are depicted in Fig. 7.2. Mediators generated are shown in *red-bordered boxes*. Complement components are indicated by *C1*, *C2*, etc. When plasmin is formed, it tends to increase kinin formation and decrease the coagulation cascade. XIIa, Factor XIIa, see text. (Adapted from Dale, M.M., Foreman, J.C., Fan, T-P. (Eds) 1994. Textbook of Immunopharmacology, third ed. Blackwell Scientific, Oxford.)

to *migrate* out of the blood vessel and into the extravascular space. This process is regulated by the successive activation of different families of *adhesion molecules* on the inflamed endothelium (*selectins, intercellular adhesion molecule* [ICAM] and *integrins*) which engage corresponding *counter-ligands* on the neutrophil, capturing it as it rolls along the surface, stabilising its interaction with the endothelial cells with the aid of PECAM (*platelet endothelial cell adhesion molecule*), and enabling it to migrate out of the vessel

Neutrophils are attracted to invading pathogens by chemicals, a process known as *chemotaxis*. Some of these (such as the tripeptide formyl-Met-Leu-Phe) are released by the microorganism, whereas others, such as C5a, are produced locally or in some cases released from nearby cells such as macrophages (e.g. chemokines such as IL-8).

Neutrophils can engulf, kill and digest microorganisms. Together with eosinophils, they have surface receptors for C3b, which acts as an opsonin that forms a link between neutrophil and invading bacterium (an even more effective link may be made by antibodies). Neutrophils kill microorganisms by internalising them into vacuoles. An NADPH oxidase enzyme on the leukocyte surface raises the pH of the normally acidic vacuole to ensure optimal enzymatic digestion of the organism by neutral proteases. Toxic oxygen radicals are also produced by this enzyme, but it is now believed that these are less important in microbial killing (see Segal, 2016). If a neutrophil is inappropriately activated, these biochemical weapons may be turned inadvertently on the host, causing tissue damage (an example being in the acute respiratory distress syndrome,[ARDS]). When neutrophils have exhausted their potential, they undergo apoptosis and are cleared by phagocytic macrophages, a process known as *efferocytosis*. It is this mass of live and apoptotic neutrophils that constitutes 'pus'.

Mast cells

Another important type of 'sentinel' cells is mast cells. These express TLRs, but also have surface receptors both for IgE and for the complement-derived anaphylatoxins C3a and C5a. Ligands acting at these receptors trigger mediator release, as does direct cellular damage. One of the main substances released is histamine; others include *heparin, leukotrienes,* PGD_2, *platelet-activating factor (PAF), nerve growth factor* and some interleukins and proteases. Unusually, mast cells have preformed packets of cytokines

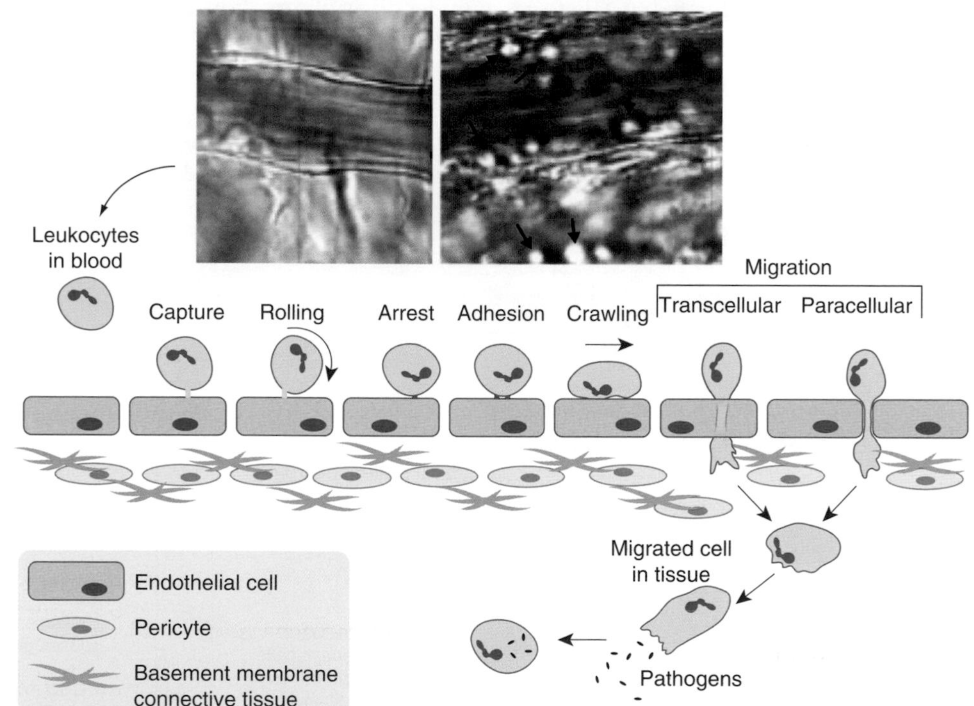

Fig. 7.2 Simplified diagram of the events leading up to polymorphonuclear leukocyte (PMN) migration in a local acute inflammatory reaction. In response to activation of pattern recognition receptors, tissue macrophages release the pro-inflammatory cytokines IL-1 and TNF-α. These act on the endothelial cells of postcapillary venules, causing exudation of fluid and expression of adhesion factors that recognise counter-ligands on blood-borne neutrophils. Free-flowing neutrophils in the blood are first 'captured' by *selectins* on activated endothelial cells. These cells then roll along the endothelium before their progress is arrested by the action of *integrins* and they adhere to the vessel wall. The activated cells then 'crawl' along the endothelium until they find a suitable site for transmigration. In a minority of cases, neutrophils can actually move through endothelial cells (*transcellular transmigration*) but they mainly migrate through the junction between endothelial cells (*paracellular transmigration*). Further adhesion molecules then guide the cell through the gaps. The migrating cells must also migrate through gaps in the layer of pericytes (contractile cells) that surround the venules as well as the basement membrane (comprised of connective tissue). Chemotactic gradients formed by the release of substances released by or from the pathogen guide the cell to its target where it can kill and/or phagocytose the invader. Neutrophils characteristically die after this event, in which case they enter apoptosis and are phagocytosed by macrophages, resolving the inflammatory event. *Photo inset:* Photomicrograph of a normal, un-inflamed microcirculation in the mesenteric bed of mouse *(left-hand panel)* and following a period of inflammation *(right-hand panel).* The arrows indicate neutrophils adhering to the endothelium as well as some that have already transmigrated. (Diagram modified from Nourshargh, S., Hordijk, P.L., Sixt, M., 2010. Breaching multiple barriers: leukocyte motility through venular walls and the interstitium. Nature Rev. Mol. Cell Biol. 11, 366–378. Picture courtesy Drs S. Yazid, G. Leoni and D. Cooper.)

that they can release instantaneously (by Ca^{2+}-mediated exocytosis; see Ch. 4) when stimulated. This makes them extremely effective triggers of the inflammatory response.

Monocytes/macrophages

Monocytes (a fascinating and multi-functional cell if ever there was one, see Guilliams et al., 2018, if interested) follow polymorphs into inflammatory lesions after a delay (sometimes several hours). Migration also depends upon adhesion molecule binding similar to that seen with neutrophils, although monocyte chemotaxis utilises additional chemokines, such as *MCP-1*[3] (which, reasonably enough, stands for *monocyte chemoattractant protein-1*) and *RANTES* (which very *unreasonably* stands for *regulated on activation normal T cell expressed and secreted*; immunological nomenclature has excelled itself here!).

Once in tissues, blood monocytes differentiate into *macrophages*, supplementing the tissue-resident macrophage population.[4] The newly differentiated cell may acquire different phenotypes including *M1*, *M2* or – more controversially – *regulatory (Mreg)*, depending upon its activation and function. The M1 phenotype is generally regarded as a pro-inflammatory cell, whereas M2 is probably more involved in tissue repair and healing (although the validity of these simplistic distinctions remains debatable: see Martinez and Gordon, 2014, and Orecchioni et al., 2019). Macrophages therefore have a remarkable range of abilities, being not only a jack-of-all-trades but also a master of many.

Activation of monocyte/macrophage TLRs stimulates the generation and release of chemokines and other cytokines that act on vascular endothelial cells, attract other leukocytes to the area and give rise to systemic manifestations of the inflammatory response such as fever (many of these inflammatory mediators have pyrogenic properties).

Macrophages also engulf tissue debris and dead cells, as well as phagocytosing and killing most (but unfortunately not all) microorganisms. They also play an important part in *antigen presentation*. When stimulated by **glucocorticoids,** macrophages can additionally secrete *annexin 1* (a potent anti-inflammatory polypeptide; see Ch. 33), which controls the development of the local inflammatory reaction helping to limit any collateral damage.

Dendritic cells

These, along with monocytes and macrophages, represent members of the 'mononuclear phagocyte system' (see Guilliams et al., 2014). They are present in many tissues, especially those that subserve a barrier function (e.g. the skin, where they are sometimes referred to as *Langerhans cells* after their discoverer). As a key 'sentinel cell' they can detect the presence of pathogens and when thus activated they can migrate into lymphoid tissue, where they play a crucial part in antigen presentation.

Eosinophils

These cells have similar capacities to neutrophils but, like mast cells, are also 'armed' with a battery of substances stored in their granules, which, when released, kill multicellular parasites (e.g. helminths). These include *eosinophil cationic protein*, a *peroxidase* enzyme, the *eosinophil major basic protein* and a *neurotoxin*. The eosinophil is considered by many to be of primary importance in the pathogenesis of the late phase of asthma where, it is suggested, secreted granule proteins cause damage to bronchiolar epithelium (see Ch. 28). Indeed, the recent success of drugs targeting IL-5 (a key inducer of eosinophil differentiation and activation) and its receptor in severe asthma testifies to its pathological role in this complex disease (see Pelaia et al., 2020).

Basophils

Basophils are very similar in many respects to mast cells. Except in certain inflammatory diseases, such as viral infections and myeloproliferative disorders, the basophil content of the tissues is generally tiny and in health they form only <0.1% of circulating white blood cells. Their role is primarily in the control of parasitic infection.

Vascular endothelial cells

Originally considered to be 'passive' lining cells, vascular endothelial cells (see also Chs 22 and 23) are now known to play an active part in inflammation. Small arteriole endothelial cells secrete nitric oxide (NO), causing relaxation of the underlying smooth muscle (see Chs 19 and 21), vasodilatation and increased delivery of plasma and blood cells to the inflamed area. The endothelial cells of the postcapillary venules regulate plasma exudation and thus the delivery of plasma-derived mediators. Vascular endothelial cells express several adhesion molecules (the ICAM and selectin families), as well as a variety of receptors, including those for histamine, acetylcholine and IL-1. In addition to NO, the cells can synthesise and release other vasodilator agents such as PGI_2 and PGE_2, the vasoconstrictor agent endothelin, plasminogen activator, PAF and several cytokines. Endothelial cells also participate in the angiogenesis that occurs during inflammatory resolution, chronic inflammation and cancer (see Chs 6 and 57).

Platelets

Platelets are involved primarily in coagulation and thrombotic phenomena (see Ch. 23) but also play a part in inflammation. They have low-affinity receptors for IgE and may contribute to the first phase of allergic asthma (see Ch. 28). In addition to generating thromboxane $(TX)A_2$ and PAF, they can generate free radicals and pro-inflammatory cationic proteins. *Platelet-derived growth factor* contributes to the repair processes that follow inflammatory responses or damage to blood vessels.

Natural killer cells

Natural killer (NK) cells are a specialised type of lymphocyte. In an unusual twist to the receptor concept, NK cells kill targets (e.g. virus-infected or tumour cells) that *lack* ligands for inhibitory receptors on the NK cells themselves. These ligands are known as *major histocompatibility complex* (MHC) molecules, and any cells lacking these become a target for NK-cell attack, a strategy sometimes dubbed the 'mother turkey strategy'.[5] MHC

[3]Human immunodeficiency virus-1 binds to the surface CD4 glycoprotein on monocytes/macrophages but is able to penetrate the cell only after binding also to MCP-1 and RANTES receptors. This is a case where the innate immune system inadvertently aids the enemy.

[4]Literally 'big eaters', compared with neutrophils, originally called *microphages* or 'little eaters'.

[5]Citing the zoologist Schliedt in his book *River Out of Eden*, Richard Dawkins explains that the 'rule of thumb a mother turkey uses to recognise nest robbers is a dismayingly brusque one; in the vicinity of the nest, attack anything that moves unless it makes a noise like a baby turkey'.

proteins (also called *HLA* in leukocytes) are expressed on the surface of most host cells.

There are three major classes of MHC molecules. From our viewpoint, the most significant are the Class I MHC proteins which are involved in the host response to intracellular pathogens such as viruses, and the Class II group which are more concerned with defence against extracellular threats such as those posed by bacteria or parasites. MHC molecules are specific for a particular individual, enabling the NK cells to avoid damaging their host's cells. NK cells also have other functions: they are equipped with Fc receptors and, in the presence of antibodies directed against a target cell, they can kill the cell by antibody-dependent cellular cytotoxicity.

THE ADAPTIVE IMMUNE RESPONSE

The adaptive response provides the cellular basis of an 'immunological memory'. It provides a more powerful defence than the innate response, as well as being highly specific for the invading pathogen. Here we will provide only a simplified outline, stressing those aspects relevant for an understanding of drug action; for more detailed coverage, see textbooks in the *References and Further Reading* section at the end of this chapter.

The key cellular players in the adaptive response are the *lymphocytes*.[6] These are long-lived cells derived from precursor stem cells within the bone marrow. Following release into the blood and maturation, they dwell in the lymphoid tissues such as the lymph nodes and spleen. Here, they are poised to detect, intercept and identify the foreign proteins presented to them by antigen-presenting cells (APCs) such macrophages or dendritic cells. The three main groups of lymphocytes are:

- *B cells*, which mature in the bone marrow. They are responsible for antibody production, i.e. the *humoral* immune response.
- *T cells*, which mature in the thymus. They are important in the induction phase of the immune response and in *cell-mediated* immune reactions.
- *NK cells*. These are really part of the innate system. They are activated by *interferons* and release cytotoxic granules that destroy target cells identified as 'foreign' or abnormal.

T and B lymphocytes express antigen-specific receptors that recognise and react with virtually all the foreign proteins and polysaccharides we are likely to encounter during our lifetime. This receptor repertoire is generated randomly and so could recognise 'self' proteins as well as foreign antigens, with devastating results. However, *tolerance* to self-antigens is acquired during fetal life by apoptotic deletion of T-cell clones in the thymus that recognise the host's own tissues. Dendritic cells and macrophages involved in the innate response also have a role in preventing harmful immune reactions against the host's own cells.

The adaptive immune response occurs in two phases, termed the *induction phase* and the *effector phase*.

[6]White blood cells (WBCs) or leukocytes in blood are mostly neutrophils (50%–60%) or lymphocytes (20%–40%), with the rest being monocytes (3%–7%), eosinophils (1%–5%) and less than 1% basophils. The WBC count in a healthy adult is in the range 3.5–11 million per mL of blood – higher values may indicate chronic bacterial or viral infection; lower levels occur in anaemia or in immunosuppressed individuals (e.g. when undergoing treatment with chemotherapeutic drugs [see Ch. 57]).

The adaptive immune response

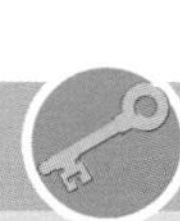

- The adaptive (specific, acquired) immunological response boosts the effectiveness of the innate responses. It has two phases, the induction phase and the effector phase, the latter consisting of (i) antibody-mediated and (ii) cell-mediated components.
- During the *induction phase*, naive T cells bearing either the CD4 or the CD8 co-receptors are presented with antigen, triggering proliferation:
  - CD8-bearing T cells develop into cytotoxic T cells that can kill virally infected cells.
  - CD4-bearing T-helper (Th) cells are stimulated by different cytokines to develop into Th1, Th2, Th9, Th17, Th22 or Treg cells.
    - *Th1* cells develop into cells that release cytokines that activate macrophages; these cells, along with cytotoxic T cells, control cell-mediated responses.
    - *Th2* cells control antibody-mediated responses by stimulating B cells to proliferate, giving rise to antibody-secreting plasma cells and memory cells.
    - *Th9* cells augment *Treg* function and are protective against parasitic infection.
    - *Th17* cells are similar to Th1 cells and are important in some human diseases such as rheumatoid arthritis.
    - *Th22* cells are involved in epithelial barrier immunity.
    - *Treg* cells restrain the development of the immune response.
- The effector phase utilises both antibody- and cell-mediated responses.
- Antibodies provide:
  - more selective complement activation
  - more effective pathogen phagocytosis
  - more effective attachment to multicellular parasites, facilitating their destruction
  - direct neutralisation of some viruses and of some bacterial toxins.
- Cell-mediated reactions provide:
  - $CD8^+$ cytotoxic T cells that kill virus-infected cells
  - cytokine-releasing $CD4^+$ T cells that enable macrophages to kill intracellular pathogens such as the tubercle bacillus
  - memory cells primed to react rapidly to a known antigen
  - help for B-cell activation.
- Inappropriately deployed immune reactions are termed *hypersensitivity reactions.*
- Anti-inflammatory and immunosuppressive drugs are used when the normally protective inflammatory and/or immune responses escape control.

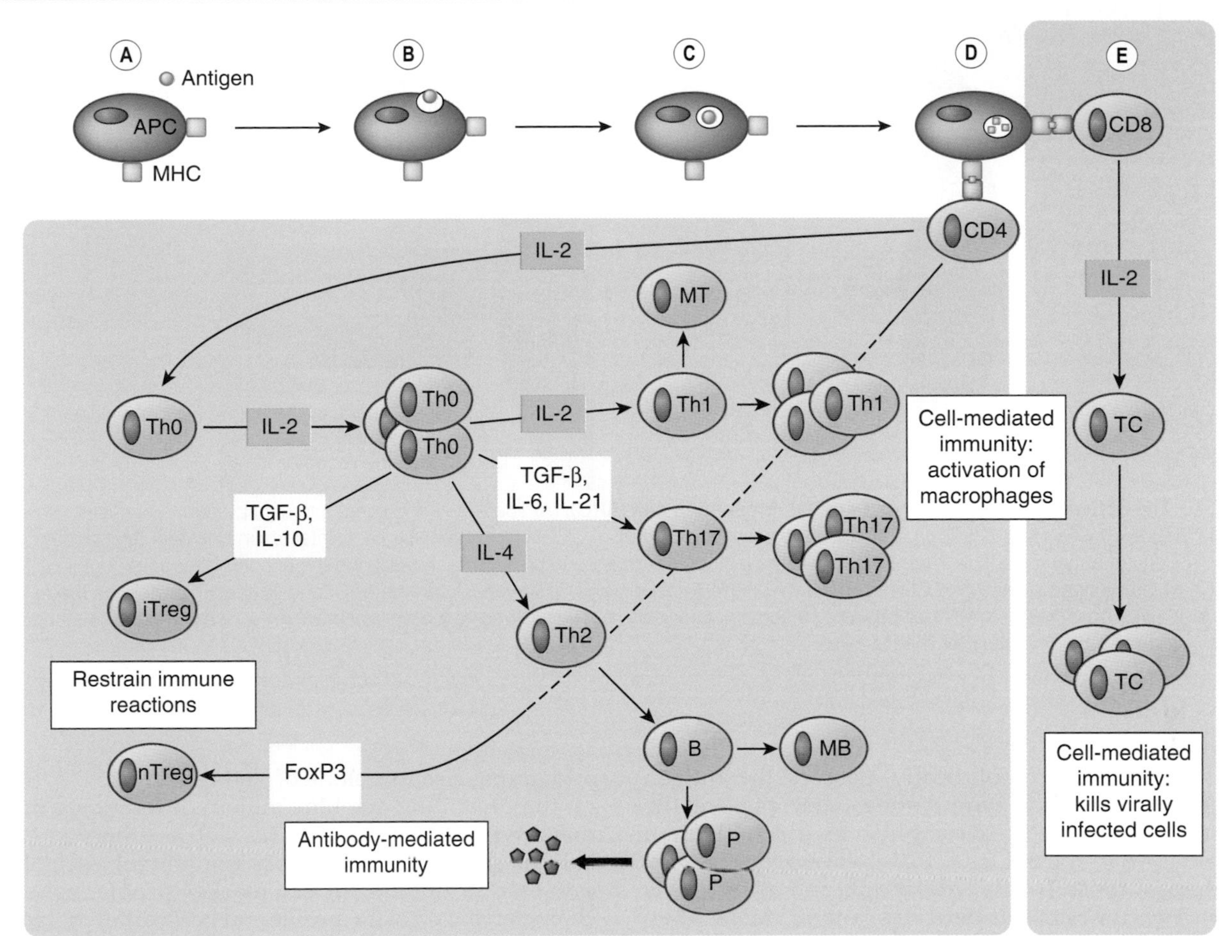

Fig. 7.3 Simplified diagram of the induction and effector phases of lymphocyte activation. APCs ingest and process antigen (A–D) before presenting fragments to naive, uncommitted CD4 (*c*luster of *d*ifferentiation 4) T cells in conjunction with MHC class II molecules, or to naive CD8 T cells in conjunction with MHC class I molecules, thus 'arming' them. Armed CD4+ T cells synthesise and express IL-2 receptors and also release this cytokine. This stimulates the cells by autocrine action, causing generation and proliferation of T-helper zero (Th0) cells. Autocrine cytokines (e.g. IL-4) cause differentiation of some Th0 cells to give Th2 cells, which are responsible for the development of antibody-mediated immune responses. These Th2 (and sometimes Th1) cells cooperate with and activate B cells to proliferate and give rise eventually to memory B cells (MB) and plasma cells (P), which secrete antibodies. The T cells that aid B cells in this way are referred to as T_{FH} (follicular homing) cells. Further stimulation by other autocrine cytokines (e.g. IL-2, 6) causes proliferation of Th0 cells to give Th1, Th17, Th9, Th22 or iTreg cells. Th1 and Th17 cells secrete cytokines that activate macrophages (responsible for some cell-mediated immune reactions). Th22 cells promote repair of damaged epithelium and augment mucosal immunity. iTreg (inducible T regulatory cell derived from Th0 precursors) and nTreg (naturally occurring T regulatory cell matured in the thymus) cells restrain and inhibit the development of the immune response, thus preventing autoimmunity and excessive immune activation. Th9 cells promote the survival and function of Treg cells. The armed CD8+ T cells (E) also synthesise and express IL-2 receptors and release IL-2, which further stimulates the cells by autocrine action to proliferate and give rise to cytotoxic T cells (TC). These can kill virally infected cells. IL-2 secreted by CD4+ cells also stimulates CD8+ cells to proliferate. Note that the 'effector phase' described in the text relates to the 'protective' action of the immune response. When the response is inappropriately deployed – as in chronic inflammatory conditions such as rheumatoid arthritis – the Th1/Th17 component of the immune response is dominant and the activated macrophages release IL-1 and TNF-α, which in turn trigger the release of the chemokines and inflammatory cytokines that play a major role in the pathology of the disease. Please see Raphael et al. (2015) and Saravia et al. (2019) for an overview of T-cell subsets in health and disease. *APC*, Antigen-presenting cell; *IL*, interleukin; *MT*, memory T cell; *MB*, memory B cell; *MHC*, major histocompatibility complex; *TC*, cytotoxic T cell; *TGF*, transforming growth factor; *P*, plasma cell; *Treg*, regulatory T cell. Th 9 and Th22 cells not detailed for clarity.

THE INDUCTION PHASE

During the induction phase, antigen is 'presented' to T cells in the lymph nodes by macrophages or large dendritic cells (Fig. 7.3). This antigen may constitute part of an invading pathogen (e.g. the coat of a bacterium) or be released by such an organism (e.g. a bacterial toxin), or it may be a vaccine, an environmental agent such as pollen, an insect bite, a foodstuff or a substance introduced experimentally to study the immune response (e.g. the injection of egg albumin into the guinea pig).

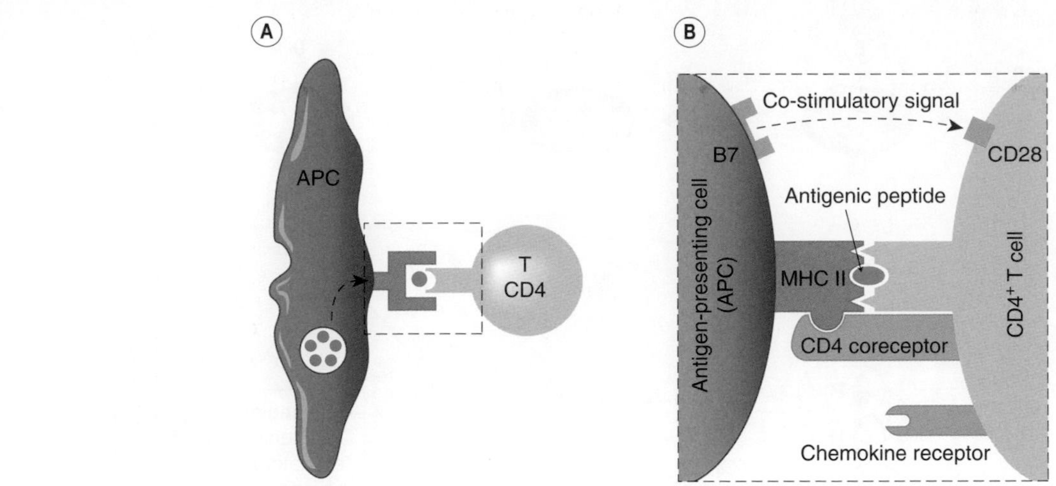

Fig. 7.4 The activation of a T cell by an antigen-presenting cell (APC). (A) The APC encounters a foreign protein, and this is proteolytically processed into peptide fragments. The activation process then involves three stages: (i) interaction between the complex of pathogen-derived antigen peptide fragments with major histocompatibility complex (MHC) class II and the antigen-specific receptor on the T cell; (B) (ii) interaction between the CD4 co-receptor on the T cell and an MHC molecule on the APC; and (iii) the B7 protein on the APC cell surface binds to CD28 on the T cell providing a co-stimulatory signal. The CD4 co-receptor, together with a T-cell chemokine receptor, constitute the main binding sites for the HIV virus (see Ch. 53).

APCs ingest and proteolytically 'process' the antigen and once they reach local lymph nodes, they 'present' the fragments on their surface to lymphocytes in combination with various MHC molecules. This is followed by complex interactions of those T cells with B cells and other T cells (Fig. 7.4). Two types of lymphocytes 'attend' APCs. They are generally distinguished by the presence, on their surface, of CD4 or CD8 receptors. These are *co-receptors* that cooperate with the main antigen-specific receptors in antigen recognition. Macrophages also carry surface CD4 proteins.

The two types of lymphocyte involved in the adaptive response are:

- Uncommitted (naive) $CD4^+$ Th lymphocytes, or Th precursor (Thp) cells, in association with class II MHC molecules.
- Naive $CD8^+$ T lymphocytes in association with class I MHC molecules.[7]

Activation of a T cell by an APC requires that several 'identification' and 'authentication' signals pass between the two cells at this 'immune synapse' (see Medzhitov and Janeway, 2000). As detailed in Fig. 7.3, following activation, the T cells both generate IL-2 and acquire IL-2 receptors. IL-2 has an autocrine[8] action, stimulating proliferation and giving rise to a clone of Th0 cells, which, depending on the prevailing cytokine milieu, differentiate into four major types of 'helper cells' (as well as others and further subtypes, which is beyond our remit here), each of which possesses a unique surface marker profile, generates a characteristic cytokine profile and has a different biological role. These characteristics are summarised in Table 7.2. Some potent anti-inflammatory drugs act by blocking the IL-2 receptor, thus preventing lymphocyte proliferation (see Ch. 25).

Knowledge of the relationship between T-cell subsets, their respective cytokine profiles and pathological conditions can be used to manipulate the immune responses for disease prevention and treatment. There are already many experimental models in which modulation of the Th1/Th2 balance with recombinant cytokines or cytokine antagonists alters the outcome of the disease.

THE EFFECTOR PHASE

During the effector phase, the activated B lymphocytes differentiate either into *plasma cells* or into *memory cells*. The B plasma cells produce specific antibodies, which are effective in the extracellular fluid, but which cannot neutralise pathogens within cells. T-cell-mediated immune mechanisms overcome this problem by activating macrophages or directly killing virus-infected host cells. Antigen-sensitive memory cells are formed when the clone of lymphocytes that are programmed to respond to an antigen is greatly expanded after the first contact with the organism. They allow a greatly accelerated and more effective response to subsequent antigen exposure. In some cases, the response is so rapid and efficient that a single exposure is often sufficient to

[7]The main reason that it is difficult to transplant organs such as kidneys from one person to another is that their respective MHC molecules are different. Lymphocytes in the recipient will react to non-self (*allogenic*) MHC molecules in the donor tissue, which is then likely to be rejected by a rapid and powerful immunological reaction.

[8]In 'autocrine' signalling the mediator acts on the cell that released it. In 'paracrine' signalling, the mediator acts on neighbouring cells, whilst in 'juxtacrine' signalling, it acts on cells in direct contact.

Table 7.2 Lymphocyte subsets, their role in host defence and relationship to inflammatory disease

Subset	Cytokine trigger	Main role in adaptive response	Main cytokines produced	Role in disease
Th0	IL-2	Precursor cells for further differentiation	–	–
Th1	IL-2	'Cell-mediated immunity' • Cytokines released from these cells: activate macrophages to phagocytose and kill microorganisms and kill tumour cells; drive proliferation and maturation of the clone into *cytotoxic T cells* that kill virally infected host cells; reciprocally inhibit Th2 cell maturation	IFN-γ, IL-2 and TNF-α	Insulin-dependent diabetes mellitus (see Ch. 31), multiple sclerosis, *Helicobacter pylori*–induced peptic ulcer (see Ch. 30), aplastic anaemia (see Ch. 24) and rheumatoid arthritis (see Ch. 25) Allograft rejection
Th2	IL-4	'Humoral immunity' • Cytokines released from these cells: stimulate B cells to proliferate and mature into plasma cells producing antibodies; enhance differentiation and activation of eosinophils and reciprocally inhibit Th1/Th17-cell functions. For this reason, they are often thought of as having a predominately anti-inflammatory action	IL-4, IL-5, TGF-β, IL-10 and IL-13	Asthma (see Ch. 28) and allergy AIDS progression is associated with loss of Th1 cells and is facilitated by Th2 responses
Th17	TGF-β, IL-6 and IL-21	A specialised type of Th1 cell	IL-17	The response to infection, organ-specific immune responses and in the pathogenesis of diseases such as rheumatoid arthritis and multiple sclerosis
Treg[a]	IL-10 and TGF-β or FOX P3 Matured in the thymus	Restraining the immune response, preventing autoimmunity and curtailing potentially damaging inflammatory responses	IL-10 and TGF-β	Failure of this mechanism can provoke excessive inflammation

[a]Two populations are commonly encountered: inducible (iTreg) and naturally occurring Treg cells (nTreg).
Th9 and Th22 cells are not included here for reasons of space but appropriate references are highlighted in Fig. 7.3 should readers wish to discover more about these 'new' additions.
FOX P3, 'Forkhead box 3', a transcriptional regulator which has a key role in regulation of the immune system; *IFN*, interferon; *IL*, interleukin; *TGF*, transforming growth factor; *TNF*, tumour necrosis factor.

ensure that the pathogen can never gain a foothold again. Vaccination and immunisation procedures make use of this invaluable phenomenon.

THE ANTIBODY-MEDIATED (HUMORAL) RESPONSE

There are five main classes of antibody – IgG, IgM, IgE, IgA and IgD – which differ from each other in certain structural respects. All are γ-globulins (immunoglobulins), which both recognise and interact specifically with antigens (i.e. proteins or polysaccharides foreign to the host), as well as activating one or more further components of the host's defence systems.

An antibody is a Y-shaped protein molecule (see Ch. 5) in which the arms of the Y (the fragment antigen binding – *Fab* portion) include a variable recognition site for specific antigens, and the invariable stem of the Y (the 'constant' *Fc* portion) activates host defences. The B cells that are responsible for antibody production recognise foreign molecules by means of surface receptors similar the immunoglobulins. Mammals harbour B-cell clones with recognition sites for an immense number of different antigens. Once they encounter a ligand that they recognise, synthesis of that particular species is greatly expanded and subsequently shed into the circulating blood forming a reservoir of circulating antibody specific for that particular antigen.

The induction of antibody-mediated responses varies with the type of antigen. With most antigens, a cooperative process between Th2 cells and B cells is generally necessary to produce a response. B cells can also present antigen to T cells which then release cytokines that act further on the B cell. The anti-inflammatory glucocorticoids (see Chs 25 and 33) and the immunosuppressive drug **ciclosporin** affect the molecular events crucial to induction. The cytotoxic immunosuppressive drugs inhibit the proliferation of both B and T cells. Eicosanoids may play a part in controlling these processes as PGs of the E series can inhibit lymphocyte proliferation, probably by inhibiting the release of IL-2.

As you might guess, the ability to make antibodies has huge survival value; children born without this ability, such as those suffering from Bruton's agammaglobulinemia[9] suffer repeated infections such as pneumonia, skin infections and tonsillitis. Before the days of antibiotics, they died in early childhood, and even today they require regular replacement therapy with immunoglobulin. Apart from their ability to neutralise pathogens, antibodies can boost the effectiveness and specificity of the host's defence reaction in several ways.

Antibodies and complement

Formation of the antigen–antibody complex exposes a binding site for complement on the Fc domain. This activates the complement sequence and sets in train its attendant biological effects (see Fig. 7.1). This route to C3 activation (the 'classic pathway') provides an especially selective way of activating complement in response to a particular pathogen, because the antigen–antibody reaction that initiates it is not only a highly specific recognition event but also occurs in close association with the pathogen. The lytic property of complement can be used therapeutically: monoclonal antibodies (mAbs) and complement together can be used to rid bone marrow of cancer cells as an adjunct to chemotherapy or radiotherapy (see Ch. 57).

Antibodies and the phagocytosis of bacteria

When antibodies are attached to their antigens on microorganisms by their Fab portions, the Fc domain is exposed. Phagocytic cells (neutrophils and macrophages) express surface receptors for these projecting Fc portions, which serve as a very specific link between microorganism and phagocyte.

Antibodies and cellular toxicity

In some cases, for example, with parasitic worms, the invader may be too large to be ingested by phagocytes. Antibody molecules can form a link between parasite and the host's white cells (in this case, eosinophils), which are then able to damage or kill the parasite. NK cells in conjunction with Fc receptors can also kill antibody-coated target cells (an example of *antibody-dependent cell-mediated cytotoxicity*).

Antibodies and mast cells or basophils

Mast cells and basophils have receptors for IgE, a particular form of antibody that can attach ('fix') to their cell membranes. When this cell-fixed antibody reacts with an antigen, an entire panoply of pharmacologically active mediators is secreted. This very complex reaction is found widely throughout the animal kingdom and presumably confers clear survival value to the host. Having said that, its precise biological significance is not always entirely clear, although it may be of importance in association with eosinophil activity as a defence against parasitic worms. When inappropriately triggered by substances not inherently damaging or dangerous to the host, it is implicated in certain types of allergic reaction and seemingly contributes more to illness than to survival in the modern world.

THE CELL-MEDIATED IMMUNE RESPONSE

Cytotoxic T cells (derived from $CD8^+$ cells) and inflammatory (cytokine-releasing) Th1 cells are attracted to inflammatory sites in a similar manner to neutrophils and macrophages and are involved in cell-mediated responses (see Fig. 7.3).

Cytotoxic T cells

Armed cytotoxic T cells kill intracellular microorganisms such as viruses. When a virus infects a mammalian cell, there are two aspects to the resulting defensive response. The first step is the expression on the cell surface of peptides derived from the pathogen in association with MHC molecules. The second step is the recognition of the peptide–MHC complex by specific receptors on cytotoxic ($CD8^+$) T cells (Fig. 7.4 shows a similar process for a $CD4^+$ T cell). The cytotoxic T cells then destroy virus-infected cells by programming them to undergo apoptosis. Cooperation with macrophages may be required for killing to occur.

Macrophage activating $CD4^+$ Th1 cells

Some pathogens (e.g. Mycobacteria, Listeria) survive and actually multiply within macrophages after ingestion. Armed $CD4^+$ Th1 cells release cytokines that activate macrophages to kill these intracellular pathogens. Th1 cells also recruit macrophages by releasing cytokines that act on vascular endothelial cells (e.g. TNF-α) and chemokines (e.g. MCP-1) that attract the macrophages to the sites of infection.

A complex of microorganism-derived peptides plus MHC molecules is expressed on the macrophage surface and is recognised by cytokine-releasing Th1 cells, which then generate cytokines that enable the macrophage to deploy its killing mechanisms. Activated macrophages (with or without intracellular pathogens) are veritable factories for the production of chemical mediators: they can generate and secrete not only many cytokines but also toxic oxygen metabolites and neutral proteases that kill extracellular organisms (e.g. *Pneumocystis jiroveci* and helminths), complement components, eicosanoids, NO, a fibroblast-stimulating factor, pyrogens and the 'tissue factor' that initiates the extrinsic pathway of the coagulation cascade (see Ch. 23), as well as various other coagulation factors. This is the cell-mediated reaction that is primarily responsible for allograft rejection. Macrophages are also important in coordinating the repair processes that must occur for inflammation to resolve.

The specific cell-mediated or humoral immunological response is superimposed on the innate non-specific vascular and cellular reactions described previously, making them not only markedly more effective but also much more selective for particular pathogens.

The general events of the inflammatory and hypersensitivity reactions specified earlier vary in some tissues. In the airway inflammation of asthma for example, eosinophils and neuropeptides play a particularly significant role (see Ch. 28). In central nervous system (CNS) inflammation, there is less neutrophil infiltration and monocyte influx is delayed, possibly because of lack of adhesion molecule expression on CNS vascular endothelium and deficient generation of chemokines. It has long been known that some tissues – the CNS parenchyma, the anterior chamber of the eye and the testis – are *immunologically privileged* sites, in that a foreign antigen

[9]Mainly boys: Col. Bruton was chief of paediatrics at the Walter Reid army hospital. 'Bruton's agammaglobulinemia' is caused by a defect in a tyrosine kinase (BTK) coded on the X chromosome. BTKs promote leukocyte survival and proliferation and BTK inhibitors are proving useful in treating certain leukaemias (see Ch. 57).

introduced directly does not provoke an immune reaction (which could be very disadvantageous to the host).[10] However, introduction elsewhere of an antigen already in the CNS parenchyma will trigger the development of immune/inflammatory responses in the CNS.

SYSTEMIC RESPONSES IN INFLAMMATION

In addition to the local changes in an inflammatory site, there are commonly more general systemic manifestations of inflammatory disease. Typically, these could include fever, an increase in blood leukocytes and the release from the liver of acute-phase proteins. The latter includes *C-reactive protein, α_2-macroglobulin, fibrinogen, α_1-antitrypsin, serum amyloid A* and some complement fragments. While the function of many of these components is still a matter of conjecture, many seem to have some antimicrobial actions. C-reactive protein, for example, binds to some microorganisms, and the resulting complex activates complement. Other proteins scavenge iron (an essential nutrient for invading organisms) or block proteases, perhaps protecting the host against the worst excesses of the inflammatory response.

THE ROLE OF THE NERVOUS SYSTEM IN INFLAMMATION

It has become clear in recent years that the central, autonomic and peripheral nervous systems all play an important part in the regulation of the inflammatory response. This occurs at various levels:

- *The neuroendocrine system.* Adrenocorticotrophic hormone (ACTH), released from the anterior pituitary gland in response to endogenous circadian rhythm or to stress (and thus episodes of illness), releases cortisol from the adrenal glands. This hormone plays a crucial role in regulating immune function at all levels, hence the use of glucocorticoid drugs in the treatment of inflammatory disease. This topic is explored fully in Chapters 25 and 33.
- *The CNS.* Surprisingly, cytokines such as IL-1 can signal the development of an inflammatory response directly to the brain through receptors on the vagus nerve. This may elicit an 'inflammatory reflex' and trigger activation of a cholinergic anti-inflammatory pathway. See Sternberg (2006) and Chavan et al. (2017) for interesting discussions of this topic.
- *The autonomic nervous system.* Both the sympathetic and parasympathetic systems can modulate the development of the inflammatory response. Generally speaking, their influence is anti-inflammatory. Receptors for noradrenaline and acetylcholine (such as alpha 7 nicotinic acetylcholine receptor) are found on macrophages and many other cells involved in the immune response although the origins of these ligands are unclear. Opioid receptors are also found on inflammatory cells and they also have multiple effects on many aspects of the inflammatory response (Liang et al., 2016).
- *Peripheral sensory neurons.* Some sensory neurons release inflammatory neuropeptides when appropriately stimulated. These neurons are fine afferents (capsaicin-sensitive C and Aδ fibres; see Ch. 43) with specific receptors at their peripheral terminals. Kinins, 5-hydroxytryptamine (5-HT) and other chemical mediators generated during inflammation act on these receptors, stimulating the release of neuropeptides such as the tachykinins (neurokinin A, substance P) and calcitonin gene-related peptide (CGRP), which have pro-inflammatory or algesic actions. The neuropeptides are considered further in Chapter 17.

UNWANTED INFLAMMATORY AND IMMUNE RESPONSES AND THEIR UNINTENDED CONSEQUENCES

The immune response has to strike a delicate balance. According to one school of thought, an infection-proof immune system would be a possibility but would come at a serious cost to the host. With many millions of potential antigenic sites in the host, such a 'super-immune' system would be some 1000 times more likely to attack the host itself, triggering *autoimmune disease*. It is not uncommon to encounter patients in whom exposure to ordinarily innocuous substances such as pollen or peanuts inadvertently activates the immune system. When this happens, the ensuing inflammation itself inflicts self-harm – either acutely as in (for example) anaphylaxis or chronically in (for example) asthma or rheumatoid arthritis. In either case, appropriate anti-inflammatory or immunosuppressive therapy may be required.

A proportionate response is also required in the case of acute infection with bacterial or viral pathogens. Whilst elimination of the invading organism is clearly the desired outcome, without adequate regulation there is the risk that a sustained or exaggerated host response will pose a greater threat than the pathogen itself. Such dysregulation of the immune response is responsible for syndromes including *sepsis*, ARDS and COVID-19-associated pneumonitis (see Nedeva et al., 2019).

Unwanted immune responses, termed *allergic* or *hypersensitivity* reactions, are generally classified into four types.

Type I hypersensitivity

Also called *immediate* or *anaphylactic hypersensitivity* (often known simply as 'allergy'), type I hypersensitivity occurs in individuals who predominantly exhibit a Th2 rather than a Th1 response to antigen. In these individuals, substances that are not inherently noxious (such as grass pollen, house dust mites, certain foodstuffs or drugs, animal fur and so on) provoke the production of antibodies of the IgE type.[11] These fix onto mast cells and eosinophils. Subsequent contact with the problematic substance causes the release

[10]Cold sore sufferers can blame this phenomenon for their misery – herpes simplex virus resides in the facial nervous tissue and becomes activated following stress or environmental stimuli, for example, exposure to the sun. The virus can reside in the CNS tissue for a whole lifetime from infancy, stubbornly resistant to the attempts of our immune cells to remove it. It can be transmitted to the baby from a carrier via a kiss, before the infant's immune system can eliminate the virus (usually by 6 months old). Bonnie babies are destined to suffer forever more.

[11]Such individuals are said to be 'atopic', from a Greek word meaning 'out of place'.

of histamine, PAF, eicosanoids and cytokines. The effects may be localised to the nose (hay fever), the bronchial tree (the initial phase of asthma), the skin (urticaria) or the gastrointestinal tract. In some cases, the reaction is more generalised and produces *anaphylactic shock,* which can be severe and life-threatening. Some important unwanted effects of drugs include anaphylactic hypersensitivity responses (see Ch. 58).

Type II hypersensitivity

Also called *antibody-dependent cytotoxic hypersensitivity,* type II hypersensitivity occurs when the mechanisms outlined previously are directed against cells within the host that are (or appear to be) foreign. For example, host cells or proteins altered by drugs are sometimes mistaken by the immune system for foreign organisms and evoke antibody formation. The antigen–antibody reaction triggers complement activation (and its sequelae) and may promote attack by NK cells. Examples include alteration by drugs of neutrophils, leading to *agranulocytosis* (see Ch. 57), or of platelets, leading to *thrombocytopenic purpura* (see Ch. 23). These type II reactions are also implicated in some types of *autoimmune thyroiditis* (e.g. *Hashimoto's disease;* see Ch. 34).

Type III hypersensitivity

Also called *complex-mediated hypersensitivity,* type III hypersensitivity occurs when antibodies react with *soluble* antigens. The antigen–antibody complexes can activate complement or attach to mast cells and stimulate the release of inflammatory mediators.

An experimental example of this is the *Arthus reaction* that occurs if a foreign protein is injected subcutaneously into a rabbit or guinea pig bearing pre-existing high circulating concentrations of antibody. Within 3–8 h the area becomes red and swollen because the antigen–antibody complexes precipitate in small blood vessels and activate complement. Neutrophils are attracted and activated (by C5a) to generate toxic oxygen species and to secrete enzymes.

Mast cells are also stimulated by C3a to release mediators. Damage caused by this process is involved in *serum sickness,* which occurs when antigen persists in the blood after sensitisation, causing a severe reaction, as in the response to mouldy hay (known as *Farmer's lung*), and in certain types of autoimmune kidney and arterial disease. Type III hypersensitivity is also implicated in *lupus erythematosus* (a chronic, autoimmune inflammatory disease).

Type IV hypersensitivity

The prototype of type IV hypersensitivity (also known as *cell-mediated* or *delayed hypersensitivity*) is the *tuberculin reaction,* a local inflammatory response seen when proteins derived from cultures of the tubercle bacillus are injected into the skin of a person who has been sensitised by a previous infection or immunisation. An 'inappropriate' cell-mediated immune response is stimulated, accompanied by infiltration of mononuclear cells and the release of various cytokines. Cell-mediated hypersensitivity is also the basis of the reaction seen in some other infections (e.g. mumps and measles), as well as with mosquito and tick bites. It is also important in the skin reactions to drugs or industrial chemicals (see Ch. 58), where the chemical (termed a *hapten*) combines with proteins in the skin to form the 'foreign' substance that evokes the cell-mediated immune response (see Fig. 7.3).

In essence, inappropriately deployed T-cell activity underlies all types of hypersensitivity, initiating types I, II and III, and being involved in both the initiation and the effector phase in type IV. These reactions are the basis of the clinically important group of autoimmune diseases. Immunosuppressive drugs (see Ch. 25) and/or glucocorticoids (see Ch. 33) are routinely employed to treat such disorders.

THE OUTCOME OF THE INFLAMMATORY RESPONSE

It is important not to lose sight of the fact that the inflammatory response is a defence mechanism and not a disease per se. Its role is to restore normal structure and function to the infected or damaged tissue, and in the vast majority of cases, this is what occurs.

The healing and resolution phase of the inflammatory response is, however, an active process and does not simply 'happen' in the absence of further inflammation. Resolution utilises its own unique palette of mediators and cytokines (including various growth factors, annexin A1, lipoxins, omega-3 polyunsaturated acid-derived mediators and IL-10; see Ch. 17) to terminate residual inflammation and to promote remodelling and repair of damaged tissue.

In some cases, healing will be complete, but if there has been marked damage, repair is usually necessary, and this may result in scarring. If the pathogen persists, it is enclosed by the host in a fibrous capsule 'prison' to prevent any further damage. Alternatively, the acute inflammatory response may transform into a chronic inflammatory response. This is a slow, smouldering reaction that can continue indefinitely, destroying tissue and promoting local proliferation of cells and connective tissue. The principal cell types found in areas of chronic inflammation are mononuclear cells and abnormal macrophage-derived cells. During healing or chronic inflammation, growth factors trigger angiogenesis and cause fibroblasts to lay down fibrous tissue. Infection by some microorganisms, such as syphilis, tuberculosis and leprosy, bear the characteristic hallmarks of chronic inflammation from the start and result in the formation of macrophage aggregates called *granulomas.* The cellular and mediator components of this type of inflammation are also seen in many, if not most, chronic autoimmune and hypersensitivity diseases and are important targets for drug action.

REFERENCES AND FURTHER READING

The innate and adaptive responses

Anwar, M.A., Shah, M., Kim, J., Choi, S., 2019. Recent clinical trends in Toll-like receptor targeting therapeutics. Med. Res. Rev. 39 (3), 1053–1090.

Chavan, S.S., Pavlov, V.A., Tracey, K.J., 2017. Mechanisms and therapeutic relevance of neuro-immune communication. Immunity 46 (6), 927–942.

Delves, P.J., Roitt, I.M., 2000. The immune system. N. Engl. J. Med. 343, 108–117 37–49.

Fitzgerald, K.A., Kagan, J.C., 2020. Toll-like receptors and the control of immunity. Cell 180 (6), 1044–1066.

Gabay, C., Kushner, I., 1999. Acute phase proteins and other systemic responses to inflammation. N. Engl. J. Med. 340, 448–454.

Guilliams, M., Ginhoux, F., Jakubzick, C., et al., 2014. Dendritic cells, monocytes and macrophages: a unified nomenclature based on ontogeny. Nat. Rev. Immunol. 14 (8), 571–578.

Guilliams, M., Mildner, A., Yona, S., 2018. Developmental and functional heterogeneity of monocytes. Immunity 49 (4), 595–613.

Hughes, C.E., Nibbs, R.J.B., 2018. A guide to chemokines and their receptors. FEBS J. 285 (16), 2944–2971.

Kay, A.B., 2001. Allergic diseases and their treatment. N. Engl. J. Med. 344, 109–113 30–37.

Kennedy, M.A., 2010. A brief review of the basics of immunology: the innate and adaptive response. Vet. Clin. North Am. Small. Anim. Pract. 40, 369-379.

Li, D., Wu, M., 2021. Pattern recognition receptors in health and diseases. Signal Transduct. Target. Ther. 6 (1), 291.

Liang, X., Liu, R., Chen, C., Ji, F., Li, T., 2016. Opioid system modulates the immune function: a review. Transl. Perioper. Pain. Med. 1, 5–13.

Martinez, F.O., Gordon, S., 2014. The M1 and M2 paradigm of macrophage activation: time for reassessment. F1000Prime Rep. 6, 13.

Medzhitov, R., Janeway, C., 2000. Innate immunity. N. Engl. J. Med. 343, 338–344.

Mills, K.H., 2008. Induction, function and regulation of IL-17-producing T cells. Eur. J. Immunol. 38, 2636–2649.

Murphy, P.M., 2001. Viral exploitation and subversion of the immune system through chemokine mimicry. Nat. Immunol. 2, 116–122.

Nedeva, C., Menassa, J., Puthalakath, H., 2019. Sepsis: inflammation is a necessary evil. Front. Cell Dev. Biol. 7, 108.

Nourshargh, S., Hordijk, P.L., Sixt, M., 2010. Breaching multiple barriers: leukocyte motility through venular walls and the interstitium. Nat. Rev. Mol. Cell Biol. 11, 366–378.

Orecchioni, M., Ghosheh, Y., Pramod, A.B., Ley, K., 2019. Macrophage polarization: different gene signatures in M1(LPS+) vs. classically and M2(LPS-) vs. alternatively activated macrophages. Front. Immunol. 10, 1084.

Pelaia, C., Crimi, C., Vatrella, A., Tinello, C., Terracciano, R., Pelaia, G., 2020. Molecular targets for biological therapies of severe asthma. Front. Immunol. 11, 603312.

Raphael, I., Nalawade, S., Eagar, T.N., Forsthuber, T.G., 2015. T cell subsets and their signature cytokines in autoimmune and inflammatory diseases. Cytokine 74 (1), 5–17.

Saravia, J., Chapman, N.M., Chi, H., 2019. Helper T cell differentiation. Cell. Mol. Immunol. 16 (7), 634–643.

Segal, A.W., 2016. NADPH oxidases as electrochemical generators to produce ion fluxes and turgor in fungi, plants and humans. Open Biol. 6, 1–15.

Sternberg, E.M., 2006. Neural regulation of innate immunity: a coordinated nonspecific host response to pathogens. Nat. Rev. Immunol. 6, 318–328.

Strowig, T., Henao-Mejia, J., Elinav, E., Flavell, R., 2012. Inflammasomes in health and disease. Nature 481, 278–286.

Wills-Karp, M., Santeliz, J., Karp, C.L., 2001. The germless theory of allergic diseases. Nat. Rev. Immunol. 1, 69–75.

Zheng, D., Liwinski, T., Elinav, E., 2020. Inflammasome activation and regulation: toward a better understanding of complex mechanisms. Cell Discov. 6, 36.

Books

Dawkins, R., 1995. River Out of Eden, first ed. Weidenfeld and Nicholson, London.

Murphy, K.M., Weaver, C., Berg, L.J., 2022. Janeway's Immunobiology, tenth ed. W.W. Norton & Company, London.

Nijkamp, F.P., Parnham, M., Rossi, A.G. (Eds.), 2020. Nijkamp and Parnham's Principles of Immunopharmacology, fourth ed. Springer, London.

Serhan, C., Ward, P.A., Gilroy, D.W. (Eds.), 2010. Fundamentals of Inflammation. Cambridge University Press, New York.

8 Method and measurement in pharmacology

OVERVIEW

We emphasised in Chapters 2 to 5 that drugs, being molecules, produce their effects by interacting with other molecules. This interaction can lead to effects at all levels of biological organisation, from molecules to human populations.[1]

Gaddum, a pioneering pharmacologist, commented in 1942: 'A branch of science comes of age when it becomes quantitative.' In this chapter, we cover the principles of metrication at the various organisational levels, ranging from laboratory methods to clinical trials. Assessment of drug action at the population level is the concern of pharmacoepidemiology and pharmacoeconomics (see Ch. 1), disciplines that are beyond the scope of this book.

We consider first the general principles of bioassay and its extension to studies in human beings; we describe the development of animal models to bridge the predictive gap between animal physiology and human disease; we next discuss aspects of clinical trials used to evaluate therapeutic efficacy in a clinical setting; finally, we consider summarising multiple datasets in a meta-analysis and the principles of balancing overall benefit and risk. Experimental design and statistical analysis are central to the interpretation of all types of pharmacological data.

BIOASSAY

Bioassay, originally defined as the estimation of the concentration or potency of a substance by measurement of the biological response that it produces, has played a key role in the development of pharmacology. Quantitation of drug effects by bioassay is necessary to compare the properties of different substances, or the same substance under different circumstances. It is used:

- to measure the pharmacological activity of new or chemically undefined substances;
- to investigate the function of endogenous mediators;
- to measure drug toxicity and unwanted effects.

Bioassay plays a key role in the development of new drugs, discussed in Chapter 60.

The use of bioassay to measure the *concentration* of drugs and other active substances in the blood or other body fluids – once an important technology – has now been largely replaced by analytical chemistry techniques.

Many hormones and chemical mediators were discovered by the biological effects that they produce. For example, the ability of extracts of the posterior lobe of the pituitary to produce a rise in blood pressure and a contraction of the uterus was observed at the beginning of the 20th century. Quantitative assay procedures based on these actions enabled a standard preparation of the extract to be established by international agreement in 1935. By use of these assays, it was shown that two distinct peptides – vasopressin and oxytocin – were responsible, and they were eventually identified and synthesised in 1953. Biological assay had already revealed much about the synthesis, storage and release of the hormones, and was essential for their purification and identification. The recent growth of *biopharmaceuticals* (see Ch. 5) as therapeutic agents has relied on bioassay techniques and the establishment of standard preparations. Biopharmaceuticals, whether derived from natural sources (e.g. monoclonal antibodies, vaccines) or by recombinant DNA technology (e.g. erythropoietin), tend to vary from batch to batch, and need to be standardised with respect to their biological activity. Varying glycosylation patterns, for example, which are not detected by immunoassay techniques, may affect biological activity.

BIOLOGICAL TEST SYSTEMS

Nowadays, an important use of bioassay is to provide information that will predict the effect of the drug in the clinical situation (where the aim is to improve function in patients suffering from the effects of disease). The choice of laboratory test systems (in vitro and in vivo 'models') that provide this predictive link is an important aspect of quantitative pharmacology.

By the 1960s, pharmacologists had become adept at using isolated organs and laboratory animals (usually under anaesthesia) for quantitative experiments, and had developed the principles of bioassay to allow reliable measurements to be made with these sometimes difficult and unpredictable test systems.

These 'traditional' assay systems address drug action at the physiological level – roughly, the mid-range of the organisational hierarchy shown in Fig. 8.1. Extension of the range in both directions, towards the molecular and atomistic as well as in the opposite direction towards the clinical, has taken place since.

The introduction of radioligand binding assays (see Ch. 3) and subsequently the use of engineered cell lines expressing normal and mutated receptors and signalling molecules changed dramatically the ways in which bioassay could be used to study the molecular and cellular consequences of receptor activation. Indeed, the range of techniques for analysing drug effects at the cellular level is now very impressive and expanding rapidly. An example (Fig. 8.2) is the use of fluorescence-activated cell sorting (FACS) to measure the effect of a corticosteroid on the expression of a cell surface marker protein by human blood monocytes.

[1]Consider the effect of cocaine on organised crime, of organophosphate 'nerve gases' on the stability of dictatorships or of anaesthetics on the feasibility of surgical procedures for examples of molecular interactions that affect the behaviour of populations and societies.

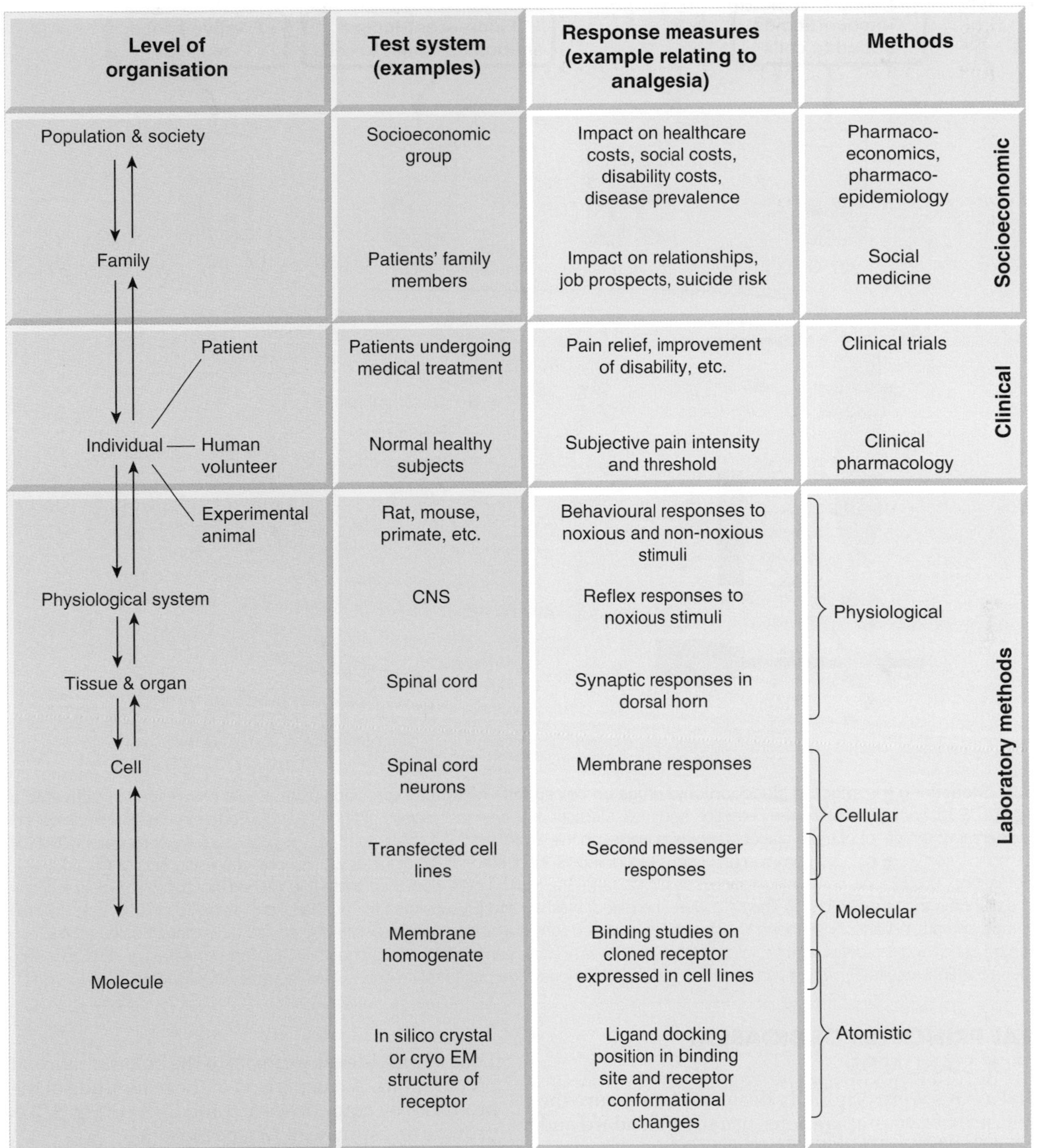

Level of organisation
Test system (examples)
Response measures (example relating to analgesia)
Methods
Population & society
Socioeconomic group
Impact on healthcare costs, social costs, disability costs, disease prevalence
Pharmaco-economics, pharmaco-epidemiology
Family
Patients' family members
Impact on relationships, job prospects, suicide risk
Social medicine
Socioeconomic
Patient
Patients undergoing medical treatment
Pain relief, improvement of disability, etc.
Clinical trials
Individual
Human volunteer
Normal healthy subjects
Subjective pain intensity and threshold
Clinical pharmacology
Clinical
Experimental animal
Rat, mouse, primate, etc.
Behavioural responses to noxious and non-noxious stimuli
Physiological system
CNS
Reflex responses to noxious stimuli
Physiological
Tissue & organ
Spinal cord
Synaptic responses in dorsal horn
Cell
Spinal cord neurons
Membrane responses
Cellular
Transfected cell lines
Second messenger responses
Molecular
Molecule
Membrane homogenate
Binding studies on cloned receptor expressed in cell lines
In silico crystal or cryo EM structure of receptor
Ligand docking position in binding site and receptor conformational changes
Atomistic
Laboratory methods

Fig. 8.1 **Levels of organisation and types of pharmacological measurement.** *CNS,* Central nervous system; *EM,* electron microscopy.

Quantitative cellular assays of this kind are now widely used in pharmacology. More recently, techniques based on X-ray crystallography, cryo electron microscopy, nuclear magnetic resonance spectroscopy and fluorescence signals have thrown much new light on drug action at the atomic and molecular levels (see reviews by Lohse et al., 2012; Nygaard et al., 2013; Safdari et al., 2018), and allow, for the first time, measurement as well as detection of the initial molecular events. These approaches have also played an important role in reducing the need to use living animals or animal tissues although it is important to be aware that many cell culture systems still rely on animal-based products and most cells still require animal sera to grow successfully in culture.

These approaches have important implications for basic understanding of drug action, and for drug design, but the need remains for measurement of drug effects at the physiological and clinical levels. Bridging the gap between events at the molecular level and at the physiological and therapeutic levels presents difficulties, because human illness cannot, in many cases, be accurately reproduced in experimental animals. The use of genetically altered animals (GAAs) to model human disease is discussed in more detail later.

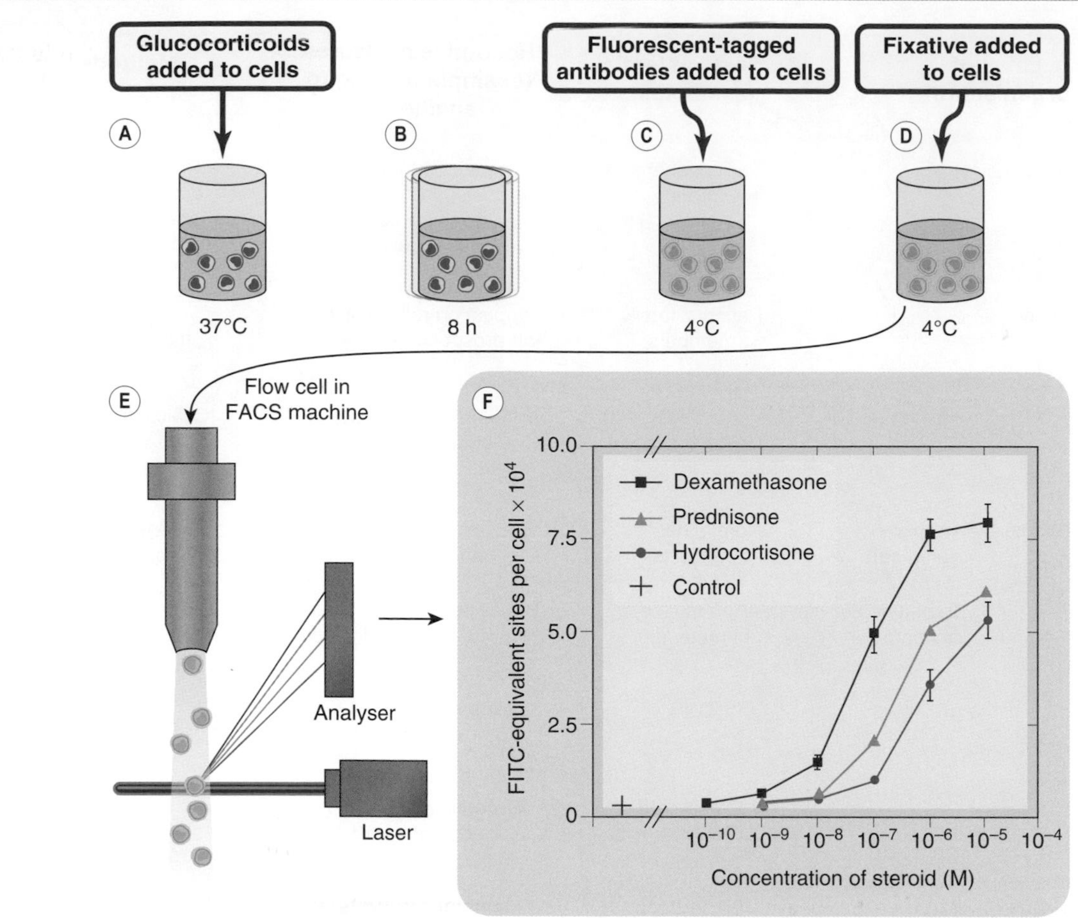

Fig. 8.2 Measuring the effect of glucocorticoid drugs on cell surface receptor expression using FACS (fluorescence-activated cell sorting). FACS technology enables the detection and measurement of fluorescent-tagged antibodies attached to structures on individual cells. In this experiment the effect of three glucocorticoids is tested on the expression of a cell surface haemoglobin scavenger receptor (CD 163). (A) Human monocytes were isolated from human venous blood and (B) incubated for 8 h alone or with various concentrations of the glucocorticoids dexamethasone, prednisone or hydrocortisone (see Chs 27 and 34). (C) The cells were then placed on ice and incubated with fluorescent-tagged antibodies to the receptor. (D) The cells were then fixed, washed and (E) subjected to FACS analysis. In this technique, cells flow through a small tube and are individually scanned by a laser. The reflected light is analysed using a series of filters (so that different coloured fluorescent tags can be used) and the data collected as *fluorescence intensity units*, compared with a standard (FITC) and expressed as 'FITC equivalents' to produce the final results (F), which can be plotted as a conventional log-concentration curve. (Data courtesy N. Goulding.)

GENERAL PRINCIPLES OF BIOASSAY

THE USE OF STANDARDS

Biological assays were originally designed to measure the *relative potency* of two preparations, usually a standard and an unknown. Maintaining stable preparations of various hormones, antisera and other biological materials as reference standards is the task of the UK National Board for Biological Standards Control. Nowadays bioassays are more commonly used to compare a new drug to a standard drug, the latter sometimes referred to as a 'prototypical' drug.

THE DESIGN OF BIOASSAYS

Given the aim of comparing the activity of two preparations, a standard (S) and an unknown (U), on a particular preparation, a bioassay must provide an estimate of the dose or concentration of U that will produce the same biological effect as that of a known dose or concentration of S. As Fig. 8.3 shows, provided that the log dose–effect curves for S and U are parallel, the ratio, M, of equiactive doses will not depend on the magnitude of response chosen. Thus M provides an estimate of the potency ratio of the two preparations. A comparison of the magnitude of the effects produced by equal doses of S and U (A_1 in Fig. 8.3) does not provide an estimate of M (see Fig. 8.3).

The main problem with all types of bioassay is that of biological variation, and the design of bioassays is aimed at:

- minimising variation
- avoiding systematic errors resulting from variation
- estimation of the limits of error of the assay result.

Historically, bioassays were performed on native tissues but it is now more common to use cell lines genetically engineered to express a specific receptor type. This has several advantages:

- expression of only a single type of receptor
- human receptors can be expressed and studied
- multiple signalling pathways can be monitored (see Ch. 3)
- signalling bias can be analysed (see Ch. 2)
- replacement of living animals

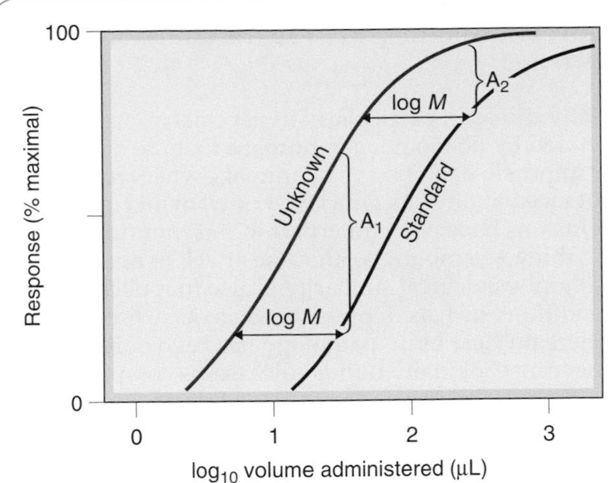

Fig. 8.3 Comparison of the potency of unknown and standard by bioassay. Note that comparing the magnitude of responses produced by the same dose (i.e. volume) of standard and unknown gives no quantitative estimate of their relative potency. (The differences, A_1 and A_2, depend on the dose chosen.) Comparison of equieffective doses of standard and unknown gives a valid measure of their relative potencies. Because the lines are parallel, the magnitude of the effect chosen for the comparison is immaterial; i.e. *log M* is the same at all points on the curves.

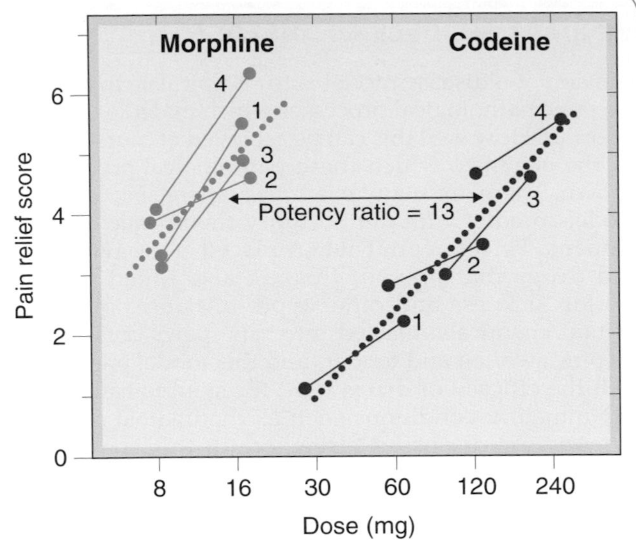

Fig. 8.4 Assay of morphine and codeine as analgesics in humans. Each of four patients (numbered *1–4*) was given, on successive occasions in random order, four different treatments (high and low morphine, and high and low codeine) by intramuscular injection, and the subjective pain relief score calculated for each. The calculated regression lines gave a potency ratio estimate of 13 for the two drugs. (After Houde, R.W., et al., 1965. In: Analgetics. Academic Press, New York.)

However, care must be taken to account for the level of recombinant receptor expression in engineered cell lines. Overexpression of receptors can result in weak partial agonist drugs appearing as 'full' agonists when the receptor reserve is larger than it would be for endogenously expressed receptors in native tissues (see Ch. 2).

Commonly, comparisons are based on analysis of *dose–response curves*, from which the matching doses of S and U are calculated. The use of a logarithmic dose scale means that the curves for S and U will normally be parallel, and the potency ratio (*M*) is estimated from the horizontal distance between the two curves (see Fig. 8.3). Assays of this type are known as *parallel line* assays, the minimal design being the 2 + 2 assay, in which two doses of standard (S_1 and S_2) and two of unknown (U_1 and U_2) are used. The doses are chosen to give responses lying on the linear part of the log dose–response curve, and are given repeatedly in randomised order, providing an inherent measure of the variability of the test system, which can be used, by means of straightforward statistical analysis, to estimate the confidence limits of the final result.

A simple example of an experiment to compare two analgesic drugs, **morphine** and **codeine** (see Ch. 43) in humans, based on a modified 2 + 2 design is shown in Fig. 8.4. Each of the four doses was given on different occasions to each of the four subjects, the order being randomised and both subject and observer being unaware of the dose given. Subjective pain relief was assessed by a trained observer, and the results showed morphine to be 13 times as potent as codeine. This, of course, does not prove its superiority, but merely shows that a smaller dose is needed to produce the same effect. Such a measurement is, however, an essential preliminary to assessing the relative therapeutic merits of the two drugs, for any comparison of other factors, such as side effects, duration of action, tolerance or dependence, needs to be done on the basis of doses that are equiactive as analgesics.

Problems arise if the two log dose–response curves are not parallel, or if the maximal responses differ, which can happen if the mechanism of action of the two drugs differs, or if one is a partial agonist (see Ch. 2). In this case it is not possible to define the relative potencies of S and U unambiguously in terms of a simple ratio and the experimenter must then face up to the fact that the comparison requires measurement of more than a single dimension of potency.

Bioassay

- Bioassay is the measurement of potency of a drug or unknown mediator from the magnitude of the biological effect that it produces.
- Bioassay normally involves comparison of the unknown preparation or novel drug with a standard. Estimates that are not based on comparison with standards are liable to vary from laboratory to laboratory.
- Comparisons are best made on the basis of dose–response curves, which allow estimates of the equiactive concentrations of unknown and standard to be used as a basis for the potency comparison. Parallel line assays follow this principle.
- The biological response may be *quantal* (the proportion of tests in which a given all-or-nothing effect is produced) or *graded*. Different statistical procedures are appropriate in each case.
- Different approaches to metrication apply according to the level of biological organisation at which the drug effect needs to be measured. Approaches range through molecular and chemical techniques, in vitro and in vivo animal studies and clinical studies on volunteers and patients, to measurement of effects at the socioeconomic level.

ANIMAL MODELS OF DISEASE

The aim of a disease model is to recapitulate in an animal the same pathological processes which underlie the human disorder. How well this can be achieved of course depends on the extent to which these pathological processes are known. There are many examples where simple intuitive models predict with fair accuracy therapeutic efficacy in humans. Ferrets vomit when placed in swaying cages, and drugs that prevent this are also found to relieve motion sickness and other types of nausea in humans. Irritant chemicals injected into rats' paws cause them to become swollen and tender, and this model predicts very well the efficacy of drugs used for symptomatic relief in inflammatory conditions such as rheumatoid arthritis in humans. As discussed elsewhere in this book, models for many important disorders, such as epilepsy, diabetes, hypertension and gastric ulceration, based on knowledge of the physiology of the condition, are available, and have been used successfully to produce new drugs, even though their success in predicting therapeutic efficacy is far from perfect.[2]

Not all animal models can be based on a known disease pathway as for many conditions, these are not known or are not fully recapitulated in a non-human species and this can lead to limitations in how well the findings in animals translate to clinical benefits. For example, even in diseases with well-established genetic origins, such as Huntington's disease or cystic fibrosis, manipulating the same genes in animals does not necessarily generate the same pathophysiological outcomes. Another challenge is how to quantify the arising consequences of the model induction and the effects of pharmacological treatments. These depend very much on the specific disorder and as much as possible aim to measure in the animal a similar readout to those which can be quantified in humans. This is where well-defined physiological changes, e.g. changes in blood pressure, or blood biomarkers, e.g. proinflammatory cytokines, are particularly helpful as well as imaging or postmortem assessment of the arising pathological changes, e.g. tumour size. Not all disorders have well-defined biomarkers particularly those involving the central nervous system, and for these models, behavioural readouts are commonly used.

Ideally, an animal model should resemble the human disease in the following ways:

- similar pathophysiological phenotype (*face validity*)
- similar causation (*construct validity*)
- similar response to treatment (*predictive validity*)

Alongside these external validity criteria, internal validity, including experiment design, reproducibility, controls and methods to avoid bias, is also critical for the reliability of data obtained using animal models.

In practice, there are many difficulties, and the shortcomings of animal models are one of the main roadblocks on the route from basic medical science to improvements in therapy. The difficulties include the following.

- Many diseases, particularly in psychiatry, are defined by phenomena in humans that are difficult or impossible to observe in animals, which rules out face validity. As far as we know, mania or delusions have no counterpart in rats, nor does anything resembling a migraine attack or autism. Pathophysiological similarity is also inapplicable to conditions such as depression or anxiety disorders, where no clear brain pathology has been defined.
- The 'cause' of many human diseases is complex or unknown. To achieve construct validity for many degenerative diseases (e.g. Alzheimer's disease, osteoarthritis, Parkinson's disease), we need to model the upstream (causative) factors rather than the downstream (symptomatic) features of the disease, although the latter are the basis of most of the simple physiological models used hitherto. The inflammatory pain model mentioned earlier lacks construct validity for rheumatoid arthritis, which is an autoimmune disease.
- Relying on response to treatment as a test of predictive validity carries the risk that drugs acting by novel mechanisms could be missed, because the model will have been selected on the basis of its responsiveness to known drugs. With schizophrenia (Ch. 47), for example, it is clear that dopamine antagonists are effective, and many of the models used are designed to assess dopamine antagonism in the brain, rather than other potential mechanisms that need to be targeted if drug discovery is to move on to address new targets.

PHARMACOLOGICAL MODELS

A common approach where a known pathology has not been established, particularly in behavioural pharmacology, has been the use of pharmacological treatments to induce a specific, quantifiable outcome in a living animal and then test if a drug treatment modifies this, e.g. *N*-methyl-D-aspartate (NMDA) receptor antagonist-induced hyperlocomotion as a model to test potential antipsychotics (see Ch. 47). Initial validation of these methods is commonly based on the ability of a known efficacious treatment to modulate the induced behaviour. These approaches can be helpful in finding drugs which act through similar mechanisms or have indirect effects on the system being altered by the pharmacologically induced readout. Most second-generation antipsychotics (see Ch. 47) and antidepressants (see Ch. 48) have been developed using this approach, however, as they do not necessarily involve relevant underlying pathology. There has also been a tendency, probably inappropriately, to use similar behavioural readouts in mechanistic studies or for evaluating drugs acting through novel mechanisms and this may be contributing to the subsequent poor translation to the clinic. Whilst pharmacological models are valuable in certain contexts, care in the interpretation of the arising data and recognition of these limitations is important.

GENETICALLY ALTERED ANIMAL MODELS

Nowadays, genetic approaches are increasingly used as an adjunct to conventional physiological and pharmacological

[2]There have been many examples of drugs that were highly effective in experimental animals (e.g. in reducing brain damage following cerebral ischaemia) but ineffective in humans (stroke victims). Similarly, substance P antagonists (Ch. 19) are effective in animal tests for analgesia, but they proved inactive when tested in humans. How many errors in the opposite direction may have occurred, we shall never know, because such drugs will never have been tested in humans.

approaches to disease modelling. Developments in the clustered regulatory interspersed short palindromic repeats (CRISPR) Cas9 gene-editing technique (Wang et al., 2013) has further accelerated the use of GAAs in research and meant that the ability to alter genes in a range of species has become much more achievable.

Animal models

- Animal models of disease are important for investigating pathogenesis and for the discovery of new therapeutic agents. Animal models generally reproduce imperfectly only certain aspects of human disease states. Models of psychiatric illness are particularly problematic.
- GAAs are produced by introducing mutations into the germ cells of animals (usually mice or zebrafish), which allow new genes to be introduced ('knockins') or existing genes to be inactivated ('knockouts') or mutated in a stable strain of animals.
- GAAs are widely used to develop disease models for drug testing. Many such models are now available. Knockout models are particularly helpful for demonstrating the role of a specific receptor in the effects of a novel drug.
- The induced mutation operates throughout the development and lifetime of the animal, and may be lethal. Techniques of conditional mutagenesis allow the abnormal gene to be switched on or off at a chosen time or within specific cell populations.

Progress in the technology for the generation of GAAs has now enabled the induction of genetic mutations in specific cell types and with specific promoters providing more control of where the modified gene is expressed.

By selective breeding, it is possible to obtain animal strains with characteristics resembling certain human diseases. Genetic models of this kind include spontaneously hypertensive rats, genetically obese mice, epilepsy-prone dogs and mice, rats with deficient vasopressin secretion and many other examples.

Genetic manipulation of the germline to generate *GAAs* (see Offermanns and Hein, 2004; Rudolph and Moehler, 1999) is important as a means of generating animal models that replicate human disease and are expected to be more predictive of therapeutic drug effects in humans. There has been a huge growth in GAA technologies in the last decade and these approaches now dominate animal models used in fundamental biology research and drug discovery. This versatile technology can be used in many different ways, for example:

- to inactivate individual genes, or mutate them to pathological forms
- to introduce new (e.g. human) genes
- to overexpress genes by inserting additional copies
- to allow gene expression to be localised to specific cell types and controlled by the experimenter

Progress from the early days of whole animal gene knockout or knockins has now largely been replaced with more sophisticated methods. It is now possible to mutate specific genes in animals to replicate known genetic mutations linked to disease. Animals can be generated to express human genes to enable more specific drug interaction studies. To avoid developmental effects, the mutated gene can be coupled to a specific promoter which is only activated by administration of an exogenous chemical activator such as doxycycline or tamoxifen. This also provides researchers with temporal control of when the mutated gene is expressed. It is also now possible to restrict the expression of the mutated gene to specific cell types, and genome editing technologies such as CRISPR Cas9 have enabled more sophisticated genetic manipulations to be achievable. Whilst mice are still the most widely used species for studying mammalian biology, other vertebrates (e.g. zebrafish) and invertebrates (*Drosophila*, *Caenorhabditis elegans*) are increasingly being used for drug screening purposes. CRISPR Cas9 has made genetic modifications more easily applicable to other species including rats.

Examples of such models include mice that overexpress mutated forms of the *amyloid precursor protein* or presenilins, which has been linked to the pathogenesis of Alzheimer's disease (see Ch. 40). When they are a few months old, these mice develop pathological lesions and cognitive changes resembling Alzheimer's disease although it should also be noted that recent trials of drugs which inhibit amyloid pathology have been disappointing in the clinic. Another neurodegenerative condition, Parkinson's disease (see Ch. 40), has been modelled in mice that overexpress *synuclein*, a protein found in the brain inclusions that are characteristic of the disease. Mice with mutations in tumour suppressor genes and oncogenes (see Ch. 6) are widely used as models for human cancers. Mice in which the gene for a particular adenosine receptor subtype has been inactivated show distinct behavioural and cardiovascular abnormalities, such as increased aggression, reduced response to noxious stimuli and raised blood pressure. GAAs can, however, be misleading in relation to human disease. For example, the gene defect responsible for causing cystic fibrosis (a disease affecting mainly the lungs in humans), when reproduced in mice, causes a disorder that mainly affects the intestine.

REDUCING USE OF ANIMALS IN RESEARCH

Animal models remain an important approach for fundamental research, drug discovery and the development of new treatments including in toxicology. However, developments in nonanimal alternatives or replacement of mammalian models with less sentient species are important for the principles of the 3Rs (reduce, refine and replace). Today, much more of the early screening of novel molecules is undertaken in silico and using high-throughput cell-based assays (see Ch. 60). It is also possible to screen for potential toxicity using in vitro assays and identify potential problems before progressing to in vivo models. Future studies may also make more use of 'organs on a chip' which provide a better model of the complexity of multicell types found in tissues than cell cultures but without needing to obtain these from an animal. These are relatively new technologies but offer the exciting prospect of creating model systems of human organs derived from human cells and hence the potential to improve the translation of findings to the clinic.

It remains unlikely that any of these methods will replace the need for animal models in the near future, but they can reduce the numbers of animals being used by providing early indications of compounds which are unlikely to be successful due to adverse effects and refine the choice of compounds to take into animal tests. Current progress in new approach methodologies is described by Fischer et al. (2020).

PHARMACOLOGICAL STUDIES IN HUMANS

Studies involving human subjects range from experimental pharmacodynamic or pharmacokinetic investigations to formal clinical trials. Non-invasive recording methods, such as *functional magnetic resonance imaging* (FMRI) to measure regional blood flow in the brain (a surrogate for neuronal activity) and *ultrasonography* to measure cardiac performance, have greatly extended the range of what is possible. The scientific principles underlying experimental work in humans designed (for example) to check whether mechanisms that operate in other species also apply to humans, or to take advantage of the much broader response capabilities of a person compared with a rat, are the same as for animals, but the ethical and safety issues are paramount. Ethics committees associated with all medical research centres tightly control the type of experiment that can be done, weighing up not only safety and ethical issues, but also the scientific importance of the proposed study. At the other end of the spectrum of experimentation on humans are formal *clinical trials*, often involving thousands of patients, aimed at answering specific questions regarding the efficacy and safety of new drugs.

CLINICAL TRIALS

Clinical trials are an important and highly specialised form of biological assay, designed specifically to measure therapeutic efficacy and adverse effects in human participants. The need to use patients for experimental purposes raises serious ethical considerations, and imposes many restrictions. Here, we discuss some of the basic principles involved in clinical trials; the role of such trials in the course of drug development is described in Chapter 60. Appropriate statistical techniques are fundamental to the conduct of medical research studies, and we refer readers to Bland (2015) for a more detailed account.

A clinical trial is a method for comparing objectively, through a prospective interventional study, the results of two or more therapeutic options. For new drugs, this is carried out during phases II and III of clinical development (see Ch. 60). It is important to realise that, until about 60 years ago, methods of treatment were chosen on the basis of clinical impression, personal experience and expert opinion rather than objective testing.[3] Although many drugs, with undoubted effectiveness, remain in use without ever having been subjected to a controlled clinical trial, any new drug is now required to have been tested in this way before being licensed for clinical use.[4]

An introduction to the principles and organisation of clinical trials is given by Hackshaw (2009). A clinical trial aims to compare the response of a test group of patients receiving a new treatment (A) with that of a control group receiving an existing 'standard' treatment (B). Treatment A might be a new drug or a new combination of existing drugs, or any other kind of therapeutic intervention, such as a surgical operation, a diet, physiotherapy and so on. The standard against which it is judged (treatment B) might be a drug or non-drug treatment that is in current clinical practice or (if there is no currently available effective treatment) a placebo or no treatment at all.

The use of controls is crucial in clinical trials. Claims of therapeutic efficacy based on reports that, for example, 16 out of 20 patients receiving drug X got better within 2 weeks are of no value (particularly so when considering self-resolving minor illnesses). Here, we need knowledge of how 20 control patients receiving a different treatment, or none at all, would have fared. In a *parallel-group design*, the controls are provided by a separate group of patients from those receiving the test treatment, but sometimes a *crossover design* is possible in which the same patients are switched from test to control treatment and vice versa, and the results compared. Randomisation is essential to avoid bias in assigning individual patients to test or control groups. Hence, the *randomised controlled clinical trial* is now regarded as *the* essential tool for assessing clinical efficacy of new drugs.

Concern inevitably arises over the ethics of assigning patients at random to particular treatment groups (or to no treatment). However, the reason for setting up a trial is that doubt exists whether the test treatment offers greater or lesser benefit than the control treatment, and there is genuine clinical equipoise in treatment selection. All would agree on the principle of informed consent,[5] whereby each patient must be told the nature and risks of the trial, and agree to participate on the basis that they will be randomly and unknowingly assigned to either the test or the control group. The regularly updated 'Declaration of Helsinki' sets

[3]Not exclusively. James Lind conducted a controlled trial in 1753 on 12 mariners, which showed that oranges and lemons offered protection against scurvy. However, 40 years passed before the British Navy acted on his advice, and a further century before the US Navy did.

[4]It is fashionable in some quarters to argue that to require evidence of efficacy of therapeutic procedures in the form of a controlled trial runs counter to the doctrines of 'holistic' medicine. This is a fundamentally antiscientific view, for science advances only by generating predictions from hypotheses and by subjecting the predictions to experimental test. 'Alternative' medical procedures, such as homeopathy or 'detox', have rarely been rigorously tested, and where they have, they generally lack efficacy. Standing up for the scientific approach is the *evidence-based medicine* movement (see Sackett et al., 1996), which sets out strict criteria for assessing therapeutic efficacy, based on randomised controlled clinical trials, and urges scepticism about therapeutic doctrines whose efficacy has not been so demonstrated.

[5]Even this can be contentious, because patients who are unconscious, patients with dementia or patients with intellectual disability are unable to give such consent, yet no one would want to preclude trials that might offer improved therapies to these needy patients. Clinical trials in children are particularly problematic but are necessary if the treatment of childhood diseases is to be placed on the same evidence base as is judged appropriate for adults. There are many examples where experience has shown that children respond differently from adults, and there is now an expectation that pharmaceutical companies should perform trials in children and vulnerable or older patients if the disease condition is relevant to these groups. If a trial uses very strict inclusion and exclusion criteria for participants, the resulting dataset may fail to be informative or generalisable to wider clinical practice.

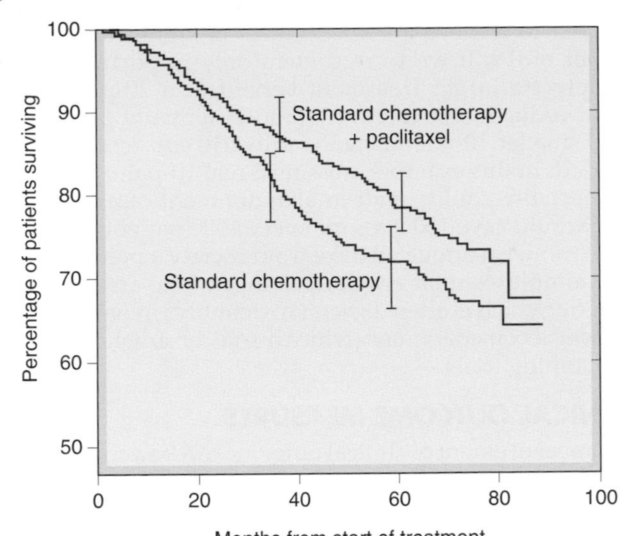

Fig. 8.5 Disease-free survival curves followed for 8 years in matched groups of breast cancer patients treated with a standard chemotherapy regime alone (629 patients), or with addition of paclitaxel (613 patients), showing a highly significant ($p = 0.006$) improvement with paclitaxel. Error bars represent 95% confidence intervals. (Redrawn from Martín M, Rodríguez-Lescure A, Ruiz A, et al., Randomized phase 3 trial of fluorouracil, epirubicin, and cyclophosphamide alone or followed by paclitaxel for early breast cancer. 2008. J. Natl. Cancer Inst. 100, 805–814.)

out the widely accepted ground rules governing research on human subjects.

Unlike the kind of bioassay discussed earlier, the large-scale clinical trial does not normally give any information about potency or the form of the dose–response curve, but merely compares the response produced by two or more stipulated therapeutic regimens. Survival curves provide one commonly used measure. Fig. 8.5 shows rates of disease-free survival in two groups of breast cancer patients treated with conventional chemotherapy with and without the addition of paclitaxel (see Ch. 57). The divergence of the curves shows that paclitaxel significantly improved the clinical response. Additional questions may be posed, such as the incidence and severity of side effects, or whether the treatment is better or worse in particular subgroups of patients, but only at the expense of added complexity, risk of bias and sample size. The investigator must decide in advance, using a protocolised approach, what dose to use and how often to give it, and the trial will reveal only whether the chosen regimen performed better or worse than the control treatment. Unless different doses are compared, it will not say whether increasing or decreasing the dose would have improved the response.

A considerable amount of preliminary or fundamental design work (including a pilot or feasibility assessment) has to be completed prior to embarking on a clinical trial that measures patient outcomes with a new drug. The basic question or (null) hypothesis posed by a clinical trial is thus simpler than that addressed by most conventional bioassays. However, the recruitment and follow-up of clinical trial participants, with strict safeguards against bias, are immeasurably more complicated, time-consuming and expensive than that of any laboratory-based assay. Observational studies may therefore be more practical or appropriate for assessing rare adverse effects where large sample sizes and long-term follow-up are needed.

RISK OF BIAS IN RANDOMISED CONTROLLED TRIALS

There are four main areas where rigorous procedures can be implemented to guard against the threat of bias:

1. random allocation of participants to ensure that treatment groups are equally balanced
2. adherence to the specified interventions
3. blinded assessment of outcomes
4. rigorous follow-up aimed at collecting the full dataset with minimal missing data

If two treatments, A and B, are being compared on a series of selected patients, the simplest form of randomisation is to allocate each patient to A or B by reference to a series of random numbers, toss of a coin or even drawing lots. In a properly randomised trial, neither the patient nor the investigator should have any influence on which treatment the patient will end up receiving, thus making the patient distribution fairly balanced at baseline. One difficulty, particularly if the groups are small, is that the two groups may turn out to be ill-matched with respect to characteristics such as age, sex or disease severity. *Stratified randomisation* avoids the difficulty by dividing the subjects into age, sex, severity, or other categories, random allocation to A or B being used within each category. It is possible to treat two or more characteristics of the trial population in this way, but the number of strata can quickly become large, and the process is self-defeating when the number of subjects in each becomes too small. As well as avoiding error resulting from imbalance of groups assigned to A and B, stratification can also allow more sophisticated conclusions to be reached. B might, for example, prove to be better than A in a particular group of patients even if it is not significantly better overall.

Strict adherence to the treatment protocol can be difficult if the drug has to be taken on a daily basis over months and years. Participants may not be able to follow the treatment schedule, or they may move on to try different therapies if they feel that the trial intervention has failed to help. Here, researchers can monitor delivery of the treatment and adherence to specified schedules, and implement various statistical methods such as 'intention to treat' and 'per protocol' analysis to address deviations from the plan.

The double-blind technique, whereby neither subject nor investigator is aware at the time of the assessment which treatment is being used, is intended to minimise subjective bias. It has been repeatedly shown that, with the best will in the world, subjects and investigators both contribute to bias if they know which treatment is which. Awareness of the specific trial intervention may lead to changes in clinical management, or to biased reporting and measurement of outcomes. Although the use of a double-blind technique is an important safeguard, this is not always possible. A dietary regimen, for example, can seldom be disguised; with drugs, pharmacological effects may reveal to patients what they are taking and predispose them to report accordingly.[6] In general, however, the

[6]The distinction between a true pharmacological response and a beneficial clinical effect produced by the knowledge (based on the pharmacological effects that the drug produces) that an active drug is being administered is not easy to draw, and we should not expect a mere clinical trial to resolve such a tricky semantic issue.

double-blind procedure, with precautions if necessary to disguise such clues as the taste or appearance of the two drugs, is used whenever possible.[7] If full blinding of participants and investigators is not possible, one option is to measure outcomes using assessors who are unaware of the treatments being used (an example would be an open-label trial with blinded endpoint assessment by an external independent committee).

High-quality clinical trials have pre-specified follow-up time points where outcomes are measured in a defined manner. Study results may be incomplete and potentially biased if patients drop out of the study or fail to attend follow-up because the intervention did not improve their symptoms. Inadequate follow-up or missing data means that important outcomes (such as serious adverse events) may not have been detected.

THE SIZE OF THE SAMPLE

Feasibility, ethical and financial considerations mean that the trial should involve the minimum number of subjects required to adequately answer the clinical question. Much statistical thought has gone into the problem of deciding in advance how many subjects will be required to produce a clinically useful – and statistically meaningful – result (a *power* calculation).

Judgements on the appropriate sample size should be based on whether the aim is to demonstrate that two treatments are equivalent (e.g. new treatment is non-inferior to the one that is currently in use), or whether the aim is to demonstrate a significant difference between interventions. Two types of erroneous conclusion are possible, referred to as *type I* and *type II errors*. A type I error occurs if the results show a difference between A and B when none actually exists (false-positive). A type II error occurs if no difference is found although A and B do actually differ (false-negative). A major factor that determines the size of sample needed is the degree of certainty the investigator seeks in avoiding either type of error. The probability of incurring a type I error is expressed as the *significance* of the result. To say that A and B are different at the $p < 0.05$ level of significance means that the probability of obtaining a false-positive result (i.e. incurring a type I error) is less than 1 in 20. For most purposes, this level of significance is considered acceptable as a basis for drawing conclusions.

The probability of detecting a genuine difference that exists between interventions and avoiding a type II error is termed the *power* of the trial. We tend to regard type II errors more leniently than type I errors, and it is often acceptable to design trials with a power of 0.8–0.9, which means that there is an 80%–90% chance of detecting a real effect. A larger sample size will confer greater power or ability to detect any difference that exists, with correspondingly more precise estimates of treatment effect.

The second factor that determines the sample size required is the magnitude of difference between A and B that is regarded as clinically important. For example, to detect that a given treatment reduces the mortality in a certain condition by at least 10 percentage points, say from 50% (in the control group) to 40% (in the treated group), would require 850 subjects, assuming that we wanted to achieve a $p < 0.05$ level of significance and a power of 0.9. If we were content only to power the trial to detect a larger treatment benefit of a 20-percentage point reduction in mortality (and potentially fail to pick up a smaller 10-point benefit), only 210 subjects would be needed. In this example, missing a real 10-point reduction in mortality could result in abandonment of a treatment that would save 100 lives for every 1000 patients treated – an extremely serious mistake from society's point of view. This simple example emphasises the need to assess clinical benefit (which is often difficult to quantify) in parallel with statistical considerations (which are fairly straightforward) in planning trials.

CLINICAL OUTCOME MEASURES

The measurement of clinical outcome can be a complicated business, and both ethics committees and funders of clinical trials are placing much greater emphasis on outcomes that are important to patients and health services, rather than pharmacological or physiological endpoints. With rising disease burden in ageing populations, commissioners of health services are more preoccupied with assessing the cost-effectiveness of therapeutic procedures in terms of improved length and quality of life, and societal and (health) economic benefit. Various scales for assessing 'health-related quality of life' have been devised and tested (see Walley and Haycocks, 1997); these may be combined with measures of life expectancy to arrive at the measure 'quality-adjusted life years' (QALYs) as an overall measure of therapeutic efficacy, which attempts to combine both survival time and relief from suffering in assessing overall benefit.[8] The cost per QALY gained with a new treatment is a critical consideration in allocation of healthcare funds.

However, measuring long-term patient benefit may take years, so objective clinical effects, such as lowering of blood pressure, improved airway conductance or change in white cell count, continue to be used as outcome measures. These *surrogate markers* reflect pathophysiological changes of which the patient is most likely unaware, but can readily be measured in smaller, short-term trials. In many cases such changes correlate well with clinical outcome as it affects the patient; not always, though. Regulatory authorities are therefore rightly cautious about accepting surrogate end points as a measure of actual patient benefit, unless there is clear evidence that changes in the surrogate marker have a direct robust relationship with important outcomes.

PLACEBOS

A placebo is a dummy medicine containing no active ingredient (or alternatively, a dummy surgical procedure, diet or other kind of therapeutic intervention), which the patient believes is (or could be, in the context of a

[7]Maintaining the blind can be problematic. In a crossover trial of sildenafil (known to the lay public as the little blue pill Viagra) for limb ischaemia, all the patients were able to correctly guess the time that they were on sildenafil rather than placebo. Unsurprisingly, almost 90% asked to continue with the trial medication after the research study had finished.

[8]As may be imagined, trading off duration and quality of life raises issues about which many of us feel decidedly squeamish. Not so economists, however. They approach the problem by asking such questions as: 'How many years of life would you be prepared to sacrifice in order to live the rest of your life free of the disability you are currently experiencing?' Or, even more disturbingly: 'If, given your present condition, you could gamble on surviving free of disability for your normal lifespan, or (if you lose the gamble) dying immediately, what odds would you accept?' Imagine being asked this by your doctor. 'But I only wanted something for my sore throat', you protest weakly.

controlled trial) the real thing. The 'placebo response' (see review by Enck et al., 2013) is widely believed to be a powerful therapeutic effect,[9] producing a significant beneficial effect in about one-third of patients. While many clinical trials include a placebo group that shows improvement, few have compared this group directly with untreated controls, particularly where the natural history of the disease is symptom resolution without any intervention. The role of placebo is a topic of major debate, with some arguing that placebo has limited effect, except perhaps in trials involving pain or nausea (Hróbjartsson and Gøtzsche, 2010), while others have reported clinically meaningful effects with placebo (Howick et al., 2013). There are also growing numbers of pragmatic trials where the new treatment is compared against 'standard or usual' care, rather than the artificial construct of a placebo dummy pill that has no relationship to typical clinical practice.

The risks of placebo therapies should not be underestimated. The use of active medicines may be delayed. The necessary element of deception[10] risks undermining the confidence of patients in the integrity of doctors. A state of 'therapy dependence' may be produced in people who are not ill, because there is no way of assessing whether a patient still 'needs' the placebo.

META-ANALYSIS

It is possible, using statistical techniques, to combine the data obtained in several individual trials in order to gain greater power and to compare consistency of findings between studies. This procedure, known as *meta-analysis*, can be very useful in arriving at a conclusion on the basis of several trials, of which some claimed superiority of the intervention over the control while others did not. The meta-analysis is usually based on a systematic review using defined search strategies, study selection and quality assessment criteria. This approach to summarising the overall body of evidence is certainly preferable to the 'take your pick' approach adopted by most human beings when confronted with diverse data sets. Statistical models involving multiple treatment comparisons in network meta-analysis can help determine which particular medicine, of several available drug options, has the greater chance of success.

The main drawback in any meta-analysis is susceptibility to selective reporting of results, hidden data and 'publication bias'. Negative studies (or unfavourable findings) are less likely to be reported than positive studies, partly because they are considered less interesting or, more seriously, because publication would harm the interests of the organisation that performed the trial.[11]

The published clinical trials literature contains reports of many trials that are poorly designed and unreliable. The Cochrane Collaboration (www.cochrane.org) sifts carefully through the literature and produces *systematic reviews* that collate and combine data only from trials (of drugs and other therapeutic interventions) that meet strict quality criteria. About 8600 such 'gold-standard' summaries are available, and provide the most reliable evaluation of trials data on a wide range of interventions.

Clinical trials

- A clinical trial is a special type of bioassay done to compare the clinical efficacy of a new drug or intervention with that of a standard treatment (or a placebo).
- At its simplest, the aim is a straight comparison of unknown (A) with standard (B) at a single-dose level. The result may be: 'B better than A', 'B worse than A', or 'No difference detected'. Efficacy, not potency, is compared.
- To avoid bias, clinical trials should ideally be:
  - *controlled* (comparison of A with B, rather than study of A alone);
  - *randomised* (assignment of subjects to A or B on a random basis);
  - *double-blind* (neither the subject nor the assessor knows whether A or B is being used).
- Type I errors (concluding that A is better than B when the difference is actually due to chance) and type II errors (concluding that A is not different from B because a real difference has escaped detection) can occur; the likelihood of either kind of error decreases as the methodological quality, sample size and number of end-point events are increased.
- Interim analysis of data, carried out by an independent group, may be used as a basis for determining if a trial should continue. Premature termination of the trial may occur if the interim data are already strongly conclusive (of major benefit or serious harm), or if a clear result is unlikely to be reached (futility).
- All experiments on human subjects require approval by an independent ethics committee.
- Clinical trials require very careful planning and execution, and are inevitably expensive.
- Clinical outcome measures may comprise:
  - physiological measures (e.g. blood pressure, liver function tests, airways function);
  - subjective assessments (e.g. pain relief, mood);
  - long-term outcome (e.g. survival or freedom from recurrent disease);
  - overall '*quality of life*' measures;
  - '*QALYs*', which combine survival with quality of life.
- Meta-analysis is a statistical technique used to pool the data from several independent trials.

CLINICAL CONSIDERATION OF BENEFIT AND RISK

There are many different ways of quantifying and presenting the benefits and risks of drugs in clinical use. One useful approach is to *compare* from clinical trial data the

[9]Its opposite, the *nocebo effect*, describes the adverse effects reported with dummy medicines.

[10]Surprisingly, deception may not even be necessary. Kaptchuk et al. (2010) found that symptoms of irritable bowel syndrome were improved slightly more in patients given inert sugar pills, described as such by the physician, than in patients given no pills. The effect was, however, small, and the patients were encouraged to think that the pills might engage 'mind-body healing processes'.

[11]To reduce this bias, measures are now in place to ensure that most clinical trials are registered and the results publicly disclosed.

proportion of test and control patients who will experience (A) a defined level of clinical benefit (e.g. survival beyond 2 years, pain relief to a certain predetermined level, slowing of cognitive decline by a given amount) and (B) adverse effects of defined degree. These estimates of proportions of patients showing beneficial or harmful reactions can be expressed as *number needed to treat* (NNT; i.e. the number of patients who need to be treated in order for one to show the given effect, whether beneficial or adverse). For example, in a recent study of pain relief by antidepressant drugs compared with placebo, the findings were as follows: for benefit (a defined level of pain relief), NNT = 3; for minor unwanted effects, NNT = 3; for major adverse effects, NNT = 22. Thus of 100 patients treated with the drug, on average 33 will experience pain relief, 33 will experience minor unwanted effects, and 4 or 5 will experience major adverse effects. *This format of presenting benefit and harm* information is helpful in guiding therapeutic choices. One advantage of this type of analysis is that it can take into account the underlying disease severity in quantifying benefit. Thus if drug A halves the mortality of an often fatal disease (reducing it from 50% to 25%, say), the NNT to save one life is 4; if drug B halves the mortality of a rarely fatal disease (reducing it from 5% to 2.5%, say), the NNT to save one life is 40. Notwithstanding other considerations, drug A is judged to be more valuable than drug B, even though both reduce mortality by one-half. Furthermore, the clinician must realise that to save one life with drug B, 40 patients must be exposed to a risk of adverse effects, whereas only four are exposed for each life saved with drug A.

REFERENCES AND FURTHER READING

General references

Bland, J.M., 2015. An Introduction to Medical Statistics, fourth ed. Oxford University Press, Oxford.

Colquhoun, D., 1971. Lectures on Biostatistics. Oxford University Press, Oxford.

Hróbjartsson, A., Gøtzsche, P.C., 2010. Placebo interventions for all clinical conditions. Cochrane Database Syst. Rev. CD003974.

Walley, T., Haycocks, A., 1997. Pharmacoeconomics: basic concepts and terminology. Br. J. Clin. Pharmacol. 43, 343–348.

Yanagisawa, M., Kurihara, H., Kimura, S., et al., 1988. A novel potent vasoconstrictor peptide produced by vascular endothelial cells. Nature 332, 411–415.

Molecular methods

Lohse, M.J., Nuber, S., Hoffmann, C., 2012. Fluorescence/ bioluminescence resonance energy transfer techniques to study G protein-coupled receptor activation and signaling. Pharmacol. Rev. 64, 299–336.

Nygaard, R., Zou, Y., Dror, R.O., et al., 2013. The dynamic process of β(2)-adrenergic receptor activation. Cell 152 (3), 532–542.

Safdari, H.A., Pandey, S., Shukla, A.K., Dutta, S., 2018. Illuminating GPCR signaling by cryo-EM. Trends Cell Biol. 28, 591–594.

Animal models

Fischer, I., Milton, C., Wallace, H., 2020. Toxicity testing is evolving. Toxicol. Res (Camb). 9, 67–80.

Offermanns, S., Hein, L., et al., 2004. Transgenic Models in Pharmacology. Handbook of Experimental Pharmacology, Vol. 159. Springer-Verlag, Heidelberg.

Rudolph, U., Moehler, H., 1999. Genetically modified animals in pharmacological research: future trends. Eur. J. Pharmacol. 375, 327–337.

Wang, H., Yang, H., Shivalila, C.S., et al., 2013. One-step generation of mice carrying mutations in multiple genes by CRISPR/Cas-mediated genome engineering. Cell 153, 910–918.

Clinical trials

Enck, P., Bigel, U., Schedlowski, M., Rief, W., 2013. The placebo response in medicine: minimize, maximize or personalize? Nat. Rev. Drug Discov. 12, 191–204.

Hackshaw, A., 2009. A Concise Guide to Clinical Trials. Wiley Blackwell, Oxford.

Howick, J., Friedemann, C., Tsakok, M., et al., 2013. Are treatments more effective than placebos? A systematic review and meta-analysis. PLoS One 8, e62599.

Kaptchuk, T.J., Friedlander, E., Kelley, J.M., et al., 2010. Placebos without deception: a randomized controlled trial in irritable bowel syndrome. PLoS One 5 (12), e15591.

Sackett, D.L., Rosenburg, W.M.C., Muir-Gray, J.A., et al., 1996. Evidence-based medicine: what it is and what it isn't. Br. Med. J. 312, 71–72.

Absorption and distribution of drugs

9

OVERVIEW

The physical processes of diffusion, penetration of membranes, binding to plasma protein and partition into fat and other tissues underlie the absorption and distribution of drugs. These processes are described, followed by more specific coverage of the process of drug absorption and related practical issue of routes of drug administration, and of the distribution of drugs into different bodily compartments. Drug interactions caused by one drug altering the absorption or distribution of another are described. There is a short final section on special drug delivery systems designed to deliver drugs efficiently and selectively to their sites of action.

INTRODUCTION

Drug disposition is divided into four stages designated by the acronym 'ADME':

- **A**bsorption from the site of administration
- **D**istribution within the body
- **M**etabolism
- **E**xcretion from the body

General aspects of drug absorption and distribution are considered here, together with routes of administration. Absorption and distribution of inhaled general anaesthetics (a special case) are described in Chapter 41. Metabolism and excretion are covered in Chapter 10. We begin with a description of the physical processes that underlie drug disposition.

PHYSICAL PROCESSES UNDERLYING DRUG DISPOSITION

Drug molecules move around the body in two ways:

- bulk flow (i.e. in the bloodstream, lymphatics or cerebrospinal fluid, or during passage through the gastrointestinal tract)
- diffusion (i.e. molecule by molecule, over short distances).

The chemical nature of a drug makes no difference to its transfer by bulk flow. The cardiovascular system provides a rapid long-distance distribution system. In contrast, diffusional characteristics differ markedly between different drugs. In particular, ability to cross hydrophobic diffusion barriers is strongly influenced by lipid solubility. Aqueous diffusion is part of the overall mechanism of drug transport, because it is this process that delivers drug molecules to and from the non-aqueous barriers. The rate of diffusion of a substance depends mainly on its molecular size, the *diffusion coefficient* being inversely proportional to the square root of molecular weight. Consequently, while large molecules diffuse more slowly than small ones, the variation with molecular weight is modest. Classical 'small molecule' drugs mainly fall within the molecular weight range 200–1000 Da, and variations in aqueous diffusion rate have only a small effect on their overall pharmacokinetic behaviour, whereas biopharmaceuticals are typically much larger molecules (see Ch. 5). Thus, the molecular weight of a monoclonal antibody drug is approximately 150 kDa and of a small interfering RNA drug approximately 16 kDa, so diffusion can be an important limitation to the rate of onset of action of biopharmaceutical drugs.

For small molecule drugs, we can treat the body as a series of interconnected, well-stirred compartments, within each of which the drug concentration is uniform. It is movement *between* compartments, generally involving penetration of non-aqueous diffusion barriers, which determines where, and for how long, a drug will be present in the body after it has been administered. The analysis of drug movements with the help of a simple compartmental model is discussed in Chapter 11.

THE MOVEMENT OF DRUG MOLECULES ACROSS CELL BARRIERS

Cell membranes form the barriers between aqueous compartments in the body. A single layer of membrane separates the intracellular from the extracellular compartments. An epithelial barrier, such as the gastrointestinal mucosa or renal tubule, consists of a layer of cells tightly connected to each other so that molecules must traverse at least two cell membranes (inner and outer) to pass from one side to the other. The anatomical disposition and permeability of vascular endothelium (the cell layer that separates intravascular from extravascular compartments) varies from one tissue to another. Gaps between endothelial cells are packed with a loose matrix of proteins that act as filters, retaining large molecules and letting smaller ones through. The cut-off of molecular size is not exact: water permeates rapidly whereas molecules of 80,000–100,000 Da permeate very slowly. In some regions, especially the *blood–brain barrier* (see later) and the placenta, there are tight junctions between the cells, and the endothelium is encased in an impermeable layer of periendothelial cells (*pericytes*). These features prevent potentially harmful molecules from penetrating to brain or fetus and have major consequences for drug distribution and activity.

In other organs (e.g. the liver and spleen), endothelium is discontinuous, allowing free passage between cells. In the liver, hepatocytes form the barrier between intra- and extravascular compartments and take on several endothelial cell functions. Fenestrated ('windowed') endothelium occurs in endocrine glands, facilitating transfer to the bloodstream of hormones or other molecules through pores in the endothelium. Formation of fenestrated endothelium is controlled by a specific endocrine gland-derived vascular endothelial growth factor (dubbed EG-VEGF). Endothelial cells lining postcapillary venules have specialised functions relating to leukocyte migration and inflammation, and the sophistication of the intercellular junction can be appreciated from the observation that leukocyte migration can occur without any detectable leak of water or small ions (see Ch. 7).

There are three main ways by which small molecules cross cell membranes (Fig. 9.1):

- by diffusing directly through the lipid;
- by combination with a *solute carrier* (SLC) or other membrane transporter;
- by diffusing through aqueous pores formed by special membrane glycoproteins (*aquaporins*) that traverse the lipid;
- further, small quantities of macromolecules may cross cell barriers by *pinocytosis* – 'cell drinking' (see later).

Of these routes, diffusion through lipid and carrier-mediated transport are particularly important in relation to pharmacokinetic mechanisms.

Diffusion through aquaporins is probably important in the transfer of gases such as carbon dioxide, but the pores are too small in diameter (about 0.4 nm) to allow most drug molecules (which usually exceed 1 nm in diameter) to pass through. Consequently, drug distribution is not notably abnormal in patients with genetic diseases affecting aquaporins. Pinocytosis involves invagination of part of the cell membrane and the trapping within the cell of a tiny vesicle containing extracellular constituents. The vesicle contents can then be released within the cell or extruded from its other side. This mechanism may be important for the transport of some macromolecules, but not for small molecules.

DIFFUSION THROUGH LIPID

Non-polar molecules (in which electrons are uniformly distributed) dissolve freely in membrane lipids, and consequently diffuse readily across cell membranes, in contrast to polar molecules in which electrons are distributed non-uniformly. Weak acids and weak bases may exist in either ionised (highly polar) or non-ionised state depending on pH (see later). The number of molecules crossing the membrane per unit area in unit time is determined by the *permeability coefficient*, *P*, and the concentration difference across the membrane. Permeant molecules must be present within the membrane in sufficient numbers and must be mobile within the membrane if rapid permeation is to occur. Thus, two physicochemical factors contribute to *P*, namely *solubility* in the membrane (which can be expressed as a partition coefficient for the substance distributed between the membrane phase and the aqueous environment) and *diffusivity*, which is a measure of the mobility of molecules within the lipid and is expressed as a diffusion coefficient. The diffusion coefficient varies only modestly between conventional drugs, as noted earlier, so the most important determinant of membrane permeability for conventional low-molecular-weight drugs is the partition coefficient (Fig. 9.2). Many pharmacokinetic characteristics of a drug – such as rate of absorption from the gut, penetration into different tissues and the extent of renal elimination – can be predicted from knowledge of its lipid solubility.

Diffusion through lipid
Diffusion through aqueous channel
Carrier
EXTRACELLULAR
MEMBRANE
INTRACELLULAR

Fig. 9.1 Routes by which solutes can traverse cell membranes. (Molecules can also cross cellular barriers by pinocytosis.)

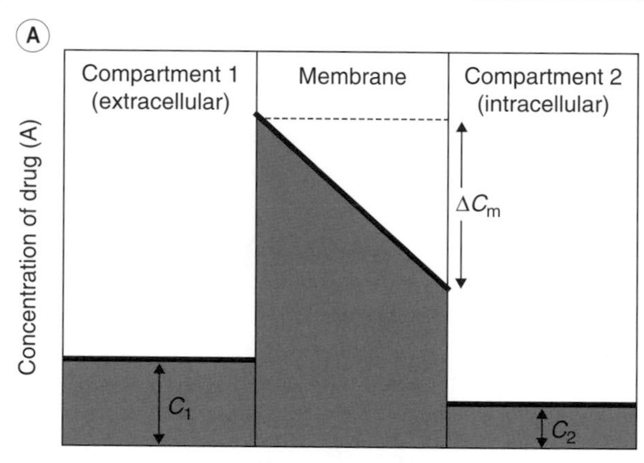

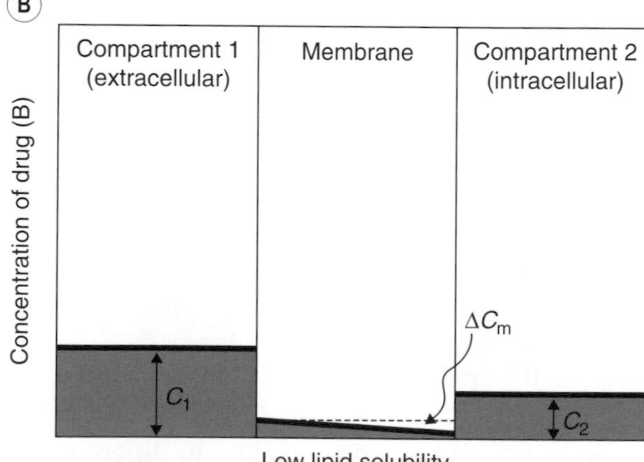

Fig. 9.2 The importance of lipid solubility in membrane permeation. (A) and (B) show the concentration profile in a lipid membrane separating two aqueous compartments. A lipid-soluble drug (A) is subject to a much larger transmembrane concentration gradient (ΔC_m) than a lipid-insoluble drug (B). It therefore diffuses more rapidly, even though the aqueous concentration gradient (C_1–C_2) is the same in both cases.

ION TRAPPING

Ionisation and membrane permeability affect not only the rate at which drugs permeate membranes but also the steady-state distribution of drug molecules between aqueous compartments. Lipid-soluble molecules diffuse into cells where they can be metabolised (e.g. by esterases); this may liberate a functionally important charged (and hence impermeant) metabolite, which is consequently trapped within the cell. This has been extensively exploited, notably in probing the function of intracellular mediators such as Ca^{2+} using fluorescent indicators such as fura-2, which is loaded into cells as an uncharged ester and trapped intracellularly as the charged form (see, for example, Fig. 4.2). The same approach has been used recently by pharmaceutical chemists seeking to target drugs (several of which are in development) to intracellular sites of action within monocytes and macrophages using esterase-sensitive chemical motifs conjugated to a drug such as a histone deacetylase inhibitor. This forms a prodrug (see later) that delivers the drug to cells of the monocyte macrophage lineage which selectively express human carboxylesterase-1, the charged active drug product being trapped in the monocyte cytoplasm, which is its site of action (Needham et al., 2011).

pH and ionisation

One important complicating factor in relation to membrane permeation is that many drugs are weak acids or bases, and therefore exist in both un-ionised and ionised form, the ratio of the two forms varying with pH. For a weak base, B, the ionisation reaction is:

$$BH^+ \xrightarrow{K_a} B + H^+$$

and the dissociation constant pK_a is given by the Henderson–Hasselbalch equation

$$pK_a = pH + \log_{10}\frac{[BH^+]}{[B]}$$

For a weak acid, AH:

$$AH \overset{K_a}{\rightleftharpoons} A^- + H^+$$

$$pK_a = pH + \log_{10}\frac{[AH]}{[A^-]}$$

In either case, the ionised species, BH^+ or A^-, has very low lipid solubility and is virtually unable to permeate membranes except where a specific transport mechanism exists. The lipid solubility of the uncharged species, B or AH, depends on the chemical nature of the drug; for many drugs, the uncharged species is sufficiently lipid-soluble to permit rapid membrane permeation, although there are exceptions (e.g. aminoglycoside antibiotics; see Ch. 52) where even the uncharged molecule is insufficiently lipid-soluble to cross membranes appreciably. This is usually because of hydrogen-bonding groups (such as hydroxyl in sugar moieties in aminoglycosides) that render the uncharged molecule hydrophilic.

pH partition and ion trapping

If a pH difference exists between body compartments, this can alter the steady-state distribution of drugs that are weak acids or weak bases via its influence on their ionisation. Fig. 9.3 shows how a weak acid (e.g. **aspirin**, pK_a 3.5) and a weak base (e.g. **pethidine**, pK_a 8.6) would be distributed at equilibrium between three body compartments, namely plasma (pH 7.4), alkaline urine (pH 8) and gastric juice (pH 3). Within each compartment, the ratio of ionised to un-ionised drug is governed by the pK_a of the drug and the pH of that compartment. It is assumed that the un-ionised species can cross the membrane, and therefore reaches an equal concentration in each compartment. The ionised species is assumed not to cross at all. The result is that, at equilibrium, the total (ionised + un-ionised) concentration of the drug will be different in each compartment, with an acidic drug being concentrated in the compartment with high pH ('ion trapping'), and vice versa. The concentration gradients produced by ion trapping can theoretically be very large if there is a large pH difference between compartments. Thus, aspirin would be concentrated more than 4-fold with respect to plasma in an alkaline renal tubule, and about 6000-fold in plasma with respect to the acidic gastric contents. Such large gradients are not achieved in reality for two main reasons. First, assuming total impermeability of the charged species is not realistic, and even a small permeability will attenuate considerably the concentration difference that can be reached. Second, body compartments rarely approach equilibrium. Neither the gastric contents nor the renal tubular fluid stands still, and the resulting bulk flow of drug molecules reduces the concentration gradients well below the theoretical equilibrium conditions. The pH partition mechanism nonetheless correctly explains some of the qualitative effects of pH changes in different body compartments on the pharmacokinetics of weakly acidic or basic drugs, particularly in relation to renal excretion and to penetration of the blood–brain barrier.

pH partition is not the main determinant of the site of absorption of drugs from the gastrointestinal tract. This is because the enormous absorptive surface area of the villi and microvilli in the ileum compared with the much smaller absorptive surface area in the stomach is of overriding importance. Thus absorption of an acidic drug such as aspirin is promoted by drugs that accelerate gastric emptying (e.g. **metoclopramide**) and slowed by drugs that slow gastric emptying (e.g. **propantheline**), even though the acidic pH of the stomach contents favours absorption of weak acids. Values of pK_a for some common drugs are shown in Fig. 9.4.

There are several important consequences of pH partition:

- Free-base trapping of some antimalarial drugs (e.g. **chloroquine**, see Ch. 55) in the acidic environment in the food vacuole of the malaria parasite contributes to the disruption of the haemoglobin digestion pathway that underlies their toxic effect on the parasite.
- Urinary acidification accelerates excretion of weak bases and retards that of weak acids (see Ch. 10).
- Urinary alkalinisation has the opposite effects: it reduces excretion of weak bases and increases excretion of weak acids.
- Increasing plasma pH (e.g. by administration of sodium bicarbonate) causes weakly acidic drugs to be extracted from the central nervous system (CNS) into the plasma. Conversely, reducing plasma pH (e.g. by administration of a carbonic anhydrase

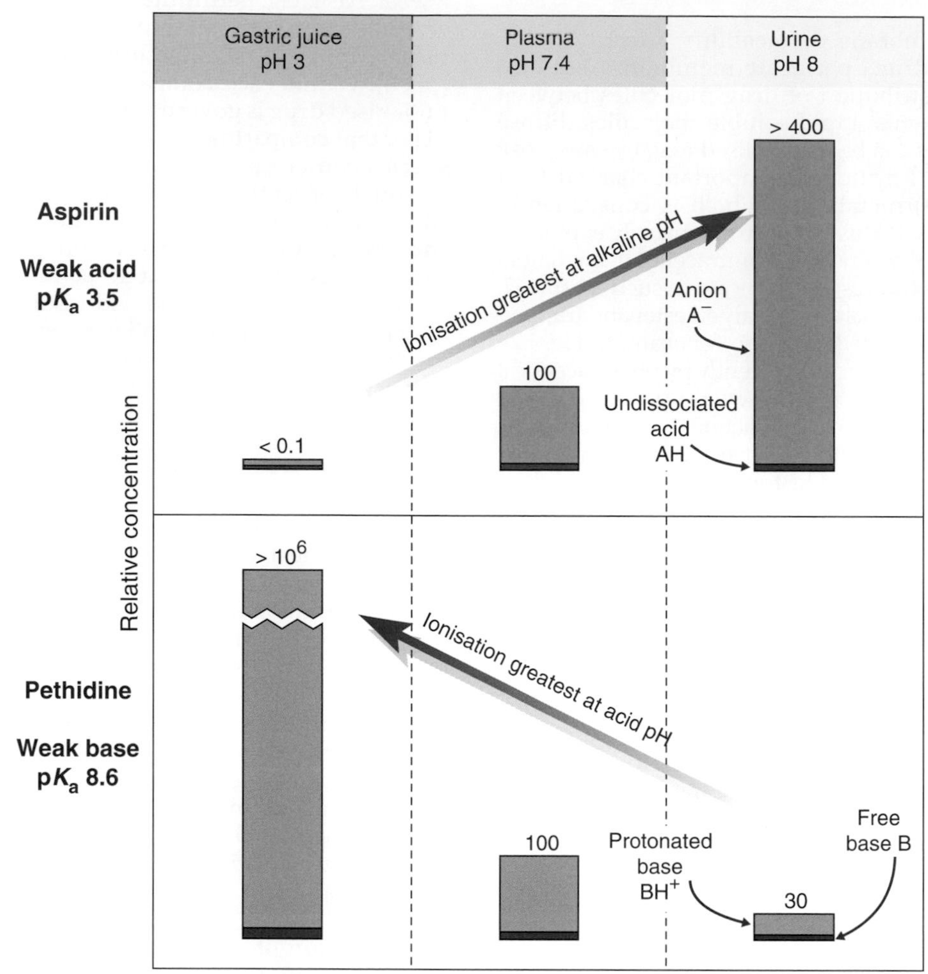

Fig. 9.3 Theoretical partition of a weak acid (aspirin) and a weak base (pethidine) between aqueous compartments (urine, plasma and gastric juice) according to the pH difference between them. Numbers represent relative concentrations (total plasma concentration = 100). It is assumed that the uncharged species in each case can permeate the cellular barrier separating the compartments, and therefore reaches the same concentration in all three. Variations in the fractional ionisation as a function of pH give rise to the large total concentration differences with respect to plasma.

inhibitor such as **acetazolamide**, see Ch. 29) causes weakly acidic drugs to become concentrated in the CNS, potentially increasing their neurotoxicity. This has practical consequences in choosing a means to alkalinise urine in treating aspirin overdose: bicarbonate and acetazolamide each increase urine pH and hence increase salicylate elimination, but bicarbonate reduces whereas acetazolamide increases distribution of salicylate to the CNS.

CARRIER-MEDIATED TRANSPORT

Many cell membranes possess specialised transport mechanisms that regulate entry and exit of physiologically important molecules, such as sugars, amino acids, neurotransmitters and metal ions. They are broadly divided into *SLC transporters* and *ATP-binding cassette (ABC) transporters*. The former facilitate passive movement of solutes down their electrochemical gradient, while the latter are active pumps fuelled by ATP. Over 300 human genes are believed to code these transporters, most of which act mainly on endogenous substrates, but some also transport foreign chemicals ('xenobiotics') including drugs. The role of such transporters in neurotransmitter function is discussed in Chapters 14, 15 and 37.

Organic cation transporters and organic anion transporters

Two structurally related SLCs of importance in drug distribution are the organic cation transporters (OCTs – see e.g. Ciarimboli, 2008 and 2021) and organic anion transporters (OATs – see e.g. Nosaki and Izumi, 2020). The carrier molecule consists of a transmembrane protein that binds one or more molecules or ions, changes conformation and releases its cargo on the other side of the membrane. Such systems may operate purely passively, without any energy source; in this case, they merely facilitate the process of transmembrane equilibration of a single transported species in the direction of its electrochemical gradient. The OCTs translocate dopamine, choline and various drugs including **vecuronium**, **quinine** and **procainamide**. They are 'uniporters' (i.e. each protein transporter molecule

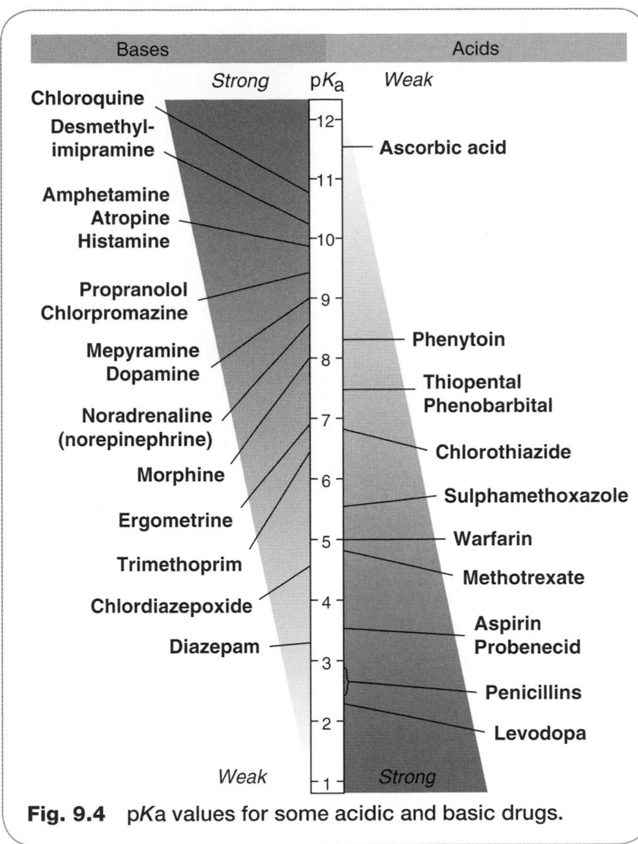

Fig. 9.4 p*K*a values for some acidic and basic drugs.

binds one solute molecule at a time and transports it down its gradient). OCT2 (present in proximal renal tubules) concentrates drugs such as **cisplatin** (an important anticancer drug; see Ch. 57) in these cells, resulting in its selective nephrotoxicity; related drugs (e.g. **carboplatin**, **oxaliplatin**) are not transported by OCT2 and are less nephrotoxic; competition with **cimetidine** for OCT2 offers possible protection against cisplatin nephrotoxicity (Fig. 9.5). Other SLCs are coupled to the electrochemical gradient of Na^+ or other ions across the membrane, generated by ATP-dependent ion pumps (see Ch. 4); in this case, transport can occur against an electrochemical gradient. It may involve exchange of one molecule for another ('antiport') or transport of two molecules together in the same direction ('symport'). The OATs are responsible for the renal secretion of urate, prostaglandins, several vitamins and *p*-amino hippurate, and for drugs such as **probenecid**, many antibiotics, antiviral, non-steroidal anti-inflammatory and antineoplastic drugs. Uptake is driven by exchange with intracellular dicarboxylic acids (mainly α-ketoglutarate, partly derived from cellular metabolism and partly by co-transport with Na^+ entering cells down its concentration gradient). Metabolic energy is provided by ATP for Na^+/K^+ exchange. Carrier-mediated transport, because it involves a binding step, shows the characteristic of saturation.

Carriers of this type are ubiquitous, and many pharmacological effects are the result of interference with them. Thus some nerve terminals have transport mechanisms that accumulate specific neurotransmitters or their precursors, and there are many examples of drugs that act by inhibiting these transport mechanisms (see Chs 14, 15, 37, 48 and 49). From a general pharmacokinetic point of view, however, the main sites where SLCs, including OCTs and OATs, are expressed and carrier-mediated drug transport is important are:

- the blood–brain barrier
- the gastrointestinal tract
- the renal tubule
- the biliary tract
- the placenta

P-glycoprotein transporters

P-glycoproteins (P-gp; P for 'permeability'), which belong to the ABC transporter superfamily, are the second important class of transporters and are responsible for multidrug resistance in cancer cells, many of which express an ATP-dependent pump with broad specificity called multidrug resistance protein 1 (mdr1) – see Chapter 57. This is expressed in animals, fungi and bacteria and may have evolved as a defence mechanism against toxins. P-gps are present in renal tubular brush border membranes, in bile canaliculi, in astrocyte foot processes in brain microvessels[1] and in the gastrointestinal tract. They play an important part in the absorption, distribution and elimination of many drugs, and are often co-located with SLC drug carriers, so that a drug that has been concentrated by, for example, an OAT transporter in the basolateral membrane of a renal tubular cell may then be extruded by a P-gp in the lumenal membrane (see Ch. 29).

Polymorphic variation in the genes coding SLCs and P-gp contributes to individual genetic variation in responsiveness to different drugs, and competition between drugs for the same transporter cause drug–drug interactions (see Lund et al., 2017, Nosaki and Izumi, 2020 and Yoshida et al., 2013, for reviews). OCT1 transports several drugs, including **metformin** (used to treat type 2 diabetes; see Ch. 31), into hepatocytes (in contrast to OCT2 which is expressed in renal proximal tubular cells, see previously). Metformin acts partly through effects within hepatocytes, and single nucleotide polymorphisms (SNPs) that impair the function of OCT1 influence its effectiveness (Fig. 9.6). This is but one example of many genetic influences on drug effectiveness or toxicity via altered activity of carriers that influence drug disposition. Furthermore, induction or competitive inhibition of transporter molecules can occur in the presence of a second ligand that binds the carrier, so there is a potential for drug–drug interaction (see Fig. 9.5 and Ch. 12).

Plasma protein and tissue partition of drugs

In addition to the processes so far described, which govern the transport of drug molecules across the barriers between different aqueous compartments, two additional factors have a major influence on drug distribution and elimination. These are:

- binding to plasma proteins
- partition into body fat and other tissues

[1]This accounts for some strain and species differences. For example, Collie dogs lack the multidrug resistance gene (*MDR1*), that encodes a P-gp which extrudes toxins from the cerebrospinal fluid across the blood–brain barrier. This has consequences for veterinary medicine because **ivermectin** (an anthelminthic drug; see Ch. 56) is severely neurotoxic in the many breeds with Collie ancestry.

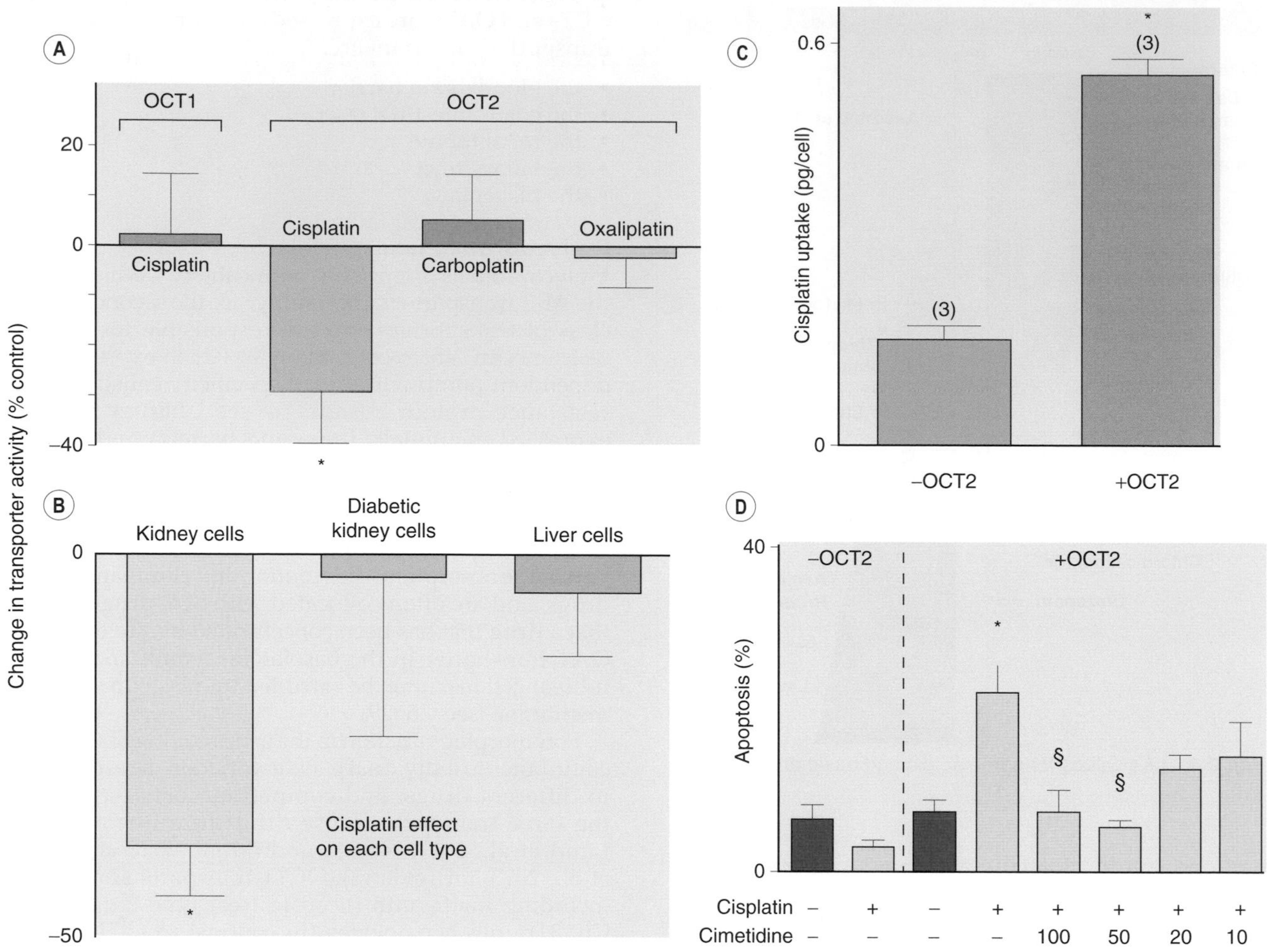

Fig. 9.5 Human organic cation transporter 2 (OCT2) mediates cisplatin nephrotoxicity. OCT2 is expressed in kidney whereas OCT1 is expressed in liver. Cisplatin (100 μmol/L) influences the activity of OCT2 but not of OCT1, each expressed in a cultured cell line (A), whereas the less nephrotoxic drugs carboplatin and oxaliplatin do not. Cisplatin similarly influences OCT2 activity in fresh human kidney tubule cells but not in fresh hepatocytes or kidney cells from patients with diabetes who are less susceptible to cisplatin nephrotoxicity (B). Cisplatin accumulates in cells that express OCT2 (C) and causes cell death (D). Cimetidine competes with cisplatin for OCT2 and concentration dependently protects against cisplatin-induced apoptosis (D) – cimetidine concentrations are in μmol/L. (Data redrawn from Ciarimboli, G., et al., 2005. Am. J. Pathol. 167, 1477–1484.)

Movement of drugs across cellular barriers

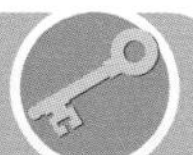

- To traverse cellular barriers (e.g. gastrointestinal mucosa, renal tubule, blood–brain barrier, placenta), drugs have to cross lipid membranes.
- Drugs cross lipid membranes mainly (a) by passive diffusional transfer and (b) by carrier-mediated transfer.
- The main factor that determines the rate of passive diffusional transfer across membranes is a drug's lipid solubility.
- Many drugs are weak acids or weak bases; their state of ionisation varies with pH according to the Henderson–Hasselbalch equation.
- With weak acids or bases, only the uncharged species (the protonated form for a weak acid, the unprotonated form for a weak base) can diffuse across lipid membranes; this gives rise to pH partition.
- pH partition means that weak acids accumulate in compartments of relatively high pH, whereas weak bases do the reverse.
- Carrier-mediated transport is mediated by solute carriers (SLCs), which include OCTs and OATs, and P-gps, which are ABC transporters in the renal tubule, blood–brain barrier and gastrointestinal epithelium. These are important in determining the distribution of many drugs, are prone to genetic variation and are targets for drug–drug interactions.

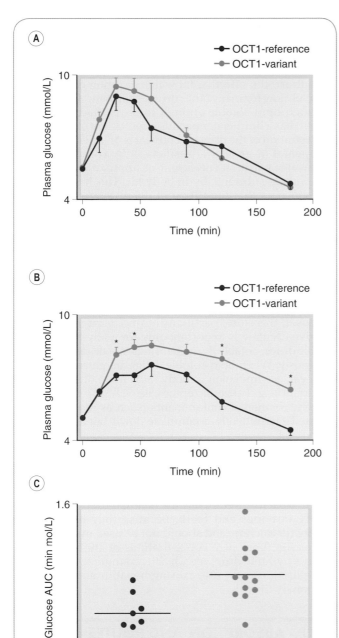

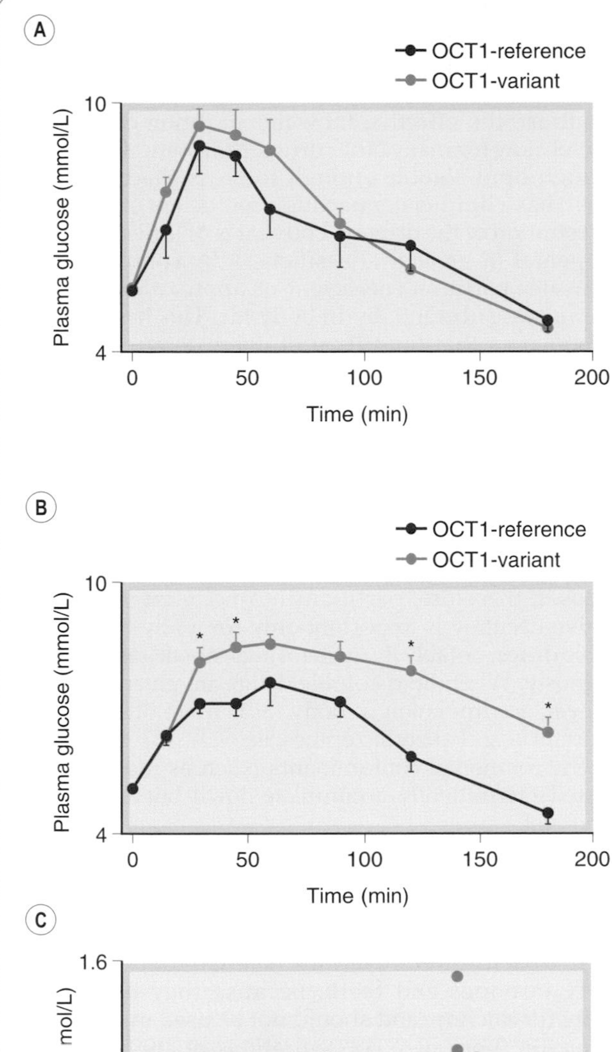

Fig. 9.6 Genetic variants of organic cation transporter 1 (OCT1) are associated with different responses to metformin in healthy humans. (A) An oral glucose tolerance test (OGTT) gave similar plasma glucose responses in control subjects with only reference *OCT1* alleles versus subjects with at least one reduced function *OCT1* allele. (B) In contrast, after metformin treatment, the OGTT response was less in the same reference subjects than in those with reduced function *OCT1* alleles – i.e. the effect of metformin was blunted in the variant-allele group. (C) Glucose exposure estimated by area under the glucose time curves was significantly lower in subjects with only reference *OCT1* alleles, $p = 0.004$. (Data redrawn from Yan Shu, et al., 2007. J. Clin. Invest. 117, 1422–1431.)

BINDING OF DRUGS TO PLASMA PROTEINS

At therapeutic concentrations in plasma, many drugs exist mainly in bound form. The fraction of drug that is unbound and pharmacologically active in plasma can be less than 1%, the remainder being associated with plasma protein. Seemingly small differences in protein binding (e.g. 99.5% vs 99.0%) can have large effects on free drug concentration and drug effect. Such differences are common between human plasma and plasma from species used in preclinical drug testing and must be taken into account when estimating a suitable dose for 'first time in human' studies during drug development. The most important plasma protein in relation to drug binding is albumin, which binds many acidic drugs (e.g. warfarin, non-steroidal anti-inflammatory drugs, sulfonamides) and a smaller number of basic drugs (e.g. tricyclic antidepressants and chlorpromazine). Other plasma proteins, including β-globulin and a circulating acid glycoprotein that increases in inflammatory disease, have also been implicated in the binding of certain basic drugs such as quinine.

The amount of a drug that is bound to protein depends on three factors:

- the concentration of free drug
- its affinity for the binding sites
- the concentration of protein

As a first approximation, the binding reaction can be regarded as a simple association of the drug molecules with a finite population of binding sites, analogous to drug–receptor binding (see Ch. 2):

$$\underset{\text{free drug}}{D} + \underset{\text{binding site}}{S} \rightleftharpoons \underset{\text{complex}}{DS}$$

The usual concentration of albumin in plasma is approximately 0.6 mmol/L (4 g/100 mL). With two sites per albumin molecule, the drug-binding capacity of plasma albumin would therefore be about 1.2 mmol/L. For most drugs, the total plasma concentration required for a clinical effect is much less than 1.2 mmol/L, so with usual therapeutic doses the binding sites are far from saturated, and the concentration bound [DS] varies nearly in direct proportion to the free concentration [D]. Under these conditions, the fraction bound, [DS]/([D] + [DS]), is independent of the drug concentration. However, some drugs, for example, **tolbutamide** (see Ch. 31), act at plasma concentrations at which its binding to plasma albumin approaches saturation (i.e. on the flat part of the binding curve). This means that increasing the dose increases the free (pharmacologically active) concentration disproportionately. This is illustrated in Fig. 9.7.

Plasma albumin binds many different drugs at one or another of a limited number of binding sites, so competition can occur between drugs. If two drugs (A and B) compete in this way, administration of drug B can reduce the protein binding, and hence increase the free plasma concentration, of drug A. To do this, drug B needs to occupy an appreciable fraction of the binding sites. Few therapeutic drugs affect the

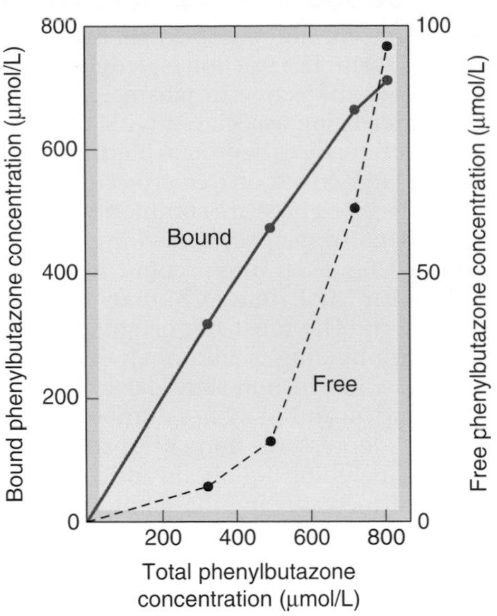

Fig. 9.7 Binding of phenylbutazone to plasma albumin. The graph shows the disproportionate increase in free concentration as the total concentration increases, owing to the binding sites approaching saturation. (Data from Brodie, B., Hogben, C.A.M., 1957. J. Pharm. Pharmacol. 9, 345.)

binding of other drugs because they occupy, at therapeutic plasma concentrations, only a tiny fraction of the available sites. *Sulfonamides* (see Ch. 52) are an exception, because they occupy about 50% of the binding sites at therapeutic concentrations and so can cause harmful effects by displacing other drugs or, in premature babies, bilirubin (see later). Much has been made of binding interactions of this kind as a source of untoward drug interactions in clinical medicine, but this type of competition is less important than was once thought (see Ch. 12).

Binding of drugs to plasma proteins

- Plasma albumin binds mainly acidic drugs (approximately two molecules per albumin molecule).
- Saturable binding can lead to a non-linear relation between dose and free (active) drug concentration, but the effective concentration range of most therapeutic drugs is below that at which this would be important.
- Binding to plasma protein is a source of species variation, important in interpreting preclinical pharmacology studies and estimating the first-in-human dose.
- β-Globulin and acid glycoprotein also bind some drugs in plasma.
- Extensive protein binding slows drug elimination (metabolism and/or glomerular filtration).
- Competition between drugs for protein binding can lead to clinically significant drug interactions, but this is uncommon.

PARTITION INTO BODY FAT AND OTHER TISSUES

Fat potentially provides a large reservoir for non-polar drugs. In practice, this is important for many general anaesthetics (see Ch. 41), which are relatively lipid soluble. In contrast, the effective fat:water partition coefficient is relatively low for many other drugs. Morphine, for example, although lipid-soluble enough to cross the blood–brain barrier, has a lipid:water partition coefficient of only 0.4, so sequestration of the drug by body fat is of little importance. **Thiopental** (a general anaesthetic[2]), by comparison, has a fat:water partition coefficient of approximately 10 and accumulates substantially in body fat. This has important consequences that limit its usefulness as an intravenous anaesthetic to short-term initiation ('induction') of anaesthesia, and it has been replaced by propofol even for this indication in many countries (see Ch. 41).

The second factor that limits the accumulation of drugs in body fat is its low blood supply – less than 2% of the cardiac output. Consequently, drugs are delivered slowly to body fat, and the theoretical equilibrium distribution between fat and body water is delayed. For practical purposes, therefore, partition into body fat when drugs are given acutely is important only for a few highly lipid-soluble drugs, notably the general anaesthetics as mentioned previously. When lipid-soluble drugs are given *chronically*, however, accumulation in body fat is more often clinically important (e.g. benzodiazepines; see Ch. 45). Some drugs and environmental contaminants (such as insecticides), if ingested intermittently, accumulate slowly but progressively in body fat.

Fat is not the only tissue in which drugs can accumulate. **Chloroquine** – an antimalarial drug (see Ch. 55) – has a high affinity for melanin and is taken up by the retina, which is rich in melanin granules, accounting for chloroquine's ocular toxicity. Tetracyclines (see Ch. 52) accumulate slowly in bones and teeth, because they have a high affinity for calcium, and should not be used in children for this reason. Very high concentrations of **amiodarone** (an antidysrhythmic drug; see Ch. 20) accumulate in liver and lung during chronic use, causing hepatitis and interstitial pulmonary fibrosis.

DRUG ABSORPTION AND ROUTES OF ADMINISTRATION

The main routes of drug administration and elimination are shown schematically in Fig. 9.8. Absorption is defined as the passage of a drug from its site of administration into the plasma. It is important for all routes of administration except intravenous injection, where it is complete by definition. There are instances, such as topical administration of a steroid cream to skin or inhalation of a bronchodilator aerosol to treat asthma (see Ch. 28), where absorption as just defined is not required for the drug to act, but in most cases the drug must enter plasma before reaching its site of action.

The main routes of administration are:

- oral (drug is swallowed)

[2]Also known as sodium pentothal or 'truth serum'. This barbiturate, at sub-narcosis doses, can reduce an individual's resolve and make them more compliant to suggestions – at least in the movies.

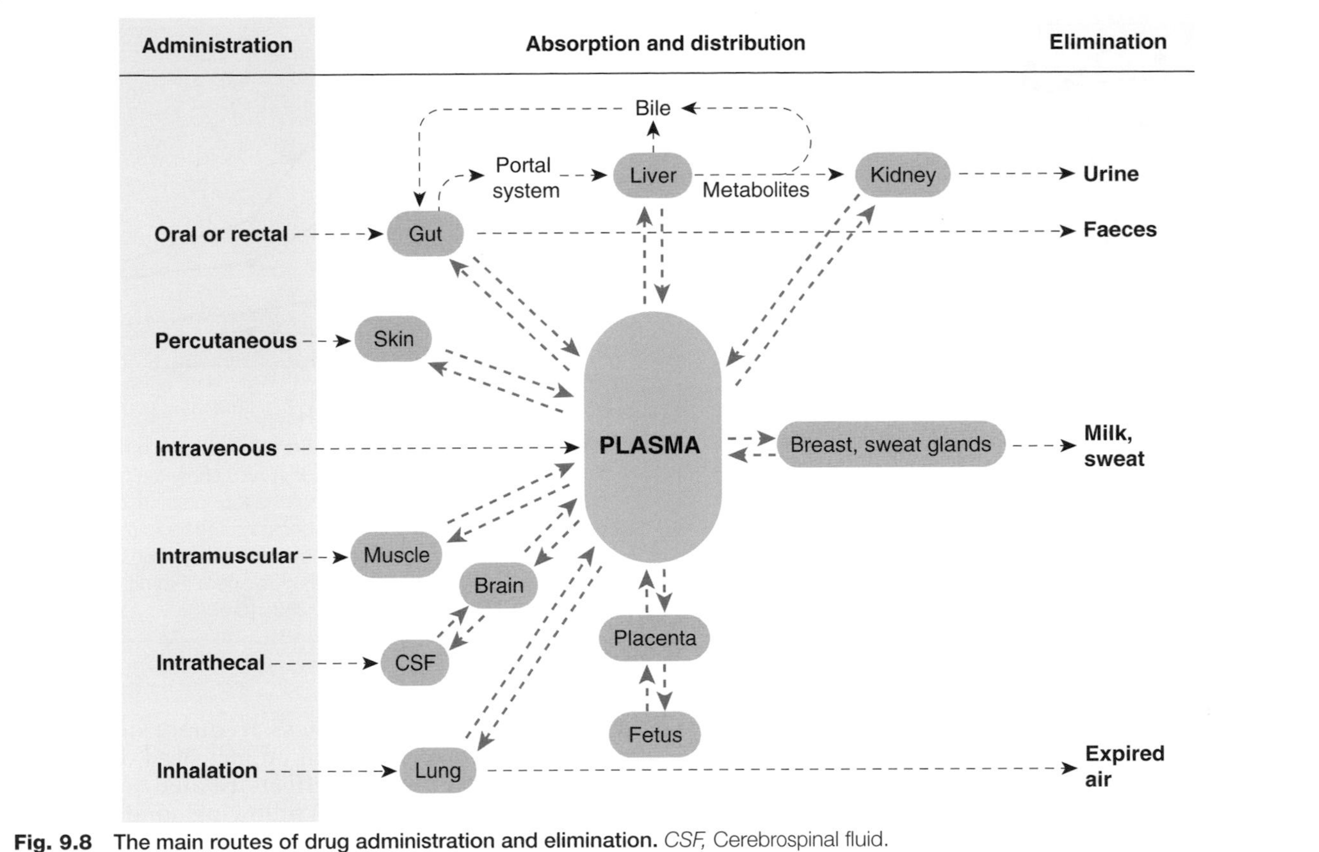

Fig. 9.8 The main routes of drug administration and elimination. *CSF,* Cerebrospinal fluid.

- sublingual or buccal (drug is kept in contact with the oral mucosa)
- rectal
- application to other epithelial surfaces (e.g. skin, conjunctiva, vagina and nasal mucosa)
- inhalation
- injection
  - subcutaneous
  - intramuscular
  - intravenous
  - intrathecal
  - intravitreal

ORAL ADMINISTRATION

Most small molecule drugs are taken by mouth and swallowed. Little absorption occurs until the drug enters the small intestine, although non-polar drugs applied to the buccal mucosa or under the tongue are absorbed directly from the mouth (e.g. organic nitrates, see Ch. 20, and buprenorphine, see Ch. 42). Peptides and proteins are subject to digestion, so the oral route is not generally suitable to biopharmaceuticals, and despite ingenious pharmaceutical approaches to circumvent these problems, success has been limited (Dubey et al., 2021).

DRUG ABSORPTION FROM THE INTESTINE

For most drugs, the mechanism of absorption is the same as for other epithelial barriers, namely, passive transfer at a rate determined by the ionisation and lipid solubility of the drug molecules. Fig. 9.9 shows the absorption of various weak acids and bases as a function of pK_a. As expected, strong bases of pK_a 10 or higher are poorly absorbed, as are strong acids of pK_a less than 3, because they are fully ionised. The arrow poison **curare** used by South American indigenous tribes contains quaternary ammonium compounds that block neuromuscular transmission (see Ch. 14). These strong bases are poorly absorbed from the gastrointestinal tract, so the meat from animals killed in this way was safe to eat.

In some instances, intestinal drug absorption depends on carrier-mediated transport rather than simple lipid diffusion. Examples include **levodopa**, used in treating Parkinson's disease (see Ch. 40), which is taken up by the carrier that normally transports phenylalanine, and **fluorouracil** (see Ch. 57), a cytotoxic drug that is transported by the carrier for pyrimidines (thymine and uracil). Iron is absorbed via specific carriers in the epithelial cell membranes of jejunal mucosa, and calcium is absorbed by a vitamin D-dependent carrier.

FACTORS AFFECTING GASTROINTESTINAL ABSORPTION

Typically, about 75% of a drug given orally is absorbed in 1–3 h, but numerous factors alter this, some physiological and some to do with the formulation of the drug. The main factors are:

- gut content (e.g. fed vs fasted)
- gastrointestinal motility
- splanchnic blood flow
- particle size and formulation
- physicochemical factors, including some drug–drug interactions

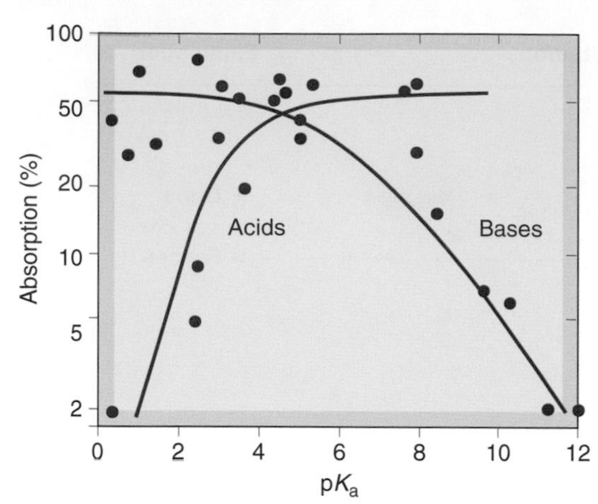

Fig. 9.9 Absorption of drugs from the intestine, as a function of p*K*a, for acids and bases. Weak acids and bases are well absorbed; strong acids and bases are poorly absorbed. (Redrawn from Schanker, L.S., et al., 1957. *J. Pharmacol. Exp. Therap.* 120, 528.)

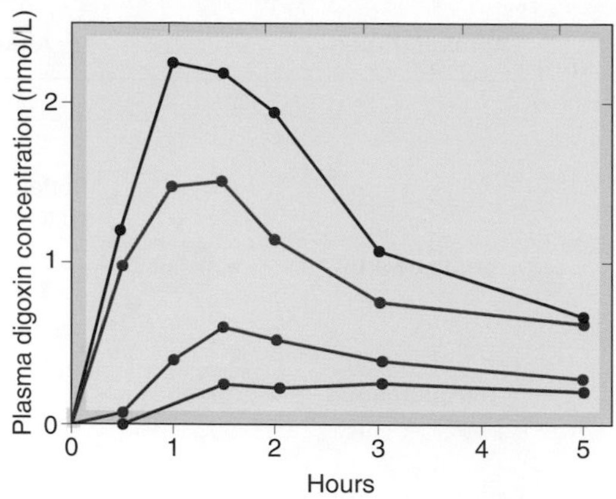

Fig. 9.10 Variation in oral absorption among different formulations of digoxin. The four curves show the mean plasma concentrations attained for the four preparations, each of which was given on separate occasions to four subjects. The large variation has caused the formulation of digoxin tablets to be standardised since this study was published. (From Lindenbaum, J., et al., 1971. N. Engl. J. Med. 285, 1344.)

- genetic polymorphisms in, and drug–drug competition for, transporters

The influence of feeding, which influences both gut content and splanchnic blood flow, is routinely examined in early phase clinical trials (the pharmacokinetic measure of interest is T_{max}, the time after dosing at which the plasma concentration of the drug is maximal, C_{max}), and prescribing advice tailored accordingly. Gastrointestinal motility has a large effect. Many disorders (e.g. migraine, diabetic neuropathy) cause gastric stasis and slow drug absorption. Drug treatment can also affect motility, either reducing it (e.g. drugs that block muscarinic receptors; see Ch. 14) or increasing it (e.g. **metoclopramide**, an antiemetic used in migraine to facilitate absorption of analgesic; see Chs 16, 30 and 42). Excessively rapid movement of gut contents (e.g. in some forms of diarrhoea) can impair absorption. Several drugs (e.g. **propranolol**) reach a higher plasma concentration if they are taken after a meal, probably because food increases splanchnic blood flow. Conversely, splanchnic blood flow is greatly reduced by exercise and by hypovolaemia or heart failure, with a resultant reduction of drug absorption.

Particle size and formulation have major effects on absorption. In 1971, patients in a New York hospital were found to require unusually large maintenance doses of **digoxin** (see Ch. 20). In a study on healthy volunteers, it was found that standard digoxin tablets from different manufacturers resulted in different plasma concentrations (Fig. 9.10), even though the digoxin content of the tablets was the same, probably in part because of differences in particle size.

Therapeutic drugs are formulated to produce desired absorption characteristics. Capsules may be designed to remain intact for some hours after ingestion in order to delay absorption, or tablets may have a resistant coating to give the same effect. In some cases, a mixture of slow- and fast-release particles is included in a capsule to produce rapid but sustained absorption. More elaborate pharmaceutical systems include modified-release preparations that permit less frequent dosing. Such preparations not only permit an increased dose interval but also reduce adverse effects related to high peak plasma concentration (C_{max}) following administration of a conventional formulation.

When drugs are swallowed, the intention is usually that they should be absorbed and cause a systemic effect, but there are exceptions. **Vancomycin** is very poorly absorbed and is administered orally to eradicate toxin-forming *Clostridium difficile* from the gut lumen in patients with pseudomembranous colitis (an adverse effect of broad-spectrum antibiotics caused by appearance of this organism in the bowel). **Mesalazine** is a formulation of 5-aminosalicylic acid in a pH-dependent acrylic coat that degrades in the terminal ileum and proximal colon, and is used to treat inflammatory bowel disease affecting this part of the gut. **Olsalazine** is a prodrug (see later) consisting of a dimer of two molecules of 5-aminosalicylic acid that is cleaved by colonic bacteria in the distal bowel and is used to treat patients with distal colitis.

Bioavailability and bioequivalence

To access the systemic circulation, a drug given orally must not only penetrate the intestinal mucosa, it must also run a gauntlet of inactivating enzymes in the gut wall and liver, referred to as 'presystemic' or 'first-pass' metabolism. The term *bioavailability* is used to indicate the fraction (F) of an orally administered dose that reaches the systemic circulation as intact drug, taking into account both absorption and local metabolic degradation. F is measured by determining the plasma drug concentration versus time curves in a group of subjects following oral and (on a separate occasion) intravenous administration (the fraction absorbed following an intravenous dose is 1 by definition). The area under the plasma concentration time curves (AUC) provides an integrated measure of drug exposure, taking into account time as well as concentration, and F is estimated as $AUC_{oral}/AUC_{intravenous}$. Bioavailability is not a characteristic solely of the drug preparation: variations in enzyme activity of gut wall or liver, in gastric pH or intestinal motility all affect it. Because of this, one cannot speak strictly of the bioavailability of a particular preparation, but only of that preparation in a given individual on a particular occasion, and *F* determined in a group of healthy volunteer subjects may differ substantially from the value determined in patients with diseases of gastrointestinal or circulatory systems.

Bioavailability relates only to the total proportion of the drug that reaches the systemic circulation and neglects the rate of absorption. If a drug is completely absorbed in 30 min, it will reach a much higher peak plasma concentration (and have a more dramatic effect) than if it were absorbed over several hours. Regulatory authorities – which have to make decisions about the licensing of products that are 'generic equivalents' of patented products – require evidence of 'bioequivalence' based on the maximum concentration achieved (C_{max}) and time between dosing and C_{max} (T_{max}) as well as $AUC_{(0-t)}$. For most drugs, $AUC_{(0-t)}$ and C_{max} must each lie between 80% and 125% of a marketed preparation for the new generic product to be accepted as bioequivalent to the comparator, which is usually the market leader (EMEA, 2010).

OROMUCOSAL (SUBLINGUAL OR BUCCAL) ADMINISTRATION

Absorption directly from the oral cavity is sometimes useful when a rapid response is required, particularly when the drug is either unstable at gastric pH or rapidly metabolised by the liver. **Glyceryl trinitrate** and **buprenorphine** (mentioned earlier) are examples of drugs that are often given sublingually (see Chs 20 and 42, respectively). Buccal midazolam is as effective and safe as intravenous or rectal diazepam in terminating early *status epilepticus* (see Ch. 46) in children (Brigo et al., 2015). Times from arrival in the emergency department to drug administration and to seizure cessation are shortened and the drug is easier to administer. Drugs absorbed from the mouth pass directly into the systemic circulation without entering the portal system, and so escape first-pass metabolism by enzymes in the gut wall and liver.

RECTAL ADMINISTRATION

Rectal administration is used for drugs that are required to produce either a local effect (e.g. anti-inflammatory drugs such as **mesalazine** suppositories or enemas for use in ulcerative colitis; see Ch. 30) or systemic effects. Absorption following rectal administration may be unreliable but can be rapid and more complete than following oral administration, since only a fraction of the capillary drainage returns to the systemic circulation via the portal vein. This route can be useful in patients who are vomiting or are unable to take medication by mouth (e.g. postoperatively or during palliative care), but rectal administration has not been widely adopted even when there is a seemingly good rationale and suppositories are commercially available, for example, ergotamine-containing suppositories for treating migraine attacks – a condition where gastric stasis and vomiting can limit the effectiveness of oral tablets (see Ch. 42).

APPLICATION TO EPITHELIAL SURFACES

CUTANEOUS ADMINISTRATION

Cutaneous administration is used when a local effect on the skin is required (see Ch. 26). Appreciable absorption may nonetheless occur and lead to systemic effects; absorption is sometimes exploited therapeutically, for example, in local application of rub-on gels of non-steroidal anti-inflammatory agents such as **ibuprofen** (see Ch. 25).

Most drugs are absorbed very poorly through unbroken skin. However, a number of organophosphate insecticides (see Ch. 14), which need to penetrate an insect's cuticle to work, are absorbed through skin, and accidental poisoning occurs in farm workers.

A case is recounted of a 35-year-old florist in 1932. 'While engaged in doing a light electrical repair job at a work bench he sat down in a chair on the seat of which some "Nico-Fume liquid" (a 40% solution of free nicotine) had been spilled. He felt the solution wet through his clothes to the skin over the left buttock, an area about the size of the palm of his hand. He thought nothing further of it and continued at his work for about 15 min, when he was suddenly seized with nausea and faintness … and found himself in a drenching sweat. On the way to hospital he lost consciousness.' He survived, just, and then 4 days later: 'On discharge from the hospital he was given the same clothes that he had worn when he was brought in. The clothes had been kept in a paper bag and were still damp where they had been wet with the nicotine solution.' The sequel was predictable. He survived again but felt thereafter 'unable to enter a greenhouse where nicotine was being sprayed'. Transdermal dosage forms of nicotine are now used to reduce the withdrawal symptoms that accompany stopping smoking (see Ch. 50).

Transdermal dosage forms, in which the drug is incorporated in a stick-on patch applied to the skin, are used increasingly, and several drugs – for example **oestrogen** and **testosterone** for hormone replacement (see Ch. 35) – are available in this form. Such patches produce a steady rate of drug delivery and avoid presystemic metabolism. **Fentanyl** is available in a patch to treat intermittent breakthrough pain (see Ch. 43). However, the method is suitable only for lipid-soluble drugs and is relatively expensive.

NASAL SPRAYS

Some peptide hormone analogues, for example, **antidiuretic hormone** (see Ch. 33) and **gonadotrophin-releasing hormone** (see Ch. 35), are given as nasal sprays, as is **calcitonin** (see Ch. 36). Absorption is believed to take place through mucosa overlying nasal-associated lymphoid tissue. This is similar to the mucosa overlying Peyer's patches in the small intestine, which is also unusually permeable.

EYE DROPS

Many drugs are applied as eye drops (see Ch. 27), relying on absorption through the epithelium of the conjunctival sac to produce their effects. Desirable local effects within the eye can be achieved without causing systemic side effects; for example, **dorzolamide** is a carbonic anhydrase inhibitor that is given as eye drops to lower ocular pressure in patients with glaucoma. It achieves this without affecting the kidney (see Ch. 29), thus avoiding the acidosis that is caused by oral administration of acetazolamide. Some systemic absorption from the eye occurs, however, and can result in unwanted effects (e.g. bronchospasm in asthmatic patients using **timolol** eye drops for glaucoma).

ADMINISTRATION BY INHALATION

Inhalation is the route used for volatile and gaseous anaesthetics, the lung serving as the route of both administration and elimination (see Ch. 41). The rapid exchange resulting from the large surface area and blood flow makes it possible to achieve rapid adjustments of plasma concentration. The pharmacokinetic behaviour of inhalation anaesthetics is discussed in Chapter 41.

Drugs used for their effects on the lung are also given by inhalation, usually as an aerosol mist of liquid droplets or sometimes of solid particles. Glucocorticoids (e.g. **beclometasone dipropionate**) and bronchodilators (e.g. **salbutamol** and **formoterol**; see Ch. 28) are given in this way to achieve high local concentrations in the lung while minimising systemic effects. However, drugs given by inhalation in this way are usually partly absorbed into the circulation, and systemic side effects (e.g. tremor following salbutamol) can occur. Chemical modification of a drug may minimise such absorption. For example, **ipratropium**, a muscarinic-receptor antagonist (see Chs 14 and 28), is a quaternary ammonium ion analogue of atropine. It is used as an inhaled bronchodilator because its poor absorption prolongs its local action and reduces the likelihood of systemic adverse effects.

ADMINISTRATION BY INJECTION

Intravenous injection is the fastest and most certain route of drug administration. Bolus injection rapidly produces a high concentration of drug, first in the right heart and pulmonary vessels and then in the systemic circulation. The peak concentration reaching the tissues depends critically on the rate of injection. Administration by intravenous infusion using a mechanical pump avoids the uncertainties of absorption from other sites, while avoiding high peak plasma concentrations caused by bolus injection.

Subcutaneous or intramuscular injection of drugs usually produces a faster effect than oral administration, but the rate of absorption depends greatly on the site of injection and on local blood flow. The rate-limiting factors in absorption from the injection site are:

- diffusion through the tissue
- removal by local blood flow

Absorption from a site of injection (sometimes but not always desirable, see later) is increased by increased blood flow. *Hyaluronidase* (an enzyme that breaks down the intercellular matrix, thereby increasing diffusion) also increases drug absorption from the site of injection. Conversely, absorption is reduced in patients with circulatory failure (shock) in whom tissue perfusion is reduced (see Ch. 21).

METHODS FOR DELAYING ABSORPTION

It may be desirable to delay absorption, either to produce a local effect or to prolong systemic action. For example, addition of adrenaline (epinephrine) to a local anaesthetic reduces absorption of the anaesthetic into the general circulation, usefully prolonging the anaesthetic effect (see Ch. 44). Formulation of insulin with protamine and zinc produces a long-acting form (see Ch. 31). Even longer-acting insulin analogues are now available that can provide basal insulin levels with once daily dosing. These include **insulin glargine**, **insulin detemir** and **insulin degladec.** The longest acting of these, insulin degladec, has one amino acid deleted and a lysine residue is conjugated to a long-chain fatty acid via a g-L-glutamyl spacer. This analogue provides basal insulin for up to 42 h after a single injection - a useful property in managing diabetic patients with cognitive impairment at home via visiting nurses who may not be able to call at the same time each day. Procaine penicillin (see Ch. 52) is a poorly soluble salt of **penicillin**; when injected as an aqueous suspension, it is slowly absorbed and exerts a prolonged action. Esterification of steroid hormones (e.g. medroxyprogesterone acetate, testosterone propionate; see Ch. 35) and antipsychotic drugs (e.g. fluphenazine decanoate; see Ch. 47) increases their solubility in oil and slows their absorption when they are injected in an oily solution.

Another method used to achieve slow and continuous absorption of certain steroid hormones (e.g. **oestradiol**; see Ch. 35) is the subcutaneous implantation of the drug substance formulated as a solid pellet. The rate of absorption is proportional to the surface area of the implant.

INTRATHECAL INJECTION

Injection of a drug into the subarachnoid space via a lumbar puncture needle is used for some specialised purposes. **Methotrexate** (see Ch. 57) is administered in this way in the treatment of certain childhood leukaemias to prevent relapse in the CNS. Regional anaesthesia can be produced by intrathecal administration of a local anaesthetic such as **bupivacaine** (see Ch. 44); opioid analgesics can also be used in this way (see Ch. 43). **Baclofen** (a GABA analogue; see Ch. 38) is used to treat disabling muscle spasms. It has been administered intrathecally to minimise its adverse peripheral effects. Some antibiotics (e.g. aminoglycosides) cross the blood–brain barrier very slowly, and in rare clinical situations where they are essential (e.g. nervous system infections with bacteria resistant to other antibiotics) can be given intrathecally or directly into the cerebral ventricles via a reservoir. **Nusinersen**, an antisense oligonucleotide used to treat spinal muscular atrophy (see Chs 5 and 40), is administered intrathecally and this route may become increasingly important in view of the therapeutic potential of biopharmaceuticals in neurological disorders and the access problem posed to these agents by the blood–brain barrier.

INTRAVITREAL INJECTION (SEE CH. 27)

Ranibizumab (monoclonal antibody fragment that binds to vascular endothelial growth factor; see Ch. 21) or a fusion protein, **aflibercept,** are given by intravitreal injection by ophthalmologists treating patients with wet age-related macular degeneration, macular oedema and choroidal neovascularisation. Intravitreal implants that slowly release corticosteroids (such as **fluocinolone** or **dexamethasone**) over a period of months are used in macular oedema.

Drug absorption and bioavailability

- Drugs of very low lipid solubility, including those that are strong acids or bases, are generally poorly absorbed from the gut.
- Exceptions (e.g. **levodopa**) are absorbed by carrier-mediated transfer.
- Absorption from the gut depends on many factors, including:
  - gastrointestinal motility
  - gastrointestinal pH
  - particle size
  - physicochemical interaction with gut contents (e.g. chemical interaction between calcium and tetracycline antibiotics)
  - genetic polymorphisms in drug transporters and competition for transporters.
- Bioavailability is the fraction of an ingested dose of a drug that gains access to the systemic circulation. It may be low because absorption is incomplete, or because the drug is metabolised in the gut wall or liver before reaching the systemic circulation ('pre-systemic metabolism').
- Bioequivalence implies that if one formulation of a drug is substituted for another, no clinically untoward consequences will ensue.

DISTRIBUTION OF DRUGS IN THE BODY

BODY FLUID COMPARTMENTS

Body water is distributed into four main compartments (Fig. 9.11). Water constitutes 50% to 70% of body weight, being rather less in women than in men.

Extracellular fluid comprises the blood plasma (about 4.5% of body weight), interstitial fluid (16%) and lymph (1.2%). Intracellular fluid (30%–40%) is the sum of the fluid contents of all cells in the body. Transcellular fluid (2.5%) includes the cerebrospinal, intraocular, peritoneal, pleural and synovial fluids and digestive secretions. The fetus may also be regarded as a special type of transcellular compartment. Within each of these aqueous compartments, drug molecules usually exist both in free solution and in bound form; furthermore, drugs that are weak acids or bases will exist as an equilibrium mixture of the charged and uncharged forms, the position of the equilibrium depending on the pH of the fluid and pK_a of the drug.

The equilibrium pattern of distribution between the various compartments will therefore depend on:

- permeability across tissue barriers
- binding within compartments
- pH partition
- fat:water partition

To enter the transcellular compartments from the extracellular compartment, a drug must cross a cellular barrier, a particularly important example being the blood-brain barrier.

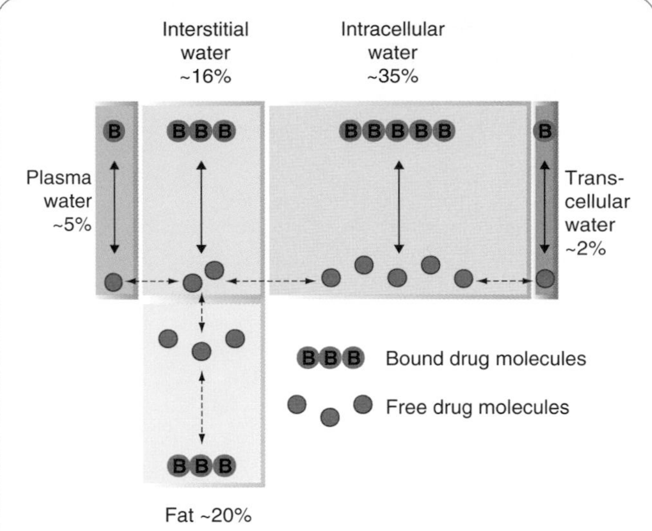

Fig. 9.11 The main body fluid compartments, expressed as a percentage of body weight. Drug molecules exist in bound or free form in each compartment, but only the free drug is able to move between the compartments.

THE BLOOD–BRAIN BARRIER

The concept of the blood–brain barrier was introduced by Paul Ehrlich to explain his observation that intravenously injected dye stained most tissues but not the brain. The barrier consists of a continuous layer of endothelial cells joined by tight junctions and surrounded by pericytes. Several efflux pumps extrude substrate molecules, including water-soluble drugs that penetrate into CSF. The brain is consequently inaccessible to many drugs of low lipid solubility, and efforts have been made to improve central nervous sustem pharmacotherapy by modulating permeability proteins in the blood brain barrier (reviewed by Miller et al 2008). However, inflammation can disrupt the integrity of the blood–brain barrier (Fig. 9.12) and activity of efflux pumps; consequently, penicillin (see Ch. 52) can be given intravenously (rather than intrathecally) to treat bacterial meningitis, which is accompanied by intense inflammation. Loperamide, an opioid agonist used for its effect on the ileum in treating diarrhoea (see Ch. 30), is another drug that does cross the blood–brain barrier but is very rapidly pumped out so is in effect confined to the periphery. In some parts of the CNS, including the *chemoreceptor trigger zone*, the barrier is leaky. This enables **domperidone**, an antiemetic dopamine-receptor antagonist (see Chs 30 and 40) that does not penetrate the blood–brain barrier but does access the chemoreceptor trigger zone, to be used to prevent the nausea caused by dopamine agonists such as **apomorphine** when these are used to treat advanced Parkinson's disease. This is achieved without loss of efficacy, because dopamine receptors in the basal ganglia are accessible only to drugs that have traversed the blood–brain barrier.

Methylnaltrexone bromide, naloxegol and **naldemedine** are peripherally acting μ-opioid-receptor antagonists which do not cross the blood–brain barrier. They are used in treating opioid-induced constipation in patients requiring opioids as part of palliative care (see Ch. 43). **Alvimopan** is similar and used in treating postoperative ileus. These drugs have limited gastrointestinal absorption and do not cross the blood–brain barrier, so do not block the desired opioid effects in the CNS.

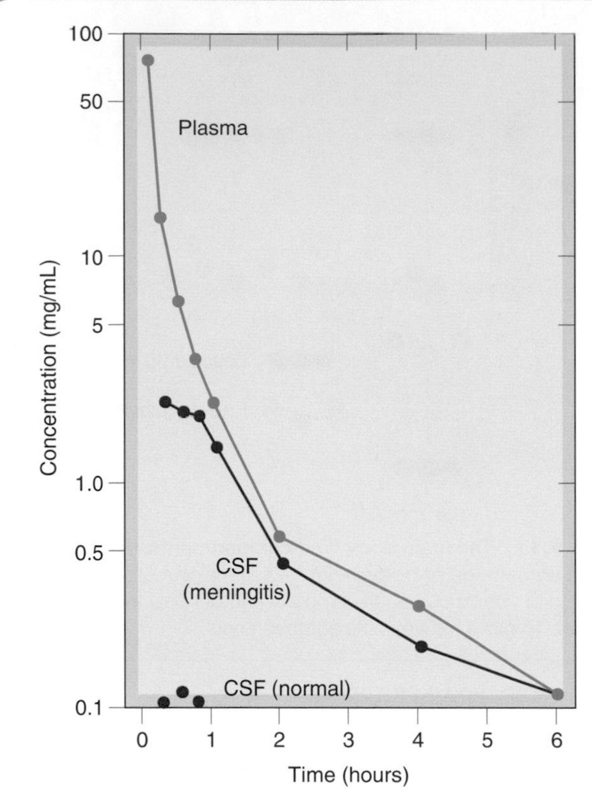

Fig. 9.12 Plasma and cerebrospinal fluid concentrations of an antibiotic (thienamycin) following an intravenous dose (25 mg/kg). In normal rabbits, no drug reaches the cerebrospinal fluid (CSF), but in animals with experimental *Escherichia coli* meningitis the concentration of drug in CSF approaches that in the plasma. (From Patamasucon, P., McCracken Jr, G.H., 1973. Antimicrob. Agents Chemother. 3, 270.)

Several peptides, including bradykinin, increase blood–brain barrier permeability. There is interest in exploiting this and other possible interventions to improve penetration of anticancer drugs during treatment of brain tumours and other neurological diseases. Despite considerable ongoing effort (see e.g. Marcucci et al., 2021) this has not yet led to routine clinical application.

VOLUME OF DISTRIBUTION

The apparent volume of distribution, V_d (see Ch. 11), is defined as the volume that would contain the total body content of the drug (Q) at a concentration equal to that present in the plasma (C_p):

$$V_d = \frac{Q}{C_p}$$

It is important to avoid identifying a given range of V_d too closely with a particular anatomical compartment. Drugs may act at very low concentrations in the key compartment that provides access to their receptors. For example, insulin has a measured V_d similar to the volume of plasma water but exerts its effects on muscle, fat and liver cells via receptors that are exposed to interstitial fluid but not to plasma (see Ch. 31).

DRUGS LARGELY CONFINED TO THE PLASMA COMPARTMENT

The plasma volume is about 0.05 L/kg body weight. A few drugs, such as **heparin** (see Ch. 23), are confined to plasma because the molecule is too large to cross the capillary wall easily. More often, retention of a drug in the plasma following a single dose reflects strong binding to plasma protein. It is, nevertheless, the free drug in the interstitial fluid that exerts a pharmacological effect. Following repeated dosing, equilibration occurs and measured V_d increases. Some dyes bind exceptionally strongly to plasma albumin, as with Evans blue, such that its V_d has been used experimentally to measure plasma volume.

DRUGS DISTRIBUTED IN THE EXTRACELLULAR COMPARTMENT

The total extracellular volume is about 0.2 L/kg body weight, and this is the approximate V_d for many polar compounds, such as vecuronium (see Ch. 14), **gentamicin** and **carbenicillin** (see Ch. 52). These drugs cannot easily enter cells because of their low lipid solubility, and they do not traverse the blood–brain or placental barriers freely. Many macromolecular biopharmaceuticals, notably monoclonal antibodies (see Ch. 5), distribute in the extracellular space and access receptors on cell surfaces but do not readily enter cells. Nucleic acid-based biopharmaceuticals work intracellularly and are often provided with special delivery systems (see Ch. 5) that facilitate access to the cell interior.

DISTRIBUTION THROUGHOUT THE BODY WATER

Total body water represents about 0.55 L/kg. This approximates the distribution of many drugs that readily cross cell membranes, such as **phenytoin** (see Ch. 46) and **ethanol** (see Ch. 50). The binding of drugs outside the plasma compartment, or partitioning into body fat, increases V_d beyond the volume of total body water. Consequently, there are also many drugs with V_d greater than the total body volume, such as morphine (see Ch. 43), tricyclic antidepressants (see Ch. 48) and **haloperidol**

Drug distribution

- The major compartments are:
  - plasma (5% of body weight)
  - interstitial fluid (16%)
  - intracellular fluid (35%)
  - transcellular fluid (2%)
  - fat (20%).
- Volume of distribution (V_d) is defined as the volume of solvent that would contain the total body content of the drug (Q) at a concentration equal to the measured plasma concentration (C_p), $V_d = Q/C_p$.
- Lipid-insoluble drugs are mainly confined to plasma and interstitial fluids; most do not enter the brain following acute dosing.
- Lipid-soluble drugs reach all compartments and may accumulate in fat.
- For drugs that accumulate outside the plasma compartment (e.g. in fat or by being bound to tissues), V_d may exceed total body volume.

(see Ch. 47). Such drugs are not efficiently removed from the body by haemodialysis, which filters blood plasma and is therefore unhelpful in managing overdose with such agents.

DRUG INTERACTIONS CAUSED BY ALTERED ABSORPTION (SEE CH. 12 FOR A GENERAL APPROACH TO DRUG–DRUG INTERACTIONS)

Gastrointestinal absorption is slowed by drugs that inhibit gastric emptying, such as atropine or opiates, or accelerated by drugs that hasten gastric emptying (e.g. metoclopramide; see Ch. 30). Alternatively, drug A may interact physically or chemically with drug B in the gut in such a way as to inhibit absorption of B. For example, Ca^{2+} and Fe^{2+} each forms insoluble complexes with **tetracycline** that retard their absorption; **colestyramine**, a bile acid-binding resin, binds several drugs (e.g. warfarin, digoxin), preventing their absorption if administered close in time to one another. The addition of **adrenaline** (**epinephrine**) to local anaesthetic injections causes vasoconstriction which slows the absorption of the anaesthetic, thus prolonging its local effect (see Ch. 44). Physiologically based modelling is now beginning to be used to predict quantitatively the effects of genetic polymorphisms of drug transporters in intestine and hepatocytes and of drug–drug interactions due to competition for these transporters (see e.g. Nosaki and Izumi, 2020; Yoshida et al., 2013).

DRUG INTERACTIONS CAUSED BY ALTERED DISTRIBUTION (SEE CH. 12 FOR A GENERAL APPROACH TO DRUG INTERACTIONS)

Altered distribution as a consequence of altered protein binding

One drug may alter the distribution of another, by competing for a common binding site on plasma albumin or tissue protein, but such interactions are seldom clinically important unless accompanied by a separate effect on drug elimination (see Chs 10 and 12). Displacement of a drug from binding sites in plasma or tissues transiently increases the concentration of free (unbound) drug, but this is followed by increased elimination, so a new steady state results in which total drug concentration in plasma is reduced but the free drug concentration is similar to that before introduction of the second 'displacing' drug. Consequences of potential clinical importance include:

- Harm from the transient increase in concentration of free drug before the new steady state is reached.
- If dose is being adjusted according to measurements of total plasma concentration, it must be appreciated that the target therapeutic concentration range will be altered by co-administration of a displacing drug.
- When the displacing drug additionally reduces elimination of the first, so that the free concentration is increased not only acutely but also chronically at the new steady state, severe toxicity may ensue.

Although many drugs have appreciable affinity for plasma albumin, and therefore might potentially be expected to interact in these ways, there are rather few instances of clinically important interactions of this type. Protein-bound drugs that are given in large enough dosage to act as displacing agents include various *sulfonamides* and **chloral hydrate**; trichloroacetic acid, a metabolite of chloral hydrate, binds very strongly to plasma albumin. Displacement of bilirubin from albumin by such drugs in jaundiced premature neonates can have clinically disastrous consequences: bilirubin metabolism is undeveloped in the premature liver, and unbound bilirubin can cross the immature blood–brain barrier and cause kernicterus (staining of the basal ganglia by bilirubin). This causes a distressing and permanent disturbance of movement known as choreoathetosis, characterised by involuntary writhing and twisting movements in the child.

Phenytoin dose is adjusted according to measurement of its concentration in plasma, and such measurements do not routinely distinguish bound from free phenytoin (i.e. they reflect the total concentration of drug). Introduction of a displacing drug in an epileptic patient whose condition is stabilised on phenytoin (see Ch. 46) reduces the total plasma phenytoin concentration owing to increased elimination of free drug, but there is no loss of efficacy because the concentration of unbound (active) phenytoin at the new steady state is unaltered. If it is not appreciated that the therapeutic range of plasma concentrations has been reduced in this way, an increased dose may be prescribed, causing harm.

Drugs that alter protein binding sometimes additionally reduce elimination of the displaced drug, causing clinically important interactions. *Salicylates* displace **methotrexate** from binding sites on albumin and reduce its secretion into the nephron by competition with the OAT (see Ch. 10). **Quinidine** and several other antidysrhythmic drugs including **verapamil** and **amiodarone** (see Chs 20 and 21) displace digoxin from tissue-binding sites while simultaneously reducing its renal excretion; they consequently can cause severe dysrhythmias through digoxin toxicity.

Altered distribution as a consequence of competition for shared transporters

Drugs may compete for shared transport mechanisms (see earlier). Carrier mediated transport by SLC and ABC mechanisms is implicated not only in drug distribution (e.g. the OAT that excludes penicillin from the CNS; and see Ch. 12) but also in drug absorption, excretion and access to metabolising enzymes in the liver (e.g. Figs 9.5 and 9.6 and see Ch. 10). There is currently a major interest in new approaches better to predict transporter-mediated drug-drug interactions such as measurement of endogenous substrates as biomarkers for transporter function (see Muller et al., 2018, for a review).

SPECIAL DRUG DELIVERY SYSTEMS

Several approaches are used or in development to improve drug delivery to the target tissue. They include:

- prodrugs
- antibody–drug conjugates
- packaging in liposomes
- coated implantable devices

PRODRUGS

Prodrugs are inactive precursors that are metabolised to active metabolites; they are described in Chapter 10 and are reviewed by Huttunen et al. 2011. Some of the examples in clinical use confer no obvious benefits and have been found to be prodrugs only retrospectively, not having been designed with this in mind. However, some do have advantages. For example, the cytotoxic drug **cyclophosphamide** (see Ch. 57) becomes active only after it has been metabolised in the liver; it can therefore be taken orally in therapeutic doses without causing serious damage to the gastrointestinal epithelium. Levodopa is absorbed from the gastrointestinal tract and crosses the blood–brain barrier via an amino acid transport mechanism before conversion to active dopamine in nerve terminals in the basal ganglia (see Ch. 40). **Zidovudine** is phosphorylated to its active triphosphate metabolite only in cells containing the appropriate viral enzyme, hence conferring selective toxicity towards cells infected with HIV (see Ch. 53). **Valaciclovir** and **famciclovir** are each ester prodrugs, respectively of **aciclovir** and of **penciclovir**. Their bioavailability is greater than that of aciclovir and penciclovir, which are themselves prodrugs that are converted into active metabolites in virally infected cells (see Ch. 53). **Diacetyl morphine** ('heroin') is a prodrug that penetrates the blood–brain barrier even faster than its active metabolites morphine and 6-monoacetyl morphine (see Ch. 43), accounting for increased 'buzz' and hence abuse potential.

Delivering nucleic acid-based drugs (antisense oligonucleotides and small interfering RNA drugs) to their intracellular sites of action is a major issue with this class of biopharmaceutical (see Ch. 5). Conjugating these agents with *N*-acetylgalactosamine (GalNAc) that binds to specific surface transporters permits drug delivery to hepatocytes. The asialoglycoprotein receptor (ASGR) is a lectin that is abundantly expressed on the cell surface of hepatocytes and binds terminal galactose and *N*-acetylgalactosamine (GalNAc) residues (as part of the host defence mechanism against gram-negative bacteria), leading to selective hepatocyte uptake of the conjugated drug which is converted to the oligonucleotide in the cytoplasm (Prakash et al., 2016).

Other problems could theoretically be overcome by using suitable prodrugs, for example, instability of drugs at gastric pH, direct gastric irritation (aspirin was synthesised in the 19th century in a deliberate attempt to produce a prodrug of salicylic acid that would be tolerable when taken by mouth), failure of a drug to cross the blood–brain barrier and so on. While the optimistic prodrug designer 'will have to bear in mind that an organism's normal reaction to a foreign substance is to burn it up for food', the successes mentioned previously in delivering nucleic acid drugs to hepatocytes are notable (see Ch. 5).

ANTIBODY–DRUG CONJUGATES

One of the aims of cancer chemotherapy is to improve the selectivity of cytotoxic drugs (see Ch. 57). One approach which has led to a surge of licensed agents (12 currently licensed by the FDA and counting) is to attach the drug or toxin to an antibody directed against a tumour-specific antigen, which will bind selectively to tumour cells (Thomas et al., 2016). **Ado-trastuzumab emtansine, brentuximab vedotin** and **gemtuzumab ozogamicin** are three examples which have now been in clinical use for some years (see Ch. 57). Ado-trastuzumab emtansine is trastuzumab, a HER2-targeted antibody, covalently complexed via a linker molecule with a microtubule inhibitor, DM1. It is used, as a single agent, for the treatment of selected patients with HER2-positive, metastatic breast cancer. Trastuzumab binds to HER2 in the tumour, inhibiting HER2 receptor signalling and delivering the microtubule inhibitory drug DM1 (a maytansine derivative) to its site of action in the tumour. Randomised clinical trials demonstrated improved progression-free and overall survival compared with an active comparator group. Brentuximab vedotin is an antibody–drug conjugate used to treat selected lymphomas. It selectively targets tumour cells expressing the CD30 antigen, a defining marker of Hodgkin's disease and some other T-cell lymphomas. Likewise, gemtuzumab ozogamicin is a CD33 mAb-cytotoxic agent conjugate targeting myeloid progenitor cells for treatment of CD33-positive relapsed or refractory acute myeloid leukaemia. It has been reintroduced into the clinic after earlier safety concerns were addressed, resulting in its reappearance on the market.

PACKAGING IN LIPOSOMES

Liposomes are vesicles 0.1–1 μm in diameter produced by sonication of an aqueous suspension of phospholipids. They can be filled with non-lipid-soluble drugs, which are retained until the liposome is disrupted. Liposomes are taken up by reticuloendothelial cells, especially in the liver. They are also concentrated in malignant tumours, and several liposomal chemotherapeutic formulations are commercially available (see Yingchoncharoeu et al., 2016). Amphotericin, an antifungal drug used to treat systemic mycoses (see Ch. 54), is available in a liposomal formulation that is less nephrotoxic and better tolerated than the conventional form, albeit considerably more expensive. A long-acting form of doxorubicin encapsulated in liposomes is available for the treatment of malignancies (including ovarian cancer and myeloma), and paclitaxel is available in an albumin nanoparticle preparation used to treat breast cancer (see Ch. 57). A liposomal preparation of cytarabine is available for intrathecal treatment of lymphomatous meningitis, and a liposomal formulation of vincristine is available for selected patients with acute lymphoblastic leukaemia.

COATED IMPLANTABLE DEVICES

Impregnated coatings have been developed that permit localised drug delivery from implants. Examples include hormonal delivery to the endometrium from intrauterine devices (see Ch. 35) or Depo-Provera subcutaneous protection, and delivery of antithrombotic and antiproliferative agents (drugs or radiopharmaceuticals) to the coronary arteries from *stents* (expansile tubular devices inserted via a catheter after a diseased coronary artery has been dilated with a balloon – see Ch. 21). Stents reduce the occurrence of re-stenosis, but this can still occur at the margin of the device. Coating stents with drugs such as **sirolimus** (a potent immunosuppressant; see Ch. 25) embedded in a surface polymer prevents this important clinical problem.

REFERENCES AND FURTHER READING

Drug absorption, distribution and bioequivalence

EMEA, 2010. Guideline on the Investigation of Bioequivalence. Available at: http://www.ema.europa.eu/docs/en_GB/document_library/Scientific_guideline/2010/01/WC500070039.pdf.

Lund, M., Petersen, T.S., Dalhoff, K.P., 2017. Clinical implications of P-glycoprotein modulation in drug-drug interactions. Drugs 77, 859–883.

Nosaki, Y., Izumi, S., 2020. Recent advances in preclinical in vitro approaches toward quantitative prediction of hepatic clearance and drug-drug interactions involving organic anion transporting polypeptide (OATP) 1B transporters. Drug Metabol. Pharmacokinet. 35, 56–70.

Yoshida, K., Maeda, K., Sugiyama, Y., 2013. Hepatic and intestinal drug transporters: prediction of pharmacokinetic effects caused by drug-drug interactions and genetic polymorphisms. Ann. Rev. Pharmacol. Toxicol. 53, 581–612.

Drug distribution (including blood–brain barrier)

Ciarimboli, G., 2008. Organic cation transporters. Xenobiotica 38, 936–971.

Ciarimboli, G., 2021. Regulation mechanisms of expression and function of organic cation transporter 1. Front. Pharmacol. 11, 1-9.

Marcucci, F., Corti, A., Ferreri, A.J.M., 2021. Breaching the blood-brain tumor barrier for tumor therapy. Cancers 13, 2931.

Miller, D.S., Bauer, B., Hartz, A.M.S., 2008. Modulation of P-glycoprotein at the blood–brain barrier: opportunities to improve central nervous system pharmacotherapy. Pharmacol. Rev. 60, 196–209.

Muller, F., Sharma, A., Fromm, M.F., 2018. Biomarkers for in vivo assessment of transporter function. Pharmacol. Rev. 70, 246–277.

Drug delivery and routes of administration

Brigo, F., Nardone, R., Tezzon, F., Trinka, E., 2015. Nonintravenous midazolam versus intravenous or rectal diazepam for the treatment of early status epilepticus: a systematic review with meta-analysis. Epilepsy Behav. 49, 325–336.

Dubey, S.K., Parab, S., Dabholkar, N., et al., 2021. Oral peptide delivery: challenges and the way ahead. Drug Discov. Today 26, 931–950.

Huttunen, K.M., Raunio, H., Rautio, J., 2011. Prodrugs - from serendipity to rational design. Pharmacol. Rev. 63, 750–771.

Needham, L.A., Davidson, A.H., Bawden, L.J., Belfield, A., 2011. Drug targeting to monocytes and macrophages using esterase-sensitive chemical motifs. J. Pharmacol. Exp. Ther. 339, 132–142.

Prakash, T.P., Yu, J., Migawa, M.T., et al., 2016. Comprehensive structure activity relationship of triantennary *N*-acetylgalactosamine conjugated antisense oligonucleotides for targeted delivery to hepatocytes. J. Med. Chem. 59, 2718–2733.

Thomas, A., Teichner, B.A., Hassan, R., 2016. Antibody-drug conjugates for cancer therapy. Lancet Oncol. 17 (6), e254–e262.

Yingchoncharoeu, P., Kanilowski, D.S., Richardson, D.R., 2016. Lipid-based drug delivery systems in cancer therapy: what is available and what is yet to come. Pharmacol. Rev. 63, 701–787.

10 Drug metabolism and elimination

OVERVIEW

We describe phases 1 and 2 of drug metabolism, emphasising the importance of the cytochrome P450 monooxygenase system. We then cover the processes of biliary excretion and enterohepatic recirculation of drugs and of drug–drug interactions caused by induction or inhibition of metabolism. Drug and drug metabolite elimination by the kidney and drug–drug interactions due to effects on renal elimination are then considered.

INTRODUCTION

Drug elimination is the irreversible loss of drug from the body. It occurs by two processes: *metabolism* and *excretion*. Metabolism consists of anabolism and catabolism, that is, respectively, the build-up and breakdown of substances by enzymic conversion of one chemical entity to another within the body, whereas excretion consists of elimination from the body of drug or drug metabolites. The main excretory routes are:

- the kidneys
- the hepatobiliary system
- the lungs (important for volatile/gaseous anaesthetics)

Most drugs leave the body in the urine, either unchanged or as polar metabolites. Some drugs are secreted into bile via the liver, but most of these are then reabsorbed from the intestine. There are, however, instances (e.g. **rifampicin**; see Ch. 52) where faecal loss accounts for the elimination of a substantial fraction of unchanged drug in healthy individuals, and faecal elimination of drugs such as **digoxin** that are normally excreted in urine (see Ch. 20) becomes progressively more important in patients with advancing renal impairment. Excretion via the lungs occurs only with highly volatile or gaseous agents (e.g. general anaesthetics; see Ch. 41). Small amounts of some drugs are also excreted in secretions such as milk or sweat. Elimination by these routes is quantitatively negligible compared with renal excretion, although excretion into milk can sometimes be important because of effects on the baby (www.fpnotebook.com/ob/Pharm/MdctnsInLctn.htm, Accessed 25 October 2021).

Lipophilic substances are not eliminated efficiently by the kidney (see later). Consequently, most lipophilic drugs are metabolised to more polar products, which are then excreted in urine. Drugs are metabolised predominantly in the liver, especially by the cytochrome P450 (CYP) system. Some P450 enzymes are extrahepatic and play an important part in the biosynthesis of steroid hormones (see Ch. 33) and eicosanoids (see Ch. 17), but here we are concerned with catabolism of drugs by the hepatic P450 system.

DRUG METABOLISM

Animals have evolved complex systems that detoxify foreign chemicals ('xenobiotics'), including carcinogens and toxins present in poisonous plants. Drugs are a special case of such xenobiotics and, like plant alkaloids, they often exhibit *chirality* (i.e. there is more than one stereoisomer), which affects their overall metabolism. Drug metabolism involves two kinds of reaction, known as phase 1 and phase 2, which often occur sequentially. Both phases decrease lipid solubility, thus increasing renal elimination.

PHASE 1 REACTIONS

Phase 1 reactions (e.g. oxidation, reduction or hydrolysis) are catabolic, and the products are often more chemically reactive and hence, paradoxically, sometimes more toxic or carcinogenic than the parent drug. Phase 1 reactions often introduce a reactive group, such as hydroxyl, into the molecule, a process known as 'functionalisation'. This group then serves as the point of attack for the conjugating system to attach a substituent such as glucuronide (Fig. 10.1), explaining why phase 1 reactions often precede phase 2 reactions. The liver is especially important in phase 1 reactions. Many hepatic drug-metabolising enzymes, including CYP enzymes, are embedded in the smooth endoplasmic reticulum. They are often called 'microsomal' enzymes because, on homogenisation and differential centrifugation, the endoplasmic reticulum is broken into very small fragments that sediment only after prolonged high-speed centrifugation in the microsomal fraction. To reach these metabolising enzymes in life, a drug must cross the plasma membrane. Polar molecules do this less readily than non-polar molecules except where there are specific transport mechanisms (see Ch. 9), so intracellular metabolism is important for lipid-soluble drugs, while polar drugs are, at least partly, excreted unchanged in the urine.

THE P450 MONOOXYGENASE SYSTEM

Nature, classification and mechanism of P450 enzymes

Cytochrome P450 enzymes are the most versatile protective biocatalysts in nature, catalysing a vast array of reactions. They are haem proteins, comprising a large family ('superfamily') of related but distinct enzymes, each referred to as CYP followed by a defining set of numbers and a letter. P450 enzymes (reviewed by Guengerich, 2019, and Nair et al., 2016) differ from one another in amino acid sequence, in sensitivity to inhibitors and inducing agents (see later) and in the specificity of the reactions that they catalyse. Different members of the family have distinct, but often overlapping, substrate specificities. Purification and cloning of P450 enzymes form the basis of the current classification, which is based on amino acid sequence similarities. Not all 57 human CYPs are involved in drug metabolism, but it has been estimated that CYP enzymes in families 1–3

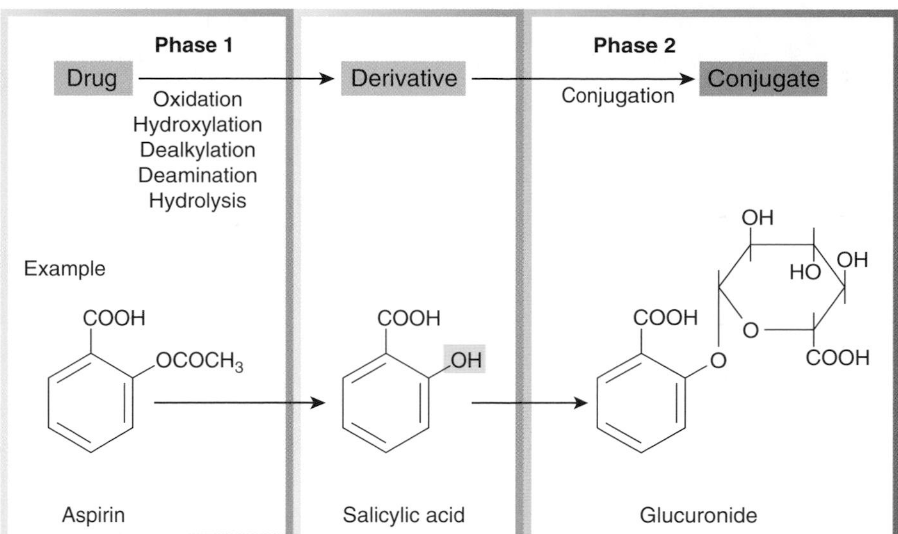

Fig. 10.1 The two phases of drug metabolism. In the example, *aspirin* reacts with water (H_2O) – a hydrolysis reaction – to form *salicylic acid* + acetic acid (CH_3COOH), and *glucuronide* is then transferred to salicylic acid by uridine diphosphate (UDP)-glucuronyl transferase to form the glucuronide product (details of the reactions not shown).

mediate 70%–80% of all phase 1-dependent metabolism of clinically used small-molecule drugs (Ingelman-Sundberg, 2004). Twelve CYPs accounted for 93.0% of drug metabolism of 1839 known drug-metabolising reactions in a large international database (Preissner et al., 2013). CYPs 1A2, 3A4, 2D6, 2C9 and 2C19 were responsible for approximately 60% of drug metabolism. Examples of therapeutic drugs that are substrates for some important P450 isoenzymes are shown in Table 10.1, and a useful table of drug substrates, inhibitors and inducers of CYP subtypes is provided by Indiana University (Cytochrome P450 Drug Interaction Table - Drug Interactions (iu.edu): https://drug-interactions.medicine.iu.edu/MainTable.aspx, accessed 03 January 2023).

Drug oxidation by the monooxygenase P450 system requires drug (substrate, 'DH'), P450 enzyme, molecular oxygen, nicotinamide adenine dinucleotide phosphate (NADPH) and NADPH–P450 reductase (a flavoprotein). The mechanism involves a complex cycle (Fig. 10.2), but the outcome of the reaction is quite simple, namely the addition of one atom of oxygen (from molecular oxygen) to the drug to form a hydroxylated product (DOH), the other atom of oxygen being converted to water. (Hydroxylation is a chemical process that introduces a hydroxyl group into an organic molecule, whereas hydrolysis involves a reaction with a water molecule - see later.)

P450 enzymes have unique spectral properties, and the reduced forms combine with carbon monoxide to form a pink compound (hence 'P') with absorption peaks near 450 nm (range 447–452 nm). The first clue that there is more than one form of CYP came from the observation that treatment of rats with 3-methylcholanthrene (3-MC), an inducing agent (see later), causes a shift in the absorption maximum from 450 to 448 nm - the 3-MC-induced isoform of the enzyme absorbs light maximally at a slightly shorter wavelength than the un-induced enzyme.

P450 and biological variation

There are important variations in the expression and regulation of P450 enzymes between species. For instance, the pathways by which certain dietary heterocyclic amines (formed when meat is cooked) generate genotoxic products involves one member of the P450 superfamily (CYP1A2) that is constitutively present in humans and rats (which develop colon tumours after treatment with such amines) but not in cynomolgus monkeys (which do not). Such species differences have crucial implications for the choice of species to be used for toxicity and carcinogenicity testing during the development of new drugs for use in humans.

Within human populations, there are major sources of inter-individual variation in P450 enzymes that are of great importance in therapeutics. These include genetic polymorphisms (alternative sequences at a locus within the DNA strand - alleles - that persist in a population through several generations; see Ch. 12). Environmental factors are also important, since enzyme inhibitors and inducers are present in the diet and environment. For example, a component of grapefruit juice inhibits drug metabolism (leading to potentially disastrous consequences, including cardiac dysrhythmias), whereas Brussels sprouts and cigarette smoke induce P450 enzymes. Components of the herbal medicine St John's wort (see Ch. 48) induce CYP450 isoenzymes as well as P-glycoprotein (P-gp; see Ch. 9). Drug interactions based on one drug altering the metabolism of another are common and clinically important (see Ch. 12). Predicting such potential interactions as an aid to personalising treatment (see Ch. 12) depends on the subject's phenotype at the time of treatment. Investigating this directly is difficult and expensive, so the simpler approach of genotyping has been advocated, but the correlation between genotype and phenotype is often poor (reviewed by Waring, 2020).

Not all drug oxidation reactions involve the hepatic P450 system. Some drugs are metabolised in plasma (e.g. hydrolysis of **suxamethonium** by plasma cholinesterase;

Table 10.1 Examples of drugs that are substrates of P450 isoenzymes

Isoenzyme P450	Drug(s)
CYP1A2	Caffeine, paracetamol (→NAPQI), tacrine, theophylline
CYP2B6	Cyclophosphamide, methadone
CYP2C8	Paclitaxel, repaglinide
CYP2C19	Omeprazole, phenytoin
CYP2C9	Ibuprofen, tolbutamide, warfarin
CYP2D6	Codeine, debrisoquine, S-metoprolol
CYP2E1	Alcohol, paracetamol
CYP3A4, 5, 7	Ciclosporin, nifedipine, indinavir, simvastatin

NAPQI, *N*-acetyl-*p*-amino-benzoquinone imine – the metabolite responsible for paracetamol toxicity in overdose.
Adapted from the Department of Medicine, Indiana University. Drug interactions: Flockhart table. https://drug-interactions.medicine.iu.edu/MainTable.aspx. Accessed 03 January 2023.

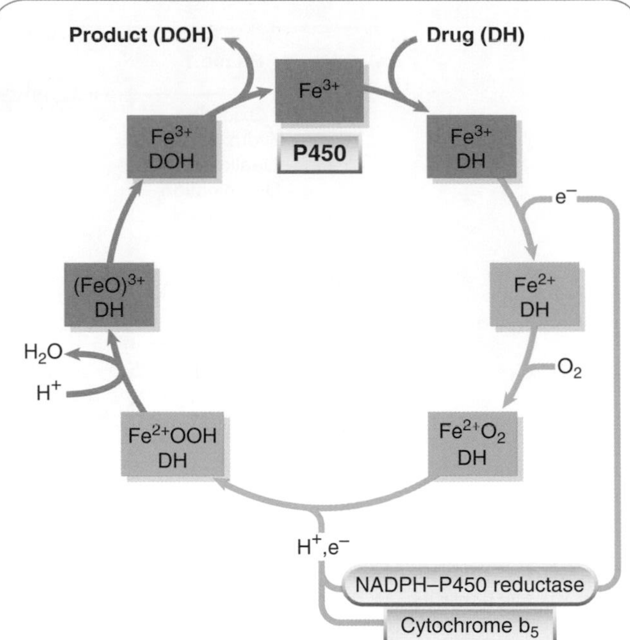

Fig. 10.2 The monooxygenase P450 cycle. Each of the *pink* or *blue* rectangles represents one single molecule of cytochrome P450 (P450) undergoing a catalytic cycle. Iron in P450 is in either the ferric *(pink rectangles)* or ferrous *(blue rectangles)* state. P450 containing ferric iron (Fe^{3+}) combines with a molecule of drug (DH) and receives an electron from NADPH–P450 reductase, which reduces the iron to Fe^{2+}. This combines with molecular oxygen, a proton and a second electron (either from NADPH–P450 reductase or from cytochrome b_5) to form an $Fe^{2+}OOH$–DH complex. This combines with another proton to yield water and a ferric oxene $(FeO)^{3+}$–DH complex. $(FeO)^{3+}$ extracts a hydrogen atom from DH, with the formation of a pair of short-lived free radicals (see text), liberation from the complex of oxidised drug *(DOH)*, and regeneration of P450 enzyme. *NADPH*, Nicotinamide adenine dinucleotide phosphate.

see Ch. 14), lung (e.g. various prostanoids; see Ch. 17) or gut (e.g. **tyramine, salbutamol**; see Chs 15 and 28). **Ethanol** (see Ch. 50) is metabolised by a soluble cytoplasmic enzyme, alcohol dehydrogenase, in addition to CYP2E1. Other P450-independent enzymes involved in drug oxidation include xanthine oxidase, which inactivates **6-mercaptopurine** (see Ch. 57), and monoamine oxidase, which inactivates many biologically active amines (e.g. **noradrenaline**, tyramine, 5-hydroxytryptamine; see Chs 15 and 16).

HYDROLYTIC REACTIONS

Hydrolysis, which is a chemical reaction in which water participates as nucleophile, breaking a chemical bond (e.g. hydrolysis of **aspirin**; see Fig. 10.1), occurs in plasma and in many tissues. Both ester and (less readily) amide bonds are susceptible to hydrolytic cleavage.

Reduction

Reduction is much less common in phase 1 metabolism than oxidation; keto- groups in **warfarin** (see Ch. 23) are, however, reduced to hydroxyl groups by CYP2A6, yielding inactive alcohols, in addition to oxidation by CYP2C9 with the production of inactive hydroxylated metabolites (the main route of its inactivation).

PHASE 2 REACTIONS

Phase 2 reactions are synthetic ('anabolic') and involve conjugation (i.e. attachment of a substituent group), which usually results in inactive products, although there are exceptions (e.g. the active sulphate metabolite of **minoxidil**, a potassium channel activator used to treat severe hypertension (see Ch. 21) and (as a cream) to promote hair growth (see Ch. 26)). Phase 2 reactions take place mainly in the liver. If a drug molecule or phase 1 product has a suitably reactive 'handle' (e.g. a hydroxyl, thiol or amino group), it is susceptible to conjugation. The chemical group inserted may be glucuronyl (Fig. 10.3), sulphate, methyl or acetyl. The tripeptide glutathione conjugates drugs or their phase 1 metabolites via its sulfhydryl group, as in the detoxification of **paracetamol** (see Fig. 58.1). Glucuronidation involves the formation of a high-energy phosphate ('donor') compound, uridine diphosphate glucuronic acid (UDPGA), from which glucuronic acid is transferred to an electron-rich atom (N, O or S) on the substrate, forming an amide, ester or thiol bond. Uridine diphosphate (UDP)-glucuronyl transferase, which catalyses these reactions, has very broad substrate specificity embracing many drugs and other foreign molecules. Several important endogenous substances, including bilirubin and adrenal corticosteroids, are conjugated by the same pathway.

Acetylation and methylation reactions occur with acetyl-coenzyme A (CoA) and S-adenosyl methionine, respectively, acting as the donor groups. Many conjugation reactions occur in the liver, but other tissues, such as lung and kidney, are also involved.

STEREOSELECTIVITY

Many clinically important drugs, such as **sotalol** (see Ch. 20), **warfarin** (see Ch. 23) and **cyclophosphamide** (see Ch. 57), are mixtures of stereoisomers, the components of which differ not only in their pharmacological effects but also in their metabolism, which may follow completely distinct pathways

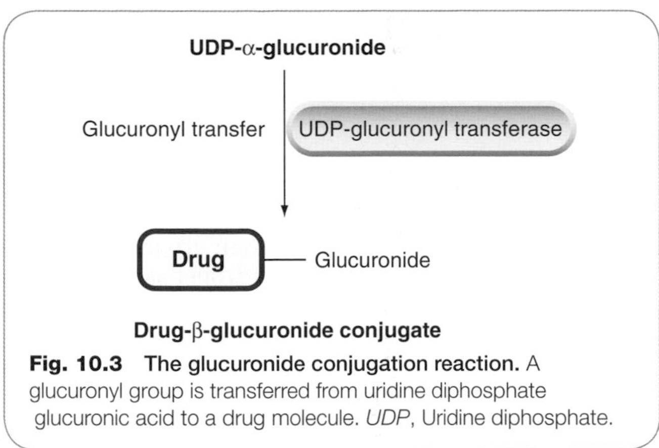

Fig. 10.3 The glucuronide conjugation reaction. A glucuronyl group is transferred from uridine diphosphate glucuronic acid to a drug molecule. *UDP*, Uridine diphosphate.

(Campo et al., 2009). Several clinically important drug interactions involve stereospecific inhibition of metabolism of one drug by another. In some cases, drug toxicity is mainly linked to one of the stereoisomers, not necessarily the pharmacologically active one. Where practicable, regulatory authorities urge that new drugs should consist of single isomers to lessen these complications.[1]

INHIBITION OF P450

Inhibitors of P450 differ in their selectivity towards different isoforms of the enzyme, and are classified by their mechanism of action. Some drugs compete for the active site but are not themselves substrates (e.g. **quinidine** is a potent competitive inhibitor of CYP2D6 but is not a substrate for it). Non-competitive inhibitors include drugs such as **ketoconazole**, which forms a tight complex with the Fe^{3+} form of the haem iron of CYP3A4, causing reversible non-competitive inhibition. So-called mechanism-based inhibitors require oxidation by a P450 enzyme. Examples include the oral contraceptive **gestodene** (CYP3A4) and the anthelmintic drug **diethylcarbamazine** (CYP2E1). An oxidation product (e.g. a postulated epoxide intermediate of gestodene) binds covalently to the enzyme, which then destroys itself ('suicide inhibition'; see Hakkola et al., 2020).

INDUCTION OF MICROSOMAL ENZYMES

A number of drugs, such as **rifampicin** (see Ch. 52), **ethanol** (see Ch. 50) and **carbamazepine** (see Ch. 46), increase the activity of microsomal oxidase and conjugating systems, especially when administered repeatedly. Many carcinogenic chemicals, e.g. benzpyrene and 3-MC, also have this effect, which can be substantial; Fig. 10.4 shows a nearly 10-fold increase in the rate of benzpyrene metabolism 2 days after a single dose. The effect is referred to as *induction* and is the result of increased synthesis and/or reduced breakdown of microsomal drug metabolising enzymes, notably CYP enzymes and UDP-glucuronyl transferase (Hakkola et al., 2020).

Enzyme induction can increase drug toxicity and carcinogenicity because several phase 1 metabolites are toxic or carcinogenic: paracetamol is an important example of a drug with a highly toxic CYP-metabolite *N*-acetyl-*p*-amino-benzoquinone imine (NAPQI; see Ch. 58, Fig. 58.1).

Enzyme induction is exploited therapeutically by administering **phenobarbital** to premature babies to induce glucuronyl transferase, thereby increasing bilirubin conjugation and reducing the risk of *kernicterus* (staining and neurological damage of the basal ganglia by bilirubin; see Ch. 9).

The first inducing agents to be studied were polycyclic aromatic hydrocarbons (e.g. 3-MC). These bind to the ligand-binding domain of a soluble cytoplasmic protein, termed the *aryl hydrocarbon receptor (AHR)*. Formation of this complex results in dissociation of chaperone molecules and transport of the activated receptor to the nucleus by an AHR nuclear translocator. In the nucleus it binds to response elements in the DNA, thereby promoting transcription of genes including *CYP1A1*. In addition to aryl hydrocarbons, AHR is also activated or inhibited by several endogenous indoles including kynurenine, and regulating CYP enzymes influences immunity, stem cell maintenance and cell differentiation. Activation of the AHR leads to down-regulation of proinflammatory cytokines, including interleukin-17 (IL-17), and influences skin barrier function. Consequently, AHR is a potential target for therapeutic drugs, and the FDA recently approved one agent (**tapinarof**) that binds and activates AHR as a topical therapy for plaque psoriasis (see Ch. 26).

In addition to enhanced transcription, some inducing agents (e.g. ethanol, which induces CYP2E1 in humans) also work by stabilising mRNA or P450 protein.

Recently, the constitutive androstane receptor (CAR) and pregnane X receptor (PXR) have been recognised as more important than AHR in the context of clinically important drug–drug interactions in humans. Like the AHR, these function as ligand activated transcription factors and have large flexible ligand-binding pockets, conferring promiscuity with regards to ligand binding. After transfer to the nucleus, they form heterodimers with the retinoid X receptor (RXR), bind DNA and act as transcription factors, increasing transcription of mRNA coding for CYP3A4 and many other proteins important in drug metabolism (reviewed by Hakkola et al., 2020).

PRESYSTEMIC ('FIRST-PASS') METABOLISM

Following oral administration, some drugs are extracted so efficiently by the liver or gut wall that the amount reaching the systemic circulation is considerably less than the amount absorbed. This is known as presystemic (or 'first-pass') metabolism and reduces bioavailability (see Ch. 9), even when a drug is well absorbed. Presystemic metabolism is important for many therapeutic drugs (Table 10.2 shows some examples), and is a problem because:

- A much larger dose of the drug is needed when it is taken by mouth than when it is given parenterally.
- Marked individual variations occur in the extent of first-pass metabolism, both in the activities of drug-metabolising enzymes and also as a result of variations in hepatic or intestinal blood flow. Hepatic blood flow can be reduced in disease (e.g. heart failure) or by drugs, such as β-adrenoceptor antagonists, which impair the clearance of chemically unrelated drugs, such as lidocaine, that are subject to presystemic metabolism due

[1]Well intentioned – although the usefulness of expensive 'novel' entities that are actually just the pure active isomer of well-established and safe racemates has been questioned, and enzymic interconversion of stereoisomers may subvert such sophisticated chemical design.

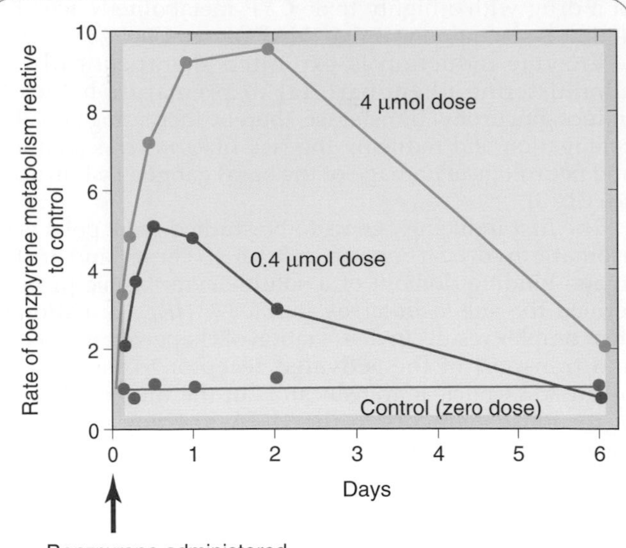

Fig. 10.4 Induction of hepatic metabolism of benzpyrene by substrate. Young rats were given benzpyrene (intraperitoneally) in the doses shown, and the benzpyrene-metabolising activity of liver homogenates was measured at times up to 6 days. (From Conney, A.H., et al., 1957. J. Biol. Chem. 228, 753.)

Table 10.2 Examples of drugs that undergo substantial pre-systemic ('first-pass') elimination

Aspirin	Metoprolol
Glyceryl trinitrate	Morphine
Isosorbide dinitrate	Propranolol
Levodopa	Salbutamol
Lidocaine	Verapamil

to a high hepatic extraction ratio. Intestinal blood flow is strongly influenced by eating and by the composition of the meal - especially by its fat content - and studies on the pharmacokinetic effects of food are routine in the development of orally administered drugs.

PHARMACOLOGICALLY ACTIVE DRUG METABOLITES

In some cases (Table 10.3), a drug becomes pharmacologically active only after it has been metabolised. For example, **azathioprine**, an immunosuppressant drug (see Ch. 25), is metabolised to **mercaptopurine**; and **enalapril**, an angiotensin-converting enzyme inhibitor (see Ch. 21), is hydrolysed to its active form **enalaprilat**. Such drugs, in which the parent compound lacks activity of its own, are known as *prodrugs*. These are sometimes designed deliberately to overcome problems of drug delivery (see Ch. 9). Metabolism can alter the pharmacological actions of a drug qualitatively. **Aspirin** inhibits platelet function and has anti-inflammatory activity (see Chs 23 and 25). It is hydrolysed to salicylic acid (see Fig. 10.1), which has anti-inflammatory but not antiplatelet activity.

In other instances, metabolites have pharmacological actions similar to those of the parent compound (e.g. benzodiazepines, many of which form long-lived active metabolites that cause sedation to persist after the parent drug has disappeared; see Ch. 45). There are also cases in which metabolites are responsible for toxicity. Bladder toxicity of **cyclophosphamide**, which is caused by its toxic metabolite acrolein (see Ch. 57), is an example. Methanol and ethylene glycol both exert their toxic effects via metabolites formed by alcohol dehydrogenase. Poisoning with these agents is treated with ethanol (or with a more potent inhibitor), which competes for the active site of the enzyme.

Drug metabolism

- Phase 1 reactions involve oxidation, reduction and hydrolysis. They:
  - often form more chemically reactive products, which can be pharmacologically active, toxic or carcinogenic.
  - often involve a monooxygenase system in which cytochrome P450 (CYP) enzymes play a key role.
- Phase 2 reactions involve conjugation (e.g. glucuronidation) of a reactive group (often inserted during phase 1 reaction) and usually lead to inactive and polar products that are readily excreted in urine.
- Some conjugated products are excreted via bile and may be excreted in the faeces or may be reactivated in the intestine and reabsorbed ('enterohepatic circulation').
- Induction of P450 enzymes can greatly accelerate hepatic drug metabolism. It can increase the toxicity of drugs with toxic metabolites and is an important cause of drug–drug interaction, as is enzyme inhibition.
- Presystemic metabolism in liver or gut wall reduces the bioavailability of several drugs when they are administered by mouth.

DRUG INTERACTIONS DUE TO ENZYME INDUCTION OR INHIBITION

INTERACTIONS CAUSED BY ENZYME INDUCTION

Enzyme induction is an important cause of drug interaction. The slow onset of induction and slow recovery after withdrawal of the inducing agent, together with the potential for selective induction of one or more CYP isoenzymes, contribute to the insidious nature of the clinical problems that induction presents. Adverse clinical outcomes from such interactions are very diverse, including graft rejection as a result of loss of effectiveness of immunosuppressive treatment, seizures due to loss of anticonvulsant effectiveness, unwanted pregnancy from loss of oral contraceptive action and thrombosis (from loss of effectiveness of warfarin) or bleeding (from failure to recognise the need to reduce warfarin dose when induction wanes after an inducing agent is discontinued). Over 200 drugs cause enzyme induction and thereby decrease the pharmacological activity of a range of other drugs. Some examples are given in Table 10.4, and further examples are given at

Table 10.3 Some drugs that produce active or toxic metabolites

Inactive (prodrugs)	Active drug	Active metabolite	Toxic metabolite	See Chapter
Azathioprine →		Mercaptopurine		25
Cortisone →		Hydrocortisone		33
Prednisone →		Prednisolone		33
Enalapril →		Enalaprilat		21
Zidovudine →		Zidovudine trisphosphate		53
Cyclophosphamide →		Phosphoramide mustard →	Acrolein	57
	Diazepam - - →	Oxazepam		45
	Morphine →	Morphine 6-glucuronide		43
	Halothane →		Trifluoroacetic acid	41
	Methoxyflurane →		Fluoride	41
	Paracetamol →		*N*-acetyl-*p*-amino-benzoquinone imine	25, 58

Table 10.4 Examples of drugs that induce drug-metabolising enzymes

Drugs inducing enzyme action	Examples of drugs with metabolism affected
Phenobarbital	Warfarin
Rifampicin	Oral contraceptives
Griseofulvin	Corticosteroids
Phenytoin	Ciclosporin
Ethanol	Paracetamol (increased toxicity)
Carbamazepine	Oral contraceptives, corticosteroids

the Indiana University website cited earlier. Because the inducing agent is often itself a substrate for the induced enzymes, the process can result in slowly developing tolerance. This pharmacokinetic kind of tolerance is generally less marked than pharmacodynamic tolerance, for example, to opioids (see Ch. 43), but it is clinically important when starting treatment with the antiepileptic drug **carbamazepine** (see Ch. 46). Treatment starts at a low dose to avoid toxicity (because liver enzymes are not induced initially) and is gradually increased over a period of a few weeks, during which it induces its own metabolism.

Fig. 10.5 shows how the antibiotic **rifampicin**, given for 3 days, reduces the effectiveness of **warfarin** as an anticoagulant. Conversely, enzyme induction can increase the toxicity of a second drug if the toxic effects are mediated via an active metabolite. **Paracetamol** (**acetaminophen**) toxicity is a case in point (see Fig. 58.1): this is caused by its CYP metabolite *N*-acetyl-*p*-amino-benzoquinone imine (NAPQI). Consequently, the risk of serious hepatic injury following paracetamol overdose is increased in patients in whom CYP has been induced, for example, by chronic alcohol consumption.

INTERACTIONS CAUSED BY ENZYME INHIBITION

As with induction, interactions caused by enzyme inhibition are hard to anticipate from first principles. If in doubt about the possibility of an interaction, it is best to look it up (e.g. in the *British National Formulary*, which has an invaluable appendix on drug interactions indicating which are of known clinical importance).

Enzyme inhibition, particularly of CYP enzymes, slows the metabolism and hence increases the action of other drugs inactivated by the enzyme. Such effects can be clinically important and are major considerations in the treatment of patients with HIV infection with combination therapy because several protease inhibitors are potent CYP inhibitors (see Ch. 53). Other examples of drugs that are enzyme inhibitors are shown in Table 10.5. To make life even more difficult, several inhibitors of drug metabolism influence the metabolism of different stereoisomers selectively. For example, **metronidazole** selectively inhibits the metabolism of the active (*S*) isomer of **warfarin**, while **omeprazole** selectively inhibits metabolism of the less active (*R*) isomer and **amiodarone** inhibits metabolism of both isomers similarly.

The therapeutic effects of some drugs are a direct consequence of enzyme inhibition (e.g. the xanthine oxidase inhibitor **allopurinol**, used to prevent gout; see Ch. 25). Xanthine oxidase metabolises several cytotoxic and immunosuppressant drugs, including **mercaptopurine** (the active metabolite of **azathioprine**), the action of which is thus potentiated and prolonged by allopurinol. **Disulfiram**, an inhibitor of aldehyde dehydrogenase that is used to produce an aversive reaction to ethanol (see Ch. 50), also inhibits metabolism of other drugs, including **warfarin**, which it potentiates. **Metronidazole**, an antimicrobial used to treat anaerobic bacterial infections and several protozoal diseases (see Chs 52 and 55), also inhibits this enzyme, and

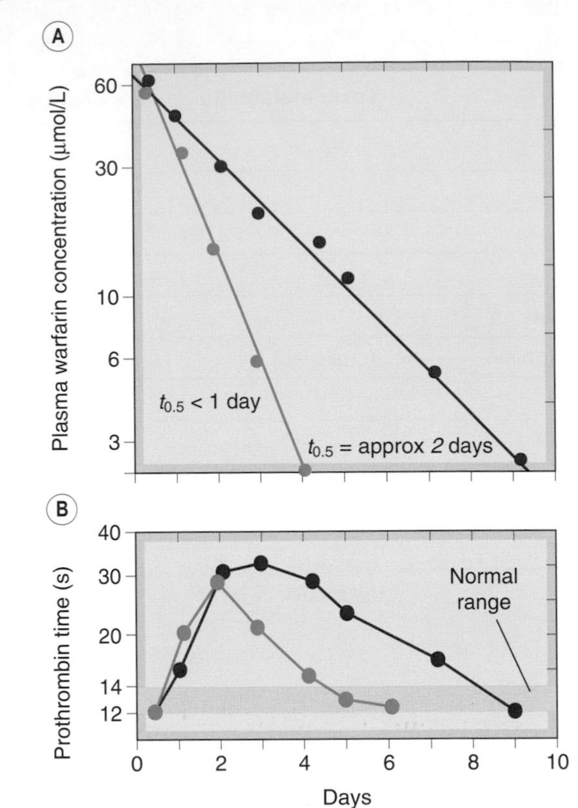

Fig. 10.5 Effect of rifampicin on the metabolism and anticoagulant action of warfarin in a healthy human volunteer. (A) Plasma concentrations of warfarin (log scale) as a function of time following a single oral dose of 5 µmol/kg body weight *(red symbols)*. After the subject was given rifampicin (600 mg daily for a few days), the same dose of warfarin showed that the plasma half-life of warfarin decreased from approximately 2 days to <1 day *(green symbols)*. (B) The effect of each single dose of warfarin on prothrombin time, before *(red curve)* and after rifampicin *(green curve)* administration. The normal range of prothrombin time is shown by the *pink stripe*. (Redrawn from O' Reilly, R.A., 1974. Ann. Intern. Med. 81, 337.)

patients prescribed it are advised to avoid alcohol for this reason.

There are also examples of drugs that inhibit the metabolism of other drugs, even though enzyme inhibition is not the main mechanism of action of the offending agents. Thus, glucocorticosteroids and **cimetidine** potentiate a range of drugs, including some antidepressant and cytotoxic drugs. Inhibition of the conversion of a prodrug to its active metabolite can result in *loss* of activity. Proton pump inhibitors (such as **omeprazole**; see Ch. 30) and the antiplatelet drug **clopidogrel** (see Ch. 23) have been widely co-prescribed, because clopidogrel is often used with other antithrombotic drugs predisposing to bleeding from the stomach - omeprazole reduces gastric acid secretion and the risk of gastric haemorrhage (see Ch. 30). Clopidogrel works through an active metabolite formed by CYP2C19 which is inhibited by omeprazole, possibly thereby reducing the antiplatelet effect. It is unclear how clinically important this may be (https://dig.pharmacy.uic.edu/faqs/2019-2/october-2019-faqs/what-is-the-clinical-relevance-of-the-clopidogrel-proton-pump-inhibitor-ppi-interaction/, Accessed 1 November 2021), but the FDA continues to warn against concomitant use of these drugs for this reason.

DRUG AND METABOLITE EXCRETION

BILIARY EXCRETION AND ENTEROHEPATIC CIRCULATION

Liver cells transfer various substances, including drugs, from plasma to bile by transport systems analogous to those of the renal tubule; these include organic cation transporters (OCTs), organic anion transporters (OATs) and P-gps (see Ch. 9). Various hydrophilic drug conjugates (particularly glucuronides) are concentrated in bile and delivered to the intestine, where the glucuronide can be hydrolysed, regenerating active drug; free drug can then be reabsorbed and the cycle repeated, a process referred to as *enterohepatic circulation*. The result is a 'reservoir' of recirculating drug that can amount to about 20% of total drug in the body, prolonging drug action. Examples where this is important include **morphine** (see Ch. 43) and **ethinylestradiol** (see Ch. 35). Several drugs are excreted to an appreciable extent in bile. **Vecuronium** (a non-depolarising muscle relaxant; see Ch. 14) is an example of a drug that is excreted mainly unchanged in bile. **Rifampicin** (see Ch. 52) is absorbed from the gut and slowly deacetylated, retaining its biological activity. Both forms are secreted in the bile, but the deacetylated form is not reabsorbed, so eventually most of the drug leaves the body in this form in the faeces.

RENAL EXCRETION OF DRUGS AND METABOLITES

RENAL CLEARANCE

Elimination of drugs by the kidneys is best quantified by the renal clearance (CL_{ren}; see Ch. 11). This is defined as the volume of plasma which contains the amount of drug that is removed from the body by the kidneys in unit time. It is calculated from the plasma concentration, C_p, the urinary concentration, C_u, and the rate of flow of urine, V_u, by the equation:

$$CL_{ren} = (C_u \times V_u)/C_p$$

CL_{ren} varies greatly for different drugs, from less than 1 mL/min to the theoretical maximum set by the renal plasma flow, which is approximately 700 mL/min, measured by *p*-aminohippuric acid (PAH) clearance (renal extraction of PAH approaches 100%).

Drugs differ greatly in the rate at which they are excreted by the kidney, ranging from **penicillin** (see Ch. 52), which is (like PAH) cleared from the blood almost completely on a single transit through the kidney, to **amiodarone** (see Ch. 20) and **risedronate** (see Ch. 36), which are cleared extremely slowly. Most drugs fall between these extremes. Three fundamental processes account for renal drug excretion:

1. glomerular filtration
2. active tubular secretion
3. passive reabsorption (diffusion from the concentrated tubular fluid back across tubular epithelium)

Table 10.5 Examples of drugs that inhibit drug-metabolising enzymes

Drugs inhibiting enzyme action	Drugs with metabolism affected
Allopurinol	Mercaptopurine, azathioprine
Chloramphenicol	Phenytoin
Cimetidine	Amiodarone, phenytoin, pethidine
Ciprofloxacin	Theophylline
Corticosteroids	Tricyclic antidepressants, cyclophosphamide
Disulfiram	Warfarin
Erythromycin	Ciclosporin, theophylline
Monoamine oxidase inhibitors	Pethidine
Ritonavir	Saquinavir

Table 10.6 Important drugs and related substances secreted into the proximal renal tubule by either the organic anion transporter (OAT) or organic cation transporter (OCT)

OAT	OCT
p-Aminohippuric acid	Amiloride
Furosemide	Dopamine
Glucuronic acid conjugates	Histamine
Glycine conjugates	Mepacrine
Indometacin	Morphine
Methotrexate	Pethidine
Penicillin	Quaternary ammonium compounds
Sulfate conjugates	Quinine
Thiazide diuretics	5-Hydroxytryptamine (serotonin)
Uric acid	Triamterene

GLOMERULAR FILTRATION

Glomerular capillaries allow drug molecules of molecular weight below about 20 kDa to pass into the glomerular filtrate. Plasma albumin (molecular weight approximately 68 kDa) is almost completely impermeant, but most drugs – with the exception of macromolecules such as **heparin** (see Ch. 23) or biopharmaceuticals (see Ch. 5) – cross the barrier freely. If a drug binds to plasma albumin, only free drug is filtered. If, like **warfarin** (see Ch. 23), a drug is approximately 98% bound to albumin, the concentration in the filtrate is only 2% of that in plasma, and clearance by filtration is correspondingly reduced.

TUBULAR SECRETION

Approximately 20% of renal plasma flow is filtered through the glomerulus in a healthy human, leaving at least 80% of delivered drug to pass on to the peritubular capillaries of the proximal tubule. Here, drug molecules are transferred to the tubular lumen by two independent and relatively non-selective carrier systems (see Ch. 9). One of these, the OAT, transports acidic drugs in their negatively charged anionic form (as well as various endogenous acids, such as uric acid), while an OCT handles organic bases in their protonated cationic form. Some important drugs that are transported by these two carrier systems are shown in Table 10.6. The OAT carrier can transport drug molecules against an electrochemical gradient and can reduce the plasma concentration nearly to zero, whereas OCT facilitates transport down an electrochemical gradient. Because at least 80% of the drug delivered to the kidney is presented to the carrier, tubular secretion is potentially the most effective mechanism of renal drug elimination. Unlike glomerular filtration, carrier-mediated transport can achieve maximal drug clearance even when most of the drug is bound to plasma protein.[2] **Penicillin** (see Ch. 52), for example, although about 80% protein-bound and therefore cleared only slowly by filtration, is almost completely removed by proximal tubular secretion, and is therefore rapidly eliminated.

Many drugs compete for the same transport systems (Table 10.6), leading to drug interactions. For example, **probenecid** was developed originally to potentiate penicillin by retarding its tubular secretion (see later).

DIFFUSION ACROSS THE RENAL TUBULAR EPITHELIUM

Water is reabsorbed as fluid traverses the tubule, the volume of urine emerging per unit of time being only about 1% of that of the glomerular filtrate. Consequently, if the tubule is freely permeable to drug molecules, some 99% of the filtered drug will be reabsorbed passively down the resulting concentration gradient. Lipid-soluble drugs are therefore excreted poorly, whereas polar drugs of low tubular permeability remain in the lumen and become progressively concentrated as water is reabsorbed. Polar drugs handled in this way include **digoxin** and aminoglycoside antibiotics. These exemplify a relatively small but important group of drugs (Table 10.7) that are not inactivated by metabolism, the rate of renal elimination being the main factor that determines their duration of action. These drugs have to be used with special care in individuals whose renal function may be impaired, including the elderly and patients with renal disease or any severe acute illness.

The degree of ionisation of many drugs – weak acids or weak bases – is pH dependent, and this markedly influences

[2]Because filtration involves isosmotic movement of both water and solutes, it does not affect the free concentration of drug in the plasma. Thus, the equilibrium between free and bound drug is not disturbed, and there is no tendency for bound drug to dissociate as blood traverses the glomerular capillary. The rate of clearance of a drug by filtration is therefore reduced directly in proportion to the fraction of the drug that is bound. In the case of active tubular secretion, this is not so because the carrier transports drug molecules unaccompanied by water. As free drug molecules are taken from the plasma, therefore, the free plasma concentration falls, causing dissociation of bound drug from plasma albumin. Secretion is only retarded slightly, even though the drug is mostly bound, because effectively 100% of the drug, both bound and free, is available to the carrier.

their renal excretion. The ion-trapping effect (see Ch. 9) means that a basic drug is more rapidly excreted in an acid urine that favours the charged form and thus inhibits reabsorption. Conversely, acidic drugs are most rapidly excreted if the urine is alkaline (Fig. 10.6).

DRUG INTERACTIONS DUE TO ALTERED DRUG EXCRETION

The main mechanisms by which one drug can affect the rate of renal excretion of another are by:

- altering protein binding, and hence filtration
- inhibiting tubular secretion
- altering urine flow and/or urine pH

INHIBITION OF TUBULAR SECRETION

Probenecid (see Ch. 25) was developed to inhibit secretion of **penicillin** and thus prolong its action. It also inhibits the excretion of other drugs, including **zidovudine** (see Ch. 53). Other drugs have an incidental probenecid-like effect and can enhance the actions of substances that rely on tubular secretion for their elimination. Table 10.8 gives some examples. Because diuretics, such as furosemide, act from within the tubular lumen, drugs that inhibit their secretion into the tubular fluid, such as non-steroidal anti-inflammatory drugs, reduce their effect.

Table 10.7 Examples of drugs that are excreted largely unchanged in the urine

Percentage	Drugs excreted
100–75	Furosemide, gentamicin, methotrexate, atenolol, digoxin
75–50	Benzylpenicillin, cimetidine, oxytetracycline, neostigmine
~50	Propantheline, tubocurarine

Table 10.8 Examples of drugs that inhibit renal tubular secretion

Drug(s) causing inhibition	Drug(s) affected
Probenecid Sulfinpyrazone Phenylbutazone Sulfonamides Aspirin Thiazide diuretics Indometacin	Penicillin Azidothymidine Indometacin
Verapamil Amiodarone Quinidine	Digoxin
Indometacin	Furosemide (frusemide)
Aspirin Non-steroidal anti-inflammatory drugs	Methotrexate

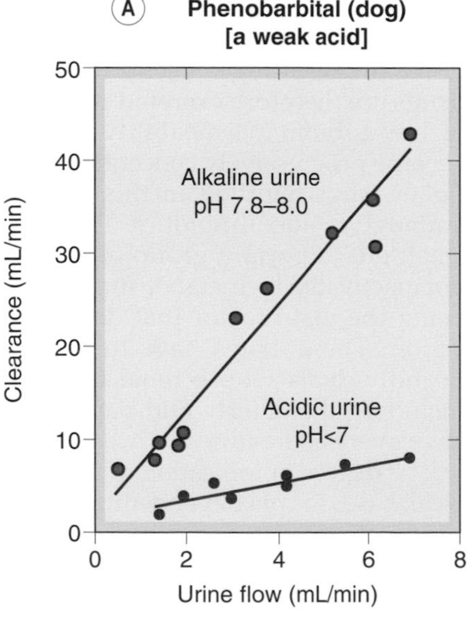

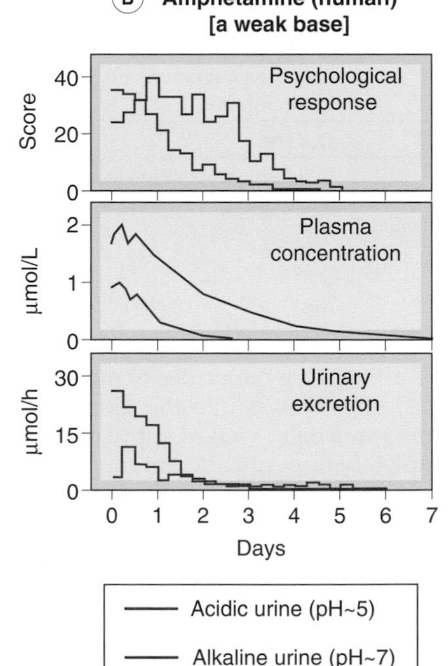

Fig. 10.6 The effect of urinary pH on drug excretion. (A) Phenobarbital clearance in the dog as a function of urine flow. Because phenobarbital is a weak acid, alkalinising the urine increases clearance about five-fold. (B) Amphetamine excretion in humans. Acidifying the urine increases the rate of renal elimination of amphetamine, reducing its plasma concentration and its effect on the subject's mental state. (Data from Gunne and Anggard, 1974. In: Torrell, T., et al. (Eds). Pharmacology and Pharmacokinetics. Plenum, New York.)

ALTERATION OF URINE FLOW AND pH

Diuretics tend to increase the urinary excretion of other drugs and their metabolites, but this is seldom immediately clinically important. Conversely, loop and thiazide diuretics indirectly *decrease* the excretion of **lithium**; they reduce body Na^+ content, to which the kidney responds by increased proximal tubular reabsorption of Na^+, and Li^+, which is handled in a similar way to Na^+. This can cause lithium toxicity in patients treated with lithium carbonate for mood disorders (see Ch. 48). The effect of urinary pH on the excretion of weak acids and bases is put to use in the treatment of poisoning with *salicylate*, but is not a cause of accidental interactions.

Elimination of drugs by the kidney

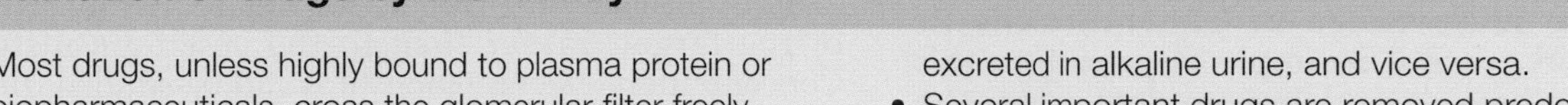

- Most drugs, unless highly bound to plasma protein or biopharmaceuticals, cross the glomerular filter freely.
- Many drugs, especially weak acids and weak bases are secreted, actively or by facilitated transport, into the renal tubule and rapidly excreted.
- Lipid-soluble drugs are passively reabsorbed down their concentration gradient across the tubular epithelium as water is reabsorbed, so are not efficiently excreted in the urine.
- Because of pH partition, weak acids are more rapidly excreted in alkaline urine, and vice versa.
- Several important drugs are removed predominantly by renal excretion and are liable to cause toxicity in elderly persons and patients with renal disease.
- There are instances of clinically important drug–drug interactions due to one drug reducing the renal clearance of another (examples include diuretics/lithium and indometacin/methotrexate), but these are less common than interactions due to altered drug metabolism.

REFERENCES AND FURTHER READING

General further reading

Coon, M.J., 2005. Cytochrome P450: nature's most versatile biological catalyst. Annu. Rev. Pharmacol. Toxicol. 45, 1–25.

Nassar, A.F., 2009. Drug Metabolism Handbook: Concepts and Applications. Wiley-Blackwell, Hoboken, NJ.

Testa, B., Krämer, S.D., 2009. The Biochemistry of Drug Metabolism. Wiley-VCH, Weinheim.

Drug metabolism

Campo, V.L., Bernardes, L.S.C., Carvalho, I., 2009. Stereoselectivity in drug metabolism: molecular mechanisms and analytical methods. Curr. Drug Metab. 10, 188–205.

Guengerich, F.P., 2019. Cytochrome P450 research and *The Journal of Biological Chemistry*. J. Biol. Chem. 294, 1671–1680.

Ingelman-Sundberg, M., 2004. Pharmacogenetics of cytochrome P450 and its applications in drug therapy: the past, present and future. Trends Pharmacol. Sci. 25, 193–200.

Nair, P.C., McKinnon, R.A., Miners, J.O., 2016. Cytochrome P450 structure-function: insights from molecular dynamics simulations. Drug Metab. Rev. 48, 434–452.

Preissner, S.C., Hoffmann, M.F., Preissner, R., Dunkel, M., Gewiess, A., Preissner, S., 2013. Polymorphic cytochrome P450 enzymes (CYPs) and their role in personalized therapy. PLoS One 8, e82562.

Waring, R.H., 2020. Cytochrome P450: genotype to phenotype. Xenobiotica 50, 9–18.

P450 enzyme induction and inhibition

Hakkola, J., Hukkanon, J., Pelkonen, O., 2020. Inhibition and induction of CTP enzymes in humans: an update. Arch. Toxicol. 94, 3671–3722.

Henderson, L., Yue, Q.Y., Bergquist, C., et al., 2002. St John's wort (*Hypericum perforatum*): drug interactions and clinical outcomes. Br. J. Clin. Pharmacol. 54, 349–356.

Drug elimination

Kusuhara, H., Sugiyama, Y., 2009. In vitro–in vivo extrapolation of transporter-mediated clearance in the liver and kidney. Drug Metab. Pharmacokinet. 24, 37–52.

11 Pharmacokinetics

OVERVIEW

We explain the importance of pharmacokinetic (PK) analysis and present a simple approach to this topic. We explain how drug clearance determines the steady-state plasma concentration during constant-rate drug administration and how the characteristics of absorption and distribution (considered in Ch. 9) plus metabolism and excretion (considered in Ch. 10) determine the time course of drug concentration in blood plasma during and following drug administration. The effect of different dosing regimens on the time course of drug concentration in plasma is explained. Population PK is mentioned briefly, and a final section considers limitations to the PK approach.

INTRODUCTION: DEFINITION AND USES OF PHARMACOKINETICS

PK is the branch of pharmacology dedicated to determining the fate of chemical substances administered to a living organism – 'what the body does to the drug'. In practice this involves the measurement and formal interpretation of changes with time of drug and drug metabolite concentrations in plasma, urine and sometimes other accessible regions of the body, in relation to dosing. It provides a framework for understanding what happens to a drug when given to an animal or human, where it goes in the body and how quickly, that enables one to understand the effects that it produces. In contrast, pharmacodynamics (PD: 'what the drug does to the body') describes events consequent on interaction of the drug with its receptor or other molecular target. The distinction is useful, although the words cause dismay to etymological purists.

Pharmacodynamic received an entry in a dictionary of 1890 ('relating to the powers or effects of drugs') whereas PK studies became possible only in the latter part of the 20th century with the development of sensitive, specific and accurate physicochemical analytical techniques, especially high-performance chromatography and mass spectrometry, for measuring drug concentrations in biological fluids. Latterly, '*in silico*' computer modelling of PK has become increasingly important as the discipline has evolved. The time course of drug concentration following dosing depends on the processes of absorption, distribution, metabolism and excretion (ADME) that we have considered qualitatively in Chapters 9 and 10.

In practice, PK usually focuses on concentrations of drug in *blood plasma*, which is easily sampled via venepuncture, since plasma concentrations are assumed usually to bear a clear relation to the concentration of drug in extracellular fluid surrounding cells that express the receptors or other targets with which drug molecules combine. This underpins what is termed the *target concentration strategy*, where biological effect is related to the *concentration* of the drug in plasma, as surrogate for the liquid environment of the target, rather than to the *dose* administered. Concentration-effect relationships can be studied directly in cell or tissue preparations in vitro, whereas in whole animal pharmacology (including human pharmacology) it is usually the dose rather than the concentration that is under direct control. Individual variation in response to a given dose of a drug is often greater than variability in response to the *plasma concentration* after that dose because plasma concentration (C_p) accounts for the individual variations in absorption, distribution and elimination. Measurements of C_p are especially useful in the early stages of drug development (see later). Concentrations of drug or drug metabolites in other body fluids (e.g. urine,[1] saliva, cerebrospinal fluid, milk) may add useful information.

For a few therapeutic drugs, plasma drug concentrations are also used in routine clinical practice to individualise dosage to achieve the desired therapeutic effect while minimising adverse effects in each individual patient – an approach known as *therapeutic drug monitoring*, often abbreviated TDM. Table 11.1 shows examples of drugs where a therapeutic range of plasma concentrations has been established, enabling TDM. Clinicians use this approach when there is a steep dose–effect relationship and little separation between doses needed to cause desired versus adverse effects – referred to as a narrow therapeutic range. However, they much prefer to use drugs where a large margin of safety permits the use of a standard dose without the discomfort, inconvenience and expense of monitoring, which entails sequential blood sampling and dose adjustment. While warfarin therapy (which relies on pharmacodynamic monitoring to optimise efficacy while minimising the risk of bleeding) was used for chronic anticoagulation for many decades, the introduction of direct oral anticoagulants that are administered in standard dose and do not require such intensive monitoring has rapidly altered practice (see Ch. 23), and analogous improvements of other drugs currently monitored by measuring their plasma concentrations (Table 11.1) will hopefully be introduced. The drugs of choice will vary according to local analytical capabilities as well as economic considerations for many years to come.

Formal interpretation of PK data consists of fitting concentration-versus-time data to a model (whether abstract or physiologically-based) and determining parameters that describe the observed behaviour. The parameters can then be used to adjust the dose regimen to achieve a desired target plasma concentration. The pharmacologically

[1]*Clinical* pharmacology became at one time so associated with the measurement of drugs in urine that the canard had it that clinical pharmacologists were the new alchemists – they turned urine into airline tickets.

Table 11.1 Examples of drugs where therapeutic drug monitoring of plasma concentrations is used clinically

Category	Example(s)	See chapter
Immunosuppressants	Ciclosporin, tacrolimus	25
Cardiovascular	Digoxin	20
Respiratory	Theophylline	28
Central nervous system	Lithium, phenytoin	48, 46
Antibacterials	Aminoglycosides	52
Anticancer drugs	Methotrexate	57

active concentration range is estimated from preclinical experiments on cells, tissues or laboratory animals, and modified as data emerge from early-phase human pharmacology trials. These often start by testing single doses of the new drug administered to successive groups of volunteers in progressively increasing doses - single ascending dose (SAD) studies (see Ch. 60). Some descriptive PK parameters can be estimated directly by inspecting the time course of drug concentration in plasma following dosing - important examples,[2] illustrated more fully later, are the *maximum plasma concentration* following a given dose of a drug administered in a defined dosing form (C_{max}) and the *time* (T_{max}) between drug administration and achieving C_{max}. Other PK parameters are estimated mathematically from experimental data; examples include *volume of distribution* (V_d) and *clearance* (CL), concepts that have been introduced in Chapters 9 and 10, respectively, and to which we return later. This approach applies both to classical low-molecular-weight drugs and to macromolecular biopharmaceuticals (see Ch. 5), although qualitative aspects of absorption, distribution and elimination are, of course, very different and PK parameters differ markedly - for example, antibodies have evolved to persist for long periods after exposure to antigen, and therapeutic antibodies commonly have low rates of clearance and long elimination half-lives in consequence.

USES OF PHARMACOKINETICS

Knowledge of the PK behaviour of drugs in animals and man is crucial in drug development, both to make sense of preclinical toxicological and pharmacological data[3] and to decide on an appropriate dose and dosing regimen for clinical trials (see Ch. 60). In particular, where possible, dose escalation during early-phase human trials of new chemical entities is now informed by real-time data on drug exposure to make decisions safely. Relevant parameters of exposure are C_{max} (especially for events related to peak concentration such as dysrhythmias) and the area under the concentration–time curve (AUC – introduced in Ch. 9, in the context of bioavailability, and see later) which may be more relevant to cumulative toxicity, for example hepatotoxicity.

Drug regulators have additionally developed concepts such as *bioavailability* and *bioequivalence* (see Ch. 9) to support the licensing of generic versions of drugs produced when originator products lose patent protection. These do not extend to biopharmaceuticals which can undergo subtle but significant post-translational modification in the cells in which they are manufactured, leading to the distinct but parallel regulatory concept of *biosimilars* (see Ch. 60).

Understanding the general principles of PK is also important in clinical practice, to understand the rationale of recommended dosing regimens, to time blood sampling correctly in relation to dosing and interpret drug concentrations for TDM, to adjust dose regimens rationally and to identify and evaluate possible drug interactions (see Chs 9 and 10). In particular, intensive care specialists and anaesthetists dealing with a severely ill patient often need to individualise the dose regimen depending on the urgency of achieving a therapeutic plasma concentration, and whether the PK behaviour of the drug is likely to be affected by illness such as renal impairment or liver disease.

SCOPE OF THIS CHAPTER

We describe:

- how total drug clearance determines steady-state plasma concentration during administration by intravenous infusion or repeated dosing;
- how drug concentration versus time can be predicted using a simple model in which the body is represented as a single well-stirred compartment, of volume V_d. This describes accumulation before steady state and the decline of concentration after dosing is discontinued, based on the elimination half-life ($t_{1/2}$);
- situations where this model is inadequate, and introduce a two-compartment model;
- situations where clearance of a drug varies with its concentration ('non-linear kinetics');
- situations (such as paediatrics) where only a few samples are available from each subject and population PK may be appropriate.

Finally, we consider some of the limitations inherent in the PK approach. More detailed accounts are provided by Atkinson et al. (2012), Birkett (2010) and Derendorf and Schmidt (2020).

DRUG ELIMINATION EXPRESSED AS CLEARANCE

The overall clearance of a drug by all routes (CL_{tot}) is the fundamental PK parameter describing drug elimination. It is defined as the volume of plasma which contains the total amount of drug that is removed from the body in unit time.

[2]Important because dose-related adverse effects often occur around C_{max}.
[3]For example, doses used in experimental animals often need to be much greater than those in humans on a 'per unit body weight' basis, because drug metabolism is commonly much more rapid in rodents – **methadone** (Ch. 43) is one of many such examples. When using animal data to estimate a 'human equivalent dose' in planning the first-in-human study, doses of low-molecular-weight drugs are normalised (so-called 'allometric scaling') to estimated body surface area rather than to body weight. Paediatricians commonly use the same approach, estimating appropriate doses for babies and young children from adult human doses in terms of dose/unit of estimated body surface area rather than dose/kg body weight.

It is thus expressed as volume per unit time, e.g. mL/min or L/h. Renal clearance (CL_{ren}), an important component of CL_{tot}, was described in Chapter 10.

The overall clearance of a drug (CL_{tot}) is the sum of clearance rates for each mechanism involved in eliminating the drug, usually renal clearance (CL_{ren}) and metabolic clearance (CL_{met}) plus any additional appreciable routes of elimination (faeces, breath, etc.). It relates the rate of elimination of a drug (in units of mass/unit time) to the plasma concentration, C_p:

$$\text{Rate of drug eliminaton} = C_p \times CL_{tot} \qquad \textbf{(11.1)}$$

Drug clearance can be determined in an individual subject by measuring the plasma concentration of the drug (in units of, say, mg/L) at intervals during a constant-rate intravenous infusion (delivering, say, X mg of drug per hour), until a steady state is approximated (Fig. 11.1A). At steady state, the rate of *input to the body is equal to the rate of elimination*, so:

$$X = C_{ss} \times CL_{tot} \qquad \textbf{(11.2)}$$

Rearranging this,

$$CL_{tot} = \frac{X}{MATH_{ss}} \qquad \textbf{(11.3)}$$

where C_{SS} is the plasma concentration at steady state, and CL_{tot} is in units of volume/time (L/h in the example given). Note that this estimate of CL_{tot}, unlike estimates based on the elimination rate constant or half-life (see later), does not depend on the applicability of any particular compartmental model.

For many drugs, clearance in an individual subject is independent of dose (at least within the range of doses used therapeutically – but see the section on saturation kinetics later for exceptions), so knowing the clearance enables one to calculate the dose rate needed to achieve a desired steady-state ('target') plasma concentration from Eq. 11.2: if the infusion rate (X) is doubled the steady-state plasma concentration is also doubled, and a plot of X (ordinate) versus C_{SS} (abscissa) is a straight line through the origin with a slope of CL_{tot} – so-called *linear kinetics*.

CL_{tot} can also be estimated by measuring plasma concentrations at intervals following a single intravenous bolus dose of, say, Q mg (Fig. 11.1B). This provides a concentration–time curve. $AUC_{0-\infty}$ is the area under the full curve relating C_p to time following a bolus dose given at time $t = 0$ (Fig 11.1B) and provides an integrated measure of tissue exposure to the drug in units of time multiplied by drug concentration. In addition to its use in determining the bioavailabilities of different routes of administration of a drug and of different drug preparations described in Chapter 9, $AUC_{0-\infty}$ provides measures of clearance and drug exposure considered here. It can be estimated graphically by summing the areas of trapezia (rectangles with a triangle on top) between adjacent data points (above) and the time axis (below) to the last measured point plus an area to account for the area after the last measured point to time zero using an estimate called the trapezoidal rule.

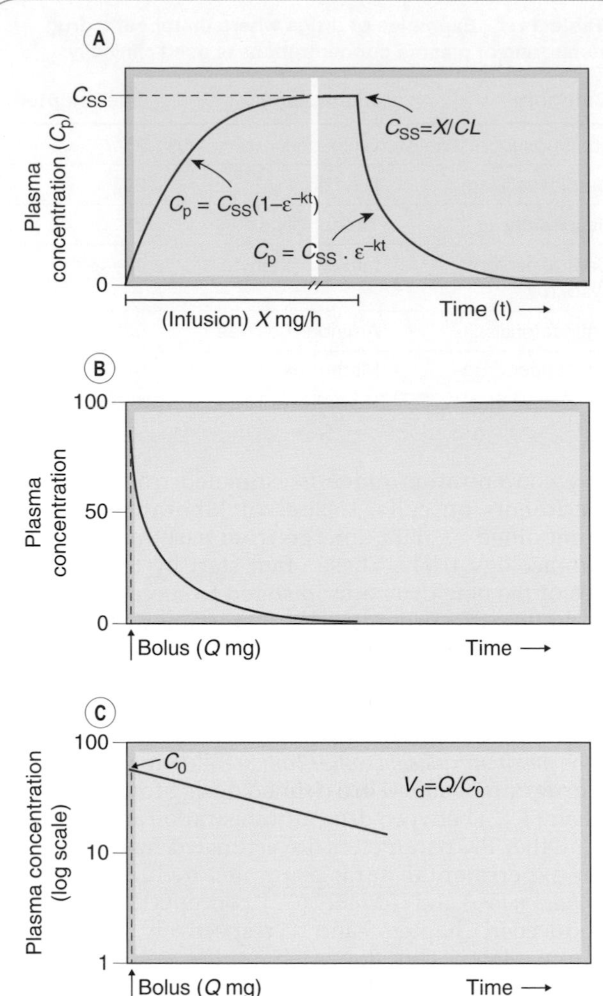

Fig. 11.1 Plasma drug concentration–time curves. (A) During a constant intravenous infusion at rate X mg/h, indicated by the horizontal bar, the plasma concentration (C_p) increases from zero to a steady-state value (C_{SS}); when the infusion is stopped, C declines from C_{SS} toward zero. The start times for the accumulation and the decay equations are set/re-set, respectively, to 0, so C_0 (C_p at time 0) is 0 for accumulation and is C_{SS} for the decline phase. (B) Following an intravenous bolus dose (Q mg), the plasma concentration rises abruptly and then declines towards zero. (C) Data from panel (B) plotted with plasma concentrations on a logarithmic scale. The straight line shows that concentration declines exponentially. Extrapolation back to the ordinate at zero time gives an estimate of C_0, the concentration at zero time, and hence of V_d, the volume of distribution.

From $AUC_{0-\infty}$, CL_{tot} is estimated from:

$$CL_{tot} = \frac{Q}{AUC_{0-\infty}} \qquad \textbf{(11.4)}$$

If plasma concentration declines exponentially after an intravenous bolus (see later) $AUC_{0-\infty}$ can be calculated from the negative of the slope of the linear decline in the natural logarithm of C_p ($\ln C_p$) versus time (see later). Since the slope is of declining concentration it is negative, so the negative of the slope is positive. It is the elimination rate constant k_{el}. $AUC_{0-\infty}$ is obtained from k_{el} and C_0 (C_p at time 0):

$$AUC_{0-\infty} = C_0/k_{el} \tag{11.5}$$

In practice, C_0 is obtained by extrapolating the linear part of a semi-logarithmic plot of the plasma concentration–time curve back to the ordinate axis (Fig 11.1C). Note that AUC has units of time - on the abscissa - multiplied by concentration (mass/volume) - on the ordinate; so CL (= $Q/AUC_{0-\infty}$) has units of volume/time as it should.

SINGLE-COMPARTMENT MODEL

Consider a highly simplified model of a human being, which consists of a single well-stirred compartment, of volume V_d (distribution volume), into which a quantity of drug Q is introduced rapidly by intravenous injection, and from which it is removed either by being metabolised or by being excreted (Fig. 11.2). For most drugs, V_d is an apparent volume rather than the volume of an anatomical compartment (see Ch. 9). It links the total amount of drug in the body to its concentration in plasma. The quantity of drug in the body immediately after it is administered as a single bolus is equal to the administered dose Q. The initial concentration, C_0, will therefore be given by:

$$C_0 = \frac{Q}{V_d} \tag{11.6}$$

In practice, as mentioned earlier, C_0 can be estimated by extrapolating the linear portion of a semilogarithmic plot of C_p against time back to its intercept at time 0 (Fig. 11.1C). C_p at any time 0 depends on CL_{tot} as well as on the dose and V_d. Many drugs exhibit linear kinetics (see earlier), where the clearance is constant (independent of plasma concentration). This occurs because the rate of elimination is directly proportional to drug concentration.

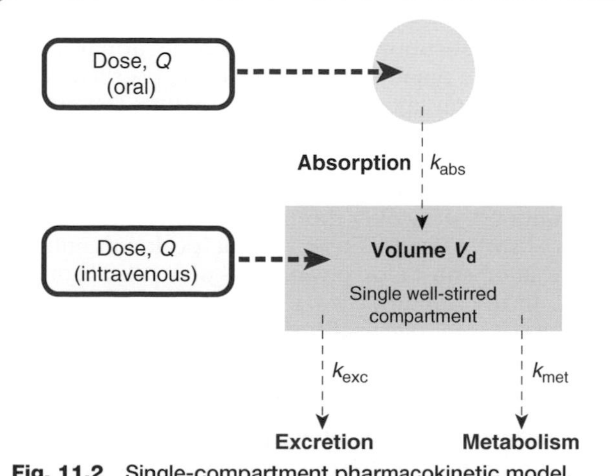

Fig. 11.2 Single-compartment pharmacokinetic model. This model is applicable if the plasma concentration falls exponentially after drug administration (as in Fig. 11.1).

This gives rise to the exponential decay 'die-away' curve characteristic of many natural processes such as cooling (described by Newton's law of cooling), radioactive decay and the oscillations of a released spring. In each case the rate of change of the variable at any time is directly proportional to the value of the variable at that time. In the case of PK the rate of change of plasma concentration (dC_p/dt), is directly proportional to C_p. This is the condition determining exponential decay:

$$C_t = C_0.e^{-kt} \tag{11.7}$$

Where k is the *elimination rate constant* k_{el}. It will be seen from this equation that C_t falls from its initial maximum value of C_0 immediately after the bolus injection (when $C_t = C_0$), since when $t = 0$ $e^{-kt} = e^0 = 1$: first rapidly then slower and slower towards a value of 0 when $t = \infty$ so $e^{-kt} = 0$), as illustrated in Fig. 11.1B and Fig. 11.3. Taking logarithms to the base e (written as ln) in Eq. 11.7 gives:

$$\ln C_t = \ln C_0 - k_{el}t \tag{11.8}$$

This is the equation of a straight line ($y = c + mx$), so plotting $\ln C_t$ against time (t) yields a straight line with slope $-k_{el}$.

The elimination rate constant k_{el} has units of 1/time and is the *fraction* of the dose present in the body that is eliminated per unit time. For example, if the rate constant is 0.1/h this implies that at each time point the elimination rate is one-tenth of the drug remaining in the body at that time per hour. Since drug present in the body is distributed as in a volume V_d, and CL_{tot} is the volume of plasma from which drug is eliminated in unit time, k_{el} is equal to the clearance as a fraction of V_d:

$$k_{el} = CL_{tot}/V_d \tag{11.9}$$

The *elimination half-life*, $t_{1/2}$, is the time taken for C_p to decrease by half (to $C_p/2$) and is equal to $\ln 2/k_{el}$, since:

$$C_t/2 = Ct.e^{-kt_{1/2}} \tag{11.10}$$

Taking logarithms:

$$\ln C_t - \ln 2 = \ln C_t - k_{el}.t_{1/2} \tag{11.11}$$

So:

$$k_{el}.t_{1/2} = \ln 2 = 0.693 \tag{11.12}$$

And:

$$t_{1/2} = 0.693/k_{el} \tag{11.13}$$

The half-life has units of time and enables one conveniently to predict the time course of C_p after the start or end of an infusion or of the rate of drug accumulation during repeated bolus administration (see later), when C_p is rising to its steady-state level or declining to zero.

When a single-compartment model is applicable, a constant-rate drug infusion (see Fig. 11.1A) causes the drug concentration in plasma (C_t) to increase from 0 at time 0 toward the steady-state value C_{SS}, the accumulation equation being:

$$C_t = C_{SS}\left(1 - e^{-kt}\right) \tag{11.14}$$

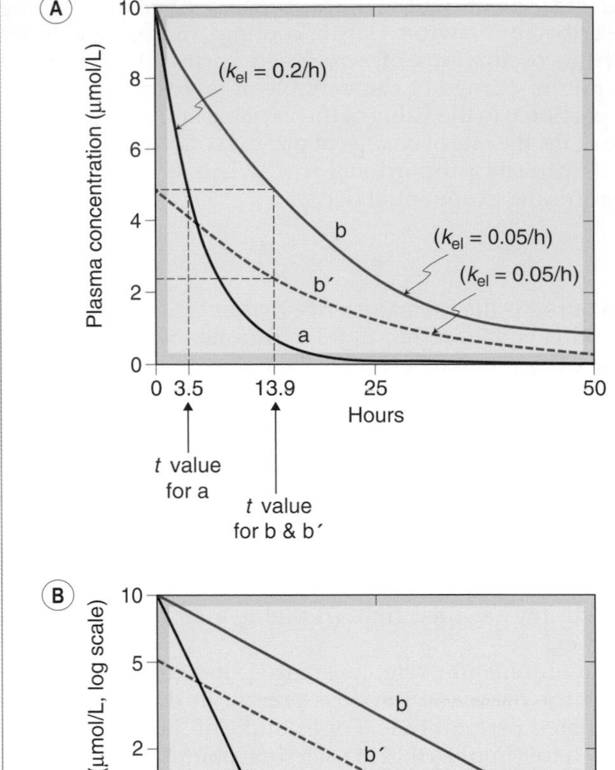

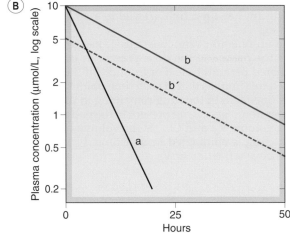

Fig. 11.3 Predicted behaviour of single-compartment model following intravenous drug administration at time 0. Drugs *a* and *b* differ only in their elimination rate constant, k_{el}. Curve *b′* shows the plasma concentration time course for a smaller dose of *b*. Note that the half-life ($t_{1/2}$) (indicated by *broken lines*) does not depend on the dose. (A) Linear concentration scale. (B) Logarithmic concentration scale.

When the infusion is discontinued at a new time 0 after steady state has been approximated (so $C_0 = C_{SS}$), the concentration falls exponentially from C_{SS} towards 0, the decay equation being $C_t = C_0.e^{-kt}$ (Eq. 11.7).

TThe accumulation curve (Eq. 11.14) is the inverse of the die-away curve (Eq. 11.7) so the rate constants (k) for accumulation and elimination are the same, as are the half-lives ($t_{1/2}$) of elimination and accumulation. One half-life after stopping the infusion, the concentration will have fallen to half the initial concentration; after two half-lives, it will have fallen to one-quarter the initial concentration; after three half-lives, to one-eighth; and so on. It is intuitively obvious that the longer the half-life, the longer the drug will persist in the body after dosing is discontinued. It is less obvious, but nonetheless true, that during chronic drug administration, the longer the half-life, the longer it will take for the drug to accumulate to its steady-state level: one half-life to reach 50% of the steady-state value, two to reach 75%, three to reach 87.5% and so on. This is extremely helpful to a clinician deciding how to start treatment. If the drug in question has a half-life of approximately 24 h, for example, it will take 3–5 days to approximate the steady-state concentration during a constant-rate infusion. If this is too slow in the face of the prevailing clinical situation, a *loading dose* may be used in order to achieve a therapeutic concentration of drug in the plasma more rapidly (see later). The size of such a dose is determined by the volume of distribution (Eq. 11.6).

REPEATED DOSING

Drugs are usually given therapeutically as repeated doses rather than single injections or a constant infusion. Repeated injections (each of dose Q) give a more complicated pattern than the smooth exponential rise during intravenous infusion, but the principle is the same (Fig. 11.4). The mean concentration will rise to a mean steady-state concentration with the same time course as during a constant rate infusion, but C_p will oscillate around the mean (through a range Q/V_d if injections are intravenous so absorption is complete). The smaller and more frequent the doses, the more closely the situation approaches that of a continuous infusion, and the smaller the swings in concentration. The exact dosage schedule, however, does not affect the mean steady-state concentration, or the rate at which it is approached. In practice, a steady state is effectively achieved after three to five half-lives. Speedier attainment of the steady state can be achieved by starting with a larger dose, as mentioned earlier. Such a loading dose is sometimes used when starting treatment with a drug with a half-life that is long in the context of the urgency of the clinical situation, as may be the case when treating cardiac dysrhythmias with drugs such as **amiodarone** or **digoxin** (see Ch. 20).

EFFECT OF VARIATION IN RATE OF ABSORPTION

If a drug is absorbed slowly from the gut or from an injection site into the plasma, it is (in terms of a compartmental model) as though it were being slowly infused at a variable rate into the bloodstream. For the purpose of kinetic modelling, the transfer of drug from the site of administration to the central compartment can be represented approximately by a rate constant, k_{abs} (see Fig. 11.2). This assumes that the rate of absorption is directly proportional, at any moment, to the amount of drug still unabsorbed, which is at best a rough approximation to reality. The effect of slow absorption on the time course of the rise and fall of the plasma concentration is shown in Fig. 11.5. The curves show the effect of spreading out the absorption of the same total amount of drug over different times. In each case, the drug is absorbed completely, but the peak concentration appears later and is lower and less sharp if absorption is slow. In the limiting case, a dosage form that releases drug at a constant rate as it traverses the ileum (see Ch. 9) approximates a constant-rate infusion. Once absorption is complete, the plasma concentration declines with the same half-time, irrespective of the rate of absorption.

For the kind of PK model discussed here, the $AUC_{0-\infty}$ is directly proportional to the total amount of drug introduced into the plasma compartment, irrespective of the rate at which it enters. Incomplete absorption, or destruction by presystemic metabolism before the drug reaches the plasma

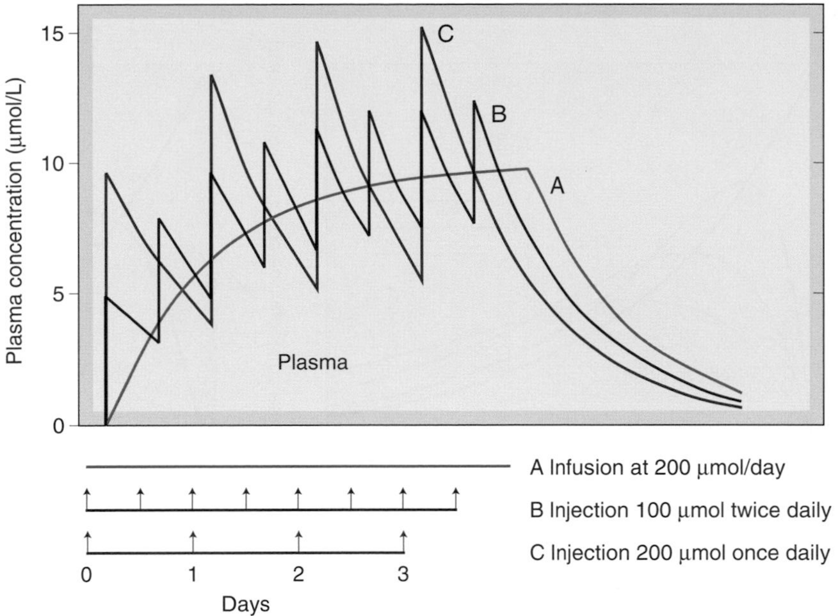

Fig. 11.4 Predicted behaviour of single-compartment model with continuous or intermittent drug administration. Smooth *curve A* shows the effect of continuous infusion for 4 days; *curve B*, the same total amount of drug given in eight equal doses; and *curve C*, the same total amount of drug given in four equal doses. The drug has a half-life of 17 h and a volume of distribution of 20 L. Note that in each case a steady state is effectively reached after about 2 days (about three half-lives), and that the mean concentration reached in the steady state is the same for all three schedules.

Pharmacokinetics

- Total clearance (CL_{tot}) of a drug is the fundamental parameter describing its elimination: the rate of elimination equals CL_{tot} multiplied by plasma concentration.
- CL_{tot} determines steady-state plasma concentration (C_{SS}): C_{SS} = rate of drug administration/CL_{tot}.
- For many drugs, disappearance from the plasma follows an approximately exponential time course. Such drugs can be described by a model where the body is treated as a single well-stirred compartment of volume V_d. V_d is an apparent volume linking the amount of drug in the body at any time to the plasma concentration.
- Elimination half-life ($t_{1/2}$) is directly proportional to V_d and inversely proportional to CL_{tot}.
- With repeated dosage or sustained delivery of a drug, the plasma concentration approaches a steady value within three to five plasma half-lives.
- In urgent situations, a loading dose may be needed to achieve therapeutic concentration rapidly.
- The loading dose (L) needed to achieve a desired initial plasma concentration C_{target} is determined by V_d: $L = C_{target} \times V_d$.
- A two-compartment model can be used when the observed kinetics are biexponential. The two components approximate the processes of transfer between plasma and tissues (α phase) and elimination from the body (β phase).
- Some drugs show non-exponential 'saturation' kinetics, with important clinical consequences, especially a disproportionate increase in steady-state plasma concentration when dose is increased.

compartment, reduces $AUC_{0-\infty}$ after oral administration (see Ch. 9). Changes in the rate of absorption, however, do not of themselves affect AUC. Again, it is worth noting that provided absorption is complete, the relation between the rate of administration and the steady-state plasma concentration (Eq. 11.3) is unaffected by k_{abs}, although the rate of rise of the increase of plasma concentration with each dose is reduced if absorption is slowed.

MORE COMPLICATED KINETIC MODELS

So far, we have considered a single-compartment PK model in which the rates of absorption, metabolism and excretion are all assumed to be directly proportional to the concentration of drug in the compartment from which transfer is occurring. This is a useful way to illustrate some basic principles but is clearly a physiological oversimplification. The characteristics of different parts of the body, such as brain, body fat and muscle, are quite different in terms of their blood supply, partition coefficients for drugs and the permeability of their capillaries to drugs. These differences, which the single-compartment model ignores, can markedly affect the time courses of drug distribution and action, and much theoretical work has gone into the mathematical analysis of more complex models (see Atkinson et al., 2012; Derendorf and Schmidt, 2020).

The two-compartment model, which introduces a separate 'peripheral' compartment to represent the tissues, in communication with the 'central' plasma compartment, more closely resembles the real situation without involving excessive complications and is conceptually useful although non-compartmental analysis is now usually preferred in drug development.

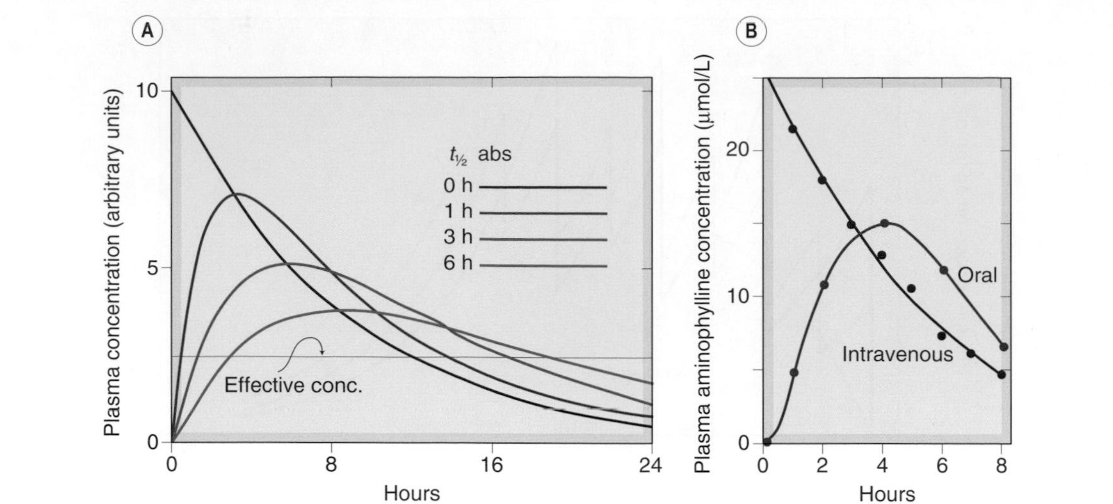

Fig. 11.5 The effect of slow drug absorption on plasma drug concentration. (A) Predicted behaviour of single-compartment model with drug absorbed at different rates from the gut or an injection site. The elimination half-time is 6 h. The absorption half-times ($t_{1/2}$ abs) are marked on the diagram. (Zero indicates instantaneous absorption, corresponding to intravenous administration.) Note that the peak plasma concentration is reduced and delayed by slow absorption, and the duration of action is somewhat increased. (B) Measurements of plasma aminophylline concentration in humans following equal oral and intravenous doses. (Data from Swintowsky, J.V., 1956. J. Am. Pharm. Assoc. 49, 395.)

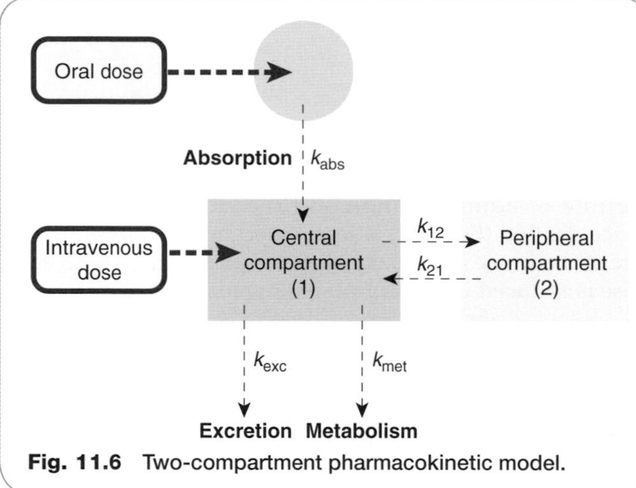

Fig. 11.6 Two-compartment pharmacokinetic model.

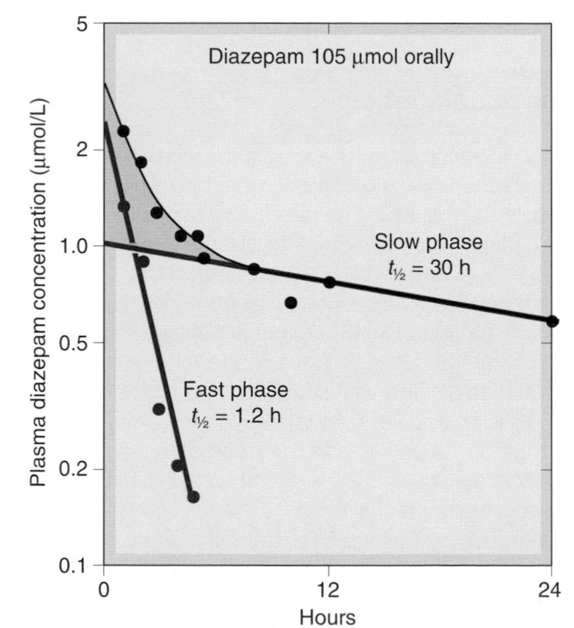

Fig. 11.7 Kinetics of diazepam elimination in humans following a single oral dose. The graph shows a semilogarithmic plot of plasma concentration versus time. The experimental data *(black symbols)* follow a curve that becomes linear after about 8 h (slow phase). Plotting the deviation of the early points *(pink shaded area)* from this line on the same coordinates *(red symbols)* reveals the fast phase. This type of two-component decay is consistent with the two-compartment model (see Fig. 11.6) and is obtained with many drugs. (Data from Curry, S.H., 1980. Drug Disposition and Pharmacokinetics. Blackwell, Oxford.)

TWO-COMPARTMENT MODEL

The two-compartment model is a widely used approximation in which the tissues are lumped together as a peripheral compartment. Drug molecules can enter and leave the peripheral compartment only via the central compartment (Fig. 11.6), which usually represents the plasma. The effect of adding a second compartment to the model is to introduce a second exponential component into the predicted time course of the plasma concentration, so that it comprises a fast and a slow phase. This pattern is often observed experimentally and is most clearly revealed when the concentration data are plotted semi-logarithmically (Fig. 11.7). If, as is often the case, the transfer of drug between the central and peripheral compartments is relatively fast compared with the rate of elimination, then the fast phase (often called the *α phase*) can be taken to represent the redistribution of the drug (i.e. drug molecules passing from plasma to tissues, thereby rapidly lowering the plasma concentration). The plasma concentration reached when the fast phase is complete, but before appreciable elimination has occurred, allows a measure of the combined distribution volumes of the two compartments; the half-time for the slow phase (the *β phase*) provides an estimate of k_{el}. If a drug is rapidly metabolised or excreted, the α and β phases are not well separated, and the calculation of separate V_d and k_{el} values for each phase is not straightforward. Problems also arise with drugs (e.g. very fat-soluble drugs) for which it is unrealistic to lump all the peripheral tissues together.

SATURATION KINETICS

In the case of some drugs, including **ethanol**, **phenytoin** and **salicylate**, the time course of disappearance of drug from the plasma does not follow the exponential or bi-exponential patterns shown in Figs 11.3 and 11.7 but is initially linear (i.e. drug is removed at a constant rate that is independent of plasma concentration). This is often called *zero-order kinetics* to distinguish it from the usual first-order kinetics that we have considered so far (these terms have their origin in chemical kinetic theory). *Saturation kinetics* is a better term, because it conveys the underlying mechanism, namely that a carrier or enzyme saturates and so as the concentration of drug substrate increases, the rate of elimination approaches a constant value. Fig. 11.8 shows the example of ethanol. It can be seen that the rate of disappearance of ethanol from the plasma is constant at approximately 4 mmol/L per hour, irrespective of dose or of the plasma concentration of ethanol. The explanation for this is that the rate of oxidation by the enzyme alcohol dehydrogenase reaches a maximum at low ethanol concentrations, because of limited availability of the cofactor NAD^+ (see Ch. 49, Figs 49.5 and 49.6).

Saturation kinetics has several important consequences (Fig. 11.9 and see Ch. 46, Fig. 46.4). One is that the duration of action is more strongly dependent on dose than is the case with drugs that do not show metabolic saturation. Another consequence is that the relationship between dose and steady-state plasma concentration is steep and unpredictable, and it does not obey the proportionality rule implicit in Eq. 11.3 for non-saturating drugs (see Fig. 49.6 for another example related to ethanol). The maximum rate of metabolism sets a limit to the rate at which the drug can be administered; if this rate is exceeded, the amount of drug in the body will, in principle, increase indefinitely and never reach a steady state (see Fig. 11.9). This does not actually happen, because there is always some dependence of the rate of elimination on the plasma concentration (usually because other, non-saturating metabolic pathways or renal excretion contribute significantly at high concentrations). Nevertheless, the steady-state plasma concentrations of drugs of this kind vary widely and unpredictably with dose. Similarly, variations in the rate of metabolism (e.g. through enzyme induction) cause disproportionately large changes in the plasma concentration. These problems are well recognised for drugs such as phenytoin, an anticonvulsant for which plasma concentration needs to be closely controlled to achieve an optimal clinical effect (see Ch. 46, Fig. 46.4). Drugs showing saturation kinetics are less predictable in clinical use than ones with first-order kinetics, so may be rejected during drug development if a pharmacologically similar candidate with first-order kinetics is available (see Ch. 60).

Uses of pharmacokinetics

- Pharmacokinetic studies performed during drug development underpin the standard dose regimens approved by regulatory agencies.
- Clinicians sometimes need to individualise dose regimens to account for individual variation in a particular patient (e.g. a neonate, a patient with impaired and changing renal function or a patient taking drugs that interfere with drug metabolism; see Ch. 10).
- Drug effect (PD) is often used for such individualisation, but there are drugs (including some anticonvulsants, immunosuppressants and antineoplastics) where a therapeutic range of plasma concentrations has been defined, and for which it is useful to adjust the dose to achieve a concentration in this range.
- Knowledge of kinetics enables rational dose adjustment. For example:
  - the frequency of dosing of a drug such as **gentamicin** eliminated by renal excretion may need to be markedly reduced in a patient with renal impairment (see Ch. 52);
  - the dose increment needed to achieve a target plasma concentration range of a drug such as **phenytoin** with saturation kinetics (see Ch. 46, Fig. 46.4) is much less than for a drug with linear kinetics.
- Knowing the approximate $t_{1/2}$ of a drug can be very useful, even if a therapeutic concentration is not known:
  - in correctly interpreting adverse events that occur some considerable time after starting regular treatment (e.g. benzodiazepines; see Ch. 45);
  - in deciding on the need or otherwise for an initial loading dose when starting treatment with drugs such as **digoxin** and **amiodarone** (see Ch. 20).
- The volume of distribution (V_d) of a drug determines the size of loading dose needed. If V_d is large (as for many tricyclic antidepressants), haemodialysis will not be an effective way of increasing the rate of elimination in treating overdose.

The opposite kind of non-linearity is also encountered during drug development, where plasma concentration increases less (rather than more than) in proportion with dose increment. This can occur when drugs are administered by mouth and an absorption carrier becomes saturated or (more commonly) when the pharmaceutical formulation fails to disperse adequately with higher doses.

Clinical applications of PK are summarised in the clinical box.

POPULATION PHARMACOKINETICS

In some situations, for example when a drug is intended for use in chronically ill children, it is desirable to obtain PK data in a patient population rather than in healthy adult volunteers. Such studies in children are inevitably limited and samples for drug analysis are often obtained opportunistically during clinical care, with limitations as to quality of the data and on the number of samples collected from each patient. Population PK addresses how best to analyse such data. Fitting data from all subjects as if there were no kinetic differences between individuals and fitting each individual's data separately and then combining the individual parameter estimates, each has obvious shortcomings. A better method is to use non-linear mixed effects modelling (NONMEM). How population studies relate to the individual requires the use of such mathematical modelling. Such analysis is used to predict individual variation whether in clinical trial or clinical practice. The uncertainties and the statistical technicalities are considerable and beyond the scope of this chapter: the interested reader is referred to Sheiner et al. (1997).

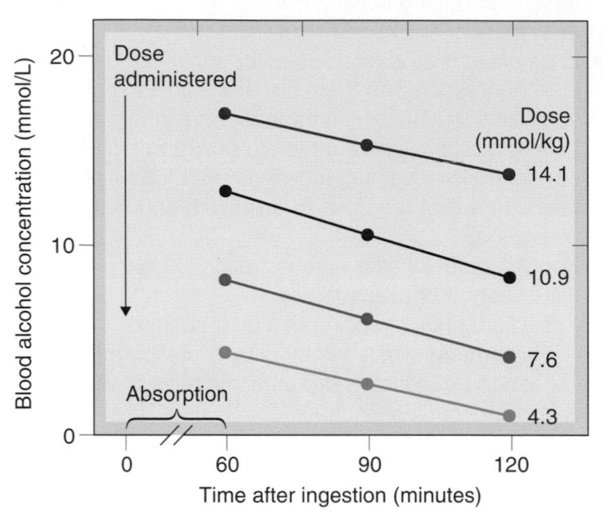

Fig. 11.8 Saturating kinetics of alcohol elimination in humans. The blood alcohol concentration falls linearly rather than exponentially, and the rate of fall does not vary with dose. (From Drew, G.C., Colquhoun, W.P., Long, H.A., 1958. Effects of small doses of alcohol on a skill resembling driving. Br. Med. J. 2, 5103.)

LIMITATIONS OF PHARMACOKINETICS

Some limitations of the PK approach will be obvious from the earlier account, such as the proliferation of parameters in even quite conceptually simple models. There are also limitations in the usefulness of monitoring drug concentrations in plasma as an approach to reducing individual variability in drug response (see Ch. 12). Two main assumptions underpin the expectation that by relating response to a drug to its plasma concentration we can reduce variability of response by accounting for PK variation – that is, variation in ADME. They are:

1. That plasma concentration of a drug bears a precise relation to the concentration of drug in the immediate environment of its target (receptor, enzyme, etc.).
2. That drug response depends uniquely on the concentration of the drug in the immediate environment of its target.

While the first of these assumptions is plausible for those few drugs that work through a target in the circulating blood (e.g. a fibrinolytic drug working on intravascular fibrin) and reasonably plausible for a drug working on an

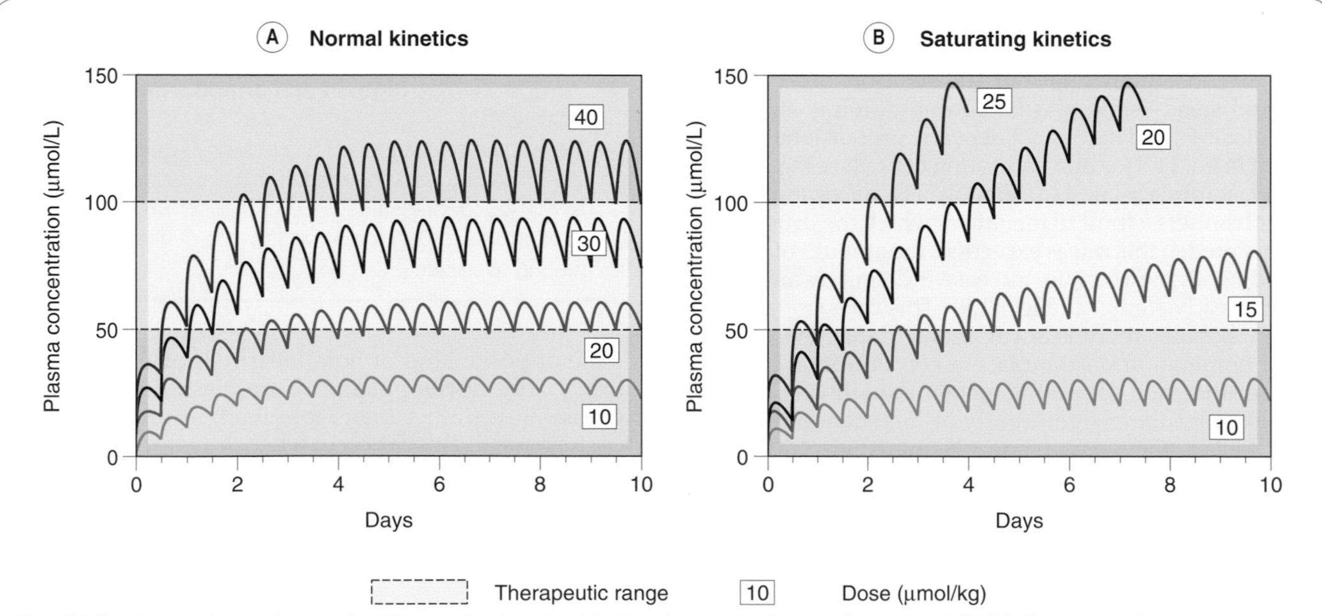

Fig. 11.9 Comparison of non-saturating and saturating kinetics for drugs given orally every 12 h. (A) The curves showing an imaginary drug, similar to the antiepileptic drug phenytoin at the lowest dose, but with linear kinetics. The steady-state plasma concentration is reached within a few days, and is directly proportional to dose. (B) Curves for saturating kinetics calculated from the known PK parameters of phenytoin (see Ch. 46). Note that no steady state is reached with higher doses of phenytoin, and that a small increment in dose results after a time in a disproportionately large effect on plasma concentration. (Curves were calculated with the Sympak pharmacokinetic modelling program written by Dr. J.G. Blackman, University of Otago.)

enzyme, ion channel or G protein–coupled or kinase-linked receptor located in the cell membrane and accessed by drug molecules dissolved in the extracellular fluid, it is less likely to be true in the case of a nuclear receptor or when an active metabolite is involved. Because of the blood–brain barrier, plasma concentrations rarely reflect local drug concentrations in the brain, so, with the exception of lithium (see Ch. 48) and of some antiepileptic drugs (see Ch. 46), monitoring of plasma concentrations has not proved to be clinically useful for drugs acting in the brain.

The second assumption is untrue in the case of drugs that form a stable covalent attachment with their target, and so produce an effect that outlives their presence in solution. Examples include the antiplatelet effects of **aspirin** and **clopidogrel** (see Ch. 23) and the effect of some monoamine oxidase inhibitors (see Ch. 48) and proton pump inhibitors (see Ch. 30). In other cases, drugs in therapeutic use act only after delay (e.g. antidepressants; see Ch. 48), or gradually induce tolerance (e.g. opioids; see Ch. 43) or physiological adaptations (e.g. corticosteroids; see Ch. 33) that alter the relation between concentration and drug effect in a time-dependent manner such that drug effect is not uniquely determined by drug concentration in the plasma.

REFERENCES AND FURTHER READING

Atkinson, A., Huang, S.M., Lertora, J., Markey, S. (Eds.), 2012. Principles of Clinical Pharmacology, third ed. Academic Press, London.

Birkett, D.J., 2010. Pocket Guide: Pharmacokinetics Made Easy. McGraw-Hill Australia, Sydney.

Derendorf, H., Schmidt, S., 2020. Rowland and Tozer's Clinical Pharmacokinetics and Pharmacodynamics. Concepts and Applications, fifth ed. Wolters Kluwer, Philadelphia.

Population Pharmacokinetics

Sheiner, L.B., Rosenberg, B., Marethe, V.V., 1997. Estimation of population characteristics of pharmacokinetic parameters from routine clinical data. J. Pharmacokinet. Biopharm. 5, 445–479.

12 Individual variation, pharmacogenomics and personalised medicine

OVERVIEW

This chapter addresses the sources of variation between individuals (inter-individual variation) in their responses to drugs. Important factors, including ethnicity, age, pregnancy, disease and drug interaction (i.e. modification of the action of one drug by another), are described. The concept of individualising drug therapy in light of genomic information ('personalised medicine') – a rapidly expanding area of clinical pharmacology – is introduced. We explain relevant elementary genetic concepts and describe briefly several single-gene pharmacogenetic disorders that affect drug responses. We then cover how pharmacogenomic tests can be used to guide the choice of therapy and adjustments to dosing regimens.

INTRODUCTION

Therapeutics would be a great deal easier if the same dose of drug always produced the same response. In reality, inter- and even intra-individual variation is often substantial and this can lead to important differences in the balance between benefit and harm of treatment. Physicians need to be aware of the sources of such variation to prescribe drugs safely and effectively. Variation can be caused by different concentrations at sites of drug action or by different responses to the same drug concentration. The first kind is called *pharmacokinetic variation* and can occur because of differences in absorption, distribution, metabolism or excretion (ADME; Chs 9 and 10). The second kind is called *pharmacodynamic variation*. Responses to some therapeutic agents, for example, most vaccines and oral contraceptives (see Ch. 35), are sufficiently predictable to permit a standard dose regimen, whereas treatment with **lithium** (see Ch. 48), antihypertensive drugs (see Ch. 21), anticoagulants (see Ch. 23) and many other drugs is individualised, doses being adjusted on the basis of monitoring the drug concentration in the plasma or a response such as change in blood pressure, together with any adverse effects.

Inter-individual variation in response to some drugs is a serious problem; if not taken into account, it can result in lack of efficacy or unexpected adverse effects. Whilst large-scale clinical trials may be able to predict the 'average' effect of a drug, clinicians also recognise that there are subgroups of individuals who have a greater likelihood for beneficial (or harmful) response than others. This is particularly relevant to life-threatening conditions (such as cancer) where optimised individual therapy guided by predictive markers may achieve striking gains in the benefit:harm ratio. Variation is partly caused by environmental factors, but studies comparing identical with non-identical twins suggest that much of the variation in response to certain drugs is genetically determined; for example, the elimination half-lives of antipyrine, a probe of hepatic drug oxidation, and of **warfarin**, an oral anticoagulant (see Ch. 23), differ much less between identical than between fraternal twins.

Genes influence pharmacokinetics by altering the expression of proteins involved in drug ADME; pharmacodynamic variation reflects differences in drug targets, G proteins or other downstream pathways whilst individual susceptibility to uncommon qualitatively distinct adverse reactions (see Ch. 58) can result from genetically determined differences in enzymes or immune mechanisms. Here, the introduction of rapid, easily accessible methods to identify genetic differences between individuals is a key consideration. It is now possible to use genetic information specific to an individual patient to preselect a drug that will be effective and not cause excessive toxicity, rather than relying on trial and error supported by physiological clues as at present – an aspiration referred to as *personalised medicine*. Thus far, this approach, which was initially over-hyped, has faced hurdles in translation to patient benefit throughout daily clinical practice. Research continues at a breakneck pace however, and the US FDA has listed over 480 pharmacogenomic biomarkers for inclusion in drug labelling information – a doubling since the last edition of this book. As one might expect, the vast majority of recommendations for pharmacogenetic testing are in relation to the critically poised benefit:harm profiles of anticancer drugs.

The Genetic Testing Registry (https://www.ncbi.nlm.nih.gov/gtr/) in the United States accepts submissions from laboratories worldwide regarding the genetic tests that are made available for the purposes of screening, diagnosis, drug/disease monitoring and treatment response. As of January 2023, the registry has recorded information on 76,531 tests covering 18,737 genes that are associated with 22,574 conditions. There is no doubt that pharmacogenetic testing can make an important contribution to therapeutics, but serious questions remain about the cost–benefit, and how this avalanche of genetic information could be effectively incorporated into daily clinical workflows.

In this chapter we first describe the most important epidemiological sources of variation in drug responsiveness, before revisiting some elementary genetics as a basis for understanding genetic disorders characterised by abnormal responses to drugs. We conclude with a brief account of currently available pharmacogenomic tests and how these are beginning to be applied to individualise drug therapy (*pharmacogenomics*). In particular, we will summarise four key roles of pharmacogenetic data in treatment decisions involving drug indication, dosage, safety and communication of risk.

Individual variation

- Variability is a serious problem; if not taken into account, it can result in:
  - lack of efficacy
  - unexpected harmful effects
- Types of variability may be classified as:
  - pharmacokinetic
  - pharmacodynamic
- The main causes of variability are:
  - age
  - genetic factors
  - immunological factors (see Ch. 58)
  - disease (especially when this influences drug elimination or metabolism, e.g. kidney or liver disease)
  - drug interactions

Table 12.1 Effect of age on plasma elimination half-lives of various drugs

Drug	Mean or range of half-life (h): Term neonate[a]	Adult	Elderly person
Drugs that are mainly excreted unchanged in the urine			
Gentamicin	10	2	4
Lithium	120	24	48
Digoxin	200	40	80
Drugs that are mainly metabolised			
Diazepam	25–100	15–25	50–150
Phenytoin	10–30	10–30	10–30
Sulfamethoxypyridazine	140	60	100

[a]Even greater differences from mean adult values occur in premature babies.

Data from Reidenberg, M.M., 1971. Renal Function and Drug Action. Saunders, Philadelphia; and Dollery, C.T., 1991. Therapeutic Drugs. Churchill Livingstone, Edinburgh.

EPIDEMIOLOGICAL FACTORS AND INTER-INDIVIDUAL VARIATION OF DRUG RESPONSE

ETHNICITY

Ethnic means 'pertaining to race', and many anthropologists are sceptical as to the value of this concept (see, for example, Cooper et al., 2003). Members of racial groups share some characteristics on the basis of common genetic and cultural heritage, but there is enormous diversity within each group. Could an Asian Indian conceivably have the same drug response as an Asian Chinese, or Japanese? Coarse and inconsistent ethnic categories based on visual impressions of outward appearance are unlikely to help in personalising medicine for individuals within diverse populations (see Po, 2007). The expanding availability of comprehensive testing for individual genetic markers helps us to move away from outdated and imprecise concepts of ethnicity.

AGE

The main reason that age affects drug action is that drug elimination is less efficient in newborn babies and in older people, so that drugs commonly produce greater and more prolonged effects at the extremes of life. Other age-related factors, such as variations in pharmacodynamic sensitivity, are also important with some drugs. Body composition changes with age, fat contributing a greater proportion to body mass in the elderly, with consequent changes in distribution volume of drugs. Elderly people typically consume more drugs than do younger adults, so the potential for drug interactions is also increased. For fuller accounts of drug therapy in paediatrics and in the elderly, see the chapters on renal and hepatic disease in Huang et al. (2021).

EFFECT OF AGE ON RENAL EXCRETION OF DRUGS

Glomerular filtration rate (GFR) in the newborn, normalised to body surface area, is only about 20% of the adult value. Accordingly, plasma elimination half-lives of renally eliminated drugs are longer in neonates than in adults (Table 12.1). In babies born at term, renal function increases to values similar to those in young adults in less than a week and continues to increase to a maximum of approximately twice the adult value at 6 months of age. Improvement in renal function occurs more slowly in premature infants. Renal immaturity in premature infants can have a substantial effect on drug elimination. For example, in premature newborn babies, the antibiotic **gentamicin** (see Ch. 52) has a plasma half-life of ≥18 h, compared with 1–4 h for adults and approximately 10 h for babies born at term. It is therefore necessary to reduce and/or space out doses to avoid toxicity in premature babies.

GFR declines slowly from about 20 years of age, falling by about 25% at 50 years and by 50% at 75 years. Fig. 12.1 shows that the renal clearance of **digoxin** in young and elderly subjects is closely correlated with creatinine clearance, a measure of GFR. Consequently, chronic administration over the years of the same daily dose of digoxin to an individual as he or she ages leads to a progressive increase in plasma concentration, and this is a common cause of glycoside toxicity in elderly people (see Ch. 20).The age-related decline in GFR is not reflected by an increase in plasma creatinine *concentration,* as distinct from creatinine *clearance.* Plasma creatinine typically remains within the normal adult range in elderly persons despite substantially diminished GFR. This is because creatinine synthesis is reduced in elderly persons because of their reduced muscle mass. Consequently, a 'normal' plasma creatinine in an elderly person does not indicate that they have a normal GFR. Failure to recognise this and reduce the dose of drugs that are eliminated by renal excretion can lead to drug toxicity.

EFFECT OF AGE ON DRUG METABOLISM

Several important enzymes, including hepatic microsomal oxidase, glucuronyltransferase, acetyltransferase and plasma esterases, have low activity in neonates, especially if premature. These enzymes take 8 weeks or longer to reach the adult level of activity. The relative lack of conjugating

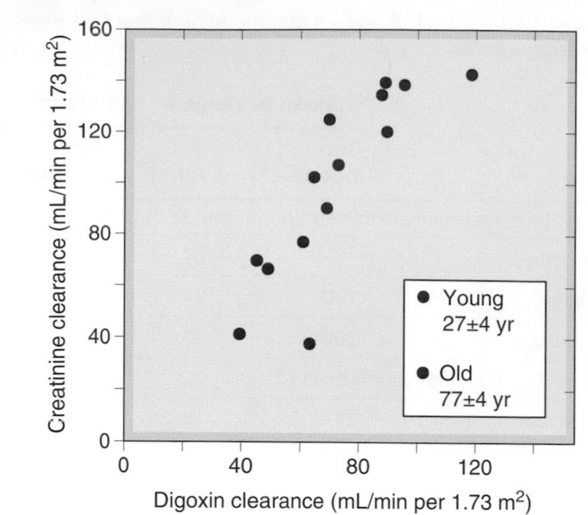

Fig. 12.1 Relationship between renal function (measured as creatinine clearance) and digoxin clearance in young and older subjects. (From Ewy, G.A., et al., 1969. Circulation 34, 452.)

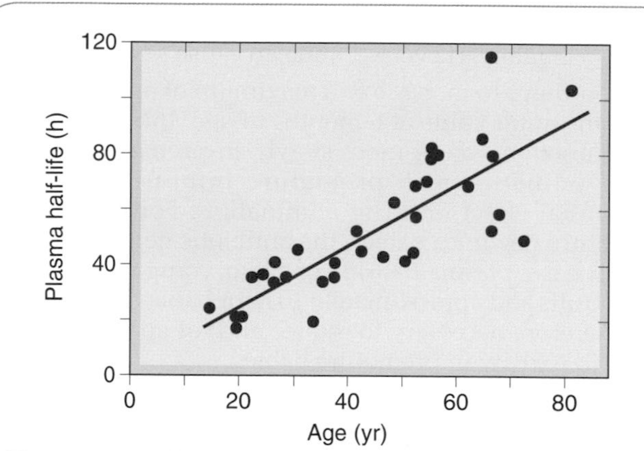

Fig. 12.2 Increasing plasma half-life for diazepam with age in 33 normal subjects. Note the increased variability as well as increased half-life with ageing. (From Klotz, U., et al., 1975. J. Clin. Invest. 55, 347.)

activity in the newborn can have serious consequences, as in *kernicterus* caused by drug displacement of bilirubin from its binding sites on albumin (see Ch. 9) and in the 'grey baby' syndrome caused by the antibiotic **chloramphenicol** (see Ch. 52). This sometimes-fatal condition, at first thought to be a specific biochemical sensitivity to the drug in young babies, actually results simply from accumulation of very high tissue concentrations of chloramphenicol because of slow hepatic conjugation. Chloramphenicol is no more toxic to babies than to adults, provided the dose is reduced to make allowance for this. Slow conjugation is also one reason why **morphine** (which is excreted mainly as the glucuronide, see Ch. 43) is not used as an analgesic in labour, because drug transferred via the placenta has a long half-life in the newborn baby and can cause prolonged respiratory depression.

The activity of hepatic microsomal enzymes declines slowly (and very variably) with age, and the distribution volume of lipid-soluble drugs increases, because the proportion of the body that is fat increases with advancing age. The increasing half-life of the anxiolytic drug **diazepam** with advancing age (Fig. 12.2) is one consequence of this. Some other benzodiazepines and their active metabolites show even greater age-related increases in half-life. Because half-life determines the time course of drug accumulation during repeated dosing (see Ch. 11), insidious effects, developing over days or weeks, can occur in elderly people and may be misattributed to age-related memory impairment rather than to drug accumulation. Even if the mean half-life of a drug is little affected, there is often a striking increase in the *variability* of half-life between individuals with increasing age (as in Fig. 12.2). This is important, because a population of older people will contain some individuals with grossly reduced rates of drug metabolism, whereas such extremes do not occur so commonly in young adult populations. Drug regulatory authorities therefore usually require studies in elderly persons as part of the evaluation of drugs likely to be used in older people (similarly for potential use in children).

AGE-RELATED VARIATION IN SENSITIVITY TO DRUGS

The same plasma concentration of a drug can cause different effects in young and old subjects. Benzodiazepines (see Ch. 45) exemplify this, producing more confusion and less sedation in elderly than in young subjects; similarly, hypotensive drugs (see Ch. 21) cause postural hypotension more commonly in elderly than in younger adult patients.

PREGNANCY

Pregnancy causes physiological changes that influence drug disposition in mother and fetus. Maternal plasma albumin concentration is reduced, influencing drug protein binding. Cardiac output is increased, leading to increased renal blood flow and GFR, and increased renal elimination of drugs. Lipophilic molecules rapidly traverse the placental barrier, whereas transfer of hydrophobic drugs is slow, limiting fetal drug exposure following a single maternal dose. The placental barrier excludes some drugs (e.g. low molecular-weight heparins; see Ch. 23) so effectively that they can be administered chronically to the mother without causing effects in the fetus. However, drugs that are transferred to the fetus are eliminated more slowly than from the mother. The activity of most drug-metabolising enzymes in fetal liver is much less than in the adult. Furthermore, the fetal kidney is not an efficient route of elimination because excreted drug enters the amniotic fluid, which is swallowed by the fetus. For a fuller account, see Huang et al. (2021).

DISEASE

Therapeutic drugs are prescribed to patients, so the effects of disease on drug response are very important, especially disease of the major organs responsible for drug metabolism and drug (and drug metabolite) excretion. Detailed consideration is beyond the scope of this book and interested readers should refer to a clinical text such as the chapters on renal and hepatic disease in Huang et al. (2021). Disease can cause pharmacokinetic or pharmacodynamic variation. Common disorders such as impaired renal or hepatic function predispose to toxicity by causing unexpectedly intense or prolonged drug effects as a result of increased drug concentration following a 'standard' dose. Drug absorption is slowed in conditions causing gastric stasis (e.g. migraine, diabetic neuropathy) and may be incomplete in patients with malabsorption owing to ileal or pancreatic disease or to oedema of the ileal mucosa caused by heart failure or nephrotic syndrome. *Nephrotic syndrome* (characterised by heavy proteinuria, oedema and a reduced concentration of albumin in plasma) alters drug absorption because of oedema of intestinal mucosa; alters drug disposition through changes in binding to plasma albumin; and causes insensitivity to diuretics such as **furosemide** that act on ion transport mechanisms in the lumenal surface of tubular epithelium (see Ch. 29), through drug binding to albumin in tubular fluid. *Hypothyroidism* is associated with increased sensitivity to several drugs (e.g. **pethidine**), for reasons that are poorly understood. *Hypothermia* (to which elderly persons, in particular, are predisposed) markedly reduces the clearance of many drugs.

Other disorders affect drug sensitivity by altering receptor or signal-transduction mechanisms (see Ch. 3). Examples include the following:

- Diseases that influence receptors:
  - *myasthenia gravis*, an autoimmune disease characterised by antibodies to nicotinic acetylcholine receptors (see Ch. 14) and increased sensitivity to neuromuscular-blocking agents (e.g. **vecuronium**) and other drugs that may influence neuromuscular transmission (e.g. *aminoglycoside antibiotics*; see Ch. 52);
  - *X-linked nephrogenic diabetes insipidus*, characterised by abnormal antidiuretic hormone (ADH; vasopressin) receptors (see Ch. 29) and insensitivity to ADH;
  - *familial hypercholesterolaemia*, an inherited disease of low-density lipoprotein receptors (see Ch. 22); the homozygous form is relatively resistant to treatment with statins (which act partly by causing increased hepatic expression of these receptors), whereas the much commoner heterozygous form responds well to statins.
- Diseases that influence signal-transduction mechanisms:
  - *pseudohypoparathyroidism*, which stems from impaired coupling of G protein–coupled receptors with adenylyl cyclase;
  - *familial precocious puberty* and *hyperthyroidism* caused by functioning thyroid adenomas, which are each caused by mutations in G protein–coupled receptors that result in the receptors remaining 'turned on' even in the absence of the hormones that are their natural agonists.

DRUG INTERACTIONS

Many patients, especially if elderly are treated continuously with one or more drugs for chronic diseases such as hypertension, heart failure, osteoarthritis and so on. Acute events (e.g. infections, myocardial infarction) are treated with additional drugs. The potential for drug interactions is therefore substantial, and drug interactions account for 5%–20% of adverse drug reactions. These may be serious (approximately 30% of fatal adverse drug reactions are estimated to be the consequence of drug interaction). Drugs can also interact with chemical entities in other dietary constituents (e.g. grapefruit juice, which down-regulates expression of CYP3A4 in the gut) and herbal remedies (such as St John's wort; see Ch. 48). The administration of one chemical entity (A) can alter the action of another (B) by one of two general mechanisms[1]:

1. Modifying the pharmacological effect of B without altering its concentration in the tissue fluid (pharmacodynamic interaction).
2. Altering the concentration of B at its site of action (pharmacokinetic interaction), as described in Chapters 9 and 10.

PHARMACODYNAMIC INTERACTION

Pharmacodynamic interaction can occur in many different ways (including those discussed under *Drug antagonism* in Ch. 2). There are many mechanisms, and some examples of practical importance are probably more useful than attempts at classification.

- β-Adrenoceptor antagonists diminish the effectiveness of β-adrenoceptor agonists such as **salbutamol** (see Ch. 15).
- Many diuretics lower plasma K^+ concentration (see Ch. 29), and thereby predispose to **digoxin** toxicity and to toxicity with *class III antidysrhythmic drugs* (see Ch. 20).
- **Sildenafil** inhibits the isoform of phosphodiesterase (type V) that inactivates cGMP (see Chs 19 and 35); consequently, it potentiates organic nitrates, which activate guanylyl cyclase, and can cause severe hypotension in patients taking these drugs.
- *Monoamine oxidase inhibitors* increase the amount of noradrenaline stored in noradrenergic nerve terminals and interact dangerously with drugs, such as **ephedrine** or **tyramine**, which release stored noradrenaline. This can also occur with tyramine-rich foods – particularly fermented cheeses such as Camembert (see Ch. 48).
- **Warfarin** competes with vitamin K, preventing hepatic synthesis of various coagulation factors (see Ch. 23). If vitamin K production in the intestine is inhibited (e.g. by antibiotics), the anticoagulant action of warfarin is increased.
- The risk of bleeding, especially from the stomach, caused by warfarin is increased by drugs that cause bleeding by different mechanisms (e.g. **aspirin**, which inhibits platelet thromboxane A_2 biosynthesis and which can damage the stomach; see Ch. 25).
- *Sulfonamides* prevent the synthesis of folic acid by bacteria and other microorganisms; **trimethoprim** inhibits its reduction to its active tetrahydrofolate form. Given together, the drugs have a synergistic action of value in treating *Pneumocystis* infection (see Chs 54 and 55).
- *Non-steroidal anti-inflammatory drugs* (NSAIDs; see Ch. 25), such as **ibuprofen** or **indometacin**, inhibit biosynthesis of prostaglandins, including renal vasodilator/natriuretic prostaglandins

---

[1]A third category of pharmaceutical interactions should be mentioned, in which drugs interact in vitro so that one or both are inactivated. No pharmacological principles are involved, just chemistry. An example is the formation of a complex between **thiopental** and **suxamethonium**, which must not be mixed in the same syringe. **Heparin** is highly charged and interacts in this way with many basic drugs; it is sometimes used to keep intravenous lines or cannulae open and can inactivate basic drugs if they are injected without first clearing the line with saline.

(prostaglandin E_2, prostaglandin I_2). If administered to patients receiving treatment for hypertension, they increase the blood pressure. If given to patients being treated with diuretics for chronic heart failure, they cause salt and water retention and hence cardiac decompensation.[2]
- Histamine H_1-receptor antagonists, such as **promethazine**, commonly cause drowsiness as an unwanted effect. This is more troublesome if such drugs are taken with alcohol, leading to accidents at work or on the road.

PHARMACOKINETIC INTERACTION

All the four major processes that determine pharmacokinetics – absorption, distribution, metabolism and excretion (ADME) – can be affected by drugs. For instance, absorption and distribution interactions can arise between compounds with shared transporters (see Ch. 9). Further details on pharmacokinetic interactions are covered in Chapters 9 and 10.

Drug interactions

- These are many and varied: if in doubt, look it up.
- Interactions may be pharmacodynamic or pharmacokinetic.
- Pharmacodynamic interactions are often predictable from the actions of the interacting drugs.
- Pharmacokinetic interactions can involve effects on:
  - absorption (see Ch. 9)
  - distribution (e.g. competition for protein binding, see Ch. 9)
  - hepatic metabolism (induction or inhibition, see Ch. 10)
  - renal excretion (see Ch. 10)

GENETIC VARIATION IN DRUG RESPONSIVENESS

A patient's response to a particular drug may be influenced by a rare genetic trait, or a complex multifactorial trait involving effects of several genetic and environmental factors. Complex traits may not adhere to typical Mendelian or familial inheritance because they involve the additive or synergistic influence of multiple gene variants that can interact with environmental factors to result in a wide spectrum of inter-individual drug response. Potential pharmacogenetic markers of variation may include measurable differences in gene expression or functional deficiencies related to genetic factors, i.e. somatic or germline mutations and chromosomal abnormalities.

Mutations are heritable changes in the base sequence of DNA. These may, or may not,[3] result in a change in the amino acid sequence of the protein for which the gene codes. *Germline* or *hereditary* mutations are those that affect the body's reproductive cells (egg or sperm) and can be passed to the next generation where they are present in all cells. In practice, tests for such germline mutations in individuals are usually made on venous blood samples that contain chromosomal and mitochondrial DNA in white blood cells. Germline genetic variations that contribute to differences in drug response and adverse effects in specific populations can be assessed in large cohort or case-control studies that use microarrays or whole genome/exome sequencing strategies to analyse several million genetic variants. The recent emergence of high-throughput genotyping technology has enabled genome-wide association studies to identify loci that are potentially linked to drug effect.

Somatic or *acquired* mutations are not present at birth but can occur in any of the body cells (except the ova and sperm) during a lifetime and are not passed on to the offspring. Whilst the vast majority of somatic mutations are thought to have no clinical consequence, those that affect key signalling pathways involved in cell growth, division and differentiation can predispose to carcinogenesis, as well as late-onset mitochondrial and neurogenerative disorders. Somatic cell mutations underlie the pathogenesis of some tumours (see Ch. 6), and the presence or absence of such somatic cell mutations guides drug selection. The genomic tests are performed on DNA from samples of the tumour obtained surgically. The tests themselves involve amplification of the relevant sequence(s) and molecular biological methods, often utilising chip technology, to identify the various polymorphisms.

Genetic variation or mutations are not always deleterious and they may confer an advantage under some environmental circumstances. A pharmacogenetically relevant example is the X-linked gene for *glucose 6-phosphate dehydrogenase* (G6PD); deficiency of this enzyme confers partial resistance to malaria (a considerable selective advantage in parts of the world where this disease is common) at the expense of susceptibility to haemolysis in response to oxidative stress in the form of exposure to various dietary constituents, including several drugs (e.g. the antimalarial drug **primaquine**; see Ch. 55). This ambiguity gives rise to the abnormal gene being preserved in future generations, at a frequency that depends on the balance of selective pressures in the environment. Thus the distribution of G6PD deficiency is similar to the geographical distribution of malaria. The situation where functionally distinct forms of a gene are common in a population is called a 'balanced' polymorphism (balanced because a disadvantage, for example in a homozygote, is balanced by an advantage, for example in a heterozygote).

---

[2]The interaction with diuretics may involve a pharmacokinetic interaction in addition to the pharmacodynamic effect described here, because NSAIDs compete with weak acids, including diuretics, for renal tubular secretion; see Chapter 10.

[3]The genetic code is said to be 'degenerate' because of presence of redundancy, where more than one set of nucleotide base triplets code for each amino acid. A 'silent' mutation with no change in the protein and consequently no change in function can stem from a base change involving a triplet that codes for the same amino acid as the original. Such mutations are neither advantageous nor disadvantageous, so they will neither be eliminated by natural selection nor accumulate in the population at the expense of the wild-type gene.

Polymorphisms are relatively common variants (alternative sequences at a locus within the DNA strand) that are found in >1% of individuals within a given population. They arise initially because of a mutation, and are stable if they are non-functional, or die out during subsequent generations if (as is usually the case) they are disadvantageous. However, if the prevailing selective pressures in the environment are favourable, leading to a selective advantage, a polymorphism may increase in frequency over successive generations. Now that genes can be sequenced readily, it has become apparent that *single nucleotide polymorphisms* ([SNPs] – DNA sequence variations that occur when a single nucleotide in the genome sequence is altered) are very common. They may entail substitution of one nucleotide for another (substitution of C for T in two-thirds of SNPs), or deletion or insertion of a nucleotide. Insertions and deletions of one or more nucleotides (other than when the change in number of nucleotides is a multiple of three) result in a 'frame shift' in translation. For example, after an insertion of one nucleotide, the first element of the next triplet in the code becomes the second and all subsequent bases are shifted one 'to the right'. Changes to the coding region of a gene may result in loss of protein synthesis, abnormal protein synthesis or an abnormal rate of protein synthesis.

On average, SNPs occur once in every 300 bases along the 3-billion base human genome, thus resulting in the presence of about 10 million SNPs. They can occur in coding (gene) and non-coding regions of the genome, and they may have a greater role in physiological function if located within a gene or in a regulatory sequence close to the gene. Whilst many SNPs do not have a clear association with health conditions, some SNPs have a demonstrable relationship with susceptibility to harmful chemicals, magnitude of drug response and likelihood of developing a disease. For example, SNPs affecting the *F5* gene can cause factor V Leiden blood-clotting disorder, which is the commonest form of inherited thrombophilia (see Ch. 23). The abnormality in the factor V clotting factor confers an increased risk of venous thrombosis in response to environmental factors such as prolonged immobility, but might perhaps have been an advantage to ancestors more at risk of haemorrhage than of thrombosis.

SINGLE-GENE PHARMACOKINETIC DISORDERS

The classical Mendelian model contrasts with the complex disease paradigm because it applies to single-gene or monogenic disorders where a mutation in a gene is the primary or sole cause of profound disruption. These are typically rare disorders where the underlying genetic variants have very high penetrance with inheritance patterns that are readily predicted in a Mendelian fashion. This was recognised for albinism (albinos lack an enzyme that is needed to synthesise the brown pigment melanin) and other 'inborn errors of metabolism' in the early part of the 20th century by Archibald Garrod, a British physician who initiated the study of biochemical genetics. Investigation of this large group of individually rare diseases has contributed to our understanding of this particular aspect of molecular pathology – familial hypercholesterolaemia and the mechanism of action of statins (see Ch. 22) is one example; further examples of single-gene disorders are given in the following.

PLASMA CHOLINESTERASE DEFICIENCY

In the 1950s Walter Kalow discovered that **suxamethonium** sensitivity is due to genetic variation in the rate of drug metabolism as a result of a Mendelian autosomal recessive trait. This short-acting neuromuscular-blocking drug is widely used in anaesthesia and is normally rapidly hydrolysed by plasma cholinesterase (see Ch. 14). About 1 in 3000 individuals fails to inactivate suxamethonium rapidly and experiences prolonged neuromuscular block if treated with it; this is because a recessive gene gives rise to an abnormal type of plasma cholinesterase. The abnormal enzyme has a modified pattern of substrate and inhibitor specificity. It is detected by a blood test that measures the effect of **dibucaine**, which inhibits the abnormal enzyme less than the normal enzyme. Heterozygotes can hydrolyse suxamethonium at a more or less normal rate, but their plasma cholinesterase has reduced sensitivity to dibucaine, intermediate between normal subjects and homozygotes. Only homozygotes express the disease: they appear completely healthy unless exposed to suxamethonium or **mivacurium** (which is also inactivated by plasma cholinesterase) but experience prolonged paralysis if exposed to a dose that would cause neuromuscular block for only a few minutes in a healthy person.[4] There are other reasons why responses to suxamethonium may be abnormal in an individual patient, notably *malignant hyperpyrexia* (see Ch. 14), a genetically determined idiosyncratic adverse drug reaction involving the ryanodine receptor (see Ch. 4). It is important to check the family history and test family members who may be affected, but the disorder is so rare that it is currently impractical to screen for it routinely before therapeutic use of suxamethonium.

ACUTE INTERMITTENT PORPHYRIA

The hepatic *porphyrias* are prototypic pharmacogenetic disorders in which patients may be symptomatic even if they are not exposed to a drug, but where many drugs can provoke very severe worsening of the course of the disease. They are inherited disorders involving the biochemical pathway of porphyrin haem biosynthesis. *Acute intermittent porphyria* is the most common acute and severe form. It is inherited as an autosomal dominant trait and is due to one of many different mutations in the gene coding *porphobilinogen deaminase* (PBGD), a key enzyme in haem biosynthesis in red cell precursors, hepatocytes and other cells. All of these mutations reduce the activity of this enzyme, and clinical features are caused by the resulting build-up of haem precursors, including porphyrins. There is a strong interplay with the environment through exposure to drugs, hormones and other chemicals. The use of sedative, anticonvulsant or other drugs in patients with undiagnosed porphyria can be lethal, although with appropriate supportive management most patients recover

[4]An apparently healthy middle-aged man saw one of the authors over several months because of hypertension; he also saw a psychiatrist because of depression. This failed to improve with other treatment and he underwent electroconvulsive therapy (ECT). Suxamethonium was used to prevent injury caused by convulsions; this usually results in short-lived paralysis but this poor man recovered consciousness some 2 days later to find himself being weaned from artificial ventilation in an intensive care unit. Subsequent analysis showed him to be homozygous for an ineffective form of plasma cholinesterase.

completely.[5] Many drugs, especially but not exclusively those that induce CYP enzymes (e.g. barbiturates, **griseofulvin**, **carbamazepine**, oestrogens – see Ch. 10), can precipitate acute attacks in susceptible individuals. Porphyrins are synthesised from δ-amino laevulinic acid (ALA), which is formed by ALA synthase in the liver. This enzyme is induced by drugs such as barbiturates, resulting in increased ALA production and, hence, increased porphyrin accumulation. As mentioned previously, the genetic trait is inherited as an autosomal dominant trait, but frank disease is approximately five times more common in women than in men, because hormonal fluctuations precipitate acute attacks. Intriguingly, acute intermittent porphyria can now be treated with **givosiran**, a small interfering RNA that reduces ALA synthase mRNA (and currently one of the world's most expensive drugs), thus alleviating the build up of neurotoxins that are implicated in porphyria attacks.

THERAPEUTIC DRUGS AND CLINICALLY AVAILABLE PHARMACOGENOMIC TESTS

Clinical tests to predict drug responsiveness were anticipated to be one of the first applications of sequencing the human genome. Although a profusion of new pharmacogenetic tests are now marketed to healthcare professionals as well as direct to consumer, the adoption and implementation in routine clinical practice have been slowed by various scientific, commercial, political and educational barriers. Reimbursement for expensive tests and drugs, whether provided by the state or by insurance schemes, depends increasingly on evidence of cost-effectiveness. Here, new pharmacogenetic tests are required to have a positive or meaningful influence on prescribing practice, such as the use of a validated alternative drug or different dosing regimen that leads to measurable improvements in patient outcomes (Khoury and Galea, 2016; Manrai et al., 2016). The need for reliable evidence regarding clinical and cost-effectiveness of any diagnostic or prognostic test has stimulated increasing numbers of randomised controlled trials of pharmacogenomics-informed prescribing strategy versus current best practice.

However, evaluation of drug response in complex multifactorial traits is a major challenge because multiple genes and genetic variants interact with environmental factors, and the genetic component may only have a modest influence on treatment effect. Much of the earlier research has been focused on striking single pathogenic variants that have readily apparent or clear-cut 'all or none' treatment effect. In reality, however, the probability of drug benefit and harm is often a continuum with a wide range of variation across individuals in a population (Manrai et al., 2016), and reliance on a single predictive genetic biomarker may not be sufficiently precise or reliable to guide treatment of serious disease. Equally, we recognise that clinicians already tailor treatment according to a multitude of biomarkers such as age, renal function, body surface area and so on. Here, healthcare providers need greater clarity regarding extent of improvement or added value from implementing new clinical pathways based on genetic information.

The clinical setting is another important factor to consider. At present, many of the largest genetic research studies are carried out in resource-rich areas with a predominantly White population. Hence, we are uncertain about the applicability of the studies to wider locations around the world, particularly with areas that have more diverse non-White populations. Equally much of the focus has been on personalising cancer treatments delivered in specialist oncology centres, where the available genetic information is directly relevant to choosing one particular type of drug or another. However, the situation is much more complex in primary care where the prescriber has to deal with patients who are burdened with polypharmacy. Multiple genetics tests of diverse medications would need to be interpreted together with the full medical history and other biomarkers.

The key steps in evaluating pharmacogenetic markers in clinical care should be confirmation of analytic validity (accuracy and reliability of the test) and determination of a robust, replicable relationship between the marker and drug response in the population (clinical validity). Clinical utility must then be demonstrated through improved efficacy or safety in patients receiving the biomarker-guided therapeutic regimens. There are also health economic considerations as to whether the genetic markers are of sufficiently high frequency in their patient population to justify the costs of screening. Policy makers and funding agencies will then have to look at feasibility of using the biomarker testing strategy in a way that does not delay patient treatment. Here, the historical approach of single-gene as needed, or 'one at a time' testing can seem slow, inefficient and costly when compared with the recent availability of pre-emptive testing for multiple genetic markers. The growing availability of rapid testing using multi-gene panels means that the individual's genetic data from a single sample can be used to inform many different treatment decisions that subsequently arise in their lifetime.

At present, pharmacogenetic evaluation can include tests for (a) variants of different human leukocyte antigens (HLAs) that have been strongly linked to susceptibilities to several severe harmful drug reactions that are likely to have arisen from an immunological interaction between the drug molecule and the major histocompatibility molecules in the patient (Chan et al., 2015) (b) genes controlling aspects of drug metabolism; and (c) genes encoding drug targets, where the concept of 'companion diagnostics' (defined by the FDA as: 'a diagnostic test used as a companion to a therapeutic drug to determine its applicability to a specific person') involves detection of a pharmacogenetic marker so that rational drug selection can be made based on the pathway related to the underlying mutation. For one drug (**warfarin**), a test would need to combine genetic information

[5]Life expectancy, obtained from parish records, of patients with porphyria diagnosed retrospectively within large kindreds in Scandinavia was normal until the advent and widespread use of barbiturates and other sedative and anticonvulsant drugs in the 20th century, when it plummeted. There is a long and useful list of drugs to avoid in the *British National Formulary*, together with the warning that drugs not on the list may not necessarily be safe in such patients!

Pharmacogenetics and pharmacogenomics

- Several inherited disorders influence responses to drugs, including single-gene conditions such as:
  - *glucose 6-phosphate dehydrogenase deficiency*, a sex-linked disorder in which affected men (or rare homozygous women) experience haemolysis if exposed to various chemicals including the antimalarial drug **primaquine**;
  - *plasma cholinesterase deficiency*, an autosomal recessive disorder that confers sensitivity to the neuromuscular blocker suxamethonium;
  - *acute intermittent porphyria*, an autosomal dominant disease more severe in women and in which severe attacks are precipitated by drugs or endogenous sex hormones that induce CYP enzymes;
- SNPs and combinations of SNPs (haplotypes) in genes coding for proteins involved in drug disposition or drug action are common and may predict drug response. Pharmacogenomic tests in blood or tissue removed surgically have established associations between several such variants and individual drug response.
- Such tests are available for:
  - several HLA variants that predict toxicity of **abacavir** and **carbamazepine**;
  - genes for several enzymes in drug metabolism including CYP2D6 and CYP2C9, DPYD and thiopurine-*S*-methyltransferase (TPMT);
  - germline and somatic mutations in growth factor receptors that predict responsiveness to cancer treatments including **imatinib** and **trastuzumab.**

about metabolism with information about its target (see Fig 12.3).

INCORPORATING PHARMACOGENETIC DATA INTO DAILY CLINICAL WORKFLOWS

One of the major challenges relates to the multiple hurdles spanning the scientific discovery of an important genetic marker to the actual delivery of a tailored treatment plan guided by this new knowledge. The wide availability of large throughput studies and electronic patient databases means that even modest genetic associations can now be readily detected. However, these discoveries come with uncertain clinical relevance, particularly with regards to strength of evidence and the actual size of the genetic contribution to treatment response, given that there are a multitude of influential physiological and environmental factors in the melee. Moreover, whilst 'clinically actionable' is the present 'buzzword' to describe important genetic information, no one knows exactly what the correct clinical action is, nor if any specific pathway is better or worse than alternative ones. This has led to discrepant or divergent treatment recommendations amongst learned bodies that assess pharmacogenomic data (Abdullah-Koolmees et al., 2020). Inevitably, the busy clinician, when considering a pharmacogenetic test, will be confronted with three key questions – is this the right situation to request a genetic test, how should the data be interpreted, and is there a universally agreed recommended course of action?

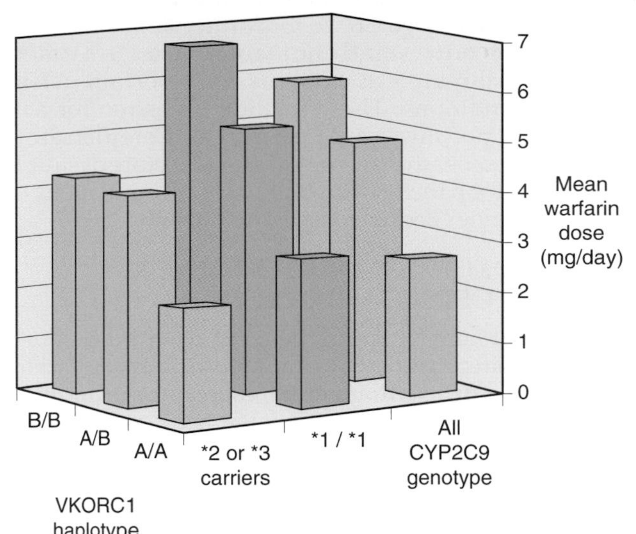

Fig. 12.3 Effect of *VKOR* haplotype and *CYP2C9* genotype on warfarin dose. A series of 186 patients on long-term warfarin treatment who had already been studied for *CYP2C9* were studied retrospectively for genetic variants of *VKOR* (Rieder et al., 2005). *VKOR* haplotype as well as *CYP2C9* genotype influenced the mean warfarin dose (which had been adjusted to achieve therapeutic International Normalised Ratio). *A*, Haplotypes 1 and 2; *B*, haplotypes 7, 8 and 9. *A/A*, *A/B* and *B/B* represent haplotype combinations. **1/*1* represents CYP2C9 wild-type homozygotes; **2* and **3* represent CYP2C9 variants. (Figure redrawn from Beitelshees, A.L., McLeod, H.L., 2006. Applying pharmacogenomics to enhance the use of biomarkers for drug effect and drug safety. TIPS 27, 498–502.)

There are a number of examples as how this might pan out in current clinical practice (for further reading, see Mehta et al., 2020).

INDICATIONS

Here, we describe examples where genetic information helps us decide whether the particular drug is indicated, or not. **Trastuzumab** ('Herceptin'; Ch. 57) is a monoclonal antibody that antagonises epidermal growth factor (EGF) by binding to one of its receptors (human EGF receptor 2 – HER2) which can occur in tumour tissue as a result of somatic mutation. It is used in patients with breast cancer whose tumour tissue is positive for this receptor.

Dasatinib and imatinib are first-line tyrosine kinase inhibitors used in haematological malignancies characterised by the presence of a Philadelphia chromosome, namely chronic myeloid leukaemia (CML) and in some adults with acute lymphocytic leukaemia (ALL). The Philadelphia chromosome results from a translocation defect when parts of two chromosomes (9 and 22) swap places; part of a 'breakpoint cluster region' (BCR) in chromosome 22 links to the 'Abelson-1' (ABL) region of chromosome 9. A mutation (T315I) in BCR/ABL confers resistance to the inhibitory effect of dasatinib and patients with this variant do not benefit from this drug. Instead, **ponatinib** is licensed in the United States for treatment of patients who have this BCR-ABL T315I mutation.

Drug treatment options for cystic fibrosis (an autosomal recessive condition involving the cystic fibrosis transfer receptor) include channel potentiators and channel correctors that are efficacious for patients who carry specific genetic mutations (see Ch. 28 for further details).

There are now small-molecule-based treatments specifically targeted at patients with certain defined inherited conditions. These include givosiran for acute intermittent porphyria (see earlier) and **eteplersen** (an antisense oligomer that acts on mRNA to restore dystrophin production) for patients with highly specific mutations that cause Duchenne/Becker muscular dystrophy.

DOSAGE ADJUSTMENT BASED ON GENETIC PREDICTORS OF DRUG METABOLISM

Here, we highlight two prominent examples where dosing schedule is can be guided by evaluation of genetic variants.

Thiopurine drugs (**tioguanine**, **mercaptopurine** and its prodrug **azathioprine**; Ch. 57) have been used for more than 50 years to treat leukaemias, and more recently to cause immunosuppression, for example, in treating inflammatory disorders involving the bowel, skin, or joints. These drugs are detoxified by thiopurine-*S*-methyltransferase (TPMT), which is present in blood cells, as well as by xanthine oxidase. Reduced starting doses are recommended for patients who have genotypes associated with reduced metabolism. Even with such testing, careful monitoring of the white blood cell count is needed because genetic testing cannot fully account for toxicity, and there are also environmental susceptibility factors.

5-FU (see Ch. 57, Fig. 57.6) and related compounds such as capecitabine and tegafur are used extensively to treat solid tumours, but have a narrow therapeutic window and serious toxicity (neutropaenia, vomiting, diarrhoea, mucocutaneous syndromes) in 10%–40% of patients, resulting in a fatality rate of about 1 in 100 overall. Approximately 80% of 5-FU is detoxified by dihydropyrimidine dehydrogenase (DPYD), which has four main clinically important genetic variants that account for 20%–30% of the cases suffering from life-threatening toxicity. Identification of the variants helps to guide dose reductions, more gradual dose increments, and even the choice of moving to a different type of chemotherapy.

SCREENING OUT PATIENTS WHO ARE HIGHLY SUSCEPTIBILE TO SERIOUS ADVERSE DRUG REACTIONS

Here, we highlight two prominent examples where evaluation of genetic variants can help us avoid prescribing drugs that can cause serious harm to certain susceptible individuals.

▾ **Abacavir** (see Ch. 53) is a reverse transcriptase inhibitor that is highly effective in treating HIV infection. Its use has been limited by severe rashes. Susceptibility to this adverse effect is closely linked to the HLA variant *HLAB*5701*, and testing for this variant is now considered a standard of care supported by prospective randomised trials (Fig. 12.4; Martin and Kroetz, 2013).

Carbamazepine (see Ch. 46) can also cause severe (life-threatening) rashes including *Stevens–Johnson syndrome* and *toxic epidermal necrolysis* (multiform rashes with painful blistering lesions and skin detachment sometimes extending into the gastrointestinal tract) and now considered to be a disease continuum distinguished chiefly by severity, based upon the percentage of body surface involved with skin detachment. These are associated with a particular HLA allele, *HLAB*1502*, which occurs more commonly in ethnic groups in Thailand, Malaysia and Taiwan (Barbarino

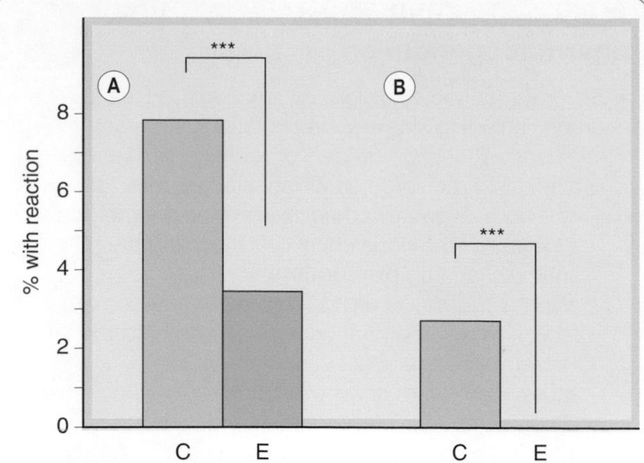

Fig. 12.4 Incidence of abacavir hypersensitivity is reduced by pharmacogenetic screening. In the PREDICT-1 study (Mallal et al., 2008), patients were randomised to standard care (*C*, control group) or prospective pharmacogenetic screening (*E*, experimental group). All the control subjects were treated with abacavir, but only those experimental subjects who were *HLA-B*5701* negative were treated with abacavir. There were two prespecified end points: clinically suspected hypersensitivity reactions (A) and clinically suspected reactions that were immunologically confirmed by a positive patch test (B). Both end points favoured the experimental group ($p < 0.0001$). (Figure redrawn from Hughes, A.R., et al., 2008. Pharmacogenet. J. 8, 365–374.)

et al., 2015), but with far lower frequencies in Korean, Japanese and White populations. Screening for this allele before starting treatment is potentially worthwhile in populations where the allele frequency is high.

COMMUNICATING THE PRESENCE OR ABSENCE OF RISK

Here, a particular drug may have been specifically tested in people with different genetic variants, and there may be information on extent of risk, if any. For instance, the product information for lacosamide (used in the treatment of epilepsy) states that there was no clinically relevant difference in lacosamide exposure when comparing extensive metabolisers against poor metabolisers according to CYP2C19 status.

CONCLUSIONS

Twin studies as well as several well-documented single-gene disorders (including Mendelian chromosomal – autosomal recessive, autosomal dominant and X-linked – and maternally inherited mitochondrial disorders) prove the concept that susceptibility to adverse drug effects can be genetically determined. Pharmacogenomic testing offers the possibility of more precise 'personalised' therapeutics for several drugs and disorders, but high-quality trial evidence of clinical utility in diverse populations is still being pursued, particularly in instances where drug response is influenced by complex multifactorial traits. This is a field of intense research activity, rapid progress and high expectations, but proving that these tests consistently add to present best practice and improve outcomes remains a key goal.

REFERENCES AND FURTHER READING

Abdullah-Koolmees, H., van Keulen, A.M., Nijenhuis, M., et al., 2020. Pharmacogenetics guidelines: overview and comparison of the DPWG, CPIC, CPNDS, and RNPGx guidelines. Front. Pharmacol. 11, 595219.

Barbarino, J.M., Kroetz, D.L., Klein, T.E., Altman, R.B., 2015. PharmGKB summary: very important pharmacogene information for human leukocyte antigen B (HLA-B). Pharmacogenet. Genomics 25, 205–221.

Chan, S.L., Jin, S., Loh, M., Brunham, L.R., 2015. Progress in understanding the genomic basis for adverse drug reactions: a comprehensive review and focus on the role of ethnicity. Pharmacogenomics 16, 1161–1178.

Cooper, R.S., Kaufman, J.S., Ward, R., 2003. Race and genomics. N. Engl. J. Med. 348, 1166–1170.

Doogue, M.P., Polasek, T.M., 2011. Drug dosing in renal disease. Clin. Biochem. Rev. 32, 69–73.

Huang, S.M., Lertora, J., Vicini, P., Atkinson Jr., A.J., 2021. Atkinson's Principles of Clinical Pharmacology, fourth ed. Academic Press, San Diego.

Ingelman-Sundberg, M., 2020. Translation of pharmacogenomic drug labels into the clinic. Current problems. Pharmacol. Res. 153, 104620.

Khoury, M.J., Galea, S., 2016. Will precision medicine improve population health? JAMA 316, 1357–1358.

Luzum, J.A., Petry, N., Taylor, A.K., et al., 2021. Moving pharmacogenetics into practice: it's all about the evidence. Clin. Pharmacol. Ther. 110, 649–661.

Mallal, S., Phillips, E., Carosi, G., et al., 2008. HLA-B*5701 screening for hypersensitivity to abacavir. N. Engl. J. Med. 358, 568–579.

Manrai, A.K., Ioannidis, J.A., Kohane, I.S., 2016. Clinical genomics: from pathogenicity claims to quantitative risk estimates. JAMA 315, 1233–1234.

Martin, M.A., Kroetz, D.L., 2013. Abacavir pharmacogenetics – from initial reports to standard of care. Pharmacotherapy 33, 765–775.

Mehta, D., Uber, R., Ingle, T., et al., 2020. Study of pharmacogenomic information in FDA-approved drug labeling to facilitate application of precision medicine. Drug Discov. Today 25, 813–820.

Phillips, K.A., Deverka, P.A., Sox, H.C., et al., 2017. Making genomic medicine evidence-based and patient-centered: a structured review and landscape analysis of comparative effectiveness research. Genet. Med. 19 (10), 1081–1091.

Po, A.L.W., 2007. Personalised medicine: who is an Asian? Lancet 369, 1770–1771.

Relling, M.V., Evans, W.E., 2015. Pharmacogenomics in the clinic. Nature 526, 343–350.

Rieder, M.J., Reiner, A.P., Gage, B.F., et al., 2005. Effect of VKORC1 haplotype on transcriptional regulation and warfarin dose. N. Engl. J. Med. 352, 2285–2293.

Wadman, M., 2005. Drug targeting: is race enough? Nature 435, 1008–1009.

13 Chemical mediators and the autonomic nervous system

OVERVIEW

The network of chemical signals and associated receptors by which cells in the body communicate with one another provides many targets for drug action, and has always been a focus of attention for pharmacologists. Chemical transmission in the peripheral autonomic nervous system, and the various ways in which the process can be pharmacologically subverted, is the main focus of this chapter, but the mechanisms described operate also in the central nervous system (CNS). In addition to neurotransmission, we also consider briefly the less clearly defined processes, collectively termed neuromodulation, by which many mediators and drugs exert control over the function of the nervous system. The relative anatomical and physiological simplicity of the peripheral nervous system has made it the proving ground for many important discoveries about chemical transmission, and the same general principles apply to the CNS (see Ch. 37). For more detail than is given here, see Robertson et al. (2012) and Kandel et al. (2021).

HISTORICAL ASPECTS

Studies initiated on the peripheral nervous system have been central to the understanding and classification of many major types of drug action, so it is worth recounting a little history. Excellent accounts are given by Bacq (1975), Valenstein (2005) and Burnstock (2009).

Experimental physiology became established as an approach to the understanding of the function of living organisms in the middle of the 19th century. The peripheral nervous system, and particularly the autonomic nervous system, received a great deal of attention. The fact that electrical stimulation of nerves could elicit a whole variety of physiological effects – from blanching of the skin to arrest of the heart – presented a real challenge to comprehension, particularly of the way in which the signal was passed from the nerve to the effector tissue. In 1877, Du Bois-Reymond was the first to put the alternatives clearly: 'Of known natural processes that might pass on excitation, only two are, in my opinion, worth talking about – either there exists at the boundary of the contractile substance a stimulatory secretion … or the phenomenon is electrical in nature.' The latter view was generally favoured. In 1869, it had been shown that an exogenous substance, **muscarine**, could mimic the effects of stimulating the vagus nerve, and that **atropine** could inhibit the actions both of muscarine and of nerve stimulation. In 1905, Langley showed the same for **nicotine** and **curare** acting at the neuromuscular junction. Most physiologists interpreted these phenomena as stimulation and inhibition of the nerve endings, respectively, rather than as evidence for chemical transmission. Hence the suggestion of T.R. Elliott, in 1904, that **adrenaline** (**epinephrine**) might act as a chemical transmitter mediating the actions of the sympathetic nervous system was coolly received, until Langley, the Professor of Physiology at Cambridge and a powerful figure at that time, suggested, a year later, that transmission to skeletal muscle involved the secretion by the nerve terminals of a substance related to nicotine.

One of the key observations for Elliott was that degeneration of sympathetic nerve terminals did not abolish the sensitivity of smooth muscle preparations to adrenaline (which the electrical theory predicted) but actually enhanced it. The hypothesis of chemical transmission was put to direct test in 1907 by Dixon, who tried to show that vagus nerve stimulation released from a dog's heart into the blood a substance capable of inhibiting another heart. The experiment failed, and the atmosphere of scepticism prevailed.

It was not until 1921, in Germany, that Loewi showed that stimulation of the vagosympathetic trunk connected to an isolated and cannulated frog's heart could cause the release into the cannula of a substance ('Vagusstoff') that, if the cannula fluid was transferred from the first heart to a second, would inhibit the second heart. This is a classic and much-quoted experiment that proved extremely difficult for even Loewi to perform reproducibly. In an autobiographical sketch, Loewi tells us that the idea of chemical transmission arose in a discussion that he had in 1903, but no way of testing it experimentally occurred to him until he dreamt of the appropriate experiment one night in 1920. He wrote some notes of this very important dream in the middle of the night, but in the morning could not read them. The dream obligingly returned the next night and, taking no chances, he went to the laboratory at 3 a.m. and carried out the experiment successfully. Loewi's experiment may be, and was, criticised on numerous grounds (it could, for example, have been potassium rather than a neurotransmitter that was acting on the recipient heart), but a series of further experiments proved him to be right. His findings can be summarised as follows:

- Stimulation of the vagus caused the appearance in the perfusate of the frog heart of a substance capable of producing, in a second heart, an inhibitory effect resembling vagus stimulation.
- Stimulation of the sympathetic nervous system caused the appearance of a substance capable of accelerating a second heart. By fluorescence measurements, Loewi concluded later that this substance was adrenaline.
- Atropine prevented the inhibitory action of the vagus on the heart but did not prevent release of Vagusstoff. Atropine thus prevented the effects, rather than the release, of the transmitter.
- When Vagusstoff was incubated with ground-up heart muscle, it became inactivated. This effect is now known to be due to enzymatic destruction of acetylcholine (ACh) by cholinesterase.

- **Physostigmine**, which potentiated the effect of vagus stimulation on the heart, prevented destruction of Vagusstoff by heart muscle, providing evidence that the potentiation is due to inhibition of cholinesterase, which normally destroys the transmitter substance ACh.

A few years later, in the early 1930s, Dale showed convincingly that ACh was also the transmitter substance at the neuromuscular junction of striated muscle and at autonomic ganglia. One of the keys to Dale's success lay in the use of highly sensitive bioassays, especially the leech dorsal muscle, for measuring the amount of ACh that had been released. Chemical transmission at sympathetic nerve terminals was demonstrated at about the same time as cholinergic transmission and by very similar methods. Cannon and his colleagues at Harvard first showed unequivocally the phenomenon of chemical transmission at sympathetic nerve endings, by experiments in vivo in which tissues made supersensitive to adrenaline by prior sympathetic denervation were shown to respond, after a delay, to the transmitter released by stimulation of the sympathetic nerves to other parts of the body. The chemical identity of the transmitter, tantalisingly like adrenaline but not identical to it, caused confusion for many years, until, in 1946, von Euler showed it to be the non-methylated derivative **noradrenaline** (**norepinephrine**).

THE AUTONOMIC NERVOUS SYSTEM

The autonomic nervous system for a long time occupied centre stage in the pharmacology of chemical transmission.

BASIC ANATOMY AND PHYSIOLOGY

The autonomic nervous system (see Robertson et al., 2012) consists of three main anatomical divisions: *sympathetic*, *parasympathetic* and *enteric* nervous systems. The sympathetic and parasympathetic systems (Fig. 13.1) provide a link between the CNS and peripheral organs. The enteric nervous system comprises the intrinsic nerve plexuses of the gastrointestinal tract, which are closely interconnected with the sympathetic and parasympathetic systems.

The autonomic nervous system conveys all the outputs from the CNS to the rest of the body, except for the motor innervation of skeletal muscle. The enteric nervous system has sufficient integrative capabilities to allow it to function independently of the CNS, but the sympathetic and parasympathetic systems are agents of the CNS and cannot function without it. The autonomic nervous system is largely outside the influence of voluntary control. The main processes that it regulates, to a greater or lesser extent, are:

- contraction and relaxation of vascular and visceral smooth muscle
- all exocrine and certain endocrine secretions
- the heartbeat

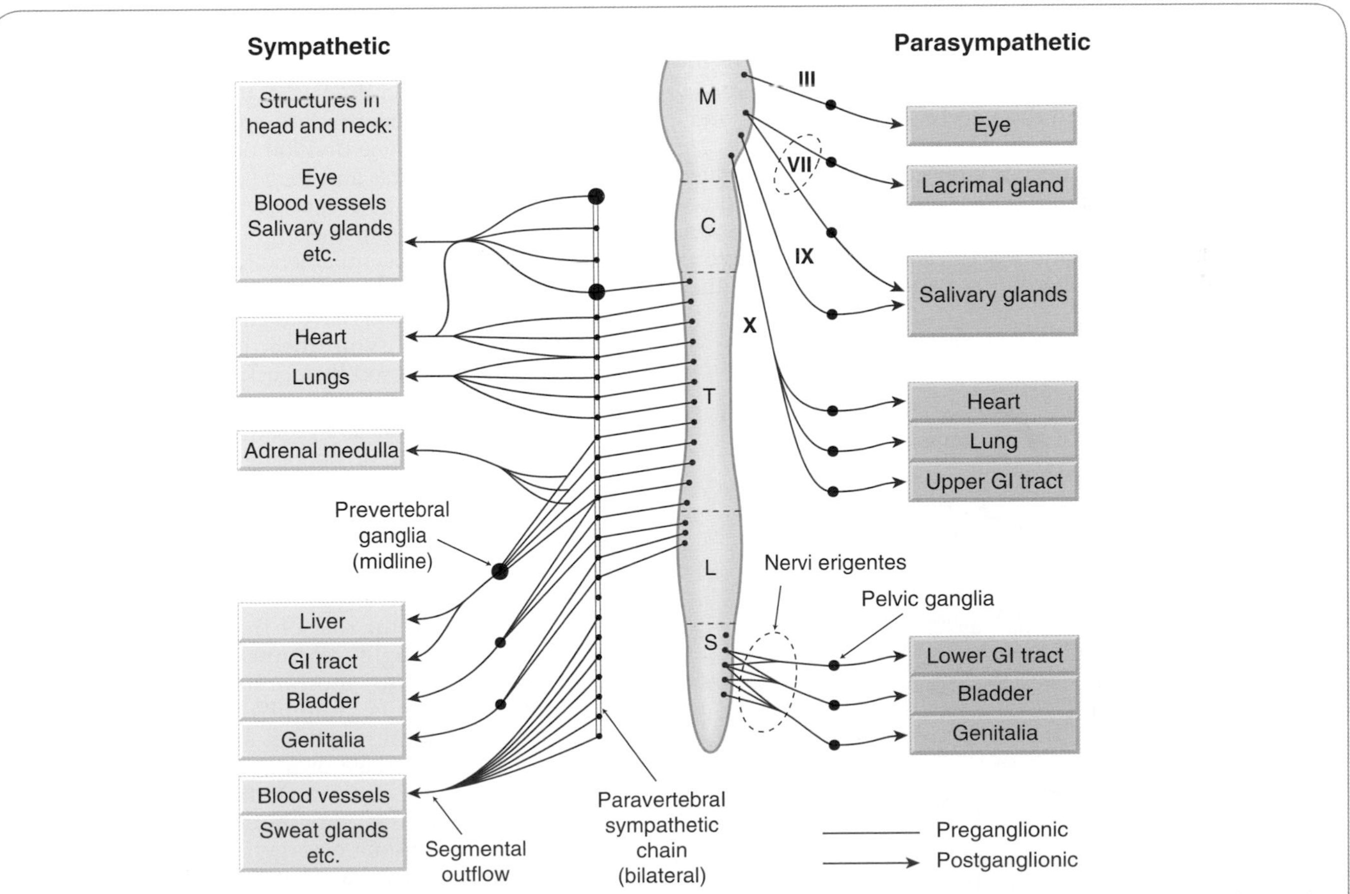

Fig. 13.1 Basic plan of the mammalian autonomic nervous system. *C*, Cervical; *GI*, gastrointestinal; *L*, lumbar; *M*, medullary; *S*, sacral; *T*, thoracic.

- energy metabolism, particularly in liver and skeletal muscle

A degree of autonomic control also affects many other systems, including the kidney, immune system and somatosensory system. The autonomic efferent pathway consists of two neurons arranged in series, whereas in the somatic motor system a single motor neuron connects the CNS to the skeletal muscle fibre (Fig. 13.2). The two neurons in the autonomic pathway are known, respectively, as *preganglionic* and *postganglionic*. In the sympathetic nervous system, the intervening synapses lie in *autonomic* ganglia, which are outside the CNS, and contain the nerve endings of preganglionic fibres and the cell bodies of postganglionic neurons. In parasympathetic pathways, the postganglionic cells are mainly found in the target organs, discrete parasympathetic ganglia (e.g. the ciliary ganglion) being found only in the head and neck.

The cell bodies of the sympathetic preganglionic neurons lie in the *lateral horn* of the grey matter of the thoracic and lumbar segments of the spinal cord, and the fibres leave the spinal cord in the spinal nerves as the *thoracolumbar sympathetic outflow*. The preganglionic fibres synapse in the *paravertebral chains* of sympathetic ganglia, lying on either side of the spinal column. These ganglia contain the cell bodies of the postganglionic sympathetic neurons, the axons of which rejoin the spinal nerve. Many of the postganglionic sympathetic fibres reach their peripheral destinations via the branches of the spinal nerves. Others, destined for abdominal and pelvic viscera, have their cell bodies in a group of unpaired *prevertebral ganglia* in the abdominal cavity. The only exception to the two-neuron arrangement is the innervation of the adrenal medulla. The catecholamine-secreting cells of the adrenal medulla are, in effect, modified postganglionic sympathetic neurons, and the nerves supplying the gland are equivalent to preganglionic fibres.

The parasympathetic nerves emerge from two separate regions of the CNS. The *cranial outflow* consists of preganglionic fibres in certain cranial nerves, namely the *oculomotor nerve* (carrying parasympathetic fibres destined for the eye), the *facial* and *glossopharyngeal nerves* (carrying fibres to the salivary glands and the nasopharynx) and the *vagus nerve* (carrying fibres to the thoracic and abdominal viscera). The ganglia lie scattered in close relation to the target organs; the postganglionic axons are very short compared with those of the sympathetic system. Parasympathetic fibres destined for the pelvic and abdominal viscera emerge as the *sacral outflow* from the spinal cord in a bundle of nerves known as the *nervi erigentes* (because stimulation of these nerves evokes genital erection – a fact of some importance to those responsible for artificial insemination of livestock). These fibres synapse in a group of scattered *pelvic ganglia*, whence the short postganglionic fibres run to target tissues such as the bladder, rectum and genitalia. The pelvic ganglia carry both sympathetic and parasympathetic fibres, and the two divisions are not anatomically distinct in this region.

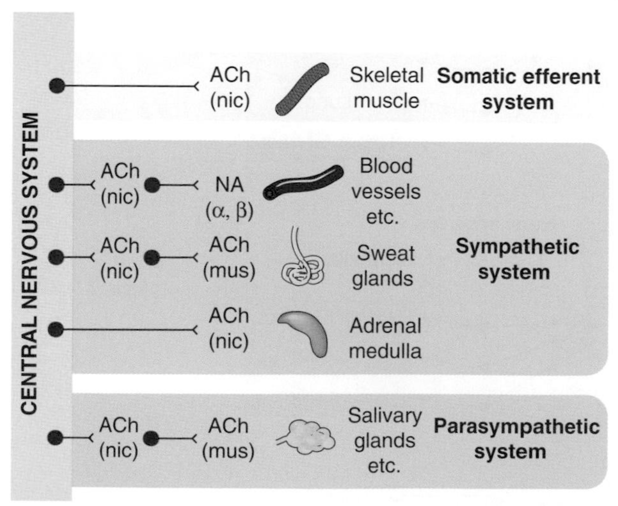

Fig. 13.2 Acetylcholine and noradrenaline as transmitters in the peripheral nervous system. The two main types of acetylcholine (ACh) receptor, nicotinic (nic) and muscarinic (mus) (see Ch. 14) and two types of adrenoceptor, α and β (see Ch. 15), are indicated. *NA*, Noradrenaline (norepinephrine).

The enteric nervous system (reviewed by Furness et al., 2014) consists of the neurons whose cell bodies lie in the intramural plexuses in the wall of the intestine. It is estimated that there are more cells in this system than in the spinal cord, and functionally they do not fit simply into the sympathetic/parasympathetic classification. Incoming nerves from both the sympathetic and the parasympathetic systems terminate on enteric neurons, as well as running directly to smooth muscle, glands and blood vessels. Some enteric neurons function as mechanoreceptors or chemoreceptors, providing local reflex pathways that can control gastrointestinal function without external inputs. The enteric nervous system is pharmacologically more complex than the sympathetic or parasympathetic systems, involving many neuropeptide and other transmitters (such as 5-hydroxytryptamine, nitric oxide and ATP; see Ch. 30).

In some places (e.g. in the visceral smooth muscle of the gut and bladder, and in the heart), the sympathetic and the parasympathetic systems produce opposite effects, but there are others where only one division of the autonomic system operates. The *sweat glands* and most *blood vessels*, for example, have only a sympathetic innervation, whereas the *ciliary muscle* of the eye has only a parasympathetic innervation. *Bronchial smooth muscle* has only a parasympathetic (constrictor) innervation (although its tone is highly sensitive to circulating adrenaline). *Resistance arteries* (see Ch. 21) have a sympathetic vasoconstrictor innervation but no parasympathetic innervation; instead, the constrictor tone is opposed by a background release of nitric oxide from the endothelial cells (see Ch. 19). There are other examples, such as the *salivary glands*, where the two systems produce similar, rather than opposing, effects.

It is therefore a mistake to think of the sympathetic and parasympathetic systems simply as physiological opponents. Each serves its own physiological function and can be more or less active in a particular organ or tissue according to the need of the moment. Cannon rightly emphasised the general role of the sympathetic system in evoking 'fight or flight' reactions in an emergency, but emergencies are rare for most animals. In everyday life, the autonomic nervous system functions continuously to control specific local functions, such as adjustments to postural changes, exercise or ambient temperature. The popular concept of a continuum from the extreme 'rest and digest' state (parasympathetic active, sympathetic quiescent) to the extreme emergency fight or flight state (sympathetic active, parasympathetic quiescent) is an oversimplification, albeit one that provides the student with a generally reliable *aide memoire*.

Table 13.1 lists some of the more important autonomic responses in humans.

Table 13.1 The main effects of the autonomic nervous system

Organ	Sympathetic effect	Adrenoceptor type[a]	Parasympathetic effect	Cholinoceptor type[a]
Heart				
Sinoatrial node	Rate ↑	β_1	Rate ↓	M_2
Atrial muscle	Force ↑	β_1	Force ↓	M_2
Atrioventricular node	Automaticity ↑	β_1	Conduction velocity ↓	M_2
			Atrioventricular block	M_2
Ventricular muscle	Automaticity ↑	β_1	No effect	M_2
	Force ↑			
Blood vessels				
ARTERIOLES				
Large coronary	Constriction	α_1, α_2	No effect	—
Small coronary	Dilatation	β_2	No effect	—
Muscle	Dilatation	β_2	No effect	—
Viscera, skin, brain	Constriction	α_1	No effect	—
Erectile tissue	Constriction	α_1	Dilatation	M_3[b]
VEINS	Constriction	α_1, α_2	No effect	—
	Dilatation	β_2	No effect	—
Viscera				
BRONCHI				
Smooth muscle	No sympathetic innervation, but dilated by circulating adrenaline (epinephrine)	β_2	Constriction	M_3
Glands	No effect	—	Secretion	M_3
GASTROINTESTINAL TRACT				
Smooth muscle	Motility ↓	α_1, α_2, β_2	Motility ↑	M_3
Sphincters	Constriction	α_1, α_2, β_2	Dilatation	M_3
Glands	No effect	—	Secretion	M_3
		—	Gastric acid secretion	M_1
BLADDER	Relaxation	β_2	Contraction	M_3
	Sphincter contraction	α_1	Sphincter relaxation	M_3
UTERUS				
Pregnant	Contraction	α_1	Variable	—
Non-pregnant	Relaxation	β_2		
MALE SEX ORGANS	Ejaculation	α_1	Erection	M_3[b]
Eye				
Pupil	Dilatation	α_1	Constriction	M_3
Ciliary muscle	Relaxation (slight)	β_2	Contraction	M_3
Skin				
Sweat glands	Secretion (mainly cholinergic via M_3 receptors)	—	No effect	—
Pilomotor	Piloerection	α_1	No effect	—
Salivary glands	Secretion	α_1, β_1, β_2	Secretion	M_3
Lacrimal glands	No effect	—	Secretion	M_3
Kidney	Renin secretion	β_1	No effect	—
Liver	Glycogenolysis	α_1, β_2	No effect	—
	Gluconeogenesis			
Adipose tissue[c]	Lipolysis	β_3	No effect	—
	Thermogenesis			
Pancreatic islets[c]	Insulin secretion ↓	α_2	No effect	—

[a]The adrenoceptor and cholinoceptor types shown are described more fully in Chapters 14 and 15. Transmitters other than acetylcholine and noradrenaline contribute to many of these responses (see Table 13.2).
[b]Vasodilator effects of M_3 receptors are due to nitric oxide release from endothelial cells (see Ch. 19).
[c]No direct innervation. Effect mediated by circulating adrenaline released from the adrenal medulla.

Basic anatomy and physiology of the autonomic nervous system

Anatomy

- The autonomic nervous system comprises three divisions: *sympathetic*, *parasympathetic* and *enteric*.
- The basic (two-neuron) pattern of the sympathetic and parasympathetic systems consists of a *preganglionic* neuron with a cell body in the CNS and a *postganglionic* neuron with a cell body in an autonomic ganglion.
- The parasympathetic system is connected to the CNS via:
  - cranial nerve outflow (III, VII, IX, X)
  - sacral outflow.
- Parasympathetic ganglia usually lie close to or within the target organ.
- Sympathetic outflow leaves the CNS in thoracic and lumbar spinal roots. Sympathetic ganglia form two paravertebral chains, plus some midline ganglia.
- The enteric nervous system consists of neurons lying in the intramural plexuses of the gastrointestinal tract. It receives inputs from sympathetic and parasympathetic systems, but can act on its own to control the motor and secretory functions of the intestine.

Physiology

- The autonomic system controls smooth muscle (visceral and vascular), exocrine (and some endocrine) secretions, rate and force of contraction of the heart and certain metabolic processes (e.g. glucose utilisation).
- Sympathetic and parasympathetic systems have opposing actions in some situations (e.g. control of heart rate, gastrointestinal smooth muscle), but not in others (e.g. salivary glands, ciliary muscle).
- Sympathetic activity increases in stress ('fight or flight' response), whereas parasympathetic activity predominates during satiation and repose. Both systems exert a continuous physiological control of specific organs under normal conditions, when the body is at neither extreme.

TRANSMITTERS IN THE AUTONOMIC NERVOUS SYSTEM

The two main neurotransmitters that operate in the autonomic system are **acetylcholine** and **noradrenaline**, whose sites of action are shown diagrammatically in Fig. 13.2. This diagram also shows the type of postsynaptic receptor with which the transmitters interact at the different sites (discussed more fully in Chs 14 and 15). Some general rules apply:

- All autonomic nerve fibres leaving the CNS release ACh, which acts on *nicotinic receptors* (although in autonomic ganglia a minor component of excitation is due to activation of *muscarinic receptors*; see Ch. 14).
- All postganglionic parasympathetic fibres release ACh, which acts on *muscarinic receptors*.
- All postganglionic sympathetic fibres (with one important exception) release noradrenaline, which may act on either α or β *adrenoceptors* (see Ch. 15). The exception is the sympathetic innervation of sweat glands, where transmission is due to ACh acting on muscarinic receptors. In some species, but not humans, vasodilatation in skeletal muscle is produced by cholinergic sympathetic nerve fibres.

ACh and noradrenaline are the grandees among autonomic transmitters and are central to understanding autonomic pharmacology. However, many other chemical mediators are also released by autonomic neurons (see later in this chapter), and their functional significance is gradually becoming clearer.

Transmitters of the autonomic nervous system

- The principal transmitters are **acetylcholine** (ACh) and **noradrenaline.**
- Preganglionic neurons are cholinergic, and ganglionic transmission occurs via nicotinic ACh receptors (nAChRs) (although excitatory muscarinic ACh receptors are also present on postganglionic cells).
- Postganglionic parasympathetic neurons are cholinergic, acting on muscarinic receptors in target organs.
- Postganglionic sympathetic neurons are mainly noradrenergic, although a few are cholinergic (e.g. sweat glands).
- Transmitters other than noradrenaline and ACh (NANC transmitters) are also abundant in the autonomic nervous system. The main ones are nitric oxide and vasoactive intestinal peptide (VIP) (parasympathetic), ATP and neuropeptide Y (NPY) (sympathetic). Others, such as 5-hydroxytryptamine, γ-aminobutyric acid (GABA) and dopamine, also play a role.
- Co-transmission, release of more than one transmitter from a nerve ending, is a general phenomenon.

SOME GENERAL PRINCIPLES OF CHEMICAL TRANSMISSION

The essential processes in chemical transmission – the release of mediators, and their interaction with receptors on target cells – are described in Chapters 4 and 3, respectively. Here we consider some general characteristics of chemical transmission of particular relevance to pharmacology. Many of these principles apply also to the CNS and are taken up again in Chapter 37.

PRESYNAPTIC MODULATION

The presynaptic terminals that synthesise and release transmitter in response to electrical activity in the nerve fibre are often themselves sensitive to transmitter substances and to other substances that may be produced locally in tissues (for review see Boehm and Kubista, 2002). Such presynaptic effects most commonly act to inhibit transmitter release, but may enhance it. Fig. 13.3A shows the inhibitory effect of adrenaline on the release of ACh (evoked by electrical stimulation) from the postganglionic parasympathetic nerve terminals of the intestine. The release of noradrenaline from nearby sympathetic nerve terminals can also inhibit release of ACh. Noradrenergic and cholinergic nerve terminals often lie close together in the myenteric plexus, so the opposing effects of the sympathetic and parasympathetic systems result not only from the opposite effects of the two transmitters on the smooth muscle cells, but also from the inhibition of ACh release by noradrenaline acting on the parasympathetic nerve terminals. A similar situation of mutual presynaptic inhibition exists in the heart, where noradrenaline inhibits ACh release and ACh also inhibits noradrenaline release. These are examples of *heterotropic interactions*, where one neurotransmitter affects the release of another. *Homotropic interactions* also occur, where the transmitter, by binding to presynaptic autoreceptors, affects the nerve terminals from which it is being released. This type of *autoinhibitory feedback* acts powerfully at noradrenergic nerve terminals (see Starke et al., 1989). Fig. 13.3B shows that in normal mice, noradrenaline release increases only slightly as the number of stimuli increases from 1 to 64. In transgenic mice lacking a specific type of presynaptic α_2 adrenoceptor (see Ch. 15), the amount released by the longer stimulus train is greatly increased, although the amount released by a single stimulus is unaffected. This is because with one or a few stimuli, there is no opportunity for autoinhibitory feedback to develop, whereas with longer trains the inhibition operates powerfully. A similar autoinhibitory feedback occurs with many transmitters, including ACh and 5-hydroxytryptamine.

In both the noradrenergic and cholinergic systems, the presynaptic autoreceptors are pharmacologically distinct from the postsynaptic receptors (see Fig. 13.4 and Chs 14 and 15), and there are drugs that act selectively, as agonists or antagonists, on the pre- or postsynaptic receptors.

Cholinergic and noradrenergic nerve terminals respond not only to ACh and noradrenaline, as described earlier, but also to other substances that are released as co-transmitters, such as ATP and NPY, or derived from other sources, including nitric oxide, prostaglandins, adenosine, dopamine, 5-hydroxytryptamine, GABA, opioid peptides, endocannabinoids and many other substances. The description of the autonomic nervous system represented in Fig. 13.2 is undoubtedly oversimplified. Fig. 13.4 shows some of the main presynaptic interactions between autonomic neurons and summarises the many chemical influences that regulate transmitter release from noradrenergic neurons.

Presynaptic receptors regulate transmitter release mainly by affecting Ca^{2+} entry into the nerve terminal (see Ch. 4), but also by other mechanisms (see Kubista and Boehm, 2006). Most presynaptic receptors are of the G protein–coupled type (see Ch. 3), which control the function of calcium channels and potassium channels either through a direct interaction of G proteins with the channels or by second messengers that regulate the state of phosphorylation of the channel proteins. Transmitter release is inhibited when calcium channel opening is inhibited, or when potassium channel opening is increased (see Ch. 4); in many cases, both mechanisms operate simultaneously. Presynaptic regulation by receptors linked directly to ion channels (ionotropic receptors; see Ch. 3) rather than to G proteins also occurs (see Dorostkar and Boehm, 2008). nAChRs are particularly important in this respect. They can either facilitate or inhibit the release of other transmitters, such as glutamate (see Ch. 38), and most of the nAChRs expressed in the CNS are located presynaptically. Another example is the $GABA_A$ receptor, whose action is to inhibit transmitter release (see Chs 4 and 37). Other ionotropic receptors, such

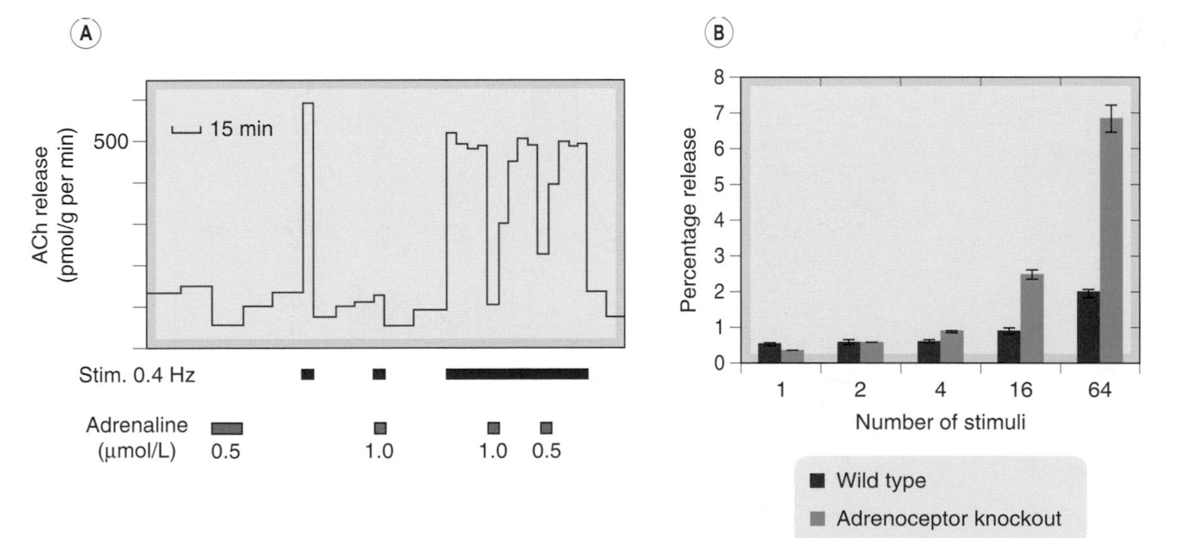

Fig. 13.3 Examples of presynaptic inhibition. (A) Inhibitory effect of adrenaline on acetylcholine (ACh) release from postganglionic parasympathetic nerves in the guinea pig ileum. The intramural nerves were stimulated electrically where indicated, and the ACh released into the bathing fluid determined by bioassay. Adrenaline strongly inhibits ACh release. (B) Noradrenaline (NA) release from mouse hippocampal slices in response to trains of electrical stimuli. *Red bars* show normal (wild-type) mice. *Blue bars* show α_2-adrenoceptor knockout mice. The lack of presynaptic autoinhibition in the knockout mice results in a large increase in release with a long stimulus train but does not affect release by fewer than four stimuli, because the autoinhibition takes a few seconds to develop. This example is taken from a study of brain noradrenergic nerves, but similar findings have been made on sympathetic nerves. (Panel [A] from Vizi, E.S., 1979. Prog. Neurobiol. 12, 181; panel [B] redrawn from Trendelenburg, et al., 2001. Naunyn Schmiedeberg's Arch. Pharmacol. 364, 117–130.)

as those activated by ATP and 5-hydroxytryptamine (see Chs 16 and 39), have similar effects on transmitter release.

POSTSYNAPTIC MODULATION

Chemical mediators often act on postsynaptic structures, including neurons, smooth muscle cells, cardiac muscle cells, and so on, in such a way that their excitability or spontaneous firing pattern is altered. In many cases, as with presynaptic modulation, this is caused by changes in calcium and/or potassium channel function. We give only a few examples here.

- The slow excitatory effect produced by various mediators, including ACh and peptides such as

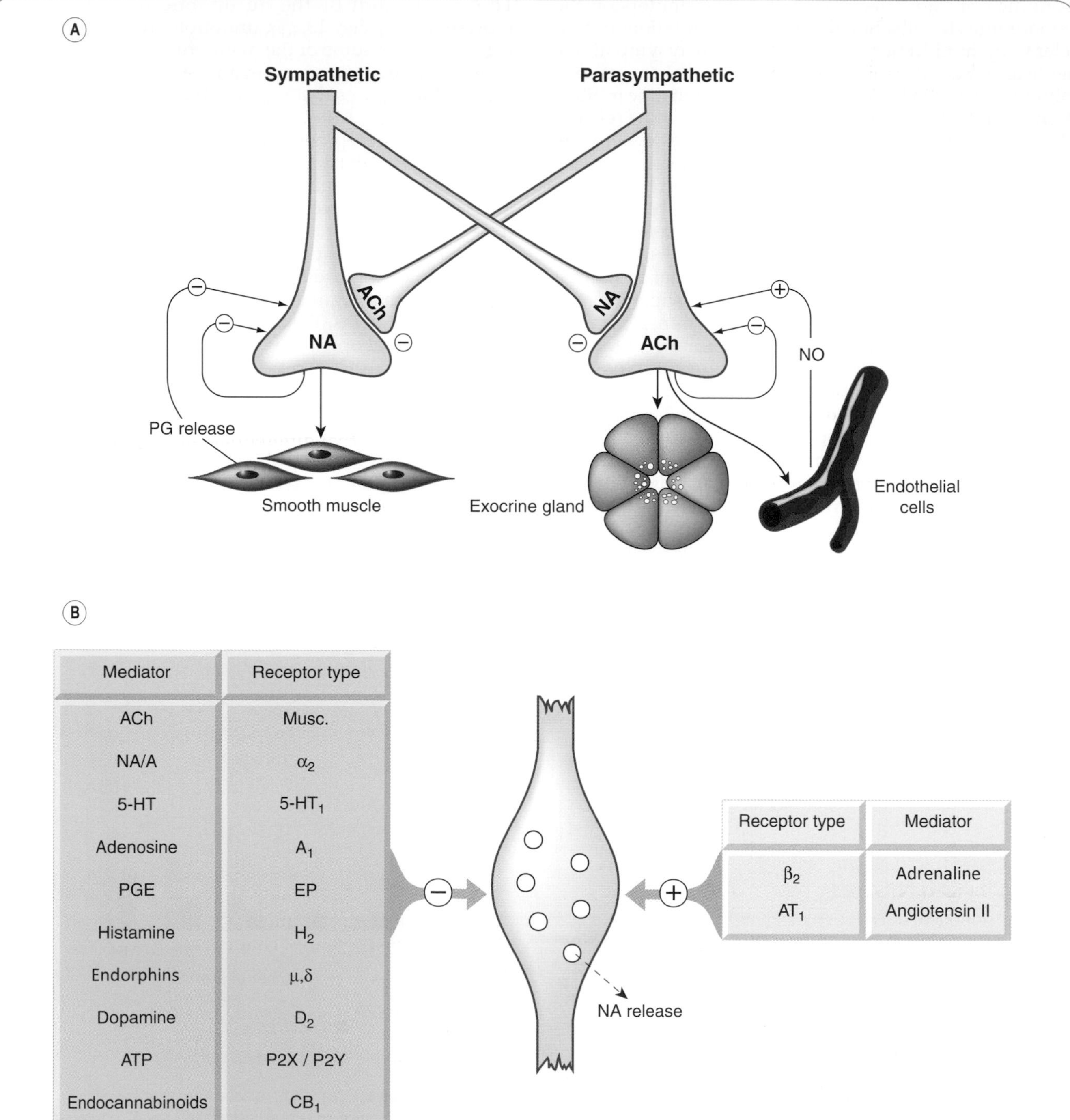

Fig. 13.4 Presynaptic regulation of transmitter release from noradrenergic and cholinergic nerve terminals. (A) Postulated homotropic and heterotropic interactions between sympathetic and parasympathetic nerves. (B) Some of the known inhibitory and facilitatory influences on noradrenaline release from sympathetic nerve endings. *ATP,* Adenosine triphosphate; *5-HT,* 5-hydroxytryptamine; *ACh,* acetylcholine; *NA,* noradrenaline; *NO,* nitric oxide; *PG,* prostaglandin; *PGE,* prostaglandin E.

Neuromodulation and presynaptic interactions

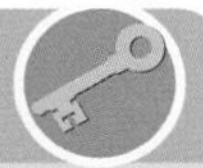

- As well as functioning directly as neurotransmitters, chemical mediators may regulate:
  - presynaptic transmitter release
  - neuronal excitability.
- Both are examples of *neuromodulation* and generally involve second messenger regulation of membrane ion channels.
- Presynaptic receptors may inhibit or increase transmitter release, the former being more important.
- Inhibitory *presynaptic autoreceptors* occur on noradrenergic and cholinergic neurons, causing each transmitter to inhibit its own release (*autoinhibitory feedback*).
- Many endogenous mediators (e.g. GABA, prostaglandins, opioid and other peptides), as well as the transmitters themselves, exert presynaptic control (mainly inhibitory) over autonomic transmitter release.

substance P, results mainly from a decrease in K^+ permeability. Conversely, the inhibitory effect of various opioid peptides in the gut is mainly due to increased K^+ permeability.

- **NPY**, is released as a co-transmitter with noradrenaline at many sympathetic nerve endings and acts on smooth muscle cells to enhance the vasoconstrictor effect of noradrenaline, thus greatly facilitating transmission.

The pre- and postsynaptic effects described previously are often described as *neuromodulation*, because the mediator acts to increase or decrease the efficacy of synaptic transmission without participating directly as a transmitter. Many neuropeptides, for example, affect membrane ion channels in such a way as to increase or decrease excitability and thus control the firing pattern of the cell. Neuromodulation is loosely defined but, in general, involves slower processes (taking seconds to days) than neurotransmission (which occurs in milliseconds), and operates through cascades of intracellular messengers (see Ch. 3) rather than directly on ligand-gated ion channels.

TRANSMITTERS OTHER THAN ACETYLCHOLINE AND NORADRENALINE

As mentioned earlier, ACh and noradrenaline are not the only autonomic transmitters. The rather grudging realisation that this was so dawned many years ago when it was noticed that autonomic transmission in many organs could not be completely blocked by drugs that abolish responses to these transmitters. The dismal but tenacious term *non-adrenergic non-cholinergic* (NANC) transmission was coined. Later, fluorescence and immunocytochemical methods showed that neurons, including autonomic neurons, contain many potential transmitters, often several in the same cell. Compounds now known to function as NANC transmitters include ATP, VIP, NPY and nitric oxide (Fig. 13.5 and Table 13.2), which function at postganglionic nerve terminals, as well as substance P, 5-hydroxytryptamine, GABA and dopamine, which play a role in ganglionic transmission (see Lundberg, 1996, for a comprehensive review).

CO-TRANSMISSION

It is the rule rather than the exception that neurons release more than one transmitter or modulator (see Lundberg, 1996), each of which interacts with specific receptors and produces effects, often both pre- and postsynaptically. The example of noradrenaline/ATP co-transmission at sympathetic nerve endings is shown in Fig. 13.5, and the best-studied examples and mechanisms are summarised in Table 13.2 and Figs 13.6 and 13.7.

What, one might well ask, could be the functional advantage of co-transmission, compared with a single transmitter acting on various different receptors? The possible advantages include the following:

- One constituent of the cocktail (e.g. a peptide) may be removed or inactivated more slowly than the other (e.g. a monoamine), and therefore reach targets further from the site of release and produce longer-lasting effects. This appears to be the case, for example, with ACh and gonadotrophin-releasing hormone in sympathetic ganglia.
- The balance of the transmitters released may vary under different conditions. At sympathetic nerve terminals, for example, where noradrenaline and NPY are stored in separate vesicles, NPY is preferentially released at high stimulation frequencies, so that differential release of one or other mediator may result from varying impulse patterns. Differential effects of presynaptic modulators are also possible; for example, activation of β adrenoceptors inhibits ATP release while enhancing noradrenaline release from sympathetic nerve terminals.

TERMINATION OF TRANSMITTER ACTION

Chemically transmitting synapses other than the peptidergic variety invariably incorporate a mechanism for disposing rapidly of the released transmitter, so that its action remains brief and localised. At cholinergic synapses (see Ch. 14), the released ACh is inactivated very rapidly in the synaptic cleft by *acetylcholinesterase*. In most other cases (see Fig. 13.8), transmitter action is terminated by active reuptake into the presynaptic nerve, or into smooth muscle. Such reuptake depends on transporter proteins (see Ch. 4), each being specific for a particular transmitter. The major class (Na^+/Cl^- co-transporters), whose molecular structure and function are well understood (see Torres et al., 2003; Gether et al., 2006), consists of a family of membrane proteins, each possessing 12 transmembrane helices. Different members of the family show selectivity for each of the main monoamine transmitters (e.g. the noradrenaline [norepinephrine] transporter [NET]; the serotonin transporter [SERT], which transports 5-hydroxytryptamine; and the dopamine transporter [DAT]) (see Manepalli et al., 2012). These transporters are important targets for psychoactive drugs, particularly antidepressants (see Ch. 48), anxiolytic drugs (see Ch. 45) and stimulants (see Ch. 49). Transporters for glycine and GABA belong to the same family.

Vesicular transporters (see Ch. 4), which load synaptic vesicles with transmitter molecules, are closely related to plasma membrane transporters. Membrane transporters usually act as co-transporters of Na^+, Cl^- and

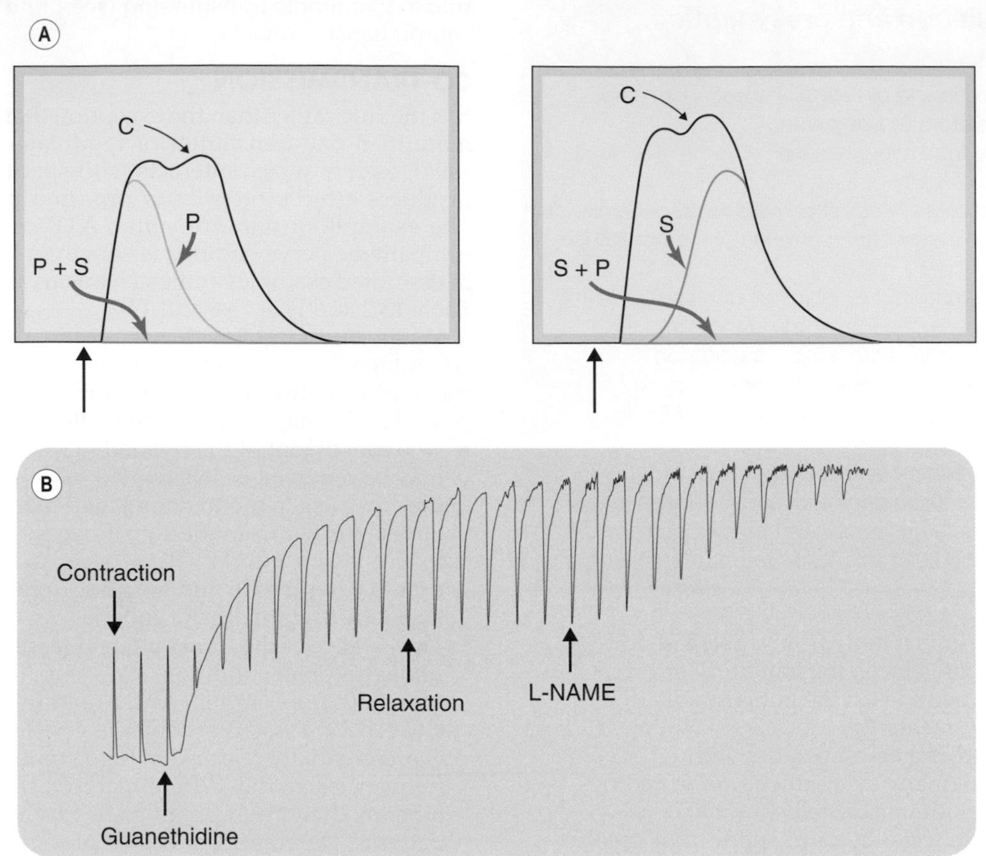

Fig. 13.5 ATP and nitric oxide as neurotransmitters. (A) Noradrenaline and ATP are co-transmitters released from the same nerves in the guinea pig vas deferens. Contractions of the tissue are shown in response to a single electrical stimulus causing excitation of sympathetic nerve endings. With no blocking drugs present, a twin-peaked response is produced *(C)*. The early peak is selectively abolished by the ATP antagonist suramin *(S)*, while the late peak is blocked by the α_1-adrenoceptor antagonist prazosin *(P)*. The response is completely eliminated when both drugs are present. (B) Noradrenaline and nitric oxide are neurotransmitters in the rat anococcygeus muscle but are probably released from different nerves. The nerves innervating the muscle were stimulated with brief trains of pulses. Initially, nerve stimulation evoked rapid contractions by releasing noradrenaline. Application of guanethidine blocked stimulus-evoked noradrenaline release and raised the tone of the preparation revealing nerve-evoked relaxations that were blocked by L-NAME, an inhibitor of nitric oxide synthesis. (Panel [A] reproduced with permission from von Kugelglen, I., Starke, K., 1991. Trends Pharmacol. Sci. 12, 319–324; data in panel [B] are from a student practical class at Glasgow Caledonian University, courtesy of A. Corbett.)

transmitter molecules, and it is the inwardly directed 'downhill' gradient for Na^+ that provides the energy for the inward 'uphill' movement of the transmitter. The simultaneous transport of ions along with the transmitter means that the process generates a net current across the membrane, which can be measured directly and used to monitor the transport process. Very similar mechanisms are responsible for other physiological transport processes, such as glucose uptake (see Ch. 31) and renal tubular transport of amino acids. Because it is the electrochemical gradient for sodium that drives the inward transport of transmitter molecules, a reduction of this gradient can reduce or even reverse the flow of transmitter. This is probably not important under physiological conditions, but when the nerve terminals are depolarised or abnormally loaded with sodium (e.g. in ischaemic conditions), the resulting non-vesicular release of transmitter (and inhibition of the normal synaptic reuptake mechanism) may play a significant role in the effects of ischaemia on tissues such as heart and brain (see Chs 20 and 40). Studies with transgenic 'knockout' mice (see Torres et al., 2003) show that the store of releasable transmitter is substantially depleted in animals lacking the membrane transporter, showing that synthesis is unable to maintain the store if the recapture mechanism is disabled. As with receptors (see Ch. 3), many genetic polymorphisms of transporter genes occur in humans, finding associations with various neurological, cardiovascular and psychiatric disorders has provided insight into their aetiology and may explain altered responsiveness to drugs (see Reynolds et al., 2014).

As we shall see in subsequent chapters, both plasma membrane and vesicular transporters are targets for various drugs, and defining the physiological role and pharmacological properties of these molecules has been the focus of much research.

Table 13.2 Examples of non-adrenergic non-cholinergic transmitters and co-transmitters in the peripheral nervous system

Transmitter	Location	Function
Non-peptides		
ATP	Postganglionic sympathetic neurons	Fast depolarisation/contraction of smooth muscle cells (e.g. blood vessels, vas deferens)
GABA, 5-HT	Enteric neurons	Peristaltic reflex
Dopamine	Some sympathetic neurons (e.g. kidney)	Vasodilatation
Nitric oxide	Pelvic nerves Gastric nerves	Erection Gastric emptying
Peptides		
Neuropeptide Y	Postganglionic sympathetic neurons	Facilitates constrictor action of noradrenaline; inhibits noradrenaline release (e.g. blood vessels)
VIP	Parasympathetic nerves to salivary glands NANC innervation of airways smooth muscle	Vasodilatation; co-transmitter with acetylcholine Bronchodilatation
Gonadotrophin-releasing hormone	Sympathetic ganglia	Slow depolarisation; co-transmitter with acetylcholine
Substance P	Sympathetic ganglia, enteric neurons	Slow depolarisation; co-transmitter with acetylcholine
Calcitonin gene-related peptide	Non-myelinated sensory neurons	Vasodilatation; vascular leakage; neurogenic inflammation

ATP, Adenosine triphosphate; *GABA,* gamma-aminobutyric acid; *5-HT,* 5-hydroxytryptamine; *NANC,* non-adrenergic non-cholinergic; *VIP,* vasoactive intestinal peptide.

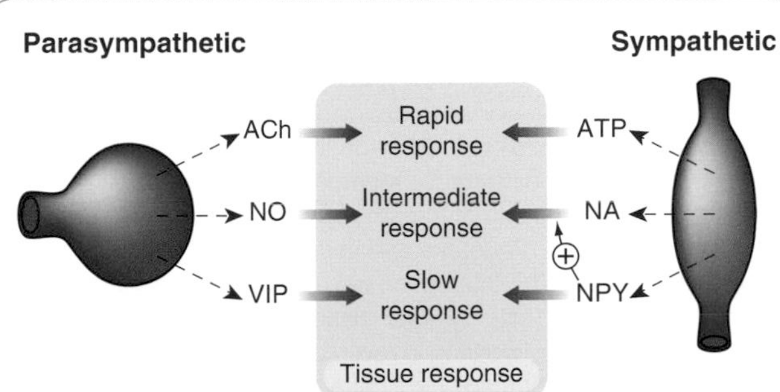

Fig. 13.6 The main co-transmitters at postganglionic parasympathetic and sympathetic neurons. The different mediators generally give rise to fast, intermediate and slow responses of the target organ. *ACh,* Acetylcholine; *ATP,* adenosine triphosphate; *NA,* noradrenaline; *NO,* nitric oxide; *NPY,* neuropeptide Y; *VIP,* vasoactive intestinal peptide.

DENERVATION SUPERSENSITIVITY

It is known, mainly from the work of Cannon on the sympathetic system, that if a nerve is cut and its terminals are allowed to degenerate, the structure supplied by it becomes supersensitive to the transmitter substance released by the terminals. Thus skeletal muscle, which normally responds to injected ACh only if a large dose is given directly into the arterial blood supply, will, after denervation, respond by contracture to much smaller amounts. Other organs, such as salivary glands and blood vessels, show similar supersensitivity to ACh and noradrenaline when the postganglionic nerves degenerate, and there is evidence that pathways in the CNS show the same phenomenon.

Several mechanisms contribute to denervation supersensitivity, and the extent and mechanism of the phenomenon varies from organ to organ. Reported mechanisms include the following (see Luis and Noel, 2009).

- Proliferation of receptors. This is particularly marked in skeletal muscle, in which the number of ACh receptors increases 20-fold or more after denervation; the receptors, normally localised to the endplate region of the fibres (see Ch. 14), spread over the whole surface. Elsewhere, increases in receptor number are much smaller, or absent altogether.
- Loss of mechanisms for transmitter removal. At noradrenergic synapses, the loss of neuronal uptake of noradrenaline (see Ch. 15) contributes substantially to denervation supersensitivity. At cholinergic synapses, a partial loss of cholinesterase occurs (see Ch. 14).
- Increased postjunctional responsiveness. Smooth muscle cells become partly depolarised and hyperexcitable after denervation (due in part to reduced Na^+-K^+-ATPase activity; see Ch. 4) and this phenomenon contributes appreciably to their supersensitivity. Increased Ca^{2+} signalling, resulting in enhanced excitation–contraction coupling, may also occur.

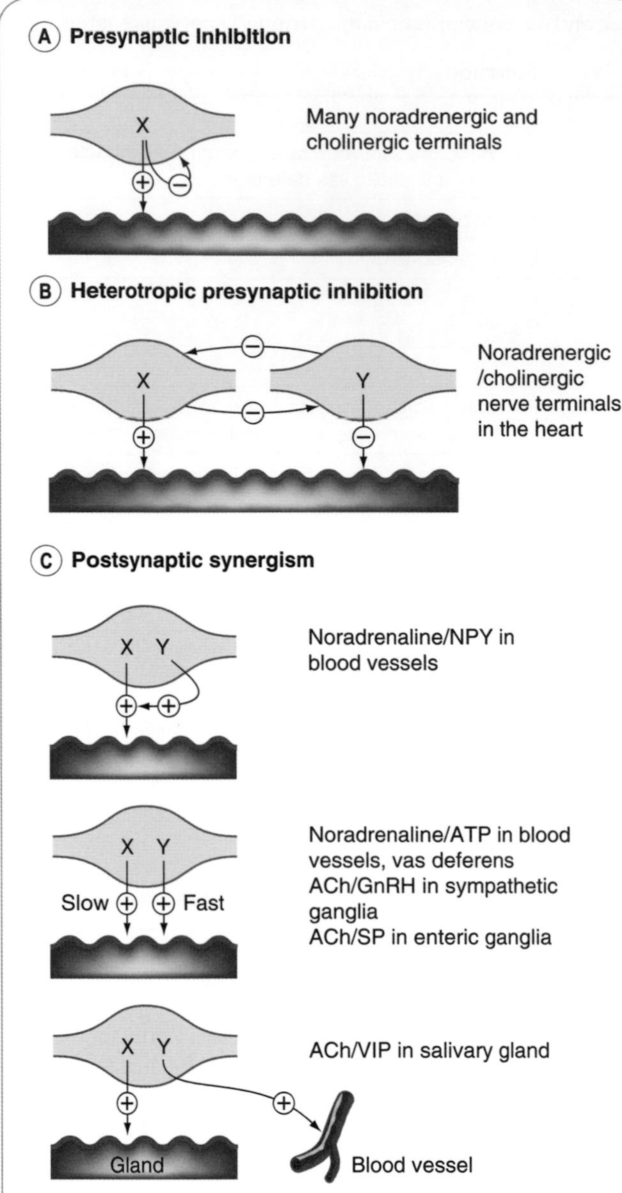

Fig. 13.7 Co-transmission and neuromodulation – some examples. (A) Presynaptic inhibition. (B) Heterotropic presynaptic inhibition. (C) Postsynaptic synergism. *ACh,* Acetylcholine; *ATP,* adenosine triphosphate; *GnRH,* gonadotrophin-releasing hormone (luteinising hormone-releasing hormone); *NPY,* neuropeptide Y; *SP,* substance P; *VIP,* vasoactive intestinal peptide.

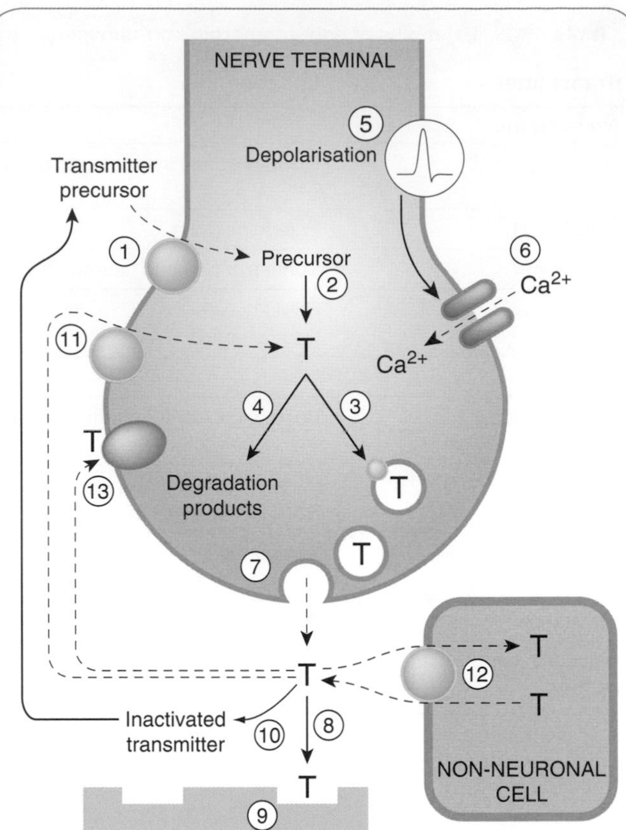

Fig. 13.8 The main processes involved in synthesis, storage and release of amine and amino acid transmitters. *1,* Uptake of precursors; *2,* synthesis of transmitter; *3,* uptake/transport of transmitter into vesicles; *4,* degradation of surplus transmitter; *5,* depolarisation by propagated action potential; *6,* influx of Ca^{2+} in response to depolarisation; *7,* release of transmitter by exocytosis; *8,* diffusion to postsynaptic membrane; *9,* interaction with postsynaptic receptors; *10,* inactivation of transmitter; *11,* reuptake of transmitter or degradation products by nerve terminals; *12,* uptake and release of transmitter by non-neuronal cells; and *13,* interaction with presynaptic receptors. The transporters *(11 and 12)* can release transmitter under certain conditions by working in reverse. These processes are well characterised for many transmitters (e.g. acetylcholine, monoamines, amino acids, ATP). Peptide mediators differ in that they may be synthesised and packaged in the cell body rather than the terminals.

Supersensitivity can occur, but is less marked, when transmission is interrupted by processes other than nerve section. Pharmacological block of ganglionic transmission, for example, if sustained for a few days, causes some degree of supersensitivity of the target organs, and long-term blockade of postsynaptic receptors also causes receptors to proliferate, leaving the cell supersensitive when the blocking agent is removed. Phenomena such as this are of importance in the CNS, where such supersensitivity can cause 'rebound' effects when drugs that impair synaptic transmission are given for some time and then discontinued.

BASIC STEPS IN NEUROCHEMICAL TRANSMISSION: SITES OF DRUG ACTION

Fig. 13.8 summarises the main processes that occur in a classical chemically transmitting synapse, and provides a useful basis for understanding the actions of the many different classes of drug, discussed in later chapters, that act by facilitating or blocking neurochemical transmission.

All the steps shown in Fig. 13.8 (except for transmitter diffusion, step 8) can be influenced by drugs. For example, the enzymes involved in synthesis or inactivation of the transmitter can be inhibited, as can the transport systems responsible for the neuronal and vesicular uptake of the transmitter or its precursor. The actions of the great majority of drugs that act on the peripheral nervous system (see Chs 14 and 15) and the CNS fit into this general scheme.

REFERENCES AND FURTHER READING

General references

Bacq, Z.M., 1975. Chemical Transmission of Nerve Impulses: A Historical Sketch. Pergamon Press, Oxford.

Burnstock, G., 2009. Autonomic neurotransmission: 60 years since sir henry dale. Ann. Rev. Pharmacol. 49, 1–30.

Furness, J.B., Callaghan, B.P., Rivera, L.R., Cho, H.J., 2014. The enteric nervous system and gastrointestinal innervation: integrated local and central control. Adv. Exp. Med. Biol. 817, 39–71.

Kandel, E.R., Koester, J.D., Mack, S.H., Siegelbaum, S.A., 2021. Principles of Neural Science, sixth ed. Elsevier, New York.

Luis, E.M.Q., Noel, F., 2009. Mechanisms of adaptive supersensitivity in vas deferens. Auton. Neurosci. 146, 38–46.

Robertson, D.W., Biaggioni, I., Burnstock, G., Low, P.A., Paton, J.F.R. (Eds.), 2012. Primer on the Autonomic Nervous System, third ed. Academic Press, London.

Valenstein, E.S., 2005. The War of the Soups and the Sparks. Columbia University Press, New York.

Presynaptic modulation

Boehm, S., Kubista, H., 2002. Fine tuning of sympathetic transmitter release via ionotropic and metabotropic receptors. Pharm. Rev. 54, 43–99.

Dorostkar, M.M., Boehm, S., 2008. Presynaptic ionotropic receptors. Handb. Exp. Pharmacol. 184, 479–527.

Kubista, H., Boehm, S., 2006. Molecular mechanisms underlying the modulation of exocytotic noradrenaline release via presynaptic receptors. Pharm. Ther. 112, 213–242.

Starke, K., Gothert, M., Kilbinger, H., 1989. Modulation of neurotransmitter release by presynaptic autoreceptors. Physiol. Rev. 69, 864–989.

Co-transmission

Lundberg, J.M., 1996. Pharmacology of co-transmission in the autonomic nervous system: integrative aspects on amines, neuropeptides, adenosine triphosphate, amino acids and nitric oxide. Pharmacol. Rev. 48, 114–192.

Transporters

Gether, U., Andersen, P.H., Larsson, O.M., et al., 2006. Neurotransmitter transporters: molecular function of important drug targets. Trends Pharmacol. Sci. 27, 375–383.

Manepalli, S., Surratt, C.K., Madura, J.D., Nolan, T.L., 2012. Monoamine transporter structure, function, dynamics, and drug discovery: a computational perspective. AAPS J. 14, 820-831.

Reynolds, G.P., McGowan, O.O., Dalton, C.F., 2014. Pharmacogenomics in psychiatry: the relevance of receptor and transporter polymorphisms. Br. J. Clin. Pharmacol. 77, 654–672.

Torres, G.E., Gainetdinov, R.R., Caron, M.G., 2003. Plasma membrane monoamine transporters: structure, regulation and function. Nat. Rev. Neurosci. 4, 13–25.

14 Cholinergic transmission

OVERVIEW

This chapter is concerned mainly with cholinergic transmission in the periphery, and the ways in which drugs affect it. We describe the different types of acetylcholine (ACh) receptors and their functions, as well as the synthesis, release and degradation of ACh. Drugs that act on ACh receptors, many of which have clinical uses, are described, as are drugs that inhibit cholinesterase enzymes. Cholinergic mechanisms in the central nervous system (CNS) and their relevance to dementia are discussed in Chapters 39 and 40.

MUSCARINIC AND NICOTINIC ACTIONS OF ACETYLCHOLINE

The discovery of the pharmacological action of ACh came, paradoxically, from work on adrenal glands, extracts of which were known to produce a rise in blood pressure owing to their content of adrenaline (epinephrine). In 1900, Reid Hunt found that after adrenaline had been removed from such extracts, they produced a fall in blood pressure instead of a rise. He established that this was likely due to the presence of ACh, the physiological role of which became apparent when Loewi, Dale and their colleagues demonstrated its transmitter role in the 1930s.

Analysing the pharmacological actions of ACh in 1914, Dale distinguished two types of activity, which he designated as *muscarinic* and *nicotinic* because they mimicked, respectively, the effects of **muscarine**, the active principle of the poisonous mushroom *Amanita muscaria*, and of **nicotine**. Muscarinic actions closely resemble the effects of parasympathetic stimulation (see Table 13.1). After the muscarinic effects have been blocked by **atropine**, larger doses of ACh produce nicotine-like effects, which include:

- stimulation of all autonomic ganglia
- stimulation of voluntary muscle
- secretion of adrenaline from the adrenal medulla.

The muscarinic and nicotinic actions of ACh are demonstrated in Fig. 14.1. Bolus intravenous doses of ACh produce a transient fall in blood pressure due to arteriolar vasodilatation and slowing of the heart – muscarinic effects that are abolished by atropine. A large dose of ACh given after atropine produces nicotinic effects: an initial rise in blood pressure due to a stimulation of sympathetic ganglia and consequent vasoconstriction, and a secondary rise resulting from secretion of adrenaline.

Dale's pharmacological classification corresponds closely to the main physiological functions of ACh in the body. The muscarinic actions correspond to those of ACh released at postganglionic parasympathetic nerve endings, with two significant exceptions:

1. ACh causes generalised vasodilatation, even though most blood vessels have no parasympathetic innervation. This is an indirect effect: ACh (like many other mediators) acts on vascular endothelial cells to release **nitric oxide** (see Chs 19 and 21), which relaxes smooth muscle. The physiological function of this is uncertain, because ACh is not normally present in circulating blood.
2. ACh evokes secretion from sweat glands, which are innervated by cholinergic fibres of the sympathetic nervous system (see Table 13.1).

The nicotinic actions correspond to those of ACh acting on autonomic ganglia of the sympathetic and parasympathetic systems, the motor endplate of voluntary muscle and the secretory cells of the adrenal medulla.

ACETYLCHOLINE RECEPTORS

Although Dale himself dismissed the concept of receptors as sophistry rather than science, his functional classification provided the basis for distinguishing muscarinic and nicotinic receptors, the two major classes of ACh receptor (see Ch. 3 and Southan et al., 2016). Many important therapeutic drugs target these receptors, and despite their long and distinguished history, recent advances continue to open new opportunities for drug development in both muscarinic (Kruse et al., 2014; He et al., 2015) and nicotinic (Dinely et al., 2015) fields, especially for CNS indications (see Chs 39 and 40).

NICOTINIC RECEPTORS

All nicotinic ACh receptors (nAChRs) are pentameric structures that function as ligand-gated ion channels (see Fig. 3.4). nAChRs fall into three main classes – the muscle, ganglionic and CNS types – whose subunit compositions are summarised in Table 14.1. Muscle receptors are confined to the skeletal neuromuscular junction; ganglionic receptors are responsible for fast transmission at sympathetic and parasympathetic ganglia; and CNS-type receptors are widespread in the brain, and are heterogeneous with respect to their molecular composition and location (see Ch. 39). Most of the CNS-type nAChRs are located presynaptically and serve to facilitate or inhibit the release of other mediators, such as glutamate and dopamine.

The five subunits that form the receptor–channel complex are similar in structure, and so far 17 different members of the family have been identified and cloned, designated α (10 types), β (4 types) and γ, δ and ε (1 of each). The five subunits each possess four membrane-spanning helical domains, and one of these helices (M_2) from each subunit defines the central pore (see Ch. 3). nAChR subtypes generally contain

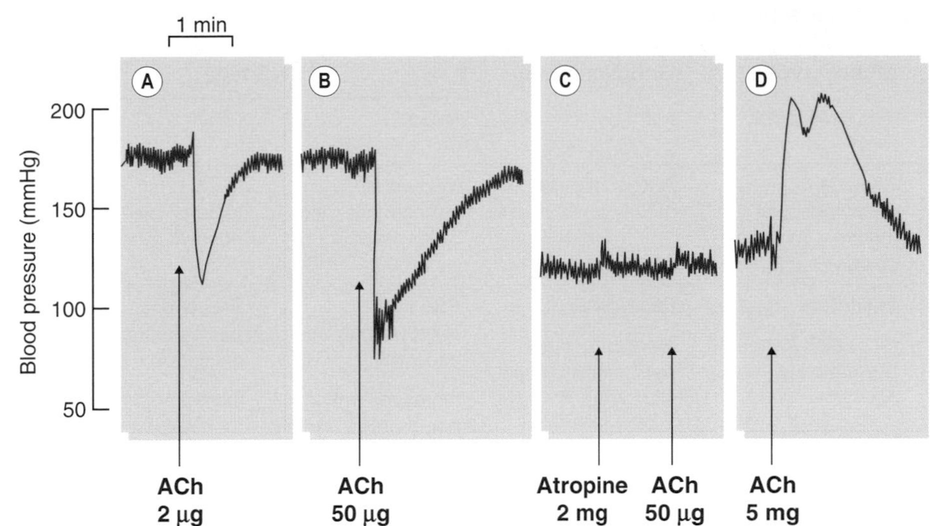

Fig. 14.1 Dale's experiment showing that acetylcholine (ACh) produces two kinds of effect on blood pressure. Arterial pressure was recorded with a mercury manometer in a cat with spinal cord intact but brainstem control centres surgically disconnected. (A) ACh causes a fall in blood pressure due to vasodilatation. (B) A larger dose also produces bradycardia. Both (A) and (B) are muscarinic effects. (C) After atropine (muscarinic antagonist), the same dose of ACh has no effect. (D) Still under the influence of atropine, a much larger dose of ACh causes a rise in blood pressure due to stimulation of sympathetic ganglia, accompanied by tachycardia, followed by a secondary rise due to release of adrenaline from the adrenal gland, resulting from its action on nicotinic receptors. (From Burn, J.H., 1963. Autonomic Pharmacology. Blackwell, Oxford.)

both α and β subunits, the exception being the homomeric α_7 subtype found mainly in the brain (see Ch. 39). The adult muscle receptor has the composition α2β1ε1δ1, while the main ganglionic subtype is α2β3 (for more detail on which subunits are present in the different subtypes see Southan et al., 2016). The two binding sites for ACh (both of which need to be occupied to cause the channel to open) reside at the interface between the extracellular domain of each of the α subunits and its neighbour.

The patch clamp technique has enabled the function of the nAChR-channel complex to be studied in their physiological environment at the molecular level (see Bouzat and Sine, 2018, for a review). As explained in Chapter 3 nicotinic agonists open a pore, approximately 0.7 nm diameter, that penetrates the central core of the pentameric complex and, when the receptor complex is activated, permits cation flux across the cell membrane (see Fig. 3.4). The channel conductance produced by different agonists is the same, whereas the mean channel lifetime varies according to the efficacy of the agonist. The mean open time is determined mainly by the closing rate constant α for the reaction $AR \rightleftarrows AR^*$, where A is the agonist and R* is the activated conformation of the receptor (see Fig. 2.1). This rate constant varies from drug to drug.

The diversity of the nAChR family (for details see Kalamida et al., 2007), which emerged from cloning studies in the 1980s, took pharmacologists somewhat by surprise. Although they knew that the neuromuscular and ganglionic synapses differed pharmacologically and suspected that cholinergic synapses in the CNS might be different again, the molecular diversity goes far beyond this, and its functional significance is only slowly emerging.

The different action of agonists and antagonists on neuromuscular, ganglionic and brain synapses is of practical importance and mainly reflects the differences between the muscle and neuronal nAChRs (Table 14.1).

MUSCARINIC RECEPTORS

Muscarinic receptors (mAChRs) are typical G protein–coupled receptors (see Ch. 3), and five molecular subtypes (M_1–M_5) are known. The odd-numbered members of the group (M_1, M_3, M_5) couple with G_q to activate the inositol phosphate pathway (see Ch. 3), while the even-numbered receptors (M_2, M_4) act through G_i to open potassium (K_{ir}) channels, causing membrane hyperpolarisation which inhibits voltage-dependent Ca^{2+}-channels, and to inhibit adenylyl cyclase. G_q- and G_i-coupled muscarinic receptors also activate the mitogen-activated protein kinase pathway. The location and pharmacology of the various receptor subtypes are summarised in Table 14.2.

M_1 receptors ('neural') are found mainly on CNS and peripheral neurons and on gastric parietal cells. They mediate excitatory effects, for example, the slow muscarinic excitation mediated by ACh in sympathetic ganglia (see Ch. 13) and central neurons. This excitation is produced by a decrease in K^+ conductance, which causes membrane depolarisation. Deficiency of this kind of ACh-mediated effect in the brain is possibly associated with dementia (see Ch. 40), although transgenic M_1-receptor knockout mice show only slight cognitive impairment. M_1 receptors are also implicated in the increase of gastric acid secretion following vagal stimulation (see Ch. 30).

M_2 receptors ('cardiac') occur in the heart, and on the presynaptic terminals of peripheral and central neurons. They exert inhibitory effects, mainly by increasing K^+ conductance and by inhibiting calcium channels (see Ch. 4). M_2-receptor activation is responsible for cholinergic inhibition of the heart, as well as presynaptic inhibition in the CNS and periphery (see Ch. 13). They are also co-expressed with M_3 receptors in visceral smooth muscle and contribute to the smooth-muscle-stimulating effect of muscarinic agonists in several organs.

Table 14.1 Nicotinic receptor subtypes[a]

	Muscle type	Ganglion type	CNS type		Notes
Main molecular form	$(\alpha1)_2\beta1\delta\varepsilon$ (adult form)	$(\alpha3)_2(\beta2)_3$	$(\alpha4)_2(\beta2)_3$	$(\alpha7)_5$	–
Main synaptic location	Skeletal neuromuscular junction: mainly postsynaptic	Autonomic ganglia: mainly postsynaptic	Many brain regions: pre- and postsynaptic	Many brain regions: pre- and postsynaptic	–
Membrane response	Excitatory Increased cation permeability (mainly Na^+, K^+)	Excitatory Increased cation permeability (mainly Na^+, K^+)	Pre- and postsynaptic excitation Increased cation permeability (mainly Na^+, K^+)	Pre- and postsynaptic excitation Increased cation permeability	$(\alpha7)_5$ receptor produces large Ca^{2+} entry, evoking transmitter release
Agonists	Acetylcholine Carbachol Succinylcholin	Acetylcholine Carbachol Nicotine Epibatidine Dimethylphenyl-piperazinium	Nicotine Epibatidine Acetylcholine Varenicline[b]	Epibatidine Dimethylphenyl-piperazinium Varenicline[b]	–
Antagonists	Tubocurarine Pancuronium Atracurium Vecuronium α-Bungarotoxin α-Conotoxin	Mecamylamine Trimetaphan Hexamethonium α-Conotoxin	Mecamylamine Methylaconitine	α-Bungarotoxin α-Conotoxin Methylaconitine	–

[a]This table shows only the main subtypes expressed in mammalian tissues. Several other subtypes are expressed in selected brain regions, and also in the peripheral nervous system and in non-neuronal tissues. For further details, see Chapter 39 and review by Kalamida et al. (2007).
[b]Varenicline is used as an aid to smoking cessation. It acts as a partial agonist on $(\alpha4)_2(\beta2)_3$ receptors and a full agonist on $(\alpha7)_5$ receptors (see Ch. 50).

M_3 receptors (*glandular/smooth muscle*) produce mainly excitatory effects, i.e. stimulation of glandular secretions (salivary, bronchial, sweat, etc.) and contraction of visceral smooth muscle. M_3 receptor activation also causes relaxation of some smooth muscles (mainly vascular) via the release of nitric oxide from neighbouring endothelial cells (see Ch. 19). M_3 receptors occur also in specific locations in the CNS (see Ch. 39).

M_4 and M_5 receptors are largely confined to the CNS, and their functional role is not well understood, although mice lacking these receptors do show behavioural changes.

Cytokine secretion from lymphocytes and other cells is regulated by M_1 and M_3 receptors, while M_2 and M_4 receptors affect cell proliferation in various situations, opening up the possibility of new therapeutic roles for mAChR ligands (see Wessler and Kirkpatrick, 2020).

The agonist binding region is highly conserved between the different subtypes, so attempts to develop selective agonists and antagonists have had limited success. Most known agonists are non-selective, although an experimental compound, **McNA343**, is selective for M_1 receptors. **Cevimeline**, a relatively selective M_3-receptor agonist, is used clinically (see further in the chapter). It is possible that new mAChR ligands (see Jakubik and El-Fakahany, 2020) known as positive allosteric modulators (PAMs, see Ch. 3, Fig. 3.7) will allow better subtype selectivity for drugs acting on this important class of receptors, for example, by targeting CNS muscarinic receptors without producing unwanted cardiovascular effects (see Ch. 40).

There is more subtype selectivity among antagonists. Although most of the classic muscarinic antagonists (e.g. **atropine**, **hyoscine**) are non-selective, **pirenzepine** (previously used for peptic ulcer disease) is selective for M_1 receptors, and **darifenacin** (used for urinary incontinence in adults with detrusor muscle instability, known as 'overactive bladder') is selective for M_3 receptors. **Gallamine**, once used as a neuromuscular-blocking drug, is also a selective, although weak, allosteric M_2 receptor antagonist.[1] Toxins from the venom of the green mamba have been discovered to be highly selective mAChR antagonists (see Table 14.2).

[1]Unlike most other antagonists, gallamine acts *allosterically* (i.e. at a site distinct from the ACh binding site).

Acetylcholine receptors

- Main subdivision is into nicotinic (nAChR) and muscarinic (mAChR) subtypes.
- nAChRs are directly coupled to cation channels, and mediate fast excitatory synaptic transmission at the neuromuscular junction, autonomic ganglia and various sites in the CNS. Muscle and neuronal nAChRs differ in their molecular structure and pharmacology.
- mAChRs and nAChRs occur presynaptically as well as postsynaptically, and function to regulate transmitter release.
- mAChRs are G protein–coupled receptors causing:
  - Gq: activation of phospholipase C (hence formation of diacylglycerol and inositol trisphosphate as second messengers, releasing Ca^{2+} from the endoplasmic reticulum).
  - Gi: activation of potassium channels and/or inhibition of calcium channels; inhibition of adenylyl cyclase.
- All mAChRs are activated by ACh and blocked by **atropine.** They mediate ACh effects at postganglionic parasympathetic synapses (mainly heart, smooth muscle and glands), and contribute to ganglionic excitation. They occur in many parts of the CNS.
- There are three main types of mAChR:
  - M_1 receptors ('neural') producing slow excitation of ganglia. They are selectively blocked by **pirenzepine.**
  - M_2 receptors ('cardiac') causing decrease in cardiac rate. They are selectively blocked by **gallamine.** M_2 receptors also mediate presynaptic inhibition.
  - M_3 receptors ('glandular') causing secretion, contraction of visceral smooth muscle, vascular relaxation. **Cevimeline** is a selective M_3 agonist.
- Two further mAChR subtypes, M_4 and M_5, occur mainly in the CNS.

PHYSIOLOGY OF CHOLINERGIC TRANSMISSION

The physiology of cholinergic neurotransmission is described in detail by Nicholls et al. (2012). The main ways in which drugs can affect cholinergic transmission are shown in Fig. 14.2.

ACETYLCHOLINE SYNTHESIS AND RELEASE

ACh is synthesised within the nerve terminal from choline, which is taken up into the nerve terminal by a specific transporter (see Ch. 13), similar to those that operate for many transmitters but which transports the precursor, choline, not ACh, so it is not important in terminating the action of the transmitter. The concentration of choline in the blood and body fluids is normally about 10 µmol/L, but in the immediate vicinity of cholinergic nerve terminals it increases, probably to about 1 mmol/L, when the released ACh is hydrolysed, and more than 50% of this choline is normally recaptured by the nerve terminals. Free choline within the nerve terminal is acetylated by a cytosolic enzyme, *choline acetyltransferase* (CAT), which transfers the acetyl group from acetyl coenzyme A. The rate-limiting process in ACh synthesis appears to be choline transport, which is determined by the extracellular choline concentration and hence is linked to the rate at which ACh is being released (see Fig. 14.2). *Cholinesterase* is present in the presynaptic nerve terminals, and ACh is continually being hydrolysed and resynthesised. Inhibition of the nerve terminal cholinesterase causes the accumulation of surplus ACh in the cytosol, which is not available for release by nerve impulses (although it is able to leak out via the choline carrier). Most of the ACh synthesised, however, is packaged into synaptic vesicles, in which its concentration is extraordinarily high (about 100 mmol/L), and from which release occurs by exocytosis triggered by Ca^{2+} entry into the nerve terminal (see Ch. 4).

Cholinergic vesicles accumulate ACh actively, by means of a specific transporter belonging to the family of amine transporters described in Chapter 13. Accumulation of ACh is coupled to the large electrochemical gradient for protons that exists between acidic intracellular organelles and the cytosol; it is blocked selectively by the experimental drug **vesamicol**. Following its release, ACh diffuses across the synaptic cleft to combine with receptors on the postsynaptic cell. Some of it succumbs on the way to hydrolysis by *acetylcholinesterase* (AChE), an enzyme that is bound to the basement membrane that lies between the pre- and postsynaptic membranes. At fast cholinergic synapses (e.g. the neuromuscular and ganglionic synapses), but not at slow ones (smooth muscle, gland cells, heart, etc.), the released ACh is hydrolysed very rapidly (within 1 ms), so that it acts only very briefly.

At the neuromuscular junction, which is a highly specialised synapse, a single nerve impulse releases about 300 synaptic vesicles (altogether about 3 million ACh molecules) from the nerve terminals supplying a single muscle fibre. Each nerve terminal contains a total of approximately 3 million synaptic vesicles. The synaptic vesicles are the structural basis for the release of ACh from the nerve terminal in packets ('quanta'). Approximately 2 million of the ACh molecules released by a single impulse combine with receptors, of which there are about 30 million on each muscle fibre, the rest of the released ACh being hydrolysed without reaching a receptor. The ACh molecules remain bound to receptors for, on average, about 2 ms, and are quickly hydrolysed after dissociating. The result is that transmitter action is very rapid in onset and very brief in duration, which is important for a synapse that initiates speedy muscular responses and transmits signals faithfully at high frequency. Muscle cells are much larger than neurons and require much more synaptic current to generate an action potential. Thus all the chemical events happen on a larger scale than at a neuronal synapse; the number of transmitter molecules in a quantum, the number of quanta released, and the number of receptors activated by each quantum are all 10–100 times greater. Our brains would be huge, but not very clever, if their synapses were built on the industrial scale of the neuromuscular junction.

PRESYNAPTIC MODULATION

ACh release is regulated by mediators, including ACh itself, acting on presynaptic receptors, as discussed in Chapter 13. At postganglionic parasympathetic nerve endings, inhibitory M_2 receptors participate in autoinhibition of ACh release; other mediators, such as noradrenaline, also inhibit the release of ACh (see Ch. 13). At the neuromuscular junction, however, presynaptic nAChRs facilitate ACh

Table 14.2 Muscarinic receptor subtypes[a]

	M_1 ('neural')	M_2 ('cardiac')	M_3 ('glandular/ smooth muscle')	M_4	M_5
Main locations	Autonomic ganglia (including intramural ganglia in stomach) Gastric oxyntic glands (acid secretion) Glands: salivary, lacrimal, etc. Cerebral cortex	Heart: atria CNS: widely distributed	Exocrine glands: salivary, etc. Smooth muscle: gastrointestinal tract, eye, airways, bladder Blood vessels: endothelium	CNS	CNS: very localised expression in substantia nigra Salivary glands Iris/ciliary muscle
Cellular response	↑ IP_3, DAG Depolarisation Excitation (slow epsp) ↓ K^+ conductance	↓ cAMP Inhibition ↓ Ca^{2+} conductance ↑ K^+ conductance	↑ IP_3 Stimulation ↑ $[Ca^{2+}]_i$	↓ cAMP Inhibition	↑ IP_3 Excitation
Functional response	CNS excitation (? improved cognition) Gastric secretion	Cardiac inhibition Neural inhibition Central muscarinic effects (e.g. tremor, hypothermia)	Gastric, salivary secretion Gastrointestinal smooth muscle contraction Ocular accommodation Vasodilatation	Enhanced locomotion	Not known
Non-selective agonists (see also Table 14.3)	Acetylcholine Carbachol Oxotremorine Pilocarpine Bethanechol				
Selective agonists	McNA343		Cevimeline		
Non-selective antagonists (see also Table 14.4)	Atropine Dicycloverine Tolterodine Oxybutynin Ipratropium				
Selective antagonists	Pirenzepine Mamba toxin MT7	Gallamine	Darifenacin Solifenacin	Mamba toxin MT3	

[a]This table shows only the predominant subtypes expressed in mammalian tissues. For further details, see Chapter 39 and review by Kalamida et al. (2007).
DAG, Diacylglycerol; *epsp*, excitatory postsynaptic potential; *IP_3*, inositol trisphosphate.

release, a mechanism that may allow the synapse to function reliably during prolonged high-frequency activity. In the brain, as mentioned previously, presynaptic nAChRs either facilitate or inhibit the release of other mediators.

ELECTRICAL EVENTS IN TRANSMISSION AT FAST CHOLINERGIC SYNAPSES

ACh, acting on the postsynaptic membrane of a nicotinic (neuromuscular or ganglionic) synapse, causes a large increase in its permeability to cations, particularly to Na^+ and K^+, and to a lesser extent Ca^{2+}. The resulting inflow of Na^+ depolarises the postsynaptic membrane. This transmitter-mediated depolarisation is called an *endplate potential* (*epp*) in a skeletal muscle fibre, or a *fast excitatory postsynaptic potential* (*fast epsp*) at the ganglionic synapse. In a muscle fibre, the localised epp spreads to adjacent, electrically excitable parts of the muscle fibre; if its amplitude reaches the threshold for excitation, an action potential is initiated, which propagates to the rest of the fibre and evokes a contraction (see Ch. 4).

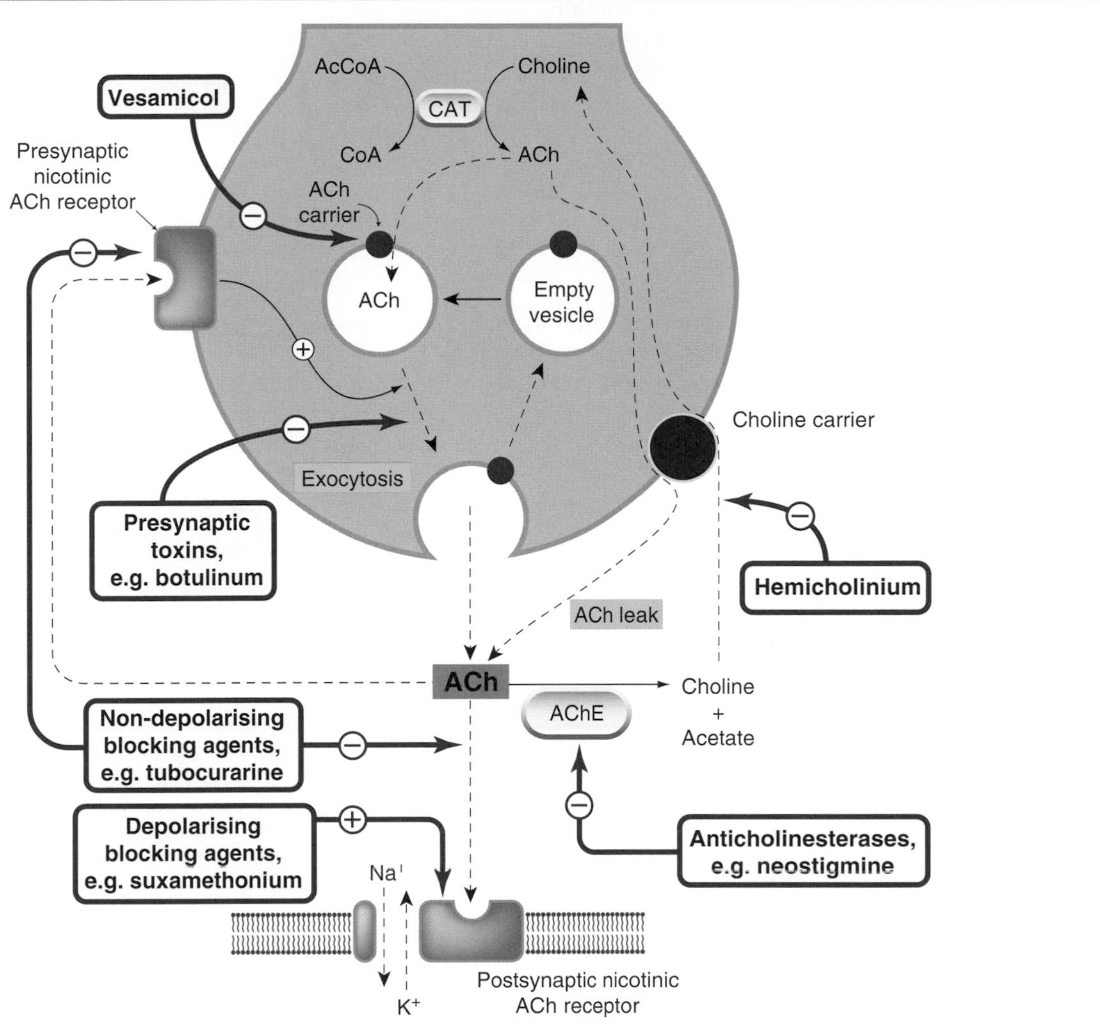

Fig. 14.2 Events and sites of drug action at a nicotinic cholinergic synapse. Acetylcholine (ACh) is shown acting postsynaptically on a nicotinic receptor controlling a cation channel (e.g. at the neuromuscular or ganglionic synapse), and also on a presynaptic nicotinic receptor that acts to facilitate ACh release during sustained synaptic activity. The nerve terminal also contains acetylcholinesterase (not shown); when this is inhibited, the amount of free ACh, and the rate of leakage of ACh via the choline carrier, is increased. Under normal conditions, this leakage of ACh is insignificant. At muscarinic cholinergic junctions (e.g. heart, smooth muscle and exocrine glands), both postsynaptic and presynaptic (inhibitory) receptors are of the muscarinic type. *AcCoA,* Acetyl coenzyme A; *AChE,* acetylcholinesterase; *CAT,* choline acetyltransferase; *CoA,* coenzyme A.

In a nerve cell, depolarisation of the soma or a dendrite by the fast epsp causes a local current to flow. This depolarises the axon hillock region of the cell, where, if the epsp is large enough, an action potential is initiated. Fig. 14.3 shows that **tubocurarine**, a drug that blocks postsynaptic nACh receptors, reduces the amplitude of the fast epsp until it no longer initiates an action potential, although the cell is still capable of responding when it is stimulated electrically. Most ganglion cells are supplied by several presynaptic axons, and it requires simultaneous activity in more than one to make the postganglionic cell fire (integrative action). At the neuromuscular junction, only one nerve fibre supplies each muscle fibre – like a relay station in a telegraph line the synapse ensures faithful 1:1 transmission despite the impedance mismatch between the fine nerve fibre and the much larger muscle fibre. The amplitude of the epp is normally more than enough to initiate an action potential – indeed, transmission still occurs when the epp is reduced by 70%–80%, showing a large margin of safety so that fluctuations in transmitter release (e.g. during repetitive stimulation) do not affect transmission.

Transmission at the ganglionic synapse is more complex than at the neuromuscular junction. Although the primary event at both is the depolarisation (fast epsp or epp, respectively) produced by ACh acting on nAChRs, this is followed in the ganglion by a succession of much slower postsynaptic responses:

- A *slow inhibitory (hyperpolarising) postsynaptic potential (slow ipsp),* lasting 2–5 s. This mainly reflects a muscarinic (M_2)-receptor-mediated increase in K^+ conductance, but other transmitters, such as dopamine and adenosine, also contribute.
- A *slow epsp,* which lasts for about 10 s. This is produced by ACh acting on M_1 receptors, which close K^+ channels.
- A *late slow epsp,* lasting for 1–2 min. This is thought to be mediated by a peptide co-transmitter,

substance P in some ganglia, and a gonadotrophin-releasing hormone-like peptide in others (see Ch. 13). Like the slow epsp, it is produced by a decrease in K^+ conductance.

Cholinergic transmission

- Acetylcholine (ACh) synthesis:
  - requires choline, which enters the neuron via carrier-mediated transport
  - choline is acetylated to form ACh by choline acetyl transferase, a cytosolic enzyme found only in cholinergic neurons. Acetyl coenzyme A provides the acetyl groups.
- ACh is packaged into synaptic vesicles at high concentration by carrier-mediated transport.
- ACh release occurs by Ca^{2+}-mediated exocytosis. At the neuromuscular junction, one presynaptic nerve impulse releases 100–500 vesicles.
- At the neuromuscular junction, ACh acts on nicotinic receptors to open cation channels, producing a rapid depolarisation (endplate potential), which normally initiates an action potential in the muscle fibre. Transmission at other 'fast' cholinergic synapses (e.g. ganglionic) is qualitatively similar.
- At 'fast' cholinergic synapses, ACh is hydrolysed within about 1 ms by acetylcholinesterase, so a presynaptic action potential produces only one postsynaptic action potential.
- Transmission mediated by muscarinic receptors is much slower in its time course, and synaptic structures are less clearly defined. In many such situations, ACh functions as a *modulator* (i.e. where the mediator acts indirectly to alter the efficiency of transmission rather than as a direct transmitter – see Ch. 13).
- Main mechanisms of pharmacological block: inhibition of choline uptake, inhibition of ACh release, block of postsynaptic receptors or ion channels, persistent postsynaptic depolarisation.

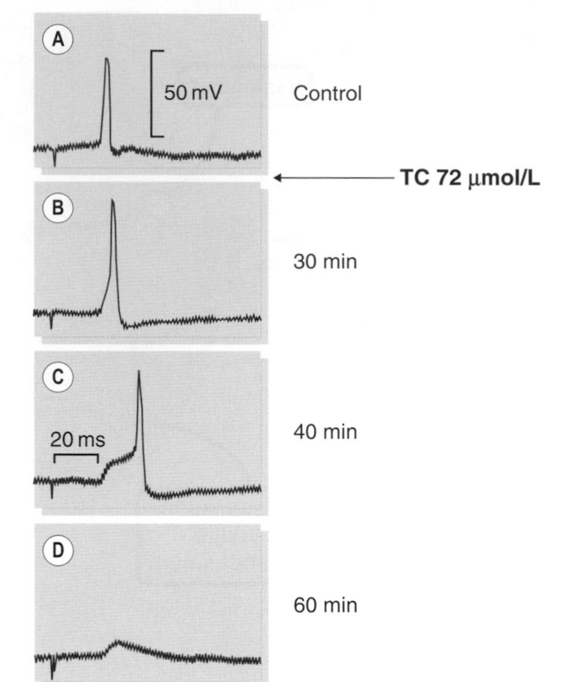

Fig. 14.3 Cholinergic transmission in an autonomic ganglion cell. Records were obtained with an intracellular microelectrode from a guinea pig parasympathetic ganglion cell. The artefact at the beginning of each trace shows the moment of stimulation of the preganglionic nerve. Tubocurarine (TC), an acetylcholine antagonist, causes the excitatory postsynaptic potential to become smaller. In record (C), it only just succeeds in triggering the action potential, and in (D) it has fallen below the threshold. Following complete block, antidromic stimulation (not shown) will still produce an action potential (cf. depolarisation block, Fig. 14.4). (From Blackman, J.G., et al., 1969. J. Physiol. 201, 723.)

DEPOLARISATION BLOCK

Depolarisation block occurs at cholinergic synapses when the excitatory nAChRs are persistently activated, and it results from a decrease in the electrical excitability of the postsynaptic cell. This is shown in Fig. 14.4. Application of nicotine to a sympathetic ganglion activates nAChRs, causing a depolarisation of the cell, which at first initiates action potential discharge. After a few seconds, this discharge ceases and transmission is blocked. The loss of electrical excitability is shown by the fact that electrical stimuli also fail to produce an action potential. The main reason for the loss of electrical excitability during a period of maintained depolarisation is that the voltage-sensitive sodium channels (see Ch. 4) become inactivated (i.e. refractory) and no longer able to open in response to a brief depolarising stimulus.

A second type of effect is also seen in the experiment shown in Fig. 14.4. After nicotine has acted for several minutes, the cell partially repolarises and its electrical excitability returns but, despite this, transmission remains blocked. This type of secondary, *non-depolarising block* occurs also at the neuromuscular junction if repeated doses of the depolarising drug **suxamethonium**[2] (see later) are used. The main factor responsible for the secondary block (known clinically as *phase II block*) appears to be receptor desensitisation (see Ch. 2). This causes the depolarising action of the blocking drug to subside, but transmission remains blocked because the receptors are desensitised to ACh.

EFFECTS OF DRUGS ON CHOLINERGIC TRANSMISSION

As shown in Fig. 14.2, drugs can influence cholinergic transmission either by acting on postsynaptic ACh receptors as agonists or antagonists (see Tables 14.1 and 14.2), or by affecting the release or destruction of endogenous ACh.

In the rest of this chapter, we describe the following groups of drugs, subdivided according to their site of action:

[2]Also known as **succinylcholine**.

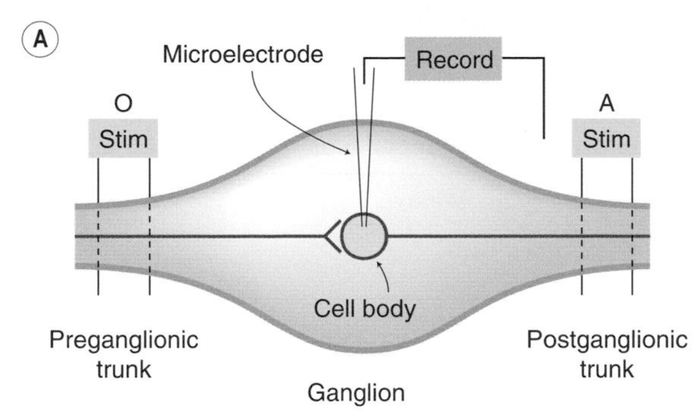

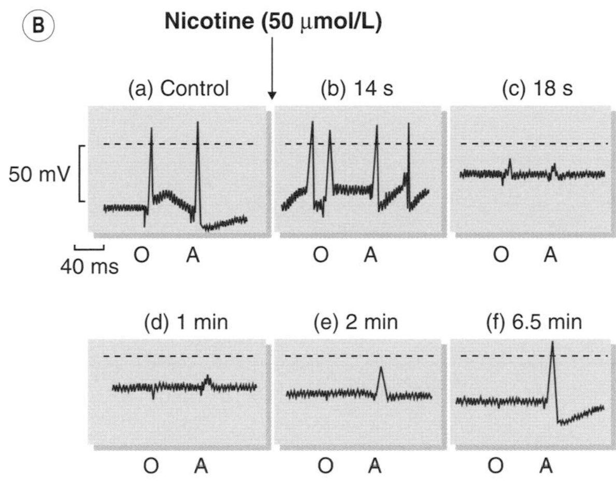

Fig. 14.4 Depolarisation block of ganglionic transmission by nicotine. (A) System used for intracellular recording from sympathetic ganglion cells of the frog, showing the location of orthodromic *(O)* and antidromic *(A)* stimulating (stim) electrodes. Stimulation at *O* excites the cell via the cholinergic synapse, whereas stimulation at *A* excites it by electrical propagation of the action potential. (B) The effect of nicotine. *(a)* Control records. The membrane potential is −55 mV (dotted line = 0 mV), and the cell responds to both *O* and *A*. *(b)* Shortly after adding nicotine, the cell is slightly depolarised and spontaneously active, but still responsive to *O* and *A*. *(c and d)* The cell is further depolarised, to −25 mV, and produces only a vestigial action potential. The fact that it does not respond to *A* shows that it is electrically inexcitable. *(e and f)* In the continued presence of nicotine, the cell repolarises and regains its responsiveness to *A*, but it is still unresponsive to *O* because the ACh receptors are desensitised by nicotine. (From Ginsborg, B.L., Guerrero, S., 1964. J. Physiol. 172, 189.)

- muscarinic agonists
- muscarinic antagonists
- ganglion-stimulating drugs
- ganglion-blocking drugs
- neuromuscular-blocking drugs
- anticholinesterases and other drugs that enhance cholinergic transmission

DRUGS AFFECTING MUSCARINIC RECEPTORS

MUSCARINIC AGONISTS

Structure–activity relationships

Muscarinic agonists, as a group, are often referred to as *parasympathomimetic*, because the main effects that they produce in the whole animal resemble those of parasympathetic stimulation. The structures of ACh and related choline esters are given in Table 14.3. They are agonists at both mAChRs and nAChRs, but act more potently on mAChRs (see Fig. 14.1). **Bethanechol**, **pilocarpine** and **cevimeline** are the main ones used clinically.

The key features of the ACh molecule are the quaternary ammonium group, which bears a positive charge, and the ester group, which bears a partial negative charge and is susceptible to rapid hydrolysis by cholinesterase. Variants of the choline ester structure (see Table 14.3) have the effect of reducing the susceptibility of the compound to hydrolysis by cholinesterase and altering the relative activity on mAChRs and nAChRs.

Carbachol and **methacholine** are less rapidly hydrolysed by cholinesterase enzymes than is ACh. They are used as experimental tools. Bethanechol, which is a hybrid of these two molecules, is stable to hydrolysis and selective for mAChRs, and has been used clinically (see clinical box, later). Pilocarpine is a partial agonist and shows some selectivity in stimulating secretion from sweat, salivary, lacrimal and bronchial glands, and contracting iris smooth muscle, with weak effects on gastrointestinal smooth muscle and the heart.

Effects of muscarinic agonists

The main actions of muscarinic agonists are readily understood in terms of the parasympathetic nervous system.

Cardiovascular effects

These include cardiac slowing and a decrease in cardiac output due mainly to the reduced heart rate. There is also a decreased force of contraction of the atria (the ventricles have only a sparse parasympathetic innervation and a low sensitivity to muscarinic agonists). Generalised vasodilatation also occurs (mediated by nitric oxide, NO; see Ch. 19) and, combined with the reduced cardiac output, produces a fall in arterial pressure (see Fig. 14.1). Parasympathetic regulation of the heart is discussed in Chapter 20 (see Fig. 20.7).

Smooth muscle

Smooth muscle generally *contracts* in direct response to muscarinic agonists, in contrast to their indirect effect via NO on vascular smooth muscle. Peristaltic activity of the gastrointestinal tract is increased, which can cause colicky pain, and the bladder and bronchial smooth muscle also contract.

Sweating, lacrimation, salivation and bronchial secretion

Muscarinic agonists stimulate exocrine glands. The combined effect of bronchial secretion and constriction can interfere with breathing. **Methacholine** is used as an inhaled challenge agent in the investigation of airways responsiveness.

Effects on the eye

The ocular effects of muscarinic agents are clinically important. The parasympathetic nerves to the eye supply the constrictor pupillae muscle and the ciliary muscle. The constrictor pupillae is important not only for adjusting the pupil in response to changes in light intensity, but also in regulating the intraocular pressure. The effects of drugs that

Table 14.3 Muscarinic agonists

Compound	Structure	Receptor specificity		Hydrolysis by cholinesterase	Clinical uses
		Muscarinic	Nicotinic		
Acetylcholine		+++	+++	+++	None
Carbachol		++	+++	–	None
Methacholine		+++	+	++	None
Bethanechol		+++	–	–	Treatment of bladder and gastrointestinal hypotonia[a]
Muscarine		+++	–	–	None[b]
Pilocarpine		++	–	–	Glaucoma
Oxotremorine		++	–	–	None
Cevimeline		++[c]	–	–	Sjögren's syndrome (to increase salivary and lacrimal secretion)

[a]Essential to check that bladder neck is not obstructed.
[b]Cause of one type of mushroom poisoning.
[c]Selective for M_3 receptors.

influence cholinergic transmission on the eye are described in more detail in Chapter 27.

Clinical use

Currently there are few important clinical uses of muscarinic agonists, although hopes remain that new more selective agents may prove useful in various CNS disorders. **Pilocarpine** can be used as eye drops (see Ch. 27) and it or the M_3-selective agonist **cevimeline** are used to increase salivary and lacrimal secretion in patients with dry eyes and dry mouth, e.g. following irradiation or in patients with Sjögren's syndrome, an autoimmune disorder characterised by dryness of mouth and eyes. Cholinesterase inhibitors (see later) were used in the past to potentiate endogenous parasympathetic muscarinic effects on bowel and bladder, as stimulant laxatives or to stimulate bladder emptying.

MUSCARINIC ANTAGONISTS

mAChR antagonists (*parasympatholytic drugs*; Table 14.4) are competitive antagonists whose chemical structures usually contain ester and basic groups in the same relationship as ACh, but with a bulky aromatic group in place of the acetyl group. The two naturally occurring compounds, **atropine** and **hyoscine** (also known as **scopolamine**), are alkaloids found in solanaceous plants. The deadly nightshade (*Atropa belladonna*) contains mainly atropine, whereas the thorn apple (*Datura stramonium*) contains mainly hyoscine. These are tertiary ammonium compounds that are sufficiently lipid-soluble to be readily absorbed from the gut or conjunctival sac and, importantly, to penetrate the blood–brain barrier. Analogues containing quaternary rather than tertiary ammonium groups have peripheral actions very similar to those of atropine but, because of their exclusion from the brain, lack central actions. Clinically important examples include **hyoscine butylbromide** and **propantheline**. Other muscarinic antagonists in clinical use are described later.

Effects of muscarinic antagonists

All muscarinic antagonists produce similar peripheral effects, although some show a degree of selectivity, for example, for the heart or bladder, reflecting heterogeneity among mAChRs.

The main effects of atropine are:

Inhibition of secretions

Salivary, lacrimal, bronchial and sweat glands are inhibited by very low doses of atropine, producing uncomfortably dry eyes, mouth and skin. Gastric secretion is only slightly reduced. Mucociliary clearance in the bronchi is inhibited, so that residual secretions tend to accumulate in the lungs. **Ipratropium** (see later) lacks this latter undesired effect.

Effects on heart rate

Atropine causes tachycardia through block of cardiac mAChRs. The tachycardia is modest, up to 80–90 beats/min in humans, since it has no effect on the sympathetic system, working by inhibition of tonic parasympathetic activity. Tachycardia is most pronounced in young people, in whom vagal tone at rest is highest; it is often absent in the elderly. At very low doses, atropine causes a paradoxical bradycardia, possibly due to a central action. Arterial

Table 14.4 Muscarinic antagonists[a]

Compound	Pharmacological properties	Notes
Atropine	Non-selective antagonist Well absorbed orally CNS stimulant	Belladonna alkaloid Main side effects: urinary retention, dry mouth, blurred vision Dicycloverine (dicyclomine) is similar and used mainly as an antispasmodic agent
Glycopyrronium	Similar to atropine	Quaternary ammoniun compound Reduces secretions and salivation in palliative care, perioperative patients, and children with chronic neurological conditions. Also available as inhaler for chronic obstructive pulmonary disease
Hyoscine	Similar to atropine CNS depressant	Belladonna alkaloid (also known as scopolamine) Causes sedation; other side effects as atropine
Hyoscine butylbromide	Similar to atropine but poorly absorbed and lacks many CNS effects Significant ganglion-blocking activity	Quaternary ammonium derivative Similar drugs include atropine methonitrate, propantheline
Tiotropium	Similar to atropine methonitrate Does not inhibit mucociliary clearance from bronchi	Quaternary ammonium compound Ipratropium similar
Tropicamide	Similar to atropine May raise intraocular pressure	Used topically (eye drops) as a mydriatic
Cyclopentolate	Similar to tropicamide	–
Darifenacin	Selective for M_3 receptors	Used to treat unstable bladder and associated urge incontinence. Causes fewer adverse effects than unselective muscarinic antagonists
Solifenacin	Selective for M_3 receptors	Similar to darifenacin
Tolterodine	Selective for M_3 and M_2 receptors	Similar to darifenacin and solifenacin

[a]For chemical structures, see Southan, C., Sharman, J.L., Benson, H.E., et al., 2016. The IUPHAR/BPS Guide to Pharmacology in 2016: towards curated quantitative interactions between 1300 protein targets and 6000 ligands. Nucl. Acids Res. 44 (Database Issue), D1054–D1068.
CNS, Central nervous system.

blood pressure and the response of the heart to exercise are unaffected.

Effects on the eye

These are described in Chapter 27.

Effects on the gastrointestinal tract

Gastrointestinal motility is inhibited by atropine, although this requires larger doses than the other effects listed and is not complete since excitatory transmitters other than ACh are important in normal function of the myenteric plexus (see Ch. 13). Atropine-like drugs such as **hyoscine butylbromide** relax intestinal spasm and are used for symptomatic relief in pathological conditions in which there is gastrointestinal spasm, as well as in gastrointestinal imaging to improve resolution. **Pirenzepine**, owing to its selectivity for M_1 receptors, inhibits gastric acid secretion in doses that do not affect other systems.

Effects on other smooth muscle

Atropine relaxes bronchial, biliary and urinary tract smooth muscle. Reflex bronchoconstriction (e.g. during anaesthesia) is prevented, whereas bronchoconstriction caused by mediators such as histamine and leukotrienes (see Ch. 28) is unaffected. **Ipratropium** and **tiotropium**, quaternary ammonium antimuscarinic drugs, are administered by inhalation as bronchodilators (see Ch. 28). Biliary and urinary tract smooth muscle are only slightly affected in normal individuals, probably because transmitters other than ACh (see Ch. 13) are important in these organs; nevertheless, atropine and similar drugs commonly worsen urinary hesitancy and can precipitate urinary retention in elderly men with prostatic enlargement. **Oxybutynin**, **tolterodine** and **darifenacin** (M_3-selective) act on the bladder to inhibit micturition and are used for treating overactive bladder. They produce unwanted effects typical of muscarinic antagonists, such as dry mouth, constipation and blurred vision, but these are less severe than with less selective drugs.

Effects on the CNS

Atropine produces mainly excitatory effects on the CNS. At low doses, this causes mild restlessness; higher doses cause agitation and disorientation. In atropine poisoning, which occurs in young children who eat deadly nightshade berries, marked excitement and irritability result in hyperactivity and a considerable rise in body temperature, which is accentuated by the loss of sweating. The central effects are the result of blocking mAChRs in the brain and are less marked or absent with quaternary ammonium drugs such as hyoscine butylbromide, propantheline, ipratropium and tiotropium that have limited access beyond the blood–brain barrier. The central effects of muscarinic antagonists are opposed by anticholinesterase drugs (see later) such as **physostigmine**, which have been used to treat atropine poisoning. Hyoscine in low doses causes marked sedation but has similar effects to atropine in high dosage. Hyoscine has a central antiemetic effect and is used to prevent motion sickness; hyoscine hydrobromide is also effective for this indication, presumably because the blood–brain barrier is deficient in the location of the chemoreceptor trigger zone (see Ch. 30 on antiemetic drugs). Muscarinic antagonists also affect the extrapyramidal system, reducing the involuntary movement and rigidity of patients with Parkinson's disease (see Ch. 40) and counteracting the unwanted extrapyramidal effects caused by many antipsychotic drugs (see Ch. 47).

Drugs acting on muscarinic receptors

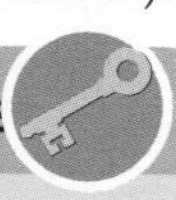

Muscarinic agonists

- Important compounds include **acetylcholine**, **carbachol**, **methacholine**, **muscarine** and **pilocarpine.** They vary in muscarinic/nicotinic selectivity, and in susceptibility to cholinesterase.
- Main effects are bradycardia and vasodilatation (endothelium-dependent), leading to fall in blood pressure; contraction of visceral smooth muscle (gut, bladder, bronchi, etc.); exocrine secretions (e.g. salivation); pupillary constriction and ciliary muscle contraction, leading to constriction of the pupil and reduced intraocular pressure.
- Main use is in treatment of glaucoma (especially **pilocarpine**) see Chapter 27.
- Most agonists currently in therapeutic use show little receptor subtype selectivity; **cevimeline**, a selective M_3 agonist, is an exception.
- PAMs offer prospects for more selective clinical agents.

Muscarinic antagonists

- The main drugs are **atropine, hyoscine butylbromide, ipratropium, tiotropium** and the M_3-selective drugs **oxybutynin, tolterodine** and **darifenacin.**
- Main effects are inhibition of secretions; tachycardia, pupillary dilatation and paralysis of accommodation; relaxation of smooth muscle (gut, bronchi, biliary tract, bladder); CNS effects (mainly excitatory with **atropine**; depressant, including amnesia, with **hyoscine**), including antiemetic effect and antiparkinsonian effect.

Clinical use

The main uses of muscarinic antagonists are summarised in the clinical box.

Clinical uses of muscarinic antagonists

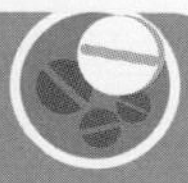

Cardiovascular

- Treatment of sinus bradycardia (e.g. after myocardial infarction; see Ch. 20): for example, **atropine.**

Ophthalmic

- To dilate the pupil: for example **tropicamide** or **cyclopentolate** eye drops (see Ch. 27).

Neurological

- Prevention of motion sickness: for example, **hyoscine hydrobromide.**
- Parkinsonism (see Ch. 40), especially to counteract movement disorders caused by antipsychotic drugs (see Ch. 47): for example, **orphenadrine.**

Respiratory

- Asthma and chronic obstructive pulmonary disease (see Ch. 28): **ipratropium** or **tiotropium** by inhalation.

Palliative care

- Bowel colic and excessive salivation/respiratory secretion: hyoscine or glycopyrronium.

Anaesthetic premedication

- To dry secretions: for example, **atropine**, **hyoscine.** (Current anaesthetics are relatively non-irritant, see Ch. 41, so this is less important than in the past.)

Gastrointestinal

- To facilitate endoscopy and gastrointestinal radiology by relaxing gastrointestinal smooth muscle (antispasmodic action; see Ch. 30): for example, **hyoscine butylbromide.**
- As an antispasmodic in irritable bowel syndrome or colonic diverticular disease: for example, **dicycloverine** (**dicyclomine**).

Urinary tract

- To relieve symptoms of overactive bladder: for example, **oxybutynin**, **tolterodine**, **darifenacin.**

DRUGS AFFECTING AUTONOMIC GANGLIA

GANGLION STIMULANTS

Most nAChR agonists act on either neuronal (ganglionic and CNS) nAChRs or on striated muscle (motor endplate) receptors but not, apart from nicotine and ACh, on both (Table 14.5).

Nicotine and **lobeline** are tertiary amines found in the leaves of tobacco and lobelia plants, respectively. Nicotine belongs in pharmacological folklore, as it was the substance on the tip of Langley's paintbrush causing stimulation of muscle fibres when applied to the endplate region, leading him to postulate in 1905 the existence of a 'receptive substance' on the surface of the fibres (see Ch. 13). **Epibatidine**, found in the skin of poisonous frogs, is a highly potent nicotinic agonist selective for ganglionic and CNS receptors. It was found, unexpectedly, to be a powerful analgesic (see Ch. 43), although its autonomic side effects

Table 14.5 Nicotinic receptor agonists and antagonists

Drug	Main site	Type of action	Notes
Agonists			
Nicotine	Autonomic ganglia	Stimulation then block	See Ch. 50
	CNS	Stimulation	
Lobeline	Autonomic ganglia	Stimulation	—
	Sensory nerve terminals	Stimulation	
Epibatidine	Autonomic ganglia	Stimulation	Isolated from frog skin
	CNS		Highly potent
			No clinical use
Varenicline	CNS	Stimulation	Used for nicotine addiction (see Ch. 50)
	Autonomic ganglia		
Suxamethonium	Neuromuscular junction	Depolarisation block	Used clinically as muscle relaxant
Decamethonium	Neuromuscular junction	Depolarisation block	No clinical use
Antagonists			
Hexamethonium	Autonomic ganglia	Transmission block	No clinical use
Trimetaphan	Autonomic ganglia	Transmission block	Short acting; iv infusion was used to control blood pressure during aortic aneurysm surgery
Tubocurarine	Neuromuscular junction	Transmission block	Now rarely used
Pancuronium	Neuromuscular junction	Transmission block	Widely used as muscle relaxants in anaesthesia
Atracurium			
Vecuronium			

CNS, Central nervous system.

ruled out its clinical use. **Varenicline**, a synthetic agonist relatively selective for CNS receptors, is used (as is nicotine itself) to treat nicotine addiction (see Ch. 50). Otherwise, these drugs are used only as experimental tools.

Nicotinic agonists cause complex peripheral responses associated with generalised stimulation of autonomic ganglia. The effects of nicotine on the gastrointestinal tract and sweat glands are familiar to neophyte smokers (see Ch. 50), although usually insufficient to act as an effective deterrent.

GANGLION-BLOCKING DRUGS

Ganglion-blocking drugs are used experimentally to study autonomic function. In the middle of the last century, Paton and Zaimis investigated a series of linear bisquaternary compounds and found that compounds with five or six carbon atoms in the methylene chain linking the two quaternary groups produced ganglionic block.[3] **Hexamethonium** is obsolete clinically but famous as the first effective antihypertensive drug.

Ganglion block can occur by several mechanisms:

- By interference with ACh release, as at the neuromuscular junction (see Ch. 13).
- By prolonged depolarisation. Nicotine (see Fig. 14.4) blocks ganglia after initial stimulation, as does ACh itself if cholinesterase is inhibited.
- Interfering with the postsynaptic action of ACh, by blocking neuronal nAChRs or the associated ion channels.

Effects of ganglion-blocking drugs

The effects of ganglion-blocking drugs are diverse, because both divisions of the autonomic nervous system are blocked indiscriminately. The description by Paton of 'hexamethonium man' cannot be bettered:

He is a pink-complexioned person, except when he has stood in a queue for a long time, when he may get pale and faint. His handshake is warm and dry. He is a placid and relaxed companion; for instance he may laugh but he can't cry because the tears cannot come. Your rudest story will not make him blush, and the most unpleasant circumstances will fail to make him turn pale. His collars and socks stay very clean and sweet. He wears corsets and may, if you meet him out, be rather fidgety (corsets to compress his splanchnic vascular pool, fidgety to keep the venous return going from his legs). He dislikes speaking much unless

[3]Based on their structural similarity to ACh, these compounds were originally assumed to compete with ACh for its binding site. However, they are now known to act mainly by blocking the ion channel rather than the receptor itself.

helped with something to moisten his dry mouth and throat. He is long-sighted and easily blinded by bright light. The redness of his eyeballs may suggest irregular habits and in fact his head is rather weak. But he always behaves like a gentleman and never belches or hiccups. He tends to get cold and keeps well wrapped up. But his health is good; he does not have chilblains and those diseases of modern civilisation, hypertension and peptic ulcer, pass him by. He gets thin because his appetite is modest; he never feels hunger pains and his stomach never rumbles. He gets rather constipated so that his intake of liquid paraffin is high. As old age comes on, he will suffer from retention of urine and impotence, but frequency, precipitancy and strangury (i.e. an intensely painful sensation of needing to pass urine coupled with an inability to do so) will not worry him. One is uncertain how he will end, but perhaps if he is not careful, by eating less and less and getting colder and colder, he will sink into a symptomless, hypoglycaemic coma and die, as was proposed for the universe, a sort of entropy death.

(From Paton, W.D.M., 1954. The principles of ganglion block. Lectures on the Scientific Basis of Medicine, Vol. 2.)

In practice, the main effect is a marked fall in arterial blood pressure on standing upright ('postural hypotension') resulting mainly from block of sympathetic ganglia. This causes vasodilatation and loss of cardiovascular reflexes so that the heart rate fails to increase in compensation for the fall in blood pressure. Venoconstriction, which occurs normally when a subject stands up and prevents a fall in central venous pressure and cardiac output, is reduced leading to faintness or syncope.

Drugs acting on autonomic ganglia

Ganglion-stimulating drugs

- Compounds include nicotine, dimethylphenylpiperazinium (DMPP).
- Both sympathetic and parasympathetic ganglia are stimulated, so effects are complex, including tachycardia and increase of blood pressure; variable effects on gastrointestinal motility and secretions; increased bronchial, salivary and sweat secretions. Additional effects result from stimulation of other neuronal structures, including sensory and noradrenergic nerve terminals.
- Ganglion stimulation is followed by depolarisation block.
- Nicotine also has important CNS effects (see Ch. 50).
- Therapeutic uses are limited to assisting smoking cessation (nicotine, varenicline).

Ganglion-blocking drugs

- Compounds include hexamethonium, tubocurarine (also nicotine).
- Block all autonomic ganglia and enteric ganglia. Main effects: postural hypotension and loss of cardiovascular reflexes, inhibition of secretions, gastrointestinal paralysis, impaired micturition.
- Clinically obsolete (historically: the first therapeutic drugs for treating hypertension).

NEUROMUSCULAR-BLOCKING DRUGS

Drugs can block neuromuscular transmission either by acting presynaptically to inhibit ACh synthesis or release or by acting postsynaptically.

Neuromuscular block is an important adjunct to general anaesthesia (see Ch. 41). The drugs used for this purpose all work postsynaptically, either (a) by blocking ACh receptors (or in some cases the ion channel) or (b) by activating ACh receptors and thus causing persistent depolarisation of the motor endplate. **Suxamethonium** is the only depolarising blocker in clinical use, while all of the other drugs used clinically are *non-depolarising agents*.

NON-DEPOLARISING BLOCKING AGENTS

In 1856, Claude Bernard, in a famous experiment, showed that 'curare' causes paralysis by blocking neuromuscular transmission, rather than by abolishing nerve conduction or muscle contractility. Curare is a mixture of naturally occurring alkaloids found in various South American plants and used as arrow poisons by South American Indians. The most important component is **tubocurarine**, itself now rarely used in clinical medicine, being superseded by synthetic drugs with improved properties. The most important are **pancuronium**, **vecuronium**, **cisatracurium** and **mivacurium** (Table 14.6), which differ mainly in their duration of action. These substances are all quaternary ammonium compounds, so are poorly absorbed[4] (they are administered intravenously) and generally are efficiently excreted by the kidneys. They do not cross the placenta, which is important in relation to their use in obstetric anaesthesia.

Mechanism of action

Non-depolarising blocking agents act as competitive antagonists (see Ch. 2) at the nACh receptors of the endplate.

The amount of ACh released by a nerve impulse normally exceeds by several-fold what is needed to elicit an action potential in the muscle fibre (see Ch. 3). It is therefore necessary to block 70%–80% of the receptor sites before transmission actually fails. In any individual muscle fibre, transmission is all-or-nothing, so graded degrees of block represent a varying proportion of muscle fibres failing to respond. In this situation, where the amplitude of the epp in all the fibres is close to threshold (just above in some, just below in others), small variations in the amount of transmitter released, or in the rate at which it is destroyed, will have a large effect on the proportion of fibres contracting, so the degree of block is liable to vary according to various physiological circumstances (e.g. stimulation frequency, temperature and cholinesterase activity), which otherwise have little effect on the efficiency of transmission.

Non-depolarising blocking agents also block facilitatory presynaptic autoreceptors, and thus inhibit the release of ACh during repetitive stimulation of the motor nerve, contributing to the phenomenon of 'tetanic fade', used by anaesthetists to monitor postoperative recovery of neuromuscular transmission.

Effects of non-depolarising blocking drugs

The effects of non-depolarising neuromuscular-blocking agents are mainly due to motor paralysis, although some

[4]Animals killed by curare-tipped arrows are safe to eat because of this.

Table 14.6 Characteristics of neuromuscular-blocking drugs[a]

Drug	Speed of onset	Duration of action	Main side effects	Notes
Tubocurarine	Slow (>5 min)	Long (1–2 h)	Hypotension (ganglion block plus histamine release) Bronchoconstriction (histamine release)	Plant alkaloid, now rarely used Alcuronium is a semisynthetic derivative with similar properties but fewer side effects
Pancuronium	Intermediate (2–3 min)	Long (1–2 h)	Slight tachycardia Hypertension	The first steroid-based compound Better side effect profile than tubocurarine Widely used Pipecuronium is similar
Vecuronium	Intermediate	Intermediate (30–40 min)	Few side effects	Widely used Occasionally causes prolonged paralysis, probably owing to active metabolite Rocuronium is similar, with faster onset
Atracurium	Intermediate	Intermediate (<30 min)	Transient hypotension (histamine release)	Unusual mechanism of elimination (spontaneous non-enzymic chemical degradation in plasma); degradation slowed by acidosis Widely used Doxacurium is chemically similar but stable in plasma, giving it long duration of action Cisatracurium is the pure active isomeric constituent of atracurium, more potent but with less histamine release
Mivacurium	Fast (~2 min)	Short (~15 min)	Transient hypotension (histamine release)	Chemically similar to atracurium but rapidly inactivated by plasma cholinesterase (therefore longer acting in patients with liver disease or with genetic cholinesterase deficiency (see Ch. 12)
Suxamethonium	Fast	Short (~10 min)	Bradycardia (muscarinic agonist effect) Cardiac dysrhythmias (increased plasma K^+ concentration – avoid in patients with burns or severe trauma) Raised intraocular pressure (nicotinic agonist effect on extraocular muscles) Postoperative muscle pain	Acts by depolarisation of endplate (nicotinic agonist effect) – the only drug of this type still in use Paralysis is preceded by transient muscle fasciculations Short duration of action owing to hydrolysis by plasma cholinesterase (prolonged action in patients with liver disease or genetic deficiency of plasma cholinesterase) Used for brief procedures (e.g. tracheal intubation, electroconvulsive shock therapy) Rocuronium has similar speed of onset and recovery, with fewer unwanted effects

[a]For chemical structures, see Hardman, J.G., Limbird, L.E., Gilman, A.G., Goodman-Gilman A. et al., 2001. Goodman and Gilman's Pharmacological Basis of Therapeutics, 10th ed. McGraw-Hill, New York.

of the drugs also produce clinically significant autonomic effects by blocking ganglionic transmission.

The first muscles to be affected are the extrinsic eye muscles (causing double vision), reminiscent of the disease myasthenia gravis, which is caused by autoantibodies directed against nAChR (see later), and the small muscles of the face, limbs and pharynx (causing difficulty in swallowing). Respiratory muscles are the last to be affected and the first to recover. An experiment in 1947 in which a heroic volunteer was fully curarised while conscious under artificial ventilation established this orderly paralytic march and showed that consciousness and awareness of pain were quite normal even when paralysis was complete.[5]

[5]The risk of patients waking up paralysed during surgery, and subsequently recalling this (awareness during anaesthesia), is a serious concern.

Unwanted effects

An important unwanted effect of tubocurarine is a fall in arterial pressure, due to (a) sympathetic ganglion block and (b) histamine release from mast cells (see Ch. 17), which can also give rise to bronchospasm in sensitive individuals. This is unrelated to nAChRs but also occurs with **atracurium** and **mivacurium** as well as with some pharmacologically unrelated drugs such as morphine (see Ch. 42). Other non-depolarising blocking drugs lack these adverse effects. **Pancuronium** also blocks mAChRs, particularly in the heart, causing tachycardia.

Pharmacokinetic aspects

Neuromuscular-blocking drugs are given intravenously. They differ in their rates of onset and recovery (Fig. 14.5 and Table 14.6).

Most non-depolarising blocking agents are metabolised by the liver or excreted unchanged in the urine, exceptions being **atracurium**, which hydrolyses spontaneously in plasma, and **mivacurium**, which, like **suxamethonium** (see later), is hydrolysed by plasma cholinesterase. Their duration of action varies between about 15 min and 1–2 h (see Table 14.6), by which time the patient regains enough strength to cough and breathe properly. The route of elimination is important, because many patients undergoing anaesthesia have impaired renal or hepatic function, which can enhance or prolong paralysis to an important degree.

Atracurium, although stable when stored at an acid pH, was designed to be chemically unstable at physiological pH, splitting into two inactive fragments by cleavage at one of the quaternary nitrogen atoms. It has a short duration of action, which is unaffected by renal or hepatic function. Because of the marked pH dependence of its degradation, however, its action is shortened during respiratory alkalosis caused by hyperventilation.

Rapid postoperative recovery of muscle strength after surgery is important to minimise respiratory complications. The cholinesterase inhibitor **neostigmine** (Table 14.7) is often used to reverse the action of non-depolarising drugs postoperatively. Co-administration of atropine is necessary to prevent unwanted parasympathomimetic effects.

Anticholinesterase drugs *overcome* the blocking action of non-depolarising agents because released ACh, protected from hydrolysis, can diffuse further within the synaptic cleft and so access a wider area of postsynaptic membrane. The chances of an ACh molecule finding an unoccupied receptor before being hydrolysed are thus increased. This diffusional effect seems to be more important than a truly competitive interaction, for it is unlikely that appreciable dissociation of the antagonist can occur in the short time for which the ACh is present. In contrast, depolarisation block is either unaffected by anticholinesterase drugs or even increased via potentiation of the depolarising action of endogenous ACh.

An alternative approach for reversal of neuromuscular blockade induced by **rocuronium** or **vecuronium** is the use of a synthetic cyclodextrin, **sugammadex**, a macromolecule that selectively binds steroidal neuromuscular-blocking drugs as an inactive complex in the plasma (Nicholson et al., 2007). The complex is excreted unchanged in the urine. Sugammadex rapidly reverses block with few unwanted effects.

DEPOLARISING BLOCKING AGENTS

Suxamethonium is the only depolarising agent used clinically. There are several differences in the pattern of neuromuscular block produced by depolarising and non-depolarising mechanisms:

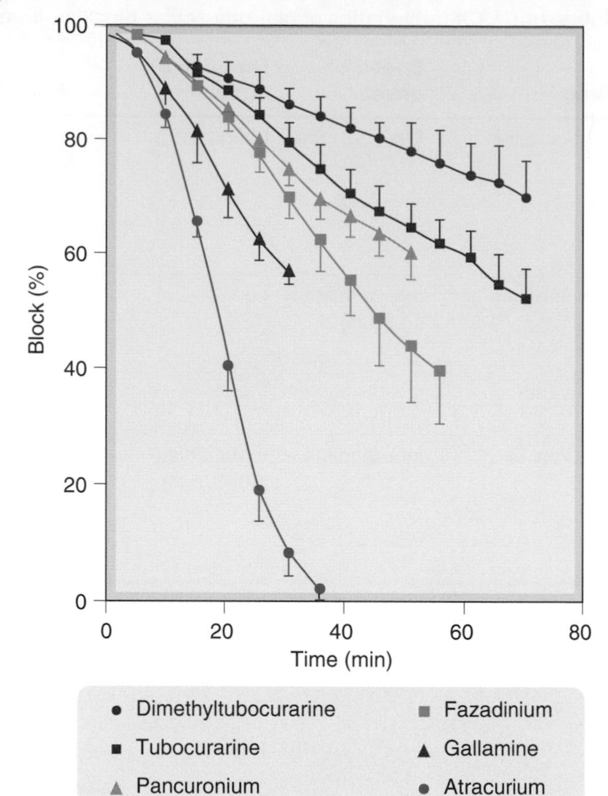

Fig. 14.5 Rate of recovery from various non-depolarising neuromuscular-blocking drugs in humans. Drugs were given intravenously to patients undergoing surgery, in doses just sufficient to cause 100% block of the tetanic tension of the indirectly stimulated adductor pollicis muscle. Recovery of tension was then followed as a function of time. (From Payne, J.P., Hughes, R., 1981. Br. J. Anaesth. 53, 45.)

- Fasciculation, seen with suxamethonium (see Table 14.6) as a prelude to paralysis, does not occur with non-depolarising drugs. Its severity is linked to postoperative muscle pain experienced after suxamethonium.
- *Tetanic fade* (see earlier in the chapter) occurs with non-depolarising blocking drugs, but not with suxamethonium, which does not block presynaptic nAChRs.

Unwanted effects and dangers of suxamethonium

Suxamethonium has several adverse effects (see Table 14.6), but remains in use for short-lasting procedures because of the rapid recovery that follows its intravenous administration.

Bradycardia

This is preventable by atropine and is due to a direct muscarinic action.

Potassium release

The increase in cation permeability of the motor endplates causes a net loss of K^+ from muscle, and thus a small rise in plasma K^+ concentration. This is not usually important, but may be an issue following trauma, burns or injuries causing muscle denervation (Fig. 14.6). Denervation increases the rise in plasma K^+ caused by suxamethonium because it causes ACh receptors to spread to regions of the muscle fibre away from the endplates (see Ch. 13), so that a much larger area of membrane is sensitive to suxamethonium. The resulting hyperkalaemia can be enough to cause ventricular dysrhythmia or cardiac arrest.

Increased intraocular pressure
Extraocular muscles are unusual in containing a population of fibres with nAChRs distributed along their length, rather than localised at motor endplates; these respond to suxamethonium with a sustained contracture, applying pressure to the eyeball. It is particularly important to avoid this if the eyeball has been injured.

Prolonged paralysis
The action of suxamethonium, given as an intravenous bolus to achieve relaxation during tracheal intubation, normally lasts for only 2–6 min, because the drug is hydrolysed by plasma cholinesterase. Its action is prolonged by various factors that reduce the activity of this enzyme:

- Genetic variants of plasma cholinesterase with reduced activity (see Ch. 12). Severe deficiency, enough to increase the duration of action to 2 h or more, occurs in approximately 1 in 3500 individuals. Rarely, the enzyme is completely absent, and paralysis lasts for many hours. Biochemical testing of enzyme activity in the plasma and its sensitivity to inhibitors is used clinically to diagnose this problem; genotyping is possible but as yet not practicable for routine screening to prevent the problem.
- Anticholinesterase drugs. The topical use of organophosphates to treat glaucoma (see Ch. 27) can inhibit plasma cholinesterase and prolong the action of suxamethonium. Competing substrates for plasma cholinesterase (e.g. **procaine**, **propanidid**) can also have this effect.
- Neonates may have low plasma cholinesterase activity and experience prolonged paralysis if treated with suxamethonium.

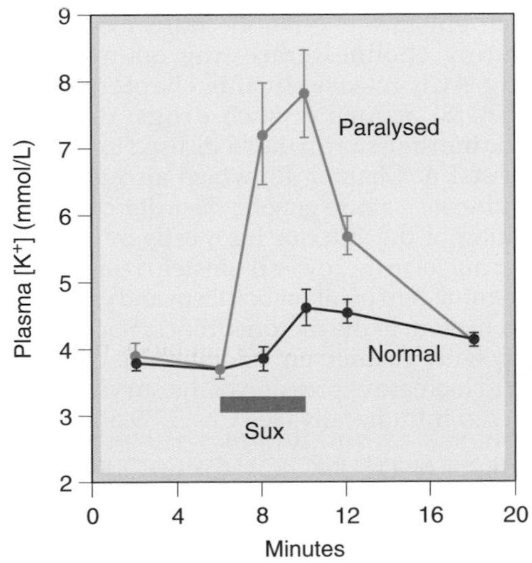

Fig. 14.6 Effect of suxamethonium (Sux) on plasma potassium concentration in humans. Blood was collected from veins draining paralysed and non-paralysed limbs of seven injured patients undergoing surgery. The injuries had resulted in motor nerve degeneration, and hence denervation supersensitivity of the affected muscles. (From Tobey, R.E., et al., 1972. Anaesthesiology 37, 322.)

Malignant hyperpyrexia
This is a rare inherited condition, due to a mutation of the Ca^{2+} release channel of the sarcoplasmic reticulum (the ryanodine receptor, see Ch. 4), which results in intense muscle spasm and a dramatic rise in body temperature in response to certain drugs (see Ch. 12). Suxamethonium is now the commonest culprit. The condition carries a high mortality (about 65%) and is treated by administration of **dantrolene**, a drug that inhibits muscle contraction by preventing Ca^{2+} release from the sarcoplasmic reticulum.

Neuromuscular-blocking drugs

- Substances that block neuronal choline uptake: for example, **hemicholinium** (not used clinically).
- Substances that block acetylcholine release: **aminoglycoside antibiotics**, **botulinum toxin.**
- Drugs used to cause paralysis during anaesthesia comprise:
  - Depolarising neuromuscular-blocking agents: **suxamethonium**, short-acting and used during induction of anaesthesia and intubation of the airway.
  - Non-depolarising neuromuscular-blocking agents: **tubocurarine**, **pancuronium**, **atracurium**, **vecuronium**, **mivacurium.** These block nicotinic acetylcholine receptors and differ mainly in duration of action; they are used to maintain neuromuscular relaxation throughout a surgical operation, or in patients in an intensive care unit who may otherwise experience muscular spasm or involuntary movement.
- Important characteristics of non-depolarising and depolarising blocking drugs:
  - Non-depolarising block is reversible by anticholinesterase drugs, depolarising block is not.
  - Steroidal ('curonium') drugs (**rocuronium**, **vecuronium**) are reversed by **sugammadex.**
  - Depolarising block produces initial fasciculations and often postoperative muscle pain.
  - **Suxamethonium** is hydrolysed by plasma cholinesterase and is normally very short-acting but may cause long-lasting paralysis in subjects with genetic cholinesterase-deficiency.
- Main side effects: early curare derivatives caused ganglion block, histamine release and hence hypotension and bronchoconstriction; newer non-depolarising blocking drugs have fewer side effects; **suxamethonium** may cause bradycardia, cardiac dysrhythmias due to K^+ release (especially in burned or injured patients), increased intraocular pressure or (in rare genetically susceptible individuals) malignant hyperthermia.

DRUGS THAT ACT PRESYNAPTICALLY

DRUGS THAT INHIBIT ACETYLCHOLINE SYNTHESIS

The steps in the synthesis of ACh in the presynaptic nerve terminals are shown in Fig. 14.2. The rate-limiting process appears to be the transport of choline into the nerve terminal. **Hemicholinium** blocks this transport and thereby inhibits ACh synthesis. It is useful as an experimental tool but has no clinical applications. Its blocking effect on transmission develops slowly, as the existing stores of ACh become depleted. **Vesamicol**, which acts by blocking ACh transport into synaptic vesicles, has a similar effect.

DRUGS THAT INHIBIT ACETYLCHOLINE RELEASE

ACh release by a nerve impulse involves the entry of Ca^{2+} into the nerve terminal; the increase in $[Ca^{2+}]_i$ stimulates exocytosis and increases the rate of quantal release (see Fig. 14.2). Agents that inhibit Ca^{2+} entry include Mg^{2+} and various aminoglycoside antibiotics (e.g. **streptomycin** and **gentamicin**; see Ch. 52), which can unpredictably prolong muscle paralysis when used clinically in patients treated with neuromuscular-blocking agents as an adjunct to general anaesthesia.

Two potent neurotoxins, **botulinum toxin** and **β-bungarotoxin**, act specifically to inhibit ACh release. Botulinum toxins are of particular scientific and medical interest (see review by Pirazzini et al., 2017). They are a family of proteins produced by the anaerobic bacillus *Clostridium botulinum*, an organism that can multiply in preserved food and can cause botulism, an extremely serious type of food poisoning.[6] Novel botulinum neurotoxins are being discovered by next generation sequencing and their pharmacology is a current focus of interest. The potency of botulinum toxin is extraordinary, the minimum lethal dose in a mouse being less than 10^{-12} g – only a few million molecules. It belongs to the group of potent bacterial exotoxins that includes tetanus and diphtheria toxins. These possess two subunits, one of which binds to a membrane receptor and is responsible for cellular specificity. By this means, the toxin enters the cell, where the other subunit produces the toxic effect. Botulinum toxins are peptidases that cleave specific proteins involved in exocytosis (*synaptobrevins, syntaxins*, etc.; see Ch. 4), thereby producing a long-lasting block of synaptic function. Each toxin component inactivates a different functional protein – a remarkably coordinated attack by a humble bacterium on a vital component of mammalian physiology.

Botulinum poisoning causes progressive parasympathetic and motor paralysis, with dry mouth, blurred vision and difficulty in swallowing, followed by progressive respiratory paralysis. Treatment with antitoxin is effective only if given before symptoms appear, for once the toxin is bound its action cannot be reversed. Mortality is high, and recovery takes several weeks. Anticholinesterases and drugs that increase transmitter release are ineffective in restoring transmission. **Botulinum toxin**, given by local injection, has a number of clinical and cosmetic uses (a testament to Paracelsus' dictum that all drugs are poisons, the distinction lying in the dose), including:

- *blepharospasm* (persistent and disabling eyelid spasm) and other forms of unwanted movement disorder including *torsion dystonia* and *spasmodic torticollis* (twisting movements of, respectively, limbs or neck);
- *spasticity* (excessive extensor muscle tone, associated with developmental brain abnormalities or birth injury);
- *urinary incontinence* associated with bladder overactivity (given by intravesical injection);
- *squint* (given by injection into extraocular muscles);
- *hyperhidrosis* (injected intradermally into axillary skin), for excessive sweating resistant to other treatment;
- *sialorrhoea* (excessive salivary secretion);
- *headache prophylaxis* (in adults with chronic migraine and frequent headaches);
- *forehead wrinkles* (injected intradermally it removes frown lines by paralysing the superficial muscles that pucker the skin).

Injections need to be repeated every few months. Botulinum toxin is antigenic, and may lose its effectiveness due to its immunogenicity. There is a risk of more general muscle paralysis if the toxin spreads beyond the injected region.

β-Bungarotoxin is a protein contained in the venom of various snakes of the cobra family, and has a similar action to botulinum toxin, although its active component is a phospholipase rather than a peptidase. The same venoms also contain α-bungarotoxin (see Ch. 3), which blocks postsynaptic ACh receptors. These snakes evidently cover all eventualities as far as causing paralysis of their victims is concerned.

DRUGS THAT ENHANCE CHOLINERGIC TRANSMISSION

Drugs that enhance cholinergic transmission act either by inhibiting cholinesterase (the main group) or by increasing ACh release. In this chapter, we focus on the peripheral actions of such drugs; drugs affecting cholinergic transmission in the CNS, used to treat dementia, are discussed in Chapter 40, which also mentions *spinal muscular atrophy* – a rare genetic disorder characterised by degeneration of the anterior horn cells in the spinal cord and motor nuclei in the lower brainstem resulting in clinical features reminiscent of infant botulism and caused by loss of a survival protein in the motoneurones. Such patients may be treated with **nusinersen**, an antisense oligonucleotide designed to increase expression of the survival protein and administered intrathecally (see Chs 5, 39 and 40).

DISTRIBUTION AND FUNCTION OF CHOLINESTERASE

There are two distinct types of cholinesterase, namely *AChE* and *butyrylcholinesterase* (BuChE, sometimes called pseudocholinesterase), closely related in molecular structure but differing in their distribution, substrate specificity and functions. Both consist of globular catalytic subunits, which constitute the soluble forms found in plasma (BuChE) and cerebrospinal fluid (AChE). Elsewhere, the catalytic units are linked to accessory proteins, which tether them like a bunch of balloons to the basement membrane (at the neuromuscular junction) or to the neuronal membrane

[6]Among the more spectacular outbreaks of botulinum poisoning was an incident on Loch Maree in Scotland in 1922, when all eight members of a fishing party died after eating duck pâté for their lunch. Their ghillies, consuming humbler fare no doubt, survived. The innkeeper committed suicide.

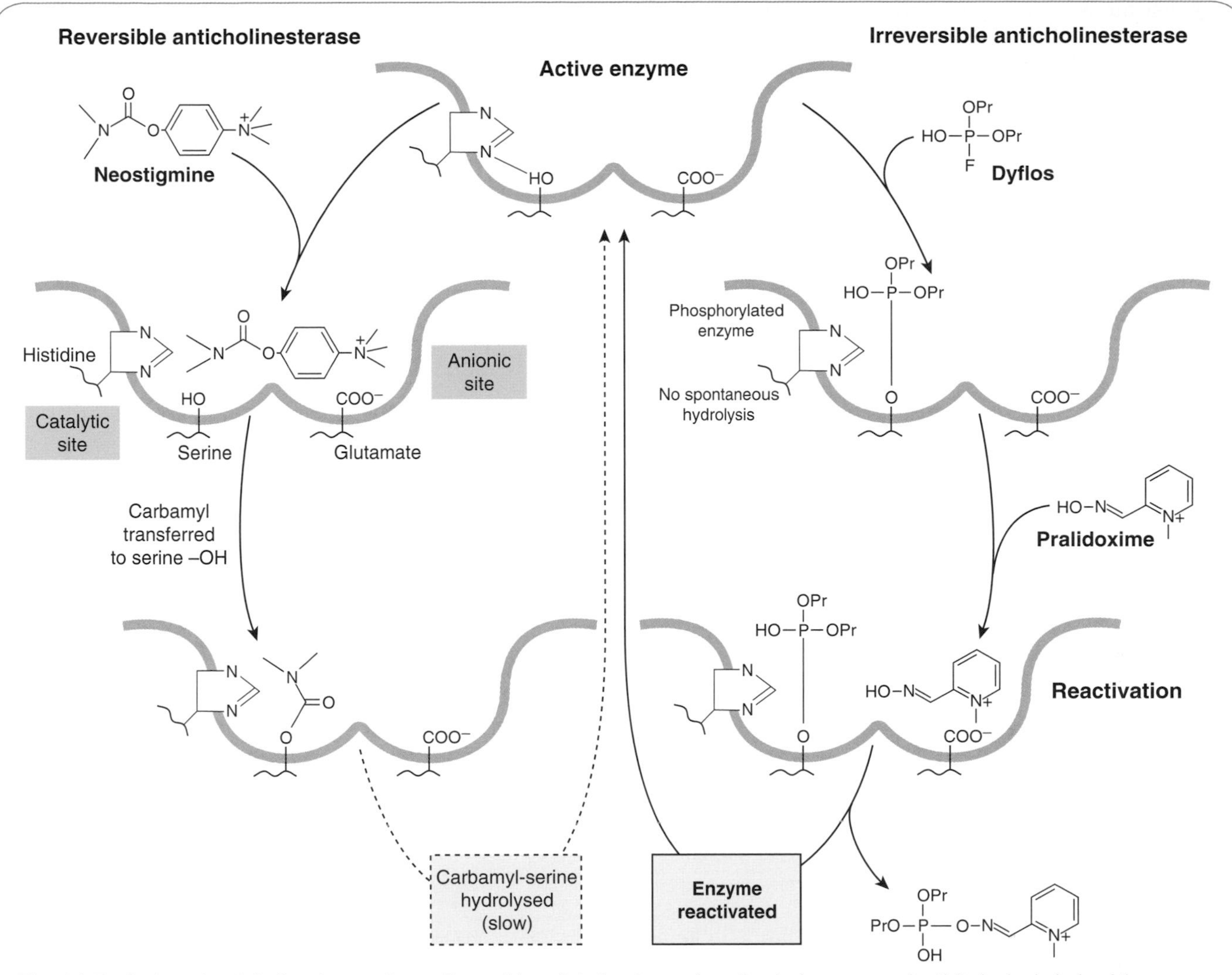

Fig. 14.7 Action of anticholinesterase drugs. Reversible anticholinesterase *(neostigmine)*: recovery of activity by hydrolysis of the carbamylated enzyme takes many minutes. Irreversible anticholinesterase *(Dyflos)*: reactivation of phosphorylated enzyme by pralidoxime. The representation of the active site is purely diagrammatic and not representative of the actual molecular structure.

at neuronal synapses (and also, oddly, to erythrocyte membranes, where the function of the enzyme is unknown).

The bound AChE at cholinergic synapses serves to hydrolyse the released transmitter and terminate its action rapidly. Soluble AChE is present in cholinergic nerve terminals, where it has a role in regulating the free ACh concentration, and from which it may be secreted; the function of the secreted enzyme is so far unclear. AChE is quite specific for ACh and closely related esters such as methacholine. Certain neuropeptides, such as substance P (see Ch. 19), are inactivated by AChE, but it is not known whether this is of physiological significance. Overall, there is poor correspondence between the distribution of cholinergic synapses and that of AChE, both in the brain and in the periphery, and AChE most probably has synaptic functions additional to disposal of ACh, although the details remain unclear (see review by Zimmerman and Soreq, 2006).

BuChE has a widespread distribution, being found in tissues such as liver, skin, brain and gastrointestinal smooth muscle, as well as in soluble form in the plasma. It is not particularly associated with cholinergic synapses, and its physiological function is unclear. It has a broader substrate specificity than AChE. It hydrolyses the synthetic substrate butyrylcholine and other esters, such as **procaine**, **suxamethonium** and **propanidid** (a short-acting anaesthetic agent; see Ch. 41), more rapidly than ACh. The plasma enzyme is important in inactivating these esters. Genetic variants of BuChE causing significantly reduced enzymic activity occur rarely, and these partly account for the variability in the duration of action of such drugs. The short duration of action of ACh given intravenously (see Fig. 14.1) results from its rapid hydrolysis in the plasma. Normally, AChE (on red cells) and BuChE (in plasma) between them keep the plasma ACh at an undetectably low level, so ACh is strictly a neurotransmitter and not a hormone.

Both AChE and BuChE belong to the class of serine hydrolases, which includes many proteases such as trypsin. The active site of AChE comprises two distinct regions (Fig. 14.7): an *anionic site* (glutamate residue), which binds the positively charged (choline) moiety of ACh, and an *esteratic (catalytic) site* (histidine + serine). As with other serine hydrolases, the acidic (acetyl) group of the substrate is transferred to the serine hydroxyl group, leaving (transiently) an acetylated enzyme molecule and a molecule of free choline. Spontaneous hydrolysis of the serine acetyl group occurs rapidly, and the overall turnover number of AChE is extremely high (over 10,000 molecules of ACh hydrolysed per second by a single active site).

DRUGS THAT INHIBIT CHOLINESTERASE

Peripherally acting anticholinesterase drugs, summarised in Table 14.7, fall into three main groups according to the nature of their interaction with the active site, which determines their duration of action. Most of them inhibit AChE and BuChE approximately equally. Centrally acting anticholinesterases such as **donepezil**, developed for the treatment of dementia, are discussed in Chapter 40.

Short-acting anticholinesterases

The only important drug of this type is **edrophonium**, a quaternary ammonium compound that binds to the anionic site of the enzyme only. The ionic bond formed is readily reversible, and the action of the drug is very brief. It has previously been used for diagnostic purposes, because improvement of muscle strength by an anticholinesterase is characteristic of myasthenia gravis (see below) but not when muscle weakness is due to other causes. However, this test has been largely superseded by measures such as repetitive nerve stimulation, and serological testing for ACh receptor antibodies.

Table 14.7 Anticholinesterase drugs

Drug	Structure	Duration of action	Main site of action	Notes
Edrophonium	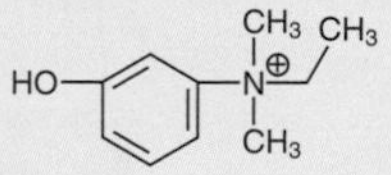	Short	NMJ	Distinguishes myasthenic from cholinergic crisis in patients with myasthenia gravis Too short-acting for therapeutic use
Neostigmine	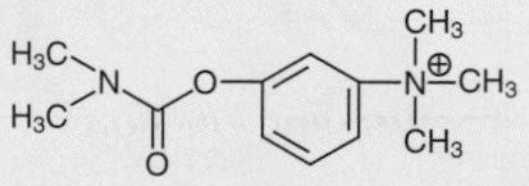	Medium	NMJ	Used intravenously to reverse competitive neuromuscular block Used orally in treatment of myasthenia gravis Visceral side effects
Physostigmine	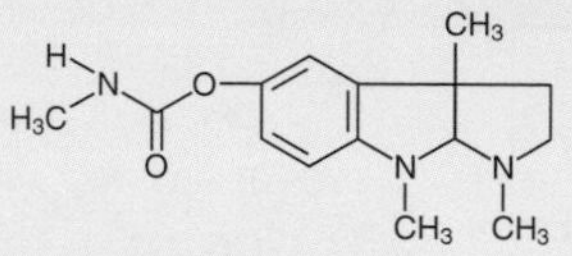	Medium	P	Used as eye drops in treatment of glaucoma
Pyridostigmine	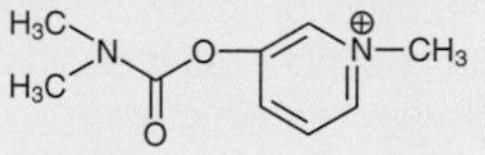	Medium	NMJ	Used orally in treatment of myasthenia gravis Better absorbed than neostigmine and has longer duration of action
Dyflos	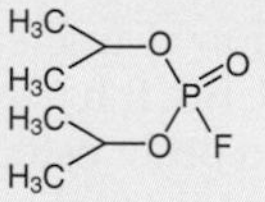	Long	P	Highly toxic organophosphate, with very prolonged action Has been used as eye drops for glaucoma
Ecothiopate	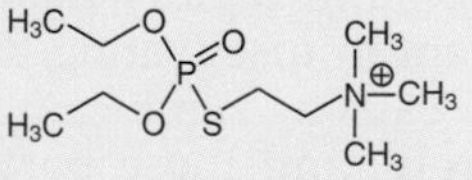	Long	P	Used as eye drops in treatment of glaucoma May cause systemic effects
Parathion	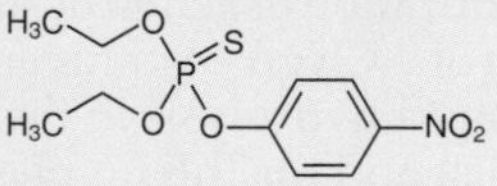	Long	–	Converted to active metabolite by replacement of sulfur by oxygen Used as insecticide but also causes poisoning in humans

Other anticholinesterase drugs developed for the treatment of dementia are described in Chapter 41.
NMJ, Neuromuscular junction; *P*, postganglionic parasympathetic junction.

Medium-duration anticholinesterases

These include **neostigmine** and **pyridostigmine**, which are quaternary ammonium compounds of clinical importance, and **physostigmine** (eserine), a tertiary amine, which occurs naturally in the Calabar bean.[7]

These drugs are all carbamyl, as opposed to acetyl, esters and all possess basic groups that bind to the anionic site in the enzyme. Transfer of the carbamyl group to the serine hydroxyl group of the esteratic site occurs as with ACh, but the carbamylated enzyme is very much slower to hydrolyse (see Fig. 14.7), taking minutes rather than microseconds. The anticholinesterase drug is therefore hydrolysed, but at a negligible rate compared with ACh, and the slow recovery of the carbamylated enzyme means that the action of these drugs is quite long-lasting.

Irreversible anticholinesterases

Irreversible anticholinesterases (see Table 14.7) are pentavalent phosphorus compounds containing a labile group such as fluoride (in **dyflos**) or an organic group (in **parathion** and **echothiophate**). This group is released, leaving the serine hydroxyl group of the enzyme phosphorylated (see Fig. 14.7). Most of these organophosphate compounds, of which there are many, were developed as weapons. **Sarin** and the more potent **VX** (10 mg of which through skin contact is said to be fatal), which acquired notoriety as an agent of state-sponsored assassination[8], are examples. Some are used as pesticides as well as for clinical use; they interact only with the esteratic site of the enzyme and have no cationic group. **Echothiophate** is an exception in having a quaternary nitrogen group designed to bind also to the anionic site on the enzyme.

The inactive phosphorylated enzyme is usually very stable. With drugs such as dyflos, no appreciable hydrolysis occurs, and recovery of enzymic activity depends on the synthesis of new enzyme molecules, a process that may take weeks. With other drugs, such as echothiophate, hydrolysis occurs over the course of a few days, so that their action is not strictly irreversible. Dyflos and parathion are volatile non-polar substances of very high lipid solubility and are rapidly absorbed through mucous membranes and even through unbroken skin and insect cuticles; the use of these agents as war gases or insecticides relies on this property. The lack of a specificity-conferring quaternary group means that most of these drugs also block other serine hydrolases (e.g. trypsin, thrombin), although their pharmacological effects result mainly from cholinesterase inhibition.

Effects of anticholinesterase drugs

Some organophosphate compounds can produce, in addition, a severe form of neurotoxicity.

Cholinesterase inhibitors affect peripheral (autonomic ganglia, neuromuscular junction and post-ganglionic parasympathetic nerves) as well as central cholinergic synapses.

Effects on autonomic cholinergic synapses

These mainly reflect enhancement of ACh activity at parasympathetic postganglionic synapses – namely increased secretions from salivary, lacrimal, bronchial and gastrointestinal glands; increased peristaltic activity; bronchoconstriction; bradycardia and hypotension; pupillary constriction; fixation of accommodation for near vision; and a fall in intraocular pressure – referred to as 'parasympathomimetic' effects. Large doses can additionally stimulate, and later block, autonomic ganglia, producing complex autonomic effects. The block, if it occurs, is a depolarisation block and is associated with a build-up of ACh in the plasma and body fluids. Neostigmine and pyridostigmine tend to affect neuromuscular transmission more than the autonomic system, whereas physostigmine and organophosphates show the reverse pattern. The reason is not clear, but therapeutic usage takes advantage of this partial selectivity.

Acute anticholinesterase poisoning (e.g. from contact with insecticides or war gases) causes severe bradycardia, hypotension and difficulty in breathing. Combined with a depolarising neuromuscular block and central effects (see later), the result may be fatal.

Effects on the neuromuscular junction

The twitch tension of a muscle stimulated via its motor nerve is increased by anticholinesterases, owing to repetitive firing in muscle fibres caused by prolongation of the epp. Normally, ACh is hydrolysed so quickly that each stimulus initiates only one action potential in the muscle fibre, but when AChE is inhibited this is converted to a short train of action potentials in the muscle fibre, and hence greater tension. Much more important is the effect produced when transmission has been blocked by a non-depolarising blocking agent such as pancuronium. In this case, addition of an anticholinesterase can dramatically restore transmission. If a large proportion of the receptors is blocked, the majority of ACh molecules will normally encounter, and be destroyed by, an AChE molecule before reaching a vacant receptor; inhibiting AChE gives the ACh molecules a greater chance of finding a vacant receptor before being destroyed, and thus increase the epp so that it reaches threshold. In myasthenia gravis (see later), transmission fails because there are too few functional ACh receptors, and cholinesterase inhibition improves transmission just as it does in the presence of a competitive antagonist.

In large doses, such as can occur in poisoning, anticholinesterases initially cause twitching of muscles. This is because spontaneous ACh release can give rise to epps that reach the firing threshold. Later, paralysis may occur due to depolarisation block, which is associated with the build-up of ACh.

Effects on the CNS

Tertiary compounds, such as physostigmine, and the non-polar organophosphates penetrate the blood–brain barrier freely and affect the brain. The result is an initial excitation, which can result in convulsions, followed by depression, which can cause unconsciousness and respiratory failure. These central effects result mainly from the activation of mAChRs and are

[7]Otherwise known as the ordeal bean. In the Middle Ages, extracts of these beans were used to determine the guilt or innocence of those accused of crime or heresy. Death implied guilt.

[8]On February 13, 2017, Kin Jong-nam, half-brother of North Korean leader Kim Jong-un, died after an assault in Kuala Lumpur International Airport. According to the authorities he was murdered by poisoning with VX, which was found on his face. The authorities further reported that one of the women suspected of applying the nerve agent experienced some physical symptoms of VX poisoning. The director of a research program of the Middlebury Institute of International Studies at Monterey stated that VX fumes would have killed the suspected attackers even if they had been wearing gloves, suggesting that the VX was applied as two non-lethal components that would mix to form VX only on the victim's face (Wikipedia, accessed June 9, 2021).

antagonised by atropine. The use of anticholinesterases to treat dementia is discussed in Chapter 40.

Cholinesterase and anticholinesterase drugs

- There are two main forms of cholinesterase: *acetylcholinesterase (AChE)*, which is mainly membrane bound, relatively specific for acetylcholine, and responsible for rapid acetylcholine hydrolysis at cholinergic synapses; and *butyrylcholinesterase* (BuChE) or pseudocholinesterase, which is relatively non-selective and occurs in plasma and many tissues. Both enzymes belong to the family of serine hydrolases.
- Anticholinesterase drugs are of three main types: short-acting (**edrophonium**), medium-acting (**neostigmine**, **physostigmine**) and irreversible (organophosphates, **dyflos**, **echothiophate**). They differ in the nature of their chemical interaction with the active site of cholinesterase.
- The effects of anticholinesterase drugs are due mainly to enhancement of cholinergic transmission at cholinergic autonomic synapses and at the neuromuscular junction. Anticholinesterases that cross the blood–brain barrier (e.g. **physostigmine**, organophosphates) also have marked CNS effects. Autonomic effects include bradycardia, hypotension, excessive secretions, bronchoconstriction, gastrointestinal hypermotility and decrease of intraocular pressure. Neuromuscular action causes muscle fasciculation and increased twitch tension and can produce depolarisation block.
- Anticholinesterase poisoning may occur from exposure to insecticides or nerve gases or to non-deliberate overdosing of patients taking it to relieve symptoms of myasthenia gravis.

Delayed neurotoxicity of organophosphates

Many organophosphates can cause a severe type of delayed peripheral nerve degeneration, leading to progressive weakness and sensory loss. This is not a problem with clinically used anticholinesterases but occasionally results from poisoning with insecticides or nerve gases. In 1931, an estimated 20,000 Americans were affected, some fatally, by contamination of fruit juice with an organophosphate insecticide, and other similar outbreaks have been recorded. The mechanism of this reaction is only partly understood, but it seems to result from inhibition of a *neuropathy target esterase* distinct from cholinesterase. Chronic low-level exposure of agricultural and other workers to organophosphorous pesticides has been associated with neurobehavioural disorders (Blanc-Lapierre et al., 2013). Other serine hydrolases apart from AChE can be secondary organophosphate targets including neuropathy target esterase, lipases and endocannabinoid hydrolases (Casida, 2017).

The main uses of anticholinesterases are summarised in the next clinical box.

Clinical uses of anticholinesterase drugs

- To reverse the action of non-depolarising neuromuscular-blocking drugs after surgery (**neostigmine**). A muscarinic antagonist (e.g. **atropine**) must be given to limit parasympathomimetic effects.
- To treat myasthenia gravis (**neostigmine** or **pyridostigmine**).
- **Edrophonium**, a short-acting drug given intravenously, has been used in the past for diagnosis of myasthenia gravis, but this method of testing is unreliable, and requires resuscitation facilities on-hand to deal with severe adverse reactions. Edrophonium test distinguishes myasthenic from cholinergic crisis in patients with myasthenia gravis with acute deterioration during treatment with a cholinesterase inhibitor.
- Alzheimer's disease (e.g. **donepezil**; see Ch. 40).

CHOLINESTERASE REACTIVATION

Spontaneous hydrolysis of phosphorylated cholinesterase is extremely slow, so poisoning with organophosphates necessitates prolonged supportive care. **Pralidoxime** (see Fig. 14.7) reactivates the enzyme by bringing an oxime group into close proximity with the phosphorylated esteratic site. This group is a strong nucleophile and lures the phosphate group away from the serine hydroxyl group of the enzyme. The effectiveness of pralidoxime in reactivating plasma cholinesterase activity in a poisoned subject is shown in Fig. 14.8. The main limitation to its use as an antidote to organophosphate poisoning is that, within a few hours, the phosphorylated enzyme undergoes a chemical change ('ageing') that renders it no longer susceptible to reactivation, so that pralidoxime must be given early in order to work. Pralidoxime does not enter the brain, but related compounds have been developed to treat the central effects of organophosphate poisoning.

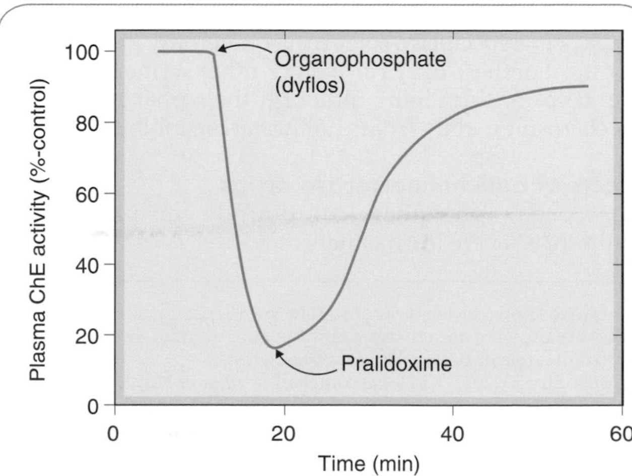

Fig. 14.8 Reactivation of plasma cholinesterase (ChE) in a volunteer subject by intravenous injection of pralidoxime.

Myasthenia gravis

The neuromuscular junction seldom fails, myasthenia gravis and the Lambert–Eaton myasthenic syndrome (see further) being two of the few disorders that affect it. Myasthenia gravis affects about 1 in 2000 individuals, often, but by no means always, young women who are susceptible to autoimmune disorders. It is characterised by weakness and increased fatigability of skeletal muscles resulting from impaired neuromuscular transmission. The tendency for transmission to fail during repetitive activity can be seen in Fig. 14.9. Muscles cannot produce prolonged contractions, resulting in the characteristic drooping eyelids and double vision on attempting to sustain lateral gaze. The effectiveness of anticholinesterase drugs in improving muscle strength in myasthenia was discovered in 1931, long before the pathophysiology of the disease was understood.

The cause of the transmission failure is an autoimmune response to nAChRs of the neuromuscular junction, first revealed in studies showing that the number of bungarotoxin-binding sites at the endplates of myasthenic patients was reduced by about 70% compared with normal. It had been suspected that myasthenia had an immunological basis, because the disease is sometimes accompanied by a tumour of the thymus gland and removal of the thymus improves the motor symptoms. Immunisation of rabbits with purified ACh receptor causes, after a delay, a disorder reminiscent of human myasthenia gravis. The presence of antibody directed against the ACh receptor protein can be detected in the serum of myasthenic patients, but the reason for the development of the autoimmune response in humans is unknown (Gilhus, 2016).

The improvement of neuromuscular function by anticholinesterase treatment (shown in Fig. 14.9) can be dramatic, but if the disease progresses too far, the number of receptors remaining may be insufficient to produce an adequate epp, and anticholinesterase drugs cease to be effective.

Alternative approaches to the treatment of myasthenia are to remove circulating antibody by plasma exchange, which is transiently effective, or, for a more prolonged effect, to inhibit antibody production with immunosuppressant drugs (e.g. **prednisolone**, **azathioprine**, **mycophenolate**, **cyclosporine** and **tacrolimus**; see Ch. 25) or thymectomy.

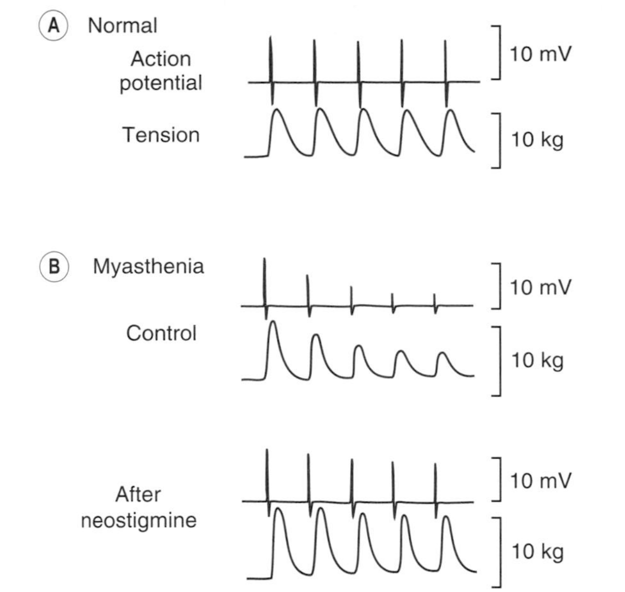

Fig. 14.9 Neuromuscular transmission in a normal and a myasthenic human subject. Electrical activity was recorded with a needle electrode in the adductor pollicis muscle, in response to ulnar nerve stimulation (3 Hz) at the wrist. In a normal subject, electrical and mechanical response is well sustained. In a myasthenic patient, transmission fails rapidly when the nerve is stimulated. Treatment with *neostigmine* improves transmission. (From Desmedt, J.E., 1962. Bull. Acad. R. Med. Belg. VII 2, 213.)

OTHER DRUGS THAT ENHANCE CHOLINERGIC TRANSMISSION

It was observed many years ago that **tetraethylammonium**, a potassium-channel blocker and ganglion-blocking drug, could reverse the neuromuscular-blocking action of tubocurarine by prolonging the action potential in the nerve terminal and hence increasing the release of transmitter evoked by nerve stimulation. Subsequently, more potent and selective potassium-channel blocking drugs, such as **amifampridine**, were developed. These drugs are not selective for cholinergic nerves but increase the evoked release of many different transmitters. Amifampridine is used to treat the muscle weakness associated with Lambert–Eaton myasthenic syndrome, a complication of certain neoplastic diseases in which ACh release is inhibited when antitumour antibodies cross react with and inhibit Ca^{2+} channels on the prejunctional membrane.

REFERENCES AND FURTHER READING

Acetylcholine receptors

Bouzat, C., Sine, S.M., 2018. Nicotinic acetylcholine receptors at the single-channel level. Br. J. Pharmacol. 175, 1789–1804.

Dinely, K.T., Pandya, A.A., Yakel, J.L., 2015. Nicotinic ACh receptors as therapeutic targets in CNS disorders. Trends Pharmacol. Sci. 36, 96–108.

Jakubik, J., El-Fakahany, E.E., 2020. Current advances in allosteric modulation of muscarinic receptors. Biomolecules 10, 325.

Kalamida, D., Poulas, K., Avramopoulou, V., et al., 2007. Muscle and neuronal nicotinic acetylcholine receptors: structure, function and pathogenicity. FEBS J. 274, 3799–3845.

Kruse, A.C., Kobilka, B.K., Gautam, D., et al., 2014. Muscarinic acetylcholine receptors: novel opportunities for drug development. Nat. Rev. Drug Discov. 13, 549–560.

Southan, C., Sharman, J.L., Benson, H.E., et al., 2016. The IUPHAR/BPS guide to pharmacology in 2016: towards curated quantitative interactions between 1300 protein targets and 6000 ligands. Nucleic Acids Res. 44 (Database Issue), D1054–D1068.

Cholinergic transmission

Gilhus, N.E., 2016. Myasthenia gravis. N. Engl. Med. 375, 2570–2581.

He, X., Zhao, M., Bi, X., et al., 2015. Novel strategies and underlying protective mechanisms of modulation of vagal activity in cardiovascular diseases. Br. J. Pharmacol. 172, S489–S500.

Drugs affecting the neuromuscular junction

Nicholson, W.T., Sprung, J., Jankowski, C.J., 2007. Sugammadex: a novel agent for the reversal of neuromuscular blockade. Pharmacotherapy 27, 1181–1188.

Pirazzini, M., Rossetto, O., Eleopra, R., Montecucco, C., 2017. Botulinum neurotoxins: biology, pharmacology, and toxicology. Pharmacol. Rev. 69, 200–235.

Cholinesterase

Blanc-Lapierre, A., Bouvier, G., Gruber, A., 2013. Cognitive disorders and occupational exposure to organophosphates: results from the PHYTONER Study. Am. J. Epidemiol. 177, 1086–1096.
Casida, J., 2017. Organophosphate xenobiotic toxicology. Ann. Rev. Pharmacol. Toxocol. 57, 309–327.
Zimmerman, G., Soreq, H., 2006. Termination and beyond: acetylcholinesterase as a modulator of synaptic transmission. Cell Tissue Res. 326, 655–669.

Further reading

Changeux, J.P., 2012. The nicotinic acetylcholine receptor: the founding father of the pentameric ligand-gated ion channel superfamily. J. Biol. Chem. 287, 40207–40215.
Fagerlund, M.J., Eriksson, L.I., 2009. Current concepts in neuromuscular transmission. Br. J. Anaesth. 103, 108–114.
Nicholls, J.G., Martin, A.R., Fuchs, P.A., Brown, D.A., Diamond, M.E., Weisblat, D., 2012. From Neuron to Brain, fifth ed. Sinauer, Sunderland.
Wessler, I., Kirkpatrick, C.J., 2020. Cholinergic signaling controls immune functions and promotes homeostasis. Int. Immunopharm. 83, 106345.

Noradrenergic transmission 15

OVERVIEW

Peripheral noradrenergic neurons and the structures that they innervate are fundamental components of autonomic function and are the targets of many therapeutic drugs of great clinical importance. In this chapter we describe the physiology of noradrenergic neurons and the properties of adrenoceptors (the receptors on which noradrenaline and adrenaline act) and discuss the various classes of drugs that affect them. For ease of reference, much drug-specific detail is summarised in tables.

CATECHOLAMINES

Catecholamines contain a catechol moiety (a benzene ring with two adjacent hydroxyl groups) and an amine side chain (Fig. 15.1). The most important are:

- *noradrenaline (norepinephrine)*, a transmitter released by sympathetic nerve terminals;
- *adrenaline (epinephrine)*, a hormone secreted by chromaffin cells in the adrenal medulla;
- *dopamine*, the metabolic precursor of noradrenaline and adrenaline, also a transmitter/neuromodulator in the central nervous system (CNS);
- *isoprenaline (isoproterenol)*, a synthetic derivative of noradrenaline and pharmacological tool.

CLASSIFICATION OF ADRENOCEPTORS

In 1896, Oliver and Schafer discovered that intravenous injection of extracts of adrenal gland in anaesthetised cats caused a rise in arterial pressure. Adrenaline was identified as the active principle and was shown by Dale in 1913 to cause two distinct kinds of vascular effect, namely vasoconstriction in certain vascular beds and vasodilatation in others. Dale showed that the vasoconstrictor component disappeared if the animal was first injected with an ergot derivative[1] (see Ch. 16), and noticed that adrenaline then caused a fall, instead of a rise, in arterial pressure, reminiscent of his demonstration of the separate muscarinic and nicotinic components of the action of acetylcholine (see Ch. 14). He avoided interpreting it in terms of different types of receptor, but later pharmacological work, beginning with that of Ahlquist, showed clearly the existence of several subclasses of adrenoceptor with distinct tissue distributions and actions (Table 15.1).

In 1948 Ahlquist found that the rank order of the potencies of various catecholamines, including adrenaline, noradrenaline and isoprenaline, fell into two distinct patterns, depending on what response was being measured. He postulated the existence of two kinds of receptor, α and β, defined in terms of agonist potencies as follows:

α: noradrenaline > adrenaline > isoprenaline
β: isoprenaline > adrenaline > noradrenaline

It was then recognised that certain ergot alkaloids, which Dale had studied, act as selective α-receptor antagonists and that Dale's adrenaline reversal experiment reflected the unmasking of the β effects of adrenaline by α-receptor blockade. Selective β-receptor antagonists were not developed until 1955, when their effects fully confirmed Ahlquist's original classification and also suggested the existence of further subdivisions of both α and β receptors. Subsequently it has emerged that there are two α-receptor subtypes (α_1 and α_2), each comprising three further subclasses (α_{1A}, α_{1B}, α_{1D} and α_{2A}, α_{2B}, α_{2C}) and three β-receptor subtypes (β_1, β_2 and β_3) – altogether nine distinct subtypes – all of which are typical G protein–coupled receptors (Table 15.2). Genetic variants of both β_1 and β_2 receptors occur in humans and influence the effects of agonists and antagonists (see Ahles and Engelhardt, 2014). Evidence from specific agonists and antagonists, as well as studies on receptor knockout mice, have shown that α_1 receptors are particularly important in the cardiovascular system and lower urinary tract, while α_2 receptors are predominantly neuronal, acting to inhibit transmitter release both in the brain and at autonomic nerve terminals in the periphery. The α_{2B} subtype appears to be involved in neurotransmission in the spinal cord, and α_{2C}, in regulating catecholamine release from adrenal medulla (Alexander et al., 2019), but the distinct functions of the different subclasses of α_1 and α_2 adrenoceptors remain for the most part unclear; they are frequently co-expressed in the same tissues, and may form heterodimers, making pharmacological analysis difficult.

α_2-Adrenoceptors and imidazoline (I) receptors. The antihypertensive drug **clonidine** (see later) was synthesised in the 1960s. It works in the CNS to reduce sympathetic outflow and was found to be an α_2-adrenoceptor agonist. Bousquet and his colleagues subsequently discovered that clonidine interacts not only with the α_2-adrenoceptors but also with a distinct imidazoline preferring binding site, located in the brainstem particularly in the nucleus reticularis lateralis in the rostroventral medulla oblongata. Three subtypes (I_1, I_2 and I_3) have subsequently been identified and some at least are G-protein coupled although the receptor structures have not yet been elucidated. Endogenous agonists remain enigmatic although several

[1]Dale was a new recruit in the laboratories of the Wellcome pharmaceutical company, given the job of checking the potency of batches of adrenaline coming from the factory. He tested one batch at the end of a day's experimentation on a cat that he had earlier injected with an ergot preparation. Because it produced a fall in blood pressure rather than the expected rise, he advised that the whole expensive consignment should be rejected. Unknown to him, he was given the same sample to test a few days later and reported it to be normal. How he explained this to Wellcome's management is not recorded.

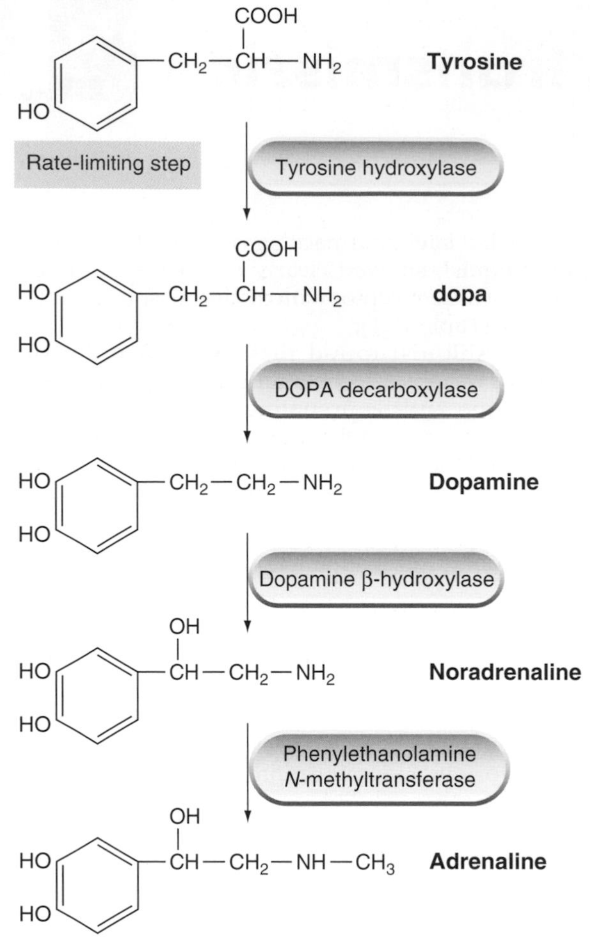

Tyrosine
Rate-limiting step
Tyrosine hydroxylase
dopa
DOPA decarboxylase
Dopamine
Dopamine β-hydroxylase
Noradrenaline
Phenylethanolamine *N*-methyltransferase
Adrenaline

Fig. 15.1 Structures of the major catecholamines.

potential candidates have been identified. Microinjection experiments showed that selective agonists at I_1 and at α_2-adrenoceptors act independently of each other to lower blood pressure but they synergise with one another when both receptors are stimulated. I_2 agonists cause analgesia and I_3 agonists, while much less studied, can produce metabolic effects by influencing insulin secretion from pancreatic B-cells. There is on-going interest in the therapeutic potential of drugs of this class (see Bousquet et al., 2020, for a review).

Each of the three main adrenoceptor subtypes is associated with a specific second messenger system (see Table 15.2). Thus α_1 receptors are coupled through Gq to phospholipase C and produce their effects mainly by the release of intracellular Ca^{2+}; α_2 receptors couple through Gi/Go to inhibit adenylyl cyclase, and thus reduce cAMP formation as well as inhibiting Ca^{2+} channels and activating K^+ channels. All three types of β receptor couple through Gs to stimulate adenylyl cyclase and downstream transduction pathways, e.g. kinases implicated in trophic actions (see Ch. 3 and further in the chapter). The main effects of adrenoceptors, and the drugs that act on them, are shown in Tables 15.1 and 15.2.

The distinction between β_1 and β_2 receptors is an important one, because β_1 receptors are found mainly in the heart, where they are responsible for the positive inotropic and chronotropic effects of catecholamines (see Ch. 20), whereas β_2 receptors are responsible for causing smooth muscle relaxation in many organs, most importantly in the lungs, where they relax the bronchioles and relieve bronchoconstriction in asthmatics (see Ch. 28). The cardiac effects can be harmful, predisposing to cardiac dysrhythmia and increasing myocardial oxygen demand (see Ch. 20); consequently, considerable efforts have been made to discover selective β_2 agonists to relax smooth muscle without affecting the heart, and selective β_1 antagonists to exert a useful blocking effect on the heart without blocking β_2 receptors at the same time (see Table 15.1). The available drugs are not completely specific and marketed selective β_1 antagonists have appreciable affinity for β_2 receptors, which can cause unwanted effects in asthmatics such as bronchoconstriction or blunted bronchodilator response to β_2 agonists.

In relation to vascular control, it is important to note that both α- and β-receptor subtypes are expressed in smooth muscle cells, nerve terminals and endothelial cells, and their role in physiological regulation and pharmacological responses of the cardiovascular system is only partly understood (see Guimaraes and Moura, 2001).

Classification of adrenoceptors

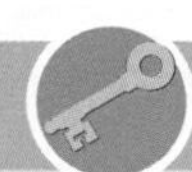

- Main pharmacological classification into α and β subtypes, based originally on order of potency among agonists, later on selective antagonists.
- Adrenoceptor subtypes:
  - two main α-adrenoceptor subtypes, α_1 and α_2, each divided into three further subtypes (α_{1A}, α_{1B}, α_{1D} and α_{2A}, α_{2B}, α_{2C})
  - three β-adrenoceptor subtypes (β_1, β_2, β_3)
  - all belong to the superfamily of G protein–coupled receptors (see Ch. 3).
- Second messengers:
  - α_1 receptors activate phospholipase C via G_q, producing inositol trisphosphate and diacylglycerol as second messengers
  - α_2 receptors modulate Ca^{2+} and K^+ channels via βα G-protein subunits and inhibit adenylyl cyclase via α_i (but cytoplasmic cAMP in nerve terminals is usually low under basal conditions, limiting the importance of this second mechanism).
  - all types of β receptor stimulate adenylyl cyclase via G_s.
- The main effects of receptor activation are:
  - α_1 receptors: vasoconstriction, relaxation of gastrointestinal smooth muscle, and hepatic glycogenolysis
  - α_2 receptors: inhibition of transmitter release (including noradrenaline and acetylcholine release from autonomic nerves) caused by opening of K^+ channels and inhibition of Ca^{2+} channels; platelet aggregation; vascular smooth muscle contraction; inhibition of insulin release
  - β_1 receptors: increased cardiac rate and force
  - β_2 receptors: bronchodilatation; vasodilatation; relaxation of visceral smooth muscle; hepatic glycogenolysis; muscle tremor
  - β_3 receptors: lipolysis and thermogenesis; bladder detrusor muscle relaxation.

Table 15.1 Distribution and actions of adrenoceptors

Tissues and effects	α_1	α_2	β_1	β_2	β_3
Smooth muscle					
Blood vessels	Constrict	Constrict/dilate	—	Dilate	—
Bronchi	Constrict	—	—	Dilate	—
Gastrointestinal tract	Relax	Relax (presynaptic effect)	—	Relax	—
Gastrointestinal sphincters	Contract	—	—	—	—
Uterus	Contract	—	—	Relax	—
Bladder detrusor	—	—	—	Relax	Relax
Bladder sphincter	Contract	—	—	—	—
Seminal tract	Contract	—	—	Relax	—
Iris (radial muscle)	Contract	—	—	—	—
Ciliary muscle	—	—	—	Relax	—
Heart					
Rate	—	—	Increase	Increase[a]	—
Force of contraction	—	—	Increase	Increase[a]	—
Other tissues/cells					
Skeletal muscle	—	—	—	Tremor Increased muscle mass and speed of contraction Glycogenolysis	Thermogenesis
Liver (hepatocytes)	Glycogenolysis	—	—	Glycogenolysis	—
Fat (adipocytes)	—	—	—	—	Lipolysis Thermogenesis
Pancreatic islets (B cells)	—	Decrease insulin secretion	—	—	—
Salivary gland	K^+ release	—	Amylase secretion	—	—
Platelets	—	Aggregation	—	—	—
Mast cells	—	—	—	Inhibition of histamine release	—
Brain stem	—	Inhibits sympathetic outflow	—	—	—
Nerve terminals					
Adrenergic	—	Decrease release	—	Increase release	—
Cholinergic	—	Decrease release	—	—	—

[a]Minor component normally but may become significant in heart failure.

Table 15.2 Characteristics of adrenoceptors

	$\alpha_{1(A,B,D)}$	$\alpha_{2(A,B,C)}$	β_1	β_2	β_3
G protein coupling	Gq	Gi/Go	G_S	G_S	G_S
Second messengers and effectors	Phospholipase C activation ↑ Inositol trisphosphate ↑ Diacylglycerol ↑ Ca^{2+}	↓ cAMP ↓ Calcium channels ↑ Potassium channels	↑ cAMP	↑ cAMP	↑ cAMP
Agonist potency order	NA > A ≫ ISO	A > NA ≫ ISO	ISO > NA > A	ISO > A > NA	ISO > NA = A
Selective agonists	Phenylephrine Midodrine Methoxamine	Clonidine (also acts through I_1 receptor)	Dobutamine Xamoterol	Salbutamol Terbutaline Salmeterol Formoterol Clenbuterol	Mirabegron
Selective antagonists	Prazosin Doxazosin	Yohimbine Idazoxan	Atenolol Metoprolol	Butoxamine	—

A, Adrenaline; *ISO*, isoprenaline; *NA*, noradrenaline.

PHYSIOLOGY OF NORADRENERGIC TRANSMISSION

THE NORADRENERGIC NEURON

Noradrenergic neurons in the periphery are postganglionic sympathetic neurons whose cell bodies are situated in sympathetic ganglia (see Ch. 13). They generally have long[2] axons that end in a series of varicosities strung along the branching terminal network. These varicosities contain numerous synaptic vesicles, which are the sites of synthesis and release of noradrenaline and of co-released mediators such as ATP and neuropeptide Y (see Ch. 13), which are stored in vesicles and released by exocytosis (see Ch. 4). In most peripheral tissues, the tissue content of noradrenaline closely parallels the density of the sympathetic innervation. With the exception of the adrenal medulla, sympathetic nerve terminals account for all the noradrenaline content of peripheral tissues. Organs such as the heart, spleen, vas deferens and some blood vessels are particularly rich in noradrenaline (5–50 nmol/g of tissue) and have been widely used for studies of noradrenergic transmission. For detailed information on noradrenergic neurons, see Robertson (2012) and Cooper et al. (2003).

NORADRENALINE AND ADRENALINE SYNTHESIS

The biosynthetic pathway for noradrenaline synthesis is shown in Fig. 15.1. The metabolic precursor for noradrenaline is *L-tyrosine*, an aromatic amino acid that is present in body fluids and is taken up by adrenergic neurons. *Tyrosine hydroxylase*, a cytosolic enzyme that catalyses the conversion of tyrosine to *dihydroxyphenylalanine* (dopa), is expressed only in catecholamine-containing cells. It is a rather selective enzyme; unlike other enzymes involved in catecholamine metabolism, it does not accept indole derivatives as substrates, and is not involved in 5-hydroxytryptamine (5-HT) synthesis. This first hydroxylation step is the main control point for noradrenaline synthesis. Tyrosine hydroxylase activity is inhibited by noradrenaline, and this provides the mechanism for the moment-to-moment regulation of the rate of synthesis; much slower regulation, taking hours or days, occurs by changes in the rate of production of the enzyme.

The tyrosine analogue **α-methyltyrosine** strongly inhibits tyrosine hydroxylase and has been used experimentally to block noradrenaline synthesis.

The next step, conversion of dopa to dopamine, is catalysed by *dopa decarboxylase*, a cytosolic enzyme that is not confined to catecholamine-synthesising cells. It is relatively non-specific and catalyses the decarboxylation of various other L-aromatic amino acids, such as *L-histidine* and *L-tryptophan*, which are precursors in the synthesis of histamine (see Ch. 17) and 5-HT (see Ch. 16), respectively. Dopa decarboxylase activity is not rate-limiting for noradrenaline synthesis and its activity does not regulate noradrenaline synthesis.

Dopamine-β-hydroxylase (DBH) is also a relatively non-specific enzyme but is restricted to catecholamine-synthesising cells. It is located in synaptic vesicles, mainly in membrane-bound form. A small amount of the enzyme is released from adrenergic nerve terminals in company with noradrenaline, representing the small proportion in a soluble form within the vesicle. Unlike noradrenaline, the released DBH is not subject to rapid degradation or uptake, so its concentration in plasma and body fluids can be used as an index of overall sympathetic nerve activity.

Many drugs inhibit DBH, including copper-chelating agents and **disulfiram** (a drug used mainly for its effect on ethanol metabolism; see Ch. 49). Such drugs can cause a partial depletion of noradrenaline stores and interference with sympathetic transmission. A rare genetic disorder, DBH deficiency, causes failure of noradrenaline synthesis resulting in severe orthostatic hypotension (see Ch. 21).

Phenylethanolamine N-*methyl transferase* (PNMT) catalyses the *N*-methylation of noradrenaline to form adrenaline. The main location of this enzyme is in the adrenal medulla, which contains a population of adrenaline-releasing (A) cells separate from the smaller proportion of noradrenaline-releasing (N) cells. The A cells, which appear only after birth, lie adjacent to the adrenal cortex, and the production of PNMT is induced by an action of the steroid hormones secreted by the adrenal cortex (see Ch. 33). PNMT is also found in a few neurons in the medulla oblongata, where adrenaline may function as a transmitter, but little is known about its role in the CNS.

In peripheral tissues, the turnover time of noradrenaline is generally about 5–15 h, but it becomes much shorter if sympathetic nerve activity is increased. Under normal circumstances, the rate of synthesis closely matches the rate of release, so that the noradrenaline content of tissues is constant regardless of how fast it is being released.

NORADRENALINE STORAGE

Most of the noradrenaline in nerve terminals and adrenal medulla is contained in vesicles; only a little is free in the cytoplasm under normal circumstances. The concentration in the vesicles is very high (0.3–1.0 mol/L) and is maintained by the *vesicular monoamine transporter* (VMAT), which shares some features of the amine transporter responsible for noradrenaline uptake into the nerve terminal (see Ch. 13) but uses the transvesicular proton gradient as its driving force. Certain drugs, such as **reserpine** (Table 15.3), block this transport and cause nerve terminals to become depleted of their vesicular noradrenaline stores. The vesicles contain two major constituents besides noradrenaline, namely ATP (about four molecules per molecule of noradrenaline) and a protein called *chromogranin A*. These substances are released along with noradrenaline, and it is generally assumed that a reversible complex, depending partly on the opposite charges on the molecules of noradrenaline and ATP, is formed within the vesicle. This would serve both to reduce the osmolarity of the vesicle contents and to reduce the tendency of noradrenaline to leak out of the vesicles within the nerve terminal.

ATP itself has a transmitter function at sympathetic nerve synapses (see Fig. 13.5; Ch. 16), being responsible for the fast-excitatory synaptic potential and the rapid phase of contraction produced by sympathetic nerve activity in many smooth muscle tissues.

NORADRENALINE RELEASE

The processes linking the arrival of a nerve impulse at a nerve terminal, Ca^{2+} entry, and the release of transmitter are described in Chapter 4. Drugs that affect noradrenaline release are summarised in Table 15.6.

[2]Just how long may be appreciated by scaling up the 20 μm diameter of a neuronal cell body to that of a golf ball (~40,000 μm diameter, a scaling factor of about 2000); proportionately the axon (length from sympathetic chain ganglion to, say, a blood vessel in the calf (approximately 1 m in humans, never mind giraffes)), will now reach about 2 km – some challenge in terms of command and control!

Table 15.3 Characteristics of noradrenaline (norepinephrine) transport systems

	Neuronal (NET)	Extraneuronal (EMT)	Vesicular (VMAT)
Transport of NA (rat heart) V_{max} (nmol g^{-1} min^{-1})	1.2	100	–
K_m (μmol/L)	0.3	250	~0.2
Specificity	NA > A > ISO	A > NA > ISO	NA = A = ISO
Location	Neuronal membrane	Non-neuronal cell membrane (smooth muscle, cardiac muscle, endothelium)	Synaptic vesicle membrane
Other substrates	Tyramine Methylnoradrenaline Adrenergic neuron-blocking drugs (e.g. guanethidine) Amphetamine[a]	(+)-Noradrenaline Dopamine 5-Hydroxytryptamine Histamine	Dopamine 5-Hydroxytryptamine Guanethidine MPP^+ (see Ch. 41)
Inhibitors	Cocaine Tricyclic antidepressants (e.g. desipramine) Phenoxybenzamine Amphetamine[a]	Normetanephrine Steroid hormones (e.g. corticosterone) Phenoxybenzamine	Reserpine Tetrabenazine

[a]Amphetamine is transported slowly, so acts both as a substrate and as an inhibitor of noradrenaline uptake.
For details, see Gainetdinov, R.R., Caron, M.G., 2003. Monoamine transporters: from genes to behaviour. Annu. Rev. Pharmacol. Toxicol. 43, 261–284.
A, Adrenaline; *EMT*, extraneuronal monoamine transporter; *ISO*, isoprenaline; *MPP*+, toxic metabolite of MPTP (see and Ch. 41); *NA*, noradrenaline; *NET*, norepinephrine transporter; *VMAT*, vesicular monoamine transporter.

An unusual feature of the release mechanism at the varicosities of noradrenergic nerves is that the probability of release, even of a single vesicle, when a nerve impulse arrives at a varicosity is very low (less than 1 in 50). A single neuron possesses many thousand varicosities, so one impulse leads to the discharge of a few hundred vesicles, scattered over a wide area. This contrasts sharply with the neuromuscular junction (see Ch. 14), where the release probability at a single terminal is high, and release of acetylcholine is sharply localised.

Regulation of noradrenaline release

Noradrenaline release is affected by a variety of substances that act on presynaptic receptors (see Ch. 13). Many different types of nerve terminal (cholinergic, noradrenergic, dopaminergic, 5-HT-ergic, etc.) are subject to this type of control, and many different mediators (acetylcholine acting through muscarinic receptors, catecholamines acting through α and β receptors, angiotensin II, prostaglandins, purine nucleotides, neuropeptides, etc.) can act on presynaptic terminals. Presynaptic modulation represents an important physiological control mechanism throughout the nervous system.

Noradrenaline, by acting on presynaptic α_2 receptors, can down-regulate its own release, and that of co-released ATP (see Ch. 13). This is believed to occur physiologically, so that released noradrenaline exerts a local inhibitory effect on the terminals from which it came – the so-called *autoinhibitory feedback* mechanism (Fig. 15.2; see Gilsbach and Hein, 2012). Agonists or antagonists affecting presynaptic receptors can have large effects on sympathetic transmission. However, the physiological significance of presynaptic autoinhibition in the sympathetic nervous system is still somewhat contentious, and there is evidence that, in most tissues, it is less influential than biochemical measurements of transmitter overflow

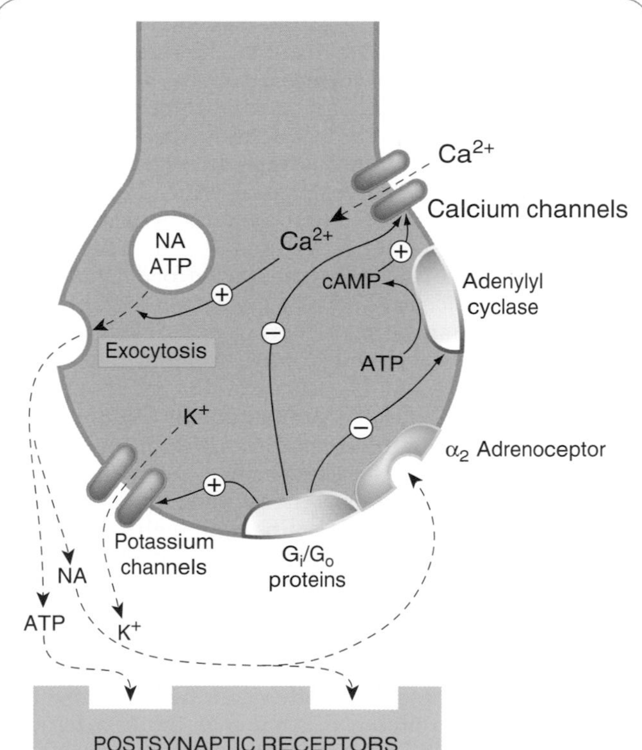

Fig. 15.2 Feedback control of noradrenaline (NA) release. The presynaptic α_2 receptor inhibits Ca^{2+} influx in response to membrane depolarisation via an action of the βγ subunits of the associated G protein on the voltage-dependent Ca^{2+} channels (see Ch. 3).

would seem to imply. Thus, although blocking autoreceptors causes large changes in noradrenaline *overflow* – the amount of noradrenaline released into the bathing solution or the bloodstream when sympathetic nerves are stimulated – the associated changes in the tissue response are often rather small. This suggests that what is measured in overflow experiments may not be the physiologically important component of transmitter release.

The inhibitory feedback mechanism operates through α_2 receptors, which inhibit adenylyl cyclase and prevent the opening of calcium channels (see Fig. 15.2). Sympathetic nerve terminals also possess β_2 receptors, coupled to activation of adenylyl cyclase, which *increase* noradrenaline release. Whether these have any physiological function is not clear.

UPTAKE AND DEGRADATION OF CATECHOLAMINES

The action of released noradrenaline is terminated mainly by reuptake of the transmitter into noradrenergic nerve terminals. Some is also sequestered by other cells in the vicinity. Circulating adrenaline and noradrenaline are degraded enzymically, but much more slowly than acetylcholine (see Ch. 14), where synaptically located acetylcholinesterase inactivates the transmitter in milliseconds. The two main catecholamine-metabolising enzymes are located intracellularly, so uptake into cells necessarily precedes metabolic degradation.

UPTAKE OF CATECHOLAMINES

The characteristics of noradrenergic transporters are summarised in Table 15.3. About 75% of the noradrenaline released by sympathetic neurons is recaptured and repackaged into vesicles. This serves to cut short the action of the released noradrenaline, as well as recycling it. The remaining 25% is captured by non-neuronal cells in the vicinity, limiting its local spread. These two uptake mechanisms depend on distinct transporter molecules. Neuronal uptake is performed by the plasma membrane noradrenaline transporter (generally known as NET, the *norepinephrine transporter*), which belongs to the family of neurotransmitter transporter proteins which include the dopamine transporter (DAT) and serotonin transporter (SERT) as well as the NET. These are specific for different amine transmitters, described in Chapter 13; and act as co-transporters of Na^+, Cl^- and the amine in question, using the electrochemical gradient for Na^+ as a driving force. Packaging into vesicles occurs through the VMAT, driven by the proton gradient between the cytosol and the vesicle contents. Extraneuronal uptake is performed by the *extraneuronal monoamine transporter* (EMT), which belongs to a large and widely distributed family of organic cation transporters (OCTs, see Ch. 9). NET is relatively selective for noradrenaline, with high affinity and a low maximum rate of uptake, and it is important in maintaining releasable stores of noradrenaline. NET is blocked by tricyclic antidepressant drugs and **cocaine**. EMT has lower affinity and higher transport capacity than NET, and transports adrenaline and isoprenaline as well as noradrenaline. The effects of several important drugs that act on noradrenergic neurons depend on their ability either to inhibit NET or to enter the nerve terminal with its help. Table 15.3 summarises the properties of neuronal and extraneuronal uptake.

METABOLIC DEGRADATION OF CATECHOLAMINES

Endogenous and exogenous catecholamines are metabolised mainly by two intracellular enzymes: *monoamine oxidase* (MAO) and *catechol-O-methyl transferase* (COMT). MAO (of which there are two distinct isoforms, MAO-A and MAO-B; see Ch. 48) is bound to the surface membrane of mitochondria. It is abundant in noradrenergic nerve terminals but is also present in liver, intestinal epithelium and other tissues. MAO converts catecholamines to their corresponding aldehydes,[3] which, in the periphery, are rapidly metabolised by *aldehyde dehydrogenase* to the corresponding carboxylic acid (3,4-dihydroxyphenylglycol being formed from noradrenaline; Fig. 15.3). MAO can also oxidise other monoamines, including dopamine and 5-HT. It is inhibited by various drugs which are used mainly for their antidepressant effects in the CNS (see Ch. 48), where these three amines all have transmitter functions (see Ch. 39). These drugs have important harmful effects that are related to disturbances of peripheral noradrenergic transmission. Within sympathetic neurons, MAO controls the content of dopamine and noradrenaline, and the releasable store of noradrenaline increases if the enzyme is inhibited. MAO and its inhibitors are discussed in more detail in Chapter 48.

The second major pathway for catecholamine metabolism involves methylation of one of the catechol hydroxyl groups by COMT to give a methoxy derivative. COMT is absent from noradrenergic neurons but present in the adrenal medulla and many other tissues. The final product formed by the sequential action of MAO and COMT is *3-methoxy-4-hydroxyphenylglycol* (MHPG; see Fig. 15.3). This is partly conjugated to sulfate or glucuronide derivatives, which are excreted in the urine and reflect noradrenaline release in brain, but most of it is converted to *vanillylmandelic acid* (VMA; see Fig. 15.3) and excreted in the urine in this form. In patients with tumours of chromaffin tissue that secrete these amines (a rare cause of high blood pressure), the urinary excretion of VMA is markedly increased, this being used as a diagnostic test for such tumours.

In the periphery, neither MAO nor COMT is primarily responsible for the termination of transmitter action, most of the released noradrenaline being quickly recaptured by NET. Circulating catecholamines are sequestered and inactivated by a combination of NET, EMT and COMT, the relative importance of these processes varying according to the agent concerned. Thus circulating noradrenaline is removed mainly by NET, whereas adrenaline is more dependent on EMT. Isoprenaline, however, is not a substrate for NET, and is removed by a combination of EMT and COMT.

In the CNS (see Ch. 39), MAO is more important as a means of terminating transmitter action than it is in the periphery, and MAO knockout mice show a greater enhancement of noradrenergic transmission in the brain than do NET knockouts, in which neuronal stores of noradrenaline are much depleted (see Gainetdinov and Caron, 2003). The main excretory product of noradrenaline released in the brain is MHPG.

DRUGS ACTING ON NORADRENERGIC TRANSMISSION

Many clinically important drugs, particularly those used to treat cardiovascular, respiratory and psychiatric disorders (see Chs 20, 21, 28, 48 and 49), work by affecting noradrenergic neuron function, acting on adrenoceptors, transporters or catecholamine-

[3]Aldehyde metabolites are potentially neurotoxic, and are thought to play a role in certain degenerative CNS disorders (see Ch. 40).

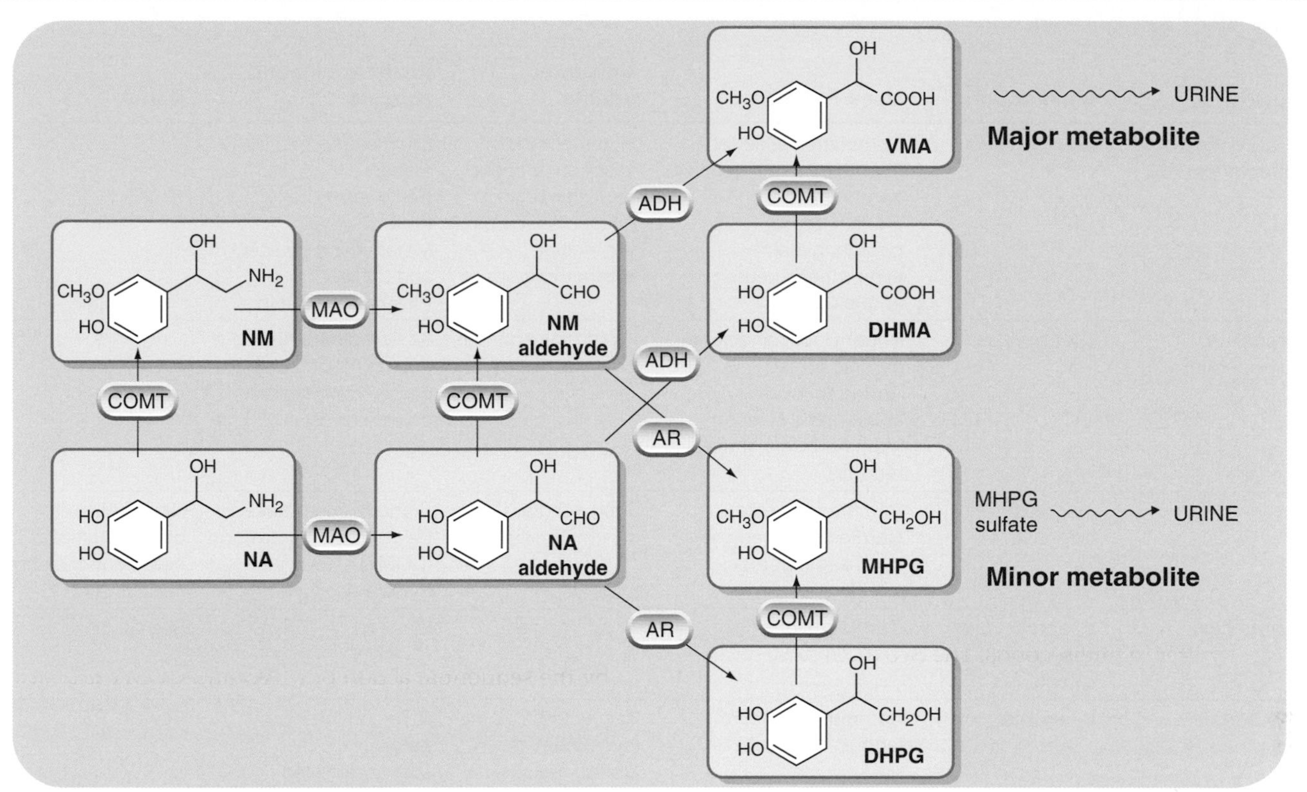

Fig. 15.3 The main pathways of noradrenaline metabolism. The oxidative branch (catalysed by aldehyde dehydrogenase [ADH]) predominates, giving vanillylmandelic acid (VMA) as the main urinary metabolite. The reductive branch (catalysed by aldehyde reductase [AR]) produces the less abundant metabolite, 3-methoxy-4-hydroxyphenylglycol (MHPG), which is conjugated to MHPG sulfate before being excreted; MHPG sulfate excretion reflects noradrenaline (NA) release in brain. *COMT,* Catechol-O-methyl transferase; *DHMA,* 3,4-dihydroxymandelic acid; *DHPG,* 3,4-dihydroxyphenylglycol; *MAO,* monoamine oxidase; *NM,* normetanephrine.

Noradrenergic transmission

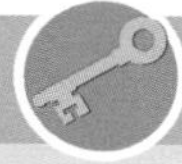

- Transmitter synthesis involves the following:
  - L-tyrosine is converted to dopa by tyrosine hydroxylase (rate-limiting step). Tyrosine hydroxylase occurs only in catecholaminergic neurons.
  - Dopa is converted to dopamine by dopa decarboxylase.
  - Dopamine is converted to noradrenaline by DBH, located in synaptic vesicles.
  - In the adrenal medulla, noradrenaline is converted to adrenaline by phenylethanolamine *N*-methyltransferase.
- Transmitter storage: noradrenaline is stored at high concentration in synaptic vesicles, together with ATP, chromogranin and DBH, which are co-released by exocytosis. Transport of noradrenaline into vesicles occurs by a reserpine-sensitive transporter, VMAT. Noradrenaline content of cytosol is normally low due to MAO in nerve terminals.
- Transmitter release occurs normally by Ca^{2+}-mediated exocytosis from varicosities on the terminal network. Non-exocytotic release occurs in response to indirectly acting sympathomimetic drugs (e.g. **tyramine** and **amphetamine**), which displace noradrenaline from vesicles. Noradrenaline escapes via the NET (reverse transport).
- Transmitter action is terminated mainly by reuptake of noradrenaline into nerve terminals via the NET transporter. NET is blocked by tricyclic antidepressant drugs and **cocaine.**
- Noradrenaline release is controlled by autoinhibitory feedback mediated by α_2 receptors.
- Co-transmission occurs at many noradrenergic nerve terminals, ATP and neuropeptide Y being frequently co-released with NA. ATP mediates the early phase of smooth muscle contraction in response to sympathetic nerve activity.

metabolising enzymes. The properties of important drugs in this category are summarised in Tables 15.4–15.6.

DRUGS ACTING ON ADRENOCEPTORS

The overall activity of these drugs is governed by their affinity, efficacy and selectivity with respect to different types of adrenoceptor, and intensive research has been devoted to developing drugs with the right properties for specific clinical indications. As a result, the pharmacopoeia is awash with adrenoceptor ligands. Many clinical needs are met, it turns out, by drugs that relax smooth muscle in different organs of the body[4] and those that block the cardiac

[4]And conversely, contracting smooth muscle is often bad news. This bald statement must not be pressed too far, but the exceptions (such as nasal decongestants and drugs acting on the eye) are surprisingly few. Even adrenaline (potentially lifesaving in cardiac arrest) dilates some vessels while constricting others to less immediately essential tissues such as skin).

Table 15.4 Adrenoceptor agonists

Drug	Main action	Uses/function	Unwanted effects	Pharmacokinetic aspects	Notes
Noradrenaline (Norepinephrine)	α/β agonist	Sometimes used for hypotension in intensive care Transmitter at postganglionic sympathetic neurons, and in CNS	Hypertension, vasoconstriction, tachycardia (or reflex bradycardia), ventricular dysrhythmias	Poorly absorbed by mouth Rapid removal by tissues Metabolised by MAO and COMT Plasma $t_{1/2}$ ~2 min	—
Adrenaline (Epinephrine)	α/β agonist	Anaphylactic shock, cardiac arrest Added to local anaesthetic solutions Main hormone of adrenal medulla	As norepinephrine	As norepinephrine Given i.m. or s.c. (i.v. infusion in intensive care settings)	
Isoprenaline	β agonist (non-selective)	Asthma (obsolete), Cardiac emergencies such as heart block, shock	Tachycardia, dysrhythmias	Some tissue uptake, followed by inactivation (COMT) Plasma $t_{1/2}$ ~2 h	Now replaced by salbutamol in treatment of asthma see Ch. 28
Dobutamine	β_1 agonist (also has weak β_2 and α_1 activity)	Cardiogenic shock	Dysrhythmias	Plasma $t_{1/2}$ ~2 min Given i.v.	See Ch. 21
Salbutamol	β_2 agonist	Asthma, premature labour	Tachycardia, dysrhythmias, tremor, peripheral vasodilatation	Given orally or by aerosol Mainly excreted unchanged Plasma $t_{1/2}$ ~4 h	See Ch. 28
Salmeterol	β_2 agonist	Asthma	As salbutamol	Given by aerosol Long acting	Formoterol is similar
Terbutaline	β_2 agonist	Asthma Delay of parturition	As salbutamol	Poorly absorbed orally Given by aerosol Mainly excreted unchanged Plasma $t_{1/2}$ ~4 h	See Ch. 28
Clenbuterol	β_2 agonist	'Anabolic' action to increase muscle strength	As salbutamol	Active orally Long acting	Illicit use in sport; see Ch. 59
Mirabegron	β_3 agonist	Symptoms of overactive bladder	Tachycardia	Active orally, given once daily	See Ch. 29
Phenylephrine	α_1 agonist	Nasal decongestion	Hypertension, reflex bradycardia	Given intranasally Metabolised by MAO Short plasma $t_{1/2}$	—
Midodrine	α_1 agonist	Treatment of severe postural hypotension due to autonomic dysfunction	Urinary retention due to stimulation of α_1 receptors of the bladder	Midodrine is pro-drug metabolised to active compound desglymidodrine	
Methoxamine	α agonist (non-selective)	Nasal decongestion	As phenylephrine	Given intranasally Plasma $t_{1/2}$ ~1 h	—
Clonidine, moxonidine, rilmenidine, lofexidine	α_2 partial agonist, + imidazoline I_1 agonists; moxonidine and rilmenidine prefer I1 receptor	Hypertension, migraine prophylaxis, vasomotor instability ('hot flushes'); lofexidine is used to reduce symptoms during opioid withdrawal	Drowsiness, hypotension, oedema and weight gain, rebound hypertension	Well absorbed orally Excreted unchanged and as conjugate	Originally licensed for use in hypertension
Dexmedetomidine	α_2 agonist	Sedation in intensive care patients, anaesthetic premedication for small animal veterinary medicine			

CNS, Central nervous system; *COMT*, catechol-*O*-methyl transferase; *MAO*, monoamine oxidase.

Table 15.5 Adrenoceptor antagonists

Drug	Main action	Uses/function	Unwanted effects	Pharmacokinetic aspects	Notes
α-Adrenoceptor antagonists					
Phenoxybenzamine	α antagonist (non-selective, irreversible) Uptake 1 inhibitor	Phaeochromocytoma	Postural hypotension, tachycardia, nasal congestion, impotence	Absorbed orally Plasma $t_{1/2}$ ~12 h	Action outlasts presence of drug in plasma, because of covalent binding to receptor
Phentolamine	α antagonist (non-selective), vasodilator	Rarely used	As phenoxybenzamine	Usually given i.v. Metabolised by liver Plasma $t_{1/2}$ ~2 h	
Prazosin	α_1 antagonist	Hypertension	As phenoxybenzamine	Absorbed orally Metabolised by liver Plasma $t_{1/2}$ ~4 h	Doxazosin and terazosin are similar but longer acting See Ch. 21
Tamsulosin	α_{1A} antagonist ('uroselective')	Prostatic hyperplasia	Failure of ejaculation	Absorbed orally Plasma $t_{1/2}$ ~5 h	Selective for α_{1A}-adrenoceptor
Yohimbine	α_2 antagonist	Not used clinically Claimed to be aphrodisiac	Excitement, hypertension	Absorbed orally Metabolised by liver Plasma $t_{1/2}$ ~4 h	
β-Adrenoceptor antagonists					
Propranolol	β antagonist High affinity for β_1 and β_2 receptors but lower affinity for β_3 receptors	Angina, hypertension, cardiac dysrhythmias, anxiety, tremor, glaucoma	Bronchoconstriction, cardiac failure, cold extremities, fatigue and depression, hypoglycaemia	Absorbed orally Extensive first-pass metabolism About 90% bound to plasma protein Plasma $t_{1/2}$ ~4 h	Timolol is similar and used mainly to treat glaucoma See Ch. 27
Alprenolol	β antagonist (non-selective) (partial agonist)	As propranolol	As propranolol	Absorbed orally Metabolised by liver Plasma $t_{1/2}$ ~4 h	Oxprenolol and pindolol are similar See Ch. 21
Metoprolol	β_1 antagonist	Angina, hypertension, dysrhythmias	As propranolol, less risk of bronchoconstriction	Absorbed orally Mainly metabolised in liver Plasma $t_{1/2}$ ~3 h	Atenolol is similar, with a longer half-life See Ch. 21
Nebivolol	β_1 antagonist Enhances nitric oxide synthesis	Hypertension	Fatigue, headache	Absorbed orally $t_{1/2}$ ~10h	–
Butoxamine	β_2-selective antagonist Weak α agonist	No clinical uses	–	–	–
Mixed (α-/β-) antagonists					
Labetalol	α/β antagonist	Hypertension in pregnancy, hypertensive emergencies	Postural hypotension, bronchoconstriction	Absorbed orally Conjugated in liver Plasma $t_{1/2}$ ~4 h	–
Carvedilol	β/α_1 antagonist	Heart failure	As for other β blockers Initial exacerbation of heart failure Renal failure	Absorbed orally $t_{1/2}$ ~10 h	Additional actions may contribute to clinical benefit. See Ch. 21

Table 15.6 Drugs that affect noradrenaline synthesis, release or uptake

Drug	Main action	Uses/function	Unwanted effects	Pharmacokinetic aspects	Notes
Drugs affecting NA synthesis					
α-Methyl-p-tyrosine	Inhibits tyrosine hydroxylase	Occasionally used in phaeochromocytoma	Hypotension, sedation	—	—
Carbidopa	Inhibits dopa decarboxylase	Used as adjunct to levodopa to prevent peripheral effects	—	Absorbed orally Does not enter brain	See Ch. 40
Methyldopa	False transmitter precursor	Hypertension in pregnancy	Hypotension, drowsiness, diarrhoea, impotence, hypersensitivity reactions	Absorbed slowly by mouth Excreted unchanged or as conjugate Plasma $t_{1/2}$ ~6 h	See Ch. 21
Droxidopa (L-dihydroxyphenylserine, L-DOPS)	Converted to NA by dopa decarboxylase, thus increasing NA synthesis and release	Neurogenic orthostatic hypotension	Not known	Absorbed orally Duration of action ~6 h	FDA approved
Drugs that release NA (indirectly acting sympathomimetic amines)					
Tyramine	NA release	No clinical uses Present in various foods	As norepinephrine	Normally destroyed by MAO in gut Does not enter brain	See Ch. 48 for interaction with MAO inhibitors
Amphetamine	NA release, MAO inhibitor, NET inhibitor, CNS stimulant	Used as CNS stimulant in narcolepsy, also (paradoxically) in hyperactive children Appetite suppressant Drug of abuse	Hypertension, tachycardia, insomnia Acute psychosis with overdose Dependence	Well absorbed orally Penetrates freely into brain Excreted unchanged in urine Plasma $t_{1/2}$ ~12 h, depending on urine flow and pH	See Ch. 49 Methylphenidate and atomoxetine are similar (used for CNS effects; see Ch. 49)
Ephedrine	NA release, β agonist, weak CNS stimulant action	Nasal decongestion	As amphetamine but less pronounced	Similar to amphetamine aspects	Interacts with MAO inhibitors; see Ch. 48
Drugs that inhibit NA release					
Reserpine	Depletes NA stores by inhibiting VMAT	Hypertension (obsolete)	As methyldopa Also depression, parkinsonism, gynaecomastia	Poorly absorbed orally Slowly metabolised Plasma $t_{1/2}$ ~100 h Excreted in milk	Antihypertensive effect develops slowly and persists when drug is stopped
Guanethidine	Inhibits NA release Also causes NA depletion and can damage NA neurons irreversibly	Hypertension (obsolete)	As methyldopa Hypertension on first administration	Poorly absorbed orally Mainly excreted unchanged in urine Plasma $t_{1/2}$ ~100 h	Action prevented by NET inhibitors
Drugs affecting NA uptake					
Imipramine	Blocks neuronal transporter (NET) Also has atropine-like action	Depression	Atropine-like side effects Cardiac dysrhythmias in overdose	Well absorbed orally 95% bound to plasma protein Converted to active metabolite (desmethylimipramine) Plasma $t_{1/2}$ ~4 h	Desipramine and amitriptyline are similar See Ch. 48
Cocaine	Local anaesthetic; blocks NET CNS stimulant	Rarely used local anaesthetic Major drug of abuse	Hypertension, excitement, convulsions, dependence	Well absorbed orally or intranasally	See Chs 44 and 50

CNS, Central nervous system; *MAO,* monoamine oxidase; *NA,* noradrenaline; *NET,* norepinephrine transporter; *VMAT,* vesicular monoamine transporter.

stimulant effects of the sympathetic nervous system; on the other hand, cardiac stimulation is generally undesirable in chronic disease.

Broadly speaking, β_2-adrenoceptor agonists are useful as smooth muscle relaxants (especially in the airways), while β_1-adrenoceptor antagonists (often called β blockers) are used mainly for their cardiodepressant effects. α_1-Adrenoceptor antagonists are used mainly for their vasodilator effects in cardiovascular indications and also for the treatment of prostatic hyperplasia. Adrenaline, with its mixture of cardiac stimulant, vasodilator and vasoconstrictor actions, is uniquely important in cardiac arrest (see Ch. 20). α_1-Adrenoceptor agonists are widely used (intranasally or systemically) as decongestants.

ADRENOCEPTOR AGONISTS

Examples of adrenoceptor agonists (also known as *directly-acting sympathomimetic* drugs) are given in Table 15.2, and the characteristics of individual drugs are summarised in Table 15.4.

Actions

The major physiological effects mediated by different types of adrenoceptor are summarised in Table 15.1.

Smooth muscle tone

All types of smooth muscle, except that of the gastrointestinal tract, contract in response to stimulation of α_1 adrenoceptors, through activation of the G_q signal transduction mechanism, leading to intracellular Ca^{2+} release as described in Chapter 4. Although vascular smooth muscle possesses both α_1 and α_2 receptors, it appears that α_1 receptors lie close to the sites of noradrenaline release (and are mainly responsible for neurally mediated vasoconstriction), while α_2 receptors lie elsewhere on the muscle fibre surface or on nerve terminals.

When α_1 agonists are given systemically to experimental animals or humans, the most important action is on vascular smooth muscle, particularly in the small arteries and arterioles in skin and splanchnic vascular beds, which are strongly constricted increasing total peripheral vascular resistance. Smooth muscle cells in the walls of large arteries and veins also contract, resulting in decreased arterial compliance and increased central venous pressure, which contribute to an increase in arterial and venous pressure and increased cardiac work. Some vascular beds (e.g. cerebral, coronary and pulmonary) are relatively little affected.

In the whole animal, baroreceptor reflexes are activated by the rise in arterial pressure produced by α_1 agonists, limiting the rise in blood pressure and causing reflex bradycardia.

Smooth muscle in the vas deferens, spleen capsule and eyelid retractor muscles (or nictitating membrane, in some species) is also stimulated by α_1 agonists, and these organs were once widely used for pharmacological studies. Contraction of the erector pili muscles literally causes the hair to stand on end in some species, and in humans causes a very unpleasant sensation like insects crawling over one's body ('formication' after the Latin word for 'ant' – pronounce with care!).

Stimulation of β receptors relaxes most kinds of smooth muscle by increasing cAMP formation (see Ch. 4). β-Receptor activation enhances Ca^{2+} extrusion and intracellular Ca^{2+} sequestration, both effects acting to reduce cytoplasmic Ca^{2+} concentration. In the vascular system, β_2-mediated vasodilatation (particularly in humans) is mainly endothelium dependent and mediated by nitric oxide (see Ch. 19). It occurs in many vascular beds and is especially marked in skeletal muscle.

The powerful inhibitory effect of the sympathetic system on gastrointestinal smooth muscle is produced by both α and β receptors, the gut being unusual in that α receptors cause relaxation in most regions other than the sphincters. Part of the effect is due to stimulation of presynaptic α_2 receptors (see later), which inhibit the release of excitatory transmitters (e.g. acetylcholine) from intramural nerves, but there are also α_1 and α_2 receptors on the muscle cells, stimulation of which hyperpolarises the cell by increasing the membrane permeability to K^+ and inhibits action potential discharge. The *sphincters* of the gastrointestinal tract are contracted by α-receptor activation.

Bronchial smooth muscle is relaxed by activation of β_2 adrenoceptors, and selective β_2 agonists are important in the treatment of asthma (see Ch. 28). Uterine smooth muscle responds similarly, and these drugs are also used to delay premature labour (see Ch. 35). Bladder detrusor muscle is relaxed by activation of β_3 adrenoceptors, and selective β_3 agonists are used to treat symptoms of overactive bladder (see Sacco and Bientinesi, 2012).

α_1 Adrenoceptors have long-lasting trophic effects stimulating smooth muscle proliferation in blood vessels and in the prostate gland. *Benign prostatic hyperplasia* (see Ch. 29) is commonly treated with α_1-adrenoceptor antagonists. 'Cross-talk' between the α_1 adrenoceptor and the growth factor signalling pathways (see Ch. 3) probably contributes to the clinical effect, in addition to immediate symptomatic improvement which is probably mediated by smooth muscle relaxation in the prostatic capsule that encases the gland.

Nerve terminals

Presynaptic adrenoceptors are present on both cholinergic and noradrenergic nerve terminals (see Chs 4 and 13). As mentioned previously, the main effect (α_2-mediated) is inhibitory; spinal α_2-adrenoceptors play an important role in pain modulation and α_2-agonists may prove to be useful to treat neuropathic pain (see Bahari and Meftafi, 2019, and Ch. 43). A weaker facilitatory action of β receptors on noradrenergic nerve terminals has also been described. Clinical uses of α_2-agonists in humans (see 'Clinical uses of adrenoceptor agonists' clinical box) are currently limited, but **dexmedetomidine** is licensed for use in intensive care patients because of its sedative and analgesic properties; its effects can be reversed by an α_2-antagonist, although this is seldom appropriate since analgesic as well as sedative effects are reversed.

Effects on cardiac structure and function

Catecholamines, acting on β_1 receptors, exert a powerful stimulant effect on the heart (see Ch. 20). Both the heart rate (*chronotropic effect*) and the force of contraction (*inotropic effect*) are increased, resulting in a markedly increased cardiac output and cardiac oxygen consumption. Cardiac efficiency (see Ch. 20) is reduced. Catecholamines can also disturb cardiac rhythm, culminating in ventricular fibrillation. (Paradoxically, but importantly, adrenaline is also used to treat ventricular fibrillation arrest as well as other forms of cardiac arrest; see Ch. 20). Fig. 15.4 shows the overall pattern of cardiovascular responses to catecholamine infusions in humans, reflecting their actions on both the heart and vascular system.

Cardiac hypertrophy occurs in response to activation of both β_1 and α_1 receptors, probably by a mechanism similar to the hypertrophy of vascular and prostatic smooth muscle. This may be important in the pathophysiology of hypertension and of cardiac failure (which is associated with sympathetic overactivity); see Chs 20 and 21.

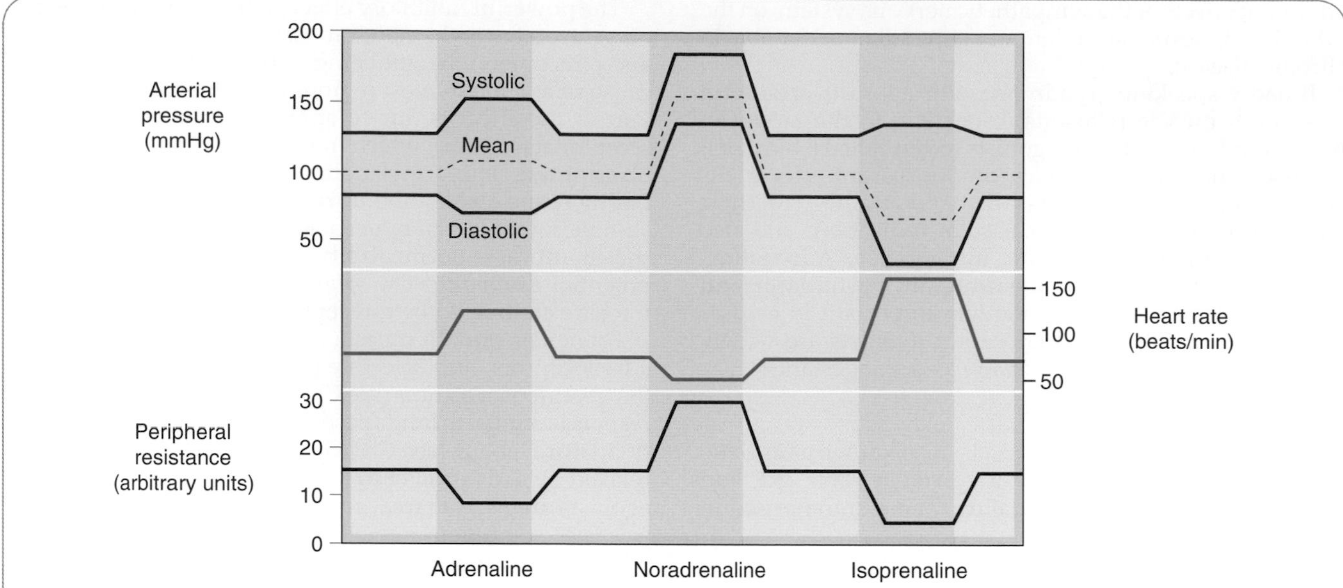

Fig. 15.4 Schematic representation of the cardiovascular effects of intravenous infusions of adrenaline, noradrenaline and isoprenaline in humans. Noradrenaline (predominantly α agonist) causes vasoconstriction and increased systolic and diastolic pressure, with a reflex bradycardia. Isoprenaline (β agonist) is a vasodilator, but strongly increases cardiac force and rate. Mean arterial pressure falls. Adrenaline combines both actions.

Beta receptors are also implicated in the pathological growth of blood vessels in severe childhood haemangiomas (see later).

Metabolism

Catecholamines convert energy stores (glycogen and fat) to freely available fuels, increasing the plasma concentration of glucose and free fatty acids. The detailed biochemical mechanisms (see review by Nonogaki, 2000) vary from species to species, but in most cases the effects on carbohydrate metabolism of liver and muscle (Fig. 15.5) are mediated through β_1 receptors and the stimulation of lipolysis and thermogenesis is produced by β_3 receptors (see Table 15.1). Activation of α_2 receptors inhibits insulin secretion, further contributing to the hyperglycaemia. The production of *leptin* by adipose tissue (see Ch. 32) is also inhibited. Adrenaline-induced hyperglycaemia in humans is blocked completely by a combination of α and β antagonists but not by either on its own.

Other effects

Skeletal muscle is affected by adrenaline, acting on β_2 receptors, although the effect is far less dramatic than that on the heart. The twitch tension of fast-contracting fibres (white muscle) is increased by adrenaline, particularly if the muscle is fatigued, whereas the twitch of slow (red) muscle is reduced. These effects depend on an action on the contractile proteins, rather than on the membrane, and the mechanism is poorly understood. In humans, adrenaline and other β_2 agonists cause a marked tremor, the shakiness that accompanies fear, excitement, withdrawal from alcohol (see Ch. 50) or the excessive use of β_2 agonists (e.g. **salbutamol**) in the treatment of asthma being examples of this. It probably results from an increase in muscle spindle discharge, coupled with an effect on the contraction kinetics of the fibres, these effects combining to produce an instability in the reflex control of muscle length. β-Receptor antagonists are sometimes used to control pathological tremor. Increased susceptibility to cardiac dysrhythmias associated with β_2 agonists is thought to be partly due to hypokalaemia, caused by an increase in K^+ uptake by skeletal muscle. β_2 Agonists also cause long-term changes in the expression of sarcoplasmic reticulum proteins that control contraction kinetics, and thereby increase the rate and force of contraction of skeletal muscle. **Clenbuterol**, an 'anabolic' drug used illicitly by athletes to improve performance (see Ch. 59), is a β_2 agonist that acts in this way.

Histamine release by human and guinea pig lung tissue in response to anaphylactic challenge (see Ch. 17) is inhibited by catecholamines, acting on β_2 receptors.

Lymphocytes and other cells of the immune system also express adrenoceptors (mainly β adrenoceptors). Lymphocyte proliferation, lymphocyte-mediated cell killing and production of many cytokines are inhibited by β-adrenoceptor agonists. The physiological and clinical importance of these effects has not yet been established, despite intense current interest in neuroimmunology (Schiller et al., 2021). For a review of the effects of the sympathetic nervous system on immune function, see Elenkov et al., 2000.

Clinical use

The main clinical uses of adrenoceptor agonists are summarised in the 'Clinical uses of adrenoceptor agonists' clinical box and Table 15.4, the most important being the use of β-adrenoceptor agonists for the treatment of asthma (see Ch. 28).

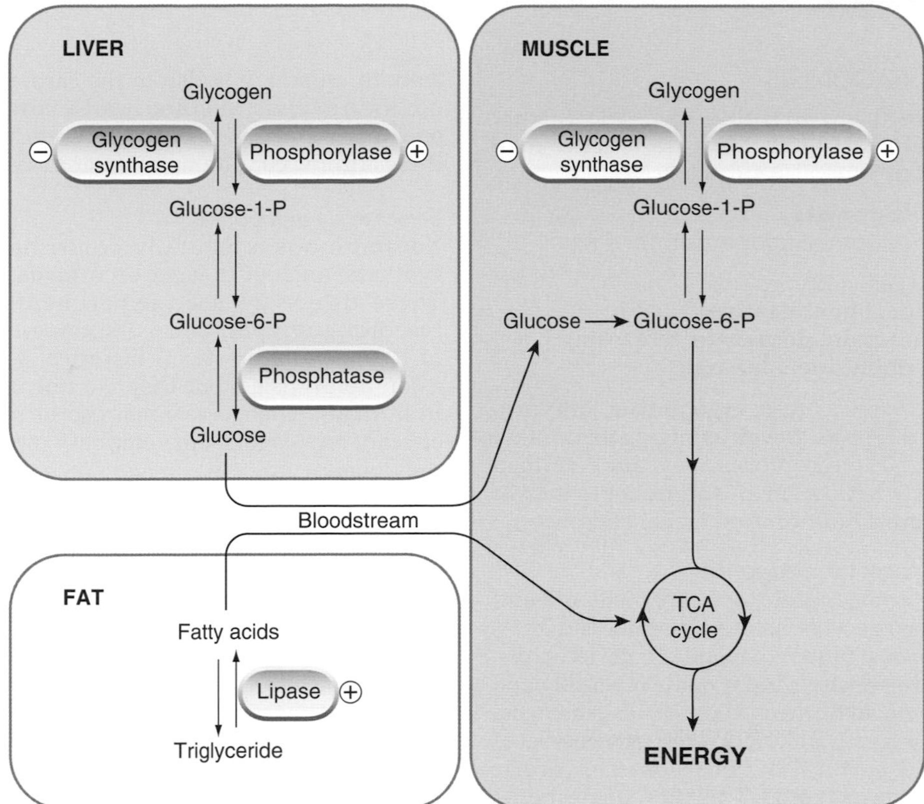

Fig. 15.5 Regulation of energy metabolism by catecholamines. The main enzymic steps that are affected by β-adrenoceptor activation are indicated by + and – signs, denoting stimulation and inhibition, respectively. The overall effect is to mobilise glycogen and fat stores to meet energy demands. *TCA,* Tricarboxylic acid.

Adrenoceptor agonists

- **Noradrenaline** and **adrenaline** show relatively little receptor selectivity.
- Selective α_1 agonists include **phenylephrine, midodrine** and **oxymetazoline.**
- α_2 agonists include **clonidine** and **α-methylnoradrenaline.** Clonidine also acts on a distinct imidazoline I_1 receptor; **moxonidine** and **rilmenidine** have greater I_1/α_2 selectivity than clonidine and cause less drowsiness than clonidine when used to treat hypertension. Methylnoradrenaline is selective for α_2 adrenoceptors over I_1. It is formed as a false transmitter from **methyldopa**, developed as a hypotensive drug (now largely obsolete, except for use during pregnancy, because it causes drowsiness).
- Selective β_1 agonists include **dobutamine.** Increased cardiac contractility may be useful clinically, but all β_1 agonists can cause cardiac dysrhythmias.
- Selective β_2 agonists include **salbutamol**, **terbutaline** and **salmeterol**; used mainly for their bronchodilator action in asthma.
- A selective β_3 agonist, **mirabegron**, is used to treat overactive bladder; β_3 agonists promote lipolysis and have potential in the treatment of obesity.

Clinical uses of adrenoceptor agonists

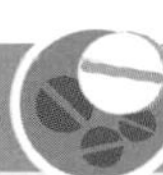

- Cardiovascular system:
  - cardiac arrest: **adrenaline**
  - cardiogenic shock (see Chs 20 and 21): **dobutamine** (β_1 agonist)
  - severe postural hypotension: **midodrine** (α_1 agonist).
- Anaphylaxis (acute hypersensitivity, see Chs 17 and 28): **adrenaline.**
- Respiratory system:
  - asthma (see Ch. 28): selective β_2-receptor agonists (**salbutamol**, **terbutaline**, **salmeterol**, **formoterol**)
  - nasal decongestion: **phenylephrine** by mouth or drops containing **xylometazoline** or **ephedrine** for short-term use.
- Miscellaneous indications:
  - **adrenaline**: with local anaesthetics to prolong their action (see Ch. 44)
  - premature labour (**salbutamol**; see Ch. 35)
  - α_2 agonists (e.g. **clonidine**, **lofexidine**): to lower blood pressure, but are now seldom prescribed. **Dexmedetomidine** is licensed for analgesia and sedation in intensive care; **lofexidine** is used as an adjunct during opioid withdrawal, to reduce menopausal flushing, especially when **oestrogen** is contraindicated as in patients with breast cancer; and to reduce frequency of migraine attacks (see Ch. 42). Tourette syndrome, characterised by multiple tics and outbursts of foul language, is an unlicensed indication
  - A β_3 agonist, **mirabegron**: to treat urgency, increased micturition frequency and incontinence (overactive bladder symptoms).

ADRENOCEPTOR ANTAGONISTS

The main drugs are listed in Table 15.2, and further information is given in Table 15.5. Most are selective for α or β receptors, and many are also subtype-selective.

α-Adrenoceptor antagonists

The main groups of α-adrenoceptor antagonists are:

- non-selective between subtypes (e.g. **phenoxybenzamine, phentolamine**)
- α_1-selective (e.g. **prazosin, doxazosin, terazosin**)
- α_2-selective (e.g. **yohimbine, idazoxan**)

In addition, *ergot derivatives* (e.g. **ergotamine, dihydroergotamine**) block α receptors as well as having many other actions, notably on 5-HT receptors. They are described in Chapter 16. Their action on α adrenoceptors is of pharmacological interest but not used therapeutically.

Non-selective α-adrenoceptor antagonists

Phenoxybenzamine is not specific for α receptors, and also antagonises the actions of acetylcholine, histamine and 5-HT. It is long lasting because it binds covalently to the receptors. **Phentolamine** is more selective, but it binds reversibly and its action is short lasting. In humans, these drugs cause a fall in arterial pressure (because of block of α-receptor-mediated vasoconstriction) and postural hypotension. The cardiac output and heart rate are increased. This is a reflex response to the fall in arterial pressure, mediated through β receptors. The concomitant block of α_2 receptors tends to increase noradrenaline release, which has the effect of enhancing the reflex tachycardia that occurs with any blood pressure-lowering agent. Phenoxybenzamine retains a niche use in preparing patients with *phaeochromocytoma* (see Ch. 21, and later) for surgery.

Labetalol and **carvedilol**[5] are mixed α_1- and β-receptor-blocking drugs, although at doses used clinically they act predominantly on β receptors. Carvedilol is used mainly to treat hypertension and heart failure (see Chs 20 and 21); labetalol is used to treat hypertension in pregnancy, as well as hypertensive emergencies (where intravenous administration is required).

Selective α_1 antagonists

Prazosin was the first selective α_1 antagonist/inverse agonist; it acts on all three subtypes of α_1 receptor (Alexander et al., 2019). Similar drugs with longer half-lives (e.g. **doxazosin, terazosin**), which have the advantage of allowing once-daily dosing, are now preferred. They are highly selective for α_1 adrenoceptors and cause vasodilatation and fall in arterial pressure, but less tachycardia than occurs with non-selective α-receptor antagonists, presumably because they do not increase noradrenaline release from sympathetic nerve terminals. Mild postural hypotension is common but is less problematic than with shorter-acting prazosin.

The α_1-receptor antagonists relax smooth muscle in the bladder neck and prostate capsule, and inhibit hypertrophy of these tissues, and are therefore useful in treating symptoms associated with *benign prostatic hypertrophy*. **Tamsulosin**, an α_{1A}-receptor antagonist, shows some selectivity for the urogenital tract, and causes less hypotension than the less selective α_1-receptor antagonists.

It is believed that α_{1A} receptors play a part in the pathological hypertrophy not only of prostatic and vascular smooth muscle, but also in the cardiac hypertrophy that occurs in hypertension and heart failure (Papay et al., 2013), and the use of selective α_{1A}-receptor antagonists to treat these chronic conditions is under investigation.

Selective α_2 antagonists

Yohimbine is a naturally occurring alkaloid; various synthetic analogues have been made, such as **idazoxan**. These drugs are used experimentally to analyse α-receptor subtypes, and yohimbine, possibly by virtue of its vasodilator effect, historically enjoyed notoriety as an aphrodisiac, but they are not used therapeutically in humans. Their occasional use to reverse the sedative effect of an α_2 agonist in veterinary medicine is mentioned previously.

α-Adrenoceptor antagonists

- Selective α_1 antagonists (e.g. **doxazosin, terazosin**) are used in treating hypertension and for benign prostatic hypertrophy. Postural hypotension, stress incontinence and impotence are unwanted effects. **Prazosin** (short acting) was the first such agent.
- **Tamsulosin** is α_{1A} selective and acts mainly on the urogenital tract. It is used to treat benign prostatic hypertrophy and may cause less postural hypotension than other α_1 agonists.
- **Yohimbine** is a selective α_2 antagonist. It is not used clinically in humans.

Clinical uses and unwanted effects of α-adrenoceptor antagonists

The main uses of α-adrenoceptor antagonists are related to their cardiovascular actions and are summarised in the 'Clinical uses of α-adrenoceptor antagonists' clinical box.

Phaeochromocytoma is a catecholamine-secreting tumour of chromaffin tissue, which causes severe and initially episodic hypertension. A combination of α- and β-receptor antagonists is the most effective way of controlling the blood pressure. The tumour may be surgically removable, and it is essential to block α and β receptors before surgery is begun, to avoid the effects of a sudden release of catecholamines when the tumour is disturbed. Phenoxybenzamine, an irreversible α antagonist which reduces the maximum of the agonist dose–response curve (see Ch. 2, Fig. 2.4B) is combined with a β-adrenoceptor antagonist for this purpose.

Clinical uses of α-adrenoceptor antagonists

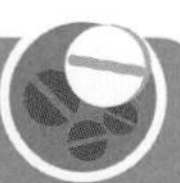

- Severe hypertension (see Ch. 21): α_1-selective antagonists (e.g. **doxazosin**) in combination with other drugs.
- Benign prostatic hypertrophy (e.g. **tamsulosin**, a selective α_{1A}-receptor antagonist).
- Phaeochromocytoma: **phenoxybenzamine** (irreversible antagonist) in preparation for surgery. A β-adrenoceptor antagonist is administered and up-titrated after α-blockade (evidenced by postural hypotension) has been established and before surgery.

[5]Carvedilol is also a biased agonist, acting through the arrestin pathway (Ch. 3).

β-Adrenoceptor antagonists

β-Adrenoceptor antagonists remain extremely therapeutically important. They were discovered in 1958, 10 years after Ahlquist had postulated the existence of β adrenoceptors. The first compound, **dichloroisoprenaline**, was a partial agonist. Further development led to **propranolol**, which is much more potent and a pure antagonist that blocks β_1 and β_2 receptors equally. The potential clinical advantages of drugs with some partial agonist activity, and/or with selectivity for β_1 receptors, led to the development of **oxprenolol** and **alprenolol** (non-selective with considerable partial agonist activity), and others, e.g. **atenolol, metoprolol** and **bisoprolol** (β_1-selective with no agonist activity). Two newer drugs are **carvedilol** (a non-selective β-adrenoceptor antagonist with additional α_1-blocking activity) and **nebivolol** (a β_1-selective antagonist with vasodilator nitric oxide-mediated activity; see Ch. 19). Both these drugs have proven more effective than conventional β-adrenoceptor antagonists in treating heart failure (see Chs 21 and 22). The characteristics of the most important compounds are set out in Table 15.5. Most clinically available β-receptor antagonists are inactive on β_3 receptors so do not affect lipolysis.

Actions

The main pharmacological actions of β-receptor antagonists can be deduced from Table 15.1. The acute effects produced in humans depend on the degree of sympathetic activity and are modest in subjects at rest. The most important effects are on the cardiovascular system and on bronchial smooth muscle (see Chs 21, 22 and 28).

In a healthy subject at rest, propranolol causes modest changes in heart rate, cardiac output or arterial pressure, but β-blockade dramatically reduces the effect of exercise or excitement on these variables (Fig. 15.6). Drugs with partial agonist activity, such as oxprenolol, increase the heart rate at rest but reduce it during exercise or excitement. Maximum exercise tolerance is considerably reduced in normal subjects, partly because of the limitation of the cardiac response, and partly because the β-mediated vasodilatation in skeletal muscle is reduced. Coronary flow is reduced, but relatively less than the myocardial oxygen consumption, so oxygenation of the myocardium is improved – of great importance in the treatment of angina pectoris (see Ch. 20). In healthy subjects, the reduction of the force of contraction of the heart is not important, in contrast to patients with heart disease (see later).

An important, and initially somewhat unexpected, effect of β-receptor antagonists is their antihypertensive action (see Ch. 21). Patients with hypertension show a gradual fall in arterial pressure that takes several days to develop fully. The mechanism is complex and involves the following:

- reduction in cardiac output;
- reduction of renin release from the juxtaglomerular cells of the kidney;
- a central action, reducing sympathetic nervous output, is less important.

Vasodilatation contributes to the antihypertensive action of those β-receptor antagonists (e.g. carvedilol and nebivolol, see earlier) that possess additional vasodilator properties.

Blockade of the facilitatory effect of presynaptic β receptors on noradrenaline release (see Table 15.1) may also contribute to the antihypertensive effect. The antihypertensive effect of β-receptor antagonists remains

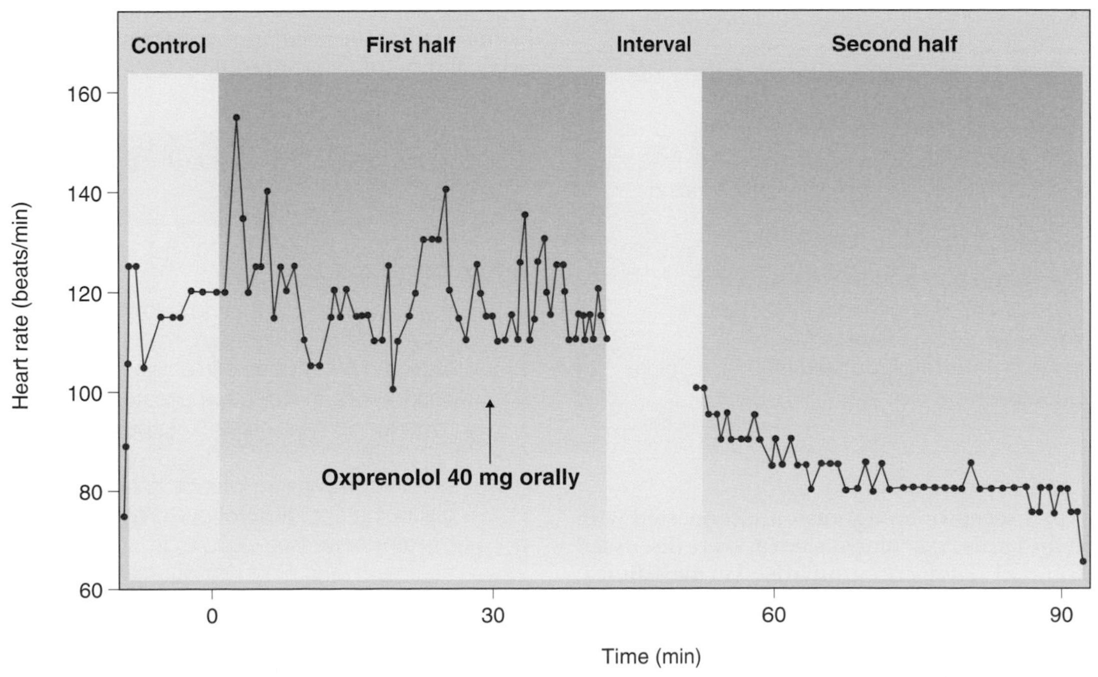

Fig. 15.6 Heart rate recorded continuously in a spectator watching a live football match, showing the effect of the β-adrenoceptor 'antagonist' oxprenolol – strictly a partial agonist. (From Taylor, S.H., Meeran, M.K., 1973. In: Burley, D.M., Fryer, J.H., Rowdel, R.K., et al. (Eds). New Perspectives in Beta-Blockade. CIBA Laboratories, Horsham.)

clinically useful. Because reflex vasoconstriction is preserved, postural and exercise-induced hypotension is less troublesome than with many other antihypertensive drugs but they are now seldom used as first-line agents in uncomplicated hypertension (see Ch. 21).

β-Receptor antagonists have several important antidysrhythmic effects on the heart (see Ch. 20).

Airways resistance in normal subjects is only slightly increased by β-receptor antagonists, and this is of no consequence. In asthmatic subjects, however, non-selective β-receptor antagonists (such as propranolol) can cause severe bronchoconstriction, which does not, of course, respond to the usual doses of drugs such as salbutamol or adrenaline. This danger is less with β_1-selective antagonists, but none is so selective in humans that the risk can be ignored.

Despite the involvement of β receptors in the hyperglycaemic actions of adrenaline, β-receptor antagonists cause only minor metabolic changes in healthy people. They do not affect the onset of hypoglycaemia following an injection of insulin, but somewhat delay the recovery of blood glucose concentration. In patients with diabetes, however, the use of β-receptor antagonists increases the likelihood of exercise-induced hypoglycaemia, because the normal adrenaline-induced release of glucose from the liver is diminished. Furthermore, β-receptor antagonists may alter the awareness of hypoglycaemia by blunting its symptoms (see Ch. 31 and further in the chapter).

β-Adrenoceptor antagonists

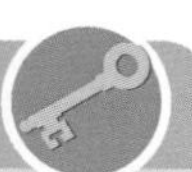

- Non-selective between β_1 and β_2 adrenoceptors: **propranolol**, **alprenolol**, **oxprenolol.**
- β_1-selective: **atenolol**, **metoprolol**, **bisoprolol**, **nebivolol.**
- **Alprenolol** and **oxprenolol** have partial agonist activity.
- Many clinical uses (see 'Clinical uses of β-adrenoceptor antagonists' clinical box).
- Important hazards are bronchoconstriction in asthmatics, and bradycardia and cardiac failure if administered to unstable patients with deteriorating cardiac function.
- Adverse effects include cold extremities, insomnia, vivid dreams, depression and fatigue.
- Some (e.g. propranolol) show rapid first-pass metabolism, hence poor bioavailability.
- Some drugs (e.g. **labetalol**, **carvedilol**) block both α and β adrenoceptors.

Clinical use

The main uses of β-receptor antagonists are connected with their effects on the cardiovascular system and are discussed in Chapters 20 and 21. They are summarised in the 'Clinical uses of β-adrenoceptor antagonists' clinical box.

The use of β-receptor antagonists in cardiac failure deserves special mention, as clinical opinion underwent a U-turn. Patients with unstable heart disease may rely on a degree of sympathetic drive to the heart to maintain an adequate cardiac output and removal of this by blocking β receptors can exacerbate cardiac failure, so using these drugs in patients with cardiac failure was considered ill-advised at best. In theory, drugs with partial agonist activity (e.g. oxprenolol, alprenolol) offer an advantage because they can, by their own agonist action, maintain a degree of β_1-receptor activation, while at the same time blunting the cardiac response to increased sympathetic nerve activity or to circulating adrenaline. Clinical trials, however, have not shown a clear advantage of these drugs measurable as a reduced incidence of cardiac failure, and one such drug (**xamoterol**, since withdrawn) with particularly marked agonist activity clearly made matters worse.

Paradoxically, β-receptor antagonists, commenced in low doses with supervised up-titration to well-compensated patients with cardiac failure, unambiguously improves survival (see Ch. 21) (Bristow, 2011). **Carvedilol**, **bisoprolol, metoprolol** and **nebivolol** are among the drugs demonstrated to improve survival in randomised controlled trials and now routinely used to treat chronic stable heart failure, in combination with other categories of drugs (see Ch. 21).

Infantile haemangioma is the commonest soft-tissue tumour in children, occurring in 3%–10% of infants and usually regressing without treatment. Approximately 12% are complicated by impingement on vital organs such as the eye and require intervention. In 2008 a chance observation that treatment of heart failure with propranolol in two young children with severe haemangiomas was associated with their regression led to clinical trials that confirmed the effectiveness of propranolol for this indication. Such use has been approved by the FDA as well as in Europe, and propranolol is now standard therapy for severe infantile haemangioma. The evidence of such marked efficacy (Léauté-Labrèze et al., 2015) highlights the importance of β-adrenoceptor-mediated trophic actions, at the least in this paediatric endothelial tumour. Milder uncomplicated forms of infantile haemangioma are sometimes treated with topical timolol or propranolol.

Clinical uses of β-adrenoceptor antagonists

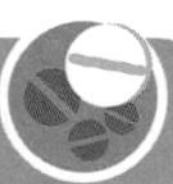

- Cardiovascular (see Chs 20 and 21):
  - angina pectoris
  - myocardial infarction, and following infarction
  - prevention of recurrent dysrhythmias (especially if triggered by sympathetic activation)
  - heart failure (in well-compensated patients)
  - hypertension (no longer first choice; see Ch. 21).
- Other uses:
  - severe/complicated infantile haemangioma
  - glaucoma (e.g. **timolol** eye drops)
  - thyrotoxicosis (see Ch. 34), as adjunct to definitive treatment (e.g. preoperatively and during initiation of carbimazole treatment)
  - anxiety (see Ch. 45), to control somatic symptoms (e.g. palpitations, tremor)
  - migraine prophylaxis (see Ch. 42)
  - benign essential tremor (a familial disorder).

Unwanted effects

The principal unwanted effects of β-receptor antagonists in therapeutic use result from their main (receptor-blocking) action.

Bronchoconstriction. As explained earlier, this is of little importance in the absence of airways disease, but in asthmatic patients the effect can be life-threatening. It is also of clinical importance in patients with other forms of obstructive lung disease (e.g. chronic bronchitis, emphysema), although the risk–benefit balance may favour cautious treatment in individual patients.

Cardiac depression. As described previously, these negative inotropes are contraindicated in acute decompensated heart failure. Patients suffering from chronic stable heart failure who are started on β-receptor antagonists may deteriorate symptomatically in the first few weeks before the beneficial effect develops (hence the advice to start at very low doses and titrate gently upwards). The desired beneficial effect in the long-term is improved left ventricular function and survival.

Bradycardia. Sinus bradycardia can progress to life-threatening heart block, particularly if β-adrenoceptor antagonists are co-administered with other antidysrhythmic drugs that impair cardiac conduction (see Ch. 20).

Hypoglycaemia. Glucose release in response to adrenaline is a safety mechanism in insulin-treated patients with diabetes and other individuals prone to hypoglycaemic attacks. The sympathetic response to hypoglycaemia produces symptoms (especially tachycardia) that warn patients of the urgent need for carbohydrate (usually in the form of a sugary drink). β-Receptor antagonists reduce these symptoms, so incipient hypoglycaemia is more likely to go unnoticed by the patient. There is a theoretical advantage in using β_1-selective agents, because glucose release from the liver is controlled by β_2 receptors.

Fatigue. This is probably due to reduced cardiac output and reduced muscle perfusion in exercise. It is a common symptom of patients taking β-adrenoceptor-blocking drugs.

Cold extremities. This is common, due to a loss of β-receptor-mediated vasodilatation in cutaneous vessels in hands and feet. Theoretically, β_1-selective drugs are less likely to produce this effect, which may also be less marked in patients treated with β-adrenoceptor antagonists with additional vasodilating properties.

Nightmares, which occur mainly with CNS-penetrant β-adrenoceptor antagonists, may be a direct result of β-receptor blockade, but the mechanism is not understood. This is an issue in the treatment of infantile haemangioma, where behavioural disturbances are sometimes of concern, and the efficacy of non–brain penetrant drugs has not been fully established.

DRUGS THAT AFFECT NORADRENERGIC NEURONS

Emphasis in this chapter is placed on peripheral sympathetic transmission. The same principles, however, are applicable to the CNS (see Ch. 39, where many of the drugs mentioned here also act). The major drugs and mechanisms are summarised in Table 15.6.

DRUGS THAT AFFECT NORADRENALINE SYNTHESIS

α-Methyltyrosine, which inhibits tyrosine hydroxylase, is used experimentally but not clinically. Indeed, few clinically important drugs affect catecholamine synthesis directly. **Carbidopa**, a hydrazine derivative of dopa which inhibits dopa decarboxylase in the periphery but does not penetrate the blood–brain barrier, is an important exception and is used as an important adjunct to levodopa in the treatment of parkinsonism (see Ch. 40).

Methyldopa, still used in the treatment of hypertension during pregnancy (see Ch. 21), is taken up by noradrenergic neurons, where it is converted to the false transmitter α-methylnoradrenaline. This is not deaminated within the neuron by MAO, so it accumulates and displaces noradrenaline from the synaptic vesicles. α-Methylnoradrenaline is released by exocytosis in the same way as noradrenaline but is less active than noradrenaline on α_1 receptors and thus is less effective in causing vasoconstriction. However, it is more active on presynaptic (α_2) receptors, so the autoinhibitory feedback mechanism operates more strongly than normal, thus reducing transmitter release. Each effect, both in the periphery and more importantly in the CNS, contributes to its hypotensive action. It produces adverse effects typical of centrally acting antiadrenergic drugs (e.g. sedation), as well as carrying 'off-target' risks of immune haemolytic anaemia (see Ch. 58) and liver toxicity, so it is now little used, except for hypertension in the second half of pregnancy where there is considerable experience of its use without harm to the unborn baby.

6-Hydroxydopamine (identical with dopamine except for an extra hydroxyl group) is a neurotoxin of the Trojan horse kind. It is taken up selectively by noradrenergic nerve terminals, where it is converted to a reactive quinone, which destroys the nerve terminal, producing a 'chemical sympathectomy'. The cell bodies survive, and eventually the sympathetic innervation recovers. The drug is useful for experimental purposes but has no clinical uses. If injected directly into the brain, it selectively destroys those nerve terminals (i.e. dopaminergic, noradrenergic and adrenergic) that take it up, but it does not reach the brain if administered systemically.

MPTP (**1-methyl-4-phenyl-1,2,3,5-tetrahydropyridine**; see Ch. 40) is a similar selective neurotoxin acting on dopaminergic neurons.

Droxidopa (**dihydroxyphenylserine**, L-DOPS) is under investigation for treating hypotension. It penetrates the blood–brain barrier and is a prodrug being converted to noradrenaline by dopa decarboxylase, bypassing the DBH-catalysed hydroxylation step. It raises blood pressure by increasing noradrenaline release.

DRUGS THAT AFFECT NORADRENALINE STORAGE

Reserpine is an alkaloid from the shrub *Rauwolfia*, which has been used in India for centuries for the treatment of mental disorders. Reserpine potently blocks the transport of noradrenaline and other amines into storage vesicles, by blocking VMAT. Noradrenaline accumulates instead in the cytoplasm, where it is degraded by MAO. The noradrenaline content of tissues drops and sympathetic transmission is blocked. Reserpine also depletes 5-HT and dopamine from neurons in the brain, where these amines are transmitters (see Ch. 39). Reserpine is now used only experimentally but was previously used in Europe and the United States as an antihypertensive drug. Its central effects, especially depression, which probably result from impairment of noradrenergic and 5-HT-mediated transmission in the brain (see Ch. 48), were a serious dose-related problem.

DRUGS THAT AFFECT NORADRENALINE RELEASE

Drugs can affect noradrenaline release in four main ways:

- by directly blocking release (noradrenergic neuron-blocking drugs)
- by evoking noradrenaline release in the absence of nerve terminal depolarisation (indirectly acting sympathomimetic drugs)
- by acting on presynaptic receptors that indirectly inhibit or enhance depolarisation-evoked release; examples include α_2 agonists (see above), angiotensin II, dopamine and prostaglandins
- by increasing or decreasing available stores of noradrenaline (e.g. reserpine, see earlier; MAO inhibitors, see Ch. 48).

NORADRENERGIC NEURON-BLOCKING DRUGS

Noradrenergic neuron-blocking drugs (e.g. **guanethidine**) were discovered in the mid-1950s when alternatives to ganglion-blocking drugs were being sought for use in the treatment of hypertension. They are of pharmacological interest but are now seldom if ever used clinically. The main effect of guanethidine is to inhibit the release of noradrenaline from sympathetic nerve terminals. It has little effect on the adrenal medulla, and none on nerve terminals that release transmitters other than noradrenaline. Related drugs include **bretylium**, **bethanidine** and **debrisoquin** (now of interest mainly as a probe for studying drug metabolism; see Ch. 12).

Actions

Drugs of this class reduce or abolish the response of tissues to sympathetic nerve stimulation.

The action of guanethidine on noradrenergic transmission is complex. It is selectively accumulated by noradrenergic nerve terminals, being a substrate for NET (see Table 15.6). Its initial activity is due to block of impulse conduction in the nerve terminals that selectively accumulate the drug – acting as a local anaesthetic selective for noradrenergic nerves, the selectivity being down to its concentration by NET in the terminals of these axons. Consequently, its action is prevented by drugs such as *tricyclic antidepressants* (see Ch. 48) that block NET.

Guanethidine is also concentrated in synaptic vesicles by means of the vesicular transporter VMAT, possibly interfering with their ability to undergo exocytosis, and displacing noradrenaline. In this way, it causes a gradual and long-lasting depletion of noradrenaline in sympathetic nerve endings, similar to the effect of reserpine.

Large doses of guanethidine cause structural damage to noradrenergic neurons, probably due to its accumulation in high concentration in the nerve terminals.

Although extremely effective in lowering standing blood pressure, they produce severe adverse effects associated with the loss of sympathetic nerve function. The most troublesome include postural hypotension, diarrhoea, nasal congestion and failure of ejaculation. They fail to lower blood pressure effectively at night, when patients are lying flat.

INDIRECTLY ACTING SYMPATHOMIMETIC AMINES

Mechanism of action and structure–activity relationships

Tyramine, **amphetamine** and **ephedrine** are structurally related to noradrenaline and, although much less potent, have qualitatively similar effects. However, rather than acting directly on adrenoceptors they mainly act indirectly by releasing endogenous noradrenaline from the sympathetic nerve endings. Drugs that act similarly and are used for their central effects (see Ch. 49) include **methylphenidate** and **atomoxetine**.

These drugs have only weak direct actions on adrenoceptors, but sufficiently resemble noradrenaline to be transported into nerve terminals by NET. Once inside the nerve terminals, they are taken up into the vesicles by VMAT, in exchange for noradrenaline, which escapes into the cytosol. Cytosolic noradrenaline escapes via NET, in exchange for the foreign monoamine, to act on postsynaptic receptors (Fig. 15.7). Exocytosis is not involved in the release process, so their actions do not require an elevation of cytoplasmic Ca^{2+}. They are not completely specific in their actions, and act partly by a direct effect on adrenoceptors, partly by inhibiting NET (thereby enhancing the effect of the released noradrenaline) and partly by inhibiting MAO.

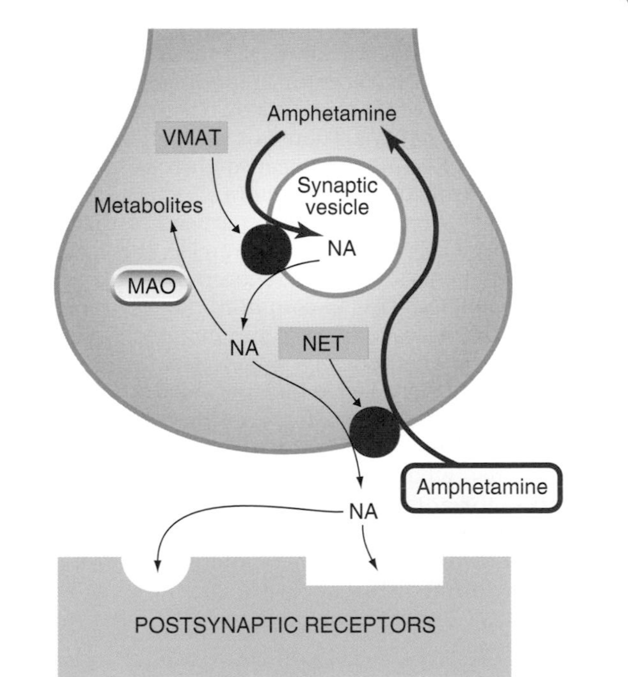

Fig. 15.7 The mode of action of amphetamine, an indirectly acting sympathomimetic amine. Amphetamine enters the nerve terminal via the noradrenaline transporter (NET) and enters synaptic vesicles via the vesicular monoamine transporter (VMAT), in exchange for noradrenaline **(NA)**, which accumulates in the cytosol. Some of the NA is degraded by monoamine oxidase (MAO) within the nerve terminal and some escapes, in exchange for amphetamine via NET, to act on postsynaptic receptors. Amphetamine also reduces NA reuptake via the transporter, so enhancing the action of the released NA.

As would be expected, the effects of these drugs are strongly influenced by other drugs that modify noradrenergic transmission. Thus, reserpine and 6-hydroxydopamine abolish their effects by depleting the terminals of noradrenaline. MAO inhibitors, on the other hand, strongly potentiate their effects by preventing inactivation, within the terminals, of the transmitter displaced from the vesicles. MAO inhibition particularly enhances the action of tyramine, because this substance is itself a substrate for MAO. Normally, dietary tyramine is destroyed by MAO in the gut wall and liver before reaching the systemic circulation. When MAO is inhibited this is prevented, and ingestion of tyramine-rich foods such as fermented cheese (e.g. ripe Brie) can then provoke a sudden and dangerous rise in blood pressure. Inhibitors of NET, such as **imipramine** (see Table 15.6) and **amphetamine**, which is transported slowly by NET, so acts both as a substrate of NET and as an inhibitor of noradrenaline uptake, interfere with the effects of indirectly acting sympathomimetic amines by preventing their uptake into the nerve terminals.

These drugs, especially amphetamine, have important effects on the CNS (see Chs 49 and 50) that depend on their ability to release not only noradrenaline, but also 5-HT and dopamine from nerve terminals in the brain. An important characteristic of the effects of indirectly acting sympathomimetic amines is that marked tolerance develops. Repeated doses of amphetamine or tyramine, for example, produce progressively smaller pressor responses. This is probably caused by depletion of the releasable store of noradrenaline. Tolerance to the central effects also develops with repeated administration.

Actions

The peripheral actions of the indirectly acting sympathomimetic amines include bronchodilatation, raised arterial pressure, peripheral vasoconstriction, increased heart rate and force of myocardial contraction and inhibition of gut motility. Their central actions account for their significant abuse potential and for limited therapeutic applications (see Chs 49, 50 and 59). Apart from ephedrine, which is still used as a nasal decongestant because its central action is minor, these drugs are no longer used for their peripheral sympathomimetic effects.

INHIBITORS OF NORADRENALINE UPTAKE

Reuptake of released noradrenaline by NET is the most important mechanism by which its action is terminated. Many drugs inhibit NET, and thereby enhance the effects of both sympathetic nerve activity and circulating noradrenaline. NET is not responsible for clearing circulating adrenaline, so these drugs do not affect responses to this amine.

The main class of drugs whose primary action is inhibition of NET are the *tricyclic antidepressants* (see Ch. 48), for example **imipramine**. These drugs have their major effect on the CNS but also cause tachycardia and cardiac dysrhythmias, reflecting their peripheral effect on sympathetic transmission. **Cocaine**, known mainly for its abuse liability (see Chs 49 and 50) and local anaesthetic activity (see Ch. 44), enhances sympathetic transmission, causing tachycardia and increased arterial pressure (and, with chronic use, cardiomyopathy and cardiac hypertrophy). Its central effects of euphoria and excitement (see Ch. 49) are probably a manifestation of the same mechanism acting via dopamine and 5-HT in the brain. It strongly potentiates the actions of noradrenaline in experimental animals or in isolated tissues provided the sympathetic nerve terminals are intact.

Many drugs that act mainly on other steps in sympathetic transmission also inhibit NET to some extent, presumably because the carrier molecule has structural features in common with other noradrenaline recognition sites, such as receptors and degradative enzymes.

The EMT, which is important in clearing circulating adrenaline from the bloodstream, is not affected by most of the drugs that block NET. It is inhibited by **phenoxybenzamine**, however, and by various *corticosteroids*. This action of corticosteroids may have some relevance to their therapeutic effect in conditions such as asthma but is probably of minor importance.

The main sites of action of drugs that affect adrenergic transmission are summarised in Fig. 15.8.

Drugs acting on noradrenergic nerve terminals

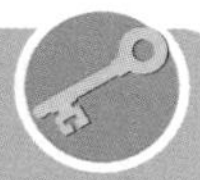

- Drugs that inhibit noradrenaline synthesis include:
  - **α-methyltyrosine**: blocks tyrosine hydroxylase; not used clinically
  - **carbidopa**: blocks peripheral dopa decarboxylase and is used to potentiate the central action of levodopa to treat Parkinson's disease (see Ch. 40)
- **α-Methyldopa** gives rise to false transmitter (α-methylnoradrenaline), which is a potent α_2 agonist, thus causing powerful presynaptic inhibitory feedback in CNS and periphery. Its use as an antihypertensive agent is now limited mainly to during pregnancy.
- **Reserpine** blocks noradrenaline accumulation in vesicles by VMAT, thus depleting noradrenaline stores and blocking transmission. Effective in hypertension but may cause severe depression, so clinically obsolete.
- Noradrenergic neuron-blocking drugs (e.g. **guanethidine**, **bethanidine**) are selectively concentrated in terminals and in vesicles (by NET and VMAT respectively), and block transmitter release, partly by local anaesthetic action. Effective in hypertension but cause severe side effects (postural hypotension, diarrhoea, nasal congestion, etc.), so now little used.
- **6-Hydroxydopamine** is selectively neurotoxic for noradrenergic neurons, because it is taken up and converted to a toxic metabolite. Used experimentally to eliminate noradrenergic neurons, not used clinically.
- Indirectly acting sympathomimetic amines (e.g. **amphetamine**, **ephedrine**, **tyramine**) are accumulated by NET and displace noradrenaline from vesicles, allowing it to escape. The effect is much enhanced by MAO inhibition, which can lead to severe hypertension following ingestion of tyramine-rich foods by patients treated with MAO inhibitors.
- Indirectly acting sympathomimetic agents are CNS stimulants. **Methylphenidate** and **atomoxetine** block NET and DAT but are not themselves transported by them so they do not displace endogenous transmitter monoamines; they are used to treat attention deficit–hyperactivity disorders (see Ch. 49).
- Drugs that inhibit NET include cocaine and **tricyclic antidepressant** drugs. Sympathetic effects are enhanced by such drugs.

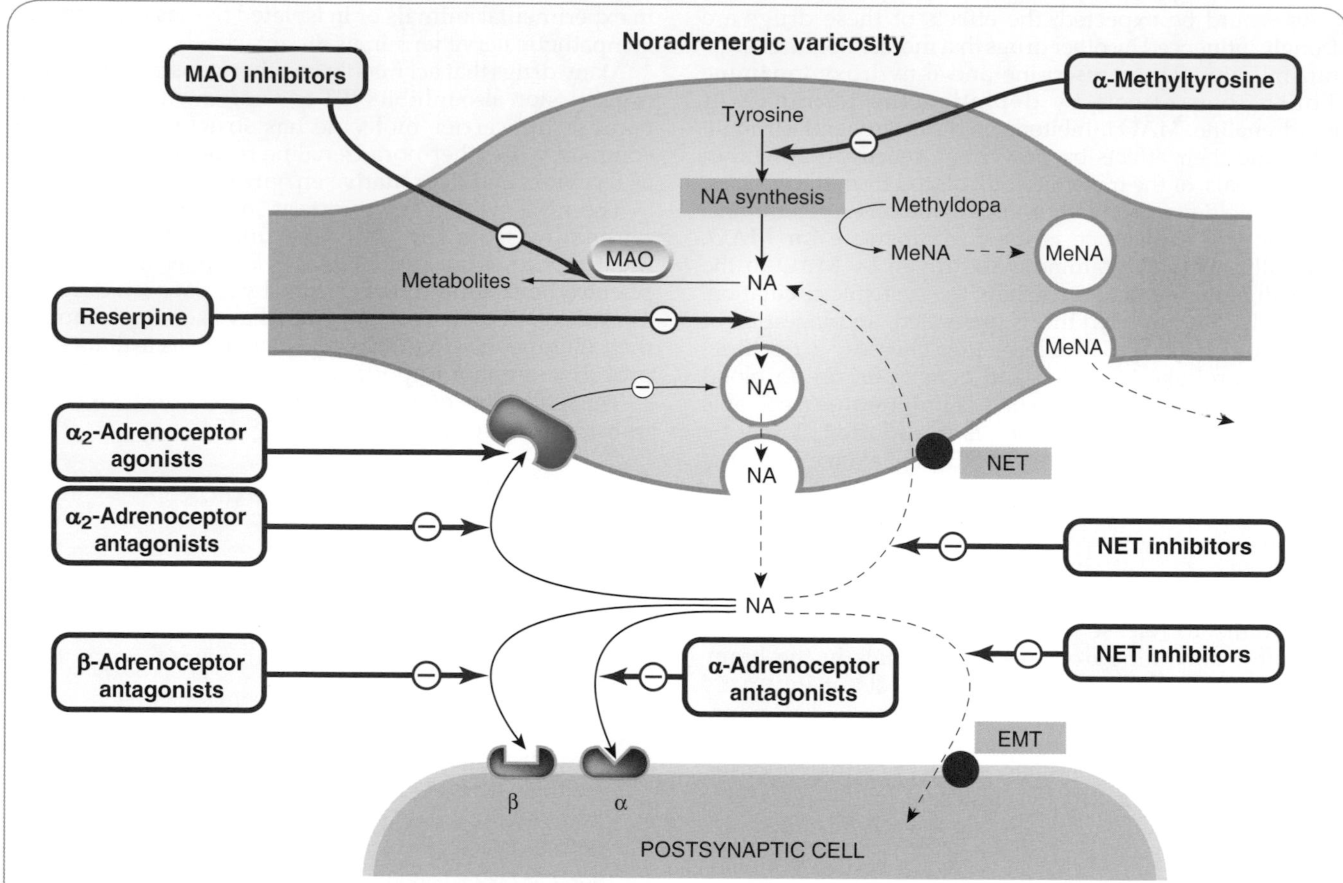

Fig. 15.8 Generalised diagram of a noradrenergic nerve terminal, showing sites of drug action. *EMT,* Extraneuronal monoamine transporter; *MAO,* monoamine oxidase; *MeNA,* methylnoradrenaline; *NA,* noradrenaline; *NET,* neuronal noradrenaline transporter.

REFERENCES AND FURTHER READING

General

Cooper, J.R., Bloom, F.E., Roth, R.H. 2003. The Biochemical Basis of Neuropharmacology, 8th edition. Oxford University Press.

Robertson, D., Biaggioni, I., Burnstock, G., Low, P.A., Paton, G.F.R. (Eds.), 2012. Primer on the Autonomic Nervous System, third ed. Academic Press, Elsevier, Amsterdam.

Adrenoceptors and imidazoline receptors

Ahles, A., Engelhardt, S., 2014. Polymorphic variants of adrenoceptors: pharmacology, physiology, and role in disease. Pharmacol. Rev. 66, 598–637.

Akinaga, J., Garcia-Sainz, J.A., Pupo, A.S., 2019. Updates in the function and regulation of a_1-adrenoceptors. Br. J. Pharmacol. 176, 2343–2357.

Alexander, S.P.H., Christopoulos, A., Davenport, A.P., et al., 2019. The concise guide to pharmacology 2019/20: G protein-coupled receptors. Br. J. Pharmacol. 176, S21-S141.

Bahari, Z., Meftafi, G.H., 2019. Spinal A_2-adrenoceptors and neuropathic pain modulation: therapeutic target. Br. J. Pharmacol. 176, 2366-2381.

Baker, J.G., Hall, I.P., Hill, S.J., 2003. Agonist and inverse agonist actions of β-blockers at the human β_2-adrenoceptor provide evidence for agonist-directed signalling. Mol. Pharmacol. 64, 1357–1369.

Bousquet, P., Hudson, A., Garcia-Sevilla, J.A., Jun-Xu, L., 2020. Imidazoline receptor system: the past, the present and the future. Pharmacol. Rev. 72, 50–79.

Gilsbach, R., Hein, L., 2012. Are the pharmacology and physiology of α_2 adrenoceptors determined by α_2-heteroreceptors and autoreceptors respectively? Br. J. Pharmacol. 165, 90–102.

Guimaraes, S., Moura, D., 2001. Vascular adrenoceptors: an update. Pharmacol. Rev. 53, 319–356.

Kahsai, A.W., Xiao, K.H., Rajagopal, S., et al., 2011. Multiple ligand-specific conformations of the beta(2)-adrenergic receptor. Nature Chem. Biol. 7, 692–700.

Papay, R.S., Ting, S., Piascik, M.T., Prasad, S.V.N., Perez, D.M., 2013. α_{1A}-Adrenergic receptors regulate cardiac hypertrophy in vivo through interleukin-6 secretion. Mol. Pharmacol. 83, 939–948.

Miscellaneous topics

Bermingham, D.P., Blakely, R.D., 2016. Kinase-dependent regulation of monoamine neurotransmitter transporters. Pharmacol. Rev. 68, 888–953.

Biaggioni, I., 2017. The pharmacology of autonomic failure: from hypotension to hypertension. Pharmacol. Rev. 69, 53–62.

Bristow, M.R., 2011. Treatment of chronic heart failure with beta-adrenergic receptor antagonists: a convergence of receptor pharmacology and clinical cardiology. Circ. Res. 109, 1176–1194.

Eisenhofer, G., Kopin, I.J., Goldstein, D.S., 2004. Catecholamine metabolism: a contemporary view with implications for physiology and medicine. Pharmacol. Rev. 56, 331–349.

Elenkov, I.J., Wilder, R.L., Chrousos, G.P., et al., 2000. The sympathetic nerve – an integrative interface between two supersystems: the brain and the immune system. Pharmacol. Rev. 52, 595–638.

Gainetdinov, R.R., Caron, M.G., 2003. Monoamine transporters: from genes to behaviour. Annu. Rev. Pharmacol. Toxicol. 43, 261–284.

Léauté-Labrèze, C., Hoeger, P., Mazereeuw-Hautier, J., et al., 2015. A randomized, controlled trial of oral propranolol in infantile hemangioma. N. Engl. J. Med. 372, 735–746.

Nonogaki, K., 2000. New insights into sympathetic regulation of glucose and fat metabolism. Diabetologia 43, 533–549.

Sacco, E., Bientinesi, R., 2012. Mirabegron: a review of recent data and its prospects in the management of overactive bladder. Ther. Adv. Urol. 4, 315–324.

Schiller, M., Ben-Shaanan, T.L., Rolls, A., 2021. Neuronal regulation of immunity: why, how and where? Nat. Rev. Immunol. 21, 20–36.

5-Hydroxytryptamine and the purines

16

OVERVIEW

In this chapter we discuss two small molecule transmitters which have a surprisingly complex pharmacology. *5-Hydroxytryptamine* (5-HT) is a local hormone of ancient lineage, widely conserved and present in many primitive animals, even those lacking nervous systems. 5-HT played an important part in the development of pharmacology as a discipline and today it is recognised as an important neurotransmitter both in the brain and in the periphery where it fulfils many other important physiological functions. We describe its synthesis, storage and release, its role in normal physiology and the pathophysiology of disorders including carcinoid syndrome and pulmonary hypertension. We also review the pharmacology of the numerous drugs that act at a large family of 5-HT receptors.

Purines are, of course, also ancient molecules. Amongst their many roles, they comprise the building blocks of DNA or RNA as well as the phosphorylated nucleotides which play a crucial role in the energy economy of the cell. In contrast to 5-HT, however, the discovery that purine nucleosides and nucleotides function as extracellular chemical mediators is relatively recent. In this chapter we discuss the basic biology of purinergic mediators, the drugs that act through purinergic signalling pathways and the receptors that transduce these effects.

5-HYDROXYTRYPTAMINE

A biologically active, low-molecular-weight factor originally detected in the 1930s in extracts of gut ('enteramine') and in blood serum ('serotonin') was eventually identified chemically in 1949 as *5-hydroxytryptamine* (5-HT) (Fig. 16.1). Today, the terms *5-HT* and *serotonin* are used interchangeably. 5-HT was subsequently found in the central nervous system (CNS) and shown to function both as a neurotransmitter and as a local hormone in the peripheral vascular system. This chapter deals with the metabolism, distribution and physiological roles of 5-HT in the periphery, and with the different types of 5-HT receptor and the drugs that act on them. Further information on the role of 5-HT in the brain, its relationship to psychiatric disorders and the actions of psychotropic drugs is presented in Chapters 39, 45, 47 and 48. The use of drugs that modulate 5-HT in the gut is dealt with in Chapter 30.

DISTRIBUTION, BIOSYNTHESIS AND DEGRADATION

The highest concentrations of 5-HT in the body are found in three organs:

- *In the wall of the intestine.* Over 90% of the total amount in the body is present in the *enterochromaffin* cells (endocrine cells with distinctive staining properties) in the gut. These cells are derived from the neural crest and resemble those of the adrenal medulla. They are found mainly in the stomach and small intestine interspersed with mucosal cells. Some 5-HT also occurs in nerve cells of the myenteric plexus, where it functions as an excitatory neurotransmitter.
- *In blood.* Platelets contain high concentrations of 5-HT. They accumulate it from the plasma by an active transport system and release it from cytoplasmic granules when they aggregate (hence the high concentration of 5-HT in serum from clotted blood; see Ch. 23).
- *In the CNS.* 5-HT is a transmitter in the CNS and is present in in most brain areas with its neuronal cell bodies localised to regions of the midbrain (see Ch. 39).

Although 5-HT is present in the diet, most of this is metabolised before entering the bloodstream. Endogenous 5-HT arises from a biosynthetic pathway similar to that of noradrenaline (see Ch. 15), except that the precursor amino acid is *tryptophan* instead of tyrosine. Tryptophan is converted to 5-hydroxytryptophan in chromaffin cells and neurons by the action of *tryptophan hydroxylase*, an enzyme confined to 5-HT-producing cells (but not present in platelets). The 5-hydroxytryptophan is then decarboxylated to 5-HT by the ubiquitous *L-aromatic acid decarboxylase*, which also participates in the synthesis of catecholamines and histamine (see Ch. 17).

Platelets (and neurons) possess a high-affinity 5-HT uptake mechanism. Platelets become loaded with 5-HT as they pass through the intestinal circulation, where the local concentration is relatively high. Because the mechanisms of synthesis, storage, release and reuptake of 5-HT are very similar to those of noradrenaline, many drugs affect both processes indiscriminately (see Ch. 15). However, *selective serotonin reuptake inhibitors* (SSRIs) have been developed and are important therapeutically as anxiolytics and antidepressants (see Chs 45 and 48). 5-HT is often stored in neurons and chromaffin cells as a co-transmitter, acting together with various peptide hormones, such as *somatostatin*, *substance P* or *vasoactive intestinal polypeptide* (see Ch. 17).

Degradation of 5-HT occurs mainly through oxidative deamination, catalysed by *monoamine oxidase A*, followed by oxidation to *5-hydroxyindoleacetic acid* (5-HIAA), the pathway again being the same as that of noradrenaline catabolism. 5-HIAA is excreted in the urine and serves as an indicator of 5-HT production in the body. This is used, for example, in the diagnosis of carcinoid syndrome (see later).

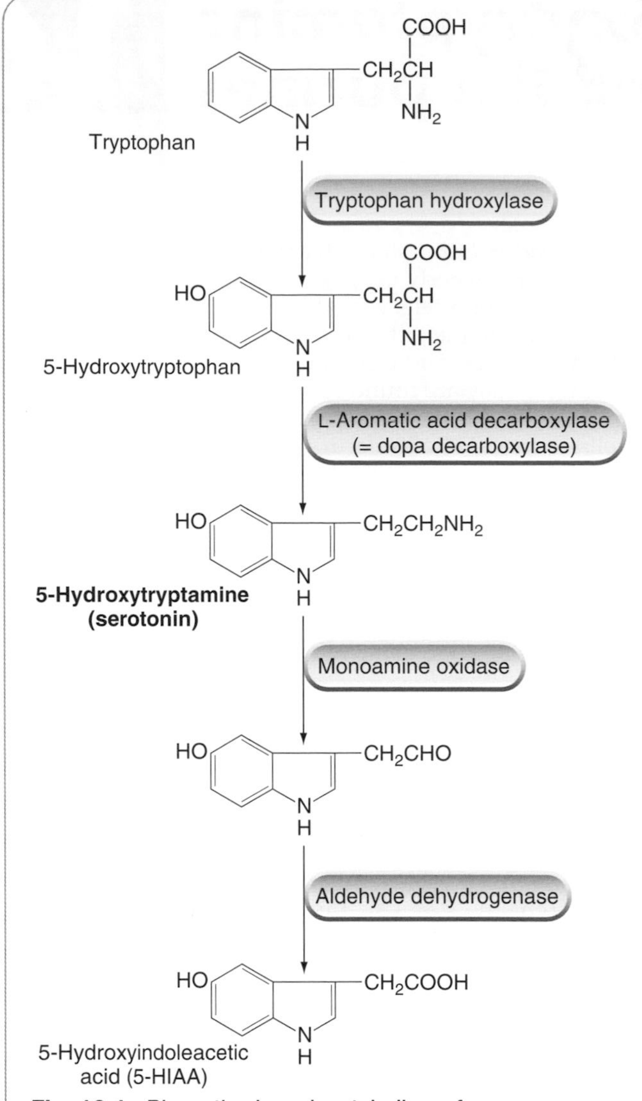

Fig. 16.1 Biosynthesis and metabolism of 5-hydroxytryptamine.

Distribution, biosynthesis and degradation of 5-hydroxytryptamine (5-HT)

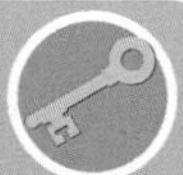

- Tissues rich in 5-HT are:
  - gastrointestinal tract (chromaffin cells and enteric neurons)
  - platelets
  - CNS.
- Metabolism closely parallels that of noradrenaline.
  - 5-HT is formed from dietary tryptophan, which is converted to 5-hydroxytryptophan by tryptophan hydroxylase, then to 5-HT by a non-specific decarboxylase.
- 5-HT is transported into cells by a specific SERT.
  - Degradation occurs mainly by monoamine oxidase, forming 5-HIAA, which is excreted in urine.

Actions and functions of 5-hydroxytryptamine (5-HT)

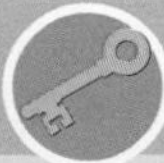

- Important actions are:
  - increased gastrointestinal motility (direct excitation of smooth muscle and indirect action via enteric neurons)
  - contraction of other smooth muscle (bronchi, uterus)
  - mixture of vascular constriction (direct and via sympathetic innervation) and dilatation (endothelium dependent)
  - platelet aggregation
  - stimulation of peripheral nociceptive nerve endings
  - excitation/inhibition of CNS neurons.
- Postulated physiological and pathophysiological roles include:
  - in periphery: peristalsis, vomiting, platelet aggregation and haemostasis, inflammation, sensitisation of nociceptors and microvascular control
  - in CNS: many postulated functions, including control of appetite, sleep, mood, hallucinations, stereotyped behaviour, pain perception and vomiting.
- Clinical conditions associated with disturbed 5-hydroxytryptamine (5-HT) include:
  - migraine, carcinoid and serotonin syndrome, pulmonary hypertension, mood disorders and anxiety.

CLASSIFICATION OF 5-HT RECEPTORS

It was realised long ago that the actions of 5-HT are not all mediated by receptors of the same type. Various pharmacological classifications have come and gone, and the nomenclature of these receptors has changed several times which makes for difficulties when reading some older papers. The current system is summarised in Table 16.1. This classification takes into account sequence data derived from cloning, signal transduction mechanisms and pharmacological specificity as well as the phenotypes of 5-HT receptor 'knock-out' mice.

Their diversity is astonishing. Currently, there are some 14 known receptor subtypes (together with an extra gene in mouse). These are divided into seven classes ($5\text{-}HT_{1-7}$), one of which ($5\text{-}HT_3$) is a ligand-gated cation channel while the remainder are G protein–coupled receptors (GPCRs; see Ch. 3). The six GPCR families are further subdivided into some 13 receptor subtypes based on their sequence and pharmacology. Most subtypes are found in all species so far examined, but there are some exceptions (the $5\text{-}HT_{5B}$ gene is found in mouse but has not been found in humans). The sequences of $5\text{-}HT_1$ and $5\text{-}HT_2$ receptors are highly conserved among species, but the $5\text{-}HT_{4-7}$ receptors are more diverse and are grouped together largely on pharmacological grounds. Most 5-HT GPCRs signal through adenylyl cyclase/cAMP, but some (the $5\text{-}HT_2$ subtype) activate phospholipase C to generate phospholipid-derived second messengers (see Ch. 3). In addition to these main subtypes, many genetic polymorphisms have been found, giving rise to four or more variants of some of these receptors. The

Table 16.1 Some significant drugs acting at the main human 5-HT receptor subtypes

Receptor	Main functions	Some significant drugs: Agonists	Antagonists	Primary signalling system
5-HT$_{1A}$	Neuronal inhibition, behavioural effects, changes in sleep, feeding, thermoregulation, memory, learning, anxiety *Implicated in periodic fever in humans*	8-OH-DPAT, cabergoline clozapine, triptans. *PA;* apomorphine, bromocriptine buspirone	Chlorpromazine, haloperidol, ketanserin, pizotifen, spiperone yohimbine	
5-HT$_{1B}$	Presynaptic inhibition, behavioural effects, changes in memory, anxiety Vasoconstriction	8-OH-DPAT, cabergoline, clozapine, dihydroergotamine; *PA;* bromocriptine, triptans	Ketanserin, methysergide, spiperone, yohimbine	G protein (Gi/Go) ↓ cAMP (may also modulate Ca^{2+} channels)
5-HT$_{1D}$	Cerebral vasoconstriction Behavioural effects: locomotion, neuroendocrine effects	8-OH-DPAT, cabergoline, clozapine, dihydroergotamine/ergotamine, triptans; *PA;* bromocriptine, pergolide	Ketanserin, methysergide, spiperone, yohimbine	
5-HT$_{1E}$	—	8-OH-DPAT, clozapine, dihydroergotamine, ergotamine, triptans	Methysergide, yohimbine	
5-HT$_{1F}$	Presynaptic inhibition	8-OH-DPAT, clozapine, dihydroergotamine, ergotamine, lasmiditan, LSD, triptans	Methysergide, yohimbine	
5-HT$_{2A}$	Neuronal excitations, behavioural effects. Smooth muscle contraction (gut, bronchi, etc.). Platelet aggregation. Vasoconstriction/vasodilatation *In humans implicated in psychiatric disorders and alcohol dependence*	Cabergoline, 8-OH-DPAT. *PA;* ergotamine, bromocriptine, methysergide	Apomorphine, chlorpromazine (*IA*), clozapine, fluoxetine, haloperidol, ketanserin, methysergide	
5-HT$_{2B}$	Cardiac development	8-OH-DPAT cabergoline LSD, methysergide. *PA;* ergotamine	Ketanserin, clozapine, yohimbine, apomorphine, tegaserod, bromocriptine	G protein (G_q/G_{11}) ↑ IP_3, Ca^{2+}
5-HT$_{2C}$	CNS, resistance to stress and epileptic seizures	Cabergoline, 8-OH-DPAT, LSD. *PA;* ergotamine, methysergide	Ketanserin, amitryptiline, methysergide clozapine (*IA*)	
5-HT$_3$ (Several subunit combinations)	Neuronal excitation (autonomic, nociceptive neurons); behavioural effects: anxiety; emesis	2-Me-5-HT, chloromethyl biguanide	Granisetron, metoclopramide, ondansetron, palonosetron, tropisetron	Ligand-gated cation channel
5-HT$_4$	Regulation of feeding, motor control, stress, resistance to seizures	Metoclopramide, cisapride; *PA*, tegaserod	Tropisetron	
5-HT$_{5A}$	Modulation of exploratory behaviour in rodents	8-OH-DPAT, LSD, triptans	Clozapine, ketanserin, methysergide, yohimbine	
5-HT$_6$	Learning and memory, modulation of neurotransmission	LSD, ergotamine, pergolide, bromocriptine	Amitryptaline, chlorpromazine, clozapine (*IA*), dihydroergotamine, ergotamine, fluoxetine, methysergide, sumatriptan	G protein (G_s) ↑ cAMP
5-HT$_7$	Thermoregulation? Circadian rhythm?	8-OH-DPAT, bromocriptine, buspirone (*PA*), cisapride, LSD	Amitryptiline, buspirone chlorpromazine (*IA*), clozapine dihydroergotamine, ketanserin, methysergide, sumatriptan yohimbine	

The list of agonists and antagonists is not exhaustive and many drugs shown are not used clinically or are not currently available in the United Kingdom (e.g. tropisetron), but are included as they are often used experimentally or referred to in the literature.

2-Me-5-HT, 2-Methyl-5-hydroxytryptamine; *5-HT*, 5-hydroxytryptamine; *8-OH-DPAT*, 8-hydroxy-2-(di-n-propylamino) tetraline; *CNS, central nervous system*; *GI*, gastrointestinal; *IA*, inverse agonist; *IP_3*, inositol trisphosphate; *LSD*, lysergic acid diethylamide; *PA*, partial agonist.

Source: www.guidetopharmacology.org

pharmacological and pathophysiological relevance of these genetic isoforms is often unclear.

Genetically altered mice lacking functional members of this receptor family have been produced (see for example Bonasera and Tecott, 2000). The functional deficits in such animals are generally quite subtle, suggesting that these receptors may serve to modulate, rather than to enable, physiological responses. With the exception of 5-HT_3-selective agents, many 5-HT receptor agonists and antagonists are relatively non-selective with respect to different receptor subtypes. This makes their pharmacology difficult to interpret and summarise. Some of the more significant drug targets include the following.

5-HT_1 receptors. Those of pharmacological significance occur mainly in the brain, the subtypes being distinguished on the basis of their regional distribution and their pharmacological specificity. Their function is mainly inhibitory. The 5-HT_{1A} subtype is particularly important in regulating 5-HT neuronal activity in the CNS and is found as an autoreceptor on the cell bodies of 5-HT neurons where activation leads to a reduction in neuronal firing. It is an important receptor in relation to mood and behaviour and 5-HT_1 'knock-out' mice exhibit defects in sleep regulation, learning ability and other CNS functions. Receptor polymorphisms may be associated with increased susceptibility to substance abuse. The 5-$HT_{1B/D/F}$ subtypes, which are expressed in neurons innervating cerebral blood vessels, are believed to be important in migraine and are the target for ***triptans*** (e.g. **sumatriptan) and the ditans** (i.e. **lasmiditan**), which together constitute an important group of drugs used to treat acute attacks (see Ch. 42). Unfortunately, the 5-HT_{1B} receptor is also present in the vasculature of the heart and elsewhere, explaining some of the unwanted effects associated with triptan therapy. In the CNS, 5-HT_{1B} receptors are found at the terminals of 5-HT neurons where activation inhibits further transmitter release provide a mechanism of negative feedback regulating endogenous 5-HT release. In an unfortunate instance of the pharmacological 'cancel culture', the hapless '5-HT_{1C}' receptor – actually the first to be cloned – has been officially declared non-existent, having been ignominiously reclassified as the 5-HT_{2C} receptor when it was found to be linked to inositol trisphosphate production rather than adenylyl cyclase.

5-HT_2 receptors. These are present in the CNS but are also particularly important in the periphery. The effects of 5-HT on smooth muscle and platelets, which have been known for many years, are mediated by the 5-HT_{2A} receptor, as are some of the behavioural effects of agents such as **lysergic acid diethylamide** (LSD). 5-HT_2 receptors are linked to phospholipase C and thus stimulate inositol trisphosphate formation. The 5-HT_{2A} subtype is functionally the most important, the others having a more limited distribution and functional role. The role of 5-HT_2 receptors in normal physiology is probably a minor one, but it becomes more prominent in pathological conditions such as asthma and vascular thrombosis (see Chs 23 and 28). Mice lacking 5-HT_2 receptors also exhibit defects in colonic motility (5-HT_{2A}), heart defects (5-HT_{2B}) and CNS disorders (5-$HT_{2A/C}$).

5-HT_3 receptors. 5-HT_3 receptors are exceptional in being membrane cation channels (see Ch. 3) and cause excitation directly, without involvement of any secondary messenger signalling system. The receptor itself consists of a homo- or hetero-pentameric assembly of distinct subunits which are designated by further subscript letters (e.g. 5-HT_{3A-E} in humans). 5-HT_3 receptors occur mainly in the peripheral nervous system, particularly on nociceptive sensory neurons (see Ch. 42) and on autonomic and enteric neurons, where 5-HT exerts a strong excitatory effect. 5-HT evokes pain when injected locally and, when given intravenously, elicits a fine display of autonomic reflexes resulting from excitation of many types of vascular, pulmonary and cardiac sensory nerve fibres. 5-HT_3 receptors also occur in the brain, particularly in the *area postrema,* a region of the medulla involved in the vomiting reflex, and selective 5-HT_3 antagonists are used as antiemetic drugs (see Ch. 30). Genetic polymorphisms in the subunits are associated with increased susceptibility to nausea and vomiting.

5-HT_4 receptors. These occur in the brain, as well as in peripheral organs such as the gastrointestinal tract, bladder and heart. Their main physiological role appears to be in the former, where they produce neuronal excitation and mediate the effect of 5-HT in stimulating peristalsis. Mice deficient in the 5-HT_4 receptor exhibit a complex phenotype including abnormal feeding behaviour in response to stress.

5-HT_5, 5-HT_6 and 5-HT_7 receptors. Less is known about these receptors. All are present in the CNS as well as other tissues. There are two genes for 5-HT_5 isoforms but only one codes for a functional receptor in humans although both may be functional in rodents. In addition to its action on 5-$HT_{1B/D}$ receptors, **sumatriptan** is also an antagonist at the 5-HT_7 receptor suggesting this receptor may also be a significant target for migraine treatment (Agosti, 2007). 5-$HT_{6/7}$ receptors are thought to be involved in various CNS functions, homeostatic and other effects of the transmitter.

PHARMACOLOGICAL EFFECTS

As one might predict from the profusion of 5-HT receptor subtypes, the biological actions of 5-HT are numerous and complex and there is considerable species variation. The main sites of action in humans are as follows.

Gastrointestinal tract. Most 5-HT receptor subtypes are present in the gut with the exception of those of the 5-$HT_{5/6}$ family. About 10% of 5-HT in the intestine is located in neurons, where it acts as a neurotransmitter, while the remainder is located in the enterochromaffin cells, which act as sensors to transduce information about the state of the gut, and which release 5-HT into the lamina propria. Broadly speaking, 5-HT receptors are present on most neuronal components of the enteric nervous system as well as smooth muscle, secretory and other cells. Their main function is to regulate peristalsis, intestinal motility, secretion and visceral sensitivity; the responses observed are complex and the reader is referred to Guzel and Mirowska-Guzel (2022) for a more comprehensive account.

The importance of 5-HT in the gut is underlined by the widespread distribution in the enteric nervous system and the intestinal mucosa, of the *serotonin uptake transporter* (SERT) which rapidly and efficiently removes extracellular 5-HT, thus limiting its action. Inhibitors of this transporter such as the SSRIs exaggerate the action of 5-HT in the gut, explaining some of the common gastrointestinal side effects of these drugs. Interestingly, there is evidence for genetic changes in this reuptake system linked to irritable bowel syndrome, which might explain the rather bewildering symptoms of the disease.

Smooth muscle. In many species (although only to a minor extent in humans), smooth muscle outside of the

5-Hydroxytryptamine (5-HT) receptors

- There are seven families (5-HT$_{1-7}$), with further subtypes of 5-HT$_1$ (A–F) and 5-HT$_2$ (A–C). Many polymorphisms and splice variants have also been observed.
- All are GPCRs, except 5-HT$_3$, which are ligand-gated cation channels.
  - 5-HT$_1$ receptors occur mainly in the CNS (all subtypes) and some blood vessels (5-HT$_{1B/D}$ subtypes). Some effects are mediated through inhibition of adenylyl cyclase, including neural inhibition and vasoconstriction. Specific agonists include triptans and ditans (used in migraine therapy) and **buspirone** (used in anxiety). Specific antagonists include **spiperone** and **methiothepin.**
  - 5-HT$_2$ receptors occur in the CNS and many peripheral sites (especially blood vessels, platelets, autonomic neurons). Neuronal and smooth muscle effects are excitatory and some blood vessels are dilated as a result of nitric oxide release from endothelial cells. 5-HT$_2$ receptors act through the phospholipase C/inositol trisphosphate pathway. Ligands include **LSD** (agonist in CNS, antagonist in periphery). Specific antagonists include **ketanserin.**
  - 5-HT$_3$ receptors occur in the peripheral nervous system, especially nociceptive afferent neurons and enteric neurons, and in the CNS. Effects are excitatory, mediated through direct receptor-coupled ion channels. **2-Methyl-5-HT** is a specific agonist. Specific antagonists include **ondansetron** and **palonosetron.** Antagonists are used mainly as antiemetic drugs but may also be anxiolytic.
  - 5-HT$_4$ receptors occur mainly in the enteric nervous system (also in the CNS). Effects are excitatory, through stimulation of adenylyl cyclase, causing increased gastrointestinal motility. Specific agonists include **metoclopramide** (used to stimulate gastric emptying).
  - 5-HT$_5$ receptors (one subtype in humans) are located in the CNS. Little is known about their role.
  - 5-HT$_6$ receptors are located in the CNS and on leukocytes. Little is known about their role in humans.
  - 5-HT$_7$ receptors are located in the CNS and the gastrointestinal tract. Little is known about their role in humans but emerging data show they may also be important in migraine.

gastrointestinal tract (e.g. uterus and bronchial tree) is also contracted by 5-HT.

Blood vessels. The effect of 5-HT on blood vessels depends on various factors, including the size of the vessel, the species and the prevailing sympathetic activity. Large vessels, both arteries and veins, are usually constricted by 5-HT, although the sensitivity varies greatly. This is the result of a direct action on vascular smooth muscle cells, mediated through 5-HT$_{2A}$ receptors. 5-HT can also cause vasodilatation indirectly by releasing nitric oxide from vascular endothelial cells (see Ch. 19) and inhibiting noradrenaline release from sympathetic nerve terminals. Dilatation of large intracranial vessels contributes to headache whereas activation of 5-HT$_{1B/D}$ receptors causes constriction, perhaps contributing to the antimigraine action of some of these drugs. If 5-HT is injected intravenously, the blood pressure initially rises, because of the constriction of large vessels, and then falls, owing to arteriolar dilatation. 5-HT may play a role in the pathology of *pulmonary hypertension* (see later in this chapter and Ch. 21).

Platelets. 5-HT causes platelet aggregation (see Ch. 23) by acting on 5-HT$_{2A}$ receptors, and these platelets can then release further 5-HT. If the endothelium is intact, 5-HT release from adherent platelets causes vasodilatation, which helps to sustain blood flow; if it is damaged however (e.g. by atherosclerosis), 5-HT causes constriction and impairs blood flow further. These effects of platelet-derived 5-HT are thought to be important in vascular disease.

Nerve endings. 5-HT stimulates nociceptive (pain-mediating) sensory nerve endings, an effect mediated mainly by 5-HT$_3$ receptors. If injected into the skin, 5-HT causes pain; when given systemically, it elicits a variety of autonomic reflexes through stimulation of afferent fibres in the heart and lungs, which further complicate interpretation of the cardiovascular response. In some species, mast cells release 5-HT when stimulated and nettle stings contain 5-HT among other mediators. 5-HT also inhibits transmitter release from adrenergic neurons in the periphery.

Central nervous system. 5-HT is an important neurotransmitter in the CNS and several important antipsychotic and antidepressant drugs act on these pathways by interfering with its disposition or action. **LSD** is a relatively non-selective 5-HT receptor agonist/partial agonist, which acts centrally as a potent hallucinogen. However, its actions are complex: 5-HT excites some neurons and inhibits others; it also acts presynaptically to inhibit transmitter release from nerve terminals and this might underlie some of the actions of serotonergic drugs in migraine. Different receptor subtypes mediate these effects.

DRUGS ACTING AT 5-HT RECEPTORS

Table 16.1 lists some significant agonists and antagonists at the different receptor types. Many are only partly selective. Our increasing understanding of the location and function of the different receptor subtypes has raised the possibility of developing compounds with improved receptor selectivity.

Important drugs that act on 5-HT receptors in the periphery include the following:

- Although not clinically useful, selective 5-HT$_{1A}$ agonists, such as 8-hydroxy-2-(di-*n*-propylamino) **tetralin** (8-OH-DPAT), are potent hypotensive agents, acting through a central mechanism. They are useful experimental drugs.
- 5-HT1$_{B/D}$ receptor agonists (e.g. the triptans) are used for treating migraine.
- 5-HT1$_F$ receptor agonists such as **lasmiditan** (e.g. the ditans) are also useful for treating migraine.
- 5-HT$_2$ receptor antagonists (e.g. **methysergide, ketanserin**) act mainly on 5-HT$_{2A}$ receptors but

may also block other 5-HT receptors, as well as α-adrenoceptors and histamine receptors (see Ch. 17). **Ergotamine** and **methysergide** belong to the 'ergot family' (see later) and have historically been used mainly for migraine prophylaxis (although rarely used these days). Other 5-HT_2 antagonists are used to control the symptoms of carcinoid tumours.
- 5-HT_3 receptor antagonists (e.g. **granisetron**, **ondansetron**, **palonosetron**) are used as antiemetic drugs (see Chs 30 and 57), particularly for controlling the severe nausea and vomiting that occur with many forms of cancer chemotherapy.
- 5-HT_4 receptor agonists that stimulate coordinated peristaltic activity (known as a 'prokinetic action') could be used for treating gastrointestinal disorders. **Metoclopramide** acts in this way, as well as by blocking dopamine receptors. Similar but more selective drugs such as **cisapride** and **tegaserod** were introduced to treat irritable bowel syndrome but were later withdrawn because of adverse cardiovascular side effects.

ERGOT ALKALOIDS

Whilst largely of historical interest today, ergot alkaloids have preoccupied pharmacologists for more than a century. As a group, they stubbornly resist classification. Many act on 5-HT receptors, but not selectively, so that their effects are complex and diverse.

Ergot, an extract of the fungus *Claviceps purpurea* that infests cereal crops, contains many active substances, and it was the study of their pharmacological properties in the early years of the 20th century that led Dale to many important discoveries concerning acetylcholine, histamine and catecholamines. Epidemics of ergot poisoning have occurred, and still occur, when contaminated grain is used for food. The symptoms include mental disturbances and intensely painful peripheral vasoconstriction leading to gangrene[1].

Chemically, ergot alkaloids are complex molecules derived from lysergic acid. The important members of the group include various naturally occurring and synthetic derivatives with different substituent groups arranged around a common nucleus; these include including **ergotamine**, **dihydroergotamine**, **ergometrine** as well as related compounds such as **bromocriptine** and **methysergide**. These compounds display diverse pharmacological actions, and it is difficult to discern any clear relationship between chemical structure and pharmacological properties.

Actions

Most of the effects of ergot alkaloids appear to be mediated through adrenoceptors, 5-HT or dopamine receptors, although some may be produced through other mechanisms. All alkaloids stimulate smooth muscle, some being relatively selective for vascular smooth muscle while others act mainly on the uterus. **Ergotamine** and **dihydroergotamine** are, respectively, a partial agonist and an antagonist at α-adrenoceptors. **Bromocriptine** is an agonist of dopamine receptors, particularly in the CNS, and **methysergide** is primarily an antagonist at 5-HT_{2A} receptors.

[1]This came to be known in the Middle Ages as *St Anthony's fire*, because it was believed that it could be cured by a visit to the Shrine of St Anthony (which conveniently happened to be in an ergot-free region of France).

The clinical use of ergot agents has diminished as more selective and safer drugs have been introduced but nevertheless, they remain important tools for pharmacologists. As one would expect of agents having so many actions, their physiological effects are complex and often rather poorly understood. **Ergotamine**, **dihydroergotamine** and **methysergide** are discussed here; further information on **ergometrine** and **bromocriptine** is given in Chapters 33, 35 and 40.

Vascular effects. When injected into an anaesthetised animal, **ergotamine** activates α-adrenoceptors, causing vasoconstriction and a sustained rise in blood pressure. At the same time, **ergotamine's** partial agonism means it reverses the pressor effect of **adrenaline** (epinephrine; see Ch. 15). The vasoconstrictor effect of **ergotamine** is responsible for the peripheral gangrene of St Anthony's fire, and probably also for some of the effects of ergot on the CNS. **Methysergide** and **dihydroergotamine** have much less vasoconstrictor effect. **Methysergide** is a potent 5-HT_{2A} receptor antagonist, whereas **ergotamine** and **dihydroergotamine** antagonise 5-HT_1 receptors, which may account for their antimigraine activity.

Clinical use. The only use of **ergotamine** is in the treatment of attacks of migraine unresponsive to simple analgesics (see Ch. 42). **Methysergide** was formerly used for migraine prophylaxis, and for treating the symptoms of carcinoid tumours, but is seldom used today. All these drugs can be used orally or by injection.

Unwanted effects. **Ergotamine** often causes nausea and vomiting, and it must be avoided in patients with peripheral vascular disease because of its vasoconstrictor action. **Methysergide** also causes nausea and vomiting, but its most serious side effect, which considerably restricts its clinical usefulness, is *retroperitoneal* and *mediastinal fibrosis*, which impairs the functioning of the gastrointestinal tract, kidneys, heart and lungs. The mechanism of this is unknown, but it is noteworthy that similar fibrotic reactions also occur in carcinoid syndrome, in which there is a high circulating level of 5-HT which may also contribute to the pathogenesis of pulmonary hypertension.

Ergot alkaloids

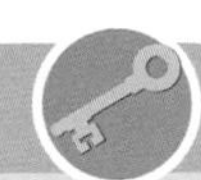

- These active substances are produced by a fungus that infects cereal crops and are responsible for occasional poisoning incidents. The most important compounds are:
  - **ergotamine**, formerly used in migraine prophylaxis, and **dihydroergotamine**
  - **ergometrine**, originally used in obstetrics to prevent postpartum haemorrhage
  - **methysergide**, formerly used to treat carcinoid syndrome, and migraine prophylaxis
  - **bromocriptine**, used in parkinsonism and endocrine disorders.
- The main sites of action are 5-HT receptors, dopamine receptors and adrenoceptors (mixed agonist, antagonist and partial agonist effects).
- Unwanted effects include nausea and vomiting, vasoconstriction (ergot alkaloids are contraindicated in patients with peripheral vascular disease).

CLINICAL CONDITIONS IN WHICH 5-HT PLAYS A ROLE

The use of 5-HT_3 antagonists for treating drug-induced emesis is discussed in Chapter 30. Modulation of 5-HT-mediated transmission in the CNS is an important mechanism of action of antidepressant and antipsychotic drugs, although the role of 5-HT in the pathophysiology of these disorders is unclear (see Chs 39, 45, 47 and 48). The role of 5-HT in migraine is dealt with in Chapter 42 and in this section, we discuss two other situations where the peripheral actions of 5-HT are believed to be important, and which are not covered elsewhere, namely *serotonin and carcinoid syndrome* and *pulmonary hypertension*.

SEROTONIN AND CARCINOID SYNDROME

Serotonin syndrome is a rare drug-induced side effect (see also Ch. 58). It is usually provoked by the administration of SSRIs particularly if there is concurrent treatment with another serotonergic agent. Fever is a common symptom; others include cardiovascular effects such as tachycardia and hypertension, neuromuscular symptoms including tremor and rigidity and mental symptoms such as confusion, agitation and anxiety (Werneke et al., 2020).

The condition seems to be increasing in frequency possibly because of the increasing number of prescriptions for monoamine oxidase inhibitors or SSRIs for depression and associated conditions, although some 'street drugs' such as *novel psychoactive substances* (NPSs), which sometimes include serotonergic agents, may provoke the condition (Schifano et al., 2021) as can some antiepileptic drugs (Prakash et al., 2021). Treatment is initiated by discontinuing the SSRI or, in some cases, administration of anti-serotonergic agents such as **cyproheptadine.** Fatalities are rare but possible if the condition is not treated.

Carcinoid syndrome is also caused by an excess of 5-HT, but in this case, a rare neuroendocrine disorder is the culprit. It manifests when malignant tumours of enterochromaffin cells, which usually arise in the small intestine and metastasise to the liver. These tumours secrete a variety of vasoactive chemical mediators: 5-HT is the most important, but neuropeptides such as substance P, and other agents such as histamine, prostaglandins and bradykinin (see Ch. 17), are also produced.

A *carcinoid crisis* occurs in only about 5% of such cases following a sudden release of these substances into the bloodstream. Sometimes this is caused by physical manipulation of the tumour or, if it is in the GI tract, when the metabolic capability of liver is overwhelmed, and these mediators enter into the systemic bloodstream. The end result is the appearance of several unpleasant symptoms, including flushing, abdominal cramps, diarrhoea, bronchoconstriction and hypotension, which may cause dizziness or fainting. More insidiously, cognitive impairment may develop and sometimes fibrotic stenosis of heart valves, leading to cardiac failure. It is reminiscent of the retroperitoneal and mediastinal fibrosis seen with **methysergide** and some other serotonergic agents and appears to be related to overproduction of 5-HT acting through 5-HT_{2B} receptors to drive the proliferation of connective tissue (Mota et al., 2016).

Clinical diagnosis can be confirmed by measuring the urinary excretion of the main metabolite of 5-HT, 5-HIAA. This may increase by as much as 20-fold when the disease is active and is raised even when the tumour is asymptomatic. 5-HT_2 antagonists, and the mixed 5-HT/histamine antagonist **cyproheptadine**, are effective in controlling some of the symptoms of carcinoid syndrome, but a more useful drug is **octreotide** (a long-acting agonist at somatostatin receptors), which suppresses hormone secretion from neuroendocrine, including carcinoid, cells (see Ch. 33) or **telotristat**, a tryptophan hydroxylase inhibitor. The condition and its treatment have been reviewed recently by Gade et al. (2020).

PULMONARY HYPERTENSION

Pulmonary hypertension (see also Ch. 21) is an incurable disease characterised by the progressive remodelling of the pulmonary vascular tree leading to a stiffening and narrowing. This leads to an inexorable rise in pulmonary arterial pressure which, if untreated (and this is difficult), inevitably leads to right heart failure and death.

There are several types of pulmonary hypertension, and in the 1990s the role of 5-HT was suggested by the fact that at least one form of the condition was precipitated by appetite suppressants (e.g. **dexfenfluramine** and **fenfluramine** and others) that were at one time widely prescribed as 'weight loss' or 'slimming' aids (and maybe are still produced by some unscrupulous manufacturers). These drugs block SERT and increase 5-HT which, acting through the $5HT_{1B}$ receptor, stimulates the growth and proliferation of pulmonary arterial smooth muscle cells and also produces a net vasoconstrictor effect in this vascular bed. *Seretonylation*, the process whereby 5-HT is linked to proteins by transglutaminase enzymes, may also be involved in the chronic stimulation of this process (Penumatsa et al., 2014). The use of SSRI antidepressants in late pregnancy may lead to pulmonary hypertension in the newborn (Masarwa et al., 2019) although the overall rate is low.

Some types of pulmonary hypertension (idiopathic and familial) are more prevalent in females and sex hormones may therefore be of relevance in the pathogenesis. The interested reader is referred to MacLean (2018) for an accessible account of the current thinking in this area, and to Chapter 21, where this topic is also discussed.

More generally, the ability of 5-HT to drive connective tissue proliferation may be important in *systemic sclerosis*, an autoimmune disorder in which fibrotic tissue proliferates in many organs including the vasculature (Sagonas and Daloussis, 2021). Such an idea is entirely consistent with the fact that serotonergic drugs such as **methysergide** can produce similar adverse effects in connective tissue.

PURINES

Nucleosides such as adenosine and nucleotides (especially ADP and ATP) will already be familiar to you because of their crucial role in DNA/RNA synthesis and energy metabolism, but it came as a surprise to the pharmacological community to learn that they also function extracellularly as signalling molecules which can produce a wide range of unrelated pharmacological effects.

The finding, in 1929, that adenosine injected into anaesthetised animals caused bradycardia, hypotension, vasodilatation and inhibition of intestinal movements foreshadowed these discoveries but the true origins of the field can really be traced to the crucial observations in 1970 by Burnstock and his colleagues, who provided first convincing evidence that ATP is a neurotransmitter (see

'Further Reading' list). After a period during which this radical idea was treated with scepticism, it has become clear that the 'purinergic' signalling system is not only of ancient evolutionary origin but participates in many physiological control mechanisms, including the regulation of coronary blood flow and myocardial function (see Chs 20 and 21), platelet aggregation and immune responses (see Chs 17 and 23), as well as neurotransmission in both the central and peripheral nervous system (see Chs 13 and 39).

The full complexity of purinergic control systems, their importance in many pathophysiological mechanisms and the therapeutic relevance of the various receptor subtypes is now emerging. As a result, there is an increasing interest in purine pharmacology and the prospect of developing novel 'purinergic' drugs for the treatment of pain and a variety of other disorders, particularly of thrombotic and inflammatory origin. Here we will focus our discussion on a few prominent areas.

PURINERGIC RECEPTORS

Fig. 16.2 summarises the mechanisms by which purines are stored, released and interconverted, and Table 16.2 lists the main receptor types through which they act and summarises what is currently known about their signalling systems, their endogenous ligands and antagonists of pharmacological interest. It should be noted, however, that the action of drugs and ligands at purinergic receptors can be confusing. In part, this is because nucleotides are rapidly degraded by ecto-enzymes and there is also evidence of interconversion of species by phosphate exchange. ATP released from cells may be rapidly dephosphorylated by tissue-specific nucleotidases, producing ADP and adenosine, both of which may produce further receptor-mediated effects. Thus, ATP may produce effects at all purinergic receptor subclasses depending upon the extent of its enzymatic conversion to ADP, AMP and adenosine. The role of intracellular ATP as a regulator of membrane potassium channels that control vascular smooth muscle (see Ch. 21) and insulin secretion (see Ch. 31) is quite distinct from these effects.

The subtypes in each family of purinergic receptors are distinguished on the basis of their molecular structure as well as their agonist and antagonist selectivity. The P2Y group is particularly problematic: several receptors have been cloned on the basis of homology with other family members, but their ligands have yet to be identified (in other words they are 'orphan receptors'). In addition, since some members of this group also recognise pyrimidines such as

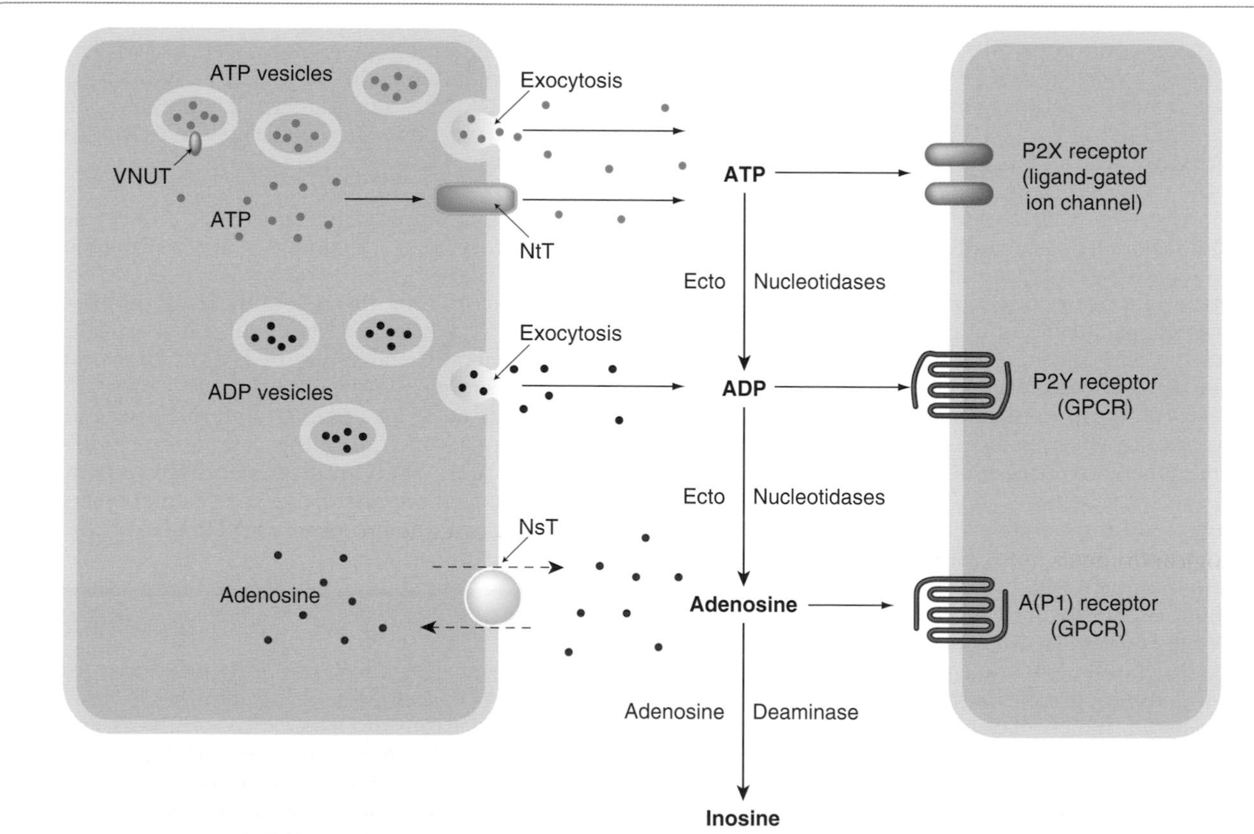

Fig. 16.2 Purines as mediators. ATP (and, in platelets, ADP) is present in the cytosol of cells (and released following cellular damage) or concentrated into vesicles by the vesicular nucleotide transporter (VNUT). Nucleotides may be released by exocytosis or through membrane channels such as pannexins (Pnx) or transporters (NtT). Once released, ATP can be converted to ADP and to adenosine by the action of ectonucleotidases. Adenosine is present in the cytosol of all cells and is released and taken up via a specific membrane transporter(s) (NsT), which is blocked by dipyridamole. Adenosine itself can be hydrolysed to inosine by the enzyme adenosine deaminase. ATP acts directly upon the P2X receptors (ligand-gated ion channels) but also upon P2Y receptors (G protein–coupled receptors [GPCRs]), the principal target for ADP. Adenosine itself acts on A receptors (also called P1 receptors), which are also GPCRs. Chapter 4 contains more details of exocytotic and other secretory mechanisms.

Table 16.2 Purinergic receptors

Receptor subtype		Principal ligands	Primary signalling system
Adenosine (also called P1)	A_1	*A*: Adenosine (high affinity). *An*: Caffeine, theophylline	G protein coupled ($G_{i/o}$): Lowers cAMP
	A_{2A}		G protein coupled (G_s): Raises cAMP
	A_{2B}	*A*: Adenosine (low affinity). *An*: Caffeine, theophylline	G protein coupled (G_s): Raises cAMP
	A_3		G protein coupled ($G_{i/o}$): Lowers cAMP
P2Y 'metabotropic'	$P2Y_1$	*A*: ADP > ATP (*A or PA*.). *An*: Suramin	G protein coupled (mainly $G_{q/11}$) Activates PLCβ mobilises Ca^{2+} Sometimes alters cAMP
	$P2Y_2$	*A*: UTP > ATP. *An*: Suramin	
	$P2Y_4$	'Pyrimidinoreceptor' *A*: UTP > ATP. *PA*: GDP	
	$P2Y_6$	'Pyrimidinoreceptor' *A*: UDP > UTP > ADP	
	$P2Y_{11}$	*A*: ATP > ADP. *An*: Suramin	
	$P2Y_{12}$	'Platelet ADP receptor' A. ADP > ATP. *An:* Clopidogrel, prasugrel, cangrelor, ticagrelor	G protein coupled (mainly $G_{i/o}$) Reduces cAMP
	$P2Y_{13}$	*A*: ADP>>ATP. *An:* Cangrelor, suramin	
	$P2Y_{14}$	*A*: UDP/UDP-glucose	
P2X 'ionotropic'	$P2X_1$	*A*: ATP. *An*: Suramin (non-selective)	Receptor-gated cation-selective ion channels
	$P2X_2$	*A*: ATP (non-selective)	
	$P2X_3$	*A*: ATP *An*: Gefapixant, sivopixant, suramin (non-selective)	
	$P2X_4$	*A*: ATP: *An*: Paroxetine	
	$P2X_5$	*Ag*: ATP: *An*: Suramin (non-selective)	
	$P2X_6$	*A*: ATP	
	$P2X_7$	*A*: ATP	

A, Agonist; *An*, antagonist; *PA*, partial agonist.
Source: www.guidetopharmacology.org

UTP and UDP as well as purines, they are sometimes classed as pyrimidinoceptors.

The three main families of purine receptor are:

- *Adenosine receptors* (A_1, A_{2A}, A_{2B} and A_3), formerly known as P1 receptors before the agonist was discovered to be adenosine. These are GPCRs that act through adenylyl cyclase/cAMP, or by direct effects on Ca^{2+} and K^+ channels, as described in Chapter 3.
- The simplest of the purines, adenosine, is found in biological fluids throughout the body. It exists free in the cytosol of all cells and is transported in by active transport from, and out to the interstitial fluid mainly by membrane transporters (of which there are several types). Little is known about the way in which this is controlled, but the extracellular concentrations are usually quite low compared with intracellular levels. Adenosine in extracellular fluid comes partly from this intracellular source and partly from hydrolysis of released ATP or ADP by nucleotidases such as CD39 and CD73. Adenosine can be inactivated by *adenosine deaminase*, yielding *inosine*, providing yet another level of control of this biologically active molecule, and another potential drug target. Virtually all cells express one or more of these adenosine receptors and so adenosine produces many pharmacological effects, both in the periphery and in the CNS.
- *P2Y metabotropic receptors* ($P2Y_{1-14}$). ADP is usually stored in vesicles in cells and released by exocytosis (see Ch. 4). It exerts its direct biological effects predominantly through the P2Y family of receptors. These are GPCRs that utilise either phospholipase C activation or cAMP as their signalling system (see Ch. 3); they respond to various adenosine nucleotides, generally preferring ATP over ADP or AMP. Some also recognise pyrimidines such as UTP.
- *P2X ionotropic receptors* ($P2X_{1-7}$), which are trimeric (in many cases heterotrimeric) ATP-gated cation channels. ATP is present in all cells in millimolar concentrations and is released if the cells are damaged (e.g. by ischaemia). The mechanism of release can be through exocytosis of vesicles containing ATP, through ATP transporters or through *pannexin* or *connexin* channels in the cell membrane. While some other actions of ATP in mammals are mediated through the P2Y receptors, it primarily exerts its action through P2X receptors. The extracellular domain of these trimeric receptors can bind three molecules of ATP. When activated by binding of two or three ATP molecules, the channels become permeable to Ca^{2+} and Na^+ ions, activating Ca^{2+}-sensitive pathways and causing membrane depolarisation. **Suramin** (a drug originally developed to treat trypanosome infections) antagonises ATP and has broad-spectrum inhibitory activity at both P2X and P2Y receptors.

THE PURINERGIC SYSTEM IN HEALTH AND DISEASE

It is now clear that the purinergic system plays an important role in the regulation of normal physiology as well as in several pathological states (Khakh and North, 2006) and we will now turn our attention to some prominent aspects of purinergic pharmacology. Adenosine, ADP and ATP are all implicated but because of the facile interconversion of purinergic species, their effects are often far from straightforward and can be difficult to understand (Chen et al., 2013). The purinergic literature has burgeoned in recent years and space does not permit us a comprehensive review. Instead, we will concentrate upon a few key areas.

Purines as mediators

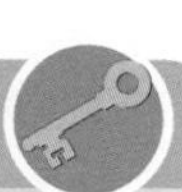

- *Adenosine* acts through A_1, A_{2A}, A_{2B} and A_3 G protein receptors, coupled to inhibition or stimulation of adenylyl cyclase. Adenosine receptors are blocked by methylxanthines such as **caffeine** and **theophylline. Dipyridamole** blocks adenosine uptake.
  - *Adenosine* affects many cells and tissues, including smooth muscle and nerve cells. It is not a conventional transmitter but may be important as a local hormone and 'homeostatic modulator'.
  - Important sites of action include the heart and the lung. Adenosine is very short-acting and is sometimes used for its antidysrhythmic effect.
- *ADP* acts through the $P2Y_{1-14}$ 'metabotropic' G protein–receptor family. These are coupled to cAMP or PLCβ.
  - Important sites of action include platelets where ADP released from granules promotes aggregation by acting on the PY_{12} receptor. This is antagonised by the drugs **clopidogrel**, **prasugrel, ticagrelor** and **cangrelor.**
- *ATP* is stored in vesicles and released by exocytosis or through membrane channels when cells are damaged. It also functions as an intracellular mediator, inhibiting the opening of membrane potassium channels.
  - ATP acts on P2X receptors: these are ligand-gated ion channels. It can also act on P2Y receptors.
  - **Clodronate** blocks **ATP** release from cells and **suramin** blocks ATP actions at most receptors.
  - Important sites of ATP action include the CNS, peripheral and central pathways and inflammatory cells.
  - When released, ATP is rapidly converted to ADP and adenosine yielding products that may act on other purinergic receptors.

THE CARDIOVASCULAR SYSTEM

Adenosine itself has a well-established role within the cardiovascular system and it is likely that all four of the adenosine receptors are involved in these effects. It inhibits cardiac pacemaker activity and atrioventricular node conduction and may be given as an intravenous bolus injection to terminate supraventricular tachycardia (see Ch. 20). Because of its short duration of action (it is destroyed or taken up within a few seconds of intravenous administration) it is considered safer than alternatives such as β-adrenoceptor antagonists or **verapamil**. The selective A_{2A} agonist **regadenoson** produces a powerful vasodilator effect and is used for diagnostic tests of cardiac function, while **dipyridamole** (a vasodilator and antiplatelet drug: see Ch. 23) blocks adenosine uptake by cells, thus effectively increasing its extracellular concentration.

Based on its ability to minimise the metabolic requirements of cells, another of adenosine's cardiovascular functions may be to act as an 'acute' defensive agent to produce vasodilation and cardioprotective effects being released immediately when tissue integrity is threatened by tissue hypoxia, ischaemia, inflammatory or other pathological changes (Guieu et al., 2020; Reiss et al., 2019). Under less extreme conditions, variations in adenosine release can control local blood flow and (through effects on the carotid bodies) tissue respiration, matching their metabolic requirements. The differential action of adenosine at A_{2A} and A_{2B} receptors in different vascular beds (Cooper et al., 2022) probably confers some regional specificity on the actions of this purine. Adenosine also regulates cholesterol trafficking through an action on its A_{2A} receptor, providing a defence against vascular damage associated with the development of plaque (Reiss et al., 2019).

ASTHMA AND INFLAMMATION

Adenosine receptors are found on all the cell types involved in asthma and inflammation (see Ch. 28). Their overall pharmacology is, however, complex (Pasquini et al., 2021): in asthma for example, activation of the A_{2A} subtype exerts a largely protective and anti-inflammatory effect, but when acting through its A_1 or A_{2B} receptor, adenosine promotes mediator release from mast cells, which causes enhanced mucus secretion, bronchoconstriction and leukocyte activation so an antagonist of the A_1 and A_{2B} receptor or an agonist of the A_{2A} receptor could represent a significant advance in this therapeutic area (see Brown et al., 2008; Burnstock et al., 2012). The role of the A_3 receptor has yet to be fully elucidated.

Methylxanthines, especially analogues of **theophylline** (see Ch. 28), are adenosine receptor antagonists and this drug is used for the treatment of asthma. Part of its beneficial activity may therefore be ascribed to its antagonism of the A_1 receptor, although methylxanthines also increase cAMP by inhibiting phosphodiesterase, and this effect also underwrites some of their pharmacological actions independently of adenosine receptor antagonism. Certain derivatives of **theophylline** are claimed to show greater selectivity for adenosine receptors over phosphodiesterase.

In contrast to the predominately anti-inflammatory effect of adenosine in airway inflammation, ATP has a pro-inflammatory role in both asthma and rheumatoid arthritis. ATP is released from stimulated, damaged or dying cells and P2X receptors are widely distributed on cells of the immune system; P2Y receptors less so. Acting through these receptors, ATP can regulate neutrophil and phagocyte chemotaxis. Activation of P2X7 (and possibly P2Y receptors) provokes the release from macrophages and mast cells of cytokines which promote local inflammatory responses in chronic inflammatory disorders (da Silva et al., 2019; Faas et al., 2017; Hechler and Gachet, 2015). Congruent with this idea is the observation that when the $P2X_7$ receptor is deleted genetically in mice they show a reduced capacity to develop chronic inflammation. Purinergic signalling also plays an important role in T-cell signalling. In asthma, adenosine, acting through its A_{2A} receptor, regulates the balance of immune cells such as to promote a less inflammatory phenotype (Junger, 2011; Wang et al., 2018). The subsequent hydrolysis of ATP to adenosine could therefore provide a counterbalancing anti-inflammatory input, by promoting resolution when the ongoing inflammation has achieved its purpose (Antonioli et al., 2022).

Inflammation is usually accompanied by pain and purines may also play a key role in nociception. ATP causes pain when injected (for example) subdermally, by activating $P2X_2$ and/or $P2X_3$ heteromeric receptors on afferent neurons involved in the transduction of nociception. The pain can be blocked by **aspirin** (see Ch. 25) suggesting the involvement of prostaglandins and also by a bisphosphonate inhibitor of ATP release (**clodronate**: see Ch. 36). There is thus considerable interest in the potential role of purinergic receptor antagonists (mainly at P2Y and P2X receptors) to treat (see Ch. 42) neuropathic and inflammatory pain (Kato et al., 2017).

Adenosine also regulates the inflammatory response elsewhere and A receptors at various locations in the eye (particularly A_{2A} receptors) have been identified as potential targets in ocular diseases, including dry eye syndrome (Guzman-Aranguez et al., 2014). Experimental A_3 antagonists have been observed to produce a beneficial effect in experimental models of colitis and may be useful in other inflammatory disorders, including rheumatoid arthritis and psoriasis (Shakya et al., 2019). Interestingly, **sulfasalazine** and **methotrexate**, which are used to treat inflammatory bowel disease (see Ch. 30), and which have other anti-inflammatory properties, stimulate the hydrolysis of ATP and AMP by ectonucleotidases to produce adenosine thereby increasing its effective local concentration and thus its actions.

PLATELETS

The secretory vesicles of blood platelets store both ATP and ADP in high concentrations and release them when the platelets are activated (see Ch. 23). One of the many effects of ADP is to promote platelet aggregation, so this system provides positive feedback and provides an important mechanism for amplifying this process. The receptor involved is $P2Y_{12}$ although the $P2Y_1$ receptor may also play a part in the overall regulation of platelet reactivity.

Exploitation of this finding has provided the best examples to date of the value of purinergic drugs. **Ticlopidine** (no longer used in UK) was the original drug of this type. This is an antagonist at platelet $P2Y_{12}$ receptors which inhibits the aggregation response. This was succeeded by **clopidogrel** and **prasugrel** (prodrugs), **cangrelor** and **ticagrelor** (allosteric antagonists). They are used, often in conjunction with aspirin, for preventing arterial thromboembolic disorders (see Ch. 23 and Laine et al., 2016) and provide superior protection to either of the agents when used individually.

PURINES AS NEUROTRANSMITTERS

The idea that such workaday metabolites as adenosine or ATP might be a member of the neurotransmitter elite was resisted for a long time but is now firmly established. ATP is contained in synaptic vesicles of both adrenergic, cholinergic and motor neurons and acts as a primary transmitter and as a co-transmitter. $P2X_2$, $P2X_4$ and $P2X_6$ are the predominant receptor subtypes expressed in neurons whereas $P2X_1$ predominates in smooth muscle.

Burnstock and his colleagues demonstrated that ATP is released on nerve stimulation in a Ca^{2+}-dependent fashion, and that exogenous ATP, in general, mimics the effects of nerve stimulation in various preparations, accounting for many of the actions produced by stimulation of nerves that are not caused by acetylcholine or noradrenaline (see Ch. 13) such as the relaxation of intestinal smooth muscle evoked by sympathetic stimulation and contraction of the bladder produced by parasympathetic nerves. ATP may function as a conventional 'fast' transmitter in autonomic ganglia and possibly the CNS, or as an inhibitory presynaptic transmitter and so the overall effect of ATP is sometimes difficult to assess.

Adenosine, produced following hydrolysis of ATP, exerts presynaptic inhibitory effects on the release of excitatory transmitters in the CNS and periphery but it is likely that this effect is only really manifest under conditions of pathological rather than physiological situations (Ziganshin et al., 2020).

SUMMARY

Despite the rather prosaic chemical nature of 5-HT and purines they have turned out to have a surprisingly complex pharmacology. 5-HT in particular utilises a quite extraordinary range of different receptors to produce its pharmacological effects whilst the mutable nature of the purines, enjoying as they do such facile interconversion, has ensured that interpretation of their pharmacology is anything but straightforward.

Notwithstanding these hinderances, huge progress in researching and developing these areas over the years has resulted in very tangible therapeutic rewards – and no doubt will continue to do so. Watch this space.

REFERENCES AND FURTHER READING

5-Hydroxytryptamine

Agosti, R.M., 2007. $5HT_{1F}$- and $5HT_7$-receptor agonists for the treatment of migraines. CNS Neurol. Disord. Drug Targets 6, 235–237.

Bonasera, S.J., Tecott, L.H., 2000. Mouse models of serotonin receptor function: towards a genetic dissection of serotonin systems. Pharmacol. Ther. 88, 133–142.

Gade, A.K., Olariu, E., Douthit, N.T., 2020. Carcinoid syndrome: a review. Cureus 12, e7186.

Guzel, T., Mirowska-Guzel, D., 2022. The role of serotonin neurotransmission in gastrointestinal tract and pharmacotherapy. Molecules 27, 1–16.

MacLean, M.M.R., 2018. The serotonin hypothesis in pulmonary hypertension revisited: targets for novel therapies (2017 Grover Conference Series). Pulm. Circ. 8 2045894018759125.
Masarwa, R., Bar-Oz, B., Gorelik, E., Reif, S., Perlman, A., Matok, I., 2019. Prenatal exposure to selective serotonin reuptake inhibitors and serotonin norepinephrine reuptake inhibitors and risk for persistent pulmonary hypertension of the newborn: a systematic review, meta-analysis, and network meta-analysis. Am. J. Obstet. Gynecol. 220, 57.e51–57.e13.
Mota, J.M., Sousa, L.G., Riechelmann, R.P., 2016. Complications from carcinoid syndrome: review of the current evidence. Ecancermedicalscience 10, 662.
Penumatsa, K., Abualkhair, S., Wei, L., et al., 2014. Tissue transglutaminase promotes serotonin-induced AKT signaling and mitogenesis in pulmonary vascular smooth muscle cells. Cell Signal. 26, 2818–2825.
Prakash, S., Rathore, C., Rana, K., Prakash, A., 2021. Fatal serotonin syndrome: a systematic review of 56 cases in the literature. Clin. Toxicol. 59, 89–100.
Sagonas, I., Daoussis, D., 2021. Serotonin and systemic sclerosis. An emerging player in pathogenesis. Joint Bone Spine 89, 105309.
Schifano, F., Chiappini, S., Miuli, A., et al., 2021. New psychoactive substances (NPS) and serotonin syndrome onset: a systematic review. Exp. Neurol. 339, 113638.
Werneke, U., Truedson-Martiniussen, P., Wikstrom, H., Ott, M., 2020. Serotonin syndrome: a clinical review of current controversies. J. Integr. Neurosci. 19, 719–727.

Purines

Antonioli, L., Pacher, P., Hasko, G., 2022. Adenosine and inflammation: it's time to (re)solve the problem. Trends Pharmacol. Sci. 43, 43–55.
Brown, R.A., Spina, D., Page, C.P., 2008. Adenosine receptors and asthma. Br. J. Pharmacol. 153 (Suppl. 1), S446–S456.
Burnstock, G., 2006. Purinergic P2 receptors as targets for novel analgesics. Pharmacol. Ther. 110, 433–454.
Burnstock, G., 2008. Purinergic receptors as future targets for treatment of functional GI disorders. Gut 57, 1193–1194.
Burnstock, G., 2012. Purinergic signalling: its unpopular beginning, its acceptance and its exciting future. Bioessays 34, 218–225.
Burnstock, G., 2017. Purinergic signalling: therapeutic developments. Front. Pharmacol. 8, 1–55.
Burnstock, G., Brouns, I., Adriaensen, D., Timmermans, J.P., 2012. Purinergic signalling in the airways. Pharmacol. Rev. 64, 834–868.
Chen, J.F., Eltzschig, H.K., Fredholm, B.B., 2013. Adenosine receptors as drug targets – what are the challenges? Nat. Rev. Drug Discov. 12, 265–286.
Cooper, S.L., Wragg, E.S., Pannucci, P., Soave, M., Hill, S.J., Woolard, J., 2022. Regionally selective cardiovascular responses to adenosine A2A and A2B receptor activation. FASEB J. 36, e22214.
da Silva, J.L.G., Passos, D.F., Bernardes, V.M., Leal, D.B.R., 2019. ATP and adenosine: role in the immunopathogenesis of rheumatoid arthritis. Immunol. Lett. 214, 55–64.
Faas, M.M., Saez, T., de Vos, P., 2017. Extracellular ATP and adenosine: the yin and yang in immune responses? Mol. Aspects Med. 55, 9–19.
Guieu, R., Deharo, J.C., Maille, B., et al., 2020. Adenosine and the cardiovascular system: the good and the bad. J. Clin. Med. 9, 1366.
Guzman-Aranguez, A., Gasull, X., Diebold, Y., Pintor, J., 2014. Purinergic receptors in ocular inflammation. Mediators Inflamm. 2014, 320906.
Hechler, B., Gachet, C., 2015. Purinergic receptors in thrombosis and inflammation. Arterioscler. Thromb. Vasc. Biol. 35, 2307–2315.
Junger, W.G., 2011. Immune cell regulation by autocrine purinergic signalling. Nat. Rev. Immunol. 11, 201–212.
Kato, Y., Hiasa, M., Ichikawa, R., et al., 2017. Identification of a vesicular ATP release inhibitor for the treatment of neuropathic and inflammatory pain. Proc. Natl. Acad. Sci. U. S. A. 114, E6297–E6305.
Khakh, B.S., North, R.A., 2006. P2X receptors as cell-surface ATP sensors in health and disease. Nature 442, 527–532.
Laine, M., Paganelli, F., Bonello, L., 2016. P2Y12-ADP receptor antagonists: days of future and past. World J. Cardiol. 8, 327–332.
Pasquini, S., Contri, C., Borea, P.A., Vincenzi, F., Varani, K., 2021. Adenosine and inflammation: here, there and everywhere. Int. J. Mol. Sci. 22, 7685.
Reiss, A.B., Grossfeld, D., Kasselman, et al., 2019. Adenosine and the cardiovascular system. Am. J. Cardiovasc. Drugs 19, 449–464.
Shakya, A.K., Naik, R.R., Almasri, I.M., Kaur, A., 2019. Role and function of adenosine and its receptors in inflammation, neuroinflammation, IBS, autoimmune inflammatory disorders, rheumatoid arthritis and psoriasis. Curr. Pharm. Des. 25, 2875–2891.
Wang, L., Wan, H., Tang, W., et al., 2018. Critical roles of adenosine A2A receptor in regulating the balance of Treg/Th17 cells in allergic asthma. Clin. Respir. J. 12, 149–157.
Ziganshin, A.U., Khairullin, A.E., Hoyle, C.H.V., Grishin, S.N., 2020. Modulatory roles of ATP and adenosine in cholinergic neuromuscular transmission. Int. J. Mol. Sci. 21, 6423.

Local hormones: histamine, lipids, peptides and proteins

17

OVERVIEW

When we discussed the function of cellular players in host defence in Chapter 7 we alluded to the crucial role of soluble chemical regulators of inflammation. In this chapter we take a closer look at these substances. We begin with some small molecule mediators: histamine and the biologically active lipids. While having a physiological role, these are also pressed into service by host defence mechanisms when necessary and are therefore important targets for anti-inflammatory drug action. These are followed by peptide and protein mediators, which are orders of magnitude larger in molecular terms. This constitutes a very diverse group including bradykinin, neuropeptides and cytokines (interleukins, chemokines and interferons), the latter of which seem to be exclusively concerned with host defence. We have included some general introductory observations on the nature and purpose of chemical messaging and, where possible, the synthesis, secretion and metabolism of these mediators. Finally, we conclude with a few remarks on mediators that down-regulate inflammation.

INTRODUCTION

The growth of pharmacology as a discipline was attended by the discovery of numerous biologically active substances. Many were initially uncharacterised, being described only as smooth muscle contracting (or relaxing) 'factors' which appeared in blood or tissues during particular physiological or pathological events. Eventually, these factors were identified chemically, some comparatively quickly while others resisted analysis for many years and so progress in a particular pharmacological area was often tied to advances in analytical methodology. For example, 5-hydroxytryptamine (see Ch. 16) and histamine, which are quite simple compounds, were identified soon after their biological properties were described. In contrast, the structural elucidation of the more complex prostaglandins, which were first discovered in the 1930s, had to await the development of the gas chromatograph–mass spectrometer (GC-MS) some 30 years later before the field could really progress.

Peptide and protein structures took even longer to solve. Substance P (11 amino acids) was also discovered in the 1930s but was not characterised until 1970 when peptide sequencing techniques had been developed. The advent of molecular biology in the 1980s greatly enhanced our analytical proficiency; for example, the 21-amino acid peptide, endothelin, was discovered and fully characterised, with the sequences of the gene and peptide published within about a year and the complete information published in a single paper (Yanagisawa et al., 1988). Techniques including high-performance liquid chromatography, solid-phase peptide synthesis and, more recently, the use of recombinant proteins as therapeutic agents (see Ch. 5) have driven development in this area. Separately, the availability of monoclonal antibodies for radioimmunoassay and immunocytochemistry has solved many quantitative problems. Transgenic animals with peptide or receptor genes deleted, overexpressed or mutated provide valuable clues about their functions, as has the use of antisense oligonucleotides, siRNA and gene editing (CRISPR-Cas9) technologies (see also Ch. 5) to silence these genes for experimental purposes. The control of precursor synthesis can now be studied indirectly by measuring mRNA at single cell resolution. The technique of *in situ hybridisation*, for example, enables the location and abundance of the mRNA to be mapped at microscopic resolution.

In summary, the molecular landscape has changed completely. Whereas the discovery of new 'small-molecule' mediators has slowed, the discovery of new protein and peptide mediators has ballooned. More than 100 cytokines have been discovered since interleukin 2 (IL-2) was first characterised in 1982 and on-going advances in analytical techniques continue to drive the discovery and identification of not only new individual signalling molecules but also whole classes of chemical mediators. Alongside the advent of cheap and readily available computing power, such techniques have additionally permitted the large-scale, integrated study of these small molecules at a systems level: the fields of proteomics, lipidomics and (more broadly) metabolomics.

WHAT IS A 'MEDIATOR'?

Like regular hormones, such as thyroxine (see Ch. 34) or insulin (see Ch. 31), a *local hormone* is simply a chemical messenger that conveys information from one cell to another.[1] Hormones such as thyroxine and insulin are released from a single endocrine gland, circulate in the blood and produce their action on other 'target' tissues. In contrast, local hormones are usually produced by cells to operate within their immediate microenvironment. The distinction is not actually completely clear-cut, however. For example, one of the 'classical' hormones, hydrocortisone, is normally released by the adrenal gland but, surprisingly, can also be produced by, and act locally upon, some other tissues such as the skin. Conversely, some cytokines, which are usually regarded as local hormones, can circulate in the blood and produce systemic actions as well.

When a local hormone is released in response to a stimulus of some kind, and produces a particular biological

[1]The term *autocrine* is sometimes used to denote a local mediator that acts on the cell from which it is released, whereas a *paracrine* mediator acts on other neighbouring cells.

effect (such as contraction of smooth muscle in response to allergen challenge), it is said to be a *mediator* of this response. Traditionally, a putative mediator[2] had to satisfy certain criteria before gaining official recognition. In the 1930s, Sir Henry Dale proposed a set of five rules to validate the credentials of mediators and these guidelines have been used as a point of reference ever since. Originally formulated as a test for putative neurotransmitters, these criteria cannot easily be applied to mediators of other responses and have thus been modified on several occasions.

Currently, the experimental criteria that establish a substance as a mediator are:

- that it should be released from local cells in sufficient amounts to produce a biological action on the target cells within an appropriate time frame;
- that application of an authentic sample of the mediator should reproduce the original biological effect;
- that interference with the synthesis, release or action (e.g. using receptor antagonists, enzyme inhibitors, 'knock-down' or 'knock-out' techniques) ablates or modulates the original biological response.

We now continue this chapter with a discussion of some prominent substances which have satisfied these stringent criteria and which are generally recognised to be important local hormones with well-defined biological properties.

HISTAMINE

In a classic study, Dale and his colleagues demonstrated that a local anaphylactic reaction (a type I or 'immediate hypersensitivity reaction' such as the response to egg albumin in a previously sensitised animal; see Ch. 7) was caused by antigen–antibody reactions in sensitised tissue and found that histamine mimicked this effect both in vitro and in vivo. Later studies confirmed that histamine is present in tissues and released (along with other mediators) during anaphylaxis.

SYNTHESIS AND STORAGE OF HISTAMINE

Histamine is a basic amine synthesised by the enzyme *histidine decarboxylase* which decarboxylates the amino acid histidine (Fig. 17.1). Histamine is widespread in the body but is present in particularly high concentrations in tissues in contact with the outside world (lungs, skin and gastrointestinal tract). At the cellular level, it is found largely in mast cells (approximately 0.1–0.2 pmol/cell) and basophils (0.01 pmol/cell), but non-mast cell histamine also occurs in enterochromaffin-like cells (ECLs) in the stomach and in histaminergic neurons in the brain (see Ch. 39). In mast cells and basophils, histamine is complexed in intracellular granules with an acidic protein and a high-molecular-weight heparin termed *macroheparin*.

HISTAMINE RELEASE

Histamine is released from mast cells during inflammatory or allergic reactions by exocytosis. Stimuli include complement components C3a and C5a (see Ch. 7), which interact with specific surface receptors, and the combination of antigen with cell-fixed immunoglobulin (Ig) E antibodies. In common with many secretory processes (see Ch. 4), histamine release is initiated by a rise in cytosolic [Ca^{2+}]. Various basic drugs, such as **morphine** and **tubocurarine**, release histamine, as does *compound 48/80*, an experimental tool often used to investigate mast cell biology. Agents that increase cAMP formation (e.g. β-adrenoceptor agonists; see Ch. 15) inhibit histamine secretion. Replenishment of secreted histamine by mast cells or basophils is a slow process, which may take days or weeks, whereas turnover of histamine in the gastric ECL is very rapid. Histamine is metabolised by diamine oxidase and/or by the methylating enzyme histamine *N*-methyltransferase (Fig. 17.1).

HISTAMINE RECEPTORS

Four types of histamine receptor, termed H_{1-4}, have been identified. All are G protein–coupled receptors (GPCRs) but their downstream signalling systems differ. H_1 and H_3 receptors, for example, elevate cAMP, whereas H_2 and H_4 receptors stimulate phospholipase C (PLC). Splice variants of H_3 and H_4 receptors have been reported. All four are implicated in the inflammatory response in some capacity and good accounts have been given by Jutel et al. (2009), with Thangam et al. (2018) focusing on how we may further translate recent insights for therapeutic benefit.

Selective antagonists of H_1, H_2 and H_3 receptors include **cetirizine**, **cimetidine** and **pitolisant**, respectively. Selective agonists for H_2 and H_3 receptors are, respectively, **dimaprit** and **(R)-methylhistamine**. Histamine H_1 antagonists are the principal antihistamines used in the treatment or prevention of inflammation (notably allergic inflammation such as hay fever). Other clinical uses of subtype antagonists may be found elsewhere in this book (e.g. Chs 25, 26, 27, 30 and 45). The pharmacology of H_4 receptors is less well developed but the evidence so far strongly suggests that the receptor also has a significant role in the inflammatory response, with eosinophils being a prominent target. Panula et al. (2015) have compiled a comprehensive review of histamine receptors and their pharmacology.

HISTAMINE ACTIONS

Smooth muscle effects. Histamine, acting on H_1 receptors, contracts the smooth muscle of the ileum, bronchi, bronchioles and uterus. The effect on the ileum is not as marked in humans as it is in the guinea pig (this tissue remains the de facto standard preparation for histamine bioassay). Histamine reduces air flow in the first phase of bronchial asthma (see Ch. 28) but H_1 antagonists are not of much benefit in the human disease. It is possible that H_4 receptors are more important (Thurmond, 2015) in mediating these resistant histamine effects in man.

Cardiovascular effects. Histamine dilates human blood vessels and increases permeability of postcapillary venules, by an action on H_1 receptors, the effect being partly endothelium dependent in some vascular beds. It also increases the rate and the output of the heart mainly by an action on cardiac H_2 receptors. It seems that this mediator is involved mainly in regulation of cardiovascular system in pathological, rather than physiological, states. Hattori et al. (2017) have reviewed the area in detail.

Gastric secretion. Histamine stimulates the secretion of gastric acid by action on H_2 receptors. In clinical terms, this is the most important action of histamine, because it is

[2]To add to the lexicographical confusion, the term *bioregulator* has recently crept into use. As this portmanteau word could cover just about any biologically active substance, it is not much use for our purposes.

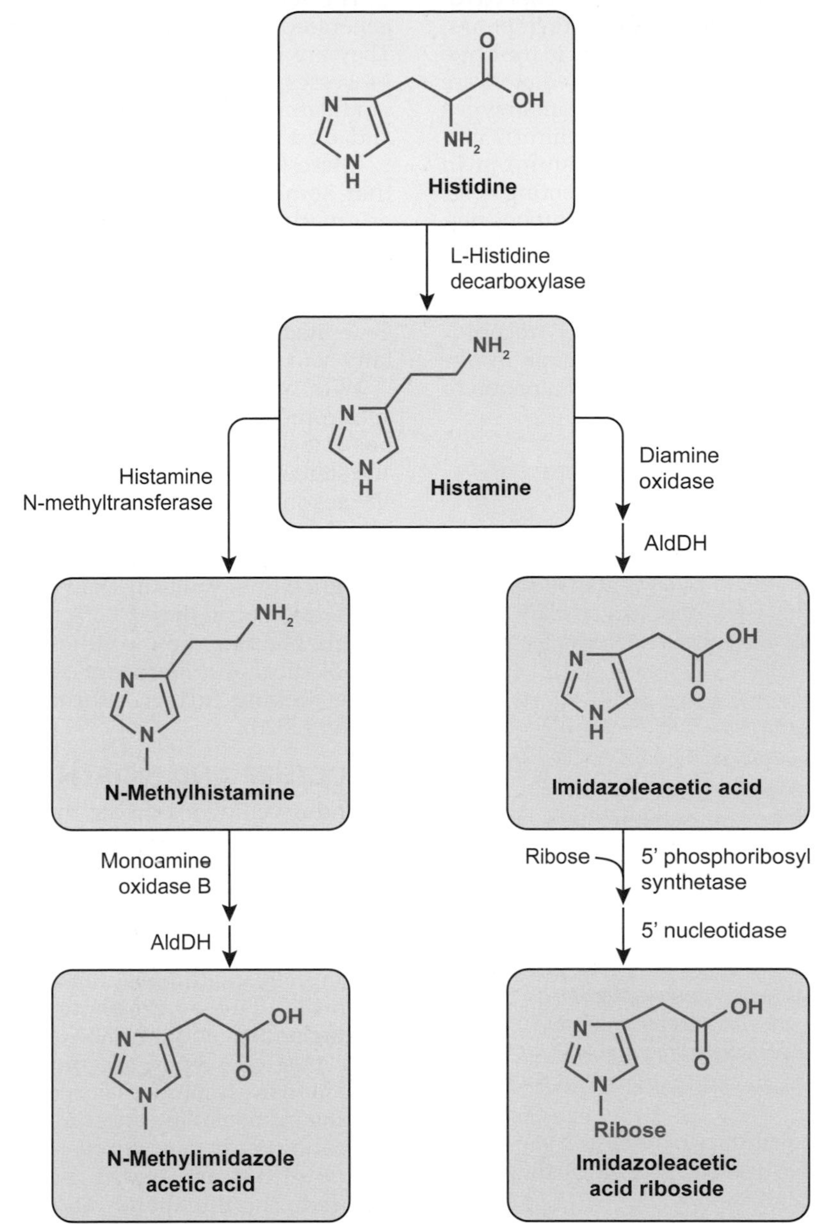

Fig. 17.1 The synthesis and metabolism of histamine. Histamine is synthesised by histidine decarboxylase, which removes the carboxyl group from histidine. Histamine can be metabolised to inactive products by several enzymes, including diamine oxidase (histaminase), and/or by the methylating enzyme histamine *N*-methyltransferase. *AldDH*, Aldehyde dehydrogenase.

implicated in the pathogenesis of peptic ulcer. It is considered in detail in Chapter 30.

Sleep/wake homeostasis. Histamine plays a key role in regulation of the sleep/wake cycle with H_1, H_2 and H_3 receptors being differentially expressed throughout the brain. Clinically, this is relevant as antagonism/inverse agonism of the H_3 receptor can be used to treat narcolepsy, a rare disorder characterised by excessive daytime sleepiness. It also explains why first-generation antihistamines (e.g. **chlorphenamine**) which can cross the blood–brain barrier are associated with drowsiness (H_1 receptors promoting wakefulness). For further information see Scammell et al. (2019) and Chapter 45.

Effects on skin. When injected intradermally, histamine causes a reddening of the skin, accompanied by a weal with a surrounding flare. This mimics the *triple response* to scratching of the skin, first described by Sir Thomas Lewis over 80 years ago. The reddening reflects vasodilatation of the small arterioles and precapillary sphincters and the weal, the increased permeability of the postcapillary venules. These effects are mainly mediated through activation of H_1 receptors. The flare is an *axon reflex*: stimulation of sensory nerve fibres evokes antidromic impulses through neighbouring branches of the same nerve, releasing vasodilators such as *calcitonin gene-related peptide* (CGRP). Histamine causes intense itch if injected into the skin or applied to a blister base, because it stimulates sensory nerve endings through an H_1-dependent mechanism. H_1 antagonists are used to control itch caused by allergic reactions, insect bites, etc.

Even though histamine release is manifestly capable of reproducing many of the inflammatory signs and symptoms, H_1 antagonists do not have much clinical utility in the acute inflammatory response per se, because other mediators are more important. Histamine is, however, important in type I hypersensitivity reactions such as allergic rhinitis and urticaria. Other significant actions of histamine in inflammation include effects on antigen-presenting cells, natural killer cells, epithelial cells and B and T lymphocytes, modulating both the innate and acquired immune response (Jutel et al., 2009; O'Mahony et al., 2011). The use of H_1 antagonists in these conditions is dealt with in Chapter 25. It is possible that the developing field of H_4 receptor pharmacology will fill in some significant gaps in our understanding of the role of histamine in inflammation in the near future (Thurmond, 2015).

Histamine

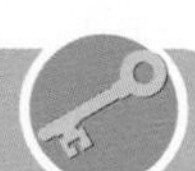

- Histamine is a basic amine, stored in mast cell and basophil granules, and secreted when C3a and C5a interact with specific membrane receptors or when antigen interacts with IgE fixed on cells triggering the high affinity IgE receptor.
- Histamine produces effects by acting on H_1, H_2, H_3 or H_4 receptors on target cells.
- The main actions in humans are:
  - stimulation of gastric secretion (H_2)
  - contraction of most smooth muscle, except blood vessels (H_1)
  - cardiac stimulation (H_2)
  - vasodilatation (H_1)
  - increased vascular permeability (H_1)
  - promoting waking (H_1) or sleep (H_3)
- Injected intradermally, histamine causes the 'triple response': *reddening* (local vasodilatation), *weal* (increased permeability of postcapillary venules) and *flare* (from an 'axon' reflex in sensory nerves releasing a peptide mediator).
- The main pathophysiological roles of histamine are:
  - as a stimulant of gastric acid secretion (treated with H_2-receptor antagonists)
  - as a mediator of type I hypersensitivity reactions such as urticaria and hay fever (treated with H_1-receptor antagonists)
  - as a regulator of sleep/wake behaviour (H_1-antagnoists being sedative in the CNS and H_3-inverse agonists promoting wakefulness).

EICOSANOIDS

GENERAL REMARKS

These bioactive lipid mediators arise from two groups of 20-carbon polyunsaturated fatty acid (PUFA) precursors: (omega) ω-6 (sometimes written n-6; a denomination determined by the position of the final carbon–carbon double bond counting from the methyl end) and ω-3 (n-3) fatty acids. Mammals cannot synthesise these *essential fatty acids* (EFAs) and they (or their immediate precursors) must therefore be present in the diet to maintain health.

The term *eicosanoids* refers to a group of mediators generated from common 20-carbon fatty acids precursors. They are implicated in the control of many physiological processes, are among the most important mediators and modulators of the inflammatory reaction (Figs 17.2 and 17.3) and are a significant target for drug action.

Interest in eicosanoids first arose in the 1930s after reports that semen contained a lipid substance, apparently originating from the prostate gland, which contracted uterine smooth muscle. Later, it became clear that *prostaglandin* (as the factor was, very reasonably, named[3]) was not a single substance but a whole family of compounds generated by virtually all cells from 20-carbon unsaturated fatty acid precursors.

With modern analytical techniques, in particular mass spectrometry–based lipidomic profiling, it has recently been possible to identify, monitor and quantify the structurally and stereochemically distinct eicosanoid and PUFA-derived species involved in both homeostasis and inflammation. These are now known to number into the hundreds, and it is manifestly clear that the 'lipidome' is more complex and biologically significant than previously thought. While exploration of all these PUFA moieties is beyond the scope of this chapter, key families and their physiological, pathological and therapeutic relevance are explored. For those seeking further information, see Han (2016) and Calder (2020).

STRUCTURE AND BIOSYNTHESIS

In land-dwelling mammals, the main eicosanoid precursor is *arachidonic acid* (5,8,11,14-eicosatetraenoic acid), an omega-6, 20-carbon unsaturated fatty acid containing four unsaturated double bonds (hence the prefix *eicosa-*, referring to the 20 carbon atoms, and *tetra*-enoic, referring to the four double bonds). The principal groups of eicosanoids are prostaglandins, *thromboxanes*, *leukotrienes*, *lipoxins* and *resolvins*. The common term *prostanoids* refers to prostaglandins and thromboxanes only.

In most cell types, arachidonic acid (which exists as arachidonate in solution) is a component of phospholipids, and the intracellular concentration of the free acid is low. Eicosanoids are not stored in cells (like histamine, for example) but are synthesised and then immediately released. The initial and rate-limiting step in eicosanoid synthesis is therefore the liberation of *arachidonate*. Usually this is a one-step process catalysed by the enzyme *phospholipase A_2* (PLA_2; see Fig. 17.3) but an alternative multi-step process involving *phospholipases C or D* in conjunction with *diacylglycerol lipase* is sometimes utilised. Several types of PLA_2 exist, but the most important is probably the highly regulated *cytosolic PLA_2* ($cPLA_2$). This enzyme not only generates arachidonic acid (and thus eicosanoids) but also lysoglyceryl-phosphorylcholine (lyso-PAF), the precursor of *platelet-activating factor* (PAF), another inflammatory mediator.

Cytosolic PLA_2 is activated by phosphorylation, and this may be triggered by signal transduction systems activated by various stimuli, such as the action of thrombin on

[3]Reasonable or not, it is a misnomer which arose through an anatomical error. In some species it is difficult to differentiate the prostaglandin-rich seminal vesicles from the prostate gland which (ironically, as we now know) contains relatively little. Nevertheless, the name stuck, outlasting the far more appropriate term *vesiglandin,* which was suggested later.

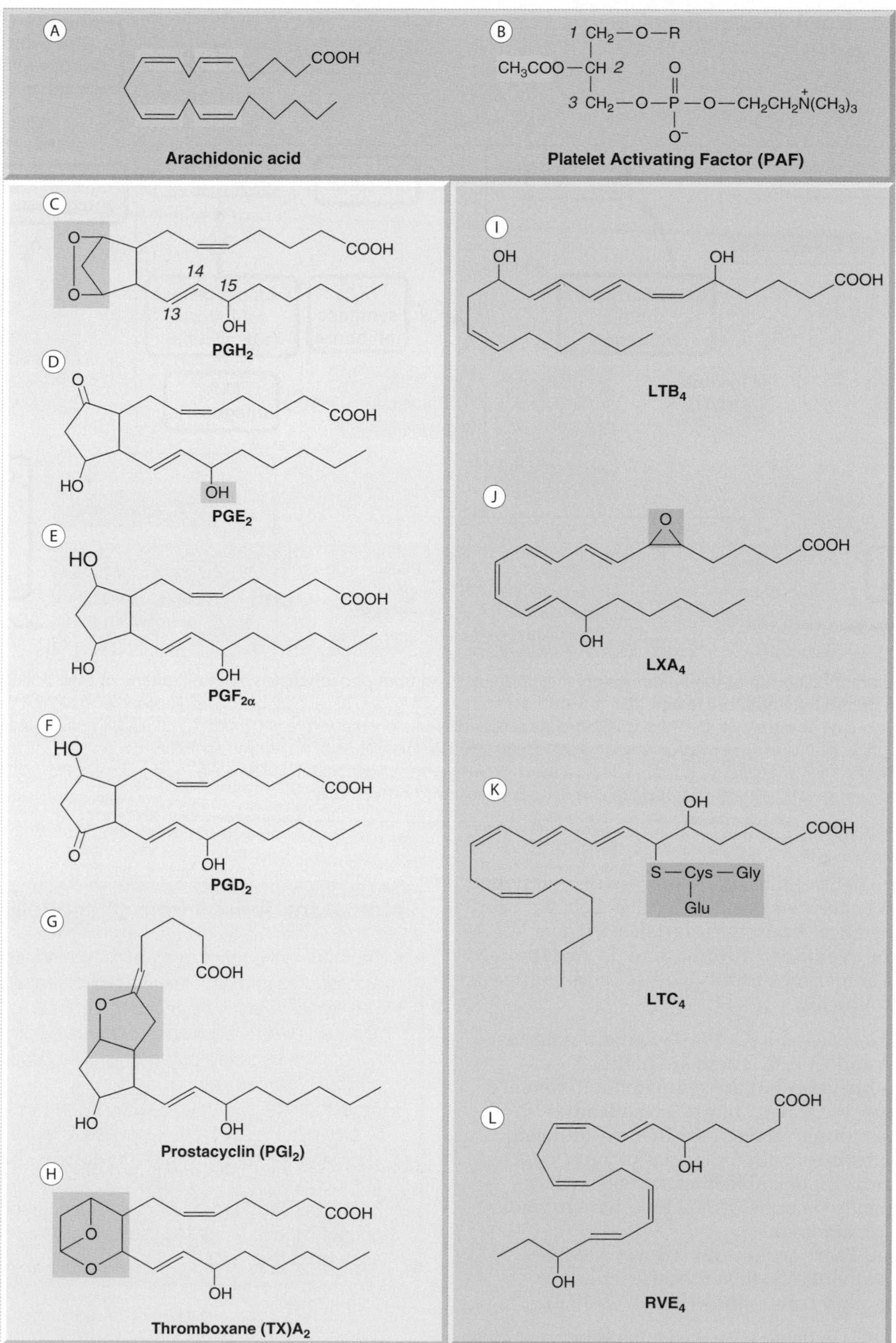

Fig. 17.2 Some key lipid mediators involved in the host defence response. (A) Arachidonic acid, an important precursor of prostanoids, leukotrienes and (some) lipoxins and resolvins. Note the conjugated double bonds *(in shaded box)*. (B) Platelet-activating factor (PAF): the location of the acetyl group at C2 is shown in the *shaded box*. R is a 6- or 8-carbon saturated fatty acid attached by an ether linkage to the carbon backbone. (C) Prostaglandin (PG)H_2, one of the labile intermediates in the synthesis of prostaglandins; note unstable ring structure *(in shaded box)* which can spontaneously hydrolyse in biological fluids if not enzymatically changed. (D) PGE_2, the 15-hydroxyl group *(in shaded box)* is crucial for the biological activity of prostaglandins and its removal is the first step in their inactivation. (E) and (F) $PGF_{2\alpha}$ and PGD_2. (G) Prostacyclin (PGI_2); note unstable ring structure (in shaded box). (H) Thromboxane (TX)A_2; note unstable oxane structure *(in shaded box)*. (I) Leukotriene (LT)B_4. (J) Lipoxin (LX)A_4; note unstable and highly reactive oxygen bridge structure *(in shaded box)*. (K) Leukotriene (LT)C_4; note conjugated glutathione moiety *(in shaded box)*. (L) Resolvin (RV)E_4.

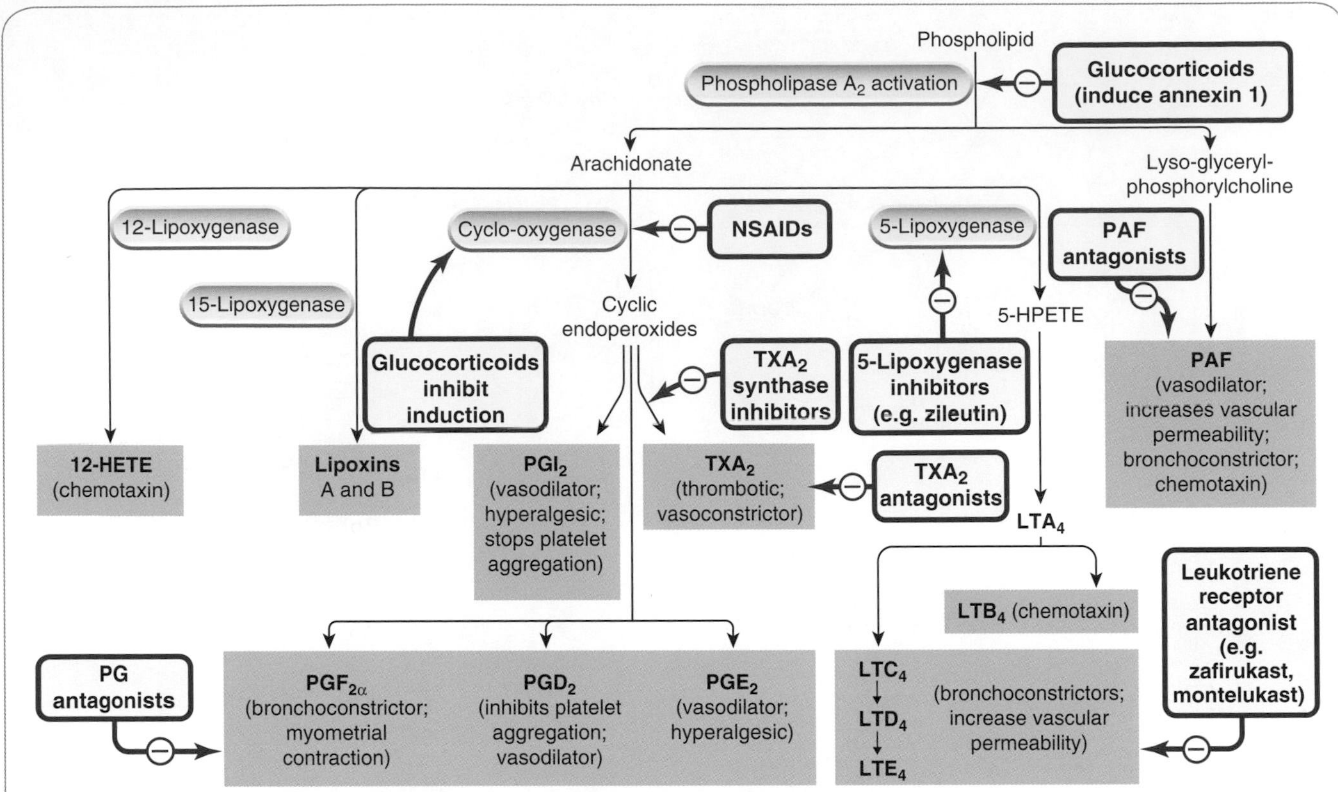

Fig. 17.3 Summary diagram of the inflammatory mediators derived from phospholipids, with an outline of their actions and the sites of action of anti-inflammatory drugs. Arachidonate metabolites are known as eicosanoids. The glucocorticoids inhibit transcription of the gene for cyclo-oxygenase (COX)-2, which is induced in cells by inflammatory mediators and induce and release annexin-A1 which down-regulates phospholipase A_2 activity, thereby limiting arachidonate release. The effects of prostaglandin (PG)E_2 depend on which of the four receptors it activates. *HETE,* Hydroxyeicosatetraenoic acid; *HPETE,* hydroperoxyeicosatetraenoic acid; *LT,* leukotriene; *NSAID,* non-steroidal anti-inflammatory drug; *PAF,* platelet-activating factor; *PGI_2,* prostacyclin; *TX,* thromboxane.

platelets, C5a on neutrophils, bradykinin on fibroblasts and antigen–antibody reactions on mast cells. Cellular injury (caused, for instance, by ischaemia) also triggers $cPLA_2$ activation. The free arachidonic acid is metabolised separately (or sometimes jointly) by several pathways, including the following.

- *Fatty acid cyclo-oxygenase* (COX). Two main isoforms exist, COX-1 and COX-2. These are highly homologous enzymes but are regulated in different and tissue-specific ways. They enzymatically combine arachidonic (and some other unsaturated fatty acid) substrates with molecular oxygen to form *cyclic endoperoxides*, unstable intermediates which can subsequently be transformed by other enzymes to different prostanoids.
- *Lipoxygenases.* There are several subtypes, which often work sequentially, to synthesise leukotrienes, lipoxins and other compounds (Figs 17.2–17.4).

Chapter 25 deals in detail with the way inhibitors of these pathways (including non-steroidal anti-inflammatory drugs (NSAIDs) and glucocorticoids) produce their anti-inflammatory effects.

We will look at the different classes of these lipid mediators separately.

Mediators derived from phospholipids

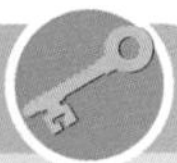

- The principal phospholipid-derived mediators are the eicosanoids (prostanoids and leukotrienes) and PAF.
- The eicosanoids are synthesised from arachidonic acid released directly from phospholipids by phospholipase A_2, or by a two-step process involving phospholipase C and diacylglycerol lipase.
- Arachidonate is metabolised by COX-1 or COX-2 to prostanoids, by 5-lipoxygenase to leukotrienes and, after further conversion, to lipoxins and other compounds.
- PAF is derived from phospholipid precursors by phospholipase A_2, giving rise to lyso-PAF, which is then acetylated to give PAF.

PROSTANOIDS

COX-1 is present in most cells as a constitutive enzyme. It produces prostanoids that act mainly as homeostatic regulators (e.g. modulating vascular responses, regulating gastric acid secretion). COX-2 is not normally present (at least in most tissues – CNS and renal tissue are important exceptions) but it is strongly induced by inflammatory stimuli and therefore generally believed to be more relevant as a target for anti-inflammatory drugs. Both enzymes catalyse the incorporation of two molecules of oxygen into two of the unsaturated double bonds in each arachidonate molecule, forming the highly unstable endoperoxides prostaglandin (PG)G_2 and PGH_2 (see Fig. 17.2). The suffix '2' indicates that the product contains only two double bonds. PGG_2 and PGH_2 are rapidly transformed in a tissue-specific manner by endoperoxide *isomerase* or *synthase* enzymes to PGE_2, PGI_2 (prostacyclin), PGD_2, $PGF_{2\alpha}$ and thromboxane (TX) A_2, which are the principal bioactive end products of this reaction. The mix of eicosanoids thus produced varies between cell types and their current activation state, depending on the particular endoperoxide isomerases or synthases present and active. In platelets, for example, TXA_2 predominates, whereas in vascular endothelium PGI_2 is the main product. Macrophages, neutrophils and mast cells synthesise a mixture of products upon stimulation. If *eicosatrienoic acid* (three double bonds) rather than arachidonic acid is the substrate for these enzymes, the resulting prostanoids have only a single double bond, for example PGE_1, while *eicosapentaenoic acid (EPA)*, which contains five double bonds, yields PGE_3. EPA, like other ω-3 PUFAs (including *docosahexaenoic acid, DHA*), is abundant in diets rich in oily fish and may, if present in sufficient amounts, represent a significant fraction of cellular fatty acids and thus constitute the major source of precursors for the COX enzyme. When this occurs, the production of the (broadly) pro-inflammatory PGE_2 and, more significantly, the generation of TXA_2 are diminished. This may partly underlie the beneficial anti-inflammatory, metabolic and cardiovascular actions that are ascribed to diets rich in this type of marine product (see also Resolvins, later, Natto et al., 2019, and Khan et al., 2021).

Another family of related compounds with a wide range of interesting biological activities has also been discovered, the *cyclopentenone prostanoids*. We do not cover these here but interested readers may refer to Lee et al. (2021) for a detailed account.

The endocannabinoid *anandamide* (see Ch. 18) is an ethanolamine derivative of arachidonic acid and, surprisingly, it can also be oxidised by COX-2 to form a range of *prostamides*. These substances are of increasing interest. They act at prostanoid receptors but often exhibit a unique pharmacology (see Urquhart et al., 2015).

CATABOLISM OF THE PROSTANOIDS

This is a multi-step process. After carrier-mediated uptake, most prostaglandins are rapidly inactivated by prostaglandin *dehydrogenase* and *reductase* enzymes. These enzymes oxidise the 15-hydroxyl group (see Fig. 17.2) and the 13–14 double bond, both of which are important for biological activity. The inactive products are further degraded by general fatty acid–oxidising enzymes and excreted in the urine. These dehydrogenase enzymes are present in high concentration in the lung, and 95% of infused PGE_2, PGE_1 or $PGF_{2\alpha}$ is inactivated after a single passage through the lungs, meaning that little normally reaches the arterial circulation and for this reason the half-life of most prostaglandins in the circulation is less than 1 minute.

TXA_2 and PGI_2 are slightly different. Both are inherently unstable and decay rapidly and spontaneously (within 30 s and 5 min, respectively) in biological fluids into inactive TXB_2 and 6-keto-$PGF_{1\alpha}$, respectively. Further metabolism then occurs, but this is less relevant to us here.

PROSTANOID RECEPTORS

There are five main classes of prostanoid receptor (see Woodward et al., 2011, and Biringer 2021), all of which are GPCRs (Table 17.1). Depending on whether their ligands are PGD, PGF, PGI, PGE or TXA species, they are termed DP, FP, IP, EP and TP receptors respectively. Some have further subtypes; for example, there are four EP receptors. Polymorphisms and other variants of these enzymes have been implicated in the pathogenesis of various diseases (see Cornejo-Garcia et al., 2016).

ACTIONS OF THE PROSTANOIDS

The prostanoids can affect most tissues and exert a bewildering variety of site- and context-dependent biological effects.

- PGD_2 causes vasodilatation in many vascular beds, inhibition of platelet aggregation, relaxation of gastrointestinal and uterine muscle and modification of release of hypothalamic/pituitary hormones. It has a bronchoconstrictor effect through a secondary action on TP receptors. It may also activate chemoattractant receptors on some leukocytes.
- $PGF_{2\alpha}$ causes uterine contraction in humans (see Ch. 35), luteolysis in some species (e.g. cattle) and bronchoconstriction in others (e.g. cats and dogs).
- PGI_2 causes vasodilatation and inhibits platelet aggregation (see Ch. 23), renin release and natriuresis through effects on tubular reabsorption of Na^+.
- TXA_2 causes vasoconstriction, platelet aggregation and bronchoconstriction (more marked in guinea pig than in humans).
- PGE_2, the predominant 'inflammatory' prostanoid has the following actions:
  - *at EP_1 receptors*, it causes contraction of bronchial, gastrointestinal and uterine smooth muscle;
  - *at EP_2 receptors*, it causes bronchodilatation, vasodilatation, stimulation of intestinal fluid secretion and relaxation of gastrointestinal smooth muscle;
  - *at EP_3 receptors*, it causes contraction of intestinal smooth muscle, inhibition of gastric acid (see Ch. 30) with increased mucus secretion, inhibition of lipolysis, inhibition of autonomic neurotransmitter release and contraction of the pregnant human uterus (see Ch. 35);
  - *at EP_4 receptors*, it causes similar effects to those of EP_2 stimulation (they were originally thought to be a single receptor). Vascular relaxation is one consequence of receptor activation, as is cervical 'ripening'. Some inhibitory effects of PGE_2 on leukocyte activation and function are probably mediated either through this receptor or EP_2.

Several clinically useful drugs act at prostanoid receptors. These include the EP agonists **misoprostol** (EP_2/EP_3), that suppresses gastric acid secretion and also acts as a potent uterine stimulant, and **dinoprostone** which aids cervical ripening and can induce labour (including via the vaginal route); the FP agonists **bimatoprost**,[4] **latanoprost, tafluprost** and **travoprost** which are used for the treatment of glaucoma (see Ch. 27); and **iloprost** and **epoprostenol** which are IP agonists used for the treatment of pulmonary hypertension (see Ch. 21). Misoprostol is also used in both medical abortion and treating postpartum bleeding in women.

Clinical uses of prostanoids

- Gynaecological and obstetric (see Ch. 35):
  - termination of pregnancy: **gemeprost** or **misoprostol** (a metabolically stable prostaglandin [PG]E analogue)
  - induction of labour: **dinoprostone** or **misoprostol**
  - postpartum haemorrhage: **carboprost.**
- Gastrointestinal:
  - to prevent ulcers associated with NSAID use: **misoprostol** (see Ch. 30).
- Cardiovascular:
  - to maintain the patency of the ductus arteriosus until surgical correction of the defect in babies with certain congenital heart malformations: **alprostadil** (PGE_1);
  - to inhibit platelet aggregation (e.g. during haemodialysis): **epoprostenol** (PGI_2), especially if **heparin** is contraindicated;
  - primary pulmonary hypertension: **epoprostenol** or **treprostinil** (PGI_2) (see Ch. 21).
- Ophthalmic:
  - open-angle glaucoma: **latanoprost** eye drops (see Ch. 27).

THE ROLE OF PROSTANOIDS IN INFLAMMATION

The inflammatory response is inevitably accompanied by the release of prostanoids. PGE_2 predominates, although PGI_2 is also important. In areas of acute inflammation, PGE_2 and PGI_2 are generated by the local tissues and blood vessels, while mast cells release mainly PGD_2. In chronic inflammation, cells of the monocyte/macrophage series also release PGE_2 and TXA_2. Together, the prostanoids exert a sort of yin-yang effect in inflammation, stimulating some responses and decreasing others. Their effects are pleiotropic and context dependent and defy simple classification. For a more thorough coverage see Dennis and Norris (2015). The most striking effects are as follows:-

- PGE_2, PGI_2 and PGD_2 are themselves powerful vasodilators but they also synergise with other inflammatory vasodilators, such as histamine and bradykinin. It is this combined dilator action on precapillary arterioles that contributes to the redness and increased blood flow in areas of acute inflammation. Prostanoids do not directly increase the permeability of the postcapillary venules but potentiate the effects on vascular leakage caused by histamine and bradykinin. Similarly, they do not themselves produce pain, but sensitise afferent C fibres (see Ch. 42) to the effects of bradykinin and other noxious stimuli. The anti-inflammatory and analgesic effects of NSAIDs stem largely from their ability to block these actions.
- Prostaglandins of the E series are also pyrogenic (i.e. they induce fever). High concentrations are found in cerebrospinal fluid during infection, and the increase in temperature (attributed to cytokines) is actually mediated by the release of PGE_2. NSAIDs exert antipyretic actions by inhibiting PGE_2 synthesis in the hypothalamus.
- Some prostaglandins have anti-inflammatory effects which are important during the resolution phase of inflammation. For example, PGE_2 decreases lysosomal enzyme release and the generation of toxic oxygen metabolites from neutrophils, as well as the release of histamine from mast cells.

As in the case of all inflammatory mediators, eicosanoids possess the intrinsic potential to be harmful to the host if their synthesis or release is dysregulated. For those interested in such 'collateral damage' mechanisms see Chapter 7 as well as articles by Theken and FitzGerald (2021) and Hammock et al. (2020) which exemplify this in the context of COVID-19.

Prostanoids

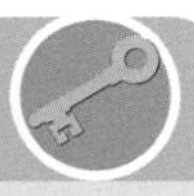

- The term *prostanoids* encompass prostaglandins and thromboxanes.
- Cyclo-oxygenases (COX) oxidise arachidonate, producing the unstable intermediates PGG_2 and PGH_2. These are enzymatically transformed to the different prostanoid species.
- There are two main COX isoforms: COX-1, a constitutive enzyme, and COX-2, which is often induced by inflammatory stimuli.
- The principal prostanoids are:
  - PGI_2 (prostacyclin), predominantly from vascular endothelium, acts on IP receptors, producing vasodilatation and inhibition of platelet aggregation.
  - Thromboxane $(TX)A_2$, predominantly from platelets, acts on TP receptors, causing platelet aggregation and vasoconstriction.
  - PGE_2 is an important mediator of inflammatory responses and also causes fever and pain.
- Other effects of PGE_2 include:
  - at EP_1 receptors: contraction of bronchial, gastrointestinal (GI) tract and uterine smooth muscle;
  - at EP_2 receptors: relaxation of bronchial, vascular and GI tract smooth muscle;

[4]Women being treated with **bimatoprost** eye drops for glaucoma were delighted with a side effect of this drug – stimulation of eyelash growth. It wasn't long before a thriving 'off-label' market had been established for its use in beauty spas. Eventually, the FDA gave in to popular lobbying and licensed a preparation specifically for this cosmetic indication.

Prostanoids—cont'd

- at EP_3 receptors: inhibition of gastric acid secretion, increased gastric mucus secretion, contraction of pregnant uterus and of gastrointestinal smooth muscle, inhibition of lipolysis and of autonomic neurotransmitter release.
- at EP_4 receptors: similar to EP_2. May mediate some inhibitory or regulatory effects on the immune response.

- $PGF_{2\alpha}$ acts on FP receptors, found in uterine (and other) smooth muscle, and corpus luteum, producing contraction of the uterus and luteolysis (in some species).
- PGD_2 is abundant in activated mast cells. It acts on DP receptors, causing vasodilatation and inhibition of platelet aggregation.

LEUKOTRIENES

Leukotrienes (*leuko-* because they are released by white cells, and *-trienes* because they contain a conjugated triene system of double bonds; see Fig. 17.2) comprise two main categories, chemoattractant (LTB_4) and cysteinyl (or *sufidopeptide*) leukotrienes (LTC_4, D_4, E_4 and F_4). Both types are synthesised from arachidonic acid by lipoxygenases. These soluble cytosolic enzymes are mainly found in lung, platelets, mast cells and white blood cells. The principal enzyme of interest is *5-lipoxygenase*. On cell activation, this enzyme translocates to the nuclear membrane, where it associates with a crucial accessory protein, affectionately termed FLAP (Five-Lipoxygenase Activating Protein). The activated 5-lipoxygenase incorporates a hydroperoxy group at C5 in arachidonic acid to form *5-hydroperoxytetraenoic acid* (5-HPETE, see Fig. 17.4), which is further converted to the unstable leukotriene (LT)A_4. This may be converted enzymatically to LTB_4 or, utilising a separate pathway involving conjugation with glutathione, to the cysteinyl-containing leukotrienes LTC_4, LTD_4, LTE_4 and LTF_4. These cysteinyl leukotrienes are produced mainly by eosinophils, mast cells, basophils and macrophages. Mixtures of these substances constitute the biological activity historically ascribed to *slow-reacting substance of anaphylaxis* (SRS-A), an elusive bronchoconstrictor factor shown many years ago to be generated in guinea pig lung during anaphylaxis, and consequently predicted to be important in asthma.

LTB_4 is produced mainly by neutrophils. Lipoxins and other active products, some of which have anti-inflammatory properties, are also produced from arachidonate by this pathway.

LTB_4 is metabolised by a unique membrane-bound cytochrome P450 enzyme in neutrophils, and then further oxidised to 20-carboxy-LTB_4. LTC_4 and LTD_4 are metabolised to LTE_4, which is excreted in the urine.

LEUKOTRIENE RECEPTORS

Leukotriene receptors are all GPCRs. They are termed *BLT* (two subtypes) if the ligand is LTB_4, and *CysLT* (two subtypes) for the cysteinyl leukotrienes (see Table 17.1).

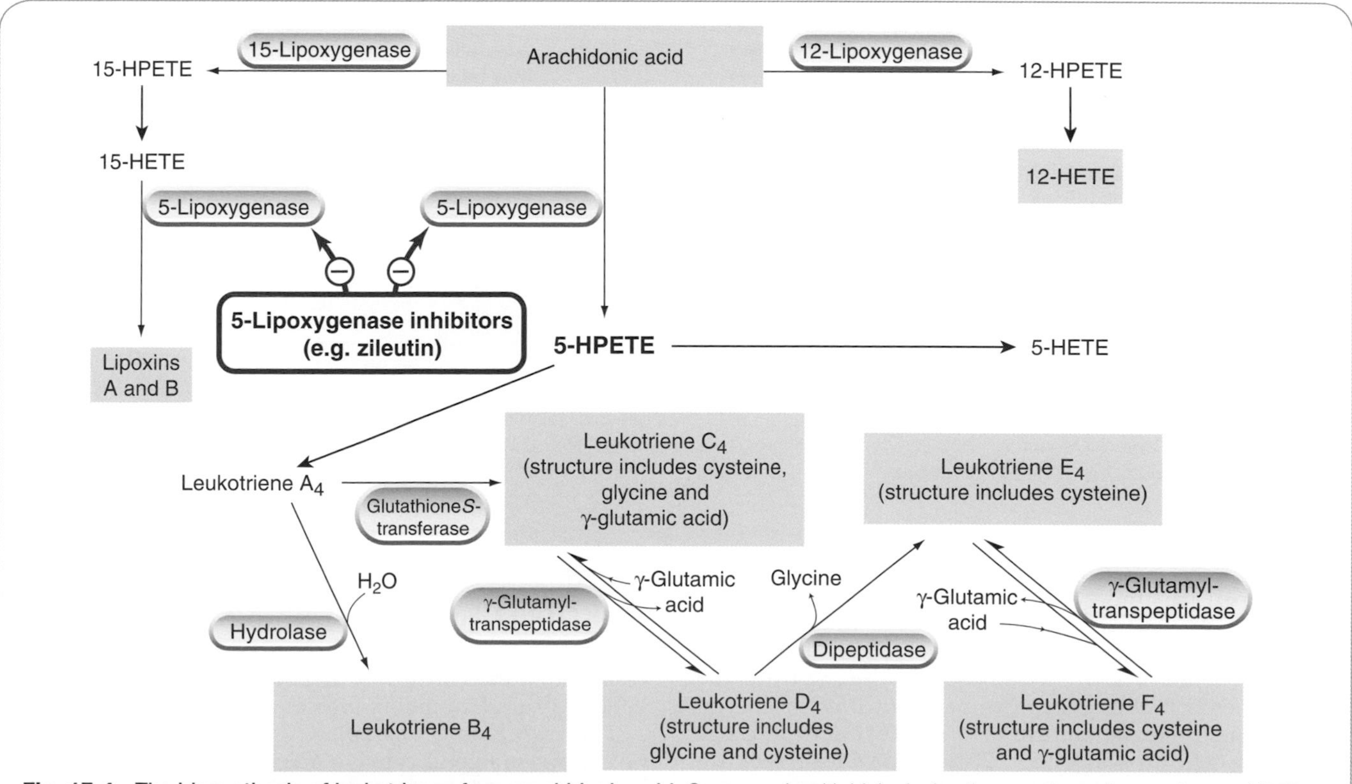

Fig. 17.4 The biosynthesis of leukotrienes from arachidonic acid. Compounds with biological action are shown in *grey boxes*. *HETE*, Hydroxyeicosatetraenoic acid; *HPETE*, hydroperoxyeicosatetraenoic acid.

Table 17.1 A simplified scheme of prostanoid and leukotriene receptor classification based upon their physiological effects

Receptor	Physiological ligands	Distribution	General physiological effects	Signalling system
IP	$PGI_2 \gg PGD_2$	Abundant in cardiovascular system, platelets, neurons and elsewhere	Generally inhibitory: e.g. smooth muscle relaxation, anti-inflammatory and anti-aggregatory effects	G_S ↑cAMP
DP_1	$PGD_2 \gg PGE_2$	Low abundance; vascular smooth muscle, platelets, CNS, airways, the eye		
EP_2	$PGE_2 > PGF_{2\alpha}$	Widespread distribution		
EP_4	$PGE_2 > PGF_{2\alpha}$	Widespread distribution		
TP	$TxA_2 = H_2 > D_2$	Abundant in cardiovascular system, platelets and immune cells. Two subtypes known with opposing actions	Generally excitatory: e.g. smooth muscle contraction, pro-inflammatory and platelet aggregatory actions	G_q/G_{11} [PLC][a] ↑Ca^{2+}
FP	$PGF_{2\alpha} > PGD_2$	Very high expression in female reproductive organs		
EP_1	$PGE_2 > PGF_{2\alpha}$	Myometrium, intestine and lung		
EP_3	$PGE_2 > PGF_{2\alpha}$	Widespread distribution throughout body; many isoforms with different G protein coupling	Generally inhibitory: e.g. smooth muscle relaxation, anti-inflammatory and anti-aggregatory effects	G_i/G_o ↓cAMP
DP_2	$PGD_2 > PGF_{2\alpha}$	Different structure to other prostanoid receptors. Widely distributed especially in immune cells		
BLT_1	LTB_4 > 20 hydroxy LTB_4	Widely distributed in leukocytes and in some endothelial cells	'High-affinity' LTB_4 receptor. Activates leukocytes and stimulates chemotaxis	G_i/G_0↓ cAMP G_q/G_{11} ↑PLC
BLT_2	LTB_4 > 20 hydroxy LTB_4	Several tissues intestine, skin and some lesions	'Low-affinity' LTB_4 receptor. May be important in GI barrier formation and airway inflammation	G_i/Gq↓ cAMP
$CysLT_1$	$LTD_4 > LTC_4 > LTE_4$	Several tissues including leukocytes, mast cells, lung, intestinal and vascular tissue	Bronchoconstriction and leukocyte activation	G_q/G_{11} ↑PLC
$CysLT_2$	$LTC_4 > LTD_4 > LTE_4$	Several tissues including leukocytes, mast cells, nasal mucosa and vascular tissue	PMN activation, inflammation, contracts some vascular smooth muscle	G_q/G_{11} ↑PLC

[a]PLC may not be involved in EP_1 signalling.
PLC, Phospholiapse C; *PMN,* polymorphonuclear leukocyte.
Data derived from Woodward, D.F., Jones, R.L., Narumiya, S., 2011. International Union of Basic and Clinical Pharmacology. LXXXIII: classification of prostanoid receptors, updating 15 years of progress. Pharmacol. Rev. 63, 471–538, and IUPHAR/BPS. Guide to Pharmacology. www.guidetopharmacology.org/.

They are all of the G_q/G_{11} family which activate PLC signalling mechanisms, although there may be other receptors that also respond to these potent mediators. Genetic variations in the enzymes that synthesise leukotrienes or in their receptors may contribute to allergy and asthma, or to the failure of drug treatment in those disorders (Thompson et al., 2016). For those seeking further information, they have been the subject of recent review by Biringer (2022).

LEUKOTRIENE ACTIONS

Cysteinyl leukotrienes have important actions on the respiratory and cardiovascular systems, as well as a more general proinflammatory effect.

The respiratory system. Cysteinyl leukotrienes are potent spasmogens, causing a dose-related contraction of human bronchiolar muscle in vitro. LTE_4 is less potent than LTC_4 and LTD_4, but its effect is much longer lasting.

All cause an increase in mucus secretion. Given by aerosol to human volunteers, they reduce specific airway conductance and maximum expiratory flow rate, the effect being more protracted than that produced by histamine (Fig. 17.5).

The cysteinyl leukotrienes are present in the sputum of chronic bronchitis patients in amounts that are biologically active. On antigen challenge, they are released from samples of human asthmatic lung in vitro, and into nasal lavage fluid in subjects with allergic rhinitis. There is evidence that they contribute to the underlying bronchial hyper-reactivity in asthmatics, and it is thought that they are among the main mediators of both the early and late phases of asthma. Yokomizo et al. (2018) have reviewed the role of these mediators as therapeutic targets.

It is therefore not surprising that CysLT-receptor antagonists such as **zafirlukast** and **montelukast** are used in the treatment of asthma and allergic rhinitis, often in conjunction with a corticosteroid. Cysteinyl leukotrienes may mediate the cardiovascular changes of acute anaphylaxis. Agents that inhibit 5-lipoxygenase are therefore obvious candidates for antiasthmatic and anti-inflammatory agents. One such drug, **zileuton**, is available in some parts of the world for the treatment of asthma.

The cardiovascular system. Small amounts of LTC_4 or LTD_4 given intravenously cause a rapid, short-lived fall in blood pressure, and significant constriction of small coronary resistance vessels. Given subcutaneously, they are equipotent with histamine in causing weal and flare. Given topically in the nose, LTD_4 increases nasal blood flow and local vascular permeability.

The role of leukotrienes in inflammation. LTB_4 is a potent chemotactic agent for neutrophils and macrophages via the BLT_1 receptor (see Ch. 7). It up-regulates membrane adhesion molecule expression on neutrophils and increases the production of superoxide anions and the release of granule enzymes. On macrophages and lymphocytes, it stimulates proliferation and cytokine release. It is found in inflammatory exudates and tissues in many inflammatory conditions, including rheumatoid arthritis, psoriasis and ulcerative colitis. BLT_1 is additionally expressed on vascular smooth muscle cells linking LTB_4 to atherogenesis and vascular injury.

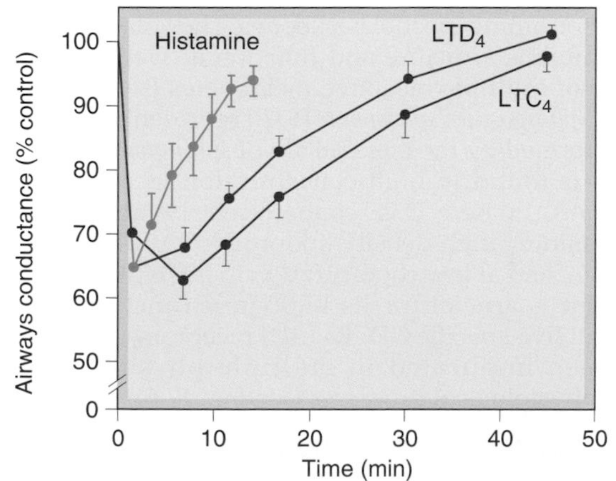

Fig. 17.5 The time course of action on specific airways conductance of the cysteinyl leukotrienes and histamine, in six normal subjects. Specific airways conductance was measured in a constant volume whole-body plethysmograph, and the drugs were given by inhalation. (From Barnes, N.C., Piper, P.J., Costello, J.F., 1984. Comparative effects of inhaled leukotriene C_4, leukotriene D_4, and histamine in normal human subjects. Thorax 39, 500–504.)

Leukotrienes

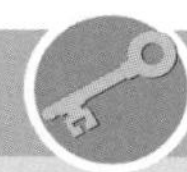

- 5-Lipoxygenase oxidises arachidonate to give 5-hydroperoxyeicosatetraenoic acid (5-HPETE), which is converted to leukotriene (LT)A_4. This, in turn, can be converted to either LTB_4 or to a series of glutathione adducts, the cysteinyl leukotrienes LTC_4, LTD_4 and LTE_4.
- LTB_4, acting on specific receptors, causes adherence, chemotaxis and activation of polymorphs and monocytes, and stimulates proliferation and cytokine production from macrophages and lymphocytes.
- The cysteinyl leukotrienes cause:
  - contraction of bronchial muscle
  - vasodilatation in most vessels, but coronary vasoconstriction
- LTB_4 is an important mediator in all types of inflammation; the cysteinyl leukotrienes are of importance in asthma and allergic rhinitis.

OTHER IMPORTANT FATTY ACID DERIVATIVES

In addition to the prostanoids and leukotrienes, PUFAs such as arachidonic acid, EPA and DHA can also be enzymatically transformed into other important lipid mediators. Trihydroxy arachidonate metabolites termed *lipoxins* (see Figs 17.2 and 17.4) are formed by the concerted action of the 5- and the 12- or 15-lipoxygenase enzymes during inflammation. Lipoxins (abbreviation Lx) act on polymorphonuclear leukocytes, through GPCRs such as ALX, also known as *formyl peptide receptor 2* (FPR2), which is also targeted by other anti-inflammatory factors such as annexin-A1 (Anx-A1) and resolvins (see later), to oppose the action of pro-inflammatory stimuli, providing what might be called 'stop signals' to halt inflammation and promote its resolution (see Jaen et al., 2021). Aspirin may generate lipoxins via an alternate biosynthetic route because COX-2 can still produce hydroxy fatty acids even when inhibited by aspirin and thus unable to synthesise prostaglandins. The formation of these aspirin-triggered or 15-epi-lipoxins via acetylation probably contributes to aspirin's anti-inflammatory effects, some of which are not completely explained through inhibition of prostaglandin generation (see Romano et al., 2015; Serhan et al., 2014).

Resolvins (abbreviation Rv) represent one member of a broader family of specialised pro-resolving mediators, often referred to as SPM. As the name implies, they are a series of compounds that fulfil a similar function to lipoxins, but unlike lipoxins, their precursor fatty acid is EPA (RvE_{1-4}) or DHA acid (RvD_{1-4}). As aforementioned, fish oils are rich in these fatty acids and it is likely that at least some of their claimed multifaceted anti-inflammatory benefit is produced through conversion to these highly active species (see Zhang and Spite, 2012, for a review of this fascinating area). RvD_1 acts through the ALX/FPR2 and GPR32 receptor systems, whereas RvE_1 acts through a GPCR called *chemerin receptor 23 (ChemR23)* to lower cAMP and release intracellular calcium. Resolvins can counteract inflammatory pain (see Oehler et al., 2017) and analogues are undergoing trials for the treatment of a variety of inflammatory conditions (Serhan and Levy, 2018). *Maresins* (abbreviation Ma) and *protectins* are dihydroxy acids generated from DHA by the actions of lipoxygenases. Maresins are predominately synthesised by macrophages and have a role in inflammatory resolution. Protectins (abbreviation P) are produced by lymphocytes and probably act to modulate the operation of the immune system among other functions. The area, which can be confusing until you come to terms with lipid structures, has been well reviewed by Sansbury and Spite (2016), Serhan and Levy (2018) and Serhan et al. (2015).

PLATELET-ACTIVATING FACTOR

Platelet-activating factor (PAF), also variously termed *PAF-acether* and *AGEPC* (acetyl-glyceryl-ether-phosphorylcholine), is a biologically active lipid that can produce effects at astonishingly low concentrations (less than 10^{-10} mol/L) through its GPCR (G_q/G_{11}; stimulates cAMP production). Although accurate since the original observation was that it was released from basophils and caused platelets to aggregate, the name 'PAF' is somewhat misleading because it acts on many different target cells and, in particular, is believed to be an important mediator in both acute and chronic allergic and inflammatory phenomena.

BIOSYNTHESIS

PAF (see Fig. 17.2) is produced by platelets in response to thrombin, and also by activated inflammatory cells. It is enzymatically synthesised from phospholipids which have an ether-linked hexadecyl or octadecyl fatty acid at C1, an unsaturated fatty acid such as arachidonic acid ester-linked at C2 and a phosphoryl choline base at C3. The action of PLA_2 removes the arachidonic acid yielding *lyso-PAF*, which is then acetylated by an *acetyltransferase* to yield the biologically active PAF. The reaction is reversible and PAF, in turn, can be inactivated by an *acetylhydrolase* yielding lyso-PAF ready for recycling. Of note, the PAF receptor is itself a potent stimulator for further PAF synthesis (indicating a feed-forward system) and PAF receptor agonists can be formed non-enzymatically by the action of free radicals on *glycerophosphocholines* (see Lordan et al., 2019).

ACTIONS AND ROLE IN INFLAMMATION

PAF can reproduce many of the signs and symptoms of inflammation. Injected locally, it produces vasodilatation (and thus erythema), increased vascular permeability and weal formation. Higher doses produce hyperalgesia. It is a potent chemoattractant for neutrophils and monocytes, and recruits eosinophils into the bronchial mucosa in the late phase of asthma (see Ch. 28). PAF also contracts both bronchial and ileal smooth muscle.

Acting predominantly in an autocrine or juxtacrine manner through its receptor, PAF activates $cPLA_2$ and stimulates arachidonate turnover in many cells. In platelets it increases TXA_2 generation, producing a shape change and the release of the granule contents. This is important in haemostasis and thrombosis (see Ch. 23).

Pathophysiologically, while elevated PAF concentrations are noted in multiple disease states, it seems directly responsible for none. Correspondingly, while several PAF antagonists (e.g. **lexipafant** and **modipafant**) exist they have not found a clear clinical niche. **Rupatadine** is a combined H_1 and PAF antagonist that is available in some parts of the world for treating allergic symptoms, but it is not clear what (if anything) its anti-PAF action adds clinically to its effect. Of note, however, the anti-inflammatory actions of the glucocorticoids may be caused, at least in part, by inhibition of PAF synthesis and it may be that competitive antagonists of PAF and/or specific inhibitors of *lyso-PAF acetyltransferase* could yet become useful modulators of inflammation (Travers et al., 2021).

Platelet-activating factor (PAF)

- PAF precursors are released from activated inflammatory cells by phospholipase A_2. After acetylation, the resultant PAF is released and acts on specific receptors in target cells.
- Pharmacological actions include vasodilatation, increased vascular permeability, chemotaxis and activation of leukocytes (especially eosinophils), activation and aggregation of platelets, and smooth muscle contraction.
- PAF is implicated in multiple inflammatory diseases but directly responsible for none.

SPHINGOSINE 1-PHOSPHATE

Sphingolipids (and the related *glycosphingolipids* and *galactosphingolipids*) are a class of lipids defined by their 18-carbon amino-alcohol backbones. They play crucial roles in membrane structure and function as well as being the source of multiple bioactive metabolites (see Gault et al., 2010). *Sphingosine 1-phosphate (S1P)* represents one of these, being formed by the metabolism of *sphingomyelin*.

S1P is found in high concentration in plasma (~0.75 nmol/mL), where it is 'chaperoned' by apolipoprotein M-containing high-density lipoprotein ($ApoM^+$ HDL) and albumin, and at low concentration in interstitial fluid. This gradient is crucial for its biological function. S1P acts through five specific GPCRs (S1P $receptors_{1-5}$; S1PRs) and has been implicated in multiple physiological and pathophysiological processes (see Fig. 17.6).

BIOSYNTHESIS AND METABOLISM

Sphingomyelinase initially generates *ceramide* from sphingomyelin which is further processed to *sphingosine* by *ceramidase*. The action of *sphingosine kinase (Sphk) isoenzymes* on this substrate results in the generation of S1P.

S1P is actively exported from cells by specific transporters (for instance *spinster 2* – don't ask!) which, supported by Sphk1 secretion to permit extracellular S1P synthesis, results in the aforementioned plasma-tissue gradient. Intracellular S1P concentrations are additionally regulated via the

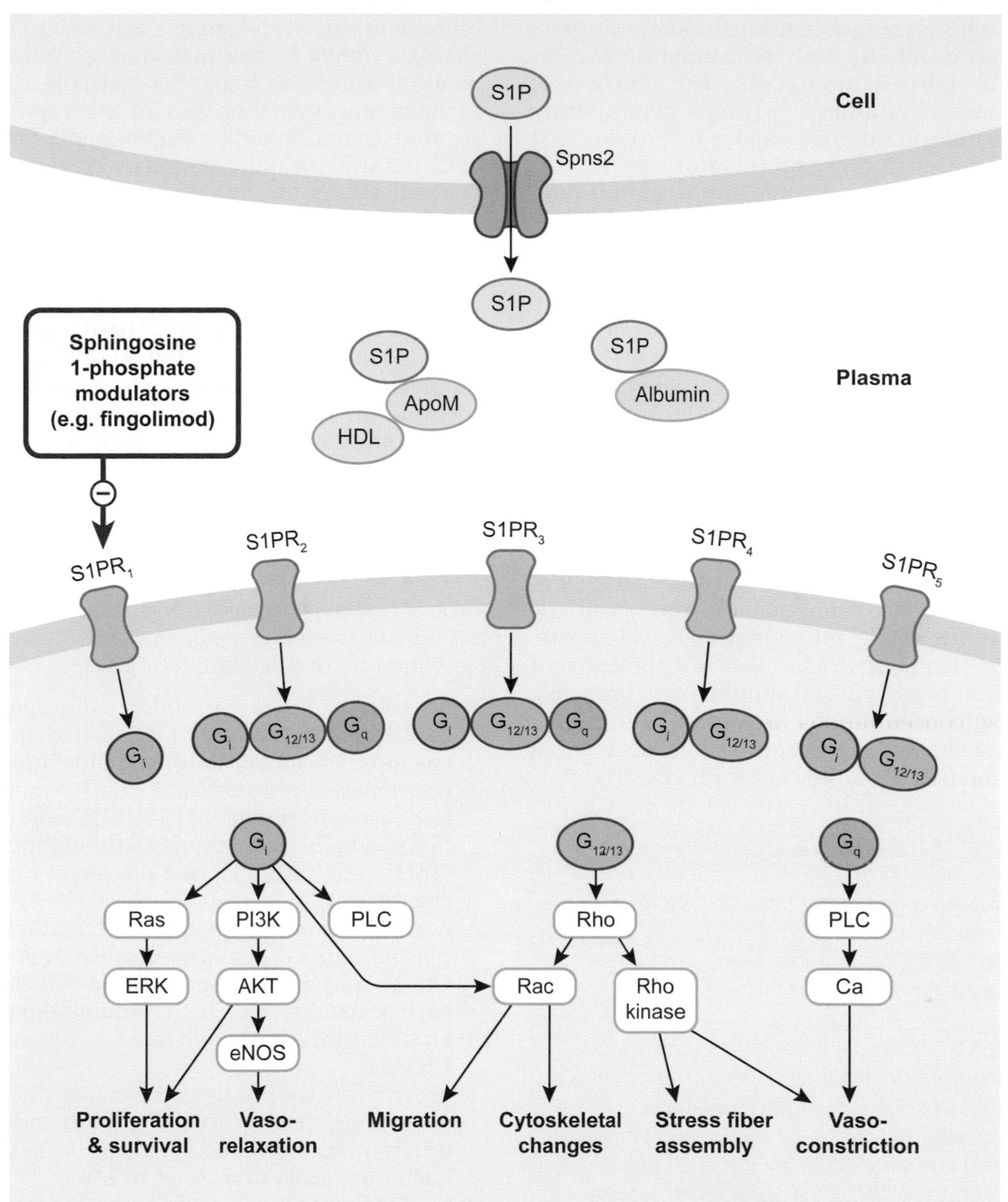

Fig. 17.6 Summary of sphingosine 1-phosphate (S1P) secretion, its cognate receptors (S1P receptors ($S1PR_{1–5}$)) and signalling pathways. S1P is produced intracellularly prior to export into the extracellular space via dedicated transporters (e.g. Spns2; Spinster-2) where it is bound by chaperones including albumin and apolipoprotein M-containing high-density lipoprotein ($ApoM^+$ HDL). While acting on five separate GPCRs, S1P's binding to $S1PR_1$ and effect on chemotaxis have received the greatest attention to date. The S1PR modulators bind this receptor on lymphocytes leading to its internalisation and loss of response to the gradient that drives egress from lymph nodes. *AKT,* Protein kinase B; *eNOS,* endothelial nitric oxide synthase; *ERK,* extracellular signal-regulated kinase; *PI3K,* phosphoinositide-3-kinase; *PLC,* phospholipase C (Based on Mendelson, K., Evans, T. & Hla, T. 2014. Sphingosine 1-phosphate signalling. Development. 141, 5–9.)

degradative *S1P phosphatases* and *S1P lyase*. *Lysophospholipid phosphatase* 3 acts on unbound extracellular SP1, converting it into sphingosine, which may then be taken up again by cells for further metabolism (Mendelson et al., 2014).

RECEPTORS AND ACTIONS

S1PRs are widely distributed cell-surface receptors. S1PR ($G_{i/o}$-coupled), the most studied and therapeutically important receptor, is found predominantly in the CNS, heart and vasculature, lung, kidney, liver and – significantly – primary and secondary lymphoid tissue including the thymus. $S1PR_{2–5}$ are found in many of the same tissues, but have more limited distribution. Signalling through S1PRs has been shown to play a key role in embryogenesis (notably neurogenesis and angiogenesis as well as pancreas and limb development), endothelial and blood–brain barrier function and the control of smooth muscle tone, both vascular and bronchial. It is however their role in mediating lymphocyte cell-trafficking and activation that is, to date, their most clinically relevant function.

$S1PR_1$ signalling mediates responsiveness to the chemotactic gradient between secondary lymphoid tissues and the efferent lymphatics such that, when its function is blocked, lymphocytes (especially naïve and

CCR7-expressing central memory T-cells) are sequestered in the lymph nodes. Antagonism additionally impairs B-cell trafficking, dendritic cell recruitment, vascular permeability and both mast cell and eosinophil degranulation and chemotaxis. $S1PR_{2-5}$ demonstrate overlapping but unique functions again broadly related to immune modulation and neural function.

S1PR modulators including **fingolimod**, **siponimod**, **ozanimod**, and **ponesimod** are consequently immunosuppressants that have found clinical utility in the treatment of multiple sclerosis (see Ch. 40). Principally exerting their action via $S1PR_1$ (but demonstrating variable selectivity for the other S1PRs which likely dictates their side effect profile), these agents are thought to exert their effect by reducing the number of circulating lymphocytes via preventing their egress from lymph nodes. They also appear to increase the proportion of T-reg (see Ch. 7) and naïve B cells, dampening inflammation. Secondary effects on the CNS including blood–brain barrier stabilisation, reduction in astrogliosis, axonal loss and demyelination may also contribute. S1PR modulators have additionally been trialled as immunosuppressants for the treatment of renal transplant, stroke, neuromuscular disorders, psoriasis and autoimmune disease (e.g. inflammatory bowel disease, systemic lupus erythematous), as well as in asthma (based on S1PR's effect on mast cells, eosinophils and bronchial muscle tone). Results have been mixed and their use limited by side effects; however, several promising avenues warrant further exploration (see McGinley and Cohen, 2021).

Sphingosine-1 phosphate (S1P)

- S1P is a sphingolipid generated from sphingomyelin via several enzymatically catalysed steps. It is actively secreted to ensure a higher gradient in blood than in tissues, thus forming a chemotactic gradient for leukocytes.
- There are five S1P receptors (S1PR) with wide-ranging expression and both developmental and physiological roles. The actions of $S1PR_1$ include regulation of lymphocyte egress from secondary lymphatic organs, chemotaxis and activation of leukocytes (including dendritic cells and eosinophils), vascular permeability and smooth muscle tone as well as maintaining CNS integrity.
- S1PR modulators are immunosuppressants and have established clinical utility in the treatment of multiple sclerosis.

PROTEIN AND PEPTIDE MEDIATORS

GENERAL PRINCIPLES

STRUCTURE

Peptide and protein mediators generally vary from 3 to about 200 amino acid residues in length, the arbitrary dividing line between peptides and proteins being about 50 residues. An important difference is that proteins need to adopt a complex folded structure to exert their specific function, whereas short peptides are, in most cases, flexible. Specific residues in proteins and peptides often undergo post-translational modifications, such as *amidation, glycosylation, acetylation, carboxylation, sulfation* or *phosphorylation*.[5] They also may contain *intramolecular* disulfide bonds, such that the molecule adopts a partially cyclic conformation, or they may comprise two or more separate chains linked by *intermolecular* disulfide bonds.

Generally speaking, larger proteins adopt restricted conformations that expose functional groups in fixed locations on their surface, which interact with multiple sites on their receptors in a 'lock-and-key' mode. To envisage flexible peptides fitting into a receptor site this way is to imagine that you can unlock your front door with a length of cooked spaghetti. These features have greatly impeded the rational design of non-peptide analogues that mimic the action of proteins and peptides at their receptors (peptidomimetics). The use of random screening methods has (somewhat to the chagrin of the rationalists) nevertheless led in recent years to the discovery of many non-peptide *antagonists* – although few *agonists* – for peptide receptors.

TYPES OF PROTEIN AND PEPTIDE MEDIATOR

Protein and peptide mediators that are secreted by cells and act on surface receptors of the same or other cells can be very broadly divided into four groups:

- neurotransmitters (e.g. endogenous opioid peptides, see Ch. 42) and neuroendocrine mediators (e.g. vasopressin, somatostatin, hypothalamic releasing hormones, adrenocorticotrophic hormone (ACTH), luteinising hormone (LH), follicle-stimulating hormone (FSH) and thyroid-stimulating hormone (TSH), see Chs 33–35) (not discussed further in this chapter);
- hormones from non-neural sources: these comprise plasma-derived peptides, notably angiotensin (see Ch. 21) and bradykinin, as well as other hormones such as insulin (see Ch. 31), endothelin (see Ch. 21), atrial natriuretic peptide (see Ch. 20) and leptin (see Ch. 32);
- growth factors: produced by many different cells and tissues that control cell growth and differentiation (especially, in adults, in the haemopoietic system; see Ch. 24);
- mediators of the immune system (cytokines, see later).

BIOSYNTHESIS AND REGULATION OF PEPTIDES

Peptide structure is, of course, directly coded in the genome, in a manner that the structure of (say) acetylcholine is not, so intracellular manufacture is by conventional protein synthesis pathways. This often begins with the manufacture of a precursor protein in which the desired final peptide sequence is embedded. Specific proteolytic enzymes excise the mature active peptide from within this peptide sequence, a process of sculpture rather than synthesis. The precursor protein is packaged into vesicles at the point of synthesis, and the

[5]Bacteria are poor at post-translational modifications, hence over half of all protein drugs (biopharmaceuticals) are generated using mammalian cell cultures (see Ch. 5).

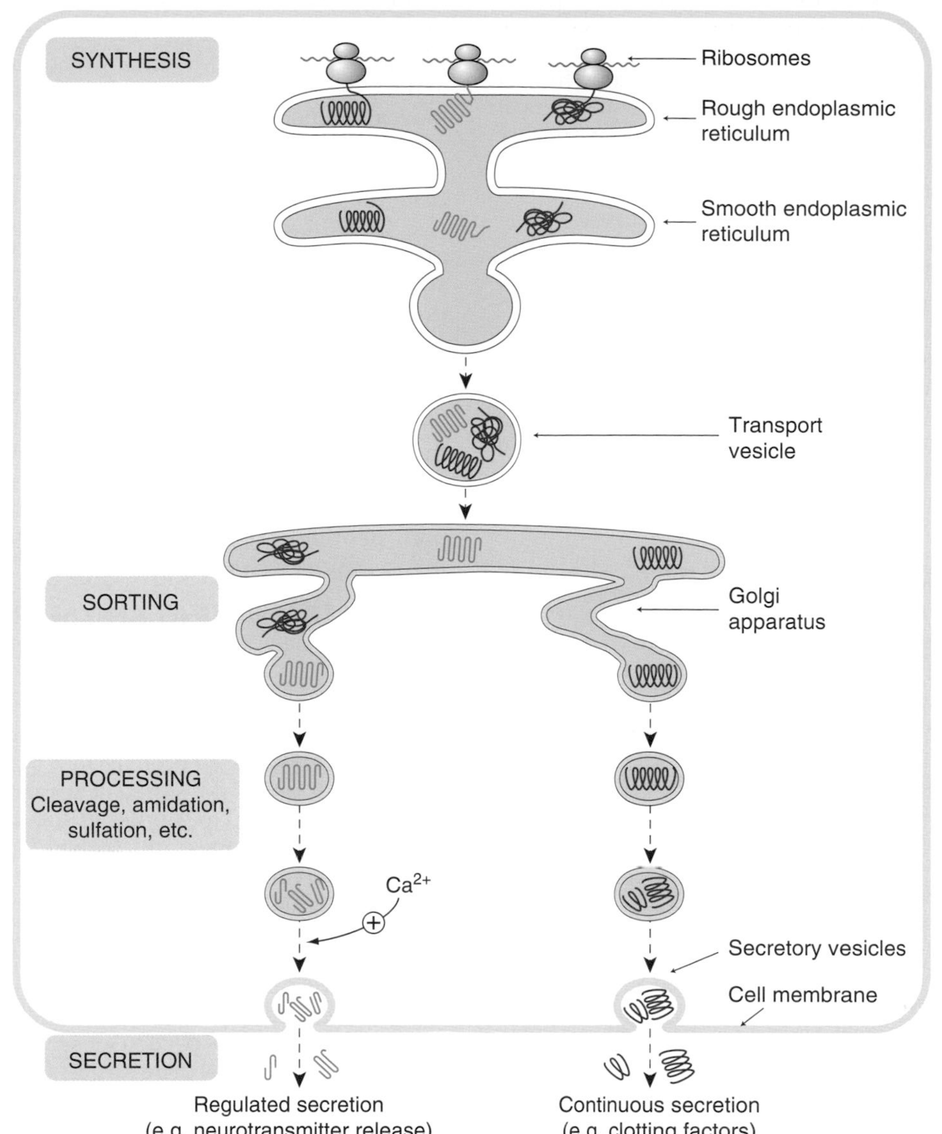

Fig. 17.7 Cellular mechanisms for peptide synthesis and release. Proteins synthesised by ribosomes are threaded through the membrane of the rough endoplasmic reticulum, from where they are conveyed in transport vesicles to the Golgi apparatus. Here, they are sorted and packaged into secretory vesicles. Processing (cleavage, glycosylation, amidation, sulfation, etc.) occurs within the transport and secretory vesicles, and the products are released from the cell by exocytosis. Constitutive secretion (e.g. of plasma proteins and clotting factors by liver cells) occurs continuously, and little material is stored in secretory vesicles. Regulated secretion (e.g. of neuropeptides or cytokines) occurs in response to increased intracellular Ca^{2+} or other intracellular signals, and material is typically stored in significant amounts in secretory vesicles awaiting release.

active peptide is formed in situ ready for release (Fig. 17.7). Thus, there is no need for specialised biosynthetic pathways, or for the uptake or recapturing mechanisms, that are important for the synthesis and release of most non-peptide mediators (e.g. 5-hydroxytryptamine; see Ch. 16).

PEPTIDE PRECURSORS

The precursor protein, or *pre-prohormone*, usually 100–250 residues in length, consists of an N-terminal *signal sequence* (peptide), followed by a variable stretch of unknown function, and a peptide-containing region that may contain several copies of active peptide fragments. Often, several different peptides are found within one precursor, but sometimes there are multiple copies of a single peptide.[6] The *signal sequence*, which is strongly hydrophobic, facilitates insertion of the protein into the endoplasmic reticulum and is then cleaved off at an early stage, yielding the *prohormone*.

The active peptides are usually demarcated within the prohormone sequence by pairs of basic amino acids (Lys-Lys or Lys-Arg), which are cleavage points for the trypsin-like proteases that release the peptides. This *endoproteolytic cleavage* generally occurs in the Golgi apparatus or the secretory vesicles. The enzymes responsible are known as *prohormone convertases*. Scrutiny of the prohormone sequence

[6]In the case of the invertebrate *Aplysia*, one protein precursor contains no fewer than 28 copies of the same short peptide.

often reveals likely cleavage points that distinguish previously unknown peptides. In some cases (e.g. *CGRP*; see later), new peptide mediators have been discovered in this way, but there are many examples where no function has yet been assigned. Whether these peptides are, like strangers at a funeral, waiting to declare their purpose or merely functionless mournful relics remains a mystery. There are also large stretches of the prohormone sequence of unknown function lying between the active peptide fragments.[7]

The abundance of mRNA coding for particular pre-prohormones, which reflects the level of gene expression, is very sensitive to physiological conditions. This type of *transcriptional control* is one of the main mechanisms by which peptide expression and release are regulated over the medium to long-term. Inflammation, for example, increases the expression, and hence the release, of various cytokines by immune cells. Sensory neurons respond to peripheral inflammation by increased expression of tachykinins (*substance P* and *neurokinins A and B*), which is important in the genesis of inflammatory pain (see Ch. 43).

DIVERSITY WITHIN PEPTIDE FAMILIES

Peptides commonly occur in families with similar or related sequences and actions. For example, the pro-opiomelanocortin (POMC) polypeptide, which has 241 amino acids, serves as a source of ACTH, melanocyte-stimulating hormones (MSHs) and β-endorphin, all of which have a role in controlling the inflammatory response (as well as other processes). There are two main mechanisms which control peptide diversity.

GENE SPLICING

Diversity of members of a peptide family can also arise by gene splicing or during post-translational processing of the prohormone. Genes contain coding regions (*exons*) interspersed with intervening non-coding (but potentially functional) regions (*introns*). When the gene is transcribed, the ensuing RNA (*heterologous nuclear RNA*, or alternatively *precursor mRNA*) is spliced to remove the introns and some of the exons, forming the final *mature mRNA* that is translated. Control of the splicing process allows a measure of cellular control over the peptides that are produced.

For example, the *calcitonin* gene codes for calcitonin itself, important in bone metabolism (see Ch. 36), and also for a completely dissimilar peptide (CGRP, involved in migraine pathogenesis, see Ch. 43). Alternative splicing allows cells to produce either pro-calcitonin (expressed in thyroid cells) or pro-CGRP (expressed in many neurons) from the same gene. Substance P and neurokinin A are two closely related tachykinins belonging to the same family and are also encoded on the same gene. Alternative splicing results in the production of two precursor proteins; one of these includes both peptides, the other includes only substance P. The ratio of the two varies widely between tissues, which correspondingly produce either one or both peptides.

POST-TRANSLATIONAL MODIFICATIONS

Many peptides, such as tachykinins and ACTH-related peptides (see Ch. 34), must undergo enzymatic *amidation* at the C-terminus to acquire full biological activity. Tissues may also generate peptides of varying length from the same primary sequence by the action of specific peptidases that cut the chain at different points. For example, *pro-cholecystokinin* (pro-CCK) contains the sequences of at least five CCK-like peptides ranging in length from 4 to 58 amino acid residues, all with the same C-terminal sequence. CCK itself (33 residues) is the main peptide produced by the intestine, whereas the brain produces mainly CCK-8. The opioid precursor *prodynorphin* similarly gives rise to several peptides with a common terminal sequence, the proportions of which vary in different tissues and in different neurons in the brain. In some cases (e.g. the inflammatory mediator bradykinin), peptide cleavage occurring after release generates a new active peptide (des-Arg^9-bradykinin), which acts on a different receptor, both peptides contributing differently to the combined inflammatory response.

PEPTIDE TRAFFICKING AND SECRETION

The basic mechanisms by which peptides are synthesised, packaged into vesicles, processed and secreted are summarised in Fig. 17.7. Two secretory pathways exist, for *constitutive* and *regulated* secretion, respectively. Constitutively secreted proteins (e.g. plasma proteins, some clotting factors) are not stored in appreciable amounts, and secretion is coupled to synthesis. Regulated secretion is, as with many hormones and transmitters, controlled by receptor-activated signals that lead to a rise in intracellular Ca^{2+}, and peptides awaiting release are stored in cytoplasmic vesicles. Specific protein–protein interactions appear to be responsible for the sorting of different proteins and their routing into different vesicles, and for choreographing their selective release. Identification of the specific 'trafficking' proteins involved in particular secretory pathways may eventually yield novel drug targets for the selective control of secretion.

Having described the general mechanisms by which peptides are synthesised, processed and released, we now describe some significant mediators that fall into this category.

BRADYKININ

Bradykinin and lysyl-bradykinin (*kallidin*) are active peptides formed by proteolytic cleavage of circulating proteins termed *kininogens* through a protease cascade pathway.

SOURCE AND FORMATION OF BRADYKININ

An outline of the formation of bradykinin from high-molecular-weight kininogen in plasma by the serine protease *kallikrein* is given in Fig. 17.8. *Kininogen* is a plasma α-globulin that exists in both high (Mr 110,000) and low (Mr 70,000) molecular-weight forms. Kallikrein itself is cleaved from the inactive precursor *prekallikrein* by the action of factor XII (Hageman factor; see Chs 7 and 23). Factor XII is activated by contact with negatively charged surfaces such as collagen, basement membrane, bacterial lipopolysaccharides, urate crystals and so on. Factor XII, prekallikrein and the

[7]When these large sequences of unknown function were discovered in our DNA, they were rather arrogantly termed 'junk DNA', not because they were rubbish, but because we didn't understand their function. It turns out 'junk DNA' is actually very important, controlling gene expression and hence cell function. It is also a significant factor in some diseases. 'Junk peptide' may yet be ascribed similar or alternate biological roles.

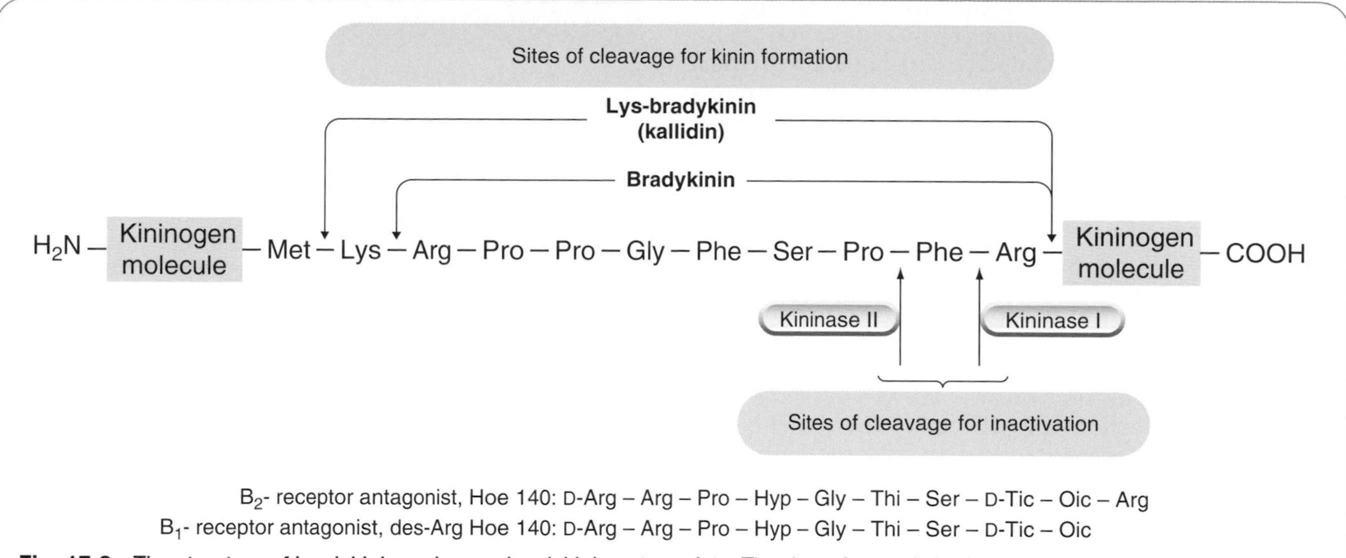

Fig. 17.8 The structure of bradykinin and some bradykinin antagonists. The sites of proteolytic cleavage of high-molecular-weight kininogen by kallikrein involved in the formation of bradykinin are shown in the upper half of the figure; the sites of cleavage associated with bradykinin and kallidin inactivation are shown in the lower half. The B_2-receptor antagonist icatibant (Hoe 140) has a pA_2 of 9, and the competitive B_1-receptor antagonist des-Arg Hoe 140 has a pA_2 of 8. The Hoe compounds contain unnatural amino acids: Thi, δ-Tic and Oic, which are analogues of phenylalanine and proline.

kininogens leak out of the vessels during inflammation because of increased vascular permeability, and exposure to negatively charged surfaces promotes the interaction of factor XII with prekallikrein. The activated enzyme then 'clips' bradykinin from its kininogen precursor. Kallikrein can also activate the complement system and can convert plasminogen to plasmin.

In addition to plasma kallikrein, there are other kinin-generating isoenzymes found in the pancreas, salivary glands, colon and skin. These *tissue kallikreins* act on both high- and low-molecular-weight kininogens and generate mainly *kallidin*, a peptide with actions similar to those of bradykinin.

METABOLISM AND INACTIVATION OF BRADYKININ

Specific enzymes that inactivate bradykinin and related kinins are called *kininases* (see Fig. 17.8). One of these, *kininase II*, is a peptidyl dipeptidase that inactivates kinins by removing the two C-terminal amino acids. This enzyme, which is bound to the luminal surface of endothelial cells, is identical to *angiotensin-converting enzyme* (ACE; see Ch. 21), which cleaves the two C-terminal residues from the inactive peptide angiotensin I, converting it to the active vasoconstrictor peptide angiotensin II. Thus, kininase II inactivates a vasodilator and activates a vasoconstrictor. Potentiation of bradykinin actions by ACE inhibitors (e.g. **ramipril**) may contribute to some side effects of these drugs (e.g. cough and angioedema).

Kinins are also metabolised by various less specific peptidases, including a serum carboxypeptidase that removes the C-terminal arginine, generating *des-Arg⁹-bradykinin*, a specific agonist at one of the two main classes of bradykinin receptor, and *neprilysin*. Neprilysin (also known as *neutral endopeptidase 24.11*, *common acute lymphoblastic leukaemia antigen* or CD10) is a predominantly membrane-bound member of the neprilysin (M13) family of metallopeptidases and is a key enzyme in the degradation of naturitic peptides. **Sacubitril**, a prodrug that is hydrolysed to form LBQ657 – a potent inhibitor of neprilysin – and licensed for the management of heart failure (see Ch. 20), also increases bradykinin concentration: a feature which contributes to both its therapeutic effect and side effect profile (see Campbell, 2018).

BRADYKININ RECEPTORS

There are two bradykinin receptors, designated B_1 and B_2. Both are GPCRs and mediate very similar effects. B_1 receptors are normally expressed at very low levels but are strongly induced in inflamed or damaged tissues by cytokines such as IL-1. B_1 receptors respond to the carboxypeptidase N (kininase I) metabolite *des-Arg^9-bradykinin* but not to bradykinin itself. A number of selective peptide and non-peptide antagonists are known. It is likely that B_1 receptors play a significant role in inflammation and hyperalgesia (see Ch. 42), and antagonists could be useful in the treatment of cough, neurological disorders and osteoarthritis (Whalley et al., 2012).

B_2 receptors are constitutively present in many normal cells and are activated by bradykinin and kallidin, but not by des-Arg^9-bradykinin. Peptide and non-peptide antagonists have been developed, the best known being the bradykinin analogue **icatibant**, used to treat acute attacks in patients with *hereditary angio-oedema* (an uncommon disorder caused by deficiency of C1-esterase inhibitor that normally restrains complement activation). Other small molecule B_2 receptor antagonists including **anatibant** and **fasitibant** have failed to demonstrate efficacy for alternate indications.

ACTIONS AND ROLE IN INFLAMMATION

Bradykinin causes vasodilatation and increased vascular permeability. Its vasodilator action is partly a result of generation of PGI_2 and release of nitric oxide (NO). It causes pain by stimulating nociceptive nerve terminals, and its action here is potentiated by prostaglandins, which are released by bradykinin. Bradykinin also contracts intestinal, uterine and bronchial smooth muscle in some species. The contraction is slow and sustained in comparison with that produced by tachykinins such as substance P (*brady-* means slow; *tachy-* means rapid). Bradykinin may also increase cell proliferation promote leukocyte activation and migration.

Although bradykinin reproduces many inflammatory signs and symptoms, its role in inflammation and allergy is not clear, partly because its effects are often component parts of a complex cascade of events triggered by other mediators. However, excessive bradykinin production contributes to the diarrhoea of gastrointestinal disorders, and in allergic rhinitis it stimulates nasopharyngeal secretion. Bradykinin also contributes to the clinical picture in *pancreatitis*,[8] although, disappointingly, B_2 antagonists worsen rather than alleviate this disorder. Physiologically, the release of bradykinin by tissue kallikrein may regulate blood flow to certain exocrine glands, and influence secretions. Bradykinin also stimulates ion transport and fluid secretion by some epithelia, including intestine, airways and gall bladder.

Bradykinin

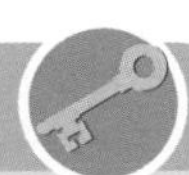

- Bradykinin (BK) is a nonapeptide 'clipped' from a plasma α-globulin, *kininogen*, by *kallikrein.*
- It is converted by *kininase I* to an active octapeptide, BK_{1-8} (des-Arg[9]-BK), and inactivated by the removal of an additional amino acid by *kininase II* (ACE) in the lung.
- Inhibition of bradykinin breakdown by angiotensin-converting enzyme or neprilysin inhibitors contributes to their side effect profile (e.g. cough and angioedema).
- Pharmacological actions:
  - vasodilatation (largely dependent on endothelial cell nitric oxide and PGI_2);
  - increased vascular permeability;
  - stimulation of pain nerve endings;
  - stimulation of epithelial ion transport and fluid secretion in airways and gastrointestinal tract;
  - contraction of intestinal and uterine smooth muscle;
  - cell proliferation, migration and activation.
- There are two main subtypes of BK receptors: B_2, which is constitutively present, and B_1, which is induced in inflammation.
- **Icatibant**, a peptide analogue of BK, is a selective competitive antagonist for B_2 receptors and is used to treat acute attacks of hereditary angioedema. Other, non-peptide antagonists for both B_1 and B_2 receptors are known and may be developed for treating inflammatory disorders.

NEUROPEPTIDES

Neuropeptides constitute a large (>100) and diverse family of small to medium-sized peptides. Many are found in the CNS, the autonomic nervous system, and peripheral sensory neurons, as well as in many peripheral tissues. They are often released as co-transmitters (see Chs 13 and 39), along with non-peptide neurotransmitters.

When released from peripheral endings of nociceptive sensory neurons (see Ch. 42), neuropeptides in some species cause *neurogenic inflammation* (Chiu et al., 2012). The main peptides involved are substance P, neurokinin A and CGRP. Substance P and neurokinin A are small (about 1100 Da) members of the *tachykinin* family with partly homologous structures. They act on mast cells, releasing histamine and other mediators, and producing smooth muscle contraction, neural activation, mucus secretion and vasodilatation. CGRP, a member of the calcitonin family (37 amino acids in length), shares these properties and is a particularly potent vasodilator. Tachykinins released from the central endings of nociceptive neurons also modulate transmission in the dorsal horn of the spinal cord, affecting sensitivity to pain (see Ji et al., 2018). All these neuropeptides act through specific GPCRs to produce their effects.

Neurogenic inflammation is implicated in the pathogenesis of several inflammatory conditions, including the delayed phase of asthma, allergic rhinitis, inflammatory bowel disease, some types of arthritis and migraine. Antagonists at the neurokinin NK_1 receptor, such as **aprepitant**, **fosaprepitant and netupitant**, are used to treat emesis, particularly that associated with some forms of cancer chemotherapy (see Ch. 57). Other important members of the neuropeptide family include *enkephalins/endorphins* (see Ch. 42) and *orexins* (see Ch. 32). The latter are the therapeutic target of **suvorexant** and **daridorexant** which, by inhibiting the binding of orexin-A and orexin-B to their OXR1 and OXR2 receptors, promote sleep (see Ch. 45).

CYTOKINES

'Cytokine' is an all-purpose functional term that is applied to protein or polypeptide mediators synthesised and released by cells of the immune system during inflammation. They are crucial for the overall coordination of the inflammatory response. Cytokines act locally by autocrine or paracrine mechanisms. Unlike conventional hormones such as insulin, concentrations in blood and tissues are almost undetectable under normal circumstances but are massively up-regulated (100–1000-fold) during inflammatory episodes. Cytokines are generally active at very low (sub-nanomolar) concentrations.

Cytokines bind to and activate specific, high-affinity receptors on target cells, that, in most cases, are also up-regulated during inflammation. Except for *chemokines*, which act on GPCRs, most cytokines act on kinase-linked receptors, regulating phosphorylation cascades that affect gene expression, such as the JAK-STAT pathway (see Ch. 25).

In addition to their own direct actions on cells, some cytokines amplify inflammation by inducing the formation of other inflammatory mediators. Others can induce receptors for other cytokines on their target cell or engage in synergistic or antagonistic interactions with other cytokines. Cytokines therefore constitute a complex chemical signalling language,

[8]A serious and painful condition in which proteolytic enzymes are released from damaged pancreatic cells, initiating proteolytic cascades that release, among other things, bradykinin.

with the final response of a particular cell involved being determined by the strength and number of different messages received concurrently at the cell surface.

Systems for classifying cytokines abound in the literature, as do diagrams depicting their complex networks of interactions with each other and with their many target cells. However, no one system of classification does justice to the complexity of cytokine biology. The terminology and nomenclature are horrendous, and a comprehensive coverage of this area is beyond the scope of this book. Table 17.2 lists some of the more significant cytokines and their biological actions. Aspiring cytokine aficionados will find further information in Liu et al. (2021), the clinically focused but renally biased Holdsworth and Gan (2015) and the IUPHAR/BPS Guide to Pharmacology. To explore the interesting history of this field, including how an understanding of cytokine biology was harnessed for therapeutic benefit, see Vilcek and Feldmann (2004) and Dinarello (2007).

More than 100 cytokines have been identified. These may be broadly categorised into four main functional groups, namely *interleukins*, *chemokines*, *interferons* and *colony-stimulating factors* (discussed separately in Ch. 24), but these demarcations are of limited use because many cytokines have multiple roles.

Using biopharmaceuticals (see Chs 5 and 25) to interfere with cytokine action has proved to be a particularly fertile area of drug development: several successful strategies have been adopted, including direct neutralisation of cytokines using antibodies and the use of 'decoy' receptor proteins that remove the biologically active pool from the circulation.

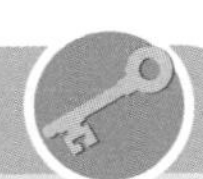

Cytokines

- Cytokines are polypeptides that are rapidly induced and released during inflammation. They regulate the action of inflammatory and immune system cells.
- The cytokine superfamily includes the *interferons*, *interleukins*, *chemokines* and *colony-stimulating factors*.
- Utilising both autocrine or paracrine mechanisms, they exert complex effects on leukocytes, vascular endothelial cells, mast cells, fibroblasts, haemopoietic stem cells and osteoclasts, controlling proliferation, differentiation and/or activation.
- Interleukin 1 (IL-1) and tumour necrosis factor-α (TNF-α) are important primary inflammatory cytokines, inducing the formation of other cytokines.
- Chemokines, such as IL-8, are mainly involved in the regulation of cell trafficking.
- Interferons IFN-α and IFN-β have antiviral activity, and IFN-α is used as an adjunct in the treatment of viral infections. IFN-γ has significant immunoregulatory function and is used in the treatment of multiple sclerosis.

INTERLEUKINS AND RELATED COMPOUNDS

The name was originally coined to describe mediators that signalled between leukocytes but, like so much else in the cytokine lexicography, it has become rather redundant, not to say misleading. The primary pro-inflammatory species are *tumour necrosis factor* (TNF)-α and *IL-1*. The principal members of the latter cytokine group consist of two agonists, IL-1α, IL-1β and, surprisingly, an endogenous soluble IL-1-receptor antagonist (IL-1ra).[9] Mixtures of these are released from macrophages and many other cells during inflammation and can initiate the synthesis and release of a cascade of secondary cytokines, among which are the chemokines. TNF and IL-1 are key regulators of almost all manifestations of the inflammatory response. A long-standing debate about which of the two is really the prime mover of inflammation ended when it was found that this varies according to the disease type. In auto-*immune* disease (e.g. rheumatoid arthritis, where the adaptive immune system is activated), TNF appears to be the predominant influence and blocking its action is therapeutically effective. In auto-*inflammatory* diseases (e.g. gout, where only the innate system is involved), IL-1 seems to be the key mediator (Dinarello et al., 2012). Both TNF-α and IL-1 are important targets for anti-inflammatory biopharmaceuticals.

Not all interleukins are pro-inflammatory: some, including transforming growth factor (TGF)-β, IL-4, IL-10 and IL-13 are potent anti-inflammatory substances. They inhibit chemokine production, and the responses driven by T-helper (Th) 1 cells, whose inappropriate activation is involved in the pathogenesis of several diseases.

CHEMOKINES

Chemokines are defined as *chemo*attractant cyto*kines* that control the migration of leukocytes, functioning as traffic coordinators during immune and inflammatory reactions. Again, the nomenclature (and the classification) is confusing because some non-cytokine mediators also control leukocyte movement (e.g. C5a, LTB_4, fMet-Leu-Phe, etc.; see Ch. 7) and many chemokines have more than one name. Furthermore, many chemokines have other actions, causing mast cell degranulation or promoting angiogenesis, for example.

More than 40 chemokines have been identified. They are all highly homologous peptides of 8–10 kDa, which are usually grouped according to the configuration of key cysteine residues in their polypeptide chain. Chemokines with one cysteine are known as *C chemokines*. If there are two adjacent cysteine residues they are termed *C–C chemokines*. Other members have cysteines separated by one (*C–X–C chemokines*) or three (*C–XXX–C chemokines*) other residues. The C–X–C chemokines (main example IL-8) act on neutrophils and are predominantly involved in acute inflammatory responses. The C–C chemokines (main examples *eotaxin*, *MCP-1* and *RANTES*) act on monocytes, eosinophils and other cells, and are involved predominantly in chronic inflammatory responses.

Chemokines generally act through GPCRs, and alteration or inappropriate expression of these is implicated in multiple sclerosis, cancer (tumorigenesis and metastasis), autoimmune and cardiovascular diseases (Raman et al., 2011). Several types of viruses (herpes virus, cytomegalovirus, pox virus and members of the retrovirus family) can manipulate the chemokine system to subvert the host's defences (Murphy, 2001). Some produce proteins that mimic host chemokines or chemokine receptors, some act as antagonists at chemokine receptors and some masquerade as growth or angiogenic factors. HIV is responsible for the most audacious exploitation: it has a protein (gp120) in its

[9] One might have expected evolution to generate more examples of endogenous receptor antagonists as physiological regulators, but apart from IL-1ra, they are only exploited as toxins directed against other species.

Table 17.2 Some examples of significant cytokines and their actions

Cytokine	Main cell source	Main target cell or biological effect	Comments
IL-1	Monocyte/macrophages, dendritic and other cells	Regulates cell migration to sites of infection, produces inflammation, fever and pain	Two original subtypes, IL-1α and IL-1β, and IL-1ra – a receptor antagonist. Target for anti-inflammatory therapy (see Ch. 25)
IL-2	T cells	Stimulates proliferation, maturation and activation of T, B and NK cells	First interleukin to be discovered
IL-4	Th2 cells	Stimulates proliferation, maturation of T and B cells and promotes IgG and E synthesis. Promotes an anti-inflammatory phenotype	A key cytokine in the regulation of the Th2 response (see Chs 7 and 25)
IL-5	Th2 cells, mast cells	Important for eosinophil activation. Stimulates proliferation, maturation of B cells and IgA synthesis	Particularly important in allergic disease
IL-6	Monocyte/macrophages and T cells	Pro-inflammatory actions including fever. Stimulation of osteoclast activity	Target for anti-inflammatory drugs (see Ch. 25)
IL-8	Macrophages, endothelial cells	Neutrophil chemotaxis, phagocytosis and angiogenesis	C–X–C chemokine (CXCL8)
IL-10	Monocytes and Th2 cells	Inhibits cytokine production and down-regulates inflammation	A predominately anti-inflammatory cytokine
IL-17	T cells and others	Stimulates Th17 cells, involved in allergic response and autoimmunity	Several subtypes. Target for anti-inflammatory drugs (see Ch. 25)
TNF-α	Mainly macrophages but also many immune and other cells	Kills tumour cells. Stimulates macrophage cytokine expression and is a key regulator of many aspects of the immune response	A major target for anti-inflammatory drugs (see Ch. 25)
TNF-β	Th1 cells	Initiates a variety of immune-stimulatory and pro-inflammatory actions in the host defence system	Now often called lymphotoxin α (LTA)
Eotaxin	Airway epithelial and other cells	Activation and chemotaxis of eosinophils. Allergic inflammation	C–C chemokine (CCL11). Three subtypes
MCP-1	Monocytes, osteoblasts/clasts, neurons and other cells	Promotes recruitment of monocytes and T cells to sites of inflammation	C–C chemokine (CC2)
RANTES	T cells	Chemotaxis of T cells. Chemotaxis and activation of other leukocytes	(CCL5)
IFN-α	Leukocytes	Activates NK cells and macrophages. Inhibits viral replication and has antitumour actions	Multiple molecular species
IFN-γ	Th1, NK cells	Stimulates Th1, and inhibits Th2, cell proliferation. Activates NK cells and macrophages	Crucial to the Th1 response (see Ch. 7)
GM–CSF	Macrophages, T cells, mast cells and others	Stimulates growth of leukocyte progenitor cells. Increases numbers of blood-borne leukocytes	Used therapeutically to stimulate myeloid cell growth (e.g. after bone marrow transplantation)
MIP-1	Macrophages/lymphocytes	Activation of neutrophils and other cells. Promotes cytokine release	C–C chemokine (CCL3). Two subtypes
TGF-β	T cells, monocytes	Induces apoptosis. Regulates cell growth	Three isoforms. Predominately anti-inflammatory action

GM–CSF, Granulocyte-macrophage colony-stimulating factor; *IFN,* interferon; *Ig,* immunoglobulin; *IL,* interleukin; *MCP,* monocyte chemoattractant protein; *MIP,* macrophage inflammatory protein; *NK,* natural killer (cell); *RANTES,* regulated on activation normal T cell expressed and secreted; *TGF,* transforming growth factor; *Th,* T-helper (cell); *TNF,* tumour necrosis factor.

envelope that recognises and binds T-cell receptors for CD4 and the chemokine co-receptors CCR5 (blocked by the HIV drug **maraviroc**) and CXCR4 to hijack its way into the cell (see Ch. 53).

INTERFERONS

So called because they interfere with viral replication, there are three main types of interferon, termed IFN-α, IFN-β and IFN-γ. 'IFN-α' is not a single substance but a family of approximately 20 proteins with similar activities. IFN-α and IFN-β have antiviral activity whereas IFN-α also has some antitumour action. Both are released from virus-infected cells and activate antiviral mechanisms in neighbouring cells. IFN-γ also induces Th1 responses (see Ch. 7). Confusingly, interferons are also grouped into three families based on their interactions with the IFN receptor subunits, peptide mapping, and sequencing homology. These consist of the *type 1 IFN* family (comprising 13 partially homologous IFN-α subtypes and a single IFN-β among others; these signal through the IFN-α receptor 1 and 2), *type II IFN family* (IFN-γ, acting on the IFN-γ receptor) and the *type III family* (IFN-λ1–3, also known as IL-29, IL-28A and IL28B). See McNab et al. (2015) and López de Padilla and Niewold (2016) for further details.

CLINICAL USE OF INTERFERONS

IFN-α is used in the treatment of chronic hepatitis B and C (although note recent advances in this field: see Ch. 53) and has some action against herpes zoster and in the prevention of the common cold. Antitumour action against some lymphomas and solid tumours has also been reported. Dose-related side effects, including influenza-like symptoms, may occur. IFN-β is used in patients with the relapsing–remitting form of multiple sclerosis, and *chronic granulomatous disease*, an uncommon chronic disease of childhood in which neutrophil function is impaired, can be treated with IFN-γ in conjunction with antibacterial drugs.

Clinical uses of interferons

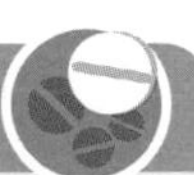

- α: chronic hepatitis B or C (in combination with **ribavirin**, however direct-acting oral antivirals e.g. **tenofovir** or **sofosbuvir** now preferred).
- Malignant disease (alone or in combination with other drugs, e.g. **cytarabine**): chronic myelogenous leukaemia (CML), hairy cell leukaemia, follicular lymphoma, metastatic carcinoid, multiple myeloma, malignant melanoma (as an adjunct to surgery), myelodysplastic syndrome.
- Conjugation with polyethylene glycol ('pegylation') results in preparations that are more slowly eliminated and are administered intermittently subcutaneously.
- β: multiple sclerosis (especially the relapsing–remitting form of this disease).
- γ: to reduce infection in children with chronic granulomatous disease.
- Inhibition of IFN action may also have therapeutic benefit, the anti-type 1 interferon receptor subunit 1 drug **anifrolumab** having efficacy in systemic lupus erythematosus.

THE 'CYTOKINE STORM'

Many cytokines release further cytokines in what is essentially a positive feedback loop. There are times when this feedback system becomes unstable, perhaps as a result of the absence of balancing anti-inflammatory factors. The result can be a massive overproduction of cytokines in response to infection or other injury. This is known as a *cytokine storm* (also called *hypercytokinemia*) and can pose a significant threat to the host. Cytokine storms may be responsible for deaths in septic shock as well as in some pandemic diseases including COVID-19 (see Fajgenbaum and June, 2020). A tragic case of volunteers suffering cytokine storms after receiving an experimental drug is related in Chapter 5.

PROTEINS AND PEPTIDES THAT DOWN-REGULATE INFLAMMATION

Inflammation is not regulated solely by factors that provoke or enhance it: it has become increasingly evident that there is another panel of mediators that function at every step to down-regulate inflammation, to check its progress and limit its duration and scope. It is the dynamic balance between these two systems that regulates the onset and resolution of inflammatory episodes, and when this breaks down, may lead also to inflammatory disease or, in extreme cases, to the cytokine storm phenomenon. Some of these counter-regulatory controllers are peptidic in nature and we have already encountered IL-1ra, TGF-β and IL-10, which are important negative regulators of inflammation. There are two other systems that are significant here because common anti-inflammatory drugs exploit their action.

Anx-A1 is a 37-kDa protein produced by many cells and especially abundant in cells of the myeloid lineage. When released, it exerts potent anti-inflammatory actions, down-regulating cell activation, cell transmigration and mediator release. It does this by acting through the GPCR ALX/FPR2, a member of the formyl peptide receptor family already discussed in the context of the anti-inflammatory lipoxins.

The significance of the Anx-A1 system is that it is activated by anti-inflammatory glucocorticoids (see Ch. 25), which increase Anx-A1 gene transcription and promote its release from cells. Interestingly, the anti-allergic cromones (**cromoglicate**, etc.; see Ch. 27) also promote the release of this protein from cells. Anx-A1 gene 'knock-out' studies have shown that this protein is important for restraining the inflammatory response, including a laboratory model of septic shock, and for its timely resolution. The anti-inflammatory glucocorticoids cannot develop their full inhibitory actions without it. A recent review of Anx-A1 biology, including its role outside of inflammation, is given by Sheikh and Solito (2018).

The *melanocortin system* also plays an important part in regulating inflammation. There are five G protein–coupled melanocortin receptors, MC_{1-5}. Endogenous ligands for these receptors, such as MSH (three types), are derived from the POMC gene, and serve a number of purposes, including regulating the development of a suntan, penile erection and the control of appetite through an action on various MC receptors.

From the point of view of host defence, the MC_3 receptor is the most important. Again, gene deletion studies have highlighted the importance of this receptor in a variety of inflammatory conditions. Interestingly, another product of the POMC gene, ACTH, was formerly used as an anti-inflammatory agent, but it was thought that its action was secondary to its ability to release endogenous cortisol from the adrenals (an MC_2 action, see Ch. 33). It is now known that it is a ligand at the MC_3 receptor, and it is likely that it owes some of its activity to this action.

An account of the importance of this field is given by Wang et al. (2019).

CONCLUDING REMARKS

In this chapter we have tried to provide an introduction to some of the key families of mediator that regulate human physiology and, in particular, contribute to host defence. Other relevant low-molecular-weight factors include the purines (see Ch. 16) and nitric oxide (see Ch. 19) which are covered elsewhere. Even from the superficial sketch presented here (and in other related parts of this book such as Ch. 7), it must be evident that the host defence response is among the most intricate of all physiological responses. Perhaps that is not surprising, given its central importance to survival.

For the same reason, it is also understandable that so many different mediators orchestrate its operation. That the activity of many of these can be blocked in experimental models with little or no obvious effect on the initiation and outcome of inflammation points to redundancy among the many component systems and goes some way to explaining why, until the advent of highly specific antibody-based therapies for inflammatory conditions, our ability to curb the worst ravages of chronic inflammatory disease was so limited.

A crucial development over recent years is the advancement of analytical techniques and their computational processing. This has allowed both the identification of new mediators (and indeed families of mediators) as well as the interrogation of human biology in health and disease at both the systems and single cell level. It is hoped that application of these techniques, allied to improved drug design and development, will continue to yield novel therapeutic leads.

REFERENCES AND FURTHER READING

Barnes, N.C., Piper, P.J., Costello, J.F., 1984. Comparative effects of inhaled leukotriene C_4, leukotriene D_4, and histamine in normal human subjects. Thorax 39, 500–504.

Biringer, R.G., 2021. A review of prostanoid receptors: expression, characterization, regulation, and mechanism of action. J. Cell Commun. Signal 15, 155–184.

Biringer, R.G., 2022. A review of non-prostanoid, eicosanoid receptors: expression, characterization, regulation, and mechanism of action. J. Cell Commun. Signal 16, 5–46.

Calder, P.C., 2020. Eicosanoids. Essays Biochem. 64, 423–441.

Campbell, D.J., 2018. Neprilysin inhibitors and bradykinin. Front. Med. 5, 257.

Chiu, I.M., von Hehn, C.A., Woolf, C.J., 2012. Neurogenic inflammation and the peripheral nervous system in host defense and immunopathology. Nat. Neurosci. 15, 1063–1067.

Chung, K.F., 2005. Drugs to suppress cough. Expert. Opin. Invest. Drugs 14, 19–27.

Cornejo-Garcia, J.A., Perkins, J.R., Jurado-Escobar, R., et al., 2016. Pharmacogenomics of prostaglandin and leukotriene receptors. Front. Pharmacol. 7, 316.

Dennis, E.A., Norris, P.C., 2015. Eicosanoid storm in infection and inflammation. Nat. Rev. Immunol. 15, 511–523.

Dinarello, C.A., 2007. Historical insights into cytokines. Eur. J. Immunol. 37 (Suppl. 1), S34–S45.

Dinarello, C.A., Simon, A., van der Meer, J.W., 2012. Treating inflammation by blocking interleukin-1 in a broad spectrum of diseases. Nat. Rev. Drug Discov. 11, 633–652.

Fajgenbaum, D.C., June, C.H., 2020. Cytokine storm. N. Engl. J. Med. 383, 2255–2273.

Gault, C.R., Obeid, L.M., Hannun, Y.A., 2010. An overview of sphingolipid metabolism: from synthesis to breakdown. Adv. Exp. Med. Biol. 688, 1–23.

Hammock, B.D., Wang, W., Gilligan, M.M., et al., 2020. Eicosanoids: the overlooked storm in coronavirus disease 2019 (COVID-19)? Am. J. Pathol. 190, 1782–1788.

Han, X., 2016. Lipidomics for studying metabolism. Nat. Rev. Endocrinol. 12, 668–679.

Hattori, Y., Hattori, K., Matsuda, N., 2017. Regulation of the cardiovascular system by histamine. Handb. Exp. Pharmacol. 241, 239–258.

Holdsworth, S.R., Gan, P.Y., 2015. Cytokines: names and numbers you should care about. Clin. J. Am. Soc. Nephrol. 10, 2243–2254.

Horuk, R., 2001. Chemokine receptors. Cytokine Growth Factor Rev. 12, 313–335.

IUPHAR/BPS. Guide to Pharmacology. Available at: www.guidetopharmacology.org/.

Jaen, R.I., Sanchez-Garcia, S., Fernandez-Velasco, M., et al., 2021. Resolution-based therapies: the potential of lipoxins to treat human diseases. Front. Immunol. 12, 658840.

Ji, R.R., Nackley, A., Huh, Y., et al., 2018. Neuroinflammation and central sensitization in chronic and widespread pain. Anesthesiology 129, 343–366.

Jutel, M., Akdis, M., Akdis, C.A., 2009. Histamine, histamine receptors and their role in immune pathology. Clin. Exp. Allergy 39, 1786–1800.

Khan, S.U., Lone, A.N., Khan, M.S., et al., 2021. Effect of omega-3 fatty acids on cardiovascular outcomes: a systematic review and meta-analysis. EClinicalMedicine 38, 100997.

Lee, B.R., Paing, M.H., Sharma-Walia, N., 2021. Cyclopentenone prostaglandins: biologically active lipid mediators targeting inflammation. Front. Physiol. 12, 640374.

Liu, C., Chu, D., Kalantar-Zadeh, K., et al., 2021. Cytokines: from clinical significance to quantification. Adv. Sci. (Weinh) 8, e2004433.

Lopez de Padilla, C.M., Niewold, T.B., 2016. The type I interferons: basic concepts and clinical relevance in immune-mediated inflammatory diseases. Gene 576, 14–21.

Lordan, R., Tsoupras, A., Zabetakis, I., et al., 2019. Forty years since the structural elucidation of platelet-activating factor (PAF): historical, current, and future research perspectives. Molecules 24, 4414.

Luster, A.D., 1998. Mechanisms of disease: chemokines – chemotactic cytokines that mediate inflammation. N. Engl. J. Med. 338, 436–445.

Mackay, C.R., 2001. Chemokines: immunology's high impact factors. Nat. Immunol. 2, 95–101.

McGinley, M.P., Cohen, J.A., 2021. Sphingosine 1-phosphate receptor modulators in multiple sclerosis and other conditions. Lancet 398, 1184–1194.

McNab, F., Mayer-Barber, K., Sher, A., et al., 2015. Type I interferons in infectious disease. Nat. Rev. Immunol. 15, 87–103.

Mendelson, K., Evans, T., Hla, T., 2014. Sphingosine 1-phosphate signalling. Development 141, 5–9.

Murphy, P.M., 2001. Viral exploitation and subversion of the immune system through chemokine mimicry. Nat. Immunol. 2, 116–122.

Natto, Z.S., Yaghmoor, W., Alshaeri, H.K., et al., 2019. Omega-3 fatty acids effects on inflammatory biomarkers and lipid profiles among diabetic and cardiovascular disease patients: a systematic review and meta-analysis. Sci. Rep. 9, 18867.

Oehler, B., Mohammadi, M., Perpina Viciano, C., et al., 2017. Peripheral interaction of resolvin D1 and E1 with opioid receptor antagonists for antinociception in inflammatory pain in rats. Front. Mol. Neurosci. 10, 242.

O'Mahony, L., Akdis, M., Akdis, C.A., 2011. Regulation of the immune response and inflammation by histamine and histamine receptors. J. Allergy Clin. Immunol. 128, 1153–1162.

Panula, P., Chazot, P.L., Cowart, M., et al., 2015. International union of basic and clinical pharmacology. XCVIII. Histamine receptors. Pharmacol. Rev. 67, 601–655.
Patel, H.B., Montero-Melendez, T., Greco, K.V., Perretti, M., 2011. Melanocortin receptors as novel effectors of macrophage responses in inflammation. Front. Immunol. 2, 41–46.
Pease, J.E., Williams, T.J., 2006. The attraction of chemokines as a target for specific anti-inflammatory therapy. Br. J. Pharmacol. 147 (Suppl. 1), S212–S221.
Raman, D., Sobolik-Delmaire, T., Richmond, A., 2011. Chemokines in health and disease. Exp. Cell Res. 317, 575–589.
Romano, M., Cianci, E., Simiele, F., et al., 2015. Lipoxins and aspirin-triggered lipoxins in resolution of inflammation. Eur. J. Pharmacol. 760, 49–63.
Sansbury, B.E., Spite, M., 2016. Resolution of acute inflammation and the role of resolvins in immunity, thrombosis, and vascular biology. Circ. Res. 119, 113–130.
Scammell, T.E., Jackson, A.C., Franks, N.P., et al., 2019. Histamine: neural circuits and new medications. Sleep 42, zsy183.
Schulze, U., Baedeker, M., Chen, Y.T., Greber, D., 2014. R&D productivity: on the comeback trail. Nat. Rev. Drug Discov. 13, 331–332.
Schulze-Topphoff, U., Prat, A., 2008. Roles of the kallikrein/kinin system in the adaptive immune system. Int. Immunopharmacol. 8, 155–160.
Serhan, C.N., Chiang, N., Dalli, J., et al., 2014. Lipid mediators in the resolution of inflammation. Cold Spring Harb. Perspect. Biol. 7, a016311.
Serhan, C.N., Dalli, J., Colas, R.A., Winkler, J.W., Chiang, N., 2015. Protectins and maresins: new pro-resolving families of mediators in acute inflammation and resolution bioactive metabolome. Biochim. Biophys. Acta 1851, 397–413.
Serhan, C.N., Levy, B.D., 2018. Resolvins in inflammation: emergence of the pro-resolving superfamily of mediators. J. Clin. Invest. 128, 2657–2669.
Sheikh, M.H., Solito, E., 2018. Annexin A1: uncovering the many talents of an old protein. Int. J. Mol. Sci. 19.
Thangam, E.B., Jemima, E.A., Singh, H., et al., 2018. The role of histamine and histamine receptors in mast cell-mediated allergy and inflammation: the hunt for new therapeutic targets. Front. Immunol. 9, 1873.
Theken, K.N., FitzGerald, G.A., 2021. Bioactive lipids in antiviral immunity. Science 371, 237–238.
Thompson, M.D., Capra, V., Clunes, M.T., et al., 2016. Cysteinyl leukotrienes pathway genes, atopic asthma and drug response: from population isolates to large genome-wide association studies. Front. Pharmacol. 7, 1–17.
Thurmond, R.L., 2015. The histamine H4 receptor: from orphan to the clinic. Front. Pharmacol. 6, 65.
Travers, J.B., Rohan, J.G., Sahu, R.P., 2021. New insights into the pathologic roles of the platelet-activating factor system. Front. Endocrinol. (Lausanne) 12, 624132.
Urquhart, P., Nicolaou, A., Woodward, D.F., 2015. Endocannabinoids and their oxygenation by cyclo-oxygenases, lipoxygenases and other oxygenases. Biochim. Biophys. Acta 1851, 366–376.
Vilcek, J., Feldmann, M., 2004. Historical review: cytokines as therapeutics and targets of therapeutics. Trends Pharmacol. Sci. 25, 201–209.
Wang, W., Guo, D.Y., Lin, Y.J., et al., 2019. Melanocortin regulation of inflammation. Front. Endocrinol. (Lausanne) 10, 683.
Whalley, E.T., Figueroa, C.D., Gera, L., et al., 2012. Discovery and therapeutic potential of kinin receptor antagonists. Expert Opin. Drug Discov. 7, 1129–1148.
Woodward, D.F., Jones, R.L., Narumiya, S., 2011. International union of basic and clinical pharmacology. LXXXIII: classification of prostanoid receptors, updating 15 years of progress. Pharmacol. Rev. 63, 471–538.
Yanagisawa, M., Kurihara, H., Kimura, S., et al., 1988. A novel potent vasoconstrictor peptide produced by vascular endothelial cells. Nature 332, 411–415.
Yokomizo, T., Nakamura, M., Shimizu, T., 2018. Leukotriene receptors as potential therapeutic targets. J. Clin. Invest. 128, 2691–2701.
Zhang, M.J., Spite, M., 2012. Resolvins: anti-inflammatory and proresolving mediators derived from omega-3 polyunsaturated fatty acids. Annu. Rev. Nutr. 32, 203–227.

Books and other resources

Cameron, M.J., Kelvin, D.J., 2013. Cytokines, Chemokines and Their Receptors. Madame Curie Bioscience Database. Landes Bioscience, Austin, Texas.
Murphy, K.M., Weaver, C., 2016. Janeway's Immunobiology, ninth ed. Taylor & Francis, London.

18 Cannabinoids

OVERVIEW

Modern pharmacological interest in cannabinoids dates from the discovery that Δ⁹-tetrahydrocannabinol (THC) is the main psychoactive component of cannabis, and took off with the discovery of specific cannabinoid receptors – termed *CB receptors* – and endogenous ligands (endocannabinoids), together with mechanisms for their synthesis and elimination. There has been a recent surge of interest in the therapeutic potential of other cannabinoids, especially cannabidiol (CBD), which lacks the psychoactive properties of THC. Here we consider plant-derived cannabinoids, cannabinoid receptors, endocannabinoids, physiological functions, pathological mechanisms, synthetic ligands and potential clinical applications. More detailed information is given by Ligresti et al. (2016) and by Pertwee (2014, 2015). The pharmacology of cannabinoids in the central nervous system (CNS) is discussed in Chapters 39, 43, 46, 49 and 50.

PLANT-DERIVED CANNABINOIDS ('PHYTOCANNABINOIDS') AND THEIR PHARMACOLOGICAL EFFECTS

Cannabis sativa, the hemp plant, has been used for its psychoactive properties for thousands of years (see Ch. 49). Its medicinal use was advocated in antiquity, but serious interest resurfaced only in 1964 with the identification of *Δ⁹-tetrahydrocannabinol* (THC; Fig. 18.1) as the main psychoactive component. Cannabis extracts contain numerous related compounds, called phytocannabinoids, most of which are insoluble in water. The most abundant phytocannabinoids are THC, *cannabidiol* (CBD) and *cannabinol*, a breakdown product formed spontaneously from THC. CBD is said to lack the psychoactive properties of THC but CBD has anticonvulsant activity in preclinical models and has been licensed for some rare but serious forms of childhood epilepsy (see Ch. 46).

CBD and THC are synthesised by distinct biochemical pathways, but CBD can be converted to THC by cyclisation by artificially smoking cigarettes impregnated with CBD (Mikeš and Waser, 1971). It has recently been suggested that CBD can be converted to THC at temperatures occurring during vaping but this still needs to be verified and any in vivo consequences investigated.

A therapeutic effect of CBD has been claimed in a remarkably wide range of preclinical models of disease states outside its licensed indications ranging from cardiovascular disease, inflammation and autoimmunity to neurodegenerative disease, renal disease and malignancy, leading unfortunately to many poorly founded claims for efficacy in human disease (see Pacher et al., 2020, for a review). Rigorous controlled clinical trials are in short supply.

PHARMACOLOGICAL EFFECTS

THC acts mainly on the CNS, producing a mixture of psychotomimetic and depressant effects, together with various centrally mediated autonomic effects. The main subjective effects in humans consist of:

- Sensations of relaxation and well-being without the accompanying recklessness and aggression sometimes caused by excessive ethanol consumption: insensitivity to risk is an important feature of alcohol intoxication and is often a factor in road accidents. Cannabis users are less accident prone in general – although acute cannabis use impairs specific driving skills, and meta-analyses show that the risks for cannabis users of car crashes are slightly, but significantly, increased (reviewed by Preuss et al., 2021).
- Feelings of sharpened sensory awareness, with sounds and sights seeming more intense and fantastic.
- These effects are similar to, but usually less pronounced than, those produced by psychotomimetic drugs such as lysergic acid diethylamide (LSD; see Ch. 49). Subjects report that time passes extremely slowly. Acute effects include feelings of paranoia especially with higher doses, although less marked than with LSD. Epidemiological studies support a connection between heavy cannabis use in adolescence and subsequent psychiatric disorder (Rubino et al., 2012). It is difficult to distinguish whether this is due to an effect common to individuals in this age group rather than an effect that is specific for susceptible individuals.

Central effects that can be directly measured in human and animal studies include:

- impairment of short-term memory and simple learning tasks – subjective feelings of confidence and heightened creativity are not reflected in actual performance;
- impairment of motor coordination (e.g. driving performance);
- catalepsy – the adoption of fixed unnatural postures;
- hypothermia;
- analgesia;
- antiemetic action (see Ch. 30);
- increased appetite.

The main peripheral effects of cannabis are:

- tachycardia, which can be prevented by drugs that block sympathetic transmission;

- vasodilatation, which is particularly marked in superficial blood vessels of the eye (scleral and conjunctival vessels), producing a bloodshot appearance which is characteristic of cannabis smokers;
- reduction of intraocular pressure;
- bronchodilatation.

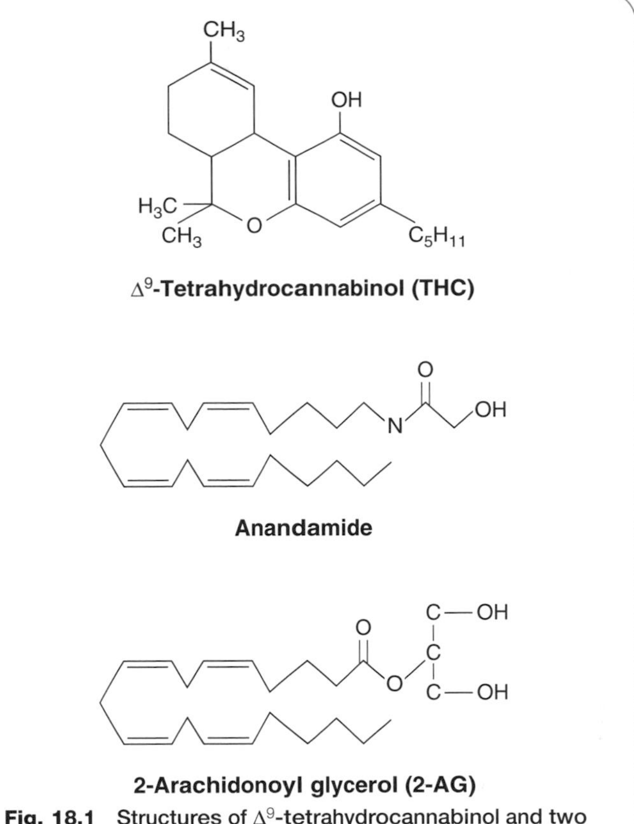

Fig. 18.1 Structures of Δ^9-tetrahydrocannabinol and two endocannabinoids.

Cannabis

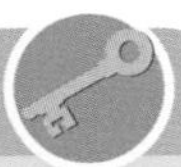

- The main psychoactive constituent is **Δ^9-tetrahydrocannabinol (THC)** which generates a pharmacologically active 11-hydroxy metabolite.
- Actions on the CNS include both depressant and psychotomimetic effects.
- Subjective experiences include euphoria and a feeling of relaxation, with sharpened sensory awareness.
- Objective tests show impairment of learning, memory and motor performance, including impaired driving ability.
- THC also shows analgesic and antiemetic activity, as well as causing catalepsy and hypothermia in animal tests.
- Peripheral actions include vasodilatation, reduction of intraocular pressure and bronchodilatation.
- Cannabinoids are less liable than opioids, **nicotine** or **alcohol** to cause dependence but may have long-term psychological effects.
- **CBD** lacks the psychoactive effects of THC but is therapeutic in some rare forms of childhood epilepsy and in a wide range of preclinical models of other diseases.

PHARMACOKINETIC ASPECTS

The effect of cannabis, taken by smoking, takes about 1 h to develop fully and lasts for 2–3 h. A small fraction of THC is converted to 11-hydroxy-THC, which is more active than THC itself and probably contributes to the pharmacological effect of smoking cannabis, but most is converted to inactive metabolites that are subject to conjugation and enterohepatic recirculation. Being highly lipophilic, THC and its metabolites are sequestered in body fat, and detectable urinary excretion continues for several weeks after a single dose.

ADVERSE EFFECTS

In acute overdose, THC is less dangerous than alcohol or opioids, producing drowsiness and confusion but not life-threatening respiratory or cardiovascular depression. Even in low doses, THC and synthetic derivatives such as **nabilone** (licensed for nausea and vomiting caused by cytotoxic chemotherapy, see later) produce euphoria and drowsiness, sometimes accompanied by sensory distortion and hallucinations. These effects, together with legal restrictions on the use of cannabis,[1] have limited the widespread therapeutic use of cannabinoids, although a cannabis extract administered by buccal spray has achieved regulatory approval in several countries as an adjunct in treating spasticity in multiple sclerosis.

In rodents, THC produces teratogenic and mutagenic effects, and an increased incidence of chromosome breaks in circulating white cells has been reported in humans. Such breaks are, however, by no means unique to cannabis, and epidemiological studies have not shown an increased risk of fetal malformation or cancer among cannabis users.

TOLERANCE AND DEPENDENCE

Tolerance to cannabis, and physical dependence, occurs only to a minor degree and mainly in heavy users. Abstinence symptoms that develop on cessation of cannabis use include nausea, agitation, irritability, confusion, tachycardia and sweating, but are relatively mild and do not result in a compulsive urge to take the drug. Psychological dependence does occur with cannabis, but it is less compelling than with the major drugs of abuse (see Ch. 50), although dependence is increasing in parallel with use of higher THC content material (Maldonado et al., 2011).

CANNABINOID RECEPTORS

Cannabinoids, being highly lipid-soluble, were originally thought to act through their physical properties when partitioned into lipid-rich neuronal membranes rather than by interaction with specific receptors. However, in 1988, saturable high-affinity binding of a tritiated cannabinoid was demonstrated in membranes prepared from homogenised rat brain. This led to the identification of specific cannabinoid

[1]Cannabis is now legal in Canada, Mexico, South Africa and Uruguay as well as in 18 states in the United States. Its use has been decriminalized in many countries (see https://en.wikipedia.org/wiki/Legality_of_cannabis#A), but not in some mid-Eastern and E Asian countries where long prison terms are imposed for possession of cannabis and related products.

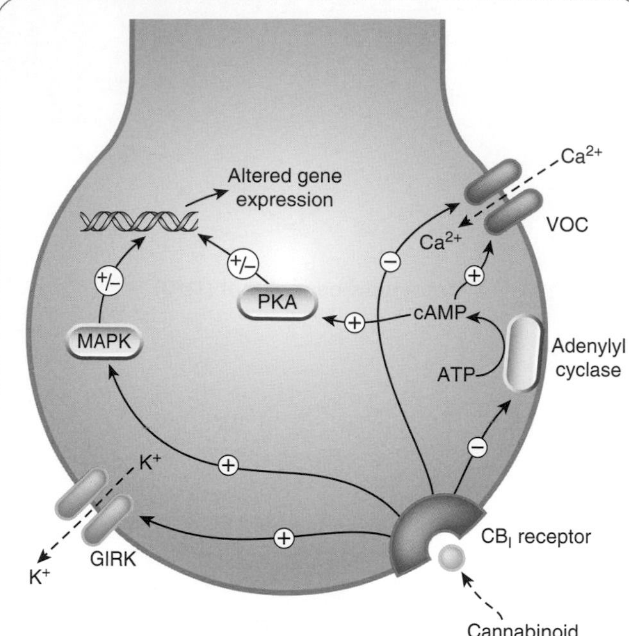

Fig. 18.2 Cellular actions of cannabinoids. CB_1 receptor activation inhibits neurotransmitter release via inhibition of Ca^{2+} entry and hyperpolarisation due to activation of potassium channels. It also alters gene expression. *GIRK*, G protein–sensitive inward-rectifying potassium channel; *MAPK*, mitogen-activated protein kinase; *PKA*, protein kinase A; *VOC*, voltage-operated calcium channel. (Redrawn from Devane, W.A., Hanu, L., Breurer, A., et al., 1992. Isolation and structure of a brain constituent that binds to the cannabinoid receptor. Science 258, 1946–1949.)

Table 18.1 Definite and possible endocannabinoids

Endocannabinoid	Selectivity
Definite endocannabinoids	
Anandamide	$CB_1 > CB_2$
2-Arachidonoyl glycerol	$CB_1 = CB_2$
Less well-established endocannabinoid candidates	
Virodhamine	$CB_2 > CB_1$
Noladin	$CB_1 \gg CB_2$
N-arachidonoyl dopamine	$CB_1 \gg CB_2$

receptors in the brain. These are now termed *CB_1 receptors* to distinguish them from the *CB_2 receptors* subsequently identified in peripheral tissues. Cannabinoid receptors are typical members of the family of G protein–coupled receptors (see Ch. 3). CB_1 receptors are linked via $G_{i/o}$ to inhibition of adenylyl cyclase and of voltage-operated calcium channels, and to activation of G protein–sensitive inwardly rectifying potassium (GIRK) channels, causing membrane hyperpolarisation (Fig. 18.2), effects similar to those mediated by opioid receptors (see Ch. 43), but with different anatomical distributions of CB_1 versus opioid receptors. CB_1 receptors are located in the plasma membrane of nerve endings and inhibit transmitter release from presynaptic terminals, which is triggered by depolarisation and Ca^{2+} entry (see Ch. 4). CB_1 receptors also influence gene expression, both directly by activating mitogen-activated protein kinase and indirectly by reducing the activity of protein kinase A as a result of reduced adenylyl cyclase activity (see Ch. 3).

CB_1 receptors are abundant in the brain, with numbers similar to those of receptors for glutamate and GABA – the main central excitatory and inhibitory neurotransmitters (see Ch. 38). They are not homogeneously distributed, being concentrated in the hippocampus (relevant to the effects of cannabinoids on memory), cerebellum (relevant to loss of coordination), hypothalamus (important in control of appetite and body temperature; see Ch. 32 and later), substantia nigra, mesolimbic dopamine pathways that have been implicated in psychological 'reward' (see Ch. 50) and in association areas of the cerebral cortex. There is a relative paucity of CB_1 receptors in the brain stem, consistent with the lack of serious depression of respiratory or cardiovascular function by cannabinoids. At a cellular level, CB_1 receptors are mainly localised presynaptically, and inhibit transmitter release, as depicted in Fig. 18.2. Like opioids, they can, however, increase the activity of some neuronal pathways by disinhibition (see Chs 37 and 43), that is by inhibiting inhibitory connections, including GABA-ergic interneurons in the hippocampus and amygdala.

In addition to their well-recognised location in the CNS, CB_1 receptors are also expressed in peripheral tissues, for example on endothelial cells, adipocytes and peripheral nerves. Cannabinoids promote lipogenesis through activation of CB_1 receptors, an action that could contribute to their effect on body weight (see DiPatrizio and Piomele, 2012).

The CB_2 receptor has only approximately 45% amino acid homology with CB_1 and is located mainly in lymphoid tissue (spleen, tonsils and thymus as well as circulating lymphocytes, monocytes and tissue mast cells). CB_2 receptors are also present on microglia – immune cells in the CNS which, when activated, contribute to chronic pain (see Ch. 43). The localisation of CB_2 receptors on cells of the immune system was unexpected but may account for inhibitory effects of cannabis on immune function. CB_2 receptors differ from CB_1 receptors in their responsiveness to cannabinoid ligands (see Table 18.1). They are linked via $G_{i/o}$ to adenylyl cyclase, GIRK channels and mitogen-activated protein kinase similarly to CB_1, but not to voltage-operated calcium channels (which are not expressed in immune cells). So far, rather little is known about their function. They are present in atherosclerotic lesions (see Ch. 22), and CB_2 agonists have potentially anti-atherosclerotic effects on macrophages and foam cells (Chiurchiu et al., 2014). The contrasting cardiovascular effects of CB_1 and CB_2 pathways are reviewed by Pacher et al. (2018).

Some endocannabinoids turned out, surprisingly,[2] to bind to sites on the cytoplasmic side of transient receptor potential channels (TRP channels), activating these ionotropic receptors and thereby stimulating nociceptive nerve endings (see Ch. 43). Other as-yet-unidentified G protein–coupled receptors are also implicated, because cannabinoids exhibit analgesic actions and activate G proteins in the brain of CB_1 knock-out mice, despite the absence of CB_1 receptors.

[2]Surprising, because capsaicin, the active principle of chili peppers, causes intense burning pain via activation of these receptors, whereas the endocannabinoid anandamide is associated with pleasure, or even bliss…so perhaps not so surprising after all!

ENDOCANNABINOIDS

The discovery of specific cannabinoid receptors led to a search for endogenous mediators. The first success was chalked up by a team that screened fractions of extracted pig brain for ability to compete with a radiolabelled cannabinoid receptor ligand (Devane et al., 1992). This led to the purification of N-*arachidonylethanolamide*, an eicosanoid mediator (see Ch. 17), the structure of which is shown in Fig. 18.1. This was christened *anandamide*.[3] Anandamide not only displaced labelled cannabinoid from synaptosomal membranes in the binding assay, but also inhibited nerve evoked twitches of mouse vas deferens, a bioassay for CB_1 receptor ligands (Fig. 18.3). A few years later, a second endocannabinoid, *2-arachidonoyl glycerol* (2-AG, see Fig. 18.1), was identified, and more recently at least three further endocannabinoid candidates – all arachidonic acid derivatives – with distinct CB_1/CB_2 receptor selectivities have been added to the list (see Table 18.1). Endocannabinoids are made 'on demand', like other eicosanoids (see Ch. 17), rather than being presynthesised and stored for release when needed.

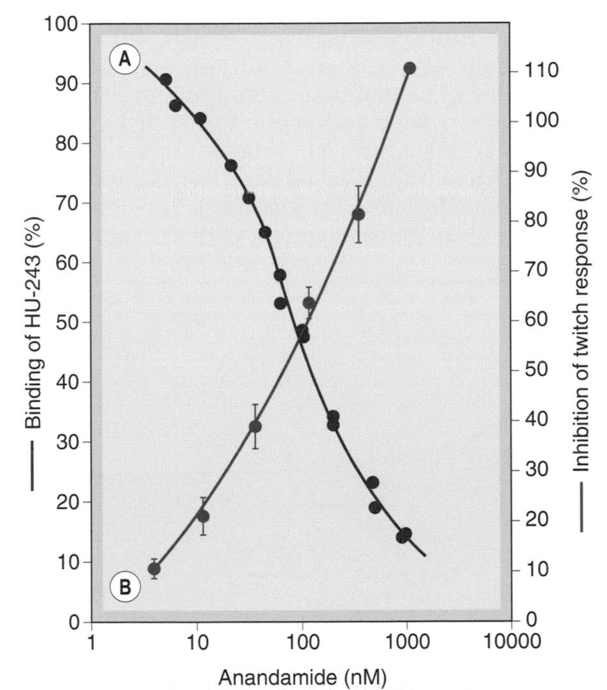

Fig. 18.3 Anandamide as an endocannabinoid. Anandamide is an endogenous cannabinoid. (A) Competitive inhibition of tritiated HU-243 (a cannabinoid receptor ligand) binding to synaptosomal membranes from rat brain by natural anandamide *(red circles, left-hand ordinate axis)*. (B) Inhibition of vas deferens twitch response (a bioassay for cannabinoids) by natural anandamide *(blue symbols, right-hand ordinate)*. Note the concordance between the binding and bioactivity. (Redrawn from Devane, W.A., Hanu, L., Breurer, A., et al., 1992. Isolation and structure of a brain constituent that binds to the cannabinoid receptor. Science 258, 1946–1949.)

[3]From a Sanskrit word meaning 'bliss' + amide.

BIOSYNTHESIS OF ENDOCANNABINOIDS

The biosynthesis of anandamide and of 2-AG is summarised in Fig. 18.4. A fuller account of biosynthesis and degradation is given by Di Marzo (2008).

Anandamide is formed by a distinct phospholipase D (PLD) selective for *N*-acyl-phosphatidylethanolamine (NAPE) but with low affinity for other membrane phospholipids, and is known as NAPE-PLD. NAPE-PLD is a zinc metallohydrolase that is stimulated by Ca^{2+} and also by polyamines. Selective inhibitors for NAPE-PLD are being sought. The precursors are produced by an as-yet-uncharacterised but Ca^{2+}-sensitive transacylase that transfers an acyl group from the *sn*-1 position of phospholipids to the nitrogen atom of phosphatidylethanolamine.

2-AG is also produced by hydrolysis of precursors derived from phospholipid metabolism. The key enzymes are two *sn*-1-selective diacylglycerol lipases (DAGL-α and DAGL-β), which belong to the family of serine lipases. Both these enzymes, like NAPE-PLD, are Ca^{2+} sensitive, consistent with intracellular Ca^{2+} acting as the physiological stimulus to endocannabinoid synthesis. The DAGLs are located presynaptically in axons during fetal development, but postsynaptically in dendrites and neuron cell bodies in adult brain. This is consistent with a role for 2-AG in neurite growth, and with a role as a retrograde mediator (see later) in adults.

Little is known about the biosynthesis of the more recent endocannabinoid candidates noladin, virodhamine and *N*-arachidonoyl dopamine. pH-dependent non-enzymatic interconversion of virodhamine and anandamide is one possibility and could result in a switch between CB_2- and CB_1-mediated responses (see Table 18.1).

TERMINATION OF THE ENDOCANNABINOID SIGNAL

Endocannabinoids are rapidly taken up from the extracellular space. Being lipid-soluble, they diffuse through plasma membranes down a concentration gradient. There is also evidence for a saturable, temperature-dependent, facilitated transport mechanism for anandamide and 2-AG, dubbed the 'endocannabinoid membrane transporter', for which selective uptake inhibitors (e.g. UCM-707) have been developed. Pathways of endocannabinoid metabolism are summarised in Fig. 18.4. The key enzyme for anandamide metabolism is a microsomal serine hydrolase known as fatty acid amide hydrolase (FAAH). FAAH converts anandamide to arachidonic acid plus ethanolamine and also hydrolyses 2-AG, yielding arachidonic acid and glycerol.

The phenotype of FAAH 'knock-out' mice gives some clues to endocannabinoid physiology; such mice have an increased brain content of anandamide and an increased pain threshold. Selective inhibitors of FAAH[4] have analgesic and anxiolytic properties in mice (see Ch. 45 for an explanation of how drugs are tested for anxiolytic properties in rodents). In contrast to anandamide, brain content of 2-AG is not increased in FAAH knock-out

[4]Several such drugs have been administered to humans (van Egmond et al., 2021). One drug, BIA 10-2474, caused severe CNS damage during a trial involving repeated dosing of healthy volunteers in Rennes, France. BIA 10-2474 is less selective than another FAAH inhibitor which was innocuous in earlier trials, inhibiting several lipases that are not targeted by the more selective drug. This suggests that promiscuous lipase inhibitors can cause metabolic dysregulation in the nervous system due to off-target toxicity (see van Esbroeck et al., 2017).

animals, indicating that another route of metabolism of 2-AG such as via monoacylglycerol lipase (MAGL; Fig 18.4) is likely to be important. Endocannabinoid pharmacology suggests that inhibitors of FAAH and/or of MAGL might have therapeutically useful effects in a wide range of disease states and several have been investigated in humans but thus far without positive outcomes (reviewed by van Egmond et al., 2021). Other possible routes of metabolism include esterification, acylation and oxidation by cyclo-oxygenase-2 to prostaglandin ethanolamides ('prostamides'), or by 12- or 15-lipoxygenase (see Ch. 17).

PHYSIOLOGICAL MECHANISMS

Stimuli that release endocannabinoids, leading to activation of CB_1 receptors and the linkage to downstream events including behavioural or psychological effects, are incompletely defined. Increased intracellular Ca^{2+} concentration is probably an important cellular trigger because, as mentioned earlier, Ca^{2+} activates NAPE-PLD and other enzymes involved in endocannabinoid biosynthesis.

Activation of CB_1 receptors is implicated in a phenomenon known as *depolarisation-induced suppression of inhibition* (DSI). DSI occurs in hippocampal pyramidal cells; when these are depolarised by an excitatory input, this suppresses the GABA-mediated inhibitory input to the pyramidal cells, implying a retrograde flow of information from the depolarised pyramidal cell to inhibitory axons terminating on it. Such a reverse flow of information from post- to presynaptic cell is a feature of other instances of neuronal plasticity, such as 'wind-up' in nociceptive pathways (see Fig. 43.2) and long-term potentiation in the hippocampus (see Figs 38.3 and 38.6). DSI is blocked by the CB_1 antagonist **rimonabant.** The presynaptic location of CB_1 receptors and cellular distributions of the DAGL and monoacyl glycerol lipase (MAGL) enzymes mentioned earlier (and see Fig. 18.4) fit nicely with the idea that the endocannabinoid 2-AG is a 'retrograde' messenger in DSI.

The neuromodulatory actions of endocannabinoids could influence a wide range of physiological activities, including nociception, cardiovascular, respiratory and gastrointestinal function. Interactions of endocannabinoids with hypothalamic hormones are believed to influence food intake and reproductive function. Mouse models lacking CB receptor subtypes (CB_1 or CB_2) support important and balanced roles of endocannabinoid signalling in male and female fertility. Such signalling is implicated in spermatogenesis, fertilisation, preimplantation development of the early embryo, implantation and postimplantation growth of the embryo (each receptor subtype is involved in specific aspects, see Battista et al., 2012). The effects of endocannabinoids on food intake (and phytocannabinoids: a strong desire for food following cannabis consumption is known colloquially as the 'munchies') are of particular interest, because of the importance of obesity (see Ch. 32).

PATHOLOGICAL INVOLVEMENT

There is evidence, both from experimental animals and from human tissue, that endocannabinoid signalling is abnormal in multiple sclerosis (see Ch. 40) and other neurodegenerative diseases. Other diseases where abnormalities of cannabinoid signalling are implicated include haemorrhagic and septic forms of hypotensive shock (see Ch. 21), advanced cirrhosis of the liver (where there is evidence that vasodilatation is mediated by endocannabinoids acting on vascular CB_1 receptors – see Bátkai et al., 2001), miscarriage (see Battista et al., 2012) and

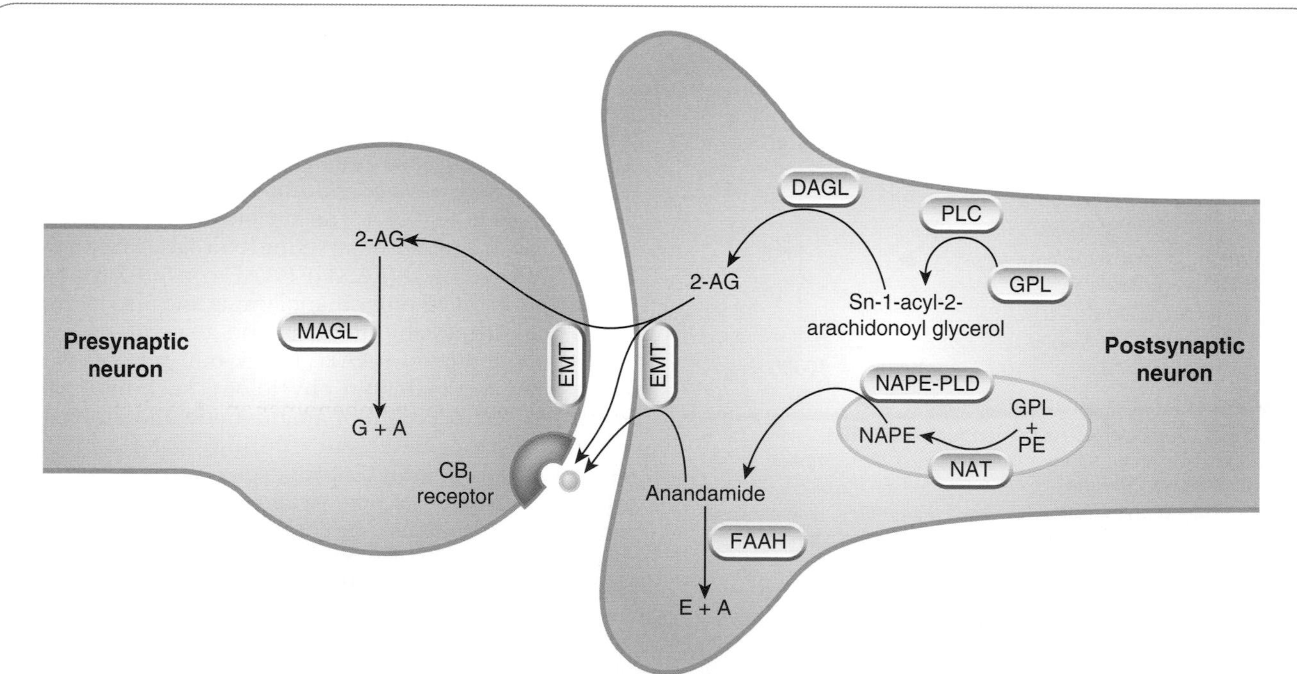

Fig. 18.4 Biosynthesis and inactivation of endocannabinoids. *2-AG,* 2-arachidonoyl glycerol; *A,* arachidonic acid; *DAGL,* diacylglycerol lipase; *E,* ethanolamine; *EMT,* endocannabinoid membrane transporter; *FAAH,* fatty acid amide hydrolase; *G,* glycerol; *GPL,* glycerophospholipid; *MAGL,* monoacyl glycerol lipase; *NAPE, N*-acyl-phosphatidylethanolamine; *NAPE-PLD, N*-acyl phosphatidylethanolamine-specific phospholipase D; *NAT, N*-acyl-transferase; *PE,* phosphatidylethanolamine; *PLC,* phospholipase C.

The endocannabinoid system

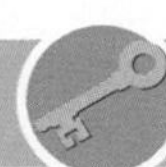

- Cannabinoid receptors (CB_1, CB_2) are G protein–coupled ($G_{i/o}$) receptors.
- CB_1 receptors are located especially on presynaptic nerve terminals. They are abundant in the CNS but not in the brainstem.
- Activation of CB_1 inhibits adenylyl cyclase and plasma membrane calcium channels, and activates potassium channels, inhibiting synaptic transmission.
- The CB_2 receptor is expressed in cells of the immune system, and its expression is also upregulated in the CNS in some pathological conditions.
- Selective agonists and antagonists have been developed for both CB_1 and CB_2 receptors.
- Endogenous ligands for CB receptors are known as endocannabinoids. They are eicosanoid mediators (see Ch. 17).
- The best-established endocannabinoids are anandamide and 2-arachidonoyl glycerol (2-AG), which have many roles and can function as 'retrograde' mediators passing information from postsynaptic to presynaptic neurons for example in DSI in hippocampal pyramidal neurons.
- The main enzyme that inactivates anandamide is FAAH.
- An 'endocannabinoid membrane transporter' transports cannabinoids from postsynaptic neurons, where they are synthesised, to the synaptic cleft, where they access presynaptic CB_1 receptors, and into presynaptic terminals, where 2-AG is metabolised.
- FAAH 'knock-out' mice have an increased brain content of anandamide and an increased pain threshold; selective inhibitors of FAAH have analgesic and anxiolytic properties, implicating endocannabinoids in nociception and anxiety.

malignant disease. It seems likely that endocannabinoid activation evolved as a protective mechanism but can become 'too much of a good thing' and actually contribute to disease progression. Consequently, there may be a place in therapeutics for drugs that potentiate or inhibit the cannabinoid system (see Pertwee, 2015, for a fuller discussion).

SYNTHETIC CANNABINOIDS

Cannabinoid receptor agonists were developed in the 1970s in the hope that they would prove useful non-opioid/non-NSAID (non-steroidal anti-inflammatory drug) analgesics (cf. Chs 43 and 25, respectively, for limitations of opioids and NSAIDs), but adverse effects, particularly sedation and memory impairment, were problematic. Nevertheless, one such drug, **nabilone**, is sometimes used clinically to reduce nausea and vomiting caused by cytotoxic chemotherapy if this is unresponsive to conventional antiemetics (see Ch. 30). Furthermore, synthetic cannabinoid receptor agonists (SCRAs; sometimes referred to as 'spice') have become major drugs of abuse especially amongst the homeless population and those in prison (see Ch. 49). The cloning of CB_2 receptors, and their absence from healthy neuronal brain cells, led to the synthesis of CB_2-selective agonists in the hope that these would lack the CNS-related adverse effects of plant cannabinoids. Several such drugs are being investigated for possible use in inflammatory and neuropathic pain.

The first selective CB_1 receptor antagonist, **rimonabant**, also has inverse agonist properties in some systems. It was licensed in Europe for treating obesity, and there were hopes that it would help promote abstinence from tobacco, but it was withdrawn because it caused psychiatric problems including depression. Synthetic inhibitors of endocannabinoid uptake and/or metabolism have shown potentially useful effects in animal models of pain, epilepsy, multiple sclerosis, Parkinson's disease, anxiety and diarrhoea.

In addition to central CB_1 receptors, hepatocyte CB_1 receptors are also implicated in obesity and in non-alcoholic fatty liver disease, and research on selective peripheral antagonists and allosteric modulators is encouraging (Nguyen et al., 2019; Rohbeck et al., 2021).

CLINICAL APPLICATIONS

Clinical uses of drugs that act on the cannabinoid system remain controversial, but in both the United Kingdom and the United States, cannabinoids have been used as antiemetics and to encourage weight gain in patients with chronic disease such as HIV/AIDS and malignancy. Cannabis extract (**nabiximols** – which contains similar amounts of THC and CBD) is used to treat spasticity, neuropathic pain and other symptoms in patients with multiple sclerosis (see Borgelt et al., 2013). Adverse events are generally mild at the doses used. Endocannabinoids have been implicated in shock and hypotension in liver disease (Malinowska et al., 2008), and modulation of this system is a potential therapeutic target. Prescription formulations of CBD are now licensed for treatment of Dravet's syndrome, Lennox-Gastaut syndrome and seizures caused by tuberous sclerosis, rare and horrible diseases of infants where uncontrollable seizures are both a symptom of disease and, via the phenomenon of excitotoxicity (see Ch. 40), causes of disease progression. A study from the group of Julius Axelrod in 1998 showed that both CBD and THC possessed neuroprotective antioxidant properties (Hampson et al., 1998), so there is enormous general interest in the long-term outcome of such treatment. Other potential clinical uses are given in the following 'Potential and actual clinical uses of cannabinoids' box.

Potential and actual clinical uses of cannabinoids

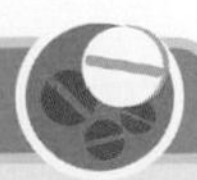

Cannabis extract (nabiximols, containing CBD and THC) is licensed as an adjunct for experts treating spasticity in multiple sclerosis.

CBD is licensed for treatment of Dravet's syndrome, Lennox-Gastaut syndrome and tuberous sclerosis complex – rare neurological diseases of infants associated with intractable seizures.

Nabilone, a synthetic cannabinoid agonist is licensed for nausea/vomiting associated with cancer chemotherapy

Cannabinoid-related drugs are undergoing evaluation for a wide range of possible indications, including:

- Agonists:
  - cancer and AIDS (to reduce weight loss)
  - neuropathic pain
  - head injury
  - glaucoma
  - Tourette syndrome (to reduce tics – rapid involuntary movements that are a feature of this disorder)
  - Parkinson's disease (to reduce involuntary movements caused as an adverse effect of **levodopa**; see Ch. 40)
- CBD
  - seizure disorders
  - anxiety
  - drug and alcohol dependence
- Antagonists:
  - obesity
  - tobacco dependence
  - drug addiction
  - alcoholism.

REFERENCES AND FURTHER READING

General reading

Freund, T.F., Katona, I., Piomelli, D., 2003. Role of endogenous cannabinoids in synaptic signaling. Physiol. Rev. 83, 1017–1066.

Ligresti, A., de Petrocellis, L., di Marzo, V., 2016. From phytocannabinoids to cannabinoid receptors and endocannabinoids: pleiotropic physiological and pathological roles through complex pharmacology. Physiol. Rev. 96, 1593–1659.

Pertwee, R.G. (Ed.), 2014. Handbook of Cannabis (Handbooks of Psychopharmacology). Oxford University Press, Oxford.

Pertwee, R.G. (Ed.), 2015. Endocannabinoids and Their Pharmacological Actions (Handbook of Experimental Pharmacology). Springer International Publications, Switzerland.

Specific aspects

Bátkai, S., Járai, Z., Wagner, J.A., et al., 2001. Endocannabinoids acting at vascular CB_1 receptors mediate the vasodilated state in advanced liver cirrhosis. Nat. Med. 7, 827–832.

Battista, N., Meccariello, R., Cobellis, G., 2012. The role of endocannabinoids in gonadal function and fertility along the evolutionary axis. Mol. Cell. Endocrinol. 355, 1–14.

Benyo, Z., Ruisanchez, E., Leszl-Ishiguro, M., 2016. Endocannabinoids in cerebrovascular regulation. Am. J. Physiol. Heart Circ. Physiol. 310, H785–H801.

Borgelt, L.M., Franson, K.L., Nussbaum, A.M., Wang, G.S., 2013. The pharmacologic and clinical effects of medical cannabis. Pharmacotherapy 33, 195–209.

Chiurchiu, V., Lanuti, M., Catanzaro, G., et al., 2014. Detailed characterization of the endocannabinoid system in human macrophages and foam cells, and anti-inflammatory role of type-2 cannabinoid receptor. Atherosclerosis 233, 55–63.

Devane, W.A., Hanu, L., Breurer, A., et al., 1992. Isolation and structure of a brain constituent that binds to the cannabinoid receptor. Science 258, 1946–1949.

Di Marzo, V., 2008. Endocannabinoids: synthesis and degradation. Rev. Physiol. Biochem. Pharmacol. 160, 1–24.

Di Marzo, V., Petrosino, S., 2007. Endocannabinoids and the regulation of their levels in health and disease. Curr. Opin. Lipidol. 18, 129–140.

DiPatrizio, N.V., Piomele, D., 2012. The thrifty lipids: endocannabinoids and the neural control of energy conservation. Trends Neurosci. 35, 403–411.

Hampson, A.J., Grimaldi, M., Axelrod, J., Wink, D., 1998. Cannabidiol and (-) D^9-tetrahydrocannabinol are neuroprotective antioxidants. Proc. Natl. Acad. Sci. USA 95, 8268–8273.

Karst, M., Salim, K., Burstein, S., et al., 2003. Analgesic effect of the synthetic cannabinoid CT-3 on chronic neuropathic pain. A randomized controlled trial. JAMA 290, 1757–1762.

Maldonado, R., Berrendero, F., Ozaita, A., et al., 2011. Neurochemical basis of cannabis addiction. Neuroscience 181, 1–17.

Malinowska, B., Lupinski, S., Godlewski, G., et al., 2008. Role of endocannabinoids in cardiovascular shock. J. Physiol. Pharmacol. 59, 91–107.

Mikeš, F., Waser, P., 1971. Marihuana components: effects of smoking on D^9-tetrahydrocannabinol and cannabidiol. Science 172, 1158–1159.

Nguyen, T., Thomas, B.F., Zhang, Y.N., 2019. Overcoming the psychiatric side effects of the cannabinoid CB1 receptor antagonists: current approaches for therapeutics development. Curr. Top. Med. Chem. 19, 1418–1435.

Pacher, P., Kogan, N.M., Mechoulam, R., 2020. Beyond THC and endocannabinoids. Annu. Rev. Pharmacol. Toxicol. 60, 637–659.

Pacher, P., Steffens, S., Hasko, G., et al., 2018. Cardiovascular effects of marijuana and synthetic cannabinoids: the good, the bad, and the ugly. Nat. Rev. Cardiol. 15, 151–166.

Preuss, U.,W., Huestis, M.A., Schneider, M., et al., 2021. Cannabis use and car crashes: a review. Front. Psychiatry 12, 643315.

Rohbeck, E., Eckel, J., Romacho, T., 2021. Cannabinoid receptors in metabolic regulation and diabetes. Physiology 36, 102–113.

Rubino, T., Zamberletti, E., Parolaro, D., 2012. Adolescent exposure to cannabis as a risk factor for psychiatric disorders. J. Psychopharmacol. 26, SI177–SI188.

Steffens, S., 2005. Low dose oral cannabinoid therapy reduces progression of atherosclerosis in mice. Nature 434, 782–786.

Taber, K.H., Hurley, R.A., 2009. Endocannabinoids: stress, anxiety and fear. J. Neuropsychiat. Clin. Neurosci. 21, 108–113.

UK MS Research Group, 2003. Cannabinoids for treatment of spasticity and other symptoms related to multiple sclerosis (CAMS study): multicentre randomised placebo-controlled trial. Lancet 362, 1517–1526.

van Egmond, N., Straub, V.M., van der Stelt, M., 2021. Targeting endocannabinoid signaling: FAAH and MAG lipase inhibitors. Annu. Rev. Pharmacol. Toxicol. 61, 441–461.

van Esbroeck, A.C.M., Janssen, A.P.A., Cognetta III, A.B., et al., 2017. Activity-based protein profiling reveals off-target proteins of the FAAH inhibitor BIA 10-2474. Science 356, 1084–1087.

19 Nitric oxide and related mediators

OVERVIEW

Nitric oxide (NO) is a ubiquitous mediator with diverse functions. It is generated from L-arginine by NO synthase (NOS), an enzyme that occurs in endothelial, neuronal and inducible isoforms. In this chapter, we concentrate on general aspects of NO, especially its biosynthesis, degradation and effects. We touch on evidence that it can act as a circulating as well as local mediator and conclude with a brief consideration of the therapeutic potential of drugs that act on the L-arginine/NO pathway. Other gaseous mediators (carbon monoxide, hydrogen sulfide)[1] are described briefly: while they have yet to yield therapeutic drugs, their pathways are possible drug targets.

INTRODUCTION

NO, a free radical gas, is formed in the atmosphere during lightning storms. Less dramatically, but with far-reaching biological consequences, it is also formed in an enzyme-catalysed reaction between molecular oxygen and L-arginine. The convergence of several lines of research led to the realisation that NO is a key signalling molecule in the cardiovascular and nervous systems, and that it has a role in host defence.

A physiological function of NO emerged when biosynthesis of this gas was shown to account for the *endothelium-derived relaxing factor* described by Furchgott and Zawadzki (1980) (Figs 19.1 and 19.2). NO is the endogenous activator of soluble guanylyl cyclase, leading to the formation of cyclic guanosine monophosphate (cGMP), an important 'second messenger' (see Ch. 3) in many cells, including neurons, smooth muscle, monocytes and platelets. Nitrogen and oxygen are neighbours in the periodic table, and NO shares several properties with O_2, in particular a high affinity for haem and other iron–sulfur groups. This is important for activation of guanylyl cyclase, which contains a haem group, for the inactivation of NO by haemoglobin and for the regulation of diffusion of NO from endothelial cells (which express the alpha chain of haemoglobin) to vascular smooth muscle.

The role of NO in specific settings is described in other chapters: the endothelium in Chapter 21, the autonomic nervous system (see Ch. 13) and as a chemical transmitter and mediator of excitotoxicity in the central nervous system (CNS) in Chapters 37–39. Therapeutic uses of organic nitrates and of nitroprusside (NO donors) are described in Chapters 20 and 21.

[1]The pure substances (NO, CO and H_2S) are gases at room temperature and usual atmospheric pressure, and when pure NO is administered therapeutically (see later), it is in the form of a gas; when formed endogenously, the gases are, of course, dissolved in intra- and extracellular fluids.

BIOSYNTHESIS OF NITRIC OXIDE AND ITS CONTROL

NOS enzymes are central to the control of NO biosynthesis. There are three isoforms: an *inducible* form (iNOS or NOS2) which is expressed in macrophages and Kupffer cells, neutrophils, fibroblasts, vascular smooth muscle and endothelial cells in response to pathological stimuli such as invading microorganisms (e.g. during sepsis, severe organ dysfunction leading to circulatory shock – see Ch. 21 – due to a dysregulated host response to infection); and two *constitutive* forms, which are present under physiological conditions in endothelium (eNOS or NOS3)[2] and in neurons (nNOS or NOS1).[3] The constitutive enzymes generate small amounts of NO, whereas NOS2 produces much greater amounts, both because of its high activity and because of its abundance in pathological states associated with cytokine release. All three NOS isoenzymes are dimeric flavoproteins, contain tetrahydrobiopterin and have homology with cytochrome P450.

The activity of constitutive isoforms of NOS is controlled by intracellular calcium–calmodulin (Fig. 19.3). L-Arginine, the substrate of NOS, is usually present in excess in endothelial cell cytoplasm, so the rate of production of NO is determined by the activity of the enzyme rather than by substrate availability. Nevertheless, very high doses of L-arginine can restore endothelial NO biosynthesis in some pathological states (e.g. hypercholesterolaemia) in which endothelial function is impaired. Possible explanations for this paradox include:

- compartmentation: i.e. existence of a distinct pool of substrate in a cell compartment with access to NOS, which can become depleted despite apparently plentiful total cytoplasmic arginine concentrations;
- competition by high concentrations of L-arginine with endogenous competitive inhibitors of NOS such as *asymmetric dimethylarginine* (ADMA; see later and Fig. 19.4), which is elevated in plasma from patients with hypercholesterolaemia;
- recoupling of electron transfer to L-arginine.

Control of constitutive NOS activity by calcium–calmodulin is exerted in two ways:

1. Many endothelium-dependent agonists (e.g. acetylcholine, bradykinin, substance P) increase the cytoplasmic concentration of calcium ions $[Ca^{2+}]_i$;

[2]NOS3 is not restricted to endothelium. It is also present in cardiac myocytes, renal mesangial cells, osteoblasts and osteoclasts, airway epithelium and, in small amounts, platelets, so the term *eNOS* is somewhat misleading.

[3]It is possible that some of the NO made in healthy animals under basal conditions is derived from the action of NOS2, just as the inducible form of cyclo-oxygenase is active under basal conditions (Ch. 17) – whether this is because there is some NOS2 expressed even when there is no pathology or because there is enough 'pathology' in healthy mammals, for example in relation to gut microflora, to induce it is a moot point.

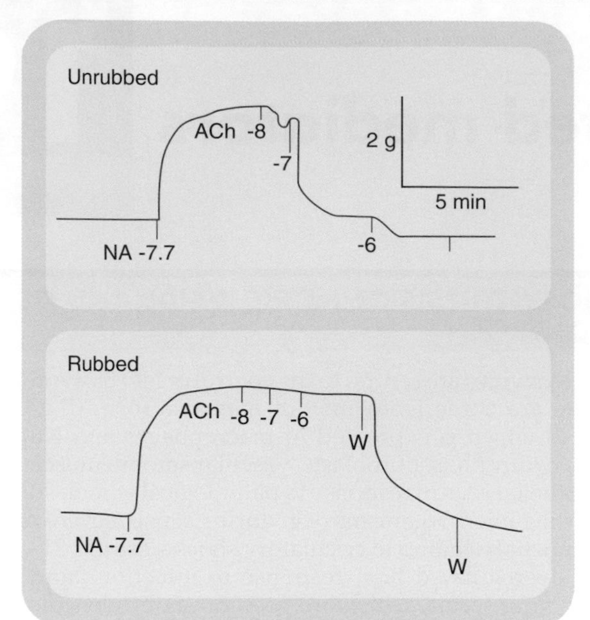

Fig. 19.1 Endothelium-derived relaxing factor. Acetylcholine (ACh) relaxes a strip of rabbit aorta precontracted with noradrenaline (NA) if the endothelium is intact *('unrubbed': upper panel)*, but not if it has been removed by gentle rubbing *('rubbed': lower panel)*. The numbers are logarithms of molar concentrations of drugs. (From Furchgott, R.F., Zawadzki, J.V., 1980. The obligatory role of endothelial cells in the relaxation of arterial smooth muscle by acetylcholine. Nature 288, 3734.)

the consequent increase in calcium–calmodulin activates NOS1 and NOS3.

2. Phosphorylation of specific residues on NOS3 controls its sensitivity to calcium–calmodulin; this can alter NO synthesis in the absence of any change in $[Ca^{2+}]_i$.

Shear stress is an important physiological stimulus to endothelial NO synthesis in resistance vessels. This is sensed by endothelial mechanoreceptors and transduced via a serine–threonine protein kinase called Akt (see Ch. 3) which is also known as protein kinase B. Agonists that increase cAMP in endothelial cells (e.g. β_2-adrenoceptor agonists) increase NOS3 activity, via protein kinase A–mediated phosphorylation[4] whereas protein kinase C *reduces* NOS3 activity by phosphorylating residues in the calmodulin-binding domain, thereby reducing the binding of calmodulin. Insulin increases NOS3 activity via tyrosine kinase activation (and also increases the expression of NOS1 in diabetic mice).

In contrast to constitutive NOS isoforms, the activity of NOS2 is effectively independent of $[Ca^{2+}]_i$, being fully activated even at the low values of $[Ca^{2+}]_i$ present under resting conditions. The enzyme is induced by bacterial lipopolysaccharide and inflammatory cytokines, notably interferon-γ, the antiviral effect of which is due to this. Tumour necrosis factor-α and interleukin-1 do not alone induce NOS2, but they each synergise with interferon-γ in this regard (see Ch. 17). Induction of NOS2 is inhibited by glucocorticoids and by several cytokines, including

[4]As explained in Chapter 4, β_2 agonists also act directly on smooth muscle cells, causing relaxation via cAMP.

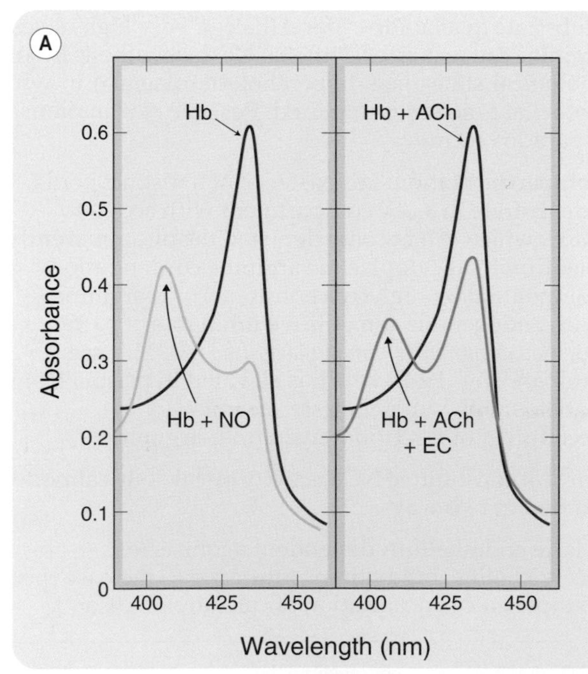

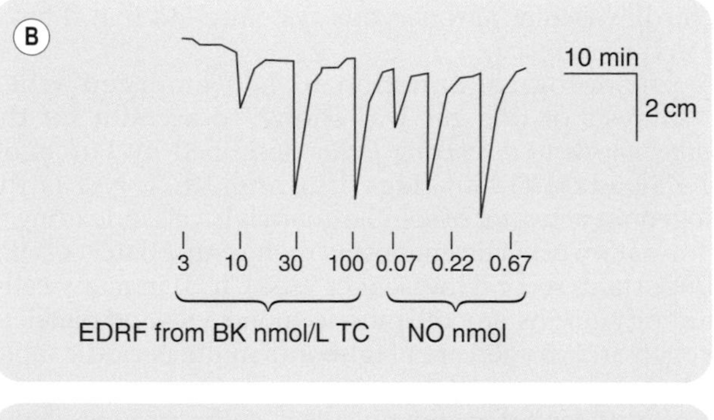

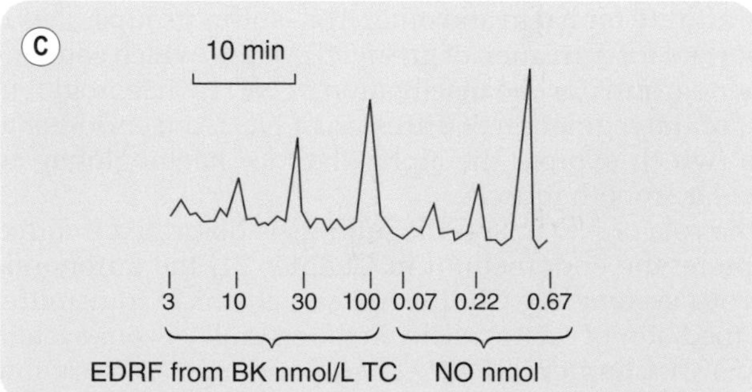

Fig. 19.2 Endothelium-derived relaxing factor (EDRF) is closely related to nitric oxide (NO). (A) EDRF released from aortic endothelial cells (EC) by acetylcholine (ACh) *(right panel)* has the same effect on the absorption spectrum of deoxyhaemoglobin (Hb) as does authentic NO *(left panel)*. (B) EDRF is released from a column of cultured ECs by bradykinin (BK; 3–100 nmol) applied through the column of cells (TC) and relaxes a de-endothelialised precontracted bioassay strip, as does authentic NO (upper trace). (C) A chemical assay of NO based on chemiluminescence shows that similar concentrations of NO are present in the EDRF released from the column of cells as in equiactive authentic NO solutions. (From Ignarro, L.J., Byrns, R.E., Buga, G.M., et al., 1987. Circ. Res. 61, 866–879; and Palmer, R.M.J., Ferrige, A.G., Moncada, S., et al., 1987. Nature 327, 524–526.)

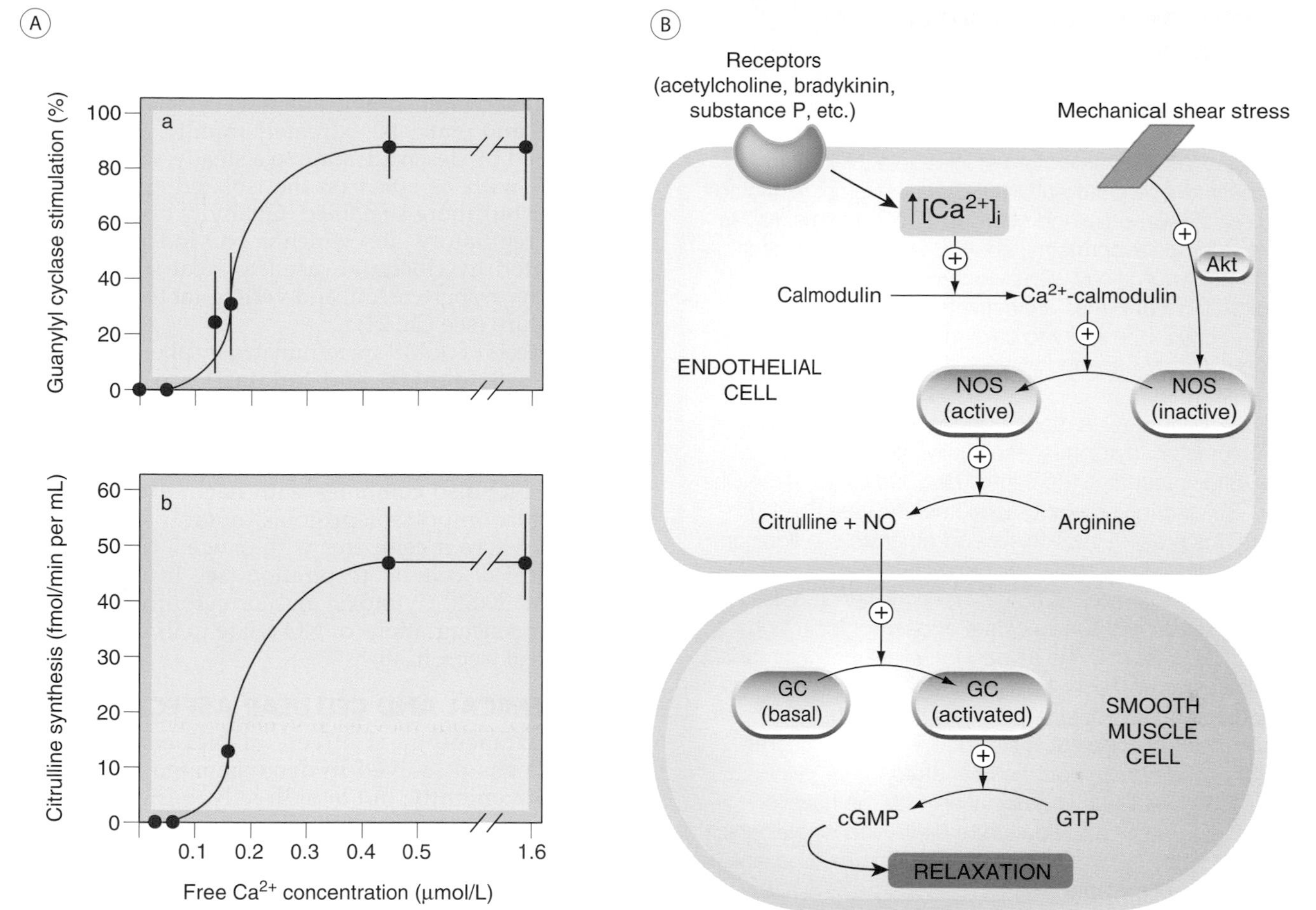

Fig. 19.3 Control of constitutive nitric oxide synthase (NOS) by calcium–calmodulin. (A) Dependence on Ca^{2+} of nitric oxide (NO) and citrulline synthesis from L-arginine by rat brain synaptosomal cytosol. Rates of synthesis of NO from L-arginine were determined by stimulation of guanylyl cyclase (GC) *(upper panel)* or by synthesis of [^{3}H]-citrulline from L-[^{3}H]-arginine *(lower panel)*. (B) Regulation of GC in smooth muscle by NO formed in adjacent endothelium. Akt is a protein kinase that phosphorylates NOS, making it more sensitive to calcium–calmodulin. (Panel [A] from Knowles, R.G., et al., 1989. Proc. Natl. Acad. Sci. U. S. A. 86, 5159–5162.)

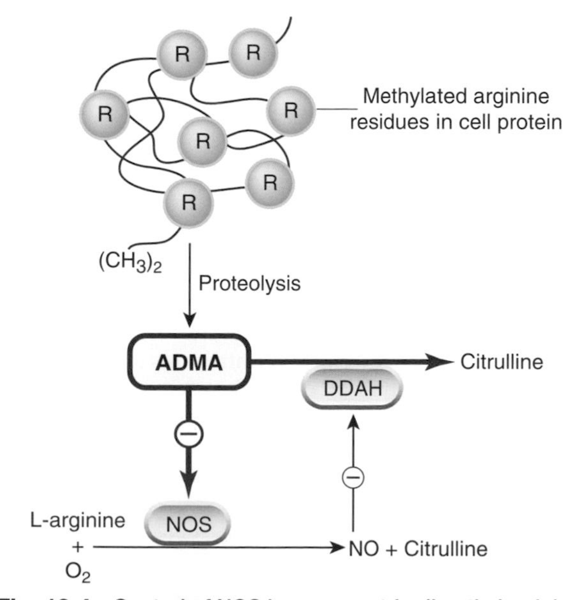

Fig. 19.4 Control of NOS by asymmetric dimethylarginine (ADMA). *DDAH,* Dimethylarginine dimethylamino hydrolase; *NO,* nitric oxide; *NOS,* nitric oxide synthase.

transforming growth factor-β. There are important species differences in the inducibility of NOS2, which is less readily induced in human than in mouse cells.

DEGRADATION AND CARRIAGE OF NITRIC OXIDE

NO reacts with oxygen to form N_2O_4, which combines with water to produce a mixture of nitric and nitrous acids. Nitrite ions are oxidised to nitrate by oxyhaemoglobin. These reactions are summarised as follows:

$$2NO + O_2 \rightarrow N_2O_4 \quad \mathbf{(19.1)}$$

$$N_2O_4 + H_2O \rightarrow NO_3^- + NO_2^- + 2H^+ \quad \mathbf{(19.2)}$$

$$NO_2^- + HbO \rightarrow NO_3^- + Hb \quad \mathbf{(19.3)}$$

Low concentrations of NO are relatively stable in air, because the rate of reaction shown in Eq. 19.1 depends on the square of the NO concentration, so small amounts of NO produced in the lung escape degradation and can be

Nitric oxide: synthesis, inactivation and carriage

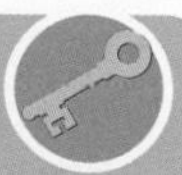

- NO is synthesised from L-arginine and molecular O_2 by NOS.
- NOS exists in three isoforms: inducible (NOS2) and constitutive 'endothelial' (NOS3, which is not restricted to endothelial cells) and neuronal (NOS1) forms. NOSs are dimeric flavoproteins, contain tetrahydrobiopterin and have homology with cytochrome P450. The constitutive enzymes are activated by calcium–calmodulin. Sensitivity to calcium–calmodulin is controlled by phosphorylation of specific residues on the enzymes.
- NOS2 is induced in macrophages and other cells by inflammatory cytokines, especially interferon-γ.
- NOS1 is present in the central nervous system (see Chs 37–39) and in some autonomic nerves (see Ch. 13).
- NOS3 is present in platelets and other cells in addition to endothelium.
- NO diffuses to sites of action in neighbouring cells. This is regulated by the redox state of haemoglobin alpha which is present in the myoendothelial junctions that act as diffusion corridors across the internal elastic lamina (and in other cells): signalling can occur when the haem is in the Fe^{3+} state but is stopped – like at a red traffic light – when haem is in the Fe^{2+} state.
- NO is inactivated by combination with the haem of haemoglobin or by oxidation to nitrite and nitrate, which are excreted in urine; it is also present in exhaled air, especially in patients who have exacerbations of their asthma.
- NO can react reversibly with cysteine residues (e.g. in globin or albumin) to form stable nitrosothiols; as a result, red cells can act as an O_2-regulated source of NO. NO released in this way escapes inactivation by haem by being exported via cysteine residues in the anion exchange protein in red cell membranes.

detected in exhaled air. Exhaled NO is increased in patients who have airway inflammation. Measurement of 'fractional exhaled NO' is used in clinical services to diagnose patients with suspected asthma, and to guide drug therapy for better control of the inflamed airways.

EFFECTS OF NITRIC OXIDE

NO reacts with various metals, thiols and oxygen species, thereby modifying proteins, DNA and lipids. One of its most important biochemical effects (see Ch. 3) is activation of soluble guanylyl cyclase, a heterodimer present in vascular and nervous tissue as two distinct isoenzymes. Guanylyl cyclase synthesises the second messenger cGMP. NO activates the enzyme by combining with its haem group, and many physiological effects of low concentrations of NO are mediated by cGMP. These effects are prevented by inhibitors of guanylyl cyclase (e.g. 1H-[1,2,4]-oxadiazole-[4,3-α]-quinoxalin-1-one, better known as 'ODQ'), which are useful investigational tools. NO activates soluble guanylyl cyclase in intact cells (neurons and platelets) extremely rapidly, and activation is followed by desensitisation to a steady-state level. This contrasts with its effect on the isolated enzyme, which is slower but more sustained. Guanylyl cyclase contains another regulatory site, which is NO independent. This is activated by **riociguat**, used to treat some forms of pulmonary hypertension, and **vericiguat** for treatment of heart failure (see Ch. 21).

The effects of cGMP are terminated by phosphodiesterase enzymes. **Sildenafil** and **tadalafil** are inhibitors of phosphodiesterase type V. They are used to treat erectile dysfunction and work by potentiating NO actions in the corpora cavernosa of the penis by this mechanism (see Ch. 35). NO also combines with haem groups in other biologically important proteins, notably cytochrome c oxidase, where it competes with oxygen, contributing to the control of cellular respiration (see Erusalimsky and Moncada, 2007). Cytotoxic and/or cytoprotective effects of higher concentrations of NO relate to its chemistry as a free radical (see Ch. 40).

BIOCHEMICAL AND CELLULAR ASPECTS

The pharmacological effects of NO can be studied with NO gas dissolved in deoxygenated salt solution. More conveniently, but less directly, various donors of NO, such as **nitroprusside**, S-*nitrosoacetylpenicillamine* (SNAP) or S-*nitrosoglutathione* (SNOG), have been used as surrogates. This has pitfalls; for example, ascorbic acid potentiates SNAP but inhibits responses to authentic NO.[5]

NO can activate guanylyl cyclase in the same cells that produce it, giving rise to autocrine effects, for example on the barrier function of the endothelium. NO also diffuses from its site of synthesis and activates guanylyl cyclase in neighbouring cells. The resulting increase in cGMP affects protein kinase G, ion channels and possibly other proteins, inhibiting $[Ca^{2+}]_i$-induced smooth muscle contraction and platelet aggregation. NO hyperpolarises vascular smooth muscle as a consequence of potassium-channel activation, and inhibits monocyte adhesion and migration, adhesion and aggregation of platelets, and smooth muscle and fibroblast proliferation. These cellular effects probably underlie the anti-atherosclerotic action of NO (see Ch. 22).

Large amounts of NO (released following induction of NOS or excessive stimulation of *N*-methyl-D-aspartate [NMDA] receptors in the brain, see Chs 39 and 40) cause cytotoxic effects, either directly or via formation of peroxynitrite. Such cytotoxicity contributes to host defence, but also to the neuronal cell death that occurs when there is overstimulation of NMDA receptors by glutamate (see Chs 38 and 40). Paradoxically, NO is also cytoprotective under some circumstances (see Ch. 40).

[5] Ascorbic acid releases NO from SNAP but accelerates NO degradation in solution, which could explain this divergence.

VASCULAR EFFECTS (SEE ALSO CH. 21)

The L-arginine/NO pathway is tonically active in resistance vessels, reducing peripheral vascular resistance and hence systemic blood pressure. Genetically altered mice that lack coding for NOS3 are hypertensive, consistent with a role for NO biosynthesis in the physiological control of blood pressure. In addition, NO derived from NOS1 is implicated in the control of basal resistance vessel tone in human forearm and cardiac muscle vascular beds (Seddon et al., 2008, 2009). NO is believed to contribute to the generalised vasodilatation that occurs during pregnancy. In addition to effects on basal resistance vessel tone and mediating the effects of endothelium-dependent vasodilator agonists such as acetylcholine and substance P, it has more recently been appreciated that NO promotes new vessel formation ('angiogenesis') and vascular remodelling (Ghimire et al., 2017; Kraehling and Sessa, 2017).

NEURONAL EFFECTS (SEE ALSO CH. 13)

NO is a non-noradrenergic non-cholinergic (NANC) neurotransmitter in many tissues (see Fig. 13.5), including the upper airways, gastrointestinal tract and corpora cavernosa of the penis (Chs 28, 30 and 35). It is implicated in the control of neuronal development and of synaptic plasticity in the CNS (Chs 37 and 40). There also appears to be a role in hippocampal and cortical long-term potentiation (LTP) through NO activation of NMDA receptors mediated by protein kinases. However, there is still considerable debate as to whether NO is protective or harmful in neurodegenerative diseases, particularly in light of the diversity of pathology that afflicts the CNS.

In the eye, NO appears to increase outflow of aqueous humour by relaxing the trabecular meshwork and Schlemm's canal (thus helping to reduce intraocular pressure in patients with glaucoma).

HOST DEFENCE (SEE CH. 7)

The cytotoxic and/or cytostatic effects of NO are implicated in primitive non-specific host defence mechanisms against numerous pathogens, including viruses, bacteria, fungi, protozoa and parasites, and against tumour cells. The importance of this is evidenced by the susceptibility of mice lacking NOS2 to *Leishmania major* (to which wild-type mice are highly resistant). Mechanisms whereby NO damages invading pathogens include nitrosylation of nucleic acids and combination with haem-containing enzymes, including the mitochondrial enzymes involved in cell respiration.

THERAPEUTIC ASPECTS

Novel therapeutic approaches under investigation to increase the bioavailability of NO include new ways to increase NOS activity; amplify the nitrate–nitrite–NO pathway, novel classes of NO donors and drugs that limit NO inactivation by reactive oxygen species; and modulate phosphodiesterases and soluble guanylyl cyclases (reviewed by Lundberg et al., 2015).

NITRIC OXIDE

Inhaling high concentrations of NO (as occurred when cylinders of nitrous oxide, N_2O, for anaesthesia were accidently contaminated) causes acute pulmonary oedema and methaemoglobinaemia, but concentrations below 50 ppm (parts per million) are not toxic. NO (5–300 ppm) inhibits bronchoconstriction (at least in guinea pigs), but the main action of low concentrations of inhaled NO in man is pulmonary vasodilatation. Inspired NO acts preferentially on ventilated alveoli, and is used therapeutically in respiratory distress syndrome, including acute hypoxic respiratory failure in newborn babies for which NO has regulatory approval in the United States. This condition is characterised by intrapulmonary 'shunting', that is, pulmonary arterial blood passing through non-ventilated alveoli and remaining deoxygenated. This causes arterial hypoxaemia and, because hypoxaemia causes pulmonary arterial vasoconstriction, acute pulmonary arterial hypertension. Inhaled NO dilates blood vessels in ventilated alveoli (which are exposed to the inspired gas) and thus reduces shunting. NO is used in intensive care units to reduce pulmonary hypertension and to improve oxygen delivery in patients with respiratory distress syndrome, but it is not known whether this improves long-term survival in these severely ill patients.

NITRIC OXIDE DONORS/PRECURSORS

Nitrovasodilators have been used therapeutically for over a century. The common mode of action of these drugs is as a source of NO (see Chs 20 and 21). There are numerous clinical trials evaluating the vascular effects of dietary inorganic nitrate ions (contained in beetroot juice) on arterial blood pressure as well as other cardiovascular parameters. These studies have yielded mixed findings; equally, trials of beetroot juice have failed to enhance exercise performance in populations as diverse as 5-km runners, basketball and tennis players and patients with heart failure.

Actions of nitric oxide

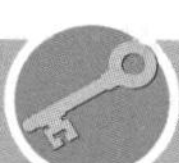

- Nitric oxide (NO) acts by:
  - combining with haem in guanylyl cyclase, activating the enzyme, increasing cGMP and thereby lowering $[Ca^{2+}]_i$;
  - combining with haem groups in other proteins (e.g. cytochrome C oxidase);
  - combining with superoxide anion to yield the cytotoxic peroxynitrite anion;
  - nitrosation of proteins, lipids and nucleic acids.
- Effects of NO include:
  - vasodilatation, inhibition of platelet and monocyte adhesion and aggregation, inhibition of smooth muscle proliferation, protection against atheroma, vascular remodelling and angiogenesis;
  - synaptic effects in the peripheral and central nervous system;
  - host defence and cytotoxic effects on pathogens;
  - cytoprotection.

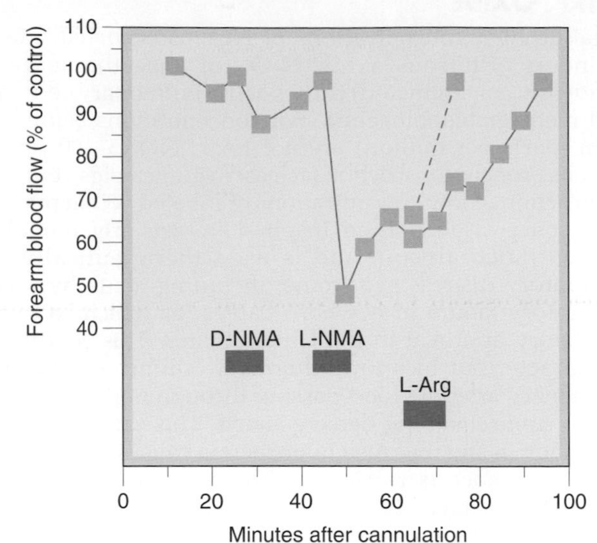

Fig. 19.5 Basal blood flow in the human forearm is influenced by nitric oxide (NO) biosynthesis. Forearm blood flow is expressed as a percentage of the flow in the non-cannulated control arm (which does not change). Brachial artery infusion of the D-isomer of the arginine analogue N^G-monomethyl-L-arginine (D-NMA) has no effect, while the L-isomer (L-NMA) causes vasoconstriction. L-arginine (L-Arg) accelerates recovery from such vasoconstriction *(dashed line)*. (From Vallance, P., Collier, J., Moncada, S., et al., 1989. Effects of endothelium-derived nitric oxide on peripheral arteriolar tone in man. Lancet 334, 997–1000.)

INHIBITION OF NITRIC OXIDE SYNTHESIS

Drugs can inhibit NO synthesis or action by several mechanisms. Certain arginine analogues compete with arginine for NOS, and the first inhibitors of NOS developed in the 1980s and 1990s were based on the L-arginine substrate. These non-selective inhibitors, for example N^G-monomethyl-L-arginine (L-NMMA) and N^G-nitro-L-arginine methyl ester (L-NAME), have been used as experimental tools and in clinical trials. Infusion of the non-selective NOS inhibitor L-NMMA into the brachial artery causes local vasoconstriction (Fig. 19.5), owing to inhibition of the basal production of NO in the infused arm, probably partly by inhibiting NOS1 in autonomic nerve fibres (Seddon et al., 2008). Intravenous L-NMMA causes vasoconstriction in renal, mesenteric, cerebral and striated muscle resistance vessels, increases blood pressure and causes reflex bradycardia.

Elucidation of the crystal structure of NOS isoforms led to development of selective inhibitors of different isoforms of NOS. Early examples of this include 7-nitroindazole, which selectively inhibits NOS1, and aminoguanidine for NOS2. A wide range of selective NOS inhibitors (for each of the three isoforms) are now available for research purposes.

NITRIC OXIDE REPLACEMENT OR POTENTIATION

Several means whereby the L-arginine/NO pathway could be enhanced are under investigation. Some of these rely on existing drugs of proven value in other contexts. The hope (as yet unproven) is that, by potentiating NO, they will prevent atherosclerosis or its thrombotic complications or have other beneficial effects attributed to NO. However, efforts to modulate NO concentrations through NO donors and use of NOS substrates have met limited clinical success; similarly, the use of general antioxidants to alleviate oxidative stress has been negative (reviewed by Tejero et al., 2019). Alternatively, oral ingestion of nitrate/nitrite (e.g. via leafy green vegetables) adds to the body stores and can generate NO through reduction in the nitrate–nitrite–NO pathway, particularly in hypoxic tissue.

CLINICAL CONDITIONS IN WHICH NITRIC OXIDE MAY PLAY A PART

The wide distribution of NOS enzymes and diverse actions of NO suggest that abnormalities in the L-arginine/NO pathway could be important in disease. Either increased or reduced production could play a part, and hypotheses abound.

We caution the reader that while there is a huge amount of pre-clinical research drawing possible associations between the NO pathway and diverse diseases, we also recognise that not all of these possibilities are likely to have genuine clinical relevance or withstand the test of time.

The ubiquity of NO in the vascular beds and NOS2 as an inducible form in response to hypoxia, infection, ischaemia and acidosis means that altered NO balance can be detected in experimental or observational studies across almost every organ system. There is increasing recognition that dysregulation of NO during serious illness can involve a deficit (e.g. of endothelial NO synthesis in microvascular areas), which at the same time is accompanied by an excess of NO on other systems that cause cardiac and macrovascular dysfunction (Lambden, 2019). For instance, it is thought that NOS3 in the sinusoidal endothelial cells of the liver confers protection against liver disease, whereas increased NOS1 contributes to harmful pathology. The complexity and interconnected nature of the NO pathways mean that clinical correlations can be hard to interpret. This creates major challenges for pharmacological targeting of specific disease processes, particularly with regards to unintended effects across other parts of the body where NO is ubiquitous.

Sepsis, and the resulting multiple organ failure, is another key example here. Whereas NO benefits host defence by killing invading organisms, excessive NO causes harmful hypotension. Disappointingly, however, L-NMMA (which blocks synthesis of all three NO isoforms) worsens survival in sepsis. The bad news continues – a haemoglobin-based nitric oxide scavenger, pyridoxalated haemoglobin polyoxyethylene, was found to increase mortality and adverse events in a phase III trial of intensive care patients with shock. There is also ongoing debate regarding the possible signals of renal failure associated with inhaled NO therapy in critically ill patients.

Established clinical uses of drugs that influence the L-arginine/NO system are summarised in the 'Nitric oxide in therapeutics' clinical box.

Nitric oxide in pathophysiology

- NO is synthesised under physiological and pathological circumstances.
- Either reduced or increased NO production can contribute to disease.
- In serious illness, there may be a complex competing interplay between excess synthesis of NO in some organs occurring at the same time as decreased production in other systems

Nitric oxide in therapeutics

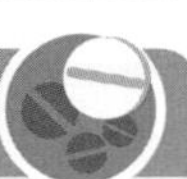

- NO donors (e.g. **nitroprusside** and organic nitrovasodilators) are well established in treatment of cardiovascular disease (see Chs 20 and 21).
- Type V phosphodiesterase inhibitors (e.g. **sildenafil**, **tadalafil**) potentiate the action of NO. They are used to treat erectile dysfunction and pulmonary hypertension (see Chs 21 and 35).
- Inhaled NO is used in intensive care of adult and neonatal respiratory distress syndrome.
- Latanoprostene bunod, an NO releasing prostaglandin F2 agonist, is licensed for treatment of glaucoma. This compound is metabolised into two components – latanoprost and butanediol mononitrate (which subsequently releases NO). It is unclear whether the NO component offers greater benefit above latanoprost alone (see Ch. 27)

RELATED MEDIATORS

NO, promoted from pollutant to 'molecule of the year',[6] was joined, similarly implausibly, by carbon monoxide (CO) – a potentially lethal exhaust gas – and by hydrogen sulfide (H_2S), which are also formed in mammalian tissues. There are striking similarities between these three gases, as well as some contrasts. All three are highly diffusible labile molecules that are rapidly eliminated from the body: NO as nitrite and nitrate in urine as well as NO in exhaled air (see earlier discussion); CO in exhaled air; H_2S as thiosulfate, sulfite and sulfate in urine (Fig. 19.6) as well as in exhaled breath. All three react with haemoglobin, and all three affect cellular energetics via actions on cytochrome C oxidase. All have vasodilator effects (although chronic exposure to CO can cause vasoconstriction), and all have anti-inflammatory and cytoprotective effects at low concentrations but cause cellular injury at higher concentrations.

HYDROGEN SULFIDE (H_2S) AND CARBON MONOXIDE (CO)

H_2S has potent pharmacological effects in the cardiovascular system, including vasorelaxation secondary to activation of vascular smooth muscle K_{ATP} channels (see Ch. 4). It also acts on the nervous system and influences nociception, selectively modulating voltage-dependent T-type Ca^{2+} channels (Elies et al., 2016). It also influences inflammatory processes. For a review of the effects of H_2S on ion channels and intracellular transduction systems see Li et al. (2011).

[6] By the American Association for the Advancement of Science in 1992.

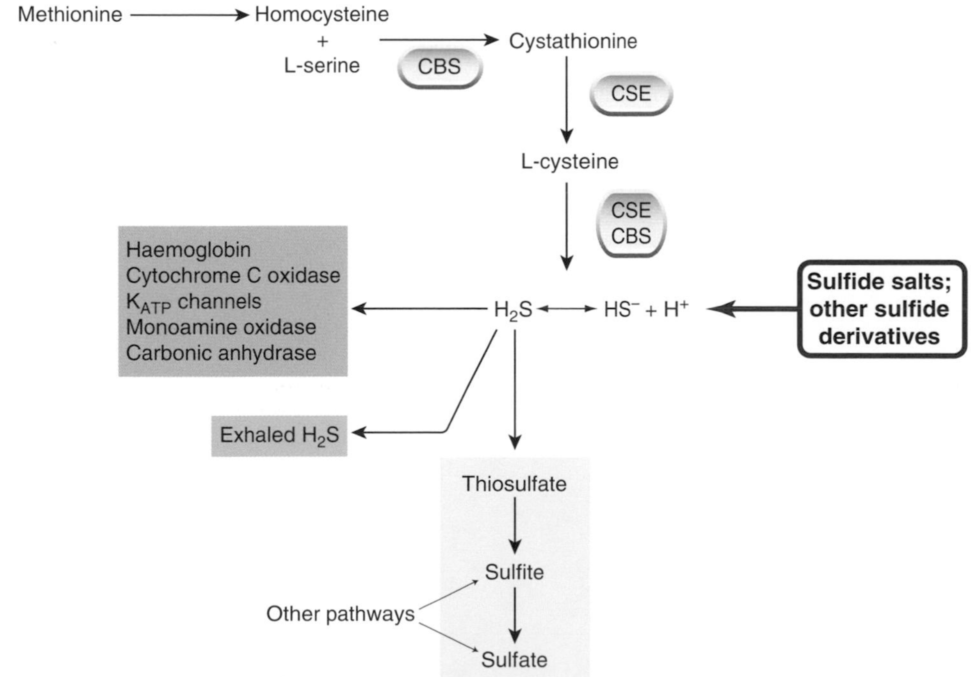

Fig. 19.6 Synthesis, sites of action and disposition of H_2S. Endogenous biosynthesis from sulphur-containing amino acids (methionine, cysteine) via actions of the regulated enzymes methionine cystathionine γ-lyase (CSE) and cystathionine β-synthase (CBS) is shown; pharmacological H_2S donors *(red-rimmed box)* may be administered exogenously. Most H_2S is probably renally excreted as sulfate *(yellow box)*. Some is eliminated in exhaled air *(green box)*. Some molecular targets of H_2S are indicated in the *blue box*. (Adapted with permission from Ritter, J.M., 2010. Human pharmacology of hydrogen sulfide: putative gaseous mediator. Br. J. Clin. Pharmacol. 69, 573–575.)

There are clinical trials of the effects of H_2S donor diseases as diverse as heart failure, ischaemic heart disease, cancer and male subfertility (Gojon et al., 2020), but none of the studies have progressed to phase III randomised trials as yet. **Otenaproxesul**, a sulfide-releasing derivative of naproxen, is moving towards phase III trials in chronic pain after demonstrating lower peptic ulcer rick than the parent naproxen compound in phase II trials. It is worth noting though that naproxcinod, a nitric-oxide releasing derivative of naproxen, failed to clear regulatory hurdles due to safety concerns.

Sodium thiosulfate, a downstream oxidation product of H_2S, has also showed therapeutic promise. Randomised trial data have indicated some efficacy in preventing chemotherapy-induced toxicity, whilst further trials are planned in a wide range of conditions (see Zhang et al., 2021, for description of potential clinical applications).

There are as yet no therapeutic drugs acting via CO pathways, but CO (perhaps surprisingly for a gas associated with lethal effects in a domestic setting) has potentially beneficial effects on cell survival, and CO-releasing molecules are under investigation (Motterlini and Foresti, 2017).

REFERENCES AND FURTHER READING

Biochemical aspects

Derbyshire, E.R., Marletta, M.A., 2012. Structure and regulation of soluble guanylate cyclase. Annu. Rev. Biochem. 81, 533–559.

Tejero, J., Shiva, S., Gladwin, M.T., 2019. Sources of vascular nitric oxide and reactive oxygen species and their regulation. Physiol. Rev. 99, 311–379.

Physiological aspects

Carlström, M., 2021. Nitric oxide signalling in kidney regulation and cardiometabolic health. Nat. Rev. Nephrol. 17, 575–590.

Erusalimsky, J.D., Moncada, S., 2007. Nitric oxide and mitochondrial signalling from physiology to pathophysiology. Arterioscler. Thromb. Vasc. Biol. 27, 2524–2531.

Furchgott, R.F., Zawadzki, J.V., 1980. The obligatory role of endothelial cells in the relaxation of arterial smooth muscle by acetylcholine. Nature 288, 3734.

Garthwaite, J., 2008. Concepts of neural nitric oxide-mediated transmission. Eur. J. Neurosci. 27, 2783–2802.

Ghimire, K., Altmann, H.M., Straub, A.C., Isenberg, J.S., 2017. Nitric oxide: what's new to NO? Am. J. Physiol. Cell Physiol. 312, C254–C262.

Kraehling, J.R., Sessa, W.C., 2017. Contemporary approaches to modulating the nitric oxide-cGMP pathway in cardiovascular disease. Circ. Res. 120, 1174–1182.

Seddon, M.D., Chowienczyk, P.J., Brett, S.E., et al., 2008. Neuronal nitric oxide synthase regulates basal microvascular tone in humans *in vivo*. Circulation 117, 1991–1996.

Seddon, M., Melikian, N., Dworakowski, R., et al., 2009. Effects of neuronal nitric oxide synthase on human coronary artery diameter and blood flow in vivo. Circulation 119, 2656–2662.

Pathological aspects

Caplin, B., Leiper, J., 2012. Endogenous nitric oxide synthase inhibitors in the biology of disease: markers, mediators, and regulators? Arterioscler. Thromb. Vasc. Biol. 32, 1343–1353.

Farah, C., Michel, L.Y.M., Balligand, J.L., 2018. Nitric oxide signalling in cardiovascular health and disease. Nat. Rev. Cardiol. 15, 292–316.

Lambden, S., 2019. Bench to bedside review: therapeutic modulation of nitric oxide in sepsis-an update. Intensive Care Med. Exp. 7, 64.

Clinical and therapeutic aspects

Lundberg, J.O., Gladwin, M.T., Weitzberg, E., 2015. Strategies to increase nitric oxide signalling in cardiovascular disease. Nat. Rev. Drug Discov. 14, 623–641.

Hydrogen sulfide and carbon monoxide as possible mediators

Elies, J., Scragg, J.L., Boyle, J.P., 2016. Regulation of the T-type Ca^{2+} channel Cav3.2 by hydrogen sulfide: emerging controversies concerning the role of H_2S in nociception. J. Physiol. (Lond.) 594, 4119–4129.

Gojon, G., Morales, G.A., 2020. SG1002 and catenated divalent organic sulfur compounds as promising hydrogen sulfide prodrugs. Antioxid Redox Signal. 33, 1010–1045.

Li, L., Rose, P., Moore, P.K., 2011. Hydrogen sulfide and cell signaling. Annu. Rev. Pharmacol. Toxicol. 51, 169–187.

Motterlini, R., Foresti, R., 2017. Biological signaling by carbon monoxide and carbon monoxide-releasing molecules. Am. J. Physiol. Cell Physiol. 312, C302–C313.

Nowaczyk, A., Kowalska, M., Nowaczyk, J., et al., 2021. Carbon monoxide and nitric oxide as examples of the youngest class of transmitters. Int. J. Mol. Sci. 22, 6029.

Zhang, M.Y., Dugbartey, G.J., Juriasingani, S., et al., 2021. Hydrogen sulfide metabolite, sodium thiosulfate: clinical applications and underlying molecular mechanisms. Int. J. Mol. Sci. 22, 6452.

20 The heart

OVERVIEW

This chapter presents an overview of cardiac function in terms of electrophysiology, contraction, oxygen consumption and coronary blood flow, autonomic control and natriuretic peptides as a basis for understanding the effects of drugs on the heart and their place in treating cardiac disease. We concentrate on drugs that act directly on the heart, namely antidysrhythmic drugs and drugs that increase the force of contraction (especially digoxin), as well as anti-anginal drugs that act indirectly by reducing cardiac work. The commonest form of heart disease is caused by atheroma in the coronary arteries, complicated by thrombosis on ruptured atheromatous plaques; drugs to treat and prevent these are considered in Chapters 22 and 23. Heart failure is mainly treated by drugs that work indirectly on the heart via actions on vascular smooth muscle, discussed in Chapter 21, by diuretics and sodium glucose transport 2 (SGLT2) inhibitors (Chs 29 and 31) and β-adrenoceptor antagonists (see Ch. 15).

INTRODUCTION

In this chapter we consider the effects of drugs on the heart under three main headings:

1. Rate and rhythm
2. Myocardial contraction
3. Metabolism and blood flow

The effects of drugs on these aspects of cardiac function are not, of course, independent of each other. For example, if a drug affects the electrical properties of the myocardial cell membrane, it is likely to influence both cardiac rhythm and myocardial contraction. Similarly, a drug that affects contraction will inevitably alter metabolism and blood flow as well. Nevertheless, from a therapeutic point of view, these three classes of effect represent distinct clinical objectives in relation to the treatment, respectively, of cardiac dysrhythmias, cardiac failure and coronary insufficiency (as occurs during angina pectoris or myocardial infarction).

PHYSIOLOGY OF CARDIAC FUNCTION

CARDIAC RATE AND RHYTHM

The chambers of the heart normally contract in a coordinated manner, pumping blood efficiently by a route determined by the valves. Coordination of contraction is achieved by a specialised conducting system. Normal *sinus rhythm* is generated by pacemaker impulses that arise in the sinoatrial (SA) node and are conducted in sequence through the atria, the atrioventricular (AV) node, bundle of His, Purkinje fibres and ventricles. Cardiac cells owe their electrical excitability to voltage-sensitive plasma membrane channels selective for various ions, including Na^+, K^+ and Ca^{2+}, the structure and function of which are described in Chapter 4. The electrophysiological features of cardiac muscle that distinguish it from other excitable tissues include:

- pacemaker activity
- absence of fast Na^+ current in SA and AV nodes, where slow inward Ca^{2+} current initiates action potentials
- long action potential ('plateau') and refractory period
- influx of Ca^{2+} during the plateau

Several of these special features of cardiac rhythm relate to Ca^{2+} currents. The heart contains *intracellular* calcium channels (i.e. ryanodine receptors and inositol trisphosphate-activated calcium channels described in Chapter 4, which are important in myocardial contraction) and voltage-dependent calcium channels in the plasma membrane, which are important in controlling cardiac rate and rhythm. The main type of voltage-dependent calcium channel in adult working myocardium is the L-type channel, which is also important in vascular smooth muscle; L-type channels are important in specialised conducting regions as well as in working myocardium.

The action potential of an idealised cardiac muscle cell is shown in Fig. 20.1A and is divided into five phases: 0 (fast depolarisation), 1 (partial repolarisation), 2 (plateau), 3 (repolarisation) and 4 (pacemaker).

Ionic mechanisms underlying these phases can be summarised as follows.

Phase 0, rapid depolarisation, occurs when the membrane potential reaches a critical firing threshold (about −60 mV), at which the inward current of Na^+ flowing through the voltage-dependent sodium channels becomes large enough to produce a regenerative ('all-or-nothing') depolarisation. This mechanism is the same as that responsible for action potential generation in neurons (see Ch. 4). Activation of sodium channels by membrane depolarisation is transient, and if the membrane remains depolarised for more than a few milliseconds, they close again (inactivation). They are therefore closed during the plateau of the action potential and remain unavailable for the initiation of another action potential until the membrane repolarises.

Phase 1, partial repolarisation, occurs as the Na^+ current is inactivated.

Phase 2, the plateau, results from an inward Ca^{2+} current. Calcium channels show a pattern of voltage-sensitive activation and inactivation qualitatively similar to sodium channels, but with a much slower time course. The plateau is assisted by a special property of the cardiac muscle membrane known as inward-going rectification, which means that the K^+ conductance falls to a low level when the membrane is depolarised. Because of this, there is little

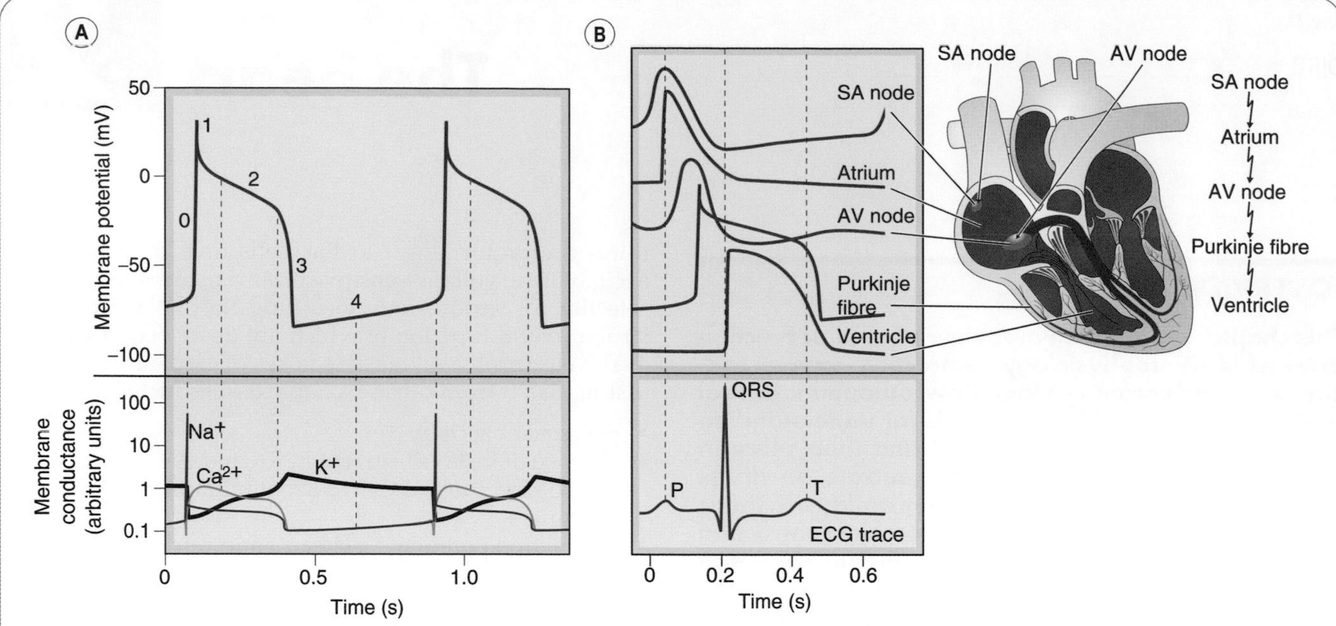

Fig. 20.1 The cardiac action potential. (A) Phases of the action potential: *(0)* rapid depolarisation; *(1)* partial repolarisation; *(2)* plateau; *(3)* repolarisation; *(4)* pacemaker depolarisation. The *lower panel* shows the accompanying changes in membrane conductance for Na^+, K^+ and Ca^{2+}. (B) Conduction of the impulse through the heart, with the corresponding electrocardiogram (ECG) trace. Note that the longest delay occurs at the atrioventricular (AV) node, where the action potential has a characteristically slow waveform. *SA*, Sinoatrial.

tendency for outward K^+ current to restore the resting membrane potential during the plateau, so a relatively small inward Ca^{2+} current suffices to maintain the plateau. A persistent sodium current (I_{Nap}) also contributes to the plateau; it is very small compared with the fast component of sodium current, but as it flows throughout the action potential it makes a substantial contribution to sodium loading during each cardiac cycle, and is a major contributor to ischaemic arrhythmias and a drug target (see later).

Phase 3, repolarisation, occurs as the Ca^{2+} current inactivates and a delayed outwardly rectifying K^+ current (analogous to, but much slower than, the K^+ current that causes repolarisation in nerve fibres; see Ch. 4) activates, causing outward K^+ current. This is augmented by another K^+ current, which is activated by high intracellular Ca^{2+} concentrations, $[Ca^{2+}]_i$, during the plateau, and sometimes also by other K^+ currents, including one through channels activated by acetylcholine (see Ch. 14 and later) and another that is activated by arachidonic acid, which is liberated under pathological conditions such as myocardial infarction.

Phase 4, the pacemaker potential, is a gradual depolarisation during diastole. Pacemaker activity is normally found only in nodal and conducting tissue. The pacemaker potential is caused by a combination of increasing inward currents and declining outward currents during diastole. It is usually most rapid in cells of the SA node, which therefore acts as pacemaker for the whole heart. Cells in the SA node have a greater background Na^+-conductance than do atrial or ventricular myocytes, leading to a greater background inward current. In addition, inactivation of voltage-dependent calcium channels wears off during diastole, resulting in increasing inward Ca^{2+} current during late diastole. Activation of T-type calcium channels during late diastole contributes to pacemaker activity in the SA node. The negative membrane potential early in diastole activates a cation channel that is permeable to Na^+ and K^+, giving rise to another inward current, called I_f.[1] An inhibitor of this current, **ivabradine**, slows the heart and is used therapeutically (see later).

Several voltage- and time-dependent outward currents play a part as well: delayed rectifier K^+ current (I_K), which is activated during the action potential, is turned off by the negative membrane potential early in diastole. Current from the electrogenic Na^+/K^+ pump also contributes to the outward current during the pacemaker potential.

Fig. 20.1B shows the action potential configuration in different parts of the heart. Phase 0 is absent in the nodal regions, where the conduction velocity is correspondingly slow (~5 cm/s) compared with other regions such as the Purkinje fibres (conduction velocity ~200 cm/s), which propagate the action potential rapidly to the ventricles. Regions that lack a fast inward current have a much longer refractory period than fast-conducting regions. With fast-conducting fibres, inactivation of the Na^+ current recovers rapidly, and the cell becomes excitable again almost as soon as it is repolarised.

The orderly pattern of sinus rhythm can be disrupted either by heart disease or by the action of drugs or circulating hormones, and an important therapeutic use of drugs is to restore a normal cardiac rhythm where it has become disturbed. The commonest cause of cardiac dysrhythmia is ischaemic heart disease, and between 25% and 50% of deaths following myocardial infarction result from *ventricular tachycardia or fibrillation* rather than directly

[1] 'f' for 'funny', because it is unusual for cation channels to be activated by hyperpolarisation; cardiac electrophysiologists have a peculiar sense of humour!

from failure of the contractile machinery due to death of cardiac myocytes.

DISTURBANCES OF CARDIAC RHYTHM

Clinically, dysrhythmias are classified according to:

- the site of origin of the abnormality - atrial, junctional or ventricular;
- whether the rate is increased (>100 beats per minute [bpm] - *tachycardia*) or decreased (<60 bpm - *bradycardia*).

They may be asymptomatic, or cause chest pain and palpitations (awareness of the heartbeat), or symptoms from cerebral hypoperfusion (faintness or loss of consciousness). Their diagnosis depends on the surface electrocardiogram (ECG), and details are beyond the scope of this book - see Hampton and Hampton (2019). The commonest types of tachyarrhythmia are *atrial fibrillation*, where the heartbeat is completely irregular, and *paroxysmal supraventricular tachycardia* (SVT), where the heartbeat is rapid but regular. Occasional ectopic beats (ventricular as well as supraventricular) are common. Sustained ventricular tachyarrhythmias are much less common but more serious; they include *ventricular tachycardia* and *ventricular fibrillation*, where the electrical activity in the ventricles is completely chaotic and cardiac output ceases. Bradyarrhythmias include various kinds of *heart block* (e.g. at the AV or SA node) and complete cessation of electrical activity ('asystolic arrest'). It is often unclear in individual patients which of the various mechanisms discussed later are directly responsible but disturbances of cardiac rhythm typically occur because of disruptions in electrical impulse formation and/or conduction (see Tse, 2016, for a detailed review on the cellular mechanisms for cardiac arrhythmias):

1. Tachycardia with greater impulse formation (through triggered activity or increased automaticity), and re-entry circuits
2. Bradycardia due to reduced automaticity at the sinus node, or impaired conduction along the pathway

Triggered activity describes premature activation of the cardiac myocytes and extra beats, due to a phenomenon known as 'after-depolarisation'. Here, fluctuations in the membrane potential can trigger additional depolarisations while repolarisation is still ongoing (known as 'early after-depolarisation'), or only after repolarisation is complete - known as 'delayed after-depolarisation' (Fig. 20.2). Important (and treatable) factors that cause after-depolarisation are hypokalaemia, hypercalcaemia, hypoxia and acidosis, usually in the context of underlying myocardial damage. Prolonged duration of the action potential, as seen in bradycardia, and long QT syndromes, which are often related drug toxicities (see later), are key factors behind early after-depolarisation and triggered activity. Recognised causes of delayed after-depolarisation include catecholamine excess (that triggers polymorphic ventricular tachycardia) and digitalis toxicity.

Some areas of the heart have pacemaker cells that spontaneously depolarise and discharge (known as 'automaticity'). The natural or physiological pacemaker in the SA node oversees the regulation of heart rate, but a number of other cardiac tissues can take on subsidiary pacemaker activity (albeit at a slower discharge rate). This

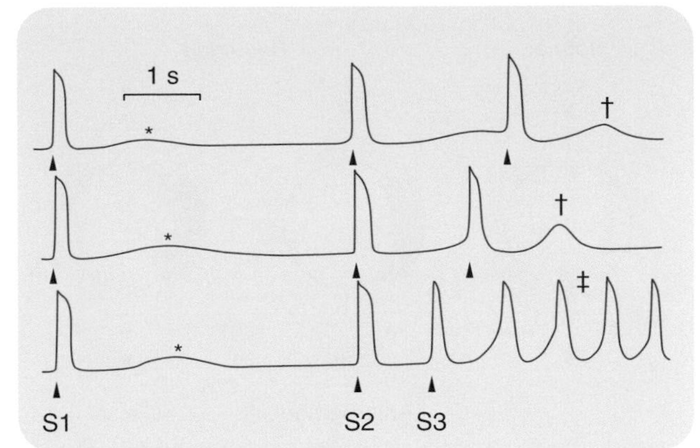

Fig. 20.2 After-depolarisation in cardiac muscle recorded from a dog coronary sinus in the presence of noradrenaline (norepinephrine). The first stimulus *(S1)* causes an action potential followed by a small after-depolarisation. As the interval *S2–S3* is decreased, the after-depolarisation gets larger (†) until it triggers an indefinite train of action potentials (‡). (Adapted from Wit, A.L., Cranefield, P.F., 1977. Circ. Res. 41, 435.)

provides a safety mechanism in the event of failure of the SA node but can also trigger tachyarrhythmias. Here, enhanced automaticity and ectopic pacemaker activity can be caused by ischaemic damage, electrolyte disturbances and sympathetic activity. For instance, catecholamines, acting on β_1 adrenoceptors (see Ch. 15), increase the rate of depolarisation during phase 4 and can provoke normally quiescent parts of the heart to take on a spontaneous rhythm. Several tachyarrhythmias (e.g. paroxysmal atrial fibrillation) can be triggered by circumstances associated with increased sympathetic activity, e.g. pain during myocardial infarction.

Normally, a cardiac action potential dies out after it has activated the ventricles because it is surrounded by refractory tissue, which it has just traversed. *Re-entry* (Fig. 20.3) describes a situation in which the impulse re-excites regions of the myocardium after the refractory period has subsided, causing continuous circulation of action potentials. It can result from anatomical anomalies or, more commonly, from myocardial damage. Re-entry underlies many types of dysrhythmia, the pattern depending on the site of the re-entrant circuit, which may be in the atria, ventricles or nodal tissue. A simple ring of tissue can give rise to a re-entrant rhythm if a transient or unidirectional conduction block is present. Normally, an impulse originating at any point in the ring will propagate in both directions and die out when the two impulses meet, but if a damaged area causes either a transient block (so that one impulse is blocked but the second can get through; see Fig. 20.3) or a unidirectional block, continuous circulation of the impulse can occur. This is known as *circus movement* and was demonstrated experimentally on rings of jellyfish tissue many years ago.

Heart block results from fibrosis of, or ischaemic damage to, the conducting system (often in the AV node). In complete heart block, the atria and ventricles beat independently of one another, the ventricles beating at a slow rate determined by whatever pacemaker picks up distal to the block. Sporadic complete failure of AV conduction causes sudden

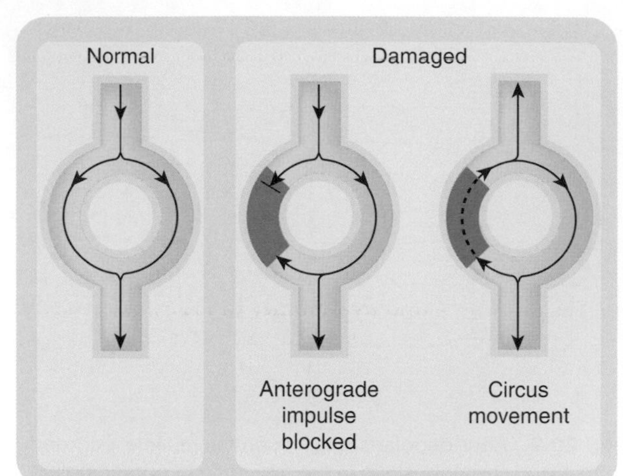

Fig. 20.3 Generation of a re-entrant rhythm by a damaged area of myocardium. The damaged area *(brown)* conducts in one direction only. This disturbs the normal pattern of conduction and permits continuous circulation of the impulse to occur.

Table 20.1 Summary of antidysrhythmic drugs (Vaughan Williams classification)

Class	Example(s)	Mechanism
Ia	Disopyramide	Sodium-channel block (intermediate dissociation)
Ib	Lidocaine	Sodium-channel block (fast dissociation)
Ic	Flecainide	Sodium-channel block (slow dissociation)
II	Atenolol	β-Adrenoceptor antagonism
III	Amiodarone, sotalol	Potassium-channel block
IV	Verapamil	Calcium-channel block

periods of unconsciousness (Stokes–Adams attacks) and is treated by implanting an artificial pacemaker.

Drug-induced ventricular arrhythmias

In the 1990s and early 2000s, a number of drugs had to be withdrawn due to their propensity for exerting *proarrhythmic* effects, notably a dangerous polymorphic form of ventricular tachycardia called (somewhat whimsically) *torsade de pointes* (because the appearance of the ECG trace is said to be reminiscent of this ballet sequence). Torsade de pointes is associated with prolongation of the QT interval, and linked to drugs that inhibit the HERG (human ether-a-go-go–related gene) repolarising potassium channel.

This pro-arrhythmic risk is most prominent in patients taking anti-arrhythmic agents (type Ia and Ic and sotalol in Table 20.1), as well as a long and varied list of other culprit drugs acting on sodium and potassium channels to prolong the QT interval. In clinical settings, the pro-arrhythmic risk is greatest when there are disturbances of electrolytes involved in repolarisation (e.g. potassium, calcium, magnesium) or serious co-morbid illnesses (such as sepsis, hypoxia and underlying cardiac damage). The drug-induced arrhythmia is similar to the congenital form seen in those with hereditary prolonged QT (e.g. Ward–Romano syndrome),[2] and 15 types of familial long QT syndrome have now been described.

The dangerous association of torsades de pointes with QT prolongation has led to regulatory requirements for 'thorough QT testing' to screen out potentially risky new compounds (e.g. those that block the hERG-related potassium channel and/or lengthen the QT). However, whilst such testing can prove highly sensitive in detecting drug-induced QT prolongation, the methods are poorly specific. QT prolongation per se is a poor surrogate for clinical outcomes – some drugs (e.g. ranolazine, verapamil) can have quite marked effect on the QT interval, but this may not actually result in ventricular arrhythmias. It has also become clear that drug-induced pro-arrhythmia risk involves not only inward potassium channels but also cardiac sodium and calcium channels that mediate the action potential. An ongoing international collaborative project is working to develop more accurate predictors of clinical risk than HERG potassium channel inhibition and QT prolongation alone, incorporating drug effects on inward fast and slow sodium, L-type calcium channels (see Roden, 2019, and Yim, 2018, for clear and detailed descriptions of this challenging and evolving topic).

Cardiac dysrhythmias

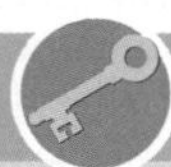

- Dysrhythmias arise because of abnormalities in electrical impulse formation and/or conduction:
  - after-depolarisation, which triggers ectopic beats
  - increased automaticity with ectopic pacemaker activity
  - re-entry circuits
  - decreased automaticity and/or heart block.
- Triggered activity from after-depolarisation can be provoked by electrolyte disturbances (calcium, potassium), ischaemia and drug toxicity.
- Increased automaticity with ectopic pacemaker activity can occur with excess sympathetic activity, ischaemia and electrolyte disturbance.
- Re-entry is facilitated when conduction is disrupted in parts of the myocardium as a result of disease.
- Heart block results from disease (e.g. fibrosis) in the conducting system, especially the AV node, or due to the use of channel-blocking drugs such as b-adrenoceptor antagonists or calcium antagonists.
- Clinically, dysrhythmias are divided:
  - according to their site of origin (supraventricular and ventricular)
  - according to whether the heart rate is increased or decreased (tachycardia or bradycardia).

[2]A 3-year-old girl began to have blackouts, which decreased in frequency with age. Her ECG showed a prolonged QT interval. When she was 18 years of age, she lost consciousness running for a bus. When she was 19, she became quite emotional as a participant in a live television audience and died suddenly. The molecular basis of this rare inherited disorder is now known. It is most commonly caused by mutations in the genes coding for potassium voltage-gated channels –KCNQ1 and KCNH2 (also known as *HERG*) – or sodium voltage-gated channel, *SCN5A*, which results in a loss of inactivation of the Na^+ current.

CARDIAC CONTRACTION

Cardiac output is the product of heart rate and mean left ventricular stroke volume (i.e. the volume of blood ejected from the ventricle with each heartbeat). Heart rate is controlled by the autonomic nervous system (see Chs 13–15 and later). Stroke volume is determined by a combination of factors, including some intrinsic to the heart itself and other haemodynamic factors extrinsic to the heart. Intrinsic factors regulate myocardial contractility via $[Ca^{2+}]_i$ and ATP, and are sensitive to various drugs and pathological processes. Extrinsic circulatory factors include the elasticity and contractile state of arteries and veins, and the volume and viscosity of the blood, which together determine cardiac load (preload and afterload, see later). Drugs that influence these circulatory factors are of paramount importance in treating patients with heart failure. They are covered in Chapter 21.

MYOCARDIAL CONTRACTILITY AND VIABILITY

The contractile machinery of myocardial striated muscle is basically the same as that of voluntary striated muscle (see Ch. 4). It involves binding of Ca^{2+} to troponin C; this changes the conformation of the troponin complex, permitting cross-bridging of myosin to actin and initiating contraction. **Levosimendan** (a drug used in some countries to treat acute decompensated heart failure; see Ch. 21), increases the force of contraction of the heart by binding troponin C and sensitising it to the action of Ca^{2+}. New drugs in development that target cardiac myosin are described later.

Many effects of drugs on cardiac contractility can be explained in terms of actions on $[Ca^{2+}]_i$, via effects on calcium channels in plasma membrane or sarcoplasmic reticulum or on the Na^+/K^+ pump, which indirectly influences the Na^+/Ca^{2+} pump (see later). Other factors that affect the force of contraction are the availability of oxygen and a source of metabolic energy such as free fatty acids.

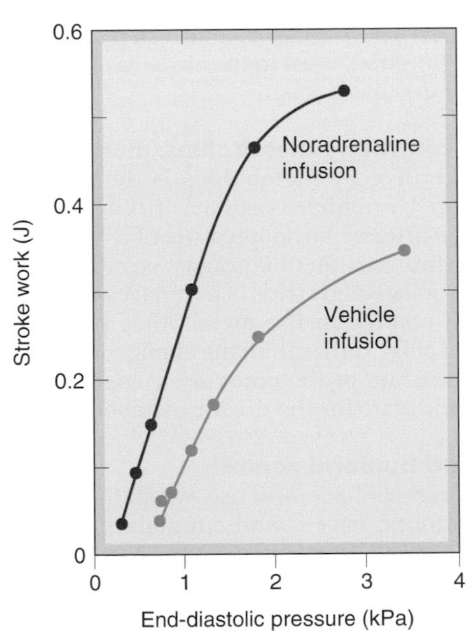

Fig. 20.4 Ventricular function curves in the dog. Infusion of physiological saline increases blood volume and hence end-diastolic pressure. This increases stroke work ('extrinsic' control) by increasing the force of contraction of the heart. This relationship is called the Starling curve. Noradrenaline has a direct action on the heart ('intrinsic' control), increasing the slope of the Starling curve. (Redrawn from Sarnoff, S.J., et al., 1960. Circ. Res. 8, 1108.)

VENTRICULAR FUNCTION CURVES AND HEART FAILURE

The force of contraction of the heart is determined partly by its intrinsic contractility (which, as described earlier, depends on $[Ca^{2+}]_i$ and availability of ATP), and partly by extrinsic haemodynamic factors that affect end-diastolic volume and hence the resting length of the muscle fibres. The end-diastolic volume is determined by the end-diastolic pressure, and its effect on stroke work is expressed in the Frank–Starling law of the heart, which reflects an inherent property of the contractile system. The Frank–Starling law can be represented as a ventricular function curve (Fig. 20.4). The area enclosed by the pressure–volume curve during the cardiac cycle provides a measure of ventricular stroke work. It is approximated by the product of stroke volume and mean arterial pressure. As Starling showed, factors extrinsic to the heart affect its performance in various ways, two patterns of response to increased load being particularly important:

- Increased cardiac filling pressure (*preload*), whether caused by increased blood volume or by venoconstriction (that returns more blood to the cardiac chambers), increases ventricular end-diastolic volume. This increases stroke volume and hence cardiac output and mean arterial pressure. Cardiac work and cardiac oxygen consumption both increase.
- Resistance vessel vasoconstriction increases *afterload.* End-diastolic volume and, hence, stroke work are initially unchanged, but constant stroke work in the face of increased vascular resistance causes reduced stroke volume and hence increased end-diastolic volume. This in turn increases stroke work, until a steady state is re-established with increased end-diastolic volume and the same cardiac output as before. As with increased preload, cardiac work and cardiac oxygen consumption both increase.

Normal ventricular filling pressure is only a few centimetres of water, on the steep part of the ventricular function curve, so a large increase in stroke work can be achieved with only a small increase in filling pressure. The Starling mechanism plays little part in controlling cardiac output in healthy subjects (e.g. during exercise), because changes in contractility, mainly as a result of changes in sympathetic nervous activity, achieve the necessary regulation without any increase in ventricular filling pressure (see Fig. 20.4). In contrast, the denervated heart in patients who have received a heart transplant relies on the Starling mechanism to increase cardiac output during exercise.

In heart failure, the cardiac output is insufficient to meet the needs of the body, initially only when these are increased during exercise but ultimately, as disease progresses, also at rest. It has many causes, most commonly ischaemic heart disease and hypertension. In patients with heart failure (see Ch. 21), the heart may be unable to deliver as much blood as the tissues require, even when its contractility is increased by sympathetic activity. Under these conditions, the basal (i.e. at rest) ventricular function curve is greatly depressed, and there is insufficient reserve, in the sense of extra contractility that can be achieved by sympathetic activity, to enable cardiac output to be maintained during exercise without a large increase in central venous pressure (see Fig. 20.4). Oedema of peripheral tissues (causing swelling of the legs) and the lungs (causing breathlessness) is an important consequence of cardiac failure. It is caused by the increased venous pressure, and retention of Na^+ (see Ch. 21).

Myocardial contraction

- Controlling factors are:
  - intrinsic myocardial contractility
  - extrinsic circulatory factors.
- Myocardial contractility depends critically on intracellular Ca^{2+}, and hence on:
  - Ca^{2+} entry across the cell membrane
  - Ca^{2+} storage in the sarcoplasmic reticulum.
- The main factors controlling Ca^{2+} entry are:
  - activity of voltage-gated calcium channels
  - intracellular Na^+, which affects Ca^{2+}/Na^+ exchange.
- Catecholamines, cardiac glycosides and other mediators and drugs influence these factors.
- Extrinsic control of cardiac contraction is through the dependence of stroke work on the end-diastolic volume, expressed in the Frank–Starling law.
- Cardiac work is affected independently by afterload (i.e. peripheral resistance and arterial compliance) and preload (i.e. central venous pressure).

MYOCARDIAL OXYGEN CONSUMPTION AND CORONARY BLOOD FLOW

Relative to its large metabolic needs, the heart is one of the most poorly perfused tissues in the body and is therefore at greater risk of ischaemic damage. Coronary flow is, under normal circumstances, closely related to myocardial oxygen consumption, and both change over a nearly 10-fold range between conditions of rest and maximal exercise. Most drugs that influence cardiac metabolism do so indirectly by influencing coronary blood flow.[3]

PHYSIOLOGICAL FACTORS

The main physiological factors that regulate coronary flow are:

- physical factors
- vascular control by metabolites
- neural and humoral control

Physical factors

During systole, the pressure exerted by the myocardium on vessels that pass through it equals or exceeds the perfusion

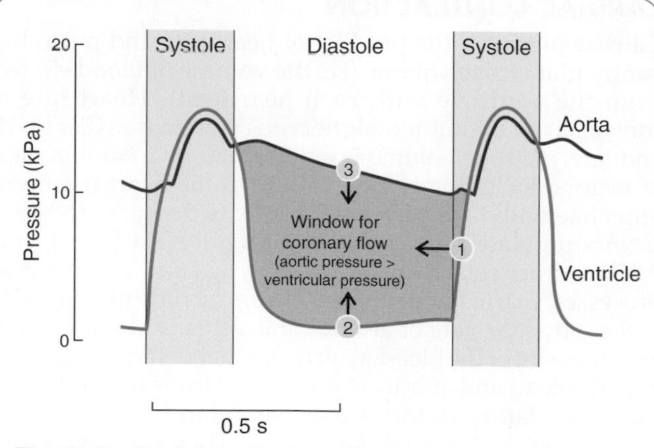

Fig. 20.5 Mechanical factors affecting coronary blood flow. The 'window' for coronary flow may be encroached on by *(1)* shortening diastole, when heart rate increases; *(2)* increased ventricular end-diastolic pressure; and *(3)* reduced diastolic arterial pressure.

pressure, so coronary flow occurs only during diastole. Diastole is shortened more than systole during tachycardia, reducing the period available for myocardial perfusion. During diastole, the effective perfusion pressure is equal to the difference between the aortic and ventricular pressures (Fig. 20.5). If diastolic aortic pressure falls or diastolic ventricular pressure increases, perfusion pressure falls and so (unless other control mechanisms can compensate) does coronary blood flow. Stenosis of the aortic valve reduces aortic pressure but increases left ventricular pressure upstream of the narrowed valve and hence reducing coronary perfusion pressure and often causes ischaemic chest pain (angina), even in the absence of coronary artery disease, by this mechanism.

Vascular control by metabolites/mediators

Vascular control by metabolites is the most important mechanism by which coronary flow is regulated. A reduction in arterial partial pressure of oxygen (P_{O_2}) causes marked vasodilatation of coronary vessels in situ but has little effect on isolated strips of coronary artery, suggesting that it is a change in the metabolites produced by the myocardial cells, rather than the change in P_{O_2} per se, that controls the state of the coronary vessels. *Adenosine* is a popular candidate for the dilator metabolite (see Ch. 16).

Neural and humoral control

Coronary vessels have a dense sympathetic innervation, but sympathetic nerves and circulating catecholamines exert only a small direct effect on the coronary circulation. Large coronary vessels possess α adrenoceptors that mediate vasoconstriction, whereas smaller vessels have β_2 adrenoceptors that have a dilator effect. Coronary vessels are also innervated by purinergic, peptidergic and nitrergic nerves, and basal coronary blood flow in patients with angiographically normal coronary arteries is reduced by about one-third by selective inhibition of NOS1 (Seddon et al., 2009). Coronary vascular responses to altered mechanical and metabolic activity during exercise or pathological events overshadow neural and endocrine effects.

[3]**Trimetazidine,** used to treat angina in some European countries, is claimed to improve cardiac metabolism by blocking fatty acid oxidation, thereby increasing the use of glucose as an energy source, which requires less oxygen per unit of energy generated. However, a large trial in patients after coronary intervention did not demonstrate significant benefit over placebo (Ferrari et al., 2020).

Coronary flow, ischaemia and infarction

- The heart has a smaller blood supply in relation to its oxygen consumption than most organs.
- Coronary flow is controlled mainly by:
  - physical factors, including transmural pressure during systole
  - vasodilator metabolites.
- Autonomic innervation is less important.
- Coronary ischaemia is usually the result of atherosclerosis and causes angina.
- Thrombosis on a fissured atheromatous plaque may result in cardiac infarction (death of a region of the myocardium) or unstable angina (occurring with less than usual exertion or at rest).
- Coronary artery spasm sometimes causes angina at rest (vasospastic angina), but less commonly on exertion.
- Cellular Ca^{2+} overload results from ischaemia and may be responsible for:
  - cell death
  - dysrhythmias.

AUTONOMIC CONTROL OF THE HEART

The sympathetic and parasympathetic systems (see Chs 13–15) each exert a tonic effect on the heart at rest and influence each of the aspects of cardiac function discussed earlier, namely rate and rhythm, myocardial contraction and myocardial metabolism and blood flow.

SYMPATHETIC SYSTEM

The main effects of sympathetic activity on the heart are:

- increased force of contraction (positive *inotropic* effect; Fig. 20.6);
- increased heart rate (positive *chronotropic* effect; Fig. 20.7);
- increased *automaticity* (i.e. tendency to generate ectopic beats);
- repolarisation and *restoration of function* following generalised cardiac depolarisation;
- reduced cardiac *efficiency* (i.e. oxygen consumption is increased more than cardiac work);
- cardiac hypertrophy (which seems to be directly mediated by stimulation of myocardial α and β adrenoceptors rather than by haemodynamic changes).

These effects mainly result from activation of β_1 adrenoceptors. The β_1 effects of catecholamines on the heart, although complex, probably all occur through activation of adenylyl cyclase resulting in increased intracellular cAMP (see Ch. 3). cAMP activates protein kinase A, which phosphorylates sites on the α_1 subunits of calcium channels. This increases the probability that the channels will open, increasing inward Ca^{2+} current and hence force of cardiac contraction (see Fig. 20.6). Activation of β_1 adrenoceptors also increases the Ca^{2+} sensitivity of the contractile machinery, possibly by phosphorylating troponin C; furthermore, it facilitates Ca^{2+} capture by the sarcoplasmic reticulum, thereby increasing the amount of Ca^{2+} available for release by the action potential. The net result of catecholamine action is to elevate and steepen the ventricular function curve (see Fig. 20.4). The increase in heart rate results from an increased slope of the pacemaker potential (see Figs 20.1 and 20.7A). Increased Ca^{2+} entry also increases automaticity because of the effect of $[Ca^{2+}]_i$ on the transient inward current, which can result in a train of action potentials following a single stimulus (see Fig. 20.2).

Activation of β_1 adrenoceptors repolarises damaged or hypoxic myocardium by stimulating the Na^+/K^+ pump. This can restore spontaneous circulation when **adrenaline** is given to patients with non-shockable rhythms during cardiac arrest.

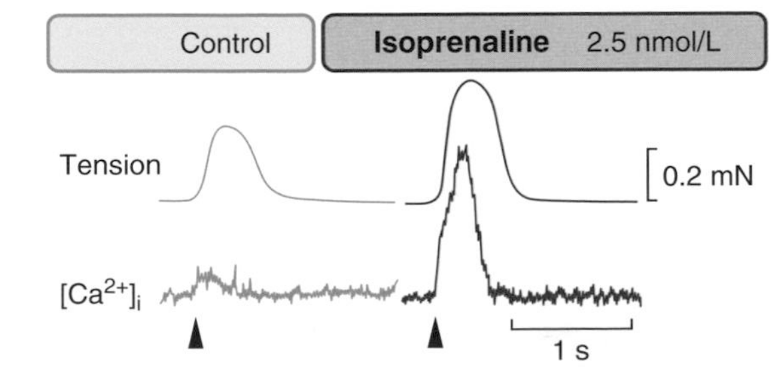

Fig. 20.6 The calcium transient in frog cardiac muscle. A group of cells was injected with the phosphorescent Ca^{2+} indicator aequorin, which allows $[Ca^{2+}]_i$ to be monitored optically. Isoprenaline causes a large increase in the tension and in the $[Ca^{2+}]_i$ transient caused by an electrical stimulus (▲). (From Allen, D.G., Blinks, J.R., 1978. Nature 273, 509.)

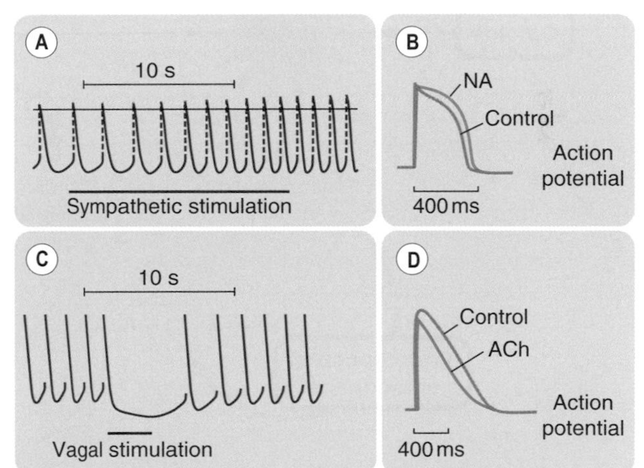

Fig. 20.7 Autonomic regulation of the heartbeat. (A) and (B) Effects of sympathetic stimulation and noradrenaline (NA). (C and D) Effects of parasympathetic stimulation and acetylcholine (ACh). Sympathetic stimulation (A) increases the slope of the pacemaker potential and increases heart rate, whereas parasympathetic stimulation (C) abolishes the pacemaker potential, hyperpolarises the membrane and temporarily stops the heart (frog sinus venosus). NA (B) prolongs the action potential, while ACh (D) shortens it (frog atrium). (Panels [A] and [C] from Hutter, O.F., Trautwein, W., 1956. J. Gen. Physiol. 39, 715; panel [B] from Reuter, H., 1974. J. Physiol. 242, 429; [D] from Giles, W.R., Noble, S.J., 1976. J. Physiol. 261, 103.)

The reduction of cardiac efficiency by catecholamines is important because it means that the oxygen requirement of the myocardium increases. This limits the use of β agonists such as adrenaline and **dobutamine** for circulatory shock (see Ch. 21). Myocardial infarction activates the sympathetic nervous system (see Fig. 20.8), which has the undesirable effect of increasing the oxygen needs of the damaged myocardium.

PARASYMPATHETIC SYSTEM

Parasympathetic activity produces effects that are, in general, opposite to those of sympathetic activation. However, in contrast to sympathetic activity, the parasympathetic nervous system has little effect on ventricular contractility, its main effects being on rate and rhythm, namely:

- cardiac slowing and reduced automaticity
- inhibition of AV conduction

These effects result from activation of muscarinic (M_2) acetylcholine receptors, which are abundant in nodal and atrial tissue but sparse in the ventricles. These receptors are negatively coupled to adenylyl cyclase and thus reduce cAMP formation, acting to inhibit the opening of L-type Ca^{2+} channels and reduce the slow Ca^{2+} current, in opposition to β_1 adrenoceptors. M_2 receptors also open a type of K^+ channel known as GIRK (G protein-activated inward rectifying K^+ channel) via production of G β/γ subunits (see Ch. 3). The resulting increase in K^+ permeability produces a hyperpolarising current that opposes the inward pacemaker current, slowing the heart and reducing automaticity (see Fig. 20.7C). Vagal activity is often increased during myocardial infarction, both in association with vagal afferent stimulation and as a side effect of opioids used to control pain, and parasympathetic effects are important in predisposing to acute dysrhythmias.

Vagal stimulation decreases the force of contraction of the atria associated with marked shortening of the action potential (see Fig. 20.7D). Increased K^+ permeability and reduced Ca^{2+} current both contribute to conduction block at the AV node, where propagation depends on the Ca^{2+} current. Shortening the atrial action potential reduces the refractory period, which can lead to re-entrant arrhythmias. Coronary vessels lack cholinergic innervation; consequently, the parasympathetic nervous system has little effect on coronary artery tone (see Ch. 14).

Autonomic control of the heart

- Sympathetic activity, acting through β_1 adrenoceptors, increases heart rate, contractility and automaticity, but reduces cardiac efficiency in relation to oxygen consumption.
- The β_1 adrenoceptors act by increasing cAMP formation, which increases Ca^{2+} currents.
- Parasympathetic activity, acting through muscarinic M_2 receptors, causes cardiac slowing, decreased force of contraction (atria only) and inhibition of AV conduction.
- M_2 receptors inhibit cAMP formation and also open potassium channels, causing hyperpolarisation.

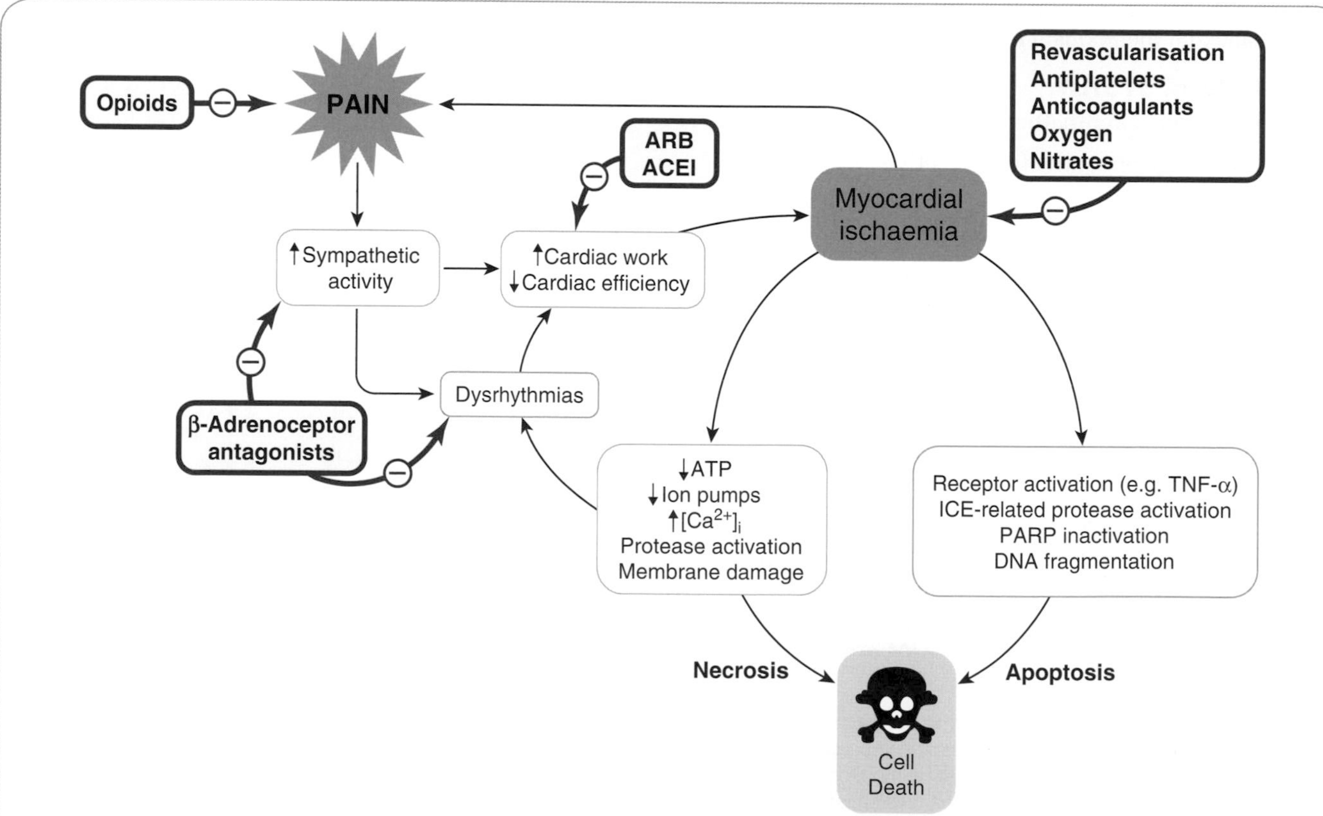

Fig. 20.8 Effects of myocardial ischaemia. This leads to cell death by one of two pathways: necrosis or apoptosis. *ACEI,* Angiotensin-converting enzyme inhibitor; *ARB,* angiotensin AT_1 receptor antagonist; *ICE,* interleukin-1-converting enzyme; *PARP,* poly-[ADP-ribose]-polymerase; *TNF-α,* tumour necrosis factor-α.

CARDIAC NATRIURETIC PEPTIDES

Cardiac natriuretic peptides are an important family of mediators that have diuretic and vasodilatory actions (see Kuwahara, 2021, for a review). Atrial cells contain secretory granules, and store and release *atrial natriuretic peptide* (ANP). The release of ANP occurs during volume overload in response to stretching of the atria, and intravenous saline infusion is sufficient to stimulate its release. B-natriuretic peptide (BNP) is released from ventricular muscle and opposes ventricular fibrosis; its plasma concentration is increased in patients with heart failure and this (or the concentration of its precursor, N-terminal pro-BNP) helps clinicians to diagnose heart failure and titrate drug treatment. C-natriuretic peptide (CNP) is stored in endothelium and is considered to have wide-ranging effects on cardiovascular structure, function and remodelling. Both ANP and BNP are inactivated by neprilysin, also known as neutral endopeptidase (NEP) (see Ch. 21). **Sacubitril**, an inhibitor of neprilysin, increases circulating BNP and ANP and, in fixed combination with **valsartan**, is effective in treating heart failure.

Broadly speaking, these natriuretic peptides have actions that oppose the renin–angiotensin–aldosterone axis. The main effects of natriuretic peptides are to increase Na^+ and water excretion by the kidney, relax vascular smooth muscle, increase vascular permeability and inhibit the release and/or actions of several vasoconstrictor or salt-retaining hormones and mediators, including aldosterone, angiotensin II, endothelin and antidiuretic hormone. They exert their effects mainly through guanylyl cyclase membrane receptors (natriuretic peptide receptors [NPRs], the main subtypes of which are designated A and B).[4]

Recombinant human BNP (**nesiritide**) is licensed in the United States for treatment of heart failure, but it has failed to gain international acceptance due to lack of benefit on hard outcomes such as hospital admissions or mortality, as well as safety concerns around hypotension.

ISCHAEMIC HEART DISEASE

Atheromatous deposits are ubiquitous in the coronary arteries of adults living in developed countries. They are asymptomatic for most of the natural history of the disease (see Ch. 22), but can progress insidiously, culminating in acute myocardial infarction and its complications, including dysrhythmia and heart failure. Details of ischaemic heart disease are beyond the scope of this book, and excellent accounts (e.g. Zipes et al., 2018) are available for those seeking pathological and clinical information. Here, we merely set the scene for understanding the place of drugs that affect cardiac function in treating this most common form of heart disease.

Important consequences of coronary atherosclerosis include:

- angina (chest pain caused by cardiac ischaemia)
- myocardial infarction

[4]The nomenclature of natriuretic peptides and their receptors is peculiarly obtuse. The peptides are named 'A' for atrial, 'B' for brain – despite being present mainly in cardiac ventricle – and 'C' for A, B, C…; NPRs are named NPR-A, which preferentially binds ANP; NPR-B, which binds CNP preferentially; and NPR-C for 'clearance' receptor, because clearance of natriuretic peptide via cellular uptake and degradation by lysosomal enzymes was previously thought to be the only definite function of this binding site.

ANGINA

Angina occurs when the oxygen supply to the myocardium is insufficient for its needs. The pain has a characteristic distribution in the chest, arm and neck, and is brought on by exertion, cold or excitement. A similar type of pain occurs in skeletal muscle when it is made to contract while its blood supply is interrupted, and Lewis showed many years ago that chemical factors released by ischaemic muscle are responsible. Possible candidates include K^+, H^+ and adenosine (see Ch. 16), all of which sensitise or stimulate nociceptors (see Ch. 43). It is possible that the same mediator that causes coronary vasodilatation is responsible, at higher concentration, for initiating pain.

Stable angina. This is predictable chest pain on exertion. It is produced by an increased demand on the heart and is usually caused by fixed narrowing(s) of the coronary vessels by atheroma, although, as explained previously, narrowing of the aortic valve ('aortic stenosis') can cause angina by reducing coronary blood flow even in the absence of coronary artery narrowing. Symptomatic therapy is directed at reducing cardiac work with organic nitrates, β-adrenoceptor antagonists and/or calcium antagonists, together with treatment of the underlying atheromatous disease, usually including a statin (see Ch. 22), and prophylaxis against thrombosis with an antiplatelet drug, such as **aspirin** (see Ch. 23).

Vasospastic angina is relatively uncommon. It can occur at rest and is caused by coronary artery spasm, often in association with atheromatous disease. Therapy is with coronary artery vasodilators (e.g. organic nitrates, calcium antagonists).

Unstable angina. This is characterised by pain that occurs with less and less exertion, culminating in pain at rest, but without complete occlusion of the vessel. Treatment is similar to that for myocardial infarction and includes imaging and consideration of revascularisation procedures. Antiplatelet drugs (aspirin and/or an ADP antagonist such as **clopidogrel, ticagrelor** or **prasugrel**; see Chs 16 and 23) reduce the risk of myocardial infarction in this setting, and anticoagulant drugs add to this benefit (see Ch. 23) at the cost of increased risk of haemorrhage. Organic nitrates (see later) are used to relieve ischaemic pain.

ACUTE CORONARY SYNDROME

The term *acute coronary syndrome* is used to describe a range of clinical presentations (unstable angina, or non-ST-segment-elevation myocardial infarction [NSTEMI] or ST-segment-elevation myocardial infarction [STEMI]) that occur when blood flow to the heart is acutely reduced (usually from thrombosis in a coronary artery). In most instances, patients have either new onset of severe chest pain or progressive worsening of their previously stable angina, culminating in pain at rest. Clinical features and test results (ECG and biochemical markers) are instrumental in making the exact diagnosis.

The pathology in acute coronary syndrome is similar amongst the three presentations, namely coronary artery occlusion from platelet–fibrin thrombus associated with a ruptured atheromatous plaque. This may be fatal, usually as a result of mechanical failure of the ventricle or from dysrhythmia. Cardiac myocytes rely on aerobic metabolism. If the supply of oxygen remains below a critical value, a sequence of events leading to cell death ensues, detected clinically by an elevation of circulating *troponin* (a biochemical marker of myocardial injury) as well as of cardiac enzymes (e.g. the cardiac isoform of creatinine kinase) and changes in the surface ECG. The sequences leading from vascular occlusion to cell death via necrosis or apoptosis (see Ch. 6) are illustrated in Fig. 20.8. The relative importance of these two pathways in causing myocardial cell death is unknown, but apoptosis may be an adaptive process in hypoperfused regions, sacrificing some jeopardised myocytes and thereby avoiding the disturbance of membrane function and risk of dysrhythmia inherent in necrosis. Consequently, it is currently unknown if pharmacological approaches to promote or inhibit this pathway could be clinically beneficial.

Prevention of irreversible ischaemic damage[5] following an episode of coronary thrombosis is crucial. Opening the occluded artery must be achieved as fast as possible. If logistically possible, *percutaneous coronary intervention* (involving a stent or balloon inserted into the coronary artery) with administration of a glycoprotein IIb/IIIa antagonist (see Ch. 23) is more effective than thrombolytic drugs, which are an alternative if percutaneous intervention is unavailable or unsuitable for the patient. The main therapeutic drugs for myocardial infarction (see Fig. 20.8) include drugs to improve cardiac function by maintaining oxygenation and reducing cardiac work, as well as treating pain and preventing further thrombosis. They are used in combination, and include:

- thrombolytic, antiplatelet and anticoagulant drugs to open the blocked artery and prevent reocclusion (see Ch. 23)
- oxygen if there is arterial hypoxia;
- opioids (given with an antiemetic) to prevent pain and reduce excessive sympathetic activity;
- organic nitrate to reduce pain from cardiac ischaemia;
- β-adrenoceptor antagonists;
- angiotensin-converting enzyme inhibitors (ACEIs) or angiotensin AT_1 receptor antagonists (ARBs; see Ch. 21).

β-Adrenoceptor antagonists reduce cardiac work and thereby the metabolic needs of the heart, and are used as soon as the patient is stable. ACEIs and ARBs also reduce cardiac work and improve survival, as does opening the coronary artery (with percutaneous intervention or thrombolytic drug) and antiplatelet treatment.

DRUGS THAT AFFECT CARDIAC FUNCTION

Drugs that have a major action on the heart can be divided into three groups.

1. Drugs that affect myocardial cells directly. These include:
   a. autonomic neurotransmitters and related drugs
   b. antidysrhythmic drugs
   c. cardiac glycosides and other inotropic drugs
   d. miscellaneous drugs and hormones; these are dealt with elsewhere (e.g. **doxorubicin**, see Ch. 57; thyroxine, see Ch. 34; glucagon, see Ch. 31)
2. *Drugs that affect cardiac function indirectly.* These have actions elsewhere in the vascular system. Some anti-anginal drugs (e.g. nitrates) fall into this category, as do many drugs that are used to treat heart failure (e.g. diuretics, ACEIs and SGLT2 inhibitors; see Ch. 21).
3. *Calcium antagonists.* These affect cardiac function by a direct action on myocardial cells and also indirectly by relaxing vascular smooth muscle.

ANTIDYSRHYTHMIC DRUGS

A classification of antidysrhythmic drugs based on their electrophysiological effects was proposed by Vaughan Williams in 1970 (Table 20.1). It provides a good starting point for discussing mechanisms, although many useful drugs do not fit neatly into this classification (Table 20.2). Antidysrhythmic drugs have at best an inconsistent track record and major safety and tolerability problems. Emergency treatment of serious dysrhythmias is usually by physical means (e.g. pacing or electrical cardioversion by applying a direct current shock to the chest or via an implanted device) rather than drugs and other devices and surgical procedures such as implantable converter defibrillators, and ablation procedures now dominate long-term dysrhythmia management as well.

There are four classes (see Table 20.1).

- Class I: drugs that block voltage-sensitive sodium channels. They are subdivided: Ia, Ib and Ic.
- Class II: β-adrenoceptor antagonists.
- Class III: drugs that substantially prolong the cardiac action potential.
- Class IV: calcium antagonists.

The phase of the action potential on which each of these classes of drug have their main effect is shown in Fig. 20.9.

MECHANISMS OF ACTION

Class I drugs

Class I drugs block sodium channels, just as local anaesthetics do, by binding to sites on the α subunit (see Ch. 44). Because this inhibits action potential propagation in many excitable cells, it has been referred to as a 'membrane-stabilising' activity, a phrase best avoided now that the ionic mechanism is understood. The characteristic effect on the action potential is to reduce the maximum rate of depolarisation during phase 0.

Table 20.2 Antidysrhythmic drugs unclassified in the Vaughan Williams system

Drug	Use
Atropine	Sinus bradycardia
Adrenaline (epinephrine)	Cardiac arrest
Isoprenaline	Heart block
Digoxin	Rapid atrial fibrillation
Adenosine	Supraventricular tachycardia
Calcium chloride	Ventricular tachycardia due to hyperkalaemia
Magnesium chloride	Ventricular fibrillation, digoxin toxicity

[5]'Irreversible' by present technologies; cell therapies based on cardiac stem cells have been attempted therapeutically, and are a beacon of hope for the future.

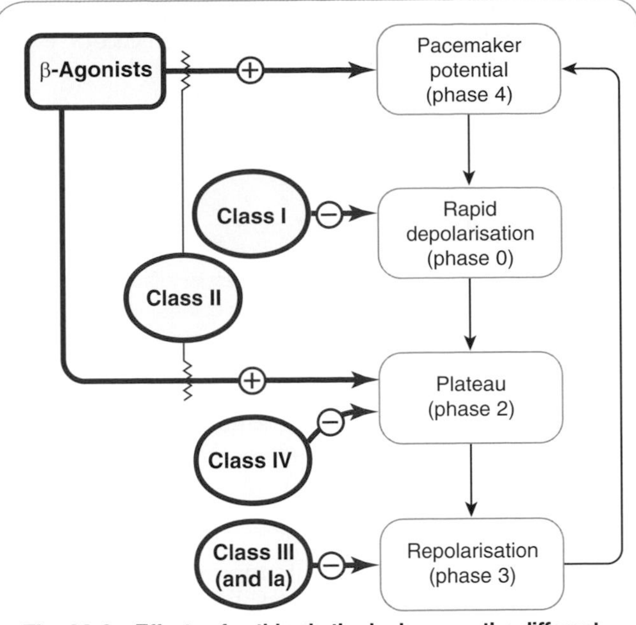

Fig. 20.9 Effects of antidysrhythmic drugs on the different phases (as defined in Fig. 20.1) of the cardiac action potential.

The reason for further subdivision of these drugs into classes Ia, Ib and Ic is that the earliest examples, **quinidine** and **procainamide** (class Ia), have different effects from many of the more recently developed drugs, even though all share the same basic mechanism of action. A partial explanation for these functional differences comes from electrophysiological studies of the characteristics of the sodium-channel block produced by different class I drugs.

The central concept is of use-dependent channel block. It is this characteristic that enables all class I drugs to block the high-frequency excitation of the myocardium that occurs in tachyarrhythmias, without preventing the heart from beating at normal frequencies. Sodium channels exist in three distinct functional states: resting, open and inactivated (see Ch. 4). Channels switch rapidly from resting to open in response to depolarisation; this is known as activation. Maintained depolarisation, as in ischaemic muscle, causes channels to change more slowly from open to inactivated, and the membrane, which is then refractory, must then be repolarised for a time to restore the channel to the resting state before it can be activated again. Class I drugs bind to channels most strongly when they are in either the open or the inactivated state, less strongly to channels in the resting state. Their action therefore shows the property of 'use dependence' (i.e. the more frequently the channels are activated, the greater the degree of block produced).

Class Ib drugs, for example, **lidocaine**, associate and dissociate rapidly within the timeframe of the normal heartbeat. The drug binds to open channels during phase 0 of the action potential (affecting the rate of rise very little but leaving many of the channels blocked by the time the action potential reaches its peak). Dissociation occurs in time for the next action potential, provided the cardiac rhythm is normal. A premature beat, however, will be aborted because the channels are still blocked. Furthermore, class Ib drugs bind selectively to inactivated channels and thus block preferentially when the cells are depolarised, for example, in ischaemia.

Class Ic drugs, such as **flecainide** and **encainide**, associate and dissociate much more slowly, thus reaching a steady-state level of block that does not vary appreciably during the cardiac cycle. They markedly inhibit conduction through the His–Purkinje system.

Class Ia, the oldest group (e.g. **quinidine**, **procainamide**, **disopyramide**), lies midway in its properties between Ib and Ic but, in addition, prolongs repolarisation, albeit less markedly than class III drugs (see later).

Class II drugs

Class II drugs comprise the β-adrenoceptor antagonists (e.g. **bisoprolol** and **metoprolol**).

Adrenaline can cause dysrhythmias by its effects on the pacemaker potential and on the slow inward Ca^{2+} current (see above). Ventricular dysrhythmias following myocardial infarction are partly the result of increased sympathetic activity (see Fig. 20.8), providing a rationale for using β-adrenoceptor antagonists in this setting. AV conduction depends critically on sympathetic activity; β-adrenoceptor antagonists increase the refractory period of the AV node and can therefore prevent recurrent attacks of SVT. The β-adrenoceptor antagonists are also used to prevent paroxysmal attacks of atrial fibrillation when these occur in the setting of sympathetic activation.

Class III drugs

The class III category was originally based on the unusual behaviour of a single drug, **amiodarone** (see later), although others with similar properties (e.g. D-**sotalol** and **vernakalant**) have since been described. All three agents have more than one mechanism of antidysrhythmic action. The special feature that defines them as class III drugs is that they substantially prolong the cardiac action potential. The mechanism of this effect is not fully understood, but it involves blocking some of the potassium channels involved in cardiac repolarisation, including the outward (delayed) rectifier. Vernakalant acts mainly on the atria and also exerts some class I effect through sodium channel blockade.

Action potential prolongation increases the refractory period, accounting for powerful and varied antidysrhythmic activity, for example, by interrupting re-entrant tachycardias and suppressing ectopic activity.

Class IV drugs

Class IV agents act by blocking voltage-sensitive calcium channels. Class IV drugs in therapeutic use as antidysrhythmic drugs (e.g. **verapamil**) act on L-type channels. Class IV drugs slow conduction in the SA and AV nodes where action potential propagation depends on inward Ca^{2+} current, slowing the heart, thus terminating SVT by causing partial AV block. They shorten the plateau of the action potential and reduce the force of contraction. Decreased Ca^{2+} entry reduces after-depolarisation and thus suppresses premature ectopic beats. Functionally distinct classes of L-type voltage-gated calcium channels are expressed in heart and vascular smooth muscle, and L-type calcium-channel blockers that act mainly on vascular smooth muscle (e.g. **nifedipine**) indirectly increase sympathetic tone via their hypotensive effect, causing reflex tachycardia.

DETAILS OF INDIVIDUAL DRUGS

Quinidine, procainamide and disopyramide (class Ia)

Quinidine and **procainamide**, now mainly of historical interest, are pharmacologically similar. **Disopyramide** resembles quinidine, but additionally possesses an atropine-like effect, distinct from its class Ia action, which can cause blurred vision, dry mouth, constipation and urinary retention. It has more negative inotropic action than quinidine but is less likely to cause hypersensitivity reactions.

Lidocaine (class Ib)

Lidocaine, also well known as a local anaesthetic (see Ch. 44), has been given by intravenous infusion, to treat and prevent ventricular dysrhythmias in the immediate aftermath of myocardial infarction or in cardiac arrest, but is less commonly used than amiodarone.

The adverse effects of lidocaine are mainly due to its actions on the central nervous system and include drowsiness, disorientation and convulsions.

Flecainide and encainide (class Ic)

Flecainide and **encainide** are efficacious in suppressing ectopic beats and tachyarrhythmias. However, in clinical trials, they unexpectedly increased the incidence of sudden death associated with ventricular fibrillation after myocardial infarction. As such, these drugs must not be used in patients who have underlying ischaemic or structural heart disease.

Clinical uses of class I antidysrhythmic drugs

- Class Ia (e.g. disopyramide)
  - ventricular dysrhythmias
  - prevention of recurrent paroxysmal atrial fibrillation triggered by vagal overactivity.
- **Class Ib** (e.g. intravenous **lidocaine**)
  - now seldom used.
- **Class Ic – use only in those who are free from underlying ischaemic or structural heart disease**
  - to prevent paroxysmal atrial fibrillation, or to restore sinus rhythm (pharmacological cardioversion) in atrial fibrillation (**flecainide**)
  - recurrent tachyarrhythmias associated with abnormal conducting pathways (e.g. Wolff–Parkinson–White syndrome).

β-Adrenoceptor antagonists (class II)

β-Adrenoceptor antagonists are described in Chapter 15. They are highly efficacious for a wide range of tachyarrhythmias and are often prescribed first line for rhythm disorders as shown in the 'Clinical uses of class II antidysrhythmic drugs (e.g. bisoprolol, metoprolol)' clinical box.

Adverse effects include worsening bronchospasm in patients with asthma, a negative inotropic effect, bradycardia and fatigue. It was hoped that the use of β_1-selective drugs (e.g. **bisoprolol**, **metoprolol**, **atenolol**) would remove the risk of bronchospasm, but their selectivity is insufficient to always achieve this goal in clinical practice, although the once-a-day convenience of several such drugs has led to their widespread use.

Clinical uses of class II antidysrhythmic drugs (e.g. bisoprolol, metoprolol)

- To reduce mortality following myocardial infarction.
- To prevent recurrence of supraventricular and ventricular tachyarrhythmias, and ectopic beats. For rate control in patients with atrial fibrillation
- In managing hyperthyroidism while control with antithyroid drugs is being established (see Ch. 34).

Class III

Amiodarone is highly effective at suppressing dysrhythmias (see the 'Clinical uses of class III antidysrhythmic drugs' clinical box). Unfortunately, several peculiarities complicate its use. It is extensively bound in tissues, has a long elimination half-life (10–100 days) and accumulates in the body during repeated dosing. For this reason, a loading dose is used, and for life-threatening dysrhythmias this is given intravenously via a central vein (it causes phlebitis if given into a peripheral vessel). Adverse effects are numerous and important; they include photosensitive rashes and a slate-grey/bluish discoloration of the skin; thyroid abnormalities (hypo- and hyper-, connected with its iodine content); pulmonary fibrosis, which is late in onset but may be irreversible; corneal deposits; and neurological and gastrointestinal disturbances, including hepatitis. Surprisingly (since it delays repolarisation and prolongs the QT interval), reports of *torsades de pointes* and ventricular tachycardia are very unusual. **Dronedarone** is a related benzofuran with somewhat different effects on individual ion channels. It does not incorporate iodine and was designed to be less lipophilic than amiodarone in hopes of reducing thyroid and pulmonary toxicities. Its elimination $t_{1/2}$ is shorter than that of amiodarone and it is indicated to maintain sinus rhythm after cardioversion of atrial fibrillation, but only as a last resort, due to safety concerns: it increased the rates of stroke, heart failure and death from cardiovascular causes in patients with permanent atrial fibrillation and risk factors for vascular events (Connolly et al., 2011). Dronedarone is contraindicated in patients with heart failure or left ventricular systolic dysfunction.

Sotalol is a non-selective β-adrenoceptor antagonist, this activity residing in the L isomer. Unlike other β antagonists, it prolongs the cardiac action potential and the QT interval by delaying the slow outward K^+ current. This class III activity is present in both L and D isomers. Racemic sotalol (the form prescribed) appears to be somewhat less effective than amiodarone in preventing chronic life-threatening ventricular tachyarrhythmias. It can cause torsades de pointes; it is used in patients in whom β-adrenoceptor antagonists are not contraindicated. Close monitoring of plasma K^+ is important for all class III drugs because of their effects on cardiac repolarisation.

Clinical uses of class III antidysrhythmic drugs

- **Amiodarone**: tachycardia associated with the Wolff–Parkinson–White syndrome. It is also effective in preventing many other supraventricular and ventricular tachyarrhythmias, but because of its serious adverse effects, amiodarone is prescribed only when other drugs (such as beta-antagonists) have failed. Intravenous amiodarone is an option for emergency treatment in life-threatening arrhythmias, or during cardiac resuscitation.
- (Racemic) **sotalol** combines class III with class II actions. It can be used in paroxysmal supraventricular dysrhythmias as well as ventricular tachycardia. However, the role of sotalol is limited because it has significant pro-arrhythmic risk.

Verapamil and diltiazem (class IV)

Verapamil is given by mouth. (Intravenous preparations are available but are seldom used because they provoke serious bradycardia and hypotension.) It has a plasma half-life of 6–8 h and is subject to quite extensive first-pass metabolism, which is more marked for the isomer that is responsible for its cardiac effects. A slow-release preparation is available for once-daily use, but it is less effective when used for prevention of dysrhythmia than the regular preparation because the bioavailability of the cardioactive isomer is reduced through the presentation of a steady low concentration to the drug-metabolising enzymes in the liver. If verapamil is added to **digoxin** in patients with poorly controlled atrial fibrillation, the dose of digoxin should be reduced and plasma digoxin concentration checked after a few days, because verapamil both displaces digoxin from tissue-binding sites and reduces its renal elimination, hence predisposing to digoxin accumulation and toxicity.

Verapamil is contraindicated in patients with Wolff–Parkinson–White syndrome (a pre-excitation syndrome caused by a rapidly conducting pathway between atria and ventricles, anatomically distinct from the physiological conducting pathway, that predisposes to re-entrant tachycardia), and is ineffective and dangerous in ventricular dysrhythmias. The adverse effects of verapamil and diltiazem are described later in the section on calcium-channel antagonists.

Diltiazem is similar to verapamil but has relatively more effect on vascular smooth muscle while producing less bradycardia (said to be 'rate neutral').

Adenosine (unclassified in the Vaughan Williams classification)

Adenosine is produced endogenously and is an important chemical mediator (see Ch. 16) with effects on breathing, cardiac and smooth muscle, vagal afferent nerves and on platelets, in addition to the effects on cardiac conducting tissue that underlie its therapeutic use. The A_1 receptor is responsible for its effect on the AV node. These receptors are linked to the same cardiac potassium channel that is activated by acetylcholine, and adenosine hyperpolarises cardiac conducting tissue and slows the rate of rise of the pacemaker potential accordingly. It is administered intravenously to terminate paroxysmal SVTs if this rhythm persists despite manoeuvres such as carotid artery massage to increase vagal tone. It has largely replaced verapamil for this purpose, because it is safer owing to its effect being short-lived as a consequence of uptake by red blood cells via a specific nucleoside transporter and metabolism by adenosine deaminase on the lumenal surface of vascular endothelium and in red cell cytoplasm. Consequently, the effects of an intravenous bolus dose of adenosine last only 20–30 s. Once SVT has terminated, the patient usually remains in sinus rhythm, even though adenosine is no longer present in plasma. Its short-lived unwanted effects include chest pain, shortness of breath, dizziness and nausea. **Regadenoson** is an A_{2A} adenosine receptor agonist that is used diagnostically in pharmacological cardiac stress testing see later). It is claimed that its selectivity and short duration of action are advantages over adenosine for this indication. It has a 2- to 3-min biological half-life and is administered as a bolus,

Theophylline and other xanthines (Chs 16 and 28) block adenosine receptors and inhibit the actions of intravenous adenosine, whereas **dipyridamole** (a vasodilator and antiplatelet drug; see later and see Ch. 23) blocks the nucleoside uptake mechanism, potentiating adenosine and prolonging its adverse effects. Both these interactions are clinically important.

Clinical uses of class IV antidysrhythmic drugs

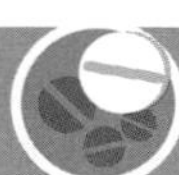

- **Verapamil** and diltiazem are used:
  - to prevent recurrence of paroxysmal SVT
  - to reduce the ventricular rate in patients with atrial fibrillation, provided they do not have Wolff–Parkinson–White or a related disorder.
- **Verapamil** was previously given intravenously to terminate SVT; it is now seldom used for this because **adenosine** is safer. (Slow-release preparations of verapamil or diltiazem are sometimes used to treat hypertension and/or angina, especially where it is desired to slow the heart rate but a β-adrenoceptor antagonist is contraindicated.)

DRUGS THAT ACT ON MYOCARDIAL CONTRACTION

CARDIAC GLYCOSIDES

Cardiac glycosides come from foxgloves (*Digitalis* spp.) and related plants. Withering wrote on the use of the foxglove in 1775: 'it has a power over the motion of the heart to a degree yet unobserved in any other medicine…' Foxgloves contain several cardiac glycosides with similar actions. Their basic chemical structure consists of three components: a sugar moiety, a steroid and a lactone ring. The lactone is essential for activity, the other parts of the molecule mainly determining potency and pharmacokinetic properties. Therapeutically the most important cardiac glycoside is **digoxin**.

Endogenous digitalis-like factors have been mooted for nearly half a century. There is evidence in mammals of an endogenous digitalis-like factor closely similar to **ouabain**, a short-acting cardiac glycoside implicated in cardiovascular function (see Schoner and Scheiner-Bobis, 2007; Blaustein et al., 2018). Endogenous cardiotonic steroids were first considered important in the regulation of renal sodium transport and arterial pressure, but have also been implicated in the regulation of cell growth, differentiation, apoptosis, fibrosis, the modulation of immunity and of carbohydrate metabolism and the control of various central nervous functions (Bagrov et al., 2009).

Actions and adverse effects

The main actions of glycosides are on the heart, but some of their adverse effects are extracardiac, including nausea, vomiting, diarrhoea and confusion. The cardiac effects are:

- cardiac slowing and reduced rate of conduction through the AV node, due to increased vagal activity;
- increased force of contraction;
- disturbances of rhythm, especially:
  - block of AV conduction;
  - increased ectopic pacemaker activity.

Adverse effects are common and can be severe. One of the main drawbacks of glycosides in clinical use is the narrow margin between effectiveness and toxicity.

Mechanism

The mechanism whereby cardiac glycosides increase the force of cardiac contraction (positive inotropic effect) is inhibition of the Na^+/K^+ pump in the cardiac myocytes. This causes increased $[Na^+]_i$, and a secondary rise in $[Ca^{2+}]_i$ (see later). Cardiac glycosides bind to a site on the extracellular aspect of the α subunit of the Na^+-K^+-ATPase and are useful experimental tools for studying this important transporter. The molecular mechanism underlying increased vagal tone (negative chronotropic effect) is unknown but could also be due to inhibition of the Na^+/K^+ pump.

Rate and rhythm

Cardiac glycosides slow, and in higher concentrations may block, AV conduction by increasing vagal outflow. Their beneficial effect in established rapid atrial fibrillation results partly from this. If ventricular rate is excessively rapid, the time available for diastolic filling is inadequate, so slowing heart rate by partly blocking AV conduction increases stroke volume and cardiac efficiency even if atrial fibrillation persists. Digoxin can terminate paroxysmal atrial tachycardia by its effect on AV conduction, although adenosine (see earlier discussion) is preferred for this indication.

Toxic concentrations of glycosides disturb sinus rhythm. This can occur at plasma concentrations of digoxin within, or only slightly above, the therapeutic range. AV block and ectopic beats can occur. Because Na^+/K^+ exchange is electrogenic, inhibition of the pump by glycosides causes depolarisation, predisposing to disturbances of cardiac rhythm. Furthermore, the increased $[Ca^{2+}]_i$ causes increased after-depolarisation, leading first to coupled beats (bigeminy), in which a normal ventricular beat is followed by an ectopic beat; ventricular tachycardia and eventually ventricular fibrillation may ensue.

Force of contraction

Glycosides cause a large increase in twitch tension in isolated preparations of cardiac muscle. Unlike catecholamines, they do not accelerate relaxation (compare Fig. 20.6 with

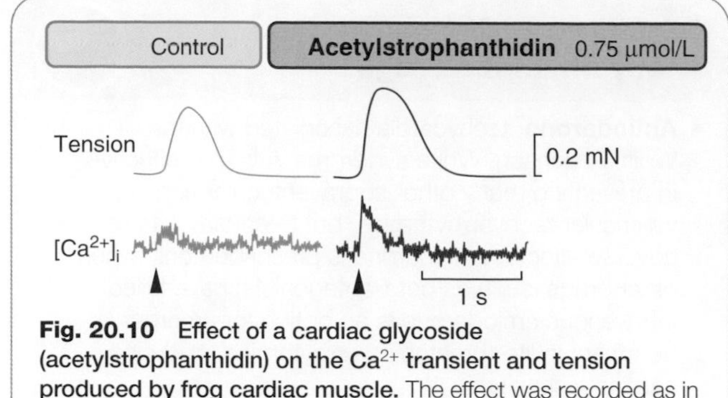

Fig. 20.10 Effect of a cardiac glycoside (acetylstrophanthidin) on the Ca^{2+} transient and tension produced by frog cardiac muscle. The effect was recorded as in Fig. 20.6. (From Allen, D.G., Blinks, J.R., 1978. Nature 273, 509.)

Fig. 20.10). Increased tension is caused by an increased $[Ca^{2+}]_i$ transient (see Fig. 20.10). The action potential is only slightly affected and the slow inward current little changed, so the increased $[Ca^{2+}]_i$ transient probably reflects a greater release of Ca^{2+} from intracellular stores. The most likely mechanism is as follows (see also Ch. 4):

1. Glycosides inhibit the Na^+/K^+ pump.
2. Increased $[Na^+]_i$ slows extrusion of Ca^{2+} via the Na^+/Ca^{2+} exchange transporter since increasing $[Na^+]_i$ reduces the inwardly directed gradient for Na^+ which drives extrusion of Ca^{2+} by Na^+/Ca^{2+} exchange.
3. Increased $[Ca^{2+}]_i$ is stored in the sarcoplasmic reticulum, and thus increases the amount of Ca^{2+} released by each action potential.

The effect of extracellular potassium

The effects of cardiac glycosides are increased if plasma $[K^+]$ decreases, because of reduced competition at the K^+-binding site on the Na^+-K^+-ATPase. This is clinically important, because many diuretics, which are often used to treat heart failure (see Ch. 29), decrease plasma $[K^+]$ thereby increasing the risk of glycoside-induced dysrhythmia.

Pharmacokinetic aspects

Digoxin is administered by mouth or, in urgent situations, intravenously. It is a polar molecule; elimination is mainly by renal excretion and involves P-glycoprotein (see Ch. 9), leading to clinically significant interactions with other drugs used to treat heart failure, such as **spironolactone**, and with antidysrhythmic drugs such as **verapamil** and **amiodarone**. Elimination half-time is approximately 36 h in patients with normal renal function, but considerably longer in elderly patients and those with overt renal failure, for whom the maintenance dose must be reduced. A loading dose is used to achieve therapeutic concentrations for rapid heart rate control in urgent situations. The therapeutic range of plasma concentrations, below which digoxin is unlikely to be effective and above which the risk of toxicity increases substantially, is rather narrow (1–2.6 nmol/L). Determination of plasma digoxin concentration is useful when lack of efficacy or toxicity is suspected.

OTHER DRUGS THAT ACT ON MYOCARDIAL CONTRACTION

Certain β_1-adrenoceptor agonists, for example **dobutamine**, are used to treat acute but potentially reversible heart

Clinical uses of cardiac glycosides (e.g. digoxin)

- To slow ventricular rate in rapid persistent atrial fibrillation. This is effective at rest but less so during exercise when vagal tone is reduced and sympathetic tone increased, limiting its usefulness.
- Treatment of heart failure in patients who remain symptomatic despite optimal use of diuretics and ACEIs (see Ch. 21).

failure (e.g. following cardiac surgery or in some cases of cardiogenic or septic shock) because of their positive inotropic action. Dobutamine, for reasons that are not well understood, produces less tachycardia than other β_1 agonists. It is used intravenously for short-term treatment of acute heart failure, or for pharmacological cardiac stress testing and echocardiography. **Glucagon** also increases myocardial contractility by increasing synthesis of cAMP, and has been used in patients with acute cardiac dysfunction caused by overdosage of β-adrenoceptor antagonists.

Inhibitors of the heart-specific subtype (type III) of phosphodiesterase, the enzyme responsible for the intracellular degradation of cAMP, increase myocardial contractility. Consequently, like β-adrenoceptor agonists, they increase intracellular cAMP and can cause dysrhythmias for the same reason. Compounds in this group include **amrinone** and **milrinone**. They improve haemodynamic indices in patients with heart failure but paradoxically worsen survival in chronic heart failure, presumably because of dysrhythmias. As with the encainide/flecainide and dronedarone examples, this disparity has had a sobering effect on clinicians and drug regulatory authorities.

Recent developments have led to phase III trials of drugs targeted at cardiac myosin. **Omecamtiv** mecarbil is a selective cardiac myosin activator that lowers the risk of hospital admissions in patients who have heart failure with reduced left ventricular ejection fraction. In contrast, **mavacamten** is a beta cardiac myosin inhibitor that decreases the excess contraction of heart muscles in patients with hypertrophic cardiomyopathy and currently under consideration by regulatory authorities for treating this disorder.

ANTI-ANGINAL DRUGS

The mechanism of anginal pain is discussed previously. Angina is managed by using drugs that improve perfusion of the myocardium or reduce its metabolic demand, or both. Two of the main groups of drugs, organic nitrates and calcium antagonists, are vasodilators and produce both these effects. The third group, β-adrenoceptor antagonists, slow the heart and hence reduce metabolic demand. Organic nitrates and calcium antagonists are described later. The β-adrenoceptor antagonists are covered in Chapter 15, and their antidysrhythmic actions are described earlier. **Ivabradine** slows the heart by inhibiting the sinus node I_f current (see earlier discussion) and is an alternative to β-adrenoceptor antagonists in patients in whom these are not tolerated or are contraindicated. Combined use of ivabradine with a β-adrenoceptor antagonist is indicated in patients whose symptoms are not adequately controlled despite an optimal dose of the β-adrenoceptor antagonist. **Ranolazine** was introduced as an adjunct to other anti-anginal drugs: it inhibits late sodium current and hence indirectly reduces intracellular calcium and force of contraction (the opposite of the effects of cardiac glycosides), without affecting heart rate; more potent and selective inhibitors of the persistent sodium current are in development. Newer anti-anginal drugs are described by Jones et al. (2013).

ORGANIC NITRATES

The ability of organic nitrates (see also Chs 19 and 21) to relieve angina was discovered by Lauder Brunton, a distinguished British physician, in 1867. He had found that angina could be partly relieved by bleeding, and knew that **amyl nitrite**, which had been synthesised 10 years earlier, caused flushing and tachycardia with a fall in blood pressure when its vapour was inhaled. He thought that the effect of bleeding resulted from hypotension and found that amyl nitrite inhalation worked much better. Amyl nitrite has now been replaced by **glyceryl trinitrate** (GTN).[6] Several related organic nitrates, of which the most important is **isosorbide mononitrate**, have a prolonged action. **Nicorandil**, a potassium-channel activator with additional nitrovasodilator activity, is sometimes combined with other anti-anginal treatment in resistant cases.

Actions

Organic nitrates relax smooth muscle (especially vascular smooth muscle, but also oesophageal and biliary smooth muscle). They relax veins, with a consequent reduction in central venous pressure (reduced preload). In healthy subjects, this reduces stroke volume; venous pooling occurs on standing and can cause postural hypotension and dizziness. Therapeutic doses have less effect on small resistance arteries than on veins, but there is a marked effect on larger muscular arteries. This reduces pulse wave reflection from arterial branches (as appreciated in the 19th century by Murrell but neglected for many years thereafter), and consequently reduces central (aortic) pressure and cardiac afterload (see Ch. 21 for the role of these factors in determining cardiac work). The direct dilator effect on coronary arteries opposes coronary artery spasm in vasospastic angina. With larger doses, resistance arteries and arterioles dilate, and arterial pressure falls. Nevertheless, coronary flow increases because of coronary vasodilatation. Myocardial oxygen consumption is reduced because of the reductions in cardiac preload and afterload. This, together with the increased coronary blood flow, causes a large increase in the oxygen content of coronary sinus blood. Studies in experimental animals have shown that GTN diverts blood from normal to ischaemic areas of myocardium. The mechanism involves dilatation of collateral vessels that bypass narrowed coronary artery segments (Fig. 20.11).

This contrasts with the effect of other vasodilators, notably **dipyridamole**, which dilate arterioles but not collaterals. Dipyridamole is at least as effective as nitrates in increasing coronary flow in normal subjects but actually worsens angina. This is probably because arterioles in an

[6]Nobel discovered how to stabilise GTN with kieselguhr, enabling him to exploit its explosive properties in dynamite, the manufacture of which earned him the fortune with which he endowed the eponymous prizes.

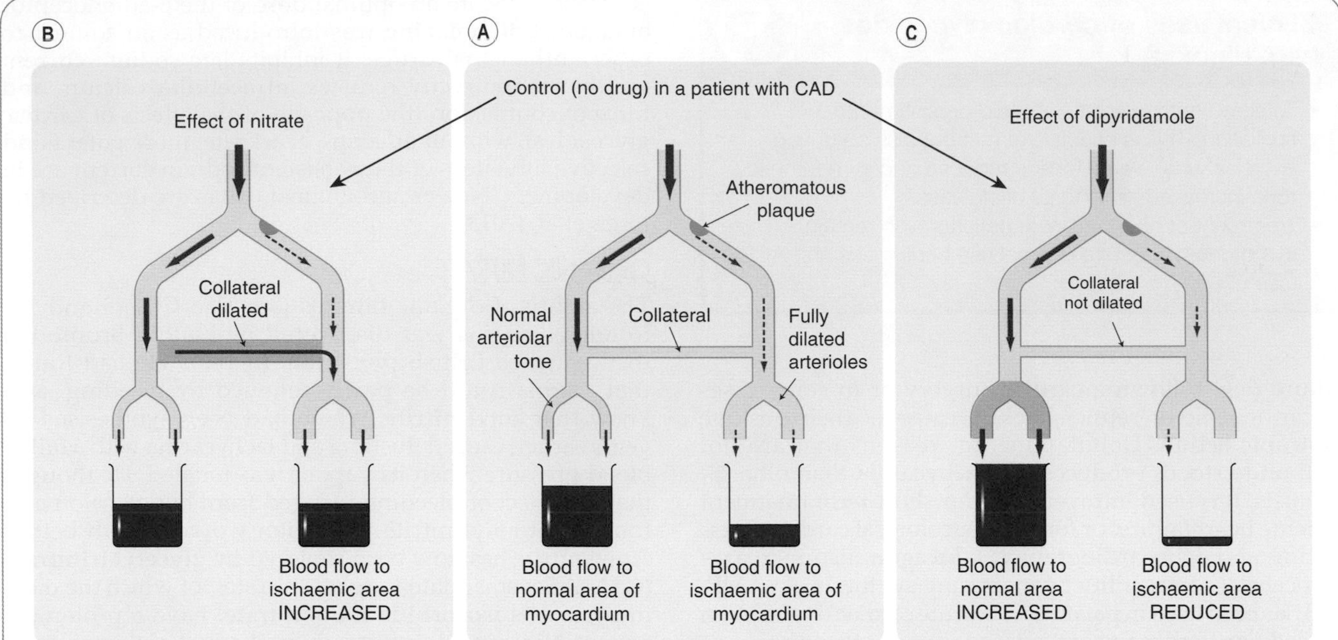

Fig. 20.11 Comparison of the effects of organic nitrates and an arteriolar vasodilator (dipyridamole) on the coronary circulation. (A) Control. (B) Nitrates dilate the collateral vessel, thus allowing more blood through to the underperfused region (mostly by diversion from the adequately perfused area). (C) Dipyridamole dilates arterioles, increasing flow through the normal area at the expense of the ischaemic area (in which the arterioles are anyway fully dilated). *CAD*, Coronary artery disease.

ischaemic region are fully dilated by the ischaemia, and drug-induced dilatation of the arterioles in normal areas has the effect of diverting blood away from the ischaemic areas (see Fig. 20.11), producing what is termed a *vascular steal*. This effect is exploited in a pharmacological 'stress test' for coronary arterial disease, in which dipyridamole is administered intravenously to patients in whom this diagnosis is suspected, while monitoring myocardial perfusion and the ECG. **Regadenoson** is an A_{2A} adenosine receptor agonist that is used similarly in pharmacological cardiac stress testing.

In summary, the anti-anginal action of nitrates involves:

- reduced cardiac work, because of reduced cardiac preload (venodilatation) and afterload (reduced arterial pressure wave reflection), leading to reduced myocardial oxygen requirement;
- redistribution of coronary flow towards ischaemic areas via collaterals;
- relief of coronary spasm.

In addition to its effects on smooth muscle, nitric oxide (NO) increases the rate of relaxation of cardiac muscle (dubbed a 'lusiotropic' action). It is probable that organic nitrates mimic this action, which could be important in patients with impaired diastolic function, a common accompaniment of hypertension and of heart failure.

Mechanism of action

Organic nitrates are metabolised with release of NO. At concentrations achieved during therapeutic use, this involves an enzymic step and possibly a reaction with tissue sulfhydryl (–SH) groups. NO activates soluble guanylyl cyclase (see Ch. 19), increasing the formation of cGMP, which activates protein kinase G (see Ch. 4) and leads to a cascade of effects in smooth muscle culminating in dephosphorylation of myosin light chains, sequestration of intracellular Ca^{2+} and relaxation.

Tolerance and unwanted effects

Repeated administration of nitrates to smooth muscle preparations in vitro results in diminished relaxation, possibly partly because of depletion of free –SH groups, although attempts to prevent tolerance by agents that restore tissue –SH groups have not been clinically useful. Tolerance to the anti-anginal effect of nitrates does not occur to a clinically important extent with ordinary formulations of short-acting drugs (e.g. GTN) but does occur with longer-acting drugs (e.g. isosorbide mononitrate) or when GTN is administered by prolonged intravenous infusion or by frequent application of slow-release transdermal patches (see later).

The main adverse effects of nitrates are a direct consequence of their main pharmacological actions and include postural hypotension and headache. This was the cause of 'Monday morning sickness' among workers in explosives factories. Tolerance to these effects develops quite quickly but wears off after a brief nitrate-free interval (which is why the symptoms appeared on Mondays and not later in the week). Formation of *methaemoglobin*, an oxidation product of haemoglobin that is ineffective as an oxygen carrier, seldom occurs when nitrates are used clinically but is induced deliberately with **amyl nitrite** in the treatment of *cyanide poisoning*, because methaemoglobin binds and inactivates cyanide ions.

Pharmacokinetic and pharmaceutical aspects

GTN is rapidly inactivated by hepatic metabolism. It is well absorbed from the mouth and is taken as a tablet under the tongue or as a sublingual spray, producing its effects within a few minutes. If swallowed, it is ineffective because of presystemic metabolism in the liver. Given sublingually, the trinitrate is converted to di- and mononitrates. Its effective duration of action is approximately 30 min. It is appreciably absorbed through the skin, and a more sustained effect can be achieved by applying it as a transdermal patch. Once a bottle of the tablets has been opened, its shelf-life is quite short because the volatile active substance evaporates; spray preparations avoid this problem.

Isosorbide mononitrate is longer acting than GTN because it is absorbed and metabolised more slowly but has similar pharmacological actions. It is not subject to first-pass metabolism in the liver and so can be swallowed rather than taken sublingually. It is usually administered in slow-release form for once-daily use in the morning, with the gradual absorption and elimination allowing a relative nitrate-free interval during the night.

Organic nitrates

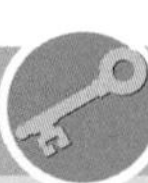

- Important compounds include **glyceryl trinitrate** and longer-acting **isosorbide mononitrate.**
- These drugs are powerful vasodilators, acting on veins to reduce cardiac preload and on arteries to reduce arterial pressure wave reflection and hence afterload.
- Act via NO, to which they are metabolised. NO stimulates formation of cGMP and hence activates protein kinase G, affecting contractile proteins (myosin light chains) and Ca^{2+} regulation.
- Tolerance occurs experimentally and is important clinically with frequent use of long-acting drugs or sustained-release preparations.
- Effectiveness in angina results partly from reduced cardiac load and partly from dilatation of collateral coronary vessels, causing more effective distribution of coronary flow. Dilatation of constricted coronary vessels is particularly beneficial in variant angina.
- Serious unwanted effects are uncommon; headache and postural hypotension may occur initially. Overdose can rarely cause methaemoglobinaemia.

Clinical uses of organic nitrates

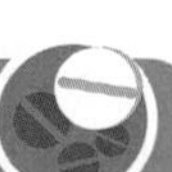

- Stable angina:
  - prevention (e.g. daily **isosorbide mononitrate**, or **glyceryl trinitrate** sublingually immediately before exertion);
  - treatment (sublingual **glyceryl trinitrate**).
- Unstable angina: intravenous **glyceryl trinitrate.**
- Acute heart failure: intravenous **glyceryl trinitrate.**
- Chronic heart failure: **isosorbide mononitrate**, with **hydralazine** in patients of African origin (see Ch. 21).

POTASSIUM-CHANNEL ACTIVATORS

Nicorandil combines activation of the potassium K_{ATP} channel (see Ch. 4) with nitrovasodilator (NO donor) actions. It is both an arterial and a venous dilator, and causes the expected unwanted effects of headache, flushing and dizziness. It is used for patients who remain symptomatic despite optimal management with other drugs, often while they await surgery or angioplasty, or if coronary intervention is not a feasible option.

β-ADRENOCEPTOR ANTAGONISTS

β-Adrenoceptor antagonists (see Ch. 15) are important in the prophylaxis of stable angina, and in treating patients with unstable angina, acting by reducing cardiac oxygen consumption. They reduce the risk of death following myocardial infarction, possibly via their antidysrhythmic action. Any effects on coronary vessel diameter are of minor importance, although these drugs are avoided in vasospastic angina because of the theoretical risk that they will increase coronary spasm. Their astonishingly diverse clinical uses are summarised in the previous clinical boxes and in Chapter 15.

CALCIUM ANTAGONISTS

The term *calcium antagonist* is used for drugs that block cellular entry of Ca^{2+} through calcium channels rather than preventing its intracellular actions (see Ch. 4). Some authors use the term *Ca^{2+} entry blockers* to make this distinction clearer. Therapeutically important calcium antagonists act on L-type channels. L-type calcium antagonists comprise three chemically distinct classes: *phenylalkylamines* (e.g. **verapamil**), *dihydropyridines* (e.g. **nifedipine, amlodipine**) and *benzothiazepines* (e.g. **diltiazem**).

Mechanism of action: types of calcium channel

The properties of voltage-gated calcium channels have been studied by voltage clamp and patch clamp techniques (see Ch. 3). Drugs of each of the three chemical classes mentioned earlier all bind the α_1 subunit of the L-type calcium channel but at distinct sites. These interact allosterically with each other and with the gating machinery of the channel to prevent its opening (see later and Fig. 20.12), thus reducing Ca^{2+} entry. Many calcium antagonists show properties of use dependence (i.e. they block most effectively in cells in which the calcium channels are most active; see the discussion of class I antidysrhythmic drugs earlier). For the same reason, they also show voltage-dependent blocking actions, blocking more strongly when the membrane is depolarised, causing calcium-channel opening and inactivation.

Dihydropyridines affect calcium-channel function in a complex way, not simply by physical plugging of the pore. Calcium channels can exist in one of three distinct states, termed *modes* (see Fig. 20.12). When a channel is in mode 0, it does not open in response to depolarisation; in mode 1, depolarisation produces a low opening probability, and each opening is brief. In mode 2, depolarisation produces a very high opening probability, and single openings are prolonged. Under normal conditions, about 70% of the channels at any one moment exist in mode 1, with only 1% or less in mode 0; each channel switches randomly and quite slowly between the three modes. Dihydropyridine

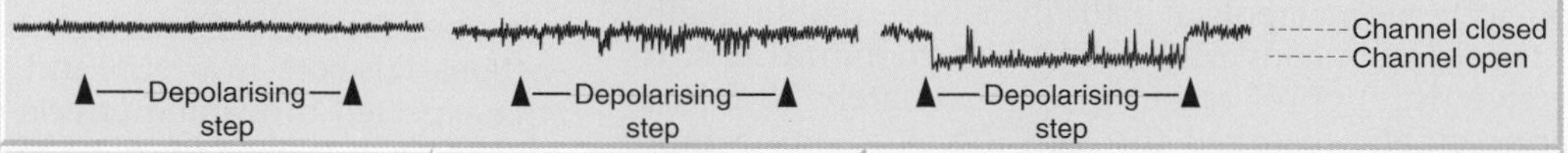

Mode	Mode 0	Mode 1	Mode 2
	Depolarising step	Depolarising step	Depolarising step (Channel closed / Channel open)
Opening probability	Zero	Low	High
Favoured by	DHP antagonists		DHP agonists
% of time normally spent in this mode	<1%	~70%	~30%

Fig. 20.12 Mode behaviour of calcium channels. The traces are patch clamp recordings (see Ch. 3) of the opening of single calcium channels *(downward deflections)* in a patch of membrane from a cardiac muscle cell. A depolarising step is imposed close to the start of each trace, causing an increase in the opening probability of the channel. When the channel is in mode 1 *(centre)*, this causes a few brief openings to occur; in mode 2 *(right)*, the channel stays open for most of the time during the depolarising step; in mode 0 *(left)*, it fails to open at all. Under normal conditions, in the absence of drug, the channel spends most of its time in modes 1 and 2, and only rarely enters mode 0. *DHP,* Dihydropyridine. (Redrawn from Hess, et al., 1984. Nature 311, 538–544.)

antagonists bind selectively to channels in mode 0, thus favouring this non-opening state, whereas agonists bind selectively to channels in mode 2 (see Fig. 20.12). This type of two-directional modulation resembles the phenomenon seen with the GABA/benzodiazepine interaction (see Ch. 45) and invites speculation about possible endogenous dihydropyridine-like mediator(s) with a regulatory effect on Ca^{2+} entry.

Ethosuximide (used to treat absence seizures; see Ch. 46) blocks T channels in thalamic and reticular neurons.

Pharmacological effects

The main effects of calcium antagonists, as used therapeutically, are on cardiac and smooth muscle. Verapamil preferentially affects the heart, whereas most of the dihydropyridines (e.g. nifedipine) exert a greater effect on smooth muscle than on the heart. Diltiazem is intermediate in its actions.

Cardiac actions

The antidysrhythmic effects of verapamil and diltiazem have been discussed earlier. Calcium antagonists can cause AV block and cardiac slowing by their actions on conducting tissues, but this is offset by a reflex increase in sympathetic activity secondary to their vasodilator action. For example, nifedipine typically causes reflex tachycardia; diltiazem causes little or no change in heart rate and verapamil slows the heart rate. Calcium antagonists also have a negative inotropic effect, from their inhibition of Ca^{2+} entry during the action potential plateau. Verapamil has the most marked negative inotropic action, and is contraindicated in heart failure, whereas amlodipine does not worsen cardiovascular mortality in patients with severe but stable chronic heart failure.

Vascular smooth muscle

Calcium antagonists cause generalised arterial/arteriolar dilatation, thereby reducing blood pressure, but do not much affect the veins. They affect all vascular beds, although regional effects vary considerably between different drugs. They cause coronary vasodilatation and are used in patients with coronary artery spasm (vasospastic angina). Other types of smooth muscle (e.g. biliary tract, urinary tract and uterus) are also relaxed by calcium antagonists, but these effects are less important therapeutically than their actions on vascular smooth muscle.

Protection of ischaemic tissues

Randomised clinical trials have been disappointing, with little or no evidence of beneficial (or harmful) effects of calcium antagonists on cardiovascular morbidity or mortality in patient groups other than patients with hypertension, in whom calcium antagonists have beneficial effects comparable with those of other drugs that lower blood pressure to similar extents (see Ch. 21). **Nimodipine** is partly selective for cerebral vasculature and there is some evidence that it reduces cerebral vasospasm following subarachnoid haemorrhage.

Pharmacokinetics

Calcium antagonists in clinical use are well absorbed from the gastrointestinal tract, and are given by mouth except for some special indications, such as following subarachnoid haemorrhage, for which intravenous preparations are available. They are extensively metabolised. Pharmacokinetic differences between different drugs and different pharmaceutical preparations are clinically important because they determine the dose interval and the intensity of some of the unwanted effects, such as headache and flushing. Amlodipine has a long elimination half-life and is given once daily, whereas nifedipine, diltiazem and verapamil have shorter elimination half-lives and are either given more frequently or are formulated in various slow-release preparations to permit once-daily dosing.

Unwanted effects

Most of the unwanted effects of calcium antagonists are extensions of their main pharmacological actions. Short-acting dihydropyridines cause flushing and headache because of their vasodilator action, and in chronic use dihydropyridines often cause ankle swelling (oedema) related to arteriolar dilatation and increased permeability of postcapillary venules. Verapamil can cause constipation, probably because of effects on calcium channels in gastrointestinal nerves or smooth muscle. Effects on cardiac rhythm (e.g. heart block) and force of contraction (e.g. worsening heart failure) were discussed earlier.

Apart from these predictable effects, calcium-channel antagonists, as a class, have few idiosyncratic adverse effects.

Calcium antagonists

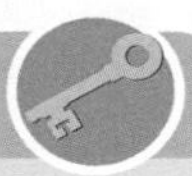

- Block Ca^{2+} entry by preventing opening of voltage-gated L-type calcium channels.
- There are three main L-type antagonists, typified by **verapamil**, **diltiazem** and dihydropyridines (e.g. **nifedipine**).
- Mainly affect heart and smooth muscle.
- **Verapamil** is relatively cardioselective, **nifedipine** is relatively smooth muscle selective, and diltiazem is intermediate.
- Vasodilator effect (mainly dihydropyridines) is mainly on resistance vessels, reducing afterload. Calcium antagonists dilate coronary vessels, which is important in vasospastic angina.
- Effects on heart (**verapamil**, **diltiazem**): antidysrhythmic action; impaired AV conduction; reduced contractility.
- Clinical uses:
  - antidysrhythmic (mainly **verapamil**)
  - angina, antidysrhythmic (e.g. **diltiazem**)
  - hypertension (mainly dihydropyridines).
- Unwanted effects include headache, constipation (**verapamil**) and ankle oedema (dihydropyridines). There is a risk of causing cardiac failure or heart block, especially with **verapamil.**

Clinical uses of calcium antagonists

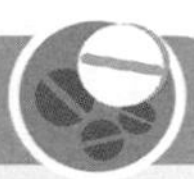

- Dysrhythmias (**verapamil, diltiazem**):
  - to slow ventricular rate in rapid atrial fibrillation
  - to prevent recurrence of SVT (intravenous administration of **verapamil** to terminate SVT attacks has been replaced by use of **adenosine**).
- Hypertension: usually a dihydropyridine (e.g. **amlodipine** or slow-release **nifedipine**; see Ch. 21).
- To prevent angina (e.g. a dihydropyridine or **diltiazem**).

REFERENCES AND FURTHER READING

Further reading

Fink, M., Noble, D., 2010. Pharmacodynamic effects in the cardiovascular system: the modeller's view. Basic Clin. Pharmacol. Toxicol. 106, 243–249.
Hampton, J.R., Hampton, J., 2019. The ECG Made Easy, ninth ed. Elsevier, Edinburgh.
Jones, D.A., Timmis, A., Wragg, A., 2013. Novel drugs for treating angina. BMJ 347, 34–37.
Zipes, D.P., Libby, P., Bonow, R.O., Mann, D.L., Tomaselli, G.F., 2018. Braunwald's Heart Disease: A Textbook of Cardiovascular Medicine, eleventh ed. Saunders/Elsevier, Philadelphia.

Physiological and pathophysiological aspects

Bagrov, A.Y., Shapiro, J.I., Fedorova, O.V., 2009. Endogenous cardiotonic steroids: physiology, pharmacology, and novel therapeutic targets. Pharmacol. Rev. 61, 9–38.
Blaustein, M.P., 2018. The pump, the exchanger, and the holy spirit: origins and 40-year evolution of ideas about the ouabain-Na(+) pump endocrine system. Am. J. Physiol. Cell Physiol. 314, C3–C26.
Eltzschig, H.K., Sitkovsky, M.V., Robson, S.C., 2012. Purinergic signaling during inflammation. N. Engl. J. Med. 367, 2322–2333.
Kuwahara, K., 2021. The natriuretic peptide system in heart failure: diagnostic and therapeutic implications. Pharmacol. Ther. 227 107863.
Noble, D., 2008. Computational models of the heart and their use in assessing the actions of drugs. J. Pharmacol. Sci. 107, 107–117.
Rockman, H.A., Koch, W.J., Lefkowitz, R.J., 2002. Seven-transmembrane-spanning receptors and heart function. Nature 415, 206–212.
Schoner, W., Scheiner-Bobis, G., 2007. Endogenous and exogenous cardiac glycosides: their roles in hypertension, salt metabolism, and cell growth. Am. J. Physiol. Cell Physiol. 293, C509–C536.
Seddon, M., Melikian, N., Dworakowski, R., et al., 2009. Effects of neuronal nitric oxide synthase on human coronary artery diameter and blood flow in vivo. Circulation 119, 2656–2662.
Tse, G., 2016. Mechanisms of cardiac arrhythmias. J. Arrhythm. 32, 75-81.
Yim, D.S., 2018. Five years of the CiPA project (2013–2018): what did we learn? Transl. Clin. Pharmacol. 26, 145–149.

Therapeutic aspects

Amuthan, R., Curtis, A.B., 2021. What clinical trials of ablation for atrial fibrillation tell us – and what they do not. Heart Rhythm O2 2, 174–186.
Connolly, S.J., Camm, J., Halperin, J.L., et al., 2011. Dronedarone in high-risk permanent atrial fibrillation. N. Engl. J. Med. 365, 2268–2276.
Ferrari, R., Ford, I., Fox, K., et al., 2020. Efficacy and safety of trimetazidine after percutaneous coronary intervention (ATPCI): a randomised, double-blind, placebo-controlled trial. Lancet 396, 830–838.
Kotecha, D., Bunting, K.V., Gill, S.K., et al., 2020. Effect of digoxin vs bisoprolol for heart rate control in atrial fibrillation on patient-reported quality of life: the RATE-AF randomized clinical trial. JAMA 324, 2497–2508.
Roden, D.M., 2019. A current understanding of drug-induced QT prolongation and its implications for anticancer therapy. Cardiovasc. Res. 115, 895–903.
Ruskin, J.N., 1989. The cardiac arrhythmia suppression trial (CAST). N. Engl. J. Med. 321, 386–388.

21 The vascular system

OVERVIEW

This chapter is concerned with the pharmacology of blood vessels. The walls of arteries, arterioles, venules and veins contain smooth muscle, the contractile state of which is controlled by circulating hormones and by mediators released locally from sympathetic nerve terminals (Ch. 15), endothelial cells and other cells resident in the vessel wall or visiting it from the circulating blood. These work mainly by regulating Ca^{2+} in vascular smooth muscle cells, as described in Chapter 4. In the present chapter, we first consider the control of vascular smooth muscle by the endothelium and by the renin–angiotensin system, followed by the actions of vasoconstrictor and vasodilator drugs. Finally, we consider briefly some of the clinical uses of vasoactive drugs in selected important diseases, namely hypertension (pulmonary as well as systemic), heart failure, shock, peripheral vascular disease and Raynaud's disease. The use of vasoactive drugs to treat angina is covered in Chapter 20.

INTRODUCTION

The actions of drugs on the vascular system can be broken down into effects on:

- total systemic ('peripheral') vascular resistance, one of the main determinants of arterial blood pressure;
- the resistance of individual vascular beds, which determines the local distribution of blood flow to and within different organs; such effects are relevant to the drug treatment of angina (see Ch. 20), Raynaud's phenomenon, pulmonary hypertension and circulatory shock;
- aortic compliance and pulse wave reflection, which are relevant to the treatment of hypertension, cardiac failure and angina;
- venous tone and blood volume (the 'fullness' of the circulation), which together determine the central venous pressure and are relevant to the treatment of cardiac failure and angina; diuretics (which reduce blood volume) are discussed in Chapter 29;
- atheroma (see Ch. 22) and thrombosis (see Ch. 23);
- new vessel formation (angiogenesis) – important, for example, in diabetic retinopathy (see Ch. 27) and in treating malignant disease (see Ch. 57).

Drug effects considered in this chapter are caused by actions on vascular smooth muscle cells. Like other muscles, vascular smooth muscle contracts when cytoplasmic Ca^{2+} ($[Ca^{2+}]_i$) rises, but the coupling between $[Ca^{2+}]_i$ and contraction is less tight than in striated voluntary or cardiac muscle (see Ch. 4). Vasoconstrictors and vasodilators act by increasing or reducing $[Ca^{2+}]_i$ and/or by altering the sensitivity of the contractile machinery to $[Ca^{2+}]_i$. Fig. 4.10 (see Ch. 4) summarises the cellular mechanisms that are involved in the control of smooth muscle contraction and relaxation. The control of vascular smooth muscle tone by various mediators is described in other chapters (noradrenaline in Ch. 15, 5-hydroxytryptamine [5-HT] in Ch. 16, prostanoids in Ch. 17, nitric oxide [NO] in Ch. 19, cardiac natriuretic peptides in Ch. 20 and antidiuretic hormone [ADH] in Ch. 33). Here we focus on endothelium-derived mediators and on the renin–angiotensin–aldosterone system (RAAS), before describing the actions of vasoactive drugs and their uses in some important clinical disorders (hypertension, heart failure, shock, peripheral vascular disease and Raynaud's disease).

VASCULAR STRUCTURE AND FUNCTION

Blood is ejected with each heartbeat from the left ventricle into the aorta, whence it flows rapidly to the organs via large conduit arteries. Successive branching leads via muscular arteries to arterioles (endothelium surrounded by a layer of smooth muscle only one cell thick) and capillaries (naked tubes of endothelium), where gas and nutrient exchanges occur. Capillaries coalesce to form postcapillary venules, venules and progressively larger veins leading, via the vena cava, to the right heart. Deoxygenated blood ejected from the right ventricle travels through the pulmonary artery, pulmonary capillaries and pulmonary veins back to the left atrium.[1] Small muscular arteries and arterioles are the main resistance vessels, while veins are capacity vessels that contain a large fraction of the total blood volume. In terms of cardiac function, therefore, arteries and arterioles regulate the *afterload*, while veins and pulmonary vessels regulate the *preload* of the ventricles (see Ch. 20).

The viscoelastic properties of large arteries determine arterial compliance (i.e. the degree to which the volume of the arterial system increases as the pressure increases). This is an important factor in a circulatory system that is driven by an intermittent pump such as the heart. Blood ejected from the left ventricle is accommodated by distension of the aorta, which absorbs the pulsations and delivers a relatively steady flow to the tissues. The greater the compliance of the aorta, the more effectively are

[1]William Harvey (physician to King Charles I) inferred the circulation of the blood on the basis of superbly elegant quantitative experiments long before the invention of the microscope enabled visual confirmation of the tiny vessels he had predicted. This intellectual triumph did his medical standing no good at all, and Aubrey wrote that 'he fell mightily in his practice', and was regarded by the vulgar as 'crack-brained'. *Plus ça change…*

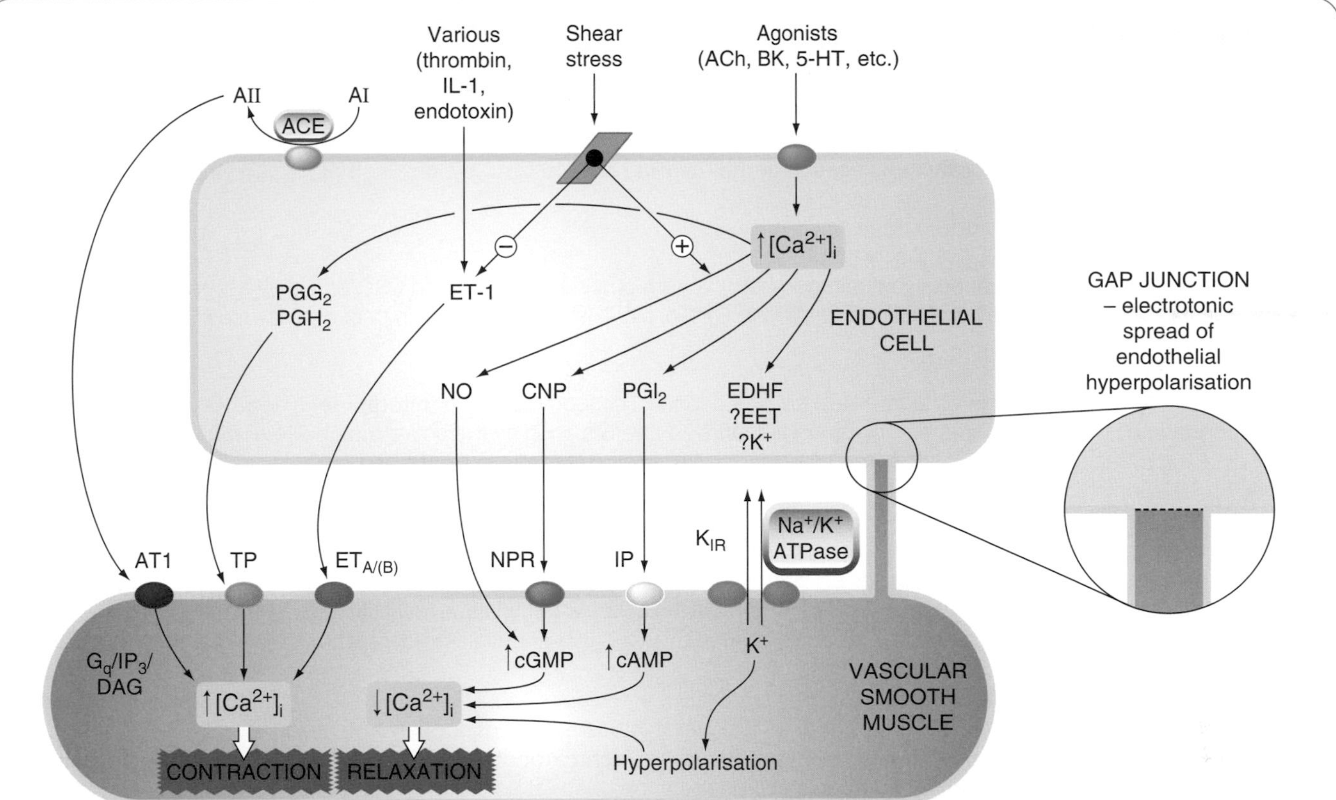

Fig. 21.1 Endothelium-derived mediators. The schematic shows some of the more important endothelium-derived contracting and relaxing mediators; many (if not all) of the vasoconstrictors also cause smooth muscle mitogenesis, while vasodilators commonly inhibit mitogenesis. *5-HT,* 5-Hydroxytryptamine; *A,* angiotensin; *ACE,* angiotensin-converting enzyme; *ACh,* acetylcholine; AT_1, angiotensin AT_1 receptor; *BK,* bradykinin; *CNP,* C-natriuretic peptide; *DAG,* diacylglycerol; *EDHF,* endothelium-derived hyperpolarising factor; *EET,* epoxyeicosatetraenoic acid; *ET-1,* endothelin-1; $ET_{A/(B)}$, endothelin A (and B) receptors; G_q, G protein; *IL-1,* interleukin-1; *IP,* I prostanoid receptor; IP_3, inosinol 1,4,5-trisphosphate; K_{IR}, inward rectifying potassium channel; *Na⁺/K⁺ ATPase,* electrogenic pump; *NO,* nitric oxide; *NPR,* natriuretic peptide receptor; *PG,* prostaglandin; *TP,* T prostanoid receptor.

fluctuations damped out,[2] and the smaller the oscillations of arterial pressure with each heartbeat (i.e. the difference between the systolic and diastolic pressure, known as the 'pulse pressure'). Reflection[3] of the pressure wave from branch points in the vascular tree also sustains arterial pressure during diastole. In young people, this helps to preserve a steady perfusion of vital organs, such as the kidneys, during diastole.

However, excessive reflection can pathologically augment aortic systolic pressure, because the less compliant the aorta, the greater the pulse wave velocity. Consequently, returning (reflected) pressure waves collide with the forward-going pulse wave from the next heartbeat earlier in the cardiac cycle. This results from stiffening of the aorta due to loss of elastin during ageing, especially in people with hypertension. Elastin is replaced by inelastic collagen. Cardiac work (see Ch. 20) can be reduced by increasing arterial compliance or by reducing arterial wave reflection (both of which decrease the pulse pressure), even if the cardiac output and mean arterial pressure are unchanged. Over the age of around 55 years, pulse pressure and aortic stiffness are important risk factors for cardiac disease.

[2]This cushioning action is called the 'Windkessel' effect. The same principle was used to deliver a steady rather than intermittent flow from old-fashioned fire pumps.

[3]Think of the waves in your bath as you sit up: down the tub, a splash down the overflow but most comes back as reflections from the foot end under the taps and interferes with the forward waves.

CONTROL OF VASCULAR SMOOTH MUSCLE TONE

In addition to the sympathetic nervous system (see Ch. 15), two important physiological systems that regulate vascular tone, namely the vascular endothelium and the renin–angiotensin system, deserve special attention.

THE VASCULAR ENDOTHELIUM

A new chapter in our understanding of vascular control opened with the discovery that vascular endothelium acts not only as a passive barrier between plasma and extracellular fluid, but also as a source of numerous potent mediators. These actively control the underlying smooth muscle as well as influencing platelet and mononuclear cell function: the roles of the endothelium in haemostasis and thrombosis are discussed in Chapter 23. Several distinct classes of mediator are involved (Fig. 21.1).

Vascular smooth muscle

- Vascular smooth muscle is controlled by mediators secreted by sympathetic nerves (see Ch. 15) and vascular endothelium, and by circulating hormones.
- Smooth muscle cell contraction is initiated by a rise in $[Ca^{2+}]_i$, which activates myosin light-chain kinase, causing phosphorylation of myosin, or by sensitisation of the myofilaments to Ca^{2+} by inhibition of myosin phosphatase (see Ch. 4).
- Agents cause contraction via one or more mechanisms:
  - release of intracellular Ca^{2+} via inositol trisphosphate,
  - depolarising the membrane, opening voltage-gated calcium channels and causing Ca^{2+} entry,
  - increasing sensitivity to Ca^{2+} via actions on myosin light-chain kinase and/or myosin phosphatase (see Ch. 4, Fig. 4.9).
- Agents cause relaxation by:
  - inhibiting Ca^{2+} entry through voltage-gated calcium channels either directly (e.g. **nifedipine**) or indirectly by hyperpolarising the membrane (e.g. potassium-channel activators such as the active metabolite of **minoxidil**);
  - increasing intracellular cAMP or cGMP; cAMP inactivates myosin light-chain kinase and facilitates Ca^{2+} efflux, cGMP opposes agonist-induced increases in $[Ca^{2+}]_i$.
- *Prostanoids* (see Ch. 17). The discovery by Bunting et al. (1976) of prostaglandin PGI_2 (prostacyclin) ushered in this era. This mediator, acting on I prostanoid (IP) receptors (see Ch. 17), relaxes smooth muscle and inhibits platelet aggregation by activating adenylyl cyclase. Endothelial cells from microvessels also synthesise PGE_2, which is a direct vasodilator and additionally inhibits noradrenaline release from sympathetic nerve terminals, while lacking the effect of PGI_2 on platelets. Prostaglandin endoperoxide intermediates (PGG_2, PGH_2) are endothelium-derived contracting factors acting via thromboxane (TX) T prostanoid (TP) receptors.
- *NO* (see Ch. 19). *Endothelium-derived relaxing factor* (EDRF) was first described in 1980, and subsequently identified as NO later on. NO activates guanylyl cyclase. It is released continuously in resistance vessels, giving rise to vasodilator tone and contributing to the physiological control of blood pressure. As well as causing vascular relaxation, it inhibits vascular smooth muscle cell proliferation, platelet adhesion and aggregation and monocyte adhesion and migration; consequently, it may protect blood vessels from atherosclerosis and thrombosis (see Chs 22 and 23).
- *Peptides.* The endothelium secretes several vasoactive peptides (see Ch. 17 for general mechanisms of peptide secretion). *C-natriuretic peptide* (CNP) (see Ch. 20) and *adrenomedullin* (a vasodilator peptide originally discovered in an adrenal tumour – phaeochromocytoma – but expressed in many tissues, including vascular endothelium) are vasodilators working, respectively, through cGMP and cAMP. *Angiotensin II*, formed by angiotensin-converting enzyme (ACE) on the surface of endothelial cells, and *endothelin* are potent endothelium-derived vasoconstrictor peptides.

In addition to secreting vasoactive mediators, endothelial cells express several enzymes and transport mechanisms that act on circulating hormones and are important targets of drug action. ACE is a particularly important example (see later, including Figs 21.2 and 21.3).

Many endothelium-derived mediators are mutually antagonistic, conjuring an image of opposing rugby football players swaying back and forth in a scrum; in moments of exasperation, one sometimes wonders whether all this makes sense or whether the designer simply could not make up their mind! An important distinction is made between mechanisms that are tonically active in resistance vessels under basal conditions, as is the case with the noradrenergic nervous system (see Ch. 15), NO (see Ch. 19) and endothelin (ET) (see later), and those that operate mainly in response to injury, inflammation, etc., as with PGI_2. Some of the latter group may be functionally redundant, perhaps representing vestiges of mechanisms that were important to our evolutionary forebears, or they may simply be taking a breather on the touchline and are ready to rejoin the fray if called on by the occurrence of some vascular insult. Evidence for such a 'back-up' role comes, for example, from mice that lack the IP receptor for PGI_2; they have a normal blood pressure and do not develop spontaneous thrombosis but are more susceptible to vasoconstrictor and thrombotic stimuli than their wild-type litter mates (Murata et al., 1997).

THE ENDOTHELIUM IN ANGIOGENESIS

As touched on in Chapter 9, the barrier function of vascular endothelium differs markedly in different organs, and its development during angiogenesis is controlled by several growth factors, including *vascular endothelial growth factor* (VEGF) and various tissue-specific factors such as endocrine gland VEGF. These are involved in repair processes and in pathogenesis (e.g. tumour growth and in neovascularisation in the eye – an important cause of blindness in patients with new vessel proliferation due to age-related macular degeneration, or diabetes mellitus; see Ch. 27). These

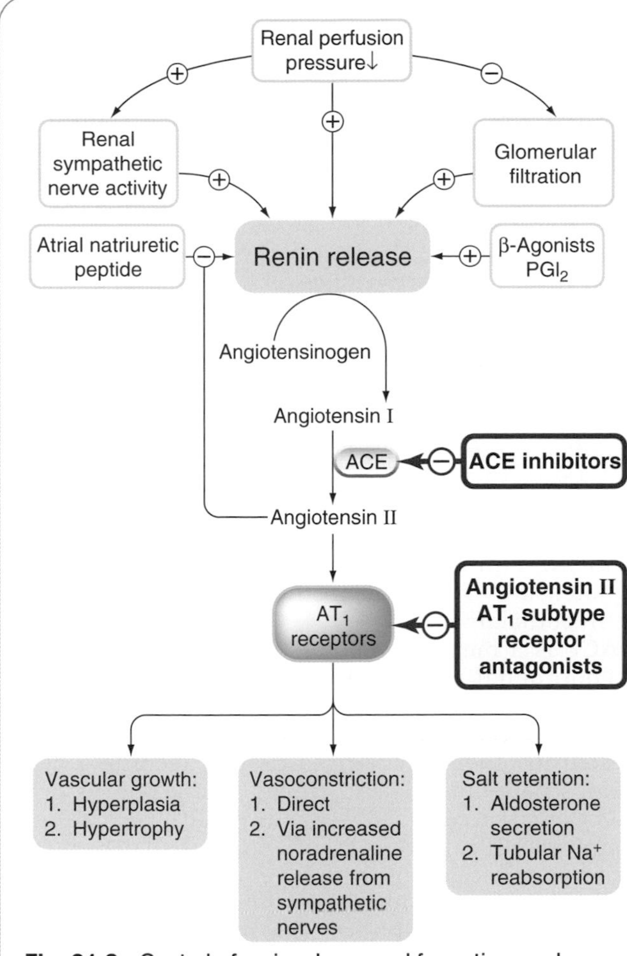

Fig. 21.2 Control of renin release and formation, and action of angiotensin II. Sites of action of drugs that inhibit the cascade are shown. *ACE*, Angiotensin-converting enzyme; *AT_1*, angiotensin II receptor subtype 1; *PGI_2*, prostaglandin I_2.

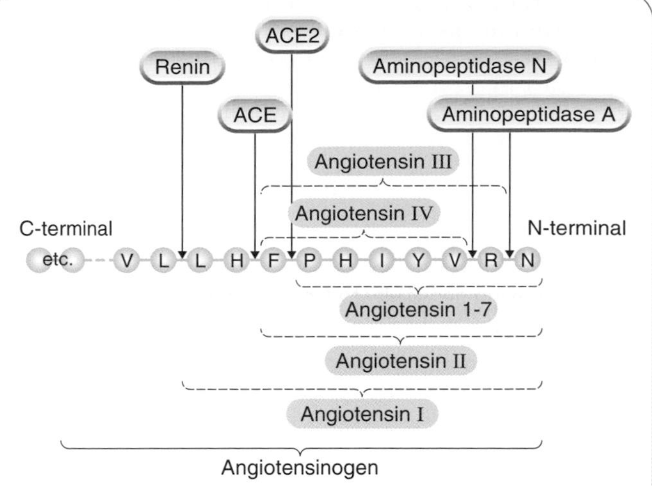

Fig. 21.3 Formation of angiotensins I–IV from the N-terminal of the precursor protein angiotensinogen. Also shown is angiotensin 17 which is a product of the action of angiotensin-converting enzyme 2 (ACE2) and opposing actins to angiotensin II.

factors and their receptors are potentially fruitful targets for drug development and new therapies (including gene therapies; see Ch. 5).

ENDOTHELIN

Discovery, biosynthesis and secretion

Hickey et al. described a vasoconstrictor factor produced by cultured endothelial cells in 1985. This was identified as *endothelin (ET)*, a 21-residue peptide, by Yangisawa, which at that time was the most potent vasoconstrictor known[4] (Barton and Yanagisawa, 2019).

There are three isoforms. ET-1 is the only ET present in endothelial cells and is also expressed in many other tissues. ET-2 is much less widely distributed: it is present in kidney and intestine. ET-3 is present in brain, lung, intestine and adrenal gland.

Stimuli of ET synthesis include many vasoactive mediators released by trauma or inflammation, including activated platelets, endotoxin, thrombin, various cytokines and growth factors, angiotensin II, ADH, adrenaline, insulin, hypoxia and low shear stress. ET concentrations are elevated in cardiac failure, hypertension, and connective tissue disorders such as scleroderma. Inhibitors of ET synthesis include NO, natriuretic peptides, PGE_2, PGI_2, heparin and high shear stress.

Endothelin receptors and responses

There are two types of ET receptors, designated ET_A and ET_B, both of which are G protein coupled (see Ch. 3). ET receptors are distributed widely across the entire body with a complex, multi-faceted range of tissue-specific expression and physiological effects that vary depend on the tissue site. For instance, the predominant overall response with ET_A is vasoconstriction through its action on smooth muscle, but ET_A also promotes inflammation and cell proliferation. In contrast, *ET_B* stimulates vasodilation (through endothelial NO release), as well as salt and water excretion in the kidney (Davenport et al., 2016).

ET-1 preferentially activates ET_A receptors. Messenger RNA for the ET_A receptor is expressed in many human tissues, including vascular smooth muscle, heart, lung and kidney. It is not expressed in endothelium. ET_A-mediated responses include vasoconstriction, bronchoconstriction and aldosterone secretion. ET_A receptors are coupled to phospholipase C, which stimulates Na^+/H^+ exchange, protein kinase C and mitogenesis, as well as causing vasoconstriction through inositol trisphosphate-mediated Ca^{2+} release (see Ch. 3). There are several partially selective ET_A-receptor antagonists of therapeutic value, including orally active non-peptide drugs (e.g. **bosentan**, a mixed ET_A/ET_B antagonist, and **ambrisentan**, ET_A selective, both of which are used in treating pulmonary arterial hypertension). ET_B receptors are activated to a similar extent by each of the three ET isoforms and, in the endothelium, are thought to mediate release of

[4]Subsequently, an 11-amino acid peptide (*urotensin*) was isolated from the brains of bony fish and found to be 50–100 times more potent than ET in some blood vessels. It and its receptor are expressed in human tissue but its function, if any, in man remains enigmatic.

vascular relaxing factors such as NO and PGI_2. ET_B is also present in vascular smooth muscle, where it initiates vasoconstriction like the ET_A receptor. ET_B receptors play a part in clearing ET-1 from the circulation, and ET antagonists with appreciable affinity for ET_B receptors consequently increase plasma concentrations of ET-1, complicating interpretation of such concentrations during experiments with these drugs.

Functions of endothelin

ET-1 is a local mediator rather than a circulating hormone, although it stimulates secretion of several hormones. ET-1 is a key player in vasoconstrictor tone and the regulation of peripheral vascular resistance in man, but ETs have several other possible functions, including roles in:

- release of various hormones, including atrial natriuretic peptide, aldosterone, adrenaline, and hypothalamic and pituitary hormones;
- natriuresis and diuresis via actions of collecting duct-derived ET-1 on ET_B receptors on tubular epithelial cells;
- renal and cerebral vasospasm;
- Organogenesis (pharyngeal arch derived organs) – ET antagonists are teratogenic in rodents.

The role of the endothelium in controlling vascular smooth muscle

- Endothelial cells release vasoactive mediators including prostacyclin (PGI_2), NO and distinct but incompletely characterised hyperpolarising factor(s) 'EDHF' (vasodilators) and ET and endoperoxide thromboxane receptor agonists (vasoconstrictors).
- Many vasodilators (e.g. acetylcholine and bradykinin) act via endothelial NO production. The NO derives from arginine and is produced when $[Ca^{2+}]_i$ increases in the endothelial cell, or the sensitivity of endothelial NO synthase to Ca^{2+} is increased (see Fig. 19.3).
- NO relaxes smooth muscle by increasing cGMP formation.
- ET is a potent and long-acting vasoconstrictor peptide released from endothelial cells by many chemical and physical factors. It is not confined to blood vessels, and it has several functional roles.

THE RENIN–ANGIOTENSIN SYSTEM

The renin–angiotensin system synergises with the sympathetic nervous system, for example, by increasing the release of noradrenaline from sympathetic nerve terminals. It stimulates aldosterone secretion and plays a central role in the control of Na^+ excretion and fluid volume, as well as of vascular tone.

The control of renin secretion (Fig. 21.2) is only partly understood. It is a proteolytic enzyme that is secreted by the *juxtaglomerular apparatus* (see Ch. 29, Fig. 29.2) in response to various physiological stimuli including reduced renal perfusion pressure, or reduced Na^+ concentration in distal tubular fluid, which is sensed by the *macula densa* (a specialised part of the distal tubule apposed to the juxtaglomerular apparatus). Renal sympathetic nerve activity, β-adrenoceptor agonists and PGI_2 all stimulate renin secretion directly, whereas angiotensin II causes feedback inhibition. Atrial natriuretic peptide (see Ch. 20) also inhibits renin secretion. Renin is cleared rapidly from plasma. It acts on *angiotensinogen* (a plasma globulin made in the liver), splitting off a decapeptide, *angiotensin I*.

Angiotensin I is inactive, but is converted by *ACE* to an octapeptide, *angiotensin II*, which is a potent vasoconstrictor. Angiotensin II is a substrate for enzymes (aminopeptidase A and N) that remove single amino acid residues, giving rise, respectively, to angiotensin III and angiotensin IV (Fig. 21.3). Angiotensin III exerts effects on the brain renin–angiotensin system to stimulate sympathetic activity and release vasopressin, thus increasing blood pressure. Angiotensin IV also has distinct actions, probably via its own receptor, including release of *plasminogen activator inhibitor-1* from the endothelium (see Ch. 23). Receptors for angiotensin IV have a distinctive distribution, including the hypothalamus.

ACE is a membrane-bound enzyme on the surface of endothelial cells, and is particularly abundant in the lung, which has a vast surface area of vascular endothelium.[5] The common isoform of ACE is also present in other vascularised tissues, including heart, brain, striated muscle and kidney, and is not restricted to endothelial cells. Consequently, local formation of angiotensin II can occur in different vascular beds, and it provides local control independent of blood-borne angiotensin II. ACE inactivates bradykinin (see Ch. 17) and several other peptides. This may contribute to the pharmacological actions of ACE inhibitors (ACEIs), as discussed later.

ACE2, a homologue of ACE, converts angiotensin II to angiotensin 1-7 (Ang 1-7) as shown in Fig. 21.3. Ang 1-7 acts on the Mas receptor (a G-protein–coupled receptor coded by the *MAS1* oncogene) opposing the effects of angiotensin II. ACE2 is widely expressed, including in cardiomyocytes, pneumocytes and endothelial cells, and potentially protects against heart failure by breaking down angiotensin II, thus reducing blood pressure and inflammatory cardiac damage. Unfortunately, the spike protein of the SARS-CoV-2 virus binds to ACE2 in the cell membrane, and uses it as a 'cellular gateway' to enter and infect cells.

Recombinant human ACE2 has been tested in humans without adverse effects while lowering plasma angiotensin II and increasing Ang 1-7 concentration. For a recent review of the therapeutic potential of enhancing ACE2/Ang 1-7 action for heart failure, see Patel et al. (2016).

The main actions of angiotensin II are mediated via AT_1 and/or AT_2 receptors, which belong to the family of G protein–coupled receptors. Effects mediated by AT_1 receptors include:

- generalised vasoconstriction, especially marked in efferent arterioles of the renal glomeruli;
- increased noradrenaline release, reinforcing sympathetic effects;

[5]Approximately that of a football field.

Table 21.1 Classification of vasoactive drugs that act indirectly

Site	Mechanism	Examples	See chapter
Vasoconstrictors			
Sympathetic nerves	Noradrenaline (norepinephrine) release Blocks noradrenaline reuptake	Tyramine Cocaine	15 50
Endothelium	Endothelin release	Angiotensin II (in part)	This chapter
Vasodilators			
Sympathetic nerves	Inhibits noradrenaline release	Prostaglandin E_2, guanethidine	17 15
Endothelium	Nitric oxide release	Acetylcholine, substance P	19
Central nervous system	Vasomotor inhibition	Anaesthetics	41
Enzymes	ACE inhibition	Captopril	This chapter

ACE, Angiotensin-converting enzyme.

- proximal tubular reabsorption of Na^+;
- secretion of aldosterone from the adrenal cortex (see Ch. 33);
- pro-inflammatory effect, growth of cardiac and vascular cells.[6]

AT_2 receptors are expressed during fetal life and in distinct brain regions in adults. They are believed to be involved in growth, development and exploratory behaviour. The cardiovascular effects of AT_2 receptors (inhibition of cell growth and lowering of blood pressure) are relatively subtle and oppose those of AT_1 receptors.

The renin–angiotensin–aldosterone pathway contributes to the pathogenesis of heart failure, and several leading classes of therapeutic drug act on it at different points (see Fig. 21.2).

VASOACTIVE DRUGS

Drugs can affect vascular smooth muscle by acting either directly on smooth muscle cells, or indirectly, for example, on endothelial cells, on sympathetic nerve terminals or on the central nervous system (CNS) (Table 21.1). Mechanisms of directly acting vasoconstrictors and vasodilators are summarised in Fig. 4.10 (see Ch. 4). Many indirectly acting drugs are discussed in other chapters (see Table 21.1). We concentrate here on agents that are not covered elsewhere.

VASOCONSTRICTOR DRUGS

The α_1-adrenoceptor agonists and drugs that release noradrenaline from sympathetic nerve terminals or inhibit its reuptake (sympathomimetic amines) are discussed in Chapter 15. Some eicosanoids (e.g. *thromboxane* A_2; see Chs 17 and 23) and several peptides, notably *ET*, *angiotensin* and *ADH*, are also predominantly vasoconstrictor. **Sumatriptan** and ergot alkaloids acting on certain 5-HT receptors ($5\text{-}HT_2$ and $5\text{-}HT_{1D}$) also cause vasoconstriction (see Ch. 42).

ANGIOTENSIN II

The physiological role of the renin–angiotensin system has been described previously. Angiotensin II is roughly 40 times as potent as noradrenaline in raising blood pressure. Like α_1-adrenoceptor agonists, it constricts mainly cutaneous, splanchnic and renal vasculature, with less effect on blood flow to brain and skeletal muscle. It has no routine clinical uses, although it has promise in the treatment of vasodilatory shock (Khanna et al., 2017), its main therapeutic importance lying in the fact that other drugs (e.g. **captopril** and **losartan**; see later) affect the cardiovascular system by reducing its production or action.

ANTIDIURETIC HORMONE

ADH (also known as vasopressin) is a posterior pituitary peptide hormone (see Ch. 33). It is physiologically important for its antidiuretic action on the kidney (see Ch. 29) but is also a powerful vasoconstrictor. Its effects are initiated by two distinct receptors (V_1 and V_2). Water retention is mediated through V_2 receptors, occurs at low plasma concentrations of ADH and involves activation of adenylyl cyclase in renal collecting ducts. Vasoconstriction is mediated through V_1 receptors (two subtypes, see Ch. 33), requires higher concentrations of ADH and involves activation of phospholipase C (see Ch. 3). ADH causes generalised vasoconstriction, including the skin, coeliac, mesenteric and coronary vessels. It also affects other (e.g. gastrointestinal and uterine) smooth muscle and causes abdominal cramps for this reason. Vasopressin or its analogue, **terlipressin**, is commonly used to treat patients with bleeding oesophageal varices and portal hypertension before more definitive endoscopic treatment; although gastroenterologists also have the option of using **octreotide** (see Ch. 33) for this. Vasopressin may also have a place in treating vasodilatory shock (see later).

[6]These effects are initiated by the G protein–coupled AT_1 receptor acting via the same intracellular tyrosine phosphorylation pathways as are used by cytokines, for example, the Jak/Stat pathway (Ch. 3).

ENDOTHELIN

ETs were discussed earlier in the context of their physiological roles; as explained previously, they have vasodilator and vasoconstrictor actions, but vasoconstriction predominates. Intravenous administration causes transient vasodilatation followed by profound and long-lived vasoconstriction. The ETs are even more potent vasoconstrictors than angiotensin II. As yet, clinical trials in a wide range of disease conditions have failed to yield consistent benefit, and ET antagonists are licensed only for their vasodilatory effects in pulmonary arterial hypertension, and scleroderma-induced digital ulcers (related to connective tissue disruption in scleroderma as well as poor blood supply from secondary Raynaud's phenomenon – see later). There are ongoing trials of ET antagonists for renal disease in diabetes (**atrasentan**) and treatment-resistant hypertension (**aprocitentan**).

Vasoconstrictor substances

- The main groups are sympathomimetic amines (direct and indirect; see Ch. 15), certain eicosanoids (especially thromboxane A_2; see Ch. 17), peptides (angiotensin II, ADH and ET) and a group of miscellaneous drugs (e.g. ergot alkaloids; see Ch. 16).
- Clinical uses include local applications (e.g. nasal decongestion, co-administration with local anaesthetics). Sympathomimetic amines and **ADH** are used in circulatory shock. **Adrenaline** is life-saving in anaphylactic shock and used in cardiac arrest. **ADH** and **terlipressin** (an analogue) are potent splanchnic vasoconstrictors given intravenously to reduce portal blood flow and stop bleeding from oesophageal varices in patients with portal hypertension caused by liver disease.

VASODILATOR DRUGS

Vasodilator drugs play a major role in the treatment of common conditions, including hypertension, cardiac failure and angina pectoris, as well as several less common but serious diseases, including pulmonary hypertension and Raynaud's disease.

DIRECT-ACTING VASODILATORS

Targets on which drugs act to relax vascular smooth muscle include plasma membrane voltage-dependent calcium channels, sarcoplasmic reticulum channels (Ca^{2+} release or reuptake) and enzymes that determine Ca^{2+} sensitivity of the contractile proteins (see Fig. 4.10).

Calcium antagonists

L-type calcium antagonists are discussed in Chapter 20.

Drugs that activate potassium channels

Some drugs (e.g. **minoxidil**, **diazoxide**) relax smooth muscle by opening K_{ATP} channels (Fig. 21.4). This hyperpolarises the cells and switches off voltage-dependent calcium channels. Potassium-channel activators work by antagonising the action of intracellular ATP on these channels.

Minoxidil (acting through an active sulfate metabolite) is an especially potent and long-acting vasodilator, used as a drug of last resort (in combination with a diuretic and β-adrenoceptor antagonist) for treating severe hypertension. It causes hirsutism (the active metabolite is actually used as a rub-on cream to treat baldness; see Ch. 26). It causes marked salt and water retention, so is usually prescribed with a loop diuretic. It causes reflex tachycardia, and a β-adrenoceptor antagonist is used to prevent this. **Nicorandil** (see Ch. 20) combines K_{ATP} channel activation with NO donor activity and is used in refractory angina.

Drugs that act via cyclic nucleotides

Cyclase activation

Many drugs relax vascular smooth muscle by increasing the cellular concentration of either cGMP or cAMP. For example, NO, nitrates and the natriuretic peptides act through cGMP (see Chs 19 and 20); riociguat and vericiguat stimulate soluble guanylyl cyclase via an NO-independent site to increase cGMP (see Ch. 19). The *β_2 agonists*, *adenosine* and *PGI_2* increase cytoplasmic cAMP (see Chs 15 and 17). *Dopamine* has mixed vasodilator and vasoconstrictor actions. It selectively dilates renal vessels, where it increases

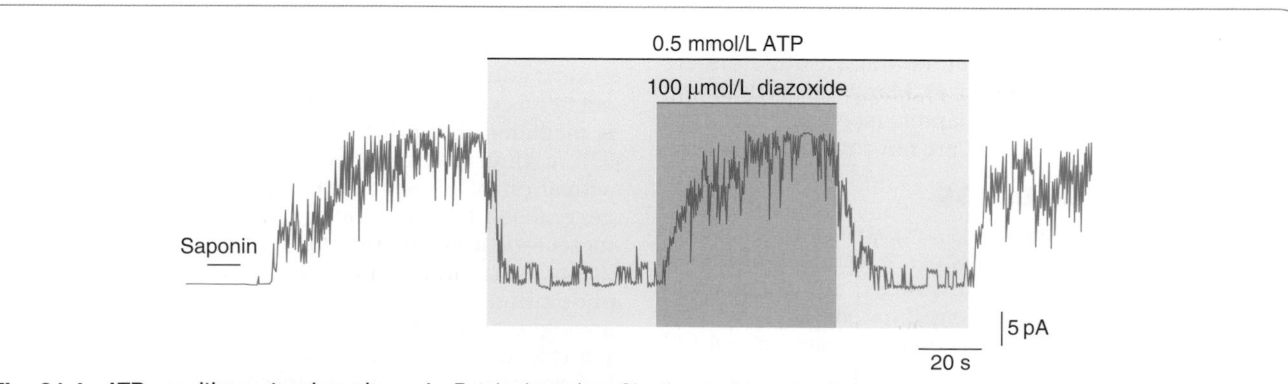

Fig. 21.4 ATP-sensitive potassium channels. Patch clamp (see Ch. 3) record from insulin-secreting pancreatic B cell: saponin permeabilised the cell, with loss of intracellular ATP, causing the channels to open (upward deflection) until they were inhibited by ATP. The addition of diazoxide, a vasodilator drug (which also inhibits insulin secretion; see text), reopens the channels. In smooth muscle, this causes hyperpolarisation and relaxation. (Redrawn from Dunne, et al., 1990. Br. J. Pharmacol. 99, 169.)

cAMP by activating adenylyl cyclase. Dopamine, when administered as an intravenous infusion, produces a mixture of cardiovascular effects resulting from agonist actions on α and β adrenoceptors, as well as on dopamine receptors. Blood pressure increases slightly, but the main effects are vasodilatation in the renal circulation and increased cardiac output. Dopamine was widely used in intensive care units in patients in whom renal failure associated with decreased renal perfusion appeared imminent; despite its beneficial effect on renal haemodynamics, clinical trials have shown that it does not improve survival in these circumstances and this use is obsolete. **Nesiritide**, a recombinant form of human B-type natriuretic peptide (BNP) (see Ch. 20), is licensed in the United States for the treatment of acutely decompensated heart failure, but efficacy data have not been impressive. However, **sacubitril**, a prodrug of an active metabolite sacubitilat, an inhibitor of neprilysin (also known as neutral endopeptidase [NEP]), increases circulating natriuretic peptides (BNP and ANP) and, in fixed combination with **valsartan**, is effective in treating chronic heart failure (see later).

Nitroprusside (nitroferricyanide) is a powerful vasodilator which acts by releasing NO (see Ch. 19). Unlike the organic nitrates, it acts equally on arterial and venous smooth muscle. Its clinical usefulness is limited because it must be given intravenously. In solution, particularly when exposed to light, nitroprusside hydrolyses with formation of cyanide. The intravenous solution must therefore be made up freshly from dry powder and protected from light. Nitroprusside is rapidly converted to thiocyanate in the body, its plasma half-life being only a few minutes, so it must be given as a continuous infusion with careful monitoring to avoid hypotension. Prolonged use causes thiocyanate accumulation and toxicity (weakness, nausea and inhibition of thyroid function); consequently, nitroprusside is useful only for short-term treatment (usually up to 72 h maximum). It is used in intensive care units for hypertensive emergencies, and to produce controlled hypotension during surgery.

Phosphodiesterase inhibition

Phosphodiesterases (PDEs; see Ch. 3) include at least 14 distinct isoenzymes. Methylxanthines (e.g. **theophylline**) and **papaverine** are non-isozyme selective PDE inhibitors (and have additional actions). Methylxanthines exert their main effects on bronchial smooth muscle and on the CNS and are discussed in Chapters 28 and 49. In addition to inhibiting PDE, some methylxanthines are also purine receptor antagonists (see Ch. 16). Papaverine is produced by opium poppies (see Ch. 43) and relaxes vascular smooth muscle. Its mechanism is poorly understood but seems to involve a combination of PDE inhibition and block of calcium channels. Selective PDE type III inhibitors (e.g. **milrinone**) increase cAMP in cardiac muscle. They have a positive inotropic effect but, despite short-term haemodynamic improvement, increase mortality in patients with heart failure, possibly by causing dysrhythmias. **Dipyridamole**, as well as enhancing the actions of adenosine (see Ch. 16), also causes vasodilatation by inhibiting PDE. Selective *PDE type V* inhibitors (e.g. **sildenafil**) inhibit the breakdown of cGMP, thereby potentiating NO signalling. It revolutionised treatment of erectile dysfunction (see Ch. 35) and is used in other situations, including pulmonary hypertension and Raynaud's phenomenon (see clinical box).

Vasodilator drugs

- Vasodilators act:
  - to increase local tissue blood flow
  - to reduce arterial pressure
  - to reduce central venous pressure
- Reduce cardiac work by reducing cardiac preload (reduced filling pressure) and afterload (reduced vascular resistance).
- Main uses are:
  - antihypertensive therapy (e.g. angiotensin II type 1 [AT_1] antagonists, calcium antagonists and α_1-adrenoceptor antagonists)
  - treatment/prophylaxis of angina (e.g. calcium antagonists, nitrates)
  - treatment of cardiac failure (e.g. ACEIs, AT_1 antagonists)
  - treatment of erectile dysfunction and Raynaud's phenomenon.

VASODILATORS WITH UNCERTAIN MECHANISM OF ACTION

Hydralazine

Hydralazine acts mainly by relaxing arteries and arterioles, causing a fall in blood pressure accompanied by reflex tachycardia and increased cardiac output. It interferes with the action of inositol trisphosphate on Ca^{2+} release from the sarcoplasmic reticulum. Its original clinical use was in hypertension and it is still used for short-term treatment of severe hypertension in pregnancy but it can cause an immune disorder resembling systemic lupus erythematosus (SLE),[7] so alternative agents are now preferred for long-term treatment of hypertension. It has a place in treating heart failure in patients of African origin in combination with a long-acting organic nitrate (see clinical box).

Ethanol

Ethanol (see Ch. 50) dilates cutaneous vessels, causing the familiar drunkard's flush. Several general anaesthetics (e.g. **propofol**) cause vasodilatation as an unwanted effect (see Ch. 41).

INDIRECTLY ACTING VASODILATOR DRUGS

Indirectly acting vasodilator drugs work by inhibiting vasoconstrictor systems, namely the sympathetic nervous system (see Ch. 15) and the renin–angiotensin–aldosterone and ET systems, or by potentiating endogenous vasodilators such as the natriuretic peptides (see Ch. 20 and further in this chapter).

The central control of sympathetically mediated vasoconstriction involves α_2 adrenoceptors and *imidazoline I_1 receptors* (see Ch. 15). **Clonidine** (an α_2-adrenoceptor agonist, now largely obsolete as an antihypertensive drug) and **moxonodine**, an I_1-receptor agonist, lower blood

[7]An autoimmune disease affecting one or more tissues, including joints, kidneys, brain, blood platelets, skin and pleural membranes (Ch. 25). Patients with hydralazine-induced lupus commonly have symptoms mimicking lupus, e.g. fever, joint pains and weight loss, with positive tests for antinuclear antibodies, but the triggering mechanism is incompletely understood.

pressure by reducing sympathetic activity centrally. In addition, many vasodilators (e.g. acetylcholine, bradykinin, substance P) exert some or all of their effects by stimulating biosynthesis of vasodilator prostaglandins or of NO (or of both) by vascular endothelium (see previously and Ch. 19), thereby causing functional antagonism of the constrictor tone caused by sympathetic nerves and angiotensin II.

Many therapeutically useful drugs block the RAAS (see Table 21.2 for a summary of selective antagonists) at one of several points:

- renin release: β-adrenoceptor antagonists inhibit renin release (see Ch. 15)
- renin activity: renin inhibitors inhibit conversion of angiotensinogen to angiotensin I
- ACE: ACEIs (see later) block conversion of angiotensin I to angiotensin II
- angiotensin II receptors: AT_1-receptor antagonists (ARBs, see later)
- aldosterone receptors: aldosterone-receptor antagonists (see later)

Renin inhibitors

Aliskiren, an orally active non-peptide renin inhibitor, was developed and registered as an antihypertensive drug. It has adverse effects that include diarrhoea (common), acute renal failure, cardiovascular events in patients with diabetes mellitus and, rarely, angioedema and severe allergic reactions.

Angiotensin-converting enzyme inhibitors

The first ACEI to be marketed was **captopril** (Fig. 21.5), an early example of successful drug design based on a chemical knowledge of the target molecule. Various small

Table 21.2 Summary of drugs that inhibit the renin–angiotensin–aldosterone system

Class	Drug[a]	Pharmacokinetics	Adverse effects[b]	Uses	Notes
ACE inhibitors	Captopril	Short acting $t_{1/2}$ ~2 h Dose 2–3 times daily	Cough Hypotension Proteinuria Taste disturbance	Hypertension Heart failure After MI	ACEIs are cleared mainly by renal excretion.
	Enalapril	Prodrug – active metabolite enalaprilat $t_{1/2}$ ~11 h Dose 1–2 times daily	Cough Hypotension Reversible renal impairment (in patients with renal artery stenosis)	As captopril	Lisinopril, perindopril, ramipril, trandolapril are similar. Some are licensed for distinct uses (e.g. stroke, left ventricular hypertrophy).
ARBs	Valsartan	$t_{1/2}$ ~6 h	Hypotension Reversible renal impairment (in patients with renal artery stenosis)	Hypertension Heart failure	ARBs are cleared by hepatic metabolism.
	Losartan	Long-acting metabolite $t_{1/2}$ ~8 h	As valsartan	As valsartan Diabetic nephropathy	Irbesartan is similar, with $t_{1/2}$ ~10–15 h.
	Candesartan	$t_{1/2}$ 5–10 h Long-acting because receptor complex is stable	As valsartan	As valsartan	Given as prodrug ester (candesartan cilexetil).
Renin inhibitor	Aliskiren	Low oral bioavailability $t_{1/2}$ 24 h	As valsartan, also diarrhoea	Essential hypertension	The FDA has warned against combining with ACEI or ARB in patients with renal impairment + diabetes mellitus.
Aldosterone antagonists	Eplerenone	$t_{1/2}$ 3–5 h	As valsartan, especially hyperkalaemia Nausea, diarrhoea	Heart failure after MI	Caution in renal impairment; monitor plasma potassium
	Spironolactone	Prodrug converted to canrenone, which has $t_{1/2}$ ~24 h	As eplerenone Also oestrogenic effects (gynaecomastia, menstrual irregularity, erectile dysfunction)	Primary hyperaldosteronism Heart failure Oedema and ascites (e.g. in hepatic cirrhosis)	

[a]All drugs listed are orally active.
[b]Adverse effects common to all drugs listed include hyperkalaemia (especially in patients with impaired renal function) and teratogenesis.
ACE, Angiotensin-converting enzyme; *ACEI*, angiotensin-converting enzyme inhibitor; *ARB*, angiotensin receptor blocker; *MI*, myocardial infarction.

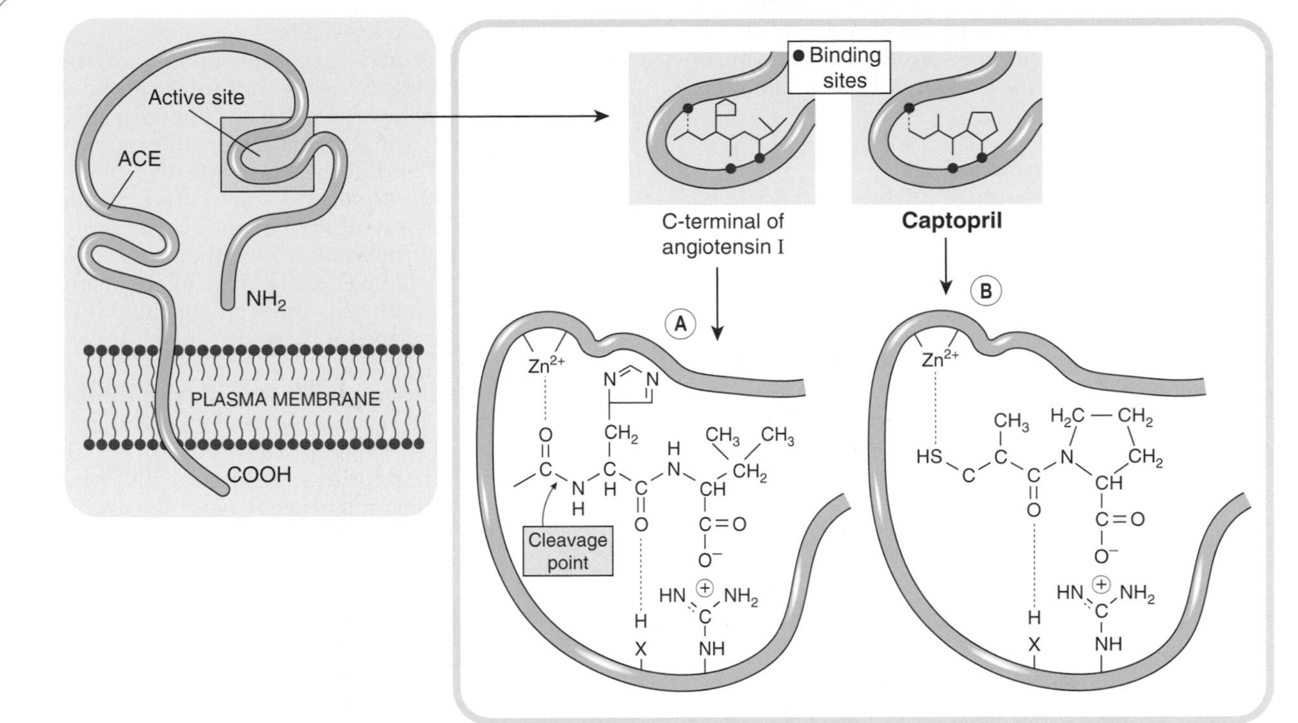

Fig. 21.5 The active site of angiotensin-converting enzyme (ACE). (A) Binding of angiotensin I. (B) Binding of the inhibitor captopril, which is an analogue of the terminal dipeptide of angiotensin I.

peptides had been found to be weak inhibitors of the enzyme.[8] Captopril was designed to combine the steric properties of such peptide antagonists in a non-peptide molecule that was active when given by mouth. Captopril has a short plasma half-life (about 2 h) and must be given two or three times daily. Many of the ACEIs developed subsequently (see Table 21.2), which are widely used in the clinic, have a longer duration of action and are administered once daily.

Pharmacological effects

ACEIs cause only a small fall in arterial pressure in healthy human subjects who are consuming the amount of salt contained in a usual Western diet, but a much larger fall in hypertensive patients, particularly those in whom renin secretion is enhanced (e.g. in patients receiving diuretics). ACEIs affect capacitance and resistance vessels and reduce cardiac load as well as arterial pressure. They act preferentially on angiotensin-sensitive vascular beds, which include those of the kidney, heart and brain. This selectivity may be important in sustaining adequate perfusion of these vital organs in the face of reduced perfusion pressure. Critical renal artery stenosis[9] represents an exception to this, where ACE inhibition results in a fall in glomerular filtration rate (see later).

Clinical uses of ACEIs are summarised in the clinical box.

[8]The lead compound was a nonapeptide derived from the venom of *Bothrops jararaca* – a South American snake. It was originally characterised as a bradykinin-potentiating peptide (ACE inactivates bradykinin; see Ch. 17).

[9]Severe narrowing of the renal artery caused, for example, by atheroma.

Clinical uses of angiotensin-converting enzyme inhibitors

- Hypertension
- Cardiac failure
- Following myocardial infarction (especially when there is ventricular dysfunction)
- Diabetic nephropathy
- Chronic renal insufficiency to prevent progression

Unwanted effects

Adverse effects (see Table 21.2) directly related to ACE inhibition are common to all drugs of this class. These include hypotension, especially after the first dose and especially in patients with heart failure who have been treated with loop diuretics, in whom the renin–angiotensin system is activated. A dry cough, possibly the result of accumulation of bradykinin (see Ch. 17), is the commonest persistent adverse effect. Kinin accumulation may also underlie *angioedema* (painful swelling in tissues which can be life-threatening if it involves the airway); this adverse effect aborted the introduction of **omapatrilat**, a combined ACEI/NEP inhibitor, and can also occur, albeit less frequently, during treatment with **sacubitril**, a selective NEP inhibitor used for chronic heart failure (see later). Patients with severe bilateral renal artery stenosis predictably develop renal failure if treated with ACEIs, because glomerular filtration is normally maintained, in the face of low afferent arteriolar pressure, by angiotensin II, which selectively constricts *efferent* arterioles. Such renal failure is reversible provided that it is recognised promptly and ACEI treatment discontinued. ACEI predispose to hyperkalaemia, which may be severe, caused by inhibition of aldosterone secretion. Monitoring of renal function and electrolytes is essential when initiating, or escalating, ACEI therapy.

Angiotensin II receptor antagonists

Losartan, **candesartan**, **valsartan** and **irbesartan** (sartans) are non-peptide, orally active AT_1 receptor antagonists (ARBs). ARBs differ pharmacologically from ACEIs (Fig. 21.6) but behave similarly to ACEIs apart from not causing cough – consistent with the 'bradykinin accumulation' explanation of this side effect, mentioned earlier. However, ACEIs are usually the preferred first-line agents as they have a more robust evidence base than ARBs. The comparison is clouded by the relative lack of head-to-head trial data, but in clinical practice, ARBs tend to be prescribed for patients who are intolerant or have not responded favourably to ACEIs.

ACE is not the only enzyme capable of forming angiotensin II, *chymase* (which is not inhibited by ACEIs) providing one alternative route. It is not known if alternative pathways of angiotensin II formation are important in vivo, but if so, then ARBs could be more effective than ACEIs when such alternative pathways are active. Again, it is not known whether any of the beneficial effects of ACEIs are bradykinin/NO mediated. It is therefore unwise to assume that ARBs will necessarily share all the therapeutic properties of ACEIs, although there is considerable overlap in the clinical indications for these drugs (see Table 21.2).

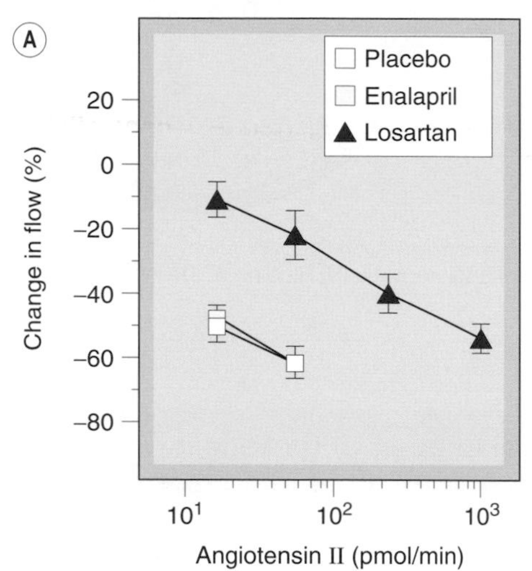

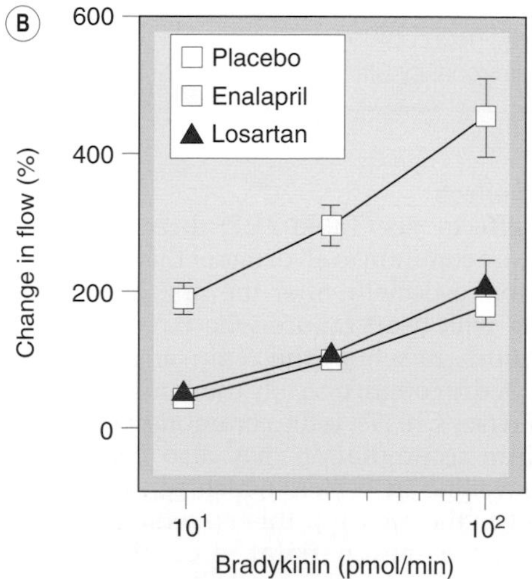

Fig. 21.6 Comparison of effects of angiotensin-converting enzyme inhibition and angiotensin receptor blockade in the human forearm vasculature. (A) Effect of brachial artery infusion of angiotensin II on forearm blood flow after oral administration of placebo, enalapril (10 mg) or losartan (100 mg). (B) Effect of brachial artery infusion of bradykinin, as in (A). (From Cockcroft, J.R., et al., 1993. J. Cardiovasc. Pharmacol. 22, 579–584.)

Neutral endopeptidase (NEP, neprilysin) inhibition

NEP (see also Ch. 20) is a zinc-dependent metalloprotease that inactivates several peptide mediators including not only natriuretic peptides (ANP and BNP) but also glucagon, enkephalins, substance P, neurotensin, oxytocin and bradykinin. In health it is expressed in many tissues including kidney, brain and lung.

Types of vasodilator drug

Directly acting vasodilators

- Calcium antagonists (e.g. **nifedipine**, **diltiazem**, **verapamil**): block Ca^{2+} entry in response to depolarisation. Common adverse effects include ankle swelling and (especially with verapamil) constipation.
- K_{ATP} channel activators (e.g. **minoxidil**): open potassium channels, hyperpolarising vascular smooth muscle cells. Ankle swelling and increased hair growth are common.
- Drugs that increase cytoplasmic cyclic nucleotide concentrations by:
  - increasing adenylyl cyclase activity, for example prostacyclin (epoprostenol), β2-adrenoceptor agonists, adenosine;
  - increasing guanylyl cyclase activity: nitrates (e.g. **glyceryl trinitrate**, **nitroprusside**) and soluble guanylyl cyclase stimulators (riociguat, vericiguat) working independently but synergistically with NO;
  - inhibiting PDE activity (e.g. **sildenafil**).

Indirectly acting vasodilators

- Drugs that interfere with the sympathetic nervous system (e.g. α_1-adrenoceptor antagonists). Postural hypotension is a common adverse effect.
- Drugs that block the renin–angiotensin system:
  - renin inhibitors (e.g. **aliskiren**)
  - ACEIs (e.g. **ramipril**); dry cough may be troublesome
  - AT_1 receptor antagonists (e.g. **losartan**).
- Drugs or mediators that stimulate endothelial NO release (e.g. acetylcholine, bradykinin).
- Drugs that block the ET system:
  - ET receptor antagonists (e.g. **bosentan**)
- Drugs that potentiate vasodilator peptides by blocking their breakdown (e.g. **sacubitril**).

Vasodilators whose mechanism is uncertain

- Miscellaneous drugs including alcohol, **propofol** (see Ch. 41) and **hydralazine.**

Clinical uses of angiotensin II subtype 1 receptor antagonists (sartans)

The AT_1 antagonists are extremely well tolerated but are teratogenic. Their uses include the following:

- Hypertension, especially in:
  - younger men, e.g. <55 years (circulating renin decreases with increasing age, and sartans are avoided during pregnancy).
- Heart failure; especially the combination of valsartan with sacubitril (NEP inhibitor).
- Chronic kidney disease, particularly with co-morbid diabetes mellitus or hypertension.

CLINICAL USES OF VASOACTIVE DRUGS

It is beyond the scope of this book to provide a detailed account of the clinical uses of vasoactive drugs, but it is nonetheless useful to consider briefly the treatment of certain important disorders, namely:

- systemic hypertension
- heart failure
- vasodilatory shock
- peripheral vascular disease
- Raynaud's disease
- pulmonary hypertension

SYSTEMIC HYPERTENSION

Systemic hypertension is a common disorder that, if not effectively treated, increases the risk of coronary artery disease, heart failure, strokes, vascular dementia, and renal failure. Until about 1950, there was no effective treatment, and the development of antihypertensive drugs has been a major success story. Systemic blood pressure is an excellent 'surrogate marker' for increased cardiovascular risk in that there is good evidence from randomised controlled trials that common antihypertensive drugs (diuretics, ACEIs, calcium antagonists) combined with lifestyle changes not only lower blood pressure but also prolong life and reduce the extra risks of cardiac complications and, especially, strokes associated with high blood pressure.

Correctable causes of hypertension include phaeochr omocytoma,[10] steroid-secreting tumours of the adrenal cortex and narrowing (coarctation) of the aorta, but most cases involve no obvious cause and are grouped as *essential hypertension* (so-called because it was originally, albeit incorrectly, thought that the raised blood pressure was 'essential' to maintain adequate tissue perfusion). Increased cardiac output may be an early feature, but by the time essential hypertension is established (commonly in middle life) there is usually increased peripheral resistance and the cardiac output is normal. Blood pressure control is intimately related to the kidneys, as demonstrated in humans requiring renal transplantation: hypertension 'goes with' the kidney from a hypertensive donor and donating a kidney from a normotensive to a hypertensive corrects hypertension in the recipient (see also Ch. 29). It seems likely that the cause of most cases of essential hypertension stems from a complex interplay of genetic, renal, endocrine, and neural factors. (Harrison et al, 2021; Meneton et al., 2005). Persistently raised arterial pressure leads to hypertrophy of the left ventricle and remodelling of resistance arteries, with narrowing of the lumen, and predisposes to atherosclerosis in larger conduit arteries.

Fig. 21.7 summarises the physiological mechanisms that control arterial blood pressure and shows sites at which antihypertensive drugs act, notably the sympathetic nervous system, the RAAS and endothelium-derived mediators. Remodelling of resistance arteries in response to raised pressure reduces the ratio of lumen diameter to wall thickness and increases the peripheral vascular resistance. The role of cellular growth factors (including

Clinical disorders for which vasoactive drugs are important

- Systemic hypertension:
  - secondary to underlying disease (e.g. renal or endocrine)
  - primary 'essential' hypertension, an important risk factor for atheromatous disease (see Ch. 22). Treatment reduces the excess risk of stroke or myocardial infarction, the main classes of drugs being (a) ACEI or AT_1 receptor antagonists, (b) calcium antagonists and (c) diuretics.
- Cardiac failure. Several diseases (most commonly ischaemic heart disease) impair the ability of the heart to deliver an output adequate to meet metabolic needs. Oedema can be improved with diuretics. Life expectancy is reduced but can be improved by treatment of haemodynamically stable patients with:
  - ACEIs or AT_1 receptor antagonists (with or without neprilysin)
  - β-adrenoceptor antagonists (e.g. **carvedilol**, **bisoprolol**)
  - aldosterone antagonists (e.g. **spironolactone**).
- Shock. Several diseases (e.g. overwhelming bacterial infections, see Ch. 52; anaphylactic reactions, see Ch. 28) lead to inappropriate vasodilatation, hypotension and reduced tissue perfusion with raised circulating concentrations of lactic acid. Pressors (e.g. **noradrenaline**) are used first-line, with vasopressin and dobutamine as second-line options.
- Peripheral vascular disease. Atheromatous plaques in the arteries of the legs are often associated with atheroma in other vascular territories. Statins (see Ch. 22) and antiplatelet drugs (see Ch. 23) are important.
- Raynaud's disease. Inappropriate vasoconstriction in small arteries in the hands causes blanching of the fingers followed by blueness and pain. **Nifedipine** or other vasodilators are used.
- Pulmonary hypertension, which can be:
  - idiopathic (a rare disorder): **epoprostenol**, **iloprost**, **bosentan** and **sildenafil** are of benefit in selected patients;
  - associated with hypoxic lung disease.

[10]Catecholamine-secreting tumours of chromaffin tissue, usually the adrenal medulla (Ch. 33).

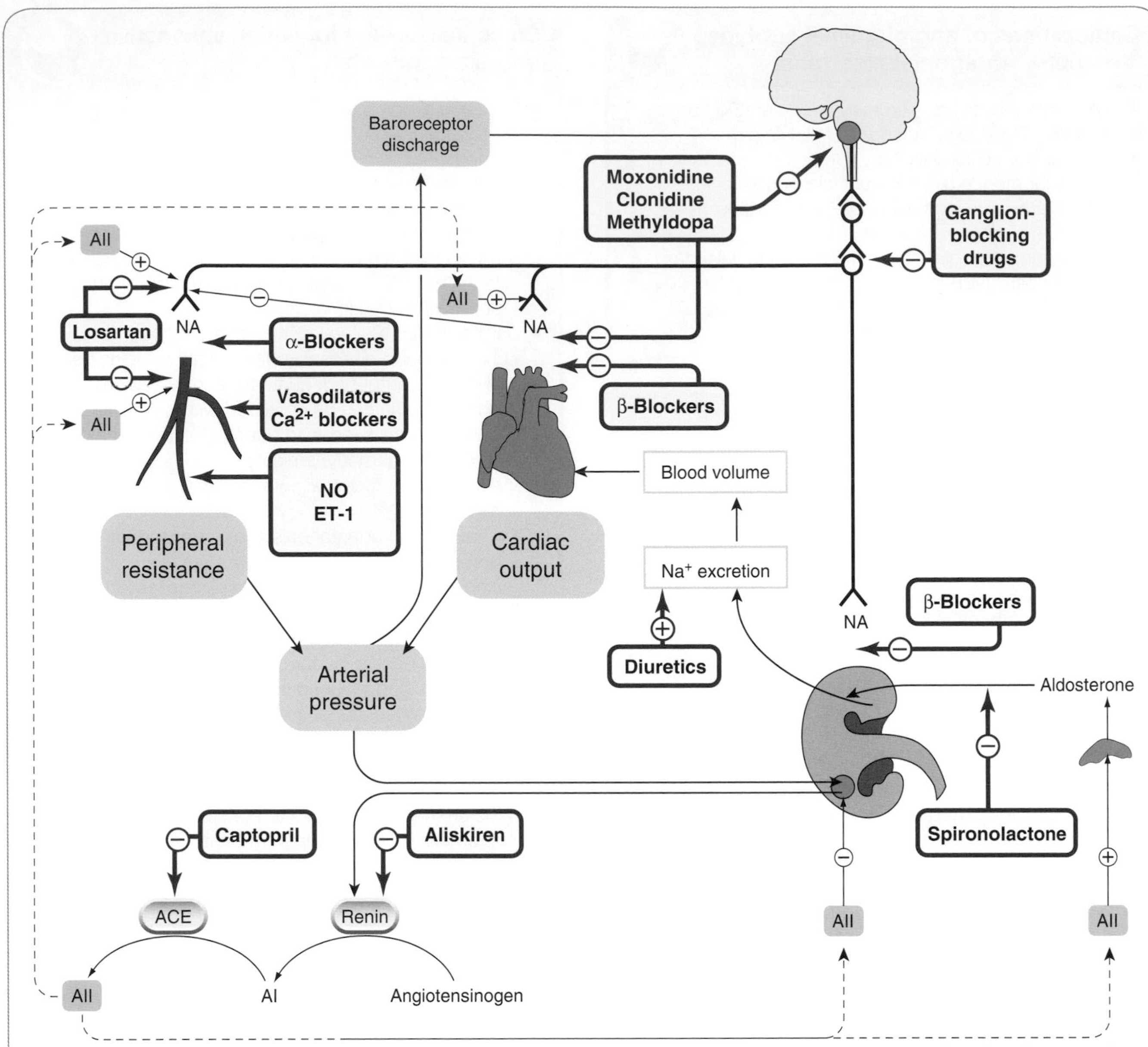

Fig. 21.7 Main mechanisms involved in arterial blood pressure regulation *(black lines)*, and the sites of action of antihypertensive drugs *(hatched boxes + orange lines)*. *ACE*, Angiotensin-converting enzyme; *AI*, angiotensin I; *AII*, angiotensin II; *ET-1*, endothelin-1; *NA*, noradrenaline; *NO*, nitric oxide.

angiotensin II) and inhibitors of growth (e.g. NO) in the evolution of these structural changes is of great interest to vascular biologists and is potentially important for ACEIs and ARBs.

Reducing arterial blood pressure greatly improves the prognosis of patients with hypertension. Controlling hypertension (which is asymptomatic) without producing unacceptable side effects is therefore an important clinical need, which is, in general, well catered for by modern drugs. Treatment involves non-pharmacological measures (e.g. increased exercise, reduced dietary salt and saturated fat with increased fruit and fibre, and weight and alcohol reduction) followed by the staged introduction of drugs, starting with those of proven benefit and least likely to produce adverse effects. Some of the drugs that were used to lower blood pressure in the early days of antihypertensive therapy, including *ganglion blockers, adrenergic neuron blockers* and **reserpine** (see Ch. 15), produced a fearsome array of adverse effects and are now obsolete. The preferred regimens have changed progressively as better-tolerated drugs have become available. A rational strategy is to start treatment with either an ACEI or an ARB in patients who are likely to have normal or raised plasma renin (i.e. younger White people), and with a calcium antagonist in older people and people of African origin (who are more likely to have low plasma renin). If the target blood pressure is not achieved but the drug is well tolerated, then a drug of the other group or a thiazide diuretic is added. It is best not to increase the dose of any one drug excessively, as this often causes adverse effects and engages homeostatic control mechanisms (e.g. renin release by a diuretic) that limit efficacy.

Table 21.3 Common antihypertensive drugs and their adverse effects

Drug	Adverse effects[a]		
	Postural hypotension	Impotence	Other
Thiazide (e.g. bendroflumethiazide) and related (e.g. chlortalidone, indapamide) diuretics	±	++	Urinary frequency, gout, glucose intolerance, hypokalaemia, hyponatraemia
ACE inhibitors (e.g. enalapril)	±	–	Cough, first-dose hypotension, teratogenicity, reversible renal dysfunction (in presence of renal artery stenosis)
AT_1 antagonists (e.g. losartan)	–	–	Teratogenicity, reversible renal dysfunction (in presence of renal artery stenosis)
Ca^{2+} antagonists (e.g. nifedipine)	–	±	Ankle oedema
β-Adrenoceptor antagonists (e.g. metoprolol)	–	+	Bronchospasm, fatigue, cold hands and feet, bradycardia
α_1-Adrenoceptor antagonists (e.g. doxazosin)	++	–	First-dose hypotension

[a]± indicates that the adverse effect occurs in special circumstances only (e.g. postural hypotension occurs with a thiazide diuretic only if the patient is dehydrated for some other reason, is taking some additional drug or suffers from some additional disorder).
ACE, Angiotensin-converting enzyme; *AT_1*, angiotensin II type 1 receptor

β-Adrenoceptor antagonists are less well tolerated than ACEIs or ARBs, and the evidence supporting their routine use is less strong than for other classes of antihypertensive drugs. They are useful for hypertensive patients with some additional indication for β blockade, such as angina or heart failure.

Addition of a third or fourth drug (e.g. to ARB/calcium antagonist combination) is often needed, and a long-acting α_1-adrenoceptor antagonist (see Ch. 15) such as once-daily **doxazosin** is one option in this setting. The α_1 antagonists additionally improve symptoms of prostatic hyperplasia (also known as benign prostatic hypertrophy) (Chs 15, 29 and 35), which is common in older men, albeit at the risk of postural hypotension, which is the main unwanted effect of these agents. **Spironolactone**, whose active metabolite canrenone is a competitive antagonist of aldosterone (see Ch. 29), has staged something of a comeback as an additional agent in treating severe hypertension. Careful monitoring of plasma K^+ concentration is required, because spironolactone inhibits urinary K^+ excretion as well as causing oestrogen-related adverse effects, but it is usually well tolerated in low doses. **Methyldopa** is now used mainly for hypertension during pregnancy because of the lack of documented adverse effects on the baby (in contrast to ACEIs, ARBs and standard β-adrenoceptor antagonists, which are contraindicated during pregnancy and therefore often avoided in women of child-bearing potential). **Clonidine** (a centrally acting α_2 agonist) is now seldom used. **Moxonidine**, a centrally acting agonist at imidazoline I_1 receptors that causes less drowsiness than α_2 agonists, is licensed for mild or moderate hypertension, but there is little evidence from clinical end-point trials to support its wider use. **Minoxidil**, combined with a diuretic and β-adrenoceptor antagonist, is sometimes effective where other drugs have failed in severe hypertension resistant to other drugs. **Fenoldopam**, a selective dopamine D_1 receptor agonist, is approved in the United States for the short-term in-hospital management of severe hypertension. Its effect is similar in magnitude to that of intravenous nitroprusside, but it lacks thiocyanate-associated toxicity and is slower in onset and offset.

Commonly used antihypertensive drugs and their main adverse effects are summarised in Table 21.3.

HEART FAILURE

Heart failure is a clinical syndrome characterised by symptoms of breathlessness and/or fatigue, usually with signs of fluid overload (oedema, raised venous pressure and crackles heard when listening to the chest). The underlying physiological abnormality (see also Ch. 20) is a cardiac output that is inadequate to meet the metabolic demands of the body, initially during exercise but, as the syndrome progresses, also at rest. It may be caused by direct damage to the myocardium itself (most commonly secondary to coronary artery disease but also other pathologies including cardiotoxic drugs such as **doxorubicin** and **trastuzumab** – see Ch. 57), or by circulatory factors such as volume overload (e.g. leaky valves, or arteriovenous shunts caused by congenital defects) or pressure overload (e.g. stenosed – i.e. narrowed – valves, systemic or pulmonary hypertension). Some of these underlying causes are surgically correctable, and in some, either the underlying disease (e.g. hyperthyroidism; see Ch. 34) or an aggravating factor, such as anaemia (see Ch. 24) or atrial fibrillation (see Ch. 20), is treatable with drugs. Here, we focus on drugs used to treat heart failure per se, irrespective of the underlying cause.

When cardiac output is insufficient to meet metabolic demand, an increase in fluid volume occurs, partly because increased venous pressure increases capillary pressure and hence formation of tissue fluid, and partly because reduced renal blood flow activates the RAAS, causing Na^+ and water retention. Irrespective of the cause, and despite major recent advances in pharmacotherapy, the outlook for adults with cardiac failure remains of concern, with up to 50% mortality after 5 years. Non-drug measures, including

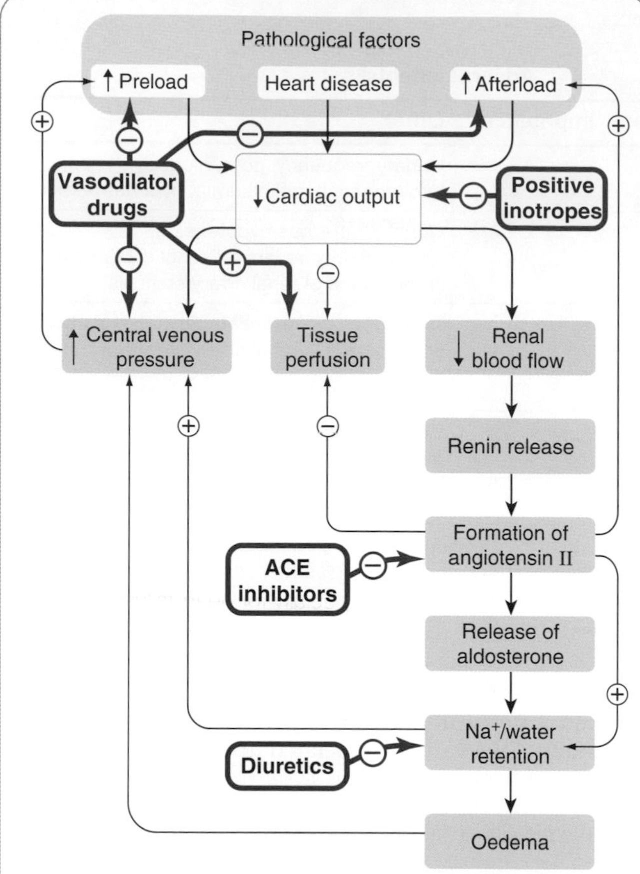

Fig. 21.8 Simplified scheme showing the pathogenesis of heart failure, and the sites of action of some of the drugs used to treat it. The symptoms of heart failure are produced by reduced tissue perfusion, oedema and increased central venous pressure. *ACE,* Angiotensin-converting enzyme.

dietary salt restriction and exercise training in mildly affected patients,[11] are important, but drugs are needed to improve symptoms of oedema, fatigue and breathlessness, and to improve prognosis.

A simplified diagram of the sequence of events is shown in Fig. 21.8. A common theme is that several of the feedbacks that are activated are 'counter-regulatory' - that is, they make the situation worse not better. This occurs because the body fails to distinguish the haemodynamic state of heart failure from haemorrhage, in which release of vasoconstrictors such as angiotensin II and ADH would be appropriate.[12] ACEIs and ARBs, β-adrenoceptor and aldosterone antagonists interrupt these counter-regulatory neurohormonal mechanisms and have each been shown to prolong life in heart failure.

Drugs used to treat heart failure act in various complementary ways to do the following.

Increase natriuresis. Diuretics, especially loop diuretics (see Ch. 29), are important in increasing salt and water excretion, especially if there is pulmonary oedema. In chronic heart failure, drugs that have been shown to improve survival were studied mainly in patients treated with diuretics.

Sodium glucose co-transporter-2 inhibitors are used in treatment of diabetes mellitus (see Ch. 31) but have also been found to reduce heart failure hospital admissions, even in patients who do not have diabetes. Several mechanisms (natriuresis, lowering of blood pressure, weight loss, post-glomerular and coronary vasodilation) have been proposed for this beneficial effect but further research is ongoing into direct action on cardiac remodelling, myocardial calcium handling and amelioration of endothelial cell dysfunction.

Inhibit the renin–angiotensin–aldosterone system/potentiate NEP. The RAAS is inappropriately activated in patients with cardiac failure, especially when they are treated with diuretics. The β-adrenoceptor antagonists inhibit renin secretion and are used as first-line agents in clinically stable patients with chronic heart failure (see clinical box). ACEIs and ARBs block the formation of angiotensin II and inhibit its action, respectively, thereby reducing vascular resistance, improving tissue perfusion and reducing cardiac afterload. They also cause natriuresis by inhibiting secretion of aldosterone and by reducing the direct stimulatory effect of angiotensin II on reabsorption of Na^+ and HCO_3^- in the early part of the proximal convoluted tubule. Most important of all, they prolong life.

Differences in the pharmacology of ACEIs and ARBs led to the hypothesis that co-administration of these drugs ('dual blockade') could confer additional benefit over increasing the dose of either given as a single agent. However, clinical trials comparing ACEI or ARB monotherapy against combined therapy found that the combined treatment had more adverse effects attributable to hypotension, and no survival benefit compared with monotherapy in patients after acute myocardial infarction.

In contrast to the disappointing experience of combining ARBs with ACEI, a fixed combination of sacubitril with valsartan is used in patients symptomatic with chronic heart failure and reduced cardiac ejection. In comparison to an ACEI (enalapril), sacubitril/valsartan usefully reduced cardiac and all-cause mortality in such patients and Jhund and McMurray (2016) argue that this combination should therefore replace an ACEI as the foundation of treatment of symptomatic heart failure.

The choice of valsartan as ARB in this combination is supported by its pharmacokinetic similarity to sacubitril. Sacubitril, sacubitrilat and valsartan are highly bound to plasma proteins (94%–97%) but sacubitril does cross the blood–brain barrier to a limited extent (0.28%). Cerebrospinal fluid (CSF) Aβ clearance in young cynomolgus monkeys is reduced by sacubitril/valsartan. Administration of the combination for 2 weeks to healthy subjects increased CSF Aβ1-38 without change in Aβ1-40 and 1-42. However, pharmacoepidemiological data have not confirmed any definitive effect on cognition thus far, and the product is subject to ongoing safety monitoring in large clinical trials.

Adverse effects and drug interactions observed during treatment with valsartan/sacubitril are in line with those of its two components. Hypotension, hyperkalaemia and renal impairment are the commonest observed adverse effects. Angioedema occurred during the pivotal controlled trial in 0.5% of patients treated with the combination,

[11]Bed rest used to be recommended but results in deconditioning, and regular exercise has been shown to be beneficial in patients who can tolerate it.

[12]Natural selection presumably favoured mechanisms that would benefit young hunter-gatherers at risk of haemorrhage; middle-aged or elderly people at high risk of heart failure are past their reproductive prime.

compared with 0.2% of patients treated with enalapril. Concomitant use of sacubitril with ACEIs is contraindicated since, consistent with the experience with omapatrilat mentioned earlier, the concomitant inhibition of NEP and ACE increases the risk of angioedema. PDE5 inhibitors (see Ch. 20), including sildenafil, which work through cGMP signalling are potentiated by sacubitril.

Angiotensin II is not the only stimulus to aldosterone secretion, and during chronic treatment with ACEIs, circulating aldosterone concentrations return towards pretreatment values (a phenomenon known as 'aldosterone escape'). This provides a rationale for combining **spironolactone** (an aldosterone antagonist; see Ch. 33) with ACEI treatment, which further reduces mortality. **Eplerenone** is an aldosterone antagonist with less oestrogen-like adverse effects than spironolactone; it too has been shown to improve survival in patients with heart failure when added to conventional therapy. Patients with impaired renal function were excluded from these trials, and careful monitoring of plasma K^+ concentration is important when they are treated with an ACEI or an ARB in combination with an aldosterone antagonist.

Block β adrenoceptors. Heart failure is accompanied by potentially harmful activation of the sympathetic nervous system as well as of the renin–angiotensin system, providing a rationale for using β-adrenoceptor antagonists. Most clinicians were very wary of this approach because of the negative inotropic action of these drugs, but when started in low doses that are increased slowly, **metoprolol, carvedilol, nebivolol** and **bisoprolol** each improve survival when added to optimal treatment in clinically stable patients with chronic heart failure.

Vasodilators. Glyceryl trinitrate (see Ch. 20) is infused intravenously to treat acute cardiac failure. Its venodilator effect reduces venous pressure, and its effects on arterial compliance and wave reflection further reduce cardiac work. The combination of hydralazine (to reduce afterload) with a long-acting organic nitrate (to reduce preload) in patients with chronic heart failure improved survival in a North American randomised controlled trial, but the results suggested that the benefit was restricted to patients of African origin. This ethnic group is genetically very heterogeneous, and it is unknown what other groups will benefit from such treatment. The future role of hydralazine/nitrate in targeting specific ethnic groups is now uncertain given that sacubitril/valsartan and sodium glucose co-transporter-2 inhibitors have demonstrable efficacy for heart failure in both White and non-White populations.

Vericiguat is an oral guanylyl cyclase stimulator that has recently received positive regulatory opinion on reduction of heart failure hospitalisations for patients with reduced ejection fraction.

Increase the force of cardiac contraction. Cardiac glycosides (see Ch. 20) are used either in patients with heart failure who also have chronic rapid atrial fibrillation (in whom it improves cardiac function by slowing ventricular rate and hence ventricular filling in addition to any benefit from its positive inotropic action) or in patients who remain symptomatic despite treatment with a diuretic and ACEI. **Digoxin** does not reduce mortality in heart failure patients in sinus rhythm who are otherwise optimally treated but does improve symptoms and reduce the need for hospital admission. In contrast, PDE inhibitors (see Ch. 20) increase cardiac output, but increase mortality in heart failure, probably through cardiac dysrhythmias. **Dobutamine** (a β_1-selective adrenoceptor agonist; see Ch. 20) is used intravenously when a rapid response is needed in the short term, for example following heart surgery. Omecamtiv, a cardiac myosin activator, is currently being evaluated for treatment of heart failure (see Ch. 20).

Drugs used in chronic heart failure

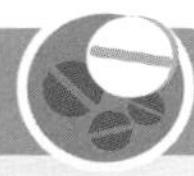

- Loop diuretics, for example **furosemide** (see Ch. 29).
- ACEIs (e.g. **ramipril**) are a first-line option.
- Angiotensin II subtype 1 receptor antagonists (e.g. **valsartan**, **candesartan**) alone or, increasingly, in combination with an NEP inhibitor (**valsartan/sacubitril**).
- β-Adrenoceptor antagonists (e.g. **metoprolol**, **bisoprolol**, **carvedilol**), introduced in low dose in stable patients, are also first-line options.
- Aldosterone-receptor antagonists (e.g. **spironolactone**, see Ch. 33; and **eplerenone**).
- **Digoxin** (see Ch. 20), especially for heart failure associated with established rapid atrial fibrillation. It is also indicated in patients who remain symptomatic despite optimal treatment.
- Organic nitrates (e.g. **isosorbide mononitrate**) reduce preload, and **hydralazine** reduces afterload. Used in combination, these prolong life in African-Americans with heart failure.
- Vericiguat is an option in symptomatic patients who have recently recovered from acute decompensated heart failure.

VASODILATORY SHOCK AND HYPOTENSIVE STATES

Shock is a medical emergency characterised by inadequate perfusion of vital organs, usually because of a very low arterial blood pressure. This leads to anaerobic metabolism and hence to increased lactate production. Mortality is very high, even with optimal treatment in an intensive care unit. Shock can be caused by various insults, including haemorrhage, burns, bacterial infections, anaphylaxis and myocardial infarction (Fig. 21.9). The common factor is reduced effective circulating blood volume (hypovolaemia) caused directly either by bleeding or by movement of fluid from the plasma to the gut lumen or extracellular fluid. The physiological (homeostatic) response to this is complex: vasodilatation in a vital organ (e.g. brain, heart or kidney) favours perfusion of that organ, but at the expense of a further reduction in blood pressure, which leads to reduced perfusion of other organs. Survival depends on a balance between vasoconstriction in non-essential vascular beds and vasodilatation in vital ones. The dividing line between the normal physiological response to blood loss and clinical shock is that in shock, tissue hypoxia produces secondary effects that magnify rather than correct the primary disturbance. Patients with established shock have profound and inappropriate vasodilatation in non-essential organs, and this is difficult to correct with vasoconstrictor drugs. The release of mediators (e.g. histamine, 5-HT, bradykinin, prostaglandins, cytokines

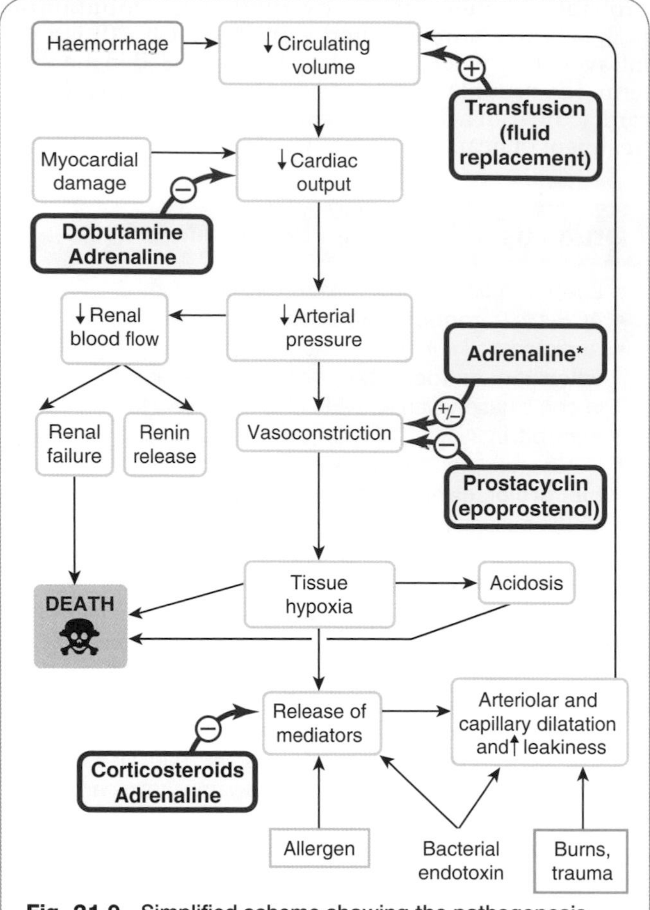

Fig. 21.9 Simplified scheme showing the pathogenesis of hypovolaemic shock. *Adrenaline causes vasodilatation in some vascular beds, vasoconstriction in others.

including interleukins and tumour necrosis factor, NO and undoubtedly many more as-yet-unidentified substances) that cause capillary dilatation and leakiness is the opposite of what is required to improve function in this setting. Mediators promoting vasodilatation in shock converge on two main mechanisms:

Activation of ATP-sensitive potassium channels in vascular smooth muscle by reduced cytoplasmic ATP and increased lactate and protons.

Increased synthesis of NO, which activates myosin light-chain phosphatase and activates K_{Ca} channels.

A third important mechanism seems to be a relative *deficiency* of ADH, which is secreted acutely in response to haemorrhage but subsequently declines, probably because of depletion within the neurohypophysis (see Ch. 33).

Patients with shock are not a homogeneous population, making it hard to perform valid clinical trials, and in contrast to hypertension and heart failure there is very little evidence to support treatment strategies based on hard clinical end points (such as improved survival). *Volume replacement* is of benefit if there is hypovolaemia; *antibiotics* are essential if there is persistent bacterial infection; **adrenaline** can be life-saving in anaphylactic shock and is also used by intensivists in managing circulatory shock of other aetiologies. Hypoperfusion leads to multiple organ failure (including renal failure), and intensive therapy specialists spend much effort supporting the circulations of such patients with cocktails of vasoactive drugs in attempts to optimise flow to vital organs. Trials of antagonists designed to block or neutralise endotoxin, interleukins, tumour necrosis factor and the inducible form of NO synthase and of recombinant human protein C have shown them to be ineffective or actually harmful. **Vasopressin** or angiotensin II may increase blood pressure even when there is resistance to adrenaline. *Corticosteroids* suppress the formation of NO and of prostaglandins but are not of proven benefit once shock is established; positive inotropic agents, including adrenaline, noradrenaline and **dobutamine**, may be used to increase blood pressure in individual patients.

PERIPHERAL VASCULAR DISEASE

When atheroma involves peripheral arteries, the first symptom is usually pain in the calves on walking (claudication), followed by pain at rest, and in severe cases gangrene of the feet or legs. Other vascular beds (e.g. coronary, cerebral and renal) are often also affected by atheromatous disease in patients with peripheral vascular disease. Treatment is mainly mechanical (open surgery or endovascular procedures to open the stenosed artery), combined with drugs that reduce the risk of ischaemic heart disease and strokes. Drug treatment includes antiplatelet drugs (e.g. **aspirin**, **clopidogrel**; see Ch. 23), a statin (e.g. **simvastatin**; see Ch. 22) and an ACEI (e.g. **ramipril**).

RAYNAUD'S DISEASE

Inappropriate vasoconstriction of small arteries and arterioles gives rise to Raynaud's phenomenon (blanching of the fingers during vasoconstriction, followed by blueness owing to deoxygenation of the static blood and redness from reactive hyperaemia following return of blood flow). This can be mild, but if severe causes ulceration and gangrene of the fingers. It can occur in isolation (Raynaud's disease) or in association with a number of other diseases, including several so-called connective tissue diseases (e.g. systemic sclerosis, SLE). Treatment of Raynaud's phenomenon hinges on stopping smoking (crucially) and on avoiding the cold; β-adrenoceptor antagonists are contraindicated. Vasodilators (e.g. **nifedipine**; see Ch. 20) are of some benefit in severe cases, and evidence from several small studies suggests sildenafil is helpful, as well as other vasodilators (e.g. PGI_2, calcitonin gene-related peptide [CGRP]) which can have surprisingly prolonged effects long outlasting their presence in the circulation, but are difficult to administer.

PULMONARY HYPERTENSION

After birth, pulmonary vascular resistance becomes much lower than systemic vascular resistance, and systolic pulmonary artery pressure in adults is normally approximately 20 mm Hg.[13]

[13]In fetal life, pulmonary vascular resistance is high; failure to adapt appropriately at birth is associated with prematurity, lack of pulmonary surfactant and hypoxaemia. The resulting pulmonary hypertension is treated by paediatric intensive care specialists with measures including replacement of surfactant and ventilatory support, sometimes including inhaled NO – see Chapter 19.

Pulmonary artery pressure is much less easy to estimate than systemic pressure, requiring echocardiography and/or cardiac catheterisation, so only more severe and symptomatic pulmonary hypertension tends to be diagnosed. Pulmonary hypertension usually causes some regurgitation of blood from the right ventricle to the right atrium. This tricuspid regurgitation can be used to estimate the pulmonary artery pressure indirectly by ultrasonography. Pulmonary hypertension may rarely be *idiopathic* (i.e. of unknown cause, a severe and progressive form), but is more commonly associated with some other disease (typically involving underlying pulmonary pathology). It can result from an increased cardiac output (such as occurs, for example, in patients with hepatic cirrhosis – where vasodilatation may accompany intermittent subclinical exposure to bacterial endotoxin – or in patients with congenital connections between the systemic and pulmonary circulations). Vasoconstriction and/or structural narrowing of the pulmonary resistance arteries increase pulmonary arterial pressure, even if cardiac output is normal. In some situations, both increased cardiac output and increased pulmonary vascular resistance are present.

Endothelial dysfunction (Chs 22 and 23) is implicated in the aetiology of pulmonary hypertension. Drugs (e.g. anorexic drugs including **dexfenfluramine**, now withdrawn) and toxins (e.g. *monocrotaline*) can cause pulmonary hypertension. Occlusion of the pulmonary arteries, for example with *recurrent pulmonary emboli* (see Ch. 23), is a further primary cause or exacerbating factor, and *anticoagulation* (see Ch. 23) is an important part of treatment. Aggregates of deformed red cells in patients with *sickle cell anaemia* (see Ch. 24) can occlude small pulmonary arteries.

Increased pulmonary vascular resistance may, alternatively, result from vasoconstriction (e.g. due to persistent hypoxia in chronic lung disease) and/or structural changes in the walls of pulmonary resistance arteries. Many of the diseases (e.g. systemic sclerosis) associated with Raynaud's phenomenon mentioned in the previous section are also associated with pulmonary hypertension. Vasoconstriction may precede cellular proliferation and medial hypertrophy which causes wall thickening in the pulmonary vasculature. Calcium antagonists (e.g. nifedipine) are used, but benefit is limited. Vasodilators with an antiproliferative action (e.g. epoprostenol, Fig. 21.10), drugs that potentiate NO such as **riociguat**, an allosteric activator of soluble guanylyl cyclase (see earlier and Ch. 19), approved for this indication in Europe and the United States, or antagonise ET – for example bosentan and **ambrisentan** – are considered to yield greater benefit.

Drugs used in treating pulmonary arterial hypertension and clinical disorders for which vasoactive drugs are important are shown in the clinical boxes.

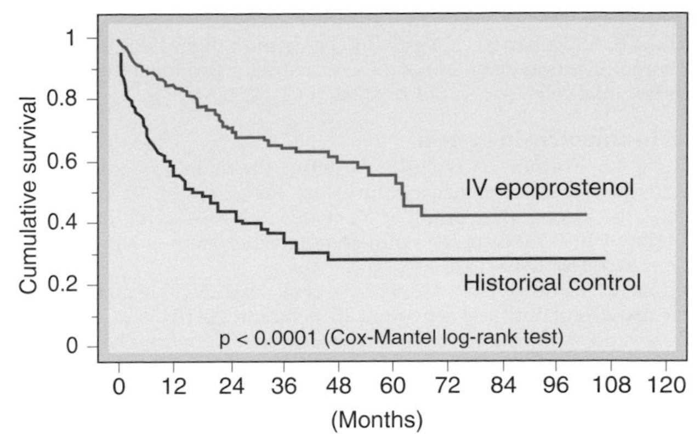

Fig. 21.10 Survival in primary pulmonary hypertension. Survival in 178 patients treated with intravenous epoprostenol versus a historical control group of 135 patients matched for disease severity. (Adapted from Sitbon, O., et al., 2002. Prog. Cardiovasc. Dis. 45, 115.)

Drugs used in pulmonary arterial hypertension

Drugs are used where indicated to treat any underlying cause. The specific aims of treatment include supportive background therapy to manage symptoms, as well targeted agents to reduce disease progression.

Management of symptoms and complications is usually achieved with:

- Oral anticoagulants (see Ch. 23)
- Diuretics (see Ch. 29)
- **Oxygen**
- **Digoxin** (see Ch. 20)

Targeted treatment to reduce pulmonary arterial pressure and progression of disease usually involves a variety of agents, including:

- Calcium-channel blockers.
- ET receptor antagonists (e.g. **bosentan**, **ambrisentan**, **sitaxentan**) by mouth for less severe stages of disease, in combination with PDE V inhibitors, **sildenafil** or **tadalafil.**
- Prostanoid analogues (**iloprost**, **treprostinil**, **beraprost**), subcutaneous or inhaled, are used for more severe stages of disease.
- **Epoprostenol** (see Ch. 17) is given as a long-term intravenous infusion and improves survival (see Fig. 23.10).
- Inhaled **NO** is administered in intensive care, for example for pulmonary hypertensive crises in newborn babies.
- Riociguat (activator of guanylyl cyclase).

REFERENCES AND FURTHER READING

Vascular endothelium (see Ch. 19 for further reading on nitric oxide)

Prostacyclin

Bunting, S., Gryglewski, R., Moncada, S., Vane, J.R., 1976. Arterial walls generate from prostaglandin endoperoxides a substance (*prostaglandin X*) which relaxes strips of mesenteric and celiac arteries and inhibits platelet aggregation. Prostaglandins 12, 897–913.

Murata, T., Ushikubi, F., Matsuoka, T., et al., 1997. Altered pain perception and inflammatory response in mice lacking prostacyclin receptor. Nature 388, 678–682.

Endothelin

Barton, M., Yanagisawa, M., 2019. Endothelin: 30 years from discovery to therapy. Hypertension 74, 1232–1265.

Davenport, A.P., Hyndman, K.A., Dhaun, N., et al., 2016. Endothelin. Pharmacol. Rev. 68, 357–418.
Hickey, K.A., Rubanyi, G., Paul, R.J., Highsmith, R.F., 1985. Characterization of a coronary vasoconstrictor produced by cultured endothelial cells. Am. J. Physiol. 248 (Pt 1), C550–C556.

Renin–angiotensin system

Lang, C.C., Struthers, A.D., 2013. Targeting the renin-angiotensin-aldosterone system in heart failure. Nat. Rev. Cardiol. 10, 125–134.
Patel, V.B., Zhong, J.C., Grant, M.B., et al., 2016. Role of the ACE2/angiotensin 1-7 axis of the renin-angiotensin system in heart failure. Circ. Res. 118, 1313–1326.
Sandner, P., Zimmer, D.P., Milne, G.T., et al., 2021. Soluble guanylate cyclase stimulators and activators. In: Schmidt, H.H.H.W., Ghezzi, P., Cuadrado, A. (Eds.), Reactive Oxygen Species: Network Pharmacology and Therapeutic Applications. Springer International Publishing, Cham.

Hypertension

Azizi, M., Rossignol, P., Hulot, J.S., 2019. Emerging drug classes and their potential use in hypertension. Hypertension 74, 1075–1083.
Harrison, D.G., Coffman, T.M., Wilcox, C.S., 2021. Pathophysiology of hypertension: the mosaic theory and beyond. Circ. Res. 128, 847–863.
Meneton, P., Jeunemaitre, X., de Wardener, H.E., MacGregor, G.A., 2005. Links between dietary salt intake, renal salt handling, blood pressure, and cardiovascular diseases. Physiol. Rev. 85, 679–715.

Heart failure

Chaudhary, A.G., Alreefi, F.M., Aziz, M.A., 2021. Emerging pharmacologic therapies for heart failure with reduced ejection fraction. CJC Open 3, 646–657.
Jhund, P.S., McMurray, J.J.V., 2016. The neprilysin pathway in heart failure: a review and guide on the use of sacubitril/valsartan. Heart 102, 1342–1347.
Pellicori, P., Khan, M.J.I., Graham, F.J., et al., 2020. New perspectives and future directions in the treatment of heart failure. Heart Fail. Rev. 25, 147–159.

Shock

Holmes, C.L., Russell, J.A., 2004. Vasopressin. Semin. Respir. Crit. Care Med. 25, 705–711.
Khanna, A., English, S.W., Wang, X.S., et al., For the ATHOS3 investigators, 2017. Angiotensin II for the treatment of vasodilatory shock. N. Engl. J. Med. 377, 419–430.

Pulmonary arterial hypertension (PAH)

Galiè, N., Channick, R.N., Frantz, R.P., et al., 2019. Risk stratification and medical therapy of pulmonary arterial hypertension. Eur. Respir. J. 53, 1801889.
Humbert, M., Ghofrani, H.A., 2016. The molecular targets of approved treatments for pulmonary arterial hypertension. Thorax 71, 73–83.
Maron, B.A., 2022. Pulmonary Hypertension. In: Libby, P., Bonow, R.O., Mann, D.L., Tomaselli, G.F., Bhatt, D.L., Solomon, S.D. (Eds.). Braunwald's Heart Disease: A Textbook of Cardiovascular Medicine, twelfth ed. Saunders/Elsevier, Philadelphia.

Atherosclerosis and lipoprotein metabolism 22

OVERVIEW

Atheromatous disease is ubiquitous and underlies the commonest causes of death (myocardial infarction caused by thrombosis – Ch. 23 – on ruptured atheromatous plaque in a coronary artery) and disability (stroke, heart failure) in industrial societies. Hypertension is one of the most important risk factors for atheroma, and is discussed in Chapter 21. Here, we consider other risk factors, especially dyslipidaemia,[1] which, like hypertension, is amenable to drug therapy. We describe briefly the processes of atherogenesis and of lipid transport as a basis for understanding the actions of lipid-lowering drugs. Agents employed therapeutically (statins, inhibitors of PCSK9,[2] fibrates and cholesterol absorption inhibitors) are described, with emphasis on the statins which, in selected patients, reduce the incidence of arterial disease and prolong life.

INTRODUCTION

In this chapter we summarise the pathological process of atherogenesis and approaches to the prevention of atherosclerotic disease. Lipoprotein transport forms the basis for understanding drugs used to treat dyslipidaemia. We emphasise the **statins**, which have been a major success story, not only lowering plasma cholesterol but also reducing cardiovascular events by approximately 25%–50% and prolonging life in people at increased risk of vascular disease. However, some patients do not tolerate them, and others fail to respond. Evidence that other drugs that influence dyslipidaemia improve clinical outcomes is less secure than for the statins, and there have been setbacks, described later, that call into question the universal reliability of changes in circulating lipid concentrations in response to drugs as surrogates predicting clinical improvement. Other classes of lipid-lowering drugs currently remain second line to statins whilst we await robust outcome data from large long-term randomised clinical trials.

ATHEROGENESIS

Atheroma is a focal disease of the intima of large and medium-sized arteries. Lesions evolve over decades, during most of which time they are clinically silent, the occurrence of symptoms signalling advanced disease. Presymptomatic lesions are often difficult to detect non-invasively, although ultrasound is useful in accessible arteries (e.g. the carotids), and associated changes such as reduced aortic compliance and arterial calcification can be detected by measuring, respectively, aortic pulse wave velocity and coronary artery calcium score (through computed tomography scans). There were no good animal models until genetically-altered mice (see Ch. 8) deficient in apolipoproteins or receptors that play key roles in lipoprotein metabolism transformed the scene. Nevertheless, most of our current understanding of atherogenesis comes from human epidemiology and pathology, and from clinical investigations.

Epidemiological studies have identified numerous risk factors for atheromatous disease. Some of these cannot be altered (e.g. a family history of ischaemic heart disease[3]), but others are modifiable (Table 22.1) and are potential targets for therapeutic drugs. Clinical trials have shown that improving risk factors can reduce the consequences of atheromatous disease. Many risk factors (e.g. type 2 diabetes, dyslipidaemia, cigarette smoking) cause endothelial dysfunction (see Ch. 21), evidenced by reduced vasodilator responses to acetylcholine or to increased blood flow (so-called flow-mediated dilatation), responses that are inhibited by drugs that block nitric oxide (NO) synthesis (see Ch. 19). Healthy endothelium produces NO and other mediators that protect against atheroma, so it is likely that metabolic cardiovascular risk factors act by causing endothelial dysfunction.

Atherogenesis involves:

1. *Endothelial dysfunction*, with altered NO (see Ch. 19) biosynthesis which predisposes to atherosclerosis.
2. *Injury* of dysfunctional endothelium, which leads to expression of adhesion molecules. This encourages monocyte attachment and migration of monocytes from the lumen into the intima. Lesions have a predilection for regions of disturbed flow such as the origins of aortic branches.
3. *Low-density lipoprotein (LDL) cholesterol* transport into the vessel wall. Endothelial cells and monocytes/macrophages generate free radicals that oxidise LDL (oxLDL), resulting in lipid peroxidation.
4. *oxLDL* uptake by macrophages via 'scavenger' receptors. Such macrophages are called *foam cells* because of their 'foamy' histological appearance, resulting from accumulation of cytoplasmic lipid, and are characteristic of atheroma. Uptake of oxLDL activates macrophages which release proinflammatory cytokines.
5. Subendothelial accumulation of foam cells and T lymphocytes to form *fatty streaks*.

[1]The term *dyslipidaemia* is preferred to *hyperlipidaemia* because a low plasma concentration of high-density lipoprotein cholesterol is a risk factor for atheromatous disease.
[2]PCSK9 stands for proprotein convertase subtilisin/kexin type 9.

[3]As we learn how to tinker with the expression of genes, even this seeming truism may turn out to be less immutable than it seemed (see Ch. 5 and later.)

Table 24.1 Modifiable risk factors for atheromatous disease

Raised low-density lipoprotein cholesterol
Reduced high-density lipoprotein cholesterol
Hypertension (Ch. 21)
Diabetes mellitus (Ch. 31)
Cigarette smoking (Ch. 50)
Obesity (Ch. 32)
Physical inactivity
Raised C-reactive protein[a]
Raised coagulation factors (e.g. factor VII, fibrinogen)
Raised homocysteine
Raised lipoprotein(a)

[a]Strongly associated with atheromatous disease but not causal of it.

6. Protective mechanisms, for example cholesterol *mobilisation from the artery wall* and transport in plasma as high-density lipoprotein (HDL) cholesterol, termed *reverse cholesterol transport*.
7. Cytokine and growth factor release by activated platelets, macrophages and endothelial cells, causing proliferation of smooth muscle and deposition of connective tissue components. This *inflammatory fibroproliferative response* leads to a dense fibrous cap overlying a lipid-rich core, the whole structure comprising the atheromatous plaque.
8. Plaque *rupture*, which provides a substrate for *thrombosis* (see Ch. 23, Figs 23.1 and 23.10). The presence of large numbers of macrophages predisposes to plaque rupture, whereas vascular smooth muscle and matrix proteins stabilise the plaque.

To understand how drugs prevent atheromatous disease, it is necessary briefly to review lipoprotein transport.

LIPOPROTEIN TRANSPORT

Lipids and cholesterol are transported in the bloodstream as complexes of lipid and protein known as *lipoproteins*. These consist of a central core of hydrophobic lipid (including triglycerides and cholesteryl esters) encased in a hydrophilic coat of polar phospholipid, free cholesterol and *apoprotein*. There are four main classes of lipoprotein, differing in the relative proportion of the core lipids and in the type of apoprotein (various kinds of apoA and apoB). Apoproteins bind to specific receptors that mediate cellular uptake of lipoprotein particles into liver, blood or other tissues. Lipoproteins differ in size and density, and this latter property, measured originally by ultracentrifugation but now commonly estimated by simpler methods, is the basis for their classification into:

- HDL particles (contain apoA1 and apoA2), diameter 7–20 nm
- LDL particles (contain apoB-100), diameter 20–30 nm
- very-low-density lipoprotein (VLDL) particles (contain apoB-100), diameter 30–80 nm
- chylomicrons (contain apoB-48), diameter 100–1000 nm

Each class of lipoprotein has a specific role in lipid transport, and there are different pathways for exogenous and endogenous lipids, as well as a pathway for reverse cholesterol transport (Fig. 22.1). In the *exogenous pathway*, cholesterol and triglycerides absorbed from the ileum are transported as chylomicrons in lymph and then blood, to capillaries in muscle and adipose tissue. Here, triglycerides are hydrolysed by lipoprotein lipase, and the tissues take up the resulting free fatty acids and glycerol. The chylomicron remnants, still containing their full complement of cholesteryl esters, pass to the liver, bind to receptors on hepatocytes and undergo endocytosis. Cholesterol liberated in hepatocytes is stored, oxidised to bile acids, secreted unaltered in bile, or can enter the endogenous pathway.

In the *endogenous pathway*, cholesterol and newly synthesised triglycerides are transported from the liver as VLDL to muscle and adipose tissue, where triglyceride is hydrolysed to fatty acids and glycerol; these enter the tissues as described previously. During this process, the lipoprotein particles become smaller but retain a full complement of cholesteryl esters and become LDL particles. LDL provides the source of cholesterol for incorporation into cell membranes and for synthesis of steroids (see Chs 33 and 35) but is also key in atherogenesis. Cells take up LDL by endocytosis via *LDL receptors* that recognise apoB-100. LDL receptors are critically important in determining the concentration of circulating LDL, and hence the development and progression of atheromatous disease; the most widely used drugs for the prevention of such disease, the statins, act by blocking the synthesis of cholesterol within hepatocytes which respond by increasing LDL receptor expression on their surface membranes (see later). A new class of drugs, monoclonal antibodies that inhibit PCSK9, also influence LDL receptor density but by a different mechanism, namely reduced lysosomal degradation of internalised LDL receptors leading to increased recycling of functional LDL receptors to the surface membrane (see later). Alternatively, inhibition of PCSK9 can be achieved using small interfering RNA (siRNA; see Ch. 5); **inclisiran** is a newly approved siRNA drug that blocks PCSK9 synthesis in the liver (see later).

Cholesterol can return to plasma from the tissues in HDL particles (reverse cholesterol transport). Cholesterol is esterified with long-chain fatty acids in HDL particles, and the resulting cholesteryl esters are transferred to VLDL or LDL particles by a transfer protein present in the plasma and known as *cholesteryl ester transfer protein* (CETP). Lipoprotein(a), or Lp(a), is a species of LDL that is associated with atherosclerosis and is localised in atherosclerotic lesions. Lp(a) contains a unique apoprotein, apo(a), with structural similarities to plasminogen (see Ch. 23). Lp(a) competes with plasminogen for its receptor on endothelial cells. Plasminogen is the substrate for plasminogen activator, which is secreted by, and bound to, endothelial cells, generating the fibrinolytic enzyme *plasmin* (see Fig. 23.10). The effect of the binding of Lp(a) is that less plasmin is generated, fibrinolysis is inhibited and thrombosis promoted.

Microsomal triglyceride transport protein (MTP) is a lipid-transfer protein present in the lumen of the endoplasmic reticulum responsible for binding and

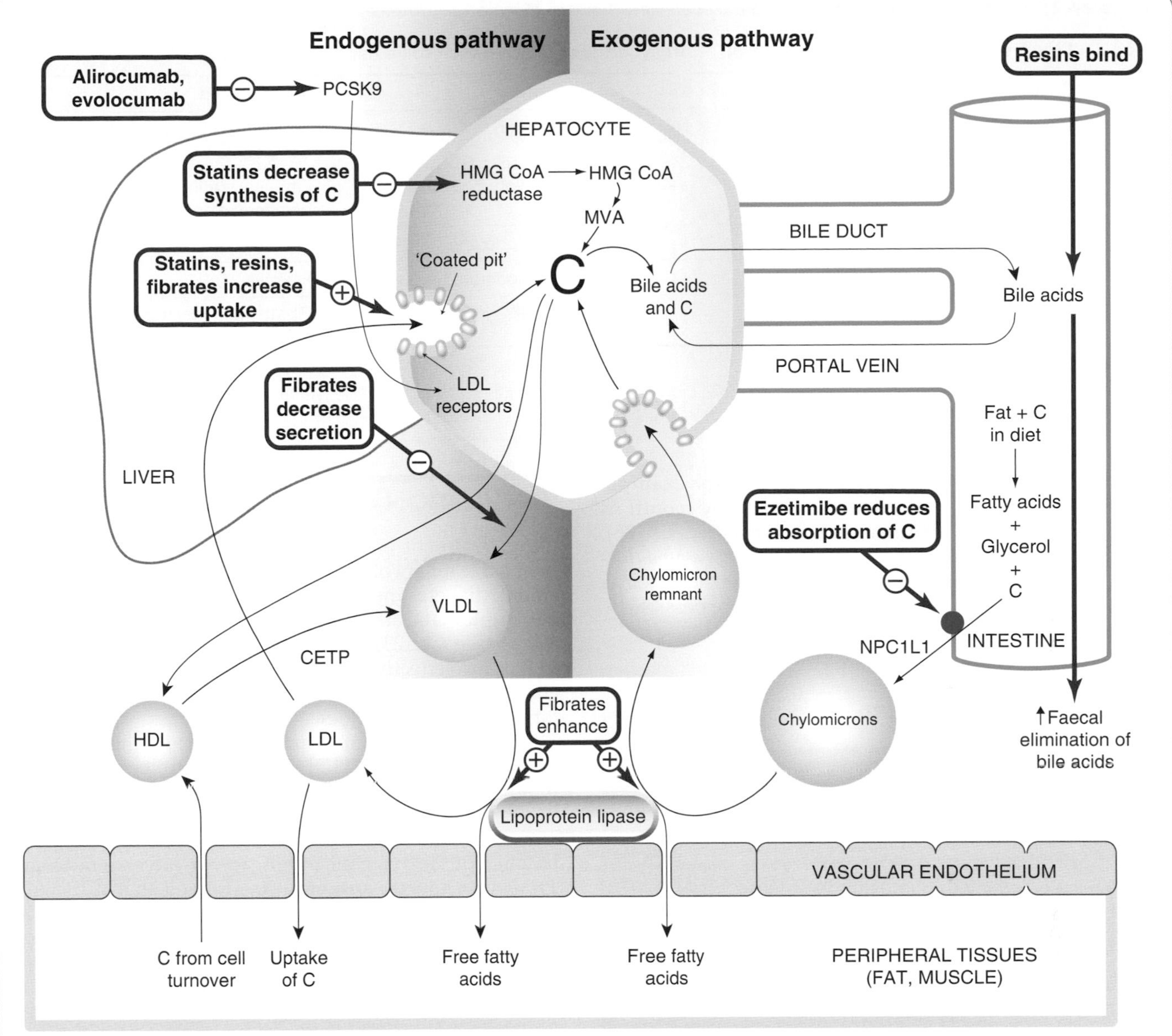

Fig. 22.1 Schematic diagram of cholesterol transport in the tissues, with sites of action of the main drugs affecting lipoprotein metabolism. *C*, Cholesterol; *CETP*, cholesteryl ester transport protein; *HDL*, high-density lipoprotein; *HMG-CoA*, 3-hydroxy-3-methylglutaryl-coenzyme A; *LDL*, low-density lipoprotein; *MVA*, mevalonate; *NPC1L1*, a cholesterol transporter in the brush border of enterocytes; *PCSK9*, proprotein convertase subtilisin/kexin 9; *VLDL*, very-low-density lipoprotein.

transfer of lipids between membranes. The inhibition of MTP interferes with apoB secretion and LDL assembly, and **lomitapide**, one such inhibitor (see later), is used in addition to diet and other measures in homozygous familial hypercholesterolaemia (FH).

DYSLIPIDAEMIA

Dyslipidaemia may be primary or secondary. The *primary* forms are due to a combination of diet and genetics (often but not always polygenic). They are classified into six phenotypes (the Frederickson classification; Table 22.2). An especially great risk of ischaemic heart disease occurs in a subset of primary type IIa hyperlipoproteinaemia caused by single-gene defects of LDL receptors; this is known as *familial hypercholesterolaemia* (FH), and the plasma total cholesterol concentration, normally <5 mmol/L, in affected adults is typically >8 mmol/L in heterozygotes and 12–25 mmol/L in homozygotes. A study of FH enabled Brown and Goldstein (1986) to define the LDL receptor pathway of cholesterol homeostasis (for which they shared a Nobel Prize). Further investigation of people with very low or very high circulating LDL-cholesterol (LDL-C) concentrations led to the discovery of inactivating and gain-of-function variants of the *PCSK9* gene (see Hall, 2013, for a popular account, and later). Drugs used to treat primary dyslipidaemia are described later.

Secondary forms of dyslipidaemia are a consequence of other conditions, such as diabetes mellitus, alcoholism, nephrotic syndrome, chronic renal failure, hypothyroidism,

Table 24.2 Frederickson/World Health Organization classification of hyperlipoproteinaemia

Type	Lipoprotein elevated	Cholesterol	Triglycerides	Atherosclerosis risk	Drug treatment
I	Chylomicrons	+	+++	NE	Volanesorsen
IIa	LDL	++	NE	High	Statin ± ezetimibe, PCSK9 inhibitor, bempedoic acid, lomitapide
IIb	LDL + VLDL	++	++	High	Fibrates, statin, PCSK9 inhibitor, bempedoic acid
III	βVLDL	++	++	Moderate	Fibrates
IV	VLDL	+	++	Moderate	Fibrates
V	Chylomicrons + VLDL	+	++	NE	Fibrate, and statin combinations

+indicates increased concentration.
LDL, Low-density lipoprotein; *NE*, not elevated; *PCSK9*, proprotein convertase subtilisin/kexin 9; *VLDL*, very-low-density lipoprotein; *βVLDL*, a qualitatively abnormal form of VLDL identified by its pattern on electrophoresis

liver disease and administration of drugs, for example **isotretinoin** (an isomer of vitamin A given by mouth as well as topically in the treatment of severe acne, see Ch. 26), **tamoxifen**, **ciclosporin**-(see Ch. 25) and *protease inhibitors* used to treat infection with human immunodeficiency virus (see Ch. 53). Secondary forms are treated where possible by correcting the underlying cause.

Lipoprotein metabolism and dyslipidaemia

Lipids, including cholesterol and triglycerides, are transported in the plasma as lipoproteins, of which there are four classes:

- Chylomicrons transport triglycerides and cholesterol from the gastrointestinal tract to the tissues, where triglyceride is split by lipoprotein lipase, releasing free fatty acids and glycerol which are taken up in muscle and adipose tissue. Chylomicron remnants are taken up in the liver, where cholesterol is stored, secreted in bile, oxidised to bile acids or converted into:
  - VLDLs, which transport cholesterol and newly synthesised triglycerides to the tissues, where triglycerides are removed as before, leaving:
  - intermediate-density lipoprotein and LDL particles with a large component of cholesterol; some LDL-C is taken up by the tissues and some by the liver, by endocytosis via specific LDL receptors.
- HDL particles adsorb cholesterol derived from cell breakdown in tissues (including arteries) and transfer it to VLDL and LDL particles via cholesterol ester transport protein (CETP).
- Dyslipidaemias can be primary, or secondary to a disease (e.g. hypothyroidism). They are classified according to which lipoprotein particle is abnormal into six phenotypes (the Frederickson classification). The higher the LDL-C and the lower the HDL cholesterol, the higher the risk of ischaemic heart disease.

PREVENTION OF ATHEROMATOUS DISEASE

Drug treatment is often justified, to supplement healthy habits. Treatment of hypertension (see Ch. 21) and, to a lesser extent, diabetes mellitus (see Ch. 31) reduces the incidence of symptomatic atheromatous disease, and antithrombotic drugs (see Ch. 23) reduce arterial thrombosis. Reducing LDL is also effective and is the main subject of this present chapter, but steps to increase HDL have also been potential targets for pharmacological attack.

Whilst regular exercise increases circulating HDL, drug treatment to increase HDL is of uncertain benefit. Fibrates modestly increase HDL and reduce LDL and triglycerides. In subjects with low HDL, inhibition of CETP can markedly increase circulating HDL, but three such drugs have failed because of lack of clinical efficacy or adverse outcomes. Trials of a fourth, **anacetrapib,** showed that it increases HDL and lowers LDL, and is associated with a modest reduction in major coronary events. However, there was no effect on overall mortality, and its development has been discontinued. It appears that whilst low HDL may be a good risk marker in certain ethnic groups for atherosclerosis, HDL itself may not prove to be a good pharmacological target (Parhofer, 2015).

LIPID-LOWERING DRUGS

Several drugs decrease plasma lipoprotein concentrations. Drug therapy is used in addition to dietary measures and correction of other modifiable cardiovascular risk factors.

The main agents used clinically are:

- statins: 3-hydroxy-3-methylglutaryl-coenzyme A (HMG-CoA) reductase inhibitors
- bempedoic acid
- PCSK9 inhibitors
- fibrates
- inhibitors of cholesterol absorption
- small molecule inhibitors

Atheromatous disease

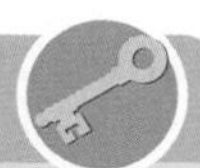

- Atheroma is a uniquely human focal disease of large- and medium-sized arteries. Atheromatous plaques occur in most people, progress insidiously over many decades and underlie the commonest causes of death (myocardial infarction) and disability (e.g. stroke) in industrialised countries.
- Fatty streaks are the earliest structurally apparent lesion and progress to fibrous and/or fatty plaques. Symptoms such as angina occur only when blood flow through the vessel is reduced below that needed to meet the metabolic demands of tissues downstream from the obstruction.
- Important modifiable risk factors include hypertension (see Ch. 21), dyslipidaemia (this chapter) and smoking (see Ch. 50).
- The pathophysiology is of chronic inflammation in response to injury. Endothelial dysfunction leads to loss of protective mechanisms, monocyte/macrophage and T-cell migration, uptake of LDL-C and its oxidation, uptake of oxidised LDL by macrophages, smooth muscle cell migration and proliferation and deposition of collagen.
- Plaque rupture leads to platelet activation and thrombosis (see Ch. 23) with the potential to cause downstream infarction of, for example, heart muscle or brain.

STATINS: HMG-COA REDUCTASE INHIBITORS

The rate-limiting enzyme in cholesterol synthesis is HMG-CoA reductase, which catalyses the conversion of HMG-CoA to mevalonic acid (see Fig. 22.1). **Simvastatin, lovastatin** and **pravastatin** are specific, reversible, competitive HMG-CoA reductase inhibitors with K_i values of approximately 1 nmol/L. **Atorvastatin** and **rosuvastatin** are long-lasting inhibitors. Decreased hepatic cholesterol synthesis upregulates LDL receptor synthesis, increasing LDL clearance from plasma into liver cells. The main biochemical effect of statins is therefore to reduce plasma LDL. There is also some reduction in plasma triglyceride and increase in HDL. Several large randomised placebo-controlled trials of the effects of HMG-CoA reductase inhibitors on morbidity and mortality have been positive.

Other actions of statins

Products of the mevalonate pathway react with protein ('lipidation', which is the addition to a protein of hydrophobic groups such as prenyl or farnesyl moieties). Several important membrane-bound enzymes (e.g. endothelial NO synthase; see Ch. 19) are modified in this way. The fatty groups serve as anchors, localising the enzyme in organelles such as caveolae and Golgi apparatus. Consequently, there is interest in actions of statins that are unrelated, or indirectly related, to their effect on plasma LDL (sometimes referred to as *pleiotropic* effects). Some of these actions are undesirable (e.g. HMG-CoA reductase guides migrating primordial germ cells, and statin use is contraindicated during pregnancy), but some offer therapeutic promise. Such potentially beneficial actions include:

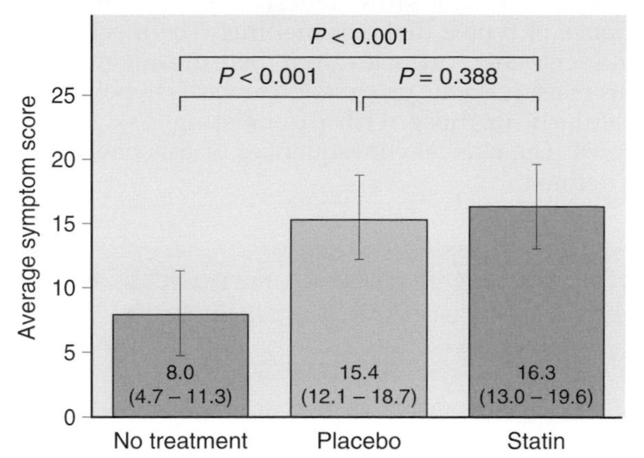

Fig. 22.2 Adverse effect symptom scores according to treatment allocation in three-way crossover trial conducted by Howard, J.P., Wood, F.A., Finegold, J.A., et al. 2021. Side effect patterns in a crossover trial of statin, placebo, and no treatment. J. Am. Coll. Cardiol. 78, 1210-1222.

- improved endothelial function
- reduced vascular inflammation
- reduced platelet aggregability
- increased neovascularisation of ischaemic tissue
- increased circulating endothelial progenitor cells
- stabilisation of atherosclerotic plaque
- antithrombotic actions
- enhanced fibrinolysis

The extent to which these effects contribute to the anti-atheromatous actions of statins is unknown.

Pharmacokinetics

Short-acting statins are given by mouth at night to reduce peak cholesterol synthesis in the early morning. They are well absorbed and extracted by the liver, their site of action, and are subject to extensive presystemic metabolism via cytochrome P450 and glucuronidation pathways. Simvastatin is an inactive lactone prodrug; it is metabolised in the liver to its active form, the corresponding β-hydroxy fatty acid.

Adverse effects

Statins are well tolerated; mild unwanted effects include muscle pain (myalgia), gastrointestinal disturbance, raised concentrations of liver enzymes in plasma, insomnia and rash. More serious adverse effects are rare but include skeletal muscle damage (myositis, which when severe is described as rhabdomyolysis) and angio-oedema. Myositis is a class effect of statins, occurring also with other lipid-lowering drugs (especially fibrates), and is dose related.[4]. However, re-instatement of statin therapy in placebo-controlled crossover trials did not find a statistically significance in symptoms with statins compared to placebo (Fig. 22.2). It is possible that the bulk of adverse symptoms associated with statins are due to the nocebo effect (worsening of symptoms due to sham or placebo), and that most patients who had stopped statins due to suspected adverse events can actually safely resume therapy.

[4]**Cerivastatin**, a potent statin introduced at relatively high dose, was withdrawn because of rhabdomyolysis occurring particularly in patients treated with gemfibrozil – discussed later in the chapter.

Statin therapy leads to a modest increase in the long-term incidence of type 2 diabetes mellitus. The mechanism for this adverse effect is unclear, but there are suggestions that statins may accelerate progression towards hyperglycaemia, particularly in those with pre-existing risk factors for diabetes. The clinical consequences of this have not been well defined.

Clinical uses of HMG-CoA reductase inhibitors (statins, e.g. simvastatin, atorvastatin)

- Secondary prevention of myocardial infarction and stroke in patients who have symptomatic atherosclerotic disease (e.g. angina, transient ischaemic attacks, or following myocardial infarction or stroke).
- Primary prevention of arterial disease in patients who are at high risk because of elevated serum cholesterol concentration, especially if there are other risk factors for atherosclerosis such as diabetes (see Ch. 31) or renal failure (see Ch. 29). Tables (available, for example, in the British National Formulary) are used to target treatment to those at greatest risk.
- **Atorvastatin** lowers serum cholesterol in patients with homozygous FH.
- In severe drug-resistant dyslipidaemia (e.g. heterozygous FH), **ezetimibe,** which inhibits cholesterol absorption, is combined with statin treatment.
- Contraindicated in pregnancy.

BEMPEDOIC ACID

Bempedoic acid is an inhibitor of ATP-citrate lyase, an enzyme upstream of HMG-CoA-reductase (Fig 22.3). It exerts its effects on the same cholesterol synthesis pathway as the statin drugs. Bempedoic acid is a dicarboxylic acid; it is a pro-drug that requires activation in the liver to a CoA thioester. There is no activation of bempedoic acid in skeletal muscle, thus potentially lowering the likelihood of myositis. Clinical trial data indicate that add-on bempedoic acid therapy can deliver further cholesterol reduction in patients who may already be on maximal statin doses. Two separate formulations are licensed, a single agent and a combination with ezetimibe (see later). Recognised adverse effects of bempedoic acid are hyperuricaemia and gout, stemming from inhibition of renal tubular organic anion transporter 2 (see Ch. 9).

INHIBITION OF PCSK9

PCSK9 is synthesised in inactive form by many tissues, including brain and liver. It is activated autocatalytically by proteolytic cleavage, which removes a section of its peptide chain that blocks its activity. When activated, it binds to LDL receptors and promotes their lysosomal degradation following LDL uptake into hepatocyte cytoplasm (see Fig. 22.1), thereby preventing recycling of LDL receptors to the surface membrane and diminishing their ability to sequester LDL. Family members who inherit a hyperactive form of the *PCSK9* gene suffer from severe hypercholesterolaemia; conversely individuals with inactivating mutations in this gene have low circulating LDL and a low incidence of atheromatous disease. Individuals homozygous for inactivated PCSK9 have very low plasma

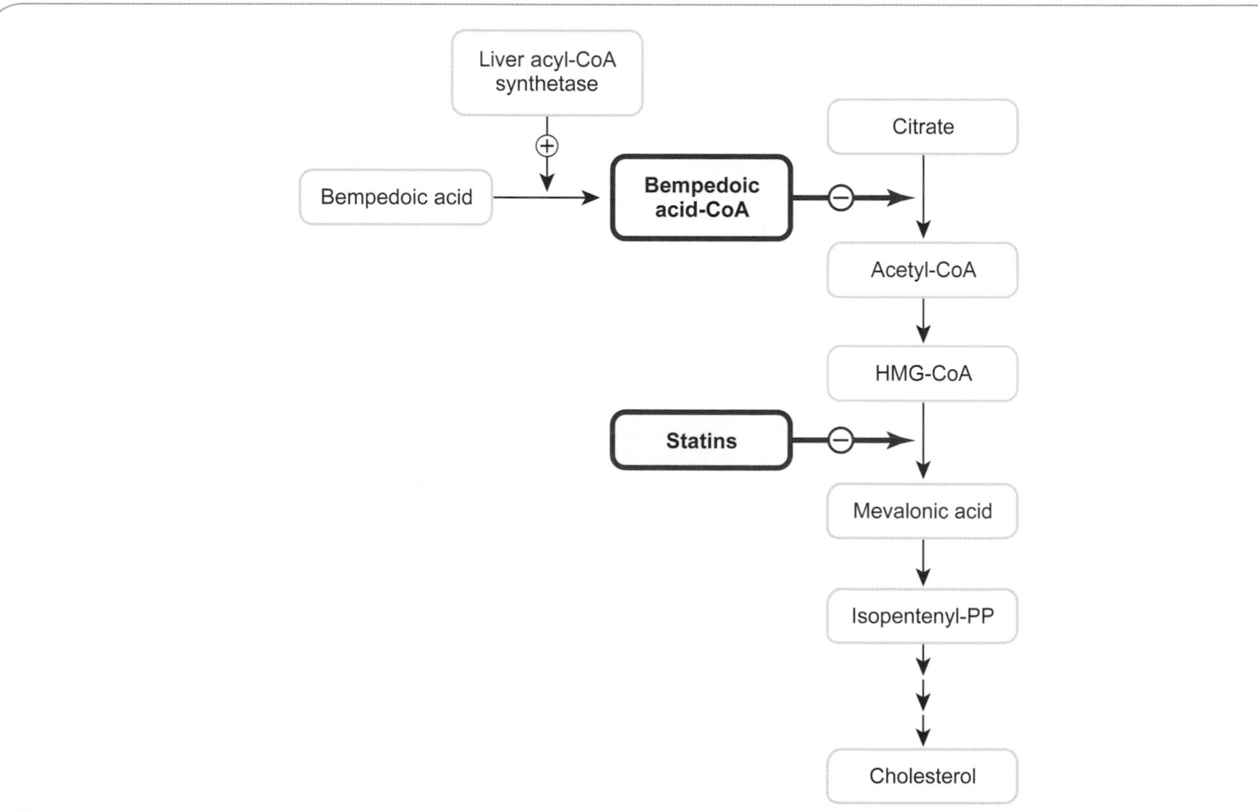

Fig. 22.3 Mechanism of action for bempedoic acid. Bempedoic acid is a pro-drug that is activated in the liver. It inhibits acetyl-CoA carboxylase and reduces subsequent production of cholesterol. *CoA*, Coenzyme A; *HMG*, 3-hydroxy-3-methylglutaryl.

concentrations of LDL and are healthy. This encouraged the development of monoclonal antibodies that block PCSK9, thereby preventing it from combining with LDL receptors and marking them down for lysosomal destruction. **Evolocumab** and **alirocumab** are now licensed for the treatment of primary hypercholesterolaemia in patients whose circulating LDL is not adequately controlled by a statin or statin/ezetimibe combination, as additional agents (or given alone to patients who do not tolerate treatment with a statin). Evolocumab is administered subcutaneously every 2–4 weeks, alirocumab every 2 weeks. Nasopharyngitis and influenza-like symptoms are common adverse effects of both agents.

INCLISIRAN

Inclisiran is a recently licensed double-stranded siRNA that inhibits PCSK9 synthesis. It works through RNA interference, with enhanced breakdown of mRNA relating to PCSK9. An N-acetylgalactosamine component recognised by hepatocyte receptors (see Chs 5 and 9) is conjugated onto the sense strand so that inclisiran has high uptake and selectivity for its site of action in the liver.

It is given by subcutaneous injection twice a year, so is potentially suitable for administration in primary care centres. There are, as yet, no major safety concerns, but more robust data will emerge with longer-term experience.

FIBRATES

Several fibric acid derivatives (fibrates) are available, including **bezafibrate**, **ciprofibrate**, **gemfibrozil**, **fenofibrate** and **clofibrate**. These markedly reduce circulating VLDL, and hence triglyceride, with a modest (approximately 10%) reduction in LDL and an approximately 10% increase in HDL. Their mechanism of action is complex (see Fig. 22.1). They are agonists at PPARα nuclear receptors[5] (see Ch. 3); in humans, the main effects are to increase transcription of the genes for lipoprotein lipase, apoA1 and apoA5. They increase hepatic LDL uptake. In addition to effects on lipoproteins, fibrates reduce plasma C-reactive protein and fibrinogen, improve glucose tolerance and inhibit vascular smooth muscle inflammation by inhibiting the expression of the transcription factor nuclear factor κB (see Ch. 3). The relative importance of these effects is uncertain, and fibrates have not been demonstrated to improve survival.

Adverse effects

Rhabdomyolysis is unusual but severe, giving rise to acute renal failure associated with excretion of muscle proteins, especially myoglobin, by the kidney. It occurs particularly in patients with renal impairment, because of reduced protein binding and impaired drug elimination. Fibrates should be avoided in such patients and also in alcoholics, who are predisposed to hypertriglyceridaemia but are at risk of severe muscle inflammation and injury.[6] Rhabdomyolysis can also be caused (rarely) by statins (see earlier), and the combined use of fibrates with this class of drugs is therefore generally inadvisable (although it is sometimes undertaken by specialists). Gastrointestinal symptoms, pruritus and rash are more common than with statins. Clofibrate predisposes to gallstones, and its use is therefore limited to patients who have had a cholecystectomy (i.e. removal of the gall bladder).

[5]Standing for peroxisome proliferator-activated receptors – don't ask! (Peroxisomes are organelles that are not present in human cells, so something of a misnomer!) Thiazolidinedione drugs used in treating diabetes act on related PPARγ receptors (see Ch. 31).

[6]For several reasons, including a tendency to lie immobile for prolonged periods followed by generalised convulsions – 'rum fits' – and delirium tremens..

Clinical uses of fibrates (e.g. gemfibrozil, fenofibrate)

- Mixed dyslipidaemia (i.e. raised serum triglyceride as well as cholesterol), provided this is not caused by excessive alcohol consumption. **Fenofibrate** is uricosuric, which may be useful where hyperuricaemia coexists with mixed dyslipidaemia.
- Severe hypertriglyceridaemia when dietary and other measures have failed.
- Combined with other lipid-lowering drugs in patients with severe treatment-resistant dyslipidaemia. This may, however, increase the risk of rhabdomyolysis.

DRUGS THAT INHIBIT CHOLESTEROL ABSORPTION

Historically, bile acid-binding resins (e.g. **colestyramine**, **colestipol**) were the only agents available to reduce cholesterol absorption and were among the few means to lower plasma cholesterol. Taken by mouth they sequester bile acids in the intestine and prevent their reabsorption and enterohepatic recirculation (see Fig. 22.1). The concentration of HDL is unchanged, and they cause an unwanted increase in triglycerides.

Decreased absorption of exogenous cholesterol and increased metabolism of endogenous cholesterol into bile acids in the liver lead to increased expression of LDL receptors on hepatocytes, and hence to increased clearance of LDL from the blood and a reduced concentration of LDL in plasma. Resins are bulky, unpalatable and often cause diarrhoea. They interfere with the absorption of fat-soluble vitamins, and of thiazide diuretics (see Ch. 29), digoxin (see Ch. 20) and warfarin (see Ch. 23), which should therefore be taken at least 1 h before or 4–6 h after the resin. With the introduction of statins, their use in treating dyslipidaemia was relegated largely to additional treatment in patients with severe disease, and (a separate use) treating bile salt-associated symptoms of pruritus (itch) and diarrhoea – see clinical box later. **Colesevelam** is available in tablet form and is less bulky (daily dose up to 4 g compared with a dose up to 36 g for colestyramine) but more expensive. Subsequently, plant sterols and stanols have been marketed; these are isolated from wood pulp and used to make margarines or yoghurts. They reduce plasma cholesterol to a small extent and are tastier than resins. Phytosterol and phytostanol esters interfere with the micellar presentation of sterols to the enterocyte surface, reducing cholesterol absorption and hence the exogenous pathway.

EZETIMIBE

Ezetimibe is one of a group of azetidinone cholesterol absorption inhibitors and is used as an adjunct to diet and statins in hypercholesterolaemia. It inhibits absorption of cholesterol (and of plant stanols) from the duodenum by blocking a transport protein (NPC1L1) in the brush border of enterocytes, without affecting the absorption of fat-soluble vitamins, triglycerides or bile acids. Because of its high potency compared with resins (a daily dose of 10 mg), it represents a useful advance as a substitute for resins as supplementary treatment to statins in patients with severe dyslipidaemia.

Ezetimibe is administered by mouth and is absorbed into intestinal epithelial cells, where it localises to the brush border, which is its presumed site of action. It is also extensively (>80%) metabolised to an active metabolite. Enterohepatic recycling results in slow elimination. The terminal half-life is approximately 22 h. It enters milk (at least in animal studies) and is contraindicated for women who are breastfeeding. It is generally well tolerated but can cause diarrhoea, abdominal pain or headache; rash and angio-oedema have been reported.

Clinical use of drugs that reduce cholesterol absorption: ezetimibe or bile acid-binding resins (e.g. colestyramine, colesevelam)

- As an addition to a statin when response has been inadequate (**ezetimibe**).
- For hypercholesterolaemia when a statin is contraindicated.
- Uses unrelated to atherosclerosis, include:
  - pruritus in patients with partial biliary obstruction (bile acid-binding resin)
  - bile acid diarrhoea, for example, caused by diabetic neuropathy (bile acid-binding resin).

MICROSOMAL TRIGLYCERIDE TRANSPORT PROTEIN (MTP) INHIBITORS

LOMITAPIDE

Lomitapide is a small molecule inhibitor of MTP that has recently been approved as an adjunct to other treatment for homozygous FH. MTP plays a key role in the assembly and release of apoB-containing lipoproteins into the circulation, and inhibition of this protein significantly lowers plasma lipid levels. This action contrasts with other lipid-lowering drugs, which mainly work by increasing LDL uptake rather than by reducing hepatic lipoprotein secretion. Lomitapide is administered orally once a day and the dose is individualised according to how it is tolerated. Gastrointestinal disturbances are common.

ANTISENSE OLIGONUCLEOTIDES

Mipomersen, the first single-stranded antisense oligonucleotide to be marketed, blocks synthesis of apoB100 and was licensed for use in patients with homozygous FH. However it was withdrawn because of hepatotoxicity.

Volanesorsen is an antisense oligonucleotide that inhibits the production of apoC-III. It is a single-stranded molecule (unlike inclisiran – see earlier). Volanesorsen binds selectively, within the 3′ untranslated region, to the apoC-III mRNA, leading to breakdown of the mRNA. In the liver, apoC-III has a role in triglyceride metabolism and inhibits the clearance of chylomicrons and lipoproteins. Decreased production of apoC-III has the beneficial effect of taking away its inhibitory effects on triglyceride clearance. Volanesorsen has been found in clinical trials to significantly reduce apoC-III and serum triglycerides, and is approved for treatment of familial chylomicron syndrome, an autosomal recessive disorder of the gene coding lipoprotein lipase with an incidence of approximately 1 per million. Thrombocytopenia is a potentially serious adverse effect.

Drugs in dyslipidaemia

The main drugs used in patients with dyslipidaemias are:

- HMG-CoA reductase inhibitors (statins, e.g. **simvastatin**): inhibit synthesis of cholesterol, increasing the expression of LDL receptors on hepatocytes and hence increasing hepatic LDL-C uptake. They reduce cardiovascular events and prolong life in people at risk, and clinically are the most important class of drugs used in dyslipidaemias. Adverse effects include myalgias (rarely, severe muscle damage) and raised liver enzymes.

  Agents that target PCSK9 (alirocumab, evolocumab, inclisiran), or bempedoic acid, are used when there is inadequate response to statins, or where statins are contraindicated or not tolerated.
- Fibrates (e.g. **gemfibrozil**): activate PPARα receptors, increase the activity of lipoprotein lipase, decrease hepatic VLDL production and enhance clearance of LDL by the liver. They markedly lower serum triglycerides, and modestly increase HDL cholesterol. Adverse effects include muscle damage.
- Agents that interfere with cholesterol absorption, usually as an adjunct to diet plus statin:
  - **ezetimibe**
  - stanol-enriched foods
  - bile acid–binding resins (e.g. colestyramine, colesevelam).
- **Lomitapide** blocks MTP and is used to treat patients with homozygous FH.
- Voranesorsen is a single-stranded antisense drug that blocks the synthesis of apoC-III. It is used to treat familial chylomicron syndrome.

REFERENCES AND FURTHER READING

Atherosclerosis and dyslipidaemia

Brown, M.S., Goldstein, J.L., 1986. A receptor-mediated pathway for cholesterol homeostasis. Science 232, 34–47.

Durrington, P.N., 2007. Hyperlipidaemia: Diagnosis and Management, third ed. Hodder Arnold, London.

Hall, S.H., 2013. Genetics: a gene of rare effect. Nature 496, 152–155.

Parhofer, K.G., 2015. Increasing HDL-cholesterol and prevention of atherosclerosis: a critical perspective. Atheroscler. Suppl. 18, 109–111.

Drug therapy

Agarwala, A., Quispe, R., Goldberg, A.C., et al., 2021. Bempedoic acid for heterozygous familial hypercholesterolemia: from bench to bedside. Drug Des. Devel. Ther. 15, 1955–1963.

Alam, U., Al-Bazz, D.Y., Soran, H., 2021. Bempedoic acid: the new kid on the block for the treatment of dyslipidemia and LDL cholesterol: a narrative review. Diabetes Ther. 12, 1779–1789.

Herrett, E., Williamson, E., Brack, K., et al., 2021. Statin treatment and muscle symptoms: series of randomised, placebo controlled n-of-1 trials. BMJ 372, n135.

Howard, J.P., Wood, F.A., Finegold, J.A., et al., 2021. Side effect patterns in a crossover trial of statin, placebo, and no treatment. J. Am. Coll. Cardiol. 78, 1210–1222.

Ruscica, M., Ferri, N., Santos, R.D., et al., 2021. Lipid lowering drugs: present status and future developments. Curr. Atheroscler. Rep. 23, 17.

Potential therapies

Giglio, R.V., Pantea Stoian, A., Al-Rasadi, K., et al., 2021. Novel therapeutical approaches to managing atherosclerotic risk. Int. J. Mol. Sci. 22, 4633.

Pećin, I., Reiner, Ž., 2021. Novel experimental agents for the treatment of hypercholesterolemia. J. Exp. Pharmacol. 13, 91–100.

23 Haemostasis and thrombosis

OVERVIEW

This chapter summarises the main features of blood coagulation, platelet function and fibrinolysis. These processes underlie haemostasis and thrombosis and provide a basis for understanding haemorrhagic disorders (e.g. haemophilia) and thrombotic diseases of both arteries (e.g. thrombotic stroke, myocardial infarction) and veins (e.g. deep vein thrombosis, pulmonary embolism). Anticoagulants, antiplatelet drugs and fibrinolytic drugs are especially important because of the prevalence of thrombotic disease.

INTRODUCTION

Haemostasis is the arrest of blood loss from damaged blood vessels, an essential survival mechanism for complex organisms in a hazardous environment. A wound causes vasoconstriction, accompanied by:

- adhesion and activation of platelets
- formation of fibrin

Platelet activation leads to the formation of a haemostatic plug, which stops the bleeding and is subsequently reinforced by fibrin. The relative importance of each process depends on the type of vessel (arterial, venous or capillary) that has been injured.

Thrombosis is the pathological formation of a 'haemostatic' plug within the vasculature in the absence of bleeding ('haemostasis in the wrong place'). Over a century ago, Rudolph Virchow defined three predisposing factors – 'Virchow's triad': *injury to the vessel wall* – for example, when an atheromatous plaque ruptures or becomes eroded; *altered blood flow* – for example, in the left atrial appendage of the heart during atrial fibrillation, or in the veins of the legs while sitting awkwardly on a long journey; and *abnormal 'coagulability'* of the blood – as occurs, for example, in the later stages of pregnancy or during treatment with certain oral contraceptives (see Ch. 35). Increased coagulability of the blood can be inherited and is referred to as *thrombophilia*. A *thrombus*, which forms in vivo, should be distinguished from a *clot*, which forms in blood in vitro (for example in a glass tube). Clots are amorphous, consisting of a diffuse fibrin meshwork in which red and white blood cells are trapped indiscriminately. By contrast, arterial and venous thrombi each have a distinct structure.

An *arterial thrombus* (Fig. 23.1) is composed of so-called white thrombus consisting mainly of platelets in a fibrin mesh. It is usually associated with atherosclerosis and can interrupt blood flow, causing ischaemia or death of tissue (infarction) downstream. Venous thrombus is composed of 'red thrombus' and consists of a small white head and a large jelly-like red tail, similar in composition to a blood clot, which streams away in the flow. Thrombus can break away from its attachment and float through the circulation, forming an embolus; venous emboli usually lodge in a pulmonary artery ('pulmonary embolism'), while a thrombus that embolises from the left heart or a carotid artery usually lodges in an artery in the brain or other organs, causing death, stroke or other disaster.

Drug therapy to promote haemostasis (e.g. antifibrinolytic and haemostatic drugs; see later) is indicated when this essential process is defective (e.g. defective or missing coagulation factors in haemophilia or following excessive anticoagulant therapy), or when it proves difficult to staunch haemorrhage following surgery or for menorrhagia (heavy menstrual periods). Drug therapy to treat or prevent thrombosis or thromboembolism is extensively used because such diseases are common as well as serious. Drugs affect haemostasis and thrombosis in three distinct ways, by influencing:

- blood coagulation (fibrin formation)
- platelet function
- fibrin removal (fibrinolysis)

BLOOD COAGULATION

COAGULATION CASCADE

Blood coagulation means the conversion of liquid blood to a clot. The main event is the conversion by thrombin of soluble *fibrinogen* to insoluble strands of *fibrin*, the last step in a complex enzyme cascade. The components (called factors) are present in blood as inactive precursors (zymogens) of proteolytic enzymes and co-factors. They are activated by proteolysis, the 'active' forms being designated by the suffix 'a'. Factors XIIa, XIa, Xa, IXa and thrombin (IIa) are all serine proteases. Activation of a small amount of one factor catalyses the formation of larger amounts of the next factor, which catalyses the formation of still larger amounts of the next, and so on; consequently, the cascade provides a mechanism of amplification.[1] As might be expected, this accelerating enzyme cascade has to be controlled by inhibitors, because otherwise all the blood in the body would solidify within minutes of the initiation of haemostasis. One of the most important inhibitors is *antithrombin III*, which neutralises all the serine proteases in the cascade. Vascular endothelium also actively limits thrombus extension (see later).

Two pathways of fibrin formation were described traditionally (termed *intrinsic* – because all the components

[1]Coagulation of 100 mL of blood requires 0.2 mg of factor VIII, 2 mg of factor X, 15 mg of prothrombin and 250 mg of fibrinogen.

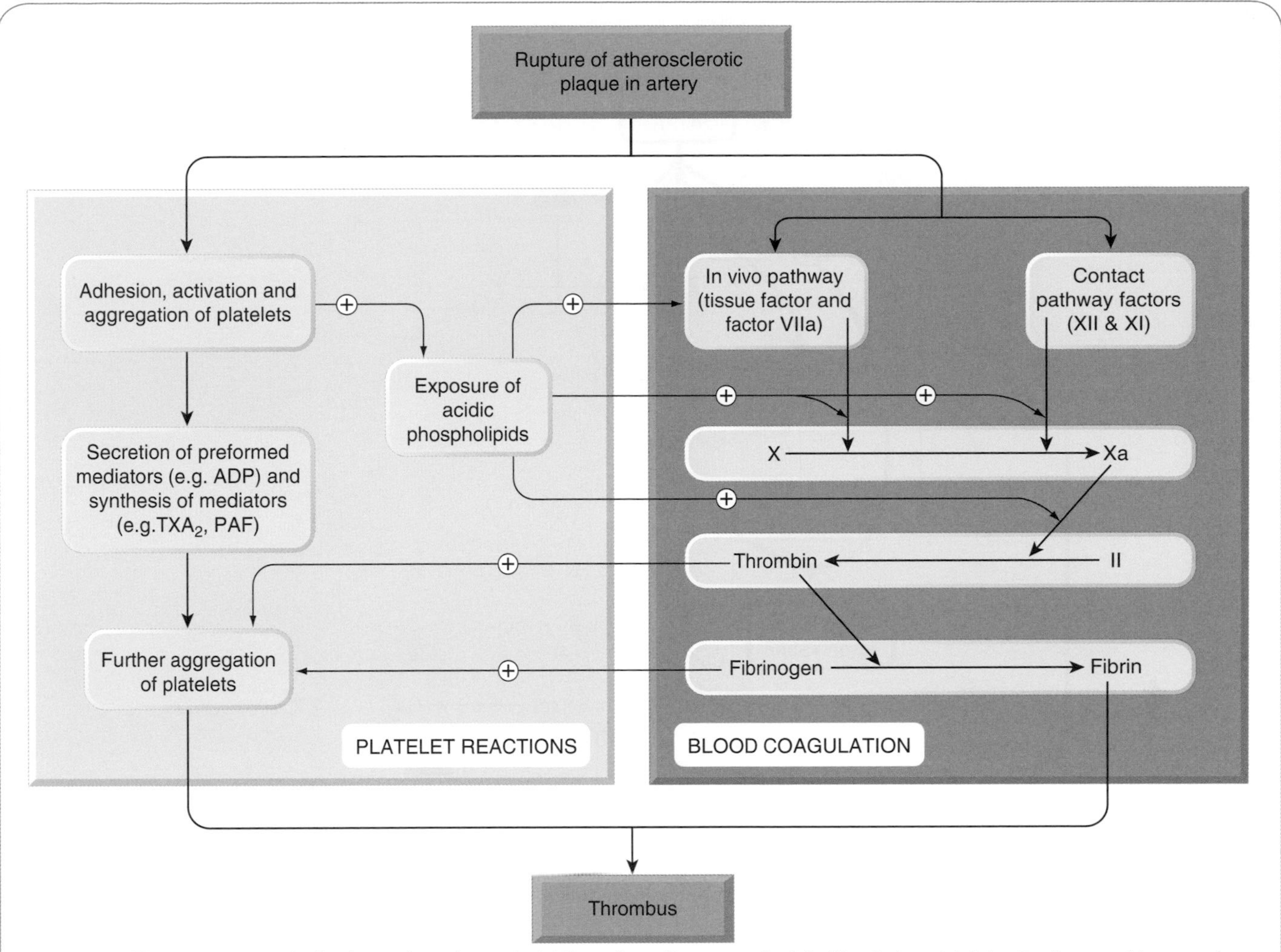

Fig. 23.1 The main events in the formation of an arterial thrombus. Exposure of acidic PLs during platelet activation provides a surface on which factors IXa and VIIa interact with factor X; factor Xa then interacts with factor II, as illustrated in more detail in Fig. 23.4. Activation of factor XII also initiates the fibrinolytic pathway, which is shown in Fig. 23.9. (A similar series of events occurs when there is vascular damage, leading to haemostasis.) *PAF*, Platelet-activating factor; *TXA2*, thromboxane A_2.

are present in the blood - and *extrinsic* - because some components come from outside the blood). The intrinsic or 'contact' pathway is activated when shed blood comes into contact with an artificial surface such as glass, but physiologically the system functions as a single in vivo *pathway* (Fig. 23.2). Tissue damage exposes blood to *tissue factor*, initiating the process and leading to production of a small amount of thrombin. This acts through several positive feedbacks (on Va, VIIIa and on platelets) that amplify and propagate the process with production of more thrombin.

'Tissue factor' is the cellular receptor for factor VII, which, in the presence of Ca^{2+}, undergoes an active site transition. This results in rapid autocatalytic activation of factor VII to VIIa. The tissue factor–VIIa complex activates factors IX and X. Acidic phospholipids (PLs) function as *surface catalysts*. They are provided during platelet activation, which exposes acidic PLs (especially phosphatidylserine), on the platelets' outwardly facing membranes, and these activate various clotting factors, closely juxtaposing them in functional complexes. Platelets also contribute by secreting coagulation factors, including factor Va and fibrinogen. Coagulation is sustained by further generation of factor Xa by IXa–VIIIa–Ca^{2+}–PL complex. This is needed because the tissue factor–VIIa complex is rapidly inactivated in plasma by tissue factor pathway inhibitor and by antithrombin III. Factor Xa, in the presence of Ca^{2+}, PL and factor Va, activates prothrombin to thrombin, the main enzyme of the cascade. The *contact* (intrinsic) pathway commences when factor XII (Hageman factor) adheres to a negatively charged surface and converges with the in vivo pathway at the stage of factor X activation (see Fig. 23.2). The proximal part of this pathway is not crucial for blood coagulation in vivo.[2] The two pathways are not entirely separate even before they converge, and various positive feedbacks promote coagulation.

[2]Mr Hageman (the patient deficient in factor XII after whom it was named) died not of excessive bleeding but of a pulmonary embolism: factor XII deficiency does not give rise to a bleeding disorder.

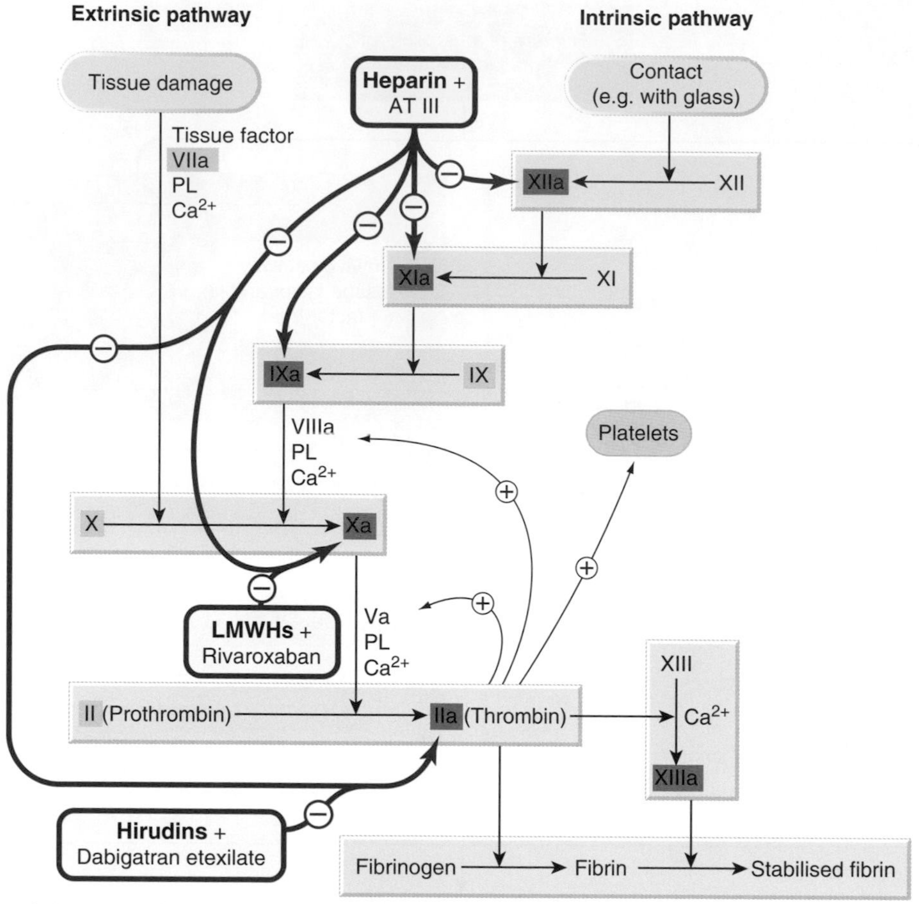

Fig. 23.2 The coagulation cascade: sites of action of anticoagulant drugs. Oral anticoagulants that inhibit vitamin K synthesis interfere with post-translational g-carboxylation of factors II, VII, IX and X (shown in blue boxes); see Fig. 23.4. Heparins activate antithrombin III. *AT III*, Antithrombin III; LMWHs, low-molecular-weight heparins; *PL*, negatively charged PL supplied by activated platelets.

Haemostasis and thrombosis

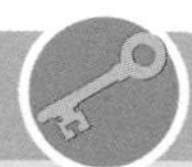

- Haemostasis is the arrest of blood loss from damaged vessels and is essential to survival. The main phenomena are:
  - platelet adhesion and activation
  - blood coagulation (fibrin formation)
- Thrombosis is a pathological condition resulting from inappropriate activation of haemostatic mechanisms:
  - venous thrombosis is usually associated with stasis of blood; a venous thrombus has a small platelet component and a large component of fibrin;
  - arterial thrombosis is usually associated with atherosclerosis, and the thrombus has a large platelet component.
- A portion of a thrombus may break away, travel as an embolus and lodge downstream, causing ischaemia and/or infarction.

THE ROLE OF THROMBIN

Thrombin (factor IIa) enzymatically cleaves fibrinogen, producing fragments that polymerise to form fibrin. It also activates factor XIII, a *fibrinoligase*, which strengthens fibrin-to-fibrin links, thereby stabilising the coagulum. In addition to coagulation, thrombin also causes platelet aggregation, stimulates cell proliferation and modulates smooth muscle contraction. Paradoxically, it can inhibit as well as promote coagulation (see later). The effects of thrombin on platelets and smooth muscle are initiated by an interaction with specific protease-activated receptors (PARs; see Ch. 3), which belong to the superfamily of G protein–coupled receptors. PARs initiate cellular responses that contribute not only to haemostasis and thrombosis, but also to inflammation and perhaps angiogenesis. Receptor activation requires cleavage by thrombin of the extracellular N-terminal domain of the receptor, revealing a new N-terminal sequence that acts as a 'tethered agonist' (see Fig. 3.8), an unusual mechanism.

VASCULAR ENDOTHELIUM IN HAEMOSTASIS AND THROMBOSIS

Vascular endothelium, the container of the circulating blood, can change focally from a non-thrombogenic to a thrombogenic structure in response to different demands. Normally, it provides a non-thrombogenic surface by virtue of membrane *heparan sulfate*, a glycosaminoglycan related to the endogenous anticoagulant heparin (see later), which is, like heparin, a co-factor for antithrombin III. Endothelium thus plays an essential role in preventing intravascular platelet activation and coagulation. However, it also plays an active part in haemostasis, synthesising and storing several key haemostatic components; von Willebrand factor,[3] tissue factor and plasminogen activator inhibitor (PAI)-1 are particularly important. PAI-1 is secreted in response to *angiotensin IV*, receptors for which are present on endothelial cells, providing a link between the renin–angiotensin system (see Ch. 21) and thrombosis. These prothrombotic factors are involved, respectively, in platelet adhesion and in coagulation and clot stabilisation. However, the endothelium is also implicated in thrombus limitation. Thus it generates anti-aggregatory prostaglandin (PG) I_2 (prostacyclin; see Ch. 17) and nitric oxide (NO; see Ch. 19); converts adenosine diphosphate (ADP), which causes platelet aggregation, to adenosine, which inhibits it (see Ch. 17); synthesises *tissue plasminogen activator* (tPA; see later); and expresses *thrombomodulin*, a receptor for thrombin. After combination with thrombomodulin, thrombin activates an anticoagulant, *protein C*. Activated protein C, helped by its co-factor protein S, inactivates factors Va and VIIa. This is functionally important, because a naturally occurring mutation of the gene coding for factor V (factor V Leiden), which confers resistance to activated protein C, results in the commonest recognised form of inherited thrombophilia.

Endotoxin and some cytokines (see Ch. 7), including tumour necrosis factor, tilt the balance of prothrombotic and antithrombotic endothelial functions towards thrombosis by causing loss of heparan (see earlier) and increased expression of tissue factor, and alter endothelial NO function. If other mechanisms limiting coagulation are also faulty or become exhausted, *disseminated intravascular coagulation*, a serious complication of sepsis and of certain malignancies, can result.

Blood coagulation (fibrin formation)

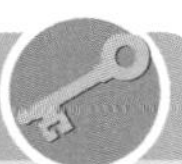

The clotting system consists of a cascade of proteolytic enzymes and co-factors.

- Inactive precursors are activated sequentially in an amplifying cascade.
- The last enzyme, thrombin, derived from prothrombin (II), converts soluble fibrinogen (I) to an insoluble meshwork of fibrin in which blood cells are trapped, forming the clot.
- There are two limbs in the cascade:
  - the in vivo (extrinsic) pathway
  - the contact (intrinsic) pathway
- Both pathways result in activation of factor X to Xa, which converts prothrombin to thrombin.
- Calcium ions and a negatively charged PL are essential for three steps, namely the actions of:
  - factor IXa on X
  - factor VIIa on X
  - factor Xa on II
- PL is provided by activated platelets adhering to the damaged vessel.
- Some factors promote coagulation by binding to PL and a serine protease factor; for example, factor Va in the activation of II by Xa, or VIIIa in the activation of X by IXa.
- Blood coagulation is controlled by:
  - enzyme inhibitors (e.g. antithrombin III)
  - fibrinolysis

[3]von Willebrand factor is a glycoprotein that is missing in a hereditary haemorrhagic disorder called von Willebrand disease, which is the most common of the inherited bleeding disorders. The factor is synthesised by vascular endothelial cells – indeed the presence of immunoreactive von Willebrand factor is an identifying feature of these cells in culture – and is also present in platelets.

DRUGS THAT ACT ON THE COAGULATION CASCADE

Drugs are used to correct a defect in coagulation or when there is an increased risk of unwanted coagulation, or actual thrombotic disease.

COAGULATION DEFECTS

Genetically determined deficiencies of clotting factors are not common. Examples are classic haemophilia, caused by lack of factor VIII, and an even rarer form of haemophilia (haemophilia B) caused by lack of factor IX. Intravenous factor replacement using recombinant human factor VIII or IX is given by specialists to prevent or to limit bleeding in such patients. Some patients develop antibodies that act as factor inhibitors, and their management is particularly demanding (involving, for example, induction of immune tolerance, see Ch. 7).

Acquired clotting defects are more common than hereditary ones. The causes include liver disease (many coagulation factors are synthesised in the liver), vitamin K deficiency (universal in neonates who are routinely given vitamin K prophylactically) and excessive **warfarin** therapy (see later), each of which may require treatment with vitamin K.

A human recombinant form of factor VIIa is available to treat bleeding in patients with severe bleeding disorders but can cause intravascular coagulation.

VITAMIN K

Vitamin K (for *Koagulation* in German) is a fat-soluble vitamin (Fig. 23.3) occurring naturally in plants (vitamin K_1) and as a series of bacterial menaquinones (vitamin K_2) formed in the gut (see Shearer and Newman, 2008, for a review). It is needed for the formation of clotting factors II, VII, IX and X, which are glycoproteins (GPs) with γ-carboxyglutamic acid (Gla) residues. The interaction of factors Xa and prothrombin (factor II) with Ca^{2+} and PL is shown in Fig. 23.4. γ-Carboxylation occurs after the synthesis of the amino acid chain, and the carboxylase enzyme requires reduced vitamin K as a co-factor (Fig. 23.5). Binding does not occur in the absence of γ-carboxylation. Similar considerations apply to the proteolytic activation of factor X by IXa and by VIIa (see Fig. 23.2).

There are several other vitamin K-dependent Gla proteins, including proteins C and S (mentioned earlier) and osteocalcin in bone (see Ch. 36).

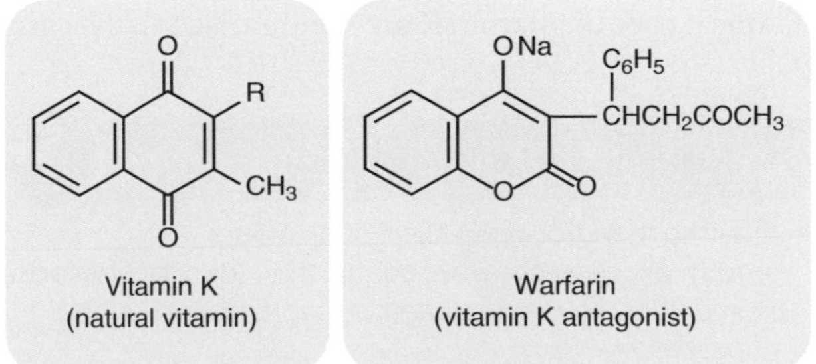

Fig. 23.3 Vitamin K and warfarin. Warfarin, a vitamin K antagonist, is an oral anticoagulant. It competes with vitamin K (note the similarity in their structures) for the reductase enzyme (vitamin K epoxide reductase component 1 [VKORC1]) that activates vitamin K and is the site of its action (see Fig. 23.5).

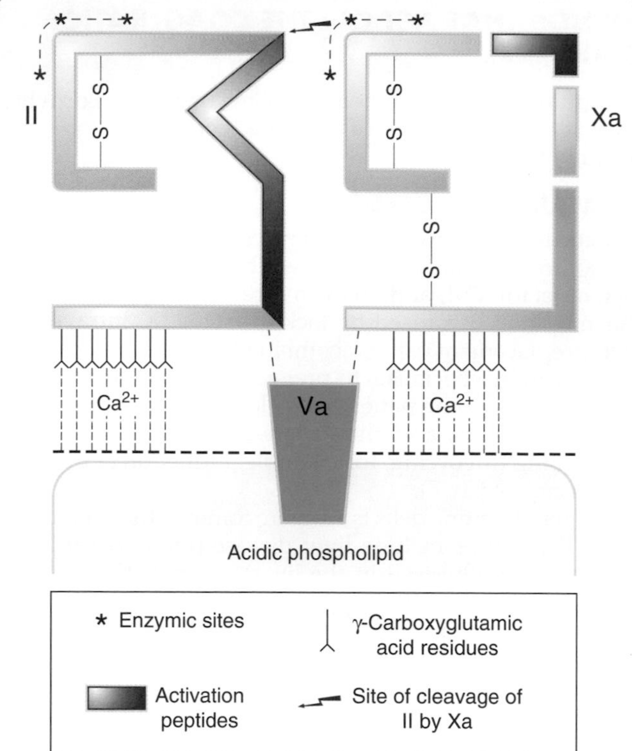

Fig. 23.4 Activation of prothrombin (factor II) by factor Xa. The complex of factor Va with a negatively charged PL surface (supplied by aggregating platelets) forms a binding site for factor Xa and prothrombin (II), which have peptide chains *(shown schematically)* that are similar to one another. Platelets thus serve as a localising focus. Calcium ions are essential for binding. Xa activates prothrombin, liberating thrombin *(shown in grey)*. (Modified from Jackson, C.M., 1978. Br. J. Haematol. 39, 1.)

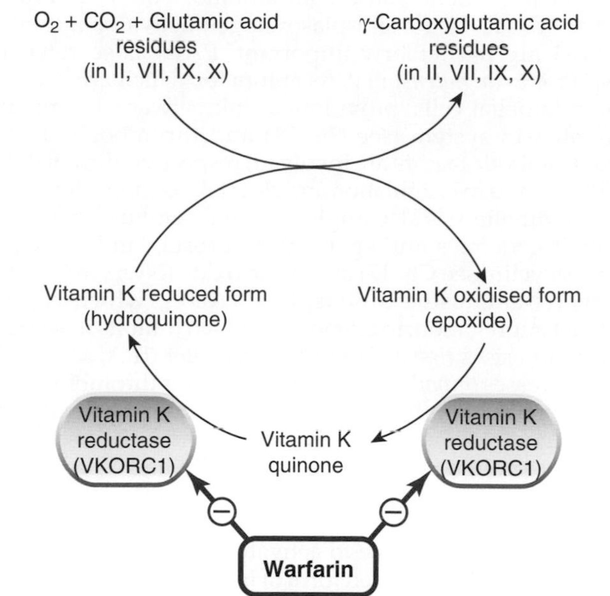

Fig. 23.5 Mechanism of vitamin K and of warfarin. After the peptide chains in clotting factors II, VII, IX and X have been synthesised, reduced vitamin K (the hydroquinone) acts as a co-factor in the conversion of glutamic acid to γ-carboxyglutamic acid. During this reaction, the reduced form of vitamin K is converted to the epoxide, which in turn is reduced to quinone and then hydroquinone by vitamin K epoxide reductase component 1 (VKORC1), the site of action of warfarin.

Administration and pharmacokinetic aspects

Natural vitamin K_1 (**phytomenadione**) may be given orally or by injection. If given by mouth, it requires bile salts for absorption, and this occurs by a saturable energy-requiring process in the proximal small intestine. A synthetic preparation, **menadiol sodium phosphate**, is also available. It is water soluble and does not require bile salts for its absorption. This synthetic compound takes longer to act than phytomenadione. There is very little storage of vitamin K in the body. It is metabolised to more polar substances that are excreted in the urine and the bile.

Clinical uses of vitamin K are summarised in the clinical box.

Clinical uses of vitamin K

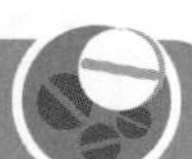

- Treatment and/or prevention of bleeding:
  - from excessive oral anticoagulation (e.g. by **warfarin**)
  - in babies: to prevent *haemorrhagic disease of the newborn*
- For vitamin K deficiencies in adults:
  - sprue, coeliac disease, steatorrhoea (excessively fatty faeces)
  - lack of bile (e.g. with obstructive jaundice)

THROMBOSIS

Thrombotic and thromboembolic disease is common and has severe consequences, including myocardial infarction, stroke, deep vein thrombosis and pulmonary embolus. The main drugs used for prophylaxis of platelet-rich 'white' arterial thrombi are the antiplatelet drugs; fibrinolytic drugs are used in addition to antiplatelet drugs for treatment of acute thrombotic events if mechanical methods of emergency opening of the artery are not available. The main drugs used to prevent or treat 'red' venous thrombi are:

- injectable anticoagulants (**heparin** and newer thrombin inhibitors);
- oral anticoagulants: direct oral anticoagulants (DOACs) are inhibitors of thrombin or of factor Xa. These have largely supplanted **warfarin** and related compounds that work indirectly by antagonising vitamin K.

Heparins and DOACs act immediately, whereas warfarin and other vitamin K antagonists take several days to exert their effect due to the presence of circulating preformed coagulation factors at the start of treatment.

HEPARIN (INCLUDING LOW-MOLECULAR-WEIGHT HEPARINS)

Heparin was discovered in 1916 by a second-year medical student at Johns Hopkins Hospital. He was attempting to extract coagulant substances from various tissues during a vacation project but found instead a powerful anticoagulant activity.[4] This was named heparin, because it was first extracted from liver.

Heparin is not a single substance but a family of sulfated glycosaminoglycans (mucopolysaccharides). It is present together with histamine in the granules of mast cells. Commercial preparations are extracted from beef lung or hog intestine and, because preparations differ in potency, assayed biologically against an agreed international standard: doses are specified in units of activity rather than of mass.

Heparin fragments (e.g. **enoxaparin, dalteparin**), referred to as low-molecular-weight heparins (LMWHs), or a synthetic pentasaccharide that inhibits factor Xa (**fondaparinux**), are longer acting than unfractionated heparin (UFH) and are usually preferred, the unfractionated product being reserved for special situations such as patients with renal failure in whom LMWHs are contraindicated.

Mechanism of action

Heparin inhibits coagulation, both in vivo and in vitro, by activating antithrombin III. Antithrombin III inhibits thrombin and other serine proteases by binding to the active site. Heparin modifies this interaction by binding, via a unique pentasaccharide sequence, to antithrombin III, changing its conformation and increasing its affinity for serine proteases.

To inhibit thrombin, it is necessary for heparin to bind to the enzyme as well as to antithrombin III; to inhibit factor Xa, it is necessary only for heparin to bind to antithrombin III. Consequently, the LMWHs increase the action of antithrombin III on factor Xa but not its action on thrombin, because the molecules are too small to bind to both enzyme and inhibitor (see Fig. 23.6).

Antithrombin III deficiency is very rare but can cause thrombophilia and unresponsiveness to heparin therapy.

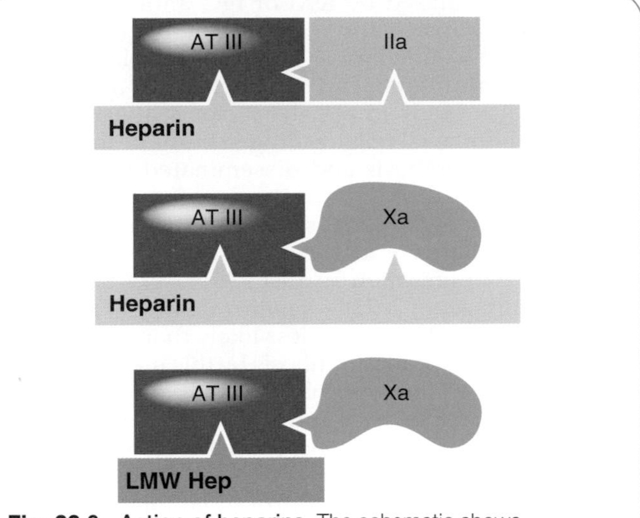

Fig. 23.6 Action of heparins. The schematic shows interactions of heparins, antithrombin III (AT III) and clotting factors. To increase the inactivation of thrombin (IIa) by AT III, heparin needs to interact with both substances *(top)*, but to speed up its effect on factor Xa it needs only to interact with AT III *(middle)*. Low-molecular-weight heparins (LMW Hep) increase the action of AT III on factor Xa *(bottom)*, but cannot increase the action of AT III on thrombin because they cannot bind both simultaneously.

Administration and pharmacokinetic aspects

Heparin is not absorbed from the gut because of its charge and high molecular weight, and it is therefore given intravenously or subcutaneously (intramuscular injections would cause haematomas).

After intravenous injection of a bolus dose, there is a phase of rapid redistribution followed by slower elimination caused by a combination of saturable processes involving binding to sites on endothelial cells and macrophages and slower non-saturable processes including renal excretion. As a result, the plasma concentration increases disproportionately with increasing dose (saturation kinetics; see Ch. 11).

Heparin acts immediately following intravenous administration, but the onset is delayed by up to 60 min when it is given subcutaneously. The elimination half-life is approximately 40–90 min. In urgent situations, it is therefore usual to start treatment with a bolus intravenous dose, followed by a constant-rate infusion. The *activated partial thromboplastin time* (APTT), or some other clotting test, is measured and the dose of heparin adjusted to achieve a value within a target range (e.g. 1.5–2.5 times control).

LMWHs are given subcutaneously. They have a longer elimination half-life than UFH, and this is independent of dose (first-order kinetics), so the effects are more predictable and dosing less frequent (once or twice a day). LMWHs do not prolong the APTT. Unlike UFH, the effect of a standard dose is sufficiently predictable that monitoring is not required routinely. LMWHs are eliminated mainly by renal excretion, and UFH is indicated in renal failure, but with this exception LMWHs are at least as safe and effective as UFH and are more convenient to use, because patients can be taught to inject themselves at home and there is generally no need for blood tests and dose adjustment.

Unwanted effects

Haemorrhage. The main hazard is haemorrhage, which is treated by stopping therapy and, if necessary, giving **protamine sulfate**. This heparin antagonist is a strongly basic protein that forms an inactive complex with heparin; it is given intravenously. The dose of protamine is estimated from the dose of heparin that has been administered recently, and it is important not to give too much, as this can itself cause bleeding. If necessary, an in vitro neutralisation test is performed first on a sample of blood from the patient to provide a more precise indication of the required dose.

Thrombosis. This is an uncommon but serious adverse effect of heparin and, as with warfarin necrosis (see below), may be misattributed to the natural history of the disease for which heparin is being administered.

Paradoxically, it is associated with a low blood platelet count: *heparin-induced thrombocytopenia* (HIT). A transitory early decrease in platelet numbers is not uncommon after initiating heparin treatment and is not clinically important. More serious thrombocytopenia that occurs 2–14 days after the start of therapy is uncommon and is referred to as type

[4]This kind of good fortune also favoured Vane and his colleagues in their discovery of PGI_2 (Ch. 17), where they were looking for one kind of biological activity and found another. More specific chemical assays (Ch. 8), for all their strengths, cannot throw up this kind of unexpected discovery.

II HIT. This is caused by IgM or IgG antibodies against complexes of heparin and a platelet-derived chemokine, platelet factor 4. Circulating immune complexes bind to circulating platelets, and cause thrombocytopenia. Antibody also binds to platelet factor 4 attached to the surface of endothelial cells, leading to immune injury of the vessel wall, thrombosis and disseminated intravascular coagulation.

A similar mechanism is believed to underlie the thrombocytopenia and thrombosis that can, rarely, complicate immunisation against SARS COV-2 (see Chs 5 and 53; Scully et al., 2021) – heparin treatment is avoided in such patients. LMWHs are less likely than UFH to cause thrombocytopenia and thrombosis by this mechanism. HIT is usually treated by substituting **danaparoid** or a direct thrombin inhibitor such as **lepirudin** instead of the heparin preparation that caused the problem. Danaparoid is a low-molecular-weight heparinoid consisting of a mixture of heparan, dermatan and chondroitin sulfates, with well-established antithrombotic activity.

Osteoporosis with spontaneous fractures has been reported with long-term (6 months or more) treatment with heparin. Its mechanism is unknown.

Hypoaldosteronism (with consequent hyperkalaemia) is uncommon but can occur with prolonged treatment. It is recommended to check plasma K^+ concentration if treatment is to be continued for >7 days.

Hypersensitivity reactions to heparin are rare.

DIRECT THROMBIN AND XA INHIBITORS

The current generation of direct thrombin inhibitors descend from *hirudins*, polypeptides from the anticoagulant present in saliva from the medicinal leech (*Hirudo medicinalis*). Unlike the heparins, they do not depend on the activation of antithrombin. The early successes, still used therapeutically, require parenteral administration. **Lepirudin** is a recombinant hirudin that binds irreversibly to both the fibrin-binding and catalytic sites on thrombin and is used for thromboembolic disease in patients with type II HIT. It is administered intravenously, the dose being adjusted depending on the APTT, and can cause bleeding or hypersensitivity reactions (rash or fever). **Bivalirudin**, another hirudin analogue, is used in combination with **aspirin** and **clopidogrel** (see later) in patients undergoing percutaneous coronary artery surgery. Treatment is initiated with an intravenous bolus followed by an infusion during and up to 4 h after the procedure. It can cause bleeding and hypersensitivity reactions.

DOACs and DOAC-reversal agents

The field of direct-acting oral anticoagulants (DOAC) had more than one false dawn, but the current agents have largely replaced warfarin in the prevention of thrombotic diseases such as deep vein thrombosis following orthopaedic surgery and embolic stroke in patients with atrial fibrillation, as well as in the treatment of thrombotic disease. These drugs do not require repeated blood testing to monitor their effect, and are less prone to interactions with other drugs or dietary constituents than is warfarin but are not suitable for patients with severe renal impairment.

Dabigatran is a synthetic serine protease inhibitor; **dabigatran etexilate**, a prodrug with a hydrophobic tail, is orally active and is licensed for prevention of venous thromboembolism following hip or knee replacement and for the prevention of stroke and systemic embolism in atrial fibrillation (see Ch. 20). It works rapidly and is administered 1–4 h after surgery and then once daily for up to a month (depending on the type of surgery), or twice daily indefinitely for the prevention of stroke. The dose is reduced in patients aged over 75 or receiving concomitant verapamil or amiodarone. **Rivaroxaban** is an orally active direct inhibitor of factor Xa rather than of thrombin. **Apixaban** and **edoxaban** are similar to rivaroxaban. Their commonest adverse effects are predictable (bleeding, anaemia). When these drugs were first introduced there was concern at the lack of specific treatments to neutralise their effects in patients who experienced severe bleeding, in contrast to the older agents such as heparin and warfarin. These concerns have now, at least partly, been met. **Idarucizumab** is a humanised monoclonal antibody fragment that binds dabigatran and its metabolites, blocking its effect, and is licensed for emergency procedures or severe bleeding caused by dabigatran. **Andexanet alpha** is a modified human factor Xa which binds rivaroxaban and apixaban, reducing their anticoagulant effect. It is used in severe bleeding caused by these agents. Whilst these approaches are highly effective, DOAC-induced severe bleeding, especially when intracerebral, continues to have a high mortality. Other adverse effects caused by DOACs include hepatotoxicity (rivaroxaban).

WARFARIN

Oral anticoagulants were discovered as an indirect result of a change in agricultural policy in North America in the 1920s. Sweet clover was substituted for corn in cattle feed, and an epidemic of deaths of cattle from haemorrhage ensued. This turned out to be caused by bishydroxycoumarin in spoiled sweet clover, and it led to the discovery of warfarin (named for the Wisconsin Alumni Research Foundation). One of the first uses to which this was put was as a rat poison, but for *nearly a century* it was the standard anticoagulant for the treatment and prevention of thromboembolic disease. By 2018, however, prescription numbers in the United States for DOACs were outnumbering those for warfarin by nearly 3:2 (https://clincalc.com/DrugStats/), although it remains commonly prescribed in the 2020s.

Warfarin (see Fig. 23.3) is the most important vitamin K antagonist; alternatives with a similar mechanism of action, for example **phenindione**, are now used only in rare patients who experience idiosyncratic off-target adverse reactions to warfarin[5] (see Ch. 12). Warfarin and other vitamin K antagonists require frequent blood tests to individualise dose, and are consequently inconvenient as well as having a low margin of safety.

---

[5]Warfarin highlights the competing philosophies of simplicity ('one size fits all') versus 'personalised medicine' or 'pharmacogenomics' (see Ch. 12). Prior to dosing with the anticoagulant, the patient can be checked by genotyping for mutations in their *VKORC1* and *CYP2C9* genes, which are involved in the coagulation cascade and metabolism of the drug. In patients possessing common mutations of these genes (particularly *VKORC1-1639G>A* and *-1173C>T*), standard doses of warfarin may cause potentially lethal bleeding or thromboembolism due to therapeutic failure. The success of the DOACs suggests that the outcome of the debate is likely to be both drug and technology dependent.

Mechanism of action

Vitamin K antagonists act only in vivo and have no effect on clotting if added to blood in vitro. They interfere with the post-translational γ-carboxylation of glutamic acid residues in clotting factors II, VII, IX and X. They do this by inhibiting *vitamin K epoxide reductase component 1* (VKORC1), thus inhibiting the reduction of vitamin K epoxide to its active hydroquinone form (see Fig. 23.5). Inhibition is competitive (reflecting the structural similarity between warfarin and vitamin K; see Fig. 23.3). The *VKORC1* gene is polymorphic (see Ch. 12), and different haplotypes have different affinities for warfarin. Genotyping to determine the *VKORC1* haplotype, combined with genotyping *CYP2C9* (see later), can be used to optimise the starting dose, reducing the variability in response to warfarin by around one-third. The effect of warfarin takes several days to develop because of the time taken for degradation of preformed carboxylated clotting factors. Onset of action thus depends on the elimination half-lives of the relevant factors. Factor VII, with a half-life of approximately 6 h, is affected first, then IX, X and II, with half-lives of 24, 40 and 60 h, respectively.

Administration and pharmacokinetic aspects

Warfarin is absorbed rapidly and completely from the gut after oral administration. It has a small distribution volume, being strongly bound to plasma albumin (see Ch. 9). The peak concentration in the blood occurs within an hour of ingestion, but because of its mechanism of action this does not coincide with the peak pharmacological effect, which occurs about 48 h later. The effect on prothrombin time (PT, see later) of a single dose starts after approximately 12–16 h and lasts 4–5 days. Warfarin is metabolised by CYP2C9, which is polymorphic (see Ch. 12). Partly in consequence of this, its half-life is very variable, being of the order of 40 h in many individuals.

Warfarin crosses the placenta and is not given in the first months of pregnancy because it is teratogenic (see Table 58.2), nor in the later stages because it can cause intracranial haemorrhage in the baby during delivery. It appears in milk during lactation. This could theoretically be important because newborn infants are naturally deficient in vitamin K. However, infants are routinely prescribed vitamin K to prevent haemorrhagic disease, so warfarin treatment of the mother does not generally pose a risk to the breastfed infant.

The therapeutic use of warfarin requires a careful balance between giving too little, leaving unwanted coagulation unchecked, and giving too much, thereby causing haemorrhage. Therapy is complicated not only because the effect of each dose is maximal some 2 days after its administration, but also because numerous medical and environmental conditions modify sensitivity to warfarin, including interactions with other drugs (see Chs 9, 10 and 12). The effect of warfarin is monitored by measuring PT, which is expressed as an *international normalised ratio* (INR).

The PT is the time taken for clotting of citrated plasma after the addition of Ca^{2+} and standardised reference thromboplastin; it is expressed as the ratio (PT ratio) of the PT of the patient to the PT of a pool of plasma from healthy subjects on no medication. Because of the variability of thromboplastins, different results are obtained in different laboratories. To standardise PT measurements internationally, each thromboplastin is assigned an international sensitivity index (ISI), and the patient's PT is expressed as an INR, where INR = (PT ratio)^{ISI}, ensuring similar results when a patient travels from, say, Birmingham to Baltimore.

The dose of warfarin is usually adjusted to give an INR of 2–4, the precise target depending on the clinical situation. The duration of treatment also varies, but for several indications (e.g. to prevent thromboembolism in chronic atrial fibrillation), treatment is long term, with the logistical challenge of providing a worldwide network of anticoagulant clinics and demands on the patient in terms of repeat visits and blood tests. Warfarin prescriptions in the United States declined from a peak of approximately 35 million in 2010 to approximately 14.5 million in 2018 (https://clincalc.com/DrugStats/Drugs/Warfarin), so it remains important, at least for now.

FACTORS THAT POTENTIATE WARFARIN

Various diseases and drugs potentiate warfarin, increasing the risk of haemorrhage.

Disease

Liver disease interferes with the synthesis of clotting factors; conditions in which there is a high metabolic rate, such as fever and thyrotoxicosis, increase the effect of anticoagulants by increasing degradation of clotting factors.

Drugs (see also Ch. 10)

Many drugs potentiate warfarin.

Agents that inhibit hepatic drug metabolism. Examples include **co-trimoxazole, ciprofloxacin, metronidazole, amiodarone** and many antifungal azoles. Stereoselective effects (warfarin is a racemate, and its isomers are metabolised differently from one another) are described in Chapter 10.

Drugs that inhibit platelet function. Aspirin increases the risk of bleeding if given during warfarin therapy, although this combination can be used safely with careful monitoring. Other non-steroidal anti-inflammatory drugs (NSAIDs) also increase the risk of bleeding, partly by their effect on platelet thromboxane synthesis (see Ch. 25), by causing gastrointestinal damage with bleeding and, in the case of some NSAIDs, also by inhibiting warfarin metabolism.

Drugs that displace warfarin from binding sites on plasma albumin. Some of the NSAIDs and **chloral hydrate** cause a transient increase in the concentration of free warfarin in plasma by competing with it for binding to plasma albumin. This mechanism seldom causes clinically important effects as explained in Chapter 9.

Drugs that inhibit reduction of vitamin K. Such drugs include the *cephalosporins*.

Drugs that decrease the availability of vitamin K. Broad-spectrum antibiotics and some *sulfonamides* (see Ch. 51) depress the intestinal flora that normally synthesise vitamin K_2; this has little effect unless there is concurrent dietary deficiency or fat malabsorption.

FACTORS THAT LESSEN THE EFFECT OF WARFARIN

Physiological state/disease

There is a decreased response to warfarin in conditions (e.g. pregnancy) where there is increased coagulation factor synthesis. Similarly, the effect of oral anticoagulants is lessened in hypothyroidism, which is associated with reduced degradation of coagulation factors.

Vitamin K. This vitamin is a component of some parenteral feeds and vitamin preparations.

Drugs that induce hepatic P450 enzymes. Enzyme induction (e.g. by **rifampicin, carbamazepine**) increases the rate of degradation of warfarin, risking under-treatment and thrombosis unless the dose of warfarin is increased. Induction wanes slowly and variably after the inducing drug is discontinued, making it difficult to adjust the warfarin dose appropriately and risking haemorrhage.

Drugs that reduce absorption. Drugs that bind warfarin in the gut, for example, **colestyramine** (see Ch. 22), reduce its absorption.

Drugs affecting blood coagulation

Procoagulant drugs: vitamin K

- Reduced vitamin K is a co-factor in the post-translational g-carboxylation of glutamic acid (Glu) residues in factors II, VII, IX and X. The γ-carboxylated glutamic acid (Gla) residues are essential for the interaction of these factors with Ca^{2+} and negatively charged PL.

Heparin, LMWHs, injectable anticoagulants that:

- Potentiate antithrombin III, a natural inhibitor that inactivates Xa and thrombin.
- Act both in vivo and in vitro.
- Anticoagulant activity results from a unique pentasaccharide sequence with high affinity for antithrombin III.
- **Unfractionated heparin (UFH)** therapy is monitored via APTT, and dose individualised. UFH is used for patients with impaired renal function.
- **LMWHs** have the same effect on factor X as heparin but less effect on thrombin; therapeutic efficacy is similar to **heparin** but monitoring and dose individualisation are not needed. Patients can administer them subcutaneously at home. They are preferred over UFH except for patients with impaired renal function.

Oral anticoagulants, e.g. direct oral anticoagulants (DOACs); warfarin

- Orally active direct thrombin inhibitors (e.g. **dabigatran etexilate**) or factor Xa inhibitors (e.g. **rivaroxaban, apixaban, edoxaban**) are used increasingly instead of warfarin and do not require laboratory monitoring/dose titration. They are licensed for preventing stroke in patients with atrial fibrillation and for preventing deep vein thrombosis after orthopaedic surgery and for the treatment of deep vein thrombosis and some cases of pulmonary embolism.
- **Warfarin** is the main vitamin K antagonist.
- Vitamin K antagonists act on VKORC1 to inhibit the reduction of vitamin K epoxide, thus inhibiting the γ-carboxylation of Glu in II, VII, IX and X.
- Vitamin K antagonists act only in vivo, and their effect is delayed until preformed clotting factors are depleted.
- Many factors modify the action of vitamin K antagonists; genetic factors (polymorphisms of *CYP2C6* and *VKORC1*) and drug interactions are especially important.
- There is wide variation in response to vitamin K antagonists; their effect is monitored by measuring the INR and the dose individualised accordingly.

UNWANTED EFFECTS OF WARFARIN

Haemorrhage (especially into the bowel or the brain) is the main hazard. Depending on the urgency of the situation, treatment may consist of withholding warfarin (for minor problems), administration of vitamin K or fresh frozen plasma or prothrombin complex concentrate (for life-threatening bleeding).

Oral anticoagulants are *teratogenic*, causing disordered bone development which is believed to be related to binding to the vitamin K–dependent protein osteocalcin.

Hepatotoxicity occurs but is uncommon.

Necrosis of soft tissues (e.g. breast or buttock) owing to thrombosis in venules is a rare but serious effect that occurs shortly after starting treatment and is attributed to inhibition of biosynthesis of protein C, which has a shorter elimination half-life than do the vitamin K–dependent coagulation factors; this results in a procoagulant state soon after starting treatment. Treatment with a heparin is usually started at the same time as warfarin, avoiding this problem.

The clinical use of anticoagulants is summarised in the box.

Clinical uses of anticoagulants

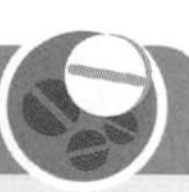

Heparin (often as **LMWH**) or a direct-acting intravenous thrombin antagonist such as **lepirudin** is used acutely. A **DOAC** or **warfarin** is used for more prolonged therapy.

Anticoagulants are used to prevent:

- deep vein thrombosis (e.g. perioperatively)
- extension of established deep vein thrombosis
- pulmonary embolism
- thrombosis and embolisation in patients with atrial fibrillation (see Ch. 20)
- thrombosis on prosthetic heart valves
- clotting in extracorporeal circulations (e.g. during haemodialysis)
- progression of myocardial damage in patients with unstable angina and during treatment of ST-elevation myocardial infarction

PLATELET ADHESION AND ACTIVATION

Platelets maintain the integrity of the circulation: a low platelet count results in *thrombocytopenic purpura*.[6]

When platelets are activated, they undergo a sequence of reactions that are essential for haemostasis, important for the healing of damaged blood vessels, and which also play a part in inflammation (see Ch. 17). Several of these reactions are redundant in the sense that if one pathway of activation is blocked another is available and many are autocatalytic providing positive feedback:

- *adhesion* following vascular damage. von Willebrand factor bridges subendothelial macromolecules and GPIb receptors on the platelet surface[7];

[6]Purpura is a purple rash caused by multiple spontaneous bleeding points in the skin. It can be caused by disease of platelets or of the microvasculature. Bleeding can also occur into other organs, including the gut and brain.

[7]Various platelet membrane glycoproteins act as receptors or binding sites for adhesive proteins such as von Willebrand factor or fibrinogen.

- *shape change*: from smooth discs to spiny spheres with protruding pseudopodia;
- *secretion* of the granule contents which include platelet agonists such as ADP and 5-hydroxytryptamine, and coagulation factors and growth factors, such as platelet-derived growth factor (PDGF);
- *biosynthesis of labile mediators* such as platelet-activating factor and thromboxane (TX)A_2 (see Ch. 17 and Fig. 23.7);
- *aggregation*, which is promoted by various agonists, including collagen, thrombin, ADP, 5-hydroxytryptamine and TXA_2, acting on specific receptors on the platelet surface; activation by

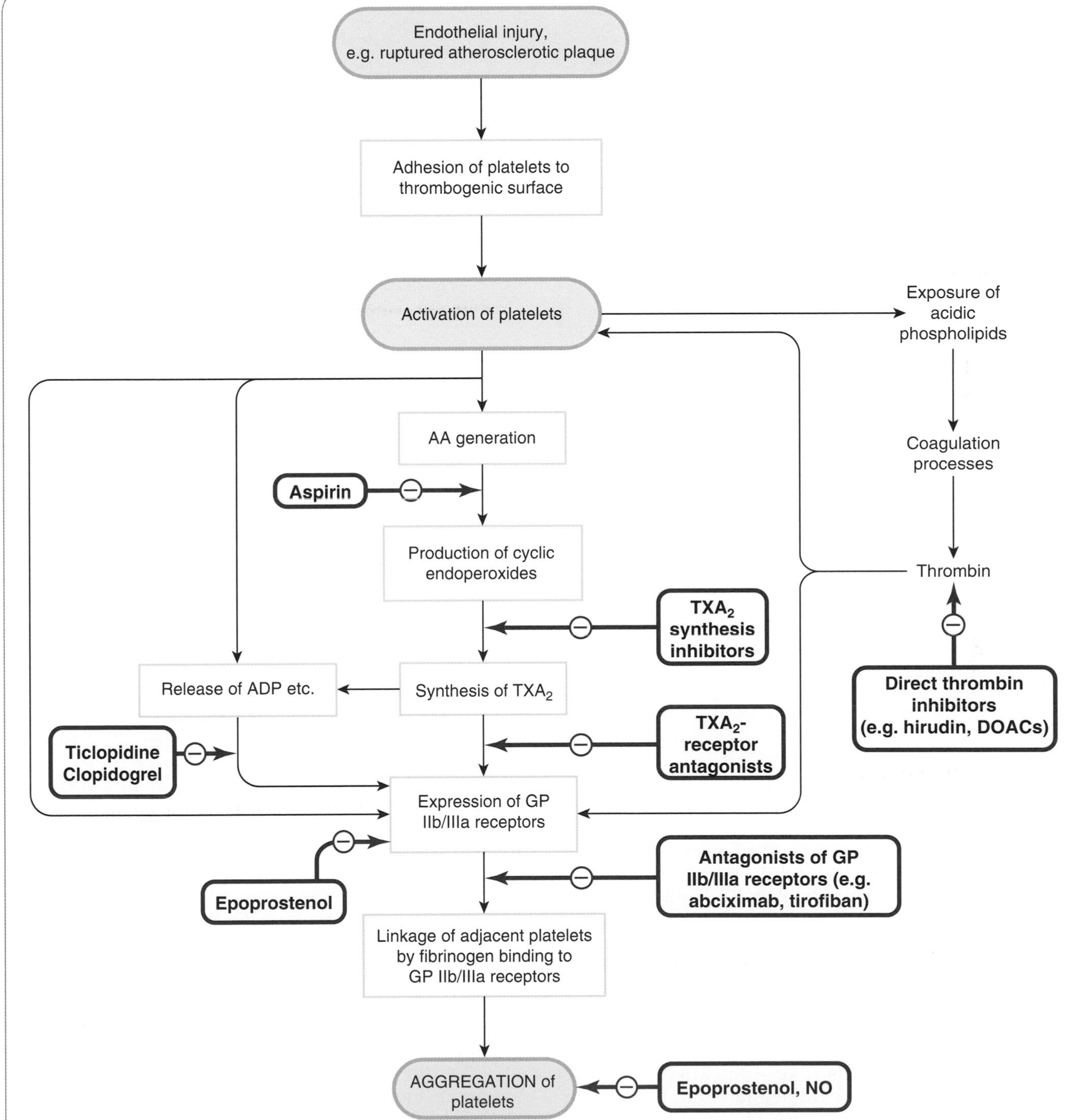

Fig. 23.7 Platelet activation. Events involved in platelet adhesion and aggregation are shown, with the sites of action of drugs and endogenous mediators. *AA*, Arachidonic acid; *ADP*, adenosine bisphosphate; *DOACs*, direct oral anticoagulants *GP*, glycoprotein; *NO*, nitric oxide; TXA_2, thromboxane A_2.

agonists leads to expression of GPIIb/IIIa receptors that bind fibrinogen, which links adjacent platelets to form aggregates;

- *exposure of acidic PL* on the platelet surface, promoting thrombin formation and further platelet activation via thrombin receptors and fibrin formation via cleavage of fibrinogen.

These processes are essential for haemostasis but may be inappropriately triggered if the artery wall is diseased, most commonly with atherosclerosis, resulting in thrombosis (see Fig. 23.7).

Platelet function

- Healthy vascular endothelium prevents platelet adhesion.
- Platelets adhere to diseased or damaged areas and become activated, changing shape and exposing negatively charged PLs and GPIIb/IIIa receptors, and synthesise and/or release various mediators, for example, thromboxane A_2 and ADP, which activate other platelets, causing aggregation.
- Aggregation entails fibrinogen binding to and bridging between GPIIb/IIIa receptors on adjacent platelets.
- Activated platelets constitute a focus for fibrin formation.
- Chemotactic factors (e.g. PF4) and growth factors (e.g. PDGF) necessary for repair, but also implicated in atherogenesis, are released during platelet activation.

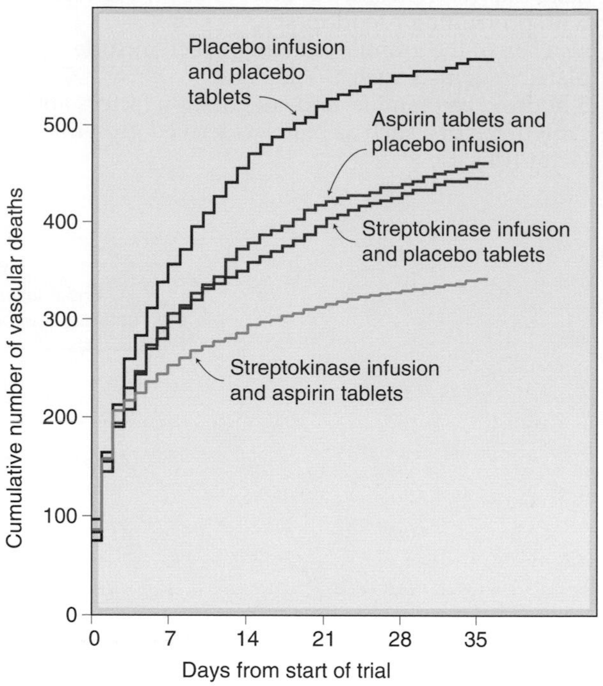

Fig. 23.8 Efficacy of aspirin and streptokinase for myocardial infarction. The curves show cumulative vascular mortality in patients treated with placebo, aspirin alone, streptokinase alone or a combined aspirin–streptokinase regimen. (ISIS-2 Trial, 1988. Lancet. ii, 350–360.)

ANTIPLATELET DRUGS

Platelets play such a critical role in thromboembolic disease that it is no surprise that antiplatelet drugs are of great therapeutic value. Clinical trials of aspirin radically altered clinical practice, and more recently drugs that block ADP receptors and GPIIb/IIIa have also been found to be therapeutically useful. Sites of action of antiplatelet drugs are shown in Fig. 23.7.

ASPIRIN

Low-dose aspirin (see Ch. 25) administered repeatedly profoundly (>95%) inhibits platelet TXA_2 synthesis, by irreversible acetylation of a serine residue in the active site of cyclo-oxygenase I (COX-1). Oral administration is relatively selective for platelets partly because of presystemic drug elimination (see Ch. 10). Unlike nucleated cells, platelets cannot synthesise proteins, so after administration of aspirin, TXA_2 synthesis does not recover fully until the affected cohort of platelets is replaced in 7–10 days. Clinical trials have demonstrated the efficacy of aspirin in several clinical settings (e.g. Fig. 23.8) and its value in the secondary prevention of cardiovascular disease is firmly established. For acute indications (progressing thrombotic stroke - so-called stroke-in-evolution - and acute myocardial infarction) treatment is started with a single dose of approximately 300 mg in order to achieve rapid substantial (>95%) inhibition of platelet thromboxane synthesis, followed by regular daily doses of 75 mg. For long-term thromboprophylaxis, a low dose (often 75 mg once daily) is used. At this dose, the risk of gastrointestinal bleeding is less than with the usual 300 mg dose given to control inflammation, but still significant, so thromboprophylaxis is reserved for people at high cardiovascular risk (e.g. survivors of myocardial infarction so-called *secondary* prevention), in whom the benefit usually outweighs the risk of gastrointestinal bleeding. Its place in *primary* prevention of cardiovascular disease and cancer is still debated (Patrono and Baigent, 2019; Ricciotti and FitzGerald, 2021).

Treatment failure can occur despite taking aspirin, and the possibility has been raised that some patients exhibit a syndrome of 'aspirin resistance', although the mechanism and possible importance of this remain controversial (see Goodman et al., 2008; Pollack and Wang, 2021). Other non-steroidal drugs (NSAIDs) that, like aspirin, inhibit platelet TXA_2 synthesis >95% (e.g. **sulfinpyrazone**, for which there is also supportive clinical trial evidence) may have antithrombotic effects. In contrast, where inhibition of platelet TXA_2 synthesis does not reach this threshold, NSAIDs, whether or not they are selective for COX-2, are prothrombotic and increase blood pressure. This is believed to be due to inhibition of COX enzymes leading to reduced synthesis of antiaggregatory and vasodilatory PGI_2 in blood vessels in the kidneys and elsewhere, and results in increased cardiovascular risk during chronic treatment with NSAIDs (see Ch. 25).

DIPYRIDAMOLE

Dipyridamole inhibits platelet aggregation by several mechanisms, including inhibition of phosphodiesterase (hence potentiating mediators that inhibit platelet function by increasing cytoplasmic cAMP or cGMP), block of adenosine uptake into red cells and endothelial cells (see Ch. 16), potentiating this vasodilator and inhibitor of platelet aggregation. Clinical effectiveness has been uncertain, but one study showed that a modified-release form of dipyridamole reduced the risk of stroke and death in patients with transient ischaemic attacks by around 15% – similar to aspirin (25 mg twice daily).[8] The beneficial effects of aspirin and dipyridamole were additive. The main adverse effects of dipyridamole are dizziness, headache and gastrointestinal disturbances; unlike aspirin, it does not appear to increase the risk of bleeding.

PURINE ($P2Y_{12}$) RECEPTOR ANTAGONISTS

$P2Y_{12}$ receptor antagonists (see Ch. 16) block the pro-aggregatory effect of ADP on platelets. **Ticlopidine** was the first to be introduced but can cause serious blood dyscrasias (neutropenia and thrombocytopenia). The main agents are currently **clopidogrel**, **prasugrel** and **ticagrelor**, each of which is combined with low-dose aspirin in patients with unstable coronary artery disease, usually for up to 1 year.

Clopidogrel and prasugrel inhibit ADP-induced platelet aggregation by irreversible inhibition of $P2Y_{12}$ receptors (see Ch. 16) to which they link via a disulfide bond, whereas ticagrelor is a reversible but non-competitive inhibitor of the $P2Y_{12}$ receptor.

Pharmacokinetics and unwanted effects

Clopidogrel is well absorbed when administered by mouth, and in urgent situations is given orally as a loading dose of 300 mg followed by maintenance dosing of 75 mg once daily. It is a prodrug and is converted into its active sulfhydryl metabolite by CYP enzymes in the liver including CYP2C19. Patients with variant alleles of *CYP2C19* (rapid or poor metabolisers) are at increased risk of therapeutic failure from lack of efficacy or from bleeding. There is a potential for interaction with other drugs, such as **omeprazole** (see Ch. 30), that are metabolised by CYP2C19 and current labelling recommends against use with proton pump inhibitors for this reason. Strong inducers such as **rifampicin** increase the concentration of active metabolite and risk of bleeding. Prasugrel and ticagrelor are also given as a loading dose followed by maintenance once-daily dosing.

These drugs predictably increase the risk of haemorrhage over and above that caused by aspirin given alone. Clopidogrel can cause dyspepsia, rash or diarrhoea. The serious blood dyscrasias caused by ticlopidine are very rare with clopidogrel. Prasugrel can cause rash or, rarely, hypersensitivity reactions and angioedema. Ticagrelor can cause dyspnoea (perhaps related to the role of adenosine signalling in the carotid bodies, see Ch. 28) or, less commonly, gastrointestinal symptoms.

Clinical use

Clopidogrel was slightly more effective than aspirin as a single agent in reducing a composite outcome of ischaemic stroke, myocardial infarction or vascular death in one large trial; it can be used instead of aspirin for secondary prevention in patients with symptomatic atheromatous disease who are intolerant of aspirin. Clinical trials of adding clopidogrel to aspirin in patients with acute coronary syndromes and (in a megatrial of over 45,000 patients) in patients with acute myocardial infarction (COMMIT Collaborative Group, 2005) demonstrated that combined treatment reduces mortality. Treatment with clopidogrel for this indication is given for 4 weeks. Prasugrel is more effective than clopidogrel in acute coronary syndromes, but more often causes serious bleeding. Pretreatment with clopidogrel and aspirin followed by longer-term therapy is also effective in patients with ischaemic heart disease undergoing percutaneous coronary interventions. Treatment of acute coronary syndrome with ticagrelor as compared with clopidogrel significantly reduces mortality for unknown reasons.

GLYCOPROTEIN IIB/IIIA RECEPTOR ANTAGONISTS

Antagonists of the GPIIb/IIIa receptor have the theoretical attraction that they inhibit all pathways of platelet activation because these all converge on activation of GPIIb/IIIa receptors. A hybrid murine–human monoclonal antibody Fab fragment directed against the GPIIb/IIIa receptor, which rejoices in the catchy little name of **abciximab**,[9] is licensed for use in high-risk patients undergoing coronary angioplasty, as an adjunct to heparin and aspirin. It reduces the risk of restenosis at the expense of an increased risk of bleeding. Immunogenicity limits its use to a single administration.

Tirofiban is a synthetic non-peptide and **eptifibatide** is a cyclic peptide based on the Arg–Gly–Asp ('RGD') sequence that is common to ligands for GPIIb/IIIa receptors. Neither is absorbed if administered by mouth. Given intravenously as an adjunct to aspirin and a heparin preparation, they reduce early events in acute coronary syndrome, but long-term oral therapy with GPIIb/IIIa receptor antagonists is not effective and may be harmful. Unsurprisingly, they increase the risk of bleeding.

OTHER ANTIPLATELET DRUGS

Epoprostenol (PGI_2), an agonist at prostanoid IP receptors (see Ch. 17), causes vasodilatation as well as inhibiting platelet aggregation. It can be added to blood entering the dialysis circuit in order to prevent thrombosis during haemodialysis, especially in patients in whom heparin is contraindicated. It is also used in severe pulmonary hypertension (see Ch. 21) and circulatory shock associated with meningococcal septicaemia. It is unstable under physiological conditions and has a half-life of around 3 min, so it is administered as an intravenous infusion. A more stable analogue of PGI_2, **iloprost**, is administered by inhalation of a nebulised solution to patients with severe pulmonary artery hypertension. Adverse effects related to

[8]This dose regimen of aspirin is unconventional, being somewhat lower than the 75 mg once daily commonly used in thromboprophylaxis.

[9]The convention for naming monoclonals is as follows: momab = -**mo**use **m**onoclonal **a**nti**b**ody; -umab = human; -zumab = humanised; -ximab = chimeric – a kind of mythical mouse–man nightmare.

the vasodilator action of either of these prostanoids include flushing, headache and hypotension.

The clinical use of antiplatelet drugs is summarised in the clinical box.

Antiplatelet drugs

- **Aspirin** inhibits cyclo-oxygenase irreversibly. In chronic use, low doses (75 mg once daily) very effectively (>95%) inhibit platelet thromboxane (TX)A_2 synthesis and reduce the risk of thrombosis. Treatment is started with a single larger dose (300 mg) in acute settings in order to achieve rapid inhibition of platelet thromboxane synthesis.[10]
- ADP antagonists are combined with low-dose aspirin in treating patients with unstable coronary artery disease. **Clopidogrel** is a prodrug. Given by mouth, it irreversibly inhibits $P2Y_{12}$ receptors and thereby inhibits platelet responses to ADP. Its clinical effect is additive with **aspirin. Prasugrel** has a similar mechanism. **Ticagrelor** is reversible but non-competitive. **Prasugrel** and **ticagrelor** are more effective than licensed doses of **clopidogrel**, but more likely to cause haemorrhage.
- Antagonists of GPIIb/IIIa receptors include a monoclonal antibody (**abciximab**) and several synthetic molecules (e.g. **tirofiban**). They inhibit diverse agonists, for example, ADP and TXA_2, because different pathways of activation converge on GPIIb/IIIa receptors. They are administered intravenously for short-term treatment.
- **Dipyridamole** inhibits phosphodiesterase and red cell adenosine uptake. It is used in addition to aspirin in some patients with stroke or transient ischaemic attack.
- **Epoprostenol** (synthetic PGI_2) is chemically unstable. Given as an intravenous infusion, it acts on I prostanoid (IP) receptors on vascular smooth muscle and platelets (see Ch. 17), stimulating adenylyl cyclase and thereby causing vasodilatation and inhibiting aggregation caused by any pathway (e.g. ADP or TXA_2). It is used to prevent clotting during haemodialysis in patients who cannot be treated with heparin, and to treat pulmonary arterial hypertension (see Ch. 21). **Iloprost** is a less unstable analogue of PGI_2 and can be administered by inhalation of a nebulised solution to treat pulmonary hypertension.

[10]Its antithrombotic action is the main basis for the saying 'An aspirin a day keeps the doctor away' – although aspirin also has anticancer properties, particularly against colon cancer. However, its chronic use in primary prevention is seldom justified because of the bleeding it can cause.

FIBRINOLYSIS (THROMBOLYSIS)

When the coagulation system is activated, the fibrinolytic system is also set in motion via several endogenous *plasminogen activators*, including tPA, urokinase-type plasminogen activator, kallikrein and neutrophil elastase. tPA is inhibited by a structurally related lipoprotein, *lipoprotein(a)*, increased plasma concentrations of which constitute an independent risk factor for myocardial infarction (see Ch. 22). Plasminogen is deposited on the

Clinical uses of antiplatelet drugs

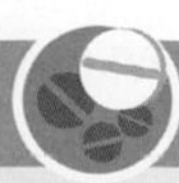

The main drug is **aspirin**. Other drugs with distinct actions (e.g. **dipyridamole**, **clopidogrel**, **ticagrelor**) can have additive effects, or be used in patients who are intolerant of **aspirin**. Uses of antiplatelet drugs relate mainly to arterial thrombosis and include:

- acute myocardial infarction
- prevention of myocardial infarction in patients at high risk, including a history of myocardial infarction, angina or intermittent claudication
- following coronary artery bypass grafting
- unstable coronary syndromes (a $P2Y_{12}$ antagonist such as **clopidogrel, prasugrel** or **ticagrelor** is added to **aspirin**)
- following coronary artery angioplasty and/or stenting. Intravenous glycoprotein IIb/IIIa antagonists, e.g. **abciximab**, are used in some patients in addition to **aspirin.**
- transient cerebral ischaemic attack ('ministrokes') or thrombotic stroke, to prevent recurrence (**dipyridamole** can be added to **aspirin**)
- atrial fibrillation, if oral anticoagulation is contraindicated; or, by specialists, in high-risk situations in combination with anticoagulant

Other antiplatelet drugs such as **epoprostenol** (PGI_2; see Ch. 17) have specialised clinical applications, e.g. in *haemodialysis* or *haemofiltration* (see Ch. 29) or in *pulmonary hypertension* (see Ch. 21), where an analogue, **iloprost**, can be administered by inhalation of a nebulised solution.

fibrin strands within a thrombus. Plasminogen activators are serine proteases and are unstable in circulating blood. They diffuse into thrombus and cleave plasminogen, a zymogen present in plasma, to release plasmin locally (Fig. 23.9). Plasmin is a trypsin-like protease that digests fibrin as well as fibrinogen, factors II, V and VIII and many other proteins; any plasmin that escapes into the circulation is inactivated by plasmin inhibitors, including PAI-1 (see Ch. 21), which protect us from digesting ourselves from within.

Drugs affect this system by increasing or inhibiting fibrinolysis (*fibrinolytic* and *antifibrinolytic* drugs, respectively).

FIBRINOLYTIC DRUGS

Fig. 23.9 summarises the interaction of the fibrinolytic system with the coagulation cascade and platelet activation, and the action of drugs that modify this. Several fibrinolytic (thrombolytic) drugs are used clinically, principally to reopen the occluded arteries in patients with acute myocardial infarction[11] or stroke, less commonly in

[11]Fibrinolytic drugs are now less widely used in acute myocardial infarction since many units throughout the world provide an emergency angioplasty service (the blocked artery is identified angiographically, opened with a balloon catheter and, if necessary, kept open by means of a stent; see Ch. 21). The important thing is to open the thrombosed artery as swiftly as possible. If facilities are available to do this mechanically, this is at least as good as using a lytic drug. Surgical intra-arterial thrombectomy is also being introduced for acute stroke treatment.

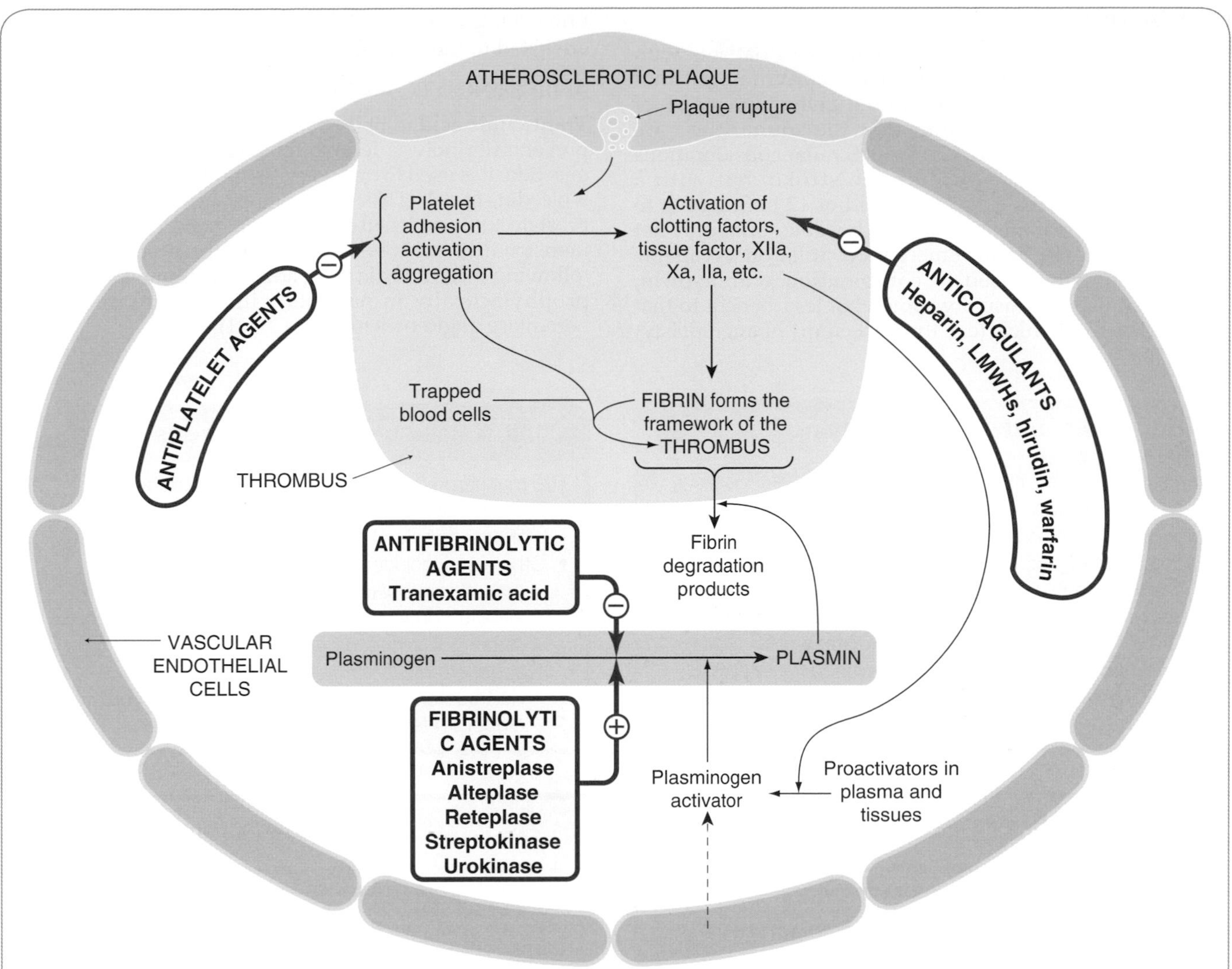

Fig. 23.9 Fibrinolytic system. The schematic shows interactions with coagulation and platelet pathways and sites of action of drugs that modify these systems. For more details of platelet activation and the coagulation cascade, refer to Figs 23.1, 23.2 and 23.7. *LMWHs*, Low-molecular-weight heparins.

patients with life-threatening venous thrombosis or pulmonary embolism.

Streptokinase is a plasminogen activating protein extracted from cultures of streptococci. Infused intravenously, it reduces mortality in acute myocardial infarction, and this beneficial effect is additive with aspirin (see Fig. 23.8). Its action is blocked by antibodies, which appear 4 days or more after the initial dose: its use should not be repeated after this time has elapsed.[12]

Alteplase and **duteplase** are, respectively, single- and double-chain recombinant tPA. They are more active on fibrin-bound plasminogen than on plasma plasminogen and are therefore said to be 'clot selective'. Recombinant tPA is not antigenic and can be used in patients likely to have antibodies to streptokinase. Because of their short half-lives, these drugs must be given as intravenous infusions. **Reteplase** is similar but has a longer elimination half-life, allowing for bolus administration and making for simplicity of administration. It is available for clinical use in myocardial infarction.

UNWANTED EFFECTS AND CONTRAINDICATIONS

The main hazard of all fibrinolytic agents is bleeding, including gastrointestinal haemorrhage and haemorrhagic stroke. If serious, this can be treated with **tranexamic acid** (see later), fresh plasma or coagulation factors. Streptokinase can cause allergic reactions and low-grade fever. Streptokinase causes a burst of plasmin formation, generating vasodilator kinins (see Ch. 17), and can cause hypotension by this mechanism.

Contraindications to the use of these agents are active internal bleeding, haemorrhagic cerebrovascular disease, bleeding diatheses, pregnancy, uncontrolled hypertension, invasive procedures in which haemostasis is important and recent trauma – including vigorous cardiopulmonary resuscitation.

[12]A once-in-a-lifetime drug!.

CLINICAL USE

Several large placebo-controlled studies in patients with myocardial infarction have shown convincingly that fibrinolytic drugs reduce mortality if given within 12 h of the onset of symptoms, and that the sooner they are administered the better is the result. Similar considerations apply to their use in thrombotic stroke, but with a compressed time scale of 3 h instead of 12 h. Scanning to exclude haemorrhagic stroke is advisable, although not always practicable in an emergency situation. Available fibrinolytic drugs, used in combination with aspirin, provide similar, but usually somewhat less, benefit to that obtained by mechanical (e.g. thrombectomy or angioplasty) unblocking procedures. Other uses of fibrinolytic agents are listed in the clinical box.

ANTIFIBRINOLYTIC AND HAEMOSTATIC DRUGS

Tranexamic acid inhibits plasminogen activation and thus prevents fibrinolysis. It can be given orally or by intravenous injection. It is used to treat various conditions in which there is bleeding or risk of bleeding, such as haemorrhage following prostatectomy or dental extraction, in menorrhagia (excessive menstrual blood loss) and for life-threatening bleeding following thrombolytic drug administration. It is also used prophylactically in patients with the rare disorder of hereditary angio-oedema (see Ch. 21).

Fibrinolysis and drugs modifying fibrinolysis

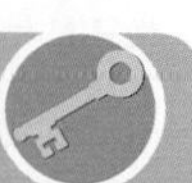

- A fibrinolytic cascade is initiated concomitantly with the coagulation cascade, resulting in the formation within the coagulum of plasmin, an enzyme which digests fibrin.
- Various agents promote the formation of plasmin from its precursor plasminogen, for example **streptokinase**, and tPAs such as **alteplase, duteplase** and **reteplase.** Most are infused intravenously; reteplase can be given as a bolus injection.
- Some drugs (e.g. **tranexamic acid**) inhibit fibrinolysis.

Clinical uses of fibrinolytic drugs

The main drugs are tPAs, for example **alteplase**.

- The main use is in acute myocardial infarction, within 12 h of onset (the earlier the better!).
- Other uses include:
  - *acute thrombotic stroke* within 3 h of onset (tPA), in selected patients
  - clearing *thrombosed shunts* and *cannulae*
  - *acute arterial thromboembolism*
  - life-threatening *deep vein thrombosis* and *pulmonary embolism* (**streptokinase**, given promptly)

REFERENCES AND FURTHER READING

Blood coagulation and anticoagulants

Hirsh, J., O'Donnell, M., Weitz, J.I., 2005. New anticoagulants. Blood 105, 453–463.

Koenig-Oberhuber, M.F., 2016. New antiplatelet drugs and new oral anticoagulants V. Br. J. Anaesth. 117 (Suppl. 2), ii74–ii84.

Martin, F.A., Murphy, R.P., Cummins, P.M., 2013. Thrombomodulin and the vascular endothelium: insights into functional, regulatory, and therapeutic aspects. Am. J. Physiol. Heart Circ. Physiol. 304 (12), H1585–H1597.

Shearer, M.J., Newman, P., 2008. Metabolism and cell biology of vitamin K. Thromb. Haemost. 100, 530–547.

Endothelium, platelets and antiplatelet agents

Chew, D.P., Bhatt, D., Sapp, S., et al., 2001. Increased mortality with oral platelet glycoprotein IIb/IIIa antagonists: a meta-analysis of phase III multicenter trials. Circulation 103, 201–206.

COMMIT Collaborative Group, 2005. Addition of clopidogrel to aspirin in 45 852 patients with acute myocardial infarction: randomised placebo-controlled trial. Lancet 366, 1607–1621.

Goodman, T., Ferro, A., Sharma, P., 2008. Pharmacogenetics of aspirin resistance: a comprehensive systematic review. Br. J. Clin. Pharmacol. 66, 222–232.

Patrono, C., Baigent, C., 2019. Role of aspirin in primary prevention of cardiovascular disease. Nat. Rev. Cardiol. 16, 675–686.

Patrono, C., Coller, B., FitzGerald, G.A., et al., 2004. Platelet-active drugs: the relationships among dose, effectiveness, and side effects. Chest 126, 234S–264S.

Pollack, C.V., Wang, T.Y., 2021. Evolution of clinical thinking and practice regarding aspirin: what has changed and why? Am. J. Cardiol. 144, S10–S14.

Wallentin, L., Becker, R.C., Budaj, A., et al., 2009. Ticagrelor versus clopidogrel in patients with acute coronary syndromes. N. Engl. J. Med. 361, 1045–1057.

Wiviott, S.D., Braunwald, E., McCabe, C.H., et al., 2007. For the TRITON-TIMI 38 Investigators. Prasugrel versus clopidogrel in patients with acute coronary syndromes. N. Engl. J. Med. 357, 2001–2015.

Clinical and general aspects

Aster, R.H., 1995. Heparin-induced thrombocytopenia and thrombosis. N. Engl. J. Med. 332, 1374–1376.

Diener, H., Cunha, L., Forbes, C., et al., 1996. European Stroke Prevention Study 2. Dipyridamole and acetylsalicylic acid in the secondary prevention of stroke. J. Neurol. Sci. 143, 1–14.

Goldhaber, S.Z., 2004. Pulmonary embolism. Lancet 363, 1295–1305.

Kyrle, P.A., Eichinger, S., 2005. Deep vein thrombosis. Lancet 365, 1163–1174.

Levine, M., 1995. A comparison of low-molecular-weight heparin administered primarily at home with unfractionated heparin administered in the hospital for proximal deep vein thrombosis. N. Engl. J. Med. 334, 677–681.

Markus, H.S., 2005. Current treatments in neurology: stroke. J. Neurol. 252, 260–267.

Ricciotti, E., FitzGerald, G.A., 2021. Aspirin in the prevention of cardiovascular disease and cancer. Ann. Rev. Med. 72, 473–495.

Scully, M., Singh, D., Lown, R., et al., 2021. Pathologic antibodies to platelet factor 4 after ChAdOx1 nCOV-19 vaccination. N. Engl. J. Med. 384, 2202–2211.

Haematopoietic system and treatment of anaemia

24

OVERVIEW

This chapter briefly reviews the haematopoietic system, emphasising the control of red cell generation ('erythropoiesis'), and summarises the different kinds of anaemia. These are caused by nutrient deficiencies, lack of bone marrow stimulation, bone marrow depression (as in aplastic anaemia) or increased red cell destruction ('haemolytic' anaemias). We then describe the main agents used to treat these and also some non-malignant diseases of white blood cells (leukocytes) and platelets. Malignant diseases of white blood cells (leukaemias) are covered in Chapter 57. Antiplatelet drugs are considered in Chapter 23. Here we describe haematopoietic growth factors and conclude by mentioning drugs used to treat sickle cell anaemia and paroxysmal nocturnal haemoglobinuria (PNH).

INTRODUCTION

In this chapter, we briefly review the haematopoietic system and different types of anaemia due to blood loss, deficiency of nutrients, lack of erythropoietin (the hormone that stimulates erythropoiesis) or increased destruction of red cells (haemolytic anaemias). Nutritional deficiencies of *iron, vitamin B_{12}* or *folic acid* are common and important, and most of this chapter is devoted to these haematinic agents (i.e. nutrients needed for healthy haematopoiesis) and related drugs.

Treatment of many forms of bone marrow depression is mainly supportive for example by transfusions of red blood cells or platelets or, in patients with neutropenic sepsis, by administration of antibiotics. However, *haematopoietic growth factors* (especially *epoietins* – preparations based on the natural hormone erythropoietin) transformed the treatment of patients with chronic kidney disease who are deficient in erythropoietin which, in adults, is made and secreted mainly by the kidneys. It has also been used, notoriously, in competitive sport (see Ch. 59). More recently, advances in understanding of the control of erythropoietin secretion by hypoxia inducible factors (HIFs), notably by $HIF_{1\alpha}$, look set to underpin further improvements in the treatment of anaemia in patients with kidney disease and potentially of wider indications including vascular disease and, via HIF *inhibition* (e.g. **belzutifan** for the treatment of von Hippel–Lindau [VHL] syndrome), and malignant diseases (see Ch. 57).

Other haematopoietic factors known as *colony-stimulating factors* (CSFs) – varieties of cytokine (see Ch. 17) – increase the numbers of circulating white blood cells and are used therapeutically.

Finally, we mention two drugs (**hydroxycarbamide** and **crisanlizumab**) that provide mechanistic insights as well as clinical benefit in sickle cell anaemia and **eculizumab** that provides insights as well as clinical benefits in PNH. Gene editing (see Ch. 5) and cell-based therapies offer a glimpse of possible future cures for sickle cell disease, the thalassaemias and related genetically determined haemoglobinopathies.

THE HAEMATOPOIETIC SYSTEM

The main components of the haematopoietic system are the blood, bone marrow, lymph nodes and thymus, with the spleen, liver and kidneys as important accessory organs. Blood consists of formed elements (red and white blood cells and platelets) and plasma. This chapter deals mainly with red cells, which carry oxygen in the blood vessels from the lungs to the tissues, where it is needed for aerobic metabolism. Their oxygen-carrying power depends on their haemoglobin content. White blood cells are of central importance in response to infection and other danger signals (see Ch. 7) and platelets are essential for haemostasis (see Ch. 23).

Erythropoiesis and its control. The most important site of formation of red blood cells in adults is the bone marrow, whereas the spleen acts as their slaughterhouse. The lifetime of a red cell is normally about 120 days, and red cell loss in healthy adults – about 2×10^{10} cells per day – is precisely balanced by production of new cells. As mentioned previously, the kidneys (and, in fetal life, the liver) manufacture *erythropoietin*, the hormone that stimulates red cell production. In healthy individuals the anatomical site with the lowest tissue concentration of oxygen is the renal medulla which utilises anaerobic metabolism for its energy supply. The low oxygen is a consequence of the anatomical arrangement of the blood supply to the medulla via vascular loops called the vasa recta. This arrangement results in counter-current exchange of plasma and a low blood flow to the deepest part of the medulla with a short-circuiting of extracellular fluid and oxygen between vasa recta vessels entering and leaving the medulla. This preserves the osmotic gradient that permits the kidney to excrete either a dilute or a concentrated urine (see Ch. 29).

The red cell content of blood is expressed as the *haematocrit*, defined as the fraction of the blood that is occupied by red cells expressed as a percentage, or as the *haemoglobin concentration* expressed nowadays (at least in European countries) in molar terms based on the molecular mass of haemoglobin and the total volume of blood in the sample – as though the haemoglobin was uniformly distributed throughout the blood sample rather than being confined within the red blood cells. The normal ranges of these measures differ between men and women, who lose blood during their reproductive years by menstruation and in childbirth.

Oxygen sensing. It has been known since early in the 20th century that the haematocrit in each sex is precisely

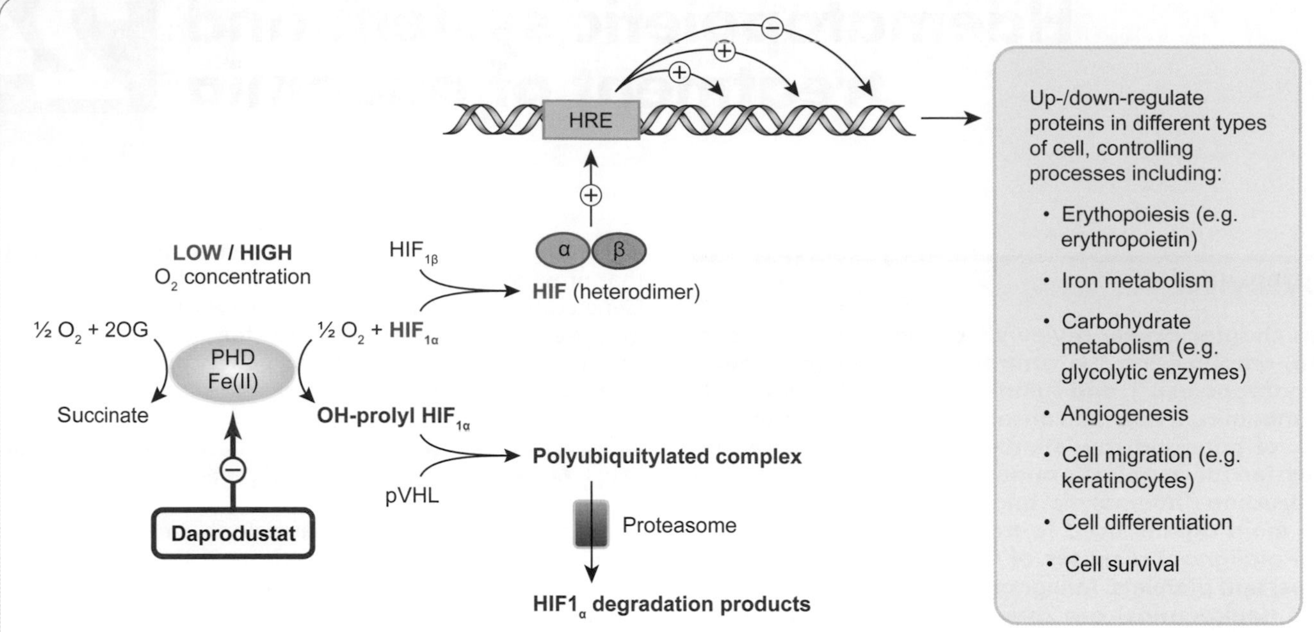

Fig 24.1 Oxygen-sensitive control of erythropoiesis by PHD/HIF. O_2 combines with Fe(II) in the active site of PHD, the oxygen sensor. At high tissue O_2 concentrations *(red)* PHD hydroxylates one or other of two prolyl residues in $HIF_{1\alpha}$ while converting 2OG to succinate. Hydroxylation of $HIF_{1\alpha}$ creates a high affinity binding site for pVHD which complexes with it and promotes polyubiquitylation, tagging the complex for destruction by proteasomes. Consequently, the concentration of $HIF_{1\alpha}$ available for combination with $HIF_{1\beta}$ to form the active HIF dimer is low when O_2 concentration is high. The affinity of PHD for O_2 is such that when the tissue O_2 concentration falls ($pO_2 < 40$ mm Hg – blue in the figure) there is a steep decline in the rate of hydroxylation of $HIF_{1\alpha}$, consequently $HIF_{1\alpha}$ increases, dimerises with $HIF_{1\beta}$ to form HIF which acts in the nucleus on chromosomal HRE to control the rate of production of erythropoietin and of other proteins involved in the response to hypoxia. *2OG*, 2-Oxoglutarate; *HIF*, hypoxia inducible factor (subunits 1a and 1b); *HRE*, HIF-response element; *PHD*, prolyl hydroxylase domain-containing protein; *pVHL*, von Hippel–Lindau protein.

controlled by oxygen,[1] but the details of how cells sense and respond to oxygen availability have only been worked out more recently. A transcription factor known as HIF combines with a 33-base pair chromosomal erythropoietin response element to stimulate synthesis of messenger RNA for erythropoietin synthesis. HIF is a heterodimer with α- and β- subunits, and $HIF_{1\alpha}$ plays a critical role in responsiveness to oxygen. It is synthesised in many kinds of cell – rather than just in cells that secrete erythropoietin – but in well-oxygenated cells it is rapidly oxidised by a prolyl hydroxylase domain-containing protein (PHD) which is a dioxygenase enzyme that hydroxylates one or other of two proline residues in $HIF_{1\alpha}$ while adding the other atom of oxygen from molecular O_2 to 2-oxoglutarate (α-ketoglutarate) converting this to succinate (Fig. 24.1).

PHD (also known as EGLN prolyl hydroxylase because of its homology with a gene of the nematode worm *Caenorhabditis elegans*) is the oxygen sensor responsible for the integrated physiological response to tissue hypoxia which includes increased erythropoietin production. It has a non-haem Fe^{2+} atom at its active site which combines with molecular oxygen. Hydroxylation of one or both prolyl residues in $HIF_{1\alpha}$ creates a high-affinity binding site for VHL[2] protein (pVHL). pVHL acts as recognition protein for ubiquitin ligase which tags the pVHL/$HIF_{1\alpha}$ complex with ubiquitin molecules ('polyubiquitylation') for destruction by proteasomes in the cytoplasm.

PHD has an affinity for oxygen that quantitatively explains oxygen sensitivity in the physiological range of the cellular environment. It works not as a stimulus to $HIF_{1\alpha}$ synthesis in the absence of oxygen but as the means to its elimination in the presence of oxygen (Fig 24.1). Under conditions of low cellular oxygen concentration $HIF_{1\alpha}$ elimination is suppressed, so it accumulates, is transported to the cell nucleus, dimerises with $HIF_{1\beta}$ and the resulting HIF_1 combines with response elements that control not only erythropoietin synthesis but a very large number of other genes (>3000) as well: it is now known that HIF is a master regulator of many integrated mechanisms including iron metabolism, anaerobic carbohydrate metabolism, cell migration and neovascularisation.

[1]Discovered by Mabel Purefoy FitzGerald, the only woman scientist in an expedition to Pike's Peak. The men stayed in luxury in an accommodation near the summit while she was assigned to less comfortable quarters lower down, whence she studied the relationship between the altitude of various communities – the determinant of the partial pressure of oxygen in the inhaled air – and the mean haematocrit of the inhabitants. She demonstrated a very sensitive steep linear relationship within each sex. The circumstances are described by Sir Peter Ratcliffe in his 2019 Nobel lecture (https://www.youtube.com/watch?v=-Q0OGLCzKEE). He shared the prize with Gregg L. Semenza and William Kaelin 'for their discoveries of how cells sense and adapt to oxygen availability'.

[2]VHL disease is a rare single-gene disorder in which pVHD is defective. It is characterised by vascular tumours in the retina, cerebellum, brainstem, kidneys and neuro-endocrine tissue (phaeochromocytomas; see Ch. 15) and in some patients by increased haematocrit.

Hypoxia may be generalised (as at high altitude where the inhaled air contains only a low oxygen content or in diseases of the lungs – see Ch. 28) or tissue hypoxia may be limited to an anatomical region as in vasoocclusive disease (see Chs 21 and 22) and in poorly vascularised regions of solid tumours (see Ch. 57) or healing wounds. There is thus therapeutic potential in either *potentiating* HIF to treat some forms of anaemia or tissue ischaemia (e.g. by blocking the degradation of $HIF_{1\alpha}$ by inhibiting PHD, see later) or in *blocking* its action, as an anti-cancer strategy (see Ch. 57).

Leukopoiesis and thrombopoiesis. Granulocyte-CSF (GCSF), macrophage-CSF (MCSF) and granulocyte-macrophage-CSF (GMCSF) regulate the production of leukocytes; they stimulate precursor cells in the bone marrow to divide and differentiate for release into the bloodstream. Several preparations of GCSF are used therapeutically – see later. Antagonists of GMCSF are being investigated as potential anti-inflammatory and anti-cancer agents. *Thrombopoietin*, a glycoprotein produced by the liver and kidneys, stimulates platelet formation by acting on thrombopoietin receptors on megakaryocytes, the precursors of platelets. The receptor is linked to the JAK/STAT signalling pathway (see Ch. 3, Fig 3.17) and promotes platelet generation and release into the circulation. Thrombopoietin is not used therapeutically, but other drugs that are agonists at the thrombopoietin receptor are available for therapeutic use – see later.

TYPES OF ANAEMIA

Anaemia is characterised by a reduced haemoglobin content in the blood. It may cause fatigue but, especially if it is chronic, is often surprisingly asymptomatic. The commonest cause is blood loss resulting from menstruation, drug treatment (e.g. with **aspirin** or other non-steroidal anti-inflammatory drugs; see Ch. 25) or pathological processes such as colonic carcinoma or (especially in developing countries) parasitic infestation (see Ch. 56). Pregnancy and child-bearing are important physiological drains on iron reserves. There are several different types of anaemia based on indices of red cell size and haemoglobin content and microscopical examination of a stained blood smear:

- *hypochromic, microcytic anaemia* (small red cells containing low haemoglobin concentration; caused by chronic blood loss giving rise to iron deficiency)
- *macrocytic anaemia* (large red cells, few in number)
- *normochromic normocytic anaemia* (fewer normal-sized red cells, each with a normal haemoglobin content)
- mixed pictures

Further evaluation may include determination of concentrations of ferritin, iron, vitamin B_{12} and folic acid in serum, and microscopic examination of smears of bone marrow. This leads to more precise diagnostic groupings of anaemias into:

- Deficiency of nutrients necessary for haematopoiesis, most importantly:
  - iron
  - folic acid and vitamin B_{12}
  - pyridoxine and vitamin C
- Depression of the bone marrow, commonly caused by:
  - drug toxicity (e.g. cytotoxic drugs, **clozapine**)
  - exposure to radiation, including radiotherapy
  - diseases of the bone marrow (e.g. idiopathic aplastic anaemia, leukaemias)
  - reduced production of, or responsiveness to, erythropoietin (e.g. chronic renal failure, rheumatoid arthritis, AIDS)
- Excessive destruction of red blood cells (i.e. haemolytic anaemia); this has many causes, including *haemoglobinopathies* (such as sickle cell anaemia), adverse reactions to drugs and immune reactions that have gone awry.

HAEMATINIC AGENTS

The use of haematinic agents is often only an adjunct to treatment of the underlying cause of the anaemia – for example, surgery for colon cancer (a common cause of iron deficiency) or antihelminthic drugs for patients with hookworm (a frequent cause of anaemia in parts of Africa and Asia; see Ch. 56). Sometimes treatment consists of stopping an offending drug, for example a non-steroidal anti-inflammatory drug that is causing blood loss from the gastrointestinal tract (see Ch. 25).

IRON

Iron is a transition metal with two important properties relevant to its biological role, namely its ability to exist in several oxidation states and to form stable coordination complexes.

The body of a 70-kg man contains about 4 g of iron, 65% of which circulates in the blood as haemoglobin. About one-half of the remainder is stored in the liver, spleen and bone marrow, chiefly as *ferritin* and *haemosiderin*. The iron in these molecules is available for haemoglobin synthesis. The rest, which is not available for haemoglobin synthesis, is present in myoglobin, cytochromes and various enzymes.

The distribution and turnover of iron in an average adult man are shown in Table 24.1 and Fig. 24.2. The corresponding values in a woman are approximately 45% less. Because most of the iron in the body is either part of – or destined to be part of – haemoglobin, the most obvious clinical result of iron deficiency is anaemia, and the only indication for therapy with iron is for treatment or prophylaxis of iron deficiency anaemia.

Haemoglobin is made up of four protein chain subunits (globins), each of which contains one haem moiety. Haem consists of a tetrapyrrole porphyrin ring containing ferrous (Fe^{2+}) iron. Each haem group can carry one oxygen molecule, which is bound reversibly to Fe^{2+} and to a histidine residue in the globin chain. This reversible binding is the basis of oxygen transport.

IRON TURNOVER AND BALANCE

The normal daily requirement for iron is approximately 5 mg for men and 15 mg for growing children and for menstruating women. A pregnant woman needs between 2 and 10 times this amount because of the demands of the fetus and increased requirements of the mother.[3] The average diet

[3]Each pregnancy 'costs' the mother 680 mg of iron, equivalent to 1300 mL of blood, owing to the demands of the fetus, plus requirements of the expanded blood volume and blood loss at delivery.

Table 24.1 Distribution of iron in the body of a healthy 70-kg man

Protein	Tissue	Iron content (mg)
Haemoglobin	Erythrocytes	2600
Myoglobin	Muscle	400
Enzymes (cytochromes, catalase, guanylyl cyclase, etc.)	Liver and other tissues	25
Transferrin	Plasma and extracellular fluid	8
Ferritin and haemosiderin	Liver	410
	Spleen	48
	Bone marrow	300

Data from Jacobs, A., Worwood, M., 1982. Chapter 5. In: Hardisty, R.M., Weatherall, D.J. (Eds). Blood and Its Disorders. Blackwell Scientific, Oxford.

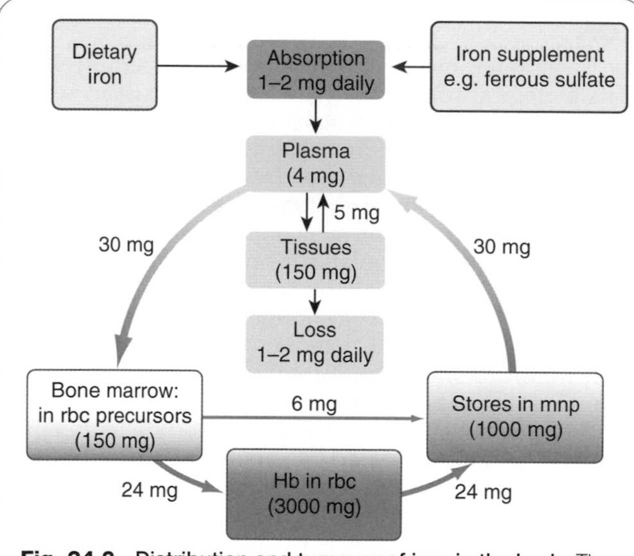

Fig. 24.2 Distribution and turnover of iron in the body. The quantities by the arrows indicate the usual amounts transferred each day. The transfer of 6 mg from red cell precursors to phagocytes represents aborted cells that fail to develop into functional red blood cells. *Hb*, Haemoglobin; *mnp*, mononuclear phagocytes (mainly in liver, spleen and bone marrow); *rbc*, red blood cells.

in Western Europe provides 15–20 mg of iron daily, mostly in meat. Iron in meat is generally present as haem, and about 20%–40% of haem iron is available for absorption.

Humans are adapted to absorb haem iron. It is thought that one reason why modern humans have problems in maintaining iron balance (there are an estimated 500 million people with iron deficiency in the world) is that the change from hunting to grain cultivation 10,000 years ago led to cereals, which contain little utilisable iron, replacing meat in the diet. Non-haem iron in food is mainly in the ferric state, and this needs to be converted to ferrous iron for absorption. Iron salts have low solubility at the neutral pH of the small intestine; however, in the stomach, iron dissolves and binds to a mucoprotein carrier. In the presence of ascorbic acid, fructose and various amino acids, iron is detached from the carrier, forming soluble low-molecular-weight complexes that enable it to remain in soluble form in the intestine. Ascorbic acid stimulates iron absorption partly by forming soluble iron–ascorbate chelates and partly by reducing ferric iron to the more soluble ferrous form. **Tetracycline** (see Ch. 52) forms an insoluble iron chelate, impairing absorption of both substances.

The amount of iron in the diet and the various factors affecting its availability are thus important determinants in absorption, but the regulation of iron absorption is a function of the intestinal mucosa, influenced by the body's iron stores. Because there is no mechanism whereby iron excretion is regulated, the absorptive mechanism has a central role in iron balance as it is the sole mechanism by which body iron is controlled.

Iron absorption takes place in the duodenum and upper jejunum and is a two-stage process involving uptake across the brush border into the mucosal cells, followed by transfer into the plasma. The second stage, which is rate limiting, is energy dependent. Haem iron in the diet is absorbed as intact haem, and the iron is released in the mucosal cell by the action of haem oxidase. Non-haem iron is absorbed in the ferrous state. Within the cell, ferrous iron is oxidised to ferric iron, which is bound to an intracellular carrier, a transferrin-like protein; the iron is then either held in storage in the mucosal cell as *ferritin* (if body stores of iron are high) or passed on to the plasma (if iron stores are low).

Iron is carried in the plasma bound to *transferrin*, a β-globulin with two binding sites for ferric iron. The binding sites are normally only approximately 30% saturated. Plasma contains 4 mg of iron at any one time, but the daily turnover is about 30 mg (see Fig. 24.2). Most of the iron that enters the plasma is derived from macrophages which have engulfed and processed time-expired erythrocytes. Intestinal absorption and mobilisation of iron from storage depots contribute only small amounts. Most of the iron that leaves the plasma each day is used for haemoglobin synthesis by red cell precursors (erythroblasts). These have receptors that bind transferrin, releasing it again when its cargo of iron has been captured.

Iron is stored in two forms: soluble ferritin and insoluble *haemosiderin*. Ferritin is present in all cells, the macrophages of liver, spleen and bone marrow containing especially high concentrations. It is also present in plasma. The precursor of ferritin, *apoferritin*, is a protein of molecular weight 450,000, composed of 24 identical polypeptide subunits that enclose a cavity in which up to 4500 iron atoms can be stored. Apoferritin takes up ferrous iron, oxidises it and deposits the ferric iron in its core. In this form, it constitutes ferritin, the primary storage form of iron, from which the iron is most readily available. The lifespan of this iron-laden protein is only a few days. Haemosiderin is a degraded form of ferritin in which the iron cores of several ferritin molecules have aggregated, following partial disintegration of the outer protein shells.

Iron is not the most soluble of metals, hence its need to bind to transferrin (whilst transferring around the body) and ferritin for use inside cells (ferritin is found mostly inside cells but can exist in the plasma too, functioning to transport iron into cells). Ferritin in plasma contains very little iron, as two-thirds of the body's iron deposits are found within red blood cells, with more ferritin in the body than free unbound iron. The slow turnover of iron absorbed from the diet, transferred around the body by transferrin, then held in cellular storage by ferritin, means that the majority of total useful iron is held in erythrocytes, and their rapid turnover is the main source of liberated iron. Iron bound to plasma ferritin is, however, in equilibrium with the storage ferritin in cells, and its concentration in plasma (normal range 40–100 ng/mL) provides a clinically useful indicator of total body iron stores: values below 40 ng/mL despite normal haemoglobin, red cell morphology, serum iron concentration and transferrin saturation signal mild iron deficiency, with values below 20 and 10 ng/mL signalling moderate and severe iron deficiency, respectively.

The body has no means of actively excreting iron. Small amounts leave the body through shedding of mucosal cells containing ferritin, and even smaller amounts leave in the bile, sweat and urine. A total of about 1 mg is lost daily. Control of iron balance is therefore critically dependent on the active absorption mechanism in the intestinal mucosa, which is influenced by the iron stores in the body. Iron balance is summarised in Fig. 24.2. Since red cells contain approximately 0.6 mg iron per mL of blood, a loss of only a few millilitres of blood per day substantially increases dietary iron requirement.

ADMINISTRATION OF IRON

Iron is usually given orally, e.g. as **ferrous sulfate**. Other salts for oral administration are **ferrous succinate**, **gluconate** or **fumarate**.

Parenteral administration of iron (e.g. as **iron-dextran**, **iron-sucrose, ferric carboxymaltose** or **ferric derisomaltose**) by injection or intravenous infusion may be necessary in individuals who are not able to absorb oral iron because of malabsorption syndromes, or as a result of surgical procedures or inflammatory conditions involving the gastrointestinal tract. It is also used for patients who do not tolerate oral preparations, and patients with chronic renal failure or with chemotherapy-induced anaemia who are receiving treatment with erythropoietin (see later). Iron-dextran can be given by deep intramuscular injection or slow intravenous infusion; iron-sucrose is given by slow intravenous infusion. A small initial dose is given because of the risk of anaphylactoid reaction (see Ch. 58). Depending on the preparation used and clinical setting it can be infused as a single total dose (e.g. ferric carboxymaltose) or in divided doses. Ongoing treatment is monitored as needed by measuring haemoglobin and serum iron concentrations.

Unwanted effects

The unwanted effects of oral iron administration are dose related and include nausea, abdominal cramps and diarrhoea. Parenteral iron can cause anaphylactoid reactions (see Ch. 58). Free Fe^{3+} is toxic and causes mitochondrial damage and oxidative stress. Iron is an important nutrient for several pathogens and there is concern that excessive iron could worsen the clinical course of infection. Iron treatment is usually avoided during infection for this reason.

Acute iron toxicity, usually seen in young children who have swallowed attractively coloured iron tablets in mistake for sweets, can result in severe necrotising gastritis with vomiting, haemorrhage and diarrhoea, followed by circulatory collapse.

Clinical use of iron

See clinical box.

Clinical uses of iron

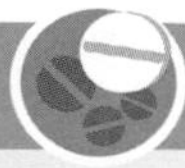

To treat iron deficiency anaemia, which can be caused by:

- *chronic blood loss* (e.g. with menorrhagia, hookworm, colon cancer – the cause must be diagnosed and treated specifically in addition to iron treatment);
- *increased demand* (e.g. in pregnancy and early infancy);
- *inadequate dietary intake* (uncommon in developed countries);
- *inadequate absorption* (e.g. following gastrectomy, or in diseases such as coeliac disease, where the intestinal mucosa is damaged by an immunologically based intolerance to the wheat protein gluten).
- Prophylactic use is sometimes appropriate.
- Parenteral iron (as **iron dextran**, **iron sucrose**, **ferric carboxymaltose** or **ferric derisomaltose**) is used if oral preparations are not tolerated or unsuccessful, and is also used in conjunction with an erythropoietin preparation in the management of patients with chronic renal failure or with chemotherapy-induced anaemia (see Ch. 57).

Iron overload

Chronic iron toxicity or iron overload occurs in chronic haemolytic anaemias requiring frequent blood transfusions, such as the *thalassaemias* (a large group of genetic disorders of globin chain synthesis) and *haemochromatosis* (a genetic iron storage disease with increased iron absorption, resulting in damage to liver, islets of Langerhans, joints and skin).[4]

The treatment of acute and chronic iron toxicity involves the use of iron chelators such as **desferrioxamine**. These form complexes with ferric iron which are excreted in the urine. Desferrioxamine is not absorbed from the gut. For treating chronic iron overload (e.g. in thalassaemia), it must be given by slow subcutaneous infusion several times a week. For acute iron overdose of oral iron tablets, it is given intramuscularly or intravenously as well as intragastrically to sequester unabsorbed iron. **Deferiprone** is an orally absorbed iron chelator, used as an alternative treatment for iron overload in patients with thalassaemia major who are unable to tolerate desferrioxamine. Agranulocytosis and other blood dyscrasias are serious potential adverse effects. **Deferasirox** is similar but can cause gastrointestinal bleeding.

[4]'Bronze diabetes' – where chronic iron overload causing dark skin and diabetes mellitus from damage to the pancreatic islets of Langerhans, is treated by repeated bleeding, one of the few modern uses of this once near-universal 'remedy'; polycythaemia vera (caused by mutations in erythroid progenitors that increase their proliferation) is another.

Iron

- Iron is important for the synthesis of haemoglobin, myoglobin, cytochromes and other enzymes. Ferric iron (Fe^{3+}) must be converted to ferrous iron (Fe^{2+}) for absorption in the gastrointestinal tract.
- Absorption involves active transport into mucosal cells in the duodenum and jejunum (the upper ileum), from where it can be transported into the plasma and/or stored intracellularly as ferritin.
- Total body iron is controlled exclusively by absorption; in iron deficiency, more is transported into plasma than is stored as ferritin in jejunal mucosa.
- Iron loss occurs mainly by sloughing of ferritin-containing mucosal cells which are eliminated in the faeces.
- Iron in plasma is bound to transferrin, and most is used for erythropoiesis. Some is stored as ferritin in other tissues. Iron from time-expired erythrocytes enters the plasma for reuse.
- The main oral therapeutic preparations are **ferrous sulfate, ferrous fumarate** or **ferrous gluconate**; parenteral preparations include **iron-sucrose, iron dextran, ferric carboxymaltose** or **ferric derisomaltose.** These can be given by intravenous infusion when oral iron is not tolerated or ineffective.
- Unwanted effects include gastrointestinal disturbances. Severe toxic effects occur if large doses are ingested; such acute poisoning can be treated with **desferrioxamine**, an iron chelator, as can chronic iron overload in diseases such as thalassaemia.

FOLIC ACID AND VITAMIN B_{12}

Vitamin B_{12} and folic acid are essential constituents of the human diet, being necessary for DNA synthesis and consequently for cell proliferation. Their biochemical actions are interdependent (see 'Vitamin B_{12} and folic acid)' key point box), and treatment with folic acid corrects some, but not all, of the features of vitamin B_{12} deficiency. Deficiency of either vitamin B_{12} or folic acid affects tissues with a rapid cell turnover, particularly bone marrow, but vitamin B_{12} deficiency also causes important neuronal disorders, which are not corrected (or may even be made worse) by treatment with folic acid. Deficiency of either vitamin causes *megaloblastic haematopoiesis,* in which there is disordered erythroblast differentiation and defective erythropoiesis in the bone marrow. Large abnormal erythrocyte precursors appear in the marrow, each with a high RNA:DNA ratio as a result of decreased DNA synthesis. The circulating abnormal erythrocytes ('macrocytes' – i.e. large red blood cells) are large fragile cells, often distorted in shape. Mild leukopenia and thrombocytopenia (i.e. low white blood cell and platelet counts) usually accompany the anaemia, and the nuclei of polymorphonuclear (PMN) leukocytes are structurally abnormal (hypersegmented – as young PMNs mature, their nuclei acquire 'lobes' in the form of discrete bulges, leading to hypersegmentation in post-mature cells. The nuclei of megaloblasts – the precursors of macrocytic red cells in patients with B_{12} or folate deficiency – are functionally asynchronous and feebly active, compared with the cells' low haemoglobin content). Neurological disorders caused by deficiency of vitamin B_{12} include peripheral neuropathy and dementia, as well as *subacute combined degeneration*[5] of the spinal cord. Folic acid deficiency is caused by dietary deficiency as in alcoholics, and especially if there is increased demand, e.g. during pregnancy – particularly important because of the link between folate deficiency and neural tube defects in the baby (see Ch. 58) – or because of chronic haemolysis in patients with haemoglobinopathies such as *sickle cell anaemia* (see later). Vitamin B_{12} deficiency, in contrast, is usually due to decreased absorption (see later).

FOLIC ACID

Some aspects of folate structure and metabolism are dealt with in Chapters 51 and 57, because several important antibacterial and anticancer drugs are antimetabolites that interfere with folate synthesis in microorganisms or tumour cells. Liver and green vegetables are rich sources of folate. In healthy non-pregnant adults, the daily requirement is about 0.2 mg daily, but this is increased during pregnancy. Healthy fetal neural development in particular requires sufficient folate in the mother's diet to prevent fetal neural tube defects.

Mechanism of action

Reduction of folic acid, catalysed by *dihydrofolate reductase* in two stages, yields *dihydrofolate* (FH_2) and *tetrahydrofolate* (FH_4), co-factors which transfer methyl groups (1-carbon transfers) in several important metabolic pathways. FH_4 is essential for DNA synthesis because of its role as co-factor in the synthesis of purines and pyrimidines. It is also necessary for reactions involved in amino acid metabolism.

FH_4 is important for the conversion of deoxyuridylate monophosphate (DUMP) to deoxythymidylate monophosphate (DTMP). This reaction is rate limiting in mammalian DNA synthesis and is catalysed by thymidylate synthetase, with FH_4 acting as methyl donor (see Fig 57.6).

Pharmacokinetic aspects

Therapeutically, folic acid is given orally and is absorbed in the ileum. Methyl-FH_4 is the form in which folate is usually carried in blood and which enters cells. It is functionally inactive until it is demethylated in a vitamin B_{12}-dependent reaction (see later). Folate is taken up into hepatocytes and bone marrow cells by active transport. Within the cells, folic acid is reduced and formylated before being converted to the active polyglutamate form. **Folinic acid**, a synthetic FH_4, is converted much more rapidly to the polyglutamate form.

Unwanted effects

Unwanted effects do not occur even with large doses of folic acid – except in the presence of vitamin B_{12} deficiency, when administration of folic acid may improve the anaemia while possibly exacerbating the neurological degeneration. It is therefore important to determine whether a megaloblastic anaemia is caused by folate or vitamin B_{12} deficiency and treat accordingly.

---

[5]'Combined' because the lateral as well as the dorsal columns are involved, giving rise to motor as well as sensory symptoms.

Clinical uses of folic acid and vitamin B_{12} (hydroxocobalamin)

Folic acid

- Treatment of megaloblastic anaemia resulting from folate deficiency, which can be caused by:
  - *poor diet* (common in alcoholic individuals)
  - *malabsorption syndromes*
  - drugs (e.g. **phenytoin**).
- Treatment or prevention of toxicity from **methotrexate**, a folate antagonist (see Chs 25 and 57).
- Prophylactically in individuals at hazard from developing folate deficiency, for example:
  - *pregnant women* and *before conception* (especially if there is a risk of birth defects)
  - *premature infants*
  - patients with *severe chronic haemolytic anaemias*, including haemoglobinopathies (e.g. sickle cell anaemia).

Vitamin B_{12} (hydroxocobalamin)

- Treatment of *pernicious anaemia* and other causes of vitamin B_{12} deficiency.
- Prophylactically after surgical operations that remove the site of production of intrinsic factor (the stomach) or of vitamin B_{12} absorption (the terminal ileum).

VITAMIN B_{12}

Vitamin B_{12}, also called cobalamin, corrects pernicious anaemia. The vitamin B_{12} preparation used therapeutically is **hydroxocobalamin,** derived from cultured microorganisms. The principal dietary sources are meat (particularly liver, where it is stored), eggs and dairy products. For activity, cobalamins must be converted to *methylcobalamin* (methyl-B_{12}) or *5′-deoxyadenosylcobalamin* (ado-B_{12}). The average European diet contains 5–25 μg of vitamin B_{12} per day, and the daily requirement is 2–3 μg. Absorption requires *intrinsic factor* (a glycoprotein secreted by gastric parietal cells). Vitamin B_{12}, complexed with intrinsic factor, is absorbed by active transport in the terminal ileum. Healthy stomach secretes a large excess of intrinsic factor, but in patients with pernicious anaemia (an autoimmune disorder where the lining of the stomach atrophies), or following total gastrectomy, the supply of intrinsic factor is inadequate to maintain vitamin B_{12} absorption in the long term. Surgical removal of the terminal ileum, for example to treat Crohn's disease (see Ch. 30), can also impair B_{12} absorption.

Vitamin B_{12} is carried in the plasma by binding proteins called *transcobalamins*. It is stored in the liver, the total amount in the body being about 4 mg. This store is so large compared with the daily requirement, that if vitamin B_{12} absorption stops suddenly – as after a total gastrectomy – it takes 2–4 years for evidence of deficiency to become manifest.

Mechanism of action

Vitamin B_{12} is required for two main biochemical reactions in humans.

The conversion of methyl-FH_4 to FH_4. The metabolic activities of vitamin B_{12} and folic acid are linked in the synthesis of DNA. It is also through this pathway that folate/vitamin B_{12} treatment can lower plasma homocysteine concentration. Because increased homocysteine concentrations may have undesirable vascular effects (see Ch. 22, Table 22.1), this has potential therapeutic and public health implications. The reaction involves conversion of both methyl-FH_4 to FH_4 and homocysteine to methionine. The enzyme that accomplishes this *(homocysteine–methionine methyltransferase)* requires vitamin B_{12} as co-factor and methyl-FH_4 as methyl donor. The methyl group from methyl-FH_4 is transferred first to B_{12}, and then to homocysteine to form methionine. Vitamin B_{12} deficiency thus traps folate in the inactive methyl-FH_4 form, thereby depleting the folate polyglutamate coenzymes needed for DNA synthesis. Vitamin B_{12}–dependent methionine synthesis additionally affects the synthesis of folate polyglutamate coenzymes because the preferred substrate for polyglutamate synthesis is formyl-FH_4, and the conversion of FH_4 to formyl-FH_4 requires a formate donor such as methionine.

Isomerisation of methylmalonyl-coenzyme A (CoA) to succinyl-CoA. This isomerisation reaction is part of a route by which propionate is converted to succinate. Through this pathway, cholesterol, odd-chain fatty acids, some amino acids and thymine can be used for gluconeogenesis or for energy production via the tricarboxylic acid (TCA) cycle. Coenzyme B_{12} (ado-B_{12}) is an essential co-factor, so methylmalonyl-CoA accumulates in vitamin B_{12} deficiency. This distorts the pattern of fatty acid synthesis in neural tissue and may be the basis of neuropathy in vitamin B_{12} deficiency.

Administration of vitamin B_{12}

When vitamin B_{12} is used therapeutically (as **hydroxocobalamin**), it is usually given by injection[6] because, as explained earlier, vitamin B_{12} deficiency commonly results from malabsorption. Patients with pernicious anaemia require life-long therapy, with maintenance injections every 3 months following a loading dose. Replacement of hydroxocobalamin does not cause unwanted effects.

HAEMATOPOIETIC GROWTH FACTORS

Every 60 s, a human being must generate about 120 million granulocytes and 150 million erythrocytes, as well as numerous mononuclear cells and platelets.[7] The cells responsible for this remarkable productivity are derived from a relatively small number of self-renewing, pluripotent stem cells laid down during embryogenesis. Maintenance of haematopoiesis necessitates a balance between self-renewal of the stem cells on the one hand, and differentiation into

[6]At least in Anglo-Saxon countries; in France, very large doses of vitamin B_{12} are given by mouth to achieve sufficient absorption for therapeutic efficacy despite the absence of intrinsic factor. Either method is a great improvement on eating the prodigious quantities of raw liver required by Minot and Murphy's 'liver diet' of 1925!

[7]That's your entire genome replicated faithfully for at least 200 million new blood cells every minute!

Vitamin B_{12} and folic acid

Both vitamin B_{12} and folic acid are needed for DNA synthesis. Deficiencies particularly affect erythropoiesis, causing macrocytic megaloblastic anaemia.

Folic acid (vitamin B9)

- There is active uptake of folic acid into cells and reduction to tetrahydrofolate (FH_4) by dihydrofolate reductase; extra glutamates are then added.
- Folate polyglutamate is a co-factor (a carrier of 1-carbon units) in the synthesis of purines and pyrimidines (especially thymidylate).

Vitamin B_{12} (hydroxocobalamin)

- Vitamin B_{12} needs intrinsic factor (a glycoprotein) secreted by gastric parietal cells for absorption in the terminal ileum.
- It is stored in the liver.
- It is required for:
  - conversion of methyl-FH_4 (inactive form of FH_4) to active formyl-FH_4, which, after polyglutamation, is a co-factor in the synthesis of purines and pyrimidines;
  - isomerisation of methylmalonyl-CoA to succinyl-CoA.
- Deficiency occurs most often in pernicious anaemia, which results from malabsorption caused by lack of intrinsic factor from the stomach. It causes neurological disease as well as anaemia.
- Vitamin B_{12} is given by injection every 3 months to treat pernicious anaemia.

the various types of blood cell on the other. The factors involved in controlling this balance are the *haematopoietic growth factors*, which direct the division and maturation of the progeny of these cells down to eight possible lines of development (Fig. 24.3). These cytokine growth factors are highly potent glycoproteins, acting at concentrations of 10^{-12} to 10^{-10} mol/L. They are present in plasma at very low concentrations under basal conditions, but on stimulation their concentrations can increase within hours by 1000-fold or more. *Erythropoietin* regulates the red cell line, and the signal for its production is blood loss and/or low tissue oxygen tension (see earlier). *CSFs* regulate the myeloid divisions of the white cell line, and the main stimulus for their production is infection (see also Ch. 7).

Recombinant erythropoietin (**epoetin**)[8] and recombinant granulocyte CSF (**filgrastim**, **lenograstim**, **pegfilgrastim**) are used clinically (see later); *thrombopoietin* has been manufactured in recombinant form but there are concerns about effects on tumour progression (it activates a cell surface protein that is an oncogene product) and it has been associated with severe immunologically mediated adverse effects. **Romiplostim** is a fusion protein that is an agonist at the thrombopoietin receptor and licensed for use by specialists for patients with immune (idiopathic) thrombocytopenic purpura (ITP) refractory to other treatments such as glucocorticoids, immunoglobulins and splenectomy. It is administered subcutaneously.

[8]One of the earliest therapeutic agents to be produced by recombinant technology, by Amgen in 1989 – a huge commercial success, heralding the emergence of the biotechnology industry – albeit with some anxious moments (see Fig. 24.4).

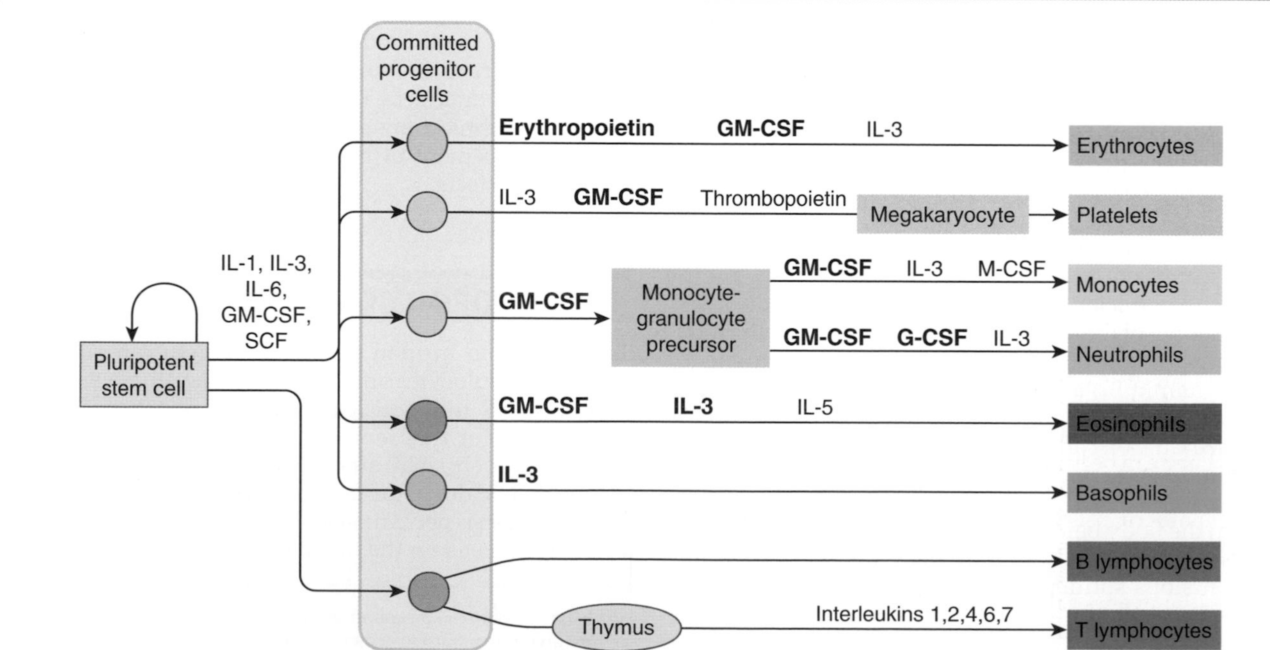

Fig. 24.3 Haematopoietic growth factors in blood cell differentiation. Various preparations of the factors shown in bold are in clinical use (see text). Most T cells generated in the thymus die by apoptosis; those that emerge are either CD4 or CD8 T cells. The colours used for the mature blood cells reflect how they appear in common staining preparations (and after which some are named). *CSF,* Colony-stimulating factor; *G-CSF,* granulocyte CSF; *GM-CSF*, granulocyte–macrophage CSF; *IL-1,* interleukin-1; *IL-3,* interleukin-3 or multi-CSF; *M-CSF,* macrophage CSF; *SCF,* stem cell factor. (See also Ch. 7.)

Eltrombopag is a small molecule agonist at thrombopoietin receptors, given by mouth, and licensed for use under expert supervision for adult and child ITP patients. It has also been used for patients with thrombocytopenia and cirrhosis associated with hepatitis C to increase platelet count to enable antiviral treatment (McHutchison et al., 2007). More recently it was licensed by the FDA for patients with aplastic anaemia unresponsive to immunosuppressive treatment in whom, interestingly, it increases cell counts of red and white blood cells as well as platelets and may produce a prolonged beneficial effect (Desmond et al., 2014).

Some of the other haematopoietic growth factors (e.g. interleukin-3, interleukin-5 and various other cytokines) are covered in Chapter 7.

ERYTHROPOIETIN

Erythropoietin is a glycoprotein produced in juxtatubular fibroblast cells in the kidney and also in macrophages; it stimulates committed erythroid progenitor cells to proliferate and generate erythrocytes (see Fig. 24.3). Recombinant human erythropoietins (epoietins) are made in cultured mammalian cells because their pharmacokinetic properties depend critically on the degree of glycosylation, a post-translational modification that occurs in mammalian but not so predictably in bacterial cells. They are used to treat anaemia caused by erythropoietin deficiency, for example in patients with chronic kidney disease, AIDS or cancer. Epoietins exist in several forms (alpha, beta, theta and zeta) with plasma half-lives of about 5 h. They are administered by injection three times weekly for convenience as this is the usual frequency of haemodialysis. **Darbepoetin**, a hyperglycosylated form, has a longer half-life (20–70 h) and can be administered less frequently, every 1–4 weeks; **methoxy polyethylene glycol-epoetin beta** is another preparation with an even longer half-life. Epoetin and darbepoetin are given intravenously or subcutaneously, the response being greater after subcutaneous injection and faster after intravenous injection.

Epoietins are reaching the end of patent protection and 'biosimilar' products have been licensed. Unlike the situation for small-molecule chemical entities where criteria for bioequivalence are relatively uncontroversial – see Chapter 9 – biologically produced macromolecules may vary markedly with seemingly minor changes in manufacture and have many opportunities to form immunologically distinct products during cell culture (see Ch. 5).

Unwanted effects

Transient influenza-like symptoms are common. Hypertension is also common and can cause encephalopathy with headache, disorientation and sometimes convulsions. Iron deficiency can be induced because more iron is required for the enhanced erythropoiesis. Blood viscosity increases as the haematocrit rises, increasing the risk of thrombosis, especially during dialysis. While anaemia in patients with chronic renal disease is associated with an increased risk of cardiovascular events, it has not been shown that correction of renal anaemia by treatment with epoetin -alpha or -beta or with darbepoetin with iron reduces this risk, and indeed there is evidence that normalisation of haemoglobin concentration in such patients may worsen cardiovascular risk especially of stroke (Drüeke et al., 2006; Pfeffer et al., 2009; Singh et al., 2006).

There have been reports of a devastating chronic condition known as pure red cell aplasia (PRCA), connected with the development of neutralising antibodies directed against erythropoietin which inactivate the endogenous hormone as well as the recombinant product (Berns, 2013). This has been a huge concern with indirect implications for quality control between batches of biological products and, indirectly, for the licensing of biosimilar products. Before 1998, only three cases of PRCA in association with epoetin treatment had been published. In that year, in response to concerns about transmitting bovine spongiform encephalopathy ('mad cow disease'), the formulation of the leading brand was changed, human serum albumin (used to stabilise the product) being replaced by polysorbate 80 and glycine. The incidence of PRCA increased abruptly (Fig 24.4), with approximately 250 documented cases by 2002, many of whom died or became completely dependent on blood transfusions. A large proportion had been treated with the new formulation. The mechanism whereby the manufacturing change led to the change in immunogenicity remains a matter of debate (Locatelli et al., 2007), but the packaging and storage were changed again in 2003, since when the incidence of PRCA has declined abruptly to baseline level (Fig. 24.4). The moral is that immunogenicity is unpredictable and can be caused by seemingly minor changes in manufacture or storage (Kuhlmann and Marre, 2010).

Clinical use

Iron or folate deficiency must be corrected before starting treatment. Parenteral iron preparations are often needed

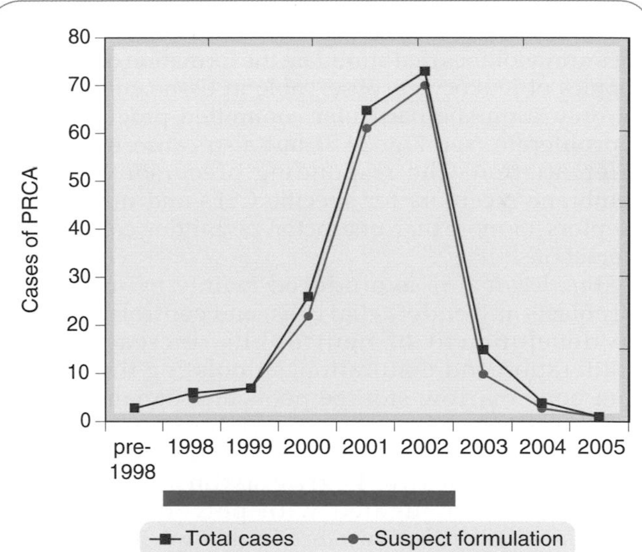

Fig. 24.4 Incidence of pure red cell aplasia (PRCA) in relation to introduction in 1998 of a changed formulation of the leading brand of epoetin. The incidence increased markedly and the suspect formulation *(blue)* accounted for almost all of the cases that were positive for anti-erythropoietin antibody *(red)*; the formulation and instructions for its administration and storage were changed again in 2003 with an abrupt subsequent decline in PRCA. The period when the suspect formulation was in use is indicated by the *blue rectangle*. (Redrawn from Kuhlmann, M., Marre, M., 2010. Lessons learned from biosimilar epoietins and insulins. Br. J. Diab. Vasc. Dis. 10, 90–97.)

(see earlier). Haemoglobin must be monitored and maintained within the range 10–12 g/dL (i.e. less than the normal range) to minimise the unwanted cardiovascular effects described earlier. The clinical use of epoetin is given in the clinical box.

New directions in treating the anaemia of chronic kidney disease

As explained earlier, while epoetins with iron are very effective in increasing the haemoglobin concentration when treating the anaemia of chronic kidney disease, it is of concern that this does not correct and indeed may exacerbate the increased cardiovascular risk of such patients. This is currently mitigated by selecting a target haemoglobin below the normal range found in healthy people but achieving and maintaining this is exacting and may leave patients symptomatic. The anaemia of chronic renal disease is multifactorial with the important contribution of reduced erythropoietin combined with abnormal iron metabolism and increased iron loss particularly in patients requiring chronic haemodialysis. It is possible that potentiating HIF could favourably influence iron metabolism as well as increase endogenous erythropoietin, since HIF also controls other aspects of iron metabolism. Inhibition of PHD increases $HIF_{1\alpha}$ by reducing its degradation (Fig 24.1), and an oral inhibitor, daprodustat was approved in 2023 by the FDA, and is the first oral treatment for anaemia caused by chronic kidney disease. It is not yet known if its use will be associated with improved cardiovascular outcomes compared with epoietin (Chen et al., 2019a, 2019b). Other HIF prolyl hydroxylase inhibitors are also undergoing phase 3 studies.

COLONY-STIMULATING FACTORS

CSFs are cytokines that stimulate the formation of maturing colonies of leukocytes, observable in tissue culture. They not only stimulate particular committed progenitor cells to proliferate (see Fig. 24.3) but also cause irreversible differentiation. The responding precursor cells have membrane receptors for specific CSFs and may express receptors for more than one factor, permitting collaborative interactions.

Granulocyte CSF is produced mainly by monocytes, fibroblasts and endothelial cells, and controls primarily the development of neutrophils, increasing their proliferation and maturation, stimulating their release from bone marrow storage pools and enhancing their function. Recombinant forms (**filgrastim**, which is not glycosylated, and glycosylated **lenograstim**) are used therapeutically. **Pegfilgrastim** is a derivative of filgrastim conjugated with polyethylene glycol ('pegylated') which slows its elimination, increasing its duration of action.

Thrombopoietin, made in liver and kidney, stimulates proliferation and maturation of megakaryocytes to form platelets. Recombinant thrombopoietin has been a tempting but horribly deceptive therapeutic target. Thrombocytopenia occurs in an autoimmune disorder known as immune (previously 'idiopathic') thrombocytopenic purpura (ITP) which is associated with a risk of severe spontaneous haemorrhage. Thrombocytopenia is also a predictable and limiting toxicity of many chemotherapeutic regimens in oncology (see Ch. 57), so a means to mitigate this would be a valuable prize. Recombinant thrombopoietin, seemingly the logical answer to this need, was manufactured and increased platelet counts in healthy volunteers and patients with mild chemotherapy-induced thrombocytopenia. But in early trials on healthy subjects, repeated dosing of a pegylated product caused the appearance of neutralising antibodies and consequently prolonged thrombocytopenia (Li et al., 2001), driving home the message from experience with erythropoietin (see Fig. 24.4) that subtle differences between biological products and natural mediators can lead to very serious immunologically mediated adverse effects. **Eltrombopag** (a small-molecule agonist administered orally) and **romiplostim** (a dimerised fusion protein analogue) are licensed as safe and effective therapeutic options for use in ITP. They bind to and activate thrombopoietin receptors which signal via the JAK/STAT pathway. Romiplostim is administered by subcutaneous injection. Both of these agonists are approved for treatment of patients with ITP who have not responded to other treatments such as immunosuppression by glucocorticoids (see Ch. 33), or splenectomy; eltrombopag is also used to increase platelet counts for aplastic anaemia and increases white and red blood cell counts as well as platelets in some such patients.

Administration and unwanted effects

Filgrastim and lenograstim are given subcutaneously or by intravenous infusion. Pegfilgrastim is administered subcutaneously. Gastrointestinal effects, fever, bone pain, myalgia and rash are recognised adverse effects; less common effects include pulmonary infiltrates and enlargement of liver or spleen.

Haematopoietic growth factors

Erythropoietin

- A hormone synthesised in the kidney and deficient in chronic kidney failure.
- Stimulates red cell production via receptors on the surface of red cell precursors.
- Its synthesis is controlled by HIF, a heterodimer controlled by PHD, the physiological oxygen sensor of the oxygen concentration of tissues. HIF is a transcription factor produced in many cell types and which controls a large number of genes implicated in responses to hypoxia.
- Is available, as epoetin or as a hyperglycosylated form **darbepoetin**, to treat patients with anaemia caused by chronic renal failure. The target haemoglobin concentration is lower than the normal range in healthy individuals because full correction of anaemia in such patients increases cardiovascular risk.
- Can cause transient flu-like symptoms, hypertension, iron deficiency (via increased utilisation) and increased blood viscosity.

Granulocyte CSF

- Stimulates neutrophil progenitors.
- Is available as **filgrastim**, **pegfilgrastim** or **lenograstim**; it is given parenterally.

Clinical uses of epoetin

- Anaemia of chronic *renal failure.* Inhibition of the physiological oxygen sensor is an alternative way to treat the anaemia of renal disease. One such inhibitor, **daprodustat**, is administered orally and was licensed recently.
- Anaemia during *chemotherapy* for cancer.
- Prevention of the anaemia that occurs in *premature infants* (unpreserved formulations are used because benzyl alcohol, used as a preservative, has been associated with a fatal toxic syndrome in neonates).
- To increase the yield of autologous blood before *blood donation.*
- Anaemia of *AIDS* (exacerbated by **zidovudine** which is used as an anti-viral).

Clinical uses of the colony-stimulating factors

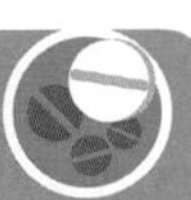

CSFs are used in specialist centres. Granulocyte colony stimulating factors are used:

- To reduce the severity/duration of neutropenia induced by cytotoxic drugs during:
  - intensive *chemotherapy* necessitating autologous *bone marrow rescue*
  - following *bone marrow transplant.*
- To harvest progenitor cells.
- To expand the number of harvested progenitor cells ex vivo before reinfusing them.
- For persistent neutropenia in advanced HIV infection.
- In aplastic anaemia.

Naturally occurring *thrombopoietin* stimulates megakaryocytes to produce platelets. It is not used clinically, but, as mentioned above, agonists at thrombopoietin receptors, e.g. a small molecule drug **eltrombopag** which is effective when given orally, are licensed for use in children and adults with ITP unresponsive to other treatments. Eltrombopag is also effective in some patients with aplastic anaemia increasing red and white blood cell production as well as platelet production.

HAEMOLYTIC ANAEMIA

Anaemia associated with increased red cell destruction can arise from genetic causes (e.g. sickle cell disease, thalassaemia, PNH) or a variety of non-genetic causes such as autoimmunity, infections and adverse drug reactions.

Sickle cell anaemia is caused by a mutation in the gene that codes the β-globin chain of adult haemoglobin (haemoglobin A), resulting in a single amino acid substitution. The abnormal haemoglobin (haemoglobin S) can polymerise when deoxygenated, changing the physical properties of the red cells (which deform to a sickle shape, hence the name) and damaging their cell membranes. P-selectin, a mediator stored in endothelial cells and platelets, is released and interacts with P-selectin glycoprotein ligand 1 (PSGL-1), causing the cells to adhere to vessel walls. This can block the microcirculation, causing tissue hypoxia and painful vaso-occlusive crises. Haemolysis also reduces the availability of nitric oxide (see Ch. 19) (Schaer et al., 2013). Polymerisation, as well as the severity of the disease, is markedly reduced when other forms of haemoglobin (A2 or/and F) are present.

PNH is a rare and previously untreatable form of haemolytic anaemia caused by clonal expansion of haematopoietic stem cells with somatic mutations that prevent formation of glycophosphatidylinositol (GPI), which anchors many proteins to the cell surface, rendering the cell susceptible to complement-mediated haemolysis. In addition to anaemia, patients with PNH suffer from other features, including thrombosis, attacks of abdominal pain and pulmonary hypertension (see Ch. 21).

DRUGS USED TO TREAT HAEMOLYTIC ANAEMIAS

As in most forms of haemolytic anaemia, treatment is symptomatic (e.g. analgesia for painful crises in patients with sickle cell disease) and supportive, e.g. oxygen therapy, blood transfusion when essential, treatment of iron overload and provision of adequate folate to support increased red cell turnover. Haemolytic anaemia associated with autoantibodies may respond to treatment with glucocorticoids (see Ch. 33). Here we mention specific treatments for two haemolytic diseases, ***sickle cell anaemia*** and ***PNH***, that are of particular clinical importance and pharmacological interest.

Hydroxycarbamide (also known as **hydroxyurea**) is a cytotoxic drug that has been used for decades to lower red cell and platelet counts in patients with *polycythaemia rubra vera* (a myeloproliferative disorder affecting especially the red cell lineage) or to treat chronic myeloid leukaemia. It is additionally used for sickle cell disease and reduces the frequency of painful crises (Charache et al., 1995; Wang et al., 2011; Weatherall, 2011). Hydroxycarbamide inhibits DNA synthesis by inhibiting *ribonucleotide reductase* and is S-phase specific (see Ch. 6). It increases circulating haemoglobin F, while reducing haemoglobin S. Hydroxycarbamide metabolism gives rise to nitric oxide, which may contribute to its beneficial effect in sickle cell disease. Some of its beneficial effect in reducing painful crises could relate to anti-inflammatory effects secondary to its cytotoxic action. Hydroxycarbamide is administered by mouth once daily at a rather lower starting dose than is used for treating malignant disease; reduced doses are used in patients with impaired renal function. The blood count and haemoglobin F are monitored and the dose adjusted accordingly. Once stabilised, treatment may be continued indefinitely.

Myelosuppression, nausea and rashes are the commonest adverse effects. Animal studies demonstrated teratogenicity and potential adverse effects on spermatogenesis. When used to treat malignant disease there is an increased risk of second malignancy, but this has not been observed when treating patients with sickle cell disease.

Crizanlizumab is a humanised monoclonal antibody that binds to P-selectin and blocks its interaction with PSGL-1 (see earlier). Administered intravenously each month it reduces the frequency of painful vaso-occlusive crises compared with placebo among patients with sickle cell disease, regardless of concomitant use of hydroxyurea (Ataga et al., 2017). A subsequent phase 3 study confirmed efficacy with an approximately 40% reduction in crises and crizanlizumab has been approved in the Unites States and Europe.

Treatment of paroxysmal nocturnal haemoglobinuria (PNH). **Eculizumab**, licensed for the treatment of PNH, is a humanised monoclonal antibody that blocks the complement protein C5 (see Ch. 7). In a double-blind, randomised, controlled trial of 87 patients, treatment with eculizumab dramatically reduced haemolysis and transfusion requirement during 6 months of treatment (Fig. 24.5). Patients must be inoculated against meningococcal infection before treatment. It is administered by intravenous infusion weekly for 4 weeks and then approximately every 2 weeks. Serious adverse effects include infection, notably meningococcal infection (the complement system is important in killing *N. meningitidis* organisms which are capsulated Gram-negative diplococci – see Ch. 52), but are uncommon. The commonest adverse effects are headache and back pain.

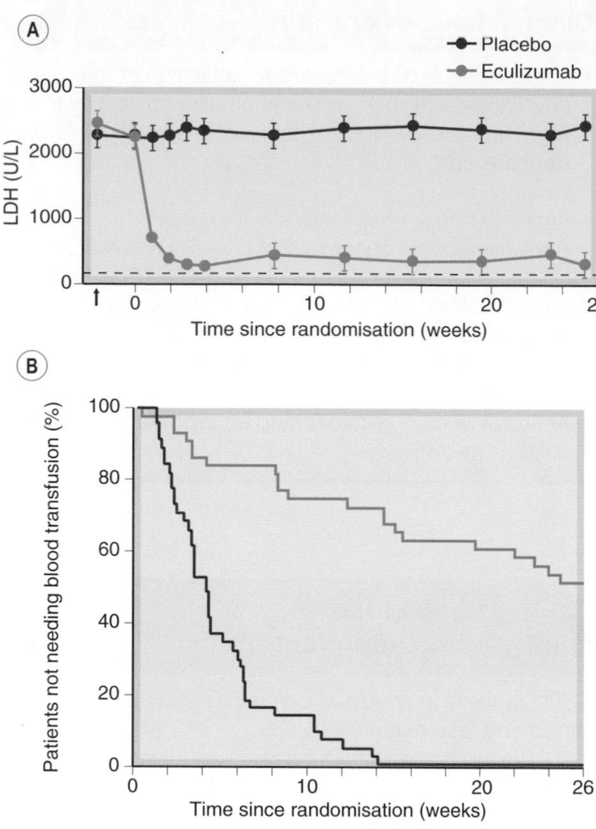

Fig. 24.5 Effect of eculizumab in patients with paroxysmal nocturnal haemoglobinuria (PNH). (A) Effect on plasma lactate dehydrogenase (LDH) activity, a measure of haemolysis. The horizontal dotted line shows the upper limit of normal. The arrow shows the baseline level at screening ($n = 44$ in the placebo group, $n = 43$ in the eculizumab group; $p < 0.001$). (B) Kaplan–Meier curves for the time to first transfusion during treatment in the same patients shown in (A) ($p < 0.001$). (Redrawn from Hillmen, P., Young, N.S., Schubert, J., et al., 2006. The complement inhibitor eculizumab in paroxysmal nocturnal hemoglobinuria. N. Engl. J. Med. 355, 1233–1243.)

REFERENCES AND FURTHER READING

General

Fishbane, S., 2009. Erythropoiesis-stimulating agent treatment with full anemia correction: a new perspective. Kidney Int. 75, 358–365.

Fishman, S.M., Christian, P., West, K.P., 2000. The role of vitamins in the prevention and control of anaemia. Public Health Nutr. 3, 125–150.

Ivan, M., Kaelin, W.G., 2017. The EGLN-HIF O2-sensing system: multiple inputs and feedbacks. Mol. Cell 66, 772–779.

Kurzrock, R., 2005. Thrombopoietic factors in chronic bone marrow failure states: the platelet problem revisited. Clin. Cancer Res. 11, 1361–1367.

Iron and iron deficiency

Andrews, N.C., 1999. Disorders of iron metabolism. N. Engl. J. Med. 341, 1986–1995.

Provan, D., Weatherall, D., 2000. Red cells, II: acquired anaemias and polycythaemia. Lancet 355, 1260–1268.

Toh, B.H., van Driel, I.R., Gleeson, P.A., 1997. Pernicious anaemia. N. Engl. J. Med. 337, 1441–1448.

Epoetins and HIF prolyl hydroxylase inhibitors

Berns, J.S., 2013. Pure red cell aplasia due to anti-erythropoietin antibodies. Available at: http://www.uptodate.com/contents/pure-red-cell-aplasia-due-to-anti-erythropoietin-antibodies.

Chen, N., Hao, C., Peng, X., et al., 2019a. Roxadustat for anemia in patients with kidney disease not receiving dialysis. N. Engl. J. Med. 381,1001–1010.

Chen, N., Hao, C., Liu, B.C., et al., 2019b. Roxadustat treatment for anemia in patients undergoing long-term dialysis. N. Engl. J. Med. 381, 1011–1022.

Drüeke, T., Locatelli, F., Clyne, N., et al., for the CREATE Investigators, 2006. Normalization of hemoglobin level in patients with chronic kidney disease and anemia. N. Engl. J. Med. 355, 2071–2084.

Kuhlmann, M., Marre, M., 2010. Lessons learned from biosimilar epoietins and insulins. Br. J. Diab. Vasc. Dis. 10, 90–97.

Locatelli, F., Del Vecchio, L., Pozzoni, P., 2007. Pure red-cell aplasia "epidemic" – mystery completely revealed? Perit. Dial. Int. 27 (Suppl. 2), S303–S307.

Pfeffer, M.A., for the TREAT investigators, et al., 2009. A trial of darbepoetin alfa in type 2 diabetes and chronic kidney disease. N. Engl. J. Med. 361, 2019–2034.
Singh, A.K., Szczech, L., Tang, K.L., et al., for the CHOIR Investigators, 2006. Correction of anemia with epoetin alfa in chronic kidney disease. N. Engl. J. Med. 355, 2085–2098.

Colony-stimulating factors

Desmond, R., Townsley, D.M., Dumitriu, D., et al., 2014. Eltrombopag restores trilineage hematopoiesis in refractory severe aplastic anemia that can be sustained on discontinuation of the drug. Blood 123, 1818–1825.
Li, J., Yang, C., Xia, Y., et al., 2001. Thrombocytopenia caused by the development of antibodies to thrombopoietin. Blood 98, 3241–3248.
Lieschke, G.J., Burges, A.W., 1992. Granulocyte colony-stimulating factor and granulocyte–macrophage colony-stimulating factor. N. Engl. J. Med. 327 (1–35), 99–106.
McHutchison, J.G., Dusheiko, G., Shiffman, M.L., et al., 2007. Eltrombopag for thrombocytopenia in patients with cirrhosis associated with hepatitis C. N. Engl. J. Med. 357, 2227–2236.
Mohle, R., Kanz, L., 2007. Hematopoietic growth factors for hematopoietic stem cell mobilization and expansion. Semin. Hematol. 44, 193–202.

Haemolytic anaemias

Ataga, K.I., Kutlar, A., Kanter, J., et al., 2017. Crizanlizumab for the prevention of pain crises in sickle cell disease. N. Engl. J. Med. 376, 429–439.
Charache, S., Terrin, M.L., Moore, R.D., et al., 1995. Effect of hydroxyurea on the frequency of painful crises in sickle-cell-anemia. N. Engl. J. Med. 332, 1317–1322.
Hillmen, P., Young, N.S., Schubert, J., et al., 2006. The complement inhibitor eculizumab in paroxysmal nocturnal hemoglobinuria. N. Engl. J. Med. 355, 1233–1243.
Schaer, D.J., Buehler, P.W., Alayash, A.I., Belcher, J.D., Vercellotti, G.M., 2013. Hemolysis and free hemoglobin revisited: exploring hemoglobin and hemin scavengers as a novel class of therapeutic proteins. Blood 121, 1276–1284.
Wang, W.C., Ware, R.E., Miller, S.T., et al., 2011. For the BABY HUG investigators. Hydroxycarbamide in very young children with sickle-cell anaemia: a multicentre, randomised, controlled trial (BABY HUG). Lancet 377, 1663–1672.
Weatherall, D.J., 2011. Hydroxycarbamide for sickle-cell anaemia in infancy. Lancet 377, 1628–1630.

25 Anti-inflammatory and immunosuppressant drugs

OVERVIEW

The inflammatory response – essentially a manifestation of the immune system in action – is a protective response, but there are occasions when it is activated inappropriately or outlasts its usefulness. In such cases, we may turn to the anti-inflammatory and immunosuppressive drugs for remedial action. This chapter deals with the main groups of these drugs, together with their therapeutic uses in a range of different inflammatory and immune disorders. While generally associated with conditions such as rheumatoid arthritis, inflammation forms a significant component of many, if not most, of the diseases encountered in the clinic; consequently, anti-inflammatory drugs are extensively employed in virtually all branches of medicine. In UK alone, 1.4 billion items of this type were dispensed in 2020/21 and since some of the drugs in this category are available without prescription from pharmacy counters, the true figure is probably much higher.

INTRODUCTION

Anti-inflammatory drugs may be divided conveniently into five major groups:

- Drugs that inhibit the cyclo-oxygenase (COX) enzyme(s) – the *non-steroidal anti-inflammatory drugs* (NSAIDs) and the *coxibs.*
- Antirheumatoid drugs – the so-called *disease-modifying antirheumatic drugs* (DMARDs). This group comprises some synthetic drugs, 'synthetic (s) DMARDs', anticytokine and other biopharmaceutical agents, referred to as 'biologic (b) DMARDs'.
- The glucocorticoids.
- Drugs specifically used to control gout.
- Antihistamines used for the treatment of allergic inflammation.

In this chapter we first describe the therapeutic effects, mechanism of action and unwanted effects common to NSAIDs and then deal in a little more detail with **aspirin**, **paracetamol**, **ibuprofen** as well as drugs that are selective for COX-2. The antirheumatoid drugs comprise a varied group comprising both synthetic and biopharmaceuticals as well as immunosuppressant drugs that are also used to treat other autoimmune diseases and prevent rejection of organ transplants. The glucocorticoids are covered in Chapters 4 and 33 but are briefly discussed in this chapter. Finally, we consider drugs that are used to control gout and the histamine H_1 receptor antagonists, which are used to treat acute allergic conditions.

CYCLO-OXYGENASE INHIBITORS

This group includes the 'traditional' (in the historical sense) NSAIDs[1] as well as the coxibs, which are more selective for COX-2. NSAIDs, sometimes called *aspirin-like drugs* or *antipyretic analgesics*, are among the most widely used of all medicines. There are now more than 50 different examples on the global market; common examples are listed in Table 25.1 and some significant NSAID structures are depicted in Fig. 25.1. It has been estimated that these drugs constitute 5%–10% of all prescriptions and are taken daily by more than 30 million people worldwide (McEvoy et al., 2021).

NSAIDs provide symptomatic relief from fever, pain and swelling in chronic joint disease such as occurs in osteo- and rheumatoid arthritis, as well as in more acute inflammatory conditions such as fractures, sprains, sports and other soft tissue injuries. They are also useful in the treatment of postoperative, dental and menstrual pain, as well as headaches and migraine. Several NSAIDs are available over the counter and are widely used to treat minor aches and pains and other ailments and some are available in different formulations including tablets, injections and gels. Virtually all these drugs, particularly the 'traditional' NSAIDs, can have significant unwanted effects, especially in the elderly. Newer agents generally provoke fewer adverse effects.

While there are differences between individual NSAIDs, their primary pharmacology is related to their shared ability to inhibit the fatty acid COX enzyme(s), thereby inhibiting the biosynthesis of prostaglandins and thromboxanes. As explained in Chapter 17, there are two common isoforms of this enzyme, COX-1 and COX-2 (although there may be further isoforms as yet uncharacterised). While they are closely related (>60% sequence identity) and catalyse the same reaction, there are important differences between the expression and role of these two isoforms. COX-1 is a constitutive enzyme expressed in most tissues, including blood platelets. It has a 'housekeeping' role in the body, being involved principally in tissue homeostasis. It is, for example, responsible for the production of prostaglandins involved in gastric cytoprotection (see Ch. 30), platelet aggregation (see Ch. 23), renal blood flow autoregulation (see Ch. 29) and the initiation of parturition (see Ch. 35).

In contrast, COX-2 is induced in inflammatory cells when they are activated by (for example) the inflammatory cytokines – interleukin (IL)-1 and tumour necrosis factor (TNF)-α (see Ch. 17). Thus, the COX-2 isoform is therefore generally considered to be mainly responsible for the production of the prostanoid mediators of inflammation (Vane and Botting, 2001). There are, however, some significant exceptions. COX-2 is constitutively expressed in the kidney, generating prostacyclin (prostaglandin I_2),

[1]Here, we use the term *NSAID* to include the coxibs but this convention is not always followed in the literature.

Table 25.1 Comparison of some common anti-inflammatory cyclo-oxygenase inhibitors

Type	Drug	Indication	COX selectivity	Comments
Propionates	Dexibuprofen	OA, MS, D, H&M	NT	Active enantiomer of ibuprofen
	Dexketoprofen	PO, D, H&M	NT	Isomer of ketoprofen
	Fenoprofen	RA, OA, MS, PO	Non-selective	Prodrug; activated in liver (not UK)
	Felbinac	MS, OA	NT	Metabolite of fenbufen
	Flurbiprofen	RA, OA, MS, PO, D, H&M	Very COX-1 selective	—
	Ibuprofen	RA, OA, MS, PO, D, H&M	Weakly COX-1 selective	Many formulations; available OTC in pharmacies; suitable for children
	Ketoprofen	RA, OA, G, MS, PO, D	Weakly COX-1 selective	Suitable for mild disease
	Naproxen	RA, OA, G, MS, PO, D	Weakly COX-1 selective	Possibly CV safe?
	Tiaprofenic acid	RA, OA, MS	NT	—
Indoles and derivatives	Acemetacin	RD, OA, MS, PO	NT	Ester of indometacin
	Indometacin	RA, OA, G, MS, PO, D	Weakly COX-1 selective	Suitable for moderate to severe disease
	Sulindac	RA, OA, G, MS	Weakly COX-2 selective	Prodrug
Oxicams	Meloxicam	RA, OA, AS	Moderately COX-2 selective	Possibly fewer gastrointestinal effects
	Piroxicam	RA, OA, AS	Weakly COX-2 selective	—
	Tenoxicam	RA, OA, MS	NT	—
Sulfonyl and sulfonamide coxibs	Celecoxib	RA, OA, AS	Moderately COX-2 selective	Fewer gastrointestinal effects
	Etoricoxib	RA, OA, G, AS	Very COX-2 selective	—
	Parecoxlb	PO	NT	Prodrug activated in liver
Phenylacetates	Aceclofenac	RA, OA, AS	NT	—
	Diclofenac	RA, OA, G, MS, PO, H&M	Weakly COX-2 selective	Moderate potency. Various salts
Fenamates	Mefenamic acid	RA, OA, PO, D	NT	Moderate activity
	Tolfenamic acid	H&M	NT	—
Miscellaneous	Ketorolac	PO	Highly COX-1 selective	Mainly ocular use
	Nabumetone	RA, OA	NT	Prodrug activated in liver
	Etodolac	RA, OA	Moderately COX-2 selective	Possibly fewer GI effects
Salicylates	Aspirin	Mainly CV usage	Weakly COX-1 selective	Component of many OTC preparations Unsuitable for children

The chemical classes of these NSAIDs are also shown because sometimes they are referred to in this manner.
AS, Ankylosing spondylitis; *COX,* cyclo-oxygenase; *CV,* cardiovascular; *D,* dysmenorrhoea; *G,* acute gout; *GI,* gastrointestinal; *H&M,* headache and migraine; *MS,* musculoskeletal injuries and pain; *NT,* not tested; *OA,* osteoarthritis; *OTC,* over-the-counter; *PO,* postoperative pain; *RA,* rheumatoid arthritis.
Data from British National Formulary, 2021, and COX selectivity data, where tested, from Warner, T.D.,et al, 1999. Proc Natl. Acad. Sci. USA 96, 7563-7568; Warner, T.D., Mitchell, J.A., 2004. FASEB J. 18, 790–804; and Warner, T.D., Mitchell, J.A., 2008. Lancet 371, 270–273.

which plays a part in renal homeostasis (see Ch. 29), and also in the central nervous system (CNS), where its function is not yet clear.

Although NSAIDs differ in toxicity and degree of patient acceptability and tolerance, with certain provisos, their pharmacological actions are broadly similar. **Aspirin** has other qualitatively different pharmacological actions and **paracetamol** is an interesting exception to the general NSAID stereotype (see later). Some notes on the relative selectivity of several NSAIDs and coxibs are provided in Table 25.1.

MECHANISM OF ACTION

In 1971, Vane and his colleagues demonstrated that the NSAIDs inhibit prostaglandin biosynthesis by a direct action on the COX enzyme and established the hypothesis

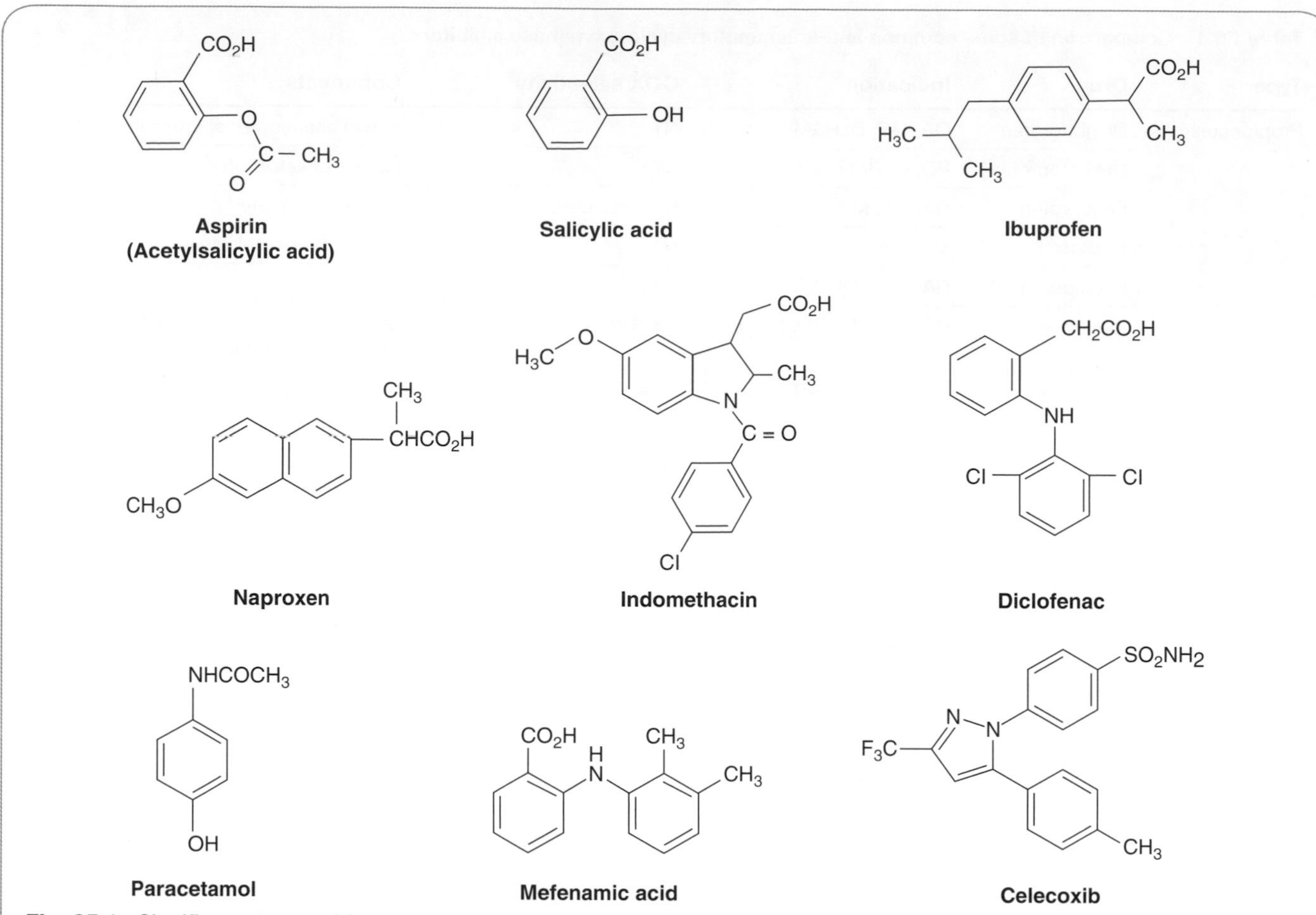

Fig. 25.1 Significant structural features of some non-steroidal anti-inflammatory drugs (NSAIDs) and coxibs. Aspirin contains an acetyl group that is responsible for the inactivation of the cyclo-oxygenase (COX) enzyme. **Salicylic acid** is the end product when **aspirin** is de-acetylated but oddly has anti-inflammatory activity in its own right. **Paracetamol** is a commonly used analgesic agent also of simple structure. Most 'classic' NSAIDs are carboxylic acids including **ibuprofen**. Coxibs (**celecoxib** shown here as an example), however, often contain sulfonamide or sulfone groups. These are thought to be important in determining the selectivity of the molecule as they impede access to the hydrophobic channel in the COX-1 enzyme (see Fig. 25.2).

that this single action explained the vast majority of their therapeutic actions and side effects. This has since been confirmed by numerous studies.

COX enzymes are bifunctional, having two distinct catalytic activities. A *dioxygenase* step is followed by a second, *peroxidase*, reaction (see Ch. 17). Both COX-1 and COX-2 are haem-containing enzymes that exist as homodimers attached to intracellular membranes. Interestingly, only one monomer is catalytically active at one time. Binding of NSAIDs to one COX monomer can inhibit the catalytic activity of the entire dimeric complex.

Most NSAIDs inhibit only the initial dioxygenation reaction. They are generally rapid 'competitive reversible' inhibitors of COX-1, but there are differences in their kinetics. Inhibition of COX-2 is generally more time dependent and the inhibition is often irreversible.

Structurally, COX-1 and COX-2 are very similar; both contain a hydrophobic 'channel' into which the arachidonic or other substrate fatty acids dock so that the oxygenation reaction can proceed. To block these enzymes, NSAIDs enter this channel, forming hydrogen bonds with an arginine residue at position 120, thus preventing substrate fatty acids from entering the catalytic domain. However, a single amino acid change (isoleucine to valine at position 523) in the structure of the entrance of this channel in COX-2 results in a 'bulge' in the channel that is not found in COX-1. This is important in understanding why some drugs, especially those with large sulfur-containing side groups (such as **celecoxib**), are more selective for the COX-2 isoform (Fig. 25.2). **Aspirin** is, however, an anomaly. It enters the active site and acetylates a serine at position 530, irreversibly inactivating COX. This is the basis for aspirin's long-lasting effects on platelets. Interestingly, aspirin-inactivated COX-2 can still generate some hydroxyacids but is unable produce the endoperoxide intermediate required for prostanoid synthesis.

PHARMACOLOGICAL ACTIONS

All the NSAIDs have actions very similar to those of **aspirin**, the archetypal NSAID which was introduced into clinical medicine in the 1890s. Their pharmacological profile is listed in the key points box.

Most traditional NSAIDs inhibit both COX-1 and COX-2, although their relative potency against the two isoforms differs. It is believed that the anti-inflammatory action (and probably most analgesic and antipyretic actions) of

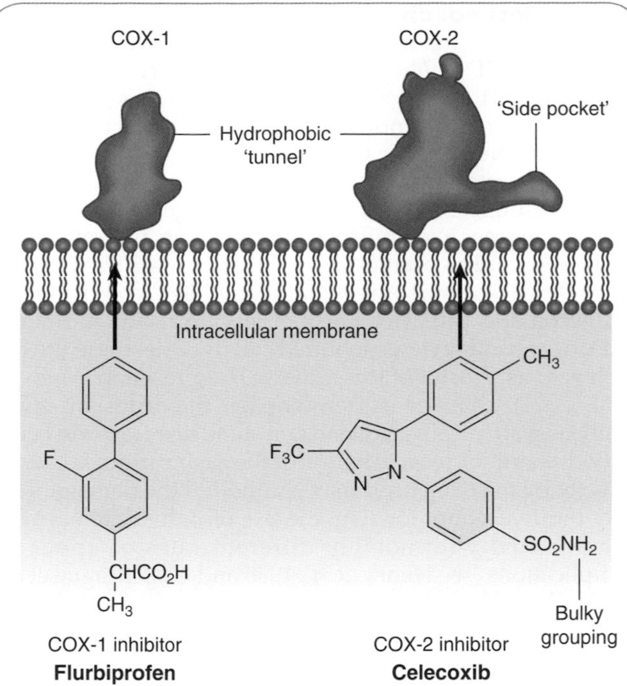

Fig. 25.2 Schematic diagram comparing the binding sites of cyclo-oxygenase (COX)-1 and COX-2. The illustration shows the differences in non-steroidal anti-inflammatory (NSAID) binding sites in the two isoforms. Note that the COX-2 binding site is characterised by a 'side pocket' that can accommodate the relatively 'bulky' groups, such as the sulfonamide moiety of **celecoxib**, which would impede its access to the COX-1 site. Other NSAIDs, such as **flurbiprofen** (shown here), can enter the active site of either enzyme. (After Luong, C., Miller, A., Barnett, J., et al., 1996. Flexibility of the NSAID binding site in the structure of human cyclooxygenase-2. Nat. Struct. Biol. 3, 927–933.)

the NSAIDs are related to inhibition of COX-2, while their physiological effects are largely a result of their inhibition of COX-1. Unfortunately, it is the latter which are often responsible for the unwanted effects of these drugs, particularly those affecting the gastrointestinal (GI) tract. Compounds with a selective inhibitory action on COX-2 show fewer GI side effects, however are by no means as well tolerated as was once hoped.

ANTI-INFLAMMATORY EFFECTS

As described in Chapter 17, many mediators coordinate inflammatory and allergic reactions. The NSAIDs reduce those components in which prostaglandins, mainly derived from COX-2, play a significant part. These include not only the characteristic vasodilatation of inflammation (because of reduced synthesis of vasodilator prostaglandins) but also the oedema because vasodilatation facilitates and potentiates the action of mediators that increase the permeability of postcapillary venules, such as histamine.

Other actions besides inhibition of COX may contribute to the anti-inflammatory effects of some NSAIDs. Reactive oxygen radicals produced by neutrophils and macrophages are implicated in tissue damage in some conditions, and some NSAIDs (e.g. **sulindac**) have oxygen radical-scavenging effects as well as COX inhibitory activity, so may decrease tissue damage. **Aspirin** also inhibits expression of the transcription factor nuclear factor kappa B (NFκB) (see Ch. 3), which has a key role in the transcription of the genes for inflammatory mediators. Reports have also emerged of an NSAID binding site on sulfotransferase enzymes (Wang et al., 2017) but the significance of this to the regulation of inflammation has yet to be established.

While NSAIDs suppress the signs and symptoms of inflammation, they have little or no action on the underlying chronic disease itself. As a class, they are generally also without direct effect on other aspects of inflammation, such as cytokine/chemokine release, leukocyte migration and lysosomal enzyme release, which contribute to tissue damage in chronic inflammatory conditions such as rheumatoid arthritis, vasculitis and nephritis. As such they are often a treatment but rarely a cure.

ANTIPYRETIC EFFECTS

Neurons in the hypothalamus control the balance between heat production and heat loss, thereby regulating normal body temperature. Fever occurs when there is a disturbance of this hypothalamic 'thermostat', which raises body temperature. NSAIDs reset this thermostat. Once there has been a return to the normal 'set point', the temperature-regulating mechanisms (dilatation of superficial blood vessels, sweating, etc.) then operate to reduce temperature.

The NSAIDs exert their antipyretic action largely through inhibition of prostaglandin production in the hypothalamus (see Lee and Simmons 2018). During infection, bacterial endotoxins cause the release from macrophages of IL-1 (see Ch. 17). In the hypothalamus this cytokine stimulates the generation of E-type prostaglandins that, through the EP3 receptor, elevate the temperature set point. COX-2 may have a role here, because IL-1 induces this enzyme in the hypothalamic vascular endothelium. There is some evidence that prostaglandins are not the only mediators of fever, hence NSAIDs may have an additional antipyretic effect through mechanisms as yet undiscovered. Normal body temperature in healthy humans is not affected by NSAIDs.[2]

ANALGESIC EFFECTS

The NSAIDs are effective against mild or moderate pain, especially that arising from inflammation or tissue damage. Two sites of action have been identified.

Peripherally, NSAIDs decrease production of prostaglandins that sensitise nociceptors to inflammatory mediators such as bradykinin (see Chs 17 and 43) and they are therefore effective in arthritis, bursitis, pain of muscular and vascular origin, toothache, dysmenorrhoea, the pain of postpartum states and the pain of cancer metastases in bone. All conditions are associated with increased local prostaglandin synthesis probably as a consequence of COX-2 induction. Alone, or in combination with paracetamol or opioids, they decrease postoperative pain and, in some cases, can reduce the requirement for opioids by as much as one-third (see Thybo et al., 2019 as a recent example). Their ability to relieve headache may be related to the reduction in vasodilator prostaglandins acting on the cerebral vasculature (see Ch. 42).

[2]With possible exception of paracetamol, which has been used clinically to lower body temperature during surgery.

In addition to these peripheral effects, there is a second, less well-characterised (at least in humans) central action in the spinal cord and possibly elsewhere in the CNS. Peripheral inflammatory lesions increase COX-2 expression and prostaglandin release within the cord itself, facilitating transmission from afferent pain fibres to relay neurons in the dorsal horn (see Ch. 43 and Vuilleumier et al., 2018).

UNWANTED EFFECTS

Although generally well tolerated, the overall burden of unwanted side effects from NSAIDs is high, probably reflecting the fact that they are used extensively, often for extended periods of time in an un-supervised manner (being available over the counter), and often by the more vulnerable elderly population. When used for joint diseases (which usually necessitates fairly large doses and sustained treatment), there is a high incidence of side effects – particularly related to the GI tract and cardiovascular system, but also in the liver, kidney, spleen, blood and bone marrow. They may also contribute to less organ-specific pathology such as falls in the elderly, where enhanced surveillance and protective pharmacological strategies are warranted to mitigate risk (see Wongrakpanich et al., 2018). The rule for prescribing NAIDS is consequently to use the lowest dose for the shortest possible period of time.

Because prostaglandins are involved in gastric cytoprotection, platelet aggregation, renal vascular autoregulation and induction of labour, all NSAIDs share a broadly similar profile of mechanism-dependent side effects on these processes, although there may be other additional unwanted effects peculiar to individual members of the group. Of note, the relative risk of given side effects (such as cardiovascular events) also appears to vary within the class: information which should influence prescription choice dependent on the indication and recipient. COX-2-selective drugs have less, but not negligible, GI toxicity.

Therapeutic effects of COX inhibitors

Important NSAIDs include **aspirin**, **ibuprofen**, **naproxen**, **indometacin**, **piroxicam** and **paracetamol**. These drugs inhibit COX enzymes, and therefore prostanoid synthesis, in inflammatory cells. Inhibition of the COX-2 isoform is probably crucial for their therapeutic actions. Agents with more selective inhibition of COX-2 (and thus fewer adverse effects on the GI tract) include **celecoxib** and **etoricoxib**. Class effects include:

- *An anti-inflammatory action*: the decrease in prostaglandin E_2 and prostacyclin reduces vasodilatation and, indirectly, oedema. Accumulation of inflammatory cells is not directly reduced.
- *An analgesic effect*: decreased prostaglandin generation means less sensitisation of nociceptive nerve endings to inflammatory mediators such as bradykinin and 5-hydroxytryptamine. Relief of headache is probably a result of decreased prostaglandin-mediated vasodilatation.
- *An antipyretic effect*: interleukin 1 releases prostaglandins in the CNS, where they elevate the hypothalamic set point for temperature control, thus causing fever.

Gastrointestinal disturbances

Adverse GI events are the commonest unwanted effects of the NSAIDs. They are believed to result mainly from inhibition of gastric COX-1, which synthesises prostaglandins that normally inhibit acid secretion and protect the mucosa (see Ch. 30).

Mild symptoms of gastric discomfort ('dyspepsia') and nausea result from gastric mucosal damage, which in some cases progresses to manifest gastric bleeding, ulceration and perforation. It has been estimated that 34%–46% of users of NSAIDs will sustain some GI damage which, while it may be asymptomatic, can carry a risk of morbidity and mortality. Indeed, a recent review identified 400–1000 deaths in the UK each year as a result of this adverse drug reaction (McEvoy et al., 2021). Damage is seen whether the drugs are given orally or systemically. However, in some cases (aspirin being a good example), local irritation of the gastric mucosa caused directly by the drug itself may compound the damage. This may partly account for why the use of individual NSAIDs is associated with notably different rates of upper GI complications (see Henry et al., 1996 and Castellsague et al., 2012). Oral administration of 'replacement' prostaglandin analogues such as **misoprostol**, or more commonly co-prescription of proton-pump inhibitors (PPI) or histamine H2-receptor antagonists (see Ch. 30), is now routinely employed to diminish the gastric damage produced by NSAIDs, especially in high risk individuals.

Based on extensive experimental evidence, it had been predicted that COX-2-selective agents would provide good anti-inflammatory and analgesic actions with less gastric damage compared to standard NSAIDs. Whilst borne out in large clinical trials of drugs such as celecoxib, the results have not been as clear-cut as had been hoped. Whilst the risk is reduced it is not eliminated and the need for PPI or alternate gastro-protective strategies is not removed (see Bakhriansyah et al., 2017). COX-2-selective agents are also associated with an increased burden of alternate side effects (notably cardiovascular, famously leading to the withdrawal of some agents such as **rofecoxib**). The actual situation following therapy is complex because the degree to which the two COX isoforms are inhibited depends not only upon the intrinsic activity of the drug but the relative inhibitory kinetics. Warner and Mitchell (2008) have suggested that the degree to which NSAIDs inhibit COX-1 at the concentration at which they inhibit COX-2 by 80% is the best measure of 'selectivity'. Newer strategies to ameliorate the gastrointestinal side effects of NSAIDs include the addition of nitric oxide (NO) generating moieties (NO-NSAIDS or COX-inhibiting NO-donating drugs; CINODs) or, perhaps more promisingly, the linkage of hydrogen sulfide (H2S) releasing molecules to NSAIDs (or their derivatives, see Wallace et al., 2020). None are currently on the market.

Damage to the small intestine and colon (NSAID enteropathy) may also occur following NSAID treatment, is difficult to prevent pharmacologically and can lead to significant morbidity and mortality, especially if anticoagulants are co-prescribed (Lanas et al., 2015). It is not clear if a COX-dependent mechanism is involved.

Hypersensitivity reactions

Approximately 5%–15% of patients exposed to NSAIDs experience hypersensitivity reactions: in fact, some authors believe that the NSAIDs are the most significant cause of drug-induced hypersensitivity reactions surpassing the β-lactam antibiotics (Blanca-Lopez et al., 2019). One manifestation of this is *NSAID-sensitive asthma* or what is now described as NSAID-exacerbated respiratory disease (NERD), characterized by moderate-to-severe asthma, often in association with chronic rhinosinusitis and nasal polyps. The exact mechanism is unknown, but inhibition of COX and overproduction of cysteinyl leukotrienes is implicated (see Ch. 28) and pre-existing viral infections may predispose (Woo et al., 2020). **Aspirin** is the worst offender but in some, although not all, patients there is cross-reaction with other NSAIDs (except possibly selective COX-2 inhibitors).

Another manifestation of hypersensitivity, skin rashes, is also a common idiosyncratic unwanted effect of NSAIDs, particularly with **mefenamic acid** (10%–15% frequency) and **sulindac** (5%–10% frequency). They vary from mild erythematous, urticarial and photosensitivity reactions to more serious and potentially fatal diseases including *Stevens–Johnson syndrome* (a blistering rash that extends into the gut, see Ch. 58), and its more severe form, *toxic epidermal necrolysis*[3] (fortunately very rare). The mechanism is unclear. See (Laidlaw and Cahill, 2017) for further reading.

Adverse renal effects

Therapeutic doses of NSAIDs taken for short periods in otherwise healthy individuals pose little threat to kidney function, but in susceptible patients they cause acute renal insufficiency, which is reversible on discontinuing the drug (see Ch. 58). This occurs because of inhibition of the biosynthesis of PGE_2 and PGI_2 (prostacyclin) which are involved in the maintenance of renal blood flow, specifically in the PGE_2-mediated compensatory vasodilatation that occurs in response to the action of noradrenaline (norepinephrine) or angiotensin II (see Ch. 29). Neonates and the elderly are especially at risk, as are patients with heart, liver or kidney disease, or a reduced circulating blood volume. Concurrent use of drugs affecting the renin-angiotensin system (such as ACE-inhibitors), diuretics or calcineurin inhibitors is an additional risk factor. Whilst classically thought to be reversible on discontinuation of the drug there is now evidence that long term NSAID use may contribute to chronic renal impairment.

Prolonged NSAID consumption, especially NSAID abuse,[4] can cause analgesic nephropathy characterised by interstitial nephritis and renal papillary necrosis (see Ch. 29). **Phenacetin** (now withdrawn) was the main culprit; paracetamol, one of its major metabolites, is much less toxic. NSAIDs may also drive electrolyte and acid-base disorders (for instance hyperkalaemia and Type 4 renal tubular acidosis) and elicit the nephrotic syndrome. For comprehensive reviews of the effects of NSAIDs on the kidneys (see Horl, 2010 and Baker and Perazella, 2020).

Cardiovascular side effects

Though aspirin is widely used clinically for its long-lasting antiplatelet action (see later) other NSAIDs lack this property, being associated with an increased rate of thrombotic cardiovascular events (stroke and myocardial infarction), even with short term use. The risk is associated with the relative degree of COX-2 versus COX-1 inhibition, with agents displaying higher COX-2 selectivity (for instance the coxibs) being the worst offenders. The biology underlying this effect is still debated, however undoubtedly relates to disturbance of the thrombotic tone exerted by vascular endothelial cell-derived anti-thrombotic prostacyclin (generated via COX-1 and COX-2) and platelet-derived pro-thrombotic and vasoconstrictive thromboxane A2 (generated via COX-1 alone) (see Mitchell et al., 2019).

NSAIDS oppose the effects of some antihypertensive drugs and also raise blood pressure in patients not taking antihypertensive drugs, thus therefore predisposing to adverse cardiovascular events through a second mechanism. Astonishingly, given the fact that some of these drugs have been in use for half a century or more, this was only recognised as a serious issue during trials of the aforementioned COX-2 inhibitor **rofecoxib** in the early 2000's. NSAID's hypertensive effect is dose- and time-dependent and rarely occurs with short-term (i.e. days) administration. Its aetiology is multi-factorial and includes suppression of vasodilatory prostacyclin release as well as modulation of renin release, itself regulated by prostaglandins acting on cells of the macula densa region. The resultant sodium and thus water retention also explains why NSAIDs may precipitate or worsen heart failure. An additional explanation for the blood pressure rise relates to inhibition of renal COX-2 that controls the methylarginine system, itself suppressing the release of cardiotoxic asymmetrical dimethyl arginate (ADMA) by the constitutive nitric oxide synthase (NOS) enzyme (see Kirby et al., 2016 and Ch. 19). It is now known that (with the exception of low-dose aspirin) these effects are common to most NSAIDs, especially following prolonged use. Patients with pre-existing cardiovascular disease are at particular risk. Some drugs (e.g. **naproxen**) appear to be better tolerated in this respect than others (e.g. **diclofenac**) (see Schjerning et al., 2020).

Other unwanted effects

Other, much less common, unwanted effects of NSAIDs include CNS effects, bone marrow disturbances and liver disorders, the last being more likely if there is already renal impairment.[5] **Paracetamol** overdose causes liver failure. All NSAIDs (except selective COX-2 inhibitors and **paracetamol** in therapeutic doses) prevent platelet aggregation to some extent and therefore may prolong bleeding. Again, **aspirin** is the main problem in this regard and risk is significantly heightened if anti-coagulants are co-prescribed.

General unwanted effects of cyclo-oxygenase (COX) inhibitors

Unwanted effects, many stemming from inhibition of the constitutive housekeeping enzyme COX-1 isoform, are common, particularly in the elderly, and include the following:

- *Dyspepsia, nausea, vomiting* and *other GI effects.* Gastric and intestinal damage may occur with chronic

[3]A horrible condition where skin peels away in sheets as if scalded.

[4]So called because the availability of NSAIDs (often in combination with other substances, such as caffeine) in over-the-counter proprietary medicines has tempted some people to consume them in prodigious quantities, for every conceivable malady. Swiss workers manufacturing watches used to share analgesics in the same way as sweets or cigarettes!

[5]An odd side effect of the NSAID diclofenac came to light when a team of scientists investigated the curious decline in the vulture population of the Indian subcontinent. These birds feed on dead cattle some of which had been treated with diclofenac for veterinary reasons. Apparently, residual amounts of the drug in the carcasses proved uniquely toxic to this species.

General unwanted effects of cyclo-oxygenase (COX) inhibitors—cont'd

use, with risk of haemorrhage, ulceration and perforation which can be life-threatening. The cause is suppression of gastroprotective prostaglandins in the gastric mucosa.
- *Adverse cardiovascular effects.* These are multi-faceted and occur with effectively all non-steroidal anti-inflammatory drugs (NSAIDs) and coxibs. Hypertension and increased thrombotic risk drive increased rates of stroke and myocardial infarction. Heart failure is worsened.
- *Hypersensitivity reactions.* NSAIDs are now probably the leading cause of hypersensitivity reactions. Common manifestations include skin reactions and exacerbation of asthma. The mechanism(s) are not fully elucidated but probably involve increasing leukotriene production.
- *Renal effects.* Result from inhibition of prostaglandins (especially I_2/E_2) involved in regulation of renal blood flow and electrolyte resorption. Exert both direct effects (e.g. papillary necrosis) on the kidney and secondary (e.g. fluid retention, raised blood pressure).
- '*Analgesic-associated nephropathy*'. This can occur following long-term high-dose regimes of NSAIDs and is often irreversible.
- *Liver disorders, bone marrow depression.* Transient elevation of liver enzymes may occur with high doses of some NSAIDs. Bone marrow depression is relatively uncommon.

SOME IMPORTANT NSAIDs AND COXIBS

Table 25.1 lists commonly used NSAIDs, and the clinical uses of the NSAIDs are summarised in the clinical box. We now look at some of the more significant drugs in a little more detail focusing on those with unusual pharmacological properties or those which are readily available at pharmacies and thus (although unprescribed) are consumed in large quantities.

Clinical uses of non-steroidal anti-inflammatory drugs (NSAIDs)

NSAIDs are widely used but cause serious adverse effects (especially GI, renal, pulmonary and cardiovascular effects related to their main pharmacological actions, as well as idiosyncratic effects). Elderly patients and those with pre-existing disorders are at particular risk. The main uses are:
- *Antithrombotic*: e.g. **aspirin** (Ch. 25) for patients at high risk of arterial thrombosis (e.g. following myocardial infarction). Other NSAIDs that cause less profound inhibition of platelet thromboxane synthesis than does **aspirin** *increase* the risk of thrombosis and should be avoided in high-risk individuals if possible.
- *Analgesia* (e.g. for headache, dysmenorrhea, backache, bony metastases, postoperative pain):
  - short-term use: e.g. **aspirin**, **paracetamol**, **ibuprofen**;
  - chronic pain: more potent, longer-lasting drugs (e.g. **naproxen**, **piroxicam**) often combined with a low-potency opioid (e.g. **codeine**, Ch. 42);

Clinical uses of non-steroidal anti-inflammatory drugs (NSAIDs)—cont'd

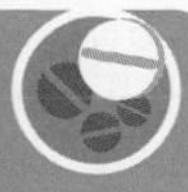

  - to reduce the requirement for narcotic analgesics (the NSAID **ketorolac** is sometimes given postoperatively for this purpose).
- *Anti-inflammatory*: e.g. **ibuprofen**, **naproxen** for symptomatic relief in rheumatoid arthritis, gout, soft tissue disorders.
- *Antipyretic*: **paracetamol.**

ASPIRIN

Aspirin (acetylsalicylic acid) was among the earliest drugs to be synthesised and is still one of the most widely consumed drugs worldwide.[6] It is also a common ingredient in proprietary over-the-counter medicines (although increasingly less so). The drug itself is relatively insoluble, but its sodium and calcium salts dissolve readily in aqueous solutions.

While **aspirin** was originally an anti-inflammatory/analgesic workhorse, it is seldom used for this purpose now (except perhaps in migraine), having been supplanted by other, better tolerated, NSAIDs. Today, its main clinical use is as a cardiovascular drug because of its ability to provide a prolonged suppression of platelet COX-1 and hence reduce aggregation (see Ch. 23).

While inhibition of platelet function is a feature of most NSAIDs, the effect of **aspirin** is longer lasting because it irreversibly acetylates platelet COX enzymes. While these proteins can be replaced in most cells, platelets, lacking a nucleus (and hence the cellular machinery for making new proteins), are not able to do so, remaining inactivated for their lifetime (approximately 10 days). Since a proportion of platelets is replaced each day from the bone marrow, this inhibition gradually abates but a small daily dose of **aspirin** (e.g. 75 mg/day) is all that is required to suppress platelet function to levels which benefit patients at risk for myocardial infarction and other cardiovascular problems (see Ch. 22). The view that even patients not at risk would benefit from taking the drug prophylactically (primary prevention) was challenged in a meta-analysis (Baigent et al., 2009) suggesting that in the general population, the risk from GI bleeding outweighed the protective action. The current guidance reflects this, recommending **aspirin** only as a secondary prevention treatment restricted to patients who have experienced, e.g., an ischaemic episode or who suffer from angina.

The use of **aspirin** has also been canvassed for other conditions. The most significant include:

- *Cancer* – especially colonic and rectal cancer: **aspirin** (and some COX-2 inhibitors) may reduce the incidence of several types of cancer although one always has to be aware of the GI risk (see Wong, 2019). Their effect may be related to their anti-inflammatory effect or their inhibitory action on

[6]Indeed, many people do not seem to regard it as a 'drug' at all. Many studies of human platelet aggregation have been ruined by the failure of volunteers to declare their consumption of aspirin.

platelets, which are thought to be involved in the metastasis of some cancers.
- *Alzheimer's disease* (see Ch. 40): epidemiological evidence suggests that **aspirin** might be beneficial in reducing the rate of cognitive decline in cases of Alzheimer's disease, but not the rate of age-related decline in normal patients (see Weng et al., 2021). However, other studies have been less encouraging.

Pharmacokinetic aspects

Aspirin, being a weak acid, is undissociated (i.e. not ionised) in the acid environment of the stomach, thus facilitating its passage across the mucosa. Most absorption, however, occurs in the ileum, because of the extensive surface area of the microvilli.

Aspirin is rapidly (within 30 min) hydrolysed by esterases in plasma and tissues, particularly the liver, yielding **salicylate**. This compound itself has anti-inflammatory actions (indeed, it was the original anti-inflammatory from which **aspirin** was derived); the mechanism is not clearly understood, although it may depend upon inhibition of the NFκB system (see Ch. 3) and only secondarily on COX inhibition. Oral **salicylate** is no longer used for treating inflammation, although it is a component of some topical preparations. Approximately 25% of the salicylate is oxidised; some is conjugated to give the glucuronide or sulfate before excretion, and about 25% is excreted unchanged, the rate of excretion being higher in alkaline urine (see Ch. 10).

The plasma half-life of **aspirin** will depend on the dose, but the duration of action is not directly related to the plasma half-life because of the irreversible nature of the action of the acetylation reaction by which it inhibits COX activity.

Unwanted effects

Salicylates (e.g. **aspirin**, **diflunisal** and **sulfasalazine**) may produce both local and systemic toxic effects. In addition to the general unwanted effects of NSAIDs outlined earlier, there are certain specific unwanted effects including *Reye's syndrome*, a rare disorder of children that is characterised by hepatic encephalopathy following an acute viral illness, which carries a 20%–40% mortality. Since the withdrawal of **aspirin** for paediatric use, the incidence of this iatrogenic disease has fallen dramatically.

Salicylism, characterised by tinnitus (high pitched ringing in the ears), vertigo, decreased hearing and sometimes also nausea and vomiting, occurs with overdosage of any **salicylate,** and acute **salicylate** poisoning (which occurs mainly in children and attempted suicides) constitutes a medical emergency. The mechanism is a major disturbance of acid–base and electrolyte balance. **Salicylates** uncouple oxidative phosphorylation (mainly in skeletal muscle), leading to hyperthermia, increased oxygen consumption and thus increased production of carbon dioxide. This stimulates respiration, which is also increased by a direct action of the drugs on the respiratory centre. The resulting hyperventilation causes a respiratory alkalosis that is normally compensated by renal mechanisms involving increased bicarbonate excretion. Larger doses actually cause a depression of the respiratory centre, less CO_2 is exhaled and therefore it increases in the blood. Because this is superimposed on a reduction in plasma bicarbonate, an uncompensated respiratory acidosis will occur. This may also be complicated by a metabolic acidosis, which results from the accumulation of metabolites of pyruvic, lactic and acetoacetic acids (an indirect consequence of uncoupled oxidative phosphorylation). Hyperthermia secondary to the increased metabolic rate is also likely to be present, and dehydration may follow repeated vomiting. In the CNS, initial stimulation with excitement is followed eventually by coma and respiratory depression. Bleeding can also occur, mainly as a result of depressed platelet aggregation.

Drug interactions

Aspirin may cause a potentially hazardous increase in the effect of **warfarin**, partly by displacing it from plasma protein binding sites (see Ch. 11) thereby increasing its effective concentration and partly because its effect on platelets further interferes with haemostasis (see Ch. 23). **Aspirin** also antagonises the effect of some antihypertensive and uricosuric agents such as **probenecid** and **sulfinpyrazone**. Because low doses of **aspirin** may, on their own, reduce urate excretion (see Ch. 29), it should not be used in gout.

Aspirin

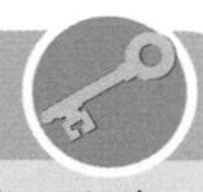

Aspirin (acetylsalicylic acid) is the oldest NSAID. It acts by irreversibly inactivating COX-1 and COX-2.

Therapeutic effects
- In addition to its anti-inflammatory actions, **aspirin** strongly inhibits platelet aggregation, and its main clinical use now is in the therapy of cardiovascular disease.
- It is given orally and is rapidly absorbed; 75% is metabolised in the liver.
- Elimination of its metabolite **salicylate** follows first-order kinetics with low doses (half-life 4 h), and saturation kinetics with high doses (half-life over 15 h).

Unwanted effects:
- With therapeutic doses: GI symptoms, often including some gastric bleeding (usually slight and asymptomatic). Hypersensitivity reactions.
- With larger doses: dizziness, deafness and tinnitus ('salicylism'); compensatory respiratory alkalosis may occur.
- With toxic doses (e.g. from self-poisoning): uncompensated metabolic acidosis may occur, particularly in children.
- **Aspirin** has been linked with a rare but serious post-viral encephalitis (Reye's syndrome) in children and is not used in paediatric patients.
- If given concomitantly with warfarin, **aspirin** can cause a potentially hazardous increase in the risk of bleeding.

PARACETAMOL

Paracetamol (called **acetaminophen** in the United States) is one of the most commonly used non-narcotic analgesic–antipyretic agents and is also a component of many over-the-counter proprietary preparations. In some ways, the drug constitutes an anomaly: while it is an excellent analgesic (see Chs 42 and 43) and antipyretic, its anti-inflammatory action is slight. It is also substantially free of the gastric and platelet side effects of the other NSAIDs. For these reasons, **paracetamol** is sometimes not classified as an NSAID at all and it's co-administration with traditional NSAIDs is both safe and effective, leading to enhanced analgesia dependent on the context of their use (see Hyllested et al., 2002). Paracetamol is also often combined with weak opioids such as **codeine** for the same reason.

The antipyretic and analgesic activities are still not fully understood. Multiple mechanisms have been suggested and include inhibition of prostaglandin biosynthesis in the CNS (where low peroxide concentrations allow paracetamol to act as a reducing agent on COX), activation of descending serotonergic pathways and increased cannabinoid receptor activation (see also Ch. 43 and Anderson, 2008).

Pharmacokinetic aspects

Paracetamol is well absorbed when given orally, with peak plasma concentrations reached in 30–60 min. The plasma half-life of therapeutic doses is 2–4 h, but with toxic doses it may be extended to 4–8 h. **Paracetamol** is inactivated in the liver, being conjugated to give the glucuronide or sulfate. Intravenous preparations of paracetamol are now available but should largely be reserved for those who cannot take the drug orally, clinical studies repeatedly demonstrating no difference in efficacy.

Unwanted effects

With therapeutic doses, side effects are few and uncommon, although allergic skin reactions sometimes occur. It is possible that regular intake of large doses over a long period may cause kidney damage. More seriously, toxic doses (<150 mg/kg, subject to modification by other clinical features) cause potentially fatal hepatotoxicity, and nephrotoxicity. This occurs when normal conjugation reactions are saturated, and the drug is metabolised instead by mixed function oxidases. The resulting toxic metabolite, *N*-acetyl-*p*-benzoquinone imine (NAPQI), is normally inactivated by conjugation with glutathione, but when this becomes depleted, the toxic intermediate accumulates in the liver and the kidney tubules and causes necrosis. Chronic, but not acute, alcohol consumption can exacerbate paracetamol toxicity by inducing the liver microsomal enzymes producing the toxic metabolite, but the situation here is complex (see Prescott, 2000). Paracetamol dosing should be adjusted in those weighing less than 50 kg.

The initial symptoms of acute **paracetamol** poisoning are nausea and vomiting, the hepatotoxicity being a delayed manifestation that occurs 24–72 h later. Further details of the toxic effects are given in Chapter 58. If the patient is seen sufficiently soon after ingestion, the liver damage can be prevented by administering agents that increase glutathione formation in the liver, principally **N-acetylcysteine** (NAC) via the intravenous route. If more than 8 h have passed since the ingestion of a large dose, then NAC, which itself can cause adverse effects (anaphylactoid reactions in 10%-50%), is less likely to be useful. Regrettably, ingestion of large amounts of **paracetamol** is a common method of suicide.

Paracetamol

Paracetamol is a commonly used drug that is widely available over the counter. It has potent analgesic and antipyretic actions but much weaker anti-inflammatory effects than other NSAIDs. Its COX inhibitory action seems to be mainly restricted to the CNS enzyme.

- It is given orally (preferentially) or intravenously and metabolised in the liver (half-life 2–4 h).

Paracetamol—cont'd

- Toxic doses cause nausea and vomiting, then, after 24–72 h, potentially fatal liver damage by saturating normal conjugating enzymes, causing the drug to be converted by mixed function oxidases to NAPQI. If not inactivated by conjugation with glutathione, this compound reacts with cellular proteins causing tissue damage.
- Agents that increase glutathione (principally intravenous **acetylcysteine**) can prevent liver damage if given early.

IBUPROFEN

Ibuprofen, the 'founder' member of the proprionic acid family of drugs, was first introduced in 1969. Although it has a different type of chemical structure from the salicylates it acts in the same manner by inhibiting COX enzymes. It is a racemic compound but only the S(+) enantiomer is fully active: the R(−) enantiomer is converted to the S(+) enantiomer in the body. It is a non-selective COX inhibitor.

Because of its excellent safety record, **ibuprofen** soon became the most commonly prescribed NSAID and was eventually made available in pharmacies without prescription. It is a versatile drug, being available in various formulations including tablets, liquids, gels for topical application and sterile intravenous formulations. It is now probably the most widely consumed of all the NSAIDs and is used for many indications including dental and postoperative pain, osteo and rheumatoid arthritis, dysmenorrhea, sprains, headache and migraine.

Ibuprofen is well absorbed orally with peak serum concentrations peaking at 1–2 h after administration (cited in Bushra and Aslam, 2010). The plasma half-life is 1.8–2.0 h; metabolism mainly occurs in the liver by hydroxylation and carboxylation followed by conjugation and the drug is completely excreted within 24 h. Very little drug is excreted unchanged. The drug is extensively bound to plasma proteins (about 99%) but unlike many NSAIDs does not displace **warfarin** from its biding sites, making concurrent use of the two drugs easier to manage.

Adverse effects

While considered a 'safe' NSAID, ibuprofen has fundamentally the same mechanism-dependent adverse effect profile as all the other drugs of this type, with GI effects, platelet effects and renal actions being the most prominent.

COXIBS

Coxibs are generally offered to patients for whom treatment with conventional NSAIDs would pose a high probability of serious GI side effects. However, these may still occur with coxibs, perhaps because COX-2 has been implicated in the healing of pre-existing ulcers, so inhibition could delay recovery from earlier lesions. As is the case with all NSAID treatment, cardiovascular risk should be assessed prior to long-term treatment. Several coxibs have been withdrawn following claims of cardiovascular and other toxicity, but three drugs are currently available for clinical use in the United Kingdom and others may be available elsewhere.

Celecoxib and etoricoxib

Celecoxib and **etoricoxib** are used for symptomatic relief in the treatment of osteoarthritis and rheumatoid arthritis and some other conditions.

Both are administered orally and have similar pharmacokinetic profiles, being well absorbed with peak plasma concentrations being achieved within 1–3 h. They are extensively (>99%) metabolised in the liver, and plasma protein binding is high (>90%). Common unwanted effects may include headache, dizziness, rashes and peripheral oedema caused by fluid retention. Because of the potential role of COX-2 in the healing of ulcers, patients with pre-existing disease should avoid the drugs.

Parecoxib

Parecoxib is a prodrug of **valdecoxib**. The latter drug has now been withdrawn, but **parecoxib** is licensed for the short-term treatment of postoperative pain. It is given by intravenous or intramuscular injection and is rapidly and virtually completely (>95%) converted into the active **valdecoxib** by enzymatic hydrolysis in the liver.

Maximum blood levels are achieved within approximately 30–60 min, depending on the route of administration. Plasma protein binding is high. The active metabolite, **valdecoxib**, has a plasma half-life of about 8 h and is converted in the liver to various inactive metabolites. Skin reactions, some of them serious, have been reported with **valdecoxib**, and patients should be monitored carefully. The drug should also be given with caution to patients with impaired renal function, and renal failure has been reported in connection with this drug. Postoperative anaemia may also occur.

ANTIRHEUMATOID DRUGS

Rheumatoid arthritis is one of the commonest chronic inflammatory conditions in developed countries, and a common cause of disability.[7] Affected joints become swollen, painful, deformed and immobile. One in three patients with rheumatoid arthritis is likely to become severely disabled. The disease also has cardiovascular and other systemic manifestations which carry an increased risk of mortality. The degenerative joint changes, which are driven by an autoimmune reaction, are characterised by inflammation, proliferation of the synovium and erosion of cartilage and bone. Davis and Matteson (2012) have reviewed the classification and treatment of this miserable and disabling affliction.

The primary inflammatory cytokines, IL-1 and (especially) TNF-α, have a major role in the disease (see Ch. 7). A simplified scheme showing the development of rheumatoid arthritis and the sites of action of therapeutic drugs is given in Fig. 25.3.

DISEASE-MODIFYING ANTIRHEUMATIC DRUGS

Unlike the NSAIDs, which only reduce the symptoms of these disorders, these drugs aim to halt or reverse the underlying disease itself, hence the name 'disease-modifying antirheumatic drugs'[8] (or more conveniently, 'DMARDs'). While originally a heterologous group of synthetic drugs with different chemical structures and mechanisms of action this group has recently been expanded to include the anti-cytokine and other agents. For this reason, this group of drugs is nowadays divided into 'conventional synthetic (cs) DMARDS' and the 'biological (b) DMARDs'. We will consider these groups in turn.

CONVENTIONAL SYNTHETIC DISEASE-MODIFYING ANTIRHEUMATIC DRUGS

The csDMARDs (Table 25.2) include **chloroquine** and other antimalarials, **methotrexate**, **sulfasalazine**, **penicillamine**, **gold compounds**, as well as various immunosuppressant drugs such as **leflunomide**. This group also comprises a subclass of these drugs which include the *Janus associated tyrosine kinase* (JAK) inhibitors **tofacitinib** and **baricitinib** and which are referred to as *targeted sDMARDs* (tsDMARDs) and which are discussed separately below. Glucocorticoids are also included in the sDMARD category by some reviewers but will not be considered in depth in this chapter. The reader is referred to Chapters 3 and 33 for more information on these drugs.

Although still licensed in the UK, revision of the *European League Against Rheumatism* (EULAR) treatment guidelines in 2016 suggested that **leflunomide** and **gold compounds** should no longer be used, and so they will not be considered further here.

Despite the evident success of the newer anticytokine bDMARDs, many authors believe that there is little overall difference in efficacy between the bDMARDs and the sDMARDs although many features of their pharmacology such as their side effect profile and pharmacokinetics are evidently so different (Chatzidionysiou et al., 2017; Ramiro et al., 2017).

The antirheumatoid action of csDMARDs was discovered through a mixture of serendipity and clinical intuition. When they were introduced, nothing was known about their mechanism of action and decades of in vitro experiments have generally resulted in further bewilderment. When successful, csDMARDs generally improve symptoms and reduce disease activity in rheumatoid arthritis, as measured by reduction in the number of swollen and tender joints, pain score, disability score, X-ray appearance and serum concentration of acute-phase proteins and of *rheumatoid factor* (an immunoglobulin M (IgM) antibody against host IgG).

The csDMARDs are sometimes referred to as *second-line drugs*, with the implication that they are only resorted to when other therapies (e.g. NSAIDs) fail, but csDMARD therapy may be initiated as soon as a definite diagnosis has been reached to reduce permanent joint damage and hence future disability. Their clinical effects are usually slow (months) in onset, and it is usual to provide NSAID 'cover' during this induction phase. If therapy is successful (and the success rate is variable), concomitant NSAID (or glucocorticoid) therapy can be reduced. Some csDMARDs (e.g. **methotrexate**) have a place in the treatment of other chronic inflammatory diseases, whereas others (e.g. **penicillamine**) are not thought to have a general anti-

[7]The term *arthritis* simply refers to inflammatory joint disorders. Clinically, more than 50 distinguishable types are recognised. To the lay person though, arthritis usually denotes either *osteoarthritis* or *rheumatoid arthritis*. These are often confused although they are entirely separate entities.

[8]Historically classified as such because, unlike NSAIDs, they lowered the erythrocyte sedimentation rate (ESR) – a marker of acute inflammation linked to increased plasma fibrinogen. Today, other acute phase reactants such as C-reactive protein (CRP) are generally preferred by rheumatologists as biochemical markers of disease activity.

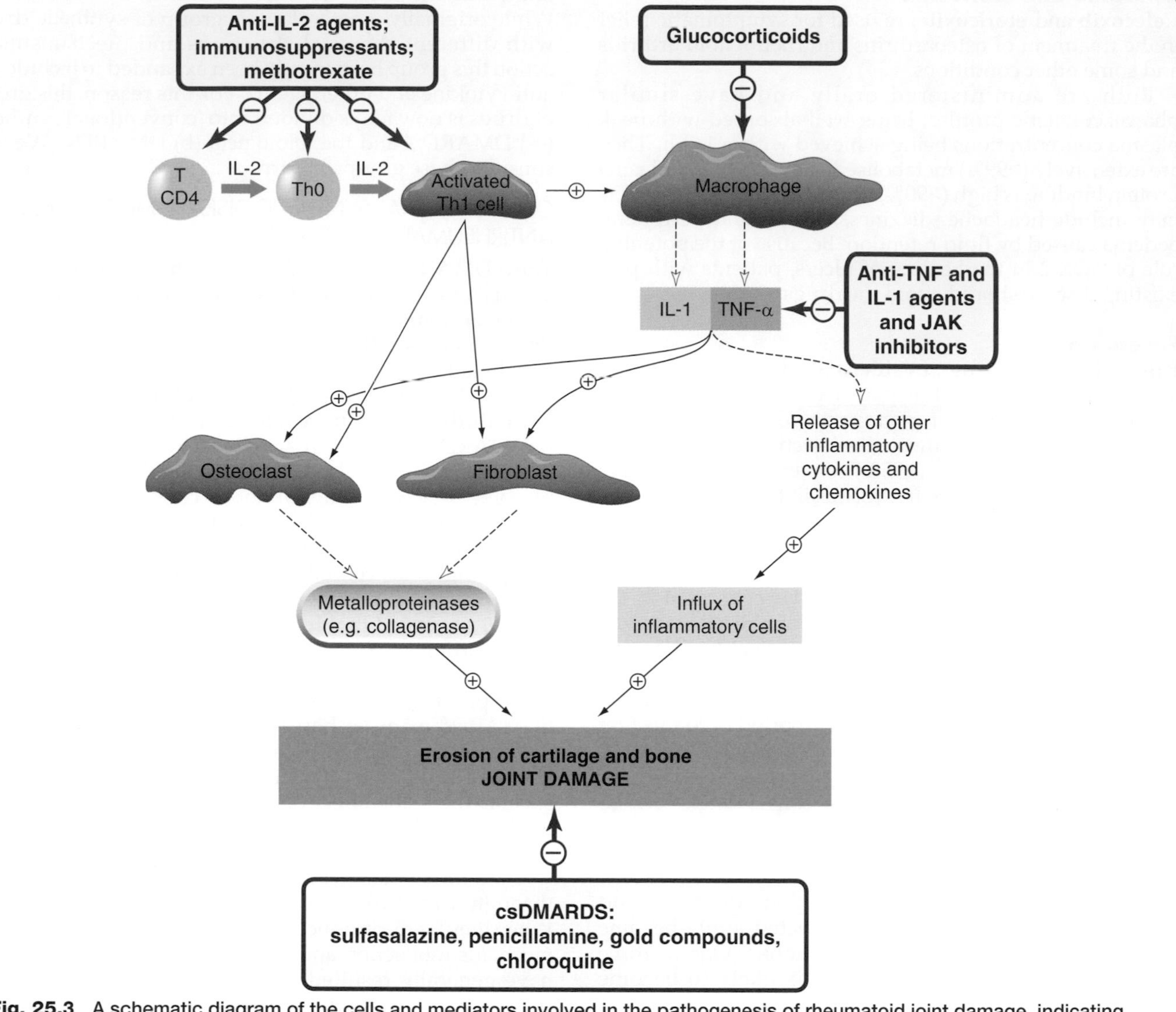

Fig. 25.3 A schematic diagram of the cells and mediators involved in the pathogenesis of rheumatoid joint damage, indicating the sites of action of disease-modifying antirheumatic drugs (conventional synthetic DMARDs, targeted synthetic DMARDs and biological DMARDs) and other drugs. For details of the anti–tumour necrosis factor (TNF), interleukin (IL)-1 and IL-2 receptor agents, see Chapter 7 and Table 25.4. The details of the cytokine receptors and the Janus associated tyrosine kinase (JAK) signalling pathways have been omitted for clarity.

inflammatory action. The putative mechanisms of action of csDMARDs have been reviewed by Cutolo (2002) and Chandrashekara (2013).

We will now look at some of the common csDMARDs in a little more detail.

Methotrexate

Methotrexate is a folic acid antagonist with cytotoxic and immunosuppressant activity (see Ch. 57). It has a useful and reliable antirheumatoid action and is a common first-choice drug. It has a more rapid onset of action than other DMARDs, but treatment must be closely monitored because of bone marrow depression, leading to a drop in white cell and platelet counts (potentially fatal) and liver cirrhosis. It is, however, superior to most other DMARDs in terms of efficacy and patient tolerance and is often given in conjunction with the anticytokine drugs.

Its mechanism of action is unrelated to its effect on folic acid (which is routinely co-administered to prevent blood disorders) but may well be connected with its ability to block adenosine uptake (see Ch. 16 and Chan and Cronstein, 2010).

Sulfasalazine

Sulfasalazine, another common first-choice sDMARD in the United Kingdom, produces remission in active rheumatoid arthritis and is also used for chronic inflammatory bowel disease (see Ch. 30). It probably acts partly by inhibiting COX and lipoxygenase pathways or by scavenging toxic free radicals, but it also reduces the release of IL-8 from colonic myofibroblasts, suggesting an additional immunosuppressive mechanism (Lodowska et al., 2015). The drug is a complex of a sulfonamide (**sulfapyridine**) and **salicylate** and is split into its component parts by bacteria in the colon. It is poorly absorbed after oral administration.

Table 25.2 Some common 'synthetic disease-modifying' and immunosuppressive drugs used in the treatment of the arthritides

Type	Drug	Indication	Comments
Antimalarials	Chloroquine	Moderate RA, SLE	Used when other therapies fail
	Hydroxychloroquine sulfate	Moderate RA, SLE	Also useful for some skin disorders
Immunomodulators	Methotrexate	Moderate to severe RA, PS, JRA	A 'first-choice' drug. Also used in Crohn's disease and cancer treatment. Often used in combination with other drugs
	Azathioprine	RA, IBS	Used when other therapies fail. Also used in transplant rejection, IBS and eczema
	Ciclosporin	Severe RA, AD, PA	Used when other therapies fail, in some skin diseases and transplant rejection
	Cyclophosphamide	Severe RA	Used when other therapies fail
NSAID	Sulfasalazine	RA, PA, JRA	A 'first-choice' drug. Also used in ulcerative colitis
Penicillin metabolite	Penicillamine	Severe RA	Many side effects. Long latency of action

AD, Atopic dermatitis; *IBS,* inflammatory bowel disease; *JRA,* juvenile rheumatoid arthritis; *NSAID,* non-steroidal anti-inflammatory drug; *PA,* psoriatic arthritis; *PS,* psoriasis; *RA,* rheumatoid arthritis; *SLE,* systemic lupus erythematosus.
Data from various sources, including the British National Formulary, 2021.

Sulfasalazine is generally well tolerated but common side effects include GI disturbances, malaise and headache. Skin reactions and leukopenia can occur but are reversible on stopping the drug. The absorption of folic acid is sometimes impaired; this can be countered by giving folic acid supplements. A reversible decrease in sperm count has also been reported. As with other sulfonamides, bone marrow depression and anaphylactic-type reactions may occur in a few patients. Haematological monitoring may be necessary.

Penicillamine

Penicillamine is *dimethylcysteine;* it is produced by hydrolysis of **penicillin** and appears in the urine after treatment with that drug. The D-isomer is used in the therapy of rheumatoid disease. About 75% of patients with rheumatoid arthritis respond to **penicillamine**. Therapeutic effects are seen within weeks but do not reach a plateau for several months. **Penicillamine** is thought to modify rheumatoid disease partly by decreasing the immune response and IL-1 generation, and/or partly by preventing the maturation of newly synthesised collagen. However, the precise mechanism of action is still a matter of conjecture. The drug has a highly reactive thiol group and also has metal-chelating properties, which are put to good use in the treatment of *Wilson's disease* (pathological copper deposition causing neurodegeneration and liver disease) and heavy metal poisoning.

Penicillamine is given orally, but only about half the dose is absorbed. It reaches peak plasma concentrations in 1–2 h and is excreted in the urine. Treatment is initiated with low doses and increased only gradually to minimise the unwanted effects, which occur in about 40% of patients and which may necessitate cessation of therapy. Rashes and stomatitis are the most common unwanted effects but may resolve if the dosage is lowered. Anorexia, fever, nausea and vomiting and disturbances of taste (the last related to the chelation of zinc) are seen, but often disappear with continued treatment. Proteinuria occurs in 20% of patients and should be monitored. Haematological monitoring is also required when treatment is initiated. Thrombocytopenia may require reduction in the dose. Leukopenia and aplastic anaemia are absolute contraindications, as are autoimmune conditions (e.g. thyroiditis, myasthenia gravis).

Antimalarial drugs

Hydroxychloroquine and chloroquine are 4-aminoquinoline drugs used mainly in the prevention and treatment of malaria (see Ch. 55), but they are also used as DMARDs. **Chloroquine** is usually reserved for cases where other treatments have failed. They are also used to treat another autoimmune disease, lupus erythematosus, but are contraindicated in patients with psoriatic arthropathy because they exacerbate the skin lesions. The related antimalarial, **mepacrine**, is also sometimes used for discoid (cutaneous) lupus. The antirheumatic effects do not appear until a month or more after the drug is started, and only about half the patients treated respond. The administration, pharmacokinetic aspects and unwanted effects of **chloroquine** are dealt with in Chapter 55; screening for ocular toxicity is particularly important.

IMMUNOSUPPRESSANT DRUGS

Immunosuppressants are used in the therapy of autoimmune disease and also to prevent and/or treat transplant rejection. Because they impair the immune response, they also carry the hazard of a decreased response to infections and may facilitate the emergence of malignant cell lines. However, the relationship between these adverse effects and potency in preventing graft rejection varies with different drugs. The clinical use of immunosuppressants is summarised in the clinical box.

Immunosuppressants

- Clonal proliferation of T-helper cells can be decreased through inhibition of transcription of IL-2: **ciclosporin, tacrolimus, sirolimus** and **pimecrolimus** and glucocorticoids act in this way.
  - **Ciclosporin**-like drugs bind to cytosolic proteins (immunophilins) which inhibit calcineurin triggering changes in gene transcription.
  - They are given orally or intravenously; a common adverse effect is nephrotoxicity.
- For glucocorticoid actions, see separate box.
- Lymphocyte proliferation is also blocked by inhibitors of DNA synthesis such as:
  - **azathioprine**, through its active metabolite **mercaptopurine**;
  - **mycophenolate mofetil**, through inhibition of de novo purine synthesis.

Most of these drugs act during the induction phase of the immunological response, reducing lymphocyte proliferation (see Ch. 7), although others also inhibit aspects of the effector phase. There are three main groups:

- drugs that inhibit IL-2 production or action (e.g. **ciclosporin**, **tacrolimus** and related drugs);
- drugs that inhibit cytokine gene expression (e.g. corticosteroids);
- drugs that inhibit purine or pyrimidine synthesis (e.g. **azathioprine**, **mycophenolate mofetil**).

Ciclosporin

Ciclosporin is a naturally occurring compound first identified in a fungus. It is a cyclic peptide of 11 amino acid residues (including some not found in animals) with potent immunosuppressive activity but no effect on the acute inflammatory reaction per se. Its unusual activity, which (unlike earlier immunosuppressants) does not entail cytotoxicity, was discovered in 1972 and was crucial for the development of transplant surgery (for a detailed review, see Borel et al., 1996). The drug has numerous actions but those of relevance to immunosuppression are:

- decreased clonal proliferation of T cells, primarily by inhibiting IL-2 synthesis and possibly also by decreasing expression of IL-2 receptors;
- reduced induction and clonal proliferation of cytotoxic T cells from $CD8^+$ precursor T cells;
- reduced function of the effector T cells responsible for cell-mediated responses (e.g. decreased delayed-type hypersensitivity);
- some reduction of T cell-dependent B-cell responses.

The main action is a relatively selective inhibitory effect on IL-2 gene transcription, although a similar effect on interferon (IFN)-γ and IL-3 has also been reported. Normally, interaction of antigen with a T-helper (Th) cell receptor results in increased intracellular Ca^{2+} (Chs 2 and 7), which in turn stimulates *calcineurin*, a phosphatase. This activates various transcription factors that initiate IL-2 expression. **Ciclosporin** binds to *cyclophilin*, a cytosolic protein member of the immunophilin family (a group of proteins that act as intracellular receptors for such drugs). The drug–immunophilin complex binds to, and inhibits, calcineurin and thus acts in opposition to the many protein kinases involved in signal transduction (see Ch. 3), preventing activation of Th cells and production of IL-2 (see Ch. 7).

Ciclosporin itself is poorly absorbed by mouth but can be given orally in a more readily absorbed formulation, or by intravenous infusion. After oral administration, peak plasma concentrations are usually attained in about 3–4 h. The plasma half-life is approximately 24 h. Metabolism occurs in the liver, and most of the metabolites are excreted in the bile. **Ciclosporin** accumulates in most tissues at concentrations three to four times that seen in the plasma. Some of the drug remains in lymphomyeloid tissue and remains in fat depots for some time after administration has stopped.

The commonest and most serious unwanted effect of **ciclosporin** is nephrotoxicity, which is thought to be unconnected with calcineurin inhibition. It may be a limiting factor in the use of the drug in some patients (see also Ch. 58). Hepatotoxicity and hypertension can also occur. Less important unwanted effects include anorexia, lethargy, hirsutism, tremor, paraesthesia (tingling sensation), gum hypertrophy (especially when co-prescribed with calcium antagonists for hypertension; see Ch. 21) and GI disturbances. **Ciclosporin** has no depressant effects on the bone marrow.

Tacrolimus

Tacrolimus is a macrolide antibiotic of fungal origin with a very similar mechanism of action to **ciclosporin**, but higher potency. The main difference is that the internal receptor for this drug is not cyclophilin but a different immunophilin termed FKBP (FK-binding protein, so called because **tacrolimus** was initially termed FK506). The **tacrolimus**–FKBP complex inhibits calcineurin with the effects described previously. It is not used for arthritis but mainly in organ transplantation and severe atopic eczema (see Ch. 26). **Pimecrolimus** (used topically to treat atopic eczema) acts in a similar way. **Sirolimus** (used to prevent organ rejection after transplantation, and also in coating on cardiac stents to prevent restenosis; see Ch. 20) also combines with an immunophilin but activates a protein kinase to produce its immunosuppressant effect.

Tacrolimus can be given orally, by intravenous injection or as an ointment for topical use in inflammatory disease of the skin. It is 99% metabolised by the liver and has a half-life of approximately 7 h. The unwanted effects of **tacrolimus** are similar to those of **ciclosporin** but are more severe. The incidence of nephrotoxicity and neurotoxicity is higher, but that of hirsutism is lower. GI disturbances and metabolic disturbances (hyperglycaemia) can occur. Thrombocytopenia and hyperlipidaemia have been reported but decrease when the dosage is reduced.

Azathioprine

Azathioprine interferes with purine synthesis and is cytotoxic. It is widely used for immunosuppression, particularly for control of autoimmune diseases such as rheumatoid arthritis and to prevent tissue rejection in transplant surgery. This drug is metabolised to **mercaptopurine**, an analogue that inhibits DNA synthesis (see Ch. 57). Because it inhibits clonal proliferation during the induction phase of the immune response (see Ch. 7) through a cytotoxic action on dividing cells, both cell-mediated and antibody-mediated immune reactions are depressed by this drug. As is the case with **mercaptopurine** itself, the main unwanted effect is depression of the bone marrow. Other toxic effects are nausea and vomiting, skin eruptions and a mild hepatotoxicity.

Cyclophosphamide

Cyclophosphamide is a potent immunosuppressant that is mainly used to treat cancer. Its mechanism of action is explained in Chapter 57. It has substantial toxicity and is therefore generally reserved for serious cases of rheumatoid arthritis in which all other therapies have failed.

Mycophenolate mofetil

Mycophenolate mofetil is a semisynthetic derivative of a fungal antibiotic and is used for preventing organ rejection. In the body, it is converted to mycophenolic acid, which restrains proliferation of both T and B lymphocytes and reduces the production of cytotoxic T cells by inhibiting inosine monophosphate dehydrogenase. This enzyme is crucial for de novo purine biosynthesis in both T and B cells (other cells can generate purines through another pathway), so the drug has a fairly selective action.

Mycophenolate mofetil is given orally and is well absorbed. Magnesium and aluminium hydroxides impair absorption, and colestyramine reduces plasma concentrations. The metabolite mycophenolic acid undergoes enterohepatic cycling and is eliminated by the kidney as the inactive glucuronide. Unwanted GI effects are common.

Glucocorticoids

The therapeutic action of the glucocorticoids involves both their inhibitory effects on the immune response and their anti-inflammatory actions. These are described in Chapters 3 and 33, and their sites of action on cell-mediated immune reactions are indicated in Fig. 25.3.

Glucocorticoids are immunosuppressant chiefly because, like **ciclosporin**, they restrain the clonal proliferation of Th cells, through decreasing transcription of the gene for IL-2. However, they also decrease the transcription of many other cytokine genes (including those for TNF-α, IFN-γ, IL-1 and many other interleukins) in both the induction and effector phases of the immune response. The synthesis and release of anti-inflammatory proteins (e.g. IL-10, annexin 1, protease inhibitors) are also increased. These effects are mediated through inhibition of the action of transcription factors, such as activator protein-1 and NFκB as well as through the action of liganded glucocorticoid receptor in the cytosol of target cells (see Ch. 3).

Clinical uses of immunosuppressant drugs

Immunosuppressant drugs are used by specialists, often in combination with glucocorticoid and/or cytotoxic drugs:

- To slow the progress of rheumatoid and other arthritic diseases including psoriatic arthritis, ankylosing spondylitis, juvenile arthritis: *DMARDs*, e.g. **methotrexate**, **ciclosporin**; *cytokine modulators* (e.g. **adalimumab**, **etanercept**, **infliximab**) are used when the response to methotrexate or other DMARDs has been inadequate.
- To suppress rejection of transplanted organs, e.g. **ciclosporin**, **tacrolimus**, **sirolimus.**
- To suppress graft-versus-host disease following bone marrow transplantation, e.g. **ciclosporin.**
- In autoimmune disorders including idiopathic thrombocytopenic purpura, some forms of haemolytic anaemias and of glomerulonephritis and myasthenia gravis.
- In severe inflammatory bowel disease (e.g. **ciclosporin** in ulcerative colitis, **infliximab** in Crohn's disease).
- In severe skin disease (e.g. **pimecrolimus**, **tacrolimus** topically for atopic eczema uncontrolled by maximal topical glucocorticoids; **etanercept**, **infliximab** for very severe plaque psoriasis which has failed to respond to **methotrexate** or **ciclosporin**).

Miscellaneous drugs

Sitting (admittedly rather uncomfortably) in the sDMARD group of drugs is **apremilast**, a phosphodiesterase (type 4) inhibitor. By elevating levels of cAMP in cells it can suppress the generation and release of proinflammatory mediators. It is generally used for the treatment of psoriatic arthritis and only used in patients who do not respond adequately to other treatment.

TARGETED SYNTHETIC DISEASE-MODIFYING ANTIRHEUMATIC DRUGS

The biological activity of inflammatory cytokines is transduced by their receptors (several types) which in turn (with the important exception of TNF) activate members of the *JAK* or *TYK* (tyrosine kinase) family of molecules. There are four members of the JAK family, JAK 1–4 (see Ch. 3), and these in turn can interact with members of the *signal transducer and activation of transcription (STAT)* family of transcription factors (six in total) thus activating the JAK–STAT signalling pathway which modulates gene translation/transcription.

Gain of function and other mutations in JAK family members are associated with a variety of rheumatological and other inflammatory disorders strongly suggesting a functional link between the activation of the JAK–STAT pathway and inflammatory pathologies and based upon this idea, inhibitors of JAK kinases such as **tofacitinib, baricitinib** and **upadacitinib** were developed for use in inflammatory and other pathologies (see Bertsias, 2020, and Table 25.3).

Table 25.3 JAK inhibitors in rheumatic disorders

Drug	Target	Cytokines inhibited[a]	Clinical use	Side effects
Tofacitinib	JAK 1	IL-2, IL-6, IL-15, IFNα.	RA (moderate–severe); PA, UC. Often used in combination with methotrexate	Anaemia, cough, GI symptoms, nausea, joint problems
	JAK 3	IL-2, IL-15		
Baricitinib	JAK 1	IL-2, IL-6, IL-15, IFNα.	RA (moderate–severe); often used in combination with methotrexate	Dyslipidaemia, nausea, thrombocytosis
	JAK 2	IL-6, IFNα, GMCSF, EPO		
Upadacitinib	JAK 1	IL-2, IL-6, IL-15, IFNα.	RA	Dyslipidaemia, nausea, fever, neutropoenia

[a]Only the key proinflammatory cytokines/growth factors are included in this table.
EPO, Erythropoietin; *GMCSF*, granulocyte-macrophage colony stimulating factor; *IFN*, interferon; *IL*, interleukin; *JAK*, Janus associated tyrosine kinase; *RA*, rheumatoid arthritis; *UC*, ulcerative colitis.
Data from various sources, including Bertias, 2020, and the British National Formulary, 2021.)

Since any interference with the immune system is likely to adversely affect the host response to infection and cytokines activate different JAK kinases, the question of which of these proinflammatory mediators was inhibited by these drugs became rather significant and there were clearly some concerns about indiscriminate inhibition of these signalling pathways.

The first of these drugs to be introduced into clinical practice was **tofacitinib** in 2012. This is a non-selective compound which inhibited JAK1 and JAK3 which was effective in reducing the action of the 'γ-chain cytokines' such as IL-2, IL-6, IL-15 and IFNγ (JAK1) and IL-2, IL-4 and IL-15 (JAK3). Later, **baricitinib** which selectively targeted JAK1 and JAK2 was approved. This drug blocked, in addition, several growth factors such as granulocyte-macrophage colony-stimulating factor (GM-CSF) and erythropoietin (EPO). Concerns about the effect of these drugs on haematological function (through inhibition of JAK2) led to the subsequent introduction of **upadacitinib,** a selective JAK1 inhibitor.

The chief adverse effects of this family of drugs include, as might be anticipated, a reduction of host response to infectious diseases and possibly activation of latent infections such as TB. Various other side effects such as nausea, joint pains fever and dyslipidaemia are commonly reported (see Table 25.3).

BIOLOGIC DISEASE-MODIFYING ANTIRHEUMATIC DRUGS, ANTICYTOKINE DRUGS AND OTHER BIOPHARMACEUTICALS

The *biopharmaceuticals* in this section represent the greatest technological and conceptual breakthrough in the treatment of severe chronic inflammation for decades (see Maini, 2005). These drugs are engineered recombinant antibodies and other proteins (see Ch. 5). As such, they are difficult and expensive to produce, and this limits their use. In the United Kingdom (in the National Health Service), they are generally restricted to patients who do not respond adequately to other DMARD therapy, and they are administered only under specialist supervision. Some are usually administered in combination with **methotrexate**, which apparently provides a synergistic anti-inflammatory action.

The characteristics and indications of some current biopharmaceuticals are shown in Table 25.4. The effect of two of these agents on rheumatoid arthritis is shown in Fig. 25.4. Many neutralise soluble cytokines. **Adalimumab**, **certolizumab pegol**, **golimumab**, **etanercept** and **infliximab** target TNF-α; **anakinra** and **canakinumab** target IL-1; **sarilumab** and **tocilizumab**, IL-6 and **ustekinumab**, IL-12 and -23. **Abatacept**, **alemtuzumab**, **basiliximab**, **belatacept**, **daclizumab** and **natalizumab** target T cells, disrupting either activation, proliferation or emigration. **Rituximab** and **belimumab** target B cells directly. While they are not used for treating arthritis, **basiliximab**, **belatacept** and **daclizumab** are included in the table as they act to prevent the rejection of transplanted organs in a similar way – by suppressing T-cell proliferation.

There is some debate over the precise nature of the target of the anti-TNF agents. Some target both soluble and membrane-bound forms of TNF whereas others are more selective. Antibodies that target membrane-bound TNF (e.g. **infliximab** and **adalimumab**) may kill the host cell by complement-induced lysis. This produces a different quality of effect than simple sequestration of the soluble mediator (by, for example, **etanercept**). This fact is probably the reason why some of these drugs exhibit a slightly different pharmacological profile despite ostensibly acting through the same mechanism (see Arora et al., 2009, for further details).

As proteins, none of these drugs can be given orally. Administration is usually by subcutaneous injection or intravenous infusion and their pharmacokinetic profiles vary enormously. Dosing regimes differ but, for example, **anakinra** is usually given daily; **efalizumab** and **etanercept** once or twice per week; **adalimumab**, **certolizumab pegol**, **infliximab** and **rituximab** every 2 weeks; and **abatacept**, **belimumab**, **golimumab**, **natalizumab** and **tocilizumab** every month. Sometimes a loading dose of these drugs is given as a preliminary to regular administration.

Usually, these biopharmaceuticals are only given to severely affected patients or to those in whom other therapies have failed. For reasons that are not entirely clear, a proportion of these patients (about 30%) do not respond and therapy is generally discontinued if no therapeutic benefit is evident within 2–4 weeks. Some studies suggest that if treatment is begun using drugs such as **infliximab** in combination with **methotrexate** this failure rate is reduced

Table 25.4 Some biopharmaceuticals used in the treatment of inflammatory diseases

Target	Drug	Type	Mode of action	Indication
Soluble TNF	Adalimumab	Humanised mAb	Immunoneutralisation	RA (moderate–severe), PA, AS, PP, CD
	Certolizumab pegol	Pegylated ab fragment	Immunoneutralisation	RA[a] (moderate–severe)
	Golimumab	Humanised mAb	Immunoneutralisation	RA (moderate–severe), PA, PS
	Infliximab	Chimeric neutralising ab	Immunoneutralisation	RA[a] (moderate–severe), PA, AS, PP
	Etanercept	Fusion protein decoy receptor	Neutralisation	RA[a] (moderate–severe), PA, AS, PP
Soluble IL-1	Anakinra	Recombinant version of IL-1 ra	Neutralisation	RA[a] (moderate–severe)
	Canakinumab	Humanised mAb	Immunoneutralisation	GA
Soluble IL-6	Tocilizumab	Humanised mAb	Blocks IL-6 receptor	RA[a] (moderate–severe)
	Sarilumab	Humanised mAb	Blocks IL-6 receptor	RA[a] (moderate–severe)
Soluble IL-12 and -23	Ustekinumab	Humanised mAb	Immunoneutralisation	PA, PP (severe), CD, UC
Soluble IL-17	Secukinumab	Humanised mAb	Immunoneutralisation	AS, PA
T cells	Abatacept	Fusion protein	Prevents co-stimulation of T cells	RA[a] (moderate–severe)
	Alemtuzumab	Humanised mAb	Binds to CD 52 causing cell lysis	MS
	Basiliximab	Chimeric mAb	IL-2 receptor antagonists	Immunosuppression for transplantation surgery
	Belatacept	Fusion protein	Prevents activation of T cells	
	Natalizumab	Humanised mAb	VLA-4 on lymphocytes (neutralises)	MS
	Ocrelizumab	Humanised mAb	Blocks CD-20 on lymphocytes	MS
	Vedolizumab	Humanised mAb	Target alpha4beta7 integrin on T cells	CD, UC
B cells	Belimumab	Humanised mAb	Immunoneutralises B cell-activating factor	SLE
	Rituximab	Chimeric mAb	Causes B cells lysis	RA[a] (moderate–severe), some malignancies

[a]Used in conjunction with methotrexate.
ab, Antibody; *AS*, ankylosing spondylitis; *CD*, Crohn's disease; *GA*, gouty arthritis; *IL*, interleukin; *mAb*, monoclonal antibody; *MS*, multiple sclerosis; *PA*, psoriatic arthritis; *PP*, plaque psoriasis (e.g. skin); *PS*, psoriasis; *RA*, rheumatoid arthritis; *SLE*, systemic lupus erythematosus; *TNF*, tumour necrosis factor; *UC*, ulcerative collitis.
Data from various sources, including the British National Formulary, 2021.

and a superior final therapeutic outcome achieved (van der Kooij et al., 2009).

Cytokines are crucial to the regulation of host defence systems (see Ch. 17), and leukocytes are key players in its successful functioning. One might predict, therefore, that anticytokine or antileukocyte therapy – like any treatment that interferes with immune function – may precipitate latent infections (e.g. tuberculosis or hepatitis B) or encourage opportunistic infections. Reports suggest that this is a problem with some of these agents (e.g. **adalimumab**, **etanercept**, **infliximab**, **natalizumab** and **rituximab**). The area has been reviewed by Bongartz et al. (2006). Another unexpected, but fortunately rare, effect seen with these drugs is the onset of psoriasis-like syndrome (Fiorino et al., 2009). Hypersensitivity, injection site reactions or mild GI symptoms may be seen with any of these drugs.

DRUGS USED IN GOUT

Gout (also known as *gouty arthritis*) is a metabolic disease in which urate crystals are deposited in tissues, usually because plasma urate concentration is raised. Sometimes this is linked to overindulgence in alcoholic beverages, especially beer, or purine-rich foods such as offal (urate is a product of purine metabolism). Increased cell turnover in

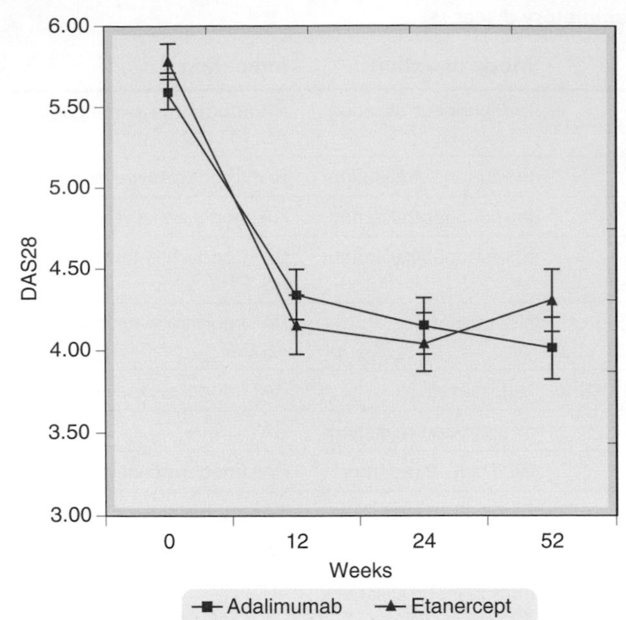

Fig. 25.4 The effect of anticytokine biopharmaceuticals on rheumatoid arthritis. In this figure, adalimumab (a humanised monoclonal antibody that neutralises tumour necrosis factor (TNF)) and etanercept (a fusion protein decoy receptor that binds to TNF) were used to treat patients with active rheumatoid arthritis. The Y-axis measures a composite disease activity scores obtained from clinical assessment of 28 joints (DAS28: the lower the score, the less swollen and painful the joints). (From Jobanputra et al., 2012.)

haematological malignancies, particularly after treatment with cytotoxic drugs (see Ch. 57), and impaired excretion of uric acid by drugs such as ordinary therapeutic doses of **aspirin** (see earlier) are other causes. It is characterised by extremely painful intermittent attacks of acute arthritis produced by the deposition of the crystals in the synovial tissue of distal joints, such as the big toe, as well as the external ear – the common theme being that these tissues are generally relatively cool, favouring crystal deposition. An inflammatory response is evoked, involving activation of the kinin, complement and plasmin systems (see Chs 7 and 17), generation of prostaglandins, lipoxygenase products such as leukotriene B_4 (see Ch. 17), and local accumulation of neutrophil granulocytes. These engulf the crystals by phagocytosis, releasing tissue-damaging toxic oxygen metabolites and subsequently causing lysis of the cells with release of proteolytic enzymes. Urate crystals also induce the production of IL-1 and possibly other cytokines.

Drugs used to treat gout act in the following ways:

- by decreasing uric acid synthesis **allopurinol** (the main prophylactic drug) or **febuxostat**;
- by increasing uric acid excretion (*uricosuric agents*: **probenecid**, **sulfinpyrazone**; see Ch. 29);
- by inhibiting leukocyte migration into the joint (**colchicine**);
- as an 'IL-1-dependent' disease, biopharmaceuticals such as **anakinra** may be useful;
- by exerting a general anti-inflammatory and analgesic effect (NSAIDs and occasionally glucocorticoids).

Their clinical uses are summarised in the clinical box.

Drugs used in gout and hyperuricaemia

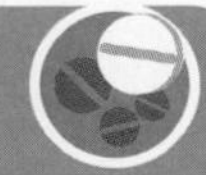

To treat acute gout:
- An NSAID, e.g. **ibuprofen**, **naproxen.**
- **Colchicine** is useful if NSAIDs are contraindicated.
- A glucocorticoid, e.g. **hydrocortisone** (oral, intramuscular or intra-articular) is an alternative to an NSAID.

For prophylaxis
- **Allopurinol**; (must not be started until the patient is asymptomatic):
  - a uricosuric drug (e.g. **probenecid**, **sulfinpyrazone**), for patients allergic to **allopurinol**
- **Rasburicase** by intravenous infusion for prevention and treatment of acute hyperuricaemia in patients with haematological malignancy at risk of rapid lysis.

Allopurinol

Allopurinol is an analogue of *hypoxanthine* that reduces the synthesis of uric acid by competitive inhibition of xanthine oxidase (Fig. 25.5). The drug is first converted by xanthine oxidase to *alloxanthine*, which persists in the tissue for a considerable time, and is an effective non-competitive inhibitor of the enzyme. Some inhibition of de novo purine synthesis also occurs.

Allopurinol reduces the concentration of the relatively insoluble urates and uric acid in tissues, plasma and urine, while increasing the concentration of their more soluble precursors, the xanthines and hypoxanthines. The deposition of urate crystals in tissues (tophi) is reversed, and the formation of renal urate stones is inhibited. **Allopurinol** is the drug of choice in the long-term treatment of gout, but it actually exacerbates inflammation and pain in an acute attack (see later). **Febuxostat** has a similar mechanism of action and pharmacology.

Allopurinol is given orally and is well absorbed. Its half-life is 2–3 h: its active metabolite alloxanthine (see Fig. 25.5) has a half-life of 18–30 h. Renal excretion is a balance between glomerular filtration and **probenecid**-sensitive tubular reabsorption.

Acute attacks of gout occur commonly during the early stages of therapy (possibly as a result of physicochemical changes in the surfaces of urate crystals as these start to re-dissolve), so treatment with **allopurinol** is never initiated during an acute attack and is usually initially combined with an NSAID. Unwanted effects are otherwise few. GI disturbances, allergic reactions (mainly rashes) and some blood problems can occur but usually disappear if the drug is stopped. Potentially fatal skin diseases such as toxic epidermal necrolysis and Stevens–Johnson syndrome are rare – but devastating.

Allopurinol increases the effect of mercaptopurine, an antimetabolite used in cancer chemotherapy, which is

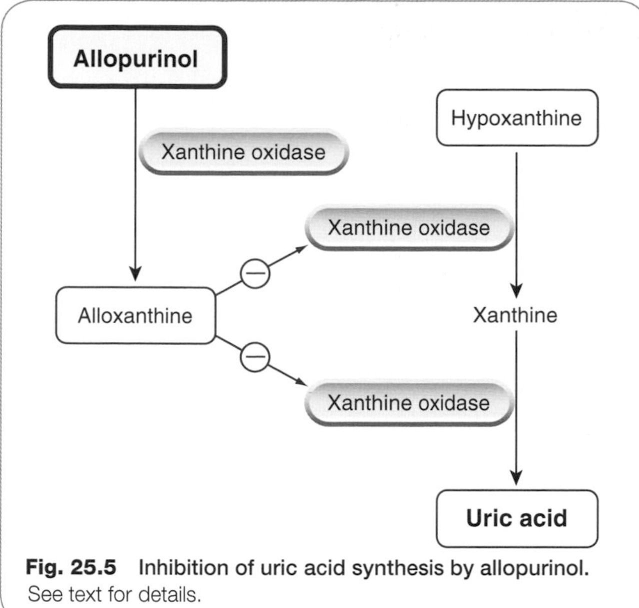

Fig. 25.5 Inhibition of uric acid synthesis by allopurinol. See text for details.

inactivated by xanthine oxidase (see Ch. 57), and also that of **azathioprine** (see Table 25.2), which is metabolised to mercaptopurine. **Allopurinol** also enhances the effect of another anticancer drug, **cyclophosphamide** (see Ch. 57). The effect of warfarin is increased because its metabolism is inhibited.

Uricosuric agents

Uricosuric drugs increase uric acid excretion by a direct action on the renal tubule (see Ch. 29). They remain useful as prophylaxis for patients with severe recurrent gout who may not tolerate **allopurinol**. Drugs in this class include **probenecid** and **sulfinpyrazone** (which also has NSAID activity). **Benzbromarone** has a role in the treatment of patients with renal impairment. Treatment with uricosuric drugs is initiated together with an NSAID, as in the case of **allopurinol**. However, **aspirin** and salicylates antagonise the action of uricosuric drugs and should not be used concurrently.

Although not strictly speaking in this group, **rasburicase**, a preparation containing the enzyme uric acid oxidase, is sometimes used for aggressive treatment of gout. It oxidises uric acid in the blood to allantoin, which is more soluble and thus more readily excreted.

Colchicine

Colchicine is an alkaloid extracted from the autumn crocus. It has a beneficial effect in gouty arthritis and can be used both to prevent and to relieve acute attacks. It prevents migration of neutrophils into the joint apparently by binding to tubulin, resulting in the depolymerisation of the microtubules and reduced cell motility. **Colchicine**-treated neutrophils exhibit erratic locomotion often likened to a 'drunken walk'. **Colchicine** may also prevent the production, by neutrophils that have phagocytosed urate crystals, of a putative inflammatory glycoprotein. Other mechanisms may also be important in bringing about its effects. At higher doses than are used to treat gout, **colchicine** inhibits mitosis, carrying a risk of serious bone marrow depression. As such it has a narrow therapeutic index and is extremely dangerous in overdose.

Colchicine is given orally and is excreted partly in the GI tract and partly in the urine.

The acute unwanted effects of **colchicine** during therapy are largely GI and include nausea, vomiting and abdominal pain. Severe diarrhoea[9] may be a problem, and with large doses, or prolonged treatment, its antimitotic action may cause serious side effects, including GI haemorrhage, kidney damage, bone marrow depression and peripheral neuropathy.

ANTAGONISTS OF HISTAMINE

As we explained in Chapter 17, histamine was first identified as a mediator of anaphylaxis by Dale and his colleagues in the early 20th century and later shown to be particularly released during other immune reactions. Mast cells are a prominent source of this mediator and release it into the local environment in response to a variety of immunological and other stimuli. Evidently therefore, there was a potential for developing drugs which inhibited histamine generation or action for the treatment of allergic inflammation.

Antihistamines were introduced by Bovet and his colleagues in the 1930s, before the discovery of the four histamine receptor subtypes described in Chapter 17. By convention, the generic term 'antihistamine' usually refers only to the H_1-receptor antagonists that are used for treating various inflammatory and allergic conditions, and it is these drugs that are discussed in this section

Details of some typical systemic H_1-receptor antagonists are shown in Table 25.5. There are several others that are primarily used topically (e.g. in nasal sprays or eye drops) in the treatment of hay fever and other allergic symptoms. These include **antazoline**, **azelastine**, **epinastine**, **olopatadine** and **emedastine**. In addition to their H_1 antagonist activities, some antihistamines (e.g. **ketotifen**) may also have 'mast cell stabilising' and other anti-inflammatory properties unrelated to histamine antagonism (see Assanasen and Naclerio, 2002).

Pharmacological actions

Conventionally, the antihistamines are divided into 'first-generation' drugs, which cross the blood–brain barrier and, by acting at histamine receptors in the CNS, often have sedating actions, and 'second-generation' drugs, which, broadly speaking, do not. Some of the original second-generation agents (e.g. **terfenadine**) exhibited some cardiac toxicity (e.g. *torsade de pointes*, see Ch. 20). While the risk was extremely low, it was increased when the drug was taken with grapefruit juice or with agents that inhibit cytochrome P450 in the liver (see Chs 10 and 58). These drugs were therefore withdrawn and replaced by 'third-generation cardio-safe' drugs (often active metabolites of the original drugs, e.g. **fexofenadine**).

Pharmacologically, most of the effects of the H_1-receptor antagonists follow from the actions of histamine outlined in Chapter 17. In vitro, for example, they decrease histamine-mediated contraction of the smooth muscle

[9]Because the therapeutic margin is so small, it used to be said by rheumatologists that 'patients must run before they can walk'!

Table 25.5 Comparison of some commonly used systemic antihistamines (H_1 antagonists)

Type	Drug	Common anti-allergic use	Comments
'Sedating'	Alimemazine	U	Strong sedative action. Sometimes used for anaesthetic premedication
	Chlorphenamine	AE, H, U	—
	Cinnarizine	—	Also used to treat nausea, vomiting, motion sickness
	Clemastine	H, U	—
	Cyclizine	—	Also used to treat nausea, vomiting, motion sickness
	Cyproheptadine	H, U	Also used for migraine
	Hydroxyzine	U	May cause QT interval prolongation
	Ketotifen	H	Mast cell 'stabilising' properties
	Promethazine	H, U, AE	Strong sedative action. Also used to control nausea and vomiting
'Non-sedating'	Acrivastine	H, U	—
	Bilastine	H, U	—
	Cetirizine	H, U	—
	Desloratadine	H, U	Metabolite of loratadine. Long-lasting action
	Fexofenadine	H, U	'Cardio-safe' metabolite of terfenadine
	Levocetirizine	H, U	Isomer of cetirizine
	Loratadine	H, U	—
	Mizolastine	H, U	May cause QT interval prolongation
	Rupatadine	H, U	Also antagonises PAF (see Ch. 17)

AE, Allergic emergency (e.g. anaphylactic shock); *H*, hay fever; *PAF*, platelet activating factor; *S*, sedation; *U*, urticaria and/or pruritus.
Data from various sources, including the British National Formulary, 2021.

of the bronchi, the intestine and the uterus. They inhibit histamine-induced increases in vascular permeability and bronchospasm in the guinea pig in vivo but are unfortunately of little value in allergic bronchospasm in humans. The clinical uses of H_1-receptor antagonists are summarised in the clinical box.

Clinical uses of histamine H_1-receptor antagonists

- Allergic reactions (see Ch. 7):
  - non-sedating drugs (e.g. **fexofenadine**, **cetirizine**) are used for allergic rhinitis (hay fever) and urticaria
  - topical preparations may be used for insect bites
  - injectable formulations are useful as an adjunct to **adrenaline** (**epinephrine**) for severe drug hypersensitivity reactions and emergency treatment of anaphylaxis.
- As antiemetics (see Ch. 30):
  - prevention of motion sickness (e.g. **cyclizine**, **cinnarizine**)
  - other causes of nausea, especially labyrinthine disorders
  - for sedation (see Ch. 45, e.g. **promethazine**).

The CNS 'side effects' of some older H_1-receptor antagonists are sometimes more clinically useful than the peripheral H_1-antagonist effects (e.g. **chlorphenamine**; see Table 25.5). When used to treat allergies, the sedative effects are generally unwanted, but there are other occasions (e.g. when taking an overnight flight) when they are more desirable. Even under these circumstances, other CNS effects, such as dizziness and fatigue, are unwelcome. Other centrally acting antihistamines are antiemetic and are used to prevent motion sickness (e.g. **promethazine**; see Ch. 30).

Several H_1-receptor antagonists show weak blockade of $\alpha 1$ adrenoceptors (e.g. **promethazine**). **Cyproheptadine** is a 5-HT antagonist as well as an H_1-receptor antagonist and **rupatadine** is also a platelet activating factor (PAF) antagonist.

Pharmacokinetic aspects

Most orally active H_1-receptor antagonists are well absorbed and remain effective for 3–6 h, although there are some prominent exceptions (e.g. **loratadine**, which is converted to a long-acting metabolite). Most appear to be widely distributed throughout the body, but some do not penetrate the blood–brain barrier, for example the non-sedating drugs mentioned previously (see Table 25.5). They are mainly metabolised in the liver and excreted in the urine.

Many antihistamines have peripheral antimuscarinic side effects. The commonest of these is dryness of the mouth, but blurred vision, constipation and retention of urine can also occur. Unwanted effects that are not mechanism based are also seen; GI disturbances are fairly common, while allergic dermatitis can follow topical application.

POSSIBLE FUTURE DEVELOPMENTS IN ANTI-INFLAMMATORY THERAPY

Undoubtedly the most exciting area of current development is in biopharmaceuticals (see Ch. 5). The success of the anti-TNF and other biological agents has been very gratifying and development of therapeutic antibodies that neutralise inflammogens or block key leukocyte receptors or adhesion molecules is likely to continue unabated and, as research progresses, may also include RNA or other drugs (Ch. 5). The main problem with this sector is the cost of these drugs and lack of oral availability. This places a strain on healthcare budgets and often prevents them from being used as a first-line therapy. The recent availability of 'biosimilars' to originator biologics offers some hope and hopefully, ways will be found to reduce the cost of production and development of these important medicines.

Clearly therefore, a low-cost alternative to a neutralising anti-TNF antibody would be a welcome development. *TNF-converting enzyme* (TACE; at least two forms) cleaves membrane-bound TNF thus releasing the soluble active form into the blood, and so might be an attractive target. A number of putative small-molecule inhibitors of this enzyme are effective in animal models but have not transferred well to the clinic so far although there remains general optimism about this general approach. The area has recently been reviewed by Murumkar et al. (2020).

The disconcerting realisation that all NSAIDs (and coxibs) have cardiovascular side effects has raised further questions about our existing therapeutic arsenal.[10] In an attempt to circumvent this and other, unwanted effects of conventional NSAIDs (such as GI toxicity) several attempts have been made to derivatise these drugs in some way so as to reduce their potential for adverse effects. Based upon impeccable research and very encouraging animal data this has been achieved by attaching NO-donating or other, 'protective' groups such as H_2S (another gaseous mediator with protective properties) to standard drugs such as **naproxen**. One of these drugs (**naproxcinod**, an NO-releasing derivative of **naproxen**) is undergoing further clinical trials at the request of the FDA (see Wallace et al., 2015; Costa et al., 2020). However, Kirkby et al. (2016) have proposed that simple arginate salts of NSAIDs may lack the unwanted cardiovascular side effects of their parent drugs. Thus the quest for a 'safe' NSAID continues.

Taking a totally different approach are attempts to use, as anti-inflammatory drugs, the endogenous mediators which normally terminate inflammation under physiological conditions (see Ch. 17). Conceptually, this would be expected to have many advantages as such agents would not be expected to subvert the normal functioning of the immune system in the same way as those drugs referred to in this chapter. There have been some encouraging preclinical findings, but as yet, no agent has actually reached the market. The area has been reviewed recently by Park et al. (2020).

[10]This does not, of course, apply to low-dose aspirin.

REFERENCES AND FURTHER READING

NSAIDs and coxibs

Anderson, B.J., 2008. Paracetamol (acetaminophen): mechanisms of action. Paediatr. Anaesth. 18, 915–921.

Baker, M., Perazella, M.A., 2020. NSAIDs in CKD: are they safe? Am. J. Kidney Dis. 76, 546–557.

Bakhriansyah, M., Souverein, P.C., de Boer, A., et al., 2017. Gastrointestinal toxicity among patients taking selective COX-2 inhibitors or conventional NSAIDs, alone or combined with proton pump inhibitors: a case-control study. Pharmacoepidemiol. Drug Saf. 26, 1141–1148.

Baigent, C.L., Blackwell, L., Collins, R., et al., 2009. Aspirin in the primary and secondary prevention of vascular disease: collaborative meta-analysis of individual participant data from randomised trials. Lancet 373, 1849–1860.

Baron, J.A., Sandler, R.S., Bresalier, R.S., et al., 2006. A randomized trial of rofecoxib for the chemoprevention of colorectal adenomas. Gastroenterology 131, 1674–1682.

Blanca-Lopez, N., Soriano, V., Garcia-Martin, E., Canto, G., Blanca, M., 2019. NSAID-induced reactions: classification, prevalence, impact, and management strategies. J. Asthma Allergy 12, 217–233.

British National Formulary, 2021. London: BMJ Group and Pharmaceutical Press. Available at: http://www.medicinescomplete.com.

Bushra, R., Aslam, N., 2010. An overview of clinical pharmacology of Ibuprofen. Oman Med. J. 25, 155–1661.

Castellsague, J., Riera-Guardia, N., Calingaert, B., et al., 2012. Individual NSAIDs and upper gastrointestinal complications: a systematic review and meta-analysis of observational studies (the SOS project). Drug Saf. 35, 1127–1146.

Conaghan, P.G., 2012. A turbulent decade for NSAIDs: update on current concepts of classification, epidemiology, comparative efficacy, and toxicity. Rheumatol. Int. 32, 1491–1502.

FitzGerald, G.A., Patrono, C., 2001. The coxibs, selective inhibitors of cyclooxygenase-2. N. Engl. J. Med. 345, 433–442.

Flower, R.J., 2003. The development of COX-2 inhibitors. Nat. Rev. Drug Discov. 2, 179–191.

Henry, D., Lim, L.L., Garcia Rodriguez, L.A., et al., 1996. Variability in risk of gastrointestinal complications with individual non-steroidal anti-inflammatory drugs: results of a collaborative meta-analysis. BMJ 312, 1563–1566.

Horl, W.H., 2010. Nonsteroidal anti-inflammatory drugs and the kidney. Pharmaceuticals (Basel) 3, 2291–2321.

Hyllested, M., Jones, S., Pedersen, J.L., et al., 2002. Comparative effect of paracetamol, NSAIDs or their combination in postoperative pain management: a qualitative review. Br. J. Anaesth. 88, 199–214.

Jobanputra, P., Maggs, F., Deeming, A., et al., 2012. A randomised efficacy and discontinuation study of etanercept versus adalimumab (RED SEA) for rheumatoid arthritis: a pragmatic, unblinded, non-inferiority study of first TNF inhibitor use: outcomes over 2 years. BMJ Open 2 (6), e001395.

Kirkby, N.S., Tesfai, A., Ahmetaj-Shala, B., et al., 2016. Ibuprofen arginate retains eNOS substrate activity and reverses endothelial dysfunction: implications for the COX-2/ADMA axis. FASEB J. 30, 4172–4179.

Laidlaw, T.M., Cahill, K.N., 2017. Current knowledge and management of hypersensitivity to aspirin and NSAIDs. J. Allergy Clin. Immunol. Pract. 5, 537–545.

Lanas, A., Carrera-Lasfuentes, P., Arguedas, Y., et al., 2015. Risk of upper and lower gastrointestinal bleeding in patients taking nonsteroidal anti-inflammatory drugs, antiplatelet agents, or anticoagulants. Clin. Gastroenterol. Hepatol. 13, 906–912 e2.

Lee, J.J., Simmons, D.L., 2018. Antipyretic therapy: clinical pharmacology. Handb. Clin. Neurol. 157, 869–881.

Luong, C., Miller, A., Barnett, J., et al., 1996. Flexibility of the NSAID binding site in the structure of human cyclooxygenase-2. Nat. Struct. Biol. 3, 927–933.

McEvoy, L., Carr, D.F., Pirmohamed, M., 2021. Pharmacogenomics of NSAID-induced upper gastrointestinal toxicity. Front. Pharmacol. 12.
Mitchell, J.A., Shala, F., Elghazouli, Y., et al., 2019. Cell-specific gene deletion reveals the antithrombotic function of COX1 and explains the vascular COX1/prostacyclin paradox. Circ. Res. 125, 847–854.
Park, J., Langmead, C.J., Riddy, D.M., 2020. New advances in targeting the resolution of inflammation: implications for specialized pro-resolving mediator GPCR drug discovery. ACS Pharmacol. Transl. Sci. 3, 88–106.
Prescott, L.F., 2000. Paracetamol, alcohol and the liver. Br. J. Clin. Pharmacol. 49, 291–301.
Schjerning, A.M., McGettigan, P., Gislason, G., 2020. Cardiovascular effects and safety of (non-aspirin) NSAIDs. Nat. Rev. Cardiol. 17, 574–584.
Thybo, K.H., Hagi-Pedersen, D., Dahl, J.B., et al., 2019. Effect of combination of paracetamol (acetaminophen) and ibuprofen vs either alone on patient-controlled Morphine consumption in the first 24 hours after total hip arthroplasty: the PANSAID randomized clinical trial. JAMA 321, 562–571.
Vane, J.R., 1971. Inhibition of prostaglandin synthesis as a mechanism of action for aspirin-like drugs. Nat. New Biol. 231, 232–239.
Vane, J.R., Botting, R.M. (Eds.), 2001. Therapeutic Roles of Selective COX-2 Inhibitors. William Harvey Press, London, p. 584.
Vuilleumier, P.H., Schliessbach, J., Curatolo, M., 2018. Current evidence for central analgesic effects of NSAIDs: an overview of the literature. Minerva. Anestesiol. 84, 865–870.
Wallace, J.L., 2000. How do NSAIDs cause ulcer disease? Baillière's best pract. Res. Clin. Gastroenterol. 14, 147–159.
Wallace, J.L., Nagy, P., Feener, T.D., et al., 2020. A proof-of-concept, phase 2 clinical trial of the gastrointestinal safety of a hydrogen sulfide-releasing anti-inflammatory drug. Br. J. Pharmacol. 177, 769–777.
Wang, T., Cook, I., Leyh, T.S., 2017. The NSAID allosteric site of human cytosolic sulfotransferases. J. Biol. Chem. 292, 20305–20312.
Warner, T.D., Giuliano, F., Vojnovic, I., et al., 1999. Nonsteroid drug selectivities for cyclo-oxygenase-1 rather than cyclo-oxygenase-2 are associated with human gastrointestinal toxicity: a full in vitro analysis. Proc. Natl. Acad. Sci. U S A. 96, 7563–7568.
Warner, T.D., Mitchell, J.A., 2004. Cyclooxygenases: new forms, new inhibitors, and lessons from the clinic. FASEB J. 18, 790–804.
Warner, T.D., Mitchell, J.A., 2008. COX-2 selectivity alone does not define the cardiovascular risks associated with non-steroidal anti-inflammatory drugs. Lancet 371, 270–273.
Weng, J., Zhao, G., Weng, L., Guan, J., Alzheimer's Disease Neuroimaging Initiative, 2021. Aspirin using was associated with slower cognitive decline in patients with Alzheimer's disease. PLoS One 16, e0252969.
Wongrakpanich, S., Wongrakpanich, A., Melhado, K., et al., 2018. A comprehensive review of non-steroidal anti-inflammatory drug use in the elderly. Aging Dis. 9, 143–150.
Woo, S.D., Luu, Q.Q., Park, H.S., 2020. NSAID-exacerbated respiratory disease (NERD): from pathogenesis to improved care. Front. Pharmacol. 11, 1147.
Wong, R.S.Y., 2019. Role of nonsteroidal anti-inflammatory drugs (NSAIDs) in cancer prevention and cancer promotion. Adv. Pharmacol. Sci, 2019, 3418975.

Antirheumatoid drugs: csDMARDs, tsDMARDs, bDMARDs and glucocorticoids

Arora, T., Padaki, R., Liu, L., et al., 2009. Differences in binding and effector functions between classes of TNF antagonists. Cytokine 45, 124–131.
Bertsias, G., 2020. Therapeutic targeting of JAKs: from hematology to rheumatology and from the first to the second generation of JAK inhibitors. Mediterr. J. Rheumatol. 31, 105–111.
Bongartz, T., Sutton, A.J., Sweeting, M.J., et al., 2006. Anti-TNF antibody therapy in rheumatoid arthritis and the risk of serious infections and malignancies: systematic review and meta-analysis of rare harmful effects in randomized controlled trials. JAMA 295, 2275–2285.
Borel, J.F., Baumann, G., Chapman, I., et al., 1996. In vivo pharmacological effects of ciclosporin and some analogues. Adv. Pharmacol. 35, 115–246.
Chan, E.S., Cronstein, B.N., 2010. Methotrexate - how does it really work? Nat. Rev. Rheumatol. 6, 175–178.
Chandrashekara, S., 2013. Pharmacokinetic consideration of synthetic DMARDs in rheumatoid arthritis. Expert Opin. Drug Metab. Toxicol. 9, 969–981.
Chatzidionysiou, K., Emamikia, S., Nam, J., et al., 2017. Efficacy of glucocorticoids, conventional and targeted synthetic disease-modifying antirheumatic drugs: a systematic literature review informing the 2016 update of the EULAR recommendations for the management of rheumatoid arthritis. Ann. Rheum. Dis. 76, 1102–1107.
Cutolo, M., 2002. Effects of DMARDs on IL-1Ra levels in rheumatoid arthritis: is there any evidence? Clin. Exp. Rheumatol. 20 (5 Suppl. 27), S26–S31.
Davis 3rd, J.M., Matteson, E.L., 2012. My treatment approach to rheumatoid arthritis. Mayo Clin. Proc. 87, 659–673.
Feldmann, M., 2002. Development of anti-TNF therapy for rheumatoid arthritis. Nat. Rev. Immunol. 2, 364–371.
Fiorino, G., Allez, M., Malesci, A., Danese, E., 2009. Review article: anti TNF-alpha induced psoriasis in patients with inflammatory bowel disease. Aliment. Pharmacol. Ther. 29, 921–927.
Lodowska, J., Gruchlik, A., Wolny, D., Wawszczyk, J., Dzierzewicz, Z., Weglarz, L., 2015. The Effect of sulfasalazine and 5-aminosalicylic acid on the secretion of interleukin 8 by human colon myofibroblasts. Acta Pol. Pharm. 72, 917–921.
Maini, R.N., 2005. The 2005 international symposium on advances in targeted therapies: what have we learned in the 2000s and where are we going? Ann. Rheum. Dis. 64 (Suppl. 4), 106–108.
Ramiro, S., Sepriano, A., Chatzidionysiou, K., et al., 2017. Safety of synthetic and biological DMARDs: a systematic literature review informing the 2016 update of the EULAR recommendations for management of rheumatoid arthritis. Ann. Rheum. Dis. 76, 1101–1136.
van der Kooij, S.M., le Cessie, S., Goekoop-Ruiterman, Y.P., et al., 2009. Clinical and radiological efficacy of initial vs delayed treatment with infliximab plus methotrexate in patients with early rheumatoid arthritis. Ann. Rheum. Dis. 68, 1153–1158.

Antihistamines

Assanasen, P., Naclerio, R.M., 2002. Antiallergic anti-inflammatory effects of H_1-antihistamines in humans. Clin. Allergy Immunol. 17, 101–139.
Simons, F.E.R., Simons, K.J., 1994. Drug therapy: the pharmacology and use of H_1-receptor-antagonist drugs. N. Engl. J. Med. 23, 1663–1670.

New directions

Costa, S., Muscara, M.N., Allain, T., et al., 2020. Enhanced analgesic effects and gastrointestinal safety of a novel, hydrogen sulfide-releasing anti-inflammatory drug (ATB-352): a role for endogenous cannabinoids. Antioxid. Redox Signal. 33, 1003–1009.
Murumkar, P.R., Ghuge, R.B., Chauhan, M., et al., 2020. Recent developments and strategies for the discovery of TACE inhibitors. Expert Opin. Drug Discov. 15, 779–801.
Ouvry, G., Berton, Y., Bhurruth-Alcor, Y., et al., 2017. Identification of novel TACE inhibitors compatible with topical application. Bioorg. Med. Chem. Lett. 27, 1848–1853.
Sharma, M., Mohapatra, J., Acharya, A., et al., 2013. Blockade of tumor necrosis factor-alpha converting enzyme (TACE) enhances IL-1-beta and IFN-gamma via caspase-1 activation: a probable cause for loss of efficacy of TACE inhibitors in humans? Eur. J. Pharmacol. 701, 106–113.
Wallace, J.L., de Nucci, G., Sulaieva, O., 2015. Toward more GI-friendly anti-inflammatory medications. Curr. Treat. Options Gastroenterol. 13, 377–385.

Skin 26

OVERVIEW

With a surface area of about 1.6–1.8 m² and a weight of about 4.5 kg in the average adult, skin qualifies as the largest and heaviest organ in the body. It is also an important target for drug therapy as well as cosmetic and other agents. Here, we look at the structure of human skin and briefly review some common skin disorders. We then discuss some of the many types of drugs that act upon, or through, this organ.

INTRODUCTION

Skin is a complex organ with many roles.[1] Firstly, it acts as a barrier. Being impermeable to water, it prevents the loss of moisture from the body as well as the ingress of water and many other substances into the body. It also cushions underlying tissues against thermal and mechanical damage and shields them from ultraviolet radiation and infection. Even if microorganisms survive in the slightly acidic environment of the skin's surface, they cannot easily cross the outer barrier of the skin. In the event that they do, they encounter specialised immunological surveillance systems comprising *Langerhans cells*, a type of dendritic cell, as well as mast cells and other immunocompetent cell types.[2]

A second function is thermoregulation. Approximately 10% of the total blood volume is contained within the dense capillary networks of the skin. Skin arterioles, controlled by the sympathetic nervous system, regulate blood flow and heat loss. Also involved in thermoregulation, and under cholinergic control, are the sweat glands (*eccrine glands*). These secrete an aqueous fluid that increases heat loss upon evaporation.

In the presence of sunlight, vitamin D_3 (cholecalciferol) is synthesised in the *stratum basale* and *stratum spinosum* of skin. Absence of this vitamin caused by inadequate exposure to the ultraviolet (UV B) component of sunlight can lead to deficiency symptoms (see Ch. 36). The dark-coloured pigment *melanin*, which protects skin against excessive and potentially damaging solar radiation and which gives skin its characteristic colour, is produced by melanocytes in the basal dermal layer. Melanin granule formation is stimulated by sunlight to match the prevailing light intensity.

Skin is also a profoundly sensory organ. It is densely innervated with neurons, including specific nerve endings that signal pain, heat and cold, and specialised receptors that detect touch (*Meissner corpuscles*) and pressure (*Pacinian corpuscles*) as well as itch – a sensation unique to skin with an interesting pharmacology. The cell bodies of cutaneous sensory nerves reside in the dorsal root ganglia.

Being highly visible, skin and its specialised appendages, hair and nails, play an important part in social and sexual signalling. As such, it is an important target for cosmetic preparations, camouflaging agents, suntan lotions, 'anti-ageing' compounds and more. Because unsightly skin can cause problems of social adjustment or even frank psychiatric illness, the distinction between a therapeutic agent and a cosmetic preparation can become blurred. This is exacerbated by controversies about the classification of 'cosmeceuticals', as they are called, which contain pharmacologically active ingredients and associated safety issues. Nevertheless, the market for such preparations is huge. According to some estimates, the global spend will rise from US $500 billion in 2018 and to over US $700 billion by 2025.

Here we look briefly at some common conditions affecting the skin and at some of the drugs used to treat them (Tables 26.1 and 26.2). In most cases, these drugs also have other uses, and their mechanisms of action are described elsewhere in the book, so the appropriate cross-references are given. Inflammation is a common feature of skin diseases, and anti-inflammatory drugs, discussed in detail in Chapter 25, are often used. In some other instances, the drugs themselves, or their particular utility, are almost unique to skin pharmacology, so they will be explained in a little more detail. Drugs used to treat skin infections and cancers are discussed in Chapters 52, 54 and 57. Of note, drugs may also precipitate dermatological problems with adverse reactions frequently manifesting in the skin. These may range from mild self-limiting rashes through to the life-threatening Stevens-Johnson syndrome and relate factors such as sun exposure (photosensitivity, for instance with tetracycline antibiotics). These are expanded upon in Chapter 58.

Topical application of drugs onto the skin can be used as a route for systemic administration (transdermal drug delivery, see Ch. 9), but also as a means of targeting therapy to treat local underlying tissues. For example, non-steroidal anti-inflammatory drugs (NSAIDs) applied topically can reduce the inflammation of underlying joints and connective tissue with less unwanted effects than those seen after systemic administration (Klinge and Sawyer, 2013). However, we will not deal in depth with this topic here.

STRUCTURE OF SKIN

Skin comprises three main layers: the outermost layer, the *epidermis*; a middle layer, the *dermis*; and the innermost

[1]As the American humourist and songwriter Alan Sherman so succinctly put it, 'Skin's the thing that if you've got it outside/It keeps your insides in'.
[2]Dendritic cells were named as such by Paul Langerhans, who discovered them in 1868 while still a medical student in Berlin. Because of their shape, he mistook them for nerve cells, but they are actually phagocytic antigen-presenting immune cells of the monocyte/macrophage lineage.

Table 26.1 Drug treatment of some common skin disorders

Disease	Class	Examples	Comments	Chapter
Acne	Antibacterials	Erythromycin, clindamycin, various antiseptic agents	For mild–moderate acne. Usually topical but sometimes systemic treatment is also used.	52
	Retinoids	Isotretinoin, adapalene, tretinoin	For more severe disease. Often combined with anti-infective agents. Sometimes systemic treatment is also used.	–
	Androgen antagonists	Co-cyprindiol	For moderate–severe disease.	35
Alopecia	Anti-androgens, vasodilators	Finasteride, minoxidil	Generally in men only.	35, 21
Hirsutism	Inhibitors of DNA/RNA synthesis	Eflornithine	Usually in women only.	57
Infections	Antibacterials	Bacitracin, metronidazole, mupirocin, neomycin sulfate, polymyxins, retapamulin, sulfadiazine, silver salts	Usually given topically but some drugs may be given orally.	52
	Antivirals	Aciclovir, penciclovir		53
	Antifungal	Amorolfine, clotrimazole, econazole, griseofulvin, ketaconazole, miconazole, terbinafine, tioconazole		54
	Antiparasite	Topical parasiticides, e.g. benzyl benzoate, dimeticone, malathion, permethrin, tazarotene	–	55/56
Pruritus	Antihistamines, topical anaesthetics and related drugs	Crotamiton, diphenhydramine, doxepin	Antihistamines may be given topically or orally. Sometimes a 'sedating' antihistamine is useful.	17
Eczema	Glucocorticoids	Mild–potentency (i.e. hydrocortisone, betamethasone esters)	May be combined with antibacterial or antifungal agent if infection is present.	25, 33
	Retinoids	Alitretinoin, acitretin	Given orally. Used only if glucocorticoid therapy has failed.	–
	Calcineurin inhibitors	Picrolimus, tacrolimus	Often topical but sometimes systemic. Used for more severe disease.	25
Psoriasis	Vitamin D analogues	Calcipotriol, calcitriol, tacalcitol	DMARDS and anticytokine drugs used for severe cases.	7, 25
	Retinoids	Acitretin, alitretinoin, tazarotene	Oral retinoids sometimes used.	–
	Glucocorticoids	Moderate–potentency (i.e. hydrocortisone butyrate, clobetasol propionate)	May be combined with antibacterial or antifungal agent if infection is present.	25, 33, 52, 54
	Calcineurin inhibitors	Picrolimus, tacrolimus	Maybe given topically or systemically. Usually used for severe cases.	25
Rosacea	Antibacterials or α_2 adrenergic agents	Doxycycline, erythromycin, metronidazole, tetracycline or brimonidine.	Glucocorticoids are contraindicated.	52
Urticaria	Antihistamines	Diphenhydramine, doxepin.	Usually given orally. Sometimes a 'sedating' antihistamine is useful.	17
Warts	Keratolytic agents and others	Formaldehyde, imiquimod, podophyllotoxin, salicylic acid, silver nitrate	Many of these substances are found in proprietary wart treatments.	–
Melanoma	Chemotherapeutic agents	Taxanes, vinca alkaloids, 5-fluorouracil, cisplatin	Biopharmaceuticals are also used, see Table 26.2.	57

DMARDs, Disease-modifying antirheumatic drugs.
Sources: BNF (2021) and others.

Table 26.2 Some biopharmaceutical drugs used for the treatment of psoriasis and other skin disorders

Drug	Type	Target	Mechanism	Disease
Brodalumab	Human-mAb	IL-17 receptor	Prevents activation of the receptor and the downstream generation of pro-inflammatory chemokines.	Plaque psoriasis (moderate–severe)
Ixekizumab	Humanised-mAb	IL-17	Binds to IL-17A protein and thus prevents the downstream generation of pro-inflammatory chemokines.	
Guselkumab	Human-mAb	IL-23	Prevents activation of the IL-23/IL-17 signalling pathway and the downstream generation of pro-inflammatory chemokines.	
Risankizumab	Humanised-mAb			
Tildrakizumab	Humanised-mAb			
Dupilumab	Human-mAb	IL-4	Inhibits binding to IL-4 receptor and hence IL-13 signalling.	Eczema (moderate-severe: and other non-dermatological conditions)
Ipilimumab	Human-mAb	CTLA-4	Activates T-cells by removing inhibitory control.	Melanoma
Nivolumab	Human-mAb	PD-1 receptor	Causes cell death	
Pembrolizumab	Humanised-mAb			

See Chapter 5 for more information on these types of drug.
Sources: BNF (2021) and others.

layer, the *subdermis*, sometimes called the *hypodermis* or *subcutis* (Fig. 26.1).

The epidermis consists largely of keratinocytes. There are four histologically distinct zones: the *stratum basale* is the innermost layer and lies adjacent to the *dermoepidermal junction*. It comprises mainly dividing keratinocytes interspersed with melanocytes. The latter cells produce granules of melanin in *melanosomes*, which are transferred to the dividing keratinocytes. As the keratinocytes divide and mature, they progress towards the skin surface. In the next layer, they form the *stratum spinosum* ('spiny' layer), so-called because *desmosomes* (intercellular protein links) begin to appear on the cells. Gradually, these cells begin to flatten, adopting a *squamous* (scaly) morphology. They lose their nuclei, and the cytoplasm acquires a granular appearance. Lying immediately above this is a thin translucent layer of tissue called the *stratum lucidum*. The outermost layer of skin is the *stratum corneum*. By now, individual keratinocytes are no longer viable because they have fused together (cornified). Most tissues have 10–30 layers of these hardened sheets of tissue. The *corneocytes*, as they are now called, are surrounded with a hydrated proteinaceous envelope. Lipid bilayers occupy the extracellular space providing a hydrophilic waterproof layer. The water and lipid content of skin is critical to its function. If the moisture content of the hydrated layer falls, the skin loses its supple properties and cracks. The keratinocytes are normally replenished about every 45 days (Bergstresser and Taylor, 1977) and so healthy skin constantly sheds the outer layer of cornified cells. If this does not occur, patches of dry skin begin to appear.

Below the epidermis lies the dermis. This layer varies in thickness. In some tissues, it is very thick (e.g. the palms and the soles of the feet) and in others, very thin (e.g. the eyelids). Histologically, the dermis comprises a *papillary layer* and a deeper *reticular layer*. The main cell types are fibroblasts. These produce and secrete important structural elements of the skin such as glycoproteins, which contribute to the hydration of the tissue, and collagen and elastin that provide strength and elasticity. Other types of cells associated with the immune system are also present (see Ch. 7). The dermis is richly endowed with blood vessels and lymphatics and densely innervated.

Hair follicles, *sebaceous glands* and *sweat glands* are embedded in the dermis. Hair follicles are lined with specialised cells that produce keratin and associated melanocytes that produce pigment for the growing hair shaft. Associated with each hair follicle is an *erector pili* muscle that causes the hair shaft to become erect. Cold, fear and other strong emotional stimuli trigger this response giving the sensation of 'goose bumps'. Sebaceous glands associated with hair follicles coat the hair with waxy substances. The growth of hair and the activity of these glands are controlled by androgens. While *eccrine* sweat glands are distributed over much of the skin surface, *apocrine* sweat glands are also associated with hair, especially in the armpits and perineum. They empty their proteinaceous secretion into the hair follicle.

The innermost layer of skin is the hypodermis or cutis. This comprises connective tissue and adipose tissue, which may be particularly thick at some anatomical locations (e.g. the abdomen).

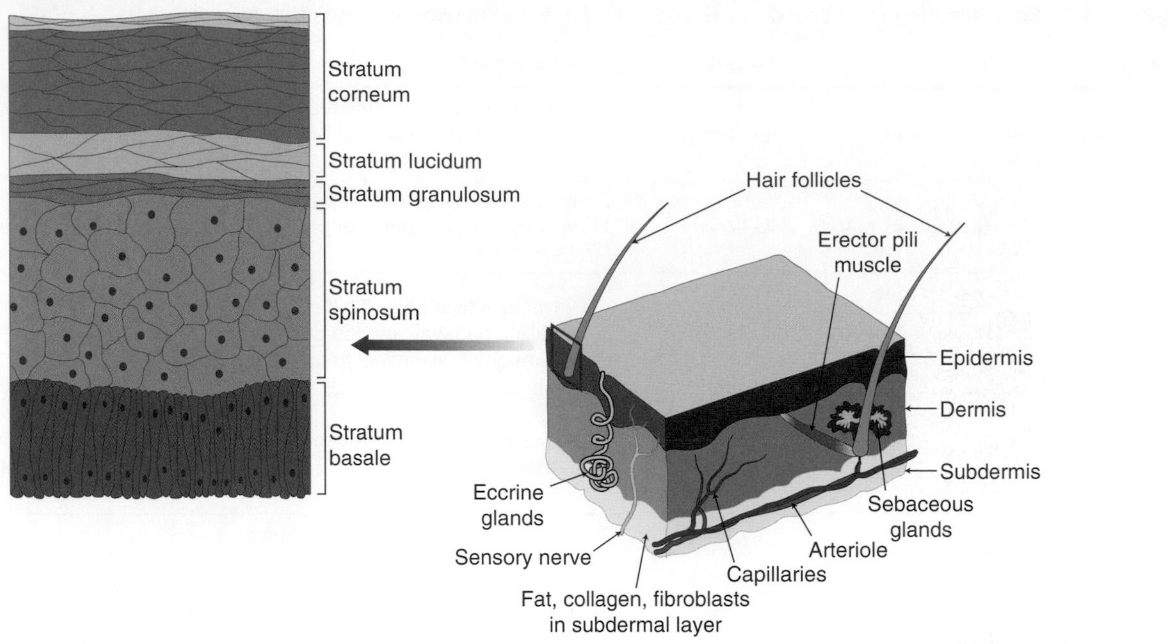

Fig. 26.1 A simplified diagram showing the structure of the skin. The skin comprises three main layers coloured differently in the right-hand drawing: epidermis *(dark red/brown)*; dermis *(pink)*; and subdermis *(yellow)*. On the left is an enlarged diagram of the complex outer, epidermal, layer. Not shown are the apocrine glands within the hair follicles.

Skin

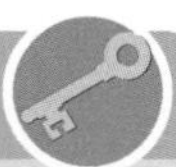

Skin is the largest and heaviest organ in the body. It is composed of three main components:

- *The epidermis.* This is the outermost layer and is composed of four layers of keratinocytes with interspersed melanocytes. Keratinocytes divide in the basal layer and migrate upwards to the skin surface where they form cornified layers. Lipids in the extracellular spaces confer water-repellent properties.
- *The dermis.* The middle layer is of variable thickness. It consists of fibroblasts that produce structural components such as collagen and elastin as well as immunocompetent cells. Hair follicles and sweat glands are also embedded in this layer and it is densely innervated with nerves, blood vessels and lymphatics.
- *The subdermis* (*hypodermis* or *hypocutis*). This comprises connective tissue and varying amounts of adipose tissue.

Skin has four main functions:

- *A barrier.* Skin prevents the egress or ingress of water, other chemicals and microorganisms. It also acts as a mechanical and thermal barrier and a shock absorber.
- *Thermoregulation.* Vasodilatation of the rich capillary network of the skin, in combination with sweating, increases the loss of heat whilst vasoconstriction has the reverse effect.
- *Vitamin D synthesis.* In the presence of sunlight, vitamin D_3 is synthesised by cells in the epidermal layer.
- *A sensory organ.* Skin contains abundant sensory receptors for touch, heat, cold, pain and itch. Information arising from these dermal receptors is one of the chief ways in which we interact with the outside world.

COMMON DISEASES OF THE SKIN

Here we briefly review some common skin disorders (see Fig. 26.2).

ACNE

The most common form of the disease occurs during puberty, especially in boys but also in girls. Changes in circulating androgens stimulate the sebaceous glands associated with hair follicles, which become enlarged and blocked with sebum and debris. The confined material may become infected, causing an inflammatory reaction that compounds the problem. Normally acne disappears after *puberty*, but some forms may persist or manifest in later life and require long-term treatment. If severe, acne can cause irreversible scarring and considerable psychological misery.

ROSACEA

The diagnostic feature of rosacea is the presence of a chronic hyperaemia of the facial skin which often adopts a characteristic pattern, spreading across the cheeks, forehead and the nose. It can sometimes cause *rhinophyma*, a condition in which the nose becomes red, the pores enlarge, and the skin becomes bumpy. Eventually the nose may actually change shape, possibly because of the formation of scar tissue. The erythema is caused by vasodilatation, and dilated blood vessels close to the surface of the skin are usually visible. The affected skin may become dry and flaky; there may be a stinging or burning sensation, and a tendency to flush in response to various stimuli, including exertion, emotional stress, heat, sunlight and spicy foods.

Rosacea affects about 10% of the population and there is a genetic basis for this disorder. It is more prevalent in women

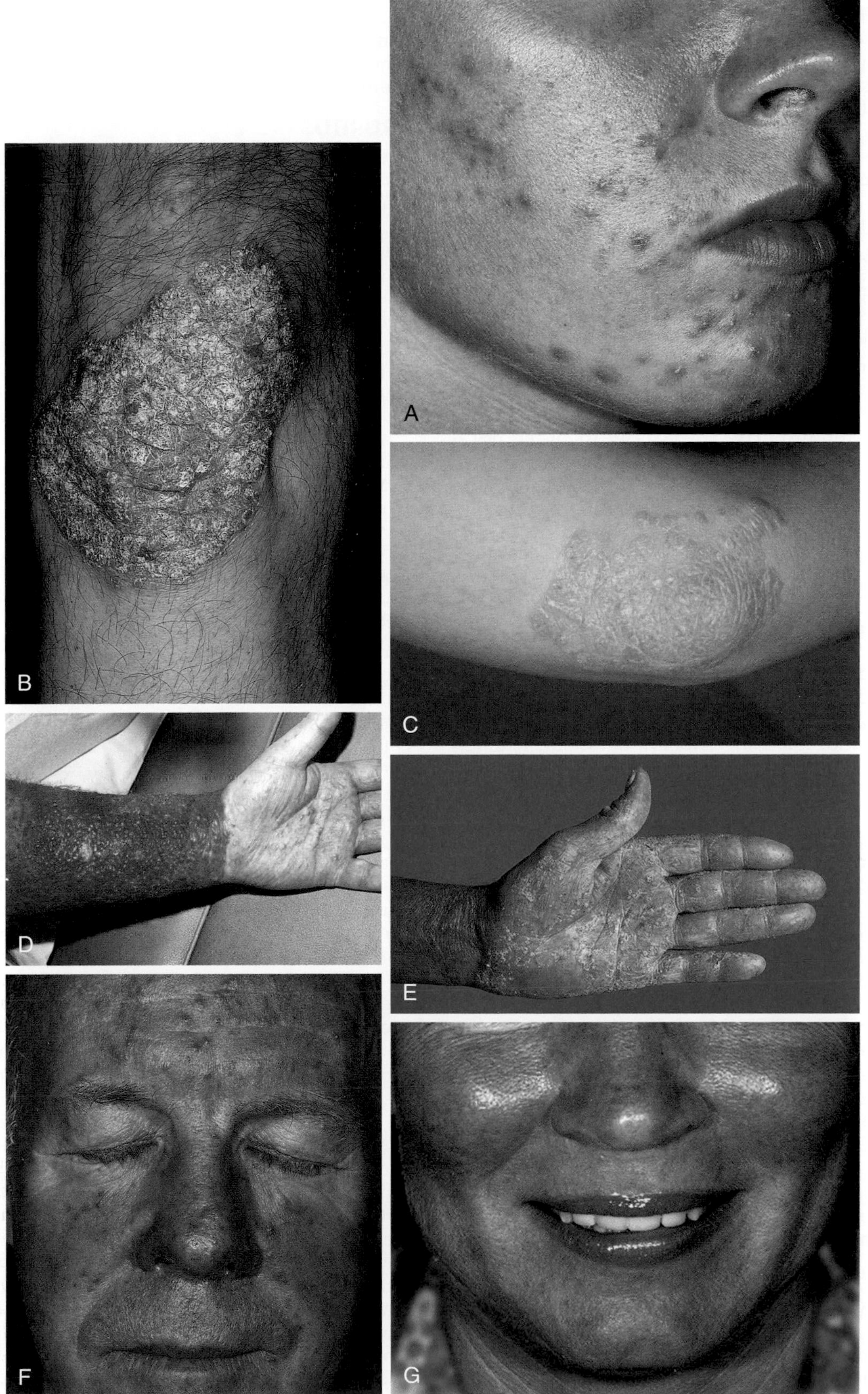

Fig. 26.2 Some common skin disorders. (A) Mild inflammatory acne. (B) Psoriasis on the knee. (C) Psoriasis on the elbow. (D) Eczematous dermatitis. (E) Eczema precipitated by allergic contact dermatitis to chromate found in cement and contact urticaria to latex in protective gloves. (F) Rosacea with pustules and erythema on the forehead, cheeks and nose. (G) Rosacea with erythema. (A and F, From Habif's Clinical Dermatology: A Color Guide to Diagnosis and Therapy, seventh ed. B, From Mosby's Pathology for Massage Therapists, second ed. C, Reproduced from Edwards L. Dermatology in Emergency Care. Churchill Livingstone, New York. D, From Buck's Step-by-Step Medical Coding, 2022 ed. E, From Dermatology Essentials, second ed. G, Courtesy of the Dr. Leonard Swinyer Collection, © 2020 University of Utah and Oregon Health & Science University.)

than men and may be exacerbated during the menopause. The condition cannot be cured, and the symptoms can be very long lasting and difficult to control, with both drug and other therapies such as *phototherapy* playing a role.

There is debate about the cause of rosacea. Although predominately inflammatory in nature, infection may be a trigger, and rosacea could be a disorder of the innate immune system in which antimicrobial peptides in the skin are indirectly responsible for the symptoms. Antibiotics or anti-inflammatory agent treatments are usually the first choices where clinical management demands drugs, but α2-agonists also play a part in controlling the erythema. Sharma et al. (2022) have recently reviewed this area.

BALDNESS AND HIRSUTISM

There are two main types of baldness, *male-pattern baldness (androgenic alopecia)* and *alopecia areata*. Androgenic alopecia is caused by rising androgen levels and so particularly affects men after puberty; it starts with bi-temporal recession and progresses. Androgens inhibit the growth of hair on the scalp but stimulate it elsewhere (e.g. the face, chest, back, etc.). Alopecia areata is a condition where hair falls out in patches. These generally come and go but may eventually coalesce, leading to total baldness. The disease seems to be of autoimmune origin.

Hirsutism is common in men (who seldom complain) but is less socially acceptable in women. Once again, rising androgen levels are the cause, stimulating the growth of hair on areas of the body where it does not normally occur in women (e.g. the face); this is commoner in some ethnic groups and seldom pathological, although it can be a symptom of androgenising endocrine tumours (such as *Sertoli–Leydig cell tumours*, which are a rare type of ovarian tumour).

ECZEMA

This is a generic term and refers to a common condition where the skin becomes dry, itchy, flaky and inflamed. The distribution is distinctive, namely on flexor surfaces such as the wrists, elbows and behind the knees (in contrast to psoriasis). There are several potential causes. *Atopic eczema* (also called *atopic dermatitis*) is the most common inflammatory skin disease, affecting about a quarter of all children and about 5% of adults. It is often seen in patients who also suffer from asthma or seasonal rhinitis (hay fever), although the long-held notion that this type of eczema is *primarily* an immunological disorder has rather little support. It tends to run in families, indicating a genetic susceptibility. *Contact dermatitis* arises when the skin becomes 'sensitised' to a particular antigen. Nickel sensitivity is a classic example: contact with the metal either provokes the production of antibodies or modifies structural elements of the epidermis so that autoantibodies are produced. This is more often seen in women because it is a common component of (less-expensive) jewellery.[3] The pathophysiology is now believed to stem from disordered barrier function leading to epidermal water loss, and a vicious cycle of itching and scratching with release of inflammatory mediators. Penetration of allergens and interaction with immunoglobulin E (IgE)-bearing Langerhans cells can add a Th2-mediated immunological component. *Xerotic eczema* refers to eczema that is produced when the skin dries out. This is more common in the winter months, especially among older people.

PRURITUS

Pruritus – itch – is a common symptom of skin diseases, but can also occur with systemic disorders, such as obstructive jaundice, or neurological disorders such as shingles (herpes zoster). Some drugs (e.g. opioids) also can cause itching. There is a complex relationship between the neural systems that detect and transduce pain and itch (see Greaves and Khalifa, 2004; Ikoma et al., 2006). Confirming the long-held notion that there may be a dedicated population of nociceptors that function as 'itch transducers', two G protein–coupled receptors (MRGPX2 and 4) that are sensitive to peptide allergens, and which are also thought to play a part in neurogenic inflammation and other disorders, have recently been identified and cloned (Cao et al., 2021; Yang et al., 2021).

Skin diseases commonly causing itch include eczema, urticaria and psoriasis. These conditions are generally accompanied by the release of inflammatory mediators in the skin from mast cells (e.g. histamine, leukotrienes, proteases and cytokines).

URTICARIA

This term refers to a range of inflammatory changes in the skin characterised by the presence of raised wheals or bumps ('nettle rash'). They are normally surrounded by a red margin and are intensely itchy. There are many known causes, including exposure to the sun (*solar urticaria*[4]), heat or cold, insect bites or stings, foodstuffs or infection, as well as some drugs. Many cases are allergic in nature while others have no known cause. A bizarre manifestation of urticaria seen in some people is *dermographia* – literally 'skin writing'. This is an exaggerated form of the 'triple response' (localised erythema, flare and wheal) seen after injecting histamine into the skin (see Ch. 17) and in this case provoked by scratching or in some cases simply rubbing or stroking the skin.

Urticaria is associated with inflammatory changes in the dermis, including mast cell degranulation and the accompanying release of mediators. It may co-exist with a related condition, *angio-oedema*, which primarily affects the blood vessels of the subdermal layer. This again relates to histamine or bradykinin release or metabolism and may be precipitated by drugs (commonly the angiotensin-converting enzyme inhibitors) as well as rare disease states such as hereditary angio-oedema (including C1 esterase inhibitor deficiency) and lymphoproliferative disorders. Urticaria can resolve relatively rapidly or can persist for weeks (*chronic urticaria*). The disorder can be difficult to manage and even glucocorticoids, which suppress most inflammatory responses, are usually ineffective. Hereditary angio-oedema management is dependent on subtype and may include recombinant C1 esterase inhibitor therapy (**conestat alfa**), bradykinin receptor antagonists (**icatibant**) and plasma kallikrein inhibitors (**ecallantide**, **lanadelumab** and **berotralstat**).

[3]However, the number of men suffering from the condition is rising because of the popularity of skin piercing. If body art is your thing, always insist on high-quality nickel-free jewellery.

[4]Not to be confused with *miliaria* (prickly heat), which is caused by blocked sweat glands.

PSORIASIS

Aside from atopic dermatitis, psoriasis is the most common inflammatory skin disease, affecting about 2%–3% of Europeans. It is an autoimmune condition and there is a genetic component. Several susceptibility loci have been identified, most of which are connected with the operation of the immune system.

Histologically, psoriasis manifests as inflammation accompanied by hyperproliferation of keratinocytes. This leads to an accumulation of scaly dead skin at the sites of the disease. The most common form is *plaque psoriasis*. This presents as areas of scaly silvery-white skin surrounded by red margins. The distribution is usually quite characteristic, with plaques first appearing on the knees and elbows. The lesions may be painful and are sometimes itchy (in fact the word 'psoriasis' originates from Greek and literally means 'itchy skin', although in contrast to eczema, itch is by no means a predominant symptom). Psoriasis can also affect the fingernails, giving a 'pitted' appearance, and/or the joints (typically but not exclusively the distal inter-phalangeal joints) or other connective tissue (*psoriatic arthritis*).

Psoriatic lesions exhibit major histological changes, including hyperproliferation of keratinocytes, vasodilatation and abnormalities in other dermal structures. The lesions are heavily infiltrated with inflammatory cells such as neutrophils but also T cells. By 2015 it had become clear that a hitherto unknown subset of T cells, Th17 cells, were present in abundance in psoriatic lesions. Th17 cells are activated by interleukin 23 (IL-23) derived from dendritic cells or monocyte/macrophages or by other cytokines to produce IL-17 (several subtypes of which IL-17A is the principal member: see Ch. 7). This cytokine is also generated by T cells, neutrophils, mast and other cell types. It stimulates keratinocytes (and other cells) to produce a panoply of other pro-inflammatory molecules. In animal models, IL-17 reproduces many of the characteristics of psoriasis and it was subsequently recognised as a major driver of the pathogenesis of this condition in humans (Kirkham et al., 2014; Martin et al., 2013) and thus a potential target for drugs that blocked either its action, generation or signalling mechanisms.

Psoriasis is generally a lifelong condition but one that can appear and disappear for no apparent reason. Stress is said to be a precipitating factor, as is dry skin. Several drugs (e.g. β-adrenoceptor antagonists, NSAIDs and **lithium**) are purported to precipitate bouts of the disease (Basavaraj et al., 2010).

Treatment is usually with anti-inflammatory or immunosuppressive drugs (see Table 26.2) but anti-cytokine biopharmaceuticals (which obviously have to be administered systemically rather than topically) can be used to treat severe manifestations of this and related diseases.

WARTS

Warts are caused by infection with one of the many types of human papilloma virus (HPV; see also Ch. 53). They are characterised by small, raised lesions with an irregular shape. As infection of the epidermis by the virus causes *hyperkeratinisation*, they also have a 'rough' feel.

The many varieties of HPV are generally tissue specific, so different strains give rise to warts at diverse anatomical locations. The most common type is usually found on hands and feet (e.g. as *verrucas*). Rather less acceptably, other types of HPV specifically infect the anogenital region, giving *anogenital warts*.

Most warts are benign in nature and disappear spontaneously after a period of time (usually weeks–months). However, some types of HPV are linked to cancers such as cervical cancer. The recent introduction of an anti-HPV vaccine has proved highly successful, reducing the incidence of this disease by 90% in young women who received the vaccine when young.

OTHER INFECTIONS

In addition to acne and rosacea, there are a number of other important bacterial skin infections that can be treated with appropriate antibiotics, either topical or systemic. These include superficial skin infections such as *erysipelas impetigo*, and *cellulitis*, which is a more deep-seated infection mainly involving the dermis and subdermis usually of the lower limbs.

Fungal infections of the skin are also a common problem. *Tinea*, *candida* and other infections (see Ch. 54) affect skin at several sites (e.g. *tinea pedis* – 'athlete's foot'). These infections are easy to catch and can be difficult to eradicate completely.

The most common viral infections affecting the skin are *herpes simplex* (cold sores) and *herpes zoster* (shingles), both of which can be treated with antiviral drugs (see Ch. 53). The most common parasite infections of the skin are head lice (*Pediculus humanus capitis*), crab lice (*Pthirus pubis*) and scabies (*Sarcoptes scabiei*).

MELANOMA

Melanoma (from a classical Greek term meaning 'black') is a malignant cancer caused by mutations in the pigment producing melanocytes, usually as a result of overexposure to UV light. A melanoma may therefore arise in the *stratum basale* layer of skin but also at other locations where these cells are found, including the inner ear and the eye. Melanoma may also develop from a *mole*, a pigmented lesion of the skin more correctly described as a type of *nevus* (birthmark). Melanoma is the most common type of skin cancer and, because of the rapidity with which it can metastasise, it is also the most dangerous, with a poor survival rate if not diagnosed and treated early. Global rates are increasing, and those with pale skins are at most risk.

Initial treatment is usually by surgical resection of the lesion, or metastatic tissue, but various other therapeutic modalities may also be useful, including dynamic phototherapy, radiotherapy, chemotherapy and immunotherapy. In the latter cases, expert supervision is essential because melanoma is notoriously adept at evading drug therapy. The pharmacology of most of the chemotherapeutic agents used (e.g. **cisplatin**, **5-fuorouracil**, **taxanes** and vinca alkaloids, protein kinase inhibitors, tissue metalloproteinase inhibitors) are dealt with in Chapter 57, but biopharmaceuticals have recently revolutionised treatment of some cases (see later). The area has been recently reviewed by Dhanyamraju and Patel (2022).

DRUGS ACTING ON SKIN

FORMULATION

Targeting drugs to the skin is both easy and difficult. Unlike most therapeutic situations, drugs can be applied directly to the diseased tissue in the form of ointments, solutions, creams, pastes or dusting powders, etc. There is an important caveat, however: since skin is a highly effective barrier, it can prevent the entry of many medicinal agents, and this can pose a therapeutic problem. To reach its site of action (often the lower layer of the epidermis or the dermis), a drug has to pass through the epidermal layer with its highly enriched lipid and aqueous environment. The transdermal delivery of drugs is therefore a highly specialised topic (see Ch. 9). Generally speaking, absorption is facilitated if the molecule is predominately hydrophobic in nature: thus, for example, glucocorticoids are often derivatised with fatty acid esters to render them more easily absorbed. The use of a waterproof *occlusion dressing* to cover the skin after applying the drug improves absorption by keeping the epidermis fully hydrated.

The vehicle in which the drug is dissolved is also important. Creams and ointments – essentially stable oil/water emulsions – can be tailored to individual drugs. For example, **tacrolimus** formulated as an ointment can be used topically on the skin, whilst an oil-in-water formulation is better for a water-soluble drug such as an NSAID. The appearance and odour of the formulated drug are also important. Most patients would rather take a tablet than apply creams that may be greasy, smelly or unsightly to large areas of their skin (see Tan et al., 2012).

The physical condition of the skin is important in maintaining its barrier function and various agents can be used to protect the skin and promote repair. These include *emollients*, which re-hydrate the skin, and *barrier creams* that help to prevent damage from irritants. Use of such agents is often indicated alongside treatment with drugs.

Assessing the pharmacokinetics (PK) of drugs absorbed from the skin is therefore quite complex and it is consequently more difficult to estimate doses of drugs given topically compared to (say) oral administration. This can be particularly problematic in the case of drugs which may cause unwanted systemic side effects if they are extensively absorbed (e.g. glucocorticoids). Many new ideas for formulating drugs for passage into and through the skin are under investigation, both for treating skin disorders and also for general systemic treatment (see for example Baveloni et al., 2021).

PRINCIPAL DRUGS USED IN SKIN DISORDERS

Many drugs in the dermatological arsenal are also used to treat other diseases and their mechanism of action is the same. The use of agents described later to treat specific skin disorders is shown in Tables 26.1 and 26.2. We refer the reader to other chapters in the book where information about these agents may be found. Other drugs, such as analogues of vitamins A and D, are rather specific to skin pharmacology.

Of note, it is relatively common practice to use mixtures of drugs in dermatological treatments. Thus anti-inflammatory glucocorticoids may be mixed with antibiotics, antiviral or keratogenic agents; coal tar derivatives mixed with emollients and so on.

ANTIMICROBIAL AGENTS

Chapters 51–56 deal in depth with the mechanism of action of this group of drugs. Antibiotics can be applied topically in diseases such as impetigo and acne or given systemically in the case of cellulitis or rosacea. Fungal infections of the skin are generally treated with topical fungicidal drugs, but oral preparations of (e.g.) **ketoconazole** may be used under some circumstances. Herpes simplex infections may be treated with topical or systemic **acyclovir** or **penciclovir**.

Drugs and the skin

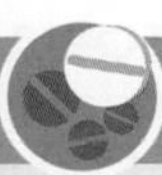

Formulation. Because the skin comprises a unique combination of hydrophobic/hydrophilic structures, many drugs are not absorbed, and special formulations may be necessary to promote penetration.

Many drugs used for skin conditions are also used to treat disorders in other organs. The main groups are:

- *Glucocorticoids.* Widely used to treat psoriasis, eczema and pruritus because of their anti-inflammatory properties. They are usually specially formulated to enhance topical penetration.
- *Antimicrobial agents.* Used topically or systemically to treat skin infections (e.g. acne, impetigo, cellulitis and rosacea).
- *Hormone antagonists.* Androgen antagonists are used topically or systemically to treat male-pattern baldness or hirsutism in women.
- *Vitamin D derivatives.* Drugs such as **calcitriol**, **calcipotriol** and **tacalcitol** are used to treat psoriasis.
- *Anticancer drugs and biopharmaceuticals* are used to treat melanoma.

Some drugs are used almost exclusively for skin disorders. These include:

- *Retinoids.* These are derivatives of vitamin A and include **tretinoin**, **isotretinoin**, **alitretinoin**, **tazarotene** and **adapalene.** They are used to treat acne, eczema and psoriasis. They are usually given topically but can be given systemically.

BIOPHARMACEUTICALS

The recognition that cytokines such as tumour necrosis factor α (TNF-α) was elevated in skin inflammation in conditions such as psoriasis led to the testing of anti-cytokine drugs such as **etanercept, adalimumab** and **infliximab** with encouraging successes. The more recent recognition of the importance of the IL-23/IL-17 axis in psoriasis has led to the introduction of a number of new biopharmaceutical agents which specifically block, immunoneutralise or otherwise affect this pathway. These agents include **brodalumab**, **ixekizumab**, **guselkumab**, **risankizumab**, **tildrakizumab** and **dupilumab** which act at different points in the pathway (see Table 26.2). These have met with great success outperforming previous biopharmaceuticals for the treatment of psoriasis when used for a year (Yasmeen et al., 2022). Fig. 26.3 shows the beneficial effect of treatment of **brodalumab** on the response of patients with moderate to severe psoriasis for periods up to 12 weeks.

IL-4, which is associated with autoimmune conditions, shares a receptor with the structurally related IL-13 and this cytokine itself has been strongly implicated in allergic conditions of various sorts. **Dupilumab**, a mAb which

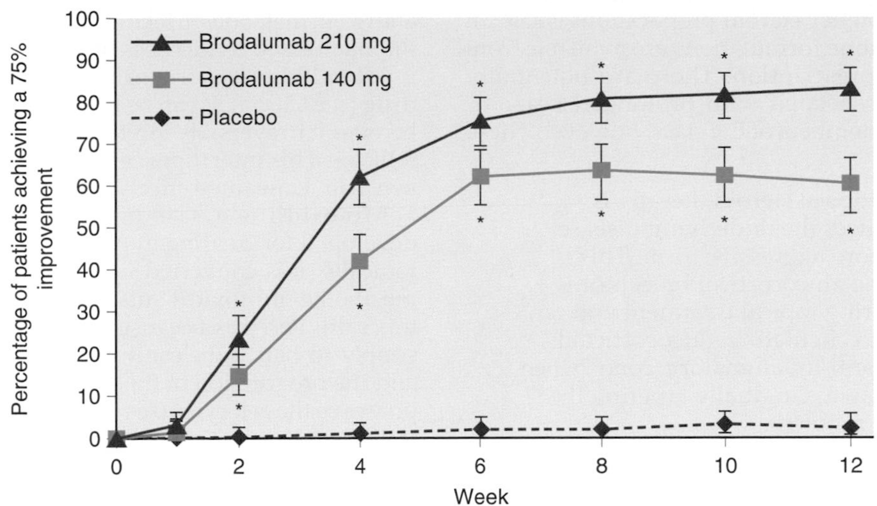

Fig. 26.3 The beneficial effect of the biopharmaceutical anti IL-17 drug brodalumab on the severity of moderate-severe psoriasis. The extent and severity of the psoriatic lesions in patients were assessed using a combined scale (PASI index) which takes into account both the extent and severity of the disease. The study was a random double-blind placebo-controlled study in which two doses of **brodalumab** (140 mg and 210 mg) were tested against a placebo for periods up to 12 weeks. In the graph, the percentage of patients responding with a 75% decrease in PASI score was plotted against time. (Adapted and modified from Papp, K.A., Reich, K., Paul, C., et al., 2016. A prospective phase III, randomized, double-blind, placebo-controlled study of brodalumab in patients with moderate-to-severe plaque psoriasis. Br. J. Dermatol. 175, 273–286..)

blocks the IL-4 receptor, has found utility in several allergic conditions, including eczema.

Biopharmaceuticals are also used in the treatment of melanoma where their overall aim is to eliminate the mutated cells. **Ipilimumab** is a human mAb which acts on T cells removing an inhibitory circuit such that they are activated and consequently more able to remove the cancerous tissue. **Nivolumab** and **pembrolizumab** are human or humanised mAbs which kill melanoma cells by acting on the 'programmed death receptor', PD-1. These biopharmaceutical drugs are commonly used in combination with other anticancer agents.

Unwanted effects.. Because cytokines are intimately involved with the operation of the immune system, one might anticipate adverse effects on the host response to infection. This is a common finding with all these agents and care must be taken to resolve any current infections prior to therapy. Other common side effects seen with some of these drugs include arthralgia, myalgia, fatigue, headache and gastrointestinal symptoms such as diarrhoea.

GLUCOCORTICOIDS AND OTHER ANTI-INFLAMMATORY AGENTS

Antihistamines (see Ch. 17) are useful when controlling mild pruritus, at least in some circumstances, e.g. eczema, insect bites and mild inflammation. Another topical drug which is useful in treating pruritus is **crotamiton**. This acts rapidly and has long-lasting effects. The mechanism of action is not known.

However, the main agents used to treat inflammation of the skin are the glucocorticoids, which are widely used to treat psoriasis and eczema and to suppress pruritus. Their general mechanism of action is described in Chapters 3, 25 and 33. Preparations used in dermatological practice are often formulated as fatty acid esters of the active drugs. This promotes their absorption through the highly hydrophobic layers of the skin but also alters their efficacy: for example, the potency of topical **hydrocortisone** on the skin is greatly enhanced by formulating it as a butyrate ester.

Although schemes around the world vary, the convention is to classify these drugs by potency. For example:

- *Mild,* e.g. **hydrocortisone**;
- *Moderate,* e.g. **alclometasone dipropionate, clobetasone butyrate, fludroxycortide** and **fluocortolone**;
- *Potent,* e.g. **beclomethasone dipropionate, betamethasone** (various esters), **fluocinolone acetonide, fluocinonide, fluticasone propionate, mometasone furoate** and **triamcinolone acetonide**;
- *Very potent,* e.g. **clobetasol propionate** and **diflucortolone valerate.**

The choice of glucocorticoid depends upon the severity of the disease and, because the thickness of skin varies from one location to the other, its anatomical site. They are sometimes combined with antibacterial or fungicidal drugs if they are to be used at the site of an infection.

The action of glucocorticoids on the skin is similar in mechanism to their effect elsewhere in the body. They are potent inhibitors of the release of inflammatory mediators from mast cells, of neutrophil activation and emigration, and immune cell activation (see Chs 7 and 25). Interestingly, and contrary to dogma, it seems that skin cells can themselves generate cortisol and there is some evidence that this ability is deficient in patients who suffer from psoriasis (Hannen et al., 2017). The topical application of glucocorticoids produces vasoconstriction in the skin causing a characteristic 'blanching' reaction.[5] The exact mechanism is unknown.

[5]This interesting observation was used by Cornell and Stoughton in 1985 as the basis for the first quantitative assay of glucocorticoid potency in man.

Unwanted effects. Generally speaking, short-term treatment with low-potency steroid preparations is safe; in fact, some **hydrocortisone** formulations are available from pharmacies without prescription. There are potentially serious side effects associated with prolonged usage or with the more potent members of the class, however. These include:

- *Steroid 'rebound'.* If topical steroid therapy is suddenly discontinued, the underlying disease often returns in a more aggressive form. This is probably because the glucocorticoid receptor is down-regulated during topical treatment and can no longer respond to circulating glucocorticoids, which maintain an anti-inflammatory 'tone', when treatment is withdrawn. Gradually tapering the drug can avoid this problem.
- *Skin atrophy.* Catabolic effects of glucocorticoids (see Ch. 33) can lead to atrophy of the skin, including stretch marks (*striae*) and small visible vessels (*telangiectases*), that is only partially reversible upon stopping treatment.
- *Systemic effects.* Systemic absorption can theoretically cause depression of the hypothalamic–pituitary–adrenal axis, as described in Chapter 33, but this does not seem to constitute a significant risk in normal clinical practice (Castela et al., 2012).
- *Spread of infection.* Because glucocorticoids suppress the immune system, there is a danger that they may encourage or reactivate infection. For this reason, they are contraindicated in acne, where there is a co-existent infection.
- *'Steroid rosacea' (skin reddening with pimples)* is a recognised problem when treating facial skin with potent glucocorticoids.

For more serious cases of eczema or psoriasis or where glucocorticoids are ineffective, topical or systemic application of immunosuppressants such as **ciclosporin, pimecrolimus** or **tacrolimus** may be successful (see Ch. 25). As described earlier, biopharmaceuticals also play an increasingly important role in the treatment of refractory cases (see Table 26.2).

DRUGS USED TO CONTROL HAIR GROWTH

Hair growth in both sexes is driven by androgens, but so is male-pattern baldness. Because of this, androgen antagonists, or compounds that modulate androgen metabolism, can be used to treat both hirsutism in women and androgenic alopecia in men.

Co-cyprindiol is a mixture of an anti-androgen, **cyproterone acetate**, and a female sex hormone, **ethinylestradiol**. Antagonising androgenic actions reduces sebum production by sebaceous glands and also hair growth (which is androgen-dependent), so it can be used for treating acne as well as hirsutism in women. Unwanted effects include venous thromboembolism, and it is contraindicated in women with a family history of cardiovascular disease.

Finasteride inhibits the enzyme (5α-reductase) that converts testosterone to the more potent androgen, dihydrotestosterone (see Ch. 35). It is used topically (usually in combination with **minoxidil**) for the treatment of androgenic alopecia, as well as orally for prostatic hypertrophy. The treatment takes months to produce real changes. Unwanted effects resulting from its action on androgen metabolism include a reduction in libido, possibly impotence and tenderness of the breasts.

Eflornithine was originally developed as an antiprotozoal drug (see Ch. 55). It can be used topically to treat hirsutism because it irreversibly inhibits *ornithine decarboxylase* in hair follicles. This interrupts cell replication and the growth of new hair. Unwanted effects include skin reactions and acne.

Minoxidil is a vasodilator drug that was originally developed for treating hypertension (see Ch. 21). Applied topically, it is converted in hair follicles to a more potent metabolite, **minoxidil sulfate** (some preparations contain this salt). Perhaps because of its ability to increase blood supply to hair follicles, it stimulates growth of new hair and the progression of the new follicle through successive phases of the cell cycle (see Ch. 6). Existing follicles, usually stalled in their resting (telogen) phase, must first be 'shed' to make way for new, rapidly growing follicles, so hair loss following initial treatment is a frequent – and presumably rather alarming – action of the drug. Other unwanted effects are few, but some local irritation may occur. Hair loss recurs when topical application is discontinued.

RETINOIDS

Disturbances in vitamin A metabolism are known to result in skin pathology. The vitamin is normally acquired in ester form from dietary sources. It is converted to *retinol* in the gut and this seems to be a storage form of the vitamin.

Vitamin A has many biological roles. As *retinal*, it is an essential component of rhodopsin and hence crucial for normal vision. However, it can also undergo an irreversible oxidation to *retinoic acid*, which has potent effects on skin homeostasis.

The retinoid drugs are derivatives of retinoic acid. The principal examples are **acitretin, adapalene, alitretinoin, isotretinoin, tretinoin**, and **tazarotene**. They are widely used (sometimes in combination with other drugs) for the treatment of acne, eczema and psoriasis. Topical application is the usual route of administration, but oral therapy is sometimes used for severe cases.

Retinoids probably act by binding to retinoid X receptor (RXR) and retinoid acid receptor (RAR) nuclear receptors (see Ch. 3 and Fig. 26.4) in their target cells, which include keratinocytes and the cells of sebaceous glands, although some have questioned this mechanism (Arechalde and Saurat, 2000). Retinoid binding proteins (RBPs) on the surface of, and within, the cell aid in transport of the molecule to its receptor and facilitate its eventual catabolism (Napoli, 2017). The main dermatological actions of retinoids include modulation of epidermal cell growth and reduction in sebaceous gland activity and sebum production. They also have pleiotropic actions on the adaptive and innate immune system, including inhibition of IL-6-induced activation of Th17 cells and Toll receptors that contribute to an anti-inflammatory effect .The area has been reviewed by Khalil et al. (2017).

Unwanted effects. After oral administration, retinoids may cause dry or flaky skin, stinging or burning sensations and joint pains, possibly because they can also activate the TRPV1 receptor (Yin et al., 2013). Retinoids are teratogenic (this is linked to the effects of retinoids on epidermal differentiation that underlie their efficacy) and can be used in women only in the presence of suitable contraception (see Chs 35 and 58). Because of their chemical relationship to retinal, retinoid drugs may cause disturbances in the

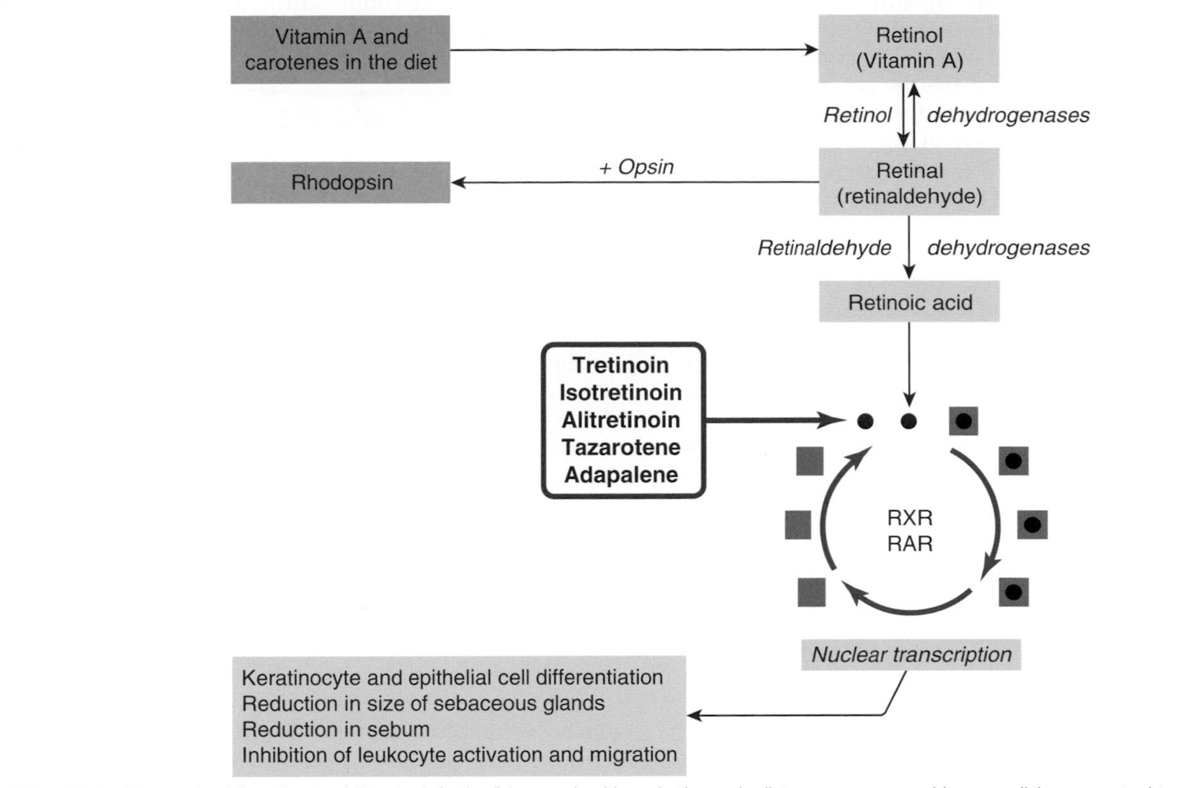

Fig. 26.4 The retinoid pathway. Vitamin A (retinol) is acquired largely through dietary sources and is reversibly converted to retinal (retinaldehyde). This may be combined with opsin to produce the visual pigment rhodopsin or irreversibly oxidised to retinoic acid. The latter species can interact with nuclear receptors (RXR and RAR; see Ch. 3) to produce changes in genes that modulate keratinocyte differentiation, reduce the size and output of sebaceous glands and exert a general anti-inflammatory action. The synthetic congeners **acitretin**, **adapalene**, **alitretinoin**, **isotretinoin**, **tazarotene** and **tretinoin** can also act at the RXR and RAR, also producing potent actions in skin disorders such as acne and psoriasis.

visual system as well as impairment of hearing. They may also incur a plethora of unwanted gastrointestinal and other effects.

VITAMIN D ANALOGUES

Vitamin D is actually a mixture of several related substances. Although classed as a 'vitamin' and therefore by implication an essential dietary factor, vitamin D_3 (cholecalciferol) is synthesised by the skin in the presence of sufficient sunlight (in fact, *phototherapy* is an important therapeutic modality in some skin disorders for this and other reasons). Other forms of the vitamin (e.g. D_2) can be obtained from the diet. The vitamin plays a crucial role in calcium and phosphate metabolism and bone formation (see Ch. 36). It also has complex pleiotropic regulatory actions on the innate and adaptive immune systems, reducing the activity of the adaptive system but increasing the activity of the innate immune system producing a net anti-inflammatory action (Charoenngam and Holick, 2020).

The biologically active metabolite *calcitriol* (see Ch. 36) is synthesised in the body by a multi-step process that requires transformations in the liver and kidney. At the molecular level, vitamin D and its analogues act though the vitamin D receptor (VDR) group of nuclear receptors (see Ch. 3) in keratinocytes, fibroblasts, Langerhans cells and sebaceous gland cells, to modulate gene transcription. Amongst the effects seen after treatment are antiproliferative and pro-differentiation actions on keratinocytes, increased apoptosis of plaque keratinocytes (Tiberio et al., 2009) and the inhibition of T-cell activation (Tremezaygues and Reichrath, 2011).

The main analogues used are **calcitriol** itself, **calcipotriol** and **tacalcitol**. Their principal clinical use is treating psoriasis. Oral administration is possible, but they are generally administered topically, sometimes in combination with a glucocorticoid.

*Unwanted effects.*There is always a concern about the possible effects of the drugs on bone and they should be avoided in patients who have problems related to calcium or bone metabolism. Topical application can lead to skin irritation.

AGENTS ACTING BY OTHER MECHANISMS

Many ancillary agents are used in dermatology, including topical antiseptics, emollients, soothing lotions and other substances. Amongst this group are '**coal tars**' or their derivatives such as **dithranol**. The former, which are poorly defined mixtures containing thousands of phenolic compounds and polycyclic aromatic hydrocarbons, are generated during the conversion of coal to coke or gas. They contain chemicals that formed the basis for many early medicines. Topical coal tar preparations have been used in dermatological practice for decades. Having anti-inflammatory, anti-pruritic and anti-infective properties, they can bring about a useful therapeutic benefit in eczema, psoriasis and some other skin conditions, and are often the first agents to be tried even though their mechanism of action was far from clear. However, recent research points to the activation of the *aryl hydrocarbon receptor* (AHR) in the skin as one possible mechanism since this leads to down-regulation of proinflammatory cytokines, including IL-17, and influences skin barrier function. Consequently, AHR is an exciting potential target for novel therapeutic drugs, and the FDA is currently evaluating one agent (**tapinarof**) that binds and activates this receptor as a topical therapy for plaque psoriasis (see Bissonnette et al., 2021). As one might expect, given their origin, coal tars contain carcinogenic substances, but in clinical use, the risk appears to be slight (Roelofzen et al., 2010).

Among other drugs unique to skin pharmacology are **salicylic acid** and **podophyllotoxin**. Topical **salicylic acid** has a *keratolytic* effect in situations when excess skin is being produced (e.g. warts), causing epidermal layers to be shed. It is a common ingredient of numerous proprietary wart removers. **Podophyllotoxin** is a toxin extracted from plants of the podophyllum family. It is usually reserved for treating anogenital warts. It is applied topically and prevents the excess growth of skin, probably because it inhibits tubulin polymerisation and hence arrests the normal cell cycle.

Another agent used for anogenital warts is **imiquimod**. This drug is an immune modifier, exerting antiproliferative effects through stimulation of pro-inflammatory cytokine release by activating innate immune cells via the Toll-like receptor 7 as well as up-regulating growth factor receptor expression. It is also used for the topical treatment of some types of pre-cancerous (e.g. actinic keratosis) and cancerous (e.g. basal cell carcinoma) skin lesions. Unwanted effects include local skin reactions.

CONCLUDING REMARKS

Despite the plethora of preparations available to treat skin disorders, there is clearly still an unfilled therapeutic need in several areas (e.g. rosacea) and, as always, reducing the unwanted effects of existing drugs is a further worthwhile objective that would greatly enhance their clinical utility. Some of the most interesting ideas have arisen from reconsidering the design of the glucocorticoids, vitamin D analogues and especially the retinoids. All these drugs act predominantly through nuclear receptors and recent thinking suggests that differentiating the mechanisms of transrepression and transactivation of genes by these drugs may be an achievable goal. Progress towards separating the useful from the unwanted effects of glucocorticoids is slowly yielding fruit (see Ch. 33 for a discussion of this), and clearly, the prospects of separating the calcaemic from the anti-inflammatory effects of vitamin D analogues (Tremezaygues and Reichrath, 2011) and improving the selectivity of retinoids (Orfanos et al., 1997) are also very attractive therapeutic goals.

It is perhaps surprising that 'itch' is still such a problem. Hopefully the recent identification of 'itch'-sensitive GPCRs mentioned earlier will impact on this area.

Biopharmaceuticals are one of the big success stories in dermatology and one can reasonably expect their numbers to increase as the search for new therapies for psoriasis, atopic dermatitis and other inflammatory conditions proceeds.

REFERENCES AND FURTHER READING

Arechalde, A., Saurat, J.H., 2000. Management of psoriasis: the position of retinoid drugs. BioDrugs 13, 327–333.

Basavaraj, K.H., Ashok, N.M., Rashmi, R., Praveen, T.K., 2010. The role of drugs in the induction and/or exacerbation of psoriasis. Int. J. Dermatol. 49, 1351–1361.

Baveloni, F.G., Riccio, B.V.F., Di Filippo, L.D., et al., 2021. Nanotechnology-based drug delivery systems as potential for skin application: a review. Curr. Med. Chem. 28, 3216–3248.

Baveloni, F.G., Riccio, B.V.F., Di Filippo, L.D., et al., 2021. Tapinarof in the treatment of psoriasis: a review of the unique mechanism of action of a novel therapeutic aryl hydrocarbon receptor-modulating agent. J. Am. Acad. Dermatol. 84, 1059–1067.

Bergstresser, P.R., Taylor, J.R., 1977. Epidermal 'turnover time'—a new examination. Br. J. Dermatol. 96, 503–509.

Cao, C., Kang, H.J., Singh, I., et al., 2021. Structure, function and pharmacology of human itch GPCRs. Nature 600, 170–175.

Castela, E., Archier, E., Devaux, S., et al., 2012. Topical corticosteroids in plaque psoriasis: a systematic review of risk of adrenal axis suppression and skin atrophy. J. Eur. Acad. Dermatol. Venereol. 26 (Suppl. 3), 47–51.

Charoenngam, N., Holick, M., 2020. Immunologic effects of vitamin D on human health and disease. Nutrients 12, 2097–2125.

Chorilli, M., 2021. Nanotechnology-based drug delivery systems as potential for skin application: a review. Curr. Med. Chem. 28, 3216–3248.

Cornell, R.C., Stoughton, R.B., 1985. Correlation of the vasoconstriction assay and clinical activity in psoriasis. Arch. Dermatol. 121, 63–67.

Dhanyamraju, P.K., Patel, T.N., 2022. Melanoma therapeutics: a literature review. J. Biomed. Res. 36, 77–97.

Di Filippo, P., Scaparrotta, A., Rapino, D., et al., 2015. Vitamin D supplementation modulates the immune system and improves atopic dermatitis in children. Int. Arch. Allergy Immunol. 166, 91–96.

Greaves, M.W., Khalifa, N., 2004. Itch: more than skin deep. Int. Arch. Allergy Immunol. 135, 166–172.

Hannen, R., Udeh-Momoh, C., Upton, J., et al., 2017. Dysfunctional skin-derived glucocorticoid synthesis is a pathogenic mechanism of psoriasis. J. Invest. Dermatol. 137, 1630–1637.

Ikoma, A., Steinhoff, M., Stander, S., Yosipovitch, G., Schmelz, M., 2006. The neurobiology of itch. Nat. Rev. Neurosci. 7, 535–547.

Khalil, S., Bardawil, T., Stephan, C., et al., 2017. Retinoids: a journey from the molecular structures and mechanisms of action to clinical uses in dermatology and adverse effects. J. Dermatolog. Treat 28, 684–696.

Kirkham, B.W., Kavanaugh, A., Reich, K., 2014. Interleukin-17A: a unique pathway in immune-mediated diseases: psoriasis, psoriatic arthritis and rheumatoid arthritis. Immunology 141, 133–142.

Klinge, S.A., Sawyer, G.A., 2013. Effectiveness and safety of topical versus oral nonsteroidal anti-inflammatory drugs: a comprehensive review. Phys. Sportsmed. 41, 64–74.

Martin, D.A., Towne, J.E., Kricorian, G., et al., 2013. The emerging role of IL-17 in the pathogenesis of psoriasis: preclinical and clinical findings. J. Invest. Dermatol. 133, 17–26.

Naldi, L., Raho, G., 2009. Emerging drugs for psoriasis. Expert Opin. Emerg. Drugs 14, 145–163.

Napoli, J.L., 2017. Cellular retinoid binding-proteins, CRBP, CRABP, FABP5: effects on retinoid metabolism, function and related diseases. Pharmacol. Ther. 173, 19–33.

Noda, S., Krueger, J.G., Guttman-Yassky, E., 2015. The translational revolution and use of biologics in patients with inflammatory skin diseases. J. Allergy Clin. Immunol. 135, 324–336.

Orfanos, C.E., Zouboulis, C.C., Almond-Roesler, B., Geilen, C.C., 1997. Current use and future potential role of retinoids in dermatology. Drugs 53, 358–388.

Papp, K.A., Reich, K., Paul, C., et al., 2016. A prospective phase III, randomized, double-blind, placebo-controlled study of brodalumab in

patients with moderate-to-severe plaque psoriasis. Br. J. Dermatol. 175, 273–286.
Roelofzen, J.H., Aben, K.K., Oldenhof, U.T., et al., 2010. No increased risk of cancer after coal tar treatment in patients with psoriasis or eczema. J. Invest. Dermatol. 130, 953–961.
Sharma, A., Kroumpouzos, G., Kassir, M., et al., 2022. Rosacea management: a comprehensive review. J. Cosmet. Dermatol. 21, 1895–1904.
Tan, X., Feldman, S.R., Chang, J., Balkrishnan, R., 2012. Topical drug delivery systems in dermatology: a review of patient adherence issues. Expert Opin. Drug Deliv. 9, 1263–1271.
Tiberio, R., Bozzo, C., Pertusi, G., et al., 2009. Calcipotriol induces apoptosis in psoriatic keratinocytes. Clin. Exp. Dermatol. 34, 972–974.
Tremezaygues, L., Reichrath, J., 2011. Vitamin D analogs in the treatment of psoriasis: where are we standing and where will we be going? Dermatoendocrinol. 3, 180–186.
Yamasaki, K., Gallo, R.L., 2011. Rosacea as a disease of cathelicidins and skin innate immunity. J. Investig. Dermatol. Symp. Proc. 15, 12–15.
Yang, F., Guo, L., Li, Y., et al., 2021. Structure, function and pharmacology of human itch receptor complexes. Nature 600, 164–169.
Yasmeen, N., Sawyer, L.M., Malottki, K., Levin, L.A., Didriksen Apol, E., Jemec, G.B., 2022. Targeted therapies for patients with moderate-to-severe psoriasis: a systematic review and network meta-analysis of PASI response at 1 year. J. Dermatolog. Treat. 33, 204–218.
Yin, S., Luo, J., Qian, A., et al., 2013. Retinoids activate the irritant receptor TRPV1 and produce sensory hypersensitivity. J. Clin. Invest. 123, 3941–3951.

27 The eye

OVERVIEW

Several unique aspects to the eye make its pharmacology both challenging and interesting. The autonomic nervous system control of the pupil and the lens is one key area that is targeted by drugs that act on the parasympathetic and the sympathetic nervous systems. Maintenance of intraocular pressure within the globe is also another area where specific pharmacological therapy such as the prostaglandin analogues has been developed. A wide range of eye drops are now available for treatment of open-angle glaucoma which is one of the most common causes of visual impairment worldwide. Targeted drug delivery is a key consideration because drops act on the external eye, cornea and anterior chambers but do not penetrate behind the lens. Systemic or intravitreal administration is required for the retina. Several pathological processes can lead to new vessel formation with subsequent complications of haemorrhage and oedema causing visual loss. Vascular endothelial growth factor (VEGF) inhibitors are given by intravitreal injection to manage conditions where new vessel formation has pathological consequences.

INTRODUCTION

The eye (Fig. 27.1), functionally analogous to a high-tech photographic camera, is a tough fluid-filled globe with an outer transparent layer (the cornea) at the front, a light receptive layer (the retina) at the back and variable-aperture and variable-focus lens at the interface between anterior and posterior chambers. The wall of the posterior chamber incorporates a dark layer of melanin-rich epithelium, so stray light is absorbed rather than being reflected within the chamber. The retina, on which light passing through the pupil is focused by refraction at the cornea and by the lens, contains the light sensitive cells (rods and cones) and the transparent nerve fibres and ganglion cells that connect the rods and cones to the optic nerve and hence to the brain where the image is interpreted.

Within this globe the anterior components are bathed in clear fluid ('aqueous humour') that helps maintain the smooth functioning of the iris and lens (Fig. 27.2). Behind the lens a clear jelly like substance ('vitreous humour') supports retinal function. The integrity and transparency of these liquid and gel-like compartments in an enclosed space are important for the pharmacology and the pathology of the eye.

The retina has high metabolic demands, and disordered blood supply is a common feature of retinal pathology. The ophthalmic artery supplies the eye via two distinct vascular networks: the choroidal network, which supplies the choroid, optic nerve head and the outer retina plus the inner layer of the macula, with the central retinal artery, which supplies almost all of the retina's inner layers of transparent nerve fibres and ganglion cells. The macula, the central area of the retina containing cones and responsible for high acuity central vision, lacks superficial retinal vessels but obtains part of its supply by diffusion from both supplies. The retinal endothelial junctions are tight, as is Bruch's membrane, the basement membrane deep to retinal pigmented epithelium. The retinal blood vessels are uniquely accessible to direct visualisation through ophthalmoscopic examination, enabling the early diagnosis of conditions that are common causes of blindness if untreated but for which effective preventive therapies are available – notably proliferative diabetic retinopathy and wet age-related macular degeneration (see later).

Eye disorders are common and range in severity from transient redness and discomfort to permanent loss of vision. Common pathological processes such as infection, inflammation and malignancy affect the eye as they do other parts of the body, but several unique aspects of ocular structure and function make its pharmacology both challenging and interesting. The close relationship between rhodopsin and its associated retinal G protein–coupled receptors is mentioned in Chapter 3; in the present chapter we emphasise aspects of therapeutic relevance.

Readers requiring a detailed account of the structure, function and pathology of the human eye are referred to *The Eye: Basic Sciences in Practice* (Forrester et al., 2020).

SPECIAL PHARMACOKINETIC CONSIDERATIONS IN THE EYE

Delivering treatment to the eye presents unique challenges. There is a scleral and conjunctival barrier at the front which limits the absorption of topical therapies and subsequent drug diffusion to the retina through the fluid-filled chambers of the eye. Systemic therapies administered by mouth or intravenously may not penetrate the tight junctions at the blood–retinal barrier. There are two parts to this barrier, with the inner retinal portion comprising of tight junctions between capillary endothelial cells, and the outer aspect involving tight junctions between retinal pigment epithelial cells. The impermeability of these barriers to certain drug formulations has led to the development of intravitreal injection (see Ch. 9), together with depot delivery systems that allow the slow dispersion of drugs introduced directly into the vitreous humour (Fig. 27.1).

Disease at the front of the eye is treated with topical agents, where possible. Formulations of eye drops are typically weak acids or bases with pH close to 7.4 and must not be irritant in nature. The blinking mechanism and release of tears means that topically delivered therapies

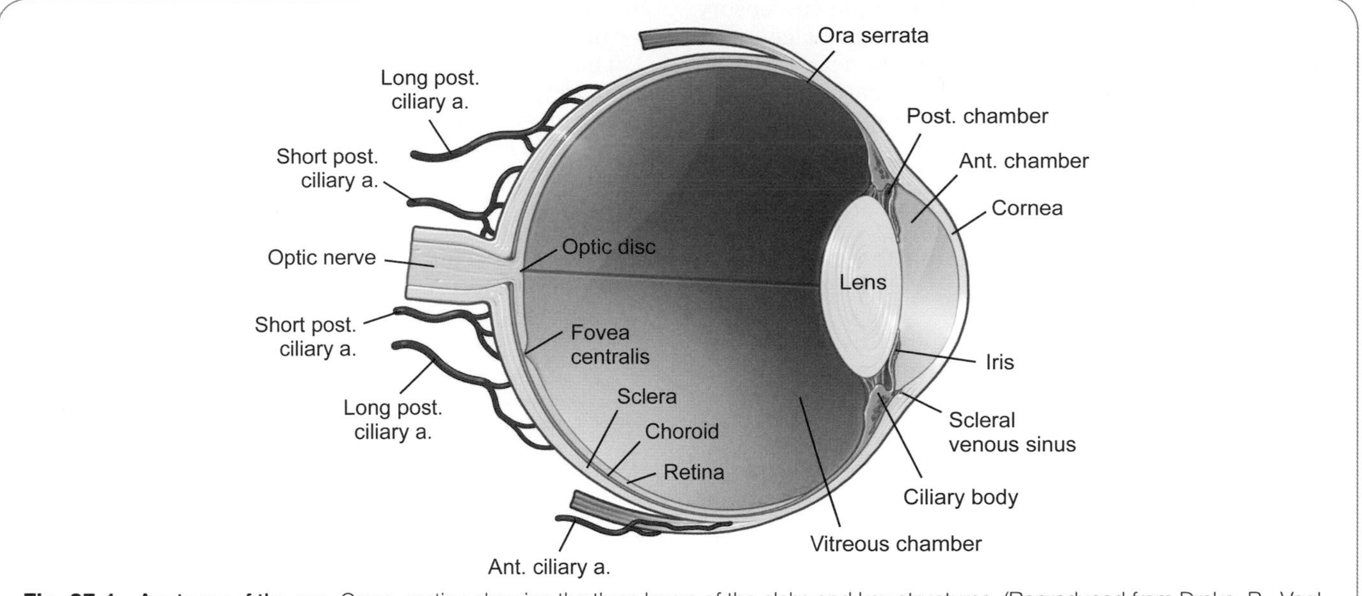

Fig. 27.1 Anatomy of the eye. Cross-section showing the three layers of the globe and key structures. (Reproduced from Drake, R., Vogl, A.W., Mitchell, A.W.. 2016. Gray's Basic Anatomy. Elsevier, London.)

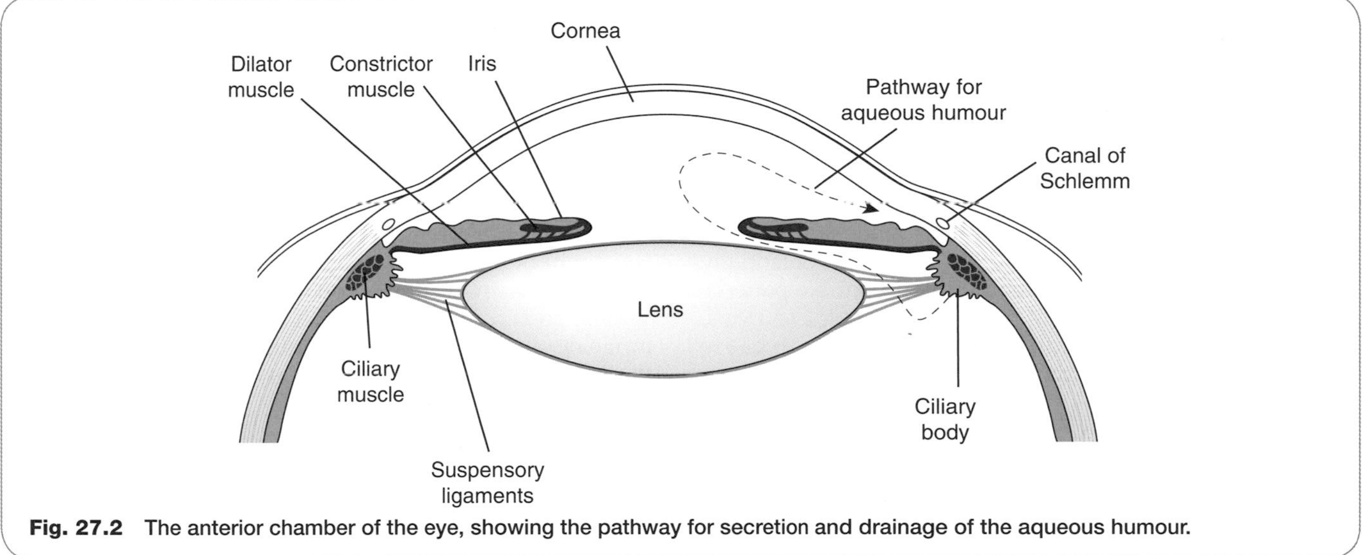

Fig. 27.2 The anterior chamber of the eye, showing the pathway for secretion and drainage of the aqueous humour.

such as eye drops remain only for a short time on the surface of the eye. A proportion of the drug will pass down the nasolacrimal duct and may be systemically absorbed to cause adverse effects such as wheezing in asthmatic patients treated with **timolol** eye drops (see further in the chapter and Ch. 15). Adherence to eye drops may be problematic particularly for formulations that have to be regularly delivered every 6–8 h, or for older patients with impaired manual dexterity. Some drops for the cornea have to be given as frequently as every hour, a problem especially overnight, for which ointments are thought to be more suitable as a depot delivery approach.

The outer part of the eye is lined by a fascial sheath known as Tenon's capsule and it is possible to inject drugs into the cavity bounded by this sheath and the sclera. This sub-Tenon or parabulbar technique can be used for local anaesthesia, e.g. cataract surgery, or corticosteroid delivery in posterior uveitis/macular oedema.

AUTONOMIC CONTROL OF THE LENS AND PUPIL, AND RELATED THERAPEUTIC DRUGS

Autonomic regulation of the **lens** is analogous to an autofocusing camera. The shape of the human lens is constantly being adjusted by the ciliary body and muscles through suspensory ligaments that bind it to the lens capsule (Fig. 27.2). This enables accommodation of the eye to distant or nearby objects, so that sharply focused images can be rendered onto the retina. Parasympathetic innervation of the **ciliary body** and the constrictor pupillae muscle is mimicked or antagonised by, respectively, muscarinic agonists and antagonists. Parasympathetic stimulation contracts the ciliary muscles, pulls the ciliary body forward and inward, thus relaxing the tension on the suspensory ligament of the **lens**. This allows the lens to bulge more, with reduction in focal length to facilitate near vision. In contrast, anticholinergic drugs that block parasympathetic stimulus relax the ciliary muscle and impair near vision due to paralysis of accommodation.

Another key component at the front of the eye is the **iris** which regulates pupillary diameter (akin to the aperture of a camera). Here, autonomic nervous system pathways regulate the amount of light entering the eye so visual perception can remain optimal within both bright and dark environments.

The diameter of the **iris** is regulated by the balance between constrictor sphincter pupillae (parasympathetic system) and the dilator pupillae (sympathetic system). Parasympathetic tone narrows the diameter of the iris (i.e. constricts the pupil) whereas the sympathetic nervous system dilates the pupil. Antimuscarinic drugs cause dilated pupils (*mydriasis*) and loss of accommodation (*cycloplegia*), and hence difficulty seeing in bright conditions and difficulty reading small print.

Dilation of the pupil enables detailed fundoscopic examination (visualising the back of the eye) and is also used in certain types of eye surgery to prevent synechiae (adhesions of the iris to the capsule of the lens) for which the long action of **atropine** is an advantage, and as an adjunct to anti-inflammatory drugs in treating inflammation of the uvea ('uveitis') which can accompany several systemic inflammatory diseases. This is usually achieved with tertiary amine muscarinic antagonists such as **tropicamide** (favoured for its rapid onset but relatively short duration of action) or **cyclopentolate** which is longer acting; atropine is longer acting still (several days). However, pupillary dilation with muscarinic antagonists can block drainage of aqueous humour into the canal of Schlemm, thus potentially triggering angle-closure glaucoma in susceptible patients (see later). **Phenylephrine** (a_1-agonist), given as eye drops, is an alternative way to dilate the pupil but can cause local irritation and systemic effects including transient hypertension. It is often used to supplement tropicamide for full dilatation.

The autonomic nervous system is also involved in regulating ocular blood flow, as well as in maintaining intraocular pressure, through its effects on aqueous humour production and outflow (Fig. 27.3). Sympathetic signalling to the blood vessels of the **ciliary body** and epithelium is a key regulator of aqueous humour production. The autonomic nervous system has an impact on the trabecular meshwork and episcleral blood vessels that drain aqueous fluid. These effects may contribute to the therapeutic effect of drugs that act on adrenoceptors in treating some forms of glaucoma (see later).

TREATMENT OF INFLAMMATION AND INFECTION IN THE EYE

Drugs for treating infection and inflammation in the eye are similar to those used elsewhere in the body, but are usually specially formulated in terms of concentration and mode of delivery.

Several antibiotics and antivirals are licensed for use in the eye, typically for treatment of conjunctivitis or corneal ulcers (often due to herpes simplex virus). Topical formulations include chloramphenicol, macrolides, aminoglycosides and quinolones (see also Ch. 52). Antivirals (see also Ch. 53) are also available – aciclovir, for instance, is used in herpes infections. Treatment of viral infections at the back of the eye is more complicated because of challenges in drug delivery (see earlier). In addition to standard oral or intravenous dosing, modified release formulations of ganciclovir or cidofovir may be delivered by intravitreal injection to achieve higher or more prolonged concentrations for treatment of cytomegalovirus retinitis – a particular issue in patients with HIV infection and AIDS.

Corticosteroids (see also Ch. 33) are used for a wide range of non-infection-related inflammatory conditions in the eye such as uveitis (see earlier) and macular oedema.

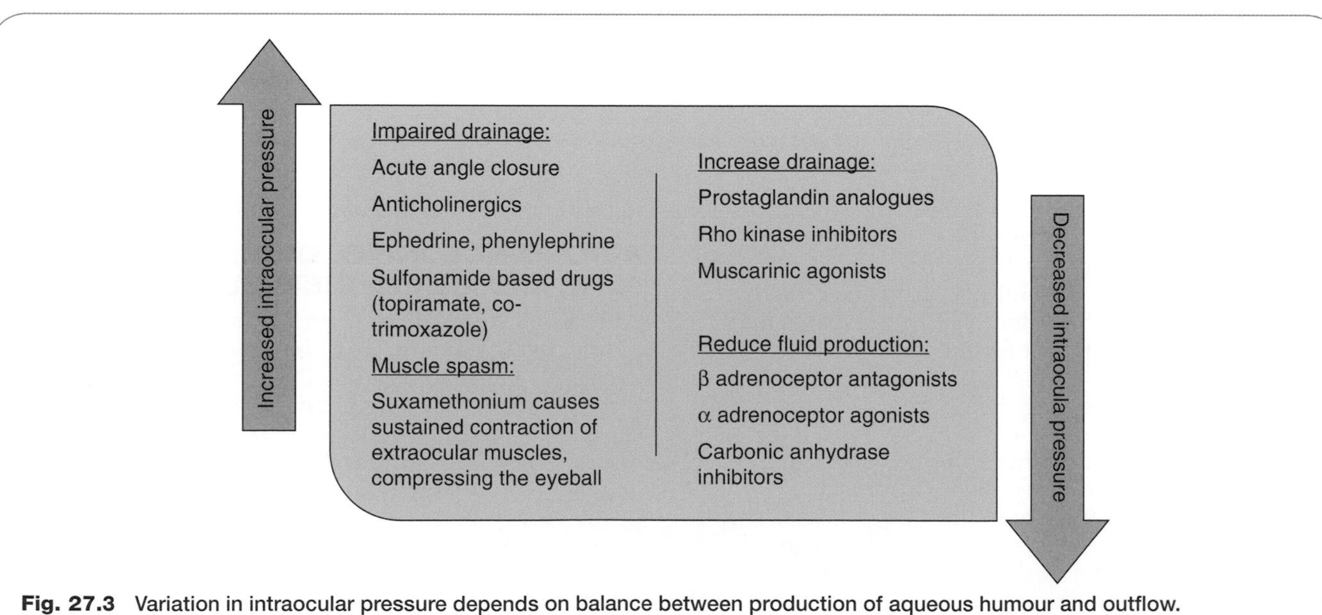

Fig. 27.3 Variation in intraocular pressure depends on balance between production of aqueous humour and outflow.

Topical preparations, for example **betamethasone** drops or ointment, can be used at the surface of the eye, and there are now modified release formulations and implants that can be introduced intravitreally so that the corticosteroid is gradually released into the posterior compartment. Examples include **dexamethasone** and **fluocinolone** vitreal implants that are used for treating conditions such as posterior uveitis, retinal vein occlusion and diabetic macular oedema. These formulations can have durations of action lasting weeks to months. However, corticosteroids can harm the eyes and are normally administered and monitored under expert supervision. In particular, they worsen the effects of herpes (especially of the cornea) and other infections, can cause acute glaucoma in susceptible individuals and can cause cataracts during prolonged use.

Topical formulations of non-steroidal anti-inflammatory drugs (e.g. **diclofenac**, **ketorolac**, see Ch. 25) are available, as are antihistamines (e.g. **azelastine**) and **cromoglicate** or **nedocromil** (see Ch. 28) for eye allergies. They are less effective than corticosteroids and may themselves cause local irritation but are sometimes used by non-experts while awaiting definitive diagnosis of a sore red eye.

CONTROL OF INTRAOCULAR PRESSURE AND TREATMENT OF GLAUCOMA

The intraocular pressure is normally about 15 mm Hg above atmospheric, which keeps the eye slightly distended. There is considerable variation in intraocular pressure, with a gradual increase during the night, as well as frequent upward spikes during the day related to mechanical stress and blood pressure. An important determinant is the production of aqueous humour, which is secreted slowly and continuously by the cells of the epithelium covering the ciliary body. Outflow drainage of the aqueous humour takes place mainly through the trabecular meshwork into the canal of Schlemm that runs around the outer margin of the iris (see Fig. 27.2). The ciliary muscle is a circular band of smooth muscle within the ciliary body and controls the flow of aqueous humour into the canal of Schlemm. A small proportion of aqueous drainage takes place through the uveoscleral outflow pathway. Here, the fluid seeps through or around ciliary muscles to reach the suprachoroidal space and sclera where it is drained through orbital veins. It is thought that prostaglandin analogues exert their effects on the uveoscleral outflow pathway to reduce intraocular pressure (see later).

Increased secretion and/or reduction in drainage causes a rise in intraocular pressure, a risk factor for primary open-angle glaucoma, the commonest form of glaucoma where drainage of aqueous humour through the trabecular meshwork is restricted.

The term *glaucoma* encompasses a group of disorders caused by damage to the retinal ganglion cells and optic nerve. This causes a distinctive appearance of the optic nerve head (the 'optic disc') called cupping of the disc and results in a loss of mid-peripheral vision. If untreated, open-angle glaucoma progresses gradually and painlessly to blindness (a 'chronic' course). This can sometimes occur when the intraocular pressure is within the normal range ('normal-tension glaucoma'), at least when measured at one or a few points in time. Drug treatment is nonetheless directed toward lowering the intraocular pressure.

Acute angle-closure glaucoma is much less common and can present as a medical/surgical emergency. The 'angle' referred to is that between the anterior outer part of the iris and the inner surface of the cornea (see the dashed arrow in Fig. 27.2 which shows the direction of flow and pathway of the aqueous humour when unimpeded). Drainage can become acutely blocked in people with a narrow angle, for example by drugs that dilate the pupil (e.g. mydriatics such as tropicamide combined with phenylephrine, see earlier); *note that tropicamide alone is rarely responsible.* In the absence of such provocation the first symptoms may arise at night when the pupils are dilated – for instance the appearance of haloes around streetlights accompanied by pain in the eyes. Treatment of both conditions is directed at lowering of intraocular pressure, and we describe the main pharmacological approaches here. Where surgery (e.g. iridectomy) is required, ongoing drug treatment is often still needed to supplement it.

PROSTAGLANDIN FP RECEPTOR AGONISTS (SEE CH. 17)

FP receptors are targeted by several prostaglandin analogues, **latanoprost, travoprost, tafluprost** and prostamide **bimatoprost,** which are used in treatment of glaucoma. Prostaglandin analogues are pro-drugs that are converted by esterases at the cornea to active forms acting on the FP receptor. The mechanism whereby this lowers intraocular pressure has not been fully elucidated but these drugs are thought to increase aqueous drainage through the uveoscleral pathway. The prostaglandin analogues are first-line eye drops for open-angle glaucoma because they offer 24-h control of intraocular pressure with once-a-day dosing, coupled with being relatively free of systemic adverse effects. However, the drugs can cause local effects through stimulation of melanocytes, e.g. eyelid pigmentation, and change in colour of the iris.

β_1 ADRENOCEPTOR ANTAGONISTS

Beta adrenoceptor antagonist eye drops (**timolol, betaxolol, levobunolol**) are widely used to reduce the production of aqueous humour. Systemic absorption that may cause bradycardia and, in asthmatic patients, bronchoconstriction is described.

α_2 ADRENOCEPTOR AGONISTS

Alpha-2-adrenoceptor agonist eye drops (e.g. **brimonidine**) decrease aqueous humour production and increase uveoscleral outflow. They are used for chronic glaucoma when β_1 adrenoceptor antagonists are inappropriate or, in combination, when treatment with a single agent was inadequate. Local symptoms such as burning sensation are common and systemic adverse effects (e.g. dry mouth) have been reported. Brimonidine eye drops are given twice a day.

CARBONIC ANHYDRASE INHIBITORS

Oral carbonic anhydrase inhibitors (e.g. **acetazolamide**, see Ch. 29) were an early treatment to lower intraocular pressure by reducing aqueous humour production and are still sometimes used for a short period to lower pressure urgently (e.g. preoperatively); however, systemic effects during chronic use led to the development of topical agents. Prostaglandin analogues and b_1 adrenoceptor antagonists subsequently became first-line glaucoma therapies, but topical carbonic anhydrase inhibitors continue to be prescribed in combination with β_1-antagonists and α-agonists (Stoner et al., 2022). The mechanism of aqueous humour secretion is not fully understood but carbonic anhydrase is implicated and it is believed that inhibitors of this enzyme reduce secretion of aqueous humour by a direct effect on ciliary epithelial carbonic anhydrase leading to reduced bicarbonate ion movement with a consequent reduction in the transport of sodium ions and fluids. Local adverse effects of the available eye drops (**brinzolamide, dorzolamide**) such as corneal erosion, conjunctival inflammation and blurred vision are common, but systemic adverse effects are not.

INHIBITORS OF RHO KINASE

The rho/rho kinase system is described in Chapter 3. Inhibitors of rho kinase lower intraocular pressure and two such drugs, **netarsudil** and **ripasudil,** have recently become available, formulated as eye drops, for the pharmacological management of glaucoma. Rho kinase influences the structure and function of the actin cytoskeleton and extracellular matrix, thus influencing the drainage channels in the trabecular meshwork of the eye. The Rho kinase inhibitors exert a beneficial effect through greater drainage of aqueous humour, thus reducing intraocular pressure. These compounds are relatively new, and their long-term tolerability and place in treatment remain to be established.

MUSCARINIC AGONISTS

Pilocarpine facilitates drainage of aqueous humour by contracting the constrictor pupillae muscles to constrict the pupil (miosis), pulling the iris away from the trabecular mesh in angle-closure glaucoma. However, pilocarpine is now seldom used in long-term treatment because of adverse local effects (excessive lacrimation, conjunctival hyperaemia, blurred vision and headache from contraction of the ciliary muscle) as well as the potential for cholinergic action systemically. Such systemic parasympathomimetic effects are rare but dose related.

Treatment of glaucoma

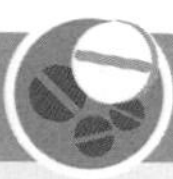

Prostaglandin analogues are the first-line drug treatment of primary open-angle glaucoma; they are often used in combined formulations with other agents. In order to help patient adherence, a wide (and sometimes bewildering) range of different permutations of compounds can be prescribed. Laser therapy is recommended for patients where eye drops have not been effective. Surgery is another option in such instances.

Tropicamide or cyclopentolate eye drops are used when mydriasis or cycloplegia is required during ophthalmic examinations or surgery.

OCULAR VASCULATURE AND VASCULAR ENDOTHELIAL GROWTH FACTOR INHIBITORS

Angiogenesis in the eye involves a complex balance of processes regulated by many cytokines, growth factors and components of the extracellular matrix. Proangiogenic factors include, most importantly, vascular endothelium–derived growth factor (VEGF), platelet-derived growth factors and fibroblast growth factor among a host of other mediators. Conversely, endostatin, thrombospondin and pigment epithelium–derived factor are considered to play an antiangiogenic role (reviewed by Selvam et al., 2018). Derangement of angiogenesis can result in serious harm. The pathological process can arise in the eye in isolation, for example with wet age-related macular degeneration (secondary to new vessels growing through Bruch's membrane) or through ischaemia secondary to retinal vessel occlusion, especially venous. Secondary processes from disease arising elsewhere in the body, such as diabetes mellitus (complicated by proliferative retinopathy, macular oedema and haemorrhage) and hypertension, are important causes of vascular damage to the eye. The new vessel proliferation and haemorrhages within the eye can cause significant impairment of vision, which may be permanent and extensive. Inhibitors of VEGF are the mainstay in the pharmacological management of pathological angiogenesis within the eye.

VEGF acts through activation of two tyrosine kinase receptors (VEGF-1 and VEGF-2) that are involved in physiological angiogenesis in the eye. Stimulation of the receptors leads to greater endothelial proliferation and migration, with new vessel formation and an increase in microvascular permeability. Pathological new vessel formation, with associated vascular fragility, leads to an increased risk of haemorrhage, with loss of vision due to blood in the chambers and retina of the eye. New vessels that form on the iris can provoke episodes of glaucoma. Enhanced microvascular permeability causes visual disturbance due to fluid leakage, oedema and swelling of the retina. Fibrovascular proliferation increases traction on the retina leading to sight threatening detachment of the retina from the posterior wall of the eye.

VEGF inhibitors are used to inhibit new vessel formation arising from these pathologies, and they are administered through intravitreal injection. Adverse effects stem from the trauma and infection risk of the procedure (endophthalmitis is a particular concern), as well as uncommon systemic problems such as hypertension and gastrointestinal disturbance as the drug is absorbed from the vitreous.

Available agents include:

Bevacizumab is a full-length humanised IgG1 monoclonal antibody that binds with high affinity to VEGF, thus blocking its activity at VEGF receptors. This drug was first made available for use in colorectal cancer but has also been found to be effective for neovascular conditions in the eye.

Ranibizumab is a monoclonal antibody fragment directed at all isoforms of VEGF-A. In contrast to bevacizumab, the formulation of ranibizumab is specifically aimed for use in the eye.

Aflibercept is a hybrid molecule consisting of the Fc segment of IgG1 structurally joined to extracellular domains from VEGF-1 and -2 receptors. Intriguingly, aflibercept was designed to have high affinity for VEGF and placental growth factor. It therefore acts as a 'decoy' molecule to soak up VEGF-A, thus reducing activation of VEGF-1 and -2 receptors at target sites in the eye (as well as in treatment of metastatic colon cancer).

Vascular endothelial growth factor (VEGF) inhibitors

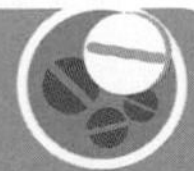

VEGF inhibitors are used in a variety of conditions where new vessel formation and proliferation, or oedema without neovascularisation, are a significant threat to vision.

- Wet age-related macular degeneration secondary to choroidal neovascularisation
- Proliferative diabetic retinopathy (as a short-term adjunct to laser photocoagulation)
- Retinal vessel occlusion
- Choroidal neovascularisation
- Retinopathy of prematurity
- Diabetic macular oedema

REFERENCES AND FURTHER READING

Aihara, M., 2021. Prostanoid receptor agonists for glaucoma treatment. Jpn. J. Ophthalmol. 65, 581–590.

Awwad, S., Mohamed Ahmed, A.H.A., Sharma, G., et al., 2017. Principles of pharmacology in the eye. Br. J. Pharmacol. 174, 4205–4223.

Cvenkel, B., Kolko, M., 2020. Current medical therapy and future trends in the management of glaucoma treatment. J. Ophthalmol. 2020, 6138132.

Dreyfuss, J.L., Giordano, R.J., Regatieri, C.V., 2015. Ocular angiogenesis. J. Ophthalmol. 2015, 892043.

Forrester, J.V., Dick, D.A., McMenamin, P.G., Roberts, F., Pearlman, E., 2020. The Eye: Basic Sciences in Practice, fifth ed. Elsevier, London.

Novack, G.D., Robin, A.L., 2016. Ocular pharmacology. J. Clin. Pharmacol. 56, 517–527.

Selvam, S., Kumar, T., Fruttiger, M., 2018. Retinal vasculature development in health and disease. Prog. Retin. Eye Res. 63, 1–19.

Stoner, A., Harris, A., Oddone, F., et al., 2022. Topical carbonic anhydrase inhibitors and glaucoma in 2021: where do we stand? Br. J. Ophthalmol. 106, 1332–1337.

28 Respiratory system

OVERVIEW

Basic aspects of respiratory physiology (regulation of airway smooth muscle, pulmonary vasculature and glands) are considered as a basis for a discussion of pulmonary disease and its treatment. We devote most of the chapter to asthma, dealing first with pathogenesis and then the main drugs used in its treatment and prevention – inhaled bronchodilators and anti-inflammatory agents. We also discuss chronic obstructive pulmonary disease (COPD), bronchiectasis as well as idiopathic pulmonary fibrosis. There are short sections on allergic emergencies, surfactants and the treatment of cough.

THE PHYSIOLOGY OF RESPIRATION

CONTROL OF BREATHING

Respiration is controlled by spontaneous rhythmic discharges from the respiratory centre in the medulla, modulated by input from pontine and higher central nervous system (CNS) centres and vagal afferents from the lungs. Various chemical factors affect the respiratory centre, including the partial pressure of carbon dioxide in arterial blood ($P_{A}CO_2$) by an action on medullary chemoreceptors, and of oxygen ($P_{A}O_2$) by an action on the chemoreceptors in the carotid bodies.

Some voluntary control can be superimposed on the automatic regulation of breathing, implying connections between the cortex and the motor neurons innervating the muscles of respiration. Bulbar poliomyelitis and certain lesions in the brain stem result in loss of the automatic regulation of respiration without loss of voluntary regulation.[1]

REGULATION OF MUSCULATURE, BLOOD VESSELS AND GLANDS OF THE AIRWAYS

Irritant receptors and non-myelinated afferent nerve fibres respond to chemical irritants and cold air, and also to inflammatory mediators. Efferent pathways controlling the airways include cholinergic parasympathetic nerves and non-noradrenergic non-cholinergic (NANC) inhibitory nerves (see Ch. 13). Bronchial hyper-responsiveness can be triggered by changes in the afferent sensory and efferent pathways, as well as the neural control networks in the brainstem (see Pincus et al., 2021, for a comprehensive review). Inflammatory mediators (see Ch. 17) and other bronchoconstrictor mediators also have a role in diseased airways.

The tone of bronchial muscle influences airway resistance, which is also affected by the state of the mucosa and activity of the submucosal mucus-secreting glands in patients with asthma and bronchitis. Airway resistance can be measured indirectly by instruments that record the volume or flow of forced expiration. FEV_1 is the forced expiratory volume in 1 second. The peak expiratory flow rate (PEFR) is the maximal flow (expressed as L/min) after a full inhalation; this is simpler to measure at the bedside than FEV_1, which it follows closely.

EFFERENT PATHWAYS

Autonomic innervation

The autonomic innervation of human airways is reviewed by van der Velden and Hulsmann (1999).

Parasympathetic innervation. Parasympathetic innervation of bronchial smooth muscle predominates. Parasympathetic ganglia are embedded in the walls of the bronchi and bronchioles, and the postganglionic fibres innervate airway smooth muscle, vascular smooth muscle and glands. Five types of muscarinic (M) receptors are present (see Ch. 14, Table 14.2). M_3 receptors are pharmacologically the most important in airways disease. They are found on bronchial smooth muscle and gland cells, and mediate bronchoconstriction and mucus secretion. M_1 receptors are localised in ganglia and on postsynaptic cells, and facilitate nicotinic neurotransmission, whereas M_2 receptors are inhibitory autoreceptors mediating negative feedback on acetylcholine release by postganglionic cholinergic nerves. Stimulation of the vagus causes bronchoconstriction – mainly in the larger airways. The possible clinical relevance of the heterogeneity of muscarinic receptors in the airways is discussed later.

A distinct population of NANC nerves (see Ch. 13) also regulates the airways. Bronchodilators released by these nerves include *vasoactive intestinal polypeptide* (Table 13.2) and *nitric oxide* (NO; see Ch. 19).

Sympathetic innervation. Sympathetic nerves innervate tracheobronchial blood vessels and glands, but not human airway smooth muscle. However, β adrenoceptors are abundantly expressed on human airway smooth muscle (as well as mast cells, epithelium, glands and alveoli) and β agonists relax bronchial smooth muscle, inhibit mediator release from mast cells and increase mucociliary clearance. In humans, β adrenoceptors in the airways are of the β_2 variety.

In addition to the efferent autonomic innervation, non-myelinated sensory fibres, linked to irritant receptors in the lungs, release tachykinins such as *substance P*, *neurokinin A* and *neurokinin B* (see Ch. 17), producing *neurogenic inflammation*.

SENSORY RECEPTORS AND AFFERENT PATHWAYS

Slowly adapting *stretch receptors* control respiration via the respiratory centre. Unmyelinated sensory *C fibres*

[1]Referred to as *Ondine curse*. Ondine was a water nymph who fell in love with a mortal. When he was unfaithful to her, the king of the water nymphs put a curse on him – that he must stay awake in order to breathe. When exhaustion finally supervened and he fell asleep, he died. Such patients are treated with mechanical ventilation. In less extreme forms, patients whose respiratory centre is relatively insensitive hypoventilate and become hypoxic when they fall asleep, leading to multiple awakenings during the night.

Regulation of airway muscle, blood vessels and glands

Afferent pathways

- Irritant receptors and C fibres respond to exogenous chemicals, inflammatory mediators and physical stimuli (e.g. cold air).

Efferent pathways

- Parasympathetic nerves cause bronchoconstriction and mucus secretion through M_3 receptors.
- Sympathetic nerves innervate blood vessels and glands, but not airway smooth muscle.
- β_2-Adrenoceptor agonists relax airway smooth muscle. This is pharmacologically important.
- Inhibitory NANC nerves relax airway smooth muscle by releasing NO and vasoactive intestinal peptide.
- Excitation of sensory nerves causes neuroinflammation by releasing tachykinins: substance P and neurokinin A.

and rapidly adapting *irritant receptors* associated with myelinated vagal fibres are also important.

Physical or chemical stimuli, acting on irritant receptors on myelinated nerve fibres in the upper airways and/or C-fibre receptors in the lower airways, cause coughing, bronchoconstriction and mucus secretion. Such stimuli include cold air and irritants such as ammonia, sulfur dioxide, cigarette smoke and the experimental tool *capsaicin* (see Ch. 43), as well as endogenous inflammatory mediators.

PULMONARY DISEASE AND ITS TREATMENT

Common symptoms of pulmonary disease include shortness of breath, wheeze, chest pain and cough with or without sputum production or haemoptysis (blood in the sputum). Ideally, treatment is of the underlying disease, but sometimes symptomatic treatment, for example of cough, is all that is possible. The lung is an important target organ of many diseases addressed elsewhere in this book, including infections (Chs 52–56), malignancy (see Ch. 57) and occupational and rheumatological diseases; drugs (e.g. **amiodarone**, **methotrexate**) can damage lung tissue and cause pulmonary fibrosis. Heart failure leads to pulmonary oedema (see Ch. 21). Thromboembolic disease (see Ch. 23) and pulmonary hypertension (see Ch. 21) affect the pulmonary circulation. In this present chapter, we concentrate on two important diseases of the airways: asthma and chronic obstructive pulmonary disease (COPD).

BRONCHIAL ASTHMA

Asthma affects about 8% of the population; it is the commonest chronic disease in children in economically developed countries and is also common in adults. It is an inflammatory condition in which there is recurrent reversible airways obstruction in response to irritant stimuli that are too weak to affect non-asthmatic subjects. The obstruction usually causes wheeze and merits drug treatment,[2] although the natural history of asthma includes spontaneous remissions. Reversibility of airways obstruction in asthma contrasts with COPD, where the obstruction is either not reversible or at best incompletely reversible by bronchodilators.

CHARACTERISTICS OF ASTHMA

Asthmatic patients experience intermittent attacks of wheezing, shortness of breath – with difficulty especially in breathing out, chest tightness and, sometimes, cough. As explained earlier, acute attacks are reversible, but the underlying pathological disorder can progress in older patients to a chronic state superficially resembling COPD.

Acute severe asthma (also known as *status asthmaticus*) is not easily reversed and causes hypoxaemia. Hospitalisation is necessary, as the condition, which can be fatal, requires prompt and energetic treatment.

Asthma is a heterogeneous disease, typically characterised by:

- chronic inflammation of the airways
- bronchial hyper-reactivity
- variable and reversible airflow limitation

Bronchial hyper-reactivity (or hyper-responsiveness) is abnormal sensitivity to a wide range of stimuli, such as irritant chemicals, cold air and bronchoconstrictor drugs. In allergic asthma, these features may be initiated by sensitisation to allergen(s), but, once established, asthma attacks can be triggered by various stimuli such as viral infection, exercise (in which the stimulus may be cold air and/or drying of the airways) and atmospheric pollutants such as sulfur dioxide. Immunological desensitisation to allergens such as pollen or dust mites is popular in some countries but is not superior to conventional inhaled drug treatment.

PATHOGENESIS OF ASTHMA

The pathogenesis of asthma involves both genetic and environmental factors, and the asthmatic attack itself consists, in many subjects, of two main phases: an immediate and a late (or delayed) phase (Fig. 28.1).

Numerous cells and mediators play a part, and the full details of the complex events involved are still a matter of debate. Disease processes in asthma are thought to involve both innate and adaptive immunity (see Boonpiyathad et al., 2019, for a comprehensive overview). The following simplified account is intended to provide a basis for understanding the rational use of drugs in the treatment of asthma.

Asthmatics have activated T cells, with a T-helper (Th)2 profile of cytokine production (see Ch. 17) in their bronchial mucosa. How these cells are activated is not fully understood, but allergens (Fig. 28.2) are one mechanism. The Th2 cytokines that are released do the following:

[2] William Osler, 19th-century doyen of American and British clinicians, wrote that 'the asthmatic pants into old age' – this at a time when the most effective drug that he could offer was to smoke stramonium cigarettes, a herbal remedy, the antimuscarinic effects of which were offset by direct irritation from the smoke. Its use persisted in English private schools into the 1950s, as one author can attest – much to the envy of his fellows!

- Attract other inflammatory granulocytes, especially eosinophils, to the mucosal surface. Interleukin (IL)-5 and granulocyte–macrophage colony-stimulating factor prime eosinophils to produce cysteinyl leukotrienes (see Ch. 17), and to release granule proteins that damage the epithelium. This damage is one cause of bronchial hyper-responsiveness.
- Promote immunoglobulin (Ig)E synthesis and responsiveness in some asthmatics (IL-4 and IL-13 'switch' B cells to IgE synthesis and cause expression of IgE receptors on mast cells and eosinophils; they also enhance adhesion of eosinophils to endothelium).

Some asthmatics, in addition to these mechanisms, are also *atopic* – that is, they make allergen-specific IgE that binds to mast cells in the airways. Inhaled allergen cross-links IgE molecules on mast cells, triggering degranulation with release of histamine and leukotriene B_4, both of which are powerful bronchoconstrictors to which asthmatics are especially sensitive because of their airway hyper-responsiveness. This provides a mechanism for acute exacerbation of asthma in atopic individuals exposed to allergen. The effectiveness of **omalizumab** (an anti-IgE antibody; see later) serves to emphasise the importance of IgE in the pathogenesis of asthma as well as in other allergic diseases. Noxious gases (e.g. sulfur dioxide, ozone) and airway dehydration can also cause mast cell degranulation. Non-steroidal anti-inflammatory drugs (NSAIDs), especially aspirin, can also precipitate asthma in sensitive individuals. Such aspirin-sensitive asthma is relatively uncommon (<10% of asthmatic subjects), and is often associated with nasal polyps

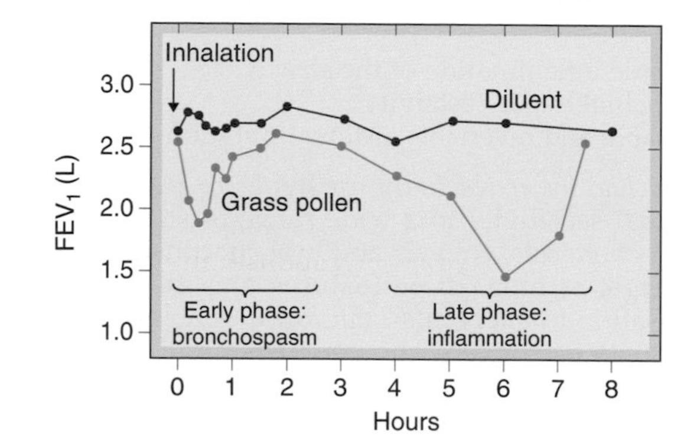

Fig. 28.1 Two phases of asthma demonstrated by the changes in forced expiratory volume in 1 second (FEV_1) after inhalation of grass pollen in an allergic subject. (From Cockcroft, D.W., 1983. Lancet ii, 253.)

Asthma is a complex heterogeneous condition with considerable variation in underlying aetiology and biological causes. Although multiple different phenotypic clusters can be considered based on clinical features, patient characteristics and physiological processes, there is no clear consensus on these classifications. In this text, we will mainly refer to the allergic and non-allergic forms.

The immediate phase of an asthma attack

In allergic asthma the immediate phase (i.e. the initial response to allergen provocation) occurs abruptly and is mainly caused by spasm of the bronchial smooth muscle. Allergen interaction with mast cell-fixed IgE causes release of histamine, leukotriene B_4 and prostaglandin (PG)D_2 (see Ch. 17).

Other mediators released include IL-4, IL-5, IL-13, macrophage inflammatory protein-1α and tumour necrosis factor (TNF)-α.

Various chemotaxins and chemokines (see Ch. 17) attract leukocytes – particularly eosinophils and mononuclear cells – setting the stage for the late phase (Fig. 28.3).

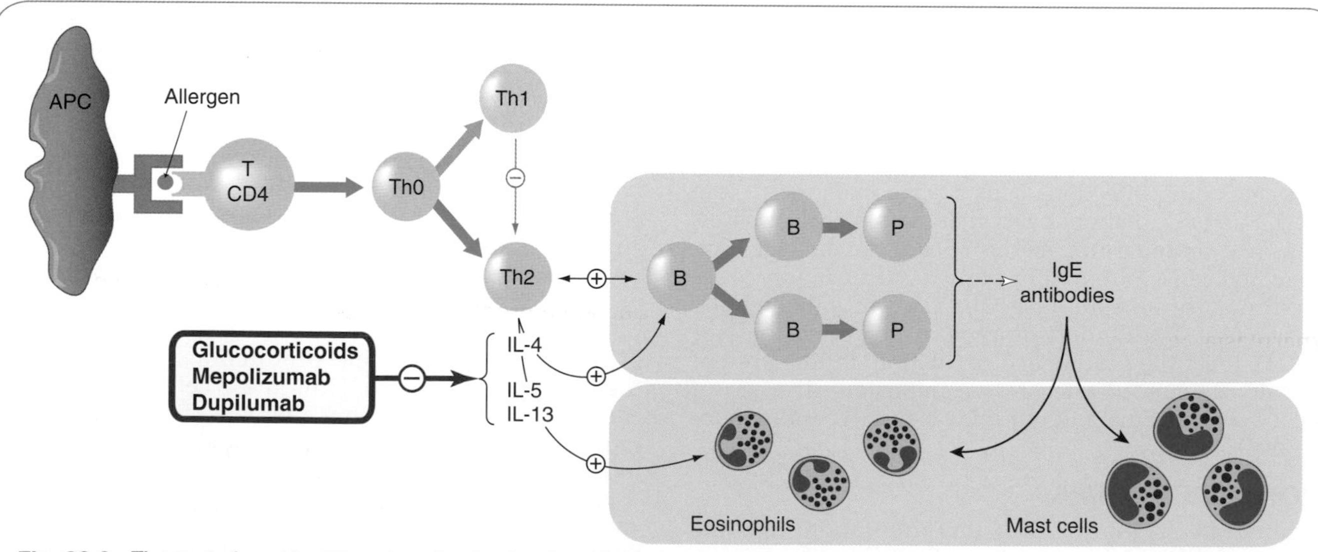

Fig. 28.2 The part played by T lymphocytes in allergic asthma. In genetically susceptible individuals, allergen *(green circle)* interacts with dendritic cells and CD4+ T cells, leading to the development of Th0 lymphocytes, which give rise to a clone of Th2 lymphocytes. These then (1) generate a cytokine environment that switches B cells/plasma cells to the production and release of immunoglobulin (Ig) E; (2) generate cytokines, such as interleukin (IL)-5, which promote differentiation and activation of eosinophils; and (3) generate cytokines (e.g. IL-4 and IL-13) that induce expression of IgE receptors. Glucocorticoids inhibit the action of the cytokines specified. *APC,* Antigen-presenting dendritic cell; *B,* B cell; *P,* plasma cell; *Th,* T-helper cell.

Asthma

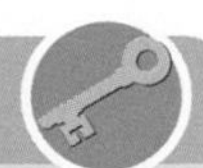

- Asthma is defined as recurrent reversible airway obstruction, with intermittent attacks of wheeze, shortness of breath, chest tightness and cough. Severe attacks cause hypoxaemia and are life-threatening.
- Typical features include:
  - airway inflammation, which causes
  - bronchial hyper-responsiveness, which in turn results in – recurrent reversible airway obstruction
- Pathogenesis involves exposure of genetically disposed individuals to allergens; activation of Th2 lymphocytes and cytokine generation promote:
  - differentiation and activation of eosinophils
  - IgE production and release
  - expression of IgE receptors on mast cells and eosinophils
- Important mediators include leukotriene B_4 and cysteinyl leukotrienes (C_4 and D_4); interleukins (IL)-4, IL-5, IL-13; and tissue-damaging eosinophil proteins.
- Antiasthmatic drugs include:
  - bronchodilators
  - anti-inflammatory agents
- Treatment is monitored by measuring forced expiratory volume in 1 second (FEV_1) or PEFR and, in acute severe disease, oxygen saturation and arterial blood gases.

The late phase

The late phase or delayed response (see Figs 28.1 and 28.3) may be nocturnal. It is, in essence, a progressing inflammatory reaction, initiation of which occurred during the first phase, the influx of Th2 lymphocytes being of particular importance. The inflammatory cells include activated eosinophils. These release cysteinyl leukotrienes, interleukins IL-3, IL-5 and IL-8 and the toxic proteins *eosinophil cationic protein*, *major basic protein* and *eosinophil-derived neurotoxin*. These play an important part in the events of the late phase, the toxic proteins causing damage and loss of epithelium. Other putative mediators of the inflammatory process in the delayed phase are adenosine (acting on the A_1 receptor; see Ch. 16), induced NO (see Ch. 19) and neuropeptides (see Ch. 17).

Growth factors released from inflammatory cells act on smooth muscle cells, causing hypertrophy and hyperplasia, and the smooth muscle can itself release proinflammatory mediators and growth factors (Chs 6 and 17). Fig. 28.4 shows schematically the changes that take place in the bronchioles. Epithelial cell loss means that irritant receptors and C fibres are more accessible to irritant stimuli - an important mechanism of bronchial hyper-reactivity.

DRUGS USED TO TREAT AND PREVENT ASTHMA

There are two categories of antiasthma drugs: *bronchodilators* and *anti-inflammatory agents*. Bronchodilators reverse the bronchospasm of the immediate phase; anti-inflammatory agents inhibit or prevent the inflammatory components of both phases (see Fig. 28.3). These two categories are not mutually exclusive: some drugs classified as bronchodilators also have some anti-inflammatory effect. In clinical practice, bronchodilator drugs are considered for use as relievers (when or if breakthrough symptoms occur), whereas anti-inflammatory agents are taken regularly as preventers or controllers of the underlying pathology.

A guideline on the management of asthma (BTS/SIGN, 2019) specifies a stepwise approach for adults and children with chronic asthma. Very mild or infrequent disease may be treated with short-acting bronchodilator (usually an inhaled short-acting β_2 agonist such as **salbutamol** or **terbutaline**, used as required), but if patients need this more than three times a week, a regular inhaled corticosteroid should be added. If the asthma remains uncontrolled, the next step is to add a long-acting bronchodilator (**salmeterol** or **formoterol**), and/or consider increased doses of inhaled corticosteroid as well as a leukotriene antagonist (such as **montelukast**). **Theophylline or tiotropium** (a long-acting muscarinic antagonist) are subsequent treatment options in patients who remain symptomatic. Addition of a regular oral corticosteroid (e.g. **prednisolone**) is recommended only in the small group of patients who do not achieve adequate control despite high-dose therapies with the other agents. Corticosteroids are the mainstay of therapy because they are the only asthma drugs that potently inhibit T-cell activation, and thus the inflammatory response, in the asthmatic airways. Omalizumab and other monoclonal antibodies (see later) are options in those with poorly controlled asthma despite optimal treatment with other agents. **Cromoglicate** (see later) has only a weak effect and is now seldom used.

BRONCHODILATORS

The main drugs used as bronchodilators are β_2-adrenoceptor agonists; others include **theophylline**, cysteinyl leukotriene receptor antagonists and muscarinic receptor antagonists.

β-Adrenoceptor agonists

The β_2-adrenoceptor agonists are dealt with in Chapter 15. Their primary effect in asthma is to dilate the bronchi by a direct action on the β_2 adrenoceptors of smooth muscle. Being physiological antagonists of bronchoconstrictors, they relax bronchial muscle whatever spasmogen is involved. They also inhibit mediator release from mast cells and TNF-α release from monocytes, and increase mucus clearance by an action on cilia.

β_2-Adrenoceptor agonists are usually given by inhalation of aerosol, powder or nebulised solution (i.e. solution that has been converted into a cloud or mist of fine droplets), but some products may be given orally or by injection. A metered-dose inhaler is used for aerosol preparations.

Two categories of β_2-adrenoceptor agonists are used in asthma:

- Short-acting agents: **salbutamol** and **terbutaline.** These are given by inhalation; they act immediately, peaking within 30 min and the duration of action is 3–5 h; they are usually used on an 'as needed' basis to control symptoms.
- Longer-acting agents: e.g. **salmeterol** and **formoterol.** These are given by inhalation, and the duration of action is 8–12 h. They are usually given regularly, twice daily, as adjunctive therapy in patients whose asthma is inadequately controlled by glucocorticoids.

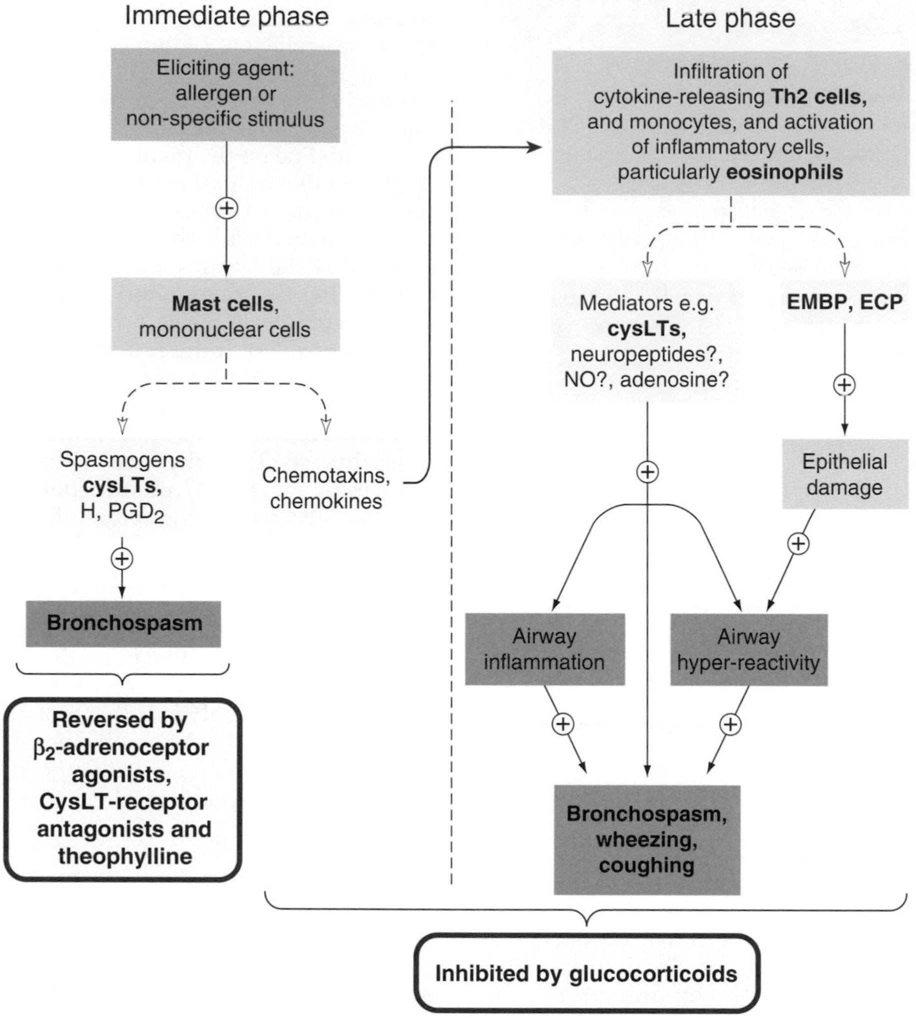

Immediate phase
Late phase
Eliciting agent: allergen or non-specific stimulus
Mast cells, mononuclear cells
Spasmogens cysLTs, H, PGD2
Chemotaxins, chemokines
Bronchospasm
Reversed by β2-adrenoceptor agonists, CysLT-receptor antagonists and theophylline
Infiltration of cytokine-releasing Th2 cells, and monocytes, and activation of inflammatory cells, particularly eosinophils
Mediators e.g. cysLTs, neuropeptides?, NO?, adenosine?
EMBP, ECP
Epithelial damage
Airway inflammation
Airway hyper-reactivity
Bronchospasm, wheezing, coughing
Inhibited by glucocorticoids

Fig. 28.3 Immediate and late phases of asthma, with the actions of the main drugs. *CysLTs*, Cysteinyl leukotrienes (leukotrienes C_4 and D_4); *ECP,* eosinophil cationic protein; *EMBP,* eosinophil major basic protein; *H,* histamine; *iNO,* induced nitric oxide. (For more detail of the Th2-derived cytokines and chemokines, see Ch. 17 and Ch. 6.)

Submucosa
Mucosa
Infiltration of inflammatory cells, (mononuclear cells, eosinophils, etc.)
Hypertrophied smooth muscle
Mononuclear cell
Oedema
Mast cell
Dilated blood vessels
Eosinophil
Epithelium
Thickened basement membrane
Mucus plug with eosinophils and desquamated epithelial cells

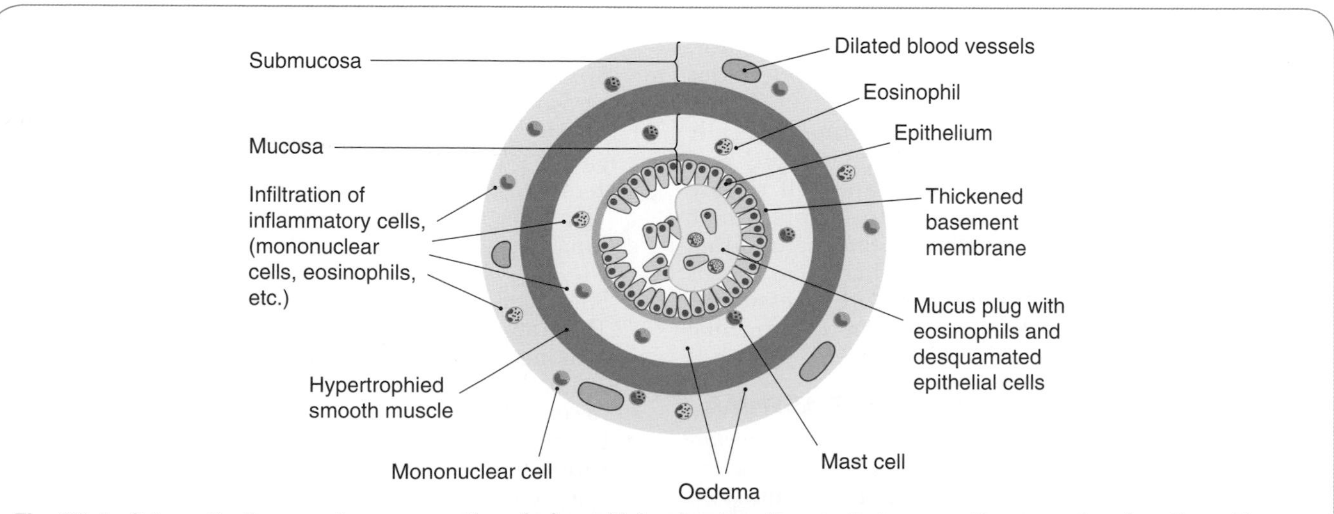

Fig. 28.4 Schematic diagram of a cross-section of a bronchiole, showing changes that occur with severe chronic asthma. The individual elements depicted are not, of course, drawn to scale.

Antiasthma drugs: bronchodilators

- β_2-Adrenoceptor agonists (e.g. **salbutamol**) are first-line drugs (for details, see Ch. 15):
  - They act as physiological antagonists of the spasmogenic mediators but have little or no effect on the bronchial hyper-reactivity.
  - Salbutamol is given by inhalation; its effects start immediately and last 3–5 h, and it can also be given by intravenous infusion in status asthmaticus.
  - **Salmeterol** or **formoterol** is given regularly by inhalation; their duration of action is 8–12 h.
- **Theophylline** (often formulated as **aminophylline**):
  - is a methylxanthine;
  - inhibits phosphodiesterase (PDE) and blocks adenosine receptors;
  - has a narrow therapeutic window: unwanted effects include cardiac dysrhythmia, seizures and gastrointestinal (GI) disturbances;
  - is a fall-back option when other safer and more established drugs have not worked. It can be given intravenously (by slow infusion) for acute severe asthma, or orally (as a sustained-release preparation) for inadequately controlled chronic asthma;
  - is metabolised in the liver by P450; liver dysfunction and viral infections increase its plasma concentration and half-life (normally approximately 12 h);
  - interacts importantly with other drugs; some (e.g. specific antibiotics) increase the half-life of **theophylline**, others (e.g. anticonvulsants) decrease it.

Unwanted effects

The unwanted effects of β_2-adrenoceptor agonists result from systemic absorption and are given in Chapter 15. In the context of their use in asthma, the commonest adverse effect is *tremor*; other unwanted effects include *tachycardia* and *cardiac dysrhythmia*.

Methylxanthines (see Chs 16 and 49)

Theophylline (1,3-dimethylxanthine), which is also used as theophylline ethylenediamine (known as **aminophylline**), is the main therapeutic drug of this class, and has long been used as a bronchodilator.[3] Here we consider it in the context of respiratory disease, its only current therapeutic use.

Mechanism of action

The mechanism of theophylline is still unclear. The relaxant effect on smooth muscle has been attributed to inhibition of PDE isoenzymes, with resultant increase in cAMP and/or cGMP (see Ch. 4, Fig. 4.10). However, the concentrations necessary to inhibit the isolated enzymes exceed the therapeutic range of plasma concentrations.

Competitive antagonism of adenosine at adenosine A_1 and A_2 receptors (see Ch. 16) may contribute, but there are other xanthines which have potent bronchodilatory effects, without any adenosine antagonist activity.

Clinical use of β_2-adrenoceptor agonists as bronchodilators

- Short-acting drugs (**salbutamol** or **terbutaline**, usually by inhalation) to prevent or treat acute symptoms in patients with reversible obstructive airways disease.
- Long-acting drugs (**salmeterol**, **formoterol**) to prevent bronchospasm (e.g. at night or with exercise) in patients requiring long-term bronchodilator therapy. Formoterol is faster acting and can also be used as an acute reliever in combination inhalers that deliver inhaled corticosteroid at the same time. This single maintenance and reliever therapy inhaler as-needed option can be used instead of the more traditional model of separate short-acting reliever (e.g. salbutamol intermittently) with regular inhaled corticosteroid.

Type IV PDE is implicated in inflammatory cells, and methylxanthines may have some anti-inflammatory effect. (**Roflumilast**, a type IV PDE inhibitor, is mentioned later in the context of COPD.)

Theophylline activates *histone deacetylase* (HDAC), which controls gene expression and may thereby reverse resistance to the anti-inflammatory effects of corticosteroids (Liao et al., 2020).

Methylxanthines stimulate the CNS (see Ch. 49) and respiratory stimulation may be beneficial in patients with COPD who suffer from reduced respiration and retention of CO_2. **Caffeine** has a special niche in treating hypoventilation of prematurity (see Ch. 49).

Unwanted effects

When theophylline is used in asthma, its other actions (CNS, cardiovascular, GI and diuretic) result in unwanted effects (e.g. insomnia, nervousness). The therapeutic plasma concentration range is 30–100 μmol/L, and adverse effects are common with concentrations greater than 110 μmol/L; thus there is a relatively narrow therapeutic window. Serious cardiovascular and CNS effects can occur when the plasma concentration exceeds 200 μmol/L. The most serious cardiovascular effect is *dysrhythmia* (especially during intravenous administration of aminophylline), which can be fatal. *Seizures* can occur with theophylline concentrations at or slightly above the upper limit of the therapeutic range, and can be fatal in patients with impaired respiration due to severe asthma. Monitoring the concentration of theophylline in plasma is useful for optimising the dose.

Pharmacokinetic aspects

Theophylline is given orally as a sustained-release preparation. Aminophylline can be given by slow intravenous injection of a loading dose followed by intravenous infusion.

Theophylline is well absorbed from the GI tract. It is metabolised by P450 enzymes in the liver; the mean elimination half-life is approximately 8 h in adults but there is wide inter-individual variation. The half-life is increased in liver disease, cardiac failure and viral

[3]Over 200 years ago, William Withering recommended 'coffee made very strong' as a remedy for asthma. Coffee contains caffeine, a related methylxanthine.

infections, and is decreased in heavy cigarette smokers (as a result of enzyme induction leading to increased clearance). Unwanted drug interactions are clinically important: its plasma concentration is decreased by drugs that induce P450 enzymes (including **rifampicin**, **phenytoin** and **carbamazepine**). The concentration is increased by drugs that inhibit P450 enzymes, such as **erythromycin**, **clarithromycin**, **ciprofloxacin**, **diltiazem** and **fluconazole**. This is important in view of the narrow therapeutic window; antibiotics such as clarithromycin are often started when asthmatics are hospitalised because of a severe attack precipitated by a chest infection, and if the dose of theophylline is unaltered, severe toxicity can result.

Muscarinic receptor antagonists

Muscarinic receptor antagonists are dealt with in Chapter 14. **Ipratropium**, given by aerosol inhalation or nebuliser, is a short-acting muscarinic antagonist that is used as a bronchodilator in acute exacerbations. Inhaled long-acting muscarinic antagonists, such as **tiotropium**, **aclidinium**, **umeclidinium** and **glycopyrrolate**, are now widely available for once-daily inhalation in COPD (see clinical box).

Ipratropium is a quaternary nitrogen compound that is derived from atropine. It does not discriminate between muscarinic receptor subtypes (see Ch. 14), and it is possible that its blockade of M_2 autoreceptors on the cholinergic nerves increases acetylcholine release and reduces the effectiveness of its antagonism at the M_3 receptors on smooth muscle. As the maximum effect occurs approximately 30 min after inhalation and persists only for 3–5 h, ipratropium has to be administered up to four times a day, thus limiting its clinical acceptability.

Long-acting muscarinic antagonists are also quaternary ammonium compounds, designed to have greater selectivity towards the M_3 receptor, and to dissociate from the receptor very slowly, producing a sustained effect with regular daily dosing. They are often used together with long-acting β_2-adrenoceptor agonists and/or inhaled corticosteroids in a combined inhaler for patients with COPD.

Clinical use of inhaled muscarinic receptor antagonists

- Ipratropium is used as an adjunct to β_2-adrenoceptor agonists in nebulised form for acute exacerbations of asthma or COPD.
- Long-acting drugs (e.g. tiotropium) are mainly indicated for regular daily use in patients with COPD; the long-term role in asthma is less certain.

Cysteinyl leukotriene receptor antagonists

Cysteinyl leukotrienes (LTC_4, LTD_4 and LTE_4) act on *CysLT₁* and *CysLT₂* receptors (see Ch. 17), both of which are expressed in respiratory mucosa and infiltrating inflammatory cells, but the functional significance of each is unclear. The 'lukast' drugs (**montelukast** and **zafirlukast**) antagonise only $CysLT_1$.

Lukasts inhibit exercise-induced asthma and decrease both early and late responses to inhaled allergen. They dilate the airways in mild asthma but are less effective than salbutamol, with which their action is additive. They reduce sputum eosinophilia, but there is no clear evidence that they modify the underlying inflammatory process in chronic asthma.

The lukasts are taken by mouth and used mainly as add-on therapy to inhaled corticosteroids and long-acting β_2 agonists. They are generally well tolerated, adverse effects consisting mainly of headache and GI disturbances.

Histamine H_1-receptor antagonists

Although mast cell mediators, including histamine, play a part in the immediate phase of allergic asthma (see Fig. 28.3) and in some types of exercise-induced asthma, histamine H_1-receptor antagonists have no routine place in therapy, although they may be modestly effective in mild atopic asthma, especially when this is precipitated by acute histamine release in patients with concomitant allergy such as severe hay fever.

ANTI-INFLAMMATORY AGENTS

Glucocorticoids

Glucocorticoids (see Ch. 33) are the main drugs used for their anti-inflammatory action in asthma. They are not bronchodilators, but prevent the progression of chronic asthma and are effective in acute severe asthma (see 'Clinical use of glucocorticoids in asthma' clinical box, later).[4]

Actions and mechanism

The basis of the anti-inflammatory action of glucocorticoids is discussed in Chapter 33. An important action, of relevance for asthma, is that they restrain clonal proliferation of Th cells by reducing the transcription of the gene for IL-2 and decrease the formation of cytokines, in particular the Th2 cytokines that recruit and activate eosinophils and are responsible for promoting the production of IgE and the expression of IgE receptors. Glucocorticoids also inhibit the generation of the vasodilators PGE_2 and PGI_2, by inhibiting induction of COX-2 (see Ch. 17). By inducing *annexin 1* (see Fig. 17.3), they could inhibit the production of leukotrienes and platelet-activating factor, although there is currently no direct evidence that annexin 1 is involved in the therapeutic action of glucocorticoids in human asthma.

Corticosteroids inhibit the allergen-induced influx of eosinophils into the lung. Glucocorticoids up-regulate β_2 adrenoceptors, decrease microvascular permeability and indirectly reduce mediator release from eosinophils by inhibiting the production of cytokines (e.g. IL-5 and granulocyte–macrophage colony-stimulating factor) that activate eosinophils. Reduced synthesis of IL-3 (the cytokine that regulates mast cell production) may explain why long-term steroid treatment eventually reduces the number of mast cells in the respiratory mucosa, and hence suppresses the early-phase response to allergens and exercise.

[4]In 1900, Solis-Cohen reported that dried bovine adrenals had anti-asthma activity. He noted that the extract did not serve acutely 'to cut short the paroxysm' but was 'useful in averting recurrence of paroxysms'. Mistaken for the first report on the effect of adrenaline, his astute observation was probably the first on the efficacy of steroids in asthma.

Glucocorticoids are sometimes ineffective, even in high doses, for reasons that are incompletely understood. Many individual mechanisms could contribute to glucocorticoid resistance. The phenomenon has been linked to the number of glucocorticoid receptors, but in some situations other mechanisms are clearly in play – for example, reduced activity of HDAC may be important in cigarette smokers.

The main compounds used are **beclometasone**, **budesonide**, **fluticasone**, **mometasone** and **ciclesonide**. These are given by inhalation with a metered-dose or dry-powder inhaler, the full effect on bronchial hyper-responsiveness being attained only after weeks or months of therapy. There are now several inhaler formulations where inhaled corticosteroids are combined together with long-acting β_2-adrenoceptor agonists and/or long-acting muscarinic antagonists (triple therapy in COPD) (Cohen et al., 2016). Oral glucocorticoids (see Ch. 33) are reserved for patients with the severest disease.

Unwanted effects

Serious unwanted effects are uncommon with inhaled steroids. Oropharyngeal candidiasis (thrush; see Ch. 54) can occur (T lymphocytes are important in protection against fungal infection), as can sore throat and croaky voice, but 'spacer' devices (plastic tubes that connect onto the mouthpiece of the inhaler on one end while the patient uses a mouthpiece or mask at the other end) decrease oropharyngeal deposition of the drug and increase airway deposition, reducing these problems. Regular high doses of inhaled glucocorticoids can produce some adrenal suppression, particularly in children, and necessitate carrying a 'steroid card' (see Ch. 33). The unwanted effects of oral glucocorticoids are given in Fig. 33.7.

Clinical use of glucocorticoids in asthma

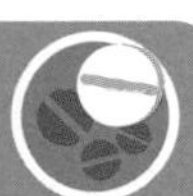

- Patients who require regular bronchodilators should also be prescribed glucocorticoid treatment (e.g. with low-dose inhaled **beclometasone**).
- More severely affected patients are treated with higher doses of inhaled corticosteroids in combination with long-acting beta-adrenoceptor agonists.
- Patients with acute exacerbations of asthma may require intravenous **hydrocortisone** followed by a course of oral **prednisolone.**
- A 'rescue course' of oral prednisolone may be needed at any stage of severity if the clinical condition is deteriorating rapidly.
- Prolonged treatment with oral prednisolone, in addition to inhaled bronchodilators and steroids, is needed by a few severely asthmatic patients.

Cromoglicate and nedocromil

These two drugs, of similar chemical structure and properties, are now hardly used for the treatment of asthma. Although very safe, they have only weak anti-inflammatory effects and a short duration of action. They are given by inhalation as aerosols or dry powders, and can also be used topically for allergic conjunctivitis or rhinitis. They are not bronchodilators, having no direct effects on smooth muscle, nor do they inhibit the actions of any of the known smooth muscle stimulants. Given prophylactically, they reduce both the immediate- and late-phase asthmatic responses and reduce bronchial hyper-reactivity.

Their mechanism of action is not fully understood. Cromoglicate is a 'mast cell stabiliser', preventing histamine release from mast cells. However, this is not the basis of its action in asthma, because compounds that are more potent than cromoglicate at inhibiting mast cell histamine release are ineffective against asthma.

Biopharmaceuticals

Anti-IgE treatment. **Omalizumab** is a humanised monoclonal anti-IgE antibody that is effective in patients with allergic asthma, as well as in chronic rhinosinusitis with nasal polyps, and in chronic spontaneous urticaria. However, omalizumab is expensive and has to be given by subcutaneous injection every 2 weeks. Its clinical role is principally for those patients with severe persistent confirmed allergic IgE-mediated asthma who have required continuous or frequent treatment with oral corticosteroids in addition to other standard therapies.

IL-5 antagonists. Eosinophilic asthma is a recognised variant for which specific therapies (such as **mepolizumab** or **reslizumab**) targeted at human IL-5 are now available. IL-5 is the key cytokine involved in growth, differentiation and activation of eosinophils (see Ch. 19). Antibodies that inhibit IL-5 signalling result in reduced production and survival of eosinophils that mediate the allergic inflammatory process in patients with asthma.

IL-4/IL-13 antagonist. Similarly, a combined inhibitor of IL-4 and IL-13 signalling (**dupilumab**) is prescribed for patients with moderate to severe eosinophilic asthma. Dupilimumab binds to the alpha subunit of the IL-4 receptor which is shared by the IL-4 and IL-13 receptor complexes. Clinical trials in asthma have found that dupilumab suppresses type 2 inflammatory biomarkers, with reductions in eotaxin-3, thymus and activation-regulated cytokine, and IgE. Intriguingly, strategies that target IL-4 or IL-13 cytokines individually have failed to yield demonstrable clinical benefits.

Thymic stromal lymphoprotein antagonist. In contrast, patients with non-allergic or non-eosinophilic asthma appear to benefit from treatment with another monoclonal antibody (**tezepelumab**) directed at thymic stromal lymphopoietin (TSLP) signalling. TSLP is a cytokine derived from epithelial cells that acts as mediator between the immune system and structural cells of the airway. This cytokine initiates several inflammatory cascades, and concentrations of TSLP are correlated with airflow limitation, asthma severity and poor response to glucocorticoids. Tezepelumab blocks its binding to its receptor. Randomised trial data demonstrate significant benefit for patients with severe asthma (irrespective of baseline eosinophilic count) with regards to pulmonary function, symptoms and reduction in exacerbations and hospital admissions.

Drugs in development

There are several novel agents targeted at mediators of eosinophilic airway inflammation (Bel and Ten Brinke, 2017), and inhibitors of prostaglandin D2 (see Fig. 28.3) are

Antiasthma drugs: glucocorticoids

Glucocorticoids (for details, see Ch. 33)

- These reduce the inflammatory component in chronic asthma and are life-saving in status asthmaticus (acute severe asthma).
- They do not prevent the immediate response to allergen or other challenges.
- The mechanism of action involves decreased formation of cytokines, particularly those generated by Th2 lymphocytes, decreased activation of eosinophils and other inflammatory cells.
- They are given by inhalation (e.g. **beclometasone**); systemic unwanted effects are uncommon at moderate doses, but oral thrush and voice problems can occur. In deteriorating asthma, an oral glucocorticoid (e.g. **prednisolone**) and/or intravenous **hydrocortisone** are also given.

currently in clinical trials (e.g. **timapiprant**) but **fevipiprant** has failed to demonstrate significant benefit in a randomised trial of patients with poorly controlled asthma.

SEVERE ACUTE ASTHMA (STATUS ASTHMATICUS)

Severe acute asthma is a medical emergency requiring hospitalisation. Treatment includes oxygen (to correct any hypoxia), inhalation of nebulised salbutamol with ipratropium and intravenous hydrocortisone followed by a course of oral prednisolone. Additional measures occasionally used include intravenous magnesium sulphate (considered to have bronchodilator effects) and, in some countries, intravenous salbutamol or aminophylline. Antibiotics are not routinely given unless there is clinical evidence of bacterial infection. Monitoring is by PEFR or FEV_1, and by measurement of arterial blood gases and oxygen saturation.

ALLERGIC EMERGENCIES

Anaphylaxis (see Ch. 7) and *angio-oedema* are emergencies involving acute airways obstruction; **adrenaline** (epinephrine) is potentially life-saving. It is administered intramuscularly (or occasionally intravenously, in specialist, intensively monitored settings). Patients at risk of acute anaphylaxis, for example, from food or insect sting allergy, may self-administer intramuscular adrenaline using a spring-loaded syringe. An antihistamine such as **chlorphenamine** may also be used if there is angio-oedema or skin rash.

Angio-oedema is the intermittent occurrence of focal swelling of the skin or intra-abdominal organs caused by plasma leakage from capillaries. Most often, it is mild and 'idiopathic', but it can occur as part of acute allergic reactions, when it is generally accompanied by urticaria – 'hives' – caused by histamine release from mast cells. If the larynx is involved, it is life-threatening; swelling in the peritoneal cavity can be very painful and mimic a surgical emergency. It can be caused by drugs, especially *angiotensin-converting enzyme inhibitors* – perhaps because they block the inactivation of peptides such as bradykinin (see Ch. 17) – and by aspirin and related drugs in patients who are aspirin sensitive (see Ch. 23). Hereditary angio-oedema is associated with lack of C1 esterase inhibitor – C1 esterase is an enzyme that degrades the complement component C1 (see Ch. 7). **Tranexamic acid** (see Ch. 23) or **danazol** (see Ch. 35) may be used to prevent attacks in patients with hereditary angioneurotic oedema, and administration of partially purified C1 esterase inhibitor or fresh plasma, with antihistamines and glucocorticoids, can terminate acute attacks. **Icatibant**, a peptide bradykinin B_2 receptor antagonist (see Ch. 17), is effective for acute attacks of hereditary angio-oedema. It is administered subcutaneously but can cause nausea, abdominal pain and nasal stuffiness.

CHRONIC OBSTRUCTIVE PULMONARY DISEASE

COPD is a major global health problem – the World Health Organization estimates that there were 3.2 million deaths from COPD in 2019, thus making it the third commonest cause of death worldwide by 2020. Cigarette smoking is the main cause, and is increasing in the developing world. Air pollution, also aetiologically important, is also increasing, and there is a huge unmet need for effective drugs. A resurgence of interest in new therapeutic approaches has yet to bear fruit but there are a number of promising avenues, in particular in defining subgroups of this rather heterogeneous disease that are responsive to particular therapeutic measures (McDonald, 2017).

Clinical features. The clinical picture starts with attacks of morning cough during the winter, and progresses to chronic cough with intermittent exacerbations, often initiated by an upper respiratory infection, when the sputum becomes purulent (i.e. yellow or green due to the presence of many pus cells – neutrophils or eosinophils). There is progressive breathlessness. Some patients have a reversible component of airflow obstruction identifiable by an improved FEV_1 following a dose of bronchodilator. Pulmonary hypertension (see Ch. 21) is a late complication, causing symptoms of heart failure (*cor pulmonale*). Exacerbations may be complicated by respiratory failure (i.e. reduced P_{AO_2}) requiring hospitalisation and intensive care. Tracheostomy and artificial ventilation, while prolonging survival, may serve only to return the patient to a miserable life.

Pathogenesis. There is fibrosis of small airways, resulting in obstruction, and/or destruction of alveoli and of elastin fibres in the lung parenchyma. The latter features are hallmarks of emphysema,[5] thought to be caused by proteases, including elastase, released during the inflammatory response. Emphysema causes respiratory failure, because it destroys the alveoli, impairing gas transfer. There is chronic inflammation (bronchitis), predominantly in small airways and lung parenchyma, characterised by increased numbers of macrophages, neutrophils and T lymphocytes. The inflammatory mediators are thought to involve T helper cell type 1 and type 17, with neutrophil and CD8 lymphocyte infiltrates in the lungs (Barnes, 2016). Mediators include a diverse range of interleukins, tumour necrosis factor and reactive oxygen species.

Principles of treatment. Stopping smoking (see Ch. 50) slows the progress of COPD. Patients should be immunised against influenza and *Pneumococcus*, because superimposed

[5]Emphysema is a pathological condition sometimes associated with COPD, in which lung parenchyma is destroyed and replaced by air spaces that coalesce to form bullae – blister-like air-filled spaces in the lung tissue.

infections with these organisms are potentially lethal. Glucocorticoids are less effective than in asthma. This contrast with asthma is puzzling, because in both diseases multiple inflammatory genes are activated, which might be expected to be turned off by glucocorticoids. Inflammatory gene activation results from acetylation of nuclear histones which opens up the chromatin structure, allowing gene transcription and synthesis of inflammatory proteins to proceed. HDAC de-acetylates histones, and suppresses the production of proinflammatory cytokines. Corticosteroids recruit HDAC to activated genes, switching off inflammatory gene transcription. Patients with COPD who do not respond to corticosteroid therapy are thought to be deficient in HDAC and nuclear factor erythroid 2-related factor (Liao et al., 2020). Inhaled steroids do not influence the progressive decline in lung function in patients with COPD, but do improve the quality of life, probably as a result of a modest reduction in hospital admissions. This is counter-balanced by the increased risk of pneumonia associated with use of inhaled corticosteroids in patients with COPD.

Long-acting bronchodilators give modest symptomatic benefit, but do not deal with the underlying inflammation. No currently licensed treatments reduce the progression of COPD or suppress the inflammation in small airways and lung parenchyma. Several new treatments that target the inflammatory process are in clinical development (Barnes, 2013). Some, such as chemokine antagonists, are directed against the influx of inflammatory cells into the airways and lung parenchyma, whereas others target inflammatory cytokines such as TNF-α. The PDE IV inhibitor **roflumilast** is licensed as an adjunct to bronchodilators for patients with severe COPD and frequent exacerbations. Other drugs that inhibit cell signalling (see Chs 3 and 6) include inhibitors of p38 mitogen-activated protein kinase, nuclear factor κβ and phosphoinositide-3 kinase-γ. More specific approaches include antioxidants, inhibitors of inducible NO synthase, and leukotriene B_4 antagonists. Other treatments have the potential to combat mucus hypersecretion, and there is a search for serine protease and matrix metalloprotease inhibitors to prevent lung destruction and the development of emphysema.

Specific aspects of treatment. Short- and long-acting inhaled bronchodilators can provide useful palliation in patients with a reversible component. The main short-acting drugs are ipratropium and salbutamol; long-acting drugs include muscarinic antagonists (e.g. **tiotropium**) which are often given together with β_2 agonists (such as **salmeterol** or **formoterol)** and/or inhaled corticosteroids (Chs 14 and 15; Cohen et al., 2016). A combination of inhaled corticosteroid with a long-acting b_2 agonist and a long-acting muscarinic antagonist is more effective than is dual therapy with a single long-acting bronchodilator. Theophylline (see Ch. 16) can be given by mouth but is of uncertain benefit. Other respiratory stimulants (e.g. **doxapram**) are sometimes used briefly in acute respiratory failure (e.g. postoperatively) but have largely been replaced by non-invasive ventilation as well as mechanical ventilatory support (intermittent positive-pressure ventilation).

Long-term oxygen therapy administered at home prolongs life in patients with severe disease and hypoxaemia (at least if they refrain from smoking – an oxygen fire is not a pleasant way to go).

Acute exacerbations. Acute exacerbations of COPD are treated with inhaled O_2 in a concentration (initially, at least) of 24%–28% O_2, that is, only just above atmospheric O_2 concentration (approximately 20%). The need for caution is because of the risk of precipitating CO_2 retention as a consequence of terminating the hypoxic drive to respiration. Blood gases and tissue oxygen saturation are monitored, and inspired O_2 subsequently is adjusted accordingly. Antibiotics such as aminopenicillins, macrolides or tetracyclines are recommended if there is evidence of infection. Inhaled bronchodilators (e.g. salbutamol and ipratropium) are prescribed for symptomatic benefit.

A systemically active glucocorticoid (intravenous hydrocortisone or oral prednisolone) is also administered, although efficacy is modest.

BRONCHIECTASIS

This is a chronic condition arising from persistent abnormalities and dilation of the bronchioles. Across the world, bronchiectasis can arise from a diverse range of lung pathologies such as COPD, tuberculosis and pneumonia. Cystic fibrosis, a genetic condition resulting in abnormal chloride ion movement, is an important cause in White populations, but rarely so in Asian or African people.

The clinical features of bronchiectasis include persistent cough, airflow limitation and recurrent chest infections that lead to permanent airway damage. The lung tissue is often colonised by antibiotic-resistant organisms, and treatment of such infections is both complex and challenging, involving nebulised as well as oral and intravenous agents (see Ch. 52).

CYSTIC FIBROSIS

Patients with cystic fibrosis have an inherited (autosomal recessive) disorder in the cystic fibrosis transmembrane conductance regulator (CFTR) protein. This has a deleterious effect on chloride channels at the plasma membrane, with severe clinical consequences on fluid and ion composition at cell surfaces of the respiratory and GI tract. In particular, there is thickening and stasis of mucus secretions with impaired clearance of the airways and progressive lung damage.

Treatment options include recombinant human DNAse to break down the thick mucus secretion. More recently, specific therapeutic agents (known as CFTR modulators) have been developed to address the deficient CFTR protein in patients with specific mutations (for example, the *F508 deletion* mutation which is the most prevalent in the UK).

Channel potentiators (e.g. **ivacaftor**) are targeted at certain CFTR gating mutations, with the aim of enhancing chloride transport by promoting opening of the channels.

Channel correctors (**lumacaftor, elexacaftor, tezacaftor**) are used in patients affected by *F508 deletion*. The drugs aim to correct deficiencies in processing and movement or trafficking of the abnormal CFTR protein so that greater number of CFTR proteins can reach the surface of the cell.

Clinical trials have demonstrated that therapy using combinations of ivacaftor and channel correctors is more efficacious than single agents alone. Combination therapy is able to achieve greater improvements in ion transport at the plasma membrane because it remedies both the quantity as well as the physiological function of CFTR.

IDIOPATHIC PULMONARY FIBROSIS

Idiopathic pulmonary fibrosis is a chronic debilitating inflammatory disorder that results in scarring of lung tissue and loss of elasticity. Lung expansion and gaseous exchange in the alveoli are impaired due to the fibrosis and consequent increased stiffness in pulmonary tissues. In the absence of a known aetiological agent, treatment is focused on the use of anti-fibrotic agents.

Pirfenidone is an immunosuppressant that reduces fibroblast proliferation and production of fibrosis-related mediators. The exact mechanism of pirfenidone is not known, but it appears to reduce fibrosis-related protein and cytokines, prevent the accumulation of inflammatory cells and inhibit expansion of extracellular matrix that is stimulated by cytokine growth factors such as transforming growth factor-β and platelet-derived growth factor (Borie et al., 2016). Clinical trials have demonstrated that pirfenidone can slow the decline in lung function and exercise capacity caused by pulmonary fibrosis.

Nintedanib is a small-molecule tyrosine kinase inhibitor that is thought to reduce inflammatory and fibrotic change in the lung. The drug acts through inhibition of signalling cascades from platelet-derived and fibroblast-derived growth factor receptors that are involved in the proliferation and differentiation of pulmonary fibroblasts and myoblasts (Borie et al., 2016). Clinical trials have demonstrated the efficacy of nintedanib in slowing the progressive loss of lung function that is seen in pulmonary fibrosis.

SURFACTANTS

Pulmonary surfactants act not by binding to specific targets but by lowering the surface tension of fluid lining the alveoli, allowing air to enter. They are effective in the prophylaxis and management of *respiratory distress syndrome* in newborn babies, especially premature babies in whom endogenous surfactant production is deficient. Examples include **beractant** and **poractant alpha**, which are derivatives of the physiological pulmonary surfactant protein. They are administered directly into the tracheobronchial tree via an endotracheal tube. (The mothers of premature infants are sometimes treated with glucocorticoids before birth in an attempt to accelerate maturation of the fetal lung and minimise incidence of this disorder.)

COUGH

Cough is a protective reflex that removes foreign material and secretions from the bronchi and bronchioles. It is a very common adverse effect of angiotensin-converting enzyme inhibitors, in which case the treatment is usually to substitute an alternative drug, often an angiotensin-receptor antagonist, less likely to cause this adverse effect (see Ch. 21). It can be triggered by inflammation in the respiratory tract, for example, by undiagnosed asthma or chronic reflux with aspiration, or by neoplasia. In these cases, cough suppressant (antitussive) drugs are sometimes useful, for example for the dry painful cough associated with bronchial carcinoma, but are to be avoided in cases of chronic pulmonary infection, as they can cause undesirable thickening and retention of sputum, and in asthma because of the risk of respiratory depression.

DRUGS USED FOR COUGH (ANTITUSSIVE DRUGS)

Opioid analgesics are sometimes prescribed but their efficacy is modest, and there are significant adverse effects (see Ch. 43). They act by inhibiting an ill-defined 'cough centre' in the brain stem and suppress cough in doses below those required for pain relief. Those used as cough suppressants have minimal analgesic actions and addictive properties.

Codeine (methylmorphine) is a weak opioid (see Ch. 43) with considerably less addiction liability than a strong opioid, and is a mild cough suppressant. It decreases secretions in the bronchioles, which thickens sputum, and inhibits ciliary activity. Constipation is common. **Dextromethorphan** (a drug with many actions, including μ-receptor and sigma-1-receptor agonist, non-selective serotonin-uptake inhibitor) and **pholcodine** (μ-receptor agonist with weak analgesic effects) have less adverse effects than codeine. Respiratory depression is a risk with all centrally acting cough suppressants. **Morphine** is used for palliative care in cases of lung cancer associated with distressing cough.

Future research developments for refractory chronic cough (where no clear precipitating cause is found) include **gefapixant**, a selective antagonist of purinergic P2X3 receptors. These receptors are thought to have a key role in the activation of sensory neurons implicated in the cough reflex.

REFERENCES AND FURTHER READING

General

Borie, R., Justet, A., Beltramo, G., et al., 2016. Pharmacological management of IPF. Respirology 21, 615–625.

Meteran, H., Sivapalan, P., Stæhr Jensen, J.U., 2021. Treatment response biomarkers in asthma and COPD. Diagnostics 11, 1668.

Pincus, A.B., Fryer, A.D., Jacoby, D.B., 2021. Mini review: neural mechanisms underlying airway hyperresponsiveness. Neurosci. Lett. 751, 135795.

van der Velden, V.H.J., Hulsmann, A.R., 1999. Autonomic innervation of human airways: structure, function, and pathophysiology in asthma. Neuroimmunomodulation 6, 145–159.

Velasquez, R., Teran, L.M., 2011. Chemokines and their receptors in the allergic airway inflammatory process. Clin. Rev. Allergy Immunol. 41, 76–88.

Asthma

Boonpiyathad, T., Sözener, Z.C., Satitsuksanoa, P., et al., 2019. Immunologic mechanisms in asthma. Semin. Immunol. 46, 101333.

BTS/SIGN (British Thoracic Society/Scottish Intercollegiate Guideline Network), 2019. British Guideline on Management of Asthma. Available at: www.brit-thoracic.org.uk/quality-improvement/guidelines/asthma/.

Wadsworth, S.J., Sandford, A.J., 2013. Personalised medicine and asthma diagnostics/management. Curr. Allergy Asthma Rep. 13, 118–129.

Chronic obstructive pulmonary disease

Barnes, P.J., 2013. New anti-inflammatory targets for chronic obstructive pulmonary disease. Nat. Rev. Drug Discov. 12, 543–559.

Barnes, P.J., 2016. Inflammatory mechanisms in patients with chronic obstructive pulmonary disease. J. Allergy Clin. Immunol. 138, 16–27.

Cohen, J.S., Miles, M.C., Donohue, J.F., Ohar, J.A., 2016. Dual therapy strategies for COPD: the scientific rationale for LAMA + LABA. Int. J. Chron. Obstruct. Pulmon. Dis. 11, 785–797.

Liao, W., Lim, A.Y.H., Tan, W.S.D., et al., 2020. Restoration of HDAC2 and Nrf2 by andrographolide overcomes corticosteroid resistance in chronic obstructive pulmonary disease. Br. J. Pharmacol. 177, 3662–3673.

McDonald, C.F., 2017. Eosinophil biology in COPD. N. Engl. J. Med. 377, 1680–1682.

Rodrigues, S.O., Cunha, C., Soares, G.M.V., et al., 2021. Mechanisms, pathophysiology and currently proposed treatments of chronic obstructive pulmonary disease. Pharmaceuticals 14, 979.

Cough

Morice, A.H., Kastelik, J.A., Thompson, R., 2001. Cough challenge in the assessment of cough reflex. Br. J. Clin. Pharmacol. 52, 365–375.
Reynolds, S.M., Mackenzie, A.J., Spina, D., Page, C.P., 2004. The pharmacology of cough. Trends Pharmacol. Sci. 25, 569–576.

Drugs and therapeutic aspects

Bel, E.H., Ten Brinke, A., 2017. New anti-eosinophil drugs for asthma and COPD: targeting the trait. Chest 152, 1276–1282.
Cazzola, M., Page, C.P., Calzetta, L., Matera, M.G., 2012. Pharmacology and therapeutics of bronchodilators. Pharmacol. Rev. 64, 450–504.
Conti, M., Beavo, J., 2007. Biochemistry and physiology of cyclic nucleotide phosphodiesterases: essential components in cyclic nucleotide signaling. Annu. Rev. Biochem. 76, 481–511.
Lewis, J.F., Veldhuizen, R., 2003. The role of exogenous surfactant in the treatment of acute lung injury. Annu. Rev. Physiol. 65, 613–642.

29 The kidney and urinary system

OVERVIEW

We set the scene with a brief outline of renal physiology based on the functional unit of the kidney – the nephron – before describing drugs that affect renal function. Emphasis is on diuretics – drugs that increase the excretion of Na^+ ions and water and reduce arterial blood pressure and cardiac work. We also mention drugs used to treat patients with renal failure and urinary tract disorders where these are not covered in other chapters.

INTRODUCTION

The main function of the kidneys is to maintain the constancy of the 'interior environment' by eliminating waste products and by regulating the volume, electrolyte content and pH of the extracellular fluid in the face of varying dietary intake and other environmental (e.g. climatic) demands. The kidneys receive approximately 20% of the cardiac output from which, in a young adult human, their glomeruli filter approximately 180 L of fluid per day, of which 99% is reabsorbed by the tubules. This results in a daily urine output of approximately 1.8 L (Table 29.1). The kidneys have important related endocrine functions including synthesis of erythropoietin (see Ch. 24), renin (see Ch. 21) and of the active form of vitamin D (see Ch. 36), and are sites of action of mediators including aldosterone (Chs 21 and 33) and antidiuretic hormone (ADH), which is also known as vasopressin (see Ch. 33).

The kidneys are targets of the familiar range of pathological processes – infectious, structural, immunological, malignant, toxic (including drug toxicities) and so on. The diverse diseases that result converge via impairment of renal function (reduced glomerular filtration rate) to a common end stage of renal failure which (if the pathological process is reversible) may be acute and recoverable or (if not) chronic and irreversible other than by transplantation. Lesser degrees of dysfunction, termed *renal impairment*, are diagnosed on the basis of reduced glomerular filtration rate which is estimated clinically from the plasma concentration of creatinine and age of the patient.

The main drugs that work on the kidney – the diuretics – are crucial in treating cardiovascular disease, especially hypertension and heart failure (Ch. 21), as well as in the management of patients with renal disease with an impaired ability to excrete salt and water. Immunosuppressant drugs (effective in several of the diseases that can cause renal failure, and crucial following renal transplantation) are covered in Chapter 25 and antibacterial drugs (used to treat renal and urinary tract infections) in Chapter 52. Several drugs that act on the autonomic nervous system influence the muscle of the bladder (the detrusor muscle) and its sphincter, and some of these are used therapeutically to improve symptoms of detrusor instability or urinary obstruction ('prostatism') (Chs 14 and 15).

The kidneys are the main organ by which drugs and their metabolites are eliminated from the body (see Ch. 10), so the dosing regimens of many drugs must be modified in patients with impaired renal function. A further challenge for clinical nephrologists is drug treatment of patients with renal failure who are being supported by artificial forms of dialysis. These are outside the scope of this book and interested readers are directed to the chapters by Golper, Udy and Lipman, and by Olyaei, Foster and Lermer in the *Oxford Textbook of Clinical* Nephrology (2015). Here we provide an introduction to renal physiology followed by coverage of the main classes of diuretics, and short sections on drugs used in renal failure and drugs used in urinary tract disorders.

OUTLINE OF RENAL FUNCTION

The glomerular filtrate in health is similar in composition to plasma, apart from the absence of protein. As it passes through the renal tubule, about 99% of the filtered water, and much of the filtered Na^+, is reabsorbed, and some substances are secreted into it from the blood.

Each kidney consists of an outer cortex, an inner medulla and the renal pelvis, which empties into the ureter. The functional unit is the nephron, of which there are approximately 1.4×10^6 in each kidney (approximately half this number in people with hypertension), with considerable variation between individuals. Nephron number declines with age, even in healthy people, accompanied by a predictable decline in renal function.

THE STRUCTURE AND FUNCTION OF THE NEPHRON

Each nephron consists of a *glomerulus, proximal tubule, loop of Henle, distal convoluted tubule* and *collecting duct* (Fig. 29.1). The glomerulus comprises a tuft of capillaries projecting into Bowman's capsule, a cup-like sack draining into the proximal tubule. Most nephrons lie largely or entirely in the cortex. The remaining 12%, called the *juxtamedullary nephrons*, have their glomeruli and convoluted tubules next to the junction of the medulla and cortex, and their loops of Henle pass deep into the medulla.

THE BLOOD SUPPLY TO THE NEPHRON

Nephrons possess the special characteristic of having two capillary beds in series with each other (see Fig. 29.1). The afferent arteriole of each cortical nephron branches to form the glomerulus; glomerular capillaries coalesce into the efferent arteriole which supplies a second capillary network

Table 29.1 Reabsorption of fluid and solute in the kidney[a]

	Filtered/ day	Excreted/ day[b]	Percentage reabsorbed
Na^+ (mmol)	25,000	150	99+%
K^+ (mmol)	600	90	93+
Cl^- (mmol)	18,000	150	99+
HCO_3^- (mmol)	4900	0	100
Total solute (mOsmol)	54,000	700	87
H_2O (L)	180	~1.5	99+

[a]Typical values for a healthy young adult: renal blood flow, 1200 mL/min (20%–25% of cardiac output); renal plasma flow, 660 mL/min; glomerular filtration rate, 125 mL/min.
[b]These are typical figures for an individual eating a Western diet. The kidney excretes more or less of each of these substances to maintain the constancy of the internal milieu, so on a low-sodium diet (for instance in the Yanamami, indigenous people of the Amazonian rain forest), NaCl excretion may be reduced to below 10 mmol/day! At the other extreme, individuals living in some fishing communities in Japan eat (and excrete) several hundred mmol/day

in the cortex, around the convoluted tubules and loops of Henle, before converging to form venules and then renal veins. By contrast, efferent arterioles of juxtamedullary nephrons lead to vessel loops (*vasa recta*) that pass deep into the medulla with the thin loops of Henle (see Fig. 29.1).

THE JUXTAGLOMERULAR APPARATUS

A conjunction of afferent arteriole, efferent arteriole and distal convoluted tubule near the glomerulus forms the juxtaglomerular apparatus (Fig. 29.2). At this site, there are specialised cells in both the afferent arteriole and the tubule. The latter, termed *macula densa* cells, respond to changes in the rate of flow and the composition of tubule fluid, and they control, probably by purinergic signalling (see Ch. 16), *renin* release from specialised granular renin-containing cells in the afferent arteriole (see Ch. 21). These cells also release renin in response to decreased pressure in the afferent arteriole. Renin, named because of its discovery during the 19th century in extracts of kidney (renal) tissue, is an enzyme that cleaves angiotensin I from angiotensinogen. Angiotensin I is converted to angiotensin II via angiotensin converting enzyme (ACE) and acts on AT_1 receptors in vascular smooth muscle to cause vasocontriction, and in the adrenal cortex to release aldosterone hence controlling vascular resistance, blood pressure, blood volume and Na^+ and K^+ balance. Renin is consequently of great importance in cardiovascular homeostasis. If it had been discovered more recently it might have been named from its biochemical action as 'angiotensinogenase'. Various

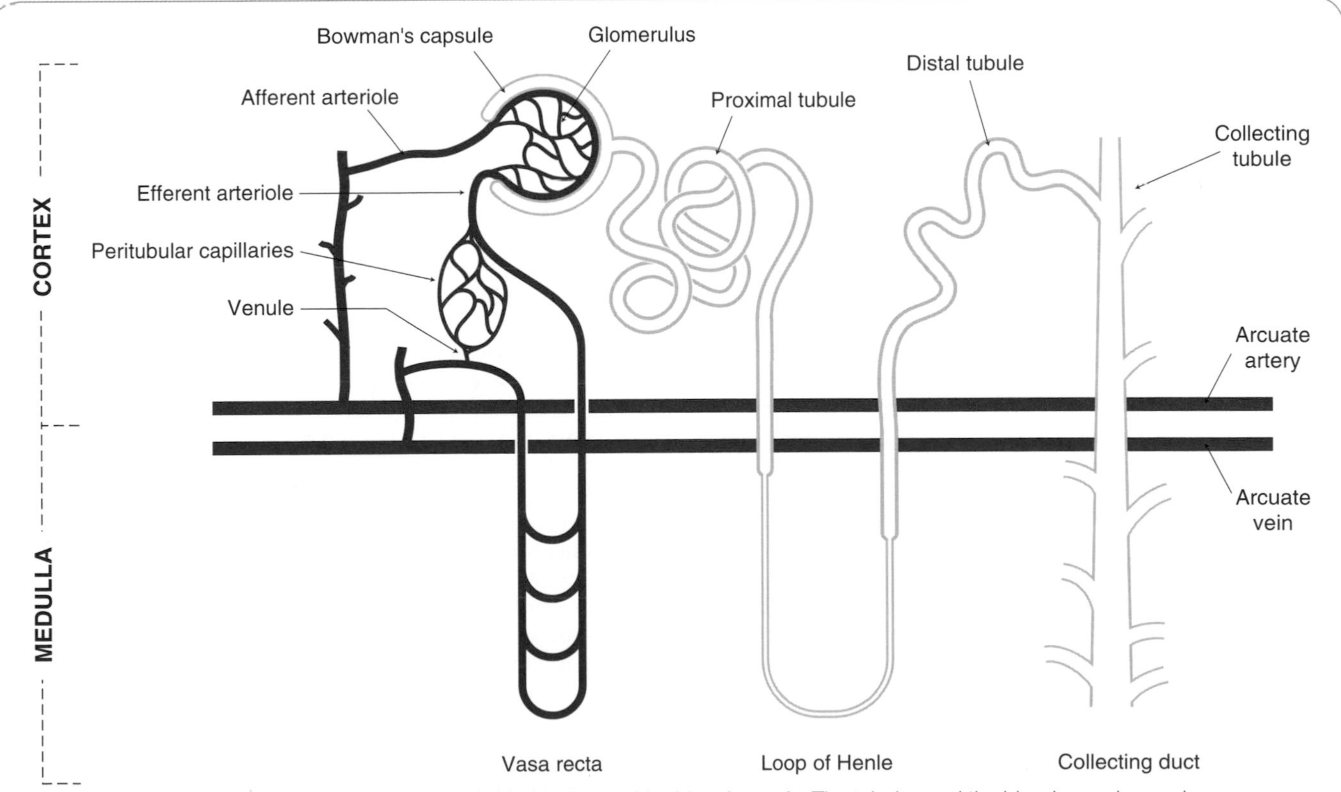

Fig. 29.1 Simplified diagram of a juxtamedullary nephron and its blood supply. The tubules and the blood vessels are shown separately for clarity. In the kidney, the peritubular capillary network surrounds the convoluted tubules, and the distal convoluted tubule passes close to the glomerulus, between the afferent and efferent arterioles. (This last is shown in more detail in Fig. 29.2.)

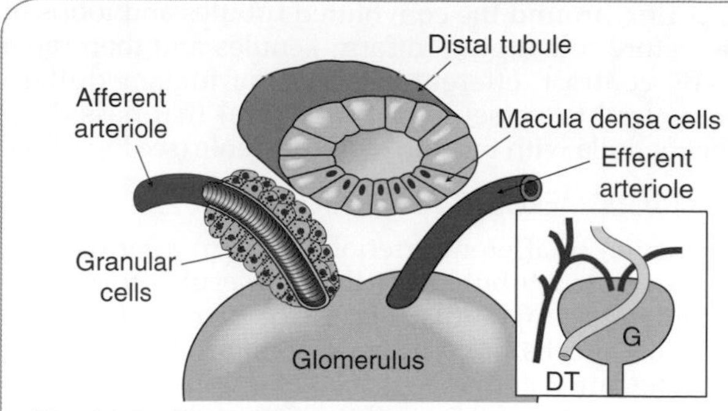

Fig. 29.2 The juxtaglomerular apparatus. The cutaway sections show the granular renin-containing cells around the afferent arteriole, and the macula densa cells in the distal convoluted tubule. The inset shows the general relationships between the structures. *DT,* Distal tubule; *G,* glomerulus.

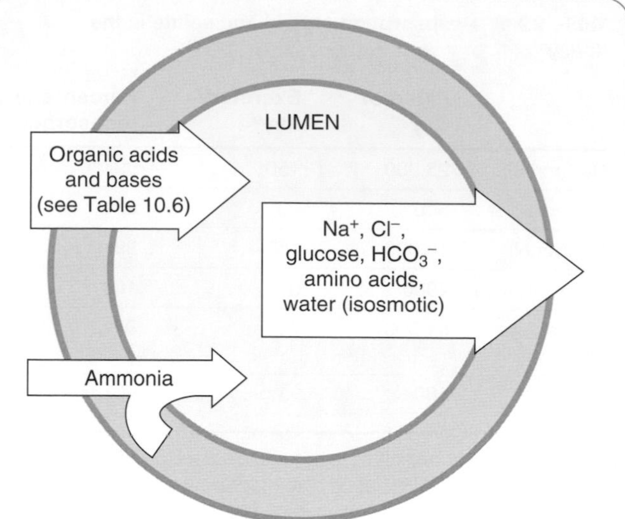

Fig. 29.3 Transport processes in the proximal convoluted tubule. The main driving force for the absorption of solutes and water from the lumen is the Na^+-K^+-ATPase in the basolateral membrane of the tubule cells. Many drugs are secreted into the proximal tubule (see Ch. 10). (Redrawn from Burg, M.B., 1985. In: Brenner, B.M., Rector, F.C. (Eds), The Kidney, third ed. WB Saunders, Philadelphia, pp. 145–175.)

chemical mediators also influence renin secretion, including β_2-adrenoceptor agonists, vasodilator prostaglandins and feedback inhibition from angiotensin II acting on AT_1 receptors (see Fig. 21.2). The role of the juxtaglomerular apparatus in the control of Na^+ balance is dealt with below.

GLOMERULAR FILTRATION

Fluid is driven from the capillaries into Bowman's capsule by hydrodynamic force opposed by the oncotic pressure of the plasma proteins, to which healthy glomerular capillaries are impermeable. All the low-molecular-weight constituents of plasma appear in the filtrate, while albumin and larger proteins are retained in the blood.

TUBULAR FUNCTION

The apex (lumenal surface) of each tubular cell is surrounded by a tight junction, as in all epithelia. This is a specialised region of membrane that separates the intercellular space from the lumen. The movement of ions and water across the epithelium can occur *through* cells (the transcellular pathway) and *between* cells through the tight junctions (the paracellular pathway). A common theme is that energy is expended to pump Na^+ out of the cell by Na^+-K^+-ATPase situated in the basolateral cell membrane and the resulting gradient of Na^+ concentration drives the entry of Na^+ from the lumen via various transporters that facilitate Na^+ entry coupled with movement of other ions, either in the same direction as Na^+, in which case they are called *symporters* or *co-transporters*, or in the opposite direction, in which case they are called *antiporters*. These transporters vary in different parts of the nephron, as described later.

THE PROXIMAL CONVOLUTED TUBULE

The epithelium of the proximal convoluted tubule is 'leaky'; i.e. the tight junctions in the proximal tubule are not so 'tight' after all, being permeable to ions and water, and permitting passive flow in either direction. This prevents the build-up of large concentration gradients; thus, although approximately 60%–70% of Na^+ reabsorption occurs in the proximal tubule, this transfer is accompanied by passive absorption of water so that fluid leaving the proximal tubule remains approximately isotonic to the glomerular filtrate.

Some of the transport processes in the proximal tubule are shown in Figs 29.3–29.5. The most important mechanism for Na^+ entry into proximal tubular cells from the filtrate occurs by Na^+/H^+ exchange (see Fig. 29.5). Intracellular carbonic anhydrase is essential for production of H^+ for secretion into the lumen. Na^+ is reabsorbed from tubular fluid into the cytoplasm of proximal tubular cells in exchange for cytoplasmic H^+. It is then transported out of the cells into the interstitium by a Na^+-K^+-ATPase (sodium pump) in the basolateral membrane. This is the main active transport mechanism of the nephron in terms of energy consumption. Reabsorbed Na^+ then diffuses into blood vessels.

Bicarbonate is normally completely reabsorbed in the proximal tubule. This is achieved by combination with protons, yielding carbonic acid, which dissociates to form carbon dioxide and water – a reaction catalysed by carbonic anhydrase present in the lumenal brush border of the proximal tubule cells (see Fig. 29.5A) – followed by passive reabsorption of the dissolved carbon dioxide.[1] The selective removal of sodium bicarbonate, with accompanying water, in the early proximal tubule causes a secondary rise in the concentration of chloride ions. Diffusion of chloride down its concentration gradient via the paracellular shunt (see Fig. 29.5A) leads, in turn, to a lumen-positive potential difference that favours reabsorption of sodium. The other mechanism involved in movement via the paracellular route is that sodium ions are secreted by Na^+-K^+-ATPase into the lateral intercellular space, somewhat raising its

[1]The reaction is reversible, and the enzyme (as any catalyst) does not alter the equilibrium, just speeds up the rate with which it is attained. The concentrations inside the cell are such that carbon dioxide combines with water to produce carbonic acid: the same enzyme (carbonic anhydrase) catalyses this as well (see Fig. 29.5A).

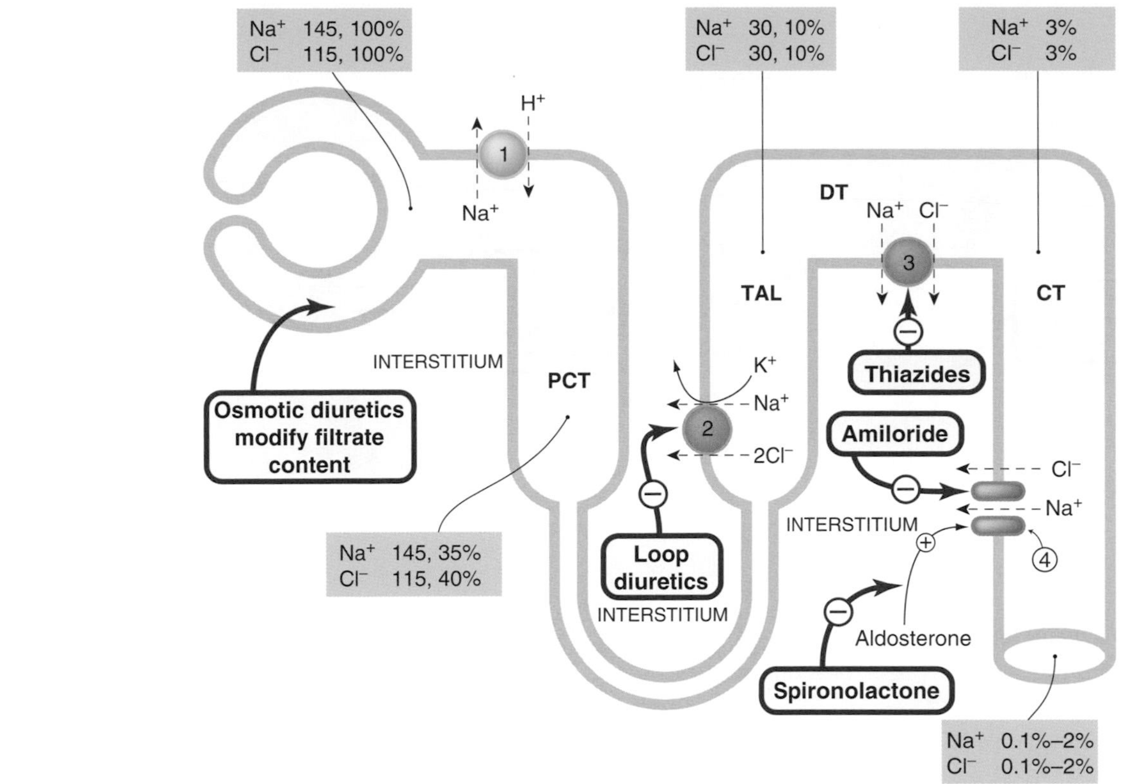

Fig. 29.4 Schematic showing the absorption of sodium and chloride in the nephron and the main sites of action of drugs. Cells are depicted as a *pink border* round the *yellow tubular lumen*. Mechanisms of ion absorption at the apical margin of the tubule cell: *(1)* Na^+/H^+ exchange; *(2)* $Na^+/K^+/2Cl^-$ co-transport; *(3)* Na^+/Cl^- co-transport; *(4)* Na^+ entry through sodium channels. Sodium is pumped out of the cells into the interstitium by the Na^+-K^+-ATPase in the basolateral margin of the tubular cells (not shown). The numbers in the boxes give the concentration of ions as millimoles per litre of filtrate, and the percentage of filtered ions still remaining in the tubular fluid at the sites specified. *CT,* Collecting tubule; *DT,* distal tubule; *PCT,* proximal convoluted tubule; *TAL,* thick ascending loop. (Data from Greger, R., 2000. Physiology of sodium transport. Am. J. Med. Sci. 319, 51–62.)

osmolality because of the 3 Na^+:2 K^+ stoichiometry of the transporter. This leads to osmotic movement of water across the tight junction (see Fig. 29.5A), in turn causing sodium and chloride ion reabsorption by convection (so-called solvent drag).

Filtered glucose is reabsorbed in the proximal tubule, being co-transported with sodium ions by *a sodium/glucose cotransporter (SGLT)*. SGLT2 is expressed early in the proximal tubule; it accounts for the reabsorption of 80%–90% of the filtered glucose and is an important drug target. It is inhibited by the gliflozins (e.g. ***canagliflozin, dapagliflozin*** and ***empagliflozin***), which improve survival in appropriately selected patients with type 2 diabetes (see Ch. 31) and heart failure (see Ch. 21). Here it is worth noting that they also improve outcome in chronic renal disease.

SGLT1 is expressed further along the proximal tubule and accounts for the reabsorption of most of the remaining glucose.

Many organic acids and bases are actively secreted into the tubule from the blood by specific transporters (Fig. 29.3 and see Table 10.6).

After passage through the proximal tubule, tubular fluid (now 30%–40% of the original volume of the filtrate) passes on to the loop of Henle.

THE LOOP OF HENLE, MEDULLARY COUNTER-CURRENT MULTIPLIER AND EXCHANGER

The loop of Henle consists of a descending and an ascending portion (see Figs 29.1 and 29.4), the ascending portion having both thick and thin segments. This part of the nephron enables the kidney to excrete urine that is either more or less concentrated than plasma, and hence to regulate the osmotic balance of the body as a whole. The loops of Henle of the juxtamedullary nephrons function as counter-current multipliers, and the vasa recta as counter-current exchangers. NaCl is actively reabsorbed in the thick ascending limb, causing hypertonicity of the interstitium. The descending limb is permeable to water, and this interstitial hypertonicity causes water to move out, so that the tubular fluid becomes progressively more concentrated as it approaches the bend.

In juxtamedullary nephrons with long loops, there is extensive movement of water out of the tubule so that the fluid eventually reaching the tip of the loop has a high osmolality – normally approximately 1200 mOsmol/kg, but up to 1500 mOsmol/kg under conditions of dehydration – compared with plasma and extracellular fluid, which is

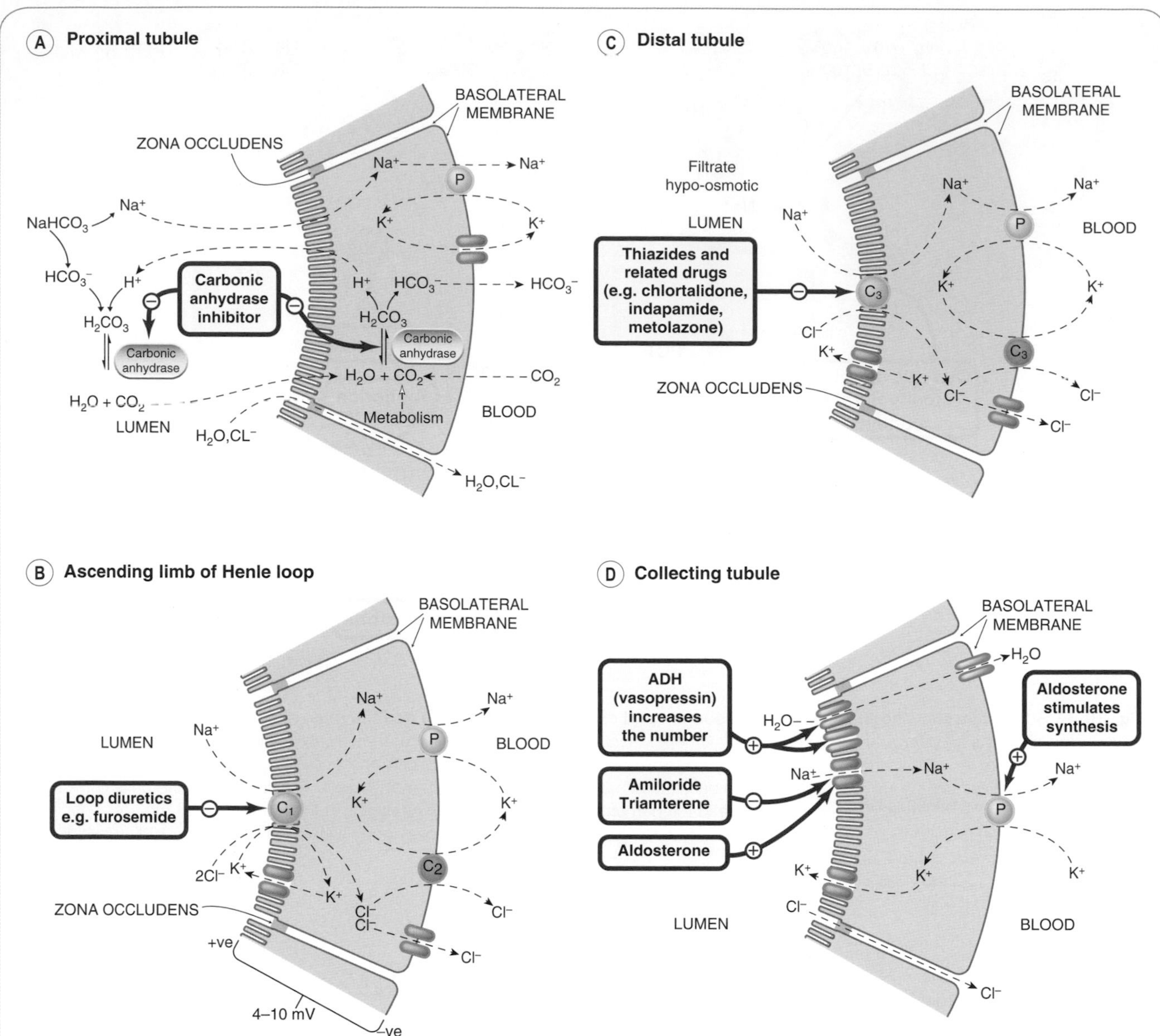

Fig. 29.5 Drug effects on renal tubular ion transport. The primary active transport mechanism is the Na^+/K^+ pump *(P)* in the basolateral membrane of cells in each location; the diagrams are simplified in that the pump exchanges three Na^+ for two K^+ ions. (A) Bicarbonate ion reabsorption in the proximal convoluted tubule, showing the action of carbonic anhydrase inhibitors. (B) Ion transport in the thick ascending limb of Henle loop, showing the site of action of loop diuretics, namely the $Na^+/K^+/2Cl^-$ co-transporter *(C_1)*. Chloride ions leave the cell both through basolateral chloride channels and by an electroneutral K^+/Cl^- co-transporter *(C_2)* which are also present in the distal tubule. (C) Salt transport in the distal convoluted tubule, showing the site of action of thiazide diuretics, namely the Na^+/Cl^- co-transporter *(C_3)*. (D) Actions of hormones and drugs on the collecting tubule. The cells are impermeable to water in the absence of antidiuretic hormone (ADH), and to Na^+ in the absence of aldosterone. Aldosterone acts on a nuclear receptor within the tubule cell and on membrane receptors. (Adapted from Greger, R., 2000. Physiology of sodium transport. Am. J. Med. Sci. 319, 51–62.)

approximately 300 mOsmol/kg.[2] The hypertonic milieu of the medulla, through which the collecting ducts of all nephrons pass on the way to the renal pelvis, is important in providing a mechanism by which the osmolarity of the urine is controlled.

The *ascending limb* has very low permeability to water; i.e. the tight junctions really are tight, enabling the build-up of a substantial concentration gradient across the wall of the tubule. It is here, in the thick ascending limb of the loop of Henle, that 20%–30% of filtered Na^+ is reabsorbed. There is active reabsorption of NaCl, unaccompanied by water, reducing the osmolality of the tubular fluid and making the interstitial fluid of the medulla hypertonic. The osmotic gradient in the medullary interstitium is the

[2]These figures are for humans; some other species, notably the desert rat, can do much better, with urine osmolalities up to 5000 mOsmol/kg.

key consequence of the counter-current multiplier system, the main principle being that small horizontal osmotic gradients stack up to produce a large vertical gradient. Urea contributes to the gradient because it is more slowly reabsorbed than water and may be added to fluid in the descending limb, so its concentration rises along the nephron until it reaches the collecting tubules, where it diffuses out into the interstitium. It is thus trapped in the inner medulla.

Ions move into cells of the thick ascending limb of the loop of Henle across the apical membrane by a $Na^+/K^+/2Cl^-$ co-transporter, driven by the Na^+ gradient produced by Na^+-K^+-ATPase in the basolateral membrane (see Fig. 29.5B). Most of the K^+ taken into the cell by the $Na^+/K^+/2Cl^-$ co-transporter returns to the lumen through apical potassium channels, but some K^+ is reabsorbed, along with Mg^{2+} and Ca^{2+}.

Reabsorption of salt from the thick ascending limb is not balanced by reabsorption of water, so tubular fluid is hypotonic with respect to plasma as it enters the distal convoluted tubule (see Fig. 29.4). The thick ascending limb is therefore sometimes referred to as the 'diluting segment'.

THE DISTAL TUBULE

In the early distal tubule, NaCl reabsorption, coupled with impermeability of the *zonula occludens* to water, further dilutes the tubular fluid. Transport is driven by Na^+-K^+-ATPase in the basolateral membrane. This lowers cytoplasmic Na^+ concentration, and consequently Na^+ enters the cell from the lumen down its concentration gradient, accompanied by Cl^-, by means of a Na^+/Cl^- co-transporter (see Fig. 29.5C).

The apical surfaces (lumen side) of distal tubular cells are permeable to Ca^{2+} via the TRPV5 channel. On the basolateral surface there is an active Na^+/Ca^{2+} transporter, and the basolateral ATP-dependent Na^+/K^+ pump produces the gradient for Ca^{2+} to be reabsorbed via a separate Na^+/Ca^{2+} basolateral antiporter. The excretion of Ca^{2+} is regulated in this part of the nephron, by *parathormone (PTH)* and *calcitriol,* both of which increase Ca^{2+} reabsorption and phosphate excretion by increasing the synthesis of several of these transporters (see Ch. 36).

THE COLLECTING TUBULE AND COLLECTING DUCT

Distal convoluted tubules empty into collecting tubules, which coalesce to form collecting ducts (see Fig. 29.1). Collecting tubules include principal cells, which reabsorb Na^+ and secrete K^+ (see Fig. 29.5D), and two populations of intercalated cells, α and β, which secrete acid and base, respectively.

The tight junctions in this portion of the nephron are impermeable to water and cations. The movement of ions and water in this segment is under independent hormonal control: absorption of NaCl by *aldosterone* (Chs 21 and 33) and absorption of water by ADH (see Ch. 33).

Aldosterone enhances Na^+ reabsorption and promotes K^+ excretion (see Fig. 29.5D). It promotes Na^+ reabsorption by:

- a rapid effect, up-regulating epithelial sodium channels in the collecting duct, increasing apical membrane permeability and hence reabsorption of sodium ions by an action on membrane aldosterone receptors.[3]
- delayed effects, via nuclear receptors (see Ch. 3), directing the synthesis of a specific protein mediator up-regulating and activating the basolateral Na^+/K^+ pump, which pumps three sodium ions out of the cell, into the interstitial fluid and two potassium ions into the cell from the interstitial fluid and stimulates synthesis of the epithelial sodium ion channel in addition to its rapid effect via the membrane receptor mentioned earlier.

ADH, diabetes insipidus and inappropriate ADH secretion (syndrome of inappropriate ADH [SIADH]). ADH is secreted by the posterior pituitary (see Ch. 33) and acts on V_2 receptors ('V' for 'vasopressin' – the alternative name for ADH) in the basolateral membranes of cells in the collecting tubules and ducts, increasing the expression of *aquaporin* (water channels; see Ch. 9) in the apical membranes (see Fig. 29.5D). This renders this part of the nephron permeable to water, allowing passive reabsorption of water as the collecting duct traverses the hyperosmotic region of the medulla, and hence the excretion of concentrated urine. Conversely, in the absence of ADH, collecting duct epithelium is impermeable to water, so hypotonic fluid that leaves the distal tubule remains hypotonic as it passes down the collecting ducts, leading to the excretion of dilute urine. Defective ADH secretion (see Ch. 33) or impaired action of ADH on the kidney results in *diabetes insipidus*, an uncommon disorder in which patients excrete large volumes of dilute urine. Excessive ADH secretion can result from various neurological disorders or from ectopic secretion by various malignant tumours. Assays for ADH in plasma are not routinely available in the clinic, so this condition is usually inferred indirectly from its characteristic effects on plasma and urine which include hyponatraemia, the production of a concentrated urine despite a low plasma osmolarity and persistent loss of Na^+ ions in the urine and referred to as the 'syndrome of inappropriate ADH' or 'SIADH'. Hyponatraemia is driven by continued drinking (from habit) despite renal water retention and can result in seizures, so dietary fluid restriction is a mainstay of management.

Ethanol (see Ch. 50) inhibits the secretion of ADH, causing a water diuresis (possibly familiar to some of our readers) as a kind of transient diabetes insipidus. **Nicotine** enhances ADH secretion (perhaps contributing to the appeal of an after-dinner cigar?).

Several drugs inhibit the action of ADH: **lithium** (used in psychiatric disorders; see Ch. 48), **demeclocycline** (a tetracycline used not as an antibiotic, but rather to treat SIADH), **colchicine** (see Ch. 25) and *vinca alkaloids* (see Ch. 57). Recently, more specific antagonists of ADH (e.g. **conivaptan**, **tolvaptan**) have been introduced for management of hyponatraemia. Any of these drugs, given in excess, can cause acquired forms of *nephrogenic* diabetes insipidus, caused by a failure of the renal collecting ducts to respond to ADH. Nephrogenic diabetes insipidus can also be caused by genetic disorders affecting the V_2 receptor or aquaporin.

ACID–BASE BALANCE

The kidneys (together with the lungs; see Ch. 28) regulate the H^+ concentration of body fluids. Acid or alkaline urine can be excreted according to need, the usual requirement being to form acid urine to eliminate phosphoric and sulfuric acids generated during the metabolism of nucleic

[3]A mechanism distinct from regulation of gene transcription, which is the classical transduction mechanism for steroid hormones (see Ch. 3).

Renal tubular function

- Protein-free glomerular filtrate enters via Bowman's capsule.
- Na^+-K^+-ATPase in the basolateral membrane is the main active transporter. It provides the Na^+-gradients (low cytoplasmic Na^+ concentrations) for passive transporters in the apical membranes which facilitate Na^+ entry (reabsorption) from the tubular fluid down a concentration gradient and in exchange for hydrogen ions (H^+).
- 60%–70% of the filtered Na^+ and >90% of HCO_3^- are absorbed in the proximal tubule.
- Glucose is reabsorbed in the proximal tubule, mainly by SGLT2. Gliflozins inhibit SGLT2 and improve survival in appropriately selected patients with type 2 diabetes mellitus (see Ch. 31) and with heart failure (see Ch. 21).
- Carbonic anhydrase is key for $NaHCO_3$ reabsorption in the proximal tubule and also for distal tubular urine acidification.
- The thick ascending limb of Henle loop is impermeable to water; 20%–30% of the filtered NaCl is actively reabsorbed in this segment.
- Ions are reabsorbed from tubular fluid by a $Na^+/K^+/2Cl^-$ co-transporter in the apical membranes of the thick ascending limb.
- $Na^+/K^+/2Cl^-$ co-transport is inhibited by loop diuretics.
- Filtrate is diluted as it traverses the thick ascending limb as ions are reabsorbed, so that it is hypotonic when it leaves.
- The tubular counter-current multiplier actively generates a concentration gradient – small horizontal differences in solute concentration between tubular fluid and interstitium are multiplied vertically. The deeper in the medulla, the more concentrated is the interstitial fluid.
- Medullary hypertonicity is preserved passively by counter-current exchange in the vasa recta.
- Na^+/Cl^- co-transport (inhibited by thiazide diuretics) reabsorbs 5%–10% of filtered Na^+ in the distal tubule.
- K^+ is secreted into tubular fluid in the distal tubule and the collecting tubules and collecting ducts.
- In the absence of ADH, the collecting tubule and collecting duct have low permeability to salt and water. ADH increases water permeability.
- Na^+ is reabsorbed from the collecting duct through epithelial sodium channels.
- These epithelial Na^+ channels are activated by aldosterone and inhibited by **amiloride** and by **triamterene.** K^+ or H^+ is secreted into the tubule in exchange for Na^+ in this distal region.

acids and of sulfur-containing amino acids consumed in the diet. Consequently, metabolic acidosis is a common accompaniment of renal failure. Altering urine pH to alter drug excretion is mentioned later.

POTASSIUM BALANCE

Extracellular K^+ concentration – critically important for excitable tissue function (see Ch. 4) – is tightly controlled through regulation of K^+ excretion by the kidney. Urinary K^+ excretion matches dietary intake, usually approximately 50–100 mmol in 24 h in Western countries. Many diuretics cause K^+ loss (see later).

Potassium ions are transported into collecting duct and collecting tubule cells from interstitial fluid by an Na^+-K^+-ATPase in the basolateral membrane which is under the control of aldosterone (see earlier), and leak into the lumen through a K^+-selective ion channel. Na^+ passes from tubular fluid through sodium channels in the apical membrane down the electrochemical gradient created by the Na^+-K^+-ATPase; a lumen-negative potential difference across the cell results, increasing the driving force for K^+ secretion into the lumen. Thus K^+ secretion is coupled to Na^+ reabsorption.

Consequently, K^+ is lost when:

- more Na^+ reaches the collecting duct, as occurs with any diuretic acting proximal to the collecting duct;
- Na^+ reabsorption in the collecting duct is increased directly (e.g. in hyperaldosteronism).

Conversely, K^+ is retained when:

- Na^+ reabsorption in the collecting duct is decreased, for example by **amiloride** or **triamterene**, which block the sodium channel in this part of the nephron, or **spironolactone**, **eplerenone**, or **finerenone**, which antagonise aldosterone (see later).

EXCRETION OF ORGANIC MOLECULES

There are distinct mechanisms (see Ch. 10, Table 10.7) for secreting organic anions and cations into the proximal tubular lumen. Secreted anions include several important drugs, for example, *thiazides*, **furosemide** and most *penicillins* and *cephalosporins* (see Ch. 52). Similarly, several secreted organic cations are important drugs, for example, **triamterene**, **amiloride**, **atropine** (see Ch. 14), **morphine** (see Ch. 43) and **quinine** (see Ch. 55). Both anion and cation transport mechanisms are, like other renal ion transport processes, indirectly powered by active transport of Na^+ and K^+, the energy being derived from Na^+-K^+-ATPase in the basolateral membrane.

Organic anions in the interstitial fluid are exchanged with cytoplasmic α-ketoglutarate by an antiport (i.e. an exchanger that couples uptake and release of α-ketoglutarate with, in the opposite direction, uptake and release of a different organic anion) in the basolateral membrane, and diffuse passively into the tubular lumen (see Fig. 29.3).

Organic cations diffuse into the cell from the interstitium and are then actively transported into the tubular lumen in exchange for H^+.

NATRIURETIC PEPTIDES

Endogenous A, B and C natriuretic peptides (ANP, BNP and CNP; see Chs 20 and 21) are involved in the regulation of Na^+ excretion. They are released from the heart in response to stretch (A and B) and from endothelium (C). They activate membrane-bound guanylyl cyclase (see Ch. 3), and cause natriuresis both by renal haemodynamic effects (increasing glomerular capillary pressure by dilating afferent and constricting efferent arterioles) and by direct tubular actions. The tubular actions include the inhibition of angiotensin II–stimulated Na^+ and water reabsorption in the proximal convoluted tubule, and of the action of ADH in promoting water reabsorption in the collecting tubule. Therapeutically, this effect has been harnessed via the inhibition of *neprilysin*, a membrane endopeptidase, by the active metabolite of **sacubitril**. Neprilysin inactivates ANP and BNP (along with other peptides, see Ch. 17), so its inhibition promotes natriuresis and sacubitril is used in combination with valsartan in the management of heart failure (see Ch. 21).

Within the kidney, the post-translational processing of ANP prohormone differs from that in other tissues, resulting in an additional four amino acids being added to the amino terminus of ANP to yield a related peptide, *urodilatin*, that promotes Na^+ excretion by acting on natriuretic peptide A receptors.

PROSTAGLANDINS AND RENAL FUNCTION

Prostaglandins (PGs; see Ch. 17) generated in the kidney influence its haemodynamic and excretory functions. The main renal prostaglandins in humans are vasodilator and natriuretic, namely PGE_2 in the medulla and PGI_2 (prostacyclin) in glomeruli. Factors that stimulate their synthesis include ischaemia, angiotensin II, ADH and bradykinin.

Prostaglandin biosynthesis is low under basal conditions. However, when vasoconstrictors (e.g. angiotensin II, noradrenaline) are released, local release of PGE_2 and PGI_2 compensates, preserving renal blood flow by their vasodilator action.

The influence of renal prostaglandins on salt balance and haemodynamics can be inferred from the effects of non-steroidal anti-inflammatory drugs (NSAIDs; which inhibit prostaglandin production by inhibiting cyclo-oxygenase; see Ch. 25). NSAIDs have little or no effect on renal function in healthy people, but predictably cause acute renal failure in clinical conditions in which renal blood flow depends on vasodilator prostaglandin biosynthesis. These include cirrhosis of the liver, heart failure, nephrotic syndrome, glomerulonephritis and extracellular volume contraction (see Ch. 58, Table 58.1). NSAIDs increase blood pressure in patients treated for hypertension by impairing PG-mediated vasodilatation and salt excretion. They exacerbate salt and water retention in patients with heart failure (see Ch. 21), partly by this same direct mechanism.[4]

DRUGS ACTING ON THE KIDNEY

DIURETICS

Diuretics increase the excretion of Na^+ and water. They decrease the reabsorption of Na^+ and an accompanying anion (usually Cl^-) from the filtrate, increased water loss being secondary to the increased excretion of NaCl (natriuresis). This can be achieved:

- by a direct action on the cells of the nephron
- indirectly, by modifying the content of the filtrate

Because a very large proportion of salt (NaCl) and water that passes into the tubule via the glomerulus is reabsorbed (see Table 29.1), even a small decrease in reabsorption can cause a marked increase in Na^+ excretion. A summary diagram of the mechanisms and sites of action of various diuretics is given in Fig. 29.4 and more detailed information on different classes of drugs in Fig. 29.5.

Most diuretics with a direct action on the nephron act from within the tubular lumen and reach their sites of action by being secreted into the proximal tubule (**spironolactone** is an exception).

DIURETICS ACTING DIRECTLY ON CELLS OF THE NEPHRON

The main therapeutically useful diuretics act on the:

- thick ascending loop of Henle
- early distal tubule
- collecting tubules and ducts

For a more detailed review of the actions and clinical uses of the diuretics, see Ellison and Subramanya (2015).

Loop diuretics

Loop diuretics (see Fig. 29.5B) are the most powerful diuretics (see Fig. 29.6 for a comparison with thiazides), capable of causing the excretion of 15%–25% of filtered Na^+. Their action is often described – in a phrase that conjures up a rather uncomfortable picture – as causing 'torrential urine flow'. The main example is **furosemide**; **bumetanide** and **torasemide** are alternative agents. These drugs act on the thick ascending limb, inhibiting the $Na^+/K^+/2Cl^-$ carrier in the lumenal membrane by combining with its Cl^- binding site.

Loop diuretics also have incompletely understood vascular actions. Intravenous administration of furosemide

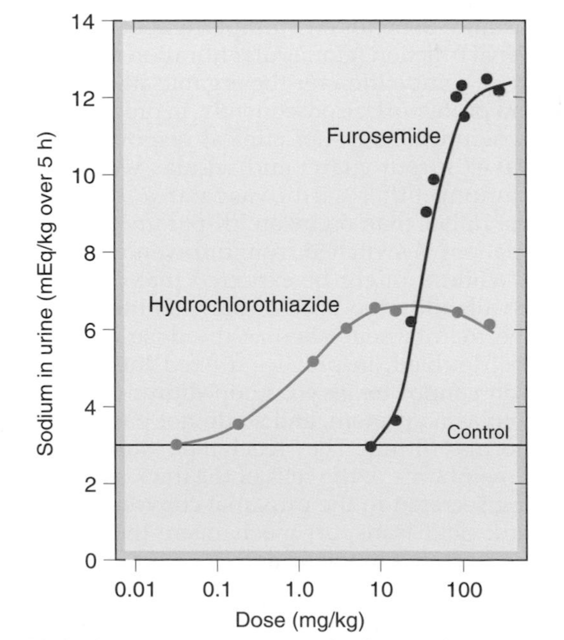

Fig. 29.6 Dose–response curves for furosemide and hydrochlorothiazide, showing differences in potency and maximum effect 'ceiling' in rat. Note that these doses are not used clinically in humans. (Adapted from Timmerman, R.J., et al., 1964. Curr. Ther. Res. 6, 88.)

[4]Additionally, NSAIDs make many of the diuretics used to treat heart failure less effective by competing with them for the organic anion transport (OAT) mechanism mentioned earlier; loop diuretics and thiazides act from within the lumen by inhibiting exchange mechanisms – see later in this chapter – so blocking their secretion into the lumen reduces their effectiveness by reducing their concentrations at their sites of action.

to patients with pulmonary oedema caused by acute heart failure (see Ch. 21) causes a therapeutically useful vasodilator effect independent of the onset of diuresis. Possible mechanisms that have been invoked include decreased vascular responsiveness to vasoconstrictors such as angiotensin II and noradrenaline; increased formation of vasodilating prostaglandins (see earlier); decreased production of the endogenous ouabain-like natriuretic hormone (Na^+-K^+-ATPase inhibitor; see Ch. 20); and potassium-channel opening effects in resistance arteries (see Ellison and Subramanya, 2015).

Loop diuretics increase the delivery of Na^+ to the distal nephron, causing loss of H^+ and K^+. Because Cl^- but not HCO_3^- is lost in the urine, the plasma concentration of HCO_3^- increases as plasma volume is reduced – a form of metabolic alkalosis therefore referred to as 'contraction alkalosis'.

Loop diuretics increase excretion of Ca^{2+} and Mg^{2+} and decrease excretion of uric acid.

Pharmacokinetic aspects

Loop diuretics are well but variably absorbed from the gastrointestinal tract and are predominantly given by mouth. They may also be given intravenously in urgent situations (e.g. acute pulmonary oedema) or when intestinal absorption is impaired, for example, as a result of reduced intestinal perfusion in patients with severe chronic congestive heart failure, who can become resistant to the action of orally administered diuretics. Given orally, they act within 1 h; given intravenously, they produce a peak effect within 30 min. Bumetanide and torasemide have greater bioavailability than furosemide, but the effect of all these drugs depends on C_{max} exceeding a threshold value, which varies markedly both within as well as between individuals, rather than on mean exposure (AUC). Patients who have a high threshold are said to be 'diuretic resistant'. Such resistance depends on multiple disease-related factors such as renal function (glomerular filtration rate), acid–base status, drug competition for the organic anion transporter (OAT) and proteinuria. Consequently, in practice physicians adjust dose on the basis of clinical response (judged by fluid intake/output charts and regular weighing of the patient among other cardiovascular and biochemical measures) rather than on mean PK parameters. Similarly, when a patient is switched from intravenous to oral loop diuretic, while it might be expected that on the basis of oral bioavailability the dose of bumetanide or torsemide should be maintained whereas the dose of furosemide should be doubled, in practice a fixed intravenous/oral conversion cannot be given. Loop diuretics are strongly bound to plasma protein, and so do not pass directly into the glomerular filtrate. They reach their site of action – the lumenal membrane of the cells of the thick ascending limb – by being secreted in the proximal convoluted tubule by the organic acid transport mechanism; the fraction thus secreted is excreted in the urine.

In nephrotic syndrome,[5] loop diuretics become bound to albumin in the tubular fluid, and consequently are not available to act on the $Na^+/K^+/2Cl^-$ carrier – another cause of diuretic resistance.

The fraction of the diuretic not excreted in the urine is metabolised, mainly in liver – **bumetanide** by cytochrome P450 pathways and **furosemide** by glucuronidation. The plasma half-life of both these drugs is approximately 90 min (longer in renal failure), and the duration of action 3–6 h. The clinical use of loop diuretics is given in the box.

Clinical uses of loop diuretics (e.g. furosemide)

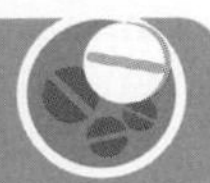

- Loop diuretics are used (cautiously!), in conjunction with dietary salt restriction and often with other classes of diuretic, in the treatment of salt and water overload associated with:
  - *acute pulmonary oedema*
  - *chronic heart failure*
  - *cirrhosis of the liver complicated by ascites*
  - *nephrotic syndrome*
  - *renal failure.*
- Treatment of *hypertension* complicated by renal impairment (thiazides are preferred if renal function is preserved).
- Treatment of *hypercalcaemia* after replacement of plasma volume with intravenous NaCl solution.

Unwanted effects

Unwanted effects directly related to the renal action of loop diuretics are common.[6] Excessive Na^+ and water loss, especially in elderly patients, can cause hypovolaemia and hypotension. Potassium loss, resulting in low plasma K^+ (hypokalaemia), and metabolic alkalosis are common. Hypokalaemia increases the effects and toxicity of several drugs (e.g. **digoxin** and type III antidysrhythmic drugs, see Ch. 20), so this is potentially a clinically important source of drug interaction. If necessary, hypokalaemia can be averted or treated by concomitant use of K^+-sparing diuretics (see later), or supplementary potassium replacement. Hypomagnesaemia is less often recognised but can also be clinically important. Hyperuricaemia is common and can precipitate acute gout (see Ch. 25). Excessive diuresis leads to reduced renal perfusion and consequent impairment of renal function (an early warning of this is a rise in plasma urea concentration).

Unwanted effects *unrelated to the renal actions* of the drugs are infrequent. Dose-related hearing loss (compounded by concomitant use of other ototoxic drugs such as aminoglycoside antibiotics) can result from impaired ion transport by the basolateral membrane of the stria vascularis in the inner ear. It occurs only at much higher doses than usually needed to produce diuresis. Adverse reactions unrelated to the main pharmacological effect (e.g. rashes, bone marrow depression) can occur.

[5]Several diseases that damage renal glomeruli impair their ability to retain plasma albumin, causing massive loss of albumin in the urine and a reduced concentration of albumin in the plasma, which can in turn cause peripheral oedema. This is referred to as nephrotic syndrome.

[6]Such unwanted effects are re-enacted in extreme form in Bartter syndrome type 1, a rare loss-of-function genetic disorder of the $Na^+/K^+/2Cl^-$ transporter, the features of which include polyhydramnios – caused by fetal polyuria – and, postnatally, renal salt loss, low blood pressure, hypokalaemic metabolic alkalosis and hypercalciuria.

Diuretics acting on the distal tubule

Diuretics acting on the distal tubule include thiazides (e.g. **bendroflumethiazide**, **hydrochlorothiazide**) – the class 'thiazides' being defined by possessing this chemical structure – and so-called 'thiazide-like' drugs (e.g. **chlortalidone**, **indapamide** and **metolazone**; see Fig. 29.5C) which act on the same molecular target but are structurally distinct. All of these agents are best thought of collectively as a single group irrespective of chemical structure, but there are pharmacokinetic differences between individual drugs, the thiazide-like drugs being cleared more slowly and hence acting throughout more of a 24-h dosing interval.

Thiazides are less powerful than loop diuretics, at least in terms of peak increase in rate of urine formation, and are preferred in treating uncomplicated hypertension (see Ch. 21). They are better tolerated than loop diuretics, and in clinical trials have been shown to reduce risks of stroke and heart attack associated with hypertension. In the largest trial (ALLHAT, 2002), chlortalidone performed as well as an angiotensin-converting enzyme (ACE) inhibitor and a calcium antagonist (see Ch. 21). Thiazides bind the Cl^- site of the distal tubular Na^+/Cl^- co-transporter, inhibiting its action and causing natriuresis with loss of sodium and chloride ions in the urine. The resulting contraction in blood volume stimulates renin secretion, leading to angiotensin formation and aldosterone secretion (see Ch. 21, see Fig. 21.9). This homeostatic mechanism limits the effect of the diuretic on blood pressure, resulting in an in vivo dose–hypotensive response relationship with only a gentle gradient during chronic dosing.

The effects of thiazides on Na^+, K^+, H^+ and Mg^{2+} balance are qualitatively similar to those of loop diuretics, but smaller in magnitude. In contrast to loop diuretics, however, thiazides reduce Ca^{2+} excretion, possibly advantageous in older patients at risk of osteoporosis and favouring thiazides over loop diuretics in this setting (Aung and Htay, 2011).

Although thiazides are milder than loop diuretics when used alone, co-administration with loop diuretics has a synergistic effect, because the loop diuretic delivers a greater fraction of the filtered load of Na^+ to the site of action of the thiazide in the distal tubule.

Thiazide diuretics have a vasodilator action. When used in the treatment of hypertension (see Ch. 21), the initial fall in blood pressure results from the decreased blood volume caused by diuresis, but vasodilatation contributes to the later phase.

Thiazide diuretics have a paradoxical effect in diabetes insipidus, where they *reduce* the volume of urine by interfering with the production of hypotonic fluid in the distal tubule, and hence reduce the ability of the kidney to excrete hypotonic urine (i.e. they reduce free water clearance).

Pharmacokinetic aspects

Thiazides and thiazide-related drugs are effective orally. All are excreted in the urine, mainly by tubular secretion, and they compete with uric acid for the OAT (see Ch. 9). Bendroflumethiazide has its maximum effect at about 4–6 h and duration is 8–12 h. Chlortalidone has a longer duration of action.

The clinical use of thiazide diuretics is given in the clinical box.

Clinical uses of thiazide/thiazide-like diuretics (e.g. bendroflumethiazide/ chlortalidone)

- *Hypertension.*
- Mild heart *failure* (loop diuretics are usually preferred).
- Severe resistant *oedema* (**metolazone**, especially, is used, together with loop diuretics).
- To prevent recurrent stone formation in idiopathic *hypercalciuria.*
- *Nephrogenic diabetes insipidus.*

Unwanted effects

Apart from an increase in *urinary frequency*, the commonest unwanted effect of thiazides is *erectile dysfunction*. This emerged in an analysis of reasons given by patients for withdrawing from blinded treatment in the Medical Research Council mild hypertension trial, where (to the surprise of the investigators) erectile dysfunction was substantially more common than in men allocated to a β-adrenoceptor antagonist or to placebo. Thiazide-associated erectile dysfunction is reversible; it is less common with the low doses used in current practice but remains a problem. *Potassium loss* can be important, as can loss of Mg^{2+}. Excretion of uric acid is decreased, and hypochloraemic alkalosis can occur.

Impaired glucose tolerance (see Ch. 31), due to inhibition of insulin secretion, is thought to result from activation of K_{ATP} channels in pancreatic islet beta-cells.[7] **Diazoxide**, a non-diuretic thiazide, also activates K_{ATP} channels, causing vasodilatation and impaired insulin secretion. **Indapamide** is said to lower blood pressure with less metabolic disturbance than related drugs, possibly because it is marketed at a lower equivalent dose.

Hyperuricaemia is common as a consequence of competition with urate for the OAT and can precipitate acute gout as with loop diuretics (see Ch. 25).

Hyponatraemia is potentially serious, especially in the elderly. Hypokalaemia can be a cause of adverse drug interaction (see previously under Loop diuretics) and can precipitate encephalopathy in patients with severe liver disease.

Adverse reactions unrelated to the main pharmacology (e.g. rashes, blood dyscrasias) are not common but can be serious.

Aldosterone antagonists

Spironolactone, **eplerenone** and **finerenone** have limited diuretic action when used singly, because distal Na^+/K^+ exchange – the site on which they act – accounts for reabsorption of only 2% of filtered Na^+. They do, however, have marked antihypertensive effects (see Ch. 21), prolong survival in selected patients with heart failure (see Ch. 21) and, in the case of finerenone (Bakris et al., 2020; Pitt et al., 2021), preserve renal function and reduce cardiovascular death in type 2 diabetic patients with chronic kidney disease

[7]The chemically related sulfonylurea group of drugs used to treat type 2 diabetes mellitus (Ch. 31) act in the opposite way, by closing K_{ATP} channels and enhancing insulin secretion.

(CKD). They can prevent hypokalaemia when combined with loop diuretics or with thiazides. They compete with aldosterone for the intracellular mineralocorticoid receptor (MR, see Ch. 33), thereby inhibiting distal Na^+ retention and K^+ secretion (see Fig. 29.5D).

Pharmacokinetic aspects

Spironolactone is well absorbed from the gut. Its plasma half-life is only 10 min, but its active metabolite, **canrenone**, has a plasma half-life of 16 h. The action of spironolactone is largely attributable to canrenone. This, in addition to the slow turnover of membrane transporters, results in a slow onset of action, occurring over several days. Eplerenone has a shorter elimination half-life than canrenone and has no active metabolites. It is administered by mouth once daily. Finerenone is administered by mouth once daily; it is inactivated by metabolism, primarily by CYP3A4.

Unwanted effects

Aldosterone antagonists predispose to hyperkalaemia, which is potentially fatal. Potassium supplements should not be co-prescribed other than in exceptional circumstances and then with close monitoring of plasma creatinine and electrolytes. Such monitoring is also needed if these drugs are used for patients with impaired renal function, especially if other drugs that can increase plasma potassium, such as *ACE inhibitors, angiotensin receptor antagonists* (sartans) (see Ch. 21) or *β-adrenoceptor antagonists* (see Ch. 15), are also prescribed - as they often are for patients with heart failure. Gastrointestinal upset is quite common. The actions of spironolactone/canrenone on progesterone and androgen receptors in tissues other than the kidney can cause gynaecomastia, menstrual disorders and testicular atrophy. Eplerenone has lower affinity for these receptors, and such oestrogen-like adverse effects are less common. Finerenone is a nonsteroidal MR antagonist: it has high potency and selectivity for the MR but no relevant affinity for androgen, progesterone, oestrogen and glucocorticoid receptors.

The clinical use of potassium-sparing diuretics is given in the clinical box.

Clinical uses of potassium-sparing diuretics

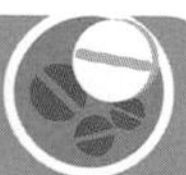

- With K^+-losing (i.e. loop or thiazide) diuretics to prevent K^+ loss, where hypokalaemia is especially hazardous (e.g. patients requiring **digoxin** or **amiodarone**; see Ch. 20).
- **Spironolactone** or **eplerenone** is used in:
  - *heart failure*, to improve survival (see Ch. 20)
  - *primary hyperaldosteronism* (Conn's syndrome)
  - *resistant essential hypertension* (especially low-renin hypertension)
  - *secondary hyperaldosteronism* caused by hepatic cirrhosis complicated by ascites.
- **Finerenone**, a non-steroidal MR antagonist, was recently approved by the FDA for use in type 2 diabetic patients with CKD to:
  - reduce the risk of *progressive renal impairment*, *cardiovascular death*, nonfatal *myocardial infarction*, and *hospitalisation* for heart failure.

Triamterene and amiloride

Like aldosterone antagonists, **triamterene** and **amiloride** have only limited diuretic efficacy, because they also act in the distal nephron, where only a small fraction of Na^+ reabsorption occurs. They act on the collecting tubules and collecting ducts, inhibiting Na^+ reabsorption by blocking lumenal sodium channels, thereby indirectly decreasing K^+ excretion (see Fig. 29.5D).

They can be given with loop diuretics or thiazides in order to maintain potassium balance.

Pharmacokinetic aspects

Triamterene is well absorbed in the gastrointestinal tract. Its onset of action is within 2 h, and its duration of action is 12–16 h. It is partly metabolised in the liver and partly excreted unchanged in the urine. Amiloride is less well absorbed and has a slower onset, with a peak action at 6 h and duration of about 24 h. Most of the drug is excreted unchanged in the urine.

Unwanted effects

The main unwanted effect, hyperkalaemia, is related to the pharmacological action of these drugs and can be dangerous, especially in patients with renal impairment or receiving other drugs that can increase plasma K^+ (see above). Gastrointestinal disturbances have been reported but are infrequent. Idiosyncratic reactions, for example, rashes, are uncommon.

Carbonic anhydrase inhibitors

Carbonic anhydrase inhibitors (see Fig. 29.5A) – for example, **acetazolamide** – increase excretion of bicarbonate with accompanying Na^+, K^+ and water, resulting in an increased flow of an alkaline urine and metabolic acidosis. These agents, although not now used as diuretics, are still used in the treatment of glaucoma to reduce the formation of aqueous humour (see Ch. 27), in some types of infantile epilepsy (see Ch. 46) and to accelerate acclimatisation to high altitude.

Urinary loss of bicarbonate depletes extracellular bicarbonate, and the diuretic effect of carbonic anhydrase inhibitors is consequently self-limiting. Acetazolamide is a sulfonamide and off-target unwanted effects such as rashes, blood dyscrasias and interstitial nephritis can occur as with other sulfonamides (see Ch. 52).

DIURETICS THAT ACT INDIRECTLY BY MODIFYING THE CONTENT OF THE FILTRATE

Osmotic diuretics

Osmotic diuretics are pharmacologically inert substances (e.g. **mannitol**) that are filtered in the glomerulus but not reabsorbed (see Fig. 29.4).[8] Their main effect is exerted in those parts of the nephron that are freely permeable to water: the proximal tubule, descending limb of the loop and (in the presence of ADH; see earlier) the collecting tubules. Passive water reabsorption is reduced by the presence of non-reabsorbable solute within the tubule; consequently, a larger volume of fluid remains within the proximal tubule. This has the secondary effect of reducing Na^+ reabsorption.

[8]In hyperglycaemia, glucose acts as an osmotic diuretic once plasma glucose exceeds the renal reabsorptive capacity (usually approximately 12 mmol/L), accounting for the cardinal symptom of polyuria in diabetes mellitus; see Chapter 31.

The main effect of osmotic diuretics is to increase the amount of water excreted, with a smaller increase in Na^+ excretion. They are sometimes used in acute renal failure, which can occur as a result of haemorrhage, injury or systemic infections. In acute renal failure, glomerular filtration rate is reduced, and absorption of NaCl and water in the proximal tubule becomes almost complete, so that more distal parts of the nephron virtually 'dry up', and urine flow ceases. Protein is deposited in the tubules and may impede the flow of fluid. Osmotic diuretics (e.g. **mannitol** given intravenously in multiple-gram doses) can limit these effects, at least if given in the earliest stages, albeit while increasing intravascular volume and cardiac pre-load.

Osmotic diuretics are also used for the emergency treatment of acutely raised intracranial or intraocular pressure. Such treatment has nothing to do with the kidney but relies on the increase in plasma osmolarity by solutes that do not enter the brain or eye, which results in efflux of water from these compartments.

Unwanted effects include transient expansion of the extracellular fluid volume (with a risk of precipitating left ventricular failure) and hyponatraemia. Headache, nausea and vomiting can occur.

Diuretics

- Normally <1% of filtered Na^+ is excreted.
- Diuretics increase the excretion of salt (NaCl or $NaHCO_3$) and water.
- Loop diuretics, thiazides and K^+-sparing diuretics are the main therapeutic drugs.
- Loop diuretics (e.g. **furosemide**) cause copious urine production. They inhibit the $Na^+/K^+/2Cl^-$ co-transporter in the thick ascending loop of Henle. They are used to treat heart failure and other diseases complicated by salt and water retention. Hypovolaemia and hypokalaemia are important unwanted effects.
- Thiazides and thiazide-like drugs (e.g. **bendroflumethiazide/chlortalidone**) have a less dramatic diuretic effect than loop diuretics. They inhibit the Na^+/Cl^- co-transporter in the distal convoluted tubule. They are used to treat hypertension, working partly through an indirect vasodilator action. Erectile dysfunction is an important adverse effect. Hypokalaemia and other metabolic effects (e.g. hyperuricaemia, hyperglycaemia) can occur, especially with high doses.
- Potassium-sparing diuretics:
  - act in the distal nephron and collecting tubules; they are weak diuretics but effective in some forms of hypertension and heart failure, and they can prevent hypokalaemia caused by loop diuretics or thiazides.
  - canrenone, the active metabolite of **spironolactone**, **eplerenone** and the nonsteroidal MR antagonist **finerenone** compete with aldosterone for the MR.
  - **amiloride** and **triamterene** act by blocking the sodium channels controlled by aldosterone's protein mediator.

DRUGS THAT ALTER THE pH OF THE URINE

It is possible, using pharmacological agents, to produce urinary pH values ranging from approximately 5 to 8.5.

Carbonic anhydrase inhibitors increase urinary pH by blocking bicarbonate reabsorption (see earlier). **Citrate** (given by mouth as a mixture of sodium and potassium salts) is metabolised via the Krebs cycle with the generation of bicarbonate, which is excreted, alkalinising the urine. This may have some antibacterial effects, as well as improving dysuria (a common symptom of bladder infection, consisting of a burning sensation while passing urine). Additionally, some citrate is excreted in the urine as such and inhibits urinary stone formation. Alkalinisation is important in preventing certain weak acid drugs with limited aqueous solubility, such as *sulfonamides* (see Ch. 52), from crystallising in the urine; it also decreases the formation of uric acid and cystine stones by favouring the charged anionic form that is more water-soluble (see Ch. 9).

Alkalinising the urine increases the excretion of drugs that are weak acids (e.g. salicylates and some barbiturates). Sodium bicarbonate is sometimes used to treat salicylate overdose (see Ch. 10).

Urinary pH can be decreased with **ammonium chloride**, but this is now rarely, if ever, used clinically.

DRUGS THAT ALTER THE EXCRETION OF ORGANIC MOLECULES

Uric acid metabolism and excretion are relevant in the treatment and prevention of gout (see Ch. 25), and a few points about its excretion are made here. Normal plasma urate concentration is approximately 0.24 mmol/L, higher concentrations predisposing to gout (see Ch. 25)

Uric acid is derived from the catabolism of purines and is present in plasma mainly as ionised urate. In humans, it passes freely into the glomerular filtrate, and most is then reabsorbed in the proximal tubule while a small amount is secreted into the tubule by the anion-secreting mechanism. The net result is excretion of approximately 8%–12% of filtered urate. The secretory mechanism is generally inhibited by low doses of drugs that affect uric acid transport (see later), whereas higher doses are needed to block reabsorption. Such drugs therefore tend to cause retention of uric acid at low doses, while promoting its excretion at higher doses. Drugs that increase the elimination of urate (*uricosuric agents*, e.g. **probenecid** and **sulfinpyrazone**) may be useful in such patients, although these have largely been supplanted by **allopurinol**, which inhibits urate synthesis (see Ch. 25).

Probenecid inhibits the anion transporter responsible for the reabsorption of urate in the proximal tubule, increasing its excretion. It has the opposite effect on penicillin, inhibiting its secretion into the tubules and raising its plasma concentration (an effect still sometimes exploited during antibiotic therapy, see Chs 10 and 52). Given orally, probenecid is well absorbed in the gastrointestinal tract, maximal concentrations in the plasma occurring in about 3 h. Approximately 90% is bound to plasma albumin. Free drug passes into the glomerular filtrate but more is actively secreted into the proximal tubule, whence it may diffuse back because of its high lipid solubility (see also Ch. 10).

Sulfinpyrazone acts similarly, but additionally inhibits cyclo-oxygenase.

The main effect of uricosuric drugs is to block urate reabsorption and lower plasma urate concentration. Both probenecid and sulfinpyrazone inhibit the secretion as well as the reabsorption of urate and, if given in subtherapeutic doses, can actually increase plasma urate concentrations.

DRUGS USED IN RENAL FAILURE

Many drugs used in chronic renal failure (e.g. antihypertensives, vitamin D preparations and **epoetin**) are covered in other chapters. Electrolyte disorders are particularly important in renal failure, notably *hyperphosphataemia* and *hyperkalaemia*, and may require drug treatment which is described briefly here.

HYPERPHOSPHATAEMIA

Phosphate metabolism is closely linked with that of calcium and is discussed in Chapter 36.

The antacid **aluminium hydroxide** (see Ch. 30) binds phosphate in the gastrointestinal tract, reducing its absorption, but may increase plasma aluminium in patients with end-stage kidney failure receiving haemodialysis treatment.[9] Calcium-based phosphate-binding agents (e.g. calcium carbonate) are widely used to treat hyperphosphatemia. They are contraindicated in hypercalcaemia or hypercalciuria but until recently have been believed to be otherwise safe. However, calcium salts may predispose to tissue calcification (including of artery walls), and calcium-containing phosphate binders may actually contribute to the very high death rates from cardiovascular disease in dialysis patients.

An anion exchange resin, **sevelamer**, lowers plasma phosphate, and is less likely than calcium carbonate to cause arterial calcification (Tonelli et al., 2010). Sevelamer is not absorbed from the gut and has an additional effect in lowering low-density lipoprotein cholesterol. It is given in gram doses by mouth three times a day with meals. Its adverse effects are gastrointestinal disturbance, and it is contraindicated in bowel obstruction.

HYPERKALAEMIA

Severe hyperkalaemia is life-threatening. Its prevalence is increased in patients with kidney failure, and by drugs that inhibit the renin–angiotensin–aldosterone axis which are widely used to slow the progression of renal impairment. Cardiac K^+-toxicity is counteracted by administering calcium chloride intravenously (see Table 20.2), and by measures that shift K^+ into the intracellular compartment, for example glucose plus insulin (see Ch. 31). **Salbutamol**, administered intravenously or by inhalation, also causes cellular K^+ uptake and is used for this indication including in children (Murdoch et al., 1991); it acts synergistically with insulin. Intravenous sodium bicarbonate moves potassium ions into cells in exchange for intracellular protons that emerge to buffer the extracellular fluid, but can paradoxically lower intracellular and transcellular pH. Removal of excessive potassium from the body can be achieved by cation exchange resins such as **sodium** or **calcium polystyrene sulfonate** administered by mouth (in combination with **sorbitol** to prevent constipation) or as an enema. There are two exchange resins (**sodium zirconium cyclosilicate** and **patiromer calcium**) licensed for alleviating hyperkalaemia in patients with CKD who require continued treatment with renin–angiotensin–aldosterone system inhibitors for comorbid hypertension or heart failure. Unlike the other resins which act mainly in the colon, sodium zirconium cyclosilicate can capture potassium ions along the entire gastrointestinal tract, with onset of action within an hour of ingestion (thus making it suitable for emergency management of hyperkalaemia). The long-term tolerability of cation exchange resins is questionable because these agents are associated with gastrointestinal upset and electrolyte abnormalities.

[9]Before Kerr identified the cause, the use of alum to purify municipal water supplies in Newcastle led to a horrible and untreatable neurodegenerative condition known as 'dialysis dementia', and also to a particularly painful and refractory form of bone disease.

DRUGS USED IN URINARY TRACT DISORDERS

Bed wetting (enuresis) is normal in young children and persists in around 5% of 10-year-olds. Nocturnal enuresis in children aged 10 years or more may warrant treatment with **desmopressin** (an analogue of ADH, given by mouth or by nasal spray for the treatment of diabetes insipidus caused by ADH deficiency due to disease of the posterior pituitary gland - see earlier discussion and Ch. 33), combined with restricting fluid intake in the evening.

Disordered micturition is also common in adults. Symptoms from benign prostatic hyperplasia may be improved by α_1-adrenoceptor antagonists, for example **doxazosin** or **tamsulosin** (see Ch. 15), or by an inhibitor of androgen synthesis such as **finasteride** (see Ch. 35).

Muscarinic receptor antagonists (see Ch. 14) such as **oxybutynin** are used for neurogenic detrusor muscle instability ('overactive bladder'), but the dose is limited by their adverse effects. A selective β_3 agonist (**mirabegron**) is also licensed for this indication (see Ch. 15) but can cause tachycardia and atrial fibrillation.

REFERENCES AND FURTHER READING

Physiological aspects

Agre, P., 2004. Aquaporin water channels (Nobel lecture). Angew. Chem. Int. Ed. Engl. 43, 4278–4290.

Gamba, G., 2015. Molecular physiology and pathophysiology of electroneutral cation-chloride cotransporters. Physiol. Rev. 85, 423–493.

Greger, R., 2000. Physiology of sodium transport. Am. J. Med. Sci. 319, 51–62.

Nigam, S.K., Bush, K.T., Martovetsky, G., 2016. The organic anion transporter (OAT) family: a systems biology perspective. Physiol. Rev. 95, 83–123.

Drugs and therapeutic aspects

Diuretics

Aung, K., Htay, T., 2011. Thiazide diuretics and the risk of hip fracture. Cochrane Database Syst. Rev. 10, CD005185.

Ellison, D.H., Subramanya, A.R., 2015. Clinical use of diuretics. In: Turner, N.N., Lameire, N., Goldsmith, D.J., et al., (Eds.), Oxford Textbook of Clinical Nephrology, fourth ed. Oxford University Press, Oxford.

Pitt, B., Filippatos, G., Agarwal, R., et al., 2021. Cardiovascular events with finerenone in kidney disease and type 2 diabetes. N. Engl. J. Med. 385, 2252–2263.

Shankar, S.S., Brater, D.C., 2003. Loop diuretics: from the Na–K–2Cl transporter to clinical use. Am. J. Physiol. Renal Physiol. 284, F11–F21.

Ca^{2+}/PO_4^- (see also Diuretics section)

Tonelli, M., Pannu, N., Manns, B., 2010. Drug therapy: oral phosphate binders in patients with kidney failure. N. Engl. J. Med. 362, 1312–1324.

Vervloet, M., Cozzolino, M., 2017. Vascular calcification in chronic kidney disease: different bricks in the wall? Kidney Int. 91, 808–817.

Antihypertensives and renal protection

ALLHAT Officers and Coordinators for the ALLHAT Collaborative Research Group, 2002. Major outcomes in high-risk hypertensive patients randomized to angiotensin-converting enzyme inhibitor or calcium channel blocker vs diuretic: the Antihypertensive and Lipid-Lowering Treatment to Prevent Heart Attack Trial (ALLHAT). JAMA 288, 2981–2997.

Bakris, G.L., Agarwal, R., Anker, S.D., et al., 2020. Effect of finerenone on chronic kidney disease outcomes in type 2 diabetes. N. Engl. J. Med. 383, 2219–2229.

Nijenhuis, T., Vallon, V., van der Kemp, A.W., et al., 2005. Enhanced passive Ca^{2+} reabsorption and reduced Mg^{2+} channel abundance explains thiazide-induced hypocalciuria and hypomagnesemia. J. Clin. Invest. 115, 1651–1658.

Sodium and potassium ion disorders

Coca, S.G., Perazella, M.A., Buller, G.K., 2005. The cardiovascular implications of hypokalemia. Am. J. Kidney Dis. 45, 233–247.

Murdoch, I.A., Dos Anjos, R., Haycock, G.B., 1991. Treatment of hyperkalaemia with intravenous salbutamol. Arch. Dis. Child. 66, 527–528.

Drug utilisation in kidney disease

Golper, T.A., Udy, A.A., Lipman, J., 2015. Drug dosing in acute kidney injury. In: Turner, N.N., Lameire, N., Goldsmith, D.J., et al., (Eds.), Oxford Textbook of Clinical Nephrology, fourth ed. Oxford University Press, Oxford.

Olyaei, A.J., Foster, T.A., Lermer, E.V., 2015. Drug dosing in chronic kidney disease. In: Turner, N.N., Lameire, N., Goldsmith, D.J., et al., (Eds.), Oxford Textbook of Clinical Nephrology, fourth ed. Oxford University Press, Oxford.

30 The gastrointestinal tract

OVERVIEW

In addition to its main function of digestion and absorption of food, the gastrointestinal (GI) tract is one of the major endocrine systems in the body. It also has its own integrative neuronal network, the enteric nervous system (see Ch. 13), which contains almost the same number of neurons as the spinal cord. It is the site of many common pathologies, ranging from simple dyspepsia to complex autoimmune conditions such as Crohn's disease, and medicines for treating GI disorders comprise some 8% of all prescriptions. In this chapter, we briefly review the physiological control of GI function and then discuss the pharmacological characteristics of drugs affecting gastric secretion and motility, and those used to treat intestinal inflammatory disease.

THE INNERVATION AND HORMONES OF THE GASTROINTESTINAL TRACT

The blood vessels and the glands (exocrine, endocrine and paracrine) of the GI tract are under both neuronal and hormonal control.

NEURONAL CONTROL

There are two principal intramural plexuses in the tract: the *myenteric plexus* (*Auerbach's plexus*) lies between the outer, longitudinal and the middle, circular muscle layers, and the *submucous plexus* (*Meissner's plexus*) lies on the lumenal side of the circular muscle layer. These plexuses are interconnected and their ganglion cells receive preganglionic parasympathetic fibres from the vagus. These are mostly cholinergic and excitatory, although a few are inhibitory. Incoming sympathetic fibres are largely postganglionic. In addition to innervating blood vessels, smooth muscle and some glandular cells directly, some sympathetic fibres terminate in these plexuses, where they inhibit acetylcholine secretion (see Ch. 13).

The neurons within the plexuses constitute the *enteric nervous system* and secrete not only acetylcholine and noradrenaline (norepinephrine), but also 5-hydroxytryptamine (5-HT), purines, nitric oxide and a variety of pharmacologically active peptides (see Chs 13–19). The enteric plexus also contains sensory neurons, which respond to mechanical and chemical stimuli.

HORMONAL CONTROL

The hormones of the GI tract include both endocrine and paracrine secretions. The endocrine secretions (i.e. substances released into the bloodstream) are mainly peptides synthesised by endocrine cells in the mucosa. Important examples include *gastrin* and *cholecystokinin* (CCK). The paracrine secretions include many regulatory peptides released from special cells found throughout the wall of the tract. These hormones act on nearby cells, and in the stomach the most important of these is *histamine*. Some of these paracrine factors also function as neurotransmitters.

Orally administered drugs are, of course, absorbed during their passage through the GI tract (see Ch. 9). Other functions of the GI tract that are important from the viewpoint of pharmacological intervention are:

- gastric secretion
- vomiting (emesis) and nausea
- gut motility and defecation
- the formation and excretion of bile

GASTRIC SECRETION

The stomach secretes about 2.5 L of gastric juice daily. The principal exocrine components are proenzymes such as *prorennin* and *pepsinogen* elaborated by the *chief* or *peptic* cells, and *hydrochloric acid* (HCl) and *intrinsic factor* (see Ch. 24) secreted by the *parietal* or *oxyntic* cells. The production of acid is important for promoting proteolytic digestion of foodstuffs, iron absorption and killing pathogens. Mucus-secreting cells also abound in the gastric mucosa. Bicarbonate ions are secreted and trapped in the mucus, creating a gel-like protective barrier that maintains the mucosal surface at a pH of 6–7 in the face of a much more acidic environment (pH 1–2) in the lumen. Alcohol and bile can disrupt this protective layer. Locally produced 'cytoprotective' prostaglandins (PGs) stimulate the secretion of both mucus and bicarbonate.

Disturbances in these secretory and protective mechanisms are thought to be involved in the pathogenesis of *peptic ulcer*, and indeed in other types of gastric damage such as *gastro-oesophageal reflux disease* (GORD[1]) and injury caused by non-steroidal anti-inflammatory drugs (NSAIDs).

THE REGULATION OF ACID SECRETION BY PARIETAL CELLS

Disturbances of acid secretion are important in the pathogenesis of peptic ulcer and constitute a particular target for drug action. The secretion of the parietal cells is an isotonic solution of HCl (150 mmol/L) with a pH less than 1, the concentration of hydrogen ions being more than a million times higher than that in the plasma. To produce this, Cl^- is actively transported into *canaliculi* in the cells that communicate with the lumen of the gastric glands and thus with the stomach itself. This is accompanied by K^+ secretion, which is then exchanged for H^+ from within the cell by a K^+-H^+-ATPase (the 'proton pump', Fig. 30.1). Within the

[1]Or GERD in the United States, to reflect the different spelling of *esophageal*.

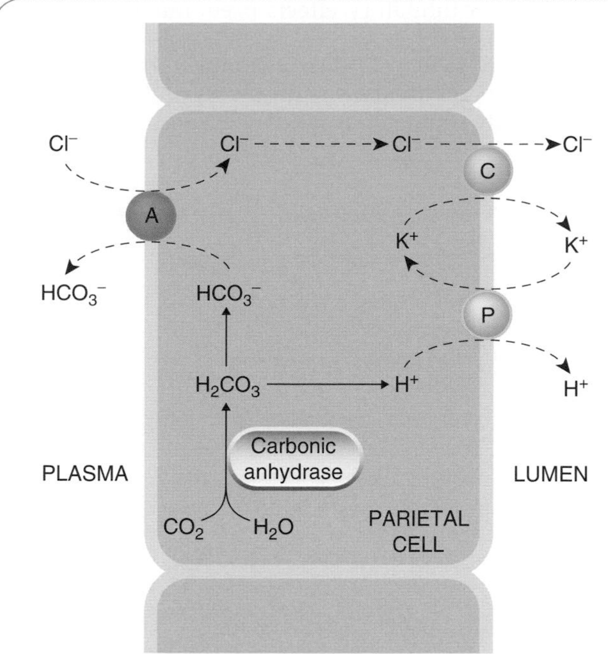

Fig. 30.1 A schematic illustration of the secretion of hydrochloric acid by the gastric parietal cell. Secretion involves a proton pump *(P)*, which is an H^+-K^+-ATPase; a symport carrier *(C)* for K^+ and Cl^-; and an antiport *(A)*, which exchanges Cl^- and HCO_3^-. An additional Na^+/H^+ antiport situated at the interface with the plasma may also have a role (not shown).

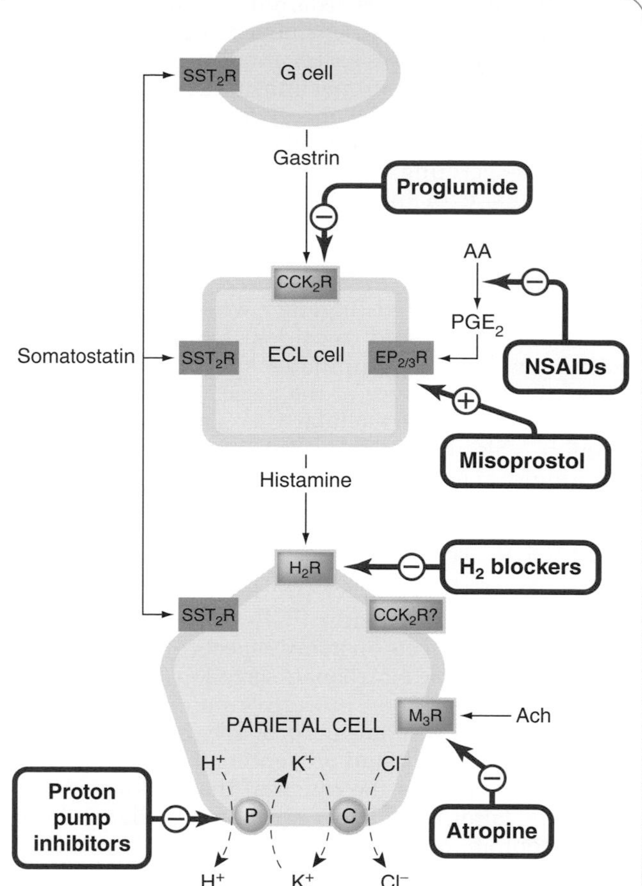

Fig. 30.2 Schematic diagram showing the regulation of the acid-secreting gastric parietal cell, illustrating the site of action of drugs influencing acid secretion. The initial step in controlling physiological secretion is the release of gastrin from G cells. This acts through its gastrin/cholecystokinin (CCK_2) receptor on mast cell-like histamine-secreting enterochromaffin (ECL) cells to release histamine and may also have a secondary direct effect on parietal cells themselves, although this is not entirely clear. Histamine acts on parietal cell H_2 receptors to elevate cAMP that activates the secretion of acid by the proton pump. Direct vagal stimulation also provokes acid secretion and released acetylcholine directly stimulates M_3 receptors on parietal cells. The influence of somatostatin on G cells, ECL cells and parietal cells is inhibitory. Local (or therapeutically administered) prostaglandins exert inhibitory effects predominately on ECL cell function. Receptors depicted in *red* have inhibitory effects on cell secretion, whilst those in *blue* stimulate cell secretion. *AA*, Arachidonic acid; *ACh*, acetylcholine; *C*, symport carrier for K^+ and Cl^-; *CCK_2*, gastrin/cholecystokinin receptor; *NSAIDs*, non-steroidal anti-inflammatory drugs; *P*, proton pump (H^+-K^+-ATPase); *PGE_2*, prostaglandin E_2.

cell, carbonic anhydrase catalyses the combination of carbon dioxide and water to give carbonic acid, which dissociates into H^+ and bicarbonate ions. The latter exchanges across the basal membrane of the parietal cell for Cl^-. The principal mediators that directly - or indirectly - control parietal cell acid output are:

- histamine (a stimulatory local hormone)
- gastrin (a stimulatory peptide hormone)
- acetylcholine (a stimulatory neurotransmitter)
- PGE_2 and PGI_2 (local hormones that inhibit acid secretion)
- somatostatin (an inhibitory peptide hormone)

HISTAMINE

Histamine is discussed in Chapter 17, and only those aspects of its pharmacology relevant to gastric secretion will be dealt with here. Neuroendocrine cells abound in the stomach and the dominant type is the *ECL cell* (enterochromaffin-like). These are histamine-containing cells similar to mast cells, which lie close to the parietal cells. They sustain a steady basal release of histamine, which is further increased by gastrin and acetylcholine. Histamine acts in a paracrine fashion on parietal cell H_2 receptors, increasing intracellular cAMP. These cells are responsive to histamine concentrations that are below the threshold required for vascular H_2 receptor activation.

GASTRIN

Gastrin is a polypeptide of 34 residues but also exists in shorter forms. It is synthesised by *G cells* in the gastric antrum and secreted into the portal blood, acting as a circulating hormone. Its main action is stimulation of acid secretion by ECL cells through its action at gastrin/CCK_2 receptors,[2] which elevate intracellular Ca^{2+}. Gastrin receptors also occur on the parietal cells but their significance in the control of physiological secretion is controversial. CCK_2 receptors are blocked by **proglumide** and **netazepide**, both of which are undergoing clinical trials in gastrointestinal disease (Fig. 30.2).

[2]These two peptides share the same, biologically active, C-terminal pentapeptide sequence.

Gastrin also stimulates histamine synthesis by ECL cells and indirectly increases pepsinogen secretion, stimulates blood flow and increases gastric motility. Release of gastrin is controlled by both neuronal transmitters and blood-borne mediators, as well as by the chemistry of the stomach contents. Amino acids and small peptides directly stimulate the gastrin-secreting cells, as do milk and solutions of calcium salts, explaining why it is inappropriate to use calcium-containing salts as antacids.

ACETYLCHOLINE

Acetylcholine, released (together with a battery of other neurotransmitters and peptides) from postganglionic cholinergic neurons, stimulates specific muscarinic M_3 receptors on the surface of the parietal cells (see Ch. 14), thereby elevating intracellular Ca^{2+} and stimulating acid secretion. It also has complex effects on other cell types; by inhibiting somatostatin release from *D cells*, it potentiates its action on parietal cell acid secretion.

PROSTAGLANDINS

Most cells of the GI tract produce PGs (see Ch. 17), the most important being PGE_2 and PGI_2. PGs exert 'cytoprotective' effects on many aspects of gastric function including increasing bicarbonate secretion ($EP_{1/2}$ receptors), increasing the release of protective mucin (EP_4 receptor), reducing gastric acid output, probably by acting on $EP_{2/3}$ receptors on ECL cells and preventing the vasoconstriction (and thus damage to the mucosa) that follows injury or insult. The latter is probably an action mediated through $EP_{2/4}$ receptors. **Misoprostol** (see later) is a synthetic PG that probably exploits many of these effects to bring about its therapeutic action.

SOMATOSTATIN

This peptide hormone is released from *D cells* at several locations within the stomach. By acting at its somatostatin $(SST)_2$ receptor, it exerts paracrine inhibitory actions on gastrin release from G cells, histamine release from ECL cells, as well as directly on parietal cell acid output.

THE COORDINATION OF FACTORS REGULATING ACID SECRETION

The regulation of the parietal cell is complex, and many local hormones probably play a role in the fine-tuning of the secretory response. The generally accepted model today is that the *gastrin–ECL–parietal cell axis* is the dominant mechanism for controlling acid secretion. According to this idea (see Fig. 30.2), which is supported by the majority of genetically altered mouse studies, the initial step in controlling physiological secretion is the release of gastrin from G cells. This acts through its CCK_2 receptor on ECL cells to release histamine and may also have a secondary direct effect on parietal cells themselves, although this has been disputed. Histamine acts on H_2 receptors on parietal cells to elevate cAMP and to activate the secretion of protons as described.

Direct vagal stimulation can also provoke acid secretion (the basis for 'stress ulcers') through a release of acetylcholine, which directly stimulates M_3 receptors on parietal cells. Somatostatin probably exerts a tonic inhibitory influence on G cells, ECL and parietal cells, and local (or therapeutically administered) PGs, acting through $EP_{2/3}$ receptors, exert inhibitory effects predominantly on ECL cell function.

This control system is clearly complex, but prolonged exposure of tissues to excess acid secretion is dangerous and must be tightly regulated (see Schubert and Peura, 2008).

Secretion of gastric acid, mucus and bicarbonate

The control of the GI tract is through nervous and humoural mechanisms.

- Acid is secreted from gastric parietal cells by a proton pump (K^+-H^+-ATPase).
- The three endogenous secretagogues for acid are histamine, acetylcholine and gastrin.
- PGE_2 and PGI_2 inhibit acid, stimulate mucus and bicarbonate secretion, and dilate mucosal blood vessels.
- Somatostatin inhibits all phases of parietal cell activation.

The genesis of peptic ulcers involves:

- infection of the gastric mucosa with *Helicobacter pylori*;
- an imbalance between mucosal-damaging (acid, pepsin) and mucosal-protecting (mucus, bicarbonate, PGE_2 and PGI_2 and nitric oxide) agents.

DRUGS USED TO INHIBIT OR NEUTRALISE GASTRIC ACID SECRETION

The principal clinical indications for reducing acid secretion are *peptic ulceration* (both duodenal and gastric), *GORD* (in which gastric secretion causes damage to the oesophagus) and the *Zollinger–Ellison syndrome* (a rare hypersecretory condition caused by a gastrin-producing tumour). If untreated, GORD can cause a dysplasia of the oesophageal epithelium which may progress to a potentially dangerous pre-cancerous condition called *Barrett oesophagus*.

The reasons why peptic ulcers develop are not fully understood, although infection of the stomach mucosa with *Helicobacter pylori*[3] – a Gram-negative bacillus that causes chronic gastritis – is now generally considered to be a major cause (especially of duodenal ulcer) and forms the usual basis for therapy. Treatment of *H. pylori* infection is discussed later.

Many non-specific NSAIDs (see Ch. 25) cause gastric bleeding and erosions by inhibiting cyclo-oxygenase I, the enzyme responsible for synthesis of protective PGs. More selective cyclo-oxygenase II inhibitors such as **celecoxib** appear to cause less stomach damage (but see Ch. 25 for a discussion of this issue).

Therapy of peptic ulcer and reflux oesophagitis aims to decrease the secretion of gastric acid with H_2 receptor antagonists or proton pump inhibitors, and/or to neutralise secreted acid with antacids. These treatments are often coupled with measures to eradicate *H. pylori*.

[3]*H. pylori* infection in the stomach has also been classified as a class 1 (definite) carcinogen for gastric cancer.

HISTAMINE H_2 RECEPTOR ANTAGONISTS

The discovery and development of histamine H_2-blocking drugs by Black and his colleagues in 1972 was a major breakthrough in the treatment of gastric ulcers – a condition that could hitherto only be treated by (sometimes rather heroic) surgery.[4] Indeed, the ability to distinguish between histamine receptor subtypes using pharmacological agents was, in itself, a major intellectual achievement since there was no direct evidence for the existence of these receptors until the advent of selective antagonists. H_2 receptor antagonists competitively inhibit histamine actions at all H_2 receptors, but their main clinical use is as inhibitors of gastric acid secretion. They can inhibit histamine- and gastrin-stimulated acid secretion; pepsin secretion also falls with the reduction in volume of gastric juice. These agents not only decrease both basal and food-stimulated acid secretion by 90% or more, but numerous clinical trials indicate that they also promote healing of gastric and duodenal ulcers. However, relapses are likely to follow cessation of treatment.

The main drugs used are **cimetidine**, **ranitidine** (sometimes in combination with **bismuth**), **nizatidine** and **famotidine**. There is little clinically relevant difference between them. The effect of cimetidine on gastric secretion in human subjects is shown in Fig. 30.3. The clinical use of H_2 receptor antagonists is explained in the clinical box.

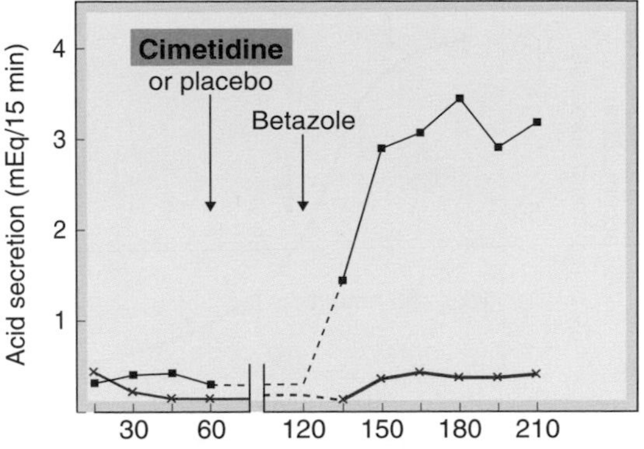

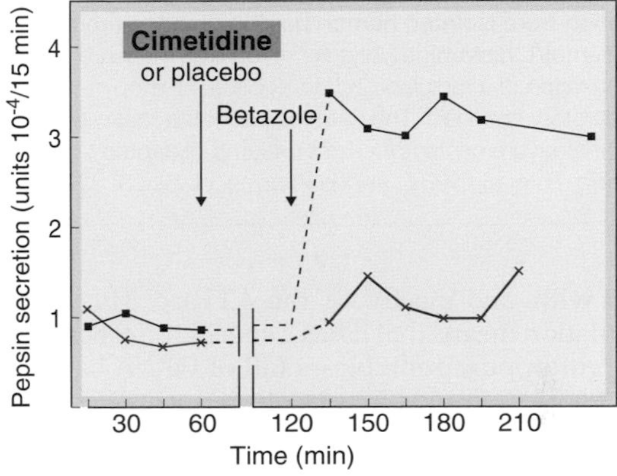

Fig. 30.3 The effect of cimetidine on betazole-stimulated gastric acid and pepsin secretion in humans. Either cimetidine or a placebo was given orally 60 min prior to a subcutaneous injection (1.5 mg/kg) of betazole, a relatively specific histamine H_2-receptor agonist that stimulates gastric acid secretion. (Modified from Binder, H.J., Donaldson, R.M., Jr., 1978. Effect of cimetidine on intrinsic factor and pepsin secretion in man. Gastroenterology 74, 371–375.)

Clinical use of agents affecting gastric acidity

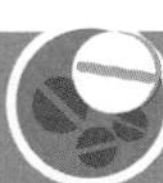

- Histamine H_2 receptor antagonists (e.g. **famotidine**):
  - peptic ulcer
  - reflux oesophagitis.
- Proton pump inhibitors (e.g. **omeprazole**, **lansoprazole**):
  - peptic ulcer
  - reflux oesophagitis
  - as one component of therapy for *H. pylori* infection
  - *Zollinger–Ellison* syndrome (a rare condition caused by gastrin-secreting tumours).
- Antacids (e.g. magnesium trisilicate, aluminium hydroxide, alginates):
  - dyspepsia
  - symptomatic relief in *peptic ulcer* or (**alginate**) *oesophageal reflux.*
- **Bismuth chelate**:
  - as one component of therapy for *H. pylori* infection.

Pharmacokinetic aspects and unwanted effects

The drugs are generally given orally and are well absorbed, although preparations for intramuscular and intravenous use are also available (except **famotidine**). Dosage regimens vary depending on the condition under treatment. Low-dosage over-the-counter formulations of **cimetidine**, **ranitidine** and **famotidine** are available from pharmacies for short-term use, without prescription.

Unwanted effects are rare. Diarrhoea, dizziness, muscle pains, alopecia, transient rashes, confusion in the elderly and hypergastrinaemia have been reported. **Cimetidine** sometimes causes gynaecomastia in men and, rarely, a decrease in sexual function. This is probably caused by a modest affinity for androgen receptors. **Cimetidine** (but not other H_2 receptor antagonists) also inhibits cytochrome P450 and can retard the metabolism (and thus potentiate the action) of a range of drugs including oral anticoagulants and tricyclic antidepressants.

PROTON PUMP INHIBITORS

The first proton pump inhibitor was **omeprazole**, which irreversibly inhibits the H^+-K^+-ATPase (the proton pump), the terminal step in the acid secretory pathway (see Figs 30.1 and 30.2). Both basal and stimulated gastric acid secretion (Fig. 30.4) is reduced. The drug comprises a racemic mixture of two enantiomers. As a weak base, it accumulates in the acid environment of the canaliculi of the stimulated parietal cell where it is converted into an achiral form and is then able

[4]This era has been referred to as the 'BC' – before cimetidine – era of gastroenterology (Schubert and Peura, 2008)! It is an indication of the clinical importance of the development of this drug.

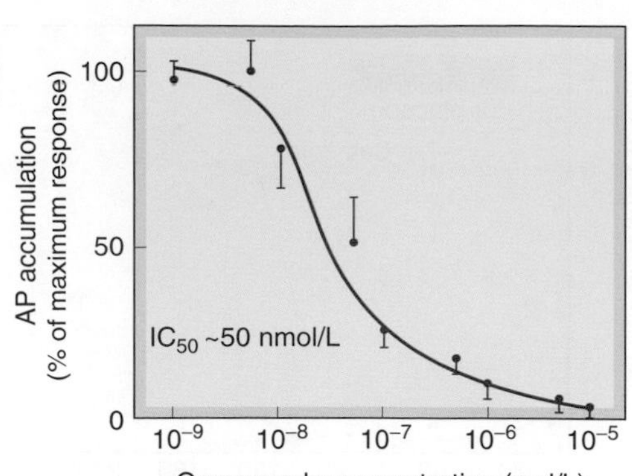

Fig. 30.4 The inhibitory action of omeprazole on acid secretion from isolated human gastric glands stimulated by 50 μmol/L histamine. Acid secretion was measured by the accumulation of a radiolabelled weak base, aminopyrine (AP), in the secretory channels. The data represent the mean and standard error of measurements from eight patients. (Adapted from Lindberg, P., et al., 1987. Trends Pharmacol. Sci. 8, 399–402.)

to react with, and inactivate, the ATPase. This preferential accumulation means that it has a specific effect on these cells. Other proton pump inhibitors (all of which have a similar mode of activation and pharmacology) include **esomeprazole** (the [S] isomer of omeprazole), **lansoprazole**, **pantoprazole** and **rabeprazole**. The clinical indication for these drugs is given in the clinical box (see earlier).

Pharmacokinetic aspects and unwanted effects

Oral administration is the most common route of administration, although some injectable preparations are available. **Omeprazole** is given orally, but as it degrades rapidly at low pH, it is administered as capsules containing enteric-coated granules. Following absorption in the small intestine, it passes from the blood into the parietal cells and then into the canaliculi where it exerts its effects. Increased doses give disproportionately higher increases in plasma concentration (possibly because its inhibitory effect on acid secretion improves its own bioavailability). Although its half-life is about 1 h, a single daily dose affects acid secretion for 2–3 days, partly because of the accumulation in the canaliculi and partly because it inhibits the H^+-K^+-ATPase irreversibly. With daily dosage, there is an increasing antisecretory effect for up to 5 days, after which a plateau is reached.

Unwanted effects of this class of drugs are uncommon. They may include headache, diarrhoea (both sometimes severe) and rashes. Acid suppression with proton pump inhibitors is associated with increased risk of *Clostridium difficile* diarrhoea, particularly in patients who are immunosuppressed or have been receiving antibiotics. Dizziness, somnolence, mental confusion, impotence, gynaecomastia and pain in muscles and joints have been reported. Proton pump inhibitors should be used with caution in patients with liver disease, or in women who are pregnant or breastfeeding. The use of these drugs may 'mask' the symptoms of gastric cancer.

ANTACIDS

Antacids are the simplest way to treat the symptoms of excessive gastric acid secretion. They directly neutralise acid and this also has the effect of inhibiting the activity of peptic enzymes, which practically ceases at pH 5. Given in sufficient quantity for long enough, they can produce healing of duodenal ulcers, but are less effective for gastric ulcers.

Most antacids in common use are salts of magnesium and aluminium. Magnesium salts cause diarrhoea and aluminium salts, constipation – so mixtures of these two can, happily, be used to preserve normal bowel function. Preparations of these substances (e.g. **magnesium trisilicate** mixtures and some proprietary aluminium preparations) containing high concentrations of sodium should not be given to patients on a sodium-restricted diet. Numerous antacid preparations are available; a few of the more significant are given later.

Magnesium hydroxide is an insoluble powder that forms magnesium chloride in the stomach. It does not produce systemic alkalosis, because Mg^{2+} is poorly absorbed from the gut. Another salt, magnesium trisilicate, is an insoluble powder that reacts slowly with the gastric juice, forming magnesium chloride and colloidal silica. This agent has a prolonged antacid effect, and it also adsorbs pepsin. **Magnesium carbonate** is also used.

Aluminium hydroxide gel forms aluminium chloride in the stomach; when this reaches the intestine, the chloride is released and is reabsorbed. Aluminium hydroxide raises the pH of the gastric juice to about 4, and also adsorbs pepsin. Its action is gradual, and its effect continues for several hours.[5] Colloidal aluminium hydroxide combines with phosphates in the GI tract and the increased excretion of phosphate in the faeces that occurs results in decreased excretion of phosphate via the kidney. This effect has been used in treating patients with chronic renal failure (see Ch. 30). Other preparations such as **hydrotalcite** contain mixtures of both aluminium and magnesium salts.

Alginates or **simeticone** are sometimes combined with antacids. Alginates are believed to increase the viscosity and adherence of mucus to the oesophageal mucosa, forming a protective barrier, whereas **simeticone** is an anti-foaming agent, intended to relieve bloating and flatulence.

TREATMENT OF *HELICOBACTER PYLORI* INFECTION

H. pylori infection has been implicated as a causative factor in the production of gastric and, more particularly, duodenal ulcers, as well as a risk factor for gastric cancer. Indeed, some would argue that infectious gastroduodenitis is actually the chief clinical entity associated with ulcers, and gastric cancer its prominent sequela. Certainly, eradication of *H. pylori* infection promotes rapid and long-term healing of ulcers, and it is routine practice to test for the organism in patients presenting with suggestive symptoms. If the test is positive, then the organism can generally be eradicated with a 1- or 2-week regimen of 'triple therapy', comprising a proton pump inhibitor in combination with the antibacterials **amoxicillin** and **metronidazole** or **clarithromycin** (see Ch. 52); other combinations are also used. Bismuth-containing preparations (see later) are

[5]There was a suggestion – no longer widely believed – that aluminium could trigger Alzheimer's disease. In fact, aluminium is not absorbed to any significant extent following oral administration of aluminium hydroxide, although when introduced by other routes (e.g. during renal dialysis with aluminium-contaminated solutions) it is extremely toxic.

sometimes added. While elimination of the bacillus can produce long-term remission of ulcers, reinfection with the organism can occur.

DRUGS THAT PROTECT THE MUCOSA

Some agents, termed *cytoprotective*, are said to enhance endogenous mucosal protection mechanisms and/or to provide a physical barrier over the surface of the ulcer.

Bismuth chelate

Bismuth chelate (tripotassium dicitratobismuthate) is sometimes used in combination regimens to treat *H. pylori*. It has toxic effects on the bacillus and may also prevent its adherence to the mucosa or inhibit its bacterial proteolytic enzymes. It is also believed to have other mucosa-protecting actions, by mechanisms that are unclear, and is widely used as an over-the-counter remedy for mild GI symptoms. Very little is absorbed, but if renal excretion is impaired, the raised plasma concentrations of bismuth can result in encephalopathy.

Unwanted effects include nausea and vomiting and blackening of the tongue and faeces.

Sucralfate

Sucralfate is a complex of aluminium hydroxide and sulfated sucrose, which releases aluminium in the presence of acid. The residual complex carries a strong negative charge and binds to cationic groups in proteins, glycoproteins, etc. It can form complex gels with mucus, an action that is thought to decrease the degradation of mucus by pepsin and to limit the diffusion of H^+ ions. Sucralfate can also inhibit the action of pepsin and stimulate secretion of mucus, bicarbonate and PGs from the gastric mucosa. All these actions contribute to its mucosa-protecting action.

Sucralfate is given orally and about 30% is still present in the stomach 3 h after administration. In the acid environment, the polymerised product forms a tenacious paste, which can sometimes produce an obstructive lump (known as a *bezoar*[6]) that gets stuck in the stomach. It reduces the absorption of a number of other drugs, including fluoroquinolone antibiotics, **theophylline**, **tetracycline**, **digoxin** and **amitriptyline**. Because it requires an acid environment for activation, antacids given concurrently or prior to its administration will reduce its efficacy.

Unwanted effects are few, the most common being constipation. Less common effects apart from bezoar formation include dry mouth, nausea, vomiting, headache and rashes.

Misoprostol

PGs of the E and I series have a generally homeostatic protective action in the GI tract, and a deficiency in endogenous production (after ingestion of an NSAID, for example) may contribute to ulcer formation. **Misoprostol** is a stable analogue of PGE_1. It is given orally and is used to promote the healing of ulcers or to prevent the gastric damage that can occur with chronic use of NSAIDs. It exerts a direct action on the ECL cell (and possibly parietal cell also; see Fig. 30.2), inhibiting the basal secretion of gastric acid as well as the stimulation of production seen in response to food, pentagastrin and caffeine. It also increases mucosal blood flow and augments the secretion of mucus and bicarbonate.

Unwanted effects include diarrhoea and abdominal cramps; uterine contractions can also occur, so the drug should not be given during pregnancy (unless deliberately to induce a therapeutic abortion; see Ch. 35). PGs and NSAIDs are discussed more fully in Chapter 25.

VOMITING

Nausea and vomiting are unwanted side effects of many clinically used drugs, notably those used for cancer chemotherapy but also opioids, general anaesthetics and digoxin. They also occur in motion sickness,[7] during early pregnancy and in numerous disease states (e.g. migraine) as well as bacterial and viral infections.

THE REFLEX MECHANISM OF VOMITING

Vomiting is a defensive response intended to rid the organism of toxic or irritating material. Poisonous compounds, bacterial toxins and many cytotoxic drugs (as well as mechanical distension) trigger the release, from enterochromaffin cells in the lining of the GI tract, of mediators such as 5-HT. These transmitters trigger signals in vagal afferent fibres. The physical act of vomiting is co-ordinated centrally by the *vomiting* (or *emetic*) *centre* in the medulla (Fig. 30.5). Actually, this is not a discrete anatomical location but a network of neural pathways that integrate signals arriving from other locations. One of these, in the *area postrema*, is known as the *chemoreceptor trigger zone* (CTZ). The CTZ receives inputs from the labyrinth in the inner ear through the *vestibular nuclei* (which explains the mechanism of motion sickness) and vagal afferents arising from the GI tract. Toxic chemicals in the bloodstream can also be detected directly by the CTZ because the blood–brain barrier is relatively permeable in this area. The CTZ is therefore a primary site of action of many emetic and antiemetic drugs (Table 30.1).

The vomiting centre also receives signals directly from vagal afferents, as well as those relayed through the CTZ. In addition, it receives input from higher cortical centres, explaining why unpleasant or repulsive sights or smells, or strong emotional stimuli, can sometimes induce nausea and vomiting.

The main neurotransmitters involved in this neurocircuitry are acetylcholine, histamine, 5-HT, dopamine and substance P and receptors for these transmitters have been demonstrated in the relevant areas (see Chs 13–17). It has been hypothesised that enkephalins (see Ch. 43) are also implicated in the mediation of vomiting, acting possibly at δ (CTZ) or μ (vomiting centre) opioid receptors. Substance P (see Ch. 17) acting at neurokinin-1 receptors in the CTZ, and endocannabinoids (see Ch. 18), may also be involved.

The neurobiology of nausea is much less well understood. Nausea and vomiting may occur together or separately and may subserve different physiological functions (see Andrews and Horn, 2006). From the pharmacologist's viewpoint, it is easier to control vomiting than nausea, and many effective antiemetics (e.g. 5-HT_3 antagonists) are much less successful in this regard.

[6]From the Persian word meaning 'a cure for poisoning'. It refers to the belief that a concoction made from lumps of impacted rubbish retrieved from the stomach of goats would protect against poisoning by one's enemies.

[7]In fact, the word *nausea* is derived from the Greek word meaning 'boat', with the obvious implication of associated motion sickness. *Vomiting* is derived from a Latin word and a *vomitorium* was the 'fast exit' passageway in ancient theatres. It has a certain resonance, as we think you will agree!

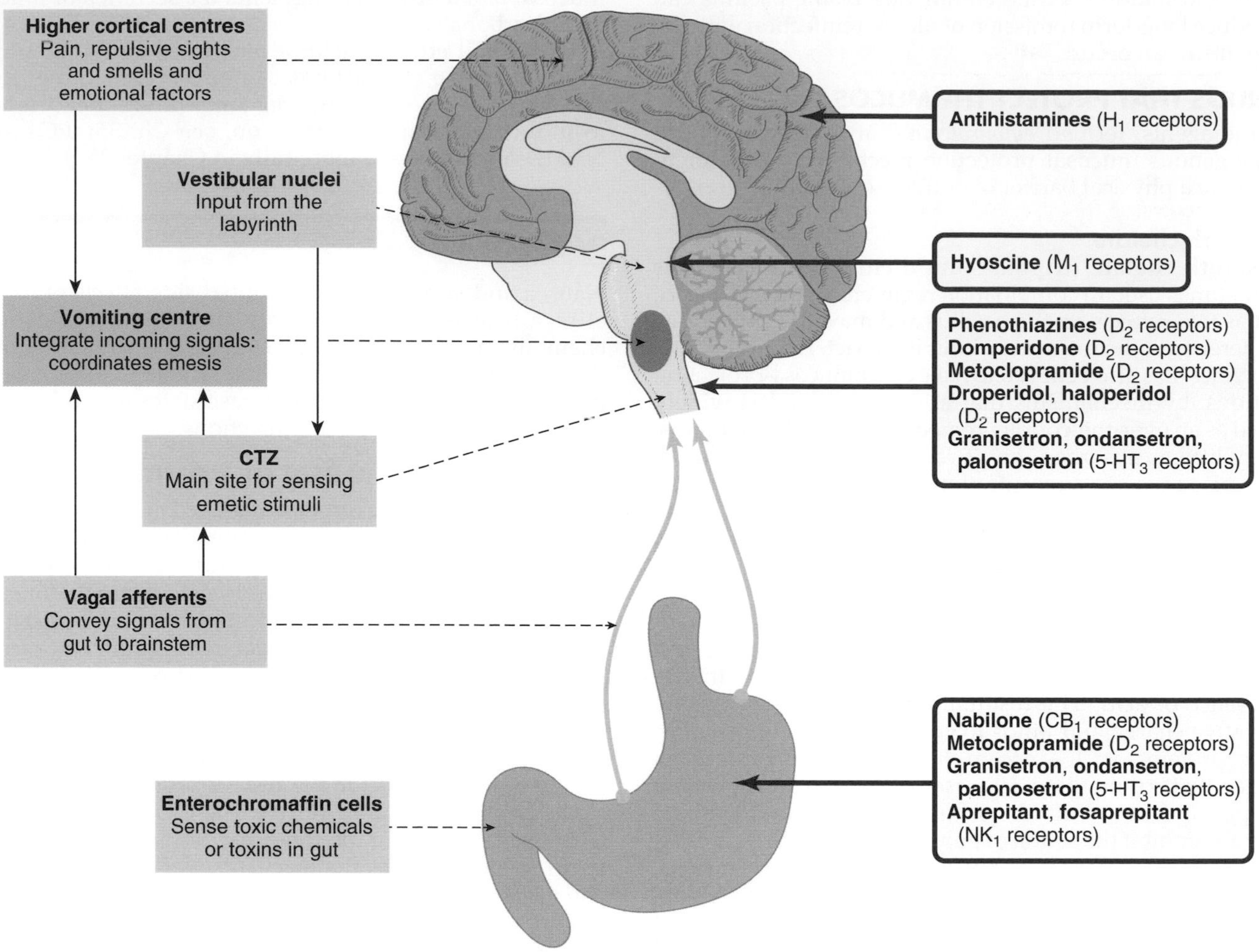

Fig. 30.5 Schematic diagram of the factors involved in the control of vomiting, with the probable sites of action of antiemetic drugs. There are three important centres located in the medulla. The chemoreceptor trigger zone (CTZ), the vomiting centre and the vestibular nuclei. The vomiting centre receives inputs from the CTZ, the gastrointestinal (GI) tract (through vagal afferent connections) and higher cortical centres and coordinates the physical act of emesis. Vagal afferents arising from the GI tract also feed into the CTZ directly as does input from the vestibular nuclei, which in turn receive inputs from the labyrinth. (Based partly on a diagram from Rojas, C., Slusher, B.S., 2012. Pharmacological mechanisms of 5-HT(3) and tachykinin NK(1) receptor antagonism to prevent chemotherapy-induced nausea and vomiting. Eur. J. Pharmacol. 684, 1–7.)

The reflex mechanism of vomiting

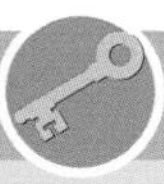

Emetic stimuli include:

- chemicals or drugs in the blood or intestine;
- neuronal input from the GI tract, labyrinth and central nervous system (CNS).

  Pathways and mediators include:
- impulses from the CTZ and various other CNS centres relayed to the vomiting centre;
- chemical transmitters such as histamine, acetylcholine, dopamine, 5-HT and substance P, acting on H_1, muscarinic, D_2, $5\text{-}HT_3$ and NK_1 receptors, respectively.

  Antiemetic drugs include:
- H_1 receptor antagonists (e.g. **cinnarizine**);
- muscarinic antagonists (e.g. **hyoscine**);
- $5\text{-}HT_3$ receptor antagonists (e.g. **ondansetron**);
- D_2 receptor antagonists (e.g. **metoclopramide**);
- cannabinoids (e.g. **nabilone**);
- neurokinin-1 antagonists (e.g. **aprepitant**, **fosaprepitant**).

  Main side effects of principal antiemetics include:
- drowsiness and antiparasympathetic effects (**hyoscine**, **nabilone** > **cinnarizine**);
- dystonic reactions (**metoclopramide**);
- general CNS disturbances (**nabilone**);
- headache, GI tract upsets (**ondansetron**).

Table 30.1 Sites of action of common antiemetic drugs

Class	Drugs	Site of action	Comments
Antihistamines	Cinnarizine, cyclizine, promethazine	H_1 receptors in the CNS (causing sedation) and possibly anticholinergic actions in the vestibular apparatus	Widely effective regardless of cause of emesis. Doxylamine/pyridoxine is licensed in pregnancy
Antimuscarinics	Hyoscine	Anticholinergic actions in the vestibular apparatus and possibly elsewhere	Mainly motion sickness
Cannabinoids	Nabilone	Probably CB_1 receptors in the GI tract	CINV in patients where other drugs have been ineffective
Dopamine antagonists	Phenothiazines: prochlorphenazine, perphenazine, trifluorphenazine, chlorpromazine	D_2 receptors in CTZ	CINV, PONV, RS
	Related drugs: droperidol, haloperidol	D_2 receptors in GI tract	CINV, PONV, RS
	Metoclopramide	D_2 receptors in the CTZ and GI tract	PONV, CINV
Glucocorticoids	Dexamethasone	Probably multiple sites of action, including the GI tract	PONV, CINV; typically used in combination with other drugs
5-HT_3 antagonists	Granisteron, ondansetron, palonosetron	5-HT_3 receptors in CTZ and GI tract	PONV, CINV
Neurokinin-1 antagonists	Aprepitant, fosapreptitant	NK_1 receptors in CTZ, vomiting centre and possibly the GI tract	CINV; given in combination with another drug

5-HT, 5-Hydroxytryptamine; *CINV,* cytotoxic drug-induced vomiting; *CNS,* central nervous system; *CTZ,* chemoreceptor trigger zone; *GI,* gastrointestinal; *PONV,* postoperative nausea and vomiting; *RS,* radiation sickness.

ANTIEMETIC DRUGS

Several antiemetic agents are available, and these are generally used for specific conditions, although there may be some overlap. Such drugs are of particular importance as an adjunct to cancer chemotherapy, where the nausea and vomiting produced by many cytotoxic drugs (see Ch. 57) can be almost unendurable.[8] In using drugs to treat the morning sickness of pregnancy, the problem of potential damage to the fetus has always to be borne in mind. In general, all drugs should be avoided during the first 3 months of pregnancy, if possible. Details of the main categories of antiemetics are given later, and their main clinical uses are summarised in the box. The clinical box and Table 30.1 give an overview of their likely sites of action and their clinical utility.

RECEPTOR ANTAGONISTS

Many H_1 (see Ch. 25), muscarinic (see Ch. 14), 5-HT_3 (see Ch. 16), dopamine (see Ch. 47) and neurokinin NK_1 receptor antagonists exhibit clinically useful antiemetic activity.

H_1 receptor antagonists

Cinnarizine, **cyclizine** and **promethazine** are the most commonly employed; they are effective against nausea and vomiting arising from many causes, including motion sickness (even in NASA space journeys!), and the presence of irritants in the stomach. They are less effective against substances that act directly on the CTZ. Promethazine or **doxylamine** are used for morning sickness of pregnancy

[8]It was reported that a young, medically qualified patient being treated by combination chemotherapy for sarcoma stated that 'the severity of vomiting at times made the thought of death seem like a welcome relief'.

Clinical use of antiemetic drugs

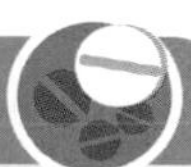

- Histamine H_1 receptor antagonists (see also clinical box in Ch. 25):
  - **Cyclizine**: motion sickness, vestibular disorders, nausea and vomiting associated with surgery and postoperative narcotic analgesic use.
  - **Cinnarizine**: motion sickness, vestibular disorders (e.g. Menière's disease).
  - **Promethazine**: severe morning sickness of pregnancy, motion sickness, vestibular disorders.
- Muscarinic receptor antagonists:
  - **Hyoscine**: motion sickness.
- Dopamine D_2 receptor antagonists:
  - Phenothiazines (e.g. **prochlorperazine**): vomiting caused by migraine, vestibular disorders, radiation, viral gastroenteritis, severe morning sickness of pregnancy.
  - **Metoclopramide**: vomiting caused by migraine, radiation, GI disorders, cytotoxic drugs, prevention of nausea and vomiting in the postoperative period.
  - **Domperidone** is less liable to cause CNS side effects in patients with Parkinson's disease as it penetrates the blood–brain barrier poorly.
- 5-HT_3 receptor antagonists (e.g. **ondansetron**): cytotoxic drugs or radiation, postoperative vomiting.
- Cannabinoids (e.g. **nabilone**): cytotoxic drugs (see Ch. 18).
- NK_1 receptor antagonists (e.g. fosaprepitant): cytotoxic drugs.

(on the rare occasions when this is so severe that drug treatment is required). Drowsiness and sedation, while possibly contributing to their clinical efficacy, are the chief unwanted effects.

Betahistine has complicated effects on histamine action, antagonising H_3 receptors but having a weak agonist activity on H_1 receptors. It is used to control the nausea and vertigo associated with *Menière's disease*.[9]

Muscarinic receptor antagonists

Hyoscine (scopolamine) is employed principally for prophylaxis and treatment of motion sickness and may be administered orally or as a transdermal patch. Dry mouth and blurred vision are the most common unwanted effects. Drowsiness also occurs, but the drug has less sedative action than the antihistamines because of poor CNS penetration.

5-HT_3 receptor antagonists

Granisetron, **ondansetron** and **palonosetron** (see Ch. 16) are of particular value in preventing and treating the vomiting and, to a lesser extent the nausea, commonly encountered postoperatively as well as that caused by radiation therapy or administration of cytotoxic drugs such as **cisplatin**. The primary site of action of these drugs is the CTZ. They may be given orally or by injection (sometimes helpful if nausea is already present). Unwanted effects such as headache and GI upsets are relatively uncommon.

Dopamine antagonists

Antipsychotic phenothiazines (see Ch. 47), such as **chlorpromazine**, **perphenazine**, **prochlorperazine** and **trifluoperazine**, are effective antiemetics commonly used for treating the more severe nausea and vomiting associated with cancer, radiation therapy, cytotoxic drugs, opioids, anaesthetics and other drugs. They can be administered orally, intravenously or by suppository. They act mainly as antagonists of the dopamine D_2 receptors in the CTZ (see Fig. 30.5) but they also block histamine and muscarinic receptors.

Unwanted effects are common and include sedation (especially chlorpromazine), hypotension and extrapyramidal symptoms including dystonias and tardive dyskinesia (see Ch. 47).

Other antipsychotic drugs, such as **haloperidol**, the related compound **droperidol** and **levomepromazine** (see Ch. 47), also act as D_2 antagonists in the CTZ and can be used for acute chemotherapy-induced emesis.

Metoclopramide and domperidone

Metoclopramide is a D_2 receptor antagonist (see Fig. 30.5), closely related to the phenothiazine group, that acts centrally on the CTZ and also has a peripheral action on the GI tract itself, increasing the motility of the oesophagus, stomach and intestine. This not only adds to the antiemetic effect but explains its use in the treatment of gastro-oesophageal reflux and hepatic and biliary disorders. As **metoclopramide** also blocks dopamine receptors elsewhere in the CNS, it produces a number of unwanted effects including disorders of movement (more common in children and young adults), fatigue, motor restlessness, spasmodic torticollis (involuntary twisting of the neck) and oculogyric crises (involuntary upward eye movements). It stimulates prolactin release (see Ch. 35) causing galactorrhoea and disorders of menstruation.

Domperidone is a similar drug used to treat vomiting due to cytotoxic therapy as well as GI symptoms. Unlike **metoclopramide**, it does not readily penetrate the blood–brain barrier and is consequently less prone to producing central side effects. However, **domperidone** is associated with a small increased risk of serious cardiac adverse effects (particularly at higher doses and in older patients), and its use is now restricted.

Both drugs are given orally, have plasma half-lives of 4–5 h and are excreted in the urine.

[9]A disabling condition named after the eponymous French physician who discovered that the nausea and vertigo that characterise this condition were associated with a disorder of the inner ear.

NK_1 receptor antagonists

Substance P causes vomiting when injected intravenously and is released by GI vagal afferent nerves as well as in the vomiting centre itself. **Aprepitant** blocks substance P (NK_1) receptors in the CTZ and vomiting centre. **Aprepitant** is given orally and is effective in controlling the late phase of emesis caused by cytotoxic drugs, with few significant unwanted effects. **Fosaprepitant** is a prodrug of **aprepitant**, which is administered intravenously.

OTHER ANTIEMETIC DRUGS

Anecdotal evidence originally suggested the possibility of using cannabinoids (see Ch. 18) as antiemetics (see Pertwee, 2001). The synthetic cannabinol **nabilone** has been found to decrease vomiting caused by agents that stimulate the CTZ and is sometimes effective where other drugs have failed. The antiemetic effect is antagonised by **naloxone**, which implies that opioid receptors may be important in the mechanism of action. Nabilone is given orally; it is well absorbed from the GI tract and is metabolised in many tissues. Its plasma half-life is approximately 120 min, and its metabolites are excreted in the urine and faeces.

Unwanted effects are common, especially drowsiness, dizziness and dry mouth. Mood changes and postural hypotension are also fairly frequent. Some patients experience hallucinations and psychotic reactions, resembling the effect of other cannabinoids (see Ch. 18).

High-dose glucocorticoids (particularly **dexamethasone**; see Chs 25 and 33) can also control emesis, especially when this is caused by cytotoxic drugs. The mechanism of action is not clear. **Dexamethasone** is typically deployed in combination with **metoclopramide** or **ondansetron** in patients receiving cytotoxics, or in postoperative nausea and vomiting.

THE MOTILITY OF THE GI TRACT

Drugs that alter the motility of the GI tract include:

- purgatives, which accelerate the passage of food through the intestine;
- agents that increase the motility of the GI smooth muscle without causing purgation;
- antidiarrhoeal drugs, which decrease motility;
- antispasmodic drugs, which decrease smooth muscle tone.

Clinical uses of drugs that affect the motility of the GI tract are summarised in the clinical box.

Drugs and GI tract motility

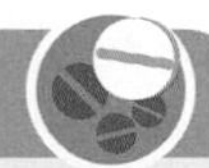

- Purgatives include:
  - bulk laxatives (e.g. **ispaghula husk**, first choice for slow action);
  - osmotic laxatives (e.g. **lactulose**);
  - faecal softeners (e.g. **docusate**);
  - stimulant purgatives (e.g. **senna**).
- Drugs used to treat diarrhoea:
  - oral rehydration with isotonic solutions of NaCl plus glucose and starch-based cereal (important in infants);
  - antimotility agents, e.g. **loperamide** (unwanted effects: drowsiness and nausea).

PURGATIVES

The transit of food through the intestine may be hastened by several different types of drugs, including laxatives, faecal softeners and stimulant purgatives. The latter agents may be used to relieve constipation or to clear the bowel prior to surgery or examination.

BULK AND OSMOTIC LAXATIVES

The *bulk laxatives* include **methylcellulose** and certain plant extracts such as **sterculia**, **agar**, **bran** and **ispaghula husk**. These agents are polysaccharide polymers that are not digested in the upper part of the GI tract. They form a bulky hydrated mass in the gut lumen promoting peristalsis and improving faecal consistency. They may take several days to work but have no serious unwanted effects.

The *osmotic laxatives* consist of poorly absorbed solutes – the saline purgatives – and **lactulose**. The main salts in use are magnesium sulfate and magnesium hydroxide. By producing an osmotic load, these agents trap increased volumes of fluid in the lumen of the bowel, accelerating the transfer of the gut contents through the small intestine. This results in an abnormally large volume entering the colon, causing distension and purgation within about an hour. Abdominal cramps can occur. The amount of magnesium absorbed after an oral dose is usually too small to have adverse systemic effects, but these salts should be avoided in small children and in patients with poor renal function, in whom they can cause heart block, neuromuscular block or CNS depression. While isotonic or hypotonic solutions of saline purgatives cause purgation, hypertonic solutions can cause vomiting. Sometimes, other sodium salts of phosphate and citrate are given rectally, by suppository, to relieve constipation.

Lactulose is a semisynthetic disaccharide of fructose and galactose. It is poorly absorbed and produces an effect similar to that of the other osmotic laxatives. It takes 2–3 days to act. Unwanted effects, seen with high doses, include flatulence, cramps, diarrhoea and electrolyte disturbance. Tolerance can develop. Another agent, **macrogol**, which consists of inert ethylene glycol polymers, acts in the same way, and is sometimes formulated together with electrolyte ions to ensure that the laxative effect does not cause marked changes in sodium, potassium and water balance.

FAECAL SOFTENERS

Docusate sodium is a surface-active compound that acts in the GI tract in a manner similar to a detergent and produces softer faeces. It is also a weak stimulant laxative. Other agents that achieve the same effect include **arachis oil**, which is given as an enema, and **liquid paraffin**, although this is now seldom used.

STIMULANT LAXATIVES

The stimulant laxative drugs act mainly by increasing electrolyte and hence water secretion by the mucosa, and by increasing peristalsis – possibly by stimulating enteric nerves. Abdominal cramping may be experienced as a side effect with almost any of these drugs.

Bisacodyl may be given by mouth but is often given by suppository. In the latter case, it stimulates the rectal mucosa, inducing defecation in 15–30 min. Glycerol suppositories act in the same manner. **Sodium picosulfate** and docusate sodium have similar actions. The former is given orally and is often used in preparation for intestinal surgery or colonoscopy.

Senna and **dantron** are **anthraquinone** laxatives. The active principle (after hydrolysis of glycosidic linkages in the case of the plant extract, senna) directly stimulates the myenteric plexus, resulting in increased peristalsis and thus defecation. **Dantron** is similar. As this drug is a skin irritant and may be carcinogenic, it is generally used only in the terminally ill.

Laxatives of any type should not be used when there is obstruction of the bowel. Overuse can lead to an atonic colon where the natural propulsive activity is diminished. In these circumstances, the only way to achieve defecation is to take further amounts of laxatives, so a sort of dependency arises.

DRUGS THAT INCREASE GASTROINTESTINAL MOTILITY

Domperidone is primarily used as an antiemetic (as described previously), but it also increases GI motility (although the mechanism is unknown).

Metoclopramide (also an antiemetic) stimulates gastric motility, causing a marked acceleration of gastric emptying. It is useful in gastro-oesophageal reflux and in disorders of gastric emptying but is ineffective in paralytic ileus.

Prucalopride is a selective 5-HT_4 receptor agonist that has marked prokinetic properties on the gut. It is generally only used when other types of laxative treatment have failed. Similarly, **tegaserod** is used to treat symptoms of constipation in those with irritable bowel syndrome (IBS) (see later).

Lubiprostone is a chloride channel-2 activator that acts on cells in the apical membrane of the small intestine to promote chloride and fluid secretion into the lumen, with associated improvements in gut motility and softer stool. It has regulatory approval for treatment of constipation due to opioids, in IBS and in patients who have failed to respond to non-drug treatment of constipation.

Naloxegol is a μ opioid-receptor antagonist that is similar to naloxone, but with the addition of a pegylated portion to prevent penetration into the CNS. **Naloxegol** counteracts the reduced GI motility and hypertonicity that is seen in opioid-induced constipation, but without exerting any adverse effect on the analgesic properties of opioid agonists centrally. **Methylnaltrexone** is a peripheral opioid-receptor antagonist that is licensed for opioid-induced constipation, and **naldemedine** is a similar compound (Nelson and Camilleri, 2016).

Elobixibat is licensed in Japan for treatment of chronic idiopathic constipation. It is an inhibitor of the ileal bile acid transporter which is responsible for re-absorption of bile salts from the terminal ileum. The suppression of bile salt reabsorption leads to greater bile acid progress into the colon, with increased water secretion and motility.

ANTIDIARRHOEAL AGENTS

There are numerous causes of diarrhoea, including underlying disease, infection, toxins and even anxiety. It may also arise as a side effect of drug or radiation therapy. The consequences range from mild discomfort and inconvenience to a medical emergency requiring hospitalisation, parenteral fluid and electrolyte replacement therapy. Globally, acute diarrhoeal disease is one of the principal causes of death in malnourished infants, especially in developing countries where medical care is less accessible and 1–2 million children die each year for want of simple counter-measures.

During an episode of diarrhoea, there is an increase in the motility of the GI tract, accompanied by an increased secretion, coupled with a decreased absorption, of fluid. This leads to a loss of electrolytes (particularly Na^+) and water. Cholera toxins and some other bacterial toxins produce a profound increase in electrolyte and fluid secretion by irreversibly activating the G proteins that couple the surface receptors of the mucosal cells to adenylyl cyclase (see Ch. 3).

There are three approaches to the treatment of severe acute diarrhoea:

- maintenance of fluid and electrolyte balance;
- use of anti-infective agents;
- use of spasmolytic or other antidiarrhoeal agents.

The maintenance of fluid and electrolyte balance by means of oral rehydration is the first priority. Wider application of this cheap and simple remedy could save the lives of many infants in the developing world. Indeed, many patients require no other treatment.

In the ileum, as in the nephron, there is co-transport of Na^+ and glucose across the epithelial cell. The presence of glucose (and some amino acids) therefore enhances Na^+ absorption and thus water uptake. Preparations of sodium chloride and glucose for oral rehydration are available in powder form, ready to be dissolved in water before use.

Many GI infections are viral in origin. Those that are bacterial generally resolve fairly rapidly, so the use of anti-infective agents is usually neither necessary nor useful. Other cases may require more aggressive therapy, however. *Campylobacter* spp. is the commonest cause of bacterial gastroenteritis in the United Kingdom, and severe infections may require **ciprofloxacin**. The most common bacterial organisms encountered by travellers include *Escherichia coli*, *Salmonella* and *Shigella*, as well as protozoa such as *Giardia* and *Cryptosporidium* spp. Drug treatment (Chs 52 and 55) may be necessary in these and other more serious infections.

TRAVELLER'S DIARRHOEA

Millions of people cross international borders each year. Many travel hopefully, but some return with GI symptoms such as diarrhoea, having encountered enterotoxin-producing *E. coli* (the most common cause) or other organisms. Most infections are mild and self-limiting, requiring only oral replacement of fluid and salt, as detailed previously. The general principles for the drug treatment of traveller's diarrhoea are detailed by Leung et al. (2019). Recent guidelines on the role of drug treatments such as antimotility agents, bismuth and antibiotics for more severe cases are listed in the Further Reading section.

ANTIMOTILITY AND SPASMOLYTIC AGENTS

The main pharmacological agents that decrease motility are opioids (see Ch. 43) and muscarinic receptor antagonists (see Ch. 14). Agents in this latter group are seldom employed as primary therapy for diarrhoea because of their actions on other systems, but small doses of **atropine** are sometimes used, combined with **diphenoxylate**. The action of **morphine**, the archetypal opiate, on the alimentary tract is complex; it increases the tone and rhythmic contractions of the intestine but diminishes propulsive activity. The pyloric, ileocolic and anal sphincters are contracted, and the tone of the large intestine is markedly increased. Its overall effect is constipating.

The main opioids used for the symptomatic relief of diarrhoea are **codeine** (a morphine congener), diphenoxylate and **loperamide** (both **pethidine** congeners that do not readily penetrate the blood–brain barrier and are used only for their actions in the gut). All may have unwanted effects, including constipation, abdominal cramps, drowsiness and dizziness. Complete loss of intestinal motility (paralytic ileus) can also occur. They should not be used in young (<4 years of age) children.

Loperamide is the drug of first choice for pharmacotherapy of traveller's diarrhoea and is a component of several proprietary antidiarrhoeal medicines. It has a relatively selective action on the GI tract and undergoes significant enterohepatic cycling. It reduces the frequency of abdominal cramps, decreases the passage of faeces and shortens the duration of the illness.

Diphenoxylate also lacks morphine-like activity in the CNS, although large doses (25-fold higher) produce typical opioid effects. Preparations of diphenoxylate usually contain atropine as well. **Codeine** and **loperamide** have antisecretory actions in addition to their effects on intestinal motility.

'Endogenous opioids', enkephalins (see Ch. 43), also play a role in regulation of intestinal secretion. **Racecadotril** is a prodrug of **thiorphan**, an inhibitor of enkephalinase. By preventing the breakdown of enkephalins, this drug reduces the excessive intestinal secretion seen during episodes of diarrhoea. It is used in combination with rehydration therapy.

Cannabinoid receptor agonists also reduce gut motility in animals, most probably by decreasing acetylcholine release from enteric nerves. There have been anecdotal reports of a beneficial effect of cannabis against dysentery and cholera.

Drugs that reduce GI motility are also useful in IBS and diverticular disease. Muscarinic receptor antagonists (see Ch. 14) used for this purpose include atropine, hyoscine, **propantheline** and **dicycloverine**. The last named is thought to have some additional direct relaxant action on smooth muscle. All produce antimuscarinic side effects such as dry mouth, blurred vision and urinary retention. **Mebeverine**, a derivative of **reserpine**, has a direct relaxant action on GI smooth muscle. Unwanted effects are few.

ADSORBENTS

Adsorbent agents are used in the symptomatic treatment of some types of diarrhoea, although properly controlled trials proving efficacy have not been carried out. The main preparations used contain kaolin, pectin, chalk, charcoal, methylcellulose and activated attapulgite (magnesium aluminium silicate). It has been suggested that these agents may act by adsorbing microorganisms or toxins, by altering the intestinal flora or by coating and protecting the intestinal mucosa, but there is no hard evidence for this. Kaolin is sometimes given as a mixture with morphine (e.g. kaolin and morphine mixture BP).

DRUGS FOR CHRONIC BOWEL DISEASE

This category comprises *IBS* and *inflammatory bowel disease* (IBD). IBS is characterised by bouts of diarrhoea (IBS-D), constipation (IBS-C) or abdominal pain, and some patients may have a mixture of symptoms (IBS-M) recurring periodically. The aetiology of IBS is uncertain, but alterations in the gut–brain axis, visceral hypersensitivity and psychological factors may play a part. Treatment is symptomatic, with a high-residue diet, **loperamide** for diarrhoea symptoms or a laxative (such as **isphagula** husk) if needed for constipation.

The serotoninergic or 5-HT pathway is thought to be one of the drivers leading to excess GI motility and secretion in IBS. Treatment of IBS-D includes the 5-HT_3 receptor antagonists **alosetron** and **ramosetron** which decrease gut motility, thus allowing more time for water reabsorption and reduction of watery stools. The opposing effect is seen with **tegaserod**, a 5-HT_4 agonist which stimulates GI motility to reduce bloating and constipation. Use of serotoninergic drugs in IBS has faced major regulatory hurdles, with both **alosetron** and **tegaserod** having been withdrawn from the US market, and then subsequently re-instated with stringent conditions.

Eluxadoline is a mixed μ and κ opioid-receptor agonist and δ-receptor antagonist that has recently been licensed for treatment of IBS with diarrhoea. The drug acts on opioid receptors in enteric neurons that regulate motility and visceral sensation in the GI tract, resulting in slowing of intestinal transit and improved stool consistency. **Eluxadoline** has low oral bioavailability and is considered to have limited potential for adverse effects on opioid receptors in the CNS (see Corsetti and Whorwell, 2016).

Linaclotide is used for symptomatic treatment of moderate to severe IBS with constipation in adults. It is a synthetic peptide that is structurally related to endogenous guanylin peptides. Linaclotide is an agonist at the guanylate cyclase-C receptor on the luminal surface of intestinal epithelium and increases the concentration of cyclic guanosine monophosphate in the intestinal cells. This results in greater secretion of chloride and bicarbonate ions and intestinal fluid, as well as more rapid intestinal transit. Clinical trials have demonstrated improvements in bowel movements and reduction in abdominal discomfort, although diarrhoea is a recognised adverse effect (see Corsetti and Whorwell, 2016). **Plecanatide** is a uroguanylin analogue that works in a similar way to **linaclotide**.

An alternative method of promoting softer stools and increasing stool frequency is to block sodium reabsorption in the small intestine. This can be achieved by inhibiting the sodium/hydrogen exchanger isoform 3, which is an antiporter found in the apical membrane of intestinal cells. **Tenapanor** (licensed in the United States) acts locally on the gut to promote sodium excretion and increased frequency of bowel movements in those with IBS-C.

Ulcerative colitis and *Crohn's disease* are forms of IBD, affecting the colon or ileum. They are autoimmune inflammatory disorders, which can be severe and progressive, requiring long-term drug treatment with anti-inflammatory and immunosuppressant drugs (see Ch. 25), and occasionally surgical resection. The following agents are commonly used.

GLUCOCORTICOIDS

Glucocorticoids are potent anti-inflammatory agents and are dealt with in Chapters 25 and 33. The drugs of choice are generally **prednisolone** or **budesonide** (although others can be used). They are administered orally or locally into the bowel by suppository or enema.

AMINOSALICYLATES

While glucocorticoids are useful for the acute attacks of IBDs, they are not ideal for long-term treatment because of their side effects. Maintenance of remission in both ulcerative colitis and Crohn's disease is generally achieved with aminosalicylates, although they are less useful in the latter condition.

Sulfasalazine consists of the sulfonamide **sulfapyridine** linked to 5-aminosalicylic acid (5-ASA). The latter forms the active moiety when it is released in the colon. Its mechanism of action is obscure. It may reduce inflammation by scavenging free radicals, by inhibiting PG and leukotriene production and/or by decreasing neutrophil chemotaxis and superoxide generation. Its unwanted effects include diarrhoea, salicylate sensitivity and interstitial nephritis. **5-ASA** is not absorbed, but the **sulfapyridine** moiety, which seems to be therapeutically inert in this instance, is absorbed, and its unwanted effects are those associated with the sulfonamides (see Ch. 52).

Newer compounds in this class, which presumably share a similar mechanism of action, include **mesalazine** (**5-ASA** itself), **olsalazine** (a **5-ASA** dimer linked by a bond that is hydrolysed by colonic bacteria) and **balsalazide** (a prodrug from which **5-ASA** is also released following hydrolysis of a diazo linkage).

OTHER DRUGS

Methotrexate and the immunosuppressants **ciclosporin**, **tacrolimus**, **azathioprine** and **6-mercaptopurine** (see Ch. 25) are also sometimes used in patients with severe IBD. The biopharmaceuticals **infliximab, adalimumab** and **golimumab**, monoclonal antibodies directed against tumour necrosis factor (TNF)-α (see Ch. 25), have also been used with success. These drugs are expensive, and their principal indication is for moderate and severe IBD that is unresponsive to glucocorticoids or immunomodulators.

Newer biopharmaceutical agents have been developed towards alternative targets in the inflammatory pathway. **Vedolizumab** is a humanised monoclonal antibody with specific binding properties for α4β7 integrin on T-helper lymphocytes that migrate to the gut. The inhibition of α4β7 integrin stops the interaction of these lymphocytes with mucosal addressin cell adhesion molecule-1 on gut epithelial cells, thus reducing the inflammatory effects in the bowel tissue that arise from trans-migration of T lymphocytes. In contrast, **ustekinumab** is targeted at the p40 protein subunit of interleukin (IL)-12 and IL-23 and prevents these cytokines from binding to IL-12Rβ1 receptors on immune cells. **Vedolizumab** and **ustekinumab** are indicated in those with moderately to severely active IBD, who have not responded to or cannot tolerate conventional treatment and other biopharmaceuticals.

The antiallergy drug sodium **cromoglicate** (see Ch. 28) is sometimes used for treating GI symptoms associated with food allergies.

DRUGS AFFECTING THE BILIARY SYSTEM

The commonest pathological condition of the biliary tract is *cholesterol cholelithiasis* – the formation of gallstones with high cholesterol content. Surgery is generally the preferred option in patients who are troubled by symptoms such as pain and infection. There are orally active drugs that dissolve non-calcified 'radiolucent' cholesterol gallstones. The principal agent is **ursodeoxycholic acid**, a minor constituent of human bile (but the main bile acid in the bear, hence *urso-*) but there is little evidence of therapeutic benefit. Diarrhoea is the main unwanted effect.

Biliary colic, the pain produced by the passage of gallstones through the bile duct, can be very intense, and immediate relief may be required. Clinical trials have demonstrated the efficacy of NSAIDs in relieving the pain of biliary colic, whilst opioid analgesics such as **morphine** and **pethidine** can also be used. Previous suggestions that morphine may have an undesirable local effect because it constricts the sphincter of Oddi and raises the pressure in the bile duct have not been borne out in clinical practice. Anticholinergic drugs (such as **dicyclomine**) are commonly employed to relieve biliary spasm and may be used in conjunction with morphine. **Glyceryl trinitrate** (see Ch. 19) can produce a marked fall of intrabiliary pressure and may be used to relieve biliary spasm.

FUTURE DIRECTIONS

The quest for novel antisecretory drugs is an ongoing task. Among the newer agents that have undergone evaluation are gastrin/CCK-2 receptor antagonists (with little success) and potassium competitive acid-blocking drugs (Inatomi et al., 2016). The latter agents work because potassium ions are exchanged for protons by the proton pump (see Fig. 30.1) and so potassium antagonists with rapid onset of action and sustained effect would represent a promising modality for inhibiting the secretion of acid. Unfortunately, the agents produced so far have not been proven conclusively to be superior to proton pump inhibitors, and currently, the available agents (**revaprazan, vonoprazan, tegoprazan**) are use in a limited number of conditions such as gastritis, erosive oesophagitis, and *H.pylori* eradication. The pharmacological therapy of IBS also remains a major challenge because of the complex interconnected networks of the gut–brain axis.

REFERENCES AND FURTHER READING

Innervation and hormones of the gastrointestinal tract

Hansen, M.B., 2003. The enteric nervous system II: gastrointestinal functions. Pharmacol. Toxicol. 92, 249–257.

Gros, M., Gros, B., Mesonero, J.E., et al., 2021. Neurotransmitter dysfunction in irritable bowel syndrome: emerging approaches for management. J. Clin. Med. 10, 3429.

Latorre, R., Sternini, C., De Giorgio, R., et al., 2016. Enteroendocrine cells: a review of their role in brain-gut communication. Neuro. Gastroenterol. Motil. 28, 620–630.

Mayer, E.A., 2011. Gut feelings: the emerging biology of gut-brain communication. Nat. Rev. Neurosci. 12, 453–466.

Gastric secretion

Binder, H.J., Donaldson Jr., R.M., 1978. Effect of cimetidine on intrinsic factor and pepsin secretion in man. Gastroenterology 74, 371–375.

Black, J.W., Duncan, W.A.M., Durant, C.J., et al., 1972. Definition and antagonism of histamine H_2-receptors. Nature 236, 385–390.

Herszényi, L., Bakucz, T., Barabás, L., et al., 2020. Pharmacological approach to gastric acid suppression: past, present, and future. Dig. Dis. 38, 104–111.

Inatomi, N., Matsukawa, J., Sakurai, Y., Otake, K., 2016. Potassium-competitive acid blockers: advanced therapeutic option for acid-related diseases. Pharmacol. Ther. 168, 12–22.

Schubert, M.L., Peura, D.A., 2008. Control of gastric acid secretion in health and disease. Gastroenterology 134, 1842–1860.

Pertwee, R.G., 2001. Cannabinoids and the gastrointestinal tract. Gut 48, 859–867.

Nausea and vomiting

Andrews, P.L., Horn, C.C., 2006. Signals for nausea and emesis: implications for models of upper gastrointestinal diseases. Auton. Neurosci. 125, 100–115.

Rojas, C., Slusher, B.S., 2012. Pharmacological mechanisms of 5-HT(3) and tachykinin NK(1) receptor antagonism to prevent chemotherapy-induced nausea and vomiting. Eur. J. Pharmacol. 684, 1–7.

Zhong, W., Shahbaz, O., Teskey, G., et al., 2021. Mechanisms of nausea and vomiting: current knowledge and recent advances in intracellular emetic signaling systems. Int. J. Mol. Sci. 22, 5797.

Motility of the gastrointestinal tract

Camilleri, M., 2021. Diagnosis and treatment of irritable bowel syndrome: a review. JAMA 325, 865–877.

Corsetti, M., Whorwell, P., 2016. Novel pharmacological therapies for irritable bowel syndrome. Expert Rev. Gastroenterol. Hepatol. 10, 807–815.

Nelson, A.D., Camilleri, M., 2016. Opioid-induced constipation: advances and clinical guidance. Ther. Adv. Chronic Dis. 7, 121–134.

Traveller's diarrhoea

Leung, A.K.C., Leung, A.A.M., Wong, A.H.C., et al., 2019. Travelers' diarrhea: a clinical review. Recent Pat. Inflamm. Allergy Drug Discov. 13, 38–48.

PHE, 2015. Managing suspected infectious diarrhoea. Quick reference guidance for primary care. Public Health England, London.

Riddle, M.S., Connor, B.A., Beeching, N.J., et al., 2017. Guidelines for the prevention and treatment of travelers' diarrhea: a graded expert panel report. J. Travel Med. 24 (Suppl. 1_1), S57–S74.

The control of blood glucose and drug treatment of diabetes mellitus

31

OVERVIEW

In this chapter we describe the endocrine control of blood glucose by pancreatic hormones, especially *insulin* but also *glucagon* and *somatostatin*, and the gut hormones (*incretins*) *glucagon-like peptide-1* (GLP-1) and *gastric inhibitory peptide* (GIP, also known as glucose-dependent insulinotropic peptide). This underpins coverage of diabetes mellitus and its treatment with insulin preparations (including insulin analogues), and other hypoglycaemic agents – metformin, sulfonylureas, α-glucosidase inhibitors, incretin mimetics such as the GLP-1 receptor agonists and gliptins (which potentiate incretins by blocking their degradation), and renal tubular sodium–glucose co-transport (SGLT) inhibitors, notably the SGLT2 inhibitors.

INTRODUCTION

Insulin is the main hormone controlling intermediary metabolism. Its most striking acute effect is to lower blood glucose. Reduced or absent secretion of insulin causes *diabetes mellitus*. It is often coupled with reduced sensitivity to its action, 'insulin resistance', which is closely related to obesity. Diabetes mellitus, recognised since ancient times, is named for the production of sugary urine in copious volumes (due to the osmotic diuretic action of the high urine glucose concentration). Diabetes is rapidly increasing to epidemic proportions (in step with obesity, see Ch. 32), and its consequences are dire – especially accelerated atherosclerosis (myocardial and cerebral infarction, gangrene or limb amputation), kidney failure, neuropathy and blindness.

In this chapter, we first describe the control of blood sugar. The second part of the chapter is devoted to the different kinds of diabetes mellitus and the role of drugs in their treatment. Diabetes, along with obesity (see Ch. 32), hypertension (see Ch. 21), dyslipidaemia (see Ch. 22), and fatty infiltration of the liver, comprise a 'metabolic syndrome', a common pathological cluster and a rapidly growing problem that is associated with many life-threatening conditions. Drugs that act on some of the many mechanisms that become deranged in metabolic syndrome, including several directed at controlling blood sugar, have been developed, but clinical success has been modest so far.

CONTROL OF BLOOD GLUCOSE

Glucose is the obligatory source of energy for the adult human brain, and physiological control of blood glucose reflects the need to maintain adequate fuel supplies in the face of intermittent food intake and variable metabolic demands. More fuel is made available by feeding than is required immediately, and excess calories are stored as glycogen or fat. During fasting, these energy stores need to be mobilised in a regulated manner. The most important regulatory hormone is *insulin*, the actions of which are described later. Increased blood glucose stimulates insulin secretion (Fig. 31.1), whereas reduced blood glucose reduces insulin secretion. The effect of glucose on insulin secretion depends on whether the glucose load is administered intravenously or by mouth. Glucose administered by mouth is more effective in stimulating insulin secretion because it stimulates release from the gut of *incretin* hormones which promote insulin secretion (see Fig. 31.1). Glucose is less effective in stimulating insulin secretion in patients with diabetes (Fig. 31.2). *Hypoglycaemia*, caused by excessive exogenous insulin, not only reduces endogenous insulin secretion but also elicits secretion of an array of 'counter-regulatory' hormones, including *glucagon*, *adrenaline* (see Ch. 15), *glucocorticoids* (see Ch. 33) and *growth hormone* (see Ch. 33), all of which increase blood glucose. Their main effects on glucose uptake and carbohydrate metabolism are summarised and contrasted with those of insulin in Table 31.1.

The kidneys also have an important role in glucose regulation. Substantial amounts of glucose (approximately 900 mmol or 160 g) are filtered each day from the plasma into the renal tubules (Abdul-Ghani et al., 2015). However, in those with normal glucose homeostasis, very little or no glucose is excreted in the urine because renal tubular SGLTs reclaim all the filtered glucose. The co-transporters are large transmembrane proteins (670 amino acids) that actively transport glucose against the concentration gradient through a mechanism that involves coupling with sodium transport (Abdul-Ghani et al., 2011). There are two SGLT variants in the kidney – SGLT2 (located in the early convoluted segment of the proximal tubule) has low affinity but high capacity and is responsible for reclaiming about 90% of the filtered renal glucose, whilst the remaining 10% is reclaimed by high-affinity, low-capacity SGLT1 (located further on in the distal straight segment of the proximal tubule; DeFronzo et al., 2012). SGLT1 is also found in the heart, lungs and gastrointestinal (GI) tract, whereas SGLT2 is principally located in the kidney so selective inhibitors of SGLT2 can promote glucose excretion without influencing glucose transport in other organs.

The evolutionary role of SGLT in the kidney has been attributed to the benefits of retaining glucose in times when starvation or food shortages were commonplace. However, when the renal capacity for glucose re-absorption is exceeded in diabetes, glucose spills over into the urine (glycosuria) and causes an osmotic diuresis (polyuria) which, in turn, results in dehydration, thirst and increased drinking (polydipsia). The chronically elevated glucose concentrations in patients with diabetes leads to up-regulation of SGLT2 expression and greater re-absorption of glucose, thus reducing glycosuria at the expense of worsening hyperglycaemia (DeFronzo et al., 2012). Because SGLT2 is a co-transporter that reabsorbs sodium ions with

Table 31.1 The effect of hormones on blood glucose

Hormone	Main actions	Main stimuli for secretion	Main effect
Main regulatory hormone			
Insulin	↑ Glucose uptake ↑ Glycogen synthesis ↓ Glycogenolysis ↓ Gluconeogenesis	Acute rise in blood glucose Incretins (GIP and GLP-1)	↓ Blood glucose
Main counter-regulatory hormones			
Glucagon	↑ Glycogenolysis ↑ Glyconeogenesis	Hypoglycaemia (i.e. blood glucose <3.9 mmol/L) (e.g. with exercise, stress, high-protein meals), etc.	↑ Blood glucose
Adrenaline (epinephrine)	↑ Glycogenolysis		
Glucocorticoids	↓ Glucose uptake ↑ Gluconeogenesis ↓ Glucose uptake and utilisation		
Growth hormone	↓ Glucose uptake		

GIP, Gastric inhibitory peptide; *GLP-1*, glucagon-like peptide-1.

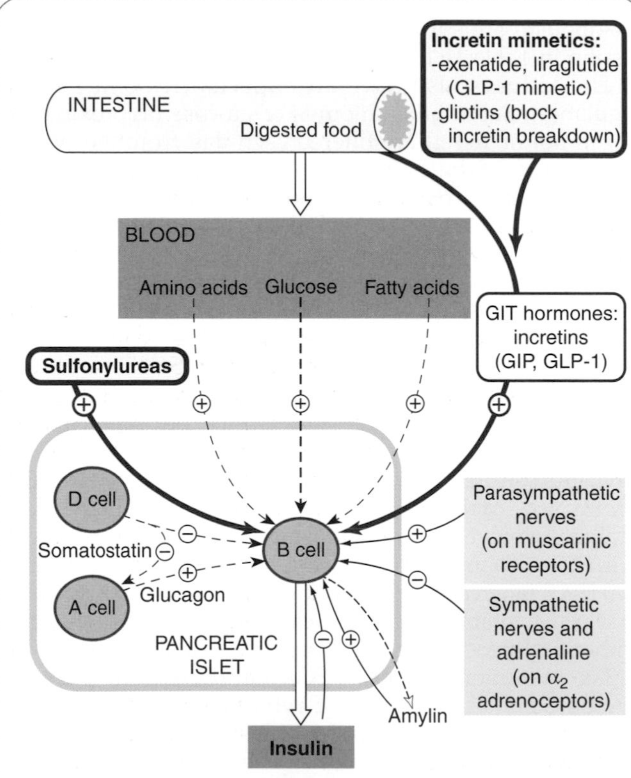

Fig. 31.1 Factors regulating insulin secretion. Blood glucose is the most important factor. Drugs used to stimulate insulin secretion are shown in *red-bordered boxes*. Glucagon potentiates insulin release but opposes some of its peripheral actions and increases blood glucose. *GIP*, Gastric inhibitory peptide; *GIT*, gastrointestinal tract; *GLP-1*, glucagon-like peptide-1.

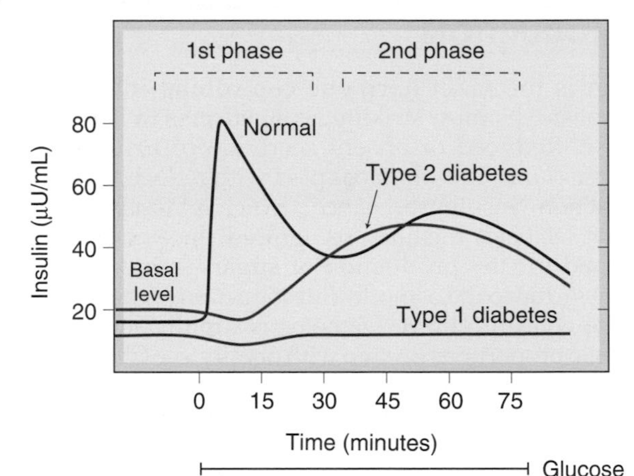

Fig. 31.2 Schematic diagram of the two-phase release of insulin in response to a constant glucose infusion. The first phase is missing in type 2 (non-insulin-dependent) diabetes mellitus, and both are missing in type 1 (insulin-dependent) diabetes mellitus. The first phase is also produced by amino acids, sulfonylureas, glucagon and gastrointestinal tract hormones. (Data from Pfeifer, M.A., Halter, J.B., Porte, D. Jr., 1981. Insulin secretion in diabetes mellitus. Am. J. Med. 70, 579–588.)

glucose, its increased expression also causes salt retention and hypertension.

PANCREATIC ISLET HORMONES

The islets of Langerhans, the endocrine part of the pancreas, contain four main types of peptide-secreting cells: β (or B) cells secrete *insulin*, α (or A) cells secrete *glucagon*, δ (or D) cells secrete *somatostatin*, PP cells secrete *pancreatic polypeptide* (PP) plus ε (or E) cells which are present in the developing

Table 31.2 Effects of insulin on carbohydrate, fat and protein metabolism

Type of metabolism	Liver cells	Fat cells	Muscle
Carbohydrate metabolism	↓ Gluconeogenesis ↓ Glycogenolysis ↑ Glycolysis ↑ Glycogenesis	↑ Glucose uptake ↑ Glycerol synthesis	↑ Glucose uptake ↑ Glycolysis ↑ Glycogenesis
Fat metabolism	↑ Lipogenesis ↓ Lipolysis	↑ Synthesis of triglycerides ↑ Fatty acid synthesis ↓ Lipolysis	
Protein metabolism	↓ Protein breakdown	–	↑ Amino acid uptake ↑ Protein synthesis

pancreas and secrete *ghrelin*, a peptide hormone that is involved in food intake and energy homeostasis (see Ch. 32).

PP is a 36-amino acid peptide closely related to neuropeptide Y (see Ch. 13) and peptide YY (see Ch. 32). It is released by eating a meal and is implicated in control of food intake (see Ch. 32). The core of each islet contains mainly the predominant β cells surrounded by a mantle of α cells interspersed with δ cells or PP cells (see Fig. 31.1). In addition to insulin, β cells secrete a peptide known as islet amyloid polypeptide or amylin, which delays gastric emptying and opposes insulin by stimulating glycogen breakdown in striated muscle, and C-peptide (see later). Glucagon opposes insulin, increasing blood glucose and stimulating protein breakdown in muscle. Somatostatin inhibits secretion of insulin and of glucagon. It is widely distributed outside the pancreas and is also released within the hypothalamus, inhibiting the release of growth hormone from the pituitary gland (see Ch. 33).

INSULIN

Insulin was the first protein for which the amino acid sequence was determined (by Sanger's group in Cambridge in 1955). It consists of two peptide chains (of 21 and 30 amino acid residues) linked by two disulfide bonds.

SYNTHESIS AND SECRETION

Like other peptide hormones (see Ch. 17), insulin is synthesised as a precursor (preproinsulin) in the rough endoplasmic reticulum. Preproinsulin is transported to the Golgi apparatus, where it undergoes proteolytic cleavage to proinsulin and then to insulin plus a fragment of uncertain function called C-peptide.[1] Insulin and C-peptide are stored in granules in β cells, and are normally co-secreted by exocytosis in equimolar amounts together with smaller and variable amounts of proinsulin.

The main factor controlling the synthesis and secretion of insulin is the blood glucose concentration (see Fig. 31.1). β Cells respond both to the absolute glucose concentration and to the rate of change of blood glucose. Other physiological stimuli to insulin release include amino acids (particularly arginine and leucine), fatty acids, the parasympathetic nervous system and *incretins* (especially *GLP-1* and *GIP*, see later). Pharmacologically, sulfonylurea drugs (see later) act by releasing insulin.

There is a steady basal release of insulin and an increase in blood glucose stimulates an additional response. This response has two phases: an initial rapid phase reflecting release of stored hormone, and a slower, delayed phase reflecting continued release of stored hormone and new synthesis (see Fig. 31.2). The response is abnormal in diabetes mellitus, as discussed later.

ATP-sensitive potassium channels (K_{ATP}; see Ch. 4) determine the resting membrane potential in β cells. Glucose enters β cells via a surface membrane transporter called Glut-2, and its subsequent metabolism via glucokinase (which is the rate-limiting glycolytic enzyme in β cells) links insulin secretion to extracellular glucose. The consequent rise in ATP within β cells blocks K_{ATP} channels, causing membrane depolarisation. Depolarisation opens voltage-dependent calcium channels, leading to Ca^{2+} influx. This triggers insulin secretion in the presence of amplifying messengers, including diacylglycerol, non-esterified arachidonic acid (which facilitates further Ca^{2+} entry) and 12-lipoxygenase products of arachidonic acid (mainly *12-S-hydroxyeicosatetraenoic acid* or 12-*S*-HETE; see Ch. 17). Phospholipases are commonly activated by Ca^{2+}, but free arachidonic acid is liberated in β cells by an ATP-sensitive Ca^{2+}-insensitive (ASCI) phospholipase A_2. Consequently, in β cells, Ca^{2+} entry and arachidonic acid production are both driven by ATP, linking cellular energy status to insulin secretion.

Insulin release is inhibited by the sympathetic nervous system (see Fig. 31.1). Adrenaline (epinephrine) increases blood glucose by inhibiting insulin release (via α_2 adrenoceptors on β-cells in the islets) and by promoting glycogenolysis via β_2 adrenoceptors in striated muscle and liver. Several peptides, including somatostatin, galanin (an endogenous K_{ATP} activator) and amylin, also inhibit insulin release.

About one-fifth of the insulin stored in the pancreas of the human adult is secreted daily. The plasma insulin concentration after an overnight fast is 20–50 pmol/L. Plasma insulin concentration is reduced in patients with type 1 (insulin-dependent) diabetes mellitus (see later), and markedly increased in patients with *insulinomas* (uncommon functioning tumours of β cells), as is C-peptide, with which it is co-released.[2] It is also raised in obesity and other normoglycaemic insulin-resistant states.

[1]Not to be confused with C-reactive peptide, which is an acute-phase reactant used clinically as a marker of inflammation (Ch. 7).

[2]Insulin for injection does not contain C-peptide, which therefore provides a means of distinguishing endogenous from exogenous insulin. This is used to differentiate insulinoma (an insulin-secreting tumour causing high circulating insulin with high C-peptide) from surreptitious injection of insulin (high insulin with low C-peptide). Deliberate induction of hypoglycaemia by self-injection with insulin is a well-recognised, if unusual, manifestation of psychiatric disorder, especially in health professionals – it has also been used in murder.

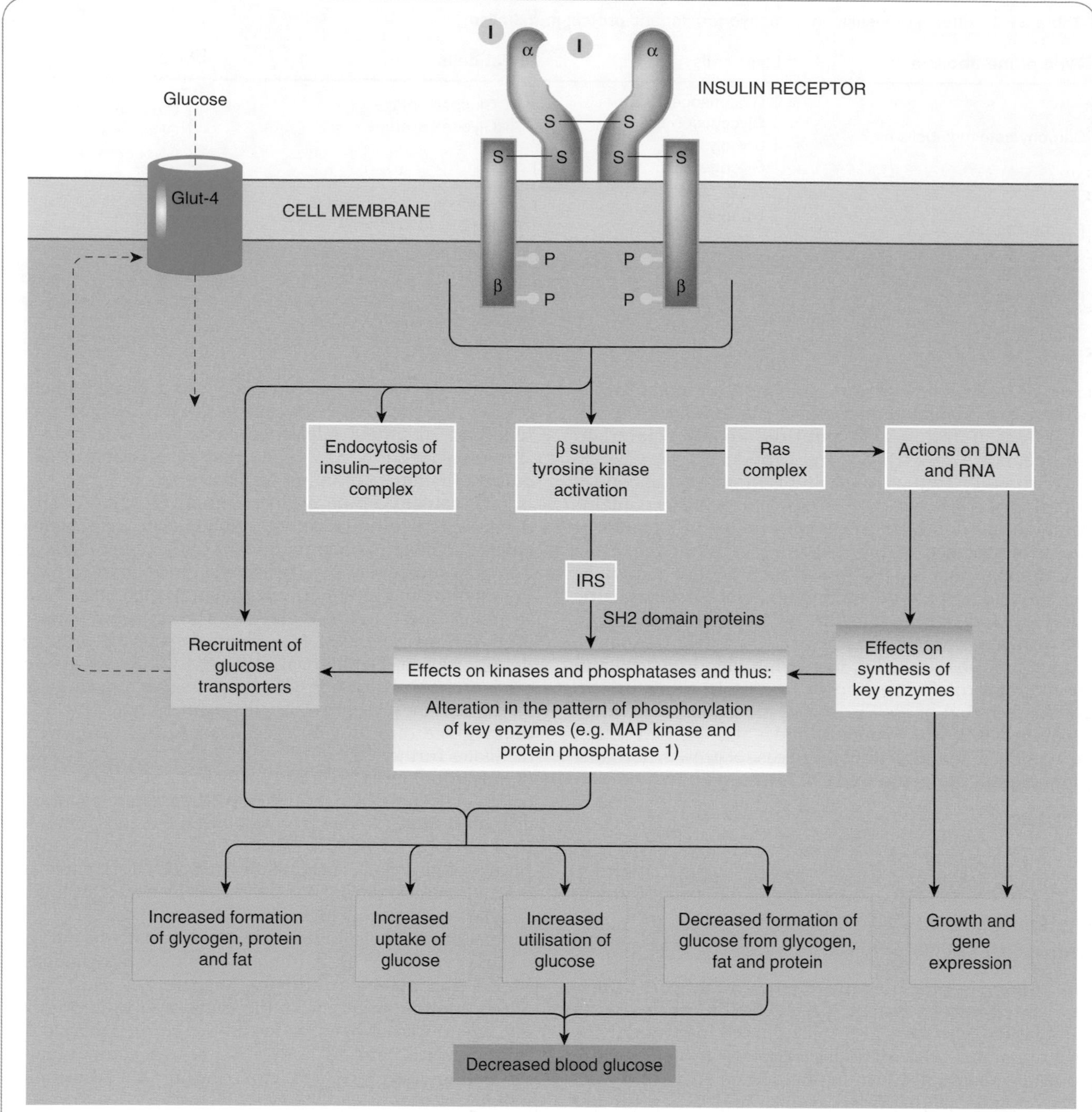

Fig. 31.3 Insulin signalling pathways. *I*, Insulin; *Glut-4*, an insulin-sensitive glucose transporter present in muscle and fat cells; *IRS*, insulin receptor substrate (several forms: 1–4).

ACTIONS

Insulin is the main hormone controlling intermediary metabolism, with actions on liver, fat and muscle (Table 31.2). It is an *anabolic hormone*: its overall effect is to conserve fuel by facilitating the uptake and storage of glucose, amino acids and fats after a meal. Acutely, it reduces blood glucose. Consequently, a fall in plasma insulin increases blood glucose. The biochemical pathways through which insulin exerts its effects are summarised in Fig. 31.3, and molecular aspects of its mechanism are discussed later.

Insulin influences glucose metabolism in most tissues, especially the liver, where it inhibits glycogenolysis (glycogen breakdown) and gluconeogenesis (synthesis of glucose from non-carbohydrate sources) while stimulating glycogen synthesis. It also increases glucose utilisation by glycolysis, but the overall effect is to increase hepatic glycogen stores.

In muscle, unlike liver, uptake of glucose is slow and is the rate-limiting step in carbohydrate metabolism. Insulin causes a glucose transporter called Glut-4, which is sequestered in vesicles, to be expressed within minutes on the surface membrane. This facilitates glucose uptake, and stimulates glycogen synthesis and glycolysis.

Insulin increases glucose uptake by Glut-4 in adipose tissue as well as in muscle. One of the main products of glucose metabolism in adipose tissue is glycerol, which is esterified with fatty acids to form triglycerides, thereby affecting fat metabolism (see Table 31.2).

Insulin increases synthesis of fatty acid and triglyceride in adipose tissue and in liver. It inhibits lipolysis, partly via dephosphorylation – and hence inactivation – of lipases (see Table 31.2). It also inhibits the lipolytic actions of adrenaline, growth hormone and glucagon by opposing their actions on adenylyl cyclase.

Insulin stimulates uptake of amino acids into muscle and increases protein synthesis. It also decreases protein catabolism and inhibits oxidation of amino acids in the liver.

Other metabolic effects of insulin include transport into cells of K^+, Ca^{2+}, nucleosides and inorganic phosphate.[3]

Long-term effects of insulin

In addition to rapid effects on metabolism, exerted via altered activity of enzymes and transport proteins, insulin has long-term actions via altered enzyme synthesis. It is an important anabolic hormone during fetal development. It stimulates cell proliferation (mitogenic action) and is implicated in somatic and visceral growth and development.

Mechanism of action

Insulin binds to a specific receptor on the surface of its target cells. The receptor is a large transmembrane glycoprotein complex belonging to the tyrosine kinase-linked type 3 receptor superfamily (see Ch. 3) and consisting of two α and two β subunits (see Fig. 31.3).

Occupied receptors aggregate into clusters, which are subsequently internalised in vesicles, resulting in down-regulation. Internalised insulin is degraded in lysosomes, but the receptors are recycled to the plasma membrane.

The signal transduction mechanisms that link receptor binding to the biological effects of insulin are complex. Receptor autophosphorylation – the first step in signal transduction – is a consequence of dimerisation, allowing each receptor to phosphorylate the other, as explained in Chapter 3.

Insulin receptor substrate (IRS) proteins undergo rapid tyrosine phosphorylation specifically in response to insulin and insulin-like growth factor-1 but not to other growth factors. The best-characterised substrate is IRS-1, which contains 22 tyrosine residues that are potential phosphorylation sites. It interacts with proteins that contain a so-called SH2 domain (see Ch. 3, Fig. 3.15), thereby passing on the insulin signal. Knock-out mice lacking IRS-1 are hyporesponsive to insulin (insulin-resistant) but do not become diabetic, because of robust β-cell compensation with increased insulin secretion. By contrast, mice lacking IRS-2 fail to compensate and develop overt diabetes, implicating the IRS-2 gene as a candidate for human type 2 diabetes (IRS proteins are reviewed by Lavin et al., 2016). Activation of phosphatidylinositol 3-kinase by the interaction of its SH2 domain with phosphorylated IRS has several important effects, including recruitment of insulin-sensitive glucose transporters (Glut-4) from the Golgi apparatus to the plasma membrane in muscle and fat cells.

The longer-term actions of insulin entail effects on DNA and RNA, mediated partly at least by the Ras signalling complex. Ras is a protein that regulates cell growth and cycles between an active GTP-bound form and an inactive GDP-bound form (see Chs 3 and 57). Insulin shifts the equilibrium in favour of the active form and initiates a phosphorylation cascade that results in activation of mitogen-activated protein kinase (MAP-kinase), which in turn activates several nuclear transcription factors, leading to the expression of genes that are involved with cell growth and with intermediary metabolism.

Insulin for treatment of diabetes mellitus is considered later in this chapter.

GLUCAGON

SYNTHESIS AND SECRETION

Glucagon is a single-chain polypeptide of 21 amino acid residues synthesised mainly in the α cell of the islets, but also in the upper GI tract. It has considerable structural homology with other GI tract hormones, including secretin, vasoactive intestinal peptide and GIP (see Ch. 30).

Amino acids (especially L-arginine) stimulate glucagon secretion, as does ingestion of a high-protein meal, but diurnal variation in plasma glucagon concentrations is less than for insulin. Glucagon secretion is stimulated by low and inhibited by high concentrations of glucose and fatty acids in the plasma. Sympathetic nerve activity and circulating adrenaline stimulate glucagon release via β adrenoceptors. Parasympathetic nerve activity also increases secretion, whereas somatostatin, released from δ cells adjacent to the glucagon-secreting α cells in the periphery of the islets, inhibits glucagon release.

Endocrine pancreas and blood glucose

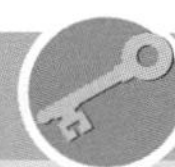

- Islets of Langerhans secrete insulin from β (or B) cells, glucagon from α cells and somatostatin from δ cells.
- Many factors stimulate insulin secretion, but the main one is blood glucose. Incretins, especially GIP and GLP-1 secreted, respectively, by K and L cells in the gut, are also important.
- Insulin is a fuel-storage hormone and also affects cell growth and differentiation. It decreases blood glucose by:
  - increasing glucose uptake into muscle and fat via Glut-4
  - increasing glycogen synthesis
  - decreasing gluconeogenesis
  - decreasing glycogen breakdown.
- Glucagon is a fuel-mobilising hormone, stimulating gluconeogenesis and glycogenolysis, also lipolysis and proteolysis. It increases blood sugar and also increases the force of contraction of the heart (positive inotrope).
- Diabetes mellitus is a chronic metabolic disorder in which there is hyperglycaemia. There is a spectrum of pathologies. Two main phenotypes are:
  - type 1 diabetes, with an absolute deficiency of insulin;
  - type 2 diabetes, with a relative deficiency of insulin associated with reduced sensitivity to its action (insulin resistance).

ACTIONS

Glucagon increases blood glucose and causes breakdown of fat and protein. It acts on specific G protein–coupled receptors to stimulate adenylyl cyclase, and its actions are somewhat similar to β-adrenoceptor–mediated actions of adrenaline. Unlike adrenaline, however, its metabolic effects are more pronounced than its cardiovascular actions.

[3]The action on K^+ is exploited in the emergency treatment of hyperkalaemia by intravenous glucose with insulin (see Ch. 29).

Glucagon is proportionately more active on liver, while the metabolic actions of adrenaline are more pronounced on muscle and fat. Glucagon stimulates glycogen breakdown and gluconeogenesis, and inhibits glycogen synthesis and glucose oxidation. Its metabolic actions on target tissues are thus the opposite of those of insulin. Glucagon increases the rate and force of contraction of the heart (positive inotropic effect; see Ch. 20), although less markedly than adrenaline.

The clinical uses of glucagon are summarised in the clinical box.

Clinical uses of glucagon

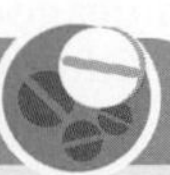

- **Glucagon** can be given intramuscularly or subcutaneously as well as intravenously.
- Treatment of *hypoglycaemia* in unconscious patients (who cannot drink); unlike intravenous glucose, it can be administered by non-medical personnel (e.g. spouses or ambulance crew). It is useful if obtaining intravenous access is difficult.
- Treatment of hypotension, *cardiac failure* or *shock* precipitated by acute overdosage of β-adrenoceptor antagonists.

SOMATOSTATIN

Somatostatin is secreted by the δ cells of the islets. It is also generated and released in the hypothalamus, where it inhibits the release of growth hormone (see Ch. 33). In the islet, it inhibits release of insulin and of glucagon. **Octreotide** is a long-acting analogue of somatostatin. It inhibits release of a number of hormones and is used clinically to relieve symptoms from mediators (such as VIP and 5-HT) secreted by several uncommon gastroentero-pancreatic endocrine tumours, and for treatment of acromegaly[4] (the endocrine disorder caused by a functioning tumour of cells that secrete growth hormone from the anterior pituitary; see Ch. 33).

AMYLIN (ISLET AMYLOID POLYPEPTIDE)

Amylin is a 37-amino acid residue peptide stored with insulin in secretory granules in β cells and is co-secreted with insulin. The role of amylin in glucose regulations stems from its effect on delaying gastric emptying and promoting satiety (see Ch. 32). **Pramlintide**, an amylin analogue with three proline substitutions that reduce its tendency to aggregate into insoluble fibrils, is approved in the United States to treat patients with type 1 diabetes and those with type 2 diabetes who use mealtime insulin but have not achieved satisfactory glucose control. It is injected subcutaneously before each major meal as an adjunct to insulin and reduces insulin requirements. Pramlintide reduces the speed of gastric emptying and decreases the postprandial rise in glucagon. Unwanted effects include hypoglycaemia and nausea – it is contraindicated in patients with loss of gastric motility (gastroparesis), a complication of diabetic autonomic neuropathy.

INCRETINS

La Barre suggested in the 1930s that crude secretin contained two active principles: 'excretin', which stimulates the exocrine pancreas, and 'incretin', which stimulates insulin release. He proposed that incretin presented possibilities for the treatment of diabetes. 'Excretin' did not catch on (perhaps not helped by an unfortunate association with other bodily functions – at least to an Anglo-Saxon ear), but 'incretin' has gone from strength to strength, and some 90 years later several incretin-based drugs are now licensed for clinical use (see later). Incretin action proved to be due to peptide hormones released from the gut, mainly *GIP* and *GLP-1*. These are both members of the glucagon peptide superfamily (see Ch. 17). GIP is a 42-amino acid peptide stored in and secreted by enteroendocrine K cells in the duodenum and proximal jejunum. GLP-1 is secreted by L cells which are more widely distributed in the gut, including in the ileum and colon as well as more proximally. Two forms of GLP-1 are secreted after a meal: GLP-1(7-37) and GLP-1(7-36) amide; these are similarly potent. Most of the circulating activity is due to GLP-1(7-36) amide. Release of GIP and GLP-1 by ingested food provides an early stimulus to insulin secretion before absorbed glucose or other products of digestion reach the islet cells in the portal blood (see Fig. 31.1). As well as stimulating insulin secretion, both these hormones inhibit pancreatic glucagon secretion and slow the rate of absorption of digested food by reducing gastric emptying. They are also implicated in control of food intake via appetite and satiety (see Ch. 32). The actions of GIP and GLP-1 are terminated rapidly by dipeptidyl peptidase-4 (DPP-4). This enzyme is a membrane glycoprotein with rather wide substrate specificity; in clinical practice, the DPP-4 inhibitors are licensed to treat diabetes (see later).

DIABETES MELLITUS

Diabetes mellitus is a chronic metabolic disorder characterised by a high blood glucose concentration – persistent hyperglycaemia (fasting plasma glucose >7.0 mmol/L, or plasma glucose >11.1 mmol/L) – caused by insulin deficiency, often combined with insulin resistance. There are a wide spectrum of aetiologies from single gene disorders through autoimmune disease, gestational diabetes, various pancreatic pathologies such as chronic alcoholic pancreatitis and many more. Two main phenotypes diabetes mellitus are:

1. **Type 1 diabetes** (previously known as insulin-dependent diabetes mellitus – IDDM – or juvenile-onset diabetes), in which there is an absolute deficiency of insulin, often caused by auto-immune destruction of the pancreatic b-cells.
2. **Type 2 diabetes** (previously known as non-insulin-dependent diabetes mellitus – NIDDM – or maturity-onset diabetes), in which there is a relative deficiency of insulin associated with reduced sensitivity to its action (insulin resistance).

Hyperglycaemia occurs because of uncontrolled hepatic glucose output and reduced uptake of glucose by skeletal muscle with reduced glycogen synthesis. Insulin deficiency causes muscle wasting through increased breakdown and reduced synthesis of proteins. Diabetic ketoacidosis (DKA) is an acute emergency that is predominantly seen in patients

[4]Octreotide is used either short term before surgery on the pituitary tumour, or while waiting for radiotherapy of the tumour to take effect, or if other treatments have been ineffective.

with type 1 diabetes. It develops in the absence of insulin because of accelerated breakdown of fat to acetyl-CoA, which, in the absence of aerobic carbohydrate metabolism, is converted to acetoacetate and β-hydroxybutyrate (which cause acidosis) and acetone (a ketone).

Various complications develop as a consequence of the metabolic derangements in diabetes, often over several years. Many of these are the result of disease of blood vessels, either large (macrovascular disease) or small (microangiopathy). Dysfunction of vascular endothelium (see Ch. 21) is an early and critical event in the development of vascular complications. Oxygen-derived free radicals, protein kinase C and non-enzymic products of glucose and albumin called *advanced glycation end products* (AGEs) have been implicated. Macrovascular disease consists of accelerated atheroma (see Ch. 22) and its thrombotic complications (see Ch. 23), which are commoner and more severe in patients with diabetes. Microangiopathy is a distinctive feature of diabetes mellitus and particularly affects the retina, kidney and peripheral nerves. Diabetes mellitus is the commonest cause of chronic renal failure, a huge and rapidly increasing problem, and a major burden to society as well as to individual patients. Co-existent hypertension promotes progressive renal damage, and treatment of hypertension slows the progression of diabetic nephropathy and reduces the risk of myocardial infarction. Angiotensin-converting enzyme inhibitors or angiotensin receptor antagonists (see Ch. 21) are more effective in preventing diabetic nephropathy than other antihypertensive drugs, perhaps because they prevent fibroproliferative actions of angiotensin II and aldosterone.

Diabetic neuropathy[5] is associated with accumulation of osmotically active metabolites of glucose, produced by the action of aldose reductase, but *aldose reductase inhibitors* have been disappointing as therapeutic drugs (see Farmer et al., 2012, for a review).

Type 1 diabetes can occur at any age, but patients are often, but by no means always, young (children or adolescents) and not obese when they first develop symptoms. There is an inherited predisposition, with a 10- to 15-fold increased incidence in first-degree relatives of an index case, and strong associations with particular histocompatibility antigens (HLA types). Identical twins are less than fully concordant, so environmental factors such as viral infection (e.g. with coxsackie virus or echovirus) are believed to be necessary for genetically predisposed individuals to express the disease. Viral infection may damage pancreatic β cells and expose antigens that initiate a self-perpetuating autoimmune process. The patient becomes overtly diabetic only when more than 90% of the β cells have been destroyed. This natural history provides a tantalising prospect of intervening in the prediabetic stage, and a variety of strategies have been mooted, including immunosuppression, early insulin therapy, antioxidants, nicotinamide and many others; so far these have disappointed, but this remains a very active field.

Type 2 diabetes is accompanied both by insulin resistance (which precedes overt disease) and by impaired insulin secretion, each of which are important in its pathogenesis. Such patients are often obese and usually, although again by no means always, present in adult life, the incidence rising progressively with age as β-cell function declines. Treatment is initially dietary, although oral hypoglycaemic drugs usually become necessary, and most patients ultimately benefit from exogenous insulin. Prospective studies have demonstrated a relentless deterioration in diabetic control[6] with increasing age and duration of disease.

Insulin secretion (basal, and in response to a meal) in a patient with type 1 or type 2 diabetes is contrasted schematically with that in a healthy control in Fig. 31.2.

There are many other less common forms of diabetes mellitus in addition to the two main ones described earlier (for example, syndromes associated with autoantibodies directed against insulin receptors which cause severe insulin resistance, functional α-cell tumours, 'glucagonomas', and many other rarities), and hyperglycaemia can also be a clinically important adverse effect of several drugs, including glucocorticoids (see Ch. 33), high doses of thiazide diuretics (see Ch. 29) and several of the protease inhibitors used to treat HIV infection (see Ch. 53).

DRUGS USED IN THE TREATMENT OF DIABETES

The main groups of drugs used are:

Agents given by injection
- Insulin, in various forms and formulations (used in type 1 and type 2 diabetes)
- Incretin mimetics (e.g. **exenatide, liraglutide, semaglutide**)

Oral agents (used in type 2 diabetes)
- Biguanides (e.g. **metformin**)
- Sulfonylureas (e.g. **tolbutamide, glibenclamide, gliclazide, glipizide**) and related drugs (e.g. **repaglinide, nateglinide**)
- Gliptins (e.g. **sitagliptin**)
- Thiazolidinediones (e.g. **pioglitazone**)

INSULIN TREATMENT

The effects of insulin and its mechanism of action are described earlier. Here we describe pharmacokinetic aspects and adverse effects, both of which are central to its therapeutic use. Insulin for clinical use was once either porcine or bovine but is now almost entirely human (made in expression systems by recombinant DNA technology, see Ch. 5). Animal insulins are liable to elicit an immune response; this is less of an issue with recombinant human insulins. Although recombinant insulin is more consistent in quality than insulins extracted from pancreases of freshly slaughtered animals, doses are still quantified in terms of units of activity, with which doctors and patients are familiar, rather than of mass.

Pharmacokinetic aspects and insulin preparations

Insulin is destroyed in the GI tract, and is ordinarily given by injection – usually subcutaneously, but intravenously or occasionally intramuscularly in emergencies. Intraperitoneal insulin can be used in special circumstances in patients with diabetes, through a continuous infusion pump, or through

[5]Neuropathy ('disease of the nerves') causes dysfunction of peripheral nerve fibres, which can be motor, sensory or autonomic. Diabetic neuropathy often causes numbness in a 'stocking' distribution caused by damage to sensory fibres, and postural hypotension and erectile dysfunction due to autonomic neuropathy.

[6]Diabetic control is not easily estimated by determination of blood glucose, because this is so variable. Instead, glycated haemoglobin (haemoglobin A_{1C}) is measured. This provides an integrated measure of control over the lifespan of the red cell: approximately 120 days. In healthy individuals, 4%–6% (20–42 mmol/mol) of haemoglobin is glycated; levels above 6.5% (48 mmol/mol) are indicative of diabetes.

ambulatory peritoneal dialysis for those with end-stage renal failure. Other potential approaches include incorporation of insulin into biodegradable polymer microspheres as a slow-release formulation, and its encapsulation with a lectin in a glucose-permeable membrane.[7] Once absorbed into plasma, insulin has an elimination half-life of approximately 10 min. It is inactivated enzymically in the liver and kidney, and 10% is excreted in the urine. Renal impairment reduces insulin requirement.

One of the main problems in using insulin is to avoid wide fluctuations in plasma concentration and thus in blood glucose. Different formulations vary in the timing of their peak effect and duration of action. *Soluble insulin* produces a rapid and short-lived effect. Longer-acting preparations are made by precipitating insulin with protamine or zinc, thus forming finely divided amorphous solid or relatively insoluble crystals, which are injected as a suspension from which insulin is slowly absorbed. These preparations include *isophane insulin* and amorphous or crystalline *insulin zinc suspensions*. Mixtures of different forms in fixed proportions are available.

More recently, modifications of insulin molecules have focused on two different areas – one being the production of molecules with a more rapid onset of action to cover mealtimes, and the other being even longer-acting formulations. Development of rapid-acting analogues is based on amino acid substitutions that promote formation of insulin monomers for faster absorption, whilst reducing the aggregation of insulin dimers and hexamers (Atkin et al., 2015). Examples of these analogues include insulin aspart, insulin lispro and insulin glulisine, which involve different amino acid switches at positions such as B28 or B29 in the insulin molecule. These analogues act more rapidly (onset of action <15 min and typically reaching peak concentrations within 40–70 min after injection) but for a shorter time than natural insulin, enabling patients to inject themselves immediately before the start of a meal rather than 30 min before eating.

Basal or longer-acting insulin analogues are designed with the opposite intention, namely to provide a constant basal insulin supply and mimic physiological postabsorptive basal insulin secretion. **Insulin glargine**, which is a clear solution, forms a microprecipitate at the physiological pH of subcutaneous tissue, and absorption from the subcutaneous site of injection is prolonged. In contrast, subcutaneous injection of **insulin detemir** causes the molecules to bind together more avidly, thus slowing the absorption into the circulation (Atkin et al., 2015). **Insulin degludec** is formed by the addition of a fatty-diacid side chain to human insulin, and the resulting molecules join up to form a depot of long multihexamers after subcutaneous injection. Monomers of insulin degludec slowly dissociate from this depot, thus giving a protracted duration of action >40 h.

Various dosage regimens are used. Some type 1 patients inject a combination of short- and intermediate-acting insulins twice daily, before breakfast and before the evening meal. Improved control of blood glucose can be achieved with the basal-bolus regimen comprising a basal insulin analogue injected once daily (often at night) and multiple daily injections of rapid-acting insulin analogues timed to be given just before meals. Insulin pumps are used in hospital to control blood glucose acutely and are also available in a portable form that delivers continuous subcutaneous infusion for outpatients. The most sophisticated forms of pump regulate the dose by means of a sensor that continuously measures blood glucose, and these programmable systems have become more widely available with significant advances in technology.

Unwanted effects

The main undesirable effect of insulin is hypoglycaemia. This is common and, if very severe, can cause brain damage or sudden cardiac death. In the Diabetes Control and Complications Trial mentioned before, intensive insulin therapy resulted in a three-fold increase in severe hypoglycaemic episodes compared with usual care. The treatment of hypoglycaemia is to take a sweet drink or snack or, if the patient is unconscious, to give intravenous glucose or intramuscular glucagon (see clinical box). Rebound hyperglycaemia ('Somogyi effect') can follow insulin-induced hypoglycaemia, because of the release of counter-regulatory hormones (e.g. adrenaline, glucagon and glucocorticoids). This can cause hyperglycaemia before breakfast following an unrecognised hypoglycaemic attack during sleep in the early hours of the morning. It is essential to appreciate this possibility to avoid the mistake of increasing (rather than reducing) the evening dose of insulin in this situation.

Clinical uses of insulin and other hypoglycaemic drugs for injection

- Patients with *type 1 diabetes* require long-term **insulin**:
  - A common regimen is basal-bolus administration using a single long-acting insulin accompanied by short-acting insulin at each mealtime. Insulin pumps have also become an option.
  - In selected patients where diabetes control is less critical, a twice-daily regimen is used; i.e. intermediate-acting preparation (e.g. **isophane insulin**) or a long-acting analogue (e.g. **glargine**) is often combined with soluble insulin or a short-acting analogue (e.g. **lispro**) taken before meals.
- **Soluble insulin** is used (intravenously) in treatment of hyperglycaemic emergencies (e.g. *diabetic ketoacidosis*).
- Approximately one-third of patients with *type 2 diabetes* ultimately require **insulin.**
- Short-term treatment of patients with type 2 diabetes or impaired glucose tolerance during intercurrent events (e.g. *operations*, *infections*, *myocardial infarction*).
- During pregnancy, for *gestational diabetes* not controlled by diet alone. Here, an infusion pump guided by continuous glucose monitoring is a suitable option.
- Emergency treatment of *hyperkalaemia* (see Ch. 29): **insulin** is given with glucose to lower extracellular K^+ via redistribution into cells.
- Glucagon-like peptide-1 **(GLP-1) agonist** for type 2 diabetes in addition to oral agents to improve control and lose weight (see Ch. 32).

[7]This could, in theory, provide variable release of insulin controlled by the prevailing glucose concentration, because glucose and glycated insulin compete for binding sites on the lectin.

Allergy to human insulin is unusual but can occur. It may take the form of local or systemic reactions. Insulin resistance as a consequence of antibody formation is rare.

Biguanides

Metformin (present in French lilac, *Galega officinalis*, which was used to treat diabetes in traditional medicine for centuries) is the only biguanide used clinically to treat type 2 diabetes, for which it is now a drug that is amongst the first choices.[8]

Actions and mechanism

The molecular target or targets through which biguanides act remain unclear, but their biochemical actions are well described, and include:

- reduced hepatic glucose production (gluconeogenesis) which is markedly increased in type 2 diabetes;
- increased glucose uptake and utilisation in skeletal muscle (i.e. reduced insulin resistance);
- reduced carbohydrate absorption from the intestine;
- increased fatty acid oxidation;
- reduced circulating low-density and very low-density lipoprotein (LDL and VLDL, respectively, see Ch. 22).

Reduced hepatic gluconeogenesis is especially important. Metformin decreases hepatic glucose production directly or indirectly by inhibiting the mitochondrial respiratory chain complex I (reviewed by Viollet et al., 2012). The resulting increase in AMP activates AMP-activated protein kinase (AMPK) which is a master regulator of energy homeostasis in eukaryotes (Myers et al., 2017). Activation of AMPK in the duodenum triggers release of GLP-1 which stimulates a gut–brain–liver vagal network that regulates hepatic glucose production (Duca et al., 2015). Chronic administration of metformin alters recirculation of bile acids and composition of the gut microbiome in type 2 leading to increased GLP-1 secretion in diabetes patients (Napolitano et al., 2014).

Metformin has a half-life of about 3 h and is excreted unchanged in the urine.

Unwanted effects

Metformin, while preventing hyperglycaemia, does *not* cause hypoglycaemia, and the commonest unwanted effects are dose-related GI disturbances (e.g. anorexia, diarrhoea, nausea), which are usually, but not always, transient. Lactic acidosis is a rare but potentially fatal toxic effect, and metformin should not be given routinely to patients with renal or hepatic disease, hypoxic pulmonary disease or shock. Such patients are predisposed to lactic acidosis because of reduced drug elimination or reduced tissue oxygenation. It should be avoided in other situations that predispose to lactic acidosis including alcohol intoxication, and some forms of mitochondrial myopathy that are associated with diabetes. Long-term use may interfere with absorption of vitamin B_{12}.

[8]Metformin had a very slow start. It was first synthesised in 1922, one of a large series of biguanides with many different pharmacological actions, which proved largely unsuitable for clinical use. Its glucose-lowering effect was noted early on but it was eclipsed by the discovery of insulin. It did not receive FDA approval until 1995.

Clinical use

Metformin is used to treat patients with type 2 diabetes. It does not stimulate appetite (rather the reverse; see earlier!) and is one of the preferred options in the majority of type 2 patients who are obese, provided they have unimpaired renal and hepatic function. It can be combined with other glucose-lowering agents if blood glucose is inadequately controlled. Potential uses outside type 2 diabetes include other syndromes with accompanying insulin resistance including polycystic ovary syndrome, non-alcoholic fatty liver disease, gestational diabetes and some forms of premature puberty.

Glucose transport inhibitors

Several SGLT2 inhibitors are licensed for use in type 2 diabetes. Examples include **canagliflozin, dapagliflozin** and **empagliflozin**.

Mechanism of action

The SGLT2 inhibitors promote glucose excretion into the urine, thereby reducing the concentration of circulating glucose. The resulting glycosuria is associated with an osmotic diuresis and salt excretion (see also Chs 21 and 29). SGLT2 inhibitors are currently being investigated for numerous other complex effects on the cardiac and renal systems, which may include reduction in oxidative stress and inflammation (described in detail by Zelniker and Braunwald, 2020).

Effects

Treatment with SGLT2 inhibitors leads to elevated amounts of glucose in the urine over sustained periods, and an associated increase in urinary volume and sodium ion excretion. Clinical trials have confirmed improvements in fasting and post-prandial glucose concentrations, and significant reduction in glycosylated haemoglobin (Zelniker and Braunwald, 2020). The natriuresis, diuresis and the caloric loss (from glucose in the urine) also lead usefully to reduction in systolic blood pressure and body weight. As such, use of SGLT2 inhibitors is now being extended to patients with heart failure, or chronic kidney disease, irrespective of whether they have diabetes or not (Zelniker and Braunwald, 2020).

Pharmacokinetic aspects

SGLT2 inhibitors are rapidly absorbed, with time to peak plasma concentrations of less than 2 h. They are highly bound to plasma proteins (>80%).

Unwanted effects

Natriuresis with diuresis can lead to increased urinary volume, hypotension and dehydration, and is accentuated with concomitant use of thiazide diuretics. The elevated glucose concentrations in the urine can lead to a significant increase in the risk of urinary tract and fungal infections such as candidal vaginitis or balanitis with SGLT2 inhibitors (Zelniker and Braunwald, 2020). However, there remains considerable debate around the uncertain association between SGLT2 inhibitors and a rare severe necrotising disease of the perineum and external genitalia (Fournier's gangrene) caused by mixed aerobic and anaerobic infection.

Safety concerns include serious adverse events such as lower limb amputations, and increased susceptibility to DKA, including specifically euglycaemic DKA. Here, the glucose-lowering effect of the SGLT2 inhibitors is thought to reduce residual endogenous insulin secretion whilst promoting glucagon production. The resulting decrease in the anti-lipolytic action of insulin leads to greater synthesis of free fatty acids which are subsequently converted to ketones by the liver. Concurrent acute illness, dehydration, decreased food intake or dietary restrictions (e.g. low carbohydrate or ketogenic diet) are important risk factors for DKA with SGLT2 inhibitors. Patients are advised to seek assistance for ketone testing, and to stop taking their SGLT2 inhibitor during acute serious illness, or before surgical procedures.

Clinical use

SGLT2 inhibitors are licensed for use in type 2 diabetes, either alone (when metformin is inappropriate) or in combination with other glucose-lowering therapies. Typically, this would involve SGLT2 use in dual or triple therapy. A potential advantage of SGLT2 inhibition in those with inadequate diabetes control is that the amount of glucose excreted in the urine will be proportionately greater in patients whose plasma glucose concentrations are high.

However, SGLT2 inhibitors are not used for glycaemic control in patients with type 1 disease because of potential harm from DKA.

The SGLT2 inhibitors are considered to have a relatively low risk of hypoglycaemia.

Incretin mimetics and related drugs

Exenatide and lixisenatide are synthetic derivatives of *exendin-4*, a peptide found in the saliva of the Gila monster (a lizard that presumably evolved this as means to disable its prey by rendering them hypoglycaemic). In contrast, other GLP-1 analogues such as liraglutide and semaglutide closely resemble human GLP-1, but with molecular modifications to enable longer duration of action.

GLP-1 agonists lower blood glucose after a meal by increasing insulin secretion, suppressing glucagon secretion and slowing gastric emptying (see earlier). They reduce food intake (by an effect on satiety, see Ch. 32) and are associated with modest weight loss. They reduce hepatic fat accumulation. Pancreatitis is a rare but potentially severe adverse effect.

GLP-1 agonists are administered by subcutaneous injection, either once daily (exenatide, **liraglutide**, **lixisenatide**) or once weekly (extended release exenatide, **albiglutide**, **dulaglutide**). Semaglutide is now available in both injectable and oral formulations.

GLP-1 agonists are used in patients with type 2 diabetes in combination with other drugs (see clinical box on uses of oral hypoglycaemic drugs).

Tirzepatide is a newly developed injectable molecule (see also Ch. 32) that has dual GLP-1 and GIP agonist activity. The additional action on GIP is thought to stimulate energy expenditure whilst reducing food intake. Randomised trials have reported significant benefits in terms of diabetes control and weight loss with tirzepatide when compared to insulin or GLP-1 analogues.

Gliptins

Gliptins (e.g. **sitagliptin**, **vildagliptin**, **saxagliptin**, **linagliptin**) are synthetic drugs that competitively inhibit DPP-4, thereby lowering blood glucose by potentiating endogenous incretins (GLP-1 and GIP, see above) which stimulate insulin secretion. They do not cause weight loss or weight gain.

They are absorbed from the gut and administered once (or, in the case of vildagliptin, twice) daily by mouth. They are eliminated partly by renal excretion and are also metabolised by hepatic CYP enzymes. They are usually well tolerated with a range of mild GI adverse effects; liver disease, heart failure (particularly with saxagliptin or alogliptin) and pancreatitis (incidence approximately 0.1%–1%) are less common but potentially serious. Gliptins can be used for type 2 diabetes in addition to other oral hypoglycaemic drugs, but not together with GLP-1 agonists because of their overlapping mechanisms

Evidence of cardiovascular efficacy or effect on mortality is inconsistent, with some GLP-1 analogues (such as liraglutide, semaglutide, dulaglutide) demonstrating a reduction in major adverse cardiac events (Gilbert and Pratley, 2020), whereas neither the gliptins nor exenatide has shown such benefits in large-scale clinical trials.

Sulfonylureas

The sulfonylureas were developed following the chance observation that a sulfonamide derivative (which was being used to treat typhoid) caused hypoglycaemia. Numerous sulfonylureas are available. The first used therapeutically were **tolbutamide** and **chlorpropamide**. Chlorpropamide has a long duration of action and a substantial fraction is excreted in the urine. It is seldom used in clinical practice because of serious adverse effects such as hypoglycaemia, flushing with alcohol and hyponatraemia. Williams (1994) comments that 'time honoured but idiosyncratic chlorpropamide should now be laid to rest' – a sentiment with which we concur. Tolbutamide, however, is still available, although far less commonly prescribed nowadays than the so-called second-generation sulfonylureas (e.g. **glibenclamide**, **gliclazide**, **glipizide**; Table 31.3) which are more potent. These second-generation drugs all contain the sulfonylurea moiety and act in the same way, but different substitutions result in differences in pharmacokinetics and hence in duration of action (see Table 31.3).

Mechanism of action

The principal action of sulfonylureas is on β cells (see Fig. 31.1), stimulating insulin secretion and thus reducing plasma glucose. High-affinity binding sites for sulfonylureas are present on the K_{ATP} channels (see Ch. 4) in the surface membranes of β cells, and the binding of various sulfonylureas parallels their potency in stimulating insulin release. Block by sulfonylurea drugs of K_{ATP} channel activation causes depolarisation of β cells, Ca^{2+} entry and insulin secretion. (Compare this with the physiological control of insulin secretion, see Fig. 31.1.)

Pharmacokinetic aspects

Sulfonylureas are well absorbed after oral administration, and most reach peak plasma concentrations within 2–4

Table 31.3 Oral hypoglycaemic sulfonylurea drugs

Drug	Relative potency[a]	Half-life (hours)	Pharmacokinetic aspects[b]	General comments
Tolbutamide	1	4	Some converted in the liver to weakly active hydroxytolbutamide; some carboxylated to inactive compound Renal excretion	Less likely to cause hypoglycaemia Usually given three times a day
Glibenclamide[c]	150	10	Some is oxidised in the liver to moderately active products and is excreted in urine; 50% is excreted unchanged in the faeces	Most likely to cause hypoglycaemia, particularly in older patients where it should be avoided The active metabolite accumulates in renal failure Once-daily dosing is possible
Gliclazide	10	10	Peak plasma concentrations at 2–6 h Mainly metabolised in liver	Well absorbed. May require twice-daily dosing
Glipizide	100	7	Peak plasma levels in 1 h Most is metabolised in the liver to inactive products, which are excreted in urine; 12% is excreted in faeces	May cause hypoglycaemia Only inactive products accumulate in renal failure

[a]Relative to tolbutamide.
[b]All are highly protein bound (90%–95%).
[c]Termed *glyburide* in the United States.

h. The duration of action varies (see Table 31.3). All bind strongly to plasma albumin and are implicated in interactions with other drugs (e.g. salicylates and sulfonamides) that compete for these binding sites (see Ch. 9). Most sulfonylureas (or their active metabolites) are excreted in the urine, so their action is increased and prolonged in the elderly and in patients with renal disease.

Most sulfonylureas cross the placenta and enter breast milk and their use is contraindicated in pregnancy and in breastfeeding.

Unwanted effects

The sulfonylureas are usually well tolerated. Unwanted effects are specified in Table 31.3. The commonest adverse effect is hypoglycaemia, which can be severe and prolonged, the highest incidence occurring with long-acting chlorpropamide and glibenclamide and the lowest with tolbutamide. Long-acting sulfonylureas are best avoided in the elderly and in patients with even mild renal impairment because of the risk of hypoglycaemia. Sulfonylureas stimulate appetite and often cause weight gain. This is a major concern in obese patients with diabetes. About 3% of patients experience GI upsets. The sulfonylureas do not appear to confer cardiovascular benefit (Flory and Lipska, 2019) and there is continued debate regarding the possibility of a detrimental effect on patients with underlying cardiovascular disease.

Drug interactions

Several drugs augment the hypoglycaemic effect of sulfonylureas. Non-steroidal anti-inflammatory drugs, warfarin, some uricosuric drugs (e.g. **sulfinpyrazone**), alcohol, monoamine oxidase inhibitors, some antibacterial drugs (including sulfonamides, **trimethoprim** and **chloramphenicol**) and some imidazole antifungal drugs have all been reported to produce severe hypoglycaemia when given with a sulfonylurea. The probable basis of most of these interactions is competition for metabolising enzymes, but interference with plasma protein binding or with transport mechanisms facilitating excretion may play some part.

Agents that decrease the action of sulfonylureas on blood glucose include high doses of thiazide diuretics (see Chs 21 and 29) and glucocorticoids, all of which can increase circulating glucose concentrations.

Clinical use

Sulfonylureas are used to treat type 2 diabetes in its early stages, but because they require functional β cells, they are not useful in type 1 or late-stage type 2 diabetes. Nowadays, the limitations of sulfonylureas (weight gain, risk of hypoglycaemia, lack of cardiovascular benefit) means that they are seldom used as first-line agents for type 2 diabetes.

OTHER DRUGS THAT STIMULATE INSULIN SECRETION

Several drugs that act, like the sulfonylureas, by blocking the sulfonylurea receptor on K_{ATP} channels in pancreatic β cells but lack the sulfonylurea moiety have been developed. These include **repaglinide** and **nateglinide** which, although much less potent than most sulfonylureas, have rapid onset and offset kinetics leading to short duration of action and a low risk of hypoglycaemia.[9] These drugs are administered shortly before a meal to reduce the postprandial rise in blood glucose in patients with type 2 diabetes that is inadequately controlled with diet and exercise. They may cause less weight gain than conventional sulfonylureas.

[9]It is ironic that these newer drugs share many of the properties of tolbutamide, the oldest, least expensive and least fashionable of the sulfonylureas.

Later in the course of the disease, they can be combined with metformin or other oral hypoglycaemic agents. Unlike glibenclamide, these drugs are relatively selective for K_{ATP} channels on β cells versus K_{ATP} channels in vascular smooth muscle.

Thiazolidinediones (glitazones): pioglitazone

The thiazolidinediones (or *glitazones*) were developed following the chance observation that a **clofibrate** analogue, **ciglitazone**, which was being screened for effects on lipids, unexpectedly lowered blood glucose. Ciglitazone caused liver toxicity, and this class of drugs (despite initial commercial success) has been dogged by adverse effects (especially cardiovascular), regulatory withdrawals and controversy. No clinical trials of these agents have demonstrated a beneficial effect on mortality, and they were licensed on the basis of statistically significant effects on haemoglobin A1c (HbA1C) (an integrated marker of longer-term glycaemic control) of uncertain clinical significance. **Pioglitazone** is the only drug of this class that remains in clinical use, its predecessors, rosiglitazone and troglitazone, having faced regulatory action because of increased risk of heart attacks and liver damage, respectively.

Effects

The effect of thiazolidinediones on blood glucose is slow in onset, the maximum effect being achieved only after 1–2 months of treatment. They act by enhancing the effectiveness of endogenous insulin, thereby reducing hepatic glucose output, and increasing glucose uptake into muscle.

They reduce the amount of exogenous insulin needed to maintain a given level of blood glucose by approximately 30%. Reduced blood glucose concentration is accompanied by reduced insulin and free fatty acid concentrations. Weight gain of 1–4 kg is common, usually stabilising in 6–12 months. Some of this is attributable to fluid retention: there is an increase in plasma volume of up to 500 mL, with a concomitant reduction in haemoglobin concentration caused by haemodilution; there is also an increase in extravascular fluid, and increased deposition of subcutaneous (as opposed to visceral) fat.

Mechanism of action

Thiazolidinediones bind to a nuclear receptor called the *peroxisome proliferator-activated receptor-γ* (PPARγ), which is complexed with retinoid X receptor (RXR; see Ch. 3).[10] It remains something of a mystery that glucose homeostasis should be so responsive to drugs that bind to receptors expressed mainly in fat cells; it has been suggested that the explanation may lie in resetting of the glucose–fatty acid (Randle) cycle by the reduction in circulating free fatty acids.

Unwanted effects

Clinical trial data have demonstrated significantly increased risk of a range of adverse events with pioglitazone, including heart failure, bone fracture, oedema and weight gain, and glitazones are now far less frequently used.

Clinical use

Pioglitazone is additive with other oral hypoglycaemic drugs in terms of effect on blood glucose, and a combination tablet with metformin is marketed.

α-Glucosidase inhibitors

Acarbose, an inhibitor of intestinal α-glucosidase, is used in type 2 diabetes inadequately controlled by diet with or without other agents. It delays carbohydrate absorption, reducing the postprandial increase in blood glucose. The commonest adverse effects are related to its main action and consist of flatulence, loose stools or diarrhoea and abdominal pain and bloating. Like metformin, it may be particularly helpful in obese type 2 patients, and it can be co-administered with metformin.

TREATMENT OF DIABETES MELLITUS

Personalised therapy of diabetes is focused on the careful balance of drug treatment aiming for near-normalisation of the HbA1C whilst avoiding hypoglycaemia. Nowadays, numerous clinical guidelines recommend target HbA1Cs which are tailored according to specific individual patient characteristics. Whilst tight control with rigorous monitoring is a cornerstone in younger patients with diabetes (mainly type 1), there are more complex considerations in older, multi-morbid patients with type 2 diabetes who are already on polypharmacy. Studies of intensive control later in the course of the disease have been disappointing, particularly with regards to older patients, where the serious harm from hypoglycaemia may outweigh any benefit from strict glucose-lowering regimens. Realistic goals in patients with type 2 diabetes are usually less ambitious than in younger type 1 patients. Dietary restriction leading to weight loss in overweight and obese patients is the cornerstone (albeit one with a tendency to crumble), combined with increased exercise. Oral agents are used to control symptoms from hyperglycaemia, as well as to limit microvascular complications, and are introduced early. Blood pressure control and statins to prevent atheromatous disease (see Ch. 22) are crucial for cardiovascular health. Here, GLP-1 analogues and SGLT2 inhibitors are currently thought to carry the greatest cardiovascular benefit amongst all the available agents (Flory and Lipska, 2019).

[10]Compare with fibrates (to which thiazolidinediones are structurally related), which bind to PPARα (see Ch. 22).

Drugs used in diabetes mellitus

Insulin and other injectable drugs

- Human **insulin** is made by recombinant DNA technology. For routine use, it is given subcutaneously (by intravenous infusion in emergencies).
- Different formulations of **insulin** differ in their duration of action:
  - rapid-acting analogues that can be given immediately before a meal, and have shorter half-lives so that post-prandial hypoglycaemia is less likely;
  - short-acting **soluble insulin**: peak action after subcutaneous dose 2–4 h and duration 6–8 h; it is the only formulation that can be given intravenously;
  - intermediate-acting insulin (e.g. **isophane insulin**); and
  - long-acting forms (e.g. **insulin glargine**).
- The main unwanted effect is hypoglycaemia.
- Altering the amino acid sequence (insulin analogues, e.g. **lispro** and **glargine**) can usefully alter **insulin** kinetics.
- **Insulins** are used for all patients with type 1 diabetes and approximately one-third of patients with type 2 diabetes.
- Injectable GLP-1 agonists are used as add-on treatment in certain patients with inadequately controlled type 2 diabetes. Unlike **insulin** they are useful in promoting weight loss.

Oral hypoglycaemic drugs

- These are used in type 2 diabetes.
- Biguanides (e.g. **metformin**):
  - have complex peripheral actions in the presence of residual insulin, increasing glucose uptake in striated muscle and inhibiting hepatic glucose output and intestinal glucose absorption;
  - reduce appetite and encourage weight loss; have low or negligible risk of hypoglycaemia;
  - are amongst the first-line choices in overweight or obese patients.
- SGLT2 inhibitors (e.g. empagliflozin)
  - promote urinary excretion of glucose;
  - have beneficial effects on weight, blood pressure, renal and cardiovascular outcomes;
  - increase the risk of dehydration and urinary tract infections, as well as rare instances of DKA.
- GLP-1 analogues – semaglutide is the only oral formulation available from this class of drugs.
- Gliptins (e.g. **sitagliptin**):
  - potentiate endogenous incretins by blocking DPP-4;
  - are added to other orally active drugs to improve control in patients with type 2 diabetes;
  - are weight-neutral; they are usually well tolerated but pancreatitis is a concern.
- Sulfonylureas and other drugs that stimulate insulin secretion (e.g. **tolbutamide**, **glibenclamide**, **nateglinide**):
  - can cause hypoglycaemia (which stimulates appetite and leads to weight gain);
  - are effective only if β cells are functional;
  - block ATP-sensitive potassium channels in β cells;
  - are well tolerated but promote weight gain and are associated with more cardiovascular disease than is **metformin.**
- Thiazolidinediones have been associated with serious cardiac toxicity. **Pioglitazone** is the only one still widely marketed; it:
  - is a PPARγ (a nuclear receptor) agonist;
  - increases insulin sensitivity and lowers blood glucose in type 2 diabetes;
  - can cause weight gain and oedema;
  - increases osteoporotic fractures.
- α-Glucosidase inhibitor, **acarbose**:
  - reduces carbohydrate absorption;
  - causes flatulence and diarrhoea.

Clinical uses of oral hypoglycaemic drugs

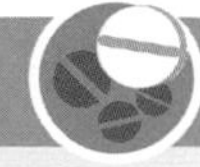

- *Type 2 diabetes mellitus*, to reduce symptoms from hyperglycaemia (e.g. thirst, excessive urination) and to reduce long-term diabetes complications ('tight' control of blood glucose may only have a small effect on cardiovascular complications in certain settings, depending on the class of drug.)
- **Metformin** is preferred, especially for obese patients unless contraindicated by factors that predispose to lactic acidosis (renal or liver failure, poorly compensated heart failure, hypoxaemia).
- SGLT2 inhibitors improve diabetes control, and are effective in reducing heart failure, hypertension and renal complications.
- GLP-1 agonists (e.g. **exenatide, lixisenatide** or **liraglutide**) are given by injection in obese patients inadequately controlled on one or two hypoglycaemic drugs. These agents are associated with the potential for weight loss or prevention of weight gain in overweight or obese patients. **Semaglutide** can be taken orally or by injection.
- DPP-4 inhibitors (gliptins, e.g. **sitagliptin**) improve control and are well tolerated and weight neutral, but outcome evidence is inconsistent. Pancreatitis and heart failure are possible adverse effects of concern.
- Drugs that act on the sulfonylurea receptor (e.g. **tolbutamide**, **glibenclamide, gliclazide**) are well tolerated but often promote weight gain. They are associated with increased hypoglycaemia and possible cardiovascular risk compared with **metformin.**
- **Pioglitazone** improves control (reduces haemoglobin A_{1C}) but increases weight, causes heart failure and fluid retention and increases risk of fractures.
- **Acarbose** (α-glucosidase inhibitor) reduces carbohydrate absorption; it causes flatulence and diarrhoea.

REFERENCES AND FURTHER READING

References

Abdul-Ghani, M.A., Norton, L., DeFronzo, R.A., 2011. Role of sodium-glucose cotransporter 2 (SGLT 2) inhibitors in the treatment of type 2 diabetes. Endocr. Rev. 32 (4), 515–531.

Abdul-Ghani, M.A., Norton, L., DeFronzo, R.A., 2015. Renal sodium-glucose cotransporter inhibition in the management of type 2 diabetes mellitus. Am. J. Physiol. Renal Physiol. 309 (11), F889–F900.

American Diabetes Association, 1993. Implications of the diabetes control and complications trial. Diabetes 42, 1555–1558.

Atkin, S., Javed, Z., Fulcher, G., 2015. Insulin degludec and insulin aspart: novel insulins for the management of diabetes mellitus. Ther. Adv. Chronic. Dis. 6 (6), 375–388.

DeFronzo, R.A., Davidson, J.A., Del Prato, S., 2012. The role of the kidneys in glucose homeostasis: a new path towards normalizing glycaemia. Diabetes Obes. Metab. 14 (1), 5–14.

Duca, F.A., Cote, C.D., Rasmussen, B.A., et al., 2015. Metformin activates a duodenal AMPK-dependent pathway to lower hepatic glucose production in rats. Nat. Med. 21, 506–511.

Flory, J., Lipska, K., 2019. Metformin in 2019. JAMA 321, 1926–1927.

Gilbert, M.P., Pratley, R.E., 2020. GLP-1 Analogs and DPP-4 inhibitors in Type 2 diabetes therapy: review of head-to-head clinical trials. Front. Endocrinol. 11, 178.

Myers, R.W., Guan, H.P., Ehrhart, J., et al., 2017. Systemic pan-AMPK activator MK-8722 improves glucose homeostasis but induces cardiac hypertrophy. Science 357, 507–511.

Napolitano, A., Miller, S., Nicholls, A.W., et al., 2014. Novel gut-based pharmacology of metformin in patients with type 2 diabetes mellitus. PLoS One 9, e100778.

Viollet, B., Guigas, B., Garcia, N.S., Leclerc, J., Foretz, M., Andreelli, F., 2012. Cellular and molecular mechanisms of metformin: an overview. Clin. Sci. 122, 253–270.

Williams, G., 1994. Management of non-insulin dependent diabetes mellitus. Lancet 343, 95–100.

Zelniker, T.A., Braunwald, E., 2020. Mechanisms of cardiorenal effects of sodium-glucose cotransporter 2 inhibitors: JACC state-of-the-art review. J. Am. Coll. Cardiol. 75, 422–434.

Further reading

Artasensi, A., Pedretti, A., Vistoli, G., et al., 2020. Type 2 diabetes mellitus: a review of multi-target drugs. Molecules 25, 1987.

Farmer, K.L., Li, C.Y., Dobrowsky, R.T., 2012. Diabetic neuropathy: should a chaperone accompany our therapeutic approach? Pharmacol. Rev. 64, 880–900.

Lavin, D.P., White, M.F., Brazil, D.P., 2016. IRS proteins and diabetic complications. Diabetologia 59, 2280–2291.

Nauck, M.A., Quast, D.R., Wefers, J., et al., 2021. GLP-1 receptor agonists in the treatment of type 2 diabetes – state-of-the-art. Mol. Metab. 46, 101102.

Obesity 32

OVERVIEW

Obesity is a growing health issue around the world and is reaching epidemic proportions in some nations. The problem is not restricted to the inhabitants of the affluent countries, to the adult population or to any one socioeconomic class. Body fat represents stored energy and obesity occurs when the homeostatic mechanisms controlling energy balance become disordered or overwhelmed. In this chapter we first outline the endogenous regulation of appetite and body mass, and then consider the main health implications of obesity and its pathophysiology. We conclude with a discussion of the drugs currently licensed for the treatment of obesity and glance at possible future pharmacological treatments for this condition.

INTRODUCTION

Survival requires a continuous provision of energy to maintain homeostasis, even when the supply of food is intermittent. Evolution has furnished a mechanism for storing excess energy latent in foodstuffs in adipose tissue as energy-dense triglycerides, such that these can be easily mobilised when food is scarce. This mechanism, controlled by the so-called *thrifty genes*, was an obvious asset to our hunter–gatherer ancestors, but in many societies a combination of sedentary lifestyle, genetic susceptibility, cultural influences and unrestricted access to an ample supply of calorie-dense foods has led to a global epidemic of obesity, or 'globesity' as it is sometimes called. Obesity is one component of a cluster of disorders described in other chapters, which often coexist in the same individual, comprising what is now described as 'metabolic syndrome' (formerly 'metabolic X syndrome'), and which constitutes a rapidly growing public health problem.

DEFINITION OF OBESITY

'Obesity' may be defined as an illness where health (and hence life expectancy) is adversely affected by excess body fat.[1] But at what point does an individual become 'obese'? The generally accepted (WHO) benchmark is the body mass index (BMI). The BMI is expressed as W/h^2, where W = body weight (in kg), h = height (in metres). Although it is not a perfect index (e.g. it does not distinguish between fat and lean mass), the BMI is generally well correlated with other measurements of body fat, and it is widely utilised as a convenient index. While there are problems in defining a 'healthy' weight for a particular population, the WHO classifies adults with a BMI of ≥25 as being overweight and those with a BMI of ≥30 as obese. Childhood obesity is more difficult to assess.

Since the BMI obviously depends on the overall energy balance, another operational definition of obesity would be that it is a multifactorial disorder of energy balance in which calorie retention over the long-term exceeds energy output.

[1]'Persons who are naturally very fat are apt to die earlier than those who are slender' observed Hippocrates.

OBESITY AS A HEALTH PROBLEM

Obesity is a growing and costly global health problem. The WHO in 2016 estimated that worldwide obesity has almost tripled since 1975 and there were more than 1.9 billion overweight adults, approximately one-third of whom – amounting to more than 13% of the world's population – were obese according to the criteria outlined earlier. National obesity levels vary enormously, being less than 4% in Japan and parts of Africa, but a staggering 40% or more in parts of Polynesia. Adult obesity levels in the United States, Europe and the United Kingdom (among others) have increased three-fold since 1980, with figures of 34% being quoted for the United States by WHO (2016) and up to 28% for the United Kingdom. The disease is not confined to adults: some 39 million children or infants under 5 years old are estimated to be overweight or obese. In the United States, the number of overweight children has doubled and the number of overweight adolescents has trebled since 1980, with the overall prevalence of obesity close to 20% (data from the US Centers for Disease Control and Prevention, https://www.cdc.gov/obesity/data/childhood.html). Ironically, obesity often coexists with malnutrition in many developing countries. All socioeconomic classes are affected. In the poorest countries, it is the top socioeconomic classes in whom obesity is prevalent, but in the affluent West it is usually the reverse. In England, for example, the rates of obesity-related hospital admission in the most deprived areas are more than two-fold higher than the least deprived areas.

Overall, more people die in the world from being overweight and obese than being underweight, and the financial burden on the healthcare system is huge. An influential report (McKinsey Global Institute, 2014) estimated the global economic burden at US$2.1 trillion in 2014, 2.9% of the global GDP – more than the cost incurred by armed violence, war and terrorism taken altogether.

Obesity often coexists with metabolic and other disorders (particularly hypertension, hypercholesterolaemia and type 2 diabetes), together comprising the *metabolic syndrome*. This carries a high risk of cardiovascular conditions, strokes, certain types of cancers (particularly hormone dependent), respiratory disorders (particularly sleep apnoea) and digestive problems, as well as osteoarthritis. Poor mobility, fear of stigmatisation and social isolation take a further toll on the mental wellbeing of people with obesity. One commentator (Kopelman, 2000) has remarked that obesity 'is beginning to replace under-nutrition and infectious diseases as the most significant contributor to ill health'. In England, this is evidenced by the substantial increase in hospitalisations, with up to a million patients in 2019–2020 admitted with a primary or secondary diagnosis of obesity.

HOMEOSTATIC MECHANISMS CONTROLLING ENERGY BALANCE

A common view, and one that is implicitly encouraged by authors of numerous self-help books as well as the enormously lucrative dieting industry, is that obesity is simply the result of bad diet or wilful overeating (hyperphagia). In truth, however, the situation is more complex. On its own, dieting seldom provides a lasting solution: the failure rate is high (probably 90%), and most dieters eventually return to their original starting weight. This suggests the operation of some intrinsic homeostatic system that aims to maintain some balance between energy intake and energy expenditure. The systems for regulating body weight are, by necessity, intricate and complex in order to cope with the challenges of the substantial day-to-day variation in food intake and physical activity. Here, the homeostatic functions exert their effects through highly sophisticated internal control mechanisms with dynamic interplay between key organs such as the brain, liver, pancreas, gut and adipose tissue.

Energy homeostasis can be affected by genetic predisposition, and subsequently vary throughout life due to the influence of hormonal changes, metabolic stress, inflammation and ageing. When exposed to the same dietary choices, some individuals will become obese whereas others will not. Studies of obesity in monozygotic and dizygotic twins have established a strong genetic influence on the susceptibility to the condition, and studies of rare mutations have led to the discovery and elucidation of the neuroendocrine pathways that match food intake with energy expenditure. These, in turn, have led to the concept that derangements in these control systems are largely responsible for the onset and maintenance of obesity.

THE ROLE OF PERIPHERAL SIGNALLING IN BODY WEIGHT REGULATION

Intensive research over several decades has helped us gradually unravel the complex homeostatic interaction among the hypothalamus, brain stem and peripheral signals regarding availability of fuel from adipose tissue and gut. At the beginning of the 20th century it was observed that patients with damage to the hypothalamus tended to gain weight. In the 1940s it was also shown that discrete lesions in the hypothalamus of rodents caused them to become obese or exhibit unusual feeding behaviour. On the basis of early (1953) observations in rats, Kennedy proposed that a hormone released from adipose tissue acted on the hypothalamus to regulate body fat and food intake. An important conceptual breakthrough came in 1994, when Friedman and his colleagues identified *leptin*[2] as the adipocyte hormone that acts on neural connections, to suppress appetite and reduce adipose tissue.

Leptin mRNA is expressed in adipocytes; its synthesis is increased by glucocorticoids, insulin and oestrogens, and is reduced by β-adrenoceptor agonists. In normal human subjects, the release of leptin is pulsatile and correlated with increasing total fat mass and BMI. Leptin acts predominantly on the hypothalamus to reduce food intake when energy stores are sufficient. The importance of leptin therapy has been emphasised in animal models and rare congenital forms of leptin deficiency (Fig. 32.1), but its value as public health intervention is limited by the fact that many obese people actually have leptin resistance rather than a genuine deficiency of leptin.

In addition to its well-recognised action on lowering blood glucose, insulin (see Ch. 31) has effects on the brain that are similar to leptin in decreasing food intake. Insulin may also stimulate leptin release although the relationship between these two hormones is complex.

In addition to leptin and insulin, several other mediators, originating mainly from the gastrointestinal (GI) tract as well as in the hypothalamus, play a crucial role in determining food intake, meal size and the feeling of satisfaction produced ('satiety').[3] Peptide hormones secreted by cells in the wall of the small intestine in response to the arrival of nutrients in the intestinal lumen (see Ch. 30) are important in this connection. Table 32.1 and Fig. 32.2 summarise the chief characteristics of these mediators.

The majority of these peptides are released either during, or in anticipation of, eating and most are inhibitory in nature, producing either satiety or satiation. Two exceptions are the gastric hormone, *ghrelin*, which promotes hunger and food intake, and leptin itself, which is controlled by the amount of adipose tissue and is thus more involved with the longer-term energy status of the individual. The main targets for these hormones are receptors on vagal afferent fibres or within the hypothalamus (or elsewhere in the central nervous system [CNS]). Here, they modulate the release of other neurotransmitters that exert a fine regulation over eating behaviour, energy expenditure and body weight. Other actions of these peptide hormones include the release of insulin by the *incretins* (see Ch. 31), which include glucagon-like peptide-1 (GLP-1) and gastric inhibitory peptide (GIP).

The small intestine has L-type enteroendocrine cells that release GLP-1 in response to glucose and fat in food and drink. The early action of GLP-1 is to stimulate insulin secretion and inhibit glucagon, thus providing a means of regulating blood glucose concentrations (see Ch. 31). However, GLP-1 receptors are found in multiple other sites and their role in tackling obesity appears to be through reduction of appetite, and promotion of satiety centrally at the hypothalamus.

There are a wide range of other gut hormones that have a signalling role in energy homeostasis, but none of them have yet to be established as therapeutic targets in wider populations. Selected examples from a lengthy list of potentially promising candidates for further research include *nesfatin 1, pancreatic peptide tyrosine tyrosine (PYY), oxyntomodulin, ghrelin and obestatin – see Miller (2019) for a detailed review.*

[2]The word is derived from the Greek *leptos*, meaning thin.

[3]The terminology can be confusing. 'Hunger' obviously refers to the desire to eat; 'satiation' is the feeling that you have eaten enough in the course of a meal. 'Satiety' refers to the feeling after a meal that you don't yet need another.

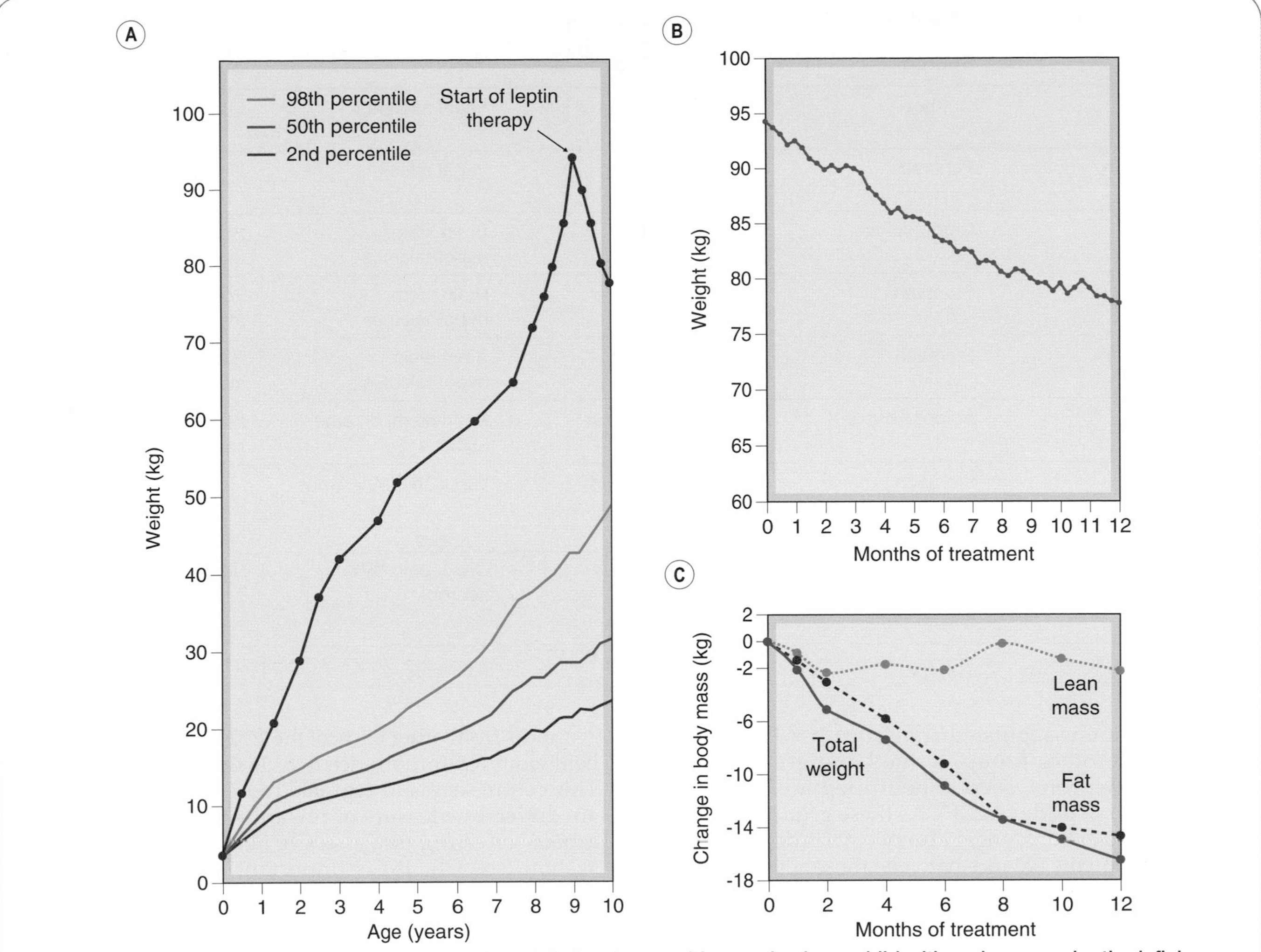

Fig. 32.1 The effect of recombinant leptin on body weight in a 9-year-old severely obese child with endogenous leptin deficiency because of a frame shift mutation in the leptin gene. Although of normal birth weight, the child began gaining weight at 4 months and was constantly demanding food. Prior to treatment, the child weighed 94.4 kg. Weight loss began after 2 weeks' treatment, and her eating pattern returned to normal. She had lost 15.6 kg of body fat after 1 year of treatment. (Data and figure adapted from Farooqi, I.S., Jebb, S.A., Langmack, G., et al., 1999. Effects of recombinant leptin therapy in a child with congenital leptin deficiency. N. Engl. J. Med. 341, 879–884.)

NEUROLOGICAL CIRCUITS THAT CONTROL BODY WEIGHT AND EATING BEHAVIOUR

CONTROL OF FOOD INTAKE

The manner in which all these hormonal and nutritional signals are processed and integrated with other viscerosensory, gustatory or olfactory information within the CNS is complex. Many sites are involved in different aspects of the process and some 50 hormones and neurotransmitters are implicated. This complex interaction between the CNS and the peripheral metabolic organs (liver, pancreas, gut, adipose tissue) needs to be tightly coordinated so that optimum weight balance is maintained. The account we present here is therefore necessarily an oversimplification: please see Roh et al. (2016) and Miller (2019) for a more complete picture of how the brain is a key player in the homeostatic regulation of energy balance.

As early lesioning studies predicted, the hypothalamus is the main brain centre that regulates appetite, feeding behaviour and energy status, although other sites in the brain, such as the nucleus accumbens (NAc), the amygdala and, especially, the nucleus tractus solitarius (NTS) in the medulla, are also crucial. Within the hypothalamus, the arcuate nucleus (ARC), situated in the floor of the third ventricle, is a key site. It receives afferent signals originating from the GI tract and contains receptors for leptin and other significant hormones. It also has extensive reciprocal connections with other parts of the hypothalamus involved in monitoring energy status, in particular the paraventricular nuclei and the ventromedial hypothalamus. Fig. 32.2 summarises in a simplified fashion some of the interactions that occur in the ARC.

Within the ARC are two groups of functionally distinct neurons that exert opposite effects on appetite. One group, termed *anorexigenic* (appetite-suppressing), secrete pro-opiomelanocortin (POMC)-derived peptides (such as α melanocyte-stimulating hormone [α-MSH]) or cocaine-

Table 32.1 Some peripheral hormones that regulate eating behaviour

Hormone	Source	Stimulus to release	Target	Effect
CCK	GI tract	During feeding or just before	Vagal afferents	Limits size of meal
Amylin, insulin, glucagon	Pancreas	During feeding or just before	Vagal afferents	Limits size of meal
PYY3–36	Ileum, colon	After feeding	Brain stem, hypothalamus	Postpones need for next meal
GLP-1	Stomach	After feeding	Brain stem, hypothalamus	Postpones need for next meal
Oxyntomodulin	Stomach	After feeding	Brain stem, hypothalamus	Postpones need for next meal
Leptin	Adipose tissue	Adiposity 'status'	Brain stem, arcuate nucleus	Longer-term regulation of food intake
Ghrelin	Stomach	Hunger, feeding	Vagus, hypothalamus	Increases food intake by increasing size and number of meals
Nesfatin 1	Hypothalamus, pancreas, adipose tissue and GI tract	Food intake	Orexigenic NPY neurons	Decreases appetite

CCK, Cholecystokinin; *GI*, gastrointestinal; *GLP-1*, glucagon-like peptide-1; *NPY*, neuropeptide Y; *PYY3–36*, peptide YY.

and amphetamine-regulated transcript (CART[4])–derived peptides. The other group, termed *orexigenic* (appetite-promoting) neurons, secrete neuropeptide Y (NPY) or agouti-related peptide (AgRP). As these groups of neurons have opposing actions, energy homeostasis depends, in the first instance, on the balance between these actions, the final effects of which are transduced by the brain stem motor system and change feeding behaviour.

Neurotransmitters such as GABA, noradrenaline, 5-hydroxytryptamine (5-HT) and dopamine also play a role in the modulation of satiety signals alongside the peptide transmitters. Noradrenaline is co-localised with NPY in some neurons and greatly potentiates its hyperphagic action. Deficit of dopamine impairs feeding behaviour, as do agonists at the 5-HT_{2C} receptor; antagonists at this receptor have the reverse effect. GABA is released from AgRP neurons and is modulated by nutritional status as well as by hormones such as leptin.

Many neural signals arising from the GI tract are integrated, and relayed on to the hypothalamus, by the NTS in the medulla. Some of these signals, including those of gustatory, olfactory, mechanical and viscerosensory signals, arise from vagal and other spinal afferents originating in the GI tract or liver. Endocrine signals have more complex signalling pathways. For example, cholecystokinin (CCK) is secreted by the duodenum in response to the process of eating and digestion of (especially fatty) foodstuffs. CCK acts locally on CCK_A receptors in the GI tract to stimulate vagal afferents and also acts on CCK_B receptors in the brain to function as a satiety factor.

Inputs from other parts of the CNS also influence feeding behaviour. Of importance to us is the input from the NAc. This centre seems to regulate those aspects of eating that are driven by pleasure or reward – the so-called 'hedonic' aspects of eating (see also Ch. 50). The endocannabinoid system (see Ch. 18) is important in this response. The hypothalamus contains large amounts of 2-arachidonyl glycerol and anandamide as well as the CB_1 receptor. Administration of endogenous or exogenous (e.g. Δ9-THC) cannabinoids provokes a powerful feeding response.[5] This system in turn may be modulated by 'stress' and other factors in the environment.

Many other hormones such as prolactin, androgens and oestrogens can modulate the activity of the hypothalamic control centres, and the situation is complex. The reader is referred to Cornejo et al. (2016) for a summary of this area.

CONTROL OF ENERGY EXPENDITURE

Balancing food intake is the energy expenditure required to maintain metabolism, physical activity and thermogenesis (heat production). The metabolic aspects include, among other things, cardiorespiratory work and the energy required by a multitude of enzymes. Physical activity increases all these, as well as increasing energy consumption by skeletal muscles. Exposure to cold also stimulates thermogenesis, and the reverse is also true. The, often dramatic (20%–40% increase), thermogenic effect of feeding itself may provide a partial protection against developing obesity.

The sympathetic nervous system (sometimes in concert with thyroid hormone) plays a significant part in energy regulation in cardiovascular and skeletal muscle function during physical activity, as well as the thermogenic

[4]So called because the administration of cocaine or amphetamine stimulates the transcription of this gene. Its expression in the hypothalamus is related to nutritional status implicating it in the control of appetite. Its receptor is unknown but it probably modulates the action of NPY and leptin.

[5]This effect is responsible for the 'munchies', a common side effect of smoking cannabis.

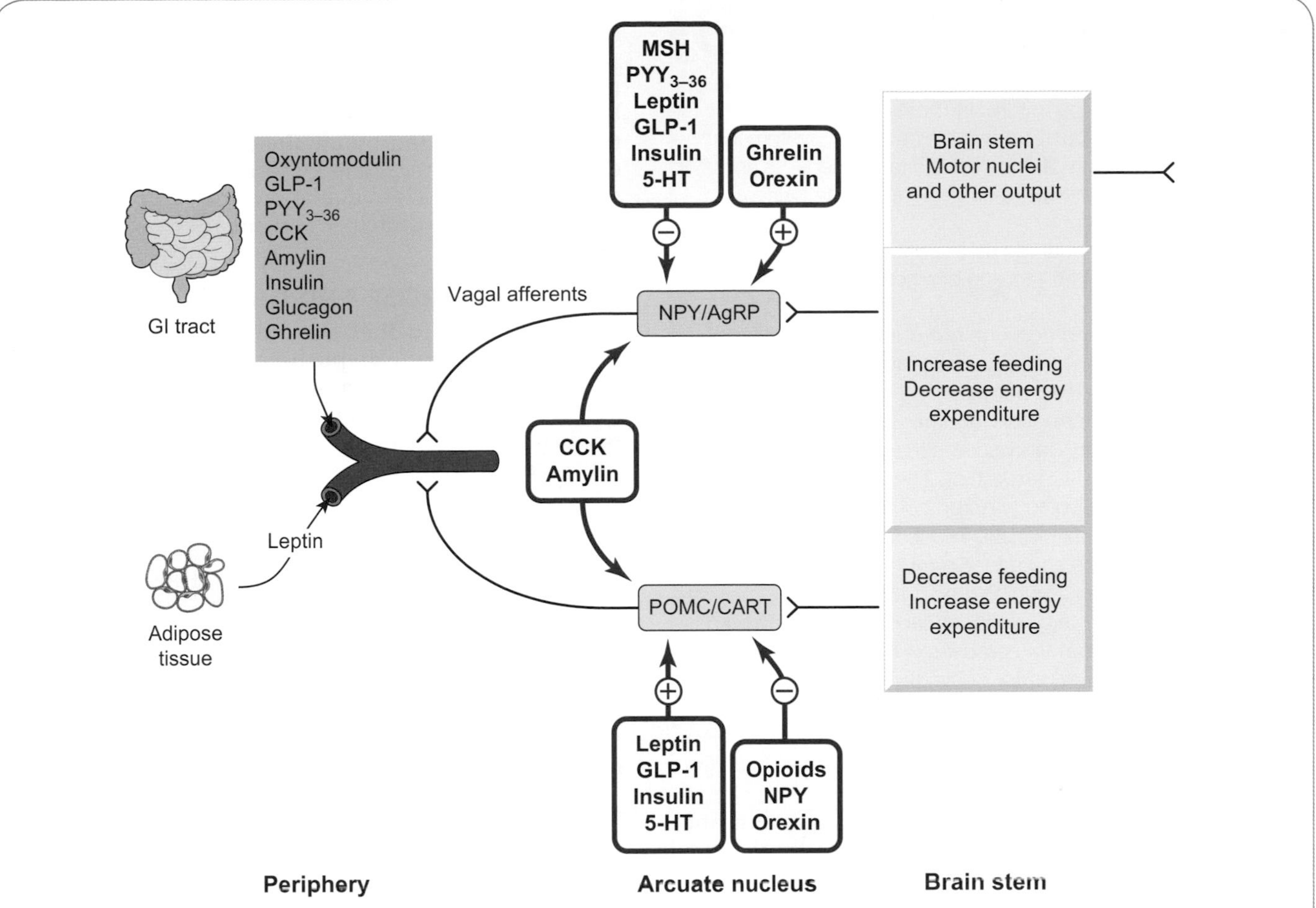

Fig. 32.2 A simplified representation of the role of peripheral hormones and other mediators in the regulation of energy balance and fat stores. The primary level of hypothalamic control is vested in two groups of neurons, with opposing actions, in the arcuate nucleus (ARC). In one group, the peptides neuropeptide Y (NPY) and agouti-related peptide (AgRP) are co-localised; the other contains the polypeptides prepro-opiomelanocortin (POMC) and cocaine- and amphetamine-related transcript (CART), which release α melanocyte-stimulating hormone (MSH). Blood-borne hormones arising from the gastrointestinal tract or adipose tissue are sensed by receptors on vagal and other afferents and are relayed through the nucleus tractus solitarius to modify the activity of these neuronal circuits. The influence of hormones on each neuronal group is indicated. Some (e.g. leptin) arise from the peripheral blood and influence the ARC neurons directly or indirectly through neuronal signals, while others (e.g. 5-hydroxytryptamine [5-HT], orexin) originate within the central nervous system itself. Activation of the NPY/AgRP group by, for example, a fall in leptin or an increase in ghrelin levels results in increased food intake and decreased energy expenditure. In the POMC/CART group of neurons, increased leptin or other hormone levels triggered by overfeeding produces a predominately inhibitory effect on feeding behaviour. Several other hormones such as cholecystokinin (CCK) and amylin also alter the properties of the ARC neurons although the mechanism is not clear. *GLP-1*, Glucagon-like peptide-1; *PYY_{3-36}*, peptide YY. (Modified from Adan, R.A., Vanderschuren, L.J., la Fleur, S.E., 2008. Anti-obesity drugs and neural circuits of feeding. Trends Pharmacol. Sci. 29, 208–217.)

response of adipose tissue and the response to cold. Adipose tissue is now recognised as an endocrine organ that secretes hormones (e.g. leptin) as well as cytokines in a complex dynamic interplay with skeletal muscle activity to regulate energy stores. Both 'white' and (especially) 'brown' fat cells (the colour is caused by the high density of mitochondria) play a major role in thermogenesis. Brown fat, which is densely innervated by the sympathetic nervous system, is abundant in rodents and human infants, but far less common in adult humans. There remains substantial uncertainty regarding the exact role of brown fat or the importance of heat-generating mitochondrial uncoupling protein (UCP-1) in human obesity.

THE PATHOPHYSIOLOGY OF HUMAN OBESITY

In most adults, body fat and body weight remain more or less constant over many years, even decades, in the face of very large variations in food intake and energy expenditure amounting to about a million calories per year. The steady-state body weight and BMI of an individual, as explained, depend upon the integration of multiple interacting regulatory pathways. How, then, does obesity occur? Why is it so difficult for the obese to lose weight and maintain the lower weight?

Energy balance

Energy balance depends on food intake, energy storage in fat and energy expenditure. In most individuals the process is tightly regulated by a homeostatic system that integrates inputs from a number of internal sensors and external factors. Important components of the system include the following:

- Hormones that signal the status of fat stores (e.g. leptin). Increasing fat storage promotes leptin release from adipocytes.
- Hormones released from the gut during feeding that convey sensations of hunger (e.g. ghrelin), satiety (e.g. CCK) or satiation (e.g. peptide YY [PYY_{3-36}]).
- This hormonal information together with neural, gustatory, olfactory and viscerosensory input is integrated in the hypothalamus. The ARC is a key site.
- Two groups of opposing neurons in the ARC sense hormonal and other signals. Those secreting POMC/CART products promote feeding while those secreting NPY/AgRP inhibit feeding. Many other CNS neurotransmitters (e.g. endocannabinoids) are involved.

The net output from this process is relayed to other sites in the brain stem motor nuclei that control feeding behaviour.

The main determinant is manifestly a disturbance of the complex homeostatic mechanisms that control energy balance, and genetic factors that underlie this disturbance. Other factors, such as the environment, food availability and lack of physical activity, also contribute. Additionally, of course, there are overlaying social, cultural and psychological aspects. The pathophysiology of obesity most likely involves disturbance(s) in any or all of the multitude of other factors involved in energy balance, thus making it difficult to achieve long-term success with drug therapy directed at single targets. We discuss here the physiological and genetic mechanisms; the role of social, cultural and psychological aspects we will leave (with a profound sigh of relief) to the psychosociologists!

FOOD INTAKE AND OBESITY

As Spiegelman and Flier (1996) point out, 'one need not be a rocket scientist to notice that increased food intake tends to be associated with obesity'. A typical obese subject will usually gain 20 kg over a decade or so. This means that there has been a daily excess of energy input over energy requirement of 30–40 kcal initially (i.e. 1.5%–2%), increasing gradually to maintain the increased body weight.

The type of food eaten, as well as the quantity, can disturb energy homeostasis. Fat is an energy-dense foodstuff, and it may be that the satiety mechanisms regulating appetite, which react rapidly to carbohydrate and protein, react too slowly to stop an individual consuming excess fat.

However, when obese individuals reduce their calorie intake as part of a diet regime, they shift into negative energy balance. When they lose weight, the resting metabolic rate decreases, and there is a concomitant reduction in energy expenditure. Thus an individual who was previously obese and is now of normal weight generally needs fewer calories to maintain that weight than an individual who has never been obese. The decrease in energy expenditure appears to be largely caused by an alteration in the conversion efficiency of chemical energy to mechanical work in the skeletal muscles. This adaptation to the caloric reduction contributes to the difficulty of maintaining weight loss by diet.

PHYSICAL EXERCISE AND OBESITY

It used to be said that the only exercise effective in combating obesity was pushing one's chair back from the table. It is now recognised that physical activity - i.e. increased energy expenditure - has a much more positive role in reducing fat storage and adjusting energy balance in the obese, particularly if associated with modification of the diet. A serendipitous natural population study provides an example. Many years ago, a tribe of Pima Indians split into two groups. One group in Mexico continued to live simply at subsistence level, eating frugally and spending most of the week in hard physical labour. They are generally lean and have a low incidence of type 2 diabetes. The other group settled in the United States - an environment with easy access to calorie-rich food and less need for hard physical work. They are, on average, 57 lb (26 kg) heavier than the Mexican group and have a high incidence of early-onset type 2 diabetes.

GENETIC FACTORS AND OBESITY

Rapid advances in genetic epidemiology have driven research towards large genome-wide association studies of obesity rather than limited or narrow observations of twins, nuclear families and adoption cohorts. It is now thought that genetic components underpin about 40%–50% of the susceptibility or predisposition to obesity in general populations. However, there are subgroups of people with severe obesity where the relative genetic contribution ('heritability') is much higher and exceeds 60%–80%. At least 15 separate genes (mainly related to the leptin-melanocortin pathway) have been implicated in monogenic or single-gene defects that contribute to obesity and can be passed on in traditional Mendelian pattern. Nevertheless, about two-thirds of the heritability surrounding BMI can be attributed to common DNA variants, of which there are potentially thousands. As more and more variants come to our attention, it becomes likely that each additional new variant may on its own only exert a modest effect on BMI, and the sum of their influence is more than the parts.

Overall, most cases of obesity will turn out to be polygenic in nature, involving a complex interaction between multiple sets of genetic sites. Single-gene defects that exert a substantial individual effect are thought to be the main underlying factor in less than 10% of people with obesity. Even then, a large population study (UK Biobank) of the melanocortin pathway has found that the accompanying polygenic contribution can significantly ameliorate the effects of the single-gene defect, thus creating substantial heterogeneity in the BMI of people carrying an MC_4 variant (see Chami et al., 2020). The potential influence of thousands of DNA variants on susceptibility to obesity, when taken in tandem with complex epigenetic, environmental and behavioural factors, makes it very difficult to develop safe and effective long-term pharmacological agents for prevention and treatment of obesity (see Bouchard, 2021, for an excellent discussion on the genetics of obesity).

PHARMACOLOGICAL APPROACHES TO THE PROBLEM OF OBESITY

The first weapons in the fight against obesity are diet and exercise. Unfortunately, these often fail or show only short-term efficacy, leaving surgical techniques (such as gastric stapling or bypass) or drug therapy as a viable alternative. *Bariatric* (weight loss) surgery is much more effective than currently licensed drugs, and is believed to work chiefly, not by mechanically limiting gastric capacity, but by its effects on gut hormone responses to feeding, acting, for example, to produce earlier satiety. This may be construed as indirect evidence for the utility of pharmacological measures designed to interrupt these messengers.

The attempt to control body weight with drugs has had a long and, regrettably, a largely undistinguished[8] history. Many types of 'anorectic' (appetite suppressant) agents have been tested in the past, including the uncoupling agent **dinitrophenol** (DNP), **amphetamine** and derivatives such as **dexfenfluramine** and **fenfluramine**. All have been withdrawn from clinical use because of serious adverse effects. DNP, an industrial chemical, is advertised online for slimmers and bodybuilders as a weight loss and 'fat-burning agent', and has caused deaths among those who use it for this purpose. It blocks mitochondrial ATP production, diverting energy metabolism to generate heat instead of ATP and increasing the overall metabolic rate, which can cause life-threatening hyperthermia.[9]

Obesity

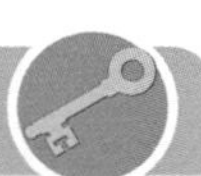

- Obesity is a multifactorial disorder of energy balance, in which long-term calorie intake exceeds energy output.
- A subject with a body mass index (BMI) (W/h^2) of 20–25 kg/m^2 is considered as having a healthy body weight, one with a BMI of 25–30 kg/m^2 as overweight, and one with a BMI >30 kg/m^2 as obese.
- Obesity is a growing problem in most rich nations; the incidence – at present approximately >30% in the United States and >20% in Europe – is increasing.
- A BMI >30 kg/m^2 significantly increases the risk of type 2 diabetes, hypercholesterolaemia, hypertension, ischaemic heart disease, gallstones and some cancers.
- The causes of obesity include:
  - dietary, exercise, social, financial and cultural factors;
  - genetic susceptibility;
  - deficiencies in the synthesis or action of leptin or other gut hormone signals;
  - defects in the hypothalamic neuronal systems responding to any of these signals;
  - defects in the systems controlling energy expenditure (e.g. reduced sympathetic activity), decreased metabolic expenditure of energy or decreased thermogenesis caused by a reduction in β_3 adrenoceptor-mediated tone and/or dysfunction of the proteins that uncouple oxidative phosphorylation.

CENTRALLY ACTING APPETITE SUPPRESSANTS

There have been many attempts to use centrally acting drugs to control appetite and this is an area which is still being actively exploited by drug hunters. Regulatory authorities in the United States and Europe have licensed the mixture of the opioid-receptor antagonist **naltrexone** and the noradrenaline–dopamine uptake–reuptake inhibitor, **bupropion** (see Ch. 50). This combination was associated with modest weight loss but there are ongoing concerns about neuropsychiatric (drowsiness, impaired mood and driving) and cardiovascular (e.g. hypertension) adverse effects. Intriguingly, a large cardiovascular trial of this product was abandoned by the academic team when potentially favourable data in the early interim phase were leaked by the pharmaceutical company. Subsequent analysis of the larger trial dataset failed to confirm these favourable findings, and a further cardiovascular trial is ongoing.

Qsymia, a mixture of an old appetite suppressant drug, **phentermine**, and an anticonvulsant, **topiramate**, was approved in the United States in 2012 despite some reservations about cardiovascular and neuropsychiatric adverse effects such as depression, anxiety and altered cognition (culminating in a negative licensing decision in Europe). The drug stimulates the synaptic release of serotonin as well as noradrenaline and dopamine (and increases GABA action).

Sibutramine (now withdrawn in most countries because of clinical trial evidence demonstrating increased cardiovascular risk) inhibits the reuptake of 5-HT and noradrenaline at the hypothalamic sites that regulate food intake.[10] Its main effects are to reduce food intake and cause dose-dependent weight loss (Fig. 32.3). It enhanced satiety and was reported to produce a reduction in waist circumference, a decrease in plasma triglycerides and very-low-density lipoproteins, but an increase in high-density lipoproteins. Like many similar drug regimes, sibutramine was much more effective when combined with lifestyle modification.

Other serotoninergic drugs have been tested with disappointing long-term findings. **Lorcaserin**, a 5-HT_{2C} receptor agonist, was approved in the United States in 2012 for use as an appetite suppressant in certain patients. It acts by increasing POMC levels in the hypothalamus. In clinical trials, it enhanced weight loss through dieting, but

[8]As the showman Bynum said: 'There's a sucker born every minute … and one born to take him' … thyroxine (to increase metabolic rate, see Ch. 34), swallowing parasites (intestinal worms compete for ingested food), amphetamines (see Ch. 59), drugs that cause malabsorption, hence leaking fat per rectum (see later in this chapter) … really!

[9]DNP is reported to have been given to Russian soldiers in the Second World War, to keep them warm.

[10]Many antidepressant drugs act by the same mechanism (see Ch. 48), and also cause weight loss by reducing appetite. However, sibutramine does not have antidepressant properties. Furthermore, depressed patients are often obese, and antidepressant drugs are used to treat both conditions (see Appolinario et al., 2004).

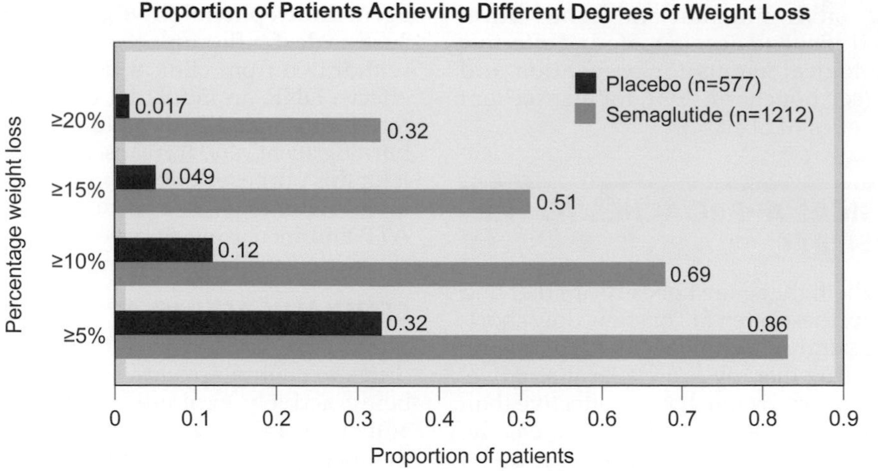

Fig. 32.3 The effect of treatment with a glucagon-like peptide-1 agonist, semaglutide 2.4 mg injected once weekly, with monthly counselling on diet and exercise. The Y axis shows percentage weight loss after 68 weeks follow-up. The X axis shows the proportions of patients achieving a particular amount of weight loss. Whilst semaglutide is clearly more effective than placebo, there remains a sizeable proportion (3 in 10) who do not achieve 10% reduction in weight with semaglutide. (Data from Wilding, J. P. H., Batterham, R. L., Calanna, S., et al. 2021. Once-weekly semaglutide in adults with overweight or obesity. N. Engl. J. Med. 384, 989–1002.)

patients regained weight after stopping the drug. It also improved blood sugar control but this did not translate into subsequent cardiovascular benefits. **Lorcaserin** was withdrawn in 2020 due to a small increased risk of cancer when compared to placebo.

The cannabinoid pathway was the target of the CB_1 receptor antagonist **rimonabant** which was originally developed to promote smoking cessation (see Ch. 18). This drug was introduced as an appetite suppressant following some encouraging clinical trials but was eventually withdrawn in the United States in 2008 because of adverse effects on mood seen in some patients. A similar fate overtook another promising CB_1 antagonist, **taranabant**.

ORLISTAT

The only drug currently (2021) available without prescription in the United Kingdom for the treatment of obesity is the lipase inhibitor **orlistat**, used with concomitant dietary and other therapy (e.g. exercise).

In the intestine, orlistat reacts with serine residues at the active sites of gastric and pancreatic lipases, irreversibly inhibiting these enzymes and thereby preventing the breakdown of dietary fat to fatty acids and glycerol. It therefore decreases absorption (and correspondingly causes faecal excretion) of some 30% of dietary fat. Given in conjunction with a low-calorie diet in obese individuals, it produces a modest but consistent loss of weight compared with placebo-treated control subjects. In a meta-analysis of 11 long-term placebo-controlled trials encompassing more than 6000 patients, orlistat was found to produce a 2.9% greater reduction in body weight than in the control group, and 12% more patients lost 10% or more of their body weight compared with the controls (Padwal et al., 2003).

Orlistat is also reported to be effective in patients suffering from type 2 diabetes and other complications of obesity. It reduces leptin levels and blood pressure, protects against weight loss–induced changes in biliary secretion, delays gastric emptying and gastric secretion and improves several important metabolic parameters without interfering with the release or action of thyroid or other important hormones (Curran and Scott, 2004). It does not induce changes in energy expenditure.

PHARMACOKINETIC ASPECTS AND UNWANTED EFFECTS

Virtually all (97%) of orlistat is excreted in the faeces (83% unchanged), with only negligible amounts of the drug or its metabolites being absorbed.

Abdominal cramps, flatus with discharge and faecal incontinence can occur, as can intestinal borborygmi (rumbling) and oily spotting. Surprisingly, in view of the possibility of these antisocial effects occurring, the drug is well tolerated. Supplementary therapy with fat-soluble vitamins may be needed. The absorption of contraceptive pills and **ciclosporin** (see Ch. 25) may be decreased. The former is not usually clinically significant but the latter is potentially more serious. Given its good safety record, orlistat is available in the UK as an over-the-counter medicine for weight loss.

GLP-1 RECEPTOR AGONISTS

Clinical trials have demonstrated the efficacy of GLP-1 receptor agonists (**liraglutide**, **semaglutide**) in lowering body weight (mainly through loss of visceral fat) in conjunction with diet and exercise (Fig. 32.3). Specific formulations of **liraglutide** (daily subcutaneous injection) and **semaglutide** (licensed as a once weekly subcutaneous injection; there is a daily oral formulation in clinical trials) are available. Higher doses of these drugs are required for treatment of obesity than the typical dose ranges used for glucose lowering in type II diabetes mellitus (see Ch. 31). GI upset (nausea, vomiting, altered bowel habit) is a recognised adverse effect that stems from GLP-1 and its action on the gut.

Recent developments include studies of agonists at two or more targets which may include GIP and glucagon receptors. **Tirzepatide** is an example of a dual GIP and GLP-1 receptor agonist with greater clinical trial efficacy in controlling blood glucose as well as promoting weight loss compared to **semaglutide** in type II diabetes. Here, it is thought that GIP

Clinical uses of anti-obesity drugs

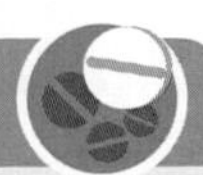

- The main treatment of obesity is a suitable sustainable diet and increased exercise.
- **Orlistat**, which causes fat malabsorption, is used together with dietary restriction in obese individuals, and also in overweight patients who have additional cardiovascular risk factors (e.g. diabetes mellitus, hypertension).
  - Orlistat therapy should be stopped after 12 weeks if the patient has not been able to lose at least 5% of their body weight from the time of drug initiation.
- **Liraglutide** and **semaglutide** are GLP-1 inhibitors that are effective in promoting weight loss as part of a diet and exercise programme; there is some evidence that **semaglutide** may be marginally more effective than **liraglutide.**
- Many centrally acting appetite suppressants (e.g. **fenfluramine**, **sibutramine**) have been withdrawn because of addiction, or other serious cardiovascular adverse effects.
- GI ('bariatric') surgery for obesity is a highly invasive procedure with potential complications but is effective for long-term management of severe obesity.

reduces food intake whilst increasing energy expenditure, thus potentially acting in tandem with GLP-1 agonism to have greater effects on body weight. Oxyntomodulin has structural similarities to proglucagon, and it has functional activity as a dual glucagon receptor and GLP-1 receptor agonist to similarly suppress appetite whilst enhancing energy use. The short half-life and high renal clearance of oxyntomodulin make it unsuitable for long-term use, but related molecules are currently being trialled.

NEW APPROACHES TO OBESITY THERAPY

As might be imagined, the quest for further effective anti-obesity agents is the subject of prodigious efforts by the pharmaceutical industry. However, this road is littered with examples of highly promising candidates that did not progress to fruition after further study (see Williams et al., 2020, for a comprehensive review)

Rare cases of leptin deficiency in patients have been successfully treated by long-term treatment with the hormone (**metreleptin**, a recombinant human leptin analogue), but this is unlikely to be of more than limited use in the future. Other strategies aim to alter the CNS levels of neurotransmitters such as NPY or melanocortins, which transduce hormonal signals regulating appetite. The tractability of the MC_4 receptor itself as a drug target, coupled with the observation that defects in MC_4 signalling are prevalent in obesity, has attracted much interest from the pharmaceutical industry. However, the polygenic nature of obesity means that **setmelanotide**, a melanocortin agonist, is only approved in the United States for rare genetic obesity disorders related to mutations in the MC_4 pathway. **Setmelanotide** can reduce body weight and hunger in certain target groups but has to be administered as a daily subcutaneous injection.

A host of other peptides have been studied, including amylin, oxyntomodulin and leptin analogues and NPY antagonists. Even vaccination against ghrelin or somatostatin has been mooted as a therapeutic strategy but none of these candidates have shown sustained benefit on their own. The complex multifactorial nature of obesity, coupled with substantial individual variation in response to single agents, has shifted the research focus towards combination therapy covering two or more targets (see Finer, 2021, and Williams et al., 2020).

All in all, it is depressing that despite all the ground-breaking work on the neuroendocrine control of feeding and body weight, so few really novel drugs with acceptable benefit:harm profiles have found their way on to the market. The lack of sustained success with pharmacological therapies has led to the emergence of bariatric surgery as a more promising long-term option for reducing complications such as hypertension and diabetes mellitus in patients with severe obesity.

REFERENCES AND FURTHER READING

Body weight regulation and obesity

Adan, R.A., Vanderschuren, L.J., la Fleur, S.E., 2008. Anti-obesity drugs and neural circuits of feeding. Trends Pharmacol. Sci. 29, 208–217.

Bouchard, C., 2021. Genetics of obesity: what we have learned over decades of research. Obesity (Silver Spring) 29, 802–820.

Chami, N., Preuss, M., Walker, R.W., et al., 2020. The role of polygenic susceptibility to obesity among carriers of pathogenic mutations in MC4R in the UK Biobank population. PLoS Med. 17, e1003196.

Cornejo, M.P., Hentges, S.T., Maliqueo, M., Coirini, H., Becu-Villalobos, D., Elias, C.F., 2016. Neuroendocrine regulation of metabolism. J. Neuroendocrinol. 28, 1–12.

Farooqi, I.S., Jebb, S.A., Langmack, G., et al., 1999. Effects of recombinant leptin therapy in a child with congenital leptin deficiency. N. Engl. J. Med. 341, 879–884.

Kopelman, P.G., 2000. Obesity as a medical problem. Nature 404, 635–643.

McKinsey Global Institute, 2014. Overcoming Obesity: An Initial Economic Analysis, p. 120. McKinsey & Company, London.

Miller, G.D., 2019. Appetite regulation: hormones, peptides, and neurotransmitters and their role in obesity. Am. J. Lifestyle Med. 13, 586–601.

Roh, E., Song, D.K., Kim, M.S., 2016. Emerging role of the brain in the homeostatic regulation of energy and glucose metabolism. Exp. Mol. Med. 48, e216.

Spiegelman, B.M., Flier, J.S., 1996. Adipogenesis and obesity: rounding out the big picture. Cell 87, 377–389.

Drugs in obesity

Appolinario, J.C., Bueno, J.R., Coutinho, W., 2004. Psychotropic drugs in the treatment of obesity: what promise? CNS Drugs 18, 629–651.

Curran, M.P., Scott, L.J., 2004. Orlistat: a review of its use in the management of patients with obesity. Drugs 64, 2845–2864.

Finer, N., 2021. Future directions in obesity pharmacotherapy. Eur. J. Intern. Med. 93, 13–20.

Padwal, R., Li, S.K., Lau, D.C., 2003. Long-term pharmacotherapy for overweight and obesity: a systematic review and meta-analysis of randomized controlled trials. Int. J. Obes. Relat. Metab. Disord. 27, 1437–1446.

West, D.B., Fey, D., Woods, S.C., 1984. Cholecystokinin persistently suppresses meal size but not food intake in free-feeding rats. Am. J. Physiol. 246, R776–R787.

Wilding, J.P.H., Batterham, R.L., Calanna, S., et al., 2021. Once-weekly semaglutide in adults with overweight or obesity. N. Engl. J. Med. 384, 989–1002.

Williams, D.M., Nawaz, A., Evans, M., 2020. Drug therapy in obesity: a review of current and emerging treatments. Diabetes Ther. 11, 1199–1216.

33 The pituitary and the adrenal cortex

OVERVIEW

The pituitary gland and the adrenal cortex release hormones that regulate salt and water balance, energy expenditure, growth, sexual behaviour and development, immune function and many other vital mechanisms. The commander-in-chief of this impressive hormonal campaign is the hypothalamus and the functioning unit is known as the *hypothalamo–pituitary–adrenal (HPA) axis*. In the first part of this chapter we review the control of pituitary function by hypothalamic hormones, and the physiological roles and clinical utilities of both anterior and posterior pituitary hormones. The second part of the chapter focuses on adrenal hormones and, in particular, the anti-inflammatory effect of glucocorticoids. This should be read in conjunction with the relevant sections of Chapters 3 and 25.

THE PITUITARY GLAND

The pituitary gland comprises three histologically distinct structures which arise from two separate embryological precursors (Fig. 33.1). The *anterior pituitary* and the *intermediate lobe* are derived from the endoderm of the buccal cavity, while the *posterior pituitary* is derived from neural ectoderm. The anterior and posterior lobes receive independent neuronal input from the hypothalamus, with which they have an intimate functional relationship.

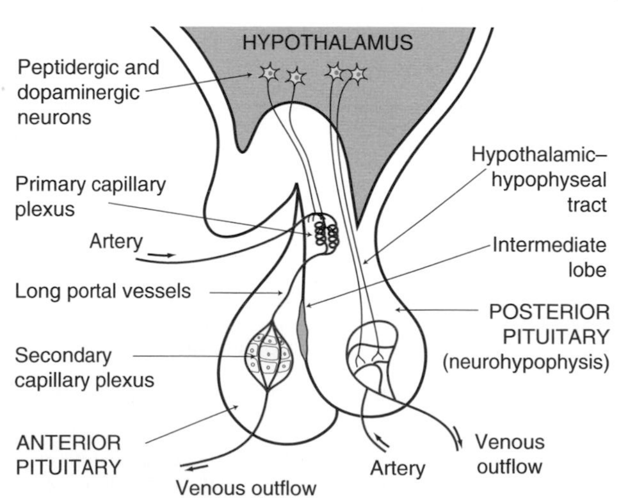

Fig. 33.1 Schematic diagram of vascular and neuronal relationships between the hypothalamus, the posterior pituitary and the anterior pituitary. The main portal vessels to the anterior pituitary lie in the pituitary stalk and arise from the primary plexus in the hypothalamus, but some (the short portal vessels) arise from the vascular bed in the posterior pituitary (not shown).

THE ANTERIOR PITUITARY GLAND

The anterior pituitary gland (*adenohypophysis*) secretes a number of hormones crucial for normal physiological function. Within this tissue are specialised cells such as *corticotrophs*, *lactotrophs* (*mammotrophs*), *somatotrophs*, *thyrotrophs* and *gonadotrophs*, which secrete hormones that regulate different endocrine organs throughout the body (Table 33.1). Interspersed among these are other cell types, including *folliculostellate cells*, which exert a nurturing and regulatory influence on the hormone-secreting endocrine cells, providing them with both structural and chemical support within the hypothalamus.

Secretion from the anterior pituitary is largely regulated by the release from the hypothalamus of, what are generally known as, 'releasing factors' – in effect, local hormones – that reach the pituitary through the bloodstream.[1] The blood supply to the hypothalamus divides to form a meshwork of capillaries, the *primary plexus*, which drains into the *hypophyseal portal vessels*. These pass through the pituitary stalk to feed a *secondary plexus* of capillaries in the anterior pituitary. Peptidergic neurons in the hypothalamus secrete a variety of releasing or inhibitory hormones directly into the capillaries of the primary capillary plexus (see Table 33.1 and Fig. 33.1). Most of these regulate the secretion of hormones from the anterior lobe, although the *melanocyte-stimulating hormones* (MSHs) are secreted mainly from the intermediate lobe.

The release of stimulatory hormones is regulated by negative feedback pathways between the hormones of the hypothalamus, the anterior pituitary and the peripheral endocrine glands. Hormones secreted from the peripheral glands exert regulatory actions on both the hypothalamus and the anterior pituitary, constituting the *long negative feedback* pathways. Anterior pituitary hormones acting directly on the hypothalamus comprise the *short negative feedback* pathway. This feedback mechanism is particularly pronounced in the HPA axis and underlies the pharmacological basis of some drug actions, which take advantage of such pronounced negative feedback loops.

The peptidergic neurons in the hypothalamus are themselves influenced by other centres within the central nervous system (CNS) and mediated through neural pathways that release dopamine, noradrenaline, 5-hydroxytryptamine and the opioid peptides (which are particularly abundant in the hypothalamus). Hypothalamic control of the anterior pituitary is also

[1]The term 'factor' was originally coined at a time when neither their structure nor their function was known. These are blood-borne messengers, and are indeed clearly hormones but the nomenclature, although irrational, lingers on. This process is common in biological nomenclature.

Table 33.1 Hormones secreted by the hypothalamus and the anterior pituitary and some related drugs

Hypothalamic factor/hormone[a]	Effect on anterior pituitary	Main effects of anterior pituitary hormone
CRF	Releases ACTH (corticotrophin) *Analogue*: tetracosactide	Stimulates secretion of adrenal cortical hormones (mainly glucocorticoids); maintains integrity of adrenal cortex.
TRH *Analogue*: protirelin	Releases TSH (thyrotrophin)	Stimulates synthesis and secretion of thyroid hormones; maintains integrity of thyroid gland.
GHRF (somatorelin) *Analogue*: sermorelin	Releases GH (somatotrophin) *Analogue*: somatropin	Regulates growth, partly directly, but also by releasing somatomedins from the liver and elsewhere; increases protein synthesis, increases blood glucose, stimulates lipolysis.
Growth hormone release-inhibiting factor (somatostatin) *Analogues*: octreotide, lanreotide, paseriotide	Inhibits the release of GH	Prevents effects of GHRF. Blocks TSH release.
GnRH *Analogues*: 'gonadorelin analogues' – buserelin, goserelin, leuprorelin, naferelin, triptorelin	Releases FSH (see Ch. 35)	Stimulates the growth of the ovum and the Graafian follicle (female) and gametogenesis (male); with LH, stimulates the secretion of oestrogen throughout the menstrual cycle and progesterone in the second half.
	Release of LH or interstitial cell-stimulating hormone (see Ch. 35)	Stimulation of ovulation and the development of the corpus luteum; with FSH, stimulation of secretion of oestrogen and progesterone in the menstrual cycle; in male, regulation of testosterone secretion.
PRF	Releases prolactin	Together with other hormones, prolactin promotes development of mammary tissue during pregnancy and stimulates milk production in the postpartum period.
Prolactin release-inhibiting factor (probably dopamine)	Inhibits the release of prolactin	Prevents effects of PRF.
MSH-releasing factor	Releases α-, β- and γ-MSH	Promotes formation of melanin, which causes darkening of skin; MSH has anti-inflammatory actions and also regulates appetite/feeding.
MSH release-inhibiting factor	Inhibits the release of α-, β- and γ-MSH	Prevents effects of MSH.

[a]These hormones are often spelled without the 'h' (e.g. corticotropin, thyrotropin, etc.) in contemporary texts. We have retained the original nomenclature in this edition.

ACTH, Adrenocorticotrophic hormone; *CRF*, corticotrophin-releasing factor; *FSH*, follicle stimulating hormone; *GH*, growth hormone; *GHRF*, growth hormone-releasing factor; *GnRH*, gonadotrophin (or luteinising hormone)-releasing hormone; *LH*, luteinising hormone; *MSH*, melanocyte-stimulating hormone; *PRF*, prolactin-releasing factor; *TRH*, thyrotrophin-releasing hormone; *TSH*, thyroid-stimulating hormone.

exerted through the *tuberohypophyseal dopaminergic pathway* (see Ch. 39), the neurons of which lie in close apposition to the primary capillary plexus. Dopamine secreted directly from dopaminergic neurons into the hypophyseal portal circulation reaches the anterior pituitary via the bloodstream, inhibiting the secretion of prolactin (see Ch. 35).

HYPOTHALAMIC HORMONES

The secretion of anterior pituitary hormones is primarily regulated by the peptide 'releasing factors' that originate from the hypothalamus. The most significant are described in more detail later. **Somatostatin** and **gonadotrophin-releasing hormone** are used therapeutically, the others have mainly diagnostic utilities or are useful research tools. Some of these peptides also function as neurotransmitters or neuromodulators elsewhere in the CNS (see Ch. 39).

SOMATOSTATIN

Somatostatin is a peptide of 14 amino acid residues, and as its name suggests ('statin'), it is inhibitory by nature. It inhibits the release of growth hormone and thyroid-stimulating hormone (TSH, thyrotrophin) from the anterior pituitary (Fig. 33.2), and insulin and glucagon

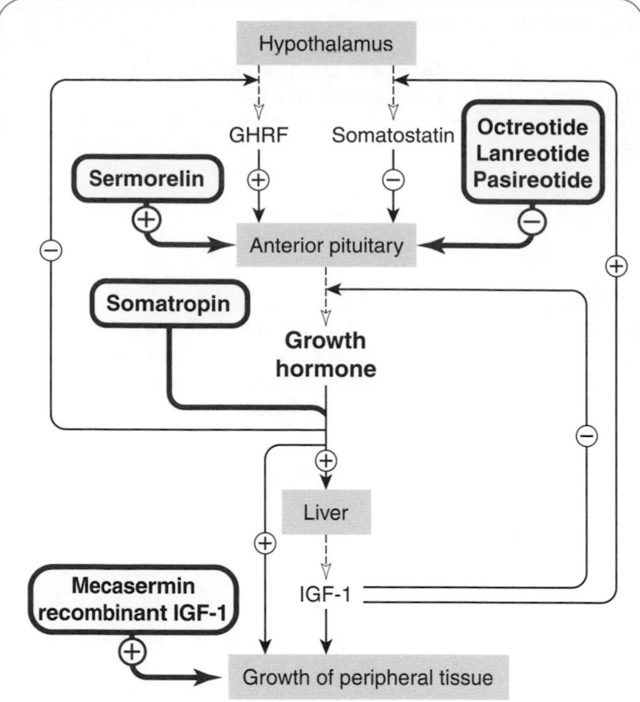

Fig. 33.2 Control of growth hormone secretion and its actions. Drugs are shown in *red-bordered boxes*. *GHRF*, Growth hormone-releasing factor; *IGF-1*, insulin-like growth factor-1.

from the pancreas. It also decreases the release of most gastrointestinal (GI) hormones and reduces gastric acid and pancreatic secretion.

Octreotide is a long-acting analogue of **somatostatin**. It is used for the treatment of *carcinoid* and other hormone-secreting tumours (see Ch. 16). It also has a place in the therapy of *acromegaly* (a condition in which there is oversecretion of growth hormone in an adult). It also constricts splanchnic blood vessels and is used to treat bleeding *oesophageal varices*. **Octreotide** is generally given subcutaneously. The peak action is at 2 h, and the suppressant effect lasts for up to 8 h.

Unwanted effects include pain at the injection site and GI disturbances. Gallstones and postprandial hyperglycaemia have also been reported and acute hepatitis or pancreatitis has occurred in a few cases.

Lanreotide and **pasireotide** have similar effects. **Lanreotide** is also used in the treatment of thyroid tumours, while **pasireotide**, which is a particularly potent analogue, is used in the treatment of *Cushing's syndrome* when surgery is inappropriate or has been ineffective.

GONADOTROPHIN-RELEASING HORMONE

Gonadotrophin- (or luteinising hormone [LH]-) releasing hormone (GnRH, previously known as LHRH) is a decapeptide that releases both *follicle-stimulating hormone* and *luteinising hormone* from gonadotrophs. **Gonadorelin**[2] and its analogues (**buserelin**, **goserelin**, **leuprorelin**, **nafarelin** and **triptorelin**) are used mainly in the treatment of infertility and some hormone-dependent tumours (see Ch. 35).

GROWTH HORMONE-RELEASING FACTOR (SOMATORELIN)

Growth hormone-releasing factor (GHRF) is a peptide with 44 amino acid residues. The main action of GHRF is summarised in Fig. 33.2.

An analogue, **sermorelin** (discontinued in some countries), has been used as a diagnostic test for growth hormone secretion. Given intravenously, subcutaneously or intranasally, it causes secretion of growth hormone within minutes and peak concentrations in 1 h. The action is selective for the somatotrophs in the anterior pituitary, and no other pituitary hormones are affected. Unwanted effects are rare.

THYROTROPHIN-RELEASING HORMONE

Thyrotrophin-releasing hormone (TRH) from the hypothalamus releases TSH from the thyrotrophs.

Protirelin (now discontinued in the United Kingdom) is a synthetic TRH that has been used for the diagnosis of thyroid disorders (see Ch. 34). Given intravenously in normal subjects, it causes an increase in plasma TSH concentration, whereas in patients with hyperthyroidism there is a blunted response because the raised blood thyroxine concentration has a negative feedback effect on the anterior pituitary. The opposite occurs with hypothyroidism, where there is an intrinsic defect in the thyroid itself.

CORTICOTROPHIN-RELEASING FACTOR

Corticotrophin-releasing factor (CRF) is a peptide that releases **adrenocorticotrophic hormone** (ACTH, corticotrophin) and β-endorphin from corticotrophs in the anterior pituitary gland. CRF acts synergistically with *antidiuretic hormone* (ADH; arginine-vasopressin, see Ch. 29), and both its action and release are inhibited by glucocorticoids (see Fig. 33.4, later). Synthetic preparations have been used to test the ability of the pituitary to secrete ACTH, and to assess whether ACTH deficiency is caused by a pituitary or a hypothalamic defect. It has also been used to evaluate hypothalamic pituitary function after therapy for Cushing's syndrome (see Fig. 33.7, later).

ANTERIOR PITUITARY HORMONES

The main hormones of the anterior pituitary are listed in Table 33.1. The gonadotrophins are dealt with in Chapter 35 and TSH in Chapter 34. The actions of the remainder are summarised here.

GROWTH HORMONE (SOMATOTROPHIN)

Growth hormone is secreted by the somatotroph cells and is the most abundant pituitary hormone. Secretion is high in the newborn, decreasing at 4 years of age to an intermediate level, which is then maintained until after puberty, after which there is a further decline. Recombinant human growth hormone (hGH), **somatropin**, is available for treating growth defects and other developmental problems.

Regulation of secretion

Secretion of growth hormone is regulated by the action of hypothalamic GHRF and modulated by somatostatin, as described earlier and outlined in Fig. 33.2. A different peptide releaser of growth hormone ('ghrelin') is released

[2]In this context, the suffix '-relin' denotes peptides that stimulate hormone release.

from the stomach and pancreas and is implicated in the control of appetite and of body weight (see Ch. 32). One of the mediators of growth hormone action, insulin-like growth factor (IGF)-1, which is released from the liver, has an inhibitory effect on growth hormone secretion by stimulating somatostatin release from the hypothalamus.

As with other anterior pituitary secretions, growth hormone release is pulsatile, and its plasma concentration may fluctuate 10- to 100-fold. These surges occur repeatedly during the day and night and reflect the dynamics of hypothalamic control. Deep sleep is a potent stimulus to growth hormone secretion, particularly in children.

Actions

The main effect of growth hormone (and its analogues) is to stimulate normal growth. To do so, it acts in conjunction with other hormones secreted from the thyroid, the gonads and the adrenal cortex. It stimulates hepatic production of the IGFs - also termed *somatomedins* - which mediate most of its anabolic actions. IGF-1 (the principal mediator) mediates many of these anabolic effects, stimulating the uptake of amino acids and increasing protein synthesis by skeletal muscle (and therefore muscle bulk) as well as by the cartilage at the epiphyses of long bones (thus influencing bone growth). Receptors for IGF-1 exist on many other cell types, including liver cells and fat cells.

Disorders of production and clinical use

Deficiency of growth hormone (or failure of its action) results in *pituitary dwarfism*. In this condition, which may result from lack of GHRF or a lack of IGF generation or action, the normal proportions of the body are maintained even though overall stature is reduced. Growth hormone is used therapeutically in these patients (often children) as well as those suffering from the short stature caused by chronic renal insufficiency or associated with the chromosomal disorder known as *Turner's syndrome* (a condition in which females are missing an X-chromosome).

Humans are insensitive to growth hormone of other species, so hGH must be used clinically. Human cadavers were the original source, but this led to the spread of *Creutzfeldt–Jakob disease*, a prion-mediated neurodegenerative disorder (see Ch. 40). hGH is now prepared by recombinant DNA technology (**somatropin**), which avoids this risk. Satisfactory linear growth can be achieved by giving **somatropin** subcutaneously, six to seven times per week, and therapy is most successful when started early.

hGH is also used illicitly by athletes (see Ch. 59) to increase muscle mass. The large doses used have serious side effects, causing abnormal bone growth and cardiomegaly. It has also been tested as a means of combating the bodily changes in senescence; clinical trials have shown increases in body mass, but no functional improvement. Human recombinant IGF-1 (**mecasermin**) is also available for the treatment of growth failure in children who lack adequate amounts of this hormone.

An excessive production of growth hormone in children results in *gigantism*. An excessive production in adults, which is usually the result of a benign pituitary tumour, results in *acromegaly*, in which there is enlargement mainly of the jaw and of the hands and feet. The dopamine agonist **bromocriptine** and octreotide may mitigate the condition. Another useful agent is **pegvisomant**, a modified analogue of growth hormone prepared by recombinant technology that is a highly selective antagonist of growth hormone actions. **Pegvisomant** is used where surgical treatment or **somatostatin** analogue therapy is negated or ineffective.

PROLACTIN

Prolactin is secreted from the anterior pituitary gland by lactotroph (mammotroph) cells. These are abundant in the gland and increase in number during pregnancy, probably under the influence of oestrogen.

Regulation of secretion

Prolactin secretion is under tonic inhibitory control by dopamine (acting on D_2 receptors on the lactotrophs) released from the hypothalamus (Fig. 33.3 and see Table 33.1). The main stimulus for release is suckling but also auditory input from infant crying noise; in rats, both the smell and the sounds of hungry pups are also effective triggers. Neural reflexes from the breast may stimulate the secretion from the hypothalamus of prolactin-releasing factor(s), possible candidates for which include TRH and **oxytocin**. Oestrogens increase both prolactin secretion and the proliferation of lactotrophs through the release, from a subset of lactotrophs, of the neuropeptide *galanin*. Dopamine antagonists (used mainly as antipsychotic drugs; see Ch. 47) are potent stimulants of prolactin release, whereas agonists such as **bromocriptine** (see Chs 39 and 47) suppress prolactin release. **Bromocriptine** is also used in Parkinson's disease (see Ch. 40).

Actions

The prolactin receptor is a single transmembrane domain receptor of the kinase linked type (see Ch. 3) related to the cytokine receptors. Several different isoforms and splice variants are known. These are found not only in the mammary gland but are widely distributed throughout the body, including the brain, ovary, heart, lungs and immune system. The main function of prolactin in women is the control of milk production. At parturition the prolactin concentration rises and lactation is initiated. Maintenance of lactation depends on suckling (see earlier), which causes a 10- to 100-fold increase in blood prolactin levels within 30 min.

Together with other hormones, prolactin is responsible for the proliferation and differentiation of mammary tissue during pregnancy. It also inhibits gonadotrophin release and/or the response of the ovaries to these trophic hormones. This is one of the reasons why ovulation does not usually occur during breastfeeding.

According to one rather appealing hypothesis, the high postpartum concentration of prolactin reflects its biological function as a 'parental' hormone. Certainly, broodiness and nest-building activity can be induced in birds, mice and rabbits by prolactin injections. Prolactin also exerts other, apparently unrelated, actions, including stimulating mitogenesis in lymphocytes. There is some evidence that it may play a part in regulating immune responses.

Modification of prolactin secretion

Prolactin itself is not used clinically. **Bromocriptine**, a dopamine receptor agonist, is used to decrease excessive prolactin secretion (*hyperprolactinaemia*). It is well absorbed orally, and peak concentrations occur after 2 h. Unwanted reactions include nausea and vomiting. Dizziness,

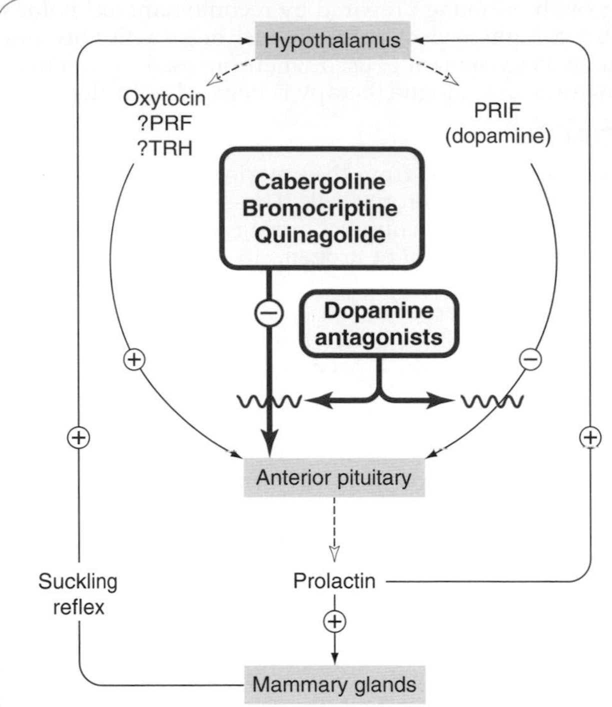

Fig. 33.3 Control of prolactin secretion. Drugs are shown in *red-bordered boxes*. *PRF*, Prolactin-releasing factor(s); *PRIF*, prolactin release-inhibiting factor(s); *TRH*, thyrotrophin-releasing hormone.

Clinical uses of bromocriptine

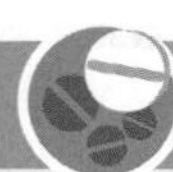

- To prevent lactation.
- To treat galactorrhoea (i.e. non-puerperal lactation in either sex), owing to excessive prolactin secretion (hyperprolactinaemia).
- To treat prolactin-secreting pituitary tumours (prolactinomas).
- In the treatment of Parkinson's disease (see Ch. 40) and of acromegaly.

constipation and postural hypotension may also occur. **Cabergoline** and **quinagolide** are similar.

ADRENOCORTICOTROPHIC HORMONE

ACTH (corticotrophin) is the anterior pituitary secretion that controls the synthesis and release of the glucocorticoids of the adrenal cortex (see Table 33.1). It is a 39-residue peptide derived from the precursor pro-opiomelanocortin (POMC) by sequential proteolytic processing. It acts on the MC_2 member of the family of melanocortin receptors (see later). Failure of ACTH action because of defects in its receptor or intracellular signalling pathways can lead to severe glucocorticoid deficiency (Chan et al., 2008). Details of the regulation of ACTH secretion are shown in Fig. 33.4.

This hormone occupies (together with cortisone) an important place in the history of inflammation therapy because of the work of Hench and his colleagues in the

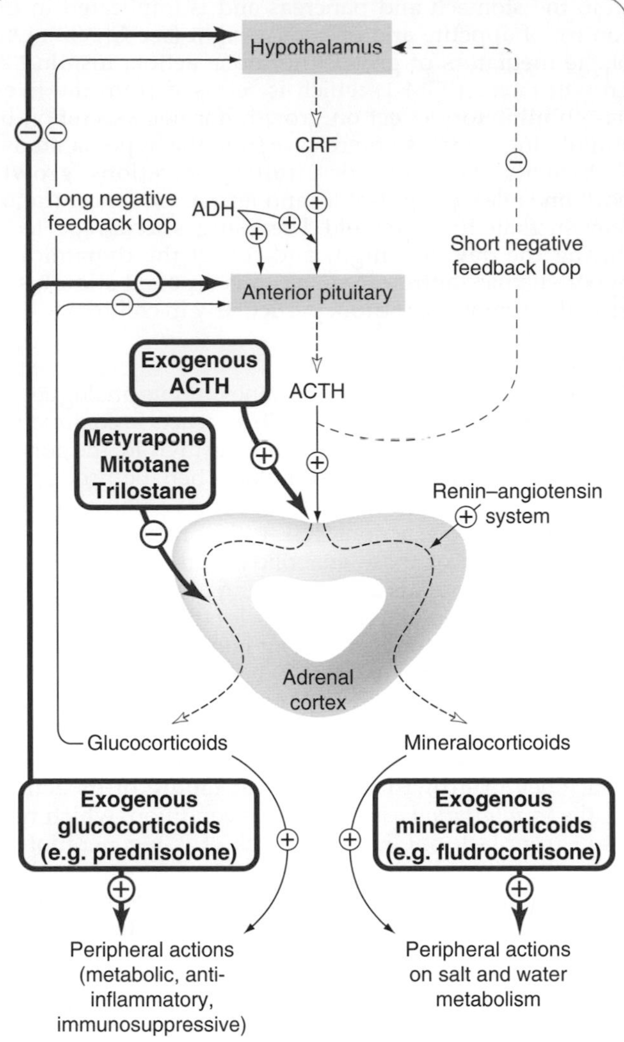

Fig. 33.4 Regulation of synthesis and secretion of adrenal corticosteroids. The long negative feedback loop is more physiologically significant than the short loop *(dashed lines)*. Adrenocorticotrophic hormone (ACTH, corticotrophin) has only a minimal effect on mineralocorticoid production. Drugs are shown in *red-bordered boxes*. *ADH*, Antidiuretic hormone (vasopressin); *CRF*, corticotrophin-releasing factor.

1940s, who first observed that both substances had anti-inflammatory effects in patients with rheumatoid disease. The effect of ACTH was thought to be secondary to stimulation of the adrenal cortex but, interestingly, the hormone also has anti-inflammatory actions in its own right, through activation of macrophage (melanocortin) MC_3 receptors (Getting et al., 2002).

ACTH itself is not often used in therapy today, because its action is less predictable than that of the corticosteroids and it may provoke antibody formation. **Tetracosactide (tetracosactrin)**, a synthetic polypeptide that consists of the first 24 N-terminal residues of human ACTH, suffers from some of the same drawbacks but is now widely used for assessing the competency of the adrenal cortex. The drug is given intramuscularly or intravenously, and the concentration of hydrocortisone in the plasma is measured by radioimmunoassay.

Actions

Acting through MC_2 receptors, **tetracosactide** and ACTH have two actions on the adrenal cortex:

- Stimulation of the synthesis and release of glucocorticoids. This action occurs within minutes of injection, and the ensuing biological actions are predominately those of the released steroids.
- A trophic action on adrenal cortical cells, and regulation of the levels of key mitochondrial steroidogenic enzymes. The loss of this effect accounts for the adrenal atrophy that results from chronic glucocorticoid administration, which suppresses ACTH secretion.

MELANOCYTE-STIMULATING HORMONE (MSH)

α-, β- and γ-MSH are peptide hormones with structural similarity to ACTH and are derived from the same precursor. Together, these peptides are referred to as *melanocortins*, because their first recognised action was to stimulate the production of melanin by specialised skin cells called *melanocytes*. As such, they play an important part in determining hair colouration, skin colour,[3] pigmentation patterns and reaction to (and protection from) ultraviolet light.

MSH acts on melanocortin receptors, of which five (MC_{1-5}) have been cloned. These are G protein–coupled receptors (GPCRs) that activate cAMP synthesis. Melanin formation is controlled by the MC_1 receptor. Excessive α-MSH production can provoke abnormal proliferation of melanocytes and may predispose those individuals to melanoma.

Melanocortins exhibit numerous other biological effects. For example, α-MSH inhibits the release of interleukin (IL)-1β and tumour necrosis factor (TNF)-α reduces neutrophil infiltration and exhibits anti-inflammatory and antipyretic activity. Levels of α-MSH are increased in the synovial fluid of patients with rheumatoid arthritis. These immunomodulatory effects are transduced by MC_1 and MC_3 receptors. Agonists at these receptors with potential anti-inflammatory activity are being sought. Central injection of α-MSH also causes changes in animal behaviour, such as increased grooming and sexual activity as well as reduced feeding through actions on MC_4 receptors, and agonists of MC_4 are under investigation as potential treatments for obesity and for erectile impotence.

Intracerebroventricular or intravenous injection of γ-MSH increases blood pressure, heart rate and cerebral blood flow. These effects are also likely to be mediated by the MC_4 receptor.

Two naturally occurring ligands for melanocortin receptors (*agouti-signalling protein* and *agouti-related peptide*, together called the *agouti*) have been discovered in human tissues. These are proteins that competitively antagonise the effect of MSH at melanocortin receptors.

[3]The Out-of-Africa model of skin colouration suggests that genetic drift in Europeans led to functional variation in MC_1 melanocortin receptor (MC_1R) as reduced UV levels resulted in less selective pressure on the MC_1R sequence.

The anterior pituitary gland and hypothalamus

- The anterior pituitary gland secretes hormones that regulate:
  - the release of *glucocorticoids* from the adrenal cortex
  - the release of *thyroid hormones*
  - the release of sex hormones: *ovulation* in the female and *spermatogenesis* in the male
  - *growth*
  - *mammary gland* structure and function
- Each anterior pituitary hormone is itself regulated by a specific hypothalamic releasing factor. Feedback mechanisms govern the release of these factors. Clinically useful drugs of this type include:
  - *GHRF* (**sermorelin**) and analogues of growth hormone (**somatrophin**)
  - *thyrotrophin-releasing factor* (**protirelin**) and TSH (thyrotrophin; used to test thyroid function)
  - **octreotide** and **lanreotide**, analogues of ***somatostatin***, which inhibit growth hormone release
  - *CRF*, used in diagnosis
  - *gonadotrophin-releasing factor, **gonadorelin** and analogues.* Used to treat infertility and some carcinomas

Adrenocorticotrophic hormone and the adrenal steroids

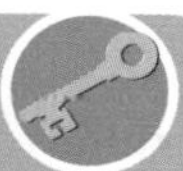

- ACTH (**tetracosactrin**, **tetracosactide**) stimulates synthesis and release of glucocorticoids (e.g. **hydrocortisone**), as well as some androgens, from the adrenal cortex.
- CRF from the hypothalamus regulates ACTH release and is regulated in turn by neural factors and negative feedback effects of plasma glucocorticoids.
- Mineralocorticoid (e.g. aldosterone) release from the adrenal cortex is controlled by the renin–angiotensin system.

POSTERIOR PITUITARY GLAND

The posterior pituitary gland (neurohypophysis) consists largely of the terminals of nerve cells originating from the *supraoptic* and *paraventricular nuclei* of the hypothalamus. Their axons form the *hypothalamic–hypophyseal tract*, and the fibres terminate in dilated nerve endings in close association with capillaries in the posterior pituitary gland (see Fig. 33.1). Peptides, synthesised in the hypothalamic nuclei, pass down these axons into the posterior pituitary, where they are stored and eventually secreted into the bloodstream.

The two main hormones of the posterior pituitary are **oxytocin** (which contracts the smooth muscle of the uterus; for details see Ch. 35) and **vasopressin** (ADH; see Chs 21 and 29). They are highly homologous cyclic nonapeptides. Several analogues have been synthesised that vary in their antidiuretic, vasopressor and oxytocic (uterine stimulant) properties.

VASOPRESSIN

Regulation of secretion and physiological role

Vasopressin released from the posterior pituitary has a crucial role in the control of the water content of the body through its action on the cells of the distal part of the nephron and the collecting tubules in the kidney (see Ch. 29). The hypothalamic nuclei that control fluid balance lie close to the nuclei that synthesise and secrete vasopressin.

One of the main stimuli for vasopressin release is an increase in plasma osmolarity (which produces a sensation of thirst). A decrease in circulating blood volume (*hypovolaemia*) is another, and here the stimuli arise from stretch receptors in the cardiovascular system or from angiotensin release. *Diabetes insipidus* is a condition in which large volumes of dilute urine are produced because vasopressin secretion is reduced or absent, or because of a reduced sensitivity of the kidney to the hormone.

Vasopressin receptors

There are three classes of receptor: V_{1A}, V_{1B} and V_2. All are GPCRs. V_2 receptors stimulate adenylyl cyclase, which mediates the main physiological actions of vasopressin in the kidney, whereas the V_{1A} and V_{1B} receptors are coupled to the phospholipase C/inositol trisphosphate system.

The receptor for oxytocin (OT receptor) is also a GPCR, which primarily signals through phospholipase C stimulation but has a secondary action on adenylyl cyclase. Vasopressin is a partial agonist at OT, but its effects are limited by the distribution of the receptor, which, as might be inferred from its classic action on the pregnant uterus, is high in the myometrium, endometrium, mammary gland and ovary. The central actions of oxytocin (and vasopressin) have also attracted the attention of sociobiologists as they are important in 'pair bonding' and the other psychosocial interactions.[4]

Actions

Renal actions

Vasopressin binds to kidney V_2 receptors in the basolateral membrane of the cells of the distal tubule and collecting ducts of the nephron. Its main effect in the collecting duct is to increase the rate of insertion of water channels (*aquaporins*) into the luminal membrane, thus increasing the permeability of the membrane to water (see Ch. 29). It also activates urea transporters and transiently increases Na^+ absorption, particularly in the distal tubule.

Several drugs affect the action of vasopressin. Non-steroidal anti-inflammatory drugs and **carbamazepine** increase, and **lithium**, **colchicine** and **vinca alkaloids** decrease, vasopressin effects. The effects of the last two agents are secondary to their action on the microtubules required for translocation of water channels. The V_2 receptor antagonists **tolvaptan and demeclocycline** (actually a tetracycline antibiotic) counteract the action of vasopressin in renal tubules and can be used to treat patients with water retention combined with urinary salt loss (and thus *hyponatraemia*) caused by excessive secretion of the hormone. This *syndrome of inappropriate ADH secretion* ('SIADH') is associated with lung or other malignancies or head injury. Specific V_2 receptor antagonists are also being investigated in the treatment of heart failure (see Ch. 22).

Other non-renal actions

Vasopressin causes contraction of smooth muscle, particularly in the cardiovascular system, by acting on V_{1A} receptors (see Ch. 22). The affinity of vasopressin for these receptors is lower than that for V_2 receptors, and smooth muscle effects are seen only with doses larger than those affecting the kidney. Vasopressin also stimulates blood platelet aggregation and mobilisation of coagulation factors. When released into the pituitary portal circulation, it promotes the release of ACTH from the anterior pituitary by an action on V_{1B} receptors (see Fig. 33.4). In the CNS, vasopressin, like oxytocin, is believed to have a role in modulating emotional and social behaviour.

Pharmacokinetic aspects

Vasopressin, and various peptidergic analogues, are used clinically either for the treatment of diabetes insipidus or as vasoconstrictors. Several analogues have been developed to (a) increase their duration of action and (b) shift the relative potency between the V_1 and V_2 receptors.

The main substances used are:

- ***vasopressin** itself:* short duration of action, weak selectivity for V_2 receptors, given by subcutaneous or intramuscular injection, or by intravenous infusion;
- ***desmopressin:*** increased duration of action, V_2-selective and thereby with fewer pressor effects, can be given by several routes including nasal spray;
- ***terlipressin:*** increased duration of action, low but protracted vasopressor action (and minimal antidiuretic properties), used to reduce bleeding (e.g. from oesophageal varices) and maintain blood pressure;
- ***felypressin:*** a short-acting vasoconstrictor that is injected with local anaesthetics such as prilocaine to prolong their action (see Ch. 44).

Vasopressin itself is rapidly eliminated, with a plasma half-life less than 10 min and a short duration of action. Tissue peptidases metabolise the hormone and 33% is removed by the kidney. Desmopressin is less subject to degradation by peptidases, and its plasma half-life is 75 min.

Unwanted effects

There are few unwanted effects, and these are mainly cardiovascular in nature: intravenous vasopressin may cause spasm of the coronary arteries with resultant angina, but this risk can be minimised if the antidiuretic peptides are administered intranasally.

THE ADRENAL CORTEX

The adrenal glands consist of two parts: the inner *medulla*, which secretes catecholamines (see Ch. 15), and the outer *cortex*, which secretes adrenal steroids. The cortex

[4]Oxytocin is released during childbirth, lactation and orgasm and has been shown to promote trust and other prosocial behaviour. This has earned it the nickname of the 'love hormone' (or, even more nauseatingly, the 'cuddle hormone') in the popular press and internet discussion groups.

The posterior pituitary gland

- The posterior pituitary gland secretes:
  - oxytocin (see Ch. 35)
  - antidiuretic hormone (**ADH, vasopressin**), which acts on V_2 receptors in the distal kidney tubule to increase water reabsorption and, in higher concentrations, on V_{1A} receptors to cause vasoconstriction. It also stimulates ACTH secretion.
- Substances available for clinical use are **vasopressin** and the analogues **desmopressin**, **felypressin** and **terlipressin.**

Clinical uses of antidiuretic hormone vasopressin) and analogues

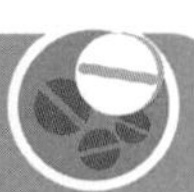

- Diabetes insipidus: **felypressin**, **desmopressin.**
- Initial treatment of bleeding oesophageal varices: **vasopressin**, **terlipressin**, **felypressin.** (**Octreotide** – a somatostatin analogue – is also used, but direct injection of sclerosant via an endoscope is the main treatment.)
- Prophylaxis against bleeding in haemophilia (e.g. before tooth extraction): **vasopressin**, **desmopressin** (by increasing the concentration of factor VIII).
- **Felypressin** is used as a vasoconstrictor with local anaesthetics (see Ch. 44).
- **Desmopressin** is used for persistent nocturnal enuresis in older children and adults.

comprises three concentric zones: the *zona glomerulosa* (the outermost layer), which elaborates mineralocorticoids; the *zona fasciculata*, which elaborates glucocorticoids; and the innermost *zona reticularis*, which produces androgen precursors. The principal adrenal steroids are those with glucocorticoid and mineralocorticoid activities.[5]Androgen secretion (see Ch. 35) by the cortex is not considered further in this chapter.

The mineralocorticoids regulate water and electrolyte balance, and the main endogenous hormone is *aldosterone*. The glucocorticoids have widespread actions on carbohydrate and protein metabolism, as well as potent regulatory effects on host defence mechanisms (see Chs 7 and 25). The adrenal gland secretes a mixture of glucocorticoids; in humans the main hormone is *hydrocortisone* (also, confusingly, known as *cortisol*), and in rodents it is *corticosterone*. The mineralocorticoid and glucocorticoid actions are not completely separated in naturally occurring steroids and some glucocorticoids have quite substantial effects on water and electrolyte balance. In fact, both hydrocortisone and aldosterone are equiactive on mineralocorticoid receptors but, in mineralocorticoid-sensitive tissues such as the kidney, the action of *11β-hydroxysteroid dehydrogenase Type 2* converts hydrocortisone to the inactive metabolite cortisone,[6] thereby preventing the tissue from responding to hydrocortisone. Interestingly, there is increasing evidence that some glucocorticoid synthesis can take place locally at extra-adrenal sites such as thymus and skin (see Talaber et al., 2015; Hannen et al., 2017) providing a fresh perspective on the local control of inflammatory processes.

With the exception of *replacement therapy*, glucocorticoids are most commonly employed for their anti-inflammatory and immunosuppressive properties (see Ch. 25). In this therapeutic context, their metabolic and other actions are seen as unwanted side effects. Synthetic steroids have been developed that exhibit a partial separation of the glucocorticoid from the mineralocorticoid actions (Table 33.2), but it has not yet been possible completely to separate the anti-inflammatory from the other actions of the glucocorticoids.

The adrenal gland is essential to life, and animals deprived of these glands are able to survive only under rigorously controlled conditions. In humans, a deficiency in corticosteroid production, termed *Addison's disease*, is characterised by muscular weakness, low blood pressure, depression, anorexia, loss of weight and hypoglycaemia. Addison's disease may have an autoimmune aetiology, or it may be secondary to destruction of the gland by chronic inflammatory conditions such as tuberculosis.

When corticosteroids are produced in excess, the clinical picture depends on which molecular species predominates. Excessive *glucocorticoid activity* results in *Cushing's syndrome*, the manifestations of which are outlined in Fig. 33.7. This can be caused by hypersecretion from the adrenal glands or by prolonged therapeutic use of glucocorticoids. An excessive production of *mineralocorticoids* results in retention of Na^+ and loss of K^+. This may be caused by hyperactivity or tumours of the adrenals (*primary hyperaldosteronism*, or *Conn's syndrome*, an uncommon but important cause of hypertension; see Ch. 22), or by excessive activation of the renin–angiotensin system such as occurs in some forms of kidney disease, cirrhosis of the liver or congestive cardiac failure (*secondary hyperaldosteronism*).

GLUCOCORTICOIDS

Synthesis and release

Glucocorticoids are not stored in the adrenal gland but are synthesised under the influence of circulating ACTH secreted from the anterior pituitary gland (see Fig. 33.4) and released in a pulsatile fashion into the blood. While glucocorticoids are continuously released, there is a well-defined circadian rhythm in the secretion in healthy humans, with the net blood concentration being highest early in the morning, gradually diminishing throughout the day and reaching a low point in the evening or night. ACTH secretion itself (also pulsatile in nature) is regulated by CRF released from the hypothalamus, and by vasopressin released from the posterior pituitary gland. The release of both ACTH and CRF, in turn, is reflexly inhibited by

[5]So named because early experimenters noticed that separate fractions of adrenal gland extracts caused changes in either blood glucose or salt and water retention.

[6]Oddly, it was cortisone that Hench originally demonstrated to have potent anti-inflammatory activity in his classic studies of 1949. The reason for this apparent anomaly is the presence in some tissues of the enzyme *11β-hydroxysteroid dehydrogenase Type 1* which can reduce cortisone to cortisol (i.e. hydrocortisone), thus restoring its biological activity.

Table 33.2 Comparison of the main corticosteroid agents used for systemic therapy (using hydrocortisone as a standard)

Compound	Relative affinity for GR	Approximate relative potency in clinical use		Duration of action after oral dose[a]	Comments
		Anti-inflammatory	Sodium retaining		
Hydrocortisone (cortisol)	1	1	1	Short	Drug of choice for replacement therapy.
Cortisone	0 (Prodrug)	0.8	0.8	Short	Inactive until converted to hydrocortisone; not used as anti-inflammatory because of mineralocorticoid effects.
Deflazacort	0 (Prodrug)	3	Minimal	Short	Converted by plasma esterases into active metabolite. Similar utility to prednisolone.
Prednisolone	2.2	4	0.8	Intermediate	Drug of choice for systemic anti-inflammatory and immunosuppressive effects.
Prednisone	0 (Prodrug)	4	0.8	Intermediate	Inactive until converted to prednisolone.
Methylprednisolone	11.9	5	Minimal	Intermediate	Anti-inflammatory and immunosuppressive.
Triamcinolone	1.9	5	None	Intermediate	Relatively more toxic than others.
Dexamethasone	7.1	27	Minimal	Long	Anti-inflammatory and immunosuppressive, used especially where water retention is undesirable (e.g. cerebral oedema); drug of choice for suppression of ACTH production.
Betamethasone	5.4	27	Negligible	Long	Anti-inflammatory and immunosuppressive, used especially when water retention is undesirable.
Fludrocortisone	3.5	15	150	Short	Drug of choice for mineralocorticoid effects.
Aldosterone	0.38	None	500	N/A	Endogenous mineralocorticoid.

[a]Duration of action (half-lives in hours): short, 8–12; intermediate, 12–36; long, 36–72. Some drugs are inactive until converted to active compounds in vivo and therefore have negligible affinity for the glucocorticoid receptor.
ACTH, Adrenocorticotrophic hormone; *GR*, glucocorticoid receptor.
Data for relative affinity obtained from Baxter, J.D., Rousseau, G.G. (Eds.), 1979. Glucocorticoid Hormone Action. Monographs on Endocrinology. Springer-Verlag, Berlin.

the ensuing rising concentrations of glucocorticoids in the blood.

Opioid peptides also exercise a tonic inhibitory control on the secretion of CRF, and psychological factors, excessive heat or cold, injury or infections can also affect the release of both vasopressin and CRF. This is the principal mechanism whereby the HPA axis is activated in response to perceived threats in the external environment.

The biosynthetic precursor of glucocorticoids is cholesterol (Fig. 33.5). The initial conversion of cholesterol to *pregnenolone* is the rate-limiting step and is regulated by ACTH. Some biosynthetic reactions can be inhibited by drugs, and these have a utility in treating Cushing's disease or adrenocortical carcinoma. **Metyrapone** prevents the β-hydroxylation at C11, and thus the formation of hydrocortisone and corticosterone. Synthesis is blocked at the 11-deoxycorticosteroid stage, leaving intermediates that have no effects on the hypothalamus and pituitary, so there is a marked increase in ACTH in the blood. **Metyrapone** can therefore be used to test ACTH production and may also be used to treat patients with Cushing's syndrome. **Trilostane** (previously used to treat Cushing's syndrome and primary hyperaldosteronism but now largely restricted to veterinary indications) blocks an earlier enzyme in the pathway – the *3β-dehydrogenase.* **Aminoglutethimide** inhibits the initial step in the biosynthetic pathway and has the same overall effect as metyrapone.

Trilostane and **aminoglutethimide** are not currently used in the United Kingdom but **ketoconazole**, an antifungal agent (see Ch. 54), also inhibits steroidogenesis and may be of value in the specialised treatment of Cushing's syndrome (Fig. 33.7). **Mitotane** suppresses glucocorticoid synthesis by a direct (and unknown) mechanism on the adrenal gland. It is chiefly used to treat advanced or inoperable adrenocortical carcinomas.

Mechanism of glucocorticoid action

The glucocorticoid effects relevant to this discussion are initiated by interaction of the drugs with specific intracellular glucocorticoid receptors (GRs)[7] belonging to the nuclear receptor superfamily (although there may be other binding proteins or sites; see Norman et al., 2004). This superfamily also includes the receptors for mineralocorticoids, the sex steroids, thyroid hormones, vitamin D_3 and retinoic acid

[7]Reader beware! The glucocorticoid receptor is also referred to as the *Type II corticosteroid receptor*, the Type I corticosteroid receptor being what we more usually call the mineralocorticoid receptor (MR).

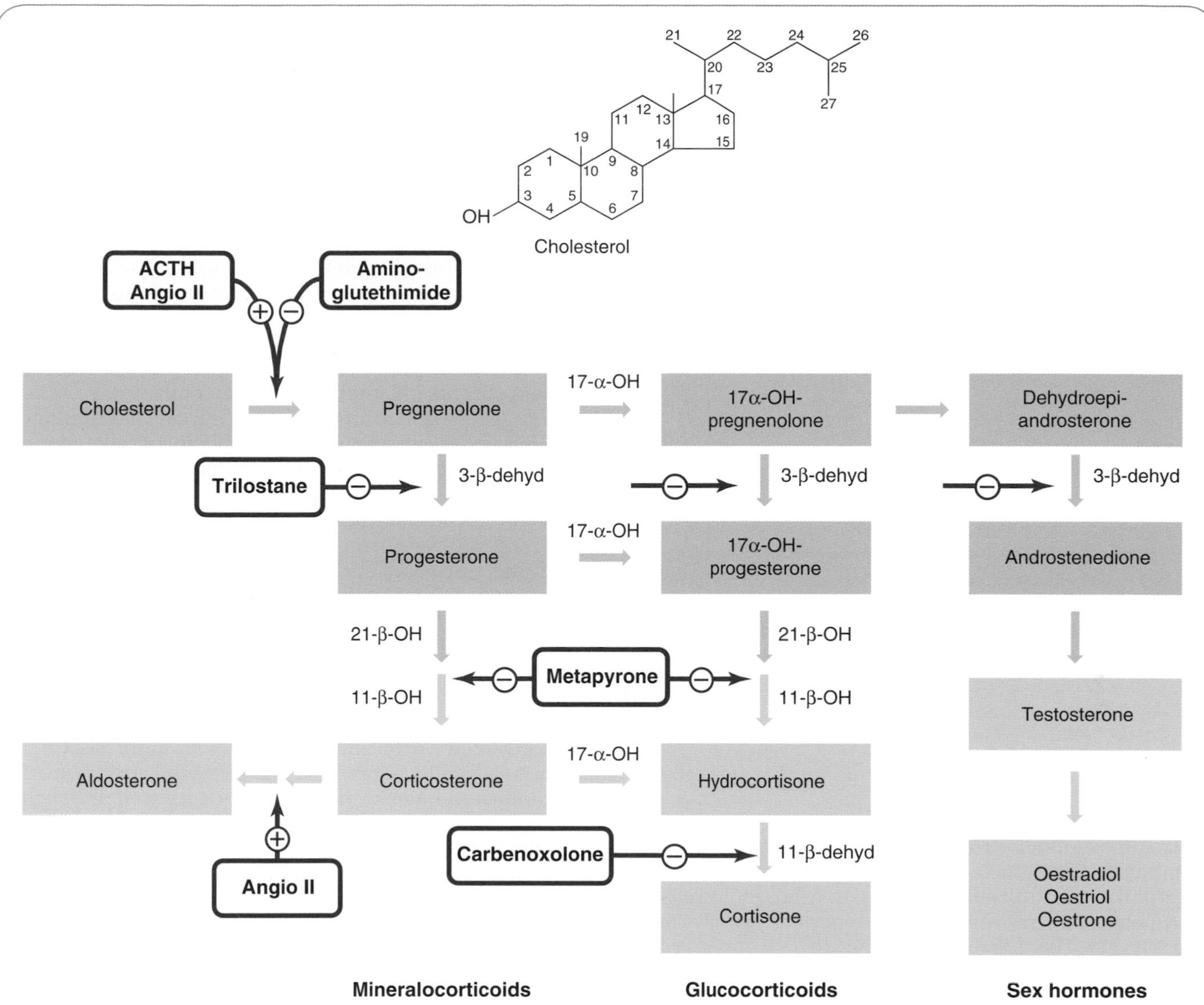

Fig. 33.5 Biosynthesis of corticosteroids, mineralocorticoids and sex hormones. All steroid hormones are synthesised from cholesterol. The biosynthetic pathway involves successive steps of hydroxylation and dehydrogenation and these are targets for drugs. Intermediates are shown in *green boxes*; interconversions occur between the pathways. *Blue boxes* indicate circulating hormones. Drugs are shown in *red-bordered boxes* adjacent to their sites of action. Glucocorticoids are produced by cells of the zona fasciculata, and their synthesis is stimulated by adrenocorticotrophic hormone (ACTH); aldosterone is produced by cells of the zona glomerulosa, and its synthesis is stimulated by angiotensin II (angio II). Metyrapone inhibits glucocorticoid synthesis; aminoglutethimide and trilostane block synthesis of all three types of adrenal steroid (see text for details). Carbenoxolone inhibits the interconversion of hydrocortisone and cortisone in the kidney. Not shown is mitotane, which suppresses adrenal hormone synthesis through an unknown mechanism. Enzymes: *17-α-OH,* 17-α-hydroxylase; *3-β-dehyd,* 3-β-dehydrogenase; *21-β-OH,* 21-β-hydroxylase; *11-β-OH,* 11-β-hydroxylase; *11-β-dehyd,* 11-β-hydroxysteroid dehydrogenase.

(see Ch. 3). The actual mechanism of transcriptional control is complex, with at least four mechanisms operating within the nucleus. These are summarised diagrammatically in Fig. 33.6.

When the nuclear actions of GRs were first discovered, it was thought that this mechanism could account for all the actions of the hormones, but a surprising discovery overturned this idea. Reichardt et al. (1998), using transgenic mice in which the GR was unable to dimerise (and therefore unable to function in the nucleus), found that glucocorticoids were still able to exert a great many biological actions. This suggested that in addition to controlling gene expression within the nucleus, the liganded receptor itself could initiate important signal transduction events while still in the cytosolic compartment (there may even be a subpopulation of receptors that reside there permanently). One such effect seems to be interaction of the receptor with the regulatory complex, NF-κB (see Fig. 33.6 and Ch. 3) and other important interactions may involve protein kinases/phosphatase signalling systems. Some of these cytosolic actions are very rapid. For example, the liganded GR-induced phosphorylation by protein kinase C (PKC) and subsequent release of the protein *Annexin A1*, which has potent inhibitory effects on leukocyte trafficking and other anti-inflammatory actions, occurs in minutes and cannot be accounted for by changes in protein synthesis; and there are many other examples of non-transcriptional activities of glucocorticoids (see Buttgereit and Scheffold, 2002; Panettieri et al., 2019).

In recent years, our understanding of the glucocorticoid field has been further enriched by the discovery of numerous isoforms and splice variants of GR, some of which are expressed in a tissue-specific manner (see Oakley and Cidlowski, 2013). This opens up a real possibility of highly selective glucocorticoid drugs in the future.

Mechanism of action of the glucocorticoids

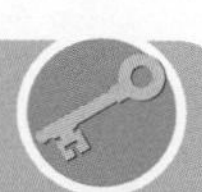

- Glucocorticoids bind intracellular receptors that then dimerise, migrate to the nucleus and interact with DNA to modify gene transcription, inducing synthesis of some proteins and inhibiting synthesis of others.
- Many acute glucocorticoid actions are mediated by signalling systems triggered by the liganded receptor in the cytosol. Some are very rapid.
- There may be different populations of receptors including membrane-bound receptors which may also transduce rapid actions.
- Tissue and splice variants of the GR are found to be distributed in a tissue-specific fashion.

Actions

General metabolic and systemic effects

The main metabolic effects are on carbohydrate and protein metabolism. The glucocorticoids cause both a decrease in the uptake and utilisation of glucose and an increase in gluconeogenesis, resulting in a tendency to hyperglycaemia (see Ch. 31). There is a concomitant increase in glycogen storage, which may be a result of insulin secretion in response to the increase in blood sugar. Overall, there is decreased protein synthesis and increased protein breakdown, particularly in muscle, and this can lead to tissue wasting. Catecholamines and some other hormones cause lipase activation through a cAMP-dependent protein kinase, the synthesis of which requires the 'permissive' presence of glucocorticoids, and several other examples of this type of hormone action have been observed. Large doses of glucocorticoids given over a long period result in the redistribution of body fat characteristic of Cushing's syndrome (Fig. 33.7).

Glucocorticoids tend to produce a negative calcium balance by decreasing Ca^{2+} absorption in the GI tract and increasing its excretion by the kidney. Together with increased breakdown of bone matrix protein this may cause osteoporosis. In higher, non-physiological concentrations, the glucocorticoids have some mineralocorticoid actions, causing Na^+ retention and K^+ loss – possibly by swamping the protective 11β-hydroxysteroid dehydrogenase and acting off-target at mineralocorticoid receptors.

Negative feedback effects on the anterior pituitary and hypothalamus

Both endogenous and exogenous glucocorticoids have a negative feedback effect on the secretion of CRF and ACTH (see Fig. 33.4), thus inhibiting the secretion of endogenous glucocorticoids and potentially causing atrophy of the adrenal cortex. If therapy is prolonged, it may take many months to return to normal function once the drugs are withdrawn.

Anti-inflammatory and immunosuppressive effects

Endogenous glucocorticoids maintain a low-level anti-inflammatory tone and are secreted in increased amounts in response to inflammatory stimuli. Consequently, adrenalectomised animals and humans with adrenal insufficiency show a heightened response to even mild insults, injuries or stresses. On this basis, it has been suggested that a failure of appropriate glucocorticoid secretion in response to injury or infection may underlie certain chronic inflammatory human pathologies.

Exogenous glucocorticoids are the anti-inflammatory drugs *par excellence*, and when given therapeutically, suppress the operation of both the innate and adaptive immune system. They reverse virtually all types of inflammatory reaction, whether caused by invading pathogens, by chemical or physical stimuli, or by inappropriately deployed immune responses such as are seen in hypersensitivity or autoimmune disease. When used prophylactically to suppress graft rejection, glucocorticoids are more efficient in suppressing the initiation and generation of the immune response than they are in preventing the operation of an established response where clonal proliferation has already occurred. Exogenous glucocorticoids are often co-administered with chemotherapeutics in cancer (see Ch. 57). This co-administration often enhanced the effectiveness of the anti-cancer agents, through a not very well understood mechanism. Of late, exogenous glucocorticoids are also administered to patients with severe **COVID-19** to reduce inflammation and sclerosis, improve lung function, and boost overall survival.

Given that glucocorticoids modify the expression of so many genes (approximately 1% of the total genome is affected), and that the extent and direction of regulation varies between tissues and even at different times during disease, you will not be surprised to learn that their anti-inflammatory effects are complex.

Actions on *inflammatory* cells include:

- decreased egress of neutrophils from blood vessels and reduced activation of neutrophils, macrophages and mast cells secondary to decreased transcription of the genes for cell adhesion factors and cytokines;
- decreased overall activation of T-helper (Th) cells, reduced clonal proliferation of T cells and a 'switch' from the Th1 to the Th2 immune response (see Ch. 7);
- decreased fibroblast function, less production of collagen and glycosaminoglycans and, under some circumstances, reduced healing and repair.

Actions on the mediators of inflammatory and immune responses (Ch. 17) include:

- decreased production of prostanoids through reduced expression of cyclo-oxygenase II and suppression of substrate arachidonic acid release;
- decreased generation of many cytokines, including IL-1, IL-2, IL-3, IL-4, IL-5, IL-6, IL-8, TNF-α, cell adhesion factors and granulocyte–macrophage

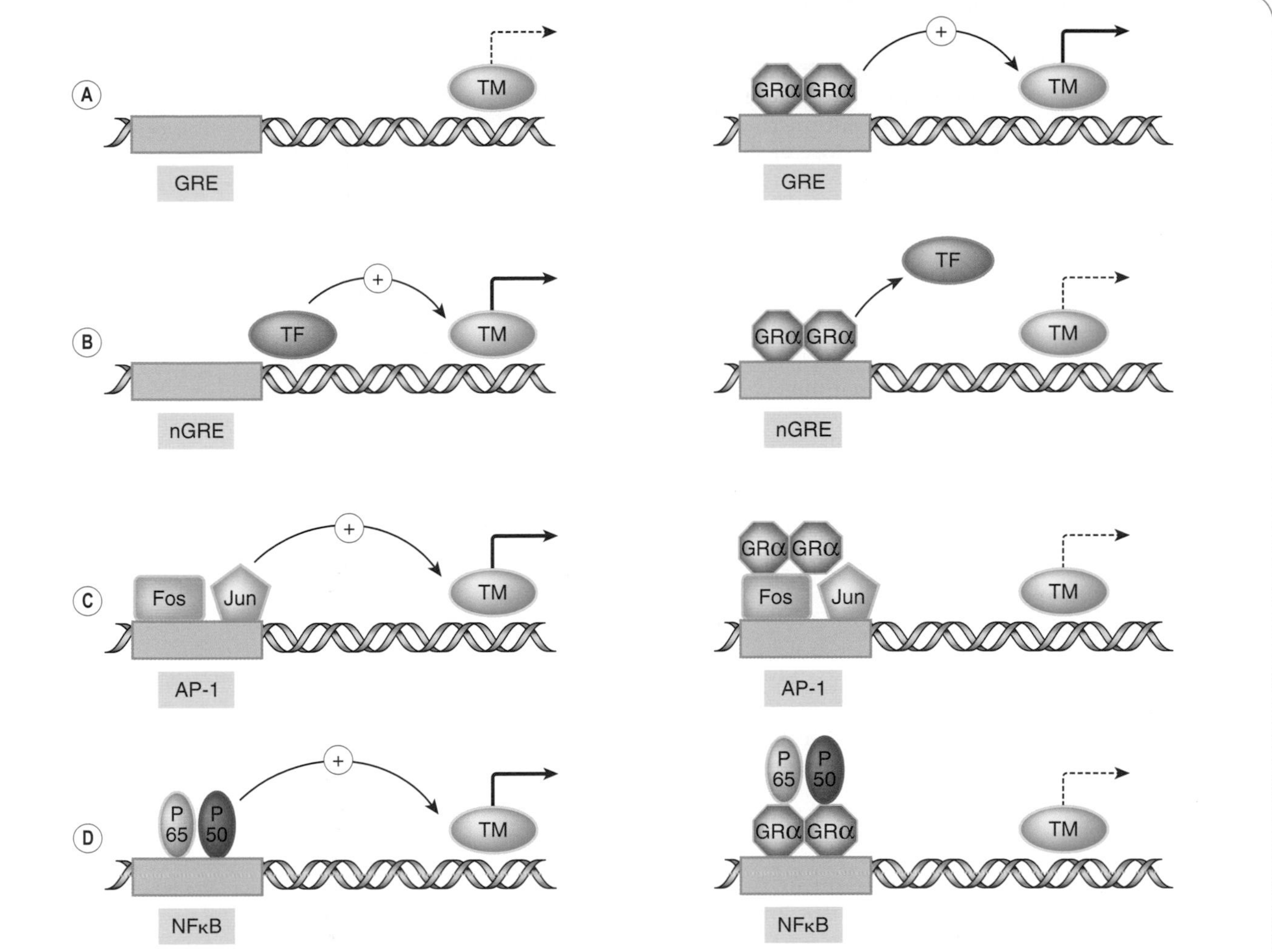

Fig. 33.6 Molecular mechanism of action of glucocorticoids. The schematic figure shows four possible ways by which the liganded glucocorticoid receptor can control gene expression following translocation into the nucleus. (A) Basic transactivation mechanism. Here, the transcriptional machinery (TM) is presumed to be operating at a low level. The liganded glucocorticoid receptor (GR) dimer binds to one or more 'positive' glucocorticoid response elements (GREs) within the promoter sequence *(shaded zone)* and upregulates transcription. (B) Basic transrepression mechanism. The TM is constitutively driven by transcription factors (TFs). In binding to the 'negative' GRE (nGRE), the receptor complex displaces these factors and expression falls. (C) Fos/Jun mechanism. Transcription is driven at a high level by Fos/Jun transcription factors binding to their AP-1 regulatory site. This effect is reduced in the presence of the GR. (D) Nuclear factor (NF)-κβ mechanism. The TFs P65 and P50 bind to the NF-κβ site, promoting gene expression. This is prevented by the presence of the GR, which binds the TFs, preventing their action (this may occur in the cytoplasm also). (For further details of the structure of the glucocorticoid receptor, see Ch. 3.) (Redrawn from Oakley, R.H., Cidlowski, J.A., 2001. The glucocorticoid receptor: expression, function and regulation of glucocorticoid responsiveness. In: Goulding, N.J., Flower, R.J. (Eds.), Milestones in Drug Therapy: Glucocorticoids. Birkhäuser Verlag, Basel.)

colony-stimulating factor. These are largely secondary to inhibition of gene transcription;

- reduction in the concentration of complement components in the plasma;
- decreased generation of nitric oxide by the inducible nitric oxide synthase 2 (NOS2) isoform;
- decreased release of histamine and other mediators from basophils and mast cells;
- decreased immunoglobulin G (IgG) production;
- increased synthesis of anti-inflammatory factors such as IL-10, IL-1-soluble receptor and Annexin 1.

Endogenous anti-inflammatory glucocorticoids circulate constantly in the blood and are increased during inflammatory episodes – or even by the anticipation of a stressful event. It is suggested (see Munck et al., 1984) that the anti-inflammatory and immunosuppressive actions of endogenous glucocorticoids play a crucial counter-regulatory role, in that they prevent excessive activation of inflammation and other powerful defence reactions that might, if unchecked, threaten homeostasis. Certainly, this view is borne out by experimental work. While these drugs are of great value in treating conditions characterised by hypersensitivity and unwanted inflammation, they carry the hazard that they are able to suppress the same defence reactions that protect us from infection and other insults.

Unwanted effects

Low-dose glucocorticoid replacement therapy is usually without problems, but serious unwanted effects occur with large doses or prolonged administration of glucocorticoids. The major effects are as follows:

- *Suppression of the response to infection or injury*: opportunistic infection can be potentially very serious unless quickly treated with antimicrobial agents along with an increase in the dose of steroid. Oral thrush (candidiasis, a fungal infection; see Ch. 54) frequently occurs when glucocorticoids are taken by inhalation, because of suppression of local anti-infective mechanisms. Wound healing is impaired, and peptic ulceration may also occur.
- *Cushing's syndrome* (see Fig. 33.7).
- *Osteoporosis*, with the attendant hazard of fractures, is one of the main limitations to long-term glucocorticoid therapy. These drugs influence bone density both by regulation of calcium and phosphate metabolism and through effects on collagen turnover. They reduce osteoblast function (which deposits bone matrix) and increase the activity of osteoclasts (which digest bone matrix). An effect on the blood supply to bone can result in avascular necrosis of the head of the femur (see Ch. 36).
- *Hyperglycaemia* produced by exogenous glucocorticoids may develop into frank (pre-) diabetes.
- *Muscle wasting* and proximal muscle weakness.
- In children, *inhibition of growth*[8] if treatment is continued for more than 6 months.
- *CNS effects:* euphoria and psychosis with short-term administration, depression with chronic treatment.
- *Other effects:* glaucoma (in genetically predisposed persons), raised intracranial pressure and an increased incidence of cataracts.

Sudden withdrawal of the drugs after prolonged therapy may result in acute adrenal insufficiency because of suppression of the patient's capacity to synthesise corticosteroids.[9] Careful procedures for phased withdrawal should be followed. Recovery of full adrenal function usually takes about 8 weeks, although it can take 18 months or more after prolonged high-dose treatment.

Pharmacokinetic aspects

There are many glucocorticoid drugs in therapeutic use. Although **cortisol** (**hydrocortisone**), the endogenous hormone, is often used, synthetic derivatives are even more common. These have different physicochemical properties as well as varying potencies and have been optimised for administration by oral, systemic or intra-articular routes or for topical application such as by aerosol directly into the respiratory tract or nose or as eye drops. They may be formulated as creams or ointments for application to the skin (see Ch. 26) or as foam enemas for the GI tract (see Ch. 30). Topical administration diminishes the likelihood of systemic toxic effects unless large quantities are used. When prolonged use of systemic glucocorticoids is necessary, therapy on alternate days may decrease suppression of the HPA axis and other unwanted effects.

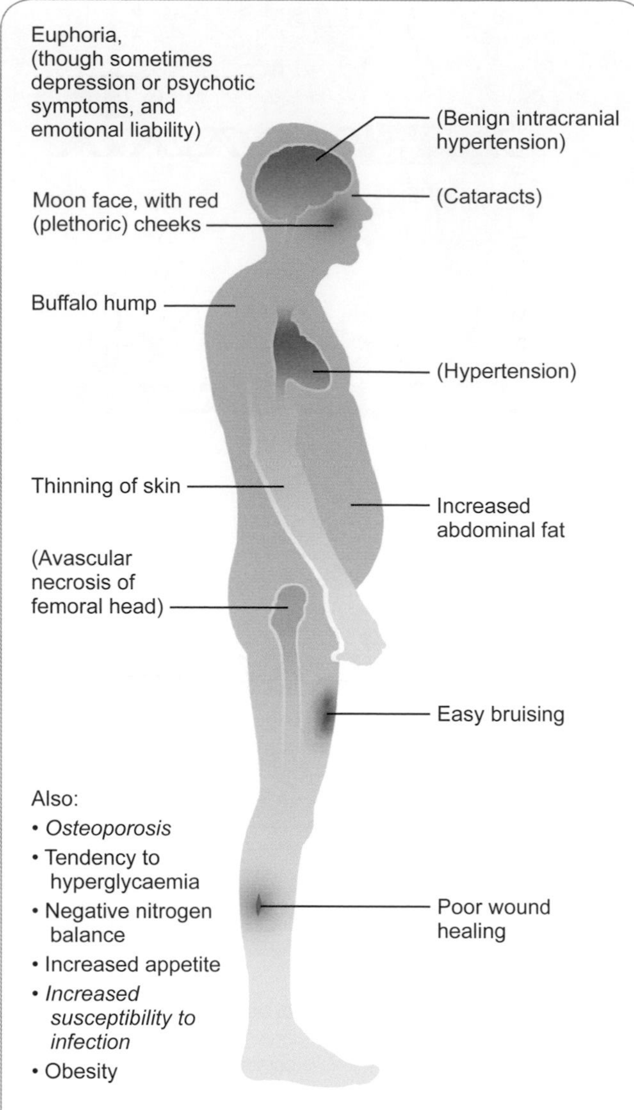

Fig. 33.7 Cushing's syndrome. This is caused by excessive exposure to endogenous glucocorticoids, by disease (e.g. an adrenocorticotrophic hormone-secreting tumour) or by prolonged administration of glucocorticoid drugs (*iatrogenic Cushing's syndrome*). *Italicised* effects are particularly common. Less frequent effects, related to dose and duration of therapy, are shown in *parentheses*. (Redrawn from Baxter, J.D., Rousseau, G.G. (Eds.), 1979. Glucocorticoid Hormone Action. Monographs on Endocrinology. Springer-Verlag, Berlin.)

Endogenous glucocorticoids are transported in the plasma bound to *corticosteroid-binding globulin* (CBG) and to albumin. About 77% of plasma **hydrocortisone** is bound to CBG, but many synthetic glucocorticoids are not bound at all. Albumin has a lower affinity for hydrocortisone but binds both natural and synthetic steroids. Both CBG-bound and albumin-bound steroids are biologically inactive. Hydrocortisone has a plasma half-life of 90 min, although many of its biological effects have a latency of 2–8 h.

As small lipophilic molecules, glucocorticoids probably enter their target cells by simple diffusion. Biological

[8]However, some of the diseases for which glucocorticoids are indicated themselves retard growth. In a classical trial, glucocorticoid treatment *increased* growth in adolescents with inflammatory bowel disease as the disease resolved (Whittington et al., 1977).

[9]Patients on long-term glucocorticoid therapy are advised to carry a card stating, 'I am a patient on STEROID TREATMENT which must not be stopped abruptly'.

inactivation, which occurs in liver cells and elsewhere, is initiated by reduction of the C4–C5 double bond. Cortisone and **prednisone** are inactive until converted in vivo by the 11β-dehydrogenase type 1 to **hydrocortisone** and **prednisolone**, respectively.

The clinical uses of systemic glucocorticoids are summarised in the clinical box. **Dexamethasone** has a special use: it is used to test HPA axis function. In the **dexamethasone** suppression test a relatively low dose of the drug is given, usually at night. This would be expected to suppress the hypothalamus and pituitary, resulting in a reduced ACTH secretion and hydrocortisone output in the plasma about 9 h later. Failure of suppression implies hypersecretion of ACTH or of glucocorticoids (Cushing's syndrome).

Actions of glucocorticoids

Common drugs used systemically include **hydrocortisone**, **prednisolone** and **dexamethasone**.

Metabolic actions

- *Carbohydrates:* decreased uptake and utilisation of glucose accompanied by increased gluconeogenesis; this causes a tendency to hyperglycaemia.
- *Proteins:* increased catabolism, reduced anabolism.
- *Lipids:* a permissive effect on lipolytic hormones and a redistribution of fat, as observed in Cushing's syndrome.

Regulatory actions

- *Hypothalamus and anterior pituitary gland:* a negative feedback action resulting in reduced release of ACTH and therefore endogenous glucocorticoids.
- *Cardiovascular system:* reduced vasodilatation, decreased fluid exudation.
- *Musculoskeletal:* decreased osteoblast and increased osteoclast activity.
- *Inflammation and immunity:*
  - in acute inflammation: decreased influx and activity of leukocytes;
  - in chronic inflammation: decreased activity of mononuclear cells, decreased angiogenesis, less fibrosis;
  - in lymphoid tissues: decreased clonal expansion of T and B cells, and decreased action of cytokine-secreting T cells. Switch from Th1 to Th2 response;
  - decreased production and action of many pro-inflammatory cytokines, including interleukins, TNF-α and granulocyte–macrophage colony-stimulating factor;
  - reduced generation of eicosanoids;
  - decreased generation of IgG;
  - decrease in complement components in the blood;
  - increased release of *anti-inflammatory* factors such as IL-10, IL-1Ra and Annexin 1.
- Overall effects: reduction in the activity of the innate and acquired immune systems, but also diminution in the protective aspects of the inflammatory response and sometimes decreased healing.

Pharmacokinetics and unwanted actions of the glucocorticoids

- Administration can be oral, topical or parenteral. Most naturally occurring glucocorticoids are transported in the blood by CBG or albumen and enter cells by diffusion. They are metabolised in the liver.
- Unwanted effects are seen mainly after prolonged systemic use as anti-inflammatory or immunosuppressive agents but not usually following replacement therapy. The most important of these are:
  - suppression of response to infection
  - suppression of endogenous glucocorticoid synthesis
  - metabolic actions (see earlier)
  - osteoporosis
  - iatrogenic Cushing's syndrome (see Fig. 33.7)

Clinical uses of glucocorticoids

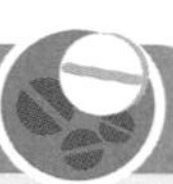

- Replacement therapy for patients with adrenal failure (*Addison's disease*).
- Anti-inflammatory/immunosuppressive therapy (see also Ch. 25):
  - in *asthma* (see Ch. 28);
  - topically in various inflammatory conditions of skin, eye, ear or nose (e.g. *eczema, allergic conjunctivitis* or *rhinitis*; see Ch. 27);
  - *hypersensitivity states* (e.g. severe allergic reactions);
  - in miscellaneous diseases with autoimmune and inflammatory components (e.g. *rheumatoid arthritis* and other 'connective tissue' diseases, *inflammatory bowel diseases*, some forms of *haemolytic anaemia*, *idiopathic thrombocytopenic purpura*);
  - to prevent graft-versus-host disease following organ or bone marrow transplantation;
  - to reduce lung inflammation and damage in intensive care COVID-19 patients.
- In neoplastic disease (see Ch. 57):
  - in combination with cytotoxic drugs in treatment of specific malignancies (e.g. *Hodgkin's disease*, *acute lymphocytic leukaemia*);
  - to reduce cerebral oedema in patients with metastatic or primary *brain tumours* (**dexamethasone**).

Mineralocorticoids

Fludrocortisone is given orally to produce a mineralocorticoid effect. This drug:

- increases Na^+ reabsorption in distal tubules and increases K^+ and H^+ efflux into the tubules;
- acts on intracellular receptors that modulate DNA transcription, causing synthesis of Na^+ channel and other proteins that mediate the effect of the drug;
- may be used together with a glucocorticoid in replacement therapy regimes.

MINERALOCORTICOIDS

The main endogenous mineralocorticoid is aldosterone. Its chief action is to increase Na^+ reabsorption by the distal tubules in the kidney, with a concomitant increase in excretion of K^+ and H^+ (see Ch. 29). An excessive secretion of mineralocorticoids, as in *Conn's syndrome*, causes marked Na^+ and water retention, with increased extracellular fluid volume and sometimes hypokalaemia, alkalosis and hypertension. Decreased mineralocorticoid secretion, as in some patients with Addison's disease, causes Na^+ loss and a marked decrease in extracellular fluid volume. There is a concomitant decrease in the excretion of K^+, resulting in hyperkalaemia.

Regulation of aldosterone synthesis and release

The regulation of the synthesis and release of aldosterone depends mainly on the electrolyte composition of the plasma and on the activity of the angiotensin II system (see Fig. 33.4 and Chs 22 and 29). Low plasma Na^+ or high plasma K^+ concentrations directly stimulate aldosterone release from the zona glomerulosa cells of the adrenal. Depletion of Na^+ also activates the renin–angiotensin system (see Ch. 22, Fig. 22.4). One of the effects of angiotensin II is to increase the synthesis and release of aldosterone (see Ch. 29, Fig. 29.5).

Mechanism of action

Like other steroid hormones, aldosterone acts through specific intracellular receptors of the nuclear receptor family. Unlike the GR, which is present in most cells, the *mineralocorticoid receptor* (also called the *corticosteroid receptor type I*) is restricted to a few tissues, such as the kidney and the transporting epithelia of the colon and bladder. Cells containing mineralocorticoid receptors also contain the 11β-hydroxysteroid dehydrogenase type 2 enzyme, which converts hydrocortisone (cortisol) into inactive cortisone, but does not inactivate aldosterone. This ensures that the cells are appropriately affected only by the mineralocorticoid hormone itself. Interestingly, this enzyme is inhibited by **carbenoxolone,** a compound derived from liquorice (and previously used to treat gastric ulcers; see Ch. 30). If this inhibition is marked, cortisol accumulates and acts on the mineralocorticoid receptor, producing an off-target effect similar to Conn's syndrome (*primary hyperaldosteronism*) except that the circulating aldosterone concentration is not raised.

As with the glucocorticoids, the interaction of aldosterone with its receptor initiates transcription and translation of specific proteins, resulting in an increase in the number of sodium channels on the apical membrane of the renal tubular cell, and subsequently an increase in the number of Na^+-K^+-ATPase molecules in the basolateral membrane (see Fig. 29.5), causing increased K^+ excretion (see Ch. 29). In addition to the genomic effects, there is evidence for a rapid *non-genomic* effect of aldosterone on Na^+ influx, through an action on the Na^+-H^+ exchanger at the apical membrane.

Clinical use of mineralocorticoids and antagonists

The main clinical use of mineralocorticoids is replacement therapy of patients with Addison's disease. The most commonly used drug is **fludrocortisone** (see Table 33.2 and Fig. 33.4), which can be taken orally to supplement the necessary glucocorticoid replacement. **Spironolactone** is a competitive antagonist of aldosterone, and it also prevents the mineralocorticoid effects of other adrenal steroids on the renal tubule (see Ch. 29). Side effects include gynaecomastia and impotence, due to **spironolactone's** ability to also partially block androgen and progesterone receptor function. It is used to treat primary or secondary hyperaldosteronism and, in conjunction with other drugs, for the treatment of resistant hypertension and of heart failure (see Ch. 22) and oedema (see Ch. 29). **Eplerenone** has a similar indication and mechanism of action, although fewer side effects as it has lower affinity for the sex hormone receptors (see Ch. 22).

NEW DIRECTIONS IN GLUCOCORTICOID THERAPY

Recent advances in the treatment of severely ill COVID-19 patients showed glucocorticoid treatment to be an effective therapy to minimise mortality rates particularly among mechanically ventilated patients but also those receiving supplemental oxygen only. The RECOVERY randomised clinical trial showed marked improvements among patients treated with systemic glucocorticoids (Horby et al., 2021), reducing lung damage and overall patient survival. It is intuitive that the first pharmacological improvements shown in COVID-19 patients would be through glucocorticoids. Indeed, glucocorticoids are highly effective in controlling inflammation, but their utility is constrained by their potentially harmful side effects. The ideal solution would be a glucocorticoid possessing the anti-inflammatory but not the unwanted metabolic or other effects.

Following the discovery of cortisol, the pharmaceutical industry pursued this ambitious goal by testing straightforward structural analogues of cortisol. While this yielded many new active and interesting compounds (several of which are in clinical use today), none achieved a true 'separation' of the glucocorticoid actions. Recently, there have been fresh attempts to accomplish this. The development of structural analogues at novel sites on the steroid template (e.g. Uings et al., 2013) has met with more success, and structural details of the receptor revealed by X-ray crystallography has enabled the design of non-steroidal receptor ligands (see, for example, Biggadike et al., 2009; He et al., 2014). Another approach has been to add other functional groups on to the steroid molecule, which alters the conformation of the liganded receptor. Fiorucci et al. (2002) attached a nitric oxide donating group to prednisolone, finding augmented efficacy and reduced unwanted effects. The compound is reported to be useful in the treatment of inflammatory bowel disease (see Schacke et al., 2007). The design of 'soft' glucocorticoids which are rapidly metabolised to inactive species, thereby limiting their capacity for producing side effects, is also being investigated (see Dobricic et al., 2017).

Many investigators in this area have been influenced by the 'dissociated steroids' or 'transrepression hypothesis': this is the notion, based upon some experimental observations, that the anti-inflammatory effects of glucocorticoids are generally caused by the *down*-regulation (*transrepression*) of genes such as those coding for cytokines, whilst the unwanted effects are usually caused by *up*-regulation (*transactivation*) of metabolic and other genes (e.g. tyrosine amino transferase and phosphoenol pyruvate carboxykinase). Because transactivation and transrepression utilise different molecular pathways (see Fig. 33.6) which depend upon different conformational states of the GR, researchers have sought **S**elective **G**lucocorticoid **R**eceptor **A**gonists (SEGRAs) that promote one set of actions without the other. The application of this idea has been reviewed by Schacke et al. (2007) and the development of compounds for treating skin and ocular conditions has been reported (Schacke et al., 2009; Spinelli et al., 2014). However, some anti-inflammatory effects of glucocorticoids do not fit neatly into this scheme (Vandevyver et al., 2013); its shortcomings have been reviewed by Clark and Belvisi (2012).

Another approach focuses upon the histone deacetylase enzymes that facilitate the transcriptional regulation of genes following nuclear receptor binding to hormone response elements (Hayashi et al., 2004). There may be a specific isoform of this enzyme that deals with gene upregulation, and if this could be inhibited, it would lessen the possibility of those unwanted effects. Barnes (2011) has reviewed this approach, particularly as it relates to the therapy of asthma. A more general review of the whole area, with particular relevance to the treatment of rheumatic diseases, has been provided by Strehl et al. (2011). Other molecular tactics that show promise include the use of GILZ (**G**lucocorticoid-**I**nduced **L**eucine **Z**ipper protein) as a therapeutic agent (Beaulieu and Morand, 2011) or exploitation of the cytosolic, non-genomic actions of these drugs (Jiang et al., 2014)

The quest for the glucocorticoid magic bullet continues.

REFERENCES AND FURTHER READING

The hypothalamus and pituitary

Chan, L.F., Clark, A.J., Metherell, L.A., 2008. Familial glucocorticoid deficiency: advances in the molecular understanding of ACTH action. Horm. Res. 69, 75–82.

Chini, B., Manning, M., Guillon, G., 2008. Affinity and efficacy of selective agonists and antagonists for vasopressin and oxytocin receptors: an 'easy guide' to receptor pharmacology. Prog. Brain Res. 170, 513–517.

Clark, A.J., Metherell, L.A., Cheetham, M.E., Huebner, A., 2005. Inherited ACTH insensitivity illuminates the mechanisms of ACTH action. Trends Endocrinol. Metab. 16, 451–457.

Drolet, G., Rivest, S., 2001. Corticotropin-releasing hormone and its receptors; an evaluation at the transcription level *in vivo*. Peptides 22, 761–767.

Freeman, M.E., Kanyicska, B., Lerant, A., Nagy, G., 2000. Prolactin: structure, function and regulation of secretion. Physiol. Res. 80, 1524–1585.

Getting, S.J., Christian, H.C., Flower, R.J., Perretti, M., 2002. Activation of melanocortin type 3 receptor as a molecular mechanism for adrenocorticotropic hormone efficacy in gouty arthritis. Arthritis Rheum. 46, 2765–2775.

Guillemin, R., 2005. Hypothalamic hormones a.k.a. hypothalamic releasing factors. J. Endocrinol. 184, 11–28.

Lamberts, S.W.J., van der Lely, A.J., de Herder, W.W., Hofland, L.J., 1996. Octreotide. N. Engl. J. Med. 334, 246–254.

Schneider, F., Tomek, W., Grundker, C., 2006. Gonadotropin-releasing hormone (GnRH) and its natural analogues: a review. Theriogenology 66, 691–709.

Thibonnier, M., Coles, P., Thibonnier, A., et al., 2001. The basic and clinical pharmacology of nonpeptide vasopressin receptor antagonists. Annu. Rev. Pharmacol. 41, 175–202.

Wikberg, J.E.S., Muceniece, R., Mandrika, I., et al., 2000. New aspects on the melanocortins and their receptors. Pharmacol. Res. 42, 393–420.

Glucocorticoids

Barnes, P.J., 2011. Glucocorticosteroids: current and future directions. Br. J. Pharmacol. 163 (1), 29–43.

Baxter, J.D., Rousseau, G.G. (Eds.), 1979. Glucocorticoid Hormone Action. Monographs on Endocrinology. Springer-Verlag, Berlin, p. 12.

Beaulieu, E., Morand, E.F., 2011. Role of GILZ in immune regulation, glucocorticoid actions and rheumatoid arthritis. Nat. Rev. Rheumatol. 7, 340–348.

Biggadike, K., Bledsoe, R.K., Coe, D.M., et al., 2009. Design and x-ray crystal structures of high-potency nonsteroidal glucocorticoid agonists exploiting a novel binding site on the receptor. Proc. Natl. Acad. Sci. U. S. A. 106, 18114–18119.

Buckingham, J.C., 1998. Stress and the hypothalamo–pituitary–immune axis. Int. J. Tissue React. 20, 23–34.

Buttgereit, F., Scheffold, A., 2002. Rapid glucocorticoid effects on immune cells. Steroids 67, 529–534.

Clark, A.R., Belvisi, M.G., 2012. Maps and legends: the quest for dissociated ligands of the glucocorticoid receptor. Pharmacol. Ther. 134, 54–67.

D'Acquisto, F., Perretti, M., Flower, R.J., 2008. Annexin-A1: a pivotal regulator of the innate and adaptive immune systems. Br. J. Pharmacol. 155, 152–169.

Dobricic, V., Jacevic, V., Vucicevic, J., et al., 2017. Evaluation of biological activity and computer-aided design of new soft glucocorticoids. Arch. Pharm. (Weinheim) 350 (5).

Fiorucci, S., Antonelli, E., Distrutti, E., et al., 2002. NCX-1015, a nitric-oxide derivative of prednisolone, enhances regulatory T cells in the lamina propria and protects against 2,4,6-trinitrobenzene sulfonic acid-induced colitis in mice. Proc. Natl. Acad. Sci. U. S. A. 99, 15770–15775.

Hannen, R., Udeh-Momoh, C., Upton, J., et al., 2017. Dysfunctional skin-derived glucocorticoid synthesis is a pathogenic mechanism of psoriasis. J. Invest. Dermatol. 137, 1630–1637.

Hayashi, R., Wada, H., Ito, K., Adcock, I.M., 2004. Effects of glucocorticoids on gene transcription. Eur. J. Pharmacol. 500, 51–62.

He, Y., Yi, W., Suino-Powell, K., et al., 2014. Structures and mechanism for the design of highly potent glucocorticoids. Cell Res. 24, 713–726.

Horby, P., Lim, W.S., Emberson, J.R., et al., 2021. Dexamethasone in hospitalized patients with COVID-19 (the RECOVERY Collaborative Group). N. Engl. J. Med. 384, 693–704.

Jiang, C.L., Liu, L., Tasker, J.G., 2014. Why do we need nongenomic glucocorticoid mechanisms? Front. Neuroendocrinol. 35, 72–75.

Kirwan, J., Power, L., 2007. Glucocorticoids: action and new therapeutic insights in rheumatoid arthritis. Curr. Opin. Rheumatol. 19, 233–237.

Munck, A., Guyre, P.M., Holbrook, N.J., 1984. Physiological functions of glucocorticoids in stress and their relation to pharmacological actions. Endocr. Rev. 5, 25–44.

Norman, A.W., Mizwicki, M.T., Norman, D.P., 2004. Steroid-hormone rapid actions, membrane receptors and a conformational ensemble model. Nat. Rev. Drug Discov. 3, 27–41.

Oakley, R.H., Cidlowski, J.A., 2001. The glucocorticoid receptor: expression, function and regulation of glucocorticoid responsiveness. In: Goulding, N.J., Flower, R.J. (Eds.), Milestones in Drug Therapy: Glucocorticoids. Birkhäuser Verlag, Basel, pp. 55–80.

Oakley, R.H., Cidlowski, J.A., 2013. The biology of the glucocorticoid receptor: new signaling mechanisms in health and disease. J. Allergy Clin. Immunol. 132, 1033–1044.

Panettieri, R.A., Schaafsma, D., Amrani, Y., et al., 2019. Non-genomic effects of glucocorticoids: an updated view. Trends Pharmacol. Sci. 40, 38–49.

Reichardt, H.M., Kaestner, K.H., Tuckermann, J., et al., 1998. DNA binding of the glucocorticoid receptor is not essential for survival. Cell 93, 531–541.

Schacke, H., Berger, M., Rehwinkel, H., Asadullah, K., 2007. Selective glucocorticoid receptor agonists (SEGRAs): novel ligands with an improved therapeutic index. Mol. Cell. Endocrinol. 275, 109–117.

Schacke, H., Zollner, T.M., Docke, W.D., et al., 2009. Characterization of ZK 245186, a novel, selective glucocorticoid receptor agonist for the topical treatment of inflammatory skin diseases. Br. J. Pharmacol. 158, 1088–1103.

Song, I.H., Gold, R., Straub, R.H., et al., 2005. New glucocorticoids on the horizon: repress, don't activate. J. Rheumatol. 32, 1199–1207.

Spinelli, S.L., Xi, X., McMillan, D.H., et al., 2014. Mapracorat, a selective glucocorticoid receptor agonist, upregulates RelB, an anti-

inflammatory nuclear factor-kappaB protein, in human ocular cells. Exp. Eye Res. 127, 290–298.
Strehl, C., Spies, C.M., Buttgereit, F., 2011. Pharmacodynamics of glucocorticoids. Clin. Exp. Rheumatol. 29, S13–S18.
Tak, P.P., Firestein, G.S., 2001. NF-kappaB: a key role in inflammatory diseases. J. Clin. Invest. 107, 7–11.
Talaber, G., Jondal, M., Okret, S., 2015. Local glucocorticoid production in the thymus. Steroids 103, 58–63.
Uings, I.J., Needham, D., Matthews, J., et al., 2013. Discovery of GW870086: a potent anti-inflammatory steroid with a unique pharmacological profile. Br. J. Pharmacol. 169, 1389–1403.
Vandevyver, S., Dejager, L., Tuckermann, J., Libert, C., 2013. New insights into the anti-inflammatory mechanisms of glucocorticoids: an emerging role for glucocorticoid-receptor-mediated transactivation. Endocrinology 154, 993–1007.
Whittington, P.F., H V Barnes, H.V., Bayless, T.M., 1977. Medical management of Crohn's disease in adolescence. Gastroenterology 72, 1338–1344.

Mineralocorticoids

Bastl, C., Hayslett, J.P., 1992. The cellular action of aldosterone in target epithelia. Kidney Int. 42, 250–264.
Jaisser, F., Farman, N., 2016. Emerging roles of the mineralocorticoid receptor in pathology: toward new paradigms in clinical pharmacology. Pharmacol. Rev. 68, 49–75.

34 The thyroid

OVERVIEW

Diseases of the thyroid gland are common, and in this chapter we deal with drug therapy used to mitigate these disorders. We set the scene by briefly outlining the structure, regulation and physiology of the thyroid, and highlight the most common abnormalities of thyroid function. We then consider the drugs that can be used to replace thyroid hormones when these are deficient or cease to function adequately, or which decrease thyroid function when this is excessive.

SYNTHESIS, STORAGE AND SECRETION OF THYROID HORMONES

The thyroid gland secretes three main hormones, which control general metabolic activities in the body: in this chapter we shall focus on two of these hormones, *thyroxine* (T_4) and *tri-iodothyronine* (T_3). The third hormone secreted by this gland is *calcitonin,* which is involved in the control of plasma [Ca^{2+}]. It is used to treat osteoporosis and other metabolic bone diseases. It is dealt with in Ch. 36. The term *thyroid hormones* will be used here solely to refer to T_4 and T_3.

Both T_3 and T_4 circulate in the blood tightly bound (>99%) to plasma proteins, mainly *thyroxine binding globulin* (TBG). The majority (~85%) of the secreted thyroid hormone is T_4. This is converted into the (three- to five-fold) more active species, T_3, in a tissue-specific manner. Both hormones are critically important for normal growth and development and for controlling energy metabolism.

The functional unit of the thyroid is the follicle or acinus. Each follicle consists of a single layer of epithelial cells surrounding a cavity, the *follicle lumen,* which is filled with a thick colloid containing *thyroglobulin*. Thyroglobulin is a large glycoprotein, each molecule of which contains about 115 tyrosine residues. It is synthesised, glycosylated and then secreted into the lumen of the follicle, where iodination of the tyrosine residues occurs. Surrounding the follicles is a dense capillary network and the blood flow through the gland is very high in comparison with other tissues. The main steps in the synthesis, storage and secretion of thyroid hormone (Fig. 34.1) are:

- uptake of plasma iodide by the follicle cells;
- oxidation of iodide and iodination of tyrosine residues of thyroglobulin;
- secretion of thyroid hormone.

UPTAKE OF PLASMA IODIDE BY THE FOLLICLE CELLS

Iodide uptake must occur against a concentration gradient (normally about 25:1) so it is an energy-dependent process. Iodide is captured from the blood and moved to the lumen by two transporters: the Na^+/I^- symporter (NIS), located at the basolateral surface of the thyrocytes (the energy being provided by Na^+/K^+-atpase), and *pendrin*[1] (PDS), an I^-/Cl^- porter in the apical membranes (Nilsson, 2001). Uptake is very rapid: labelled iodide (^{125}I) is found in the lumen within 40 s of intravenous injection. Numerous mutations have been discovered in the NIS and PDS genes and these contribute to thyroid disease in some patients.

OXIDATION OF IODIDE AND IODINATION OF TYROSINE RESIDUES

The oxidation of iodide and its incorporation into thyroglobulin (termed the *organification* of iodide) are catalysed by *thyroperoxidase*, an enzyme situated at the inner surface of the cell at the interface with the colloid. The reaction requires the presence of hydrogen peroxide (H_2O_2) as an oxidising agent. Iodination occurs after the tyrosine has been incorporated into thyroglobulin. The reaction is shown in Fig. 34.2.

Tyrosine residues are iodinated first at position 3 on the ring, forming monoiodotyrosine (MIT) and then, in some molecules, at position 5 as well, forming di-iodotyrosine (DIT). While still incorporated into thyroglobulin, these molecules are then coupled in pairs, either MIT with DIT to form T_3 or two DIT molecules to form T_4 (Figs 34.2 and 34.3). The mechanism for coupling is believed to involve a peroxidase system similar to the iodination reaction. About one-fifth of the tyrosine residues in thyroglobulin are iodinated in this way.

The iodinated thyroglobulin of the thyroid forms a large store of thyroid hormone within the gland, with a relatively slow turnover. This is in contrast to some other endocrine secretions (e.g. the hormones of the adrenal cortex), which are not stored but synthesised and released as required.

SECRETION OF THYROID HORMONE

The thyroglobulin molecule is taken up into the follicle cell by endocytosis. The endocytotic vesicles then fuse with lysosomes, and proteolytic enzymes act on thyroglobulin, releasing T_4 and T_3 to be secreted into the plasma. The surplus MIT and DIT, which are released at the same time, are scavenged by the cell and the iodide is removed enzymatically and reused.

REGULATION OF THYROID FUNCTION

Thyrotropin-releasing hormone (TRH), released from the hypothalamus in response to various stimuli, releases *thyroid-stimulating hormone* (TSH; thyrotrophin) from the anterior pituitary (Fig. 34.4), as does the synthetic tripeptide

[1]So called because it is implicated in the pathophysiology of *Pendred syndrome,* named after the eponymous English physician who first described this autosomal recessive form of familial goitre in association with sensorineural deafness.

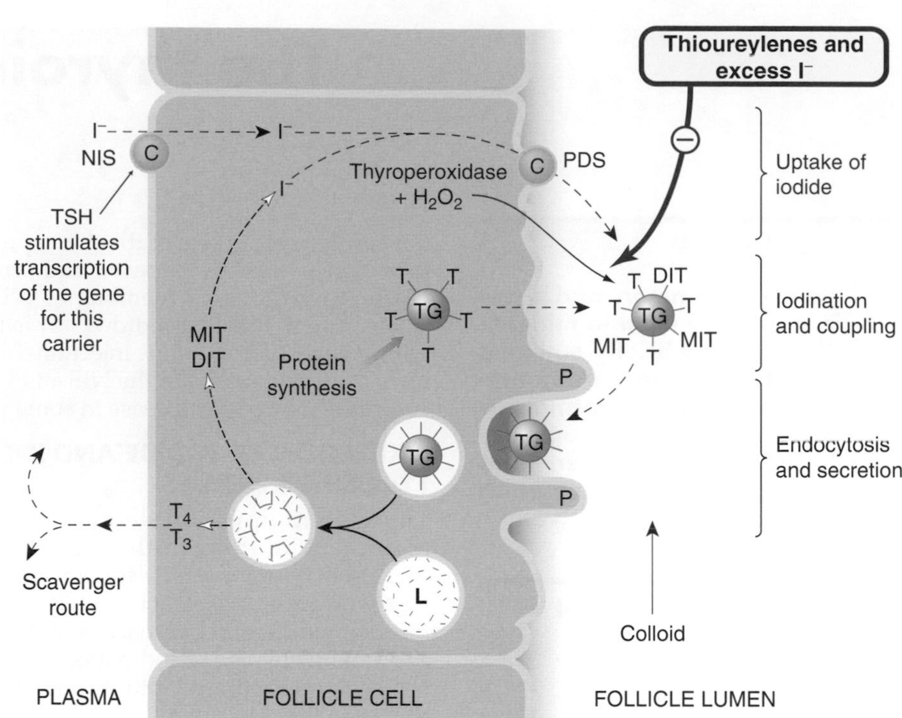

Fig. 34.1 Diagram of thyroid hormone synthesis and secretion, with the sites of action of some drugs used in the treatment of thyroid disorders. Iodide in the blood is transported by the carriers NIS and PDS through the follicular cell and into the colloid-rich lumen, where it is incorporated into tyrosines in thyroglobulin under the influence of the thyroperoxidase enzyme and monoiodotyrosine units are produced and coupled to produce the hormones (see text for details). Thyroid-stimulating hormone (thyrotropin; TSH) stimulates the endocytosis of thyroglobulin and the hormones are subsequently cleaved from the globulin by lysosomal enzymes and exported into the blood. *DIT,* Di-iodotyrosine; *L,* lysosome; *MIT,* monoiodotyrosine; *P,* pseudopod; *T,* tyrosine; T_3, tri-iodothyronine; T_4, thyroxine; *TG,* thyroglobulin.

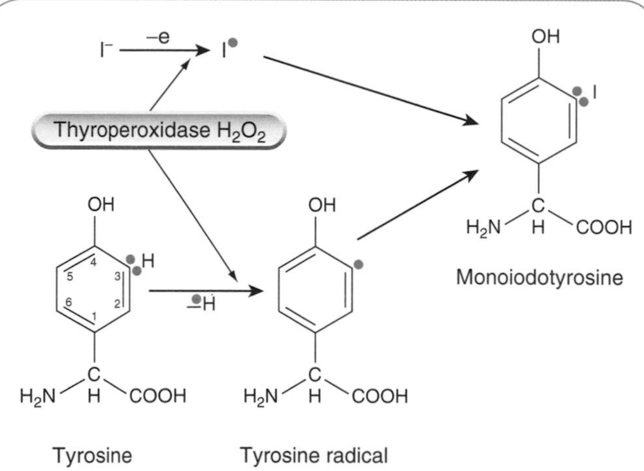

Fig. 34.2 Iodination of tyrosyl residues by the thyroperoxidase–H_2O_2 complex. This probably involves two sites on the enzyme, one of which removes an electron from iodide to give the free radical I•; another removes an electron from tyrosine to give the tyrosyl radical *(orange dot).* Monoiodotyrosine results from the addition of the two radicals.

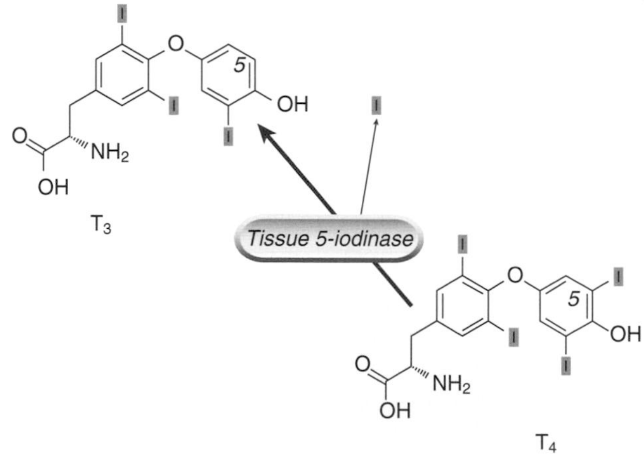

T_3

Tissue 5-iodinase

T_4

Fig. 34.3 The structures of thyroxine T_3 and T_4. The positions of the iodine residues are indicated in *orange*. T_4 is converted, in a tissue-specific manner, to the more active species T_3 by mono de-iodination at position 5 of the ring. The basic tyrosine unit is shaded in *yellow*.

protirelin (pyroglutamyl-histidyl-proline amide), which is used in this way for diagnostic purposes. TSH acts on receptors on the membrane of thyroid follicle cells through a mechanism that involves cAMP and phosphatidylinositol 3-kinase. It has a trophic action on thyroid cells and controls all aspects of thyroid hormone synthesis, mainly

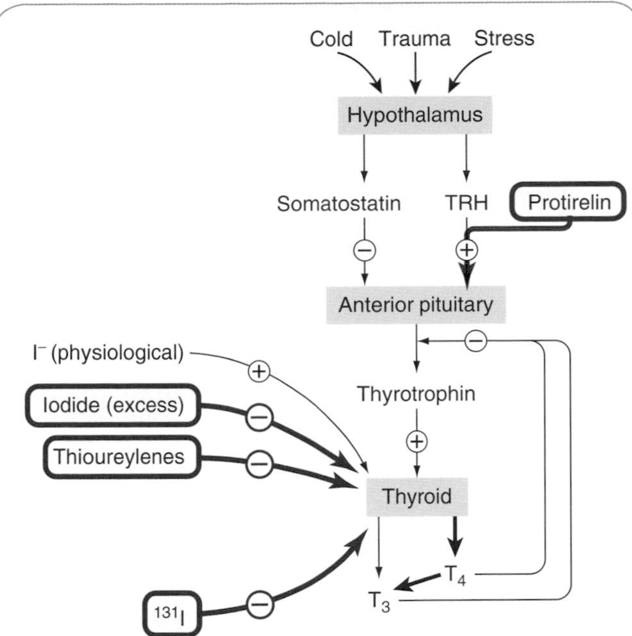

Fig. 34.4 Regulation of thyroid hormone secretion. Iodide (I^-) is essential for thyroid hormone synthesis, but excess of endogenous or exogenous iodide (30 times the daily requirement of iodine) may be used to inhibit the increased thyroid hormone production of thyrotoxicosis. Protirelin, as well as recombinant human thyrotropin-releasing hormone (TRH), is sometimes used to stimulate the system for diagnostic purposes. Larger amounts of iodine (as the ^{131}I isotope) are used for ablation of thyroid tissue (see text for details). *T_3*, Tri-iodothyronine; *T_4*, thyroxine.

by stimulating transcription of the iodide transporter genes, thereby increasing the uptake of iodide by follicle cells. This, in turn, controls all aspects of thyroid hormone synthesis including:

- the synthesis and secretion of thyroglobulin;
- the generation of H_2O_2 and the iodination of tyrosine;
- the endocytosis and proteolysis of thyroglobulin;
- the actual secretion of T_3 and T_4;
- the blood flow through the gland.

The production of TSH is also regulated by a negative feedback effect of thyroid hormones on the anterior pituitary gland and the hypothalamus; T_3 is more active than T_4 in this respect. The peptide **somatostatin** also reduces basal TSH release. The control of the secretion of TSH thus depends on a balance between the actions of T_3/T_4 and TRH (and probably also **somatostatin**) on the pituitary and most likely also at the hypothalamus. However, the relationship between T_3/T_4 concentration and TSH secretion is not linear. Small changes in thyroid hormones can produce very large changes in TSH secretion whilst large changes in TSH produce only small alterations in T_3/T_4. It is important to recognise this, as measurement of TSH is a key diagnostic tool when assessing thyroid function in patients.

The other main factor influencing thyroid function is the plasma iodide concentration. About 100 nmol of T_4 is synthesised daily, necessitating uptake by the gland of approximately 500 nmol of iodide each day (equivalent to about 70 μg of iodine). A reduced iodine intake, with reduced plasma iodide concentration, will result in a decrease of hormone production and an increase in TSH secretion. An increased plasma iodide has the opposite effect, although this may be modified by other factors. The overall feedback mechanism responds to changes of iodide slowly over fairly long periods of days or weeks, because there is a large reserve capacity for the binding and uptake of iodide in the thyroid. The size and vascularity of the thyroid are reduced by an increase in plasma iodide and this is exploited therapeutically in preparing hyperthyroid patients for surgery to the gland. Diets deficient in iodine eventually result in a continuous excessive compensatory secretion of TSH, and eventually in an increase in vascularity and (sometimes gross) hypertrophy of the gland.[2]

ACTIONS OF THE THYROID HORMONES

The physiological actions of the thyroid hormones fall into two main categories: those affecting metabolism and those affecting growth and development. Both T_3 and T_4 are extensively plasma bound and only the free concentrations of the hormones are active.

EFFECTS ON METABOLISM

The thyroid hormones produce a general increase in the metabolism of carbohydrates, fats and proteins, and regulate these processes in most tissues, T_3 being three to five times more active than T_4 in this respect (Fig. 34.5). Although the thyroid hormones directly control the activity of some of the enzymes of carbohydrate metabolism, most effects are brought about in conjunction with other hormones, such as insulin, glucagon, the glucocorticoids and the catecholamines. There is an increase in oxygen consumption and heat production, which is manifested as an increase in the measured basal metabolic rate. This reflects the action of these hormones on tissues such as heart, kidney, liver and muscle, although not on others, such as the gonads, brain or spleen. This calorigenic action is important as part of the response to a cold environment. Administration of thyroid hormone results in augmented cardiac rate and output, and increased tendency to dysrhythmias such as atrial fibrillation.

EFFECTS ON GROWTH AND DEVELOPMENT

The thyroid hormones have a critical effect on growth, partly by a direct action on cells, but also indirectly by influencing growth hormone production and potentiating its effects on its target tissues. The hormones are important for a normal response to *parathormone* (see Ch. 36) and calcitonin as well as for skeletal development; they are also essential for normal growth and maturation of the central nervous system.

MECHANISM OF ACTION

While there is some evidence for non-genomic actions (see Bassett et al., 2003), thyroid hormones act mainly through a specific nuclear receptor, TR (see Ch. 3). Two distinct genes, TRα and TRβ, code for several receptor isoforms that have distinct functions. T_4 may be regarded as a prohormone,

[2]'Derbyshire neck' was the name given to this condition in a part of the United Kingdom where sources of dietary iodine were once scarce.

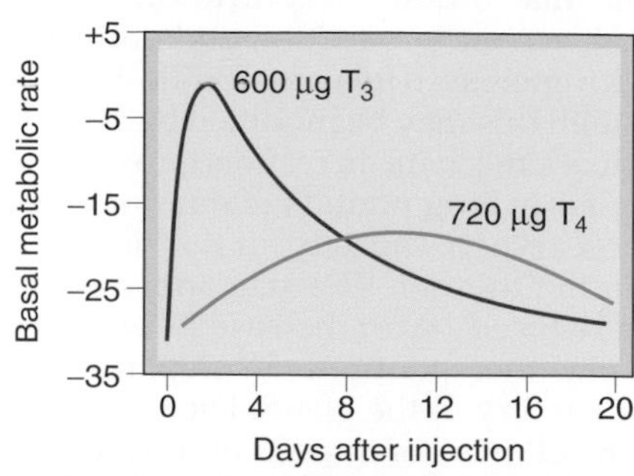

Fig. 34.5 The effect of equimolar doses of tri-iodothyronine (T_3) and thyroxine (T_4) on basal metabolic rate (BMR) in a hypothyroid subject. Note that this figure is meant only to illustrate overall differences in effect; thyroxine is not given clinically in a single bolus dose as here, but in regular daily doses so that the effect builds up to a plateau. The apparent differences in potency really represent differences in kinetics of T3 (*red line*) and T4 (*green line*), reflecting the prohormone role of T_4. (Modified from Blackburn, C.M., McConahey, W.M., Keating, F.R., Jr., Albert, A., 1954. Calorigenic effects of single intravenous doses of L-triiodothyronine and L-thyroxine in myxedematous persons. J. Clin. Invest. 33, 819–824.)

because when it enters the cell, it is converted to T_3, which then binds with high affinity to TR. This interaction is likely to take place in the nucleus, where TR isoforms generally act as a constitutive repressor of target genes. When T_3 is bound, these receptors change conformation, the co-repressor complex is released and a co-activator complex is recruited, which then activates transcription, resulting in generation of mRNA and protein synthesis. Some rare cases of thyroid hormone resistance linked to TRβ mutations have been reported (Lai et al., 2015) which can be associated with deaf mutism and colour blindness in the most severely deficient forms.

TRANSPORT AND METABOLISM OF THYROID HORMONES

Plasma concentrations of these hormones can be measured by radioimmunoassay and are approximately 1×10^{-7} mol/L (T_4) and 2×10^{-9} mol/L (T_3). Both are eventually metabolised in their target tissues by deiodination, deamination, decarboxylation and conjugation with glucuronic and sulfuric acids. The liver is a major site of metabolism, and the free and conjugated forms are excreted partly in the bile and partly in the urine. The half-life of T_3 is a few hours, whereas that of T_4 varies between 3–4 days in hyperthyroidism and 9–10 days in hypothyroidism.[3] Abnormalities in the metabolism of these hormones may occur naturally or be induced by drugs or heavy metals, and this may give rise to a variety of (uncommon) clinical conditions such as the 'low T_3 syndrome'.

ABNORMALITIES OF THYROID FUNCTION

Thyroid disorders are among the most common endocrine diseases in all age groups, including children. Subclinical thyroid disease is prevalent in the middle-aged and elderly. Thyroid disorders are accompanied by many extra-thyroidal symptoms, particularly in the heart, gastrointestinal system and skin. One (rare) cause of organ dysfunction is thyroid cancer. Many other thyroid disorders have an autoimmune basis – in fact, autoimmune thyroid disease is the commonest autoimmune disease. The reason for this is not clear, although it may be linked to a breakdown in immune tolerance to the TSH receptor, although other factors cannot be ruled out (Lee et al., 2015). It may be linked to other autoimmune conditions such as rheumatoid arthritis.

There are two main types of autoimmune thyroid disorder, *Graves' disease*[4] and *Hashimoto's disease*. Both are associated with the production of thyroid autoantibodies and immune damage to the gland itself.[5] Oddly perhaps, they result in different clinical pictures, with Graves' disease leading to thyrotoxicosis while Hashimoto's thyroiditis leads to hypoactive thyroid. Regardless of causation, thyroid dysfunction is often associated with typical gross enlargement of the gland, known as *goitre*. Like other autoimmune diseases, such thyroid disorders are more common in women than men and occur with increased frequency during pregnancy (Cignini et al., 2012).

HYPERTHYROIDISM (THYROTOXICOSIS)

In thyrotoxicosis there is excessive secretion and activity of the thyroid hormones, resulting in a high metabolic rate, an increase in skin temperature and sweating and heat intolerance. Nervousness, tremor, tachycardia and increased appetite associated with loss of weight occur. There are several types of hyperthyroidism, but only two are common: *exophthalmic* or *diffuse toxic goitre* (Graves' disease) and *toxic nodular goitre*.

Diffuse toxic goitre is an organ-specific autoimmune disease caused by autoantibodies to the TSH receptor which, when active, increase T_4 secretion. Constitutively active mutations of the TRH receptor may also be involved. As is indicated by the name, patients with exophthalmic goitre have protrusion of the eyeballs. The pathogenesis of this condition is not fully understood, but it is thought to be caused by the presence of TSH receptor–like proteins in orbital tissues. There is also an enhanced sensitivity to catecholamines. Toxic nodular goitre is caused by a benign tumour and may develop in patients with long-standing simple goitre. This condition does not usually have concomitant exophthalmos. The antidysrhythmic drug **amiodarone** (see Ch. 21) is rich in iodine and can cause either hyperthyroidism or hypothyroidism. Some iodine-containing radiocontrast agents, such as **iopanoic acid**

[3]Correcting hypothyroidism by administration of T_4 therefore takes 2–3 weeks to reach equilibrium.

[4]After a Dublin physician who connected 'violent and long continued palpitations in females' with enlargement of the thyroid gland. Their complaints of fluttering hearts and lumps in their throats had previously been attributed to hysteria.

[5]John F. Kennedy Jr suffered from Graves' disease. He inherited a propensity for autoimmune diseases from his father JFK, who himself suffered from the autoimmune *Addison's disease*, in which adrenal glands are the main organs affected. JFK's sister Eunice also suffered from Addison's disease.

and its congeners, used as imaging agents to visualise the gall bladder, may also interfere with thyroid function. The chronic use of psychotropic agents may precipitate a variety of thyroid abnormalities (Bou Khalil and Richa, 2011).

SIMPLE, NON-TOXIC GOITRE

A dietary deficiency of iodine, if prolonged, causes a rise in plasma TRH and eventually an increase in the size of the gland. This condition is known as simple or non-toxic goitre. Another cause is ingestion of *goitrogens* (e.g. from cassava root). The enlarged thyroid usually manages to produce normal amounts of thyroid hormone, although if the iodine deficiency is very severe, hypothyroidism may supervene.

HYPOTHYROIDISM

A decreased activity of the thyroid results in hypothyroidism, and in severe cases *myxoedema*. Once again, this disease is usually immunological in origin, and the manifestations include low metabolic rate, slow speech, deep hoarse voice, lethargy, bradycardia, sensitivity to cold and mental impairment. Patients also develop a characteristic thickening of the skin (caused by the subcutaneous deposition of glycosaminoglycans), which gives myxoedema its name. In Hashimoto's thyroiditis, there is an immune reaction against thyroglobulin or some other component of thyroid tissue, which can lead to both hypothyroidism and myxoedema. Genetic factors play an important role. Destruction of glandular tissue whilst treating thyroid tumours with radioiodine is another cause of hypothyroidism. Some drugs (e.g. cholecystographic agents or anti-epileptic drugs) as well as environmental 'endocrine disruptors'[6] may interfere with the normal production of thyroid hormones.

Thyroid deficiency during development, affecting 1 in 3000–4000 births, causes congenital hypothyroidism (known as *Congenital iodine deficiency syndrome*), characterised by gross restriction of growth and intellectual disability.[7]

DRUGS USED IN DISEASES OF THE THYROID

HYPERTHYROIDISM

Hyperthyroidism may be treated pharmacologically or surgically. In general, surgery is now used only when there are mechanical problems resulting from compression of the trachea by the thyroid. Under such circumstances it is usual to remove only part of the organ. Although the condition of hyperthyroidism can be controlled with antithyroid drugs, these drugs do not alter the underlying autoimmune mechanisms or improve the exophthalmos associated with Graves' disease.

RADIOIODINE

Radioiodine is a first-line treatment for hyperthyroidism (particularly in the United States). The isotope used is ^{131}I (usually as the sodium salt), and the dose generally is 5–15 mCi. Given orally, it is taken up and processed by the thyroid in the same way as the stable form of iodide, eventually becoming incorporated into thyroglobulin. The isotope emits both β and γ radiation. The γ rays pass through the tissue without causing damage, but the β particles have a very short range; they are absorbed by the tissue and exert a powerful cytotoxic action that is restricted to the cells of the thyroid follicles, resulting in significant destruction of the tissue. ^{131}I has a half-life of 8 days, so by 2 months its radioactivity has effectively disappeared. It is given as one single dose, but its cytotoxic effect on the gland is delayed for 1–2 months and does not reach its maximum for a further 2 months.

Hypothyroidism will eventually occur after treatment with radioiodine, particularly in patients with Graves' disease, but is easily managed by replacement therapy with T_4. Radioiodine is best avoided in children or pregnant patients (because of potential damage to the fetus). There is theoretically an increased risk of thyroid cancer but this has not been seen following therapeutic treatment.

The uptake of ^{131}I and other isotopes of iodine is also used diagnostically as a test of thyroid function. A tracer dose of the isotope is given orally or intravenously, and the amount accumulated by the thyroid is measured by a γ-scintillation counter placed over the gland. ^{131}I is also used for the treatment of thyroid cancer in combination with surgery, radiotherapy (external or proton-bean therapy) and/or tyrosine kinase inhibitor chemotherapeutics (**cabozantinib**, **lenvatinib**, **sorafenib**) (see Ch. 57).

The thyroid

- Thyroid hormones, tri-iodothyronine (T_3) and thyroxine (T_4), are synthesised by iodination of tyrosine residues on thyroglobulin within the lumen of the thyroid follicle.
- Hormone synthesis and secretion are regulated by TSH (thyrotropin) and influenced by plasma iodide.
- There is a large pool of T_4 in the body; it has a low turnover rate and is found mainly in the circulation.
- There is a small pool of T_3 in the body; it has a fast turnover rate and is found mainly intracellularly.
- Within target cells, T_4 is converted to T_3, which interacts with a nuclear receptor to regulate gene transcription.
- T_3 and T_4 actions:
  - stimulation of metabolism, causing increased oxygen consumption and increased metabolic rate;
  - regulation of growth and development.
- Abnormalities of thyroid function include:
  - hyperthyroidism (thyrotoxicosis): either diffuse toxic goitre or toxic nodular goitre;
  - hypothyroidism: in adults this causes myxoedema; in infants, gross restriction of growth and intellectual disability;
  - simple non-toxic goitre caused by dietary iodine deficiency, usually with normal thyroid function.

THIOUREYLENES

This group of drugs comprises **carbimazole** and **propylthiouracil**. Chemically, they are related to thiourea, and the thiocarbamide (S–C–N) group is essential for antithyroid activity.

[6]These are man-made chemicals such as pesticides or herbicides (e.g. polychlorinated biphenyls) that persist in the environment and are ingested in foodstuffs. The endocrine system is particularly sensitive to these, especially during development.

[7]An older term for this condition, *cretinism*, has been dropped.

Mechanism of action

Thioureylenes decrease the output of thyroid hormones from the gland and cause a gradual reduction in the signs and symptoms of thyrotoxicosis, with the basal metabolic rate and pulse rate returning to normal over a period of 3–4 weeks. Their mode of action is not completely understood, but there is evidence that they reduce the iodination of tyrosyl residues in thyroglobulin (see Figs 34.1 and 34.2) by inhibiting the thyroperoxidase-catalysed oxidation reactions, possibly by acting as substrates, thus competitively inhibiting the interaction with tyrosine. Propylthiouracil has the additional effect of reducing the deiodination of T_4 to T_3 in peripheral tissues.

Pharmacokinetic aspects

Thioureylenes are given orally. **Carbimazole** is rapidly converted to an active metabolite. An average dose of **carbimazole** produces more than 90% inhibition of thyroid incorporation of iodine within 12 h. The full clinical response to this and other antithyroid drugs, however, may take several weeks (Fig. 34.6), partly because T_4 has a long half-life, and also because the thyroid may have large stores of hormone, which need to be depleted before the drug's action can be fully manifest. **Propylthiouracil** is thought to act somewhat more rapidly because of its additional effect as an inhibitor of the peripheral conversion of T_4 to T_3.

Both drugs may be used during pregnancy but both can cross the placenta and may affect the fetal thyroid gland. They also appear in breast milk, but this effect is less pronounced with **propylthiouracil**, because it is more strongly bound to plasma protein. After degradation, the metabolites of these drugs are excreted in the urine. The thioureylenes may be concentrated in the thyroid.

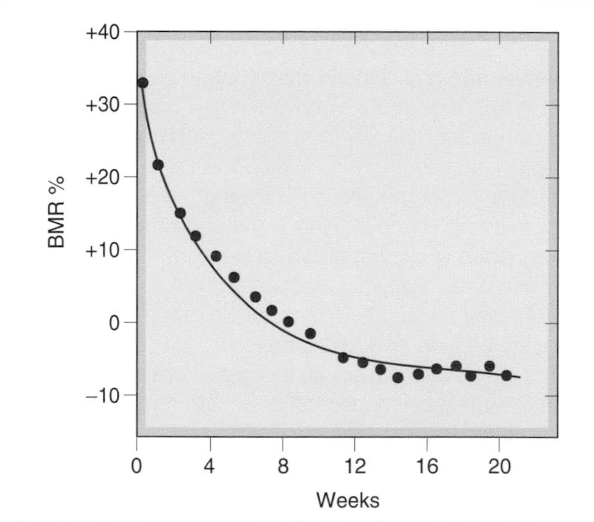

Fig. 34.6 Time course of fall of basal metabolic rate (BMR) during treatment with an antithyroid drug, carbimazole. The curve is exponential, corresponding to a daily decrease in BMR (*red line*) of 3.4%. (Modified from Furth, E.D., Becker, D.V., Schwartz, M.S., 1963. Significance of rate of response of basal metabolic rate and serum cholesterol in hyperthyroid patients receiving neomercazole and other antithyroid agents. J. Clin. Endocrinol. Metab. 23, 1130–1140.)

Unwanted effects

The most dangerous unwanted effects of thioureylene drugs are neutropenia and agranulocytosis (see Ch. 24). These are relatively rare, having an incidence of 0.1%–1.2%, and are reversible on cessation of treatment. Patients must be warned to report symptoms (especially sore throat) immediately and have a blood count. Rashes (2%–25%) and other symptoms, including headaches, nausea, jaundice and arthralgia, are common. Rare cases of fetal abnormalities have been reported with **carbimazole**.

IODINE/IODIDE

Iodine is converted in vivo to iodide (I^-), which temporarily inhibits the release of thyroid hormones. When high doses of iodine are given to thyrotoxic patients, the symptoms subside within 1–2 days. There is inhibition of the secretion of thyroid hormones and, over a period of 10–14 days, a marked reduction in vascularity of the gland, which becomes smaller and firmer. Iodine is often given orally in a solution with potassium iodide ('*Lugol iodine*'). With continuous administration, its effect reaches maximum within 10–15 days and then decreases. The mechanism of action is not entirely clear; it may inhibit iodination of thyroglobulin, possibly by reducing the H_2O_2 generation that is necessary for this process.

The main uses of iodine/iodide are for the preparation of hyperthyroid subjects for surgical resection of the gland, and as part of the treatment of severe thyrotoxic crisis (*thyroid storm*). It is also used following exposure to accidental leakage of radioactive iodine from nuclear reactors, to reduce uptake of the radioactive isotope in the thyroid. Allergic reactions can occur; these include angio-oedema, rashes and drug fever. Lacrimation, conjunctivitis, pain in the salivary glands and a cold-like syndrome are dose-related adverse effects connected to the concentration of iodide by transport mechanisms in tears and saliva.

OTHER DRUGS USED

The β-adrenoceptor antagonists, for example, **propranolol** and **nadolol** (see Ch. 15), are not antithyroid agents as such, but they are useful for decreasing many of the signs and symptoms of hyperthyroidism – tachycardia, dysrhythmias, tremor and agitation. They are used during the preparation of thyrotoxic patients for surgery, as well as in most hyperthyroid patients during the initial treatment period while the thioureylenes or radioiodine take effect, or as part of the treatment of acute hyperthyroid crisis. Eye drops containing **guanethidine**, a noradrenergic-blocking agent (see Ch. 15), are used to mitigate the exophthalmos of hyperthyroidism (which is not relieved by antithyroid drugs); it acts by relaxing the sympathetically innervated smooth muscle that causes eyelid retraction. Glucocorticoids (e.g. **prednisolone** or **hydrocortisone**) or surgical decompression may be needed to mitigate severe exophthalmia in Graves' disease.

HYPOTHYROIDISM

There are no drugs that specifically augment the synthesis or release of thyroid hormones. The only effective treatment for hypothyroidism, unless it is caused by iodine deficiency (which is treated with iodide), is to administer the thyroid hormones themselves as replacement therapy. Synthetic T_4 (official name: **levothyroxine**) and T_3 (official name: **liothyronine**), identical to the natural hormones, are given

Clinical use of drugs acting on the thyroid

Radioiodine (^{131}I)

- Hyperthyroidism (Graves' disease, multinodular toxic goitre).
- Relapse of hyperthyroidism after failed medical or surgical treatment.

Carbimazole or propylthiouracil

- Hyperthyroidism (diffuse toxic goitre); at least 1 year of treatment is needed.
- Preliminary to surgery for toxic goitre.
- Part of the treatment of thyroid storm (very severe hyperthyroidism); **propylthiouracil** is preferred, combined with a β-adrenoceptor antagonist (e.g. **propranolol**).

Thyroid hormones and iodine

- **Levothyroxine** (T_4) is the standard replacement therapy for hypothyroidism.
- **Liothyronine** (T_3), administered by slow intravenous injection, is used for myxoedema coma.
- Iodine dissolved in aqueous potassium iodide (**'Lugol iodine'**) is used short term to control thyrotoxicosis preoperatively. It reduces the vascularity of the gland.

orally. **Levothyroxine**, as the sodium salt in doses of 50–100 µg/day, is the usual first-line drug of choice. **Liothyronine** has a faster onset but a shorter duration of action and is generally reserved for acute emergencies such as the rare condition of myxoedema coma, where these properties are an advantage.

Unwanted effects may occur with overdose, and in addition to the signs and symptoms of hyperthyroidism there is a risk of precipitating angina pectoris, cardiac dysrhythmias or even cardiac failure. The effects of less severe overdose are more insidious; the patient feels well but bone resorption is increased, leading to osteoporosis (see Ch. 36).

The use of drugs to treat thyroid cancer is a specialist subject and will not be covered here. Bikas et al. (2016) and Laha et al. (2020) review the latest generation of drugs to be used for this purpose.

Finally, recombinant human TSH (rhTSH) is sometimes used for diagnostic purposes following surgery.

The use of drugs to treat disorders of the thyroid is summarised in the clinical box.

REFERENCES AND FURTHER READING

Bassett, J.H.D., Harvey, C.B., Williams, G.R., 2003. Mechanisms of thyroid hormone receptor-specific nuclear and extranuclear actions. Mol. Cell Endocrinol. 213, 1–11.

Bikas, A., Vachhani, S., Jensen, K., Vasko, V., Burman, K.D., 2016. Targeted therapies in thyroid cancer: an extensive review of the literature. Expert Rev. Clin. Pharmacol. 9, 299–1313.

Blackburn, C.M., McConahey, W.M., Keating Jr., F.R., Albert, A., 1954. Calorigenic effects of single intravenous doses of L-triiodothyronine and L-thyroxine in myxedematous persons. J. Clin. Invest. 33, 819–824.

Bou Khalil, R., Richa, S., 2011. Thyroid adverse effects of psychotropic drugs: a review. Clin. Neuropharmacol. 34, 248–255.

Cignini, P., Cafa, E.V., Giorlandino, C., et al., 2012. Thyroid physiology and common diseases in pregnancy: review of literature. J. Prenat. Med. 6, 64–71.

Furth, E.D., Becker, D.V., Schwartz, M.S., 1963. Significance of rate of response of basal metabolic rate and serum cholesterol in hyperthyroid patients receiving neomercazole and other antithyroid agents. J. Clin. Endocrinol. Metab. 23, 1130–1140.

Hadj Kacem, H., Rebai, A., Kaffel, N., et al., 2003. PDS is a new susceptibility gene to autoimmune thyroid diseases: association and linkage study. J. Clin. Endocrinol. Metab. 88, 2274–2280.

Kahaly, G.J., Dillmann, W.H., 2005. Thyroid hormone action in the heart. Endocr. Rev. 26, 704–728.

Kelly, G.S., 2000. Peripheral metabolism of thyroid hormones: a review. Altern. Med. Rev. 5, 306–333.

Kojic, K.L., Kojic, S.L., Wiseman, S.M., 2012. Differentiated thyroid cancers: a comprehensive review of novel targeted therapies. Exp. Rev. Anticancer. Ther. 12, 345–357.

Laha, D., Nilubol, N., Boufraqech, M., 2020. New therapies for advanced thyroid cancer. Front. Endocrinol. 11, 82.

Lai, S., Zhang, S., Wang, L., et al., 2015. A rare mutation in patients with resistance to thyroid hormone and review of therapeutic strategies. Am. J. Med. Sci. 350, 167–174.

Lee, H.J., Li, C.W., Hammerstad, S.S., Stefan, M., Tomer, Y., 2015. Immunogenetics of autoimmune thyroid diseases: a comprehensive review. J. Autoimmun. 64, 82–90.

Mastorakos, G., Karoutsou, E.I., Mizamtsidi, M., Creatsas, G., 2007. The menace of endocrine disruptors on thyroid hormone physiology and their impact on intrauterine development. Endocrine 3, 219–237.

McAninch, E.A., Bianco, A.C., 2016. The history and future of treatment of hypothyroidism. Ann. Intern. Med. 164, 50–56.

Nilsson, M., 2001. Iodide handling by the thyroid epithelial cell. Exp. Clin. Endocrinol. Diabetes 109, 13–17.

Roberts, C.G., Ladenson, P.W., 2004. Hypothyroidism. Lancet 363, 793–803.

Sheehan, M.T., 2016. Biochemical testing of the thyroid: TSH is the best and, oftentimes, only test needed – a review for primary care. Clin. Med. Res. 14, 83–92.

Surks, M.I., Ortiz, E., Daniels, G.H., et al., 2004. Subclinical thyroid disease: scientific review and guidelines for diagnosis and management. JAMA 291, 228–238.

Yen, P.M., 2001. Physiological and molecular basis of thyroid hormone action. Physiol. Rev. 81, 1097–1142.

Zhang, J., Lazar, M., 2000. The mechanism of action of thyroid hormones. Annu. Rev. Physiol. 62, 439–466.

35 The reproductive system

OVERVIEW

In this chapter, we describe the endocrine control of the human female and male reproductive systems as the basis for understanding drug actions in sex hormone replacement, contraception, treatment of infertility, management of labour and treatment of erectile dysfunction.

INTRODUCTION

Drugs that affect reproduction (both by preventing conception and more recently for treating infertility) transformed society in the latter half of the last century. In this chapter, we briefly summarise salient points in reproductive endocrinology as a basis for understanding the numerous important drugs that work on the male and female reproductive systems. Such drugs are used for contraception, to treat infertility, as sex hormone replacement and in obstetric practice to influence labour. They are also used to influence lifestyle (see Ch. 59). The principle of negative feedback is stressed and is central to understanding how hormones interact to control reproduction[1] – many drugs, including agents used to prevent or assist conception, work by influencing negative feedback mechanisms. The chapter concludes with a short section on erectile dysfunction. The endocrinology of transgender medicine (reviewed by T'Sjoen et al., 2019) is a specialised area and the use of puberty blockers and cross sex hormones in children and adolescents with gender dysphoria, is based on limited evidence of long-term outcomes and outside the scope of the chapter.

ENDOCRINE CONTROL OF REPRODUCTION

Hormonal control of the reproductive systems in men and women involves sex steroids from the gonads, hypothalamic mediators including the decapeptide gonadotrophin-releasing hormone (GnRH), and glycoprotein gonadotrophins from the anterior pituitary gland (see Ch. 33). Kisspeptin, a protein that is a ligand for a G protein–coupled receptor known as GPR54, initiates secretion of GnRH at puberty. GnRH is released from the hypothalamus to act on the anterior pituitary, triggering the release of luteinising hormone (LH) and follicle-stimulating hormone (FSH). These gonadotrophic hormones control sexual maturation and gametogenesis. Kisspeptin has been linked with sexual bonding. The tachykinin neurokinin B (NKB; see Ch. 17) is also implicated in controlling the secretion of GnRH in humans, with possible roles in pregnancy, sexual maturation and the menopause. It is present, together with kisspeptin and dynorphin, in the arcuate nucleus of the hypothalamus where these mediators are implicated in generating pulsatile release of GnRH. NKB is implicated in menopausal flushing and NK3 receptor block has reduced such flushing (Prague et al., 2017).

Anti-Müllerian hormone (AMH) is a homodimeric glycoprotein belonging to the transforming growth factor (TGF)-β family. It controls sexual development in the male fetus and follicle formation in adult women. It was identified functionally in the 1940s from its role in the regression of the Müllerian ducts in the male embryo, is synthesised in the Sertoli cells of the testes (see later) and the granulosa cells of the ovaries in postnatal animals and is believed to act both locally and as a blood-borne hormone on AMH receptors which are expressed in the pituitary and hypothalamus as well as the gonads and may regulate fertility (Barbotin et al., 2019). Plasma AMH concentration is increased in polycystic ovary syndrome (PCOS), a common but poorly understood condition which causes infertility due to failure to ovulate ("anovulation").

NEUROHORMONAL CONTROL OF THE FEMALE REPRODUCTIVE SYSTEM

Increased secretion of hypothalamic and anterior pituitary hormones occurs in girls at puberty and stimulates secretion of oestrogen from the ovaries. This causes maturation of the reproductive organs, development of secondary sexual characteristics and accelerated linear growth followed by closure of the epiphyses of the long bones. Sex steroids, *oestrogens* and *progesterone*, are thereafter involved in the menstrual cycle, and in pregnancy. A simplified outline is given in Figs 35.1 and 35.2.

The menstrual cycle begins with menstruation, which lasts for 3–6 days, during which the superficial layer of uterine endometrium is shed. The endometrium regenerates during the follicular phase of the cycle after menstrual flow has stopped. A releasing factor, GnRH, is secreted from peptidergic neurons in the hypothalamus which discharge in a pulsatile fashion, approximately one burst per hour. GnRH stimulates the anterior pituitary to release gonadotrophic hormones (see Fig. 35.1) – *FSH* and *LH*. These act on the ovaries to promote the development of small groups of follicles, each of which contains an ovum. One follicle develops faster than the others and forms the Graafian follicle (see Figs 35.1 and 35.2E), which secretes oestrogens, and the rest degenerate. The ripening Graafian

[1]Recognition that negative feedback is central to endocrine control was a profound insight, made in 1930 by Dorothy Price, a laboratory assistant at the University of Chicago experimenting on the effects of testosterone in rats. She referred to it as 'reciprocal influence' and it explains how many reproductive hormones seem, confusingly, to cause both an effect and its opposite if given in different doses or over different time courses.

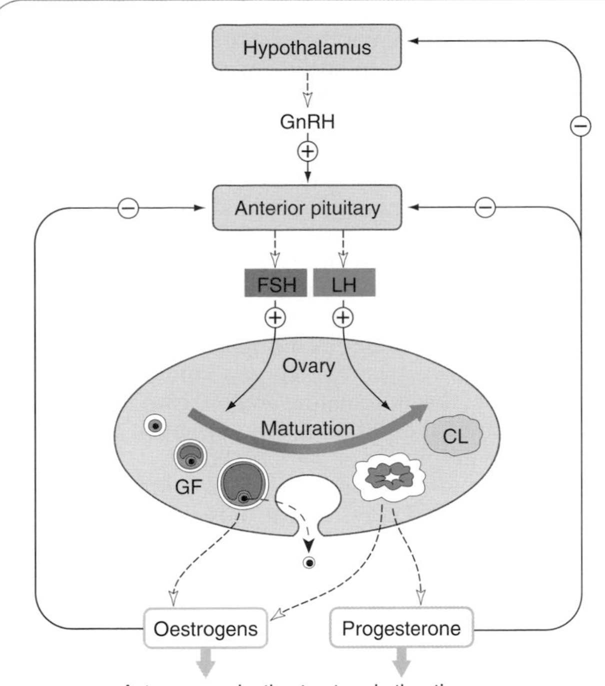

Fig. 35.1 Hormonal control of the female reproductive system. The Graafian follicle (GF) is shown developing on the *left*, then involuting to form the corpus luteum (CL) on the *right*, after the ovum (¤) has been released. *FSH*, Follicle-stimulating hormone; *GnRH*, gonadotrophin-releasing hormone; *LH*, luteinising hormone.

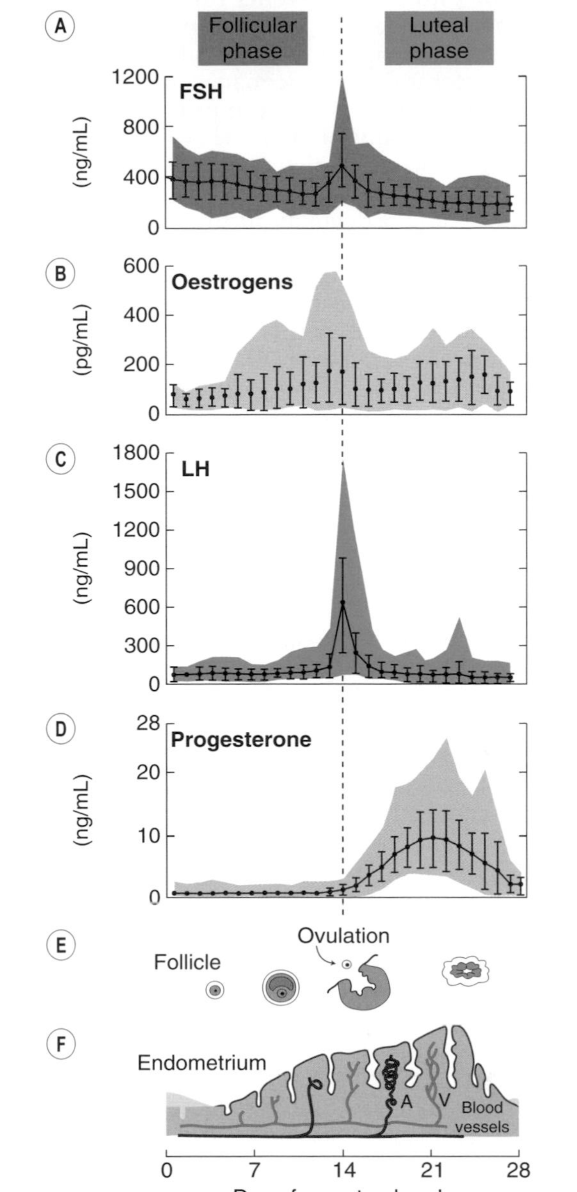

Fig. 35.2 Plasma concentrations of ovarian hormones and gonadotrophins in women during a normal menstrual cycle. Values are the mean ± standard deviation of 40 women. The *shaded areas* indicate the entire range of observations. Day 1 is the onset of menstruation. Mean plasma hormone concentrations (A–D) are shown in relation to day of menstrual cycle. (E and F) show diagrammatically the changes in the ovarian follicle and the endometrium during the cycle. Ovulation on day 14 of the menstrual cycle occurs with the mid-cycle peak of luteinising hormone (LH), represented by the *vertical dashed line*. *A*, arterioles; *FSH*, follicle-stimulating hormone; *V*, venules. (After van de Wiele, R. L., Dyrenfurth, I. 1974. Pharmacol. Rev. 25, 189–207.)

follicle consists of thecal and granulosa cells surrounding a fluid-filled core, within which lies an ovum. Oestrogens are responsible for the proliferative phase of endometrial regeneration, which occurs from day 5 or 6 until mid-cycle (see Fig. 35.2B and F). During this phase, the endometrium increases in thickness and vascularity, and at the peak of oestrogen secretion there is a prolific cervical secretion of mucus of pH 8–9, rich in protein and carbohydrate, which facilitates entry of spermatozoa. Oestrogen has a negative feedback effect on the anterior pituitary, decreasing gonadotrophin release during chronic administration of oestrogen as oral contraception (see later). In contrast, the spike of endogenous oestrogen secretion just before mid-cycle sensitises LH-releasing cells of the pituitary to the action of the GnRH and causes the mid-cycle surge of LH secretion (see Fig. 35.2C). This, in turn, causes rapid swelling and rupture of the Graafian follicle, resulting in ovulation. If fertilisation occurs, the fertilised ovum passes down the fallopian tubes to the uterus, starting to divide as it goes.

Stimulated by LH, cells of the ruptured follicle proliferate and develop into the *corpus luteum*, which secretes progesterone. Progesterone acts, in turn, on oestrogen-primed endometrium, stimulating the secretory phase of the cycle, which renders the endometrium suitable for the implantation of a fertilised ovum. During this phase, cervical mucus becomes more viscous, less alkaline, less copious and in general less welcoming for sperm (in essence, older sperm are too late at this stage). Progesterone exerts negative feedback on the hypothalamus and pituitary, decreasing the release of LH. It also has a thermogenic effect, causing a rise in body temperature of about 0.5°C at ovulation, which is maintained until the end of the cycle.

If implantation of a fertilised ovum does not occur, progesterone secretion stops, triggering menstruation. If implantation does occur the corpus luteum continues to secrete progesterone which, by its effect on the hypothalamus and anterior pituitary, prevents further ovulation. The chorion (an antecedent of the placenta) secretes human chorionic gonadotrophin (HCG), which maintains the lining of the uterus during pregnancy. Modern pregnancy tests detect HCG levels present in urine. For reasons that are not physiologically obvious, HCG has an additional pharmacological action, exploited therapeutically in treating infertility (see later), of stimulating ovulation. As pregnancy proceeds, the placenta develops further hormonal functions and secretes several hormones, including gonadotrophins, progesterone and oestrogens. Progesterone secreted during pregnancy controls the development of the secretory alveoli in the mammary gland, while oestrogen stimulates the lactiferous ducts. After parturition, oestrogen, along with prolactin (see Ch. 33), is responsible for stimulating and maintaining lactation, whereas supraphysiological doses of oestrogen suppress lactation.

Oestrogens, progestogens (progesterone-like drugs), androgens and the gonadotrophins are described later – see Fig. 35.3 for biosynthetic pathways of the steroid hormones.

Hormonal control of the female reproductive system

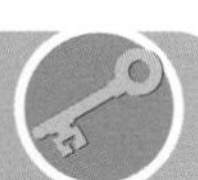

- The menstrual cycle starts with menstruation.
- GnRH, released from the hypothalamus, acts on the anterior pituitary to release FSH and LH.
- FSH and LH stimulate follicle development in the ovary. FSH is the main hormone stimulating oestrogen production. LH stimulates ovulation at mid-cycle and is the main hormone controlling subsequent progesterone synthesis and secretion from the corpus luteum.
- Oestrogen controls the proliferative phase of the endometrium and has negative feedback effects on the anterior pituitary. Progesterone controls the later secretory phase and has negative feedback effects on both the hypothalamus and anterior pituitary.
- If a fertilised ovum is implanted, the corpus luteum continues to secrete progesterone.
- After implantation, HCG from the chorion becomes important, and later in pregnancy progesterone, HCG and other hormones are secreted by the placenta.

NEUROHORMONAL CONTROL OF THE MALE REPRODUCTIVE SYSTEM

As in women, hypothalamic, anterior pituitary and gonadal hormones control the male reproductive system. A simplified outline is given in Fig. 35.4. GnRH controls the secretion of gonadotrophins by the anterior pituitary. This secretion is not cyclical as in menstruating women, although it is pulsatile in both sexes, as with other anterior pituitary hormones (see Ch. 33). There is diurnal secretion of testosterone in males (higher in the morning, lower in the evening) and purported seasonal fluctuation (higher in summer, lower in autumn). FSH is responsible for the integrity of the seminiferous tubules, and after puberty is important in gametogenesis through an action on Sertoli cells, which nourish and support developing spermatozoa. LH, which in the male is also called *interstitial cell-stimulating hormone* (ICSH), stimulates the interstitial cells (Leydig cells) to secrete androgens – in particular *testosterone*. LH/ICSH secretion begins at puberty, and the consequent secretion of testosterone causes maturation of the reproductive organs and development of secondary sexual characteristics. Thereafter, the primary function of testosterone is the maintenance of spermatogenesis and hence fertility – an action mediated by Sertoli cells. Testosterone is also important in the maturation of spermatozoa as they pass through the epididymis and vas deferens. A further action is a feedback effect on the anterior pituitary, modulating its sensitivity to GnRH and thus influencing secretion of LH/ICSH. Testosterone has marked anabolic effects, causing development of the musculature and increased bone growth which results in the pubertal growth spurt, followed by closure of the epiphyses of the long bones.

Secretion of testosterone is mainly controlled by LH/ICSH, but FSH also plays a part, possibly by releasing a factor similar to GnRH from the Sertoli cells which are its primary target. The interstitial cells that synthesise testosterone also have receptors for prolactin, which may influence testosterone production by increasing the number of receptors for LH/ICSH.

BEHAVIOURAL EFFECTS OF SEX HORMONES

As well as controlling the menstrual cycle, sex steroids affect sexual behaviour. Two types of control are recognised: *organisational* and *activational*.

Organisational control refers to the fact that sexual differentiation of the brain can be permanently altered by the presence or absence of sex steroids at key stages in development. In rats, administration of androgens to females within a few days of birth results in long-term virilisation of behaviour. Conversely, neonatal castration of male rats causes them to develop behaviourally as females. Brain development in the absence of sex steroids follows female lines, but is switched to the male pattern by exposure of the hypothalamus to androgen at a key stage of development. Similar but less complete behavioural virilisation of female offspring has been demonstrated following androgen administration in non-human primates, and probably also occurs in humans if pregnant women are exposed to excessive androgen.

The *activational* effect of sex steroids refers to their ability to modify sexual behaviour after brain development is complete. In general, oestrogens and androgens increase sexual activity in the appropriate sex. **Oxytocin**, which is important during parturition (see later), also has roles in mating and parenting behaviours, its action in the central nervous system being regulated by oestrogen (see Ch. 33).

DRUGS AFFECTING REPRODUCTIVE FUNCTION

OESTROGENS

Oestrogens are synthesised by the ovary and placenta, and in small amounts by the testis and adrenal cortex. The starting substance for synthesis of oestrogen and other steroids is cholesterol. The immediate precursors to the oestrogens are androgenic substances – androstenedione or testosterone (see Fig. 35.3). There are three main endogenous

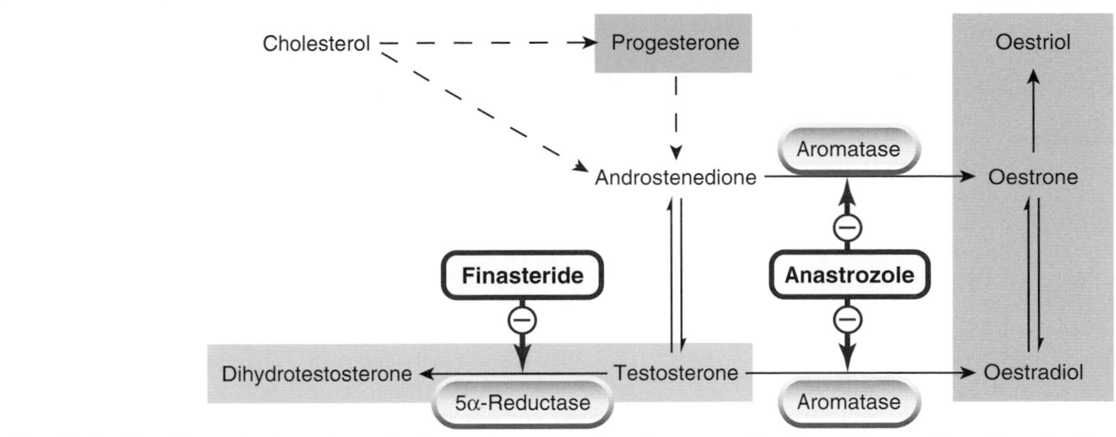

Fig. 35.3 The biosynthetic pathway for the androgens and oestrogens, with sites of drug action. (See also Fig. 33.5.) Finasteride is used in benign prostatic hyperplasia, and anastrozole, to treat breast cancer in postmenopausal women.

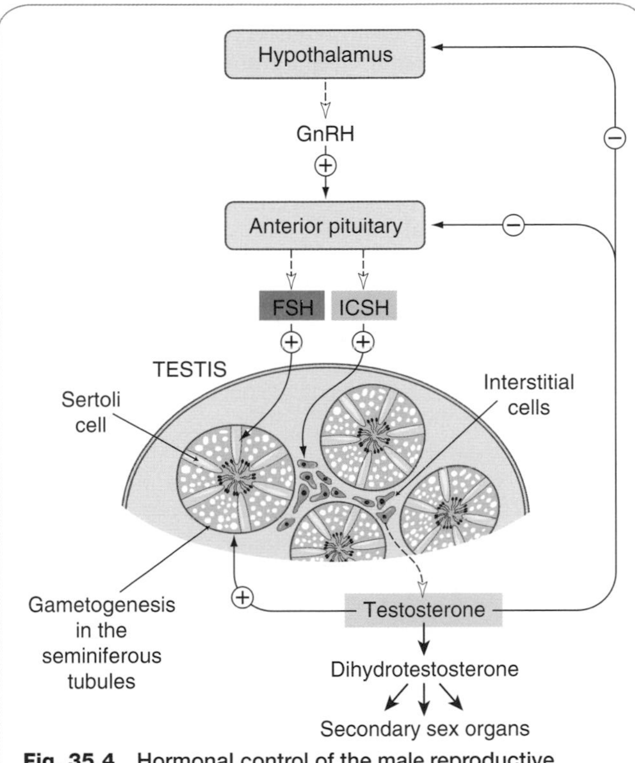

Fig. 35.4 Hormonal control of the male reproductive system. *FSH*, Follicle-stimulating hormone; *GnRH*, gonadotrophin-releasing hormone; *ICSH*, interstitial cell-stimulating hormone.

oestrogens in humans: *oestradiol*, *oestrone* and *oestriol* (see Fig. 35.3). Oestradiol is the most potent and is the principal oestrogen secreted by the ovary. At the beginning of the menstrual cycle, the plasma concentration is 0.2 nmol/L, rising to ~2.2 nmol/L in mid-cycle.

Actions

Oestrogen acts in concert with progesterone, and induces synthesis of progesterone receptors in uterus, vagina, anterior pituitary and hypothalamus. Conversely, progesterone decreases oestrogen receptor expression in the reproductive tract. *Prolactin* (see Ch. 33) also influences oestrogen action by increasing the numbers of oestrogen receptors in the mammary gland, but has no effect on oestrogen receptor expression in the uterus.

The effects of exogenous oestrogen in females depend on the state of sexual maturity when the oestrogen is administered:

- *In primary hypogonadism:* oestrogen stimulates development of secondary sexual characteristics and accelerates growth.
- *In adults with primary amenorrhoea:* oestrogen, given cyclically with a progestogen, induces an artificial cycle.
- *In sexually mature women:* oestrogen (administered with a progestogen, see later) is a contraceptive.
- *At or after the menopause:* oestrogen replacement prevents menopausal symptoms and bone loss.

Oestrogens have several metabolic actions, including mineralocorticoid (retention of salt and water) and mild anabolic actions. They increase the coagulability of blood and, in pharmacological doses, increase the risk of thromboembolism.

Mechanism of action

Oestrogen binds to nuclear receptors (see Ch. 3). There are at least two types of oestrogen receptor, termed ERα and ERβ. Binding is followed by interaction of the resultant complexes with nuclear sites and subsequent genomic effects. In addition to these 'classic' intracellular receptors, some oestrogen effects, in particular its rapid vascular actions, are initiated by interaction with membrane receptors, including a G protein–coupled oestrogen receptor (GPER), which was cloned from vascular endothelial cells and plays a part in regulating vascular tone and cell growth as well as in lipid and glucose homeostasis (Barton and Prossnitz, 2015). Acute vasodilatation caused by 17-β-oestradiol is mediated by nitric oxide, and a plant-derived (phyto-) oestrogen called **genistein** (which is selective for ERβ, as well as having quite distinct effects due to inhibition of protein kinase C) is as potent as 17-β-oestradiol in this regard (Walker et al., 2001).

Preparations

Many preparations (oral, transdermal, intramuscular, implantable and topical) of oestrogens are available for a wide range of indications. These include natural (e.g. **oestradiol**, **oestriol**) and synthetic (e.g. **mestranol**, **ethinylestradiol**, **diethylstilbestrol**) oestrogens. Oestrogens are presented either as single agents or combined with progestogen.

Pharmacokinetic aspects

Natural and synthetic oestrogens are well absorbed in the gastrointestinal (GI) tract, but after absorption the natural oestrogens are rapidly metabolised in the liver, whereas synthetic oestrogens are degraded less rapidly. There is variable enterohepatic cycling. Most oestrogens are readily absorbed from the skin and mucous membranes. They may be given as intravaginal creams or pessaries for local effect. In the plasma, natural oestrogens are bound to albumin and to a sex steroid-binding globulin. Natural oestrogens are excreted in the urine as glucuronide and sulfate metabolites.

Unwanted effects

Unwanted effects of oestrogens range from the common and tiresome to the life-threatening but rare: breast tenderness, nausea, vomiting, anorexia, retention of salt and water with resultant oedema and increased risk of thromboembolism. More details of the unwanted effects of oral contraceptives are given later.

Used intermittently for postmenopausal replacement therapy, oestrogens cause menstruation-like withdrawal bleeding. Oestrogen causes endometrial hyperplasia unless given cyclically with a progestogen. When administered to males, oestrogens result in feminisation.

There is current concern regarding environmental effects of oestrogens, including various pesticides that act on oestrogen receptors as well as oestrogens excreted in urine. Either of these sources of oestrogen can pollute groundwater and damage aquatic wildlife as well as posing risks to human health (Adeel et al., 2017; McLachlan, 2016).

Oestrogen administration to pregnant women can cause genital abnormalities in their offspring: carcinoma of the vagina was more common in young women whose mothers were given diethylstilbestrol in early pregnancy in a misguided attempt to prevent miscarriage (see Ch. 58).

The clinical uses of oestrogens and antioestrogens are summarised in the box. In addition, see the section later on postmenopausal hormone replacement therapy (HRT).

ANTIOESTROGENS, AROMATASE INHIBITORS, AND SELECTIVE OESTROGEN RECEPTOR MODULATORS (SERMs)

Raloxifene, a 'selective [o]estrogen receptor modulator' (SERM), has anti-oestrogenic effects on breast and uterus but oestrogenic effects on bone, lipid metabolism and blood coagulation. It is used for the prevention and treatment of postmenopausal osteoporosis (see Ch. 36) and reduces the incidence of oestrogen receptor-positive breast cancer similarly to **tamoxifen** but with fewer adverse events (Barrett-Connor et al., 2006; Vogel et al., 2006). The US FDA has supported its use to reduce the risk of invasive breast cancer in postmenopausal women with osteoporosis and in postmenopausal women at high risk for invasive breast cancer. Unlike oestrogen, it does not prevent menopausal flushes and menopausal symptoms are common adverse effects; it increases the risk of thromboembolic disease and is less used against osteoporosis than bisphosphonates (see Ch. 36).

Tamoxifen has an antioestrogenic action on mammary tissue but oestrogenic actions on plasma lipids, endometrium and bone. It produces mild oestrogen-like adverse effects consistent with partial agonist activity. The tamoxifen–oestrogen receptor complex does not readily dissociate, interfering with receptor recycling.

Tamoxifen upregulates TGF-β, a cytokine that retards the progression of malignancy, and that also has a role in controlling the balance between bone-producing osteoblasts and bone-resorbing osteoclasts (see Ch. 36).

The use of tamoxifen to treat and prevent breast cancer is discussed further in Chapter 57.

Blocking oestrogen synthesis provides an alternative to blocking oestrogen receptors; *aromatase inhibitors* (see Ch. 57) such as **anastrozole** block oestrogen synthesis in the adrenal (Fig. 35.3) but not in the ovary and are an alternative to receptor antagonists in postmenopausal but not in premenopausal women with breast cancer. **Clomiphene** inhibits oestrogen binding to its receptors in the anterior pituitary, so preventing negative feedback and acutely increasing secretion of GnRH and gonadotrophins; it also possesses some oestrogen agonist activity and is classified as a SERM. It is administered by mouth as a 5-day course starting around day 5 of a menstrual cycle for the treatment of infertility caused by failure of ovulation. The resulting increase in GnRH and gonadotrophin levels stimulates and enlarges the ovaries, increases oestrogen secretion and induces ovulation which can be monitored by intravaginal ultrasound. Twins are common, but multiple pregnancy is unusual.

See the clinical box on oestrogens and antioestrogens for a summary of clinical uses.

Oestrogens and antioestrogens

- The endogenous oestrogens are oestradiol (the most potent), oestrone and oestriol; there are numerous exogenous synthetic forms (e.g. **ethinylestradiol**).
- Mechanism of action involves interaction with nuclear receptors (ERα or ERβ) in target tissues, resulting in modification of gene transcription. Some of the rapid vascular and metabolic effects of oestrogens are mediated by a GPER.
- Their pharmacological effects depend on the sexual maturity of the recipient:
  - before puberty, they stimulate development of secondary sexual characteristics;
  - given cyclically in the female adult, they induce an artificial menstrual cycle and are used for contraception;
  - given at or after the menopause, they prevent menopausal symptoms and protect against osteoporosis, but increase thromboembolism.
- Antioestrogens are competitive antagonists or partial agonists. **Tamoxifen** is used in oestrogen-dependent breast cancer. **Clomiphene** induces ovulation by inhibiting the negative feedback effects on the hypothalamus and anterior pituitary.
- Selective modulators of the oestrogen receptor are oestrogen agonists in some tissues but antagonists in others. **Raloxifene** (one such drug) is used to treat and prevent osteoporosis in women who are at increased risk of breast cancer.

Clinical uses of oestrogens and antioestrogens

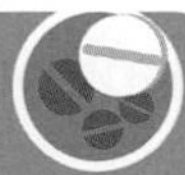

Oestrogens

- Replacement therapy:
  - primary ovarian failure (e.g. Turner's syndrome);
  - secondary ovarian failure (menopause) for flushing, vaginal dryness and to preserve bone mass. Such use should be short term because of an excess risk of thromboembolism.
- Contraception.
- Prostate and breast cancer (these uses have largely been superseded by other hormonal manipulations; see Ch. 57).

Antioestrogens/SERMs and aromatase inhibitors

- To treat oestrogen-sensitive breast cancer (**tamoxifen**, **toremifene**, **fulvestrant**).
- Aromatase inhibitors (e.g. **anastrozole**) are an alternative for breast cancer in post-menopausal women.
- To induce ovulation (**clomiphene**) in treating infertility caused by anovulation.

PROGESTOGENS

The natural progestational hormone (progestogen) is *progesterone* (see Figs 35.2 and 35.3). This is secreted by the corpus luteum in the second part of the menstrual cycle, and by the placenta during pregnancy. Small amounts are also secreted by the testis and adrenal cortex.

Progestogens act on nuclear receptors. The density of progesterone receptors is controlled by oestrogens (see earlier discussion).

Preparations

There are two main groups of progestogens:

1. The naturally occurring hormone and its derivatives (e.g. **hydroxyprogesterone**, **medroxyprogesterone**, **dydrogesterone**). Progesterone itself is virtually inactive orally, because of presystemic hepatic metabolism. Other derivatives are available for oral administration, intramuscular injection or administration via the vagina or rectum.
2. Testosterone derivatives (e.g. **norethisterone**, **norgestrel** and **ethynodiol**) can be given orally. The first two have some androgenic activity and are metabolised to give oestrogenic products. Newer progestogens used in contraception include **desogestrel** and **gestodene**; they are an option for women who experience adverse effects such as acne, depression or breakthrough bleeding with the older drugs but have been associated with higher risks of venous thromboembolic disease (see later).

Actions

The pharmacological actions of the progestogens are in essence the same as the physiological actions of progesterone described previously. Specific effects relevant to contraception are detailed later.

Pharmacokinetic aspects

Injected progesterone is bound to albumin, not to the sex steroid-binding globulin. Some is stored in adipose tissue. It is metabolised in the liver, and the products, pregnanolone and pregnanediol, are conjugated with glucuronic acid and excreted in the urine.

Unwanted effects

The unwanted effects of progestogens include weak androgenic actions. Other unwanted effects include acne, fluid retention, weight change, depression, change in libido, breast discomfort, premenstrual symptoms, irregular menstrual cycles and breakthrough bleeding. Some of the newer progestogens increase the incidence of thromboembolism.

Clinical uses of progestogens are summarised in the clinical box.

ANTIPROGESTOGENS

Mifepristone is a partial agonist at progesterone receptors. It sensitises the uterus to the action of prostaglandins (PGs). It is given orally and has a plasma half-life of 21 h. Mifepristone is used, in combination with a PG (e.g. **gemeprost**; see later), as a medical alternative to surgical termination of pregnancy (see clinical box). **Ulipristal** is a selective progesterone receptor modulator which blocks ovulation. It is available over the counter and is used for emergency contraception within 120 h of vaginal intercourse and also to reduce the size of uterine fibroids (benign tumours of the uterus) preoperatively.

Progestogens and antiprogestogens

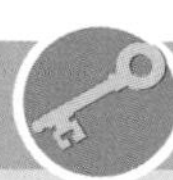

- The endogenous hormone is progesterone. Examples of synthetic drugs are the progesterone derivative **medroxyprogesterone** and the testosterone derivative **norethisterone.**
- The mechanism of action involves intracellular receptor/altered gene expression. Oestrogen stimulates synthesis of progesterone receptors, whereas progesterone inhibits synthesis of oestrogen receptors.
- Main therapeutic uses are in oral contraception and oestrogen replacement regimens, and to treat endometriosis.
- The antiprogestogen **mifepristone**, in combination with PG analogues, is an effective medical alternative to surgical termination of early pregnancy.

POSTMENOPAUSAL HORMONE REPLACEMENT THERAPY (HRT)

At the menopause, whether natural or surgically induced, ovarian function decreases and oestrogen levels fall. There is a long history of disagreement regarding the pros and cons of HRT in this context, with the prevailing wisdom undergoing several revisions over the years (see Davis et al., 2005). HRT normally involves the cyclic or continuous administration of low doses of one or more oestrogens, with or without a progestogen. Short-term HRT has some clear-cut benefits:

Clinical uses of progestogens and antiprogestogens

Progestogens

- Contraception:
  - with **oestrogen** (usually ethinylestradiol) in *combined oral contraceptive pill*;
  - as *progesterone-only contraceptive pill*;
  - as *injectable* or *implantable* progesterone-only contraception;
  - as part of an *intrauterine* contraceptive system.
- Combined with **oestrogen** for *oestrogen replacement therapy* in women with an intact uterus, to prevent endometrial hyperplasia and carcinoma.
- For endometriosis.
- In endometrial carcinoma.

Antiprogestogens

- Medical termination of pregnancy: **mifepristone** (partial agonist) combined with a PG (e.g. **gemeprost**).
- Emergency contraception (morning-after pill): **ulipristal** (selective progesterone receptor modulator), also used to reduce the size of uterine fibroids pre-operatively.

- improvement of symptoms caused by reduced oestrogen, for example, hot flushes and vaginal dryness;
- prevention and treatment of osteoporosis, but other drugs (e.g. bisphosphonates) are usually preferred (see Ch. 36).

Oestrogen replacement does not reduce the risk of coronary heart disease, despite earlier hopes, nor is there evidence that it reduces age-related decline in cognitive function. Drawbacks include:

- cyclical withdrawal bleeding;
- adverse effects related to progestogen (see later);
- increased risk of endometrial cancer if oestrogen is given unopposed by progestogen;
- increased risk of breast cancer, related to the duration of HRT use and disappearing within 5 years of stopping;
- increased risk of venous thromboembolism (risk approximately doubled in women using combined HRT for 5 years).

The web link in the reference list provides best estimates as of 2019 of risks of cancer (breast, endometrium, ovary), venous thromboembolism, stroke and coronary artery disease in relation to age and duration of HRT use.

Oestrogens used in HRT can be given orally (conjugated oestrogens, oestradiol, oestriol), vaginally (oestriol), by transdermal patch (oestradiol) or by subcutaneous implant (oestradiol). **Tibolone** is marketed for the short-term treatment of symptoms of oestrogen deficiency and for postmenopausal prophylaxis of osteoporosis in women at high risk of fracture when other prophylaxis is contraindicated or not tolerated. It has oestrogenic, progestogenic and weak androgenic activity, and can be used continuously without cyclical progesterone (avoiding the inconvenience of withdrawal bleeding).

ANDROGENS

Testosterone is the main natural androgen. It is synthesised (see Fig. 35.3 for the biosynthetic pathway) mainly by the interstitial cells of the testis, and in smaller amounts by the ovaries and adrenal cortex. Several other steroid hormones (e.g. progestogens) have some androgenic action as do a number of synthetic drugs,

Actions

In general, the effects of exogenous androgens are the same as those of testosterone and depend on the age and sex of the recipient. If prepubertal boys are given androgens, they do not reach their full predicted height because of premature closure of the epiphyses of the long bones. In boys at the age of puberty, there is rapid development of secondary sexual characteristics (i.e. growth of facial, axillary and pubic hair, deepening of the voice), maturation of the reproductive organs and a marked increase in muscular strength. There is a growth spurt with an acceleration in the usual increase in height that occurs year on year in younger children, followed by fusion of the bony epiphyses and cessation of linear growth. In adults, the anabolic effects can be accompanied by retention of salt and water. The skin thickens and may darken, and sebaceous glands become more active, predisposing to acne. Body weight and muscle mass increase, partly due to water retention. Androgens cause a feeling of well-being and an increase in physical vigour and may increase libido. Whether they are responsible for sexual behaviour as such is controversial, as is their contribution to aggressive behaviour. Supraphysiological testosterone concentrations inhibit spermatogenesis – the apparent paradox being a consequence of negative feedback of testosterone on GnRH – thereby reducing male fertility.

Mechanism of action

In most target cells, testosterone works through an active metabolite, dihydrotestosterone, to which it is converted locally by a 5α-reductase enzyme. In contrast, testosterone itself causes virilisation of the genital tract in the male embryo and regulates LH/ICSH production in anterior pituitary cells. Testosterone and dihydrotestosterone modify gene transcription by interacting with nuclear receptors.

Preparations

Testosterone can be given by subcutaneous implantation or by transdermal patches. Various esters (e.g. enanthate and propionate) are given by intramuscular depot injection. Testosterone undecanoate and mesterolone can be given orally.

Pharmacokinetic aspects

If given orally, testosterone is rapidly metabolised in the liver to androstenedione which is a weak androgen. Virtually all testosterone in the circulation is bound to plasma protein – mainly to the sex steroid-binding globulin. Approximately 90% of endogenous testosterone is eliminated as metabolites. The elimination half-life of the free hormone is short (10–20 min). Synthetic androgens are less rapidly metabolised, and some are excreted in the urine unchanged.

Androgens and the hormonal control of the male reproductive system

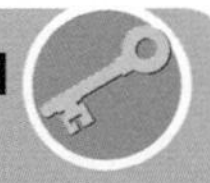

- GnRH from the hypothalamus acts on the anterior pituitary to release both FSH, which stimulates gametogenesis, and LH (also called interstitial cell-stimulating hormone), which stimulates androgen secretion.
- The main endogenous hormone is testosterone; intramuscular depot injections of testosterone esters are used for replacement therapy.
- Mechanism of action is via intracellular receptors/altered gene expression.
- Effects depend on age/sex and include development of male secondary sexual characteristics in prepubertal boys and masculinisation in women.

Clinical uses of androgens and anti-androgens

- Androgens (**testosterone** preparations) as hormone replacement in:
  - male hypogonadism due to pituitary or testicular disease.
- Anti-androgens (e.g. **flutamide**, **cyproterone**) are used as part of the treatment of prostatic cancer.
- 5α-Reductase inhibitors (e.g. **finasteride**) are used in benign prostatic hyperplasia (see Ch. 29).

Unwanted effects

The unwanted effects of androgens include decreased GnRH release during continued use, with resultant male infertility,[2] and salt and water retention leading to oedema. Adenocarcinoma of the liver has been reported. Androgens impair growth in children (via premature fusion of epiphyses), cause acne and lead to masculinisation in girls. The adverse effects of testosterone replacement and monitoring for these are reviewed by Rhoden and Morgentaler (2004).

The clinical uses of androgens are given in the clinical box.

ANABOLIC STEROIDS

Androgens can be modified chemically to alter the balance of anabolic and other effects. 'Anabolic steroids' (e.g. **nandrolone**) increase protein synthesis and muscle development disproportionately, but clinical use (e.g. in debilitating or muscle wasting disease) has been disappointing. They are used in the therapy of aplastic anaemia and (notoriously) abused by some athletes (see Ch. 59), as is testosterone itself. Unwanted effects are described previously. In addition, cholestatic jaundice, liver tumours and increased risk of coronary heart disease are recognised adverse effects of high-dose anabolic steroids.

ANTI-ANDROGENS

Both oestrogens and progestogens have anti-androgen activity, oestrogens mainly by inhibiting GnRH secretion and progestogens (some of which are weak partial agonists at androgen receptors, see earlier discussion) by competing at androgen receptors in target organs. **Cyproterone** is a derivative of progesterone and has weak progestational activity. It is a partial agonist at androgen receptors, competing with dihydrotestosterone for receptors in androgen-sensitive target tissues. Through its effect in the hypothalamus, it depresses the synthesis of gonadotrophins. It is used as an adjunct in the treatment of prostatic cancer during initiation of GnRH agonist treatment (see later). It is also used in the therapy of precocious puberty in males, and of masculinisation and acne in women. It decreases libido and has been used to treat hypersexuality in male sexual offenders.[3]

Flutamide is a non-steroidal anti-androgen used with GnRH agonists in the treatment of prostate cancer.

Drugs can have anti-androgen action by inhibiting synthetic enzymes. **Finasteride** inhibits the enzyme (5α-reductase) that converts testosterone to its active metabolite dihydrotestosterone (see Fig. 35.3). Finasteride is well absorbed after oral administration, has a half-life of about 7 h and is excreted in the urine and faeces. It is used to treat benign prostatic hyperplasia (see Ch. 29).

GONADOTROPHIN-RELEASING HORMONE (GnRH): AGONISTS AND ANTAGONISTS

GnRH is a decapeptide that controls the secretion of FSH and LH by the anterior pituitary. Secretion of GnRH is controlled by neural input from other parts of the brain, and through negative feedback by the sex steroids (Figs 35.1 and 35.5). Exogenous androgens, oestrogens and progestogens all inhibit GnRH secretion, but only progestogens exert this effect at doses that do not have marked hormonal actions on peripheral tissues, presumably because progesterone receptors in the reproductive tract are sparse unless they have been induced by previous exposure to oestrogen. **Danazol** (see later) is a synthetic steroid that inhibits release of GnRH and, consequently, of gonadotrophins (FSH and LH). **Clomiphene** is a SERM that functions mainly as an oestrogen antagonist that stimulates gonadotrophin release by inhibiting the negative feedback effects of endogenous oestrogen; it is used to treat infertility (see clinical box and Fig. 35.5).

Synthetic GnRH is termed ***gonadorelin***. Numerous analogues of GnRH, both agonists and antagonists, have been synthesised. **Buserelin**, **leuprorelin**, **goserelin** and **nafarelin** are agonists, the last being 200 times more potent than endogenous GnRH (good examples of superagonists, in that their efficacies are greater than the efficacy of the natural agonist at the receptor, GnRH).

---

[2]Large doses of androgens also adversely affect female fertility, whereas physiological concentrations of androgen are implicated in female fertility (Prizant et al., 2014).

[3]Very different doses are used for these different conditions, for example, 2 mg/day in combination with ethinylestradiol for acne, 100 mg/day for hypersexuality and up to 300 mg/day for prostatic cancer.

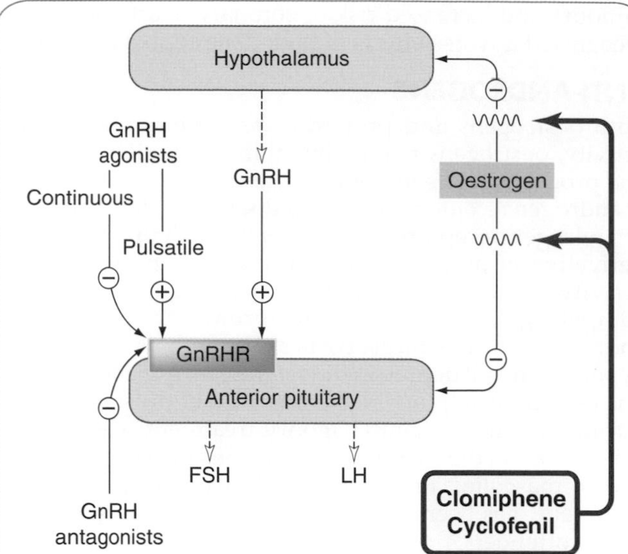

Fig. 35.5 Regulation of gonadotrophin release from the anterior pituitary. *FSH*, Follicle-stimulating hormone; *GnRHR*, gonadotrophin-releasing hormone receptor; *LH*, luteinising hormone.

Pharmacokinetics and clinical use

GnRH agonists, given by subcutaneous infusion in pulses to mimic physiological secretion of GnRH, stimulate gonadotrophin release (see Fig. 35.5) and induce ovulation. They are absorbed intact following nasal administration (see Ch. 9). Continuous use, by nasal spray or as depot preparations, stimulates gonadotrophin release transiently, but then *inhibits* gonadotrophin release (see Fig. 35.5) because of down-regulation (desensitisation) of GnRH receptors in the pituitary. GnRH analogues are given in this fashion to cause gonadal suppression in various sex hormone-dependent conditions, including prostate and breast cancers, endometriosis (endometrial tissue outside the uterine cavity) and large uterine fibroids. Continuous, non-pulsatile administration inhibits spermatogenesis and ovulation. GnRH agonists are used by specialists in infertility treatment, not to stimulate ovulation (which is achieved using gonadotrophin preparations) but to suppress the pituitary before administration of FSH or HCG.

UNWANTED EFFECTS OF GnRH ANALOGUES

The unwanted effects of GnRH agonists in women, for example, flushing, vaginal dryness and bone loss, result from hypo-oestrogenism. The initial stimulation of gonadotrophin secretion on starting treatment can transiently worsen pain from bone metastases in men with prostate cancer, so treatment is started only after the patient has received an androgen receptor antagonist such as **flutamide** (see earlier and Ch. 57).

DANAZOL

Actions and pharmacokinetics

Danazol inhibits gonadotrophin secretion (especially the mid-cycle surge), and consequently reduces oestrogen synthesis in the ovary. In men, it reduces androgen synthesis and spermatogenesis. It has androgenic activity. It is orally active and metabolised in the liver.

Danazol is used in sex hormone-dependent conditions including endometriosis, breast dysplasia (benign breast lumps) and gynaecomastia. A distinct use is to prevent attacks of swelling in hereditary angio-oedema (see Ch. 28); its mechanism when used for this indication is not known.

Unwanted effects are common, and include virilisation, GI disturbance, weight gain, fluid retention, dizziness, menopausal symptoms, muscle cramps and headache.

GONADOTROPHINS AND ANALOGUES

Gonadotrophins (FSH, LH and HCG) are glycoproteins produced and secreted by the anterior pituitary (FSH and LH, see Ch. 33) or chorion and placenta (HCG). Large amounts of gonadotrophins are present in the urine of women following the menopause, because oestrogen levels fall abolishing feedback inhibition on the pituitary, which consequently secretes large amounts of FSH and LH.[4]

Preparations

Gonadotrophins are extracted from urine of pregnant (HCG) or postmenopausal women (human menopausal gonadotrophin, which contains a mixture of FSH and LH). Recombinant FSH (**follitropin**) and LH (**lutropin**) are also available.

Pharmacokinetics and clinical use

Gonadotrophin preparations are given by injection. They are used to treat infertility caused by lack of ovulation as a result of hypopituitarism or following failure of treatment with **clomiphene**; they are also used by specialists to induce ovulation to enable eggs to be collected for in vitro fertilisation. Gonadotrophins are also sometimes used in men with infertility caused by a low sperm count as a result of hypogonadotrophic hypogonadism (a disorder that is sometimes accompanied by lifelong anosmia, i.e. lack of sense of smell). HCG has been used to stimulate testosterone synthesis in boys with delayed puberty, but testosterone is usually preferred.

Gonadotrophin-releasing hormone (GnRH) and gonadotrophins

- GnRH is a decapeptide; **gonadorelin** is the name of the synthetic form used therapeutically. **Nafarelin** is a potent analogue.
- Given in pulsatile fashion, GnRHs stimulate gonadotrophin release; given continuously, they inhibit it.
- The gonadotrophins, FSH and LH, are glycoproteins.
- Preparations of gonadotrophins (e.g. chorionic gonadotrophin) are used to treat infertility caused by failure of ovulation.
- **Danazol** is a modified progestogen that inhibits gonadotrophin production by actions on the hypothalamus and anterior pituitary.

[4]This forms the basis for the standard blood test, estimation of plasma LH/FSH concentrations, to confirm whether a woman is postmenopausal.

DRUGS USED FOR CONTRACEPTION

ORAL CONTRACEPTIVES

There are two main types of oral contraceptives:

1. Combinations of an oestrogen with a progestogen (the combined pill).
2. Progestogen alone (the progestogen-only pill).

THE COMBINED PILL

The combined oral contraceptive pill is extremely effective, at least in the absence of intercurrent illness and of treatment with potentially interacting drugs (see later). The oestrogen in most combined preparations (second-generation pills)[5] is **ethinylestradiol**, although a few preparations contain **mestranol**. The progestogen may be **norethisterone**, **levonorgestrel**, **ethynodiol**, or – in 'third-generation' pills – **desogestrel** or **gestodene**, which are more potent, have less androgenic action and cause less change in lipoprotein metabolism, but which possibly cause a greater risk of thromboembolism than do second-generation preparations. The oestrogen content is generally 20–50 μg of ethinylestradiol or its equivalent, and a preparation is chosen with the lowest oestrogen and progestogen content that is well tolerated and gives good cycle control. This combined pill is taken for 21 consecutive days followed by 7 pill-free days, which causes a withdrawal bleed. Normal cycles of menstruation usually commence fairly soon after discontinuing treatment, and permanent loss of fertility (which may be a result of early menopause rather than a long-term consequence of the contraceptive pill) is rare.

Tailored regimens with so-called 'monophasic' combined hormonal contraceptive preparations containing ethinylestradiol (unlicensed use) are an option; they offer the choice of either a shortened, or less frequent, or no hormone-free interval based on personal preference (see NICE on treatment regimens in the British National Formulary (BNF), https://bnf.nice.org.uk/treatment-summary/contraceptives-hormonal.html).

The mode of action is as follows:

- Oestrogen inhibits secretion of FSH via negative feedback on the anterior pituitary, and thus suppresses development of the ovarian follicle.
- Progestogen inhibits secretion of LH and thus prevents ovulation; it also makes the cervical mucus less suitable for the passage of sperm.
- Oestrogen and progestogen act in concert to alter the endometrium in such a way as to discourage implantation.

They may also interfere with the coordinated contractions of the cervix, uterus and fallopian tubes that facilitate fertilisation and implantation (see later).

Hundreds of millions of women worldwide have used this method since the 1960s, and in general the combined pill constitutes a safe and effective method of contraception. There are distinct health benefits from taking the pill (see later), and serious adverse effects are rare. However, minor unwanted effects constitute drawbacks to its use, and several important questions need to be considered.

Common adverse effects

The common adverse effects are:

- weight gain, owing to fluid retention or an anabolic effect, or both;
- mild nausea, flushing, dizziness, depression or irritability;
- skin changes (e.g. acne and/or an increase in pigmentation);
- amenorrhoea of variable duration on cessation of taking the pill.

Questions that need to be considered

Is there an increased risk of cardiovascular disease (venous thromboembolism, myocardial infarction, stroke)?

With second-generation pills (oestrogen content less than 50 μg), the risk of thromboembolism is small (incidence approximately 15 per 100,000 users per year, compared with 5 per 100,000 non-pregnant non-users per year or 60 episodes of thromboembolism per 100,000 pregnancies). The risk is greatest in subgroups with additional factors, such as smoking (which increases risk substantially) and long-continued use of the pill, especially in women over 35 years of age. The incidence of thromboembolic disease is approximately 25 per 100,000 users per year in users of preparations containing **desogestrel** or **gestodene**, which is still a small absolute risk compared with the risk of thromboembolism in an unwanted pregnancy. In general, provided that risk factors, e.g. smoking, hypertension and obesity, have been identified, combined oral contraceptives are safe for most women for most of their reproductive lives.

Is cancer risk affected?

Ovarian and endometrial cancer risk is *reduced*.

Is blood pressure increased?

A marked increase in arterial blood pressure occurs in a small percentage of women shortly after starting the combined oral contraceptive pill. This is associated with increased circulating angiotensinogen and disappears when treatment is stopped. Blood pressure is therefore monitored when oral contraceptive treatment is started, and an alternative contraceptive substituted if necessary.

Beneficial effects

Besides avoiding unwanted pregnancy, other desirable effects of the combined contraceptive pill include decreased menstrual symptoms such as irregular periods and intermenstrual bleeding. Iron-deficiency anaemia and premenstrual tension are reduced, as are benign breast disease, uterine fibroids and functional cysts of the ovaries.

THE PROGESTOGEN-ONLY PILL

The drugs used in progestogen-only pills include **norethisterone**, **levonorgestrel** or **ethynodiol**. The pill is taken daily without interruption. The mode of action is primarily on the cervical mucus, which is made inhospitable to sperm. The progestogen probably also hinders implantation through its effect on the endometrium (see Fig. 35.2) and on the motility and secretions of the fallopian tubes.

[5]The first-generation pills, containing more than 50 μg of oestrogen, were shown in the 1970s to be associated with an increased risk of deep vein thrombosis and pulmonary embolism.

Potential beneficial and unwanted effects

Progestogen-only contraceptives offer a suitable alternative to the combined pill for some women in whom oestrogen is contraindicated and are suitable for women whose blood pressure increases unacceptably during treatment with oestrogen. However, their contraceptive effect is less reliable than that of the combination pill and missing a dose may result in conception. Disturbances of menstruation (especially irregular bleeding) are common. Only a small proportion of women use this form of contraception, so long-term safety data are less reliable than for the combined pill.

PHARMACOKINETICS OF ORAL CONTRACEPTIVES: DRUG INTERACTIONS

Combined and progestogen-only oral contraceptives are metabolised by hepatic cytochrome P450 enzymes. Because the minimum effective dose of oestrogen is used to minimise excess risk of thromboembolism, any increase in its clearance may result in contraceptive failure, and indeed enzyme-inducing drugs can have this effect, not only for combined but also for progesterone-only pills. Such drugs include **rifampicin** and **rifabutin**, as well as **carbamazepine**, **phenytoin** and others, including the herbal preparation St John's Wort (see Ch. 48).

Oral contraceptives

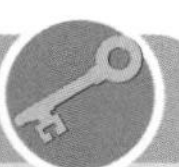

The combined pill

- The combined oestrogen plus progestogen pill is taken for 21 consecutive days out of 28; alternatively tailored regimens that offer the choice of either a shortened, or less frequent, or no hormone-free interval are an option.
- Mode of action: oestrogen inhibits FSH release and therefore follicle development; progestogen inhibits LH release and therefore ovulation, and makes cervical mucus inhospitable for sperm; together, they render the endometrium unsuitable for implantation.
- Drawbacks: weight gain, nausea, mood changes and skin pigmentation can occur.
- Serious unwanted effects are rare. A small proportion of women develop reversible hypertension; there is a small increase in the diagnosis of breast cancer, possibly attributable to earlier diagnosis, and of cervical cancer. There is an increased risk of thromboembolism with third-generation pills, especially in women with additional risk factors (e.g. smoking) and with prolonged use.
- There are several beneficial effects, not least the avoidance of unwanted pregnancy, which itself carries risks to health.

The progestogen-only pill

- The progestogen-only pill is taken continuously. It differs from the combined pill in that the contraceptive effect is less reliable and is mainly a result of the alteration of cervical mucus. Irregular bleeding is common.

OTHER DRUG REGIMENS USED FOR CONTRACEPTION

POSTCOITAL (EMERGENCY) CONTRACEPTION

Oral administration of **levonorgestrel**, alone or combined with oestrogen, is effective if taken within 72 h of unprotected intercourse and repeated 12 h later. Nausea and vomiting are common (and the pills may then be lost: replacement tablets can be taken with an antiemetic such as **domperidone**). Insertion of an intrauterine device is more effective than hormonal methods and works up to 5 days after intercourse.

LONG-ACTING PROGESTOGEN-ONLY CONTRACEPTION

Medroxyprogesterone can be given intramuscularly as a contraceptive. This is effective and safe. However, menstrual irregularities are common, and infertility may persist for many months after the final dose.

Levonorgestrel implanted subcutaneously in non-biodegradable capsules is used by approximately 3 million women worldwide. This route of administration avoids first-pass metabolism. The capsules release their progestogen content slowly over 5 years. Irregular bleeding and headache are common.

A levonorgestrel-impregnated intrauterine system provides prolonged, reliable contraception and, in contrast to standard copper containing devices, *reduces* menstrual bleeding.

THE UTERUS

The physiological and pharmacological responses of the uterus vary at different stages of the menstrual cycle and during pregnancy.

THE MOTILITY OF THE UTERUS

Uterine muscle contracts rhythmically both in vitro and in vivo, contractions originating in the muscle itself. Myometrial cells in the fundus act as pacemakers and give rise to conducted action potentials. The electrophysiological activity of these pacemaker cells is regulated by the sex hormones.

The non-pregnant human uterus contracts spontaneously but weakly during the first part of the cycle, and more strongly during the luteal phase and during menstruation. Uterine movements are depressed in early pregnancy because oestrogen, potentiated by progesterone, hyperpolarises myometrial cells. This suppresses spontaneous contractions. Towards the end of gestation, however, contractions recommence; these increase in force and frequency, and become fully coordinated during parturition. The nerve supply to the uterus includes both excitatory and inhibitory sympathetic components: adrenaline, acting on β_2 adrenoceptors, inhibits uterine contraction, whereas noradrenaline, acting on α adrenoceptors, stimulates contraction.

DRUGS THAT STIMULATE THE UTERUS

Drugs that stimulate the pregnant uterus and are important in obstetrics include **oxytocin**, **ergometrine** and PGs.

OXYTOCIN

The neurohypophyseal hormone oxytocin (an octapeptide) regulates myometrial activity, causing uterine contraction (see Ch. 33). Oxytocin release is stimulated by cervical dilatation, and by suckling; its role in parturition is incompletely understood but the fact that an antagonist (**atosiban**, see later) is effective in delaying the onset of labour implicates it in the physiology of parturition.

Oestrogen induces oxytocin receptor synthesis and, consequently, the uterus at term is highly sensitive to this hormone. Given by slow intravenous infusion to induce labour, oxytocin causes regular coordinated contractions that travel from fundus to cervix. Both the amplitude and frequency of these contractions are related to dose, the uterus relaxing completely between contractions during low-dose infusion. Larger doses further increase the frequency of the contractions, and there is incomplete relaxation between them. Still higher doses cause sustained contractions that interfere with blood flow through the placenta and cause fetal distress or death.

Oxytocin contracts myoepithelial cells in the mammary gland, which causes 'milk let-down' – the expression of milk from the alveoli and ducts. It also has a vasodilator action. A weak antidiuretic action can result in water retention, which can be problematic in patients with cardiac or renal disease, or with pre-eclampsia.[6] Oxytocin and oxytocin receptors are also found in the brain, particularly in the limbic system, and are believed to play a role in mating and parenting behaviour.

The therapeutic use of synthetic oxytocin is summarised in the clinical box.

Oxytocin can be given by intravenous injection or intramuscularly but is most often given by intravenous infusion. It is inactivated in the liver and kidneys, and by circulating placental oxytocinase.

Unwanted effects of oxytocin include dose-related hypotension, due to vasodilatation, with associated reflex tachycardia. Its antidiuretic hormone-like effect on water excretion by the kidney causes water retention and, unless water intake is curtailed, consequent hyponatraemia (see Ch. 29).

ERGOMETRINE

Ergot (*Claviceps purpurea*) is a fungus that grows on rye and contains a surprising variety of pharmacologically active substances (see Ch. 16). Ergot poisoning, which was once common, was often associated with abortion. In 1935, **ergometrine** was isolated and recognised as the oxytocic principle in ergot.

Ergometrine contracts the human uterus. This action depends partly on the contractile state of the organ. On a contracted uterus (the normal state following delivery), ergometrine has relatively little effect. However, if the uterus is inappropriately relaxed, ergometrine initiates strong contraction and reduces bleeding from the placental bed (the raw surface from which the placenta has detached). Ergometrine also has a moderate vasoconstrictor action.

The mechanism of action of ergometrine on smooth muscle is not understood. It is possible that it acts partly on α adrenoceptors, like the related alkaloid ergotamine (see Ch. 15), and partly on 5-hydroxytryptamine receptors.

The use of ergometrine is given in the clinical box, below.

Ergometrine can be given orally, intramuscularly or intravenously. It has a very rapid onset of action and its effect lasts for 3–6 h.

Ergometrine can produce vomiting, probably by an effect on dopamine D_2 receptors in the chemoreceptor trigger zone (see Ch. 31, Fig. 31.5). Vasoconstriction with an increase in blood pressure associated with nausea, blurred vision and headache can occur, as can vasospasm of the coronary arteries, resulting in angina.

PROSTAGLANDINS

PGs are discussed in detail in Chapter 17. The endometrium and myometrium have substantial PG-synthesising capacity, particularly in the second, proliferative phase of the menstrual cycle. $PGF_{2\alpha}$ is generated in large amounts and has been implicated in the ischaemic necrosis of the endometrium that precedes menstruation (although it has relatively little vasoconstrictor action on many human blood vessels, in contrast to some other mammalian species). Vasodilator PGs, PGE_2 and PGI_2 (prostacyclin), are also generated by the uterus.

In addition to their vasoactive properties, the E and F PGs contract uterine smooth muscle, whose sensitivity to these PGs increases during gestation. Their role in parturition is not fully understood, but as cyclo-oxygenase inhibitors can delay labour (see later), they probably play some part in this.

PGs also play a part in two of the main disorders of menstruation: *dysmenorrhoea* (painful menstruation) and *menorrhagia* (excessive blood loss). Dysmenorrhoea is associated with increased production of PGE_2 and $PGF_{2\alpha}$; non-steroidal anti-inflammatory drugs, which inhibit PG biosynthesis (see Ch. 25), are used to treat dysmenorrhoea. Menorrhagia, in the absence of other uterine pathology, may be caused by a combination of increased vasodilatation and reduced haemostasis. Increased generation by the uterus of PGI_2 (which inhibits platelet aggregation) could impair haemostasis as well as causing vasodilatation. Non-steroidal anti-inflammatory drugs (e.g. **mefenamic acid**) are used to treat menorrhagia as well as dysmenorrhoea.

Prostaglandin preparations

PGs of the E and F series promote coordinated contractions of the body of the pregnant uterus, while relaxing the cervix. E and F PGs reliably cause abortion in early and middle pregnancy, unlike oxytocin which generally does not cause expulsion of the uterine contents at this stage. The PGs used in obstetrics are **dinoprostone** (PGE_2), **carboprost** (15-methyl $PGF_{2\alpha}$) and **gemeprost** or **misoprostol** (PGE_1 analogues). Dinoprostone can be given intravaginally as a gel or as tablets. Carboprost is given by deep intramuscular injection. Gemeprost and misoprostol are given intravaginally.

[6]Eclampsia is a pathological condition (involving, among other things, high blood pressure, swelling and seizures) that occurs in pregnant women – it is usually preceded by milder changes ('pre-eclampsia').

Unwanted effects

Unwanted effects include uterine pain, nausea and vomiting and diarrhoea. Dinoprost can cause hypotension. When combined with mifepristone, a progestogen antagonist that sensitises the uterus to PGs, lower doses of the PGs (e.g. misoprostol) can be used to terminate pregnancy and adverse effects are reduced.

The clinical box shows the clinical uses of PGs (see also Ch. 17).

Drugs acting on the uterus

- At parturition, **oxytocin** causes regular coordinated uterine contractions, each followed by relaxation; **ergometrine**, an ergot alkaloid, causes uterine contractions with an increase in basal tone. **Atosiban**, an antagonist of oxytocin, delays labour.
- PG preparations, for example, **dinoprostone** (PGE_2) and **dinoprost** ($PGF_{2\alpha}$), contract the pregnant uterus but relax the cervix. Cyclo-oxygenase inhibitors inhibit PG biosynthesis and delay labour but are not used clinically for this indication because they delay closure of the ductus arteriosus in the fetus. They also alleviate symptoms of dysmenorrhoea and menorrhagia.
- The β_2-adrenoceptor agonists (e.g. **ritodrine**) inhibit spontaneous and oxytocin-induced contractions of the pregnant uterus.

DRUGS THAT INHIBIT UTERINE CONTRACTION

Selective β_2-adrenoceptor agonists, such as **ritodrine** or **salbutamol**, inhibit spontaneous or oxytocin-induced contractions of the pregnant uterus. These uterine relaxants are used in selected patients to prevent premature labour occurring between 22 and 33 weeks of gestation in otherwise uncomplicated pregnancies. They can delay delivery by 48 h, time that can be used to administer glucocorticoid therapy to the mother to mature the lungs of the baby and reduce neonatal respiratory distress. It has been difficult to demonstrate that any of the drugs used to delay labour improve the outcome for the baby. Risks to the mother, especially pulmonary oedema, increase after 48 h, and myometrial response is reduced, so prolonged treatment is avoided. Cyclo-oxygenase inhibitors (e.g. **indometacin**) inhibit labour, but their use could cause problems in the baby, including renal dysfunction and delayed closure of the ductus arteriosus, both of which are influenced favourably by endogenous PGs.

An oxytocin receptor antagonist, **atosiban**, provides an alternative to a β_2-adrenoceptor agonist. It is given as an intravenous bolus followed by an intravenous infusion for not more than 48 h. Adverse effects include vasodilatation, nausea, vomiting and hyperglycaemia.

Clinical uses of drugs acting on the uterus

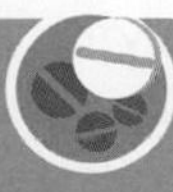

Myometrial stimulants (oxytocics)

- **Oxytocin** is infused intravenously to *induce or augment labour* when the uterine muscle is not functioning adequately. It can also be used to treat *postpartum haemorrhage.*
- **Ergometrine** is used to treat *postpartum haemorrhage.* **Carboprost** can be used if patients do not respond to **ergometrine.**
- A preparation containing both **oxytocin** and **ergometrine** is used for the management of the third stage of labour; the two agents together can also be used, before surgery, to control bleeding due to incomplete abortion.
- **Gemeprost** (intravaginally) or **misoprostol** (following mifepristone) are used to terminate pregnancy.

Myometrial relaxants

- β-Adrenoceptor agonists (e.g. **ritodrine**): to delay *preterm labour.*
- **Atosiban** (oxytocin antagonist) also delays preterm labour.

ERECTILE DYSFUNCTION

Erectile function depends on complex interactions between physiological and psychological factors. Erection is caused by vasorelaxation in the arteries and arterioles supplying the erectile tissue. This increases penile blood flow; the consequent increase in sinusoidal filling compresses the venules, occluding venous outflow and causing erection. During sexual intercourse, reflex contraction of the ischiocavernosus muscles compresses the base of the corpora cavernosa, and the intracavernosal pressure can reach several hundred millimetres of mercury during this phase of rigid erection. Innervation of the penis includes autonomic and somatic nerves. Nitric oxide (neuronal and endothelium derived) is the main mediator of erection (see Ch. 19).

Erectile function is adversely affected by several therapeutic drugs (including many antipsychotic, antidepressant and antihypertensive agents), and psychiatric and vascular disease (especially in association with endothelial dysfunction) can themselves cause erectile dysfunction, which is common in middle-aged and older men, even if they have no psychiatric or cardiovascular problems.[7] There are several organic causes, including hypogonadism, hyperprolactinaemia (see Ch. 33), arterial disease and various causes of neuropathy (most commonly diabetes), but often no organic cause is identified.

Over the centuries, there has been a huge trade in parts of various creatures that have the misfortune to bear some fancied resemblance to human genitalia, in the pathetic belief that consuming these will restore virility or act as an aphrodisiac (i.e. a drug that stimulates libido). Alcohol (see Ch. 50) 'provokes the desire but takes away the performance', and cannabis (see Ch. 18) can also release inhibitions and probably does the same. **Yohimbine** (an α_2-adrenoceptor antagonist; see Ch. 15) may have some positive effect in this regard, but trials have proved inconclusive. **Apomorphine** (a dopamine agonist) causes erections in humans as well as in rodents

[7]In randomised controlled trials, an appreciable proportion of men who discontinued treatment because of erectile dysfunction had been receiving placebo.

when injected subcutaneously, but it is a powerful emetic, a disadvantage in this context. The picture picked up somewhat when it was found that injecting vasodilator drugs directly into the corpora cavernosa causes penile erection. **Papaverine** (see Ch. 21), if necessary with the addition of **phentolamine**, was used in this way. The route of administration is not acceptable to most men but those with diabetes, in particular, are often not needle-shy, and this approach was a real boon to many such patients. **PGE$_1$** (**alprostadil**) is often combined with other vasodilators when given intracavernosally. It can also be given transurethrally as an alternative (albeit still a somewhat unromantic one) to injection. Adverse effects of all these drugs include priapism (prolonged and painful erection with risk of permanent tissue damage), which is no joke. Treatment consists of aspiration of blood and, if necessary, cautious intracavernosal administration of a vasoconstrictor such as **phenylephrine**. Intracavernosal and transurethral preparations are still available to treat erectile failure, but orally active phosphodiesterase inhibitors are now generally the drugs of choice.

PHOSPHODIESTERASE TYPE V INHIBITORS

Sildenafil, the first selective phosphodiesterase type V inhibitor (see also Chs 19 and 21), was found accidently to influence erectile function.[8] **Tadalafil** and **vardenafil** are similar. Tadalafil is longer acting than sildenafil. In contrast to intracavernosal vasodilators, phosphodiesterase type V inhibitors do not cause erection independent of sexual desire but enhance the erectile response to sexual stimulation (both physical and psychological). They have transformed the treatment of erectile dysfunction.

Mechanism of action

Phosphodiesterase V is the isoform that inactivates cGMP. Nitrergic nerves release nitric oxide (or a related nitrosothiol) which diffuses into smooth muscle cells, where it activates guanylyl cyclase. The resulting increase in cytoplasmic cGMP mediates vasodilatation via activation of protein kinase G (see Ch. 4, Fig. 4.10). Consequently, inhibition of phosphodiesterase V potentiates the effect on penile vascular smooth muscle of endothelium-derived nitric oxide and of nitrergic nerves that are activated by sexual stimulation (Fig. 35.6). Pulmonary vasculature is also affected by PDFE5 inhibitors, leading to use in pulmonary hypertension (see Ch. 21).

Pharmacokinetic aspects and drug interactions

Peak plasma concentrations of sildenafil occur approximately 30–120 min after an oral dose and are delayed by eating, so it is taken an hour or more before sexual activity. It is given as a single dose as needed. It is metabolised by CYP3A4, which is induced by **carbamazepine**, **rifampicin** and **barbiturates**, and inhibited by **cimetidine**, macrolide antibiotics, antifungal imidazolines and some antiviral drugs (such as **ritonavir**). These drugs can interact with sildenafil. Tadalafil has a longer half-life than sildenafil, so can be taken longer before sexual activity. A clinically important pharmacodynamic interaction of all phosphodiesterase V inhibitors occurs with all organic nitrates, which work through increasing cGMP (see Ch. 19) and are therefore markedly potentiated by sildenafil (see Fig. 35.6). Consequently, concurrent nitrate use, including use of **nicorandil**, contraindicates the concurrent use of any phosphodiesterase type V inhibitor.[9]

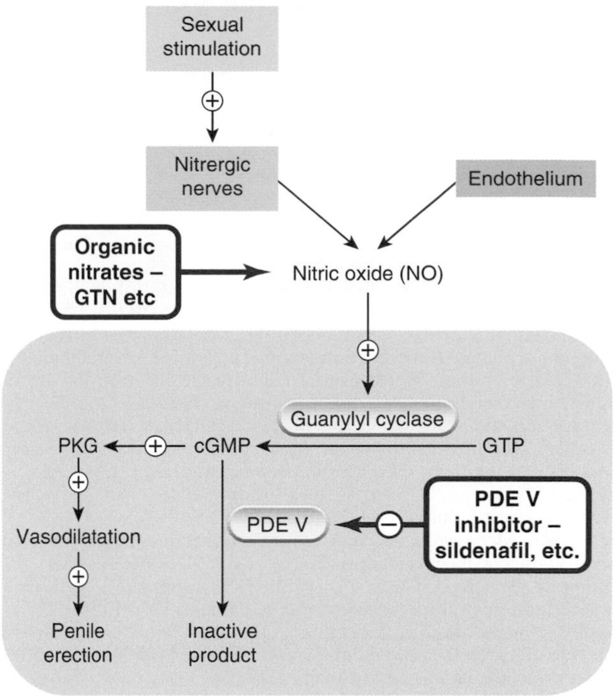

Fig. 35.6 Mechanism of phosphodiesterase V (PDE V) inhibitors on penile erection, and of the interaction of PDE V inhibitors with organic nitrates. The *large grey rectangle* denotes a vascular smooth muscle cell in the corpora cavernosa. Sexual stimulation releases nitric oxide (NO) from nitrergic nerves and this activates guanylyl cyclase, increasing cGMP production and hence activating protein kinase G (PKG), causing vasodilatation and penile erection. cGMP is inactivated by PDE V, so PDE V inhibitors (e.g. sildenafil) potentiate NO and promote penile erection. NO from organic nitrates such as glyceryl trinitrate (GTN) is also potentiated leading to generalised vasodilatation and hypotension.

Unwanted effects

Many of the unwanted effects of phosphodiesterase type V inhibitors are caused by vasodilatation in other vascular beds; these effects include hypotension, flushing and headache. Visual disturbances have occasionally been reported and are of concern because sildenafil has some action on phosphodiesterase VI, which is present in the retina and important in vision (which is also cGMP-dependent). The manufacturers advise that sildenafil should not be used in patients with hereditary retinal degenerative diseases (such as retinitis pigmentosa) because of the theoretical risk posed by this. Vardenafil is more selective for the type V isozyme than is sildenafil (reviewed by Doggrell, 2005), but is also contraindicated in patients with hereditary retinal disorders.

[8]Sildenafil was originally intended to treat angina, but bulging bedclothes were noticed in early clinical trials, providing the opportunity for the drug to be developed for a less crowded and more profitable indication than angina.

[9]This is important not only for sufferers from angina who take nitrates such as glyceryl trinitrate or isosorbide mononitrate therapeutically or prophylactically and are at risk of hypotension because of coronary artery disease, but also asymptomatic individuals who take amyl nitrate recreationally ('poppers').

REFERENCES AND FURTHER READING

Sex hormones and their control

Adeel, M., Song, X., Wang, Y., Dennis Francis, D., Yang, Y., 2017. Environmental impact of estrogens on human, animal and plant life: a critical review. Environ. Int. 99, 107–119.

Barrett-Connor, E., Mosca, L., Collins, P., et al., 2006. Effects of raloxifene on cardiovascular events and breast cancer in postmenopausal women. N. Engl. J. Med. 355, 125–137.

Barbotin, A.-L., Peigné, M., Malone, S.A., Giacobini, P., 2019. Emerging roles of anti-Müllerian hormone in hypothalamic-pituitary function. Neuroendocrinology 109, 218–229.

Barton, M., Prossnitz, E.R., 2015. Emerging roles of GPER in diabetes and atherosclerosis. Trends Endocrinol. Metab. 26, 185–192.

Chen, Z., Yuhanna, I.S., Galcheva-Gargova, Z., et al., 1999. Estrogen receptor-alpha mediates the nongenomic activation of endothelial nitric oxide synthase by estrogen. J. Clin. Invest. 103, 401–406.

Gruber, C.J., Tschugguel, W., Schneeberger, C., Huber, J.C., 2002. Production and actions of estrogens. N. Engl. J. Med. 346, 340–352.

McLachlan, J.A., 2016. Environmental signaling: from environmental estrogens to endocrine-disrupting chemicals and beyond. Andrology 4, 684–694.

Prizant, H., Gleicher, N., Sen, A., 2014. Androgen actions in the ovary: balance is key. J. Endocrinol. 222, R141–R151.

Rhoden, E.L., Morgentaler, A., 2004. Risks of testosterone-replacement therapy and recommendations for monitoring. N. Engl. J. Med. 350, 482–492.

T'Sjoen, G., Arcelus, J., Gooren, L., Klink, D.T., Tangpricha, V., 2019. The endocrinology of transgender medicine. Endocr. Rev. 40, 97–117.

Vogel, V., Constantino, J., Wickerman, L., et al., 2006. Effects of tamoxifen vs. raloxifene on the risk of developing invasive breast cancer and other disease outcomes. JAMA 295, 2727–2741.

Walker, H.A., Dean, T.S., Sanders, T.A.B., et al., 2001. The phytoestrogen genistein produces acute nitric oxide-dependent dilation of human forearm vasculature with similar potency to 17 beta-estradiol. Circulation 103, 258–262.

Contraceptives

Djerassi, C., 2001. This Man's Pill: Reflections on the 50th Birthday of the Pill. Oxford University Press, New York.

Postmenopausal aspects

Davis, S.R., Dinatale, I., Rivera-Woll, L., Davison, S., 2005. Postmenopausal hormone therapy: from monkey glands to transdermal patches. J. Endocrinol. 185, 207–222.

Hulley, S., Grady, D., Bush, T., et al., 1998. Randomized trial of estrogen plus progestin for secondary prevention of coronary heart disease in postmenopausal women. JAMA 280, 605–613.

Prague, J.K., Roberts, R.E., Comninos, A.N., 2017. Neurokinin 3 receptor antagonism as a novel treatment for menopausal hot flushes: a phase 2, randomised, double-blind, placebo-controlled trial. Lancet 389, 1809–1820.

The uterus

Norwitz, E.R., Robinson, J.N., Challis, J.R., 1999. The control of labor. N. Engl. J. Med. 341, 660–666.

Thornton, S., Vatish, M., Slater, D., 2001. Oxytocin antagonists: clinical and scientific considerations. Exp. Physiol. 86, 297–302.

Erectile dysfunction

Doggrell, S.A., 2005. Comparison of clinical trials with sildenafil, vardenafil and tadalafil in erectile dysfunction. Expert Opin. Pharmacother. 6, 75–84.

Useful Web resource

Medicines & Healthcare Products Regulatory Agency. Table 2. Detailed summary of relative and absolute risks and benefits during current use from age of menopause and up to age 69, per 1000 women with 5 years or 10 years use of HRT. Available at: https://assets.publishing.service.gov.uk/media/5d680384ed915d53b8ebdba7/table2.pdf.

36 Bone metabolism

OVERVIEW

In this chapter we consider first the cellular and biochemical processes involved in bone remodelling, and the various mediators that regulate these processes. Pathological disruption of the bony skeleton is clinically manifest in conditions such as osteoporosis, Paget's disease, osteomalacia and metastatic tumour deposits. We describe the drugs used to treat these disorders of bone, including new agents in the management of osteoporosis.

INTRODUCTION

The human skeleton undergoes a continuous process of remodelling throughout life – some bone being resorbed and new bone being laid down continuously – resulting in the complete skeleton being replaced every 10 years. Structural deterioration and decreased bone mass (osteoporosis) occur with advancing age and constitute a worldwide health problem. Other conditions that lead to treatable pathological changes in bone include nutritional deficiencies, certain endocrine disorders and malignancy. There have recently been significant advances in the understanding of bone biology, which have led in turn to several valuable new drugs.

BONE STRUCTURE AND COMPOSITION

The human skeleton consists of 80% (by mass) cortical bone and 20% trabecular bone. Cortical bone is the dense, compact outer part, and trabecular bone, the inner meshwork. The former predominates in the shafts of long bones, the latter in the vertebrae, the epiphyses of long bones and the iliac crest. Trabecular bone, having a large surface area, is metabolically more active and more affected by factors that lead to bone loss (see later).

The main minerals in bone are calcium and phosphates. More than 99% of the calcium in the body is in the skeleton, mostly as crystalline hydroxyapatite but some as non-crystalline phosphates and carbonates; together, these make up half the bone mass.

The main bone cells are *osteoblasts*, *osteoclasts* and *osteocytes*.

- Osteoblasts are bone-forming cells derived from precursor cells in the bone marrow and the periosteum: they secrete important components (particularly collagen) of the extracellular matrix of bone – which is known as *osteoid*. They also have a role in the activation of osteoclasts (Figs 36.1 and 36.2).
- Osteoclasts are multinucleated bone-resorbing cells derived from precursor cells of the macrophage/monocyte lineage.
- Osteocytes are derived from osteoblasts which, during the formation of new bone, become embedded in the bony matrix and differentiate into osteocytes. These cells form a connected cellular network that, along with nerve fibres located in bone, influences the response to mechanical loading. Osteocytes sense mechanical strain and respond by triggering bone remodelling (see later) and secreting *sclerostin*, a glycoprotein that binds to receptors on osteoblasts to suppress bone formation (McClung, 2017). **Romosozumab** is a sclerostin inhibitor that has received regulatory approval for treatment of osteoporosis (see later).
- Other important cells in bone include monocytes/macrophages, lymphocytes and vascular endothelial cells; these secrete cytokines and other mediators implicated in bone remodelling.

Osteoid is the organic matrix of bone and its principal component is collagen. Other components such as *proteoglycans*, *osteocalcin* and various phosphoproteins are also important; one of these, *osteonectin*, binds to both calcium and collagen and thus links these two major constituents of bone matrix.

Calcium phosphate crystals are deposited as hydroxyapatite $[Ca_{10}(PO_4)_6(OH)_2]$ in the osteoid, converting it into hard bone matrix.

In addition to its structural function, bone plays a major role in calcium homeostasis.

BONE REMODELLING

There has been substantial progress in our understanding of bone remodelling (see review by Kim et al., 2021).

The process of remodelling involves:

- activity of osteoblasts and osteoclasts (see Fig. 36.1);
- actions of various cytokines (see Figs 36.1 and 36.2);
- turnover of bone minerals – particularly calcium and phosphate;
- actions of several hormones: parathyroid hormone (PTH), the vitamin D family, oestrogens, growth hormone, steroids, calcitonin and various cytokines.

Diet, drugs and physical factors (exercise, loading) also affect remodelling. Bone loss – of 0.5%–1% per year – starts at age 35–40 years in both sexes and accelerates by as much as 10-fold during the menopause in women or with castration in men, and then gradually settles at 1%–3% per year. The loss during the menopause is due to increased osteoclast activity and affects mainly trabecular bone; the later loss in

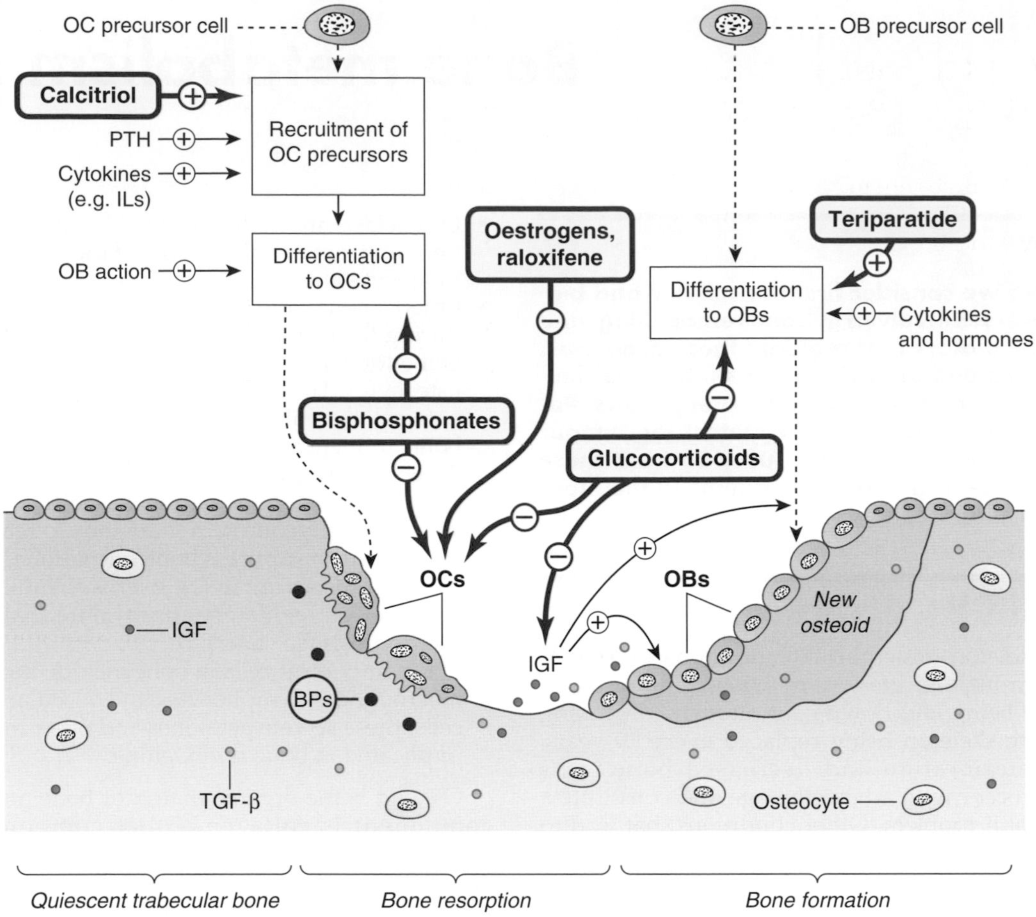

OC precursor cell
OB precursor cell
Calcitriol
PTH
Cytokines (e.g. ILs)
Recruitment of OC precursors
OB action
Differentiation to OCs
Oestrogens, raloxifene
Teriparatide
Differentiation to OBs
Cytokines and hormones
Bisphosphonates
Glucocorticoids
OCs
OBs
New osteoid
IGF
IGF
BPs
TGF-β
Osteocyte
Quiescent trabecular bone
Bone resorption
Bone formation

Fig. 36.1 The bone-remodelling cycle and the action of hormones, cytokines and drugs. *Quiescent trabecular bone:* Cytokines such as insulin-like growth factor (IGF) and transforming growth factor (TGF)-β, shown as dots, are embedded in the bone matrix. *Bone resorption* and *bone formation* are illustrated. Embedded bisphosphonates (BPs) are ingested by osteoclasts (OCs) when bone is resorbed (not shown). *IL,* Interleukin; *OB,* osteoblasts; *PTH,* parathyroid hormone.

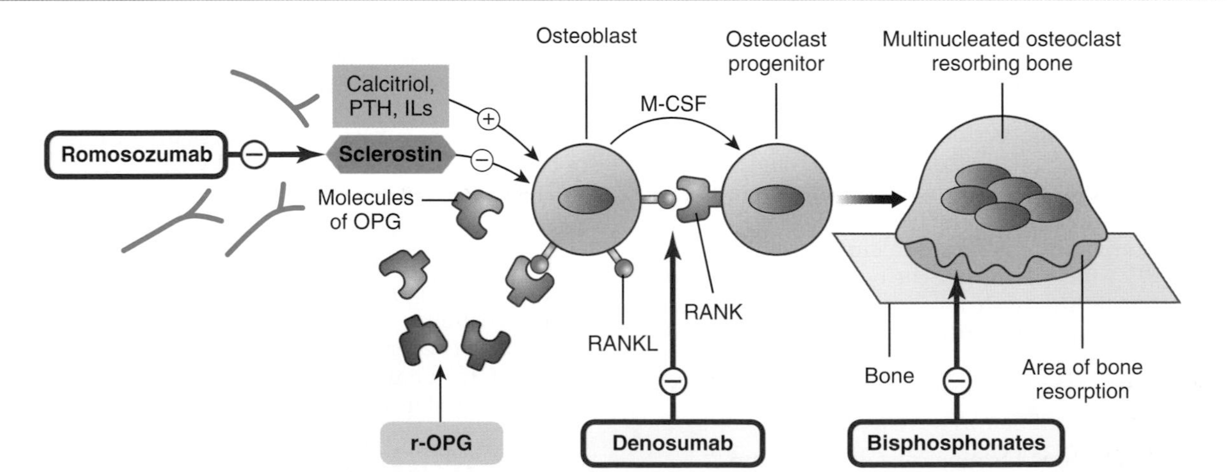

Fig. 36.2 Schematic diagram of the role of the osteoblast and cytokines in the differentiation and activation of the osteoclast and the action of drugs thereon. The osteoblast is stimulated to express a surface ligand, the RANK ligand (RANKL). RANKL interacts with a receptor on the osteoclast – an osteoclast differentiation and activation receptor termed *RANK* (receptor activator of nuclear factor κB), which causes differentiation and activation of the osteoclast progenitors to form mature osteoclasts. Bisphosphonates inhibit bone resorption by osteoclasts. Anti-RANKL antibodies (e.g. denosumab) bind RANKL and prevent the RANK–RANKL interaction. Sclerostin inhibits proliferation of osteoblasts and stimulates RANKL secretion. Romosozumab binds to and inhibits sclerostin. Drugs used clinically are in *red-bordered boxes*. *IL,* Interleukin; *M-CSF,* macrophage colony-stimulating factor; *OPG,* osteoprotegerin; *PTH,* parathyroid hormone.

both sexes with increasing age is due to decreased osteoblast numbers and affects mainly cortical bone.

THE ACTION OF CELLS AND CYTOKINES

A cycle of remodelling starts with recruitment of osteoclast precursors followed by cytokine-induced differentiation of these to mature multinucleated osteoclasts (see Fig. 36.1). The osteoclasts adhere to an area of trabecular bone, developing a ruffled border at the attachment site. They move along the bone, digging a pit by secreting hydrogen ions and proteolytic enzymes, mainly *cathepsin K*. This process gradually liberates cytokines such as insulin-like growth factor (IGF)-1 and transforming growth factor (TGF)-β, which have been embedded in the osteoid (see Fig. 36.1); these in turn recruit and activate successive teams of osteoblasts that have been stimulated to develop from precursor cells and are awaiting the call to duty (see Fig. 36.1). The osteoblasts invade the site, synthesising and secreting osteoid and secreting IGF-1 and TGF-β (which become embedded in the osteoid, as just mentioned). Some osteoblasts become embedded in the osteoid, forming osteocytes; others interact with and activate osteoclast precursors – and we are back to the beginning of the cycle.

Cytokines other than IGF-1 and TGF-β involved in bone remodelling include other members of the TGF-β family, including *bone morphogenic proteins* (BMPs), several interleukins, various hormones and members of the tumour necrosis factor (TNF) family. A member of this last family – a ligand for a receptor on the osteoclast precursor cell – is of particular importance. The receptor is termed (wait for it – biological terminology has fallen over its own feet here) *RANK*, which stands for ***r**eceptor **a**ctivator of **n**uclear factor **k**appa B* (NF-κB), NF-κB being the principal transcription factor involved in osteoclast differentiation and activation. And the ligand is termed, unsurprisingly, *RANK ligand* (RANKL).

Osteoblasts synthesise and release *osteoprotegerin* (OPG) which belongs to the same TNF receptor superfamily as RANK. In a sibling-undermining process by osteoblast and osteoclast precursor cells, OPG can function as a decoy receptor that binds to RANKL[1] (generated by the very same cells as OPG), thus inhibiting RANKL's binding to the functional receptor, RANK, on the osteoclast precursor cell (see Fig. 36.2). The ratio of RANKL to OPG is critical in the formation and activity of osteoclasts and the RANK, RANKL, OPG system is fundamental to bone remodelling (reviewed by Boyce and Xing, 2008). Denosumab is an antibody directed against RANKL that is used clinically to treat osteoporosis (see later).

THE TURNOVER OF BONE MINERALS

The main bone minerals are calcium and phosphates.

CALCIUM METABOLISM

The daily turnover of bone minerals during remodelling involves about 700 mg of calcium. Calcium has numerous roles in physiological functioning. Intracellular Ca^{2+} is part of the signal transduction mechanism of many cells (see Ch. 4), so the concentration of ionised Ca^{2+} in the extracellular fluid and the plasma, normally 1.1–1.3 mmol/L in adult humans, needs to be controlled with great precision. The plasma Ca^{2+} concentration is regulated by interactions between PTH and various forms of vitamin D (Figs 36.3 and 36.4); calcitonin also plays a part.

Calcium absorption in the intestine involves a Ca^{2+}-binding protein, the synthesis of which is regulated by calcitriol (see Fig. 36.3). It is probable that the overall calcium content of the body is regulated largely by this absorption mechanism, because urinary Ca^{2+} excretion normally remains more or less constant. However, with high blood Ca^{2+} concentrations urinary excretion increases, and with low blood concentrations urinary excretion can be reduced by PTH and calcitriol, both of which enhance Ca^{2+} reabsorption in the renal tubules (see Fig. 36.3).

PHOSPHATE METABOLISM

Phosphates are important constituents of bone and are also critically important in the structure and function of all the cells of the body. They are constituents of nucleic acids, provide energy in the form of ATP and control – through phosphorylation – the activity of many functional proteins. They also have roles as intracellular buffers and in the excretion of hydrogen ions in the kidney.

Phosphate absorption is an energy-requiring process regulated by *calcitriol*. Phosphate deposition in bone, as hydroxyapatite, depends on the plasma concentration of PTH, which, with calcitriol, mobilises both Ca^{2+} and phosphate from the bone matrix. Phosphate is excreted by the kidney; here PTH inhibits reabsorption and thus increases excretion.

Bone remodelling

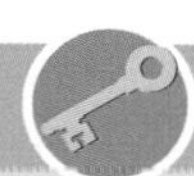

- Bone is continuously remodelled throughout life. The events of the remodelling cycle are as follows:
  - osteoclasts, having been activated by osteoblasts, resorb bone by digging pits in trabecular bone. Into these pits the bone-forming osteoblasts secrete osteoid (bone matrix), which consists mainly of collagen but also contains osteocalcin, osteonectin, phosphoproteins and the cytokines insulin growth factor (IGF) and transforming growth factor (TGF)-β;
  - the osteoid is then mineralised, i.e. complex calcium phosphate crystals (hydroxyapatites) are deposited.
- Bone metabolism and mineralisation involve the action of parathyroid hormone, the vitamin D family and various cytokines (e.g. IGF, the TGF-β family and interleukins). Declining physiological levels of oestrogens, therapeutic levels of glucocorticoids and pathologically raised concentrations of thyroid hormones can result in bone resorption not balanced by bone formation – leading to osteoporosis.

HORMONES INVOLVED IN BONE METABOLISM AND REMODELLING

The main hormones involved in bone metabolism and remodelling are PTH, members of the vitamin D family, oestrogens and calcitonin. Glucocorticoids (see Ch. 33) and thyroid hormone (see Ch. 34) also affect bone promoting catabolism of osteoid and, in excess, causing osteoporosis.

[1]RANKL is also sometimes confusingly termed *OPG ligand*.

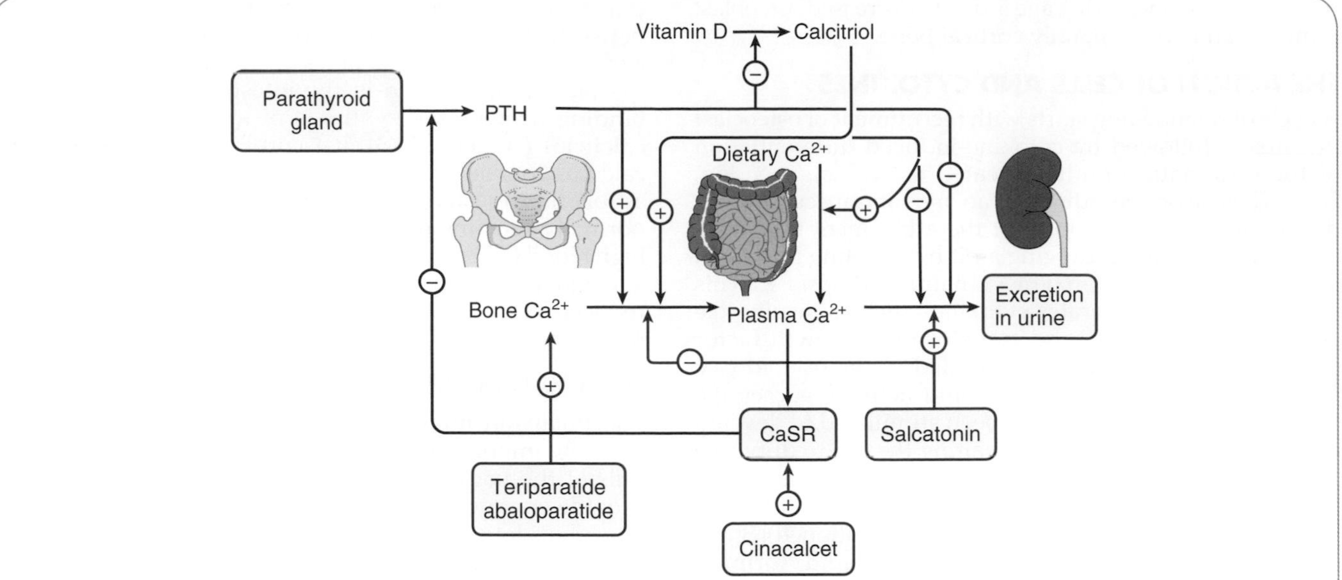

Fig. 36.3 The main factors involved in maintaining the concentration of Ca^{2+} in the plasma and the action of drugs. The calcium receptor on the parathyroid cell is a G protein–coupled receptor. Endogenous calcitonin, secreted by the thyroid, inhibits Ca^{2+} mobilisation from bone and decreases its reabsorption in the kidney, thus reducing blood Ca^{2+}. *CaSR*, Calcium-sensing receptor; *PTH*, parathyroid hormone.

PARATHYROID HORMONE

PTH, which consists of a single-chain polypeptide of 84 amino acid residues, is an important physiological regulator of Ca^{2+} metabolism. It acts on PTH type 1 receptor,[2] G protein–coupled receptors present in various tissues, especially bone - where it is expressed on osteoblast cell membranes and kidney to maintain the plasma Ca^{2+} concentration via activation of adenylyl cyclase and phospholipase C. A closely related molecule, known as PTH-related peptide (PTHrP), bears the same N-terminal end as PTH, and can activate PTH receptors in broadly similar ways (Chen, 2021). When PTH activates the osteoblast PTH type 1 receptor, osteoblasts express RANKL, which binds to RANK on osteoclasts, activating them and increasing the resorption rate.

PTH mobilises Ca^{2+} from bone, promotes its reabsorption by the kidney and stimulates the synthesis of calcitriol, which in turn increases Ca^{2+} absorption from the intestine and synergises with PTH in mobilising bone Ca^{2+} (see Figs 36.3 and 36.4). PTH promotes phosphate excretion, and thus its net effect is to increase the concentration of Ca^{2+} in the plasma and lower that of phosphate.

PTH receptors exist in two conformations (R0 and RG). Shorter duration of activation (and anabolic effect) is seen with ligands that have greater affinity for the RG conformation, whereas ligands that bind to the R0 state have a more prolonged duration of action that leads to bone resorption. Sustained elevated levels of PTH mobilise Ca^{2+} from bone and reduce renal Ca^{2+} excretion. In contrast, low intermittent therapeutic doses of PTH stimulate osteoblast activity and enhance bone formation.

[2]The type 1 receptor is the main one; the PTH type 2 receptor is also a transmembrane-spanning G protein–coupled receptor expressed in a number of tissues including central nervous system, pancreas, testis and placenta. Its functions are less well understood.

PTH is synthesised in the cells of the parathyroid glands and stored in vesicles. The principal factor controlling secretion is the concentration of ionised calcium in the plasma, low plasma Ca^{2+} stimulating secretion, high plasma Ca^{2+} decreasing it by binding to and activating a Ca^{2+}-sensing G protein–coupled surface receptor (CaSR; see Ch. 3 and Fig. 36.3). (For reviews, see Chen, 2021; Kim et al., 2021.) **Cinacalcet** increases the sensitivity of CaSR to plasma Ca^{2+}, thereby reducing PTH secretion.

Teriparatide and **abaloparatide** are shorter-chain synthetic analogues of PTH and PTHrP, respectively, licensed for treatment of osteoporosis (see later).

VITAMIN D

Vitamin D (calciferol) consists of a group of lipophilic precursors that are converted in the body into biologically active metabolites that function as true hormones, circulating in the blood and regulating the activities of various cell types (see Reichel et al., 1989). Their main action, mediated by nuclear receptors of the steroid receptor superfamily (see Ch. 3), is the maintenance of plasma Ca^{2+} by increasing Ca^{2+} absorption in the intestine, mobilising Ca^{2+} from bone and decreasing its renal excretion (see Fig. 36.3). In humans, there are two important forms of vitamin D, termed D_2 and D_3:

1. Dietary *ergocalciferol* (D_2), derived from ergosterol in plants.
2. *Cholecalciferol* (D_3), generated in the skin from 7-dehydrocholesterol by the action of ultraviolet irradiation during sun exposure, or formed from cholesterol in the wall of the intestine.

Cholecalciferol is converted to *calcifediol* (25-hydroxy-vitamin D_3) in the liver, and this is converted to a series of other metabolites of varying activity in the kidney, the most potent of which is *calcitriol* (1,25-dihydroxy-vitamin D_3); see Fig. 36.4.

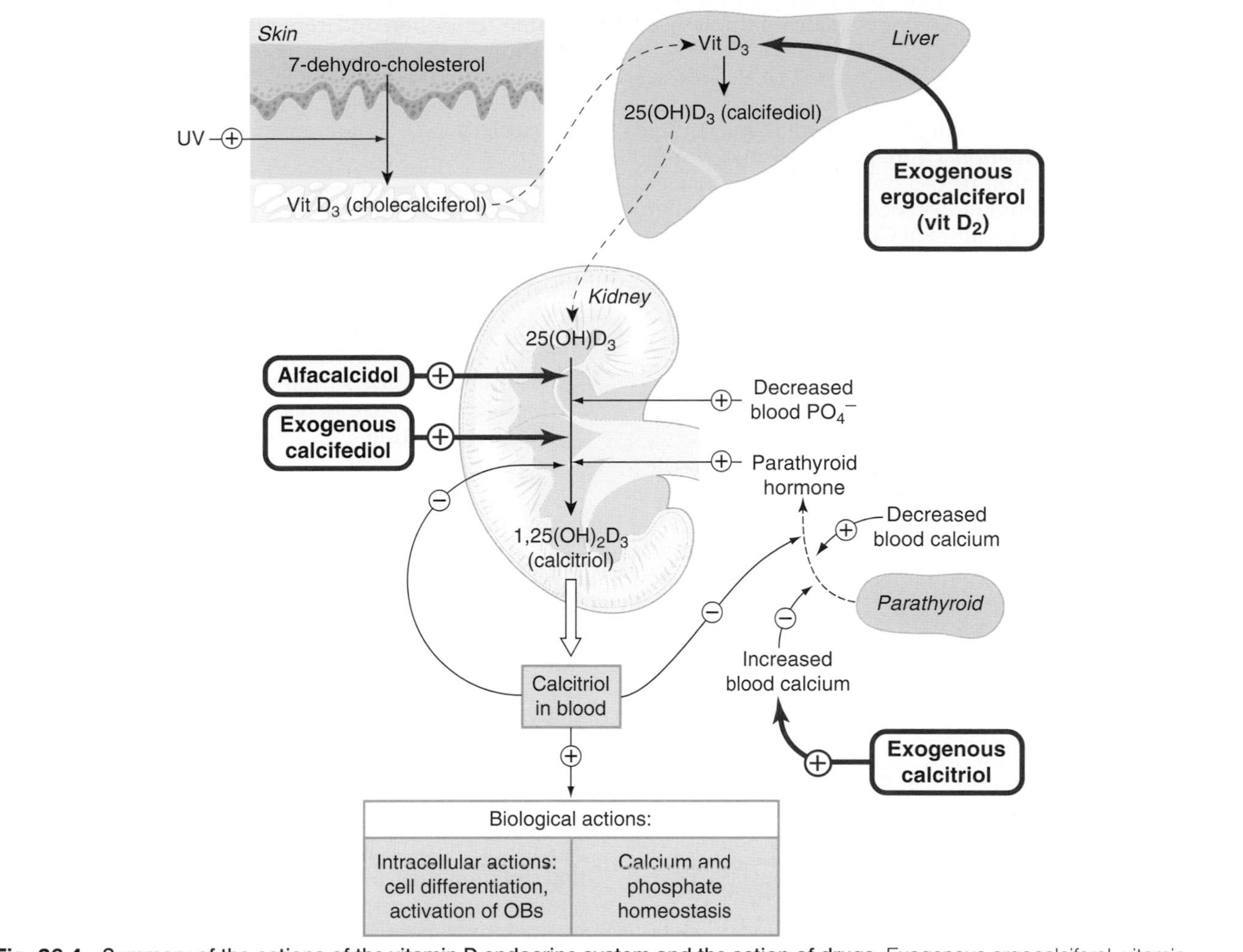

Fig. 36.4 Summary of the actions of the vitamin D endocrine system and the action of drugs. Exogenous ergocalciferol, vitamin *(vit)* D_2 (formed in plants by ultraviolet [UV] light), is converted to the corresponding D_2 metabolites in liver and kidney, as is the D_2 analogue dihydrotachysterol (not shown). Calcifediol and calcitriol are metabolites of vitamin D_3 and constitute the 'hormones' 25-hydroxy-vitamin D_3 and 1,25-dihydroxy-vitamin D_3, respectively. Alfacalcidol (1α-hydroxycholecalciferol) is 25-hydroxylated to calcitriol in the liver. *OB*, Osteoblast.

The synthesis of calcitriol from calcifediol is regulated by PTH, and is also influenced by the phosphate concentration in the plasma and by the calcitriol concentration itself through a negative feedback mechanism (see Fig. 36.4). Receptors for calcitriol are ubiquitous, and calcitriol is important in the functioning of many cell types.

The main actions of calcitriol are to stimulate absorption of Ca^{2+} and phosphate in the intestine and to mobilise Ca^{2+} from bone, but it also increases Ca^{2+} reabsorption in the kidney tubules (see Fig. 36.3). It promotes maturation of osteoclasts and stimulates their activity (see Figs 36.1 and 36.3). It decreases collagen synthesis by osteoblasts. However, the effect on bone is complex and not confined to mobilising Ca^{2+}, because in clinical vitamin D deficiency (see later section on Vitamin D Preparations), in which the mineralisation of bone is impaired, administration of vitamin D restores bone formation. One explanation may lie in the fact that calcitriol stimulates synthesis of *osteocalcin*, the Ca^{2+}-binding protein of bone matrix.

OESTROGENS

Oestrogens have an important role in maintaining bone integrity in adult women, acting on osteoblasts and osteoclasts (see Ch. 35). Oestrogen inhibits the cytokines that recruit osteoclasts and opposes the bone-resorbing, Ca^{2+}-mobilising action of PTH. It increases osteoblast proliferation, augments the production of TGF-β and BMPs and inhibits apoptosis. Withdrawal of oestrogen, as happens physiologically at the menopause, frequently leads to osteoporosis.

CALCITONIN

Calcitonin is a peptide hormone secreted by 'C' cells found in the thyroid follicles (see Ch. 34).

The main action of calcitonin is on bone; it inhibits bone resorption by binding to an inhibitory receptor on osteoclasts. In the kidney, it decreases the reabsorption of Ca^{2+} and phosphate in the proximal tubules. Its overall effect is to decrease the plasma Ca^{2+} concentration (see Fig. 36.3).

Secretion is determined mainly by the plasma Ca^{2+} concentration. A calcitonin analogue, **salcatonin**, is used clinically (see later).

OTHER HORMONES

Physiological concentrations of glucocorticoids are required for osteoblast differentiation. Higher concentrations inhibit bone formation by inhibiting osteoblast differentiation and activity, and may stimulate osteoclast action – leading to osteoporosis, which is a feature of Cushing's syndrome (see Fig. 33.7) and an important adverse effect of glucocorticoid administration (see Ch. 33).

Thyroxine stimulates osteoclast action, reducing bone density and liberating Ca^{2+}. Osteoporosis occurs in association with thyrotoxicosis, and it is important not to use excessive thyroxine for treating hypothyroidism (see Ch. 34).

Parathyroid hormone, vitamin D and bone mineral homeostasis

- The vitamin D family give rise to true hormones; precursors are converted to calcifediol in the liver, then to the main hormone, calcitriol, in the kidney.
- Calcitriol increases plasma Ca^{2+} by mobilising it from bone, increasing its absorption in the intestine and decreasing its excretion by the kidney.
- Parathyroid hormone (PTH) acts mainly on the PTH type 1 receptor on osteoblasts and in the kidney. Intermittent stimulation of PTH receptors with synthetic PTH analogues stimulates bone formation.
- Calcitonin (secreted from the thyroid) reduces Ca^{2+} resorption from bone by inhibiting osteoclast activity.

DISORDERS OF BONE

The reduction of bone mass with distortion of the microarchitecture is termed *osteoporosis*; a reduction in the mineral content is termed *osteopenia*. Dual-energy X-ray absorptiometry (DXA) and quantitative computed tomography are the standard methods for assessing osteoporosis severity and monitoring the effect of treatment (Riggs et al., 2012). Osteoporotic bone fractures easily after minimal trauma. The commonest causes of osteoporosis are postmenopausal deficiency of oestrogen and age-related deterioration in bone homeostasis. It is estimated that 50% of women and 20% of men over the age of 50 will have a fracture due to osteoporosis. With increasing life expectancy, osteoporosis has increased to epidemic proportions and is an important public health problem, affecting about 75 million people in the United States, Japan and Europe. Other predisposing factors include catabolic hormones that favour protein breakdown such as excessive thyroxine or glucocorticoid administration. Other preventable or treatable diseases of bone include *osteomalacia* and *rickets* (the juvenile form of osteomalacia), in which there are defects in bone mineralisation due to vitamin D deficiency, due to either dietary deficiency of vitamin D and lack of sunlight or renal disease resulting in reduced synthesis of the active calcitriol hormone (see Ch. 29). In *Paget's disease* there is distortion of the processes of bone resorption and remodelling as a consequence of mutation in the gene that codes for a ubiquitin-binding protein[3] called sequestosome 1 (Rea et al., 2013), which is a scaffold protein in the RANK/NF-κB signalling pathway (see earlier).

DRUGS USED IN BONE DISORDERS

Two types of agent are currently used for treatment of *osteoporosis*:

1. *Antiresorptive drugs* that decrease bone loss, e.g. bisphosphonates, calcitonin, *s*elective [o]*e*strogen *r*eceptor *m*odulators (SERMs), **denosumab**, calcium.
2. *Anabolic agents* that increase bone formation, e.g. PTH, **teriparatide.**

Rickets and *osteomalacia* are treated with vitamin D preparations.

Paget's disease of bone is common but only a small percentage of patients are symptomatic; if medical treatment is needed for symptoms such as bone pain, intermittent courses of bisphosphonates such as risedronate, **pamidronate** or **zoledronate** (see later) can provide benefit that lasts for a number of years. This is much more convenient than frequent injections of **salcatonin**, previously the only effective medical treatment.

BISPHOSPHONATES

Bisphosphonates (Fig. 36.5) are analogues of pyrophosphate, a normal constituent of tissue fluids that accumulates in bone and has a role in regulating bone resorption. Bisphosphonates inhibit bone resorption by an action mainly on the osteoclasts. They form tight complexes with calcium in the bone matrix and are released slowly as bone is resorbed by the osteoclasts, which are thus exposed to high local bisphosphonate concentrations.

Mechanism of action

Bisphosphonates reduce the rate of bone turnover. They can be grouped into two classes:

1. Simple compounds that are very similar to pyrophosphate (e.g. **etidronate, clodronate**). These are incorporated into ATP analogues that accumulate within the osteoclasts and promote their apoptosis.
2. Potent amino-bisphosphonates (e.g. **pamidronate**, **alendronate**, **risedronate**, **ibandronate**, **zoledronate**). These prevent bone resorption by interfering with the anchoring of cell surface proteins to the osteoclast membrane by prenylation, thereby preventing osteoclast attachment to bone (see Kim et al., 2021).

---

[3]Ubiquitin (Ch. 6) is a small regulatory protein present in almost all cells of the body ('ubiquitous'). It directs proteins to compartments in the cell, including the proteasome which destroys and recycles proteins. Ubiquitin-binding proteins interact with ubiquitinated targets and regulate diverse biological processes, including endocytosis, signal transduction, transcription and DNA repair.

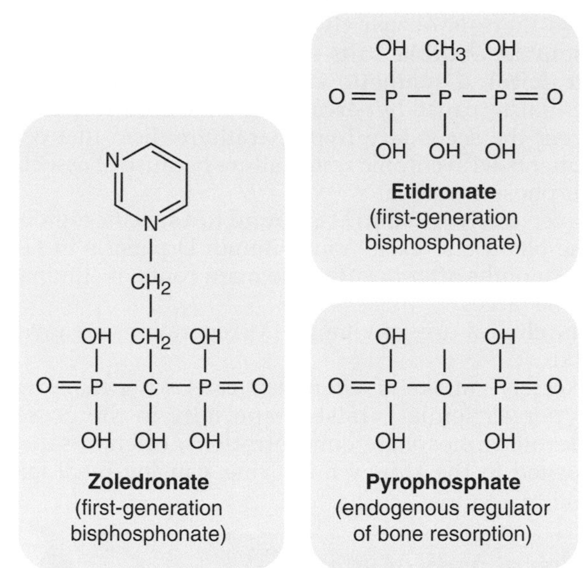

Fig. 36.5 Structure of bisphosphonates. Replacement of the oxygen atom in pyrophosphate renders the compounds enzyme-resistant. Addition of an N-containing side chain alters the mechanism of action (see text) and greatly increases potency.

Pharmacokinetic aspects

Bisphosphonates given orally are taken on an empty stomach with plenty of water in a sitting or standing position at least 30 min before breakfast because of their propensity to cause severe oesophageal problems. Pamidronate, and zoledronate are administered intravenously. They are poorly absorbed from the gut. About 50% of absorbed drug accumulates at sites of bone mineralisation, where it remains adsorbed onto hydroxyapatite crystals, potentially for months or years, until the bone is resorbed. The free drug is excreted unchanged by the kidney.

Absorption is impaired by food, particularly milk, so orally administered drugs must be taken on an empty stomach.

Unwanted effects include gastrointestinal (GI) disturbances including peptic ulcers and oesophagitis (sometimes with erosions or stricture formation). Bone pain occurs occasionally. Atypical femoral fractures are described during long-term treatment, especially of osteoporosis, and the need for continued use should be re-evaluated periodically (e.g. after 5 years). Given intravenously, some bisphosphonates (in particular zoledronate) can lead to osteonecrosis (literally 'death of bone') of the jaw, especially in patients with malignant disease; a dental check is needed before treatment, followed by any indicated remedial work before initiating treatment. After zoledronate infusion supplemental calcium and vitamin D are administered for at least 10 days.

Clinical use

Alendronate, ibandronate and risedronate are given orally for prophylaxis and treatment of osteoporosis. Etidronate is an alternative. Clodronate is used in patients with malignant disease involving bone and pamidronate is given by intravenous infusion to treat hypercalcaemia of malignancy or to treat Paget's disease. Ibandronate can also be given intravenously every 3–4 weeks in patients with breast cancer metastatic to bone, or every 3 months to treat postmenopausal osteoporosis. Zoledronate, which is given as an intravenous infusion, is used for advanced malignancy involving bone, for Paget's disease and for selected cases of osteoporosis (postmenopausal or in men) when it is administered once a year or even less frequently (see next clinical box).

Bisphosphonates

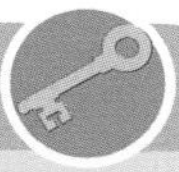

- Orally active, stable analogues of pyrophosphate, which are incorporated into remodelling bone and remain there for months to years.
- Released when osteoclast-mediated bone resorption occurs, exposing osteoclasts to their effects.
- First-generation compounds (e.g. **etidronate**) act by promoting apoptosis of osteoclasts.
- Second-generation compounds (e.g. **risedronate**) with N-containing side chains are much more potent, and prevent osteoclast action by inhibiting prenylation reactions required for membrane anchoring of functional surface proteins.
- Used long term for prevention and treatment of osteoporosis, and for symptomatic Paget's disease.
- Main unwanted effect is gastrointestinal (especially oesophageal) disturbance; a rare but serious adverse effect of the most potent drugs (notably **zoledronate**) is osteonecrosis of the jaw.

Clinical uses of bisphosphonates

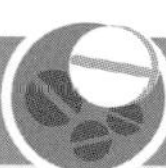

- Osteoporosis:
  - 'primary' prevention of fractures in high-risk individuals (e.g. with established osteoporosis, several risk factors for osteoporosis, chronic treatment with systemic glucocorticoids);
  - 'secondary' prevention after an osteoporotic fracture;
  - **alendronate** by mouth, given daily or once weekly in addition to calcium with vitamin D_3. **Risedronate** or **etidronate** are alternatives; **zoledronate** is given once a year by intravenous infusion; it is the most potent bisphosphonate and more likely to cause osteonecrosis of the jaw – dental check and remedial dental work are prerequisites of treatment.
- *Malignant disease* involving bone (e.g. metastatic breast cancer, multiple myeloma):
  - to reduce bone damage, pain and hypercalcaemia (e.g. **clodronate**, **ibandronate**, **zoledronate**).
- *Paget's disease* of bone (e.g. **risedronate, pamidronate, zoledronate**) administered intermittently as required in patients who are symptomatic.

OESTROGENS AND RELATED COMPOUNDS

The decline in endogenous oestrogen is a major factor in postmenopausal osteoporosis, and there is evidence that giving oestrogen as hormone replacement therapy (HRT; see Ch. 35) can ameliorate this. But HRT has actions on many systems, and newer agents (e.g. **raloxifene**; see Ch. 35) have been developed that exhibit agonist actions on some tissues and antagonist actions on others. These are termed *selective oestrogen receptor modulators* (SERMs).

RALOXIFENE

Raloxifene is a SERM that stimulates osteoblasts and inhibits osteoclasts. It also has agonist actions on the cardiovascular system, and antagonist activity on mammary tissue and the uterus.

It is well absorbed in the GI tract and undergoes extensive first-pass metabolism in the liver, yielding the glucuronide, which undergoes enterohepatic recycling. Overall bioavailability is only about 2%. Despite the low plasma concentration, raloxifene is concentrated in tissues, and is converted to an active metabolite in liver, lungs, bone, spleen, uterus and kidney. Its half-life averages 32 h. It is excreted mainly in the faeces.

Unwanted effects include hot flushes, leg cramps, flu-like symptoms and peripheral oedema. Less common are thrombophlebitis and thromboembolism. Other uncommon adverse effects are thrombocytopenia, GI disturbances, rashes, raised blood pressure and arterial thromboembolism. Raloxifene is not recommended for primary prevention of osteoporotic fractures but is one alternative to a bisphosphonate for secondary prevention in postmenopausal women who cannot tolerate a bisphosphonate.

PARATHYROID HORMONE AND ANALOGUES

PTH and fragments of PTH given in small doses paradoxically *stimulate* osteoblast activity and *enhance* bone formation, and are used to treat osteoporosis, especially in those who are receiving systemic corticosteroids. The main compound currently used is **teriparatide** – the peptide fragment (1–34) of recombinant PTH. A closely related molecule, abaloparatide (consisting of the 34 amino acids in human PTHrP), is licensed for postmenopausal women with osteoporosis who are at high risk of fracture. It is thought that the greater affinity of abaloparatide for the RG conformation of the PTH-1 receptor can result in increased bone formation without provoking bone resorption.

Teriparatide reverses osteoporosis by stimulating new bone formation. It increases bone mass, structural integrity and bone strength by increasing the number of osteoblasts and by activating those osteoblasts already in bone. It also reduces osteoblast apoptosis.

Teriparatide is given subcutaneously once daily. It is well tolerated, and serious adverse effects are few. Nausea, dizziness, headache and arthralgias can occur. Mild hypercalcaemia, transient orthostatic hypotension and leg cramps have been reported. Owing to concerns regarding long-term efficacy and safety, the maximal treatment duration of teriparatide should be limited to 24 months and must not be repeated.

VITAMIN D PREPARATIONS

Vitamin D preparations are used in the treatment of vitamin D deficiencies, bone problems associated with renal failure ('renal osteodystrophy') and hypoparathyroidism – acute hypoparathyroidism is treated with intravenous calcium and injectable vitamin D preparations.

The main vitamin D preparation used clinically is **ergocalciferol**. Other preparations are **alfacalcidol** and **calcitriol**. All can be given orally and are well absorbed unless there is obstructive liver disease (vitamin D is fat soluble, and bile salts are necessary for absorption). **Paricalcitol,** a synthetic vitamin D analogue with less potential to cause hypercalcaemia, is used to treat and prevent the secondary hyperparathyroidism that occurs in patients with chronic renal failure because of associated hyperphosphataemia.

Given orally, vitamin D is bound to a specific α-globulin in the blood and exogenous vitamin D persists in fat for many months after dosing. The main route of elimination is in the faeces.

The clinical uses of vitamin D preparations are given in the box.

Excessive intake of vitamin D causes hypercalcaemia. If hypercalcaemia persists, especially in the presence of elevated phosphate concentrations, calcium salts are deposited in the kidney and urine, causing renal failure and kidney stones.

Clinical uses of vitamin D

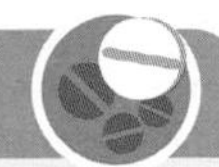

- Deficiency states: prevention and treatment of *rickets*, *osteomalacia* and vitamin D deficiency owing to *malabsorption* and *liver disease* (**ergocalciferol**).
- Hypocalcaemia caused by *hypoparathyroidism* (**ergocalciferol**).
- *Osteodystrophy* of *chronic renal failure*, which is the consequence of decreased calcitriol generation (**calcitriol** or **alfacalcidol**).

Plasma Ca^{2+} levels should be monitored during therapy with vitamin D.

BIOPHARMACEUTICALS

Denosumab is a recombinant human monoclonal antibody that inhibits RANKL, the primary signal for bone resorption (see earlier), and is particularly useful when bisphosphonates are not appropriate. It is licensed for use in men and postmenopausal women with osteoporosis who are at high risk of fracture. Denosumab can be used for prevention of skeleton-related adverse events in patients with bone metastases from solid tumours, as well as to treat bone loss in patients who are receiving hormone ablation therapy for breast or prostate cancer. Calcium and vitamin D deficiencies need to be corrected and necessary dental work needs to be undertaken before treatment with denosumab to reduce the risk of osteonecrosis of the jaw (as with potent bisphosphonates, see clinical box). It is administered as subcutaneous injections (60 mg) every 6 months for women with postmenopausal osteoporosis or men with prostate cancer at increased risk of osteoporosis because of hormone ablation, or more frequently (monthly) in patients with bone metastases. Adverse effects include altered bowel habit (diarrhoea or constipation), dyspnoea, hypocalcaemia, hypophosphataemia, infection (including respiratory, ear, cellulitis) or rash as well as (rarely) osteonecrosis of the jaw.

Romosozumab is a monoclonal antibody that binds to and inhibits sclerostin. Clinical data show that romosozumab enhances bone formation through greater recruitment of osteoprogenitor cells and increased bone matrix production by osteoblasts. There is also reduced bone resorption through inhibition of osteoclasts (McClung, 2017). The dual effect of romosozumab (Fig 36.2) is evidenced by demonstrable increases in procollagen Type I N terminal (a marker of bone formation) accompanied by reduction in type-1 collagen C-telopeptide (a marker of bone resorption).

Romosozumab is indicated for severe osteoporosis in postmenopausal women at high risk of fracture. It is given by subcutaneous injection once a month for a maximum treatment period of a year, following which patients should be offered antiresorptive therapy. There are still ongoing uncertainties surrounding possible cardiovascular risk with romosozumab, and it is currently contraindicated in women with a history of myocardial infarction or stroke.

CALCITONIN

The main preparation available for clinical use (see the clinical box) is **salcatonin** (synthetic salmon calcitonin). Synthetic human calcitonin is also available. Calcitonin is given by subcutaneous or intramuscular injection, and there may be a local inflammatory action at the injection site. It can also be given intranasally, which is more convenient but less effective. Its plasma half-life is 4–12 min, but its action lasts for several hours.

Unwanted effects include nausea and vomiting. Facial flushing may occur, as may a tingling sensation in the hands and an unpleasant taste in the mouth.

Clinical uses of calcitonin/salcatonin

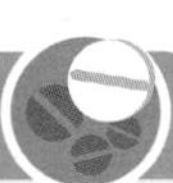

These agents are now less used.

- *Hypercalcaemia* (e.g. associated with neoplasia).
- *Paget's disease* of bone (to relieve pain and reduce neurological complications) – but it is much less convenient than an injected high-potency bisphosphonate.
- Postmenopausal and corticosteroid-induced *osteoporosis* (with other agents). Calcitonin can also be used to relieve severe back pain in patients with acute osteoporotic vertebral fractures.

CALCIUM SALTS

Calcium salts used therapeutically include **calcium gluconate** and **calcium lactate**, given orally. Calcium gluconate is also used for intravenous injection in emergency treatment of hyperkalaemia (see Ch. 29); intramuscular injection is not used because it causes local necrosis.

Calcium carbonate, an antacid and phosphate binder (see Ch. 29), is usually very poorly absorbed from the gut (an advantage since an effect within the stomach or intestine is the desired outcome for a drug intended to buffer gastric acid and to reduce ileal phosphate absorption), but there is concern that low-level systemic absorption has the potential to cause arterial calcification in patients with renal failure, especially if complicated by hyperphosphataemia (the product of calcium and phosphate ion concentrations is sometimes used clinically to estimate the risk of tissue deposition of insoluble calcium phosphate).

Unwanted effects: oral calcium salts can cause GI disturbance. Intravenous administration in emergency treatment of hyperkalaemia requires care, especially in patients receiving cardiac glycosides, the toxicity of which is influenced by extracellular calcium ion concentration (see Ch. 20).

The clinical uses of calcium salts are given in the clinical box.

Clinical uses of calcium salts

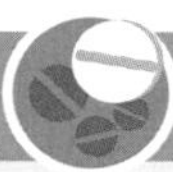

- Dietary deficiency.
- Hypocalcaemia caused by *hypoparathyroidism* or *malabsorption* (intravenous for acute tetany).
- Calcium carbonate is an antacid; it is poorly absorbed and binds phosphate in the gut. It is used to treat *hyperphosphataemia* (see Ch. 29).
- Prevention and treatment of *osteoporosis* (often with oestrogen or SERMs in women, bisphosphonate, vitamin D).
- Cardiac dysrhythmias caused by severe *hyperkalaemia* (intravenous; see Ch. 29).

CALCIMIMETIC COMPOUNDS

Calcimimetics enhance the sensitivity of the parathyroid Ca^{2+}-sensing receptor to the concentration of blood Ca^{2+}, with a consequent decrease in secretion of PTH and reduction in serum Ca^{2+} concentration. There are two types of calcimimetics:

1. Type I are agonists and include various inorganic and organic cations; Sr^{2+} is an example.
2. Type II are allosteric activators (see Ch. 3) that activate the receptor indirectly. Examples include **cinacalcet**, which is an oral preparation used for the treatment of hyperparathyroidism (see Fig. 36.3), and **etelcalcetide,** an injectable formulation that has a longer elimination half-life than cinacalcet (Hamano et al., 2017). Etelcalcetide is used to treat secondary hyperparathyroidism in patients with chronic renal failure undergoing haemodialysis. It is administered intravenously at the end of dialysis.

REFERENCES AND FURTHER READING

Bone disorders and bone remodelling

Boyce, B.F., Xing, L., 2008. Functions of RANKL/RANK/OPG in bone modeling and remodeling. Arch. Biochem. Biophys. 473, 139–146.

Chen, T., Wang, Y., Hao, Z., et al., 2021. Parathyroid hormone and its related peptides in bone metabolism. Biochem. Pharmacol. 192, 114669.

Imai, Y., Youn, M.Y., Inoue, K., 2013. Nuclear receptors in bone physiology and diseases. Physiol. Rev. 93, 481–523.

McClung, M.R., 2017. Clinical utility of anti-sclerostin antibodies. Bone 96, 3–7.

Rea, S.L., Walsh, J.P., Layfield, R., Ratajczak, T., Xu, J., 2013. New insights into the role of sequestosome 1/p62 mutant proteins in the pathogenesis of Paget's disease of bone. Endocrine Rev. 34, 501–524.

Reichel, H., Koeftler, H.P., Norman, A.W., 1989. The role of the vitamin D endocrine system in health and disease. N. Engl. J. Med. 320, 980–991.

Riggs, B.L., Khosla, S., Melton, L.J., 2012. Better tools for assessing osteoporosis. J. Clin. Invest. 122, 4323–4324.

Drugs used to treat bone disorders

Hamano, N., Komaba, H., Fukagawa, M., 2017. Etelcalcetide for the treatment of secondary hyperparathyroidism. Expert Opin. Pharmacother. 18, 529–534.
Harslof, T., Langdahl, B.L., 2016. New horizons in osteoporosis therapies. Curr. Opin. Pharmacol. 28, 38–42.
Kim, B., Cho, Y.J., Lim, W., 2021. Osteoporosis therapies and their mechanisms of action (Review). Exp. Ther. Med. 22, 1379.
van der Burgh, A.C., de Keyser, C.E., Zillikens, M.C., et al., 2021. The effects of osteoporotic and non-osteoporotic medications on fracture risk and bone mineral density. Drugs 81, 1831–1858.

Chemical transmission and drug action in the central nervous system

37

OVERVIEW

Brain function is the single most important aspect of physiology that defines human beings. Disorders of brain function, whether primary or secondary to malfunction of other systems, are a major concern of human society, and a field in which pharmacological intervention plays a key role. In this chapter we introduce some basic principles of neuropharmacology and, importantly, recognise that much of how the brain works is still not well understood and incredibly complex. This can make understanding how drugs interact with the central nervous system (CNS) challenging, particularly when trying to relate molecular mechanisms to functional effects.

INTRODUCTION

There are two reasons why understanding the action of drugs on the central nervous system (CNS) presents a particularly challenging problem. The first is that centrally acting drugs are of special significance to humankind. Not only are they of major therapeutic importance,[1] but they are also the drugs that humans most commonly administer to themselves for non-medical reasons (e.g. alcohol, tea and coffee, nicotine, cannabis, MDMA (ecstasy), opioids, cocaine, amphetamines and so on). The second reason is that the CNS is functionally far more complex than any other system in the body (also uniquely protected by a blood–brain barrier), and this makes the understanding of drug effects very much more difficult. The relationship between the behaviour of individual cells and that of the organ, as a whole, is far less direct in the brain than in other organs. Currently, the links between a drug's action at the biochemical and cellular level and its effects on brain function remain largely mysterious. Functional brain imaging is beginning to reveal relationships between brain activity in specific regions and mental function, and this tool is being used increasingly to probe drug effects. Despite sustained progress in understanding the cellular and biochemical effects produced by centrally acting drugs, and the increasing use of brain imaging to study brain function and drug effects, the gulf between our understanding of drug action at the cellular level and at the functional and behavioural level remains, for the most part, very wide.

Unlike other examples in medicine, the causes of most diseases which affect the brain remain poorly understood and the drugs used in their treatment act to modify the symptoms rather than targeting a known underlying cause. An exception to this is the relationship between dopaminergic pathways in the extrapyramidal system and the effects of drugs in alleviating or exacerbating the motor symptoms associated with Parkinson's disease (see Ch. 40).

Many CNS drugs are used to treat psychiatric disorders and the original treatments on which all current medications are based were first discovered without any knowledge of the underlying causes of the symptoms. With advances in pharmacology, we now have a good understanding of the molecular mechanisms through which these drugs exert their effects and some insights into how these relate to their clinical effects versus side effects. This knowledge has guided the development of drugs with better tolerability but the limited knowledge of the underlying pathophysiology has prevented a more rational approach to designing drugs which can prevent or cure the disorder. Studies are starting to reveal how complex genetic, environmental and psychological factors contribute to psychiatric disorders, and disease-related cognitive deficits may further contribute to the behavioural symptoms. In many CNS disorders, cognitive and emotional symptoms can develop alongside the primary illness leading to comorbid psychiatric symptoms. For example in chronic pain the affective state (mood) of the sufferer may be changed and exacerbate the painful condition. Much effort is going into pinning down the biological basis of psychiatric disorders – a necessary step to improve the design of better drugs for clinical use – but the task is daunting and progress is slow.

In this chapter we outline the general principles governing the action of drugs on the CNS. Most neuroactive drugs work by interfering with the chemical signals that underlie brain function, and the next two chapters discuss the major CNS transmitter systems and the ways in which drugs affect them.

Background information will be found in neurobiology and neuropharmacology textbooks such as Kandel et al. (2021), Nestler et al. (2020) and Stahl (2021).

CHEMICAL SIGNALLING IN THE NERVOUS SYSTEM

Brain activity is essentially mediated by electrical signals which are modulated and refined by chemical signalling to control the main functions across timescales ranging from milliseconds (e.g. returning a 100 mph tennis serve) to years (e.g. remembering how to ride a bicycle).[2] The chemical signalling mechanisms cover a correspondingly wide dynamic range, as summarised, in

[1]In England between November 2020 and October 2021, there were nearly 220 million prescriptions, costing £1.46 billion, for CNS drugs as defined by the *British National Formulary section 4*. This amounted to over three prescriptions per person across the whole population.

[2]Memory of drug names and the basic facts of pharmacology seems to come somewhere in the middle of this range (skewed towards the short end).

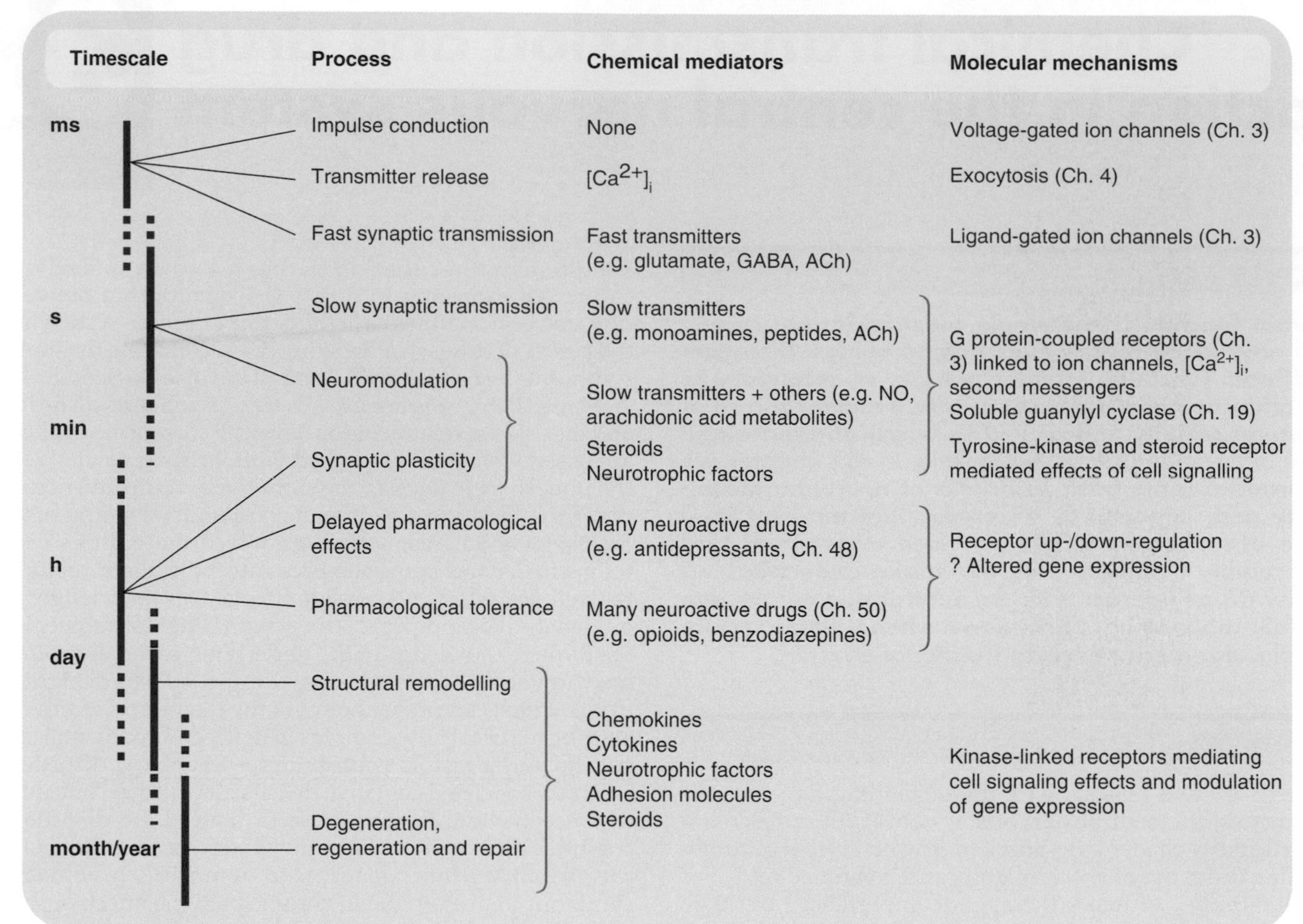

Fig. 37.1 Chemical signalling in the nervous system. Knowledge of the mediators and mechanisms becomes sparser as we move from the rapid events of synaptic transmission to the slower ones involving remodelling and alterations of gene expression. *ACh*, Acetylcholine; *CNS*, central nervous system; *NO*, nitric oxide.

a very general way, in Fig. 37.1. Currently, we understand much about drug effects on events at the fast end of the spectrum - synaptic transmission and neuromodulation - but much less about long-term adaptive processes including the interactions between chemical signalling and psychological processes. It is quite evident that the latter are of great importance for neurological and psychiatric disorders and are susceptible to drug treatment.

The original concept of neurotransmission envisaged a substance released by one neuron and acting rapidly, briefly and at short range on the membrane of an adjacent (postsynaptic) neuron, causing excitation or inhibition. The principles outlined in Chapter 13 apply to the central as well as the peripheral nervous system. It is now clear that chemical mediators within the brain also produce slow and long-lasting effects, that they can act rather diffusely, at a considerable distance from their site of release (e.g. GABA acting at extrasynaptic $GABA_A$ receptors (see Ch. 38) and monoamine transmitters (see Ch. 39) and that they can also produce other diverse effects, for example on transmitter synthesis, on the expression of receptors and on neuronal morphology, in addition to affecting the ionic conductance of the postsynaptic cell membrane. The term *neuromodulator* is often used to denote a mediator, the actions of which do not conform to the original neurotransmitter concept. The term is not clearly defined, and it covers not only the monoamine transmitters and diffusely acting neuropeptide mediators, but also mediators such as nitric oxide (NO; see Ch. 19) and arachidonic acid metabolites (see Ch. 17), which are not stored and released like conventional neurotransmitters, and may come from non-neuronal cells, particularly glia, as well as neurons. In general, *neuromodulation* relates to signalling which alters the outcome of the primary signal. This can include inducing changes in intrinsic firing activity, modulation of voltage-dependent currents, regulation of presynaptic transmitter release and longer-term adaptations including synaptic plasticity. Fig 37.2 shows a confocal microscopy image of a noradrenergic neuron illustrating the varicosities along the axon where the neuromodulator is released. Longer-term *neurotrophic* effects are involved in regulating the growth and morphology of neurons, as well as their functional properties. Table 37.1 summarises the types of chemical mediator that operate in the CNS.

Glial cells are the main non-neuronal cells in the CNS and outnumber neurons by 10 to 1. Once thought of mainly as housekeeping cells, whose function was merely to look after the fastidious neurons, glial cells, particularly astrocytes, are increasingly seen as 'inexcitable neurons' with major communications roles (see Matsas and Tsacopolous, 2013; Vasile et al., 2017). These cells express

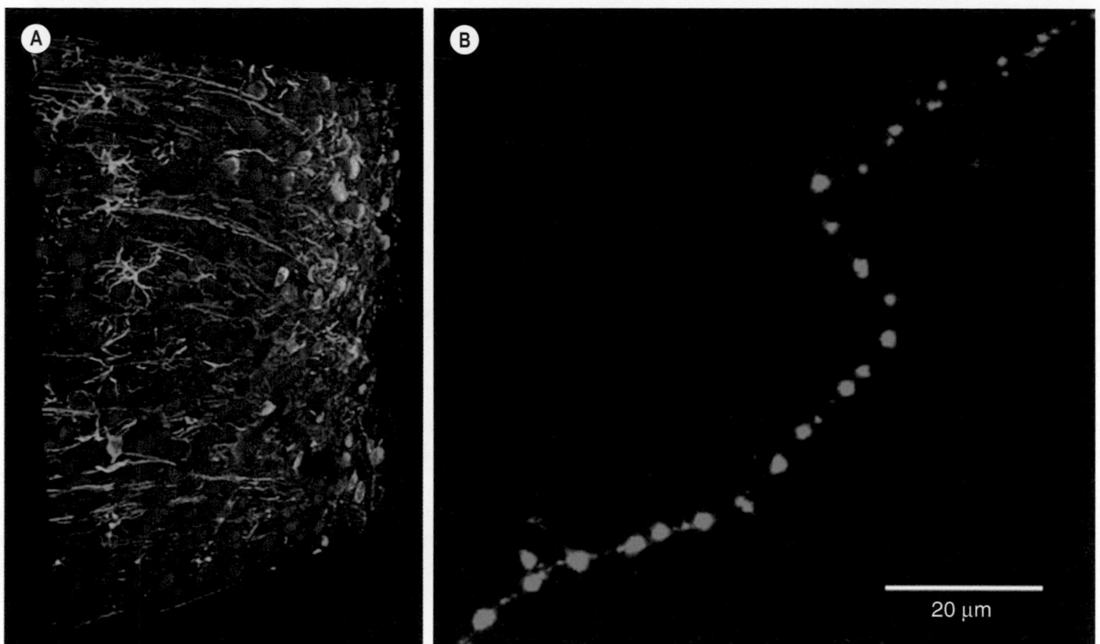

Fig. 37.2 Cellular imaging methods using fluorescence conjugated antibodies provide a means to visualise specific neuronal populations based on their expression of unique proteins. Here are selected example illustrations. (A) Confocal image of the rat prefrontal cortex illustrating glutamatergic *(green/yellow)*, GABAergic *(red)* and glia *(blue)*. (B) A single noradrenergic axon with varicosities, the sites where noradrenaline release is expected to occur. (Image A, kindly provided by Dr Abigail Benn and B, by Dr Anja Teschemacher.)

Table 37.1 Types of chemical mediators in the central nervous system

Mediator type[a]	Examples	Targets	Main functional role
Conventional small-molecule mediators	Glutamate, GABA, acetylcholine, dopamine, 5-hydroxytryptamine, etc.	Ligand-gated ion channels G protein–coupled receptors	Fast and slow synaptic neurotransmission Neuromodulation
Neuropeptides	Substance P, neuropeptide Y, endorphins, orexins, corticotrophin-releasing factor, etc.	G protein–coupled receptors	Neuromodulation
Lipid mediators	Prostaglandins, endocannabinoids	G protein–coupled receptors	Neuromodulation
'Gaseous' mediators	Nitric oxide, carbon monoxide, hydrogen sulfide, etc.	Guanylyl cyclase	Neuromodulation
Neurotrophins, cytokines	Nerve growth factor, brain-derived neurotrophic factor, interleukin-1	Kinase-linked receptors	Neuronal growth, survival and structural and functional plasticity
Steroids	Androgens, oestrogens	Nuclear and membrane receptors	Neuromodulation, neuronal metabolism, rapid and long-term effects on gene expression, structural and functional plasticity

[a]Most central nervous system pharmacology has been centred on small-molecule mediators and, less commonly, neuropeptides. Other mediator types are now being targeted for therapeutic purposes.

a range of receptors and transporters, and also release a wide variety of mediators, including glutamate, D-serine, ATP, lipid mediators and growth factors. They respond to chemical signals from neurons, and also from neighbouring astrocytes and microglial cells (the CNS equivalent of macrophages, which function much like inflammatory cells in peripheral tissues). Electrical coupling between astrocytes means they can respond in concert in a particular brain region, thus controlling the chemical environment in which the neurons operate. Although they do not conduct action potentials, and do not send signals to other parts of the body, astrocytes are otherwise very similar to neurons and play a

Chemical transmission in the central nervous system

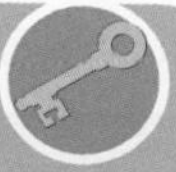

- The basic processes of synaptic transmission in the CNS are essentially similar to those operating in the periphery (see Ch. 13).
- Glial cells, particularly astrocytes, participate actively in chemical signalling, functioning essentially as 'inexcitable neurons'.
- The terms *neurotransmitter*, *neuromodulator* and *neurotrophic factor* refer to chemical mediators that operate over different timescales. In general:
  - *neurotransmitters* are released by presynaptic terminals and produce rapid excitatory or inhibitory responses in postsynaptic neurons;
  - fast neurotransmission (e.g. glutamate, GABA) operates through ligand-gated ion channels
  - slow neurotransmission (e.g. dopamine, neuropeptides, prostanoids) operate mainly through G protein–coupled receptors including pre-synaptic inhibition;
  - *neuromodulators* are released by neurons and by astrocytes, and produce slower pre- or postsynaptic responses mediated through G protein-coupled receptors;
  - *neurotrophic factors* are released by neuronal and non-neuronal cells and act on tyrosine kinase–linked receptors that regulate gene expression and control neuronal growth and phenotypic characteristics.
- The same agent (e.g. glutamate, 5-hydroxytryptamine, acetylcholine) may act through both ligand-gated channels and G protein–coupled receptors, and mediate fast and slow synaptic responses.
- Many chemical mediators, including glutamate, nitric oxide and arachidonic acid metabolites, are produced by glia as well as neurons.
- Many mediators (e.g. cytokines, chemokines, growth factors and steroids) control long-term changes in the brain (e.g. synaptic plasticity and structural remodelling) by inducing changes in gene transcription and/or modulating neurotrophic factors.

crucial communication role within the brain. Astrocytes are now thought to play an important role in synaptic plasticity and express dynamic calcium signalling events. However, despite an increasing fundamental knowledge about the role of glial cells, the development of drugs which target these mechanisms still requires more research.

TARGETS FOR DRUG ACTION

To recapitulate what was discussed in Chapters 2 and 3, neuroactive drugs act primarily on one of four types of target proteins, namely ion channels, receptors, enzymes and transport proteins. Of the four main receptor families – ionotropic receptors, G protein–coupled receptors, kinase-linked receptors and nuclear receptors – current neuroactive drugs target mainly the first two.

Since the first psychiatric drugs were discovered in the 1950s, knowledge about these targets in the CNS has accumulated rapidly, particularly as follows:

- As well as 40 or more small-molecule and peptide mediators, the importance of other 'non-classical' mediators – NO, eicosanoids, growth factors, etc. – has become apparent.
- Considerable molecular diversity of known receptor molecules and ion channels (see Ch. 3) has been revealed.
- Receptors and channels are often expressed in several subtypes, and many possess sites for allosteric modulation and exist in multiple heteromeric complexes, all of which add to the diversity of potential drug targets. In most cases, we are only beginning to discover what this diversity means at a functional level. The molecular diversity of such targets raises the possibility of developing drugs with improved selectivity of action, e.g. interacting with one kind of $GABA_A$ receptor without affecting others (see Ch. 44). The potential of these new approaches in terms of improved drugs for neurological and psychiatric diseases is large but as yet unrealised.

Our knowledge of the neurobiology of the CNS and pathophysiology of disorders such as epilepsy, neurodegenerative and psychiatric disorders is advancing and hopefully this will result in new strategies for treating these disabling conditions. Some hints of the progress which can be achieved when the underlying causes are understood can be seen with the development of the gene therapy **onasemnogene abeparvovec,** which provides a new copy of the gene that makes the human SMN protein (Ch. 40). Unfortunately though, most research is revealing just how complicated diseases of the CNS are and so there are still many challenges for the field.

DRUG ACTION IN THE CENTRAL NERVOUS SYSTEM

As already emphasised, the molecular and cellular mechanisms underlying drug action in the CNS and in the periphery have much in common. Translating from these molecular mechanisms to functional outcomes is however much more challenging for the CNS. One difficulty is the complexity of neuronal connections in the brain and the fact that much of how these neuronal networks function is not understood. In contrast to the periphery, within any region of the brain there are many different cell types and chemical mediators and the output from any single neuron arises from the integration of all these signals. Fig 37.2 illustrates this complexity in a confocal image taken from the prefrontal cortex of the rat brain where three major cell types have been visualised using specific antibodies.

The relationship between a drug's molecular effects and the functional consequences of its agonism or antagonism in the brain often causes confusion. This can be because it is assumed that the signalling mechanism associated with that receptor translates into the functional outcome, e.g. agonism of a Gi/o coupled GPCR will inhibit brain function.

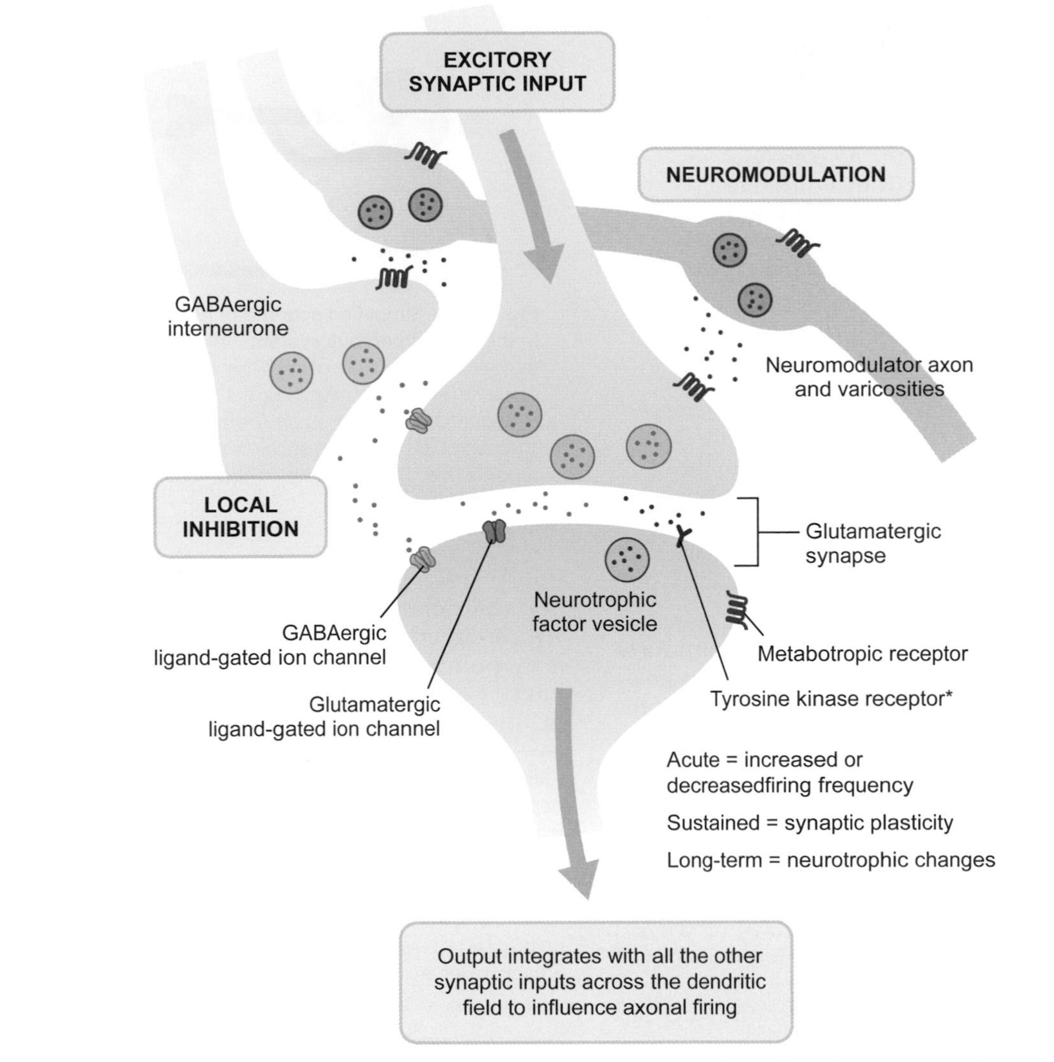

Fig 37.3 Simplified diagram of the chemical signalling at a single synapse. The amino acid transmitters together generate a balance in excitation and inhibition and this is further refined through neuromodulation. A single neuron will receive inputs across its dendritic field from both glutamatergic and GABAergic neurons as well as different neuromodulators. This figure illustrates just one of those dendritic inputs. For ease of understanding, only a single neuromodulator input is illustrated but a single neuron receives many chemical signals as well as expressing a multitude of receptors. Understanding how drugs interact within these micro- as well as macro-circuits is complicated and not fully understood.

However, there is an important step needed when relating molecular mechanisms to effects on neuronal activity and that relates to where the receptor is located. Fig 37.3 provides a schematic diagram illustrating a simple synapse with glutamatergic, GABAergic and neuromodulatory inputs. Depending on where a drug acts within this local circuit will have a major influence on the final output. For example:

- An inhibitory receptor reduces activity or transmitter release in the neuron. However, if that neuron is a GABAergic interneuron then the functional consequence will be reduced inhibition or disinhibition and an increase in activity from that region.
- An excitatory receptor increases activity or transmitter release in the neuron. However, if that neuron is a GABAergic interneuron then the consequence will be increased inhibition and a decrease in activity from that region.

Different types of interactions between neurons also add to this complexity. Fig. 37.4 provides a very simplified illustration of a neuronal network involving three neurons. In this diagram we can see different examples of the connections between neurons in the CNS including:

- *Reciprocal connections* where neuron A inputs to neuron B and neuron B also inputs to neuron A. Neuron B can modulate the function of neuron A either directly or indirectly for example via an interneuron, neuron C.
- *Presynaptic modulation of release* where either the same transmitter released by the neuron (via autoreceptors) or transmitter from a different neuron (via heteroreceptors) can alter the amount of transmitter released into the synapse. These can be inhibitory (negative feedback) or excitatory (positive feedback).
- *Multiple inputs* where any single neuron is integrating inputs from multiple chemical signals.
- Even at this grossly oversimplified level, the effects at a system level of blocking or enhancing the release or actions of one or other of the transmitters are difficult to predict and will depend greatly on the relative strength of the excitatory and inhibitory synaptic connections, and neuromodulatory inputs. Added to this complexity is the influence of glial cells, mentioned previously.

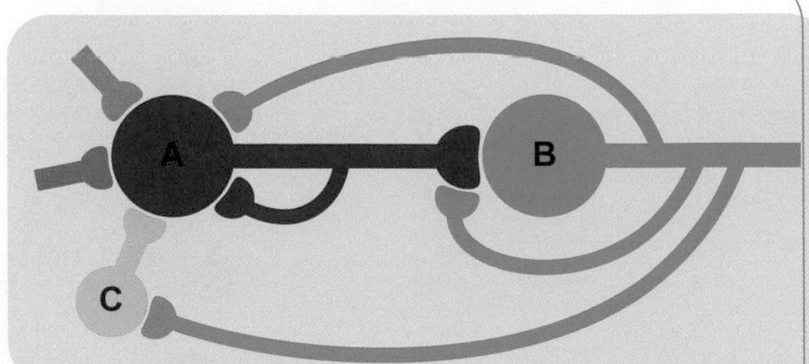

Fig. 37.4 Simplified scheme of neuronal interconnections in the central nervous system. Neurons *A*, *B* and *C* which may release excitatory or inhibitory neurotransmitters. Boutons of neuron *A* input to neuron *B*, but also neuron *A* itself. Neuron *B* also feeds back on neuron *A* either directly or indirectly via interneuron *C*. Even with such a simple network, the effects of drug-induced interference with specific transmitter systems can be difficult to predict.

The majority of drugs being used to treat CNS disorders are given over prolonged periods of time and this introduces the potential for secondary, adaptive responses set in train by any drug-induced perturbation of the system. Homeostatic responses are activated when neurotransmission is disrupted for example by an increase in transmitter release, or interference with transmitter reuptake, and countered by activation of receptor-mediated feedback mechanisms, adaptive changes such as inhibition of transmitter synthesis, enhanced transporter expression or decreased receptor expression. These changes, which can involve altered gene expression, generally take time (hours, days or weeks) to develop and are not evident in acute pharmacological experiments.

In the clinical situation, the effects of psychotropic drugs often take weeks to develop, and this has been linked to these adaptive responses rather than the immediate pharmacodynamic effects of the drug. This is well documented for antipsychotic and antidepressant drugs (see Chs 47 and 48). The development of dependence on opioids, benzodiazepines and psychostimulants is similarly gradual in onset (see Ch. 50). Thus one has to take into account not only the primary interaction of the drug with its target but also the longer-term secondary response of the brain to this primary effect; it is often this secondary response, rather than the primary effect, which is thought to lead to clinical benefit. There are also important psychological effects where the drugs change behaviour which in turn impacts on the inputs the brain receives and hence its neurochemistry, connectivity and ultimately brain morphology.

BLOOD–BRAIN BARRIER

A key factor in CNS pharmacology is the blood–brain barrier (see Ch. 9), penetration of which requires molecules to traverse the vascular endothelial cells rather than going between them. Inflammation can disrupt the integrity of the blood–brain barrier, allowing previously impermeable drugs such as **penicillin** to cross. In general, only small non-polar molecules can diffuse passively across cell membranes. Some neuroactive drugs penetrate the blood–brain barrier in this way, but many do so via transporters, which either facilitate entry into the brain or diminish it by pumping the compound from the endothelial cell interior back into the bloodstream. Drugs that gain entry in this way include **levodopa** (see Ch. 40), **valproate** (see Ch. 46) and various sedative histamine antagonists (see Ch. 17). Active extrusion of drugs from the brain occurs via P-glycoprotein, an ATP-driven drug efflux transporter, and related transporter proteins (see Ch. 9). Many antibacterial and anticancer drugs are excluded from the brain while some CNS-acting drugs – including certain opioid, antidepressant, antipsychotic and anti-epileptic drugs – are actively extruded from the brain (see Linnet and Ejsing, 2008). Variation in the activity of

Drug action in the central nervous system

- The basic types of drug target (ion channels, receptors, enzymes and transporter proteins) described in Chapter 3 apply in the CNS, as elsewhere.
- Most of these targets occur in several different molecular isoforms, giving rise to subtle differences in function and pharmacology.
- Many of the currently available neuroactive drugs are relatively non-specific, affecting several different targets at clinically relevant doses.
- The relationship between the pharmacological profile and the therapeutic effect of neuroactive drugs is often unclear. Drugs with different primary targets may be used to treat the same condition whilst the same drug may exhibit efficacy in more than one condition.
- Slowly developing secondary responses to the primary interaction of the drug with its target may be important (e.g. the delay in clinical improvements with conventional antidepressant drugs, and tolerance and dependence with opioids).

efflux transporters between individuals is an important consideration (see Chs 9 and 12).

THE CLASSIFICATION OF PSYCHOTROPIC DRUGS

Psychotropic drugs are defined as those that affect mood and behaviour. Because these indices of brain function are difficult to define and measure, there is no consistent basis for classifying psychotropic drugs. Instead, we find a confusing mêlée of terms relating to chemical structure (*benzodiazepines*, *butyrophenones*, etc.), biochemical target (*monoamine oxidase inhibitors*, *serotonin reuptake inhibitors*, etc.), behavioural effect (*hallucinogens*, *psychomotor stimulants*) or clinical use (*antidepressants*, *antipsychotic agents*, *anti-epileptic drugs*, etc.), together with a number of indefinable rogue categories (*atypical antipsychotic drugs*, *nootropic drugs*) thrown in for good measure.

Some drugs defy classification in this scheme, for example **lithium** (see Ch. 48), which is used in the treatment of bipolar disorder, and **ketamine** (see Ch. 42), which is classed as a dissociative anaesthetic and analgesic (see Ch. 42) but produces psychotropic effects rather similar to those produced by phencyclidine (PCP, see Ch. 49) and at low doses is a rapid acting antidepressant (see Ch. 48).

Table 37.2 provides a general classification of centrally acting drugs. In practice, the use of drugs in psychiatric illness frequently cuts across specific therapeutic categories. For example, antipsychotic drugs can be useful for

Table 37.2 General classification of drugs acting on the central nervous system

Class	Definition	Examples	See chapter
General anaesthetic agents	Drugs used to produce surgical anaesthesia	Isoflurane, desflurane, propofol, etomidate	41
Analgesic drugs	Drugs used clinically for controlling pain	Opiates Neuropathic pain – carbamazepine, gabapentin, amitriptyline, duloxetine	43
Anxiolytics and sedatives	Drugs that reduce anxiety and cause sleep	Benzodiazepines (e.g. diazepam, chlordiazepoxide, flurazepam, clonazepam)	45
Anti-epileptic drugs Synonym: anticonvulsants	Drugs used to reduce seizures	Carbamazepine, valproate, lamotrigine	46
Antipsychotic drugs Synonym: neuroleptics	Drugs used to relieve the symptoms of schizophrenic illness	Clozapine, haloperidol, risperidone	47
Antidepressant drugs	Drugs used to treat affective disorders including major depressive disorder and generalised anxiety disorder	Selective serotonin reuptake inhibitors, tricyclic antidepressants, monoamine oxidase inhibitors	48
Psychomotor stimulants Synonym: psychostimulants	Drugs that cause wakefulness and euphoria Treatments for attention deficit hyperactivity disorder	Amphetamine, cocaine, methylphenidate, caffeine	49
Psychotomimetic drugs Synonym: hallucinogens	Drugs that cause disturbance of perception (particularly visual hallucinations) and of behaviour in ways that cannot be simply characterised as sedative or stimulant effects Induce rapid acting antidepressant effects	Ketamine, PCP, DMT Lysergic acid, psilocybin diethylamide, mescaline, MDMA (ecstasy)	49
Cognition enhancers Synonym: nootropic drugs	Used to reduce the cognitive impairments in neurodegenerative disorders	Acetylcholinesterase inhibitors: donepezil, galantamine, rivastigmine	40
		NMDA receptor antagonists: memantine Others: piracetam, modafinil	38

DMT, N-Dimethyltryptamine; *MDMA*, 3,4-methylenedioxymethamphetamine; *NMDA*, *N*-methyl-D-aspartate; *PCP*, phenylcyclohexyl piperidine.

Table 37.3 Examples of some of the different clinical uses for CNS drugs

Drug (class)	Mechanism of action	Clinical uses[a]
Amitriptyline (tricyclic antidepressant)	Serotonin and noradrenaline re-uptake inhibitor	**Major depressive disorder** Generalised anxiety disorder Chronic pain
Pregabalin (gabapentinoid)	$\alpha 2\delta$ subunit-containing voltage-gated calcium channel inhibitor	**Epilepsy** Generalised anxiety disorder Chronic pain
Carbamazepine (anticonvulsant)	Voltage-gated sodium channel blocker	**Epilepsy** Bipolar disorder Chronic pain

[a]Bold text signifies first licensed indication.

managing both acute and chronic behavioural disorders, including being used for acute drug-induced psychosis and short-term management of agitation and aggression in dementia patients (see Ch. 47). Certain antidepressant drugs are also first-line treatment for most anxiety disorders (see Ch. 45) as well as neuropathic pain (see Ch. 43), and certain psychostimulants are effective at reducing the symptoms of ADHD (see Ch. 49). Here we adhere to the conventional pharmacological categories, but it needs to be emphasised that in clinical use these distinctions are often disregarded.[3] An illustration of the diversity of clinical uses of some exemplar drugs is given in Table 37.3.

[3]The Neuroscience based Nomenclature (NbN) is a publication and a digital application of psychiatric medications developed by the European College of Neuropsychopharmacology to classify psychiatric drugs by their pharmacology and mode of action and may become a more common way of discussing these treatments in the future (https://nbn2r.com/).

REFERENCES AND FURTHER READING

Kandel, E.R., Koester, J.D., Mack, S.H., Siegelbaum, S.A., 2021. Principles of Neural Science, sixth ed. Elsevier, New York.

Linnet, K., Ejsing, T.B., 2008. A review on the impact of P-glycoprotein on the penetration of drugs into the brain. Focus on psychotropic drugs. Eur. Neuropsychopharmacol. 18, 157–169.

Matsas, R., Tsacopolous, M., 2013. The functional roles of glial cells in health and disease: dialogue between glia and neurons. Adv. Exp. Biol. Med. 468.

Nestler, E.J., Hyman, S.E., Holzman, M., Malenka, R.C., 2020. Molecular Neuropharmacology: A Foundation for Clinical Neuroscience, fourth ed. McGraw-Hill, New York.

Prus, A., 2020. Drugs and the Neuroscience of Behavior: An Introduction to Psychopharmacology. Sage Publications, Inc, Los Angeles.

Stahl, S.M., 2021. Stahl's Essential Psychopharmacology: Neuroscientific Basis and Practical Applications, fifth ed. Cambridge University Press, Cambridge.

Vasile, F., Dossi, E., Rouach, N., 2017. Human astrocytes: structure and function in the healthy brain. Brain Struct. Funct. 222, 2017–2029.

Amino acid transmitters 38

OVERVIEW

In this chapter we discuss the major neurotransmitters in the central nervous system (CNS), namely the excitatory transmitter, glutamate and the inhibitory transmitters, γ-aminobutyric acid (GABA) and glycine. These two transmitters work together to control the level of excitability within a brain region – the excitatory/inhibitory balance. Drugs can shift the excitatory/inhibitory balance with effects ranging from loss of consciousness to seizures. It is an area in which scientific interest has been intense in recent years. Unravelling the complexities of amino acid receptors and signalling mechanisms has thrown considerable light on their role in brain function and their likely involvement in CNS disease. Drugs that target specific receptors and transporters have been developed, but translating this knowledge into drugs for therapeutic use is proving challenging. Here, we present the pharmacological principles and include recent references for those seeking more detail.

EXCITATORY AMINO ACIDS

EXCITATORY AMINO ACIDS AS CNS TRANSMITTERS

L-Glutamate is the principal and ubiquitous excitatory transmitter in the CNS.

The realisation of glutamate's importance came slowly (see Watkins and Jane, 2006). By the 1950s, work on the peripheral nervous system had highlighted the transmitter roles of acetylcholine and catecholamines and, as the brain also contained these substances, there seemed little reason to look further. The presence of **γ-aminobutyric acid** (GABA) in the brain, and its powerful inhibitory effect on neurons, was discovered in the 1950s, and its transmitter role was postulated. At the same time, work by Curtis's group in Canberra showed that glutamate and various other acidic amino acids produced a strong excitatory effect, but it seemed inconceivable that such workaday metabolites could actually be transmitters. Through the 1960s, GABA and excitatory amino acids (EAAs) were thought, even by their discoverers, to be mere pharmacological curiosities. In the 1970s, the humblest amino acid, glycine, was established as an inhibitory transmitter in the spinal cord, giving the lie to the idea that transmitters had to be exotic molecules, too beautiful for any role but to sink into the arms of a receptor. Once glycine had been accepted, the rest quickly followed. A major advance was the discovery of EAA antagonists, based on the work of Watkins in Bristol, which enabled the physiological role of glutamate to be established unequivocally, and also led to the realisation that EAA receptors are heterogeneous.

To do justice to the wealth of discovery in this field in the past 25 years is beyond the range of this book; for more detail see Bear et al. (2020). Here we concentrate on pharmacological aspects. With regard to novel drug development, many promising new compounds interacting with EAAs commenced development for the treatment of a wide range of neurological and psychiatric disorders but have failed because of lack of efficacy or adverse effects, and only a few drugs[1] have made it into clinical use. The field has yet to make a major impact on therapeutics. The major problem has been that EAA-mediated neurotransmission is ubiquitous in the brain and so agonist and antagonist drugs exert effects at many sites, giving rise not only to therapeutically beneficial effects but also to other, unwanted, harmful effects.

METABOLISM AND RELEASE OF EXCITATORY AMINO ACIDS

Glutamate is widely and fairly uniformly distributed in the CNS, where its concentration is much higher than in other tissues. It has an important metabolic role, the metabolic and neurotransmitter pools being linked by transaminase enzymes that catalyse the interconversion of glutamate and α-ketoglutarate (Fig. 38.1). Glutamate in the CNS comes mainly from either glucose, via the Krebs cycle, or glutamine, which is synthesised by glial cells and taken up by the neurons; very little comes from the periphery. The interconnection between the pathways for the synthesis of EAAs and inhibitory amino acids (GABA and glycine), shown in Fig. 38.1, makes it difficult to use experimental manipulations of transmitter synthesis to study the functional role of individual amino acids, because disturbance of any one step will affect both excitatory and inhibitory mediators.

Glutamate is stored in synaptic vesicles and released by Ca^{2+}-dependent exocytosis; specific transporter proteins account for its re-uptake by neurons and other cells, and for its accumulation by synaptic vesicles. Released glutamate is taken up into nerve terminals and neighbouring astrocytes (Fig. 38.1) by $Na^+/H^+/K^+$-dependent transporters (cf. monoamine transporters - see Ch. 13), and transported into synaptic vesicles, by a different transporter driven by the proton gradient across the vesicle membrane. Several EAA transporters have been cloned and characterised in detail (see Jensen et al., 2015). Glutamate transport can, under some circumstances (e.g. depolarisation by increased extracellular $[K^+]$), operate in reverse and constitute a source of glutamate release, a process that may occur under pathological conditions

[1]Perampanel, a non-competitive AMPA receptor antagonist, has been approved for the treatment of epilepsy (Ch. 46). Memantine, an NMDA antagonist, licensed for the treatment of moderate to severe Alzheimer's disease (Ch. 40), has been used for some time, as has the dissociative anaesthetic ketamine, an NMDA channel blocker (Ch. 41). Ketamine has also been found to have rapid-acting antidepressant effects (Ch. 48).

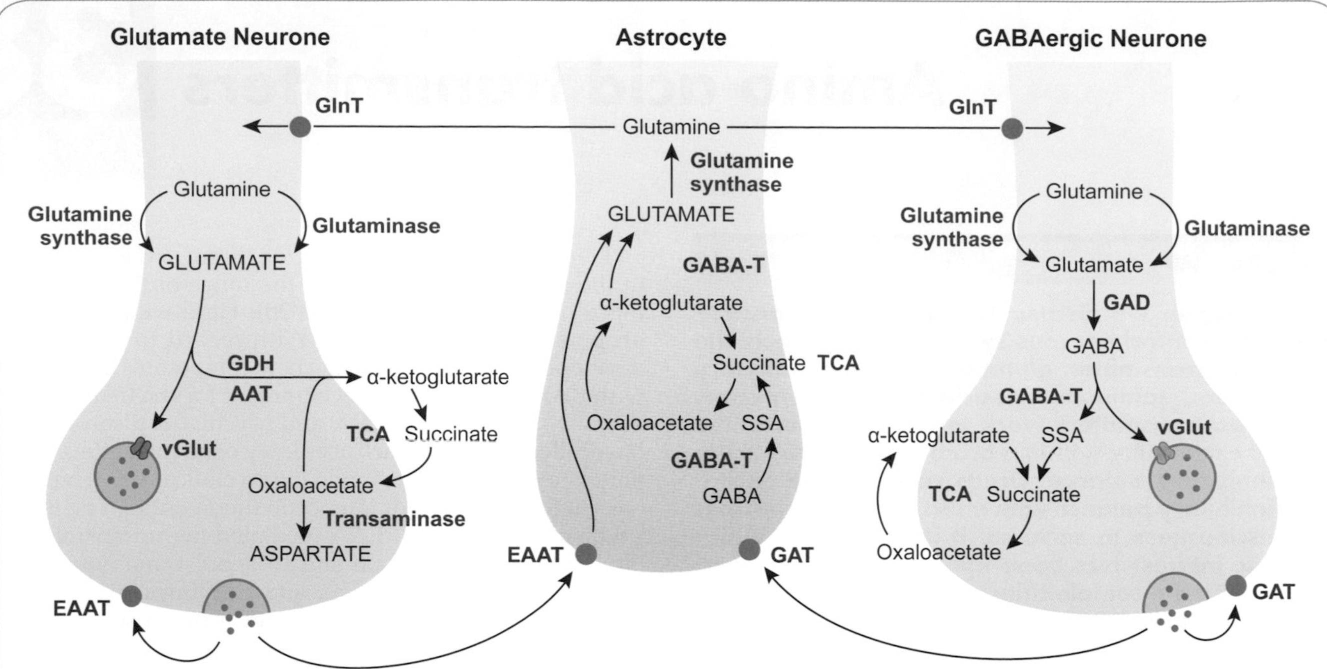

Fig. 38.1 Metabolism of transmitter amino acids in the brain. The synthesis, storage and termination of the actions of the EAA transmitters occur across neuronal and glial cells. Synthesis of the transmitter depends on the presence of key enzymes with the neurotransmitter stored into vesicles via specific vesicular transporters. Following release, neurotransmitter is taken back up into neurons and astrocytes by specific transporters. Note: although not illustrated here, the TCA takes place in the mitochondria. *AAT,* Aspartate aminotransferase; *EAAT,* excitatory amino acid transporter; *GABA,* γ-aminobutyric acid; *GABA-T,* GABA transaminase; *GAD,* glutamic acid decarboxylase; *GAT,* GABA transporter; *GDH,* glutamate dehydrogenase; *SSA,* succinic semialdehyde; *TCA,* tricarboxylic acid cycle; *vGAT,* vesicular GABA transporter; *vGlut,* vesicular glutamate transporter.

such as brain ischaemia (see Ch. 40). Glutamate taken up by astrocytes is converted to glutamine and recycled, via transporters, back to the neurons, which convert the glutamine back to glutamate (see Fig. 38.1). Glutamine, which lacks the pharmacological activity of glutamate, thus serves as a pool of inactive transmitter under the regulatory control of the astrocytes, which act as ball boys, returning the ammunition in harmless form in order to rearm the neurons.

GLUTAMATE

GLUTAMATE RECEPTOR SUBTYPES

Glutamate and related EAAs, such as aspartate and homocysteate, activate both ionotropic (ligand-gated cation channels) and metabotropic (G protein–coupled) receptors (see Ch. 3 for a general description of ionotropic and metabotropic receptors).

IONOTROPIC GLUTAMATE RECEPTORS

On the basis of studies with selective agonists and antagonists (Fig. 38.2 and Table 38.1), three main subtypes of ionotropic receptors for glutamate can be distinguished: **N-methyl-D-aspartate (NMDA)**, (*S*)-α-amino-3-hydroxy-5-methylisoxazole-4-propionic acid (**AMPA**) and **kainate**[2] receptors, named originally according to their specific agonists. These ligand-gated channels comprise four subunits, each with the 'pore loop' structure shown in Fig. 3.4 (see Ch. 3). There are some 16 different receptor subunits and their nomenclature has, until recently, been somewhat confusing.[3] Here, in this brief, general description, we use the International Union of Basic and Clinical Pharmacology (IUPHAR)-recommended terminology because it simplifies the subject considerably, but beware confusion when reading older papers. NMDA receptors are heteromers assembled from seven types of subunit (GluN1, GluN2A, GluN2B, GluN2C, GluN2D, GluN3A, GluN3B). The subunits comprising AMPA receptors (GluA1–4) and kainate receptors (GluK1–5) are closely related to, but distinct from, GluN subunits. AMPA and kainite receptors can be homomeric or heteromeric. Receptors comprising different subunits have different pharmacological and physiological characteristics, e.g. AMPA receptors lacking the GluA2 subunit have much higher permeability to Ca^{2+} than the others, which has important functional consequences (see Ch. 4). AMPA receptor subunits are also subject to other kinds of variation, namely alternative splicing, giving rise to the engagingly named *flip* and *flop* variants, RNA editing at the single amino acid level, and associated auxiliary subunits, all of which contribute yet more functional diversity to this diverse family.

[2]In the past, AMPA and kainate receptors were often lumped together as AMPA/kainate or non-NMDA receptors, but molecular studies revealed distinct subunit compositions and they should not be grouped together (see Collingridge and Abraham, 2022, for a recent review and discussion of the role of key scientists in this field).

[3]An international committee has sought to bring order to the area but, despite the logic of their recommendations, how generally accepted they will be remains to be seen (see Bettler et al., 2019, and www.guidetopharmacology.org). Scientists can get very stuck in their ways.

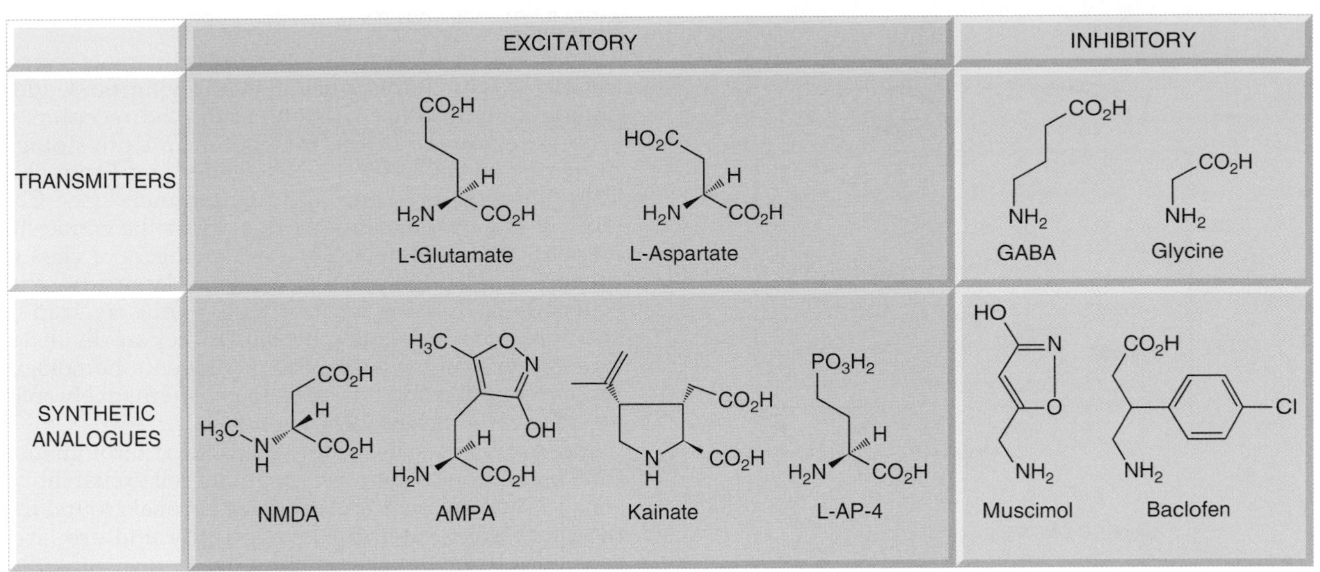

Fig. 38.2 Structures of agonists acting on glutamate, γ-aminobutyric acid (GABA) and glycine receptors. The receptor specificity of these compounds is shown in Tables 38.1 and 38.2. *AMPA*, (*S*)-α-amino-3-hydroxy-5-methylisoxazole-4-propionic acid; *L-AP4*, L-2-amino-4-phosphonopentanoic acid; *NMDA*, *N*-methyl-D-aspartic acid.

AMPA receptors, and in certain brain regions kainate receptors, serve to mediate fast excitatory synaptic transmission in the CNS – absolutely essential for our brains to function. NMDA receptors (which often coexist with AMPA receptors) contribute a slow component to the excitatory synaptic potential (Fig. 38.3B), the magnitude of which varies in different pathways. NMDA, kainate and AMPA receptors are also expressed on nerve terminals where they can enhance or reduce transmitter release.[4] AMPA receptors occur on astrocytes as well as on neurons.

Binding studies show that ionotropic glutamate receptors are most abundant in the cortex, basal ganglia and sensory pathways. NMDA and AMPA receptors are generally co-localised, but kainate receptors have a much more restricted distribution. Expression of the many different receptor subtypes in the brain also shows distinct regional differences, but we have hardly begun to understand the significance of this extreme organisational complexity.

Special features of *N*-methyl-D-aspartate receptors

NMDA receptors and their associated channels have been studied in more detail than the other types and show special pharmacological properties, summarised in Fig. 38.4, and are postulated to play a role in pathophysiological mechanisms.

- They are highly permeable to Ca^{2+}, as well as to other cations, so activation of NMDA receptors is particularly effective in promoting Ca^{2+} entry.
- They are readily blocked by Mg^{2+}, and this block shows marked voltage dependence. It occurs at physiological Mg^{2+} concentrations when the cell is normally polarised, but disappears if the cell is depolarised.
- Activation of NMDA receptors requires glycine as well as glutamate (Fig. 38.4). The binding site for glycine is distinct from the glutamate binding site, i.e. glycine is a co-agonist that acts allosterically to permit glutamate activation of the receptor (see Ch. 2), and both have to be occupied for the channel to open. This discovery by Johnson and Ascher caused a stir, because glycine had hitherto been recognised as an inhibitory transmitter, so to find it facilitating excitation ran counter to the prevailing doctrine. The concentration of glycine required depends on the subunit composition of the NMDA receptor: for some NMDA receptor subtypes, physiological variation of the glycine concentration may serve as a regulatory mechanism, whereas others are fully activated at all physiological glycine concentrations. Competitive antagonists at the glycine site (see Table 38.1) indirectly inhibit the action of glutamate. **D-serine**, somewhat surprisingly,[5] may also function as an endogenous activator of the glycine site on the NMDA receptor.
- Some endogenous polyamines (e.g. **spermine**, **spermidine**) act at an allosteric site distinct from that of glycine to facilitate channel opening. The experimental drugs **ifenprodil** and **eliprodil** block their action.
- Other allosteric sites have been identified on the NMDA receptor and positive and negative allosteric modulators with novel patterns of GluN2 subunit selectivity have been discovered (Burnell et al., 2019).

[4]In the CNS, presynaptic ligand-gated ion channels such as kainate and NMDA receptors as well as nicotinic and P2X receptors (see Ch. 39) modulate neurotransmitter release. An explanation of how this control can be either facilitatory or inhibitory is given in Schicker et al. (2008).

[5]Surprising, because it is the 'wrong' enantiomer for amino acids of higher organisms. Nevertheless, vertebrates possess specific enzymes and transporters for this D-amino acid, which is abundant in the brain.

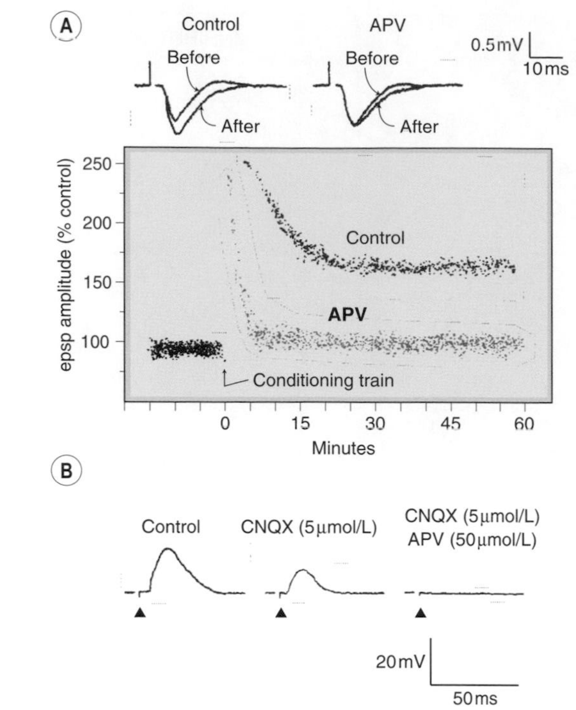

Fig. 38.3 Effects of excitatory amino acid receptor antagonists on synaptic transmission. (A) AP5 (*N*-methyl-D-aspartic acid (NMDA) antagonist) prevents long-term potentiation (LTP) in the rat hippocampus without affecting the fast excitatory postsynaptic potential (epsp). Top records show the extracellularly recorded fast epsp *(downward deflection)* before and 50 min after a conditioning train of stimuli (100 Hz for 2 s). The presence of LTP in the control preparation is indicated by the increase in epsp amplitude. In the presence of AP5 (50 μmol/L), the normal epsp is unchanged, but LTP does not occur. Lower trace shows epsp amplitude as a function of time. The conditioning train produces a short-lasting increase in epsp amplitude, which still occurs in the presence of AP5, but the long-lasting effect is prevented. (B) Block of fast and slow components of epsp by *CNQX* (6-cyano-7-nitroquinoxaline-2,3-dione; (*S*)-α-amino-3-hydroxy-5-methylisoxazole-4-propionic acid (AMPA) receptor antagonist) and 2-amino-5-phosphonovaleric acid (AP5) (NMDA receptor antagonist). The epsp *(upward deflection)* in a hippocampal neuron recorded with intracellular electrode is partly blocked by CNQX (5 μmol/L), leaving behind a slow component, which is blocked by AP5 (50 μmol/L). (A from Malinow, R., Madison, D., Tsien, R.W., 1988. Nature 335, 821; B from Andreasen, M., Lambert, J.D., Jensen, M.S., 1989. J. Physiol. 414, 317–336.)

- **Aspartate** and **homocysteate** activate NMDA receptors and may be endogenous activators in certain brain regions.
- Some well-known anaesthetic and psychotomimetic agents, such as **ketamine** (see Ch. 40) and **phencyclidine** (see Ch. 49), are selective non-competitive antagonists blocking NMDA-operated channels.

Antagonists selective for the NR2B subunit have shown promise as antidepressants (Ch. 48) with **Traxoprodil** giving a positive result in a clinical trial but unfortunately failing to progress due to side effects. Other NR2B antagonists are under development.

METABOTROPIC GLUTAMATE RECEPTORS

There are eight different metabotropic glutamate receptors (mGlu$_{1-8}$) which are unusual in showing no sequence homology with other G protein-coupled receptors (for a broad coverage of the molecular and physiological properties of mGluRs, see Niswender and Conn, 2010). They function as homo- and heterodimers[6] (see Ch. 3) cross-linked by a disulfide bridge across the extracellular domain of each protein. They are members of class C G protein-coupled receptors, possessing a large extracellular N-terminus domain that forms a Venus fly trap-like structure into which glutamate binds. They are divided into three groups on the basis of their sequence homology, G protein coupling and pharmacology. Alternatively spliced receptor variants have been reported.

mGlu receptors are widely distributed throughout the CNS on neurons, where they regulate cell excitability and synaptic transmission, and on glia. Neuronal group 1 mGlu receptors are located postsynaptically and are largely excitatory through Gq signalling. By raising intracellular [Ca^{2+}], they modify responses through ionotropic glutamate receptors (Fig. 38.6). Group 2 (somatodentritic and presynaptic) and 3 mGlu (presynaptic) receptors, and their activation, tend to reduce synaptic transmission and neuronal excitability through Gi/o signalling. They can be autoreceptors, involved in reducing glutamate release or heteroreceptors, e.g. when present on GABA-containing terminals. Selective agonists and antagonists have been developed as research tools and there have been numerous clinical trials with subtype selective compounds in a range of psychiatric and neurological disorders but they have failed to deliver on efficacy and as such the therapeutic potential of mGluRs has yet to be realised.

SYNAPTIC PLASTICITY AND LONG-TERM POTENTIATION

As well as participating in synaptic transmission, glutamate receptors play a role in long-term adaptive and pathological changes in the brain, and are of particular interest as potential drug targets.

In this context, two aspects of glutamate receptor function are of particular pathophysiological importance, namely *synaptic plasticity*, discussed here, and *excitotoxicity* (discussed in Ch. 40).

Synaptic plasticity is a general term used to describe long-term changes in synaptic connectivity and efficacy, either following physiological alterations in neuronal activity (as in learning and memory) or resulting from pathological disturbances (as in epilepsy, chronic pain or drug dependence). Synaptic plasticity underlies much of what we call 'brain function', allowing it to be influenced by past experience. Needless to say, no single mechanism is responsible; however, one significant and much-studied component is *long-term potentiation* (LTP), a phenomenon in which AMPA and NMDA receptors play a central role (Chater and Goda, 2014; Lüscher and Malenka, 2012).

LTP (see Bear et al., 2020) is a prolonged (hours in vitro, days or weeks in vivo) enhancement of synaptic transmission that occurs at various CNS synapses following a short (conditioning) burst of high-frequency

[6]It has been suggested that mGlu receptors may form heterodimers with non-mGlu receptors such as the 5-HT$_{2A}$ receptor (González-Maeso et al., 2008).

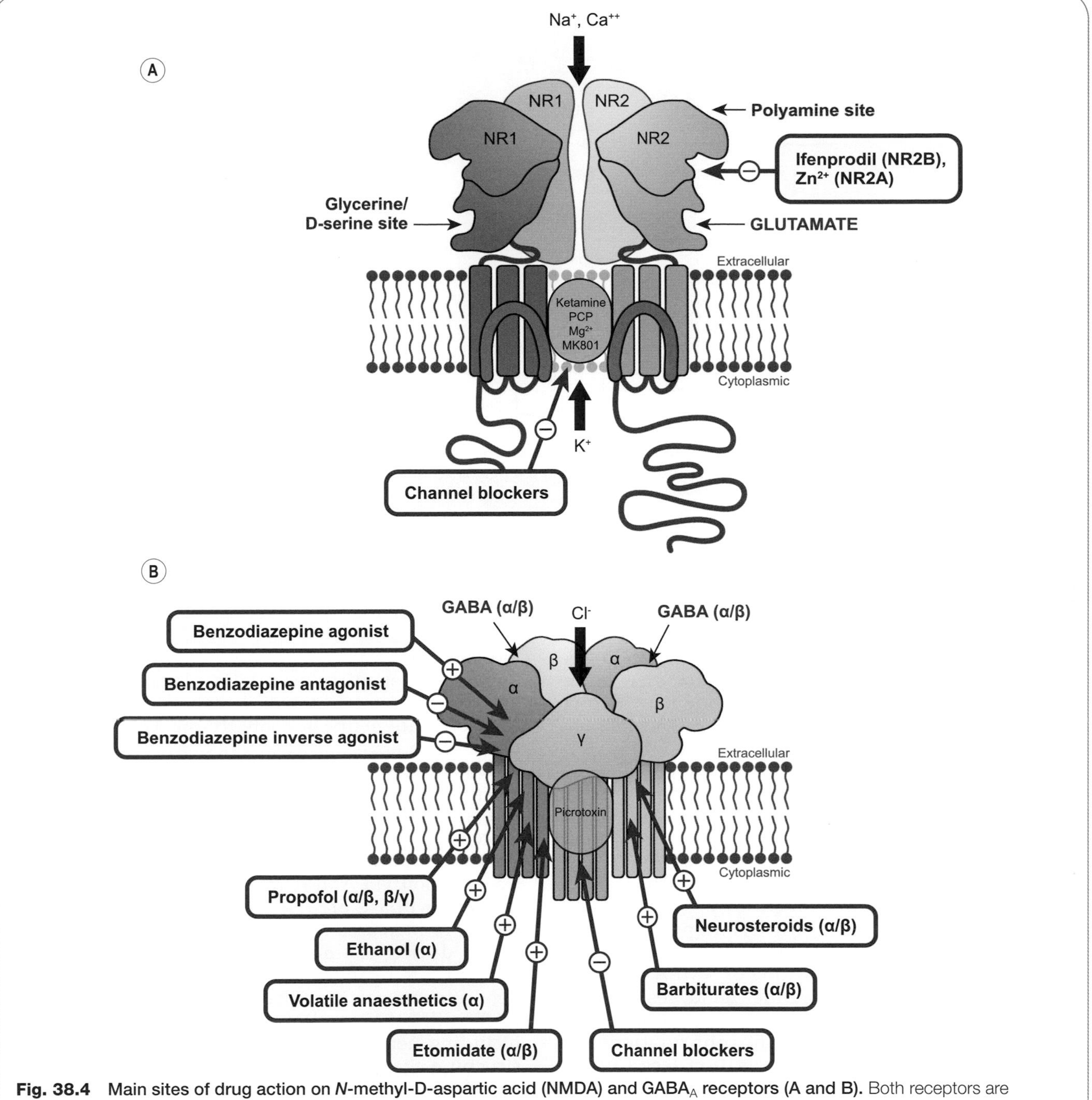

Fig. 38.4 Main sites of drug action on *N*-methyl-D-aspartic acid (NMDA) and GABA$_A$ receptors (A and B). Both receptors are multimeric ligand-gated ion channels and drugs can act as agonists or antagonists at the neurotransmitter receptor site or at modulatory sites associated with the receptor. They can also act to block the ion channel at one or more distinct sites. In the case of the GABA$_A$ receptor, the mechanism by which 'channel modulators' (e.g. ethanol, anaesthetic agents, neurosteroids) facilitate channel opening is uncertain; they may affect both ligand-binding and channel sites. The location of the different binding sites shown in the figure is not fully understood although site-directed mutagenesis studies are revealing their specific locations. Examples of the different drug classes are given in Tables 38.1 and 38.2. *GABA*, γ-Aminobutyric acid.

presynaptic stimulation. Its counterpart is *long-term depression* (LTD), which is produced at some synapses by a longer train of stimuli at lower frequency (see Connor and Wang, 2016). These phenomena have been studied at various synapses in the CNS, most especially in the hippocampus, which plays a central role in learning and memory (see Fig. 38.3). It has been argued that 'learning', in the synaptic sense, can occur if synaptic strength is enhanced following simultaneous activity in both pre- and postsynaptic neurons. LTP shows this characteristic; it does not occur if presynaptic activity fails to excite the postsynaptic neuron, or if the latter is activated independently, for instance by a different presynaptic input. The mechanisms underlying both LTP and LTD

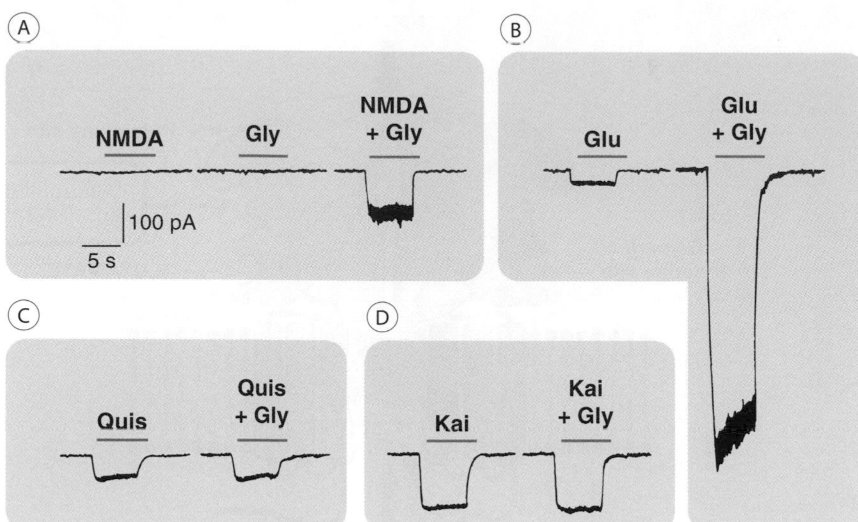

Fig. 38.5 Facilitation of *N*-methyl-D-aspartic acid (NMDA) by glycine. Recordings from mouse brain neurons in culture (whole-cell patch clamp technique). Downward deflections represent inward current through excitatory amino acid–activated ion channels. (A) NMDA (10 μmol/L) or glycine (1 μmol/L) applied separately had little or no effect, but together produced a response. (B) The response to glutamate (Glu; 10 μmol/L) was strongly potentiated by glycine (Gly; 1 μmol/L). (C and D) Responses of (*S*)-α-amino-3-hydroxy-5-methylisoxazole-4-propionic acid (AMPA) and kainate receptors to quisqualate (Quis) and kainate (Kai) were unaffected by glycine. (From Johnson, J.W., Ascher, P., 1987. Glycine potentiates the NMDA response in cultured mouse brain neurons. Nature 325, 529–531.)

differ somewhat at different synapses in the brain (see Bear et al., 2020). Here only a brief, generic view of the underlying events is given. LTP initiation may involve both presynaptic and postsynaptic components, and results from enhanced activation of postsynaptic AMPA receptors at glutamatergic synapses and (probably) to enhanced glutamate release (although the argument rumbles on about whether increased transmitter release does or does not occur in LTP; see Nicoll, 2017). The response of postsynaptic AMPA receptors to glutamate is increased due to phosphorylation of the AMPA receptor subunits by kinases such as Ca^{2+}/calmodulin-dependent protein kinase (CaMKII) and protein kinase C (PKC), thus enhancing their conductance, as well as to increase expression and trafficking of AMPA receptors to synaptic sites. LTD, on the other hand, results from modest Ca^{2+} entry into the cell activating phosphatases that reduce AMPA receptor phosphorylation and enhance AMPA receptor internalisation (see Connor and Wang, 2016).

LTP is reduced by agents that block the synthesis or effects of nitric oxide or arachidonic acid. These mediators (see Chs 17 and 19) may act as retrograde messengers through which events in the postsynaptic cell are able to influence the presynaptic nerve terminal. Endogenous cannabinoids released by the postsynaptic cell may also act as retrograde messengers to enhance glutamate release (see Chs 18 and 39). Brain-derived neurotrophic factor (BDNF) has been shown to be released from postsynaptic neurons in response to increased glutamate release and may contribute to stabilising these changes in synaptic strength (Gómez-Palacio-Schjetnan and Escobar, 2013).

Two special properties of the NMDA receptor underlie its involvement in LTP, namely voltage-dependent channel block by Mg^{2+} and its high Ca^{2+} permeability. At normal membrane potentials, the NMDA channel is blocked by Mg^{2+}; a sustained postsynaptic depolarisation produced by glutamate acting repeatedly on AMPA receptors, however, removes the Mg^{2+} block, and NMDA receptor activation then allows Ca^{2+} to enter the cell. Activation of group 1 mGlu receptors also contributes to the increase in $[Ca^{2+}]_i$. This rise in $[Ca^{2+}]_i$ in the postsynaptic cell activates protein kinases, phospholipases and nitric oxide synthase, which act jointly with other cellular processes to facilitate transmission via AMPA receptors. Initially, during the induction phase of LTP, phosphorylation of AMPA receptors increases their responsiveness to glutamate. Later, during the maintenance phase, more AMPA receptors are recruited to the membrane of postsynaptic dendritic spines as a result of altered receptor trafficking; later still, other mediators and signalling pathways including neurotrophic factors are activated, causing structural changes and leading to a permanent increase in the number of synaptic contacts.

The general descriptions of LTP and LTD given earlier are intended to provide the uninitiated reader with an overview of the topic. There are subtle differences in their forms and in the mechanisms underlying them at different synapses in the CNS. How LTP and LTD, in all of their guises, relate to different forms of memory is slowly being worked out (see Connor and Wang, 2016). Thus there is hope that drugs capable of modifying LTP and LTD may improve learning and memory.[7]

[7]In 2016, Bliss, Collingridge and Morris won the 'Brain Prize' for their seminal work on understanding memory including the role of LTP. See Bliss and Collingridge (2019) for a description of their research into LTP and the growing evidence that LTP is impaired in numerous neurological and psychiatric disorders.

Table 38.1 Properties of ionotropic glutamate receptors

	NMDA		AMPA	Kainate
Subunit composition	Tetramers consisting of GluN1–3 subunits		Tetramers consisting of GluA1–4 subunits (splice variants and RNA editing occur)	Tetramers consisting of GluK1–5 subunits
	Receptor site	***Modulatory site (glycine)***		
Endogenous agonist(s)	Glutamate Aspartate	Glycine D-Serine	Glutamate	Glutamate
Other agonist(s)[a]	NMDA	D-Cycloserine	AMPA	Kainate Domoate[b]
Antagonist(s)[a]	AP5, CPP	7-Chloro-kynurenic acid, HA-966	NBQX	NBQX ACET
Other modulators	Polyamines (e.g. spermine, spermidine) Mg^{2+}, Zn^{2+}		Cyclothiazide Perampanel Piracetam CX-516	
Channel blockers	Dizocilpine (MK801) Phencyclidine, ketamine Remacemide Memantine Mg^{2+}		—	—
Effector mechanism	Ligand-gated cation channel (slow kinetics, high Ca^{2+} permeability)	Ligand-gated cation channel (fast kinetics; channels possessing GluA2 subunits show low Ca^{2+} permeability)	Ligand-gated cation channel (fast kinetics, low Ca^{2+} permeability)	Effector mechanism
Location	Postsynaptic (some presynaptic, also glial) Wide distribution	Postsynaptic (also glial)	Pre- and postsynaptic	Location
Function	Slow epsp Synaptic plasticity (long-term potentiation, long-term depression) Excitotoxicity	Fast epsp Wide distribution	Fast epsp Presynaptic inhibition Limited distribution	Function

[a]Hansen et al. (2021) provides a detailed review of the pharmacology of ionotropic glutamate receptors including experimental compounds.
[b]A neurotoxin from mussels (see Ch. 41).
ACET, -(*S*)-1-(2-Amino-2-carboxyethyl)-3-(2-carboxy-5-phenylthiophene-3-yl-methyl)-5-methylpyrimidine-2,4-dione; *AMPA,* (*S*)-α-amino-3-hydroxy-5-methylisoxazole-4-propionic acid; *AP5,* 2-amino-5-phosphonopentanoic acid; *CPP,* 3-(2-carboxypiperazin-4-yl)-propyl-1-phosphonic acid; *CX-516,* 1-(quinoxalin-6-ylcarbonyl)-piperidine; *epsp,* excitatory postsynaptic potential; *NBQX,* 2,3-dihydro-6-nitro-7-sulfamoyl-benzoquinoxaline; *NMDA, N*-methyl-D-aspartic acid. (Other structures are shown in Fig. 39.3.)

DRUGS ACTING ON GLUTAMATE RECEPTORS

ANTAGONISTS AND NEGATIVE MODULATORS

Inotropic glutamate receptor antagonists

The main types and examples of ionotropic glutamate antagonists are shown in Table 38.1. They are selective for the main receptor types but generally not for specific subtypes. Many of these compounds, although very useful as experimental tools, are unable to penetrate the blood–brain barrier, so they are not effective when given systemically.

NMDA receptors, as discussed before, require glycine as well as NMDA to activate them, so blocking the glycine site is an alternative way to produce antagonism. **Kynurenic acid** and the more potent analogue **7-chloro-kynurenic acid** act in this way.

Another site of block is the channel itself, where substances such as ketamine, phencyclidine and **memantine** act. These agents are lipid soluble and thus able to cross the blood–brain barrier. Depending on their affinity and kinetics, these channel blocking NMDA antagonists have quite different functional effects.

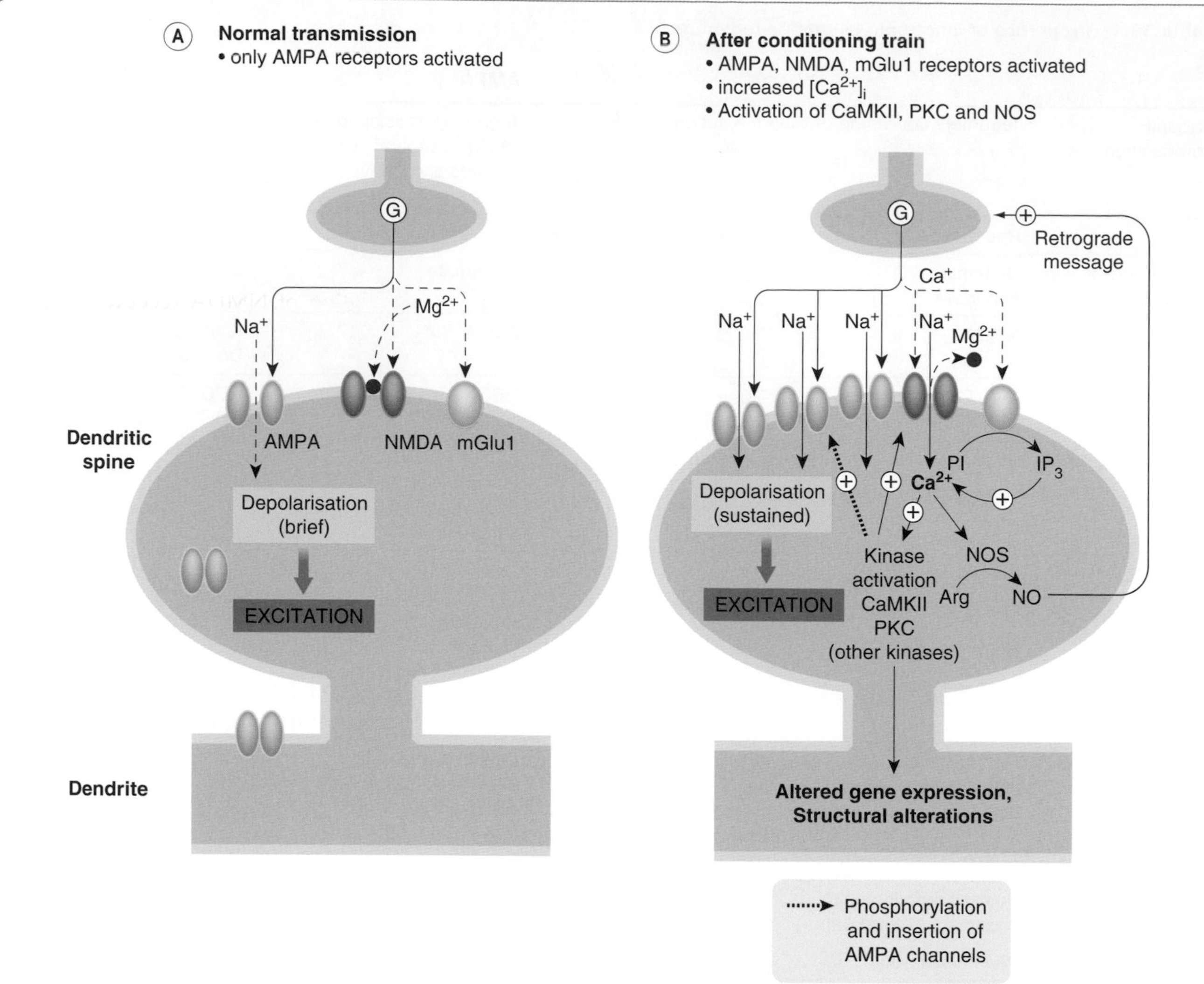

Fig. 38.6 Mechanisms of long-term potentiation. (A) With infrequent synaptic activity, glutamate (G) activates mainly (*S*)-α-amino-3-hydroxy-5-methylisoxazole-4-propionic acid (AMPA) receptors. There is insufficient glutamate to activate metabotropic receptors, and *N*-methyl-D-aspartic acid (NMDA) receptor channels are blocked by Mg^{2+}. (B) After a conditioning train of stimuli, enough glutamate is released to activate metabotropic receptors, and NMDA channels are unblocked by the sustained depolarisation. The resulting increase in $[Ca^{2+}]_i$ activates various enzymes, including the following:

- Ca^{2+}/calmodulin-dependent protein kinase (CaMKII) and protein kinase C (PKC) phosphorylate various proteins, including AMPA receptors (causing them to be trafficked to areas of synaptic contact on dendritic spines and facilitation of transmitter action) and other signal transduction molecules controlling gene transcription (not shown) in the postsynaptic cell.
- Nitric oxide synthase (NOS); release of nitric oxide (NO) facilitates glutamate release (retrograde signalling, otherwise known as NO turning back).
- Phospholipase A_2 (not shown) catalyses the formation of arachidonic acid (see Ch. 18), a retrograde messenger that increases presynaptic glutamate release.
- A phospholipase (NAPE-PLD, not shown) that catalyses production of the endocannabinoids (see Ch. 20) that act as retrograde messengers to enhance glutamate release.
- Brain-derived neurotrophic factor (BDNF) released from nerve terminals and postsynaptic structures (not shown) plays a multimodal role in the early and later stages of LTP.

Arg, Arginine; *IP_3,* inositol (1,4,5) trisphosphate; *NAPE-PLD*, N-acyl phosphatidylethanolamine-specific phospholipase D; *PI,* phosphatidylinositol.

The therapeutic potential for ionotropic glutamate receptor antagonists is diverse, including the reduction of brain damage following strokes and head injury (see Ch. 40), as well as in the treatment of epilepsy (see Ch. 46) and Alzheimer's disease (see Ch. 40). They have also been considered for indications such as drug dependence (see Ch. 50) and schizophrenia (see Ch. 47). Trials with NMDA antagonists and channel blockers have so far proved disappointing, and a serious drawback of these agents is their tendency to cause hallucinatory and other disturbances (also a feature of phencyclidine; see Ch. 49). Only two NMDA receptor antagonists, ketamine (anaesthesia, analgesia and depression; see Chs 41, 43 and 48) and memantine (Alzheimer's disease; see Ch. 40), are in clinical use. Ketamine is also used for its psychoactive properties (see Ch. 49) inducing relaxation and euphoria and at high doses an 'out-of-body' experience. It is possible that antagonists selective for NMDA receptors containing the GluN2B subunit, which is highly Ca^{2+} permeable, have reduced dissociative effects and may be better tolerated and several drugs of this type are in development as rapid-acting antidepressants (see Ch. 48).

The non-competitive AMPA receptor antagonist **perampanel** has been introduced as an antiepileptic drug (see Ch. 48). The prospects for kainate receptor antagonists appear promising – antagonists for GluK1 have shown potential for the treatment of pain, migraine, epilepsy, stroke and anxiety (see Hansen et al., 2021).

Overall, the promise foreseen for ionotropic glutamate receptor antagonists in the clinic has been less successful than was hoped. The problem may be that glutamate is such a ubiquitous and multifunctional mediator – involved, it seems, in almost every aspect of brain function – that attempting to improve a specific malfunction by flooding the brain with a compound that affects the glutamate system in some way is just too crude a strategy. The new hope is that subunit selective negative allosteric modulators may have fewer side effects than previous generations of orthosteric antagonists.

Metabotropic glutamate receptor antagonists

While antagonists that discriminate between the different groups of mGlu receptors are available, it has proven more difficult to develop selective antagonists for the subtypes within the groups. mGlu receptors, like many G protein–coupled receptors, possess allosteric modulatory sites, which can be either inhibitory or facilitatory (see Ch. 3). Antagonists or negative allosteric modulators acting at group 1 mGlu receptors have potential for the treatment of fragile X syndrome,[8] various pain states, Parkinson's disease (including the control of **levodopa**-induced dyskinesias, see Ch. 40), neuroprotection, epilepsy and drug use disorder, whereas antagonists or negative allosteric modulators of group 2 mGlu receptors have potential as cognition enhancers (see Nicoletti et al., 2011).

AGONISTS AND POSITIVE MODULATORS

Ionotropic glutamate receptors

Various agonists at ionotropic glutamate receptors that are used experimentally are shown in Table 38.1. From the clinical perspective, interest centres on the theory that positive AMPA receptor modulators may improve memory and cognitive performance. Early examples include **cyclothiazide**, **piracetam**[9] (approved for use in certain forms of epilepsy, see Ch. 46) and CX-516 (**Ampalex**). These positive allosteric modulators, known as *ampakines*, can act in subtly different ways to increase response amplitude, slow deactivation and/or attenuate desensitisation of AMPA receptor–mediated currents. They therefore increase AMPA-mediated synaptic responses and enhance LTP as well as up-regulating the production of nerve growth factors such as *brain-derived neurotrophic factor* (BDNF). Originally, ampakines were thought to have therapeutic potential as cognition enhancers (nootropics or 'smart drugs') and for the treatment of schizophrenia, depression, attention deficit hyperactivity disorder (ADHD) and Parkinson's disease (see Kadriu et al., 2021) but so far clinical trials have been disappointing. A more recently developed ampakine, CX1739, is in clinical trial for the treatment of drug-induced respiratory depression.

Inhibition of the glycine transporter GlyT1 leads to an elevation of extracellular glycine levels throughout the brain and, through potentiation of NMDA receptor-mediated responses, could be beneficial in the treatment of various neurological disorders (see Marques et al., 2020).

Metabotropic glutamate receptors

Developing selective agonists of mGlu receptors has proven to be quite difficult but selective positive allosteric modulators have been developed (see Nicoletti et al., 2011). Group 2 and 3 mGlu receptors are located presynaptically on nerve terminals and agonists at these receptors decrease glutamate release. Group 2 mGlu agonists and positive allosteric modulators were therefore thought to have therapeutic potential to decrease neuronal cell death in stroke and in the treatment of epilepsy, but to date clinical trials have been disappointing. Similarly, clinical trials with agonists and positive allosteric modulators for group 2 mGlu receptors and group 3 mGlu receptor–positive allosteric modulators have also failed to deliver on efficacy in clinical trials.

Excitatory amino acids

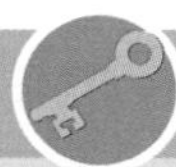

- Glutamate is the main fast excitatory transmitter in the CNS.
- Glutamate is formed mainly from the Krebs cycle intermediate α-ketoglutarate by the action of GABA transaminase.
- There are three main ionotropic glutamate receptors and eight metabotropic receptors.
- *N*-methyl-D-aspartic acid (NMDA), (*S*)-α-amino-3-hydroxy-5-methylisoxazole-4-propionic acid (AMPA) and kainate receptors are ionotropic receptors regulating cation channels.
- The channels controlled by NMDA receptors are highly permeable to Ca^{2+} and are blocked by Mg^{2+}.
- AMPA and kainate receptors are involved in fast excitatory transmission; NMDA receptors mediate slower excitatory responses and, through their effect in controlling Ca^{2+} entry, play a more complex role in controlling synaptic plasticity (e.g. long-term potentiation).
- Competitive NMDA receptor antagonists include **AP5** (2-amino-5-phosphonopentanoic acid) and **CPP** (3-(2-carboxypirazin-4-yl)-propyl-1-phosphonic acid); the NMDA-operated ion channel is blocked by **ketamine** and **memantine** with high and low affinity, respectively.

[8]Fragile X syndrome is caused by mutation of a single gene on the X chromosome. It affects about 1:4000 children of either sex, causing intellectual disability, autism and motor disturbances.

[9]Piracetam is an uncontrolled substance sold in the United States as a dietary supplement with a growing market developing for nootropic supplements and more potent ampakines for 'holistic brain hacking'.

Excitatory amino acids—cont'd

- **NBQX** (2,3-dihydro-6-nitro-7-sulfamoyl-benzoquinoxaline) is an AMPA and kainate receptor antagonist.
- NMDA receptors require low concentrations of glycine as a co-agonist, in addition to glutamate; **7-chlorokynurenic acid** blocks this action of glycine.
- NMDA receptor activation is increased by endogenous polyamines, such as **spermine**, acting on a modulatory site that is blocked by **ifenprodil.**
- The entry of excessive amounts of Ca^{2+} produced by NMDA receptor activation can result in cell death – excitotoxicity (see Ch. 40).
- Metabotropic glutamate receptors ($mGlu_1$–$_8$) are dimeric G protein–coupled receptors. $mGlu_1$ and $mGlu_5$ receptors couple through G_q to inositol trisphosphate formation and intracellular Ca^{2+} release. They play a part in glutamate-mediated synaptic plasticity and excitotoxicity. The other mGlu receptors couple to G_i/G_o and inhibit neurotransmitter release, most importantly glutamate release.
- Some specific metabotropic glutamate receptor agonists and antagonists are available, as are positive and negative allosteric modulators.

γ-AMINOBUTYRIC ACID

GABA is the main inhibitory transmitter in the brain. In the spinal cord and brain stem, glycine is also important.

SYNTHESIS, STORAGE AND FUNCTION

GABA occurs in brain tissue but not in other mammalian tissues, except in trace amounts. It is particularly abundant (about 10 μmol/g tissue) in the nigrostriatal system, but occurs at lower concentrations (2–5 μmol/g) throughout the grey matter.

GABA is formed from glutamate (see Fig. 38.1) by the action of glutamic acid decarboxylase (GAD), an enzyme found only in GABA-synthesising neurons in the brain.[10] Immunohistochemical labelling of GAD is used to map the GABA pathways in the brain. GABAergic neurons and astrocytes take up GABA via specific transporters, thus removing GABA after it has been released. GAT1 is the predominant GABA transporter in the brain and is located primarily on GABAergic nerve terminals where it recycles GABA. GAT3 is located predominantly on astrocytes around the GABAergic synapse. GABA transport is inhibited by **tiagabine** used to treat epilepsy (see Ch. 46). In astrocytes GABA can be destroyed by a transamination reaction in which the amino group is transferred to α-oxoglutaric acid (to yield glutamate), with the production of succinic semialdehyde and then succinic acid. This reaction is catalysed by GABA transaminase, an enzyme located primarily in astrocytes. It is inhibited by **vigabatrin**, another compound used to treat epilepsy (see Ch. 46).

GABA functions as an inhibitory transmitter in many different CNS pathways. About 20% of CNS neurons are GABAergic; most are short interneurons, but there are some long GABAergic tracts, e.g. from the striatum to the substantia nigra and globus pallidus (see Ch. 40). The widespread distribution of GABA - GABA serves as a transmitter at about 30% of all the synapses in the CNS - and the fact that virtually all neurons are sensitive to its inhibitory effect suggests that its function is ubiquitous in the brain. That antagonists such as **bicuculline** induce seizures illustrates the important, ongoing inhibitory role of GABA in the brain.

GABA RECEPTORS: STRUCTURE AND PHARMACOLOGY

GABA acts on two distinct types of receptor: $GABA_A$ receptors are ligand-gated ion channels permeable to chloride whereas $GABA_B$ receptors are G protein–coupled.

$GABA_A$ RECEPTORS

$GABA_A$ receptors[11] are members of the *cys-loop* family of receptors that also includes the glycine, nicotinic and $5\text{-}HT_3$ receptors (see Ch. 3). The $GABA_A$ receptors are pentamers made up of different subunits.

The reader should not despair when informed that 19 $GABA_A$ receptor subunits have been cloned (α1–6, β1–3, γ1–3, δ, ε, θ, π and ϱ1–3) and that splice variants of some subunits also exist. Although the number of possible combinations is large, only a few dozen have been shown to exist. The most common are α1β2γ2 (by far the most abundant), α2β3γ2 and α3β3γ2 subunits. To make up the pentamer, each receptor contains two α, two β and one γ subunit arranged in a circle in the sequence α–β–α–β–γ around the pore when viewed from the extracellular side of the membrane. GABA binds at each of the interfaces between the α and β subunits whereas benzodiazepines (see Ch. 45) bind at the α/γ interface. Three different benzodiazepione binding sites have been described but their functional significance is unclear at present. Receptors containing different α and γ subunits exhibit differential sensitivity to benzodiazepines and mediate different behavioural responses to these drugs. This raises the tantalising prospect of developing new agents with greater selectivity and potentially fewer side effects. The $GABA_A$ receptor should therefore be thought of as a group of receptors exhibiting subtle differences in their physiological and pharmacological properties (Olsen, 2018).

$GABA_A$ receptors are primarily located postsynaptically and mediate both fast and tonic postsynaptic inhibition. The $GABA_A$ channel is selectively permeable to Cl^- and because the equilibrium membrane potential for Cl^- is usually negative to the resting potential, increasing Cl^- permeability hyperpolarises the cell as Cl^- ions enter, thereby reducing its

[10]It has been suggested that GABA can also be synthesised in the brain from putrescine by the action of diamine oxidase and aldehyde dehydrogenase.

[11]The IUPHAR Nomenclature Committee has recommended (see Belelli et al., 2019) that the receptors previously referred to as '$GABA_C$' receptors, because they were insensitive to bicuculline, benzodiazepines and baclofen, should be subtypes of the $GABA_A$ receptor family as they are pentameric Cl^--permeable ligand-gated channels comprising homo- or heteromeric assemblies of ϱ subunits. They are referred to as $GABA_A$-rho or $GABA_A$-ϱ receptors. Their pharmacology and functional significance is slowly being worked out (see Naffaa et al., 2017).

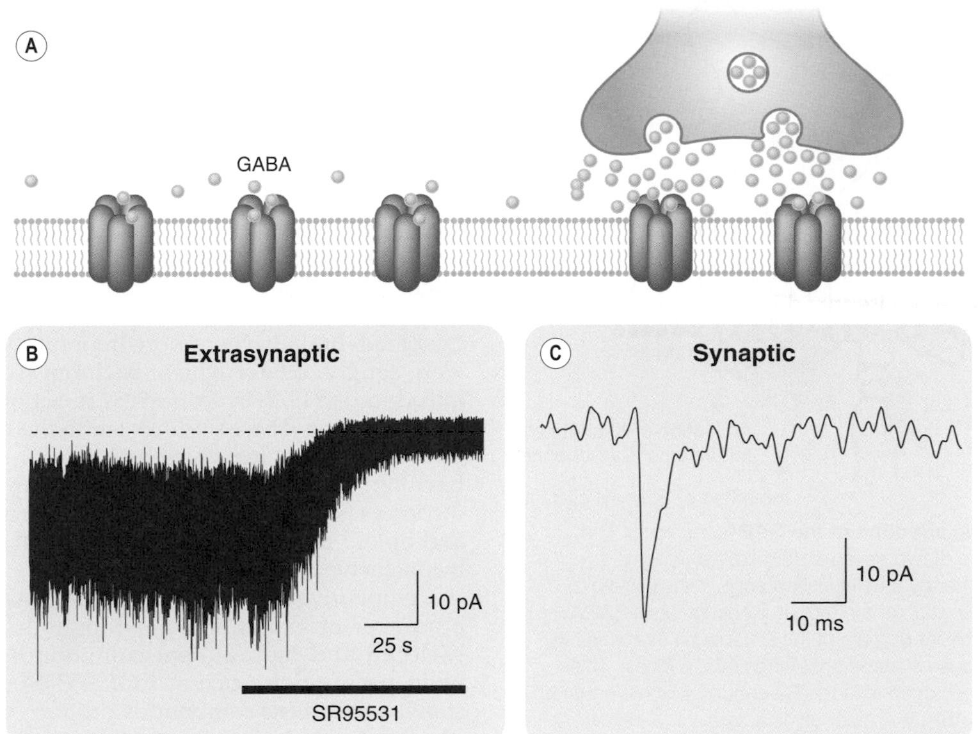

Fig. 38.7 Synaptic and extrasynaptic $GABA_A$ receptors. (A) Diagram depicting $GABA_A$ receptors at synaptic and extrasynaptic sites in the plasma membrane. The *blue dots* represent GABA molecules. (B) Tonic activation of extrasynaptic $GABA_A$ receptors gives rise to a steady-state inward current *(distance from the baseline indicated by the dashed line)* and increased 'noise' on the trace. The current is blocked on application of the $GABA_A$ receptor antagonist SR95531. (C) Phasic release of GABA from the presynaptic terminal evokes a fast synaptic current *(rapid downward deflection).* Note the different timescales in (B) and (C). *GABA*, γ-Aminobutyric acid. (Figure courtesy M. Usowicz.)

excitability.[12] In the postsynaptic cell, $GABA_A$ receptors are located both at areas of synaptic contact and extrasynaptically (Fig. 38.7, and see Farrant and Nusser, 2005). Thus GABA produces inhibition by acting both as a fast 'point-to-point' transmitter and as an 'action-at-a-distance' neuromodulator, as the extrasynaptic $GABA_A$ receptors can be tonically activated by GABA that has diffused away from its site of release. Extrasynaptic $GABA_A$ receptors contain α4 and α6 subunits as well as the δ subunit. They have higher affinity for GABA and show less desensitisation than synaptic receptors, and are also highly sensitive to general anaesthetic agents (see Ch. 41) and ethanol (see Ch. 49).

$GABA_B$ RECEPTORS

$GABA_B$ receptors (see Evenseth et al., 2020) are located pre- and postsynaptically. They are class C G protein–coupled receptors that couple through G_i/G_o to inhibit voltage-gated Ca^{2+} channels (thus reducing transmitter release), to open potassium channels (thus reducing postsynaptic excitability) and to inhibit adenylyl cyclase.

For $GABA_B$ receptors, the functional receptor is a dimer (see Ch. 3) consisting of two different seven-transmembrane subunits, B1 and B2, held together by a coil/coil interaction between their C-terminal tails. In the absence of B2, the B1 subunit does not traffic to the plasma membrane as it possesses an endoplasmic reticulum retention signal. Interaction of B1 with B2 masks the retention signal and facilitates trafficking to the membrane. Activation of the dimer results from GABA binding to the extracellular, 'Venus fly trap' domain of B1 (even although the B2 subunit possesses a similar domain) whereas it is the B2 subunit that interacts with and activates the G protein (Fig. 38.8).

DRUGS ACTING ON GABA RECEPTORS

$GABA_A$ RECEPTORS

$GABA_A$ receptors resemble NMDA receptors in that drugs may act at several different sites (see Fig. 38.4). These include:

- the GABA-binding site
- allosteric modulatory sites
- the ion channel pore

$GABA_A$ receptors are the target for several important centrally acting drugs, notably benzodiazepines (see Ch. 45), alcohol (see Ch. 49), barbiturates, neurosteroids (see Table 38.2) and many general anaesthetics (see Ch. 41). The main agonists, antagonists and modulatory substances that act on GABA receptors are shown in Table 38.2.

Muscimol, derived from a hallucinogenic mushroom, resembles GABA chemically (see Fig. 38.2) and is a

[12]During early brain development (in which GABA plays an important role), and also in some regions of the adult brain, GABA has an excitatory rather than an inhibitory effect, because the intracellular Cl^- concentration is relatively high, so that the equilibrium potential is positive to the resting membrane potential.

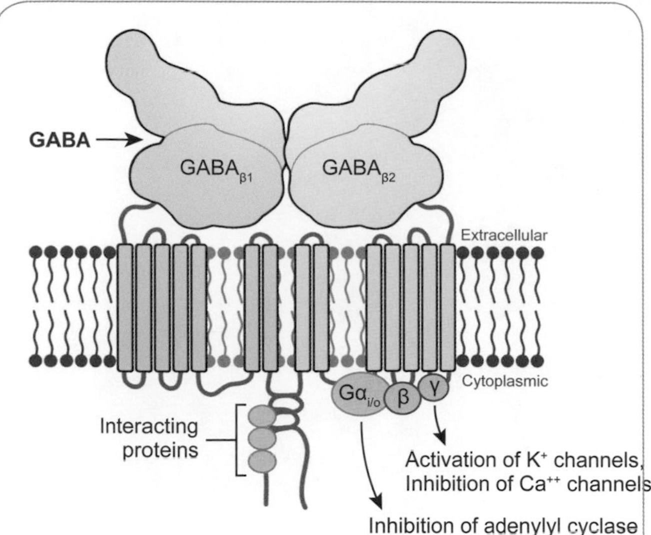

Fig. 38.8 Dimeric structure of the GABA$_B$ receptor. The receptor is made up of two seven-transmembrane domain subunits held together by a coil/coil interaction between their C-terminal tails. Activation of the receptor occurs when GABA binds to the extracellular domain of the B1 subunit (known as the Venus fly trap, because it snaps shut when GABA binds). This produces an allosteric change in the B2 subunit which is coupled to the G protein. *GABA*, γ-Aminobutyric acid.

powerful GABA$_A$ receptor agonist. A synthetic analogue, **gaboxadol,** is a partial agonist that was developed as a hypnotic drug (see Ch. 45) but has now been withdrawn. **Bicuculline**, a naturally occurring convulsant compound, is a specific antagonist that blocks the fast inhibitory synaptic potential in most CNS synapses. **Gabazine**, a synthetic GABA analogue, is similar. These compounds are useful experimental tools but have no therapeutic uses.

Benzodiazepines, which have powerful sedative, anxiolytic and anticonvulsant effects (see Ch. 45), selectively potentiate the effects of GABA on some GABA$_A$ receptors depending upon the subunit composition. They bind with high affinity to an accessory allosteric site on the GABA$_A$ receptor, in such a way that the binding of GABA is facilitated and its agonist effects are enhanced. Conversely, inverse agonists at the benzodiazepine site (e.g. Ro15-4513) reduce GABA binding and are anxiogenic and proconvulsant - they are unlikely to be therapeutically useful!

Modulators that also enhance the action of GABA, but whose site of action is less well defined than that of benzodiazepines (shown as 'channel modulators' in Fig. 38.5), include other CNS depressants such as barbiturates, anaesthetic agents (see Ch. 41) and neurosteroids. Neurosteroids (see Belelli et al., 2021) are compounds that are related to steroid hormones but that act to enhance activation of GABA$_A$ receptors - those containing δ subunits appear most sensitive. Interestingly, they include metabolites of progesterone and androgens that are formed in the nervous system and are believed to have a physiological role. Synthetic neurosteroids include **alphaxalone**, developed as an anaesthetic agent (see Ch. 41). In 2019, **allopregnanolone** (brexanolone) became the first treatment to be approved by the FDA for postpartum depression but requires a 60-h continuous infusion and is not without significant potential adverse effects including loss of consciousness.

Picrotoxin, a plant product, is a convulsant that acts by blocking the GABA$_A$ receptor chloride channel, thus blocking the postsynaptic inhibitory effect of GABA. It also blocks glycine receptors. It has no therapeutic uses.

GABA$_B$ RECEPTORS

When the importance of GABA as an inhibitory transmitter was recognised, it was thought that a GABA-like substance might prove to be effective in controlling epilepsy and other convulsive states; because GABA itself fails to penetrate the blood–brain barrier, more lipophilic GABA analogues were sought, one of which, **baclofen** (see Fig. 38.2), was introduced in 1972. Unlike GABA, its actions are not blocked by bicuculline. These findings led to the recognition of the GABA$_B$ receptor, for which baclofen is a selective agonist. Baclofen is used to treat spasticity and related motor disorders (see Ch. 46); it has been tested for treating alcohol and opioid dependence (see Ch. 49) but results so far are inconclusive.

Competitive antagonists for the GABA$_B$ receptor include a number of experimental compounds (e.g. **2-hydroxy-saclofen** and more potent compounds with improved brain penetration, such as CGP 35348). Tests in animals showed that these compounds produce only slight effects on CNS function (in contrast to the powerful convulsant effects of GABA$_A$ antagonists). The main effect observed, paradoxically, was an antiepileptic action, specifically in an animal model of absence seizures (see Ch. 46), together with enhanced cognitive performance. However, as in many areas of pharmacology, such preclinical promise has not resulted in the development of a new therapeutic drug.

γ-HYDROXYBUTYRATE

γ-Hydroxybutyrate (**sodium oxybate** or GHB) occurs naturally in the brain as a side product of GABA synthesis. As a synthetic drug it can be used to treat narcolepsy and alcoholism. In addition, it has found favour with bodybuilders, based on its ability to evoke the release of growth hormone, and with partygoers, based on its euphoric and disinhibitory effects. It is also used as an intoxicant and 'date rape' drug, but is fatal in higher doses. In common with many euphoric drugs (see Ch. 49), it activates 'reward pathways' in the brain, and its use is now illegal in most countries. GHB is an agonist at GABA$_A$ receptors containing α4 and δ subunits and a weak partial agonist at GABA$_B$ receptors. A specific GHB receptor has also been postulated but the evidence for its existence is not yet convincing.

GLYCINE

Glycine is an important inhibitory neurotransmitter in the spinal cord and brain stem. It is present in particularly high concentration (5 μmol/g) in the grey matter of the spinal cord. Applied ionophoretically to motor neurons or interneurons, it produces a hyperpolarisation that is indistinguishable from the inhibitory synaptic response. **Strychnine**, a convulsant poison that acts mainly on the spinal cord, blocks both the synaptic inhibitory response and the response to glycine. This, together with direct

Table 38.2 Properties of inhibitory amino acid receptors

	GABA$_A$				
	Receptor site	**Modulatory site (benzodiazepine)**	**Modulatory site (others)**	**GABA$_B$**	**Glycine**
Endogenous agonists	GABA	Unknown, several postulated (see text)	Various neurosteroids (e.g. progesterone metabolites)	GABA	Glycine β-Alanine Taurine
Other agonist(s)	Muscimol Gaboxadol (THIP,[a] a partial agonist)	Anxiolytic benzodiazepines (e.g. diazepam)	Barbiturates Steroid anaesthetics (e.g. alphaxalone)	Baclofen	—
Antagonist(s)	Bicuculline Gabazine	Flumazenil (inverse agonist?)	—	2-Hydroxy-saclofen CGP 35348 and others	Strychnine
Channel blocker	Picrotoxin[b]			Not applicable	—
Effector mechanism(s)	Ligand-gated chloride channel			G protein–coupled receptor; inhibition of Ca^{2+} channels, activation of K^+ channels, inhibition of adenylyl cyclase	Ligand-gated chloride channel
Location	Widespread; primarily postsynaptic			Pre- and postsynaptic Widespread	Postsynaptic Mainly in brain stem and spinal cord
Function	Postsynaptic inhibition (fast ipsp and tonic inhibition)			Presynaptic inhibition (decreased Ca^{2+} entry) Postsynaptic inhibition (increased K^+ permeability)	Postsynaptic inhibition (fast ipsp)

[a]THIP is an abbreviation of the chemical name of gaboxadol. It is reported to have preference for δ subunit-containing extrasynaptic GABA$_A$ receptors.
[b]Picrotoxin also blocks some glycine receptors.
GABA, γ-Aminobutyric acid; *ipsp*, inhibitory postsynaptic potential.

measurements of glycine release in response to nerve stimulation, provides strong evidence for its physiological transmitter role. **β-Alanine** has pharmacological effects and a pattern of distribution very similar to those of glycine, but its action is not blocked by strychnine.

The inhibitory effect of glycine is quite distinct from its role in facilitating activation of NMDA receptors (see earlier in this chapter).

The glycine receptor (see Breitinger and Breitinger, 2020.) resembles the GABA$_A$ receptor in that it is a cys-loop, pentameric ligand-gated chloride channel. There are no specific metabotropic receptors for glycine. Five glycine receptor subunits have been cloned (α1–4, β) and it appears that in the adult brain the main form of glycine receptor is a heteromeric complex of α and β subunits, probably with a stoichiometry of 2α and 3β. Homomers formed of only α subunits can form and are sensitive to glycine and strychnine, indicating that the binding site for these drugs is on the α subunit. They are also much more sensitive to channel block by **picrotoxin** than are receptors comprised of α and β subunits.

Glycine receptors are involved in the regulation of respiratory rhythms, motor control and muscle tone as well as in the processing of pain signals. Mutations of the receptor have been identified in some inherited neurological disorders associated with muscle spasm and reflex hyperexcitability. There are as yet no therapeutic drugs that act specifically by modifying glycine receptors.

Tetanus toxin, a bacterial toxin resembling **botulinum toxin** (see Ch. 14), acts selectively to prevent glycine release from inhibitory interneurons in the spinal cord, causing excessive reflex hyperexcitability and violent muscle spasms (lockjaw).[13]

[13]Botulinum toxin (also known as botox), then tetanus toxin, hold the prize for the two deadliest substances, with LD_{50}s of ~1 and 3 ng/kg. That means 1 g of each is enough to kill over 8 million people, or 975 g could potentially wipe out the entire global population!!

Glycine is removed from the extracellular space by two transporters, GlyT1 and GlyT2 (Marques et al., 2020). GlyT1 is located primarily on astrocytes and expressed throughout most regions of the CNS. GlyT2, on the other hand, is expressed on glycinergic neurons in the spinal cord, brain stem and cerebellum. The GlyT1 inhibitor **bitopertin** failed in phase III clinical trials for the treatment of negative symptoms of schizophrenia (see Ch. 47). GlyT2 inhibitors have been proposed as potential analgesics based on studies in animal models (Vandenberg et al., 2014).

Inhibitory amino acids: GABA and glycine

- GABA is the main inhibitory transmitter in the brain.
- It is present fairly uniformly throughout the brain; there is very little in peripheral tissues.
- GABA is formed from glutamate by the action of glutamic acid decarboxylase. Its action is terminated mainly by reuptake, but also by deamination, catalysed by GABA transaminase.
- There are two main types of GABA receptor: $GABA_A$ and $GABA_B$.
- $GABA_A$ receptors, which occur mainly postsynaptically, are directly coupled to chloride channels, the opening of which reduces membrane excitability.
- **Muscimol** is a specific $GABA_A$ agonist, and the convulsant **bicuculline** is an antagonist.
- Other drugs that interact with $GABA_A$ receptors and channels include:
  - benzodiazepines, which act at an allosteric binding site to facilitate the action of GABA;
  - convulsants such as **picrotoxin**, which block the anion channel;
  - neurosteroids, including endogenous progesterone metabolites;
  - CNS depressants, such as barbiturates and many general anaesthetic agents, which facilitate the action of GABA.

Inhibitory amino acids: GABA and glycine—cont'd

- $GABA_B$ receptors are heterodimeric G protein–coupled receptors. They cause pre- and postsynaptic inhibition by inhibiting Ca^{2+} channel opening and increasing K^+ conductance. **Baclofen** is a $GABA_B$ receptor agonist used to treat spasticity. $GABA_B$ antagonists are not in clinical use.
- Glycine is an inhibitory transmitter mainly in the spinal cord, acting on its own receptor, structurally and functionally similar to the $GABA_A$ receptor.
- The convulsant drug **strychnine** is a competitive glycine antagonist. Tetanus toxin acts mainly by interfering with glycine release.

CONCLUDING REMARKS

The study of amino acids and their receptors in the brain has been one of the most active fields of research in the past 30 years, and the amount of information available is prodigious. These signalling systems have been speculatively implicated in almost every kind of neurological and psychiatric disorder, and the pharmaceutical industry has put a great deal of effort into identifying specific ligands - agonists, antagonists, modulators, enzyme inhibitors, transport inhibitors - designed to influence them. While a large number of pharmacologically unimpeachable compounds have emerged, and many clinical trials have been undertaken, due to lack of efficacy and serious adverse effects, there have been few therapeutic breakthroughs. The optimistic view is that a better understanding of the particular functions of the many molecular subtypes of these targets, and the design of more subtype-specific ligands, will lead to future breakthroughs. Expectations have, however, undoubtedly dimmed in recent years.

REFERENCES AND FURTHER READING

Excitatory amino acids

Bettler, B., Collingridge, G.L., Dingledine, R., et al., 2019. Ionotropic glutamate receptors (version 2019.4) in the IUPHAR/BPS guide to pharmacology database. IUPHAR/BPS. Guide.Pharmacol. CITE 2019 (4). Available at: https://doi.org/10.2218/gtopdb/F75/2019.4.

Bliss, T.V.P., Collingridge, G.L., 2019. Persistent memories of long-term potentiation and the *N*-methyl-d-aspartate receptor. Brain Neurosci. Adv. 3 2398212819848213.

Burnell, E.S., Irvine, M., Fang, G., Sapkota, K., Jane, D.E., Monaghan, D.T., 2019. Positive and negative allosteric modulators of *N*-methyl-d-aspartate (NMDA) receptors: structure-activity relationships and mechanisms of action. J. Med. Chem. 62, 3–23.

Collingridge, G.L., Abrahams, W.C., 2022. Glutamate receptors and synaptic plasticity: the impact of Evans and Watkins. Neuropharmacology 206, 108922.

González-Maeso, J., Ang, R.L., Yuen, T., et al., 2008. Identification of a serotonin/glutamate receptor complex implicated in psychosis. Nature 452, 93–99.

Hansen, K.B., Wollmuth, L.P., Bowie, D., et al., 2021. Structure, function, and pharmacology of glutamate receptor ion channels. Pharmacol. Rev. 73, 298–487.

Jensen, A.A., Fahlke, C., Bjørn-Yoshimoto, W.E., Bunch, L., 2015. Excitatory amino acid transporters: recent insights into molecular mechanisms, novel modes of modulation and new therapeutic possibilities. Curr. Opin. Pharmacol. 20, 116–123.

Kadriu, B., Musazzi, L., Johnston, J.N., et al., 2021. Positive AMPA receptor modulation in the treatment of neuropsychiatric disorders: a long and winding road. Drug Discov. Today 26, 2816–2838.

Nicoletti, F., Bockaert, J., Collingridge, G.L., et al., 2011. Metabotropic glutamate receptors: from the workbench to the bedside. Neuropharmacology 60, 1017–1041.

Niswender, C.M., Conn, P.J., 2010. Metabotropic glutamate receptors: physiology, pharmacology, and disease. Annu. Rev. Pharmacol. Toxicol. 50, 295–322.

Watkins, J.C., Jane, D.E., 2006. The glutamate story. Br. J. Pharmacol. 147 (Suppl. 1), S100–S108.

Inhibitory amino acids

Belelli, D., Hales, T.G., Lambert, J.J., Luscher, B., et al., 2019. GABAA receptors (version 2019.4) in the IUPHAR/BPS guide to pharmacology database. IUPHAR/BPS. Guide. Pharmacol. CITE 2019 (4). Available at: https://doi.org/10.2218/gtopdb/F72/2019.4.

Belelli, D., Phillips, G.D., Atack, J.R., Lambert, J.J., 2021. Relating neurosteroid modulation of inhibitory neurotransmission to behaviour. J. Neuroendocrinol. 20, e13045.
Breitinger, U., Breitinger, H.G., 2020. Modulators of the inhibitory Glycine receptor. ACS Chem. Neurosci. 11, 1706–1725.
Evenseth, L.S.M., Gabrielsen, M., Sylte, I., 2020. The GABA B receptor-structure, ligand binding and drug development. Molecules 25, 3093.
Farrant, M., Nusser, Z., 2005. Variations on an inhibitory theme: phasic and tonic activation of $GABA_A$ receptors. Nat. Rev. Neurosci. 6, 215–229.
Felmlee, M.A., Morse, B.L., Morris, M.E., 2021. γ-Hydroxybutyric acid: pharmacokinetics, pharmacodynamics, and toxicology. AAPS J. 23, 22.
Marques, B.L., Oliveira-Lima, O.C., Carvalho, G.A., et al., 2020. Neurobiology of glycine transporters: from molecules to behavior. Neurosci. Biobehav. Rev. 118, 97–110.
Naffaa, M.M., Hung, S., Chebib, M., Johnston, G.A.R., Hanrahan, J.R., 2017. GABA-ϱ receptors: distinctive functions and molecular pharmacology. Br. J. Pharmacol. 174, 1881–1894.
Olsen, R.W., 2018. GABAA receptor: positive and negative allosteric modulators. Neuropharmacology 136, 10–22.
Vandenberg, R.J., Ryan, R.M., Carland, J.E., et al., 2014. Glycine transport inhibitors for the treatment of pain. Trends Pharmacol. Sci. 35, 423–430.

Physiological aspects

Bear, M.F., Connors, B.W., Paradiso, M.A., 2020. Neuroscience: Exploring the Brain, enhanced edition. Lippincott, Williams & Wilkins, Baltimore.
Chater, T.E., Goda, Y., 2014. The role of AMPA receptors in postsynaptic mechanisms of synaptic plasticity. Front. Cell. Neurosci. 8, 401.
Connor, S.A., Wang, Y.T., 2016. A place at the table: LTD as a mediator of memory genesis. Neuroscientist 22, 359–371.
Gómez-Palacio-Schjetnan, A., Escobar, M.L., 2013. Neurotrophins and synaptic plasticity. Curr. Top. Behav. Neurosci. 15, 117–136.
Lüscher, C., Malenka, R.C., 2012. NMDA receptor-dependent long-term potentiation and long-term depression (LTP/LTD). Cold Spring Harb. Perspect. Biol. 4, a005710.
Nicoll, R.A., 2017. A brief history of long-term potentiation. Neuron 93, 281–290.
Schicker, K.W., Dorostkar, M.M., Boehm, S., 2008. Modulation of transmitter release via presynaptic ligand-gated ion channels. Curr. Mol. Pharmacol. 1, 106–129.

39 Other transmitters and modulators

OVERVIEW

The principal 'amine' transmitters in the central nervous system (CNS), namely noradrenaline, dopamine, 5-hydroxytryptamine (5-HT, serotonin) and acetylcholine (ACh), are described in this chapter, with briefer coverage of other mediators, including histamine, melatonin and purines. The monoamines were the first CNS transmitters to be identified, and during the 1960s a combination of neurochemistry and neuropharmacology led to many important discoveries about their role, and about the ability of drugs to influence these systems. Amine mediators differ from the amino acid transmitters discussed in Chapter 38 in being localised to small populations of neurons with cell bodies in localised nuclei, which project diffusely both rostrally to cortical and other areas and in some cases caudally to the spinal cord. These amine-containing neurons are broadly associated with modulation of the primary excitatory or inhibitory signal rather than with localised synaptic excitation or inhibition.[1] More recently, 'gaseotransmitters' – such as nitric oxide (NO), carbon dioxide and hydrogen sulfide (see Ch. 19) – and endocannabinoids (see Ch. 18) have come on the scene, and they are discussed at the end of the chapter. The other major class of CNS mediators, the neuropeptides (e.g. endorphins, neurokinins and orexins), appear in later chapters in this section.

INTRODUCTION

Although we know much about the many different mediators, their cognate receptors and signalling mechanisms at the cellular level, when describing their effects on brain function and behaviour, we fall back on relatively crude terms – psychopharmacologists will be at our throats for so underrating the sophistication of their measurements – such as 'motor coordination', 'arousal', 'cognitive impairment' and 'exploratory behaviour'. The gap between these two levels of understanding still frustrates the best efforts to link drug action at the molecular level to drug action at the therapeutic level. Modern approaches, such as the use of genetically altered animal technologies (see Ch. 8) and non-invasive imaging techniques, are helping to forge links, but there is still a long way to go.

More detail on the content of this chapter can be found in Iversen et al. (2009) and Nestler et al. (2020).

[1]They are, if you like, voices from the nether regions, which make you happy or sad, sleepy or alert, cautious or adventurous, energetic or lazy, although you do not quite know why – very much the stuff of mental illness.

NORADRENALINE

The basic processes responsible for the synthesis, storage and release of noradrenaline are the same in the CNS as in the periphery (see Ch. 15). In the CNS, inactivation of released noradrenaline is by neuronal reuptake or by metabolism, largely through the *monoamine oxidase*, *aldehyde reductase* and *catechol-O-methyl transferase* mediated pathway to 3-hydroxy-4-methoxyphenylglycol (MHPG) (see Fig. 15.3).

NORADRENERGIC PATHWAYS IN THE CNS

Although the transmitter role of noradrenaline in the brain was suspected in the 1950s, detailed analysis of its neuronal distribution became possible only when a technique, based on the formation of fluorescent catecholamine derivatives when tissues are exposed to formaldehyde, was devised by Falck and Hillarp. Detailed maps of the pathway of noradrenergic, dopaminergic and serotonergic neurons in laboratory animals were produced and later confirmed in human brains. The cell bodies of noradrenergic neurons occur in small clusters in the *pons* and *medulla*, and they send extensively branching axons to many other parts of the brain and spinal cord (Fig. 39.1). The most prominent cluster is the locus coeruleus (LC), located in the pons. Although it contains only about 10,000 neurons in humans, the axons, running in a discrete *medial forebrain bundle*, give rise to many millions of noradrenergic nerve terminals throughout the cortex, hippocampus, thalamus, hypothalamus and cerebellum (Robertson et al., 2013). These nerve terminals do not form distinct synaptic contacts but appear to release transmitter somewhat diffusely. The LC also projects to the spinal cord and is involved in the descending control of pain (see Ch. 43).

Other noradrenergic neurons lie close to the LC in the pons and project to the amygdala, hypothalamus, hippocampus and other parts of the forebrain, as well as to the spinal cord. A small cluster of adrenergic neurons, which release adrenaline rather than noradrenaline, lies more ventrally in the brain stem. These cells contain phenylethanolamine *N*-methyl transferase, the enzyme that converts noradrenaline to adrenaline (see Ch. 15), and project mainly to the pons, medulla and hypothalamus. Rather little is known about them, but they are believed to be important in cardiovascular control.

FUNCTIONAL ASPECTS

Noradrenergic innervation occurs in most brain regions particularly cortical, hippocampal and hypothalamic areas and modulates a diverse range of functions from homeostasis e.g. food intake, thermogenesis, to cognitive and emotional

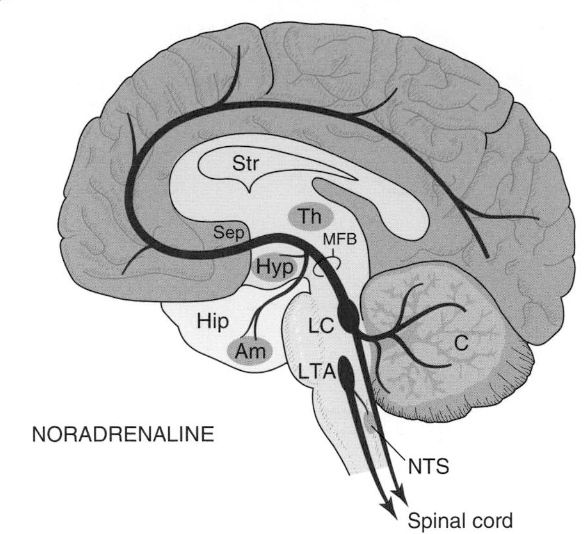

Fig. 39.1 Simplified diagram of the noradrenaline pathways in the brain. The location of the main groups of cell bodies and fibre tracts is in *solid colour*. *Light-shaded areas* show the location of noradrenergic terminals. *Am*, Amygdaloid nucleus; *C*, cerebellum; *Hip*, hippocampus; *Hyp*, hypothalamus; *LC*, locus coeruleus; *LTA*, lateral tegmental area, part of the reticular formation; *MFB*, medial forebrain bundle; *NTS*, nucleus of the tractus solitarius (vagal sensory nucleus); *Sep*, septum; *Str*, corpus striatum; *Th*, thalamus.

behaviours. With the exception of the β_3 adrenoceptor, all of the adrenoceptors (α_{1A}, α_{1B}, α_{1D}, α_{2A}, α_{2B}, α_{2C}, β_1 and β_2)[2] are expressed in the CNS (see Waterhouse and Navarra, 2019).). They are G protein–coupled receptors that interact with a variety of effector mechanisms (see Table 15.1). The role of α_1 receptors in the CNS is poorly understood. They are widely distributed, located both on postsynaptic neurons and on glial cells, and may be involved in motor control, cognition and fear. α_2 Adrenoceptors are located on noradrenergic neurons (in both somatodendritic and nerve terminal regions where they function as inhibitory autoreceptors activated by locally released noradrenaline), as well as on postsynaptic non-noradrenergic neurons. They are involved in blood pressure control (see later), sedation (α_2 agonists such as **medetomidine** are used as anaesthetics in veterinary practice) and analgesia. β_1 Receptors are found in the cortex, striatum and hippocampus whereas β_2 receptors are largely found in the cerebellum. They have been implicated in the long-term effects of antidepressant drugs but quite how remains a mystery (see Ch. 48).

Arousal and mood

Attention has focused mainly on the LC, which is the source of most of the noradrenaline released in the brain, and from which neuronal activity can be measured by implanted electrodes. LC neurons are silent during sleep, and their activity increases with behavioural arousal. 'Wake-up' stimuli of an unfamiliar or threatening kind excite these neurons much more effectively than familiar stimuli. Amphetamine-like drugs, which release catecholamines in the brain, increase wakefulness, alertness and exploratory activity (although, in this case, firing of LC neurons is actually reduced by feedback mechanisms; see Ch. 48). In contrast, activation of somatodentritic α_2 autoreceptors in the LC leads to sedation.

There is a close relationship between mood and state of arousal, and the ability of noradrenaline to directly alter 5-HT activαity (via α_1-adrenoceptors in the raphe) means that any treatment which alters noradrenaline levels will also impact on 5-HT (Ch. 48). The role of noradrenaline and dopamine in attentional processes is also thought to be important in the efficacy of treatments for attention deficit hyperactivity disorder (ADHD) (Ch. 49).

Blood pressure regulation

The role of central, as well as peripheral, noradrenergic synapses in blood pressure control is shown by the action of hypotensive drugs such as **clonidine** and **methyldopa** (see Chs 15 and 21), which decrease the discharge of sympathetic nerves emerging from the CNS. They cause hypotension when injected locally into the medulla or fourth ventricle, in much smaller amounts than are required when the drugs are given systemically. Noradrenaline and other α_2-adrenoceptor agonists have the same effect when injected locally. Noradrenergic synapses in the medulla probably form part of the baroreceptor reflex pathway, because stimulation or antagonism of α_2 adrenoceptors in this part of the brain has a powerful effect on the activity of baroreceptor reflexes.

Ascending noradrenergic fibres run to the hypothalamus, and descending fibres run to the lateral horn region of the spinal cord, acting to increase sympathetic discharge in the periphery. It has been suggested that these regulatory

Noradrenaline in the central nervous system

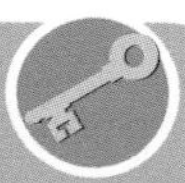

- The mechanisms for synthesis, storage, release and reuptake of noradrenaline in the central nervous system (CNS) are essentially the same as in the periphery, as are the receptors (see Ch. 15).
- Noradrenergic cell bodies occur in discrete clusters, mainly in the pons and medulla, one important such cell group being the LC.
- Noradrenergic pathways, running mainly in the medial forebrain bundle and descending spinal tracts, terminate diffusely in the cortex, hippocampus, hypothalamus, cerebellum and spinal cord.
- The actions of noradrenaline are mediated through α_1, α_2, β_1 and β_2 adrenoceptors.
- Noradrenergic transmission is believed to be important in:
  - the 'arousal' system, controlling wakefulness and alertness;
  - blood pressure regulation;
  - control of mood and cognition (functional deficiency contributing to depression).
- Psychotropic drugs that act partly or mainly on noradrenergic transmission in the CNS include antidepressants and **amphetamine.** Some antihypertensive drugs (e.g. **clonidine**, **methyldopa**) act mainly on noradrenergic transmission in the CNS.

[2]The α_{1C} receptor was subsequently found to be identical to α_{1A} receptor.

neurons may release adrenaline rather than noradrenaline as inhibition of phenylethanolamine *N*-methyl transferase, the enzyme that converts noradrenaline to adrenaline, interferes with the baroreceptor reflex.

DOPAMINE

Drugs which modulate dopamine transmission are important in the treatment of several common disorders of brain function, notably Parkinson's disease, schizophrenia and attention deficit disorder, as well as in drug dependence and certain endocrine disorders.

The distribution of dopamine in the brain is more restricted than that of noradrenaline. Dopamine is most abundant in the *corpus striatum*, a part of the extrapyramidal motor system concerned with the coordination of movement (see Ch. 40), and high concentrations also occur in certain parts of the frontal cortex, limbic system and hypothalamus (where its release into the pituitary blood supply inhibits secretion of prolactin; see Ch. 33).

The synthesis of dopamine follows the same route as that of noradrenaline (see Fig. 15.1), namely conversion of tyrosine to dopa (the rate-limiting step), followed by decarboxylation to form dopamine. Dopaminergic neurons do not express dopamine β-hydroxylase, and thus do not convert dopamine to noradrenaline.

Dopamine is largely recaptured, following its release from nerve terminals, by a specific dopamine transporter, one of the large family of monoamine transporters (see Ch. 15). It is metabolised by monoamine oxidase and catechol-*O*-methyl transferase (Fig. 39.2), the main products being *dihydroxyphenylacetic acid* (DOPAC) and *homovanillic acid* (HVA), the methoxy derivative of DOPAC. The brain content of HVA is often used in animal experiments as an index of dopamine turnover. Drugs that cause the release of dopamine increase HVA, often without changing the content of dopamine. DOPAC and HVA, and their sulfate conjugates, are excreted in the urine, which provides an index of dopamine release in human subjects.

6-Hydroxydopamine, which selectively destroys dopaminergic nerve terminals, is used as a research tool. It is taken up by the dopamine transporter and converted to a reactive metabolite that causes oxidative cytotoxicity.

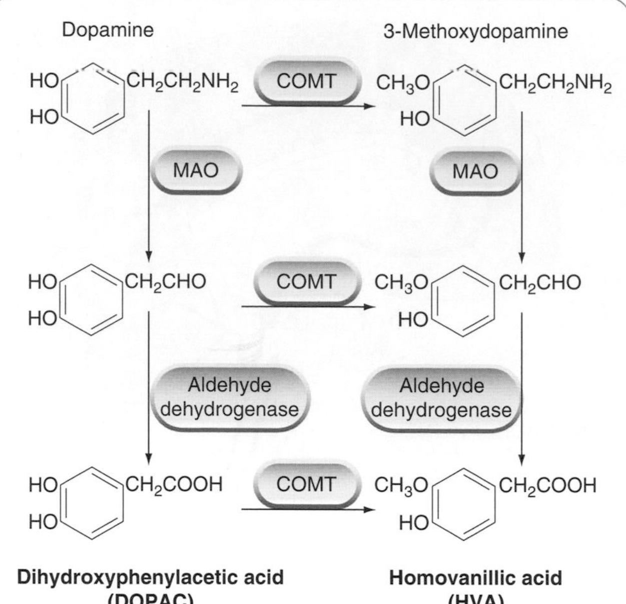

Fig. 39.2 The main pathways for dopamine metabolism in the brain. *COMT*, Catechol-*O*-methyl transferase; *MAO*, monoamine oxidase.

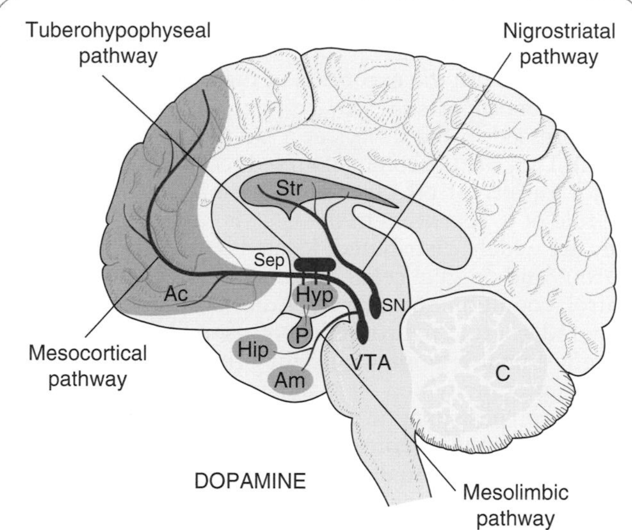

Fig. 39.3 Simplified diagram of the dopamine pathways in the brain, drawn as in Fig. 39.1. The pituitary gland (P) is shown, innervated with dopaminergic fibres from the hypothalamus. *Ac*, Nucleus accumbens; *SN*, substantia nigra; *VTA*, ventral tegmental area; other abbreviations as in Fig. 39.1.

DOPAMINERGIC PATHWAYS IN THE CNS

There are four main dopaminergic pathways in the brain (Fig. 39.3):

1. The **nigrostriatal pathway**, accounting for about 75% of the dopamine in the brain, consists of cell bodies largely in the substantia nigra whose axons terminate in the corpus striatum. These fibres run in the medial forebrain bundle along with other monoamine-containing fibres. The abundance of dopamine-containing neurons in the human striatum can be appreciated from the image shown in Fig. 39.4, which was obtained by injecting a dopa derivative containing radioactive fluorine, and scanning for radioactivity 3 h later by positron emission tomography (PET) scanning.
2. The **mesolimbic pathway**, whose cell bodies occur in the midbrain ventral tegmental area (VTA), adjacent to the substantia nigra, and whose fibres project via the medial forebrain bundle to parts of the limbic system, especially the *nucleus accumbens* and the *amygdaloid nucleus*.
3. The **mesocortical pathway**, whose cell bodies also lie in the VTA and which project via the medial forebrain bundle to the frontal cortex.
4. The **tuberohypophyseal** (or **tuberoinfundibular**) system is a group of short neurons running from the ventral hypothalamus to the median eminence

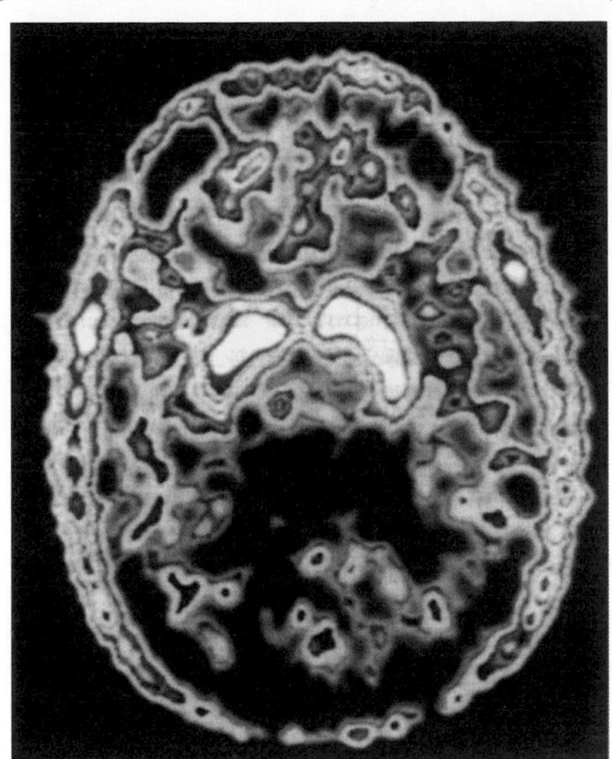

Fig. 39.4 Dopamine in the basal ganglia of a human subject. The subject was injected with 5-fluoro-dopa labelled with the positron-emitting isotope ^{18}F, which was localised 3 h later by the technique of positron emission tomography. The isotope is accumulated *(white areas)* by the dopa uptake system of the neurons of the basal ganglia, and to a smaller extent in the frontal cortex. It is also seen in the scalp and temporalis muscles. (From Garnett, E.S., Firnau, G., Nahmias, C., 1983. Dopamine visualized in the basal ganglia of living man. Nature 305, 137–138.)

and pituitary gland, the secretions of which they regulate.

There are also dopaminergic neurons in other brain regions and in the retina. For a more complete description, see Björklund and Dunnett (2007). The functions of the main dopaminergic pathways are discussed later.

DOPAMINE RECEPTORS

Two types of receptors, D_1 and D_2, were originally distinguished on pharmacological and biochemical grounds. Gene cloning revealed further subgroups, D_1 to D_5. The original D_1 family now includes D_1 and D_5, while the D_2 family consists of D_2, D_3 and D_4 (Table 39.1). Splice variants, leading to long and short forms of D_2, and genetic polymorphisms, particularly of D_4, have subsequently been identified (see Beaulieu and Gainetdinov, 2011).

All belong to the family of G protein–coupled transmembrane receptors described in Chapter 3. D_1 and D_5 receptors link through G_s to stimulate adenylyl cyclase and activate protein kinase A (PKA). PKA mediates many of the effects of D_1 and D_5 receptors by phosphorylating a wide array of proteins, including voltage-activated sodium, potassium and calcium channels, as well as ionotropic glutamate and GABA receptors. D_2, D_3, and D_4 receptors link through G_i/G_o and activate potassium channels as well as inhibiting calcium channels and adenylyl cyclase, and can also affect other cellular second messenger cascades (see Ch. 3). When intracellular cAMP is increased through activation of D_1 receptors, activating PKA, DARPP-32 (a *cAMP-regulated phosphoprotein* also known as *protein phosphatase 1 regulatory subunit 1B*) is phosphorylated. Phosphorylated DARPP-32 inhibits protein phosphatase-1, thus acting in concert with protein kinases as an amplifying mechanism favouring protein phosphorylation. In general, activation of D_2 receptors opposes the effects of D_1 receptor activation.

Dopamine receptors are expressed in the brain in distinct but overlapping areas. D_1 receptors are the most abundant and widespread in areas receiving a dopaminergic innervation (namely the striatum, limbic system, thalamus and hypothalamus; see Fig. 39.3), as are D_2 receptors, which also occur in the pituitary gland. D_2 receptors are found not only on dopaminergic neurons (on the soma, dendrites and nerve terminals), where they function as inhibitory autoreceptors activated by locally released dopamine, but also on glutamatergic, GABAergic and cholinergic nerve terminals (see De Mei et al., 2009). D_3 receptors occur in the limbic system but not in the striatum. The D_4 receptor is much more weakly expressed, mainly in the cortex and limbic systems.

Dopamine receptors also mediate various effects in the periphery (mediated by D_1 receptors), notably renal vasodilatation and increased myocardial contractility (dopamine itself has been used clinically in the treatment of circulatory shock; see Ch. 23).

FUNCTIONAL ASPECTS

The functions of dopaminergic pathways divide broadly into:

- motor control (nigrostriatal system)
- behavioural and cognitive effects (mesolimbic and mesocortical systems)
- endocrine control (tuberohypophyseal system)

Dopamine and motor systems

Ungerstedt showed, in 1968, that bilateral ablation of the substantia nigra in rats, which destroys the nigrostriatal neurons, causes profound catalepsy, the animals becoming so inactive that they die of starvation unless artificially fed. Parkinson's disease (see Ch. 40) is a disorder of motor control, associated with a deficiency of dopamine in the nigrostriatal pathway.

In treating CNS disorders, it is often desired that a certain receptor type be activated or inhibited only in one part of the brain, but the problem is that drugs are rarely brain-region selective and will affect a given receptor type throughout the brain. For example, many antipsychotic drugs (see Ch. 47) are D_2 receptor antagonists, exerting a beneficial effect by blocking D_2 receptors in the mesolimbic pathway. However, their D_2 antagonist property also gives rise to their major side effect, which is to cause movement disorders, by simultaneously blocking D_2 receptors in the nigrostriatal pathway.

Behavioural effects

Administration of **amphetamine** to rats, which releases both dopamine and noradrenaline, causes a cessation of normal

Table 39.1 Dopamine receptors

		D_1 type		D_2 type		
	Functional role	D_1	D_5	D_2	D_3	D_4
Distribution						
Cortex	Arousal, mood	+++	–	++	–	+
Limbic system	Emotion, stereotypic behaviour	+++	+	++	+	+
Striatum	Prolactin secretion	+++	+	++	+	+
Ventral hypothalamus and anterior pituitary	Prolactin secretion	–	–	++	+	–
Agonists[a]						
Dopamine		FA	FA	FA	FA	FA
Apomorphine		FA	PA	PA	PA	PA
Bromocriptine		PA	FA	FA	PA	Ant
Quinpirole		Inactive	Inactive	FA	FA	FA
Antagonists						
Chlorpromazine		++	++	++	++	++
Haloperidol		++	+	+++	++	+++
Spiperone		++	+	+++	+++	+++
Sulpiride		–	–	++	++	+
Clozapine		+	+	+	+	++
Aripiprazole		–	–	+++ (PA)	–	++
Raclopride		–	–	+++	++	+
Signal transduction		G_s coupled – activates adenylyl cyclase		G_i/G_o coupled – inhibits adenylyl cyclase, activates K^+ channels, inhibits Ca^{2+} channels, may also activate phospholipase C		
Effect		Mainly postsynaptic inhibition		Pre- and postsynaptic inhibition Stimulation/inhibition of hormone release		

[a]Agonists generally exhibit lower potency at D_1 and D_5 receptors compared with D_2, D_3 and D_4 receptors.
Ant, Antagonist; *FA*, full agonist; *PA*, partial agonist.
Data based on that contained in the IUPHAR/BPS Guide to Pharmacology database www.guidetopharmacology.org.

'ratty' behaviour (exploration and grooming), and the appearance of repeated 'stereotyped' behaviour (rearing, gnawing and so on) unrelated to external stimuli. These amphetamine-induced motor disturbances in rats probably reflect hyperactivity in the nigrostriatal dopaminergic system, and are prevented by dopamine antagonists and by destruction of dopamine-containing cell bodies in the midbrain, but not by drugs that inhibit the noradrenergic system.

Amphetamine and **cocaine** have direct effects on mesolimbic dopamine due to their inhibition of the dopamine transporter but other drugs of abuse (see Chs 49 and 50) have also been shown to indirectly activate mesolimbic dopaminergic 'reward' pathways to produce feelings of euphoria in humans, e.g. disinhibition of GABAergic interneurons in the VTA by mu-opioid receptor agonists. The main receptor involved appears to be D_1, and genetically altered mice lacking D_1 receptors behave as though generally demotivated, with reduced food intake and insensitivity to amphetamine and cocaine.

Neuroendocrine function

The tuberohypophyseal dopaminergic pathway (see Fig. 39.3) inhibits prolactin secretion via dopamine release. This system is of clinical importance. Many antipsychotic drugs (see Ch. 47), by blocking D_2 receptors, increase prolactin secretion and can cause breast development and lactation, even in males. **Bromocriptine**, a dopamine-receptor agonist derived from ergot, is used clinically to suppress prolactin secretion by tumours of the pituitary gland.

Growth hormone production is increased in normal subjects by dopamine, but bromocriptine paradoxically inhibits the excessive secretion responsible for acromegaly (probably because it desensitises dopamine receptors, in contrast to the physiological release of dopamine, which is pulsatile) and has a useful therapeutic effect, provided it is given before excessive growth has taken place. It is now rarely used, as other agents are more effective (see Ch. 33). Bromocriptine and other dopamine agonists, such as **cabergoline**, enhance libido and sexual performance.

Vomiting

Pharmacological evidence strongly suggests that dopaminergic neurons have a role in the production of nausea and vomiting. Thus nearly all dopamine-receptor agonists (e.g. bromocriptine) and **levodopa** (see Ch. 40) cause nausea and vomiting as side effects, while many dopamine antagonists (e.g. phenothiazines, **metoclopramide**; see Ch. 30) have antiemetic activity. D_2 receptors occur in the area of the medulla (the chemoreceptor trigger zone) associated with the initiation of vomiting (see Ch. 30) and are assumed to mediate this effect.

Dopamine in the central nervous system

- Dopamine is a neurotransmitter as well as being the precursor for noradrenaline. It is degraded in a similar fashion to noradrenaline, giving rise mainly to DOPAC and HVA, which are excreted in the urine.
- There are four main dopaminergic pathways:
  - nigrostriatal pathway, important in motor control;
  - mesolimbic pathway, running from groups of cells in the midbrain to parts of the limbic system, especially the nucleus accumbens, involved in emotion and drug-induced reward;
  - mesocortical pathway, running from the midbrain to the cortex, involved in emotion;
  - tuberohypophyseal neurons, running from the hypothalamus to the pituitary gland, whose secretions they regulate.
- There are five dopamine-receptor subtypes. D_1 and D_5 receptors are linked to stimulation of adenylyl cyclase. D_2, D_3 and D_4 receptors are linked to activation of K^+ channels and inhibition of Ca^{2+} channels as well as to inhibition of adenylyl cyclase.
- D_2 receptor antagonism has been implicated in treating the positive symptoms of schizophrenia.
- Parkinson's disease is associated with a loss of nigrostriatal dopaminergic neurons.
- Hormone release from the anterior pituitary gland is regulated by dopamine, especially prolactin release (inhibited) and growth hormone release (stimulated).
- Dopamine acts on the chemoreceptor trigger zone to cause nausea and vomiting.

5-HYDROXYTRYPTAMINE

The occurrence and functions of 5-HT (serotonin) in the periphery are described in Chapter 16. Interest in 5-HT as a possible CNS transmitter dates from 1953, when Gaddum found that **lysergic acid diethylamide** (LSD), a powerful hallucinogen (see Ch. 49), acted as a 5-HT antagonist on peripheral tissues,[3] and suggested that its central effects might also be related to this action. The presence of 5-HT in the brain was demonstrated a few years later. Even though brain 5-HT accounts for only about 1% of the total body content, 5-HT is an important CNS transmitter (see Iversen et al., 2009). 5-HT is involved in various physiological processes, including sleep, appetite, thermoregulation and pain perception as well as in disorders such as migraine, depression, mania, anxiety, obsessive–compulsive disorders, schizophrenia, autism and drug abuse.

In its formation, storage and release, 5-HT resembles noradrenaline. Its precursor is tryptophan, an amino acid derived from dietary protein, the plasma content of which varies considerably according to food intake and time of day. 5-HT does not cross the blood–brain barrier and is synthesised in the CNS. Tryptophan is actively taken up into neurons, converted by tryptophan hydroxylase to 5-hydroxytryptophan (see Fig. 16.1), and then decarboxylated by a non-specific amino acid decarboxylase to form 5-HT. Tryptophan hydroxylase can be selectively and irreversibly inhibited by ***p*-chlorophenylalanine** (PCPA). Availability of tryptophan and the activity of tryptophan hydroxylase are thought to be the main factors that regulate 5-HT synthesis. The decarboxylase is very similar, if not identical, to dopa decarboxylase, and does not play any role in regulating 5-HT synthesis. Following release, 5-HT is largely recovered by neuronal uptake, through a specific transporter (see Ch. 3) similar to, but not identical with, those that take up noradrenaline and dopamine. 5-HT reuptake is specifically inhibited by *selective serotonin reuptake inhibitors* (SSRIs) such as **fluoxetine** and, less specifically, by many of the drugs that inhibit catecholamine uptake (e.g. *tricyclic antidepressants*). SSRIs (see Chs 45 and 48) constitute an important group of antidepressant and anxiolytic drugs. 5-HT is degraded almost entirely by monoamine oxidase (Fig. 16.1), which converts it to 5-hydroxyindole acetaldehyde, most of which is then dehydrogenated to form 5-hydroxyindole acetic acid (5-HIAA) and excreted in the urine.

5-HT PATHWAYS IN THE CNS

The distribution of 5-HT-containing neurons (Fig. 39.5) resembles that of noradrenergic neurons. The cell bodies are grouped in the pons and upper medulla, close to the midline (raphe), and are often referred to as raphe nuclei. The rostrally situated nuclei project, via the medial forebrain bundle, to many parts of the cortex, hippocampus, basal ganglia, limbic system and hypothalamus. The caudally situated cells project more to the cerebellum, medulla and spinal cord.

5-HT RECEPTORS IN THE CNS

The main 5-HT receptor types are shown in Table 16.1. All are G protein–coupled receptors except for 5-HT_3, which is a ligand-gated cation channel (see later). All are expressed in the CNS, and their functional roles have been extensively analysed. With some 14 identified subtypes plus numerous splice variants, and a large number of pharmacological tools of relatively low specificity, assigning clear-cut functions to 5-HT receptors is not simple. Our present state of knowledge is described by Sharp and Barnes (2020).

[3]LSD has subsequently been shown to act centrally as a 5-HT2A agonist.

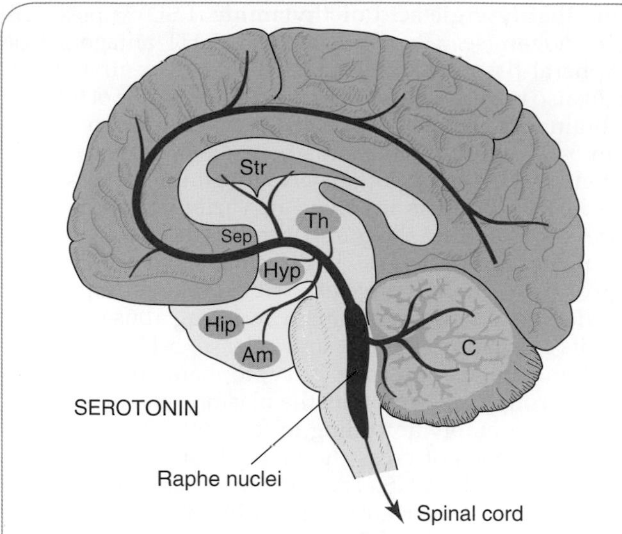

Fig. 39.5 Simplified diagram of the 5-hydroxytryptamine pathways in the brain, drawn as in Fig. 39.1. Abbreviations as in Fig. 39.1.

Certain generalisations can be made:

- 5-HT_1 receptors (5-HT_{1A}, 5-HT_{1B}, 5-HT_{1D}, 5-HT_{1E}, 5-HT_{1F})[3] are predominantly inhibitory in their effects. 5-HT_{1A} receptors are expressed on the soma and dendrites of 5-HT neurons in the raphe nuclei and are activated by locally released 5-HT. This inhibitory effect tends to limit the rate of firing of these cells. They are also widely distributed post-synaptically in the limbic system and are believed to mediate the therapeutic effects of drugs used to treat anxiety and depression (see Chs 45 and 48).
- 5-HT_{1B} and 5-HT_{1D} receptors are found mainly as presynaptic inhibitory receptors on both 5-HT-containing and other nerve terminals in the basal ganglia and cortex. Agonists acting on 5-HT_{1B} and 5-HT_{1D} receptors such as **sumatriptan** are used to treat migraine (see Ch. 16).
- 5-HT_2 receptors (5-HT_{2A}, 5-HT_{2B} and 5-HT_{2C}) are abundant in the cortex and limbic system, where they are located at both pre- and postsynaptic sites. They can exert excitatory or inhibitory effects by enhancing the release of glutamate and GABA. They are the target of some antidepressants (see Ch. 48) and antipsychotic drugs (see Ch. 47) as well as various hallucinogenic drugs (see Ch. 49). **Lorcaserin**, a 5-HT_{2C} agonist is an anti-obesity drug (see Ch. 32). The use of 5-HT_2 receptor antagonists such as **methysergide** in treating migraine is discussed in Chapter 42.
- 5-HT_3 receptors are pentameric ligand-gated cation channels that can be either homomeric or heteromeric complexes of different 5-HT_3 receptor subunits (see Peters et al., 2005). While 5-HT_{3A} and 5-HT_{3B} subunits are the most extensively studied, the roles of other subunits remain to be fully investigated (see Jensen et al., 2008). In the brain, 5-HT_3 receptors are found in the *area postrema* (a region of the medulla involved in vomiting; see Ch. 30) and other parts of the brain stem, extending to the dorsal horn of the spinal cord. They are also present in certain parts of the cortex, as well as in the peripheral nervous system. They are excitatory ionotropic receptors, and specific antagonists (e.g. **granisetron** and **ondansetron**; see Chs 16 and 30) are used to treat nausea and vomiting.
- 5-HT_4 receptors are important in the gastrointestinal (GI) tract (see Chs 16 and 31), and are also expressed in the brain, particularly in the limbic system, basal ganglia, hippocampus and substantia nigra. They are located at both pre- and postsynaptic sites. They exert a presynaptic facilitatory effect, particularly on ACh release, thus enhancing cognitive performance (see Chs 40 and 49). Activation of medullary 5-HT_4 receptors opposes the respiratory depressant actions of opioids (see Ch. 43).
- There are two 5-HT_5 receptors, 5-HT_{5A} and 5-HT_{5B}. In the human, only 5-HT_{5A} is functional. Antagonists may have anxiolytic, antidepressant and antipsychotic activity in animal models.
- 5-HT_6 receptors occur primarily in the CNS, particularly in the hippocampus, cortex and limbic system. Blockade of 5-HT_6 receptors increases glutamate and ACh release and 5HT_6-antagonists are considered potential drugs to improve cognition or relieve symptoms of schizophrenia.
- 5-HT_7 receptors occur in the hippocampus, cortex, amygdala, thalamus and hypothalamus. They are found on the soma and axon terminals of GABAergic neurons. They are also expressed in blood vessels and the GI tract. Likely CNS functions include thermoregulation and endocrine regulation, as well as suspected involvement in mood, cognitive function and sleep. The antipsychotic drug, **lurasidone** (see Ch. 47), has slightly higher affinity for 5-HT_7 receptors than for D_2 receptors. Selective antagonists are being developed for clinical use in a variety of potential indications.

FUNCTIONAL ASPECTS

The precise localisation of 5-HT neurons in the brain stem has allowed their electrical activity to be studied in detail and correlated with direct neurochemical measures and behavioural and other effects produced by drugs thought to affect 5-HT-mediated transmission. 5-HT cells show an unusual, highly regular, slow discharge pattern, and are strongly inhibited by 5-HT_1 receptor agonists, suggesting a local inhibitory feedback mechanism.

In vertebrates, certain physiological and behavioural functions relate particularly to 5-HT pathways, namely:

- hallucinations and behavioural changes
- sleep, wakefulness and mood
- feeding behaviour
- control of sensory transmission (especially pain pathways; see Ch. 43)

Hallucinatory effects

Many hallucinogenic drugs (e.g. LSD; see Ch. 49) are agonists or partial agonists at 5-HT_{2A} receptors. It is

[3]There is no 5-HT_{1C} receptor. The original 5-HT_{1C} receptor has been reclassified as 5-HT_{2C}.

suggested that a loss of cortical inhibition underlies the hallucinogenic effect. Many antipsychotic drugs (see Ch. 47) are antagonists at 5-HT_{2A} receptors in addition to blocking dopamine D_2 receptors. The psychostimulant properties of **MDMA** (3,4-methylenedioxymethamphetamine, see Ch. 49) are due partly to its ability to release 5-HT. MDMA is taken up by the serotonin transporter, and displaces 5-HT from storage vesicles – a mechanism analogous to the action of amphetamine on noradrenergic nerve terminals (see Ch. 15).

Sleep, wakefulness and mood

Lesions of the raphe nuclei, or depletion of 5-HT by PCPA administration, abolish sleep in experimental animals, whereas microinjection of 5-HT at specific points in the brain stem induces sleep. 5-HT_7 receptor antagonists inhibit 'rapid-eye-movement' (REM) sleep and increase the latency to onset of REM sleep. Attempts to cure insomnia in humans by giving 5-HT precursors (tryptophan or 5-hydroxytryptophan) have, however, proved unsuccessful. There is strong evidence that 5-HT, as well as noradrenaline, may be involved in the control of mood (see Ch. 48), and the use of tryptophan to enhance 5-HT synthesis has been tried in depression, with equivocal results.

Feeding and appetite

In experimental animals, 5-HT_{1A} agonists such as 8-hydroxy-2-(di-n-propylamino)-tetralin (8-OH-DPAT) cause hyperphagia, leading to obesity. Antagonists acting on 5-HT_{2C} receptors, including several antipsychotic drugs used clinically, also increase appetite and cause weight gain. However, antidepressant drugs that inhibit 5-HT uptake (see Ch. 48) cause loss of appetite, as does the 5-HT_{2C} receptor agonist **lorcaserin**.

Sensory transmission

After lesions of the raphe nuclei or administration of PCPA, animals show exaggerated responses to many forms of sensory stimulus. They are startled much more easily, and also quickly develop avoidance responses to stimuli that would not normally bother them. It appears that the normal ability to disregard irrelevant forms of sensory input requires intact 5-HT pathways. The 'sensory enhancement' produced by hallucinogenic drugs may be partly due to loss of this gatekeeper function of 5-HT. 5-HT also exerts an inhibitory effect on transmission in the pain pathway, both in the spinal cord and in the brain, and there is a synergistic effect between 5-HT and analgesics such as **morphine** (see Ch. 43). Thus depletion of 5-HT by PCPA, or selective lesions to the descending 5-HT-containing neurons that run to the dorsal horn, antagonise the analgesic effect of morphine, while inhibitors of 5-HT uptake have the opposite effect.

Other roles

Other roles of 5-HT include various autonomic and endocrine functions, such as the regulation of body temperature, blood pressure and sexual function. Further information can be found in Iversen et al. (2009).

CLINICALLY USED DRUGS

Several classes of drugs used clinically influence 5-HT-mediated transmission. They include:

- 5-HT reuptake inhibitors, such as fluoxetine, used as antidepressants (see Ch. 48) and anxiolytic agents (see Ch. 45)
- 5-HT_{1D} receptor agonists, such as sumatriptan, used to treat migraine (see Ch. 42)
- 5-HT_2 antagonists, such as **pizotifen**, used to treat migraine (see Ch. 42)
- 5-HT_{1A} receptor agonists have antidepressant and anxiolytic effects (see Chs 45 and 48)
- 5-HT_3 receptor antagonists, such as ondansetron, used as antiemetic agents (see Ch. 30)
- antipsychotic drugs (e.g. clozapine, see Ch. 47), which owe their efficacy at least partly to an action on 5-HT_2 receptors

ACETYLCHOLINE

There are numerous cholinergic neurons in the CNS, and the basic processes by which ACh is synthesised, stored and released are the same as in the periphery (see Ch. 14). Various biochemical markers have been used to locate cholinergic neurons in the brain, the most useful being choline acetyltransferase, the enzyme responsible for ACh synthesis, and the transporters that capture choline and package ACh, which can be labelled by immunofluorescence. Biochemical studies on ACh precursors and metabolites are generally more difficult than corresponding studies on other amine transmitters, because the relevant substances, choline and acetate, are involved in many processes other than ACh metabolism.

CHOLINERGIC PATHWAYS IN THE CNS

ACh is very widely distributed in the brain, occurring in all parts of the forebrain (including the cortex), midbrain and brain stem, although there is little in the cerebellum. Cholinergic neurons in the forebrain and brain stem send diffuse projections to many parts of the brain (Fig. 39.6). Cholinergic neurons in the forebrain lie in a discrete area, forming the magnocellular forebrain nuclei (so called because the cell bodies are conspicuously large). Degeneration of one of these, the *nucleus basalis of Meynert*, which projects mainly to the cortex, is associated with Alzheimer's disease (see Ch. 40). Another cluster, the *septohippocampal nucleus*, provides the main cholinergic input to the hippocampus, and is also involved in memory. In addition, there are – in contrast to noradrenaline, dopamine and 5-HT-containing pathways – many local cholinergic interneurons, particularly in the corpus striatum, these being important in relation to Parkinson's disease and Huntington's chorea (see Ch. 40).

ACETYLCHOLINE RECEPTORS

ACh acts on both muscarinic (G protein–coupled) and nicotinic (ionotropic) receptors in the CNS (see Ch. 14).

The muscarinic ACh receptors (mAChRs) in the brain are predominantly of the G_q-coupled M_1 class (i.e. M_1, M_3 and M_5 subtypes; see Ch. 14). Activation of these receptors can result in excitation through blockade of M-type (KCNQ/Kv7) K^+ channels (see Delmas and Brown, 2005). G_i/G_o-coupled M_2 and M_4 receptors, however, are inhibitory through activation of inwardly rectifying K^+ channels and

5-Hydroxytryptamine in the central nervous system

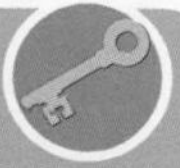

- The processes of synthesis, storage, release, reuptake and degradation of 5-HT in the brain are very similar to events in the periphery (see Ch. 16).
- Activity of the rate limiting enzyme, tryptophan hydroxylase is the main factor regulating synthesis. As the precursor, tryptophan can only be obtained from the diet, there has been some suggestion that the availability of tryptophan may also be a factor and hence why some people use dietary supplements although evidence is limited.
- Urinary excretion of 5-hydroxyindole acetic acid provides a measure of 5-HT turnover.
- 5-HT neurons are concentrated in the midline raphe nuclei in the brain stem projecting diffusely to the cortex, limbic system, hypothalamus and spinal cord, similar to the noradrenergic projections.
- Functions associated with 5-HT pathways include:
  - various behavioural responses (e.g. hallucinatory behaviour, impulsivity)
  - feeding behaviour
  - control of mood and emotion
  - control of sleep/wakefulness
  - control of sensory pathways, including nociception
  - control of body temperature
  - vomiting
- 5-HT can exert inhibitory or excitatory effects on individual neurons, acting either presynaptically or postsynaptically and, through these receptors, interacts with many other transmitter systems (De Deurwaerdere and Di Giovanni, 2021).
- The main receptor subtypes (see Table 16.1) in the CNS are 5-HT$_{1A}$, 5-HT$_{1B}$, 5-HT$_{1D}$, 5-HT$_{2A}$, 5-HT$_{2C}$ and 5-HT$_3$. Associations of behavioural and physiological functions with these receptors have been partly worked out. Other receptor types (5-HT$_{4–7}$) also occur in the CNS, but less is known about their function.
- Drugs acting selectively on 5-HT receptors or transporters include:
  - **buspirone**, a 5-HT$_{1A}$ receptor partial agonist used to treat anxiety (see Ch. 45);
  - 'triptans' (e.g. **sumatriptan**), 5-HT$_{1D}$ agonists used to treat migraine (see Ch. 16);
  - 5-HT$_2$ antagonists (e.g. **pizotifen**) used for migraine prophylaxis (see Ch. 16);
  - selective serotonin uptake inhibitors (e.g. **fluoxetine**) used to treat depression (see Ch. 48);
  - **ondansetron**, a 5-HT$_3$ antagonist, used to treat chemotherapy-induced emesis (see Chs 16 and 31);
  - **MDMA** (ecstasy), a substrate for the 5-HT transporter. It then displaces 5-HT from nerve terminals onto 5-HT receptors to produce its mood-altering effects (see Ch. 49).

inhibition of voltage-sensitive Ca^{2+} channels. mAChRs on cholinergic terminals function to inhibit ACh release, and muscarinic antagonists, by blocking this inhibition, markedly increase ACh release. Many of the behavioural effects associated with cholinergic pathways seem to be produced by ACh acting on mAChRs. Positive allosteric modulators (see Ch. 2) selective for different muscarinic receptors are under development.

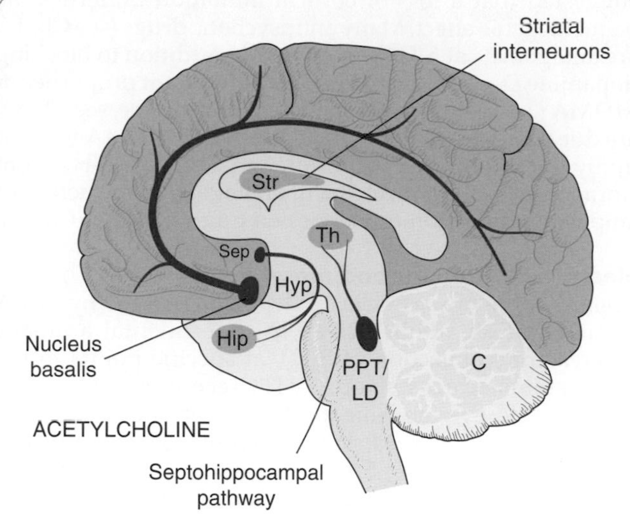

Fig. 39.6 Simplified diagram of the acetylcholine pathways in the brain, drawn as in Fig. 39.1. *PPT/LD*, Pedunculopontine and laterodorsal tegmental nuclei; other abbreviations as in Fig. 39.1.

Nicotinic ACh receptors (nAChRs) are ligand-gated cation channels permeable to Na^+, K^+ and Ca^{2+} ions (see Chs 3 and 14). They are pentamers and can be formed as homomeric or heteromeric combinations of α (α2–7) and β (β2–4) subunits (see Ch. 3; see Gotti et al., 2008) distributed widely throughout the brain (Table 39.2). Nicotine (see Ch. 49) exerts its central effects by agonist action on nAChRs. The heteromeric α4β2 and the homomeric α7 subtypes are the most extensively characterised. Subtype-specific agonists and positive allosteric modulators have been developed but initial results from clinical trials for cognitive enhancement have so far not lived up to expectation.

nAChRs are located both pre- and postsynaptically. Presynaptic nAChRs act usually to facilitate the release of other transmitters such as glutamate, dopamine and GABA.[4] Postsynaptic nAChRs mediate fast excitatory transmission, as in the periphery (see Ch. 14).

Many of the drugs that block nAChRs (e.g. **tubocurarine**; see Ch. 14) do not cross the blood–brain barrier, and even those that do (e.g. **mecamylamine**) produce only modest CNS effects. **Varenicline** is a high-affinity partial agonist for the α4β2 nAChR subtype which regulates dopamine release in the mesolimbic pathway and is used to reduce craving in smoking cessation.

FUNCTIONAL ASPECTS

The main functions ascribed to cholinergic pathways are related to arousal, reward, learning and memory and motor control. The cholinergic projection from the ventral forebrain to the cortex is thought to mediate arousal, whereas the septohippocampal pathway is involved in

[4]See Schicker et al. (2008) for a description of how presynaptic cation-selective ligand-gated channels can, under different circumstances, facilitate or enhance neurotransmitter release.

Table 39.2 Presence of nicotinic receptors of different subunit compositions in selected regions of the central nervous system

	Nicotinic receptors						
Brain region	**α7**	**α3β2**	**α3β4**	**α4β2**	**α4α5β**	**α6β2β3**	**α6α4β2β3**
Cortex	+			+	+		
Hippocampus	+		+	+	+		
Striatum				+	+	+	+
Amygdala	+			+			
Thalamus				+			
Hypothalamus	+			+			
Substantia nigra	+		+	+	+	+	
Cerebellum	+	+	+	+			
Spinal cord	+	+		+			

α7 may also form heteromeric receptors with β2 subunits. nAChRs comprising α2β2 and α3β3β4 are found in some other areas of the brain. Data taken from Gotti, C., Zoli, M., Clementi, F., 2008. Brain nicotinic acetylcholine receptors: native subtypes and their relevance. Trends Pharmacol. Sci. 27, 482–491.

learning and short-term memory (see Hasselmo, 2006). Cholinergic interneurons in the striatum are involved in motor control (see Ch. 40).

Muscarinic agonists have been shown to partially restore learning and memory deficits induced in experimental animals by lesions of the septohippocampal cholinergic pathway. **Hyoscine**, a muscarinic antagonist, impairs memory in human subjects and causes amnesia when used as preanaesthetic medication. Preliminary clinical studies suggest that another muscarinic antagonist, scopolamine, has rapid-acting antidepressant effects, possibly related to its amnesic effects (see Ch. 48).

Nicotine increases alertness and also enhances learning and memory, as do various synthetic agonists at neuronal nAChRs. Conversely, CNS-active nAChR antagonists such as mecamylamine cause detectable, although slight, impairment of learning and memory. In the dopaminergic VTA to accumbens 'reward' pathway, nicotine affects neuronal firing at the level of the cell soma in the VTA and modulates dopamine release from terminals in the nucleus accumbens to modify dopamine release in this reward pathway (see Ch. 50).

The importance of cholinergic neurons in neurodegenerative conditions such as dementia and Parkinson's disease is discussed in Chapter 40. The role of nAChRs in addiction to nicotine is described in Chapter 50 and their role in modulating pain transmission in the CNS is described in Chapter 43.

In conclusion, both nAChRs and mAChRs may play a role in learning and memory, while nAChRs also mediate behavioural arousal. Genetically altered mice lacking expression of different cholinergic receptors show very limited impairments suggesting that alternative mechanisms may be able to compensate for the loss of ACh receptor signalling.

Acetylcholine in the central nervous system

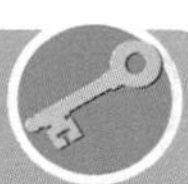

- Synthesis, storage and release of ACh in the CNS are essentially the same as in the periphery (see Ch. 14).
- ACh is widely distributed in the CNS, important pathways being:
  - basal forebrain (magnocellular) nuclei, which send a diffuse projection to most forebrain structures, including the cortex;
  - septohippocampal projection;
  - short interneurons in the striatum and nucleus accumbens.
- Certain neurodegenerative diseases, especially dementia and Parkinson's disease (see Ch. 41), are associated with abnormalities in cholinergic pathways.
- Both nicotinic and muscarinic (predominantly M_1) ACh receptors occur in the CNS. The former mediate the central effects of nicotine. Nicotinic receptors are mainly located presynaptically; there are few examples of transmission mediated by postsynaptic nicotinic receptors.
- Muscarinic receptors appear to mediate the main behavioural effects associated with ACh, namely effects on arousal, and on learning and short-term memory.
- Muscarinic antagonists (e.g. **hyoscine**) cause amnesia.

PURINES

Both adenosine and ATP act as transmitters and/or modulators in the CNS (for review, see Tozaki-Saitoh et al., 2011; Burnstock, 2018) as they do in the periphery (see Ch. 16). Mapping the pathways is difficult, because purinergic neurons are not easily identifiable histochemically. It is likely that adenosine and ATP serve as neuromodulators.

Adenosine is produced intracellularly from ATP. It is not packaged into vesicles but is released mainly by carrier-mediated transport. Because the intracellular concentration of ATP (several mmol/L) greatly exceeds that of adenosine, conversion of a small proportion of ATP results in a large increase in adenosine. ATP is packaged into vesicles and released by exocytosis as a conventional transmitter but can also leak out of cells in large amounts under conditions of tissue damage. In high concentrations, ATP can act as an excitotoxin (like glutamate; see Ch. 40) and cause further neuronal damage but it is also quickly converted to adenosine, which exerts a protective effect. These special characteristics of purine metabolism suggest that adenosine serves mainly as a safety mechanism, protecting the neurons from damage when their viability is threatened, for example by ischaemia or seizure activity. It has been suggested that adenosine deficiency may underlie a number of CNS disorders such as some epilepsies as well as Alzheimer's and Parkinson's diseases (Boison and Aronica, 2015).

Adenosine produces its effects through G protein–coupled adenosine A receptors (see Ch. 16). There are four adenosine receptors – A_1, A_{2A}, A_{2B} and A_3 – distributed throughout the CNS. The overall effect of adenosine, or of various adenosine receptor agonists, is inhibitory, leading to effects such as drowsiness and sedation, motor incoordination, analgesia and anticonvulsant activity. Xanthines, such as **caffeine** (see Ch. 49), which are antagonists at A_2 receptors, produce arousal and alertness.

For ATP there are two forms of receptor – P2X and P2Y receptors (see Ch. 16 also). P2X receptor subunits (P2X1-7) are trimeric ligand-gated cation channels that can be homomeric or heteromeric in composition. The evidence in favour of ATP acting on postsynaptic P2X receptors mediating fast synaptic transmission in the brain remains weak. P2X receptors are located on the postsynaptic cell membrane away from sites of synaptic contact, on nerve terminals and on astrocytes. Like ACh at nicotinic receptors, ATP acting on nerve terminal P2X receptors appears to play a neuromodulatory role. There are eight P2Y receptors[5]; all are G protein coupled (see Table 16.1).

While there is little doubt that purinergic signalling plays a significant role in CNS function, our understanding is still very limited (Burnstock, 2016).

HISTAMINE

Histamine is present in the brain in much smaller amounts than in other tissues, such as skin and lung, but undoubtedly serves a neurotransmitter role (see Brown et al., 2001). The cell bodies of histaminergic neurons, which also synthesise and release a variety of other transmitters, are restricted to a small part of the hypothalamus, and their axons run to virtually all parts of the brain. Unusually, no uptake mechanism for histamine is present, its action being terminated instead by enzymic methylation. Histamine's prolonged extracellular presence may explain its involvement in homeostatic process such as the sleep/wake cycle, food and water intake and temperature regulation.

Histamine acts on four types of receptors (H_{1-4}; see Ch. 17) in the brain. H_1–H_3 occur in most brain regions, H_4 has a more restricted distribution. All are G protein coupled – H_1 receptors to G_q, H_2 to G_s and H_3 and H_4 to G_i/G_o. H_3 receptors are inhibitory receptors on histamine-releasing neurons as well as on terminals releasing other neurotransmitters.

Like other monoamine transmitters, histamine is involved in many different CNS functions. Histamine release follows a distinct circadian pattern, the neurons being active by day and silent by night. H_1 receptors in the cortex and reticular activating system contribute to arousal and wakefulness, and H_1 receptor antagonists that access the CNS produce sedation (see Ch. 45). Antihistamines are widely used to control nausea and vomiting, for example, in motion sickness and middle ear disorders, as well as to induce sleep. Recent pharmaceutical industry activity has centred on the development of selective H_3 receptor antagonists, as they may have potential for the treatment of cognitive impairment associated with Alzheimer's disease (see Ch. 40), schizophrenia (see Ch. 47), ADHD (see Ch. 49) and Parkinson's disease (see Ch. 40) as well as for the treatment of narcolepsy, obesity and pain states (Hu and Chen, 2017).

OTHER CNS MEDIATORS

We now move from the familiar neuropharmacological territory of the 'classic' monoamines to some of the odder agents which challenge many of our preconceived ideas of how neurotransmission functions. Useful drugs interacting with some of these mediators are starting to be approved for clinical use.

MELATONIN

Melatonin (*N*-acetyl-5-methoxytryptamine) (reviewed by Dubocovich et al., 2010) is synthesised exclusively in the pineal, an endocrine gland that plays a role in establishing circadian rhythms. The gland contains two enzymes, not found elsewhere, which convert 5-HT by acetylation and *O*-methylation to melatonin, its hormonal product.

There are two well-defined melatonin receptors (MT_1 and MT_2) which are G protein–coupled receptors – both coupling to G_i/G_o – found mainly in the brain and retina but also in peripheral tissues (see Jockers et al., 2016). Another type (termed MT_3) has been suggested to be the enzyme quinone reductase 2 (QR2). The function of the interaction between melatonin and QR2 is unclear.

Melatonin secretion (in all animals studied, whether diurnal or nocturnal in their habits) is high at night and low by day. This rhythm is controlled by input from the retina via a noradrenergic retinohypothalamic tract that terminates in the suprachiasmatic nucleus (SCN) in the hypothalamus, a structure often termed the biological clock, which generates the circadian rhythm. Activation of MT_1 receptors inhibits neuronal firing in the SCN and prolactin secretion from the pituitary. Activation of MT_2 receptors phase shifts circadian rhythms generated within the SCN. Melatonin has antioxidant properties and may be neuroprotective in Alzheimer's disease and Parkinson's disease (see Ch. 40).

[5]Unfortunately the nomenclature for P2Y receptors has developed in a rather haphazard manner. There is compelling evidence for the existence of $P2Y_{1, 2, 4, 6, 11, 12, 13 \text{ and } 14}$ receptors, but not for others.

Given orally, melatonin is well absorbed but quickly metabolised, its plasma half-life being a few minutes. Based on its ability to reset the circadian clock, melatonin supplements has been promoted for various uses, such as controlling jet lag, improving the performance of night-shift workers, treating insomnia in the elderly and controlling sleep disorders in children with autism or as a consequence of psychostimulant use for ADHD. **Ramelteon**, an agonist at MT_1 and MT_2 receptors, is used to treat insomnia (see Ch. 45) and **agomelatine**, which also has agonist actions at MT_1 and MT_2 receptors as well as antagonist actions at 5-HT_{2C} receptors, is a novel antidepressant drug (see Ch. 48).

NITRIC OXIDE

NO as a peripheral mediator is discussed in Chapter 19. Its significance as an important chemical mediator in the nervous system has demanded a considerable readjustment of our views about neurotransmission and neuromodulation (for review, see Chachlaki et al., 2017). The main defining criteria for transmitter substances - namely that neurons should possess machinery for synthesising and storing the substance, that it should be released from neurons by exocytosis, that it should interact with specific membrane receptors and that there should be mechanisms for its inactivation - do not apply to NO. Moreover, it is an inorganic gas, not at all like the kind of molecule pharmacologists are used to. The mediator function of NO is now well established (Zhou and Zhu, 2009). NO diffuses rapidly through cell membranes, and its action is not highly localised. Its half-life depends greatly on the chemical environment, ranging from seconds in blood to several minutes in normal tissues. The rate of inactivation of NO (see Ch. 19) increases disproportionately with NO concentration, so low levels of NO are relatively stable. The presence of superoxide, with which NO reacts (see later), shortens its half-life considerably.

NO in the nervous system is produced mainly by the constitutive neuronal form of *NO synthase* (nNOS; see Ch. 19), which can be detected either histochemically or by immunolabelling. This enzyme is present in roughly 2% of neurons, both short interneurons and long-tract neurons, in virtually all brain areas, with particular concentrations in the cerebellum and hippocampus. It occurs in cell bodies and dendrites, as well as in axon terminals, suggesting that NO may be produced both pre- and postsynaptically. nNOS is calmodulin dependent and is activated by a rise in intracellular Ca^{2+} concentration, which can occur by many mechanisms (see Ch. 4), including action potential conduction and neurotransmitter action, especially by glutamate activation of *N*-methyl-D-aspartate (NMDA) receptors. NO is not stored but released as it is made. Many studies have shown that NO production is increased by activation of synaptic pathways, or by other events, such as brain ischaemia (see Ch. 40).

NO exerts pre- and postsynaptic actions on neurons as well as acting on glial cells (Garthwaite, 2008). It produces its effects in two main ways:

1. By activation of soluble guanylyl cyclase, leading to the production of cGMP, which itself or through activation of protein kinase G can affect membrane ion channels (Steinert et al., 2010). This 'physiological' control mechanism operates at low NO concentrations of about 0.1 μmol/L.
2. By reacting with the superoxide free radical to generate peroxynitrite, a highly toxic anion that acts by oxidising various intracellular proteins. This requires concentrations of 1–10 μmol/L, which are achieved in brain ischaemia.

There is good evidence that NO plays a role in synaptic plasticity (see Ch. 38), because long-term potentiation and depression are reduced or prevented by NOS inhibitors and are absent in transgenic mice in which the *nNOS* gene has been disrupted.

Based on the same kind of evidence, NO is also believed to play an important part in the mechanisms by which ischaemia causes neuronal death (see Ch. 40). There is also evidence that it may be involved in other processes, including neurodegeneration in Parkinson's disease, senile dementia and amyotrophic lateral sclerosis, and the local control of blood flow linked to neuronal activity.

Other 'gaseotransmitters'. These include carbon monoxide, hydrogen sulfide and, more recently, ammonia (see Ch. 19 and Wang, 2014). While evidence is accumulating for their roles in CNS disorders, their pharmacology is still at a very preliminary stage.

Carbon monoxide (CO) is best known as a poisonous gas present in vehicle exhaust, which binds strongly to haemoglobin, causing tissue anoxia. However, it is also formed endogenously and has many features in common with NO. Neurons and other cells contain a CO-generating enzyme, haem oxygenase, and CO, like NO, activates guanylyl cyclase. There is some evidence that CO plays a role in memory mechanisms in the hippocampus (see Cutajar and Edwards, 2007).

Hydrogen sulfide (H_2S) has been postulated to be involved in learning, memory and pain perception but then again so has almost every other neurotransmitter or neuromodulator! It has been suggested that brain H_2S concentrations are lowered in Alzheimer's and Parkinson's diseases but the relevance of such observations still needs to be worked out.

LIPID MEDIATORS

The formation of arachidonic acid, and its conversion to eicosanoids (mainly prostaglandins, leukotrienes and hydroxyeicosatetraenoic acids (HETEs) – see Ch. 17) and to endocannabinoids, anandamide and 2-arachidonoylglycerol (see Ch. 18), also takes place in the CNS.

Phospholipid cleavage, leading to arachidonic acid production, occurs in neurons in response to receptor activation by many different mediators, including neurotransmitters. The arachidonic acid so formed can act directly as an intracellular messenger, controlling both ion channels and various parts of the protein kinase cascade (see Ch. 3), producing both rapid and delayed effects on neuronal function. Both arachidonic acid itself and its products escape readily from the cell of origin and can affect neighbouring structures, including presynaptic terminals (retrograde signalling) and adjacent cells (paracrine signalling), by acting on receptors or by acting directly as intracellular messengers. Fig. 39.7 shows a schematic view of the variety of different roles these agents can play at the synapse.

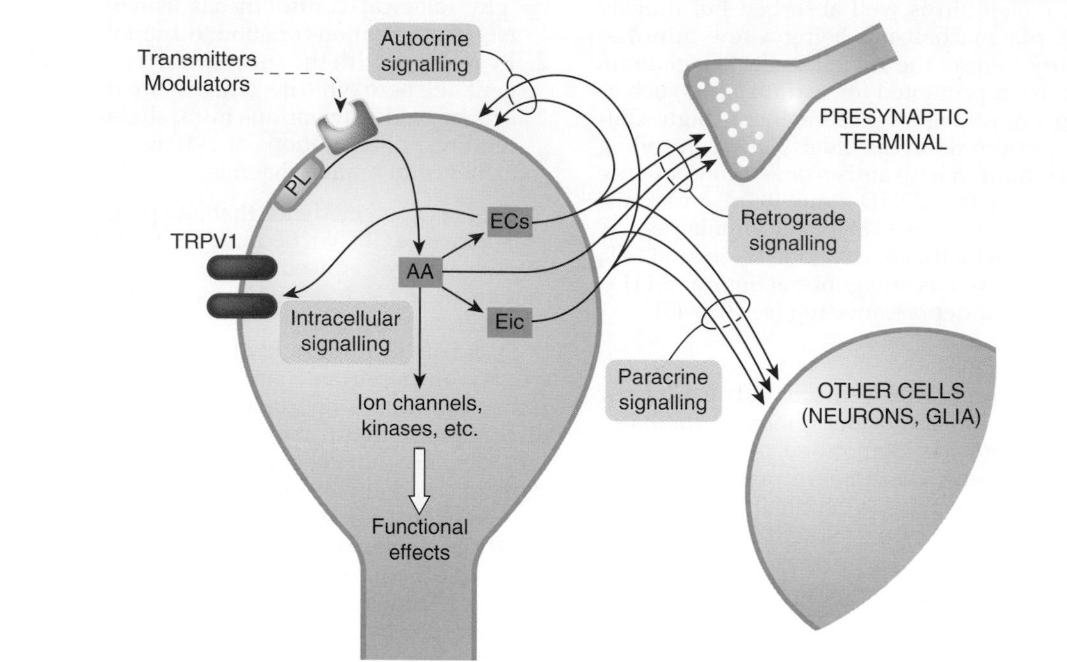

Fig. 39.7 Postulated modes of signalling by lipid mediators. Arachidonic acid (AA) is formed by receptor-mediated cleavage of membrane phospholipid. It can act directly as an intracellular messenger on ion channels or components of different kinase cascades, producing various long- and short-term effects. It can also be converted to eicosanoids (prostaglandins, leukotrienes or hydroxyeicosatetraenoic acids (HETEs)) or to the endocannabinoids (ECs), anandamide and 2-arachidonoylglycerol. ECs can also act as intracellular messengers to activate TRPV1 channels. HETEs can also act directly as intracellular messengers. All these mediators also diffuse out of the cell, and exert effects on presynaptic terminals and neighbouring cells, acting either on extracellular receptors or intracellularly. There are examples of most of these modes of signalling, but only limited information about their functional significance in the nervous system. *Eic*, Eicosanoids; *PL*, membrane phospholipid.

Arachidonic acid can be metabolised to eicosanoids, some of which (principally the HETEs) can also act as intracellular messengers acting in the same cell. Eicosanoids can also exert an autocrine effect via membrane receptors expressed by the cell (see Ch. 17). The eicosanoids play important roles in neural function including pain, temperature regulation, sleep induction, synaptic plasticity and spatial learning.

It is now generally accepted that endocannabinoids, such as anandamide and 2-arachidonylglycerol, act as retrograde synaptic messengers in the CNS (see Pertwee, 2015, and Ch. 18). They are synthesised and secreted in response to a rise in intracellular Ca^{2+} and activate presynaptic CB_1 receptors inhibiting the release of neurotransmitters such as glutamate and GABA. CB_1 receptors are widely distributed in the brain and spinal cord, not only on neurons but also on astrocytes and microglia, whereas CB_2 receptor expression is much less but may be up-regulated under pathological conditions. Agonists at CB_1 receptors have therapeutic potential for the treatment of vomiting, pain (CB_2 receptor agonists may also be effective in some pain states), muscle spasms as occur in conditions such as multiple sclerosis and anxiety, as well as in other brain disorders including Alzheimer's disease and tardive dyskinesias. Endocannabinoids released into the extracellular space are removed into cells by facilitated transport, for which inhibitors have been developed, and then metabolised (Cascio and Marini, 2015). Anandamide is metabolised by fatty acid amide hydrolase (FAAH; see Ch. 18). Inhibitors of FAAH potentiate the effects of endocannabinoids and were shown to be effective analgesics in animal models of pain (Roques et al., 2012).[6] The CB_1-receptor antagonist **rimonabant** was introduced as an anti-obesity agent but subsequently had to be withdrawn because of negative effects on mood (see Ch. 18). Endocannabinoids, besides being agonists at cannabinoid receptors, also interact with a variety of ion channels including TRPV1 channels (see Ch. 43), 5-HT3 receptors, calcium channels and potassium channels (Pertwee, 2015)

Lysophosphatidic acid and sphingosine 1-phosphate are phospholipids with important signalling functions in the brain and elsewhere throughout the body. Their effects are mediated by multiple G protein–coupled receptors (LPA1-6 and S1P1-5). Agonists at S1P1 receptors are in phase III clinical trials for the treatment of multiple sclerosis (see Ch. 40).

[6] Readers may recall the tragic phase I clinical trial of one FAAH inhibitor, BIA 10-2474, that caused sudden, severe CNS damage and resulted in one subject being brain dead and four others having permanent brain damage. In this instance the adverse effects were due to actions of the drug on other lipases.

Other transmitters and modulators

Purines

- ATP functions as a neurotransmitter, being stored in vesicles and released by exocytosis. It acts via ionotropic P2X receptors and metabotropic P2Y receptors.
- Cytosolic ATP is present at a relatively high concentration and can be released directly if neuronal viability is compromised (e.g. in stroke). Excessive release may be neurotoxic.
- Released ATP is rapidly converted to ADP, AMP and adenosine.
- Adenosine is not stored in vesicles but is released by carrier mechanisms or generated from released ATP, mainly under pathological conditions.
- Adenosine exerts mainly inhibitory effects, through A_1 and A_2 receptors, resulting in sedative, anticonvulsant and neuroprotective effects, and acting as a safety mechanism.
- Methylxanthines (e.g. **caffeine**) are antagonists at A_2 receptors and increase wakefulness.

Histamine

- Histamine fulfils the criteria for a neurotransmitter. Histaminergic neurons originate in a small area of the hypothalamus and have a widespread distribution.
- H_1, H_2 and H_3 receptors are widespread in the brain.
- The functions of histamine are not well understood, the main clues being that histaminergic neurons are active during waking hours, and H_1 receptor antagonists are strongly sedative.
- H_1 receptor antagonists are antiemetic.

Melatonin

- Melatonin is synthesised from 5-HT, mainly in the pineal gland, from which it is released as a circulating hormone.
- Secretion is controlled by light intensity, being low by day and high by night. Fibres from the retina run to the SCN ('biological clock'), which controls the pineal gland via its sympathetic innervation.
- Melatonin acts on MT_1 and MT_2 receptors in the brain.
- Agonists at melatonin receptors induce sleep and have antidepressant properties.

Other mediators

Nitric oxide

- nNOS is present in many CNS neurons, and NO production is increased by mechanisms (e.g. transmitter action) that raise intracellular Ca^{2+}.
- NO affects neuronal function by increasing cGMP formation, producing both inhibitory and excitatory effects on neurons.
- In larger amounts, NO forms peroxynitrite, which contributes to neurotoxicity.
- Inhibition of nNOS reduces long-term potentiation and long-term depression, probably because NO functions as a retrograde messenger. Inhibition of nNOS also protects against ischaemic brain damage in animal models.
- Carbon monoxide and hydrogen sulfide may also be neural mediators.

Lipid mediators

- Arachidonic acid is produced in neurons by receptor-mediated hydrolysis of phospholipid. It is converted to various eicosanoids and endocannabinoids.
- Arachidonic acid itself, as well as its active products, can produce rapid and slow effects by regulation of ion channels and protein kinase cascades. Such effects can occur in the donor cell or in adjacent cells and nerve terminals.
- Anandamide and 2-arachidonoylglycerol are endogenous activators of cannabinoid CB_1 and CB_2 receptors (see Ch. 18) and also of the TRPV1 receptor (see Ch. 43).

A FINAL MESSAGE

In the last two chapters we have taken a long and tortuous tour through the brain and its chemistry, with two questions at the back of our minds. What mediators and what receptors play a key role in what brain functions? How does the information relate to existing and future drugs that aim to correct malfunctions? Through the efforts of a huge army of researchers deploying an arsenal of powerful modern techniques, the answers to these questions are slowly being produced. The array of potential CNS targets – comprising multiple receptor subtypes, many with the added complexity of heteromeric assemblies, splice variants, etc., along with regulatory mechanisms that control their expression and localisation – continues to grow in complexity. The view that specific malfunctions in a particular system give rise to specific CNS disorders is becoming less of a reality particularly in relation to cognitive and emotional disorders. The interactions between transmitter systems and capacity within the CNS to rapidly adapt in response to drug treatments add to this complexity. In the ensuing chapters in this section we shall find that most of the therapeutic successes have come from chance discoveries that were followed up empirically; few have followed a logical, mechanism-based route to success. The optimistic view is that this is changing, and that future therapeutic discoveries will depend less on luck and more on molecular logic. But the revolution is slow in coming. One of the key problems, perhaps, is that the brain puts cells, organelles and molecules exactly where they are needed, and uses the same molecules to perform different functions in different locations. Drug discovery scientists are getting quite good at devising molecule-specific ligands (see Ch. 60), but we lack delivery systems able to target them anatomically even to macroscopic brain regions, let alone to specific cells and subcellular structures.

REFERENCES AND FURTHER READING

General references

Iversen, L.L., Iversen, S.D., Bloom, F.E., Roth, R.H., 2009. Introduction to Neuropsychopharmacology. Oxford University Press, New York.

Nestler, E.J., Hyman, S.E., Holtzman, M., Malenka, R.C., 2020. Molecular Neuropharmacology: A Foundation for Clinical Neuroscience, fourth ed. McGraw-Hill, New York.

Noradrenaline

Robertson, S.D., Plummer, N.W., de Marchena, J., Jensen, P., 2013. Developmental origins of central norepinephrine neuron diversity. Nat. Neurosci. 16, 1016–1023.

Waterhouse, B.D., Navarra, R.L., 2019. The locus coeruleus-norepinephrine system and sensory signal processing: a historical review and current perspectives. Brain Res. 1709, 1–15.

Dopamine

Beaulieu, J.-M., Gainetdinov, R.R., 2011. The physiology, signaling, and pharmacology of dopamine receptors. Pharmacol. Rev. 63, 182–217.

Björklund, A., Dunnett, S.B., 2007. Dopamine neuron systems in the brain: an update. Trends Neurosci. 30, 194–202.

De Mei, C., Ramos, M., Iitaka, C., Borrelli, E., 2009. Getting specialized: presynaptic and postsynaptic dopamine D_2 receptors. Curr. Opin. Pharmacol. 9, 53–58.

Hydroxytryptamine

De Deurwaerdere, P., Di Giovanni, G., 2021. 5-HT interaction with other neurotransmitters: an overview. Prog. Brain Res. 259, 1–5.

Jensen, A.A., Davies, P.A., Bräuner-Osborne, H., Krzywkowski, K., 2008. 3B but which 3B? And that's just one of the questions: the heterogeneity of human 5-HT_3 receptors. Trends Pharmacol. Sci. 29, 437–444.

Peters, J.A., Hales, T.G., Lambert, J.J., 2005. Molecular determinants of single-channel conductance and ion selectivity in the Cys-loop family: insights from the 5-HT_3 receptor. Trends Pharmacol. Sci. 26, 587–594.

Sharp, T., Barnes, N.M., 2020. Central 5-HT receptors and their function; present and future. Neuropharmacology 177, 108155.

Acetylcholine

Delmas, P., Brown, D.A., 2005. Pathways modulating neural KCNQ/M (Kv7) potassium channels. Nat. Rev. Neurosci. 6, 850–862.

Gotti, C., Zoli, M., Clementi, F., 2008. Brain nicotinic acetylcholine receptors: native subtypes and their relevance. Trends Pharmacol. Sci. 27, 482–491.

Hasselmo, M.E., 2006. The role of acetylcholine in learning and memory. Curr. Opin. Neurobiol. 16, 710–715.

Wess, J., 2004. Muscarinic acetylcholine receptor knockout mice: novel phenotypes and clinical implications. Annu. Rev. Pharmacol. Toxicol. 44, 423–450.

Other messengers

Boison, D., Aronica, E., 2015. Comorbidities in neurology: is adenosine the common link? Neuropharmacology 97, 18–34.

Brown, R.E., Stevens, D.R., Haas, H.L., 2001. The physiology of brain histamine. Prog. Neurobiol. 63, 637–672.

Burnstock, G., 2016. An introduction to the roles of purinergic signalling in neurodegeneration, neuroprotection and neuroregeneration. Neuropharmacology 104, 4–17.

Burnstock, G., 2018. Purine and purinergic receptors. Brain Neurosci. Adv. 2, 1–10.

Buscemi, N., Vandermeer, B., Hooton, N., et al., 2006. Efficacy and safety of exogenous melatonin for secondary sleep disorders and sleep disorders accompanying sleep restriction: meta-analysis. BMJ 332, 385–393.

Cascio, M.G., Marini, P., 2015. Biosynthesis and fate of endocannabinoids. Handb. Exp. Pharmacol. 231, 39–58.

Castillo, P.E., Younts, T.J., Chávez, A.E., Hashimotodani, Y., 2012. Endocannabinoid signaling and synaptic function. Neuron 76, 70–81.

Chachlaki, K., Garthwaite, J., Prevot, V., 2017. The gentle art of saying no: how nitric oxide gets things done in the hypothalamus. Nat. Rev. Endocrinol. 13, 521–535.

Cutajar, M.C., Edwards, T.M., 2007. Evidence for the role of endogenous carbon monoxide in memory processing. J. Cogn. Neurosci. 19, 557–562.

Dubocovich, M.L., Delagrange, P., Krause, D.N., Sugden, D., Cardinali, D.P., Olcese, J., 2010. International Union of Basic and Clinical Pharmacology. LXXV. Nomenclature, classification, and pharmacology of G protein–coupled melatonin receptors. Pharmacol. Rev. 62, 343–380.

Garthwaite, J., 2008. Concepts of neural nitric oxide-mediated transmission. Eur. J. Neurosci. 27, 2783–2802.

Hu, W., Chen, Z., 2017. The roles of histamine and its receptor ligands in central nervous system disorders: an update. Pharmacol. Ther. 175, 116–132.

Jockers, R., Delagrange, P., Dubocovich, M.L., et al., 2016. Update on melatonin receptors: IUPHAR Review 20. Br. J. Pharmacol. 173, 2702–2725.

Pertwee, R.G., 2015. Endocannabinoids and their pharmacological action. Handb. Exp. Pharmacol. 231, 1–38.

Roques, B.P., Fournié-Zaluski, M.C., Wurm, M., 2012. Inhibiting the breakdown of endogenous opioids and cannabinoids to alleviate pain. Nat. Rev. Drug Discov. 11, 292–310.

Steinert, J.R., Chernova, T., Forsythe, I.D., 2010. Nitric oxide signaling in brain function, dysfunction, and dementia. Neuroscientist 16, 435–452.

Schicker, K.W., Dorostkar, M.M., Boehm, S., 2008. Modulation of transmitter release via presynaptic ligand-gated ion channels. Curr. Mol. Pharmacol. 1, 106–129.

Tozaki-Saitoh, H., Tsuda, M., Inoue, K., 2011. Role of purinergic receptors in CNS function and neuroprotection. Adv. Pharmacol. 61, 495–528.

Wang, R., 2014. Gasotransmitters: growing pains and joys. Trends Biochem. Sci. 39, 227–232.

Zhou, L., Zhu, D.Y., 2009. Neuronal nitric oxide synthase: structure, subcellular localization, regulation and clinical implications. Nitric Oxide 20, 223–230.

Neurodegenerative diseases

40

OVERVIEW

Despite ongoing neural plasticity, dead neurons in the adult central nervous system (CNS) are not as a rule replaced,[1] nor can their terminals regenerate when their axons are interrupted. Therefore any pathological process causing neuronal death generally has irreversible consequences. At first sight, this appears to be very unpromising territory for pharmacological intervention, and indeed drug therapy is currently very limited, except in the case of Parkinson's disease (PD). Nevertheless, the incidence and social impact of neurodegenerative brain disorders in ageing populations have resulted in a massive research effort in recent years. To date there has been more success in developing drugs that treat the symptoms arising from neuronal cell loss than in developing ones that attempt to halt or reverse the degenerative processes.

In this chapter, a number of neurodegenerative conditions are described: ischaemic brain damage (stroke), dementias – Alzheimer's disease (AD), dementia associated with Lewy bodies (DLB) and vascular dementia – PD, essential tremor (ET), Huntington's disease (HD), amyotrophic lateral sclerosis (ALS), spinal muscular atrophy (SMA) and multiple sclerosis (MS).

The main topics discussed in this chapter are:

- **mechanisms responsible for neuronal death, focusing on genetic defects, protein aggregation (e.g. amyloidosis), excitotoxicity, oxidative stress and apoptosis;**
- **pharmacological approaches to neuroprotection, based on the earlier mechanisms; and**
- **pharmacological approaches to compensation for neuronal loss (applicable mainly to AD and PD).**

PROTEIN MISFOLDING AND AGGREGATION IN CHRONIC NEURODEGENERATIVE DISEASES

Protein misfolding and aggregation is considered to be the first step in many neurodegenerative diseases (see Peden and Ironside, 2012). Misfolding means the adoption of abnormal conformations, by certain normally expressed proteins, such that they tend to form large insoluble aggregates (Fig. 40.1). The conversion of the linear amino acid chain produced by the ribosome into a functional protein requires it to be folded correctly into a compact conformation with specific amino acids correctly located on its surface. This complicated stepwise sequence can easily go wrong and lead to misfolded variants that are unable to find a way back to the correct 'native' conformation. The misfolded molecules lack the normal function of the protein but can nonetheless make mischief within the cell. The misfolding often means that hydrophobic residues that would normally be buried in the core of the protein are exposed on its surface, which gives the molecules a strong tendency to stick to cell membranes and aggregate, initially as oligomers and then as insoluble microscopic aggregates (see Fig. 40.1), leading to the death of neurons. The tendency to adopt such conformations may be favoured by specific mutations of the protein in question, or by infection with prions.[2]

Misfolded conformations can be generated spontaneously at a low rate throughout life, so that aggregates accumulate gradually with age. In the nervous system, the aggregates often form distinct structures, generally known as *amyloid deposits*, that are visible under the microscope and are characteristic of neurodegenerative disease. Although the mechanisms are not clear, such aggregates, or the misfolded protein precursors, lead to neuronal death. Examples of neurodegenerative diseases that are caused by such protein misfolding and aggregation are shown in Table 40.1.

The brain possesses a variety of protective mechanisms that limit the accumulation of such protein aggregates. The main ones involve the production of 'chaperone' proteins, which bind to newly synthesised or misfolded proteins and encourage them to fold correctly, and the 'ubiquitination' reaction, which prepares proteins for destruction within the cell. Accumulation of protein deposits occurs when these protective mechanisms are unable to cope.

Protein misfolding

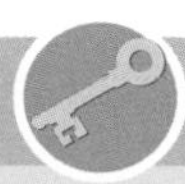

- Many chronic neurodegenerative diseases involve the misfolding of normal or mutated forms of physiological proteins. Examples include Alzheimer's disease, dementia associated with Lewy bodies, Parkinson's disease, amyotrophic lateral sclerosis and many less common diseases.
- Misfolded proteins are normally removed by intracellular degradation pathways, which may be altered in neurodegenerative disorders.
- Misfolded proteins tend to aggregate, initially as soluble oligomers, later as large insoluble aggregates that accumulate intracellularly or extracellularly as microscopic deposits, which are stable and resistant to proteolysis.
- Misfolded proteins often present hydrophobic surface residues that promote aggregation and association with membranes.
- The mechanisms responsible for neuronal death are unclear, but there is evidence that both the soluble aggregates and the microscopic deposits may be neurotoxic.

[1]It is recognised that new neurons are formed from progenitor cells (*neurogenesis*) in certain regions of the adult brain and can become functionally integrated, even in primates (see Rakic, 2002; Zhao et al., 2008). Neurogenesis in the hippocampus is thought to play a role in learning and memory but plays little if any role in brain repair. However, learning how to harness the inherent ability of neuronal progenitors (stem cells) to form new neurons is seen as a promising approach to treating neurodegenerative disorders.

[2]Such prion diseases include Creutzfeldt–Jakob's disease (CJD) and the new variant CJD. Sadly, no pharmacological treatments that prevent disease progression are yet available and treatment is aimed at ameliorating the symptoms.

MECHANISMS OF NEURONAL DEATH

Acute injury to cells causes them to undergo *necrosis*, recognised pathologically by cell swelling, vacuolisation and lysis and associated with Ca^{2+} overload of the cells and membrane damage. Necrotic cells typically spill their contents into the surrounding tissue, evoking an inflammatory response. Chronic inflammation is a feature of most neurodegenerative disorders (see Schwab and McGeer, 2008), and a possible target for therapeutic intervention.

Cells can also die by *apoptosis* (programmed cell death, see Ch. 6), a mechanism that is essential for many processes throughout life, including development, immune regulation and tissue remodelling. Apoptosis, as well as necrosis, occurs in both acute neurodegenerative disorders (such as stroke and head injury) and chronic ones (such as AD and PD). The distinction between necrosis and apoptosis as processes leading to neurodegeneration is not absolute, for challenges such as excitotoxicity and oxidative stress may be enough to kill cells directly by necrosis or, if less intense, may induce them to undergo apoptosis. Both processes therefore represent possible targets for putative neuroprotective drug therapy. Pharmacological interference with the apoptotic pathway may become possible in the future, but for the present most efforts are directed at the processes involved

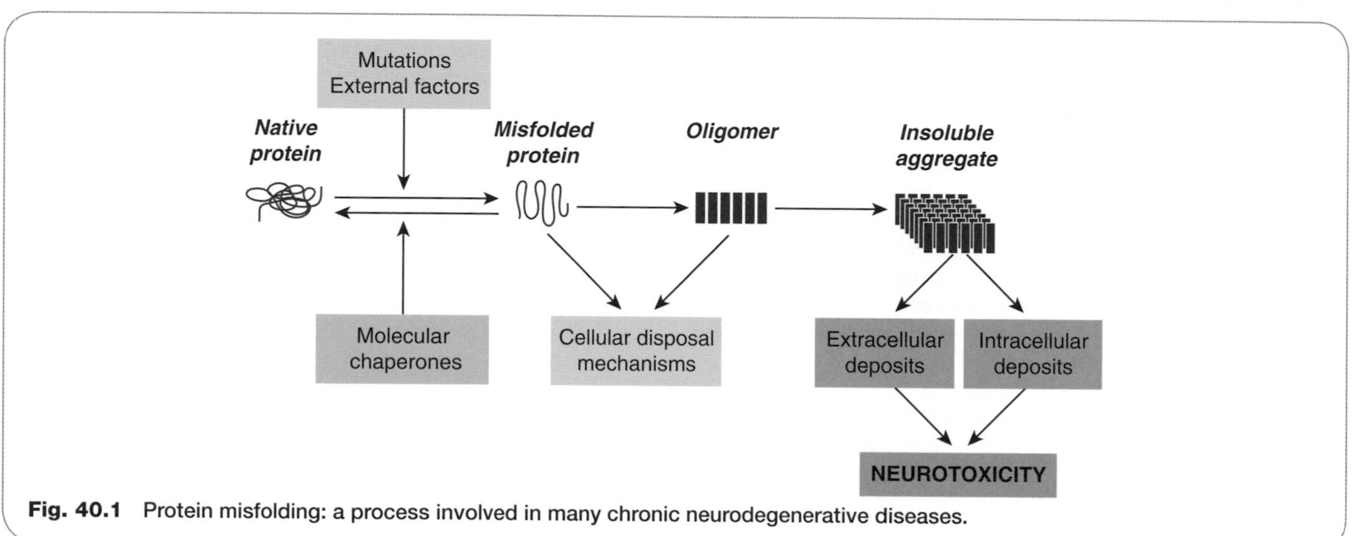

Fig. 40.1 Protein misfolding: a process involved in many chronic neurodegenerative diseases.

Table 40.1 Examples of neurodegenerative diseases associated with protein misfolding and aggregation[a]

Disease	Protein	Characteristic pathology	Notes
Alzheimer's disease	β-Amyloid (Aβ)	Amyloid plaques	Aβ mutations occur in rare familial forms of Alzheimer's disease
	Tau	Neurofibrillary tangles	Implicated in other pathologies ('tauopathies') as well as Alzheimer's disease
Dementia associated with Lewy bodies Parkinson's disease	α-Synuclein	Lewy bodies	Lewy body formation also occurs in some forms of Alzheimer's disease
Creutzfeldt–Jakob's disease	Prion protein	Insoluble aggregates of prion protein	Transmitted by infection with prion protein in its misfolded state
Huntington's disease	Huntingtin	No gross lesions	One of several genetic 'polyglutamine repeat' disorders
Amyotrophic lateral sclerosis (a form of motor neuron disease)	Superoxide dismutase	Loss of motor neurons	Mutated superoxide dismutase tends to form aggregates; loss of enzyme function increases susceptibility to oxidative stress

[a]Protein aggregation disorders are often collectively known as amyloidoses and commonly affect organs other than the brain.

in cell necrosis, and at compensating pharmacologically for the neuronal loss.

EXCITOTOXICITY

Despite its ubiquitous role as a neurotransmitter, **glutamate** is highly toxic to neurons, a phenomenon dubbed *excitotoxicity* (see Ch. 38). A low concentration of glutamate applied to neurons in culture kills the cells, and the finding in the 1970s that glutamate given orally produces neurodegeneration in vivo caused considerable alarm because of the widespread use of glutamate as a 'taste-enhancing' food additive. The Chinese restaurant syndrome - an acute attack of neck stiffness and chest pain is well known, but so far, the possibility of more serious neurotoxicity is only hypothetical.

Local injection of the glutamate receptor agonist *kainic acid* is used experimentally to produce neurotoxic lesions. It acts by excitation of local glutamate-releasing neurons, and the release of glutamate, acting on *N*-methyl-D-aspartate (NMDA) receptors, and also metabotropic receptors (see Ch. 38), leads to neuronal death.

Calcium overload is the essential factor in excitotoxicity. The mechanisms by which this occurs and leads to cell death are as follows (see also Fig. 40.2):

- Glutamate activates NMDA, (*S*)-α-amino-3-hydroxy-5-methylisoxazole-4-propionic acid (AMPA) and metabotropic glutamate receptors (sites 1, 2 and 3 in Fig. 40.2). Activation of AMPA receptors depolarises the cell, which removes the Mg^{2+} block of NMDA channels (see Ch. 38), permitting Ca^{2+} entry. Depolarisation also opens voltage-dependent calcium channels (site 4). Metabotropic receptors cause the release of intracellular Ca^{2+} from the endoplasmic reticulum. Na^+ entry further contributes to Ca^{2+} entry by stimulating Ca^{2+}/Na^+ exchange (site 5). Depolarisation inhibits or reverses glutamate uptake (site 6), thus increasing the extracellular glutamate concentration.
- The mechanisms that normally operate to counteract the rise in cytosolic free Ca^{2+} concentration, $[Ca^{2+}]_i$, include the Ca^{2+} efflux pump (site 7) and, indirectly, the Na^+ pump (site 8).
- The mitochondria and endoplasmic reticulum act as capacious sinks for Ca^{2+} and normally keep $[Ca^{2+}]_i$ under control. Loading of the mitochondrial stores beyond a certain point, however, disrupts mitochondrial function, reducing ATP synthesis, thus reducing the energy available for the membrane pumps and for Ca^{2+} accumulation by the endoplasmic reticulum. Formation of reactive oxygen species (ROS) is also enhanced. This represents the danger point at which positive feedback exaggerates the process.
- Raised $[Ca^{2+}]_i$ affects many processes, the chief ones relevant to neurotoxicity being:
  - increased glutamate release from nerve terminals;
  - activation of proteases (calpains) and lipases, causing membrane damage;
  - activation of nitric oxide synthase; while low concentrations of nitric oxide are neuroprotective, high concentrations in the presence of ROS generate peroxynitrite and hydroxyl free radicals, which damage many important biomolecules, including membrane lipids, proteins and DNA;
  - increased arachidonic acid release, which increases free radical and inflammatory mediator production and also inhibits glutamate uptake (site 6).

Glutamate and Ca^{2+} are arguably the two most ubiquitous chemical signals, extracellular and intracellular, respectively, underlying brain function, so it is disconcerting that such cytotoxic mayhem can be unleashed when they get out of control. Both are stored in dangerous amounts in subcellular organelles, like hand grenades in an ammunition store. Defence against excitotoxicity is clearly essential if our brains are to have any chance of staying alive. Mitochondrial energy metabolism provides one line of defence, and impaired mitochondrial function, by rendering neurons vulnerable to excitotoxic damage, may be a factor in various neurodegenerative conditions, including PD. Furthermore, impaired mitochondrial function can cause release of cytochrome C, which is an important initiator of apoptosis.

The role of excitotoxicity in ischaemic brain damage is well established, and it is also believed to be a factor in other neurodegenerative diseases, such as those discussed here.

There are several examples of neurodegenerative conditions caused by environmental toxins acting as agonists on glutamate receptors. *Domoic acid* is a glutamate analogue produced by mussels, which was identified as the cause of an epidemic of severe mental and neurological deterioration in a group of Newfoundlanders in 1987. On the island of Guam, a syndrome combining the features of dementia, paralysis and PD was traced to an excitotoxic amino acid, β-methylamino-alanine, in the seeds of a local plant. Discouraging the consumption of these seeds has largely eliminated the disease.

Disappointingly, intense effort, based on the mechanisms described earlier, to find effective drugs for a range of neurodegenerative disorders in which excitotoxicity is believed to play a part has had very limited success. **Riluzole** retards to some degree the deterioration of patients with ALS. Its precise mechanism of action is unclear. **Memantine** is a weak NMDA-receptor antagonist that produces slight improvement in moderate-to-severe cases of AD.

APOPTOSIS

Apoptosis can be initiated by various cell surface signals (see Ch. 6). The cell is systematically dismantled, and the shrunken remnants are removed by macrophages without causing inflammation. Apoptotic cells can be identified by a staining technique that detects the characteristic DNA breaks. Many different signalling pathways can result in apoptosis, but in all cases the final pathway resulting in cell death is the activation of a family of proteases (caspases), which inactivate various intracellular proteins. Neural survival is regulated by neuronal growth factors, including *nerve growth factor* and *brain-derived neurotrophic factor*, secreted proteins that are

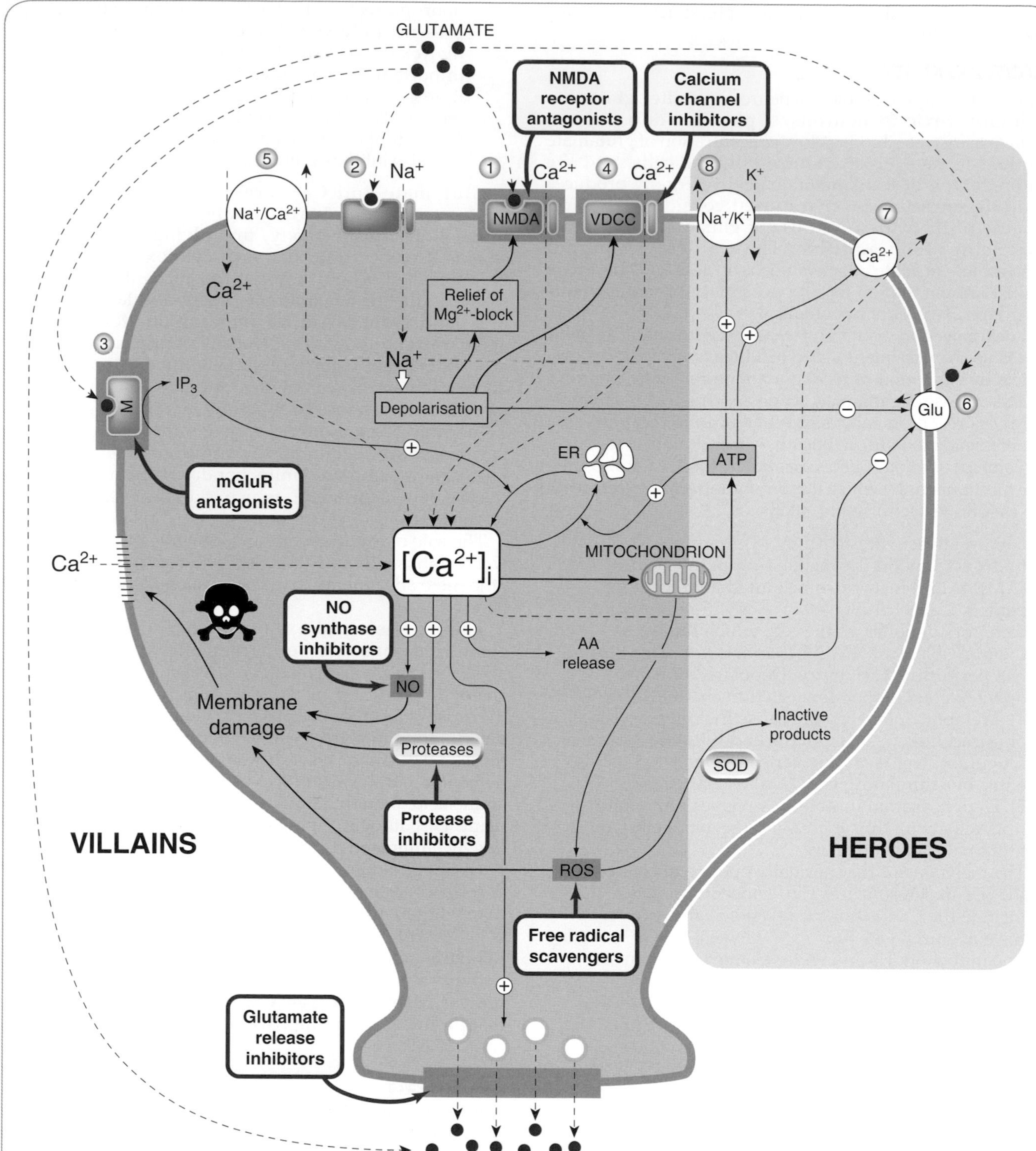

Fig. 40.2 Mechanisms of excitotoxicity. Membrane receptors, ion channels and transporters, identified by numbers 1–8, are discussed in the text. Possible sites of action of neuroprotective drugs (not yet of proven clinical value) are *highlighted*. Mechanisms on the *left* (villains) are those that favour cell death, while those on the *right* (heroes) are protective. See text for details. *AA,* Arachidonic acid; *ER,* endoplasmic reticulum; *Glu,* glutamate uptake; *IP_3,* inositol trisphosphate; *M, mGluR,* metabotropic glutamate receptor; *NMDA,* N-methyl-D-aspartate; *NO,* nitric oxide; *ROS,* reactive oxygen species; *SOD,* superoxide dismutase; *VDCC,* voltage-dependent calcium channel.

required for the survival of different populations of neurons in the CNS. These growth factors regulate the expression of the two gene products, Bax and Bcl-2, Bax being proapoptotic and Bcl-2 being antiapoptotic (see Ch. 6). Neurons also have significant expression of anti-apoptotic family member Bcl-x, but the balance of Bax and Bcl-2 are the key determinants to neuronal survival. Blocking apoptosis by interfering at specific points on these pathways represents an attractive strategy for developing neuroprotective drugs, but one that has yet to bear fruit.

OXIDATIVE STRESS

The brain has high energy needs, which are met almost entirely by mitochondrial oxidative phosphorylation, generating ATP at the same time as reducing molecular O_2 to H_2O. Under certain conditions, highly ROS, for example, oxygen and hydroxyl free radicals and H_2O_2, may be generated as side products of this process (see Barnham et al., 2004). Oxidative stress is the result of excessive production of these reactive species. They can also be produced as a byproduct of other biochemical pathways, including nitric oxide synthesis and arachidonic acid metabolism (which are implicated in excitotoxicity), as well as the P450 mono-oxygenase system (see Ch. 10). Unchecked, reactive oxygen radicals attack many key molecules, including enzymes, membrane lipids and DNA. During periods of tissue reperfusion following ischaemia (e.g. in stroke), delinquent leukocytes may exacerbate this problem by releasing their own cytotoxic oxygen products. Not surprisingly, defence mechanisms are provided, in the form of enzymes such as *superoxide dismutase* (SOD) and *catalase*, as well as antioxidants such as ascorbic acid, glutathione and α-tocopherol (vitamin E), which normally keep these reactive species in check. Some cytokines, especially tumour necrosis factor (TNF)-α, which is produced in conditions of brain ischaemia or inflammation (see Ch. 17), exert a protective effect, partly by increasing the expression of SOD. Transgenic animals lacking TNF receptors show enhanced susceptibility to brain ischaemia. Mutations of the gene encoding SOD (see Fig. 40.2) are associated with ALS, a fatal, paralytic disease resulting from progressive degeneration of motor neurons, and transgenic mice expressing mutated SOD develop a similar condition.[3] Accumulation of aggregates of misfolded mutated SOD may also contribute to neurodegeneration.

Mitochondria play a central role in energy metabolism, failure of which leads to oxidative stress. Damage to mitochondria, leading to the release of cytochrome C into the cytosol, also initiates apoptosis. Mitochondrial integrity is therefore essential for neuronal survival, and mitochondrial dysfunction is seen as a major factor in many neurodegenerative disorders (see Itoh et al., 2013). It is possible that accumulated or inherited mutations in enzymes such as those of the mitochondrial respiratory chain lead to a congenital or age-related increase in susceptibility to oxidative stress, which is manifest in different kinds of inherited neurodegenerative disorders (such as HD), and in age-related neurodegeneration.

Oxidative stress is both a cause and a consequence of inflammation (see Ch. 7), which is a general feature of neurodegenerative disease and is thought to contribute to neuronal damage (see Schwab and McGeer, 2008).

Several possible targets for therapeutic intervention with neuroprotective drugs are shown in Fig. 40.2.

[3]Surprisingly, some SOD mutations associated with ALS are more, rather than less, active than the normal enzyme. The mechanism responsible for neurodegeneration probably involves abnormal accumulation of the enzyme in mitochondria.

Excitotoxicity and oxidative stress

- Excitatory amino acids, especially glutamate, can cause neuronal death.
- Excitotoxicity is associated mainly with activation of NMDA receptors, but other types of excitatory amino acid receptors also contribute.
- Excitotoxicity results from a sustained rise in intracellular Ca^{2+} concentration (Ca^{2+} overload).
- Excitotoxicity can occur under pathological conditions (e.g. cerebral ischaemia, epilepsy) in which excessive glutamate release occurs. It can also occur when chemicals such as **kainic acid** are administered.
- Raised intracellular Ca^{2+} causes cell death by various mechanisms, including activation of proteases, formation of free radicals and lipid peroxidation. Formation of nitric oxide and arachidonic acid is also involved.
- Various mechanisms act normally to protect neurons against excitotoxicity, the main ones being Ca^{2+} transport systems, mitochondrial function and the production of free radical scavengers.
- Oxidative stress refers to conditions (e.g. hypoxia) in which the protective mechanisms are compromised, ROS accumulate and neurons become more susceptible to excitotoxic damage.
- Excitotoxicity due to environmental chemicals may contribute to some neurodegenerative disorders.
- Measures designed to reduce excitotoxicity include the use of glutamate antagonists, calcium channel-blocking drugs and free radical scavengers; none is yet proven for clinical use.
- Mitochondrial dysfunction, associated with ageing, environmental toxins and genetic abnormalities, leads to oxidative stress and is a common feature of neurodegenerative diseases.

ISCHAEMIC BRAIN DAMAGE

After heart disease and cancer, strokes are the commonest cause of death in Europe and North America, and the 70% that are non-fatal are the commonest cause of disability. Approximately 85% of strokes are *ischaemic*, usually due to cerebral arterial occlusion caused by local thrombus formation or by a circulating embolus lodging at a narrowing of the vessel. Ischaemic stroke may be preceded by transient ischaemic attacks (TIAs), or 'mini-strokes', resulting from brief episodes of inadequate blood flow. TIAs produce symptoms such as sudden limb or facial muscle weakness, inability to talk, double vision and dizziness. These symptoms usually resolve within 24 h but serve as a warning that a full stroke may occur in the near future. Measures such as taking **aspirin** or **ticagrelor** (see Ch. 23) should be taken to prevent further atherothrombotic events. The other type of stroke is *haemorrhagic*, due to rupture of a cerebral artery.

PATHOPHYSIOLOGY

Prolonged interruption of blood supply to the brain initiates the cascade of neuronal events shown in Fig. 40.2, which lead in turn to later consequences, including cerebral oedema and inflammation, which can also contribute to brain damage. Further damage can occur following reperfusion,[4] because of the production of ROS when the oxygenation is restored. Reperfusion injury may be an important component in stroke patients. These secondary processes often take hours to develop, providing a window of opportunity for therapeutic intervention. The lesion produced by occlusion of a major cerebral artery consists of a central core in which the neurons quickly undergo irreversible necrosis, surrounded by a penumbra of compromised tissue in which inflammation and apoptotic cell death develop over a period of several hours. It is assumed that neuroprotective therapies, given within a few hours, might inhibit this secondary penumbral damage.

Glutamate excitotoxicity plays a critical role in brain ischaemia. Ischaemia causes depolarisation of neurons, and the release of large amounts of glutamate. Ca^{2+} accumulation occurs, partly as a result of glutamate acting on NMDA receptors, as both Ca^{2+} entry and cell death following cerebral ischaemia are inhibited by drugs that block NMDA receptors or channels (see Ch. 38). Nitric oxide is also produced in amounts much greater than result from normal neuronal activity (i.e. to levels that are toxic rather than modulatory).

THERAPEUTIC APPROACHES

The only drug currently approved for treating ischaemic strokes is a recombinant tissue plasminogen activator, **alteplase**, given intravenously, which helps to restore blood flow by dispersing the thrombus (see Ch. 23). Clinical trials have found that it did not reduce mortality but gave significant functional benefit to patients who survive. To be effective, it must be given within about 4.5 h of the thrombotic episode. Also, it must not be given in the 15% of cases where the cause is haemorrhage rather than thrombosis, so preliminary computerised tomography (CT) scanning is essential. These stringent requirements seriously limit the use of fibrinolytic agents for treating stroke, except where specialised rapid response facilities are available. The use of intra-arterial clot retrieval devices (mechanical thrombectomy), in combination with alteplase, has yielded greater benefits and this technology is available in specialised acute stroke treatment centres.

An alternative approach would be to use neuroprotective agents aimed at rescuing cells in the penumbral region of the lesion, which are otherwise likely to die. In animal models involving cerebral artery occlusion, many drugs targeted at the mechanisms shown in Fig. 40.2 (not to mention many others that have been tested on the basis of more far-flung theories) act in this way to reduce the size of the infarct. These include glutamate antagonists, calcium and sodium-channel inhibitors, free radical scavengers, anti-inflammatory drugs, protease inhibitors and others (see Green, 2008). It seems that almost anything works in these animal models. However, of the many drugs that have been tested in over 100 clinical trials, none was effective. The dispiriting list of failures includes calcium- and sodium-channel blockers (e.g. **nimodipine**, **fosphenytoin**), NMDA-receptor antagonists (**selfotel**, **eliprodil**, **dextromethorphan**), drugs that inhibit glutamate release (adenosine analogues, **lubeluzole**), drugs that enhance GABA effects (e.g. **chlormethiazole**), 5-hydroxytryptamine (5-HT) antagonists, metal chelators and various free radical scavengers (e.g. **tirilazad**). There was hope that mGlu1-receptor antagonists or negative allosteric modulators might be effective in the treatment of ischaemic brain damage but things have gone quiet on that front recently.

Controlled clinical trials on stroke patients are problematic and very expensive, partly because of the large variability of outcome in terms of functional recovery, which means that large groups of patients (typically thousands) need to be observed for several months. The need to start therapy within hours of the attack is an additional problem.

Stroke treatment is certainly not – so far at least – one of pharmacology's success stories, and medical hopes rest more on prevention (e.g. by controlling blood pressure, taking **aspirin**, **statins** or **ticagrelor** to prevent atherosclerosis [see Ch. 23]) than on treatment.[5]

One area of promise is the use of subanaesthetic doses of **xenon**, which has NMDA-receptor antagonist properties (see Ch. 41), in combination with hypothermia to treat hypoxia-induced brain damage in neonates (Esencan et al., 2013).

Stroke

- Associated with intracerebral thrombosis or haemorrhage (less common), resulting in rapid death of neurons by necrosis in the centre of the lesion, followed by more gradual (hours) degeneration of cells in the penumbra due to excitotoxicity and inflammation.
- Spontaneous functional recovery occurs to a highly variable degree.
- Although many types of drug that interfere with excitotoxicity are able to reduce infarct size in experimental animals, none of these has so far proved efficacious in humans.
- Recombinant tissue plasminogen activator (**alteplase**), which disperses blood clots, is beneficial if it is given within 4.5 h; haemorrhagic stroke must be excluded by imaging before its administration.

DEMENTIA

Dementia is a general term describing problems with mental abilities caused by gradual changes and damage in the brain. AD is the most common type of dementia; other common types are dementia with Lewy bodies (DLB) and vascular dementia.

[4]Nevertheless, early reperfusion (within 4.5 h of the thrombosis) is clearly beneficial, based on clinical evidence with fibrinolytic drugs.

[5]Eating dark chocolate is believed to reduce the risk of stroke. Flavonoids in the chocolate may be protective due to antioxidant, anti-clotting and anti-inflammatory properties. However, this is not a reason to overindulge!

AD was originally defined as presenile dementia, but it now appears that the same pathology underlies the dementia irrespective of the age of onset. AD refers to dementia of gradual onset in adulthood, which may follow earlier brain injury, but often has no known antecedent cause. Its prevalence rises sharply with age, from about 2% in those aged 65–69 to 20% in those aged 85–89. Common symptoms of AD are difficulty remembering names and recent events, loss of executive functioning, apathy and depression. Studies have revealed specific genetic and molecular mechanisms underlying AD (see Frigero and De Strooper, 2016; Sims et al., 2020). These advances raised hopes of more effective treatments, but success has proved elusive, in part because multiple factors rather than a single cause contribute to the disease and because the symptoms of the disease become obvious only after the underlying pathology has progressed.

The symptoms of DLB include hallucinations, cognitive difficulties – although memory may be less affected in people with DLB than AD – confusion or sleepiness, impaired movement and tremors, disturbed sleep, fainting spells, unsteadiness and falls. DLB has a different aetiology from AD (see later) and in around 90% of cases occurs primarily in people with no family history of the condition.

Vascular dementia results from reduced blood flow to regions of the brain as may occur with multiple minor strokes or cardiovascular disease. Factors that increase the risk of heart disease and stroke – diabetes, high blood pressure, high cholesterol and smoking – raise the risk of vascular dementia. Symptoms include confusion, slow thinking and changes in mood or behaviour.

PATHOGENESIS OF ALZHEIMER'S DISEASE

AD is associated with brain shrinkage and loss of neurons in many brain regions, but especially in the hippocampus and basal forebrain. The loss of cholinergic neurons in the hippocampus and frontal cortex is a feature of the disease, and is thought to underlie the cognitive deficit and loss of short-term memory that occur. Two microscopic features are characteristic of the disease, namely extracellular *amyloid plaques*, consisting of amorphous extracellular deposits of β-amyloid protein (known as Aβ), and intraneuronal *neurofibrillary tangles*, comprising filaments of a phosphorylated form of a microtubule-associated protein (Tau). Both of these deposits are protein aggregates that result from misfolding of native proteins, as discussed previously. They appear also in normal brains, although in smaller numbers. The early appearance of amyloid deposits presages the development of AD, although symptoms may not develop for many years. Altered processing of amyloid protein from its precursor (*amyloid precursor protein* [APP]) has been implicated in the pathogenesis of AD. This is based on several lines of evidence, particularly the genetic analysis of certain, relatively rare, types of familial AD, in which mutations of the APP gene, or of other genes (e.g. for *presenilins* and *sortilin-related receptor 1*) that control amyloid processing, have been discovered.[6]

Amyloid deposits consist of aggregates of Aβ (Fig. 40.3), a 40- or 42-residue segment of APP, generated by the action of specific proteases (*secretases*). Aβ40 is produced normally in small amounts, whereas Aβ42 is overproduced as a result of the genetic mutations mentioned earlier. Both proteins aggregate to form *amyloid plaques*, but Aβ42 shows a stronger tendency than Aβ40 to do so, and appears to be the main culprit in amyloid formation. APP is a 770–amino acid membrane protein normally expressed by many cells, including CNS neurons. Cleavage by α-secretase releases the large extracellular domain as *soluble* APP, which is believed to serve a physiological trophic function. Formation of Aβ involves cleavage at two different points, including one in the intramembrane domain of APP, by β- and γ-secretases (see Fig. 40.3). γ-Secretase is a clumsy enzyme – actually a large intramembrane complex of several proteins – that lacks precision and cuts APP at different points in the transmembrane domain, generating Aβ fragments of different lengths, including Aβ40 and 42. Mutations in this region of the APP gene affect the preferred cleavage point, tending to favour formation of Aβ42. Mutations of the unrelated presenilin genes result in increased activity of γ-secretase, because the presenilin proteins form part of the γ-secretase complex. These different AD-related mutations increase the ratio of Aβ42:Aβ40, which can be detected in plasma, serving as a marker for familial AD. Mutations in another gene, that for the lipid transport protein ApoE4, also predispose to AD. It was originally thought that this was because mutated ApoE4 proteins are less effective in the clearance of Aβ oligomer. However, more recently the focus on ApoE4 has moved to other potential causes of AD such as tau neurofibrillary tangles (see later), microglia and astrocyte responses and blood–brain barrier disruption (Husain et al., 2021).

It is uncertain exactly how Aβ accumulation would cause neurodegeneration, and whether the damage is done by soluble Aβ monomers or oligomers or by amyloid plaques. There is evidence that the cells die by apoptosis, although an inflammatory response is also evident. Expression of Alzheimer's mutations in transgenic animals (see Götz and Ittner, 2008) causes plaque formation and neurodegeneration, and also increases the susceptibility of CNS neurons to other challenges, such as ischaemia, excitotoxicity and oxidative stress, and this increased vulnerability may be the cause of the progressive neurodegeneration in AD. However, the fact that several novel potential therapies designed to reduce Aβ production have so far proven to be ineffective in clinical trials on AD patients has led some to question the importance of amyloid plaque formation in AD (see Herrup, 2015, for a critical view).

The other main player on the biochemical stage is *Tau*, the protein of which the neurofibrillary tangles are composed (see Fig. 40.3). Its role in neurodegeneration is unclear, although similar 'tauopathies' occur in many neurodegenerative conditions (see Brunden et al., 2009; Hanger et al., 2009). Tau is a normal constituent of neurons, being associated with the intracellular microtubules that serve as tracks for transporting materials along nerve axons. In AD and other tauopathies, Tau is abnormally phosphorylated by the action of various kinases, including glycogen synthase kinase-3β (GSK-3β) and cyclin-dependent kinase 5 (CDK5), and dissociates from microtubules to be deposited intracellularly as *paired helical filaments* with a characteristic microscopic appearance. When the cells die, these filaments aggregate as extracellular *neurofibrillary tangles*. Tau phosphorylation is enhanced by the presence of Aβ, possibly by activation of kinases. Conversely, hyperphosphorylated Tau favours the formation of amyloid deposits. Whether

[6]The APP gene resides on chromosome 21, of which an extra copy is the cause of Down's syndrome, in which early AD-like dementia occurs in association with overexpression of APP.

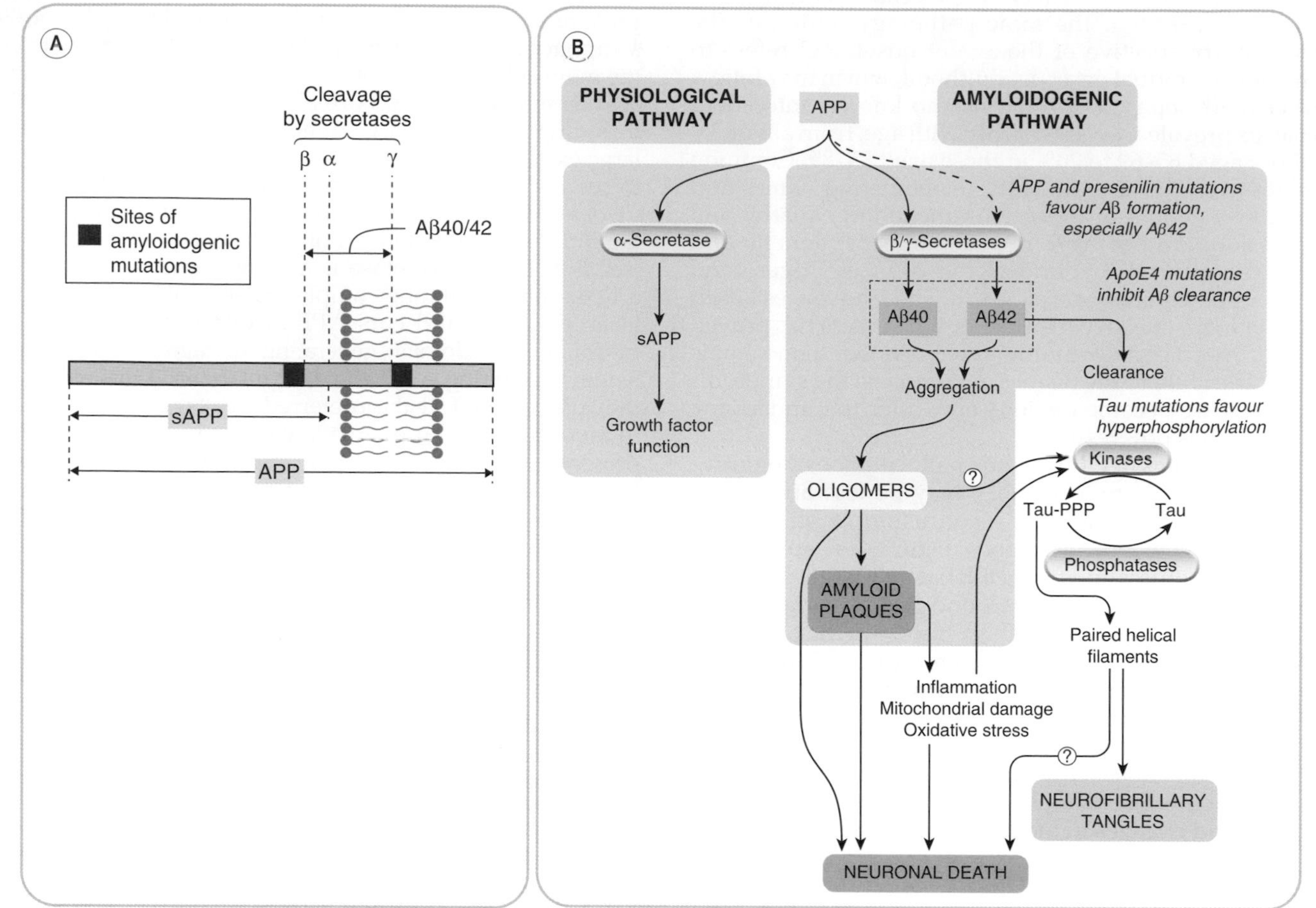

Fig. 40.3 Pathogenesis of Alzheimer's disease. (A) Structure of amyloid precursor protein (APP), showing origin of secreted APP (sAPP) and Aβ amyloid protein. The regions involved in amyloidogenic mutations discovered in some cases of familial Alzheimer's disease are shown flanking the Aβ sequence. APP cleavage involves three proteases: secretases α, β and γ. α-Secretase produces soluble APP, whereas β- and γ-secretases generate Aβ amyloid protein. γ-Secretase can cut at different points, generating Aβ peptides of varying lengths, including Aβ40 and Aβ42, the latter having a high tendency to aggregate as amyloid plaques. (B) Processing of APP. The main 'physiological' pathway gives rise to sAPP, which exerts a number of trophic functions. Cleavage of APP at different sites gives rise to Aβ, the predominant form normally being Aβ40, which is weakly amyloidogenic. Mutations in APP or presenilins increase the proportion of APP, which is degraded via the amyloidogenic pathway, and also increase the proportion converted to the much more strongly amyloidogenic form Aβ42. Hyperphosphorylated Tau results in dissociation of Tau from microtubules, misfolding and aggregation to form paired helical filaments, which enhance Aβ toxicity.

hyperphosphorylation and intracellular deposition of Tau directly harms the cell is not certain, although it is known that it impairs fast axonal transport, a process that depends on microtubules. It remains to be seen whether these pathologies drive the symptoms of the disease or arise as a consequences of other causal factors.

Loss of cholinergic neurons

Although changes in many transmitter systems have been observed, mainly from measurements on postmortem AD brain tissue, a relatively selective loss of cholinergic neurons in the basal forebrain nuclei (see Ch. 39) is characteristic. This discovery, made in 1976, implied that pharmacological approaches to restoring cholinergic function might be feasible, leading to the use of cholinesterase inhibitors to treat AD (see later).

Choline acetyl transferase activity, acetylcholine (ACh) content and acetylcholinesterase and choline transport in the cortex and hippocampus are all reduced considerably in AD but not in other disorders, such as depression or schizophrenia. Muscarinic receptor density, determined by binding studies, is not affected, but nicotinic receptors, particularly in the cortex, are reduced. The reason for the selective loss of cholinergic neurons resulting from Aβ formation is not known.

PATHOGENESIS OF DEMENTIA WITH LEWY BODIES

DLB is associated with the development of intracellular protein aggregates known as Lewy bodies in various parts of the brain. Mutations in SNCA, SNCB, GBA and ApoE genes have been implicated in DLB. Lewy bodies consist largely of α-synuclein, a synaptic protein, present in large amounts in normal brains. There is evidence that α-synuclein may act as a prion-like protein (Olanow and Brundin, 2013). α-Synuclein normally exists in an α-helical conformation. However, under certain circumstances, such as genetic duplication or triplication or genetic mutation, it can undergo a conformational change to a β-sheet-rich structure that polymerises to form toxic aggregates and amyloid plaques. It is believed that misfolding and aggregation render the protein resistant to degradation within cells, causing it to pile up in Lewy bodies.

Brain regions involved in DLB include the cerebral cortex, which controls information processing, perception, thought and language; the limbic cortex, which plays a major role in emotions and behaviour; the hippocampus, which is involved in memory processing; the midbrain and basal ganglia, involved in movement; the brain stem, which is important in regulating sleep and maintaining alertness; and olfactory pathways. Dopaminergic neurons seem to be particularly vulnerable to Lewy bodies (see Parkinson's Disease section later).

Alzheimer's disease

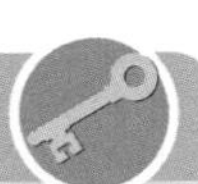

- Alzheimer's disease (AD) is a common age-related dementia, distinct from vascular dementia associated with brain infarction.
- The main pathological features of AD comprise amyloid plaques, neurofibrillary tangles and a loss of neurons (particularly cholinergic neurons of the basal forebrain).
- Amyloid plaques consist of aggregates of the Aβ fragment of amyloid precursor protein (APP), a normal neuronal membrane protein, produced by the action of β- and γ-secretases. AD is associated with excessive Aβ formation, resulting in neurotoxicity.
- Familial AD (rare) results from mutations in the APP gene, or in presenilin genes (involved in γ-secretase function), both of which cause increased Aβ formation.
- Mutations in the lipoprotein ApoE4 increase the risk of developing AD, possibly by interfering with Aβ clearance or tau-mediated neurodegeneration.
- Neurofibrillary tangles comprise intracellular aggregates of a highly phosphorylated form of a normal neuronal protein (Tau). Hyperphosphorylated Tau and Aβ act synergistically to cause neurodegeneration.
- Loss of cholinergic neurons is believed to account for much of the learning and memory deficit in AD.

THERAPEUTIC APPROACHES TO DEMENTIA

Currently, cholinesterase inhibitors (see Ch. 14) and **memantine** are the main drugs available for treating AD and DLB.

CHOLINESTERASE INHIBITORS

Tacrine was the first drug approved for treating AD but because of its hepatotoxicity and the subsequent availability of other anticholinesterase agents, use of tacrine has been discontinued. Later compounds used to treat both AD and DLB include **donepezil**, **rivastigmine** and **galantamine** (Table 40.2). Clinical trials have demonstrated modest improvements in tests of memory and cognition but no sustained effect on disease progression or improvement in other behavioural and psychological measures that affect quality of life.

Other drugs aimed at improving cholinergic function that are being investigated include other cholinesterase inhibitors and a variety of muscarinic and nicotinic receptor agonists. To date, the lack of selectivity of muscarinic orthosteric agonists has hindered their use to treat CNS disorders due to the incidence of side effects, but the hope is that positive allosteric modulators (see Ch. 3) that are selective (e.g. for the M_1 receptor) will be developed.

MEMANTINE

The other drug currently used in the treatment of AD and DLB is **memantine**, an orally active weak antagonist at NMDA receptors. It was originally introduced as an antiviral drug and resurrected as a potential inhibitor of excitotoxicity. It produces – surprisingly – a modest cognitive improvement but does not appear to be neuroprotective. It may work by selectively inhibiting excessive, pathological NMDA-receptor activation while preserving more physiological activation. It has a long plasma half-life, and its adverse effects include headache, dizziness, drowsiness, constipation, shortness of breath and hypertension as well as a raft of less common problems.

ANTI Aβ ANTIBODIES

Aducanumab was the first new treatment for AD introduced since 2003. It is a monoclonal antibody that binds to Aβ aggregates but does not target Aβ monomers. Microglia bind to the Fc region of the antibody resulting in the phagocytosis of amyloid plaques. In initial clinical trials the therapeutic benefits of aducanumab were at best modest. Its approval by the Federal Drug Administration in the United States has been controversial (Alexander et al., 2021; Walsh et al., 2021). More recently **lecanemab**, another monoclonal antibody that binds with high affinity to Aβ aggregates has shown greater promise in an initial clinical trial (van Dyck et al., 2023).

Treatment of vascular dementia focuses largely on reducing blood pressure (see Ch. 21), atherosclerosis and thrombosis (see Chs 22 and 23). Donepezil, galantamine, rivastigmine and memantine are not used to treat vascular dementia, but may be used in people who have a combination of vascular dementia and AD.

Clinical use of drugs in dementia

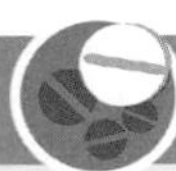

- Acetylcholinesterase inhibitors and NMDA antagonists detectably improve cognitive impairment in clinical trials but have significant adverse effects and are of limited use clinically. They have not been shown to retard neurodegeneration.
- Efficacy is monitored periodically in individual patients, and administration continued only if the drugs are believed to be working and their effect in slowing functional and cognitive deterioration is judged to outweigh adverse effects.

Acetylcholinesterase inhibitors

- **Donepezil**, **galantamine**, **rivastigmine.** Unwanted cholinergic effects may be troublesome.
- Used in mild to moderate Alzheimer's disease and dementia with Lewy bodies.

NMDA-receptor antagonists

- For example, **memantine** (see Ch. 38).
- Used in moderate-to-severe Alzheimer's disease and dementia with Lewy bodies.

Table 40.2 Cholinesterase inhibitors used in the treatment of Alzheimer's disease[a]

Drug	Type of inhibition	Duration of action and dosage	Main side effects	Notes
Donepezil	CNS, AChE selective	~24 h Once-daily oral dosage	Slight cholinergic side effects	—
Rivastigmine	CNS selective	~8 h Twice-daily oral dosage	Cholinergic side effects that tend to subside with continuing treatment	Gradual dose escalation to minimise side effects Available in a transdermal patch
Galantamine	Affects both AChE and BuChE Also enhances nicotinic ACh receptor activation by allosteric action	~8 h Twice-daily oral dosage	Slight cholinergic side effects	—

[a]Similar level of limited clinical benefit for all drugs. No clinical evidence for retardation of disease process, although animal tests suggest diminution of Aβ and plaque formation by a mechanism not related to cholinesterase inhibition.
AChE, Acetylcholinesterase; *BuChE*, butyryl cholinesterase; *CNS*, central nervous system.

Future drug development

Despite intensive research into the underlying causes of AD and DLB and the huge investment in drug development there have been few successes to date. Unravelling the mechanisms of neurodegeneration in AD and DLB has yet to result in therapies able to retard them and, with some spectacular failures having occurred in expensive clinical trials of new drugs (e.g. *verubecestat*, a β-secretase 1 [BACE1] inhibitor, and *solanezumab*, a monoclonal antibody against Aβ peptide). Fingers are crossed that aducanemab and lecanemab will be effective treatments. Descriptions of other potential therapies for AD that are still in various stages of development are provided by Cummings et al. (2017) and Yiannopoulou and Papageorgiou (2020).

For most of the disorders discussed in this chapter, including dementia, the Holy Grail, which so far eludes us, would be a drug that retards neurodegeneration. Until more is understood about the causes of the neurodegeneration, treatments may remain elusive.

Cognitive deficits occur in a number of CNS disorders including dementia, PD, schizophrenia and depression. The development of cognition-enhancing drugs that may be useful across these disorders is described in Chapter 49.

PARKINSON'S DISEASE

FEATURES OF PARKINSON'S DISEASE

PD is primarily a progressive disorder of movement that occurs mainly in the elderly. It was first described in 1817 by James Parkinson. Przedborski (2017) describes in detail how understanding of the disorder and its treatment have evolved over the subsequent 200 years.

The chief symptoms are:

- suppression of voluntary movements (*bradykinesia*), due partly to muscle rigidity and partly to an inherent inertia of the motor system, which means that motor activity is difficult to stop as well as to initiate;
- tremor at rest, usually starting in the hands ('pill-rolling' tremor), which tends to diminish during voluntary activity;
- muscle rigidity, detectable as an increased resistance in passive limb movement;
- cognitive and behavioural impairments.

Parkinsonian patients walk with a characteristic shuffling gait. They find it hard to start, and once in progress they cannot quickly stop or change direction. PD is commonly associated with dementia, depression, hallucinations, sleep disturbances and autonomic dysfunction, because the degenerative process is not confined to the basal ganglia but also affects other parts of the brain. Non-motor symptoms may appear before motor symptoms and often predominate in the later stages of the disease.

PD often occurs with no obvious underlying cause, but it may be the result of cerebral ischaemia, viral encephalitis, head injury or other types of pathological damage. The symptoms can also be drug induced, the main drugs involved being those that block dopamine receptors (e.g. antiemetic and antipsychotic drugs such as **chlorpromazine**; see Chs 30 and 47). There are rare instances of familial early-onset PD, and several gene mutations have been identified, including those encoding *synuclein* and *parkin*. Mutations in the gene encoding leucine-rich repeat kinase 2 (LRRK2) have also been associated with PD. Study of gene mutations has given some clues about the mechanism underlying the neurodegenerative process.

Neurochemical changes

PD affects the basal ganglia, and its neurochemical origin was discovered in 1960 by Hornykiewicz, who showed that the dopamine content of the substantia nigra and corpus striatum (see Ch. 39) in postmortem brains of PD patients was extremely low (usually less than 10% of normal), associated with a loss of dopaminergic neurons in the substantia nigra and degeneration of nerve terminals in the striatum.[7] Neurons containing other monoamines such as noradrenaline and 5-hydroxytryptamine are also affected. Gradual loss of dopamine occurs over several years, with symptoms of PD appearing only when the striatal dopamine content has fallen to 20%–40% of normal. Lesions of the nigrostriatal tract or chemically induced depletion of dopamine in experimental animals also produce symptoms of PD. The symptom most clearly related to dopamine deficiency is *bradykinesia*, which occurs immediately and invariably in lesioned animals. Rigidity and tremor involve more complex neurochemical disturbances of other transmitters (particularly ACh, noradrenaline, 5-hydroxytryptamine and GABA) as well as dopamine. In experimental lesions, two secondary consequences follow damage to the nigrostriatal tract, namely a hyperactivity of the remaining dopaminergic neurons, which show an increased rate of transmitter turnover, and an increase in the number of dopamine receptors, which produces a state of denervation hypersensitivity (see Ch. 13). Neurons in the striatum express mainly D_1 (excitatory) and D_2 (inhibitory) receptors (see Ch. 39), but fewer D_3 and D_4 receptors. A simplified diagram of the neuronal circuitry involved, and the pathways primarily affected in PD and HD, is shown in Fig. 40.4.

Cholinergic interneurons of the corpus striatum (not shown in Fig. 40.4) are also involved in PD and HD. ACh release from the striatum is strongly inhibited by dopamine, and it is suggested that hyperactivity of these cholinergic neurons contributes to the symptoms of PD. The opposite happens in HD, and in both conditions therapies aimed at redressing the balance between the dopaminergic and cholinergic neurons are, up to a point, beneficial.

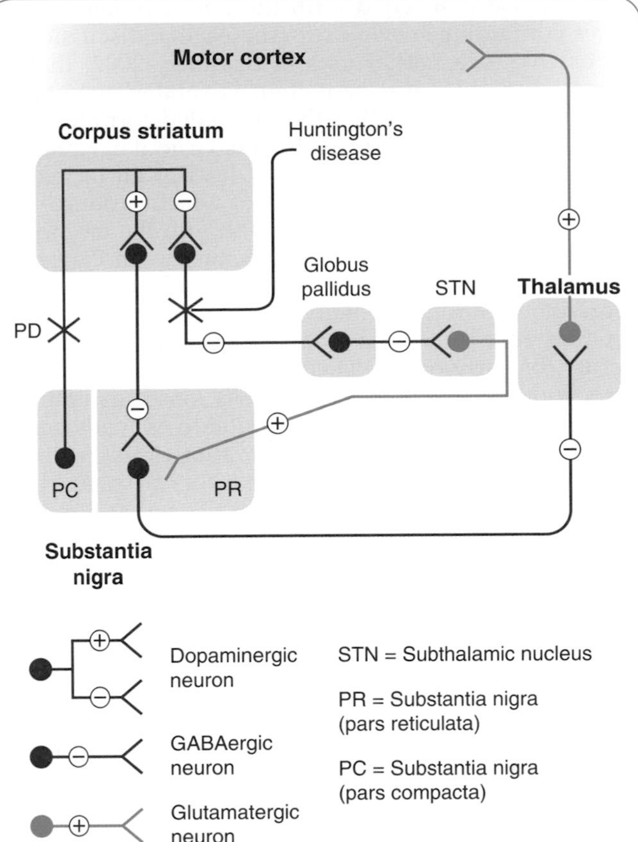

Fig. 40.4 Simplified diagram of the organisation of the extrapyramidal motor system and the defects that occur in Parkinson's disease (PD) and Huntington's disease. Normally, activity in nigrostriatal dopamine neurons causes excitation of striatonigral neurons and inhibition of striatal neurons that project to the globus pallidus. Because of the different pathways involved, the activity of *GABAergic neurons* in the *substantia nigra* is suppressed, releasing the restraint on the *thalamus* and *cortex*, causing motor stimulation. In PD, the dopaminergic pathway from the *substantia nigra (pars compacta)* to the *striatum* is impaired. In Huntington's disease, the GABAergic striatopallidal pathway is impaired, producing effects opposite to the changes in PD.

PATHOGENESIS OF PARKINSON'S DISEASE

As with other neurodegenerative disorders, the neuronal damage in PD is caused by protein misfolding and aggregation, aided and abetted by other familiar villains, namely excitotoxicity, mitochondrial dysfunction, oxidative stress, inflammation and apoptosis. Aspects of the pathogenesis and animal models of PD have been described by Duty and Jenner (2011).

Neurotoxins

New light was thrown on the possible aetiology of PD by a chance event. In 1982, a group of young drug users in California suddenly developed an exceptionally severe form of PD (known as the 'frozen addict' syndrome), and the cause was traced to the compound 1-methyl-4-phenyl-1,2,3,6-tetrahydropyridine (**MPTP**), which was a contaminant in the illegal preparation of a heroin substitute (see Langston, 1985). MPTP causes irreversible destruction of nigrostriatal dopaminergic neurons in various species, and produces a PD-like state in primates. MPTP acts by being converted to a toxic metabolite, MPP^+, by the enzyme monoamine oxidase (MAO; specifically by the MAO-B subtype that is located in glial cells; see Chs 15 and 48). MPP^+ is then taken up by the dopamine transport system, and thus acts selectively on dopaminergic neurons; it inhibits mitochondrial oxidation reactions, producing oxidative stress. MPTP appears to be selective in destroying nigrostriatal neurons and does not affect dopaminergic neurons elsewhere – the reason for this is unknown. It is also less effective in rats than in primates, yet mice show some susceptibility. **Selegiline**, a selective MAO-B inhibitor, prevents MPTP-induced neurotoxicity by blocking its conversion to MPP^+. Selegiline is also used in treating PD (see later); as well as inhibiting dopamine breakdown, it might also work by blocking the metabolic activation of a putative endogenous, or environmental, MPTP-like substance, which is involved in the causation of PD. It is possible that dopamine itself could be the culprit, because oxidation of dopamine gives rise to potentially toxic metabolites. Whether or not the action of MPTP reflects the natural pathogenesis of PD, the MPTP model is a very useful experimental tool for testing possible therapies.

Impaired mitochondrial function is a feature of the disease in humans. Various herbicides, such as **rotenone**, that selectively inhibit mitochondrial function cause a PD-like syndrome in animals. PD in humans is more common in agricultural areas than in cities, suggesting that environmental toxins could be a factor in its causation.

[7]It is emerging that other types of neuron are also affected. Here we concentrate on the dopaminergic nigrostriatal pathway as it is the most important in relation to current therapies.

PD is also associated with the development of *Lewy bodies* containing *α-synuclein* (see earlier discussion). It is possible (see Lotharius and Brundin, 2002) that the normal function of α-synuclein is related to synaptic vesicle recycling, and that the misfolded form loses this functionality, with the result that vesicular storage of dopamine is impaired. This may lead to an increase in cytosolic dopamine, degradation of which produces ROS and hence neurotoxicity. Consistent with the α-synuclein hypothesis, another mutation associated with PD (*parkin*) also involves a protein that participates in the intracellular degradation of rogue proteins.

Other gene mutations that have been identified as risk factors for early-onset PD code for proteins involved in mitochondrial function, making cells more susceptible to oxidative stress. Thus, a picture similar to AD pathogenesis is slowly emerging. Misfolded α-synuclein, facilitated by overexpression, genetic mutations or possibly by environmental factors, builds up in the cell as a result of impaired protein degradation (resulting from defective parkin) in the form of Lewy bodies, which, by unknown mechanisms, compromise cell survival. If oxidative stress is increased, as a result of ischaemia, mitochondrial poisons or mutations of certain mitochondrial proteins, the result is cell death.

Parkinson's disease

- Degenerative disease of the basal ganglia causing hypokinesia, tremor at rest and muscle rigidity, often with dementia and autonomic dysfunction.
- Associated with aggregation of α-synuclein (a protein normally involved in vesicle recycling) in the form of characteristic Lewy bodies.
- Often idiopathic but may follow stroke or virus infection; can be drug induced (antipsychotic drugs). Rare familial forms also occur, associated with various gene mutations, including α-synuclein.
- Associated with degeneration of dopaminergic nigrostriatal neurons that gives rise to the motor symptoms, as well as more general neurodegeneration resulting in dementia and depression.
- Can be induced by 1-methyl-4-phenyl-1,2,3,6-tetrahydropyridine (**MPTP**), a neurotoxin affecting dopamine neurons. Similar environmental neurotoxins, as well as genetic factors, may be involved in human Parkinson's disease.

DRUG TREATMENT OF PARKINSON'S DISEASE

Currently, the main drugs used (Fig. 40.5) are:

- **levodopa** (sometimes in combination with **carbidopa** and **entacapone**);
- dopamine agonists (e.g. **pramipexole**, **ropinirole**, **bromocriptine**);
- MAO-B inhibitors (e.g. **selegiline**, **rasagiline**);
- muscarinic ACh receptor antagonists (e.g. **orphenadrine, procyclidine** and **trihexyphenidyl**) are occasionally used.

None of the drugs used to treat PD affect the progression of the disease.

LEVODOPA

Levodopa is the first-line treatment for PD and is combined with a peripherally acting dopa decarboxylase inhibitor, such as **carbidopa** or **benserazide**, which reduces the dose needed by about 10-fold and diminishes the peripheral side effects. It is well absorbed from the small intestine, a process that relies on active transport, although much of it is inactivated by MAO in the wall of the intestine. The plasma half-life is short (about 2 h). Oral and subcutaneous slow-release preparations have been developed. Conversion to dopamine in the periphery, which would otherwise account for about 95% of the levodopa dose and cause troublesome side effects, is largely prevented by the decarboxylase inhibitor. Decarboxylation occurs rapidly within the brain, because the decarboxylase inhibitors do not penetrate the blood–brain barrier. It is not certain whether the effect depends on an increased release of dopamine from the few surviving dopaminergic neurons or on a 'flooding' of the synapse with dopamine formed elsewhere. Because synthetic dopamine agonists are equally effective, the latter explanation is more likely, and animal studies suggest that levodopa can act even when no dopaminergic nerve terminals are present. On the other hand, the therapeutic effectiveness of levodopa decreases as the disease advances, so part of its action may rely on the presence of functional dopaminergic neurons. A combination of levodopa plus a dopa decarboxylase inhibitor with a catechol-*O*-methyl transferase (COMT) inhibitor (e.g. **entacapone**, **tolcapone** or **opicapone;** see Ch. 15) to inhibit its degradation is used in patients troubled by 'end of dose' motor fluctuations.

Therapeutic effectiveness

About 80% of patients show initial improvement with levodopa, particularly of rigidity and bradykinesia, and about 20% are restored virtually to normal motor function. As time progresses, the effectiveness of levodopa gradually declines (Fig. 40.6). In a typical study of 100 patients treated with levodopa for 5 years, only 34 were better than they had been at the beginning of the trial, 32 patients having died and 21 having withdrawn from the trial. It is likely that the loss of effectiveness of levodopa mainly reflects the natural progression of the disease, but receptor down-regulation and other compensatory mechanisms may also contribute. There is no evidence that levodopa can actually accelerate the neurodegenerative process through overproduction of dopamine, as was suspected on theoretical grounds. Overall, levodopa increases the life expectancy of PD patients, probably as a result of improved motor function, although some symptoms (e.g. dysphagia, cognitive decline) are not improved.

Unwanted effects

There are two main types of unwanted effect:

1. Involuntary movements (dyskinesia), which do not appear initially but develop in the majority of patients within 2 years of starting levodopa therapy. These movements usually affect the face and limbs, and can become very severe. They occur at the

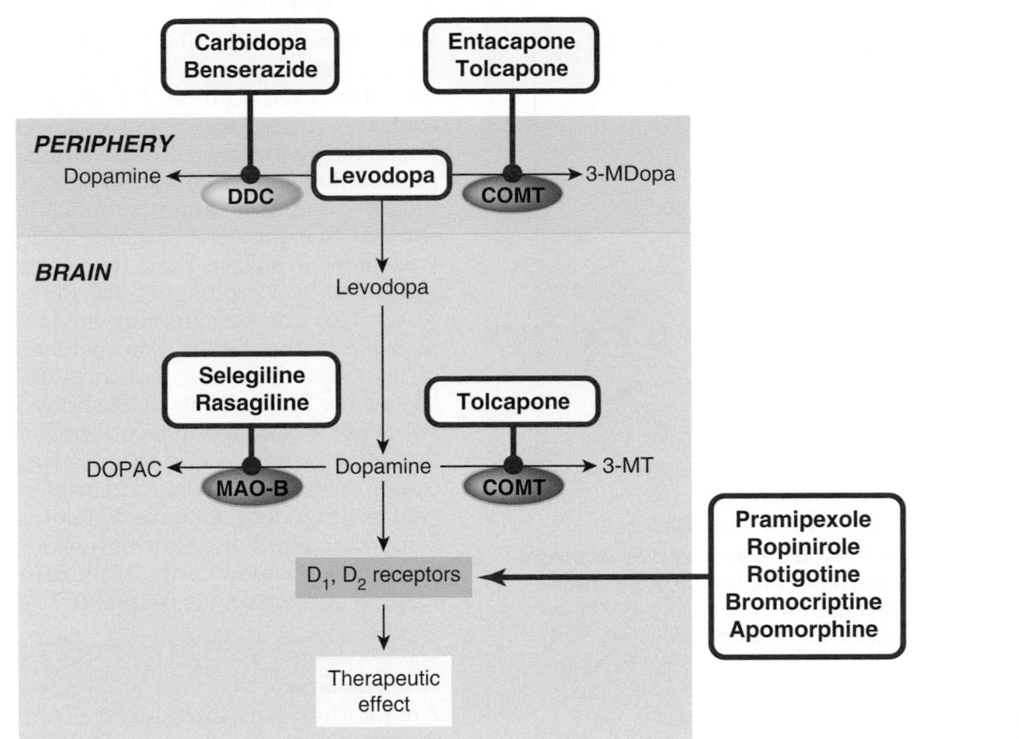

Fig. 40.5 Sites of action of drugs used to treat Parkinson's disease. *Levodopa* enters the brain and is converted to *dopamine* (the deficient neurotransmitter). Inactivation of levodopa in the periphery is prevented by inhibitors of dopa decarboxylase (DDC) and catechol-*O*-methyl transferase (COMT). Inactivation in the brain is prevented by inhibitors of COMT and monoamine oxidase-B (MAO-B). Dopamine agonists act directly on striatal dopamine receptors. *3-MDopa*, 3-Methoxydopa; *3-MT*, 3-methoxytyrosine; *DOPAC*, dihydroxyphenylacetic acid.

time of the peak therapeutic effect, and the margin between the beneficial and the dyskinetic effect becomes progressively narrower. Levodopa is short acting, and the fluctuating plasma concentration of the drug may favour the development of dyskinesias, as longer-acting dopamine agonists are less problematic in this regard.

2. Rapid fluctuations in clinical state, where bradykinesia and rigidity may suddenly worsen for anything from a few minutes to a few hours, and then improve again. This 'on–off effect' is not seen in untreated PD patients or with other anti-PD drugs. The 'off effect' can be so sudden that the patient stops while walking and feels rooted to the spot, or is unable to rise from a chair, having sat down normally a few moments earlier. As with the dyskinesias, the problem seems to reflect the fluctuating plasma concentration of levodopa, and it is suggested that as the disease advances, the ability of neurons to store dopamine is lost, so the therapeutic benefit of levodopa depends increasingly on the continuous formation of extraneuronal dopamine, which requires a continuous supply of levodopa. The use of sustained-release preparations, or co-administration of COMT inhibitors such as **entacapone**, may be used to counteract the fluctuations in plasma concentration of levodopa. Recently, **istradefylline**, an adenosine A2A receptor antagonist, has been approved as an add-on treatment to levodopa and carbidopa to reduce 'off' periods. How it produces this effect is still somewhat unclear.

In addition to these slowly developing side effects, levodopa produces several acute effects, which are experienced by most patients at first but tend to disappear after a few weeks. The main ones are as follows:

- Nausea and anorexia. **Domperidone**, a dopamine antagonist that works in the chemoreceptor trigger zone (where the blood–brain barrier is leaky) but does not gain access to the basal ganglia, may be useful in preventing this effect.
- Hypotension. Postural hypotension is a recognised problem, particularly in older patients.
- Psychological effects. Levodopa, by increasing dopamine activity in the brain, can produce a schizophrenia-like syndrome (see Ch. 47) with delusions and hallucinations. More commonly, in about 20% of patients, it causes confusion, disorientation, insomnia or nightmares.

DOPAMINE AGONISTS

Bromocriptine, **pergolide** and **cabergoline** exhibit slight selectivity for $D_{2/3}$ over D_1 receptors (see Ch. 39). Bromocriptine, which inhibits the release of prolactin from the anterior pituitary gland, was first introduced for the treatment of galactorrhoea and gynaecomastia (see Ch. 33). Although effective in controlling the symptoms of PD,

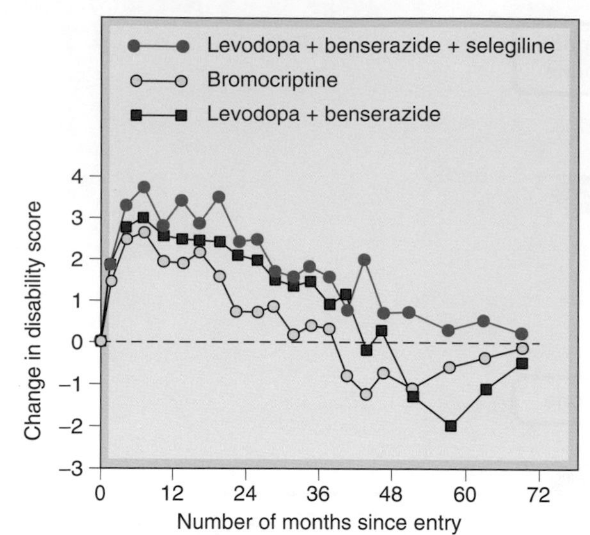

Fig. 40.6 Comparison of levodopa/benserazide, levodopa/benserazide/selegiline and bromocriptine on progression of Parkinson's disease symptoms. Patients (249–271 in each treatment group) were assessed on a standard disability rating score. Before treatment, the average rate of decline was 0.7 units/year. All three treatments produced improvement over the initial rating for 2–3 years, but the effect declined, either because of refractoriness to the drugs or disease progression. Bromocriptine appeared slightly less effective than levodopa regimens, and there was a higher drop-out rate due to side effects in this group. (From Parkinson's Disease Research Group, 1993. Br. Med. J. 307, 469–472.)

their usefulness is limited by side effects, such as nausea and vomiting, somnolence and a risk of fibrotic reactions in the lungs, retroperitoneum and pericardium. These disadvantages have led to the replacement of these drugs by **pramipexole** and **ropinirole**, which are $D_{2/3}$ selective and better tolerated, and do not show the fluctuations in efficacy associated with levodopa. They do, however, cause somnolence and sometimes hallucinations, and recent evidence suggests that they may predispose to compulsive behaviours, such as excessive gambling,[8] over-eating and sexual excess, related to the 'reward' functions of dopamine (see Ch. 50).

A disadvantage of current dopamine agonists is their short plasma half-life (6–8 h), requiring three-times daily dosage, although slow-release once-daily formulations are now available.

Rotigotine is a newer agent, delivered as a transdermal patch, with similar efficacy and side effects.

Apomorphine, given by injection, is sometimes used to control the 'off effect' with levodopa. Because of its powerful emetic action, it must be combined with an oral antiemetic drug. It has other serious adverse effects (mood and behavioural changes, cardiac dysrhythmias, hypotension) and is a last resort if other drugs fail.

MAO-B INHIBITORS

Selegiline is a selective MAO-B[9] inhibitor, which lacks the unwanted peripheral effects of non-selective MAO inhibitors used to treat depression (see Ch. 48) and, in contrast to them, does not provoke the 'cheese reaction' or interact so frequently with other drugs. Inhibition of MAO-B protects dopamine from extraneuronal degradation and was initially used as an adjunct to levodopa. Long-term trials showed that the combination of selegiline and levodopa was more effective than levodopa alone in relieving symptoms and prolonging life. Recognition of the role of MAO-B in neurotoxicity suggested that selegiline might be neuroprotective rather than merely enhancing the action of levodopa, but clinical studies do not support this. A large-scale trial (see Fig. 40.6) showed no difference when selegiline was added to levodopa/benserazide treatment. Selegiline is metabolised to amphetamine, and sometimes causes excitement, anxiety and insomnia. **Rasagiline**, a very similar drug, does not have this unwanted effect, and may somewhat retard disease progression, as well as alleviating symptoms (Olanow et al., 2009). **Safinamide** inhibits both MAO-B and dopamine reuptake.

OTHER DRUGS USED IN PARKINSON'S DISEASE

Amantadine

Amantadine was introduced as an antiviral drug and discovered by accident in 1969 to be beneficial in PD. Many possible mechanisms for its action have been suggested based on neurochemical evidence of increased dopamine release, inhibition of amine uptake or a direct action on dopamine receptors. More recently block of NMDA receptors by stabilising closed states of the channel has been described and this may be a novel target for antiparkinsonian drugs.

Amantadine is less effective than levodopa or bromocriptine in treating PD, but it is effective in reducing the dyskinesias induced by prolonged levodopa treatment.

Acetylcholine antagonists

For more than a century, until levodopa was discovered, atropine and related drugs were the main form of treatment for PD. Muscarinic ACh receptors exert an inhibitory effect on dopaminergic nerve terminals, suppression of which compensates for a lack of dopamine. The side effects of muscarinic antagonists (see Ch. 14) – dry mouth, constipation, impaired vision, urinary retention – are troublesome, and they are now rarely used, except to treat parkinsonian symptoms in patients receiving antipsychotic drugs (which are dopamine antagonists and thus nullify the effect of levodopa; see Ch. 47). Drugs used are **orphenadrine**, **procyclidine** and **trihexyphenidyl**.

Adjuncts to therapy

A range of drugs can be used to treat the non-motor symptoms associated with PD. These include cholinesterase inhibitors and memantine for dementia (see earlier), antidepressants for depression (see Ch. 48), quetiapine, clozapine and pimavanserin for hallucinations (see Ch. 47),

---

[8]In 2008 a plaintiff was awarded $8.2 million damages by a US court, having become a compulsive gambler (and losing a lot of money) after taking pramipexole for PD – a side effect of which the pharmaceutical company had been aware.

[9]MAO-B in the brain is located mainly in glial cells, and also in 5-HT neurons (although, surprisingly, it does not appear to be expressed in dopamine neurons).

modafinil for daytime sleepiness (see Ch. 49), clonazepam (see Ch. 45) and melatonin (see Ch. 39) for rapid-eye-movement (REM) sleep disturbances.

NEW PHARMACOLOGICAL APPROACHES

Potential new treatments for PD at various stages of clinical trial are reviewed by Oertel and Schulz (2016). Sadly, several candidates that showed promise in preclinical studies lacked efficacy in subsequent clinical trials (e.g. preladenant and saritozan). Active and passive immunisation against α-synuclein and inhibitors or modulators of α-synuclein aggregation may prevent the progression of the disease.

Drugs used in Parkinson's disease

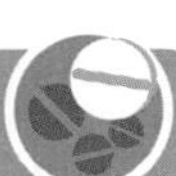

- Drugs act by counteracting deficiency of dopamine in basal ganglia or by blocking muscarinic receptors. None of the available drugs affect the underlying neurodegeneration.
- Drugs include:
  - **levodopa** (dopamine precursor; see Ch. 15), given with an inhibitor of peripheral dopa decarboxylase (e.g. **carbidopa**) to minimise side effects; sometimes a COMT inhibitor (e.g. **entacapone**) is also given, especially to patients with 'end of dose' motor fluctuations;
  - dopamine receptor agonists (**pramipexole**, **ropinirole**, **rotigotine**, **bromocriptine**); **rotigotine** is available as a transdermal patch;
  - MAO-B inhibitors (**selegiline**, **rasagiline**);
  - **amantadine** (which may enhance dopamine release);
  - **orphenadrine** (muscarinic receptor antagonist used for parkinsonism caused by antipsychotic drugs).
- Stem cell transplantation, still in early clinical development, may be effective.

NEURAL TRANSPLANTATION, GENE THERAPY AND BRAIN STIMULATION

PD is the first neurodegenerative disease for which neural transplantation was attempted in 1982, amid much publicity. Various transplantation approaches have been tried, based on the injection of dissociated fetal cells (neuroblasts) directly into the striatum. Trials in patients with PD (Barker et al., 2013) mainly involved injection of midbrain cells from aborted human fetuses. Although such transplants have been shown to survive and establish functional dopaminergic connections, this approach has fallen out of favour. Some patients have gone on to develop serious dyskinesias, possibly due to dopamine overproduction. The use of fetal material is, of course, fraught with ethical difficulties (usually cells from five or more fetuses are needed for one transplant) and hopes for the future rest mainly on developing stem cell transplants (Nishimura and Takahashi, 2013); small clinical trials are underway (Schweitzer et al., 2020).

Gene therapy (see Ch. 5) for PD is aimed at increasing the synthesis of neurotransmitters and neurotrophic factors such as:

- dopamine in the striatum – by expressing tyrosine hydroxylase or dopa decarboxylase;
- GABA in the subthalamic nucleus – by overexpression of glutamic acid decarboxylase (to reduce the excitatory input to the substantia nigra) (see Fig. 40.4);
- neurotrophic factors such as neurturin, a glial-derived neurotrophic factor (GDNF) analogue.

Electrical stimulation of the subthalamic nuclei with implanted electrodes (which inhibits ongoing neural activity, equivalent to reversible ablation) is used in severe cases, and can improve motor dysfunction in PD, but does not improve cognitive and other symptoms and does not stop the neurodegenerative process (see Okun, 2012).

ESSENTIAL TREMOR

ET is probably the most prevalent movement disorder, approximately 8 times more common than PD, but its underlying pathology is very poorly understood and there has been surprisingly little progress in this area despite its prevalence. It is characterised by a rhythmic postural or kinetic tremor at 4–12 Hz and mainly affects the upper extremities although it can progress to include other locations including the head, laryngeal muscles and lower extremities. The differences between PD-related tremor and ET are not necessarily obvious from symptom presentation but they arise from very different aetiologies. Where PD is linked to the loss of dopaminergic neurons, the neurochemical basis of ET is unknown. Based on the ability to generate tremor in an animal model using the β-carboline, harmaline, a role for GABAergic dysfunction in ET has been suggested as has a shift in the balance between excitatory/inhibitory neurotransmission but there may also be involvement of other neurotransmitters including dopamine, adenosine and noradrenaline. ET has some genetic associations and likely arises from an interaction of genetics and environmental factors (Clark and Louis, 2018).

Whilst ET may remain relatively mild and show only a slow progression and hence have limited impact on the patient, it can in other patients progress to become debilitating and make basic tasks such as eating, writing and other simple day-to-day activities challenging. It also seems to have an interesting association with emotional states and can become much more evident during periods of emotional stress.

With very limited evidence of any specific neurochemical deficit, drug treatments have relied heavily on trials with drugs used for other conditions. The most effective treatments are the β-blocker propranolol (Chs 15 and 20) and the anti-epileptic barbiturate primidone (Ch. 46), although effectiveness varies and not all patients achieve good remediation of symptoms. It is well known that alcohol is effective at reducing the amplitude and severity of the ET but this leads to a risk of patients developing alcoholism. An alternative approach to treating the central mechanisms generating ET is to target the limbs directly and injections of botulinum toxin type A into the forearm flexor and extensor muscles can improve upper limb tremor with relatively few side effects. A recent review of pharmacological approaches to treating ET discusses a wide range of drugs that have undergone clinical evaluation but there remains a pressing need for more research and understanding of the underlying pathology (Alonso-Navarro et al., 2020).

HUNTINGTON'S DISEASE

HD is an inherited (autosomal dominant) disorder resulting in progressive brain degeneration, starting in adulthood and causing rapid deterioration and death. As well as dementia, it causes severe motor symptoms in the form of choreiform (i.e. rapid, jerky involuntary) movements, especially of fingers, face or tongue. It is the commonest of a group of so-called *trinucleotide repeat* neurodegenerative diseases, associated with the expansion of the number of repeats of the CAG sequence in specific genes, and hence the number (50 or more) of consecutive glutamine residues at the N-terminal of the expressed protein (see Walker, 2007). The larger the number of repeats, the earlier the appearance of symptoms. The protein coded by the HD gene, *huntingtin*, which normally possesses a chain of fewer than 30 glutamine residues, is a soluble cytosolic protein of unknown function found in all cells. HD develops when the mutant protein contains 40 or more repeats. The long poly-Gln chains reduce the solubility of huntingtin, and favour the formation of aggregates, which are formed by proteolytic cleavage of the mutant protein, releasing N-terminal fragments that include the poly-Gln region. As with AD and PD, aggregation is probably responsible for the neuronal loss, which affects mainly the cortex and the striatum, resulting in progressive dementia and severe involuntary choreiform movements. Studies on postmortem brains showed that the dopamine content of the striatum was normal or slightly increased, while there was a 75% reduction in the activity of glutamic acid decarboxylase, the enzyme responsible for GABA synthesis (see Ch. 38). It is believed that the loss of GABA-mediated inhibition in the basal ganglia produces a hyperactivity of dopaminergic synapses, so the syndrome is in some senses a mirror image of PD (see Fig. 40.4).

The effects of drugs that influence dopaminergic transmission are correspondingly the opposite of those that are observed in PD, dopamine antagonists being effective in reducing the involuntary movements, while drugs such as levodopa and bromocriptine make them worse. Drugs used to alleviate the motor symptoms include **tetrabenazine** (an inhibitor of the vesicular monoamine transporter) (see Ch. 15) that reduces dopamine storage, dopamine antagonists such as **chlorpromazine** and **haloperidol** (see Ch. 47) and the $GABA_B$ receptor agonist **baclofen** (see Ch. 38). Other drug treatments include antidepressants, mood stabilisers (see Ch. 48) and benzodiazepines (see Ch. 45) to reduce the depression, mood swings and anxiety associated with the disorder. None of these drugs affects dementia or retards the course of the disease. Drugs (e.g. **branaplam**) and genetic approaches (e.g. antisense oligonucleotides, RNAi) that lower huntingtin levels are currently undergoing clinical investigation.

AMYOTROPHIC LATERAL SCLEROSIS

ALS is the most common form of motor neuron disease, in which degeneration of motor neurons leads to paralysis and eventual death. In ALS, degeneration occurs in both upper motor neurons, those projecting from higher centres to the spinal cord and in lower motor neurons, those projecting from the ventral horn of the spinal cord to skeletal muscle. The causes of ALS are not known, but there is evidence that both genetic and environmental factors such as exposure to bacterial toxins, heavy metals, pesticides and trauma are involved.[10] Mutations in several genes – *SOD1*, C9orf72 and NEK1 – have been associated with some cases of familial ALS (see Pochet, 2017).

The drugs currently used in ALS treatment are **riluzole** and **edaravone**. Riluzole may work by reducing glutamate release whereas edaravone may reduce oxidative stress. However, these drugs only provide limited improvement. A skeletal muscle troponin activator, **reldesemtiv**, which may slow progressive muscle weakness, has recently entered Phase 3 clinical trials. It may also be effective in spinal muscular atrophy (see later). Therapies, designed to suppress the expression of mutated genes, and stem cell therapies continue to be investigated. **Tofersen**, an antisense directed against SOD1, is currently in Phase 3 clinical trial for treatment of ALS associated with mutations of SOD1.

SPINAL MUSCULAR ATROPHY

SMA is a group of inherited neuromuscular disorders in which there is degeneration of motor neurons and progressive muscle wasting. It is the most common genetic cause of infant death. Motor neurons require expression of a protein, appropriately called *survival motorneuron protein* (SMN), for them to survive and function normally. SMA is caused by a genetic defect in the SMN-1 gene encoding for SMN. In recent years there have been several gene therapies (see Ch. 5) developed for SMA, bringing hope to families affected by these devastating disorders. **Nusinersen**, an antisense oligonucleotide sequence given by intrathecal injection, facilitates SMN expression, not from the mutated SMN-1 gene but from SMN-2, a 'backup' gene that under normal conditions, due to exon skipping, does not produce much functional SMN. Nusinersen prevents the skipping, thus allowing the cell to produce SMN. **Risdiplam**, an orally active SMN 2-directed RNA splicing modifier, increases the production of functional SMN protein. **Onasemnogene abeparvovec**,[11] an SMN-1 transgene, is a non-replicating recombinant viral vector modified to contain the cDNA of the human SMN gene. The vector carries a functional copy of the SMN1 gene into motor neurons, thus providing an alternative source of SMN protein expression in these cells.

MULTIPLE SCLEROSIS

MS is a disease associated with demyelination of nerve axons and neuronal degeneration resulting in lesions that may occur throughout the CNS. Symptoms usually start to develop between 20 and 30 years of age and depend upon the location of the lesions. Common symptoms include problems with vision, dizziness, balance, walking, fatigue, incontinence, muscle stiffness and painful muscle spasms. MS can also affect cognitive processing and mood. It affects almost three times as many women as men. There are two forms of the disease, *relapse–remitting*, in which sufferers have attacks of symptoms which subsequently fade away

[10]Intense physical exercise has been suggested to be one potential environmental factor and there are examples of leading sportspersons succumbing to the disease in later life, for example, the late Joost van der Westhuizen, the great South African scrum half, the late Doddie Weir, who played for Scotland and the British and Irish Lions, and Rob Burrow, who played rugby league for England and Great Britain.

[11]Onasemnogene is currently the world's most expensive medicine, costing £1.79m for a one-off treatment.

partially or completely but then relapse at a later date, and *primary progressive*, in which the symptoms persist and increase over time. Relapse–remitting may, however, develop into secondary progressive in later life. The cause of MS is unknown; like other neurodegenerative conditions it may result from a combination of predisposing genetic factors (Hollenbach and Oksenberg, 2015) and exposure to environmental factors such as infection.

MS has long been considered an autoimmune demyelinating disease, although the proteins, lipids and gangliosides in myelin that act as antigens have not been identified. Inflammation (see Ch. 25), enhanced permeability of blood–brain barrier, demyelination and axonal degeneration are common pathological features. It is, however, still unclear whether MS is a primary autoimmune disease that affects the CNS or a neurodegenerative disease with secondary inflammatory demyelination (see Trapp and Nave, 2008). Current therapies are aimed at moderating the acute inflammatory components of MS (Table 40.3), but they are limited in effectiveness. They may reduce the rate of clinical deterioration and incidence of relapses but by and large they do not reverse the neurodegeneration that has occurred. Several (**natalizumab**, **alemtuzumab**, **daclizumab** and **ocrelizumab**) are monoclonal antibodies that target specific proteins expressed on B and T lymphocytes to limit their spread into the brain and spinal cord where they attack the myelin sheath around motor nerves. Monoclonal antibody therapy does, however, carry the risk of serious autoimmune complications (see Ch. 5) that need to be monitored. The pathological mechanisms underlying the neurodegeneration, which renders the disease irreversible, are still not well understood but may hold the key to finding disease-curing treatments. Symptomatic treatment of MS includes **baclofen** and **nabiximols**, a botanical extract of cannabis containing tetrahydrocannabinol (THC) and cannabidiol (CBD) (see Ch. 18), for spasticity; and **fampridine** (a potassium-channel blocker that enhances action potential propagation in demyelinated axons) for a modest improvement in walking speed.

Table 40.3 Disease-modifying treatments for multiple sclerosis

Drug	Mechanism of action	Route(s) and frequency of administration	Notes
Glatiramer acetate	A random polymer (approx. 6 kDa) of four amino acids thought to interfere with the immune response to myelin	Subcutaneous (usually administered daily)	Reduces relapses
Dimethyl fumarate	Unknown	Oral (twice a day)	Reduces relapse rate and slows progression
Fingolimod, ponesimod, siponimod	Inhibit cytotoxic CD8 expressing T cells Fingolimod phosphate and siponimod are agonists at S1P receptors whereas ponesimod has agonist/partial agonist activity	Oral (daily)	Reduce the rate of relapses Increased risk of progressive multifocal leukoencephalopathy and serious ventricular arrhythmias
Beta interferons (IFN-β) (see Ch. 17)	Modulation of immune function	Subcutaneous (three times a week) Intramuscular (once a week)	Reduce relapses by approximately 30% but not all patients respond
Natalizumab (see Ch. 25)	Humanised monoclonal antibody targeting α4-integrin (see Table 25.3)	Intravenous infusion (every 4 weeks)	Slows the progression of disability in relapsing MS May cause progressive multifocal leukoencephalopathy in some cases
Alemtuzumab (see Chs 25 and 57 and Table 25.3)	Humanised monoclonal antibody targeting CD52 on B and T lymphocytes	Intravenous infusion (5-day short courses, 12 months apart)	Also used in the treatment of lymphocytic leukaemia
Daclizumab (see Ch. 25)	Humanised monoclonal antibody targeting CD25, the alpha subunit of the IL-2 receptor on T cells	Subcutaneous (once a month)	Risk of serious liver toxicity; this drug is now restricted to patients who are not suitable for other therapies
Ocrelizumab	Humanised monoclonal antibody targeting CD20 on B lymphocytes	Intravenous infusion (every 6 months after initial treatments)	Superior to beta-interferon in relapsing and progressive MS
Teriflunomide	Immunosuppressant. Active metabolite of leflunomide (see Ch. 25)	Oral (once a day)	Modest efficacy in reducing relapse
Cladribine	Purine nucleoside analogue that has immunosuppressant effects through depletion of lymphocytes	Oral therapy given as two short courses in a 2-year period	Used in rapidly evolving or severe relapsing–remitting MS. Also has a role in hairy cell leukaemia

MS, Multiple sclerosis.

Drug treatment of multiple sclerosis

Several new and efficacious agents have emerged in the treatment of multiple sclerosis (MS), but these treatments also bring with them a significant risk of serious adverse effects. As the severity and course of MS vary substantially amongst individuals, selection of appropriate therapy must consider not only the benefit and harm of the proposed agents, but also the patient's clinical condition and co-morbidities.

Prompt use of disease-modifying therapies is recommended in patients who have clinical and/or radiological evidence of active disease. Examples of therapeutic options for patients with active relapsing–remitting MS are:

- Drugs of moderate efficacy such as **interferon-beta** or **glatiramer acetate** by injection. **Teriflunomide** or **dimethylfumarate** can be used if oral therapy is preferred.
- Drugs of high efficacy such as **natalizumab** or **alemtuzumab** may be considered in those with more active disease.

There is limited evidence for interferon in progressive MS, but **ocrelizumab** is an emerging option for primary progressive disease.

Drugs that are used to manage symptoms or disease complications in MS include **baclofen** (for muscle spasticity) and **amitriptyline** (for emotional lability).

REFERENCES AND FURTHER READING

General mechanisms of neurodegeneration

Barnham, K.J., Masters, C.L., Bush, A.I., 2004. Neurodegenerative diseases and oxidative stress. Nat. Rev. Drug Discov. 3, 205–214.

Brunden, K., Trojanowski, J.O., Lee, V.M.Y., 2009. Advances in Tau-focused drug discovery for Alzheimer's disease and related tauopathies. Nat. Rev. Drug Discov. 8, 783–793.

Hanger, D.P., Anderton, B.H., Noble, W., 2009. Tau phosphorylation: the therapeutic challenge for neurodegenerative disease. Trends Mol. Med. 15, 112–119.

Itoh, K., Nakamura, K., Iijima, M., Sesaki, H., 2013. Mitochondrial dynamics in neurodegeneration. Trends Cell Biol. 23, 64–71.

Peden, A.H., Ironside, J.W., 2012. Molecular pathology in neurodegenerative diseases. Curr. Drug Targets 13, 1548–1559.

Zhao, C., Deng, W., Gage, F.H., 2008. Mechanisms and functional implications of adult neurogenesis. Cell 132, 645–660.

Stroke

Esencan, E., Yuksel, S., Tosun, Y.B., Robinot, A., Solaroglu, I., Zhang, J.H., 2013. Xenon in medical area: emphasis on neuroprotection in hypoxia and anesthesia. Med. Gas Res. 3, 4.

Green, A.R., 2008. Pharmacological approaches to acute ischaemic stroke: reperfusion certainly, neuroprotection possibly. Br. J. Pharmacol. 153 (Suppl. 1), S325–S338.

Alzheimer's disease

Alexander, G.C., Knopman, D.S., Emerson, S.S., et al., 2021. Revisiting FDA approval of aducanumab. N. Engl. J. Med. 385, 769–771.

Cummings, J., Lee, G., Mortsdorf, T., Ritter, A., Zhong, K., 2017. Alzheimer's disease drug development pipeline. Alzheimers Dement. (N Y) 3, 367–384.

Frigero, C., De Strooper, B., 2016. Alzheimer's disease mechanisms and emerging roads to novel therapeutics. Ann. Rev. Neurosci. 39, 57–79.

Götz, J., Ittner, L.M., 2008. Animal models of Alzheimer's disease and frontotemporal dementia. Nat. Rev. Neurosci. 9, 532–544.

Herrup, K., 2015. The case for rejecting the amyloid cascade hypothesis. Nat. Neurosci. 18, 794–799.

Husain, M.A., Laurent, B., Plourde, M., 2021. APOE and Alzheimer's disease: from lipid transport to physiopathology and therapeutics. Front. Neurosci. 15, 630502.

Rakic, P., 2002. Neurogenesis in the primate cortex: an evaluation of the evidence. Nat. Rev. Neurosci. 3, 65–71.

Schwab, C., McGeer, P.L., 2008. Inflammatory aspects of Alzheimer's disease and other neurodegenerative disorders. J. Alzheimer Dis. 13, 359–369.

Sims, R., Hill, M., Williams, J., 2020. The multiplex model of the genetics of Alzheimer's disease. Nat. Neuroscience 23, 311–322.

van Dyck, C.H., Swanson, C.J., Aisen, P., et al., 2023. Lecanemab in early Alzheimer's disease. N. Engl. J. Med. 388, 9–21.

Walsh, S., Merrick, R., Milne, R., Brayne, C., 2021. Aducanumab for Alzheimer's disease? BMJ 374, n1682.

Yiannopoulou, K.G., Papageorgiou, S.G. 2020. Current and future treatments in Alzheimer disease: an update. J. Cent. Nerv. Syst. Dis. 12, 1179573520907397.

Parkinson's disease

Barker, R.A., Barrett, J., Mason, S.L., Björklund, A., 2013. Fetal dopaminergic transplantation trials and the future of neural grafting in Parkinson's disease. Lancet Neurol. 12, 84–91.

Duty, S., Jenner, P., 2011. Animal models of Parkinson's disease: a source of novel treatments and clues to the cause of the disease. Br. J. Pharmacol. 164, 1357–1391.

Langston, W.J., 1985. MPTP and Parkinson's disease. Trends Neurosci. 8, 79–83.

Lotharius, J., Brundin, P., 2002. Pathogenesis of Parkinson's disease: dopamine, vesicles and α-synuclein. Nat. Rev. Neurosci. 3, 833–842.

Nishimura, K., Takahashi, J., 2013. Therapeutic application of stem cell technology toward the treatment of Parkinson's disease. Biol. Pharm. Bull. 36, 171–175.

Oertel, W., Schulz, J.B., 2016. Current and experimental treatments of Parkinson disease: a guide for neuroscientists. J. Neurochem. 139 (S1), 325–337.

Okun, M.S., 2012. Deep-brain stimulation for Parkinson's disease. N. Engl. J. Med. 367, 1529–1538.

Olanow, C.W., Brundin, P., 2013. Parkinson's disease and alpha synuclein: is Parkinson's disease a prion-like disorder? Mov. Disord. 28, 31–40.

Olanow, C.W., Rascol, O., Hauser, R., et al., 2009. A double-blind, delayed-start trial of rasagiline in Parkinson's disease. N. Engl. J. Med. 139, 1268–1278.

Przedborski, S., 2017. The two-century journey of Parkinson disease research. Nat. Rev. Neurosci. 18, 251–259.

Schweitzer, J.S., Song, B., Herrington, T.M., et al., 2020. Personalized iPSC-derived dopamine progenitor cells for Parkinson's disease. N. Engl. J. Med. 382 (20), 1926–1932.

Essential tremor

Alonso-Navarro, H., García-Martín, E., Agúndez, J.A.G., Jiménez-Jiménez, F.J., 2020. Current and future neuropharmacological options for the treatment of essential tremor. Curr. Neuropharmacol. 18, 518–537.

Clark, L.N., Louis, E.D., 2018. Essential tremor. Handb. Clin. Neurol. 147, 229–239.

Huntington's disease

Walker, F.O., 2007. Huntington's disease. Lancet 369, 218–228.

Amyotrophic lateral sclerosis

Pochet, R., 2017. Genetics and ALS: cause for optimism. Cerebrum 2017, 1–13.

Multiple sclerosis

Hollenbach, J.A., Oksenberg, J.R., 2015. The immunogenetics of multiple sclerosis: a comprehensive review. J. Autoimmun. 64, 13–25.

Trapp, B.D., Nave, K.A., 2008. Multiple sclerosis: an immune or neurodegenerative disorder. Ann. Rev. Neurosci. 31, 247–269.

41 General anaesthetic agents

OVERVIEW

General anaesthesia aims to provide balanced anaesthesia, meeting the requirements of amnesia, analgesia and muscle relaxation tailored for the intended medical procedure. In this chapter we describe the pharmacology of the main general anaesthetic agents in current use, which fall into two groups: intravenous agents and inhalation agents (gases and volatile liquids). General anaesthetics are given systemically and exert their main effects on the central nervous system (CNS), in contrast to local anaesthetics (see Ch. 44). Different general anaesthetic agents provide varying amounts of the components of balanced anaesthesia but they are rarely used in isolation nowadays. Sedative and anxiolytic drugs (see Ch. 45), analgesic drugs (see Ch. 43) and neuromuscular-blocking drugs (see Ch. 14) are normally co-administered. Although we now take them for granted, general anaesthetics are the drugs that paved the way for modern surgery. Without them, much of modern medicine would be impossible.

Detailed information on the clinical pharmacology and use of anaesthetic agents can be found in specialised textbooks (e.g. Thompson et al., 2019).

INTRODUCTION

It was only when inhalation anaesthetics were first discovered, in 1846, that most surgical operations became a practical possibility. Until that time, surgeons relied on being able to operate on struggling patients at lightning speed, and most operations were limited to amputations.

The use of **nitrous oxide** to relieve the pain of surgery was suggested by Humphrey Davy in 1800. He was the first person to make nitrous oxide, and he tested its effects on several people, including himself and the Prime Minister, noting that it caused euphoria, analgesia and loss of consciousness. The use of nitrous oxide, billed as 'laughing gas', became a popular fairground entertainment and came to the notice of an American dentist, Horace Wells, who had a tooth extracted under its influence, while he himself squeezed the inhalation bag. Ether also first gained publicity in a disreputable way, through the spread of 'ether frolics', at which it was used to produce euphoria among the guests. William Morton, also a dentist and a student at Harvard Medical School, used it successfully to extract a tooth in 1846 and then suggested to Warren, the illustrious chief surgeon at Massachusetts General Hospital, that he should administer it for one of Warren's operations. Warren grudgingly agreed, and on 16 October 1846 a large audience was gathered in the main operating theatre[1]; after some preliminary fumbling, Morton's demonstration was a spectacular success. 'Gentlemen, this is no humbug' was the most gracious comment that Warren could bring himself to make to the assembled audience.

In the same year, James Simpson, Professor of Midwifery at Edinburgh University, used chloroform to relieve the pain of childbirth, bringing on himself fierce denunciation from the clergy, one of whom wrote: 'Chloroform is a decoy of Satan, apparently offering itself to bless women; but in the end it will harden society and rob God of the deep, earnest cries which arise in time of trouble, for help.' Opposition was effectively silenced in 1853, when Queen Victoria gave birth to her seventh child under the influence of chloroform, and the procedure became known as *anaesthésie à la reine*.

The second half of the 20th century saw the introduction into clinical practice of a number of new general anaesthetic agents, most notably **isoflurane** and **propofol**, that were markedly superior to earlier agents such as **nitrous oxide** and **thiopental**. Despite the need for further improvement the pipeline has all but dried up in the 21st century, with only **fospropofol** being introduced.

MECHANISM OF ACTION OF ANAESTHETIC DRUGS

Unlike most drugs, anaesthetics, which include substances as diverse as simple gases (e.g. **nitrous oxide** and **xenon**), halogenated hydrocarbons (e.g. **isoflurane**), barbiturates (e.g. **thiopental**) and steroids (e.g. **alphaxalone**), belong to no recognisable chemical class. At one time it appeared that the shape and electronic configuration of the molecule were relatively unimportant, and the pharmacological action required only that the molecule had certain physicochemical properties. We now know much more about how different anaesthetics interact with neuronal membrane proteins and have come to realise that there are multiple mechanisms by which anaesthesia can be produced and that different anaesthetics work by different mechanisms.

As the concentration of an anaesthetic is increased, the switch from being conscious to unconscious occurs over a very narrow concentration range (approximately 0.2 of a log unit). This is a much steeper concentration–response curve than that seen with drugs that interact as agonists or antagonists at classical receptors (see Ch. 2).

LIPID SOLUBILITY

Overton and Meyer, at the turn of the 20th century, showed a close correlation between anaesthetic potency and lipid solubility in a diverse group of simple and unreactive organic compounds that were tested for their ability to immobilise tadpoles. This led to a bold theory, formulated by Meyer in 1937: 'Narcosis commences when any chemically indifferent substance has attained a certain molar concentration in the lipids of the cell'.

[1]Now preserved as the Ether Dome, a museum piece at Massachusetts General Hospital.

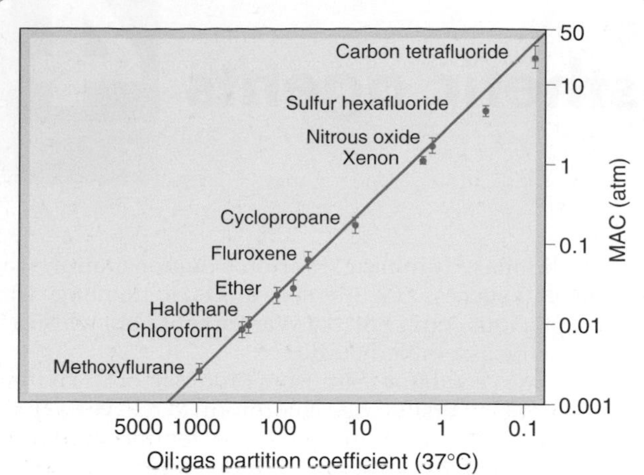

Fig. 41.1 Correlation of anaesthetic potency with oil:gas partition coefficient. Anaesthetic potency in humans is expressed as minimum alveolar partial pressure (MAC) required to produce surgical anaesthesia. There is a close correlation with lipid solubility, expressed as the oil:gas partition coefficient. (From Halsey, M.J., 1989. Physicochemical properties of inhalation anaesthetics. In: Nunn, J.F., Utting, J.E., Brown, B.R. (Eds), General Anaesthesia. Butterworth, London.)

The relationship between anaesthetic activity and lipid solubility has been repeatedly confirmed for a diverse array of agents. Anaesthetic potency in humans is usually expressed as the minimal alveolar concentration (MAC) required to abolish the response to surgical incision in 50% of subjects. Fig. 41.1 shows the correlation between MAC (inversely proportional to potency) and lipid solubility, expressed as the oil:gas partition coefficient, for a wide range of inhalation anaesthetics. The Overton–Meyer studies did not suggest any particular mechanism, but revealed an impressive correlation, for which any theory of anaesthesia needs to account. Oil:gas partition was assumed to predict partition into membrane lipids, consistent with the suggestion that anaesthesia results from an alteration of membrane function.

How the simple introduction of inert foreign molecules into the lipid bilayer could cause a functional disturbance was not explained. Two possible mechanisms, namely volume expansion and increased membrane fluidity, were suggested and tested experimentally, but both are now largely discredited and attention has swung from lipids to proteins, the correlation of potency with lipid solubility being explained by molecules of anaesthetic binding to hydrophobic pockets within specific membrane protein targets.

EFFECTS ON ION CHANNELS

Following early studies that showed that anaesthetics can bind to various proteins as well as lipids, it was found that anaesthetics affect several different types of ion channels (see Franks, 2008). For most anaesthetics, there are no known competitive antagonists, so this approach to identify sites of action is denied. Therefore the main criterion for identifying putative mechanisms of action of general anaesthetics is that, for a cellular effect to be relevant to the anaesthetic or analgesic actions of these agents, it must occur at therapeutically relevant concentrations.

Cys-loop ligand-gated ion channels. Almost all anaesthetics (with the exceptions of **cyclopropane**, **ketamine** and **xenon**[2]) potentiate the action of GABA at $GABA_A$ receptors (Antkowiak and Rudolph, 2016). As described in detail in Chapters 3 and 38, $GABA_A$ receptors are ligand-gated Cl^- channels made up of five subunits (generally comprising two α, two β and one γ or δ subunit). General anaesthetics target sites on the $GABA_A$ receptor and act as positive allosteric modulators of GABA activation (see Ch. 38). Recent ultrastructural studies of $GABA_A$ receptors have revealed that propofol and etomidate bind in cavities at the interface between the transmembrane domains of the β and α subunits whereas barbiturates bind at two other sites between the γ and β subunits and the α and β subunits as depicted in Fig. 41.2 (see Kim and Hibbs, 2021). Mutation studies suggest that volatile anaesthetics may also bind to a site at the interface between α and β subunits (see Franks, 2008).

A further level of complexity arises because there are different subtypes of each subunit (see Ch. 38). Different subunit compositions give rise to subtly different subtypes of $GABA_A$ receptor and these may be involved in different aspects of anaesthetic action. $GABA_A$ receptors clustered at the synapse have different pharmacological and kinetic properties from those that are distributed elsewhere across the cell (extrasynaptic receptors; see Ch. 38). Extrasynaptic $GABA_A$ receptors contain α4 and α6 subunits as well as the δ subunit, and anaesthetics appear to have a greater potentiating effect on these extrasynaptic $GABA_A$ receptors.

General anaesthetics also affect other neuronal cys-loop ligand-gated channels such as those activated by glycine (see Ch. 38), acetylcholine and 5-hydroxytryptamine (see Ch. 39). Their actions on these channels are similar to those on $GABA_A$ receptors but the relative importance of such actions to general anaesthesia is still to be determined.

Two-pore domain K^+ channels. These belong to a family of 'background' K^+ channels that modulate neuronal excitability. They are homomeric or heteromeric assemblies of a family of structurally related subunits (Bayliss and Barrett, 2008). Channels made up of TREK1, TREK2, TASK1, TASK3 or TRESK (see Ch. 4, Table 4.2) subunits can be directly activated by low concentrations of volatile and gaseous anaesthetics, thus reducing membrane excitability (see Franks, 2008). This may contribute to the analgesic, hypnotic and immobilising effects of these agents. Two-pore domain K^+ channels do not appear to be affected by intravenous anaesthetics.

NMDA receptors. **Glutamate**, the major excitatory neurotransmitter in the CNS, activates three main classes of ionotropic receptor – α-amino-3-hydroxy-5-methyl-4-isoxazolepropionic acid (AMPA), kainate and *N*-methyl-D-aspartate (NMDA) receptors (see Ch. 38). NMDA receptors are an important site of action for anaesthetics such as **nitrous oxide**, **xenon** and **ketamine** which act, in different ways, to reduce NMDA receptor–mediated responses. Xenon appears to inhibit NMDA receptors by competing with glycine for its regulatory site on this receptor whereas ketamine blocks the pore of the channel (see Ch. 38). Other inhalation anaesthetics may also exert effects on the NMDA receptor in addition to their effects on other proteins such as the $GABA_A$ receptor.

Other ion channels. Anaesthetics may also exert actions at cyclic nucleotide-gated K^+ channels and K_{ATP} channels. Some general anaesthetics inhibit certain subtypes of voltage-gated Na^+ channels. Inhibition of presynaptic

[2]There is some controversy about whether or not xenon potentiates $GABA_A$ responses, but at present the weight of evidence suggests it does not.

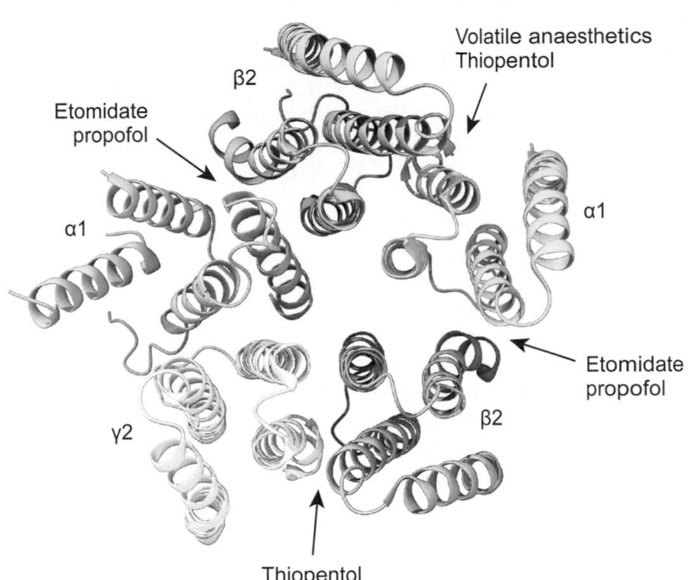

Fig. 41.2 Schematic of the putative binding sites in the clefts between the transmembrane domains of the subunits of the $GABA_A$ receptor. The view is from the extracellular side looking down and shows the transmembrane domains *(coloured helices)*. A more detailed description of the structure of a similar ligand-gated ion channel, the nicotinic acetylcholine receptor, is given in Fig 3.4. (Adapted from Kim, J.J., Hibbs, R.E, 2021. Direct structural insights into $GABA_A$ receptor pharmacology. Trends Biochem. Sci. 46, 502–517.)

Na^+ channels may give rise to the inhibition of transmitter release at excitatory synapses.

It may be overly simplistic to think of each anaesthetic as having only one mechanism of action: individual anaesthetics differ in their actions and affect cellular function in several different ways, so a single mechanism is unlikely to be sufficient.

Theories of anaesthesia

- Many simple, unreactive compounds produce general anaesthesia, the extreme example being the inert gas **xenon.**
- Anaesthetic potency is closely correlated with lipid solubility (Overton–Meyer correlation), not with chemical structure.
- Earlier theories of anaesthesia postulated interaction with the lipid membrane bilayer. Recent work favours interaction with membrane ion channels.
- Most anaesthetics enhance the activity of inhibitory $GABA_A$ receptors and other cys-loop ligand-gated ion channels. Other important effects are the activation of a subfamily of potassium channels (the two-pore domain K^+ channels) and inhibition of excitatory NMDA receptors.

EFFECTS ON THE NERVOUS SYSTEM

At the cellular level, the effects of anaesthetics are to enhance tonic inhibition (through enhancing the actions of GABA), reduce excitation (opening K^+ channels) and inhibit excitatory synaptic transmission (by depressing transmitter release and inhibiting ligand-gated ion channels). Effects on axonal conduction are relatively unimportant.

The anaesthetised state comprises several components, including *unconsciousness*, loss of reflexes (*muscle relaxation*) and *analgesia*. Much effort has gone into identifying the brain regions on which anaesthetics act to produce these effects. The most sensitive regions appear to be the midbrain reticular formation, thalamic sensory relay nuclei and, to a lesser extent, parts of the cortex. Inhibition of these regions results in unconsciousness and analgesia. Some anaesthetics - particularly volatile anaesthetics - cause inhibition at the spinal level, producing a loss of reflex responses to painful stimuli, although, in practice, neuromuscular-blocking drugs (see Ch. 14) are used as an adjunct to produce muscle relaxation rather than relying on the anaesthetic alone. Anaesthetics, even in low concentrations, cause short-term amnesia. It is likely that interference with hippocampal function produces this effect, because the hippocampus is involved in short-term memory, and certain hippocampal synapses are highly susceptible to inhibition by anaesthetics.

As the anaesthetic concentration is increased, all brain functions are progressively affected, including motor control and reflex activity, respiration and autonomic regulation. Therefore it is not possible to identify a critical 'target site' in the brain responsible for all the phenomena of anaesthesia.

High concentrations of any general anaesthetic affect all parts of the CNS, causing profound inhibition which, in the absence of artificial respiration, leads to death from respiratory failure. The margin between surgical anaesthesia and potentially fatal respiratory and circulatory depression is quite narrow, requiring careful monitoring by the anaesthetist and adjustment of the level of anaesthesia.

EFFECTS ON THE CARDIOVASCULAR AND RESPIRATORY SYSTEMS

Most anaesthetics decrease cardiac contractility, but their effects on cardiac output and blood pressure vary because of concomitant actions on the sympathetic nervous system and vascular smooth muscle. **Isoflurane** and other halogenated anaesthetics inhibit sympathetic outflow, reduce arterial and venous tone and thus decrease arterial pressure and venous pressure. By contrast, **nitrous oxide** and **ketamine** increase sympathetic discharge and plasma noradrenaline concentration and, if used alone, increase heart rate and maintain blood pressure.

Halogenated anaesthetics cause ventricular extrasystoles. The mechanism involves sensitisation to adrenaline. Electrocardiogram monitoring shows that extrasystolic beats occur commonly in patients under anaesthesia, with no harm coming to the patient. If catecholamine secretion is excessive, however (*par excellence* in phaeochromocytoma, a neuroendocrine tumour that secretes catecholamines into the circulation; see Ch. 15), there is a risk of precipitating ventricular fibrillation.

With the exception of **nitrous oxide, ketamine** and **xenon**, all anaesthetics depress respiration markedly and increase arterial P_{CO_2}. Nitrous oxide has much less effect, in part because its low potency prevents very deep anaesthesia from being produced with this drug. Some inhalation anaesthetics are pungent, particularly **desflurane**, which is liable to cause coughing, laryngospasm and bronchospasm, so desflurane is not used for induction of anaesthesia but only for maintenance.

Pharmacological effects of anaesthetic agents

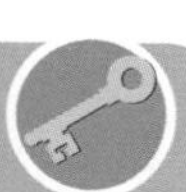

- Anaesthesia involves three main neurophysiological changes: unconsciousness, loss of response to painful stimulation and loss of reflexes (motor and autonomic).
- At supra-anaesthetic doses, all anaesthetic agents can cause death by loss of cardiovascular reflexes and respiratory paralysis.
- At the cellular level, anaesthetic agents affect synaptic transmission and neuronal excitability rather than axonal conduction. GABA-mediated inhibitory transmission is enhanced by most anaesthetics. The release of excitatory transmitters and the response of the postsynaptic receptors are also inhibited.
- Although all parts of the nervous system are affected by anaesthetic agents, the main targets appear to be the cortex, thalamus, hippocampus, midbrain reticular formation and spinal cord.
- Most anaesthetic agents (with the exception of **ketamine**, **nitrous oxide** and **xenon**) produce similar neurophysiological effects and differ mainly in respect of their pharmacokinetic properties and toxicity.
- Most anaesthetic agents cause cardiovascular depression by effects on the myocardium and blood vessels, as well as on the nervous system. Halogenated anaesthetic agents are likely to cause cardiac dysrhythmias, accentuated by circulating catecholamines.

INTRAVENOUS ANAESTHETIC AGENTS

Even the fastest-acting inhalation anaesthetics take a few minutes to act and cause a period of excitement before anaesthesia is induced. Intravenous anaesthetics act more rapidly, producing unconsciousness in about 20 s, as soon as the drug reaches the brain from its site of injection. These drugs (e.g. **propofol, thiopental** and **etomidate**) are normally used for induction of anaesthesia. They are preferred by many patients because injection avoids any unpleasantness that may be associated with the use of a face mask to administer the anaesthetic to an apprehensive individual. With propofol, recovery is also fast due to rapid metabolism.

Although many intravenous anaesthetics are not suitable for maintaining anaesthesia because their elimination from the body is relatively slow compared with that of inhalation agents, propofol can be administered either as a bolus for short procedures (<10 min) or as a continuous infusion. The duration of action of ketamine is sufficient that it can be administered as a single bolus for short procedures. Under these circumstances there is no need for an inhalation agent but a short-acting opioid such as **alfentanil** or **remifentanil** (see Ch. 43) may be co-administered to provide analgesia.

The properties of the main intravenous anaesthetics are summarised in Table 41.1.[3]

PROPOFOL

Propofol, introduced in 1983, has now largely replaced thiopental as an induction agent. It has a rapid onset of action (approximately 30 s) and a rapid rate of redistribution ($t_{1/2}$ 2–4 min), which makes it short acting. Because of its low water solubility, it is administered as an oil-in-water emulsion, which can cause pain on injection, and supports microbial growth. **Fospropofol** is a recently developed water-soluble derivative that is less painful on injection and rapidly converted by alkaline phosphatases to propofol in the body. Propofol metabolism to inactive conjugates and quinols follows first-order kinetics, in contrast to thiopental metabolism (see later), resulting in more rapid recovery and less hangover effect than occurs with thiopental. It has a cardiovascular depressant effect that may lead to hypotension and bradycardia. Respiratory depression may also occur and this may be enhanced by concurrent administration of a benzodiazepine (see Ch. 45) or an opioid (see Ch. 43). It is particularly useful for day-case surgery, especially as it causes less nausea and vomiting than do inhalation anaesthetics.

There have been reports of a propofol infusion syndrome occurring in approximately 1 in 300 patients when it has been given for a prolonged period to maintain sedation, particularly to sick patients – especially children in whom it is contraindicated in this setting – in intensive care units. This is characterised by severe metabolic acidosis, skeletal muscle necrosis (rhabdomyolysis), hyperkalaemia, lipaemia, hepatomegaly, renal failure, arrhythmia and cardiovascular collapse.

Propofol is used non-medicinally, especially by those, such as anaesthetists, who have ready access to the drug. Using propofol to obtain a sedative high is a risky business given its steep concentration–response curve.[4]

THIOPENTAL

Thiopental is the only remaining barbiturate in common use as an anaesthetic. It has very high lipid solubility, and this accounts for the speed of onset and transience

[3]**Propanidid** and **alphaxalone** were withdrawn because of allergic reactions causing hypotension and bronchoconstriction – probably attributable to the solvent cremophor – but a new formulation of alphaxalone has been reintroduced to veterinary medicine and is thought to be less allergenic.

[4]Propofol is referred to as the 'milk of amnesia'. The singer Michael Jackson died of a propofol overdose.

Table 41.1 Properties of intravenous anaesthetic agents

Drug	Speed of induction and recovery	Main unwanted effect(s)	Notes
Propofol	Fast onset, very fast recovery	Cardiovascular and respiratory depression	Rapidly metabolised Administered as a bolus or by continuous infusion Causes pain at injection site Fospropofol is a prodrug, less painful on injection
Thiopental	Fast (accumulation occurs, giving slow recovery) 'Hangover'	Cardiovascular and respiratory depression	Largely replaced by propofol Causes pain at injection site Risk of precipitating porphyria in susceptible patients
Etomidate	Fast onset, fairly fast recovery	Excitatory effects during induction and recovery Adrenocortical suppression	Less cardiovascular and respiratory depression than with thiopental Causes pain at injection site
Ketamine	Slow onset, after effects common during recovery	Psychotomimetic effects following recovery Postoperative nausea, vomiting and salivation Raised intracranial pressure	Produces good analgesia and amnesia with little respiratory depression
Midazolam	Slower than other agents	–	Amnesia, but little analgesia Little respiratory or cardiovascular depression

of its effect when it is injected intravenously. The free acid is insoluble in water, so thiopental is given as the sodium salt. On intravenous injection, thiopental causes unconsciousness within about 20 s, lasting for 5–10 min. The anaesthetic effect closely parallels the concentration of thiopental in the blood reaching the brain, because its high lipid solubility allows it to cross the blood–brain barrier without noticeable delay.

The blood concentration of thiopental declines rapidly, by about 80% within 1–2 min, following the initial peak after intravenous injection, because the drug is redistributed, first to tissues with a large blood flow (liver, kidneys, brain, etc.) and more slowly to muscle. Uptake into body fat, although favoured by the high lipid solubility of thiopental, occurs only slowly, because of the low blood flow to this tissue. After several hours, however, most of the thiopental present in the body will have accumulated in body fat, the rest having been metabolised. Recovery from the anaesthetic effect of a bolus dose occurs within about 5 min, governed entirely by redistribution of the drug to well-perfused tissues; very little is metabolised in this time. After the initial rapid decline, the blood concentration drops more slowly, over several hours, as the drug is taken up by body fat and metabolised in the liver. Consequently, thiopental produces a long-lasting hangover. Thiopental metabolism shows saturation kinetics (see Ch. 11). Because of this, large doses or repeated intravenous doses cause progressively longer periods of anaesthesia, as the plateau in blood concentration becomes progressively more elevated as more drug accumulates in the body and metabolism saturates. For this reason, thiopental is not used to maintain surgical anaesthesia but only as an induction agent. It is also still used to terminate status epilepticus if other measures fail (see Ch. 46) or (in patients with a secured airway) to lower intracranial pressure.

Thiopental binds to plasma albumin (roughly 85% of the blood content normally being bound). The fraction bound is less in states of malnutrition, liver disease or renal disease, which affect the concentration and drug-binding properties of plasma albumin, and this can appreciably reduce the dose needed for induction of anaesthesia.

If thiopental – a strongly alkaline solution – is accidently injected around rather than into a vein, or into an artery, this can cause pain, local tissue necrosis and ulceration or severe arterial spasm that can result in gangrene.

The actions of thiopental on the nervous system are very similar to those of inhalation anaesthetics, although it has little analgesic effect and can cause profound respiratory depression, even in amounts that fail to abolish reflex responses to painful stimuli. Its long after-effect, associated with a slowly declining plasma concentration, means that drowsiness and some degree of respiratory depression persist for some hours.

Thiopental, like other barbiturates, induces production of various liver enzymes, including those involved in haem synthesis, and can precipitate attacks of porphyria in patients suffering from this genetic disorder.

ETOMIDATE

Etomidate has gained favour over thiopental on account of the larger margin between the anaesthetic dose and the dose needed to produce cardiovascular depression. It is more rapidly metabolised than thiopental, and thus less likely to cause a prolonged hangover. It has no analgesic properties but causes less hypotension than propofol or thiopental. In other respects, etomidate is very similar to thiopental, although involuntary movements during induction, postoperative nausea and vomiting and pain at the injection site are problems with its use. Etomidate suppresses the production of adrenal steroids, an effect that has been associated with an increase in mortality in severely ill patients. It should be avoided in patients at risk of having adrenal insufficiency, e.g. in sepsis. It is preferable to thiopental in patients at risk of circulatory failure.

OTHER INTRAVENOUS AGENTS

KETAMINE

In human medicine **ketamine** is useful in short procedures that do not require skeletal muscle relaxation, e.g. for realignment and splinting of fractures and wound repair. It can be used in lower doses as an analgesic (see Ch. 43) and low doses have been found to induce rapid and sustained improvements in the symptoms of depression (see Ch. 48). It acts as a non-competitive channel blocker of the NMDA receptor (see Ch. 38).

In veterinary medicine, **ketamine** is commonly used for procedures in large animals and is normally given in combination with an a_2-adrenoceptor agonist, e.g. **xylazine,** or dexmedetomidine, providing rapid recumbency, immobilisation and analgesia which can also be reversed by administration of an a_2-adrenoceptor antagonist, e.g. **atipamezole**. Surgical procedures may also require the use of additional local anaesthesia.

Given intravenously, ketamine takes effect more slowly (1–2 min) than thiopental, and produces a different effect, known as 'dissociative anaesthesia', in which there is a marked sensory loss and analgesia, as well as amnesia, without complete loss of consciousness and no skeletal muscle relaxation. During induction and recovery, involuntary movements and peculiar sensory experiences often occur. Ketamine does not act simply as a CNS depressant, and it produces cardiovascular and respiratory effects quite different from those of most anaesthetics. Blood pressure and heart rate are usually increased, and respiration is unaffected by effective anaesthetic doses. This makes it relatively safe to use in low-technology healthcare situations or in accident and emergency situations where it can be administered intramuscularly if intravenous administration is not possible.[5] It is useful in patients with bronchospasm because of its bronchodilatory properties. However, ketamine, unlike other intravenous anaesthetic drugs, can increase intracranial pressure, so it should not be given to patients with raised intracranial pressure or at risk of cerebral ischaemia. Ketamine metabolism is age dependent, being faster in children and slower in the elderly.

A drawback of ketamine is that hallucinations, and sometimes delirium and irrational behaviour, may occur during recovery. These after-effects limit the usefulness of ketamine but are said to be less marked in children, and ketamine, often in conjunction with a benzodiazepine, may be used for minor procedures in paediatrics.

Ketamine is also used non-medicinally for its pronounced effects on sensory perception (see Ch. 49).

MIDAZOLAM

Midazolam, a benzodiazepine (see Ch. 45), is slower in onset and offset than the drugs discussed earlier but, like ketamine, causes less respiratory or cardiovascular depression. Midazolam is often used as an intravenous preoperative anxiolytic/sedative prior to a general anaesthetic or as a sedative during minor invasive procedures such as endoscopy or dental work, where drowsiness, sleep and amnesia are sufficient. It can be administered in combination with an analgesic such as **alfentanil**. In the event of overdose it can be reversed by **flumazenil** (see Ch. 45). **Remimazolam** is similar but has a more rapid onset and a shorter duration of action.

[5]An anaesthetist colleague tells of coming across a motorway accident where most of a victim was hidden under a mass of distorted metal but enough of a limb was available for an intramuscular injection of ketamine to be given.

Intravenous anaesthetic agents

- Most commonly used for induction of anaesthesia, followed by inhalation agent. **Propofol** can also be used to maintain anaesthesia during surgery.
- **Propofol, thiopental** and **etomidate** are most commonly used; all act within 20–30 s if given intravenously.
- **Propofol:**
  - potent;
  - rapid onset and distribution;
  - rapidly metabolised;
  - very rapid recovery, limited cumulative effect;
  - useful for day-case surgery;
  - low incidence of nausea and vomiting;
  - risk of bradycardia;
  - may induce an adverse 'propofol infusion syndrome' when administered at high doses for prolonged periods of time.
- **Thiopental:**
  - barbiturate with very high lipid solubility;
  - rapid action due to rapid transfer across blood–brain barrier; short duration (about 5 min) due to redistribution, mainly to muscle;
  - reduces intracranial pressure;
  - slowly metabolised and liable to accumulate in body fat, therefore may cause prolonged effect if given repeatedly;
  - narrow margin between anaesthetic dose and dose causing cardiovascular depression;
  - risk of tissue damage if accidently injected extravascularly or into an artery;
  - can precipitate an attack of porphyria in susceptible individuals (see Ch. 12).
- **Etomidate:**
  - similar to thiopental but more quickly metabolised;
  - less risk of cardiovascular depression;
  - may cause involuntary movements during induction and high incidence of nausea;
  - possible risk of adrenocortical suppression.
- **Ketamine:**
  - non-competitive channel blocker of NMDA receptors;
  - onset of effect is relatively slow (1–2 min);
  - powerful analgesic;
  - produces 'dissociative' anaesthesia, in which the patient may remain conscious although amnesic and insensitive to pain;
  - dysphoria and sometimes hallucinations may occur during recovery;
  - can raise intracranial pressure.
- **Midazolam:**
  - used to induce sedation, sleep and amnesia rather than full anaesthesia with loss of reflexes;
  - may be supplemented with an analgesic (e.g. alfentanil) if analgesia is required.

INHALATION ANAESTHETICS

Many inhalation anaesthetics that were once widely used, such as ether, chloroform, trichloroethylene, cyclopropane, methoxyflurane and enflurane, have now been replaced in clinical practice, particularly by **isoflurane**, **sevoflurane** and **desflurane**, which have improved pharmacokinetic properties, fewer side effects and are non-flammable. Of the older agents, **nitrous oxide** is still used (especially in obstetric practice), and **halothane** now only occasionally.

PHARMACOKINETIC ASPECTS

An important characteristic of an inhalation anaesthetic is the speed at which the arterial blood concentration, which governs the pharmacological effect in the brain, follows changes in the partial pressure of the drug in the inspired gas mixture. Ideally, the blood concentration should follow as quickly as possible, so that the depth of anaesthesia can be controlled rapidly. In particular, the blood concentration should fall to a subanaesthetic level rapidly when administration is stopped, so that the patient recovers consciousness with minimal delay. A prolonged semi-comatose state, in which vomiting is likely and respiratory reflexes are weak or absent, is particularly hazardous.

The lungs are the only quantitatively important route by which inhalation anaesthetics enter and leave the body. For modern inhalation anaesthetics, metabolic degradation is generally insignificant in determining their duration of action. Inhalation anaesthetics are all small, lipid-soluble molecules that readily cross alveolar membranes. It is therefore the rates of delivery of drug to and from the lungs, via (respectively) the inspired air and bloodstream, which determine the overall kinetic behaviour of an anaesthetic. The reason that anaesthetics vary in their kinetic behaviour is that their relative solubilities in blood, and in body fat, vary between one drug and another.

The main factors that determine the speed of induction and recovery can be summarised as follows:

- Properties of the anaesthetic:
  - blood:gas partition coefficient (i.e. solubility in blood)
  - oil:gas partition coefficient (i.e. solubility in fat)
- Physiological factors:
  - alveolar ventilation rate
  - cardiac output

SOLUBILITY OF INHALATION ANAESTHETICS

Inhalation anaesthetics can be regarded physicochemically as ideal gases: their solubility in different media is expressed as *partition coefficients*, defined as the ratio of the concentration of the agent in two phases at equilibrium.

The *blood:gas partition coefficient* is the main factor that determines the rate of induction and recovery of an inhalation anaesthetic, and the lower the blood:gas partition coefficient, the faster is induction and recovery (Table 41.2). This is because it is the partial pressure of the gas in the alveolar space that governs the concentration in the blood. The lower the blood:gas partition coefficient, the more rapidly the partial pressure of the gas in the alveolar space will equal that being administered in the inspired air (see later).

The *oil:gas partition coefficient*, a measure of fat solubility, determines the potency of an anaesthetic (as already discussed) and also influences the kinetics of its distribution in the body, the main effect being that high lipid solubility, by causing accumulation in body fat, delays recovery from anaesthesia. Values of blood:gas and oil:gas partition coefficients for some anaesthetics are given in Table 41.2.

INDUCTION AND RECOVERY

Cerebral blood flow is a substantial fraction of cardiac output (~15%), and the blood–brain barrier is freely permeable to anaesthetics, so the concentration of anaesthetic in the brain closely tracks that in the arterial blood. The kinetics of transfer of anaesthetic between the inspired air and the arterial blood therefore determine the kinetics of the pharmacological effect.

When a volatile anaesthetic is first administered, the initial breaths are diluted into the residual gas volume in the lungs, resulting in a reduction in the alveolar partial pressure of the anaesthetic as compared with the inspired gas mixture. With subsequent breaths, the alveolar partial pressure rises towards equilibrium. For an anaesthetic with a low blood:gas partition coefficient, the absorption into the blood will be slower, so with repeated breaths the partial pressure in the alveolar space will rise faster than with an agent of high blood:gas partition coefficient. Thus a smaller number of breaths (i.e. a shorter time) will be needed to reach equilibrium. Therefore, contrary to what one might intuitively suppose, the *lower* the solubility in blood, the *faster* is the process of equilibration. Fig. 41.3 shows the much faster equilibration for **nitrous oxide**, a low-solubility agent, than for **ether**, a high-solubility agent.

The rate of absorption into the blood can be enhanced by administering a volatile anaesthetic along with nitrous oxide. The rapid movement of nitrous oxide from the alveoli into the blood concentrates the volatile anaesthetic in the alveoli which will increase its movement into the blood - referred to as the *concentration effect*. Furthermore, the volume of nitrous oxide taken up from the alveoli into the blood is replaced by inspired gas, thus augmenting the delivery to the alveoli of the volatile anaesthetic and speeding its absorption – referred to as the *second gas effect*.

The transfer of anaesthetic between blood and tissues also affects the kinetics of equilibration. Fig. 41.4 shows a very simple model of the circulation, in which two tissue compartments are included. Body fat has a low blood flow but has a high capacity to take up anaesthetics, and constitutes about 20% of the volume of a non-obese human. Therefore for a drug such as **halothane**, which is about 100 times more soluble in fat than in water, the amount present in fat after complete equilibration would be roughly 95% of the total amount in the body. Because of the low blood flow to adipose tissue, it takes many hours for the drug to enter and leave the fat, which results in a pronounced slow phase of equilibration following the rapid phase associated with the blood–gas exchanges (see Fig. 41.3). The more fat-soluble the anaesthetic and the more obese the patient, the more pronounced this slow phase becomes and recovery will also be delayed.

Of the physiological factors affecting the rate of equilibration of inhalation anaesthetics, alveolar ventilation is the most important. The greater the minute volume (respiration rate × tidal volume), the faster is equilibration, particularly for drugs that have high blood:gas partition coefficients. Respiratory depressant drugs such as **morphine** (see Ch. 43) can thus retard recovery from anaesthesia. The effect of changes in cardiac output on the rate of equilibration is more complex. By reducing alveolar perfusion, a reduction of cardiac output reduces alveolar absorption of the anaesthetic, and thus

Table 41.2 Characteristics of inhalation anaesthetics

Drug	Partition coefficient		Minimum alveolar concentration (% v/v)	Induction/ recovery	Main adverse effect(s) and disadvantage(s)	Notes
	Blood:gas	Oil:gas				
Nitrous oxide	0.5	1.4	100[a]	Fast	Few adverse effects Risk of peripheral neuropathy and anaemia (with prolonged or repeated use) Accumulation in gaseous cavities	Good analgesic effect Low potency precludes use as sole anaesthetic agent – normally combined with other inhalation agents and oxygen
Isoflurane	1.4	91	1.2	Medium	Few adverse effects Possible risk of coronary ischaemia in susceptible patients	Widely used Has replaced halothane
Desflurane	0.4	23	6.1	Fast	Respiratory tract irritation, cough, bronchospasm	Used for day-case surgery because of fast onset and recovery (comparable with nitrous oxide)
Sevoflurane	0.6	53	2.1	Fast	Few reported Theoretical risk of renal toxicity owing to fluoride	Similar to desflurane
Halothane	2.4	220	0.8	Medium	Hypotension Cardiac arrhythmias Hepatotoxicity (with repeated use) Malignant hyperthermia (rare)	Little used nowadays Significant metabolism to trifluoroacetate
Enflurane	1.9	98	1.7	Medium	Risk of convulsions (slight) Malignant hyperthermia (rare)	Has declined in use May induce seizures
Ether	12.0	65	1.9	Slow	Respiratory irritation Nausea and vomiting Explosion risk	Now obsolete, except where modern facilities are lacking

[a]Theoretical value based on experiments under hyperbaric conditions.

speeds up induction, but this is partially offset by a reduction of cerebral blood flow slowing down delivery to the brain.

Recovery from anaesthesia involves the same processes as induction but in reverse, the rapid phase of recovery being followed by a slow 'hangover'. Because of these kinetic factors, the search for improved inhalation anaesthetics has focused on agents with low blood and tissue solubility. Newer drugs, which show kinetic properties similar to those of nitrous oxide but have higher potency, include **sevoflurane** and **desflurane** (see Table 41.2 and Fig. 41.3).

METABOLISM AND TOXICITY

Metabolism, although not quantitatively important as a route of elimination of inhalation anaesthetics, can generate toxic metabolites (see Ch. 58).[6] This is the main reason that agents that are now obsolete or obsolescent, such as chloroform, methoxyflurane and halothane, have been replaced by the less toxic alternatives described later.

Malignant hyperthermia is an important but rare *idiosyncratic reaction* (see Ch. 58), caused by heat production in skeletal muscle, due to excessive release of Ca^{2+} from the sarcoplasmic reticulum. The result is muscle contracture, acidosis, increased metabolism and an associated dramatic rise in body temperature that can be fatal unless treated promptly. Triggers include halogenated anaesthetics and depolarising neuromuscular-blocking drugs (see Ch. 14). Susceptibility has a genetic basis, being associated with mutations in the gene encoding the ryanodine receptor, which controls Ca^{2+} release from the sarcoplasmic reticulum (see Ch. 4). Malignant hyperthermia is treated with **dantrolene**, a muscle relaxant drug that blocks these calcium-release channels.

[6]The problem of toxicity of low concentrations of anaesthetics inhaled over long periods by operating theatre staff was at one time a cause for concern. Strict measures are now used to minimise the escape of anaesthetics into the air of operating theatres.

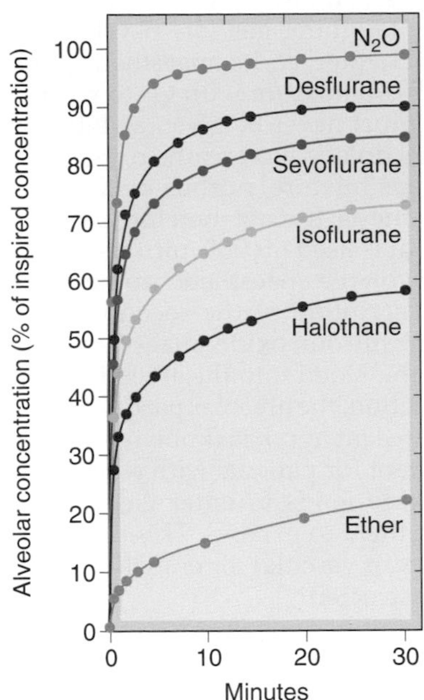

Fig. 41.3 Rate of equilibration of inhalation anaesthetics in humans. The curves show alveolar concentration (which closely reflects arterial blood concentration) as a function of time during induction. The initial rate of equilibration reflects solubility in blood. There is also a slow phase of equilibration, most marked with highly lipid-soluble drugs (ether and halothane), owing to the slow transfer between blood and fat (see Fig. 41.4). (Adapted from Yasuda, N., Lockhart, S.H., Eger, E.I. II, et al., 1991. Comparison of kinetics of sevoflurane and isoflurane in humans. Anesth. Analg. 72, 316–324.)

Pharmacokinetic properties of inhalation anaesthetics

- Rapid induction and recovery are important properties of an anaesthetic agent, allowing flexible control over the depth of anaesthesia.
- Speed of induction and recovery are determined by two properties of the anaesthetic: solubility in blood (blood:gas partition coefficient) and solubility in fat (lipid solubility).
- Agents with low blood:gas partition coefficients produce rapid induction and recovery (e.g. **nitrous oxide**, **desflurane**); agents with high blood:gas partition coefficients show slow induction and recovery.
- Agents with high lipid solubility accumulate gradually in body fat and may produce a prolonged 'hangover' if used for a long operation.
- Some halogenated anaesthetics (especially **halothane** and **methoxyflurane**) are metabolised. This is not very important in determining their duration of action but contributes to toxicity (e.g. renal toxicity associated with fluoride production with **methoxyflurane** – no longer used).

INDIVIDUAL INHALATION ANAESTHETICS

The main inhalation anaesthetics currently used in developed countries are **isoflurane**, **desflurane** and **sevoflurane**, sometimes used in combination with **nitrous oxide**. Due to its relatively rapid onset of action and pleasant smell, **sevoflurane** is used, under some circumstances, on

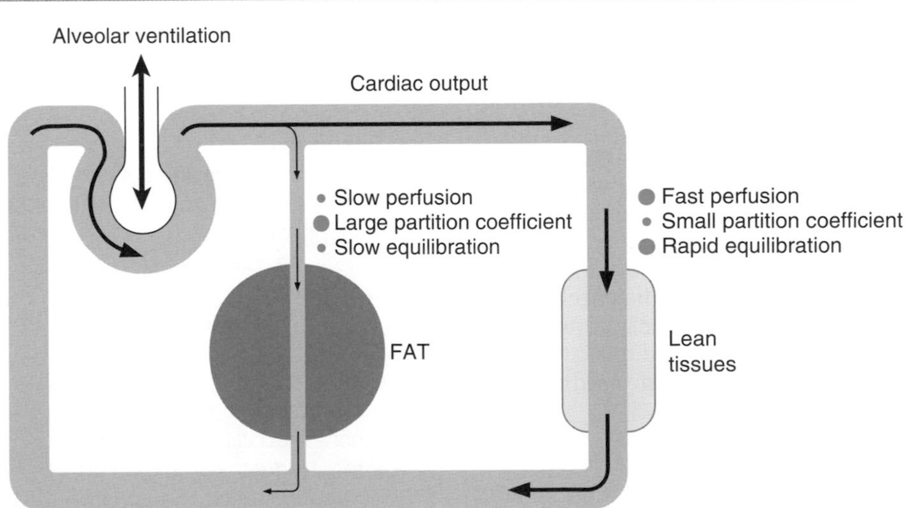

Fig. 41.4 Factors affecting the rate of equilibration of inhalation anaesthetics in the body. The body is represented as two compartments. Lean tissues, including the brain, have a large blood flow and low partition coefficient for anaesthetics, and therefore equilibrate rapidly with the blood. Fat tissues have a small blood flow and large partition coefficient, and therefore equilibrate slowly, acting as a reservoir of drug during the recovery phase.

its own to induce anaesthesia, e.g. in paediatrics or in adults frightened by the prospect of venous cannulation. **Xenon**, an inert gas shown many years ago to have anaesthetic properties, is making something of a comeback in the clinic because – not surprisingly for an inert gas – it lacks toxicity, but its relatively low potency and high cost are disadvantages. It may also be neuroprotective in neonatal hypoxia (see Ch. 40).

ISOFLURANE, DESFLURANE, SEVOFLURANE, ENFLURANE AND HALOTHANE

These volatile anaesthetics are liquids at room temperature and require the use of vaporisers for inhalational administration.

Isoflurane is a non-flammable volatile anaesthetic that is now the most widely used volatile anaesthetic. It is not appreciably metabolised and lacks the proconvulsive property of enflurane. It can cause hypotension and is a powerful coronary vasodilator. Paradoxically, this can exacerbate cardiac ischaemia in patients with coronary disease, because of the 'steal' phenomenon (see Ch. 20).

Desflurane is chemically similar to isoflurane, but its lower solubility in blood and fat means that adjustment of anaesthetic depth and recovery are faster, so it is increasingly used as an anaesthetic in obese patients undergoing bariatric surgery and for day-case surgery. It is not appreciably metabolised. It is less potent than the other halogenated general anaesthetics. At the concentrations used for induction of anaesthesia (about 10%), desflurane causes some respiratory tract irritation, which can lead to coughing and bronchospasm. Rapid increases in the depth of desflurane anaesthesia can be associated with a striking increase in sympathetic activity, which is undesirable in patients with ischaemic heart disease.

Sevoflurane resembles desflurane but is more potent and does not cause the same degree of respiratory irritation. It is partially (about 3%) metabolised, and detectable levels of fluoride are produced, although this does not appear to be sufficient to cause toxicity.

Enflurane has a moderate speed of induction but is little used nowadays. It was originally introduced as an alternative to methoxyflurane. It can cause seizures, either during induction or following recovery from anaesthesia, especially in patients suffering from epilepsy. In this connection, it is interesting that a related substance, the fluorine-substituted diethyl-ether hexafluoroether, is a powerful convulsant agent, although the mechanism is not understood.

Halothane was an important drug in the development of volatile inhalation anaesthetics, but its use has declined in favour of isoflurane due to the potential for accumulation of toxic metabolites. Halothane has a marked relaxant effect on the uterus which can cause postpartum bleeding and limits its usefulness for obstetric purposes.

NITROUS OXIDE

Nitrous oxide (N_2O, not to be confused with nitric oxide, NO) is an odourless gas. Its use as an anaesthetic is declining in the developed world. It has a global warming potential much higher than CO_2 and is regulated under the Kyoto Protocol (1997). It is the third largest contributor to the greenhouse effect in the United Kingdom.

Nitrous oxide is rapid in onset of action because of its low blood:gas partition coefficient (see Table 41.2), and is an effective analgesic in concentrations too low to cause unconsciousness. At low doses it induces euphoria, hence its nickname 'laughing gas'; its psychoactive effects are described in Chapter 49. Its anaesthetic potency is low. It is used as a 50:50 mixture with O_2 to reduce pain during childbirth. It must never be given as 100% of the inspired gas as patients do need to breathe oxygen! Even at 80% in the inspired gas mixture, nitrous oxide does not produce surgical anaesthesia. It is not therefore used on its own as an anaesthetic, but is used (as 70% nitrous oxide in oxygen) as an adjunct to volatile anaesthetics to speed up induction – see earlier description of the second gas effect. During recovery from nitrous oxide anaesthesia, the transfer of the gas from the blood into the alveoli can be sufficient to reduce, by dilution, the alveolar partial pressure of oxygen, producing transient hypoxia (known as *diffusional hypoxia*). This is important for patients with respiratory disease.

Nitrous oxide tends to enter gaseous cavities in the body causing them to expand. This can be dangerous if a pneumothorax or vascular air embolus is present, or if the intestine is obstructed.

Given for brief periods, nitrous oxide is devoid of any serious toxic effects, but prolonged or repeated exposure oxidises and inactivates vitamin B_{12}.[7] In its inactive form, vitamin B_{12} is unable to function as a co-factor for methionine synthase and this can produce peripheral neuropathy and bone marrow depression. The latter may cause anaemia and leukopenia, so its use should be avoided in patients with anaemia related to vitamin B_{12} deficiency.

Individual inhalation anaesthetics

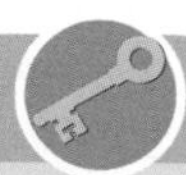

- The main agents in current use in developed countries are **isoflurane**, **desflurane** and **sevoflurane**, sometimes supplemented with **nitrous oxide.**
- As a rare but serious hazard, inhalation anaesthetics can cause malignant hyperthermia.
- **Isoflurane:**
  - similar to **enflurane** but lacks epileptogenic property
  - may precipitate myocardial ischaemia in patients with coronary disease
  - irritant to respiratory tract
- **Desflurane:**
  - similar to **isoflurane** but with faster onset and recovery
  - respiratory irritant, so liable to cause coughing and laryngospasm
  - useful for day-case surgery
- **Sevoflurane:**
  - similar to **desflurane**, with lack of respiratory irritation
- **Nitrous oxide:**
  - good analgesic properties
  - low potency as an anaesthetic, therefore must be combined with other agents
  - rapid induction and recovery
  - risk of peripheral neuropathy and bone marrow depression with prolonged administration
  - accumulates in gaseous cavities

[7]In operating theatres scavenging systems are used to prevent staff being exposed to nitrous oxide. People who overuse nitrous oxide for its euphoric effects do expose themselves to side effects associated with vitamin B_{12} deficiency (Ch. 49).

Clinical uses of general anaesthetics

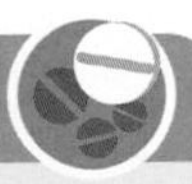

- *Intravenous anaesthetics* are used for:
  - induction of anaesthesia (e.g. **propofol** or **thiopental**);
  - maintenance of anaesthesia throughout surgery ('total intravenous anaesthesia', e.g. **propofol** sometimes in combination with muscle relaxants and analgesics).
- *Inhalational anaesthetics* (gases or volatile liquids) are used for maintenance of anaesthesia. Points to note are that:
  - volatile anaesthetics (e.g. **isoflurane**, **sevoflurane**) are delivered in air, oxygen or oxygen–nitrous oxide mixtures as the carrier gas;
  - **nitrous oxide** must always be given with oxygen;
  - because of its potential for inducing hepatotoxicity, **halothane** has largely been replaced by newer volatile anaesthetics such as **isoflurane;**
  - all inhalational anaesthetics can trigger *malignant hyperthermia* in susceptible individuals.

SEDATION AND BALANCED ANAESTHESIA

Sedation is a continuum which extends from normal consciousness to being fully unresponsive. Sedation rather than general anaesthesia is often sufficient for short, non-invasive procedures. Conscious sedation is used in dentistry and endoscopic examinations to reduce fear and anxiety, control pain and minimise excessive movement. It does not involve sleep or loss of consciousness. **Midazolam** is often administered for this purpose. Deeper procedural sedation, where the patient becomes sleepy and is less easily aroused, can be achieved by administration of **midazolam, propofol, etomidate** or **ketamine** along with an opioid analgesic (e.g. **fentanyl** or **morphine**).

In complex surgery, an array of drugs will be given at various times throughout the procedure to produce what is termed *balanced anaesthesia*. The drugs administered may include a sedative or anxiolytic premedication (e.g. a benzodiazepine, see Ch. 45), an intravenous anaesthetic for rapid induction (e.g. **propofol**), a perioperative opioid analgesic (e.g. **alfentanil** or **remifentanil**, see Ch. 43), an inhalation anaesthetic to maintain anaesthesia during surgery (e.g. **nitrous oxide** and **isoflurane**), a neuromuscular-blocking agent to produce adequate muscle relaxation (e.g. **vecuronium**, see Ch. 14) for access to the abdominal cavity for example, an antiemetic agent (e.g. **ondansetron**, see Ch. 30) and a muscarinic antagonist to prevent or treat bradycardia or to reduce bronchial and salivary secretions (e.g. **atropine** or **glycopyrrolate**, see Ch. 14). Towards the end of the procedure, an anticholinesterase agent (e.g. **neostigmine**, see Ch. 14) to reverse the neuromuscular blockade (**sugammadex**, which binds and inactivates steroidal neuromuscular-blocking drugs, can also be used for this purpose) and an analgesic for postoperative pain relief (e.g. an opioid such as **morphine** and/or a non-steroidal anti-inflammatory drug, see Ch. 43) may be used. Such combinations of drugs result in much faster induction and recovery, avoiding long (and potentially hazardous) periods of semiconsciousness, produce good analgesia and muscle relaxation and enable surgery to be carried out with less undesirable cardiorespiratory depression.

Low doses of general anaesthetics may be used to provide sedation where a local anaesthetic (see Ch. 44), administered intrathecally, is used to provide analgesia and relaxation needed to perform surgery to the lower parts of the body.

REFERENCES AND FURTHER READING

Antkowiak, B., Rudolph, U., 2016. New insights in the systemic and molecular underpinnings of general anesthetic actions mediated by γ-aminobutyric acid A receptors. Cur. Opin. Anaesth 29, 447–453.

Bayliss, D.A., Barrett, P.Q., 2008. Emerging roles for two-pore-domain potassium channels and their potential therapeutic impact. Trends Pharmacol. Sci. 29, 566–575.

Franks, N.P., 2008. General anaesthesia: from molecular targets to neuronal pathways of sleep and arousal. Nat. Rev. Neurosci. 9, 370–386.

Kim, J.J., Hibbs, R.E., 2021. Direct structural insights into $GABA_A$ receptor pharmacology. Trends Biochem. Sci. 46, 502–517.

Thompson, J., Moppett, I., Wiles, M., 2019. Smith & Aitkenhead's Textbook of Anaesthesia, seventh ed. Elsevier, London.

42 Headache

OVERVIEW

In this chapter we discuss the pharmacological treatment of headache. We first outline the spectrum of headache disorders, discuss the various drug therapies available and review their mechanisms of action. We focus particularly on the therapy of migraine, a condition which has a high morbidity.

HEADACHE

The overwhelming majority of people will suffer from headaches (*cephalalgias*) at some point in their lives. These range from the inconvenience of occasional headaches to the life-changing and debilitating effects of chronic migraine. 'Headache' is ranked among the top 10 causes of disability worldwide. While many sufferers self-treat with simple analgesics or proprietary preparations available from pharmacies, the condition can be complex and often requires careful differential diagnosis. While accounting for 4%–5% of consultations in primary care, headaches are responsible for approximately 30% of referrals to neurologists in the United Kingdom (cited in McCrone et al., 2011). In some cases, headaches may be severe enough to require hospitalisation, and according to one survey in the United States (Burch et al., 2015), headache is the fourth leading cause of visits to emergency departments.

The economic burden of headache in general, and migraine in particular, is huge. According to recent estimates, the total cost of treating headache in the United Kingdom is some £250 million per annum and the economic cost in lost productivity has been estimated to be £5–7 billion annually (cited by The Migraine Trust, 2021), although other studies have estimated that the economic cost of migraine alone could be as high as £8.8 billion (The Work Foundation 2018) and more than \$14.4 billion in the United States (McCrone et al., 2011). Despite the obvious impact on healthcare resources and national economic performance, there is little public awareness of the causes of headaches and apparently minimal time devoted to the subject during professional medical training. Three quarters of all medical schools do not even include headache in their undergraduate syllabus (The Migraine Trust, 2021).

TYPES OF HEADACHES

Although some patients may suffer from both types simultaneously, headaches are usually classified as either 'primary' or 'secondary'. The latter term refers to headaches associated with some type of underlying clinical condition such as malignancy, trauma, infections, cerebrovascular disease or trauma (e.g. subarachnoid haemorrhage), medication overuse or drug withdrawal. Today, this list of potential causes also includes 'COVID-19 headache' which seems to afflict about 10% of all patients who have caught this disease (Islam et al., 2020). In all cases of secondary headache, clinical investigations may be required to establish the root cause before choosing a treatment plan for resolving the problem.

In this chapter we will deal mainly with *primary headache* which is not caused by an underlying pathology, but which may have a genetic component or other causation (Robbins, 2021). *The International Headache Society* (IHS, 2018) has classified headaches into four main groups: *tension-type headaches*, *trigeminal autonomic cephalalgias*, *migraine* and *others*. These groups present with different clinical symptoms and, despite some overlap, often have different underlying mechanisms requiring different pharmacological approaches to treatment. We will deal with each group separately.

MIGRAINE[1]

This is the most complex of these cephalalgias. It is a common and debilitating condition affecting 10%–15% of people and is often stated to be the third most common disease in the world. Some estimates place the total number of sufferers globally at 1 billion with some 45 million years of life compromised by the misery of this disease (Nature Outlook, 2020). The WHO has classified migraine as among the 20 most disabling lifetime conditions.

Drugs used for migraine

Aspirin, ibuprofen, or other non-steroidal anti-inflammatory agents are recommended for pain relief in acute migraine, and best administered early during onset of symptoms. Antiemetics such as **metoclopramide** are given at the same time for patients who suffer with nausea.

Triptans (5-$HT_{1B/1D/F}$ agonists) are widely used for acute relief of moderate to severe migraine that has not responded to simple analgesics. The triptans are also effective in cluster headaches.

Medication overuse headaches can occur with persistent daily use of analgesics and triptans.

Regular use of prophylactic agents (such as **propranolol**, **topiramate** or **amitriptyline**) is therefore indicated for patients who suffer frequent and troubling migraine attacks. Patients who fail to respond to these oral agents can move on to injectable options such as the anti-CGRP antibodies or botulinum toxin.

[1]The word is apparently of French origin and is probably a corruption of *hemicrania*, the Latin name for the disease.

Although the causes are not completely understood, both genetic and environmental factors seem to be important. The frequency of attacks varies, with about three-quarters of *migraineurs* (as they are called) having more than one episode per month. Generally, the onset of attacks begins at puberty and wanes with increasing age. Women are twice as likely as men to suffer from the disorder, and it appears that rapidly falling oestrogen levels can precipitate bouts of migraine in susceptible subjects so that the attacks are often linked to the menstrual cycle or other reproductive events.

Migraine can be *episodic*, when the attacks are relatively infrequent, or *chronic*, if the frequency and severity become a major burden to the patient. Chronic migraine may be accompanied by comorbidities such as gastrointestinal problems or mental health issues. Pharmacotherapy of the two manifestations of migraine is a little different but it is likely that episodic attacks eventually transform into a more chronic illness unless treated.

CLINICAL SYMPTOMS

The symptomology of migraine is complex: in about a third of cases, attacks may be accompanied by an *aura* (a term taken to include any sensory changes that occur before the onset of the headache: 'classic migraine'). The onset of an attack is heralded by a *premonitory phase*, with symptoms including nausea, mood changes as well as sensitivity to light and sound (photophobia and phonophobia). These may occur hours before the onset of the *aura* phase and may be accompanied by more specific visual symptoms such as a slowly moving blind spot with associated flashing lights ('scintillating scotoma') or geometric patterns of coloured lights ('fortification spectra') or the illusion of looking through the wrong end of a telescope. The *headache* phase proper is characterised by a moderate or severe headache, starting unilaterally, but then usually spreading to both sides of the head. It may have a pulsating or throbbing quality and may be accompanied by nausea, vomiting and prostration. There may also be sensitivity to movement. This phase may persist for hours or even days. Following resolution of the headache, a *postdromal* phase may include feelings of fatigue, altered cognition or mood changes. While these different phases probably represent discrete biological events, in practice they overlap and may run in parallel. A good account of these is given by Charles (2013) and in the comprehensive review of headache disorders by the IHS (2018).

PATHOPHYSIOLOGY

The causes of migraine are incompletely understood although the pathogenesis is becoming clearer. Historically there have been three main hypotheses advanced to account for the pain and other symptoms including: the notion that inappropriate vasoconstriction and vasodilatation were responsible for the symptoms; that cortical activation accompanied by *cortical spreading depression* was the cause; or that inflammatory activation of trigeminal nerve terminals in the meninges and extracranial vessels was the primary event in a migraine attack. These are summarised and explained in more detail by Eadie (2005). It is likely that elements of all these phenomena play a role in the pathogenesis of migraine to a greater or lesser extent, but the consensus of opinion now is that the source of the pain is inflammatory activation of the *trigeminovascular system* – the sensory neurons that innervate the cerebral vessels (see Moreno-Ajona et al., 2019) – while the cortical spreading depression, triggered by changes in ion channel activity in the cortex, is responsible for the aura.

Pharmacological and other evidence strongly implicates a key role for neurotransmitters such as calcitonin gene-related peptide (CGRP) (see Ch. 43) and 5-hydroxytryptamine (5-HT) (see Ch. 16) in the onset of migraine. CGRP is a major nociceptive transmitter in the trigeminal vascular system and blood neuropeptide levels are raised in patients during episodes of migraine and fall as the condition improves or following treatment with anti-CGRP drugs (Moreno-Ajona et al., 2019). Conversely, infusion of CGRP can induce migraine attacks in susceptible people. It has long been suspected that 5-HT also plays a significant role in the pathogenesis of migraine: There is a sharp increase in the urinary excretion of the main 5-HT metabolite, 5-hydroxyindole acetic acid (5-HIAA), during a migraine attack while the blood concentration of 5-HT falls, probably because of depletion of platelet 5-HT. In addition, many selective 5-HT receptor agonists or antagonists are found to be effective in treating migraine. Originally, this was considered to be because of their ability to block the effects of 5-HT on cerebrovascular vessels. However, the consensus now is that the main site of action of these drugs is presynaptic receptors in the trigeminal neurovascular system where they inhibit the release of proinflammatory neuropeptides such as CGRP.

The symptoms associated with the premonitory phase of migraine are largely dopaminergic in origin. The onset of the aura phase coincides with the cortical spreading depression, and imaging studies have indicated widespread changes in brain perfusion during this phase. There may be *hypoperfusion* of some brain areas as well as *hyperperfusion* in others, suggesting that the physiological mechanisms that normally regulate the relationship between brain activity and blood flow become disengaged. Such *neurovascular uncoupling* is also a feature of cortical spreading depression.

Imaging studies suggest that migraine attacks are triggered by signals originating from the hypothalamus (see Haanes and Edvinsson 2019). These in turn activate the *trigeminal nucleus caudalis*, and after passing through the *trigeminal ganglion*, activated efferent C fibres dilate meningeal blood vessels, probably releasing further inflammatory mediators such as prostaglandins and nitric oxide. Activated afferent A-δ fibres signal this inflammatory state back through the trigeminal neural pathways, where it is relayed to the cortex and perceived as a painful event. Central sensitisation increases the migraineur's sensitivity to sound, light, cutaneous sensations and other normally non-painful stimuli. Many of the observed vascular and other changes may persist into the postdromal phase, which may last for hours or days.

It is noteworthy that these mechanisms do not offer a totally conclusive account of the complex symptomology of migraine, or explain how attacks are initiated or which underlying abnormality predisposes particular individuals to suffer from migraine. Some authors have identified the 'gut brain axis' (Arzani et al., 2020) or endothelial dysfunction (Paolucci et al., 2021) as being of significance. In some rare types of familial migraine, inherited mutations affecting calcium channels and Na^+-K^+-ATPase have been found, suggesting that abnormal membrane function may be responsible and **levcromakalim**, a drug which opens ATP-sensitive potassium channels, can provoke migraine

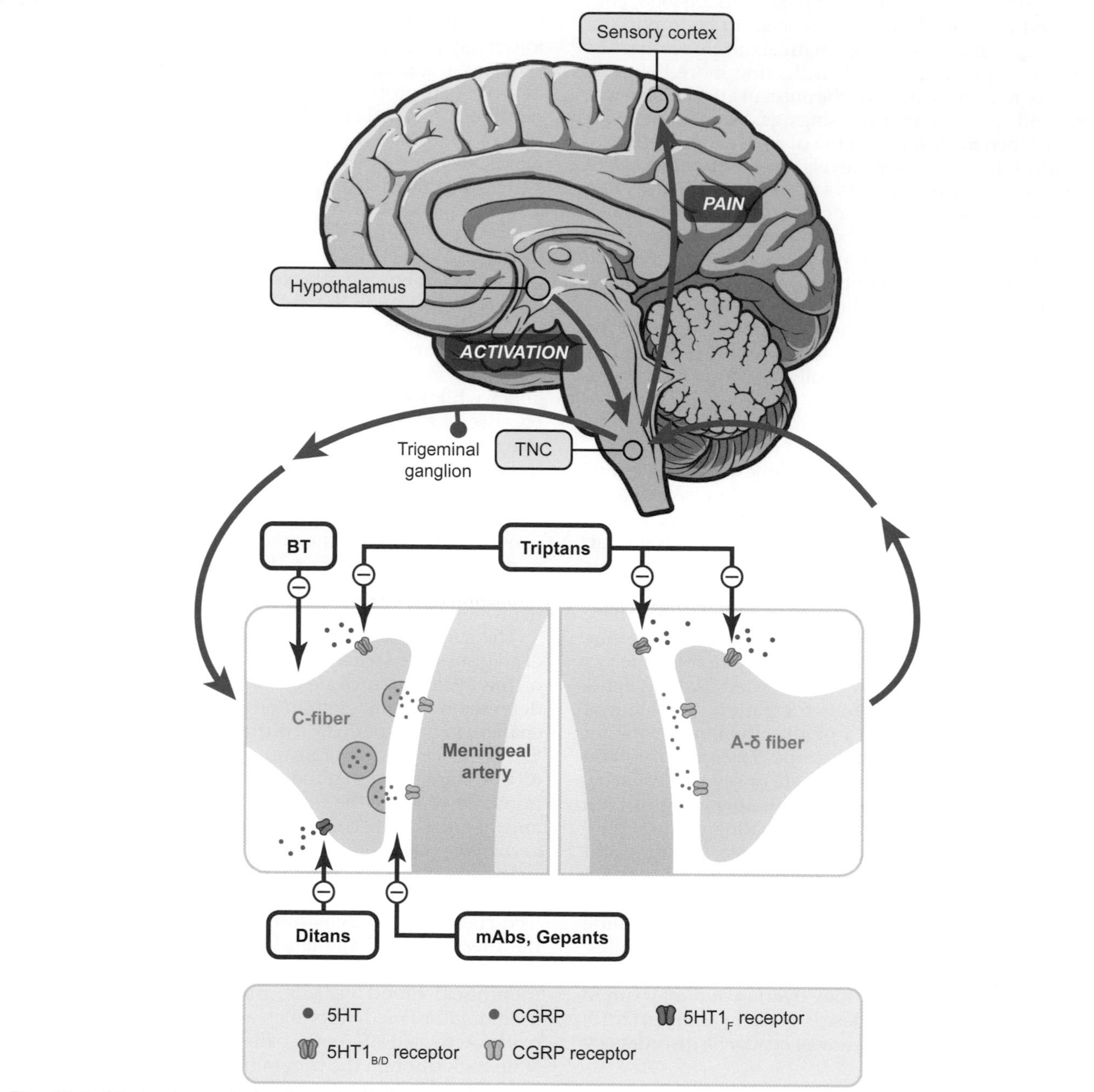

Fig. 42.1 Mechanisms of migraine pain. A diagrammatic representation of the current view of the origins of migraine pain and the sites at which antimigraine drugs act. Migraine attacks are initiated by signals arising from the hypothalamus and feeding into the *trigeminal nucleus caudalis* (TNC). These are relayed through efferent C fibres through the trigeminal ganglion (TG) to the vascular system of the meninges. These activated C fibres release calcitonin gene-related peptide (CGRP) from their terminals which dilate meningeal arteries and cause inflammation probably by releasing prostaglandins and other mediators including nitric oxide. These events activate afferent A-δ fibres which signal the sensation of pain back through the TG and TNC to the cortex. Triptans inhibit the release of CGRP by an action at presynaptic $5HT_{1B/D/F}$ receptors or by constricting the meningeal vessels through an action on $5\text{-}HT_{1B/D}$ receptors. Ditans inhibit CGRP release through an action at the $5\text{-}HT_{1F}$ presynaptic receptor. Gepants antagonise the action of CGRP at its target receptor on the vasculature or the A-δ fibre. Monoclonal antibodies (mAbs) neutralise the CGRP (or its receptor) while botulinum toxin (BT) 'denervates' the neurons.

attacks in sensitive subjects (Al-Karagholi et al., 2019). It is thought that activation of such channels in the cranial arteries and the trigeminal nerve is the cause of the pain. In most forms of migraine, however, there is no clear genetic cause.

Fig. 42.1 shows, in a diagrammatic way, our current understanding of the factors implicated in migraine pain.

TENSION-TYPE HEADACHES

These are the most common type of headache (incidence ~40%). There are several subtypes differentiated by their

Table 42.1 Drug therapy of headaches

Type of headache	Acute treatment	Prophylactic treatment
Tension headache	NSAIDs and simple analgesics (recommended only for occasional use due to risk of medication overuse headache)	Tricyclic antidepressants; SSRIs; mirtazapine
Cluster headache	Triptans; methysergide; pizotifen	Anti-CGRP mAbs; glucocorticoids
Migraine	NSAIDs and simple analgesics; triptans; ergot derivatives; gepants; ditans	β-blockers; tricyclic depressants; mirtazapine; antiepileptics; candesartan; anti-CGRP mAbs; botulinum toxin; gepants; pizotifen
Other miscellaneous headaches	NSAIDs and simple analgesics	N/A

CGRP, Calcitonin gene-related peptide; *mAb*, monoclonal antibody; *NSAID*, non-steroidal anti-inflammatory drug; *SSRI*, selective serotonin reuptake inhibitor.
Adapted and modified from Robbins, M.S., 2021. Diagnosis and management of headache: a review. JAMA 325, 1874–1885; and Headache Classification Committee of the International Headache Society (IHS), 2018. The International Classification of Headache Disorders, third ed. Cephalalgia 38, 1–211.

frequency and persistence. Attacks generally have a rapid (30 min or less) onset but can last for some days. They are more prevalent among women (especially those in their 30s) than men. The pain is of usually mild to moderate intensity and is often accompanied by a feeling of 'pressure' in the head. The headache may be bilateral or may be predominately located in the frontal or temporal region of the head and there may be associated cranial tenderness. Although they are sometimes confused with migraines, these headaches are generally not exacerbated by physical exercise, and seldom involve nausea, photophobia or phonophobia.

The underlying cause is neurobiological and is generally thought to involve activation of nociceptors in the facial musculature, provoked by some trigger mechanism. Tension headaches may be *acute* or *chronic*, with acute cases comprising the bulk of cases. Chronic tension headaches may be caused by medication overuse, or possibly depression or anxiety. Triptans are ineffective in tension-type headaches, but acute cases usually respond well to simple non-steroidal anti-inflammatory drugs (NSAIDs) (see Ch. 25), although chronic or recurrent cases may require prophylactic treatment with tricyclic antidepressants such as **amitriptyline**, selective serotonin reuptake inhibitors (SSRIs) such as **venlafaxine** or the α_2 adrenoceptor and 5-$HT_{2/3}$ antagonist **mirtazapine** (see Ch. 48).

TRIGEMINAL AUTONOMIC CEPHALALGIAS

This type of headache is caused by excessive central activation of the cranial parasympathetic system. There are several different subtypes differentiated by their frequency and persistence. *Cluster headaches* are probably the most prominent type in this group, with an incidence of <0.5% of the population and affecting more males than females. The pain which is unilateral is usually severe, often being described as 'searing', 'sharp' or 'throbbing', and may be located unilaterally in the frontal or orbital region of the head. The pain is associated with ipsilateral activation of the trigeminal nerve causing lacrimation, and other ocular symptoms including ptosis and photophobia, rhinorrhoea (running nose), facial sweating, restlessness or agitation. There may be a genetic basis for these symptoms. The attacks have a rapid (30 min) onset and can last for hours. Some patients experience attacks every other day, suggesting some circadian influence; others may experience a chronic form of the headache lasting months or years. Environmental triggers may be important: for example, some patients experience symptoms at the same time each year in response to changes in the weather (Suri and Ailani, 2021). Once again, CGRP can induce cluster headaches in susceptible subjects.

Pharmacological therapy usually consists of triptans, but more chronic manifestations may require anti-CGRP monoclonal antibody treatment or corticosteroids.

MISCELLANEOUS PRIMARY HEADACHES

This group includes headaches associated with exercise, sudden exertion, sex or coughing spasms, 'thunderclap' headache, cold stimulus headache, hypnic headache (occurring during sleep) and other headaches caused by pressure on the scalp. The causes of such headaches are generally unknown, but they often respond to simple analgesics. *New daily persistent headache* may appear suddenly and last for months and may require a treatment plan similar to migraine.

DRUG THERAPY FOR HEADACHE

Perhaps reflecting the multifactorial nature of headaches, a multitude of different drugs have been tested, and reported to be effective, in treating headaches of all types. For convenience, a summary of these appears in Table 42.1.

DRUGS ACTING ON THE 5-HT SYSTEM

Historically, this group of drugs was among the first to be utilised for the treatment of migraines and continues to be an important component of treatment regimens for both migraine and cluster headaches. They all posess $5\text{-HT}_{1A/B/D/F}$ agonist properties. The original notion that the chief target for these drugs was the vasculature has now been largely replaced by the idea that the presynaptic 5-HT receptors controlling neuropeptide release from the trigeminovascular system are more significant sites of action (Haanes and Edvinsson, 2019; Robbins, 2021).

ERGOT DERIVATIVES

Ergotamine and **dihydroergotamine** are the two most commonly used drugs in this class and among the oldest drugs to be used for treatment of migraine. They have antidopaminergic and α-adrenoceptor blocking actions as well as multiple actions at 5-HT receptors, among which (probably crucially) are 5-HT_{1D} partial agonist properties. **Methysergide** is another related drug with promiscuous actions on 5-HT receptors, including agonism at the $5\text{-HT}_{1A/B}$ and 5-HT_2 subtypes.

Clinical use

The only current use of **ergotamine** is in the treatment of attacks of migraine or cluster headaches unresponsive to simple analgesics (see Chs 25 and 43). It is sometimes given in a proprietary formulation with **caffeine** and the antihistamine/anticholinergic drug **cyclizine** which has antiemetic properties. **Methysergide** was formerly used for migraine prophylaxis, and for treating the symptoms of carcinoid tumours. It is seldom used today because of potentially serious toxicity problems, although it is sometimes still employed for the treatment of cluster headaches which are refractory to other drugs.

All these drugs can be used orally or by injection.

Unwanted effects

Ergotamine often causes nausea and vomiting, and it must be avoided in patients with peripheral vascular disease because of its vasoconstrictor action. **Methysergide** also causes nausea and vomiting, but its most serious side effect, which considerably restricts its clinical usefulness, is *retroperitoneal* and *mediastinal fibrosis*, which impairs the functioning of the gastrointestinal tract, kidneys, heart and lungs. The mechanism of this is unknown, but it is noteworthy that similar fibrotic reactions also occur in carcinoid syndrome, in which there is a high circulating level of 5-HT. In high doses, **methysergide** can cause hallucinogenic effects, possibly through an effect at 5-HT_{2A} receptors.

TRIPTANS

This important group of drugs group includes **almotriptan**, **eletriptan**, **frovatriptan**, **naratriptan**, **rizatriptan**, **sumatriptan** and **zolmitriptan**. The triptans are among the most important agents for the treatment of acute migraine and cluster headache attacks. They are usually classified as $5\text{-HT}_{1B/1D/F}$ agonists (see Ch. 16). However, selective high-affinity 5-HT_{1D} subtype agonists have proved disappointing in the clinic (see Agosti, 2007). Their principal target is probably the presynaptic $5\text{-HT}_{1B/D}$ receptors on CGRP secreting neurons but they also have vasoconstrictor actions through their action on these receptors on the meningeal vessels.

Clinical use

Triptans are mainly used to treat acute migraine but also may be given to provide prophylactic treatment of predictable (e.g. menstrual) attacks of migraine. They can also be used to treat cluster headaches. These drugs are mainly administered orally but **sumatriptan** and **zolmitriptan** are available as nasal sprays, and **rizatriptan** as a tablet that disperses on the tongue, which can be advantageous if the patient is vomiting. **Sumatriptan** is also available as an injection for subcutaneous administration.

Unwanted effects

Side effects common to many members of this group include asthenia, dizziness, drowsiness, gastrointestinal symptoms including nausea and vomiting. A major potential problem is the fact that triptans have vasoconstrictor properties and so must be used cautiously in patients who have (for example) hypertension, ischaemic heart disease, cerebrovascular disease or peripheral vascular disease.

DITANS

Lasmiditan, a new non-triptan drug, is highly effective in aborting migraine attacks (Ferrari and Rustichelli, 2021). It was approved by the FDA in 2019 but has not yet been approved in the United Kingdom. **Lasmiditan** is a selective 5HT_{1F}-receptor agonist. Interestingly, this receptor subtype is scarce in the vasculature, casting further doubt on the role of vascular changes per se in the pain experienced by migraine patients. This is significant because a major drawback to triptan therapy is vasoconstriction in other peripheral vascular beds, including the heart.

Clinical use

The drug is given orally for the treatment of acute migraine. It is not suitable for migraine prophylaxis.

Unwanted effects

While **lasmiditan** would be expected to be free of the vasoconstrictor effects of the triptans, it commonly causes other adverse effects (e.g. dizziness, drowsiness and nausea) which can be severe.

DRUGS ACTING ON THE CGRP SYSTEM

GEPANTS

Based upon the notion that CGRP is a crucial player in the pathogenesis of migraine and possibly other headaches, a group of small-molecule CGRP antagonists have been developed. These drugs, known as *gepants*, were first developed at the beginning of this century. **Telcagepant** was the first of these, but while it showed efficacy, it was discontinued because of liver toxicity problems. Two second-generation gepants, **rimegepant** and **ubrogepant**, were approved by the FDA in the United States in 2019. They are not yet approved in the United Kingdom. Both of these drugs have shown good efficacy and tolerability in trials in which they have been used acutely to treat migraine and **rimegepant** has shown efficacy as a prophylactic drug. Uniquely, the gepants may be the first specific antimigraine drugs which are effective for both acute and prophylactic treatment (Moreno-Ajona et al., 2019). Also in the process of late-stage development are the ‘third-generation’ gepants, **atogepant** and **vazegepant**.

Clinical use

These drugs are given by oral administration. **Vazegepant** (not yet approved) is designed to be administered nasally.

Unwanted effects

Unlike the triptans, the gepants lack any cardiovascular effects. However, nausea is a common feature of these drugs, sometimes accompanied by dizziness and vomiting (**rimegepant**) or dry mouth and drowsiness (**ubrogepant**).

ANTI-CGRP mAbs

An alternative approach to abolishing the actions of CGRP is to immunoneutralise the neuropeptide(s) or its receptor with neutralising monoclonal antibodies (mAbs: Abu-Zaid et al., 2020; Drellia et al., 2021). Several preparations have been approved for clinical use. These include **eptinezumab** (not UK), **fremanezumab** and **galcenezumab** (anti-neuropeptide mAbs) and **erenumab** (antireceptor mAb). These drugs are all humanised (or human) mAbs and are used for prophylactic treatment of migraine and cluster headache which does not respond to other therapy regimes. While more expensive and more difficult to administer, their effects are long-lasting (weeks) rather than hours.

Clinical use

These drugs are generally administered subcutaneously each month but **eptinezumab** (a human monoclonal antibody) is given intravenously each quarter.

Unwanted effects

These mAbs produce several common side effects which often include hypersensitivity reactions such as skin reactions and constipation. Vertigo, oedema and muscle spasms may also occur in some instances.

ANTI-INFLAMMATORY DRUGS

The notion that migraine and some other forms of headache are caused by the release of neuropeptides which in turn release prostaglandins, nitric oxide and other mediators provides a rationale for the well-established use of anti-inflammatory/analgesic drugs in headache disorders. There are several types.

NON-STEROIDAL ANTI-INFLAMMATORY AGENTS

NSAIDs (see Ch. 25) are also among the oldest drugs to be utilised for treating headaches. **Paracetamol** is one the most commonly used treatments for occasional headaches and is mostly effective. In migraine NSAIDs seem to have a variable effect, being useful for some patients but not others. **Paracetamol** is sometimes given in combination with the vasoconstrictor **isometheptene**. Among other most commonly employed NSAIDs are **ibuprofen**, **aspirin**, **naproxen** and **diclofenac**. The main mode of action of these drugs is inhibition of the synthesis of pain-producing prostaglandins which are probably released by neuropeptides.

Clinical use

Generally, therapy for migraine is begun with **aspirin** or **ibuprofen** using the other members of this group or more potent drugs such as **tolfenamic** or **mefenamic** acid if these fail.

Unwanted effects

The unwanted effects of NSAIDs are detailed in Chapter 25. The gastrointestinal side effects of these drugs are of significance because migraine is often accompanied by nausea and NSAIDs may exacerbate the issue. **Metoclopramide** (see Ch. 30) can be used to control the nausea and is sometimes given in the form of combined therapy (e.g. **metoclopramide** with **aspirin**).

GLUCOCORTICOIDS

Anti-inflammatory glucocorticoids are sometimes useful for the prophylactic treatment of cluster headaches. The pharmacology of these drugs is discussed in Chapters 3 and 25.

CENTRALLY ACTING DRUGS

ANTIHISTAMINES

Pizotifen is a non-sedating antihistamine that also has some anticholinergic actions and is also a 5-$HT_{2A/2C}$ receptor antagonist (although the anatomical site of its action is unknown). **Buclizine** is a sedating antihistamine and anticholinergic with additional antiemetic properties. It is usually administered in a proprietary formulation together with **paracetamol** and **codeine.**

Clinical use

Pizotifen is useful in some patients for the prophylactic treatment of vascular, cluster headache and migraine. **Buclizine** is used to treat acute attacks of migraine.

Unwanted effects

The typical effects of **pizotifen** include cholinergic effects such as dry mouth and also an increase in appetite and weight gain as well as central effects such as dizziness, fatigue and nausea.

ANTIEPILEPTIC DRUGS

Antiepileptic drugs have been found to be sometimes effective in prophylaxis of migraine. Commonly employed drugs include **topiramate** and **levetiracetam** (Yen et al., 2021). The general pharmacology of these drugs is discussed in Chapter 46. A reduction in glutamate transmission or enhanced $GABA_A$ activity may result in decreased cortical excitability which may be their chief mechanism of action.

TRICYCLIC ANTIDEPRESSANTS AND SSRIs

The most commonly used drugs in this group are the tricyclic drugs **amitriptyline** and **nortriptyline** and the SSRIs **venlafaxine** and **mirtazapine**.

The general pharmacology of these drugs is discussed in Chapter 48. In the prophylactic treatment for tension headaches and migraine, their hypothesised mechanism is via an increase in GABA-mediated inhibition secondary to inhibition of monoamine reuptake. However, the link between stress and tension headaches and migraine may suggest that antidepressant and anxiolytic effects may contribute to their efficacy.

CARDIOVASCULAR DRUGS

β-BLOCKERS

The β-blockers **propranolol**, **metoprolol** and **timolol** are first-line agents for migraine prophylaxis. Their general pharmacology is discussed in Chapters 15, 20 and 21, and their anxiolytic properties, in Chapter 45. Their mode of action in migraine is probably associated with a reduction of neurotransmitter release and of neuronal excitability.

Other cardiovascular drugs used in the prophylaxis of headache include calcium channel blockers (see Ch. 20) such as **verapamil** (for cluster headache) and **flunarizine** (approved in Europe and Asia for migraine; prescribed off-license in UK specialist centres). **Candesartan,** an AT1 antagonist (see Ch. 21), is sometimes prescribed for migraine prophylaxis; it reduces glutamate release and enhances GABA-ergic tone.

MISCELLANEOUS GROUP

BOTULINUM TOXIN

Botulinum toxin A is a neurotoxin produced by the gram-positive anaerobic bacterium *Clostridium botulinum* and is intensely poisonous. It produces muscular paralysis ('botulism') by inhibiting the release of acetylcholine from motor nerve terminals (see Ch. 14). The toxin is a dimer which, upon entering the cell following combination with a cell surface glycoprotein, is cleaved to release the light chain of the dimer. This moiety cleaves the SNARE 25 protein which is responsible for tethering and binding of acetylcholine vesicles to the cell membrane and forming a synaptic fusion complex prior to release (Burstein et al., 2020). The same mechanism also prevents the release of neuropeptides as well as the replenishment of normal receptors such as transient receptor potential (TRP) receptors on neurons. This produces a type of chemical denervation of the neuron.

Clinical use

The use of the drug **onabotulinumtoxin** is usually restricted to those patients in whom at least two other agents seem to be ineffective. Administration, which is a specialist procedure, entails multiple (usually about 30) discrete subcutaneous injections at sites on the scalp of the cranial musculature. Treatment is usually repeated every 3 months.

Unwanted effects

Onabotulinumtoxin is usually better tolerated than oral preventive therapies but there is a high incidence of muscular weakness in the neck with associated pain (Barbanti and Ferroni, 2017).

OTHER NON-PHARMACOLOGICAL TREATMENTS

A raft of other non-pharmacological treatments have been trialled, sometimes successfully, to treat migraines and other types of headache. These include external neuromodulation devices (see Gupta et al., 2019), acupuncture, as well as psychological approaches such as cognitive behavioural therapy (CBT), autogenic feedback and other techniques. Sometimes, these are combined with drug therapy to produce an effect superior to that which could be achieved by monotherapy.

SUMMARY

The term *headache* is a compendium definition which embraces several complex disorders which can be difficult to differentiate clinically, and which can sometimes be difficult to treat successfully.

While the foregoing chapter is of necessity rather incomplete in its coverage of the many different drugs now available, further information on these may be found in Chapters 5, 13, 16, 17, 25, 37 and 43.

REFERENCES AND FURTHER READING

Abu-Zaid, A., AlBatati, S.K., AlHossan, A.M., et al., 2020. Galcanezumab for the management of migraine: a systematic review and meta-analysis of randomized placebo-controlled trials. Cureus 12, e11621.

Agosti, R.M., 2007. 5HT1F- and 5HT7-receptor agonists for the treatment of migraines. CNS Neurol. Disord. Drug Targets 6, 235–237.

Al-Karagholi, M.A., Hansen, J.M., Guo, S., Olesen, J., Ashina, M., 2019. Opening of ATP-sensitive potassium channels causes migraine attacks: a new target for the treatment of migraine. Brain 142, 2644–2654.

Arzani, M., Jahromi, S.R., Ghorbani, Z., et al., School of Advanced Studies of the European Headache, F, 2020. Gut-brain axis and migraine headache: a comprehensive review. J. Headache Pain 21, 15.

Barbanti, P., Ferroni, P., 2017. Onabotulinum toxin A in the treatment of chronic migraine: patient selection and special considerations. J. Pain Res. 10, 2319–2329.

Burch, R.C., Loder, S., Loder, E., Smitherman, T.A., 2015. The prevalence and burden of migraine and severe headache in the United States: updated statistics from government health surveillance studies. Headache 55, 21–34.

Burstein, R., Blumenfeld, A.M., Silberstein, S.D., Manack Adams, A., Brin, M.F., 2020. Mechanism of action of onabotulinumtoxina in chronic migraine: a narrative review. Headache 60, 1259–1272.

Charles, A., 2013. The evolution of a migraine attack - a review of recent evidence. Headache 53, 413–419.

Drellia, K., Kokoti, L., Deligianni, C.I., Papadopoulos, D., Mitsikostas, D.D., 2021. Anti-CGRP monoclonal antibodies for migraine prevention: a systematic review and likelihood to help or harm analysis. Cephalalgia 41, 851–864.

Eadie, M.J., 2005. The pathogenesis of migraine - 17th to early 20th century understandings. J. Clin. Neurosci. 12, 383–388.

Ferrari, A., Rustichelli, C., 2021. Rational use of lasmiditan for acute migraine treatment in adults: a narrative review. Clin. Ther. 43, 654–670.

The Work Foundation, 2018. Society's headache: the socioeconomic impact of migraine. Available at: https://www.theworkfoundation.com/wf-reports/?society's-headache-the-socioeconomic-impact-of-migraine/.

Gupta, R., Fisher, K., Pyati, S., 2019. Chronic headache: a review of interventional treatment strategies in headache management. Curr. Pain Headache Rep. 23, 68.

Haanes, K.A., Edvinsson, L., 2019. Pathophysiological mechanisms in migraine and the identification of new therapeutic targets. CNS Drugs 33, 525–537.

Headache Classification Committee of the International Headache Society (IHS), 2018. The International Classification of Headache Disorders, third ed., vol. 38. Cephalalgia, pp. 1-211.

Islam, M.A., Alam, S.S., Kundu, S., Hossan, T., Kamal, M.A., Cavestro, C., 2020. Prevalence of headache in patients with coronavirus disease 2019 (COVID-19): a systematic review and meta-analysis of 14,275 patients. Front. Neurol. 11, 562634.

Marmura, M.J., Silberstein, S.D., Schwedt, T.J., 2015. The acute treatment of migraine in adults: the American Headache Society evidence assessment of migraine pharmacotherapies. Headache 55, 3–20.

McCrone, P., Seed, P.T., Dowson, A.J., et al., 2011. Service use and costs for people with headache: a UK primary care study. J. Headache Pain 12, 617–623.

Moreno-Ajona, D., Chan, C., Villar-Martinez, M.D., Goadsby, P.J., 2019. Targeting CGRP and 5-HT_{1F} receptors for the acute therapy of migraine: a literature review. Headache 59 (Suppl. 2), 3–19.

Nature Outlook, 2020. Headache. Nature 586, S2–S9.

Paolucci, M., Altamura, C., Vernieri, F., 2021. The role of endothelial dysfunction in the pathophysiology and cerebrovascular effects of migraine: a narrative review. J. Clin. Neurol. 17, 164–175.

Robbins, M.S., 2021. Diagnosis and management of headache: a review. JAMA 325, 1874–1885.

Suri, H., Ailani, J., 2021. Cluster headache: a review and update in treatment. Curr. Neurol. Neurosci. Rep. 21, 31.

The Migraine Trust, 2021. Facts and Figures. Available at: https://www.themigrainetrust.org/about-migraine/migraine-what-is-it/facts-figures/.

Yen, P.H., Kuan, Y.C., Tam, K.W., Chung, C.C., Hong, C.T., Huang, Y.H., 2021. Efficacy of levetiracetam for migraine prophylaxis: a systematic review and meta-analysis. J. Formos. Med. Assoc. 120, 755–764.

Analgesic drugs 43

OVERVIEW

Pain is a disabling accompaniment of many acute and chronic medical conditions, and pain control is one of the most important therapeutic priorities.

In this chapter, we discuss the neural mechanisms responsible for different types of acute and chronic pain, and the various drugs that are used to reduce the sensation of pain. The 'classic' analgesic drugs, notably opioids and non-steroidal anti-inflammatory drugs (NSAIDs; described in Ch. 25), have their origins in natural products that have been used for centuries. The original compounds, typified by morphine and aspirin, are still in widespread use, but many synthetic compounds that act by the same mechanisms have been developed. In recent years it has become apparent that chronic pains respond poorly to opioids and NSAIDs. We therefore consider various other drug classes, such as antidepressant and antiepileptic drugs, which clinical experience has shown may have efficacy in ameliorating the suffering of chronic pain.

INTRODUCTION

Pain is a subjective experience, hard to define exactly, even though we all know what we mean by it. Typically, it is a direct response to an untoward event associated with tissue damage, such as injury, inflammation or cancer, but severe pain can occur as a consequence of brain or nerve injury (e.g. following a stroke or herpes infection, and as a consequence of diabetes or multiple sclerosis) and persist long after the precipitating injury has healed (e.g. phantom limb pain). In some instances pain can arise without any obvious cause (e.g. lower back pain, fibromyalgia).

Clinically, pain is broadly categorised as 'acute' or 'chronic'. Acute pain comes on suddenly and is caused by something specific (e.g. an ankle sprain, broken bones, burns, cuts or surgery). It is sharp in nature and may last for a considerable time. It goes away when there is no longer an underlying cause for the pain. Chronic pain usually lasts longer than 3 months and may persist after the injury or illness that caused it has healed or gone away.

Acute pain, cancer pain and pain associated with inflammation generally respond to conventional analgesic drugs such as NSAIDs (see Ch. 25) and opioids. Chronic, noninflammatory pains which are very common and a major cause of disability and distress in general respond poorly to conventional analgesic drugs. All is not doom and gloom however; the good news is that a number of drugs originally developed to treat other conditions such as depression and epilepsy can reduce the suffering of chronic pains but there is still a need for more effective agents. We should think of chronic pain in terms of disordered neural function rather than simply as a 'normal' response to tissue injury. The perception of noxious stimuli (termed *nociception* by Sherrington) is not the same thing as pain, which is a subjective experience and includes a strong emotional (affective) component, especially in people suffering from chronic pain.

NEURAL MECHANISMS OF PAIN

Under normal conditions, pain is associated with impulse activity in small-diameter (C and Aδ) primary afferent fibres of peripheral nerves. These nerves have sensory endings in peripheral tissues and are activated by stimuli of various kinds (mechanical, thermal, chemical). The majority of non-myelinated (C) fibres are associated with *polymodal nociceptive* endings and convey a dull, diffuse burning pain, whereas myelinated (Aδ) fibres convey a sensation of sharp, well-localised pain. C and Aδ fibres convey nociceptive information from muscle and viscera as well as from the skin. Good accounts of the neural basis of pain can be found in McMahon et al. (2013).

With many pathological conditions, tissue injury is the immediate cause of the pain and results in the local release of a variety of chemicals that act on the nerve terminals, either activating them directly or enhancing their sensitivity to other forms of stimulation (Fig. 43.1). The pharmacological properties of nociceptive nerve terminals are discussed in more detail later in this chapter.

The cell bodies of spinal nociceptive afferent fibres lie in dorsal root ganglia; fibres enter the spinal cord via the dorsal roots, ending in the grey matter of the dorsal horn (see Fig. 43.4). Most of the nociceptive afferents terminate in the superficial region of the dorsal horn, the C fibres and some Aδ fibres innervating cell bodies in laminae I and II (also known as the *substantia gelatinosa* (SG)), while other A fibres penetrate deeper into the dorsal horn (lamina V). The SG is rich in both endogenous opioid peptides and opioid receptors, and may be an important site of action for morphine-like drugs. Cells in laminae I and V give rise to the main projection pathways from the dorsal horn to the thalamus. For a more detailed account of dorsal horn circuitry, see Todd and Koerber (2013).

Nociceptive afferent neurons release glutamate and possibly ATP as the fast neurotransmitters at their central synapses in the dorsal horn. Glutamate acting on (*S*)-α-amino-3-hydroxy-5-methylisoxazole-4-propionic acid (AMPA) receptors is responsible for fast synaptic transmission at the first synapse in the dorsal horn. There is also a slower NMDA receptor-mediated response, which is important in relation to the phenomenon of 'wind-up' (Fig. 43.2). The analgesia produced by **ketamine** most likely results from blockade of this phenomenon. The nociceptive afferent neurons also contain several neuropeptides, particularly calcitonin gene-related peptide (CGRP) and substance P. These are released

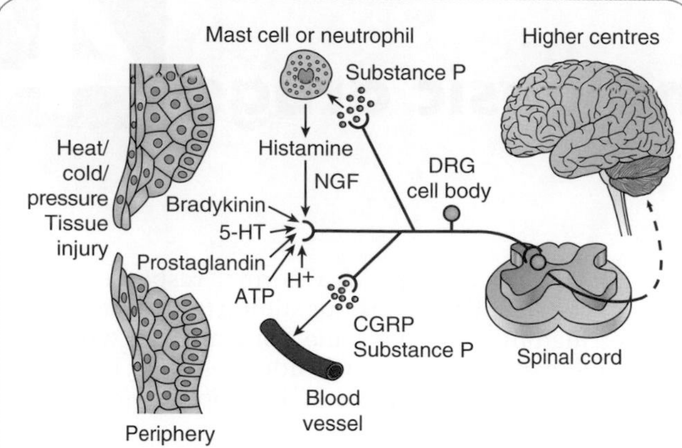

Fig. 43.1 Activation of nociceptive neurons. Various stimuli (physical and chemical), some shown here, can initiate or enhance the rate of action potential firing in nociceptive primary afferent neurons (i.e. induce pain). These afferent fibres project to the dorsal horn of the spinal cord where they synapse on neurons projecting to higher centres. *5-HT,* 5-Hydroxytryptamine; *CGRP,* calcitonin gene-related peptide; *DRG,* dorsal root ganglion; *NGF,* nerve growth factor. (Adapted from Julius, D., Basbaum, A.I., 2001. Molecular mechanisms of nociception. Nature 413, 203–210.)

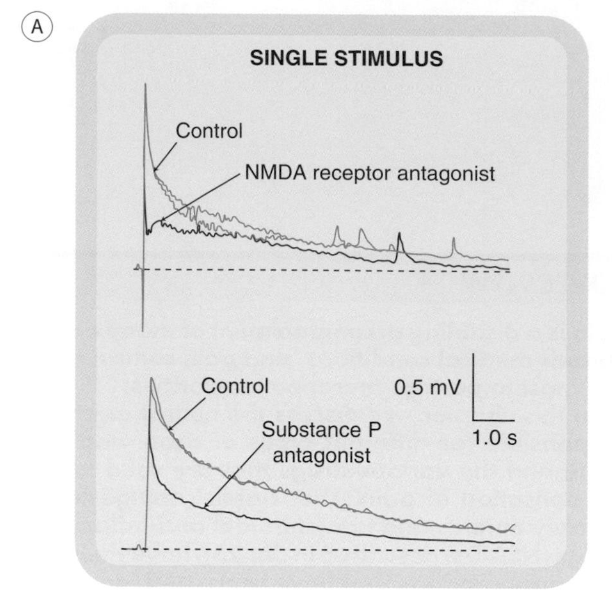

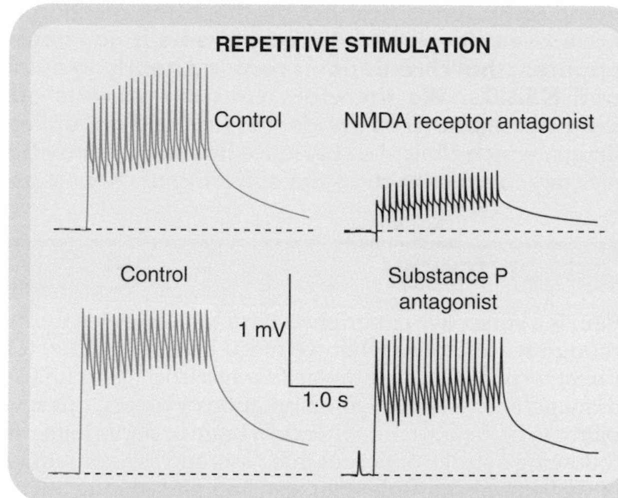

Fig. 43.2 Effect of glutamate and substance P antagonists on nociceptive transmission in the rat spinal cord. The rat paw was inflamed by ultraviolet irradiation 2 days before the experiment, a procedure that induces hyperalgesia and spinal cord facilitation. The synaptic response was recorded from the ventral root, in response to stimulation of C fibres in the dorsal root with (A) single stimuli or (B) repetitive stimuli. The effects of the NMDA receptor antagonist D-AP-5 (see ') and the substance P antagonist RP 67580 (selective for neurokinin type 2 (NK_2) receptors) are shown. The slow component of the synaptic response is reduced by both antagonists (A), as is the 'wind-up' in response to repetitive stimulation (B). These effects are much less pronounced in the normal animal. Thus both glutamate, acting on NMDA receptors, and substance P, acting on NK_2 receptors, are involved in nociceptive transmission, and their contribution increases as a result of inflammatory hyperalgesia. *NMDA, N*-methyl-D-aspartate. (Records kindly provided by L. Urban and S.W. Thompson.)

as mediators at both the central and the peripheral terminals, and play an important role in the pathology of pain. In the periphery, substance P and CGRP produce some of the features of neurogenic inflammation. CGRP antagonists are used in the treatment of migraine (see Ch. 42) but have not proved effective for other pain states. In animal models, substance P acting on NK_1 receptors was shown to be involved in wind-up and central sensitisation in the dorsal horn (see Fig. 43.2). Surprisingly, however, antagonists of substance P at NK_1 receptors turned out to be ineffective as analgesics in humans, although they do have antiemetic activity (see Ch. 30).

MODULATION IN THE NOCICEPTIVE PATHWAY

Pain resulting from trauma, inflammation or cancer is generally well accounted for in terms of nociception – an excessive noxious stimulus giving rise to an intense and unpleasant sensation. More prolonged pain and chronic pain states such as neuropathic pain are associated with aberrations of the normal physiological pathway, giving rise to the phenomena of *hyperalgesia* (an increased amount of pain associated with a mild noxious stimulus) and *allodynia* (pain evoked by a non-noxious stimulus). Some of the main mechanisms are summarised in Fig. 43.3.

HYPERALGESIA AND ALLODYNIA

Anyone who has suffered a burn or sprained ankle has experienced hyperalgesia and allodynia. Hyperalgesia involves both sensitisation of peripheral nociceptive nerve terminals and central facilitation of transmission at the level of the dorsal horn and thalamus. The peripheral component is due to the action of mediators such as bradykinin and prostaglandins acting on the nerve terminals. The central component reflects facilitation of synaptic transmission in the dorsal horn of the spinal cord (see Yaksh, 1999). The synaptic responses of dorsal horn neurons to nociceptive inputs display the phenomenon of 'wind-up' – i.e. the synaptic potentials steadily increase in amplitude with each stimulus – when repeated stimuli are delivered at physiological frequencies. This activity-dependent facilitation of transmission has features in common with the phenomenon of long-term potentiation, described in Chapter 38, and the chemical mechanisms underlying it may also be similar. In the dorsal

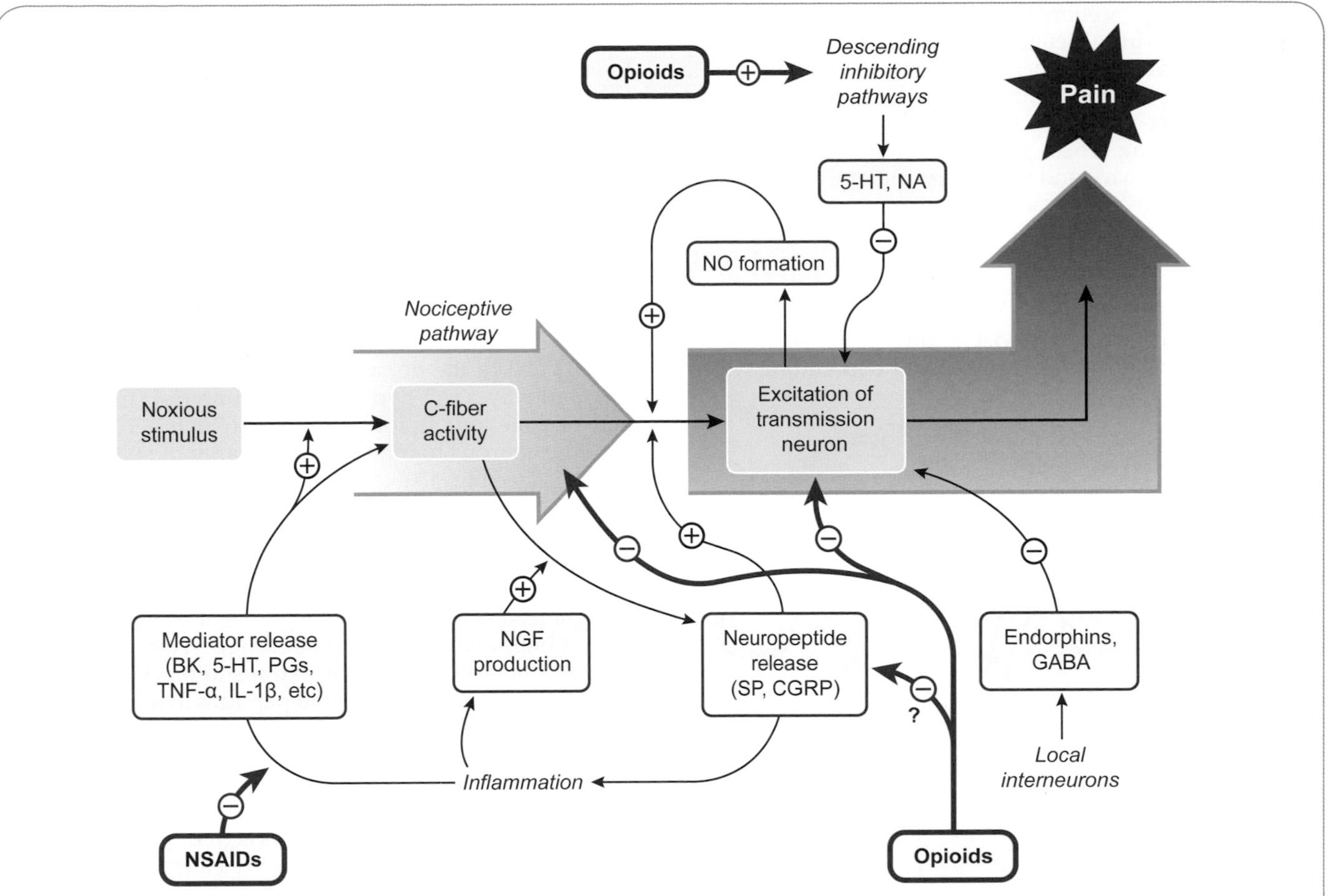

Fig. 43.3 Summary of modulatory mechanisms in the nociceptive pathway. *5-HT,* 5 Hydroxytryptamine; *BK,* bradykinin; *CGRP,* calcitonin gene-related peptide; *IL-1β,* interleukin; *NA,* noradrenaline; *NGF,* nerve growth factor; *NO,* nitric oxide; *NSAID,* non-steroidal anti-inflammatory drug; *PG,* prostaglandin; *SP,* substance P; *TNF-α,* tumour necrosis factor-α.

horn, the facilitation is blocked by NMDA receptor antagonists and also in part by antagonists of substance P and by inhibitors of nitric oxide (NO) synthesis (see Figs 43.2 and 43.3).

Substance P and CGRP released from primary afferent neurons (see Fig. 43.1) also act in the periphery, promoting inflammation by their effects on blood vessels and cells of the immune system. This mechanism, known as *neurogenic inflammation,* amplifies and sustains the inflammatory reaction and the accompanying activation of nociceptive afferent fibres.

Central facilitation is an important component of pathological hyperalgesia (e.g. that associated with inflammatory responses). The mediators responsible for central facilitation include substance P, CGRP, brain-derived neurotrophic factor (BDNF) and NO, as well as many others. For example, nerve growth factor (NGF), a cytokine-like mediator produced by peripheral tissues, particularly in inflammation, acts on a kinase-linked receptor (known as TrkA) on nociceptive afferent neurons, increasing their electrical excitability, chemosensitivity and peptide content, and also promoting the formation of synaptic contacts. Increased NGF production may be an important mechanism by which nociceptive transmission becomes facilitated by tissue damage, leading to hyperalgesia (see Mantyh et al., 2011). Increased gene expression in sensory neurons is induced by NGF and other inflammatory mediators; the up-regulated genes include those for neuropeptides and neuromodulators (e.g. CGRP, substance P and BDNF) as well as for receptors (e.g. transient receptor potential (TRP) TRPV1 and the ATP receptor P2X) and sodium channels, and have the overall effect of facilitating transmission at the first synaptic relay in the dorsal horn. BDNF released from primary afferent nerve terminals activates the kinase-linked TrkB receptor on postsynaptic dorsal horn neurons leading to phosphorylation of the NMDA subunit GluN1 and thus sensitisation of these glutamate receptors, resulting in synaptic facilitation, in the dorsal horn.

Excitation of nociceptive sensory neurons depends, as in other neurons (see Ch. 4), on voltage-gated sodium channels. Individuals who express non-functional mutations of $Na_v1.7$ are unable to experience pain. The expression and/or activity of certain sodium-channel subtypes (e.g. $Na_v1.3$, $Na_v1.7$, $Na_v1.8$ and $Na_v1.9$ channels) is increased in sensory neurons in various pathological pain states and their enhanced activity underlies the sensitisation to external stimuli that occurs in inflammatory pain and hyperalgesia (see Ch. 4 for more detail on voltage-activated sodium channels). Consistent with this hypothesis is the fact that some antiepileptic and antidysrhythmic drugs, which act by blocking sodium channels (see Chs 20 and 46), also find clinical application as analgesics.

TRANSMISSION OF PAIN TO HIGHER CENTRES

From the dorsal horn, ascending nerve axons travel in the contralateral spinothalamic tracts, and synapse on neurons in the ventral and medial parts of the thalamus, from which there are further projections to the somatosensory cortex. In the medial thalamus in particular, many cells respond specifically to noxious stimuli in the periphery, and lesions in this area cause analgesia. Functional brain imaging studies in conscious subjects have been performed to localise regions involved in pain processing. These include sensory, discriminatory areas such as primary and secondary somatosensory cortex, thalamus and posterior parts of insula as well as affective, cognitive areas such as the anterior parts of insula, anterior cingulate cortex and prefrontal cortex (see Apkarian et al., 2013).

DESCENDING INHIBITORY CONTROLS

Descending pathways (Fig. 43.4) control impulse transmission in the dorsal horn. A key part of this descending system is the *periaqueductal grey* (PAG) area of the midbrain, a small area of grey matter surrounding the central canal. In 1969, Reynolds found that electrical stimulation of this brain area in the rat caused analgesia sufficiently intense that abdominal surgery could be performed without anaesthesia and without eliciting any marked response. The responses to non-painful stimuli were unaffected. The PAG receives inputs from many other brain regions, including the hypothalamus, amygdala and cortex, and is the main pathway through which cortical and other inputs act to control the nociceptive 'gate' in the dorsal horn.

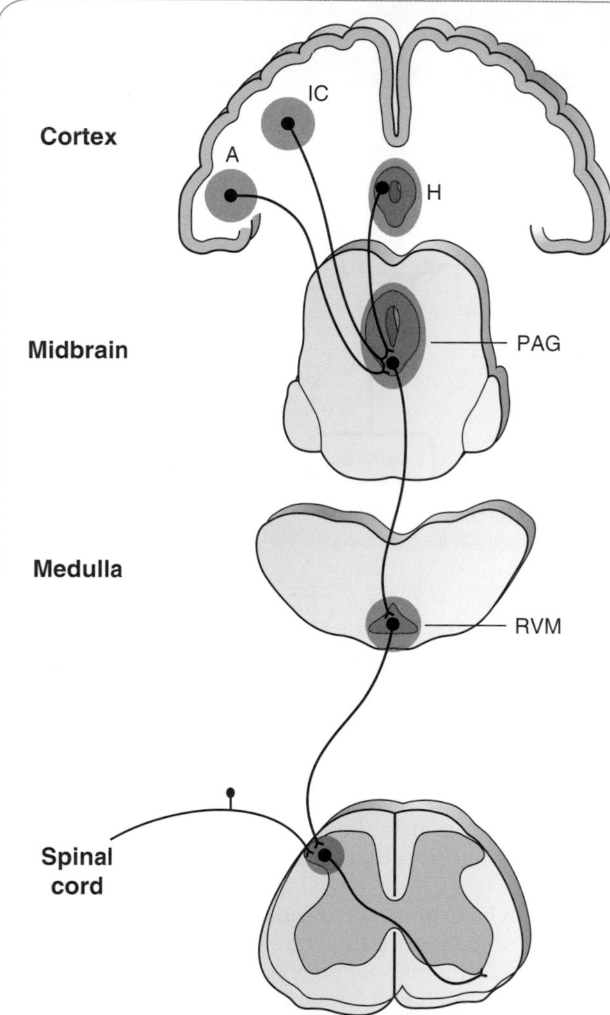

Fig. 43.4 The descending pain control system and sites of action of opioids to relieve pain. Opioids induce analgesia when microinjected into the insular cortex (IC), amygdala (A), hypothalamus (H), periaqueductal grey (PAG) region and rostroventral medulla (RVM), as well as into the dorsal horn of the spinal cord. The PAG receives input from higher centres and is the main output centre of the limbic system. It projects to the RVM. From the RVM, descending inhibitory fibres, some of which contain 5-hydroxytryptamine, project to the dorsal horn of the spinal cord. *Pink shaded areas* indicate regions expressing μ opioid receptors. The pathways shown in this diagram represent a considerable oversimplification. (Adapted from Fields, H., 2001. Pain modulation: expectation, opioid analgesia and virtual pain. Prog. Brain Res. 122, 245–253. For a fuller account of the descending pain modulating pathways, see Todd and Koerber, 2013.)

The PAG projects first to the rostroventral medulla (RVM) and thence via the dorsolateral funiculus of the spinal cord to the dorsal horn. Important transmitters in this pathway are 5-hydroxytryptamine (5-HT; serotonin) and endogenous opioid peptides, which act directly or via interneurons to inhibit the discharge of spinothalamic neurons (see Fig. 43.4).

The descending inhibitory pathway is probably an important site of action for opioid analgesics (Bagley and Ingram, 2020). Both PAG and SG are particularly rich in endogenous opioid peptide–containing neurons, and opioid antagonists such as naloxone can prevent analgesia induced by PAG stimulation, which would suggest that endogenous opioid peptides may function as transmitters in this system. The physiological role of opioid peptides in regulating pain transmission has been controversial, mainly because under normal conditions naloxone has relatively little effect on pain threshold. Under pathological conditions, however, when stress is present, naloxone causes hyperalgesia, implying that the opioid system is active.

Interneurons in the dorsal horn release GABA (see Ch. 38), which inhibits transmitter release from primary afferent terminals.

There is also a noradrenergic pathway from the *locus coeruleus* (LC; see Ch. 39), which has a similar inhibitory effect on transmission in the dorsal horn. Surprisingly, opioids inhibit rather than activate this pathway. The use of tricyclic antidepressants in managing chronic pain may involve potentiating this pathway.

It is thought that descending inhibitory purinergic pathways may release adenosine on to A_1 receptors on dorsal horn neurons to produce analgesia.

PLACEBO ANALGESIA

Placebo analgesia is the phenomenon of reduced sensation of pain when the subject believes that they have been given a drug that will suppress pain, when in fact no drug has been administered at all. It is often a substantial effect that poses problems in clinical trials of analgesic drugs. Placebo analgesia is reduced by administration of an opioid antagonist such as **naloxone**, indicating that it involves the release of endogenous opioid peptides. Brain imaging studies have revealed that the placebo response results from changes in neuronal activity in the prefrontal cortex and PAG, resulting in activation of descending inhibitory pathways to the spinal cord to suppress the processing of pain information.

Expectation can also modify the response when an analgesic drug is given. Subjects receiving an intravenous infusion of remifentanil, an opioid analgesic, showed more pain relief when they were told that they were receiving the drug than when the drug was administered without them knowing (see Bingel et al., 2012). Even more surprising was the observation that when the subjects received the same dose of remifentanil, but were told the infusion was of a substance that would exacerbate pain, they did not show any analgesic response to the opioid.

Modulation of pain transmission

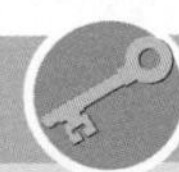

- Descending pathways from the midbrain and brain stem exert a strong inhibitory effect on dorsal horn transmission. Electrical stimulation of the midbrain PAG area causes analgesia through this mechanism.
- The descending inhibition is mediated mainly by endogenous opioid peptides, 5-HT (serotonin), noradrenaline and adenosine. Opioids cause analgesia partly by activating these descending pathways, partly by inhibiting transmission in the dorsal horn and partly by inhibiting excitation of sensory nerve terminals in the periphery.
- Repetitive C-fibre activity facilitates transmission through the dorsal horn ('wind-up') by mechanisms involving activation of NMDA and substance P receptors. This results in pain sensitisation.

CHEMICAL SIGNALLING IN THE NOCICEPTIVE PATHWAY

CHEMOSENSITIVITY OF NOCICEPTIVE NERVE ENDINGS

In most cases, stimulation of nociceptive endings in the periphery is chemical in origin. Excessive mechanical or thermal stimuli can obviously cause acute pain, but the persistence of such pain after the stimulus has been removed, or the pain resulting from inflammatory or ischaemic changes in tissues, generally reflects an altered chemical environment of the pain afferents. The current state of knowledge is summarised in Fig. 43.5.

Transient receptor potential channels – thermal sensation and pain

The *TRP* channel family comprises some 27 or more structurally related ion channels that serve a wide variety of physiological functions (see Nilius and Szallasi, 2014). Within this family are a group of channels present on sensory neurons that are activated both by thermal stimuli across a wide range of temperatures and by chemical agents (Table 43.1). With respect to pain, the most important channels are TRPV1, TRPA1 and TRPM8 (Jardin et al., 2017).

Capsaicin, the substance in chilli peppers that gives them their pungency, selectively excites nociceptive nerve terminals, causing intense pain if injected into the skin or applied to sensitive structures such as the cornea.[1] It produces this effect by activating TRPV1.[2] Agonists such as capsaicin open the channel, which is permeable to Na^+, Ca^{2+} and other cations, causing depolarisation and initiation of action potentials. The large influx of Ca^{2+} into peripheral nerve terminals also results in peptide release (mainly substance P and CGRP), causing intense vascular and other physiological responses. The Ca^{2+} influx may be enough to cause nerve degeneration (see Ch. 40). Applied topically, capsaicin reduces neuropathic and osteoarthritic pain by this mechanism, but the initial strong irritant effect is a major disadvantage.

TRPV1 responds not only to capsaicin-like agonists but also to other stimuli (see Table 43.1), including temperatures in excess of about 42°C (the threshold for pain) and proton concentrations in the micromolar range (pH 5.5 and below), which also cause pain. The receptor thus has unusual 'polymodal' characteristics and is believed to play a central role in nociception. TRPV1 is, like many other ionotropic receptors, modulated by phosphorylation, and several of the pain-producing substances that act through G protein–coupled receptors (e.g. bradykinin) work by sensitising TRPV1. A search for endogenous ligands for TRPV1 revealed, surprisingly, that **anandamide** (a lipid mediator previously identified as an agonist at cannabinoid receptors; see Ch. 18) is also a TRPV1 agonist, although less potent than capsaicin. TRPV1 knock-out mice show reduced responsiveness to noxious heat and also fail to show thermal hyperalgesia in response to inflammation. The latter observation is interesting, because TRPV1 expression is known to be increased by inflammation and this may be a key mechanism by which hyperalgesia is produced. A number of pharmaceutical companies developed TRPV1 agonists – to act as desensitising agents – and antagonists as analgesic agents. However, TRPV1 agonists were found to induce hypothermia, associated with activation of hypothalamic thermosensitive neurons, and TRPV1 antagonists were found to induce hyperthermia, consistent with a role of TRPV1 in body temperature control as well as nociception.

TRPA1 and TRPM8 respond to cold rather than heat (see Table 43.1). TRPA1 is activated in some experimental settings by noxious cold temperatures, calcium, pain-producing substances and inflammatory mediators; it can therefore also be considered to be a polymodal sensor. It may be important for the analgesic and antipyretic actions of paracetamol. TRPM8 is important in cold hypersensitivity, which is often a feature of neuropathic pain.

Kinins

When applied to sensory nerve endings, *bradykinin* and *kallidin* induce intense pain. These two closely related peptides are produced under conditions of tissue injury by the proteolytic cleavage of the active kinins from a precursor protein contained in the plasma. Bradykinin acts partly by release of prostaglandins, which strongly enhance the direct action of bradykinin on the nerve terminals (Fig. 43.6). Bradykinin acts on B_2 receptors on nociceptive neurons. B_2 receptors are coupled to activation of a specific isoform of protein kinase C (PKCε), which phosphorylates TRPV1 and facilitates opening of the TRPV1 channel.

Bradykinin is converted in tissues by removal of a terminal arginine residue to *des-Arg9 bradykinin*, which acts selectively on B_1 receptors. B_1 receptors are normally expressed at very low levels, but their expression is strongly up-regulated in inflamed tissues. Genetically modified knock-out animals lacking either type of receptor show reduced inflammatory hyperalgesia. Specific competitive antagonists for both B_1 and B_2 receptors have been developed, such as the B_2 antagonist **icatibant,** used in the treatment of angioedema, but none have yet been developed as analgesic agents.

[1]Anyone who has rubbed their eyes after cutting up chilli peppers will know this.

[2]The receptor was originally known as the vanilloid receptor because many capsaicin-like compounds are based on the structure of vanillic acid.

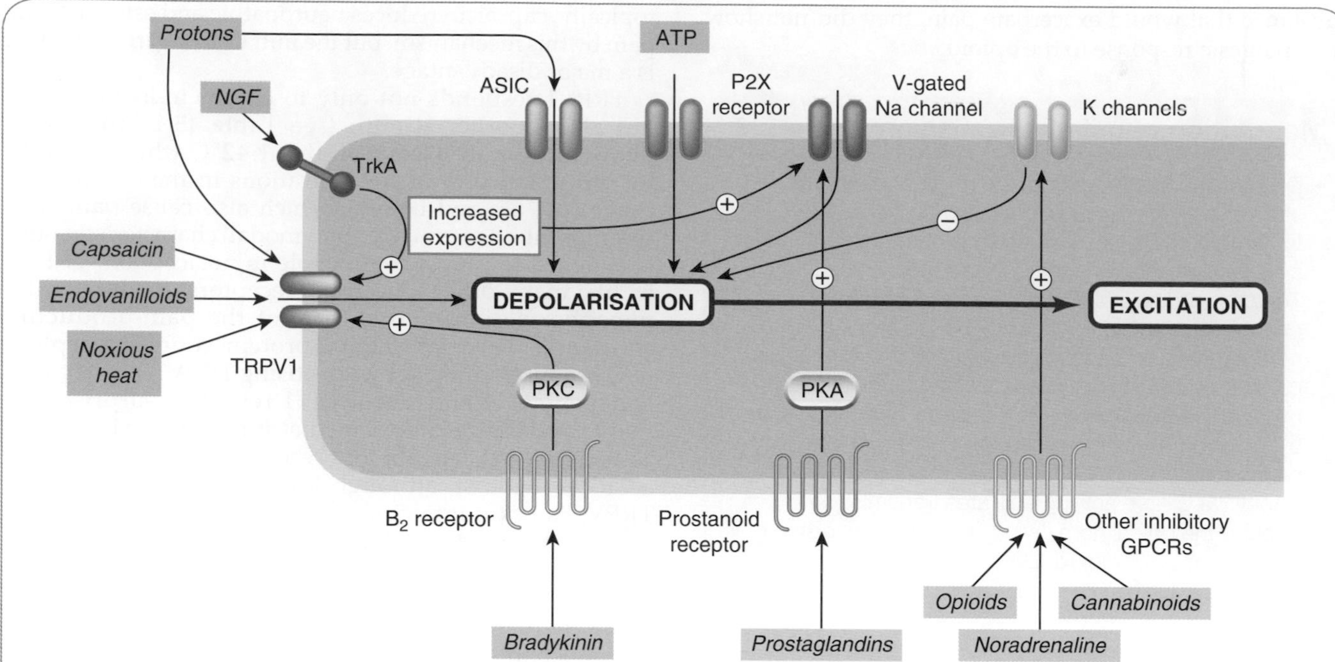

Fig. 43.5 Channels, receptors and transduction mechanisms of nociceptive afferent terminals. Only the main channels and receptors are shown. Ligand-gated channels include acid-sensitive ion channels (ASICs), ATP-sensitive channels (P2X receptors) and the capsaicin-sensitive channel (TRPV1), which is also sensitive to protons and to temperature. Various facilitatory and inhibitory G protein–coupled receptors (GPCRs) are shown, which regulate channel function through various second messenger systems. Growth factors such as nerve growth factor (NGF) act via kinase-linked receptors (TrkA) to control ion channel function and gene expression. *B_2 receptor,* Bradykinin type 2 receptor; *PKA,* protein kinase A; PKC, protein kinase C.

Table 43.1 Thermosensitive TRP channels expressed on sensory neurons

Channel type	TRPA1	TRPM8	TRPV4	TRPV3	TRPV1	TRPV2
Activation temperature (°C)	<17	8–28	>27	>33	>43	>52
Chemical activators	Icilin Wintergreen oil Mustard oil	Menthol Icilin Eucalyptol Geraniol	4αPDD	Camphor Menthol Eugenol	Capsaicin Protons Anandamide Camphor Resiniferatoxin Eugenol	Δ^9-THC

4αPDD, 4 Alpha-phorbol 12,13-didecanoate; *Δ^9-THC,* Δ^9-tetrahydrocannabinol; *TRP,* transient receptor protein.

Prostaglandins

Prostaglandins do not themselves cause pain, but they strongly enhance the pain-producing effect of other agents such as 5-HT or bradykinin (see Fig. 43.6). Prostaglandins of the E and F series are released in inflammation (see Ch. 17) and also during tissue ischaemia. Antagonists at EP_1 receptors decrease inflammatory hyperalgesia in animal models. Prostaglandins sensitise nerve terminals to other agents, partly by inhibiting potassium channels and partly by facilitating – through second messenger-mediated phosphorylation reactions (see Ch. 3) – the cation channels opened by noxious agents. It is of interest that bradykinin itself causes prostaglandin release, and thus has a powerful 'self-sensitising' effect on nociceptive afferents. Other eicosanoids, including prostacyclin, leukotrienes and the unstable hydroxyeicosatetraenoic acid (HETE) derivatives (see Ch. 17), may also be important. The analgesic effects of NSAIDs (see Ch. 25) result from inhibition of prostaglandin synthesis.

Other peripheral mediators

Pro-inflammatory cytokines such as tumour necrosis factor-α (TNF-α) and interleukin-1β (IL-1β) (described in detail in Ch. 25) are released from macrophages to activate and sensitise nociceptive neurons (see Fig. 43.3) and contribute to persistent pain states.

Various metabolites and substances are released from damaged or ischaemic cells, or inflamed tissues, including ATP, protons (produced by lactic acid), 5-HT, histamine and K^+, many of which affect nociceptive nerve terminals.

ATP excites nociceptive nerve terminals (see Fig. 43.5) by acting on homomeric $P2X_3$ receptors or heteromeric $P2X_2/P2X_3$ receptors (see Ch. 16), ligand-gated ion

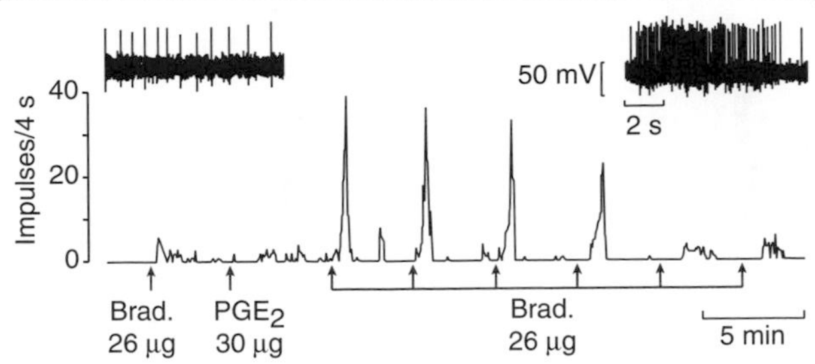

Fig. 43.6 Response of a nociceptive afferent neuron to bradykinin and prostaglandin. Recordings were made from a nociceptive afferent fibre supplying a muscle, and drugs were injected into the arterial supply. Upper records: single-fibre recordings showing discharge caused by bradykinin (Brad) alone *(left)*, and by bradykinin following injection of prostaglandin *(right)*. Lower trace: ratemeter recording of single-fibre discharge, showing long-lasting enhancement of response to bradykinin after an injection of prostaglandin E_2 (PGE_2). Prostaglandin itself did not evoke a discharge. (From Mense, S., 1981. Sensitization of group IV muscle receptors to bradykinin by 5-hydroxytryptamine and prostaglandin E_2. Brain Res. 225, 95–105.)

channels that are selectively expressed by these neurons. Down-regulation of $P2X_3$ receptors, by antisense DNA, reduces inflammatory pain.[3] Antagonists at this receptor were developed as potential analgesic drugs. In a surprising development one such $P2X_3$ antagonist, **gefapixant** (formerly known as AF-219), has been shown to be effective in treating refractory cough (see Ch. 28). Other P2X receptors ($P2X_4$ and $P2X_7$) are expressed on microglia in the spinal cord; activation results in the release of cytokines and chemokines that then act on neighbouring neurons to promote hypersensitivity. ATP and other purine mediators, such as adenosine, also play a role in the dorsal horn, and other types of purinoceptor may also be targeted by analgesic drugs in the future. Adenosine exerts dual effects – acting on A_1 receptors it causes analgesia but on A_2 receptors it does the opposite.

Low pH excites nociceptive afferent neurons partly by opening proton-activated cation channels (acid-sensitive ion channels, ASICs) and partly by activation of TRPV1. Given the acidic nature of inflamed tissue, ASICS are an exciting target for novel analgesic drug development but to date efforts in this regard have been unsuccessful (Dibas et al., 2019).

5-HT causes excitation, but studies with antagonists suggest that it plays at most a minor role. Histamine is also active but causes itching rather than pain. Both these substances are released locally in inflammation (see Chs 16 and 17).

In summary, nociceptive nerve endings can be activated or sensitised by a wide variety of endogenous mediators, the receptors for which are often up- or down-regulated under pathophysiological conditions.

[3]$P2X_3$ knock-out mice are, in contrast, fairly normal in this respect, presumably because other mechanisms take over.

Mechanisms of pain and nociception

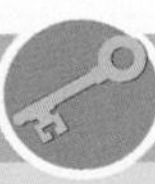

- Nociception is the mechanism whereby noxious peripheral stimuli are transmitted to the central nervous system. Pain is a subjective experience not always associated with nociception.
- Polymodal nociceptors (PMNs) are the main type of peripheral sensory neuron that responds to noxious stimuli. The majority are non-myelinated C fibres whose endings respond to thermal, mechanical and chemical stimuli.
- Chemical stimuli acting on PMNs to cause pain include bradykinin, protons, ATP and vanilloids (e.g. **capsaicin**). PMNs are sensitised by prostaglandins, which explains the analgesic effect of **aspirin**-like drugs, particularly in the presence of inflammation.
- The TRPV1 receptor responds to noxious heat as well as to **capsaicin**-like agonists.
- Nociceptive fibres terminate in the superficial layers of the dorsal horn, forming synaptic connections with transmission neurons running to the thalamus.
- PMN neurons release glutamate (fast transmitter) and various peptides that act as slow transmitters. Peptides are also released peripherally and contribute to neurogenic inflammation.

ANALGESIC DRUGS

OPIOID DRUGS

Opium is an extract of the juice of the poppy *Papaver somniferum* that contains **morphine**, the prototypic opioid agonist, and other related alkaloids. It has been used for social and medicinal purposes for thousands of years as an agent to produce euphoria, analgesia and sleep, and to prevent diarrhoea. It was introduced in Britain at the end of the 17th century, usually taken orally as 'tincture of laudanum', addiction to which acquired a certain social cachet during the next 200 years. The situation changed when the hypodermic syringe and needle were invented in the mid-19th century, and opioid addiction began to take on a more sinister significance (see Ch. 50).

The history of opioid research is reviewed by Corbett et al. (2006).

CHEMICAL ASPECTS

The structure of morphine (Fig. 43.7) was determined in 1902, and since then many semisynthetic compounds (some produced by chemical modification of morphine) and fully synthetic opioids have been developed in attempts to develop better analgesic drugs devoid of the unwanted side effects of morphine.

Morphine is a phenanthrene derivative with two planar rings and two aliphatic ring structures, which occupy a plane roughly at right angles to the rest of the molecule (see Fig. 43.7). The most important parts of the molecule for opioid activity are the free hydroxyl on the benzene ring that is linked by two carbon atoms to a nitrogen atom. Variants of the morphine molecule have been produced by substitution

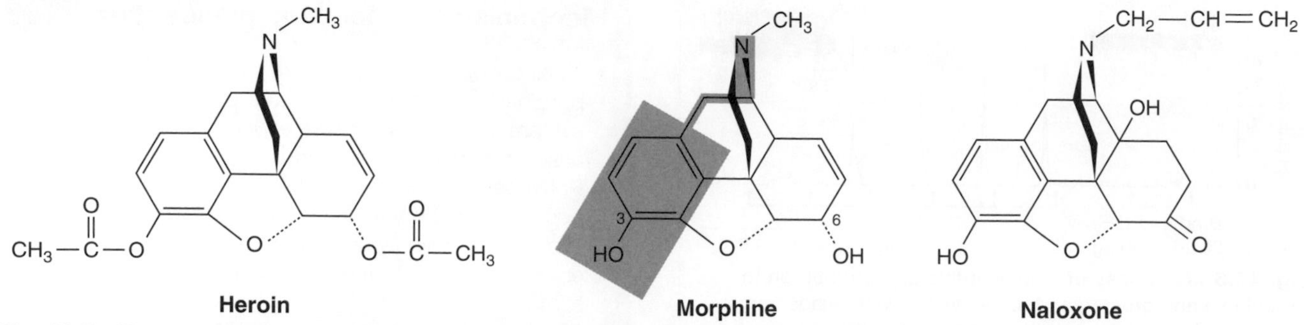

Fig. 43.7 Chemical structures of morphine and related drugs. The *shaded area* indicates the part of the morphine molecule that is structurally similar to tyrosine, the N-terminal amino acid in the endorphins. Carbon atoms 3 and 6 in the *morphine* structure are indicated. Diamorphine (heroin) is 3,6-diacetylmorphine, and morphine is metabolised by addition of a glucuronide moiety at either position 3 or position 6.

at one or both of the hydroxyls (e.g. **diamorphine**[4] 3,6-diacetylmorphine, **codeine** 3-methoxymorphine and **oxycodone**). **Pethidine** and **fentanyl** represent more dramatic changes to the basic morphine structure whereas **methadone** and the novel opioid analgesic, **oliceridine**, bear little obvious chemical relationship to morphine. Substitution of a bulky substituent on the nitrogen atom of morphine introduces antagonist activity to the molecule (e.g. **naloxone**).

Opioid analgesics

- Terminology:
  - *opioid*: any substance, whether endogenous or synthetic, that produces **morphine**-like effects that are blocked by antagonists such as **naloxone**;
  - *opiate*: compounds such as **morphine** and **codeine** that are found in the opium poppy;
  - *narcotic analgesic*: old term for opioids; *narcotic* refers to their ability to induce sleep. Unfortunately, the term narcotic has subsequently been hijacked and used inappropriately by some to refer generically to drugs of abuse (see Ch. 50).
- Important structurally related agonists include **diamorphine**, **oxycodone** and **codeine.**
- Synthetic analogues include **pethidine**, **fentanyl**, **methadone**, **buprenorphine.**
- Opioid analgesics may be given orally, by injection or intrathecally to produce analgesia.

OPIOID RECEPTORS

The proposal that opioids produce analgesia and their other effects by interacting with specific receptors first arose in the 1950s, based on the strict structural and stereochemical requirements essential for activity. It was, however, only with the development of molecules with antagonist activity (e.g. naloxone) that the notion of a specific receptor became accepted. Martin and co-workers then provided pharmacological evidence for multiple types of opioid receptors. They proposed three different types of receptor, called μ, κ and σ.[5] Subsequently, in the early 1970s, radioligand binding (see Ch. 2) was used to demonstrate the presence of μ receptors in the brain.

Why are there specific receptors in the brain for morphine, a drug that is present in the opium poppy? Hughes and Kosterlitz argued that there must be an endogenous substance or substances in the brain that activated these receptors.[6] In 1975 they reported the isolation and characterisation of the first endogenous opioid peptide ligands, the *enkephalins*. We now know that the enkephalins are two members of a larger family of endogenous opioid peptides known collectively as the *endorphins*, all of which possess a tyrosine residue at their N-terminus. The chemical structure of tyrosine includes an amine group separated from a phenol ring by two carbon atoms. This same structure (phenol-2 carbon atom chain-amine) is also contained within the morphine structure (see Fig. 43.7). It is probably just chance (good or bad luck depending on one's viewpoint) that the opium poppy synthesises a semi-rigid alkaloid molecule, morphine, part of which structurally resembles the tyrosine residue in the endogenous opioid peptides.

Following on from the discovery of the enkephalins, in vitro pharmacological studies revealed another receptor, δ, and the three recognised receptor types (μ, δ and κ) were cloned. Later, another opioid receptor that has a high a degree of amino acid sequence homology (>60%) towards the μ, δ and κ opioid receptors was identified by cloning techniques, although the antagonist, naloxone, did not bind to this new receptor. The terminology used for opioid receptors has over the years been through several revisions; in this chapter we shall use the classical terminology. The four opioid receptors, μ, δ, κ and NOP (originally referred to as opioid receptor like receptor 1 or

[4]While 'diamorphine' is the recommended International Nonproprietary Name (rINN), this drug is widely known as heroin.

[5]The σ 'receptor' is no longer considered to be an opioid receptor. It was originally postulated in order to account for the dysphoric effects (anxiety, hallucinations, bad dreams, etc.) produced by some opioids. It is now accepted that these effects result from drug-induced block of the NMDA receptor channel pore, an effect that is also produced by agents such as ketamine (see Ch. 41). Novel σ receptors – σ_1 and σ_2 subtypes – have now been cloned and characterised. They are not structurally related to other receptor types and little is known about their physiological role, but they have been suggested as novel drug targets for psychiatric disorders.

[6]It may seem obvious today that if there is a receptor then there is likely also to be an endogenous ligand for that receptor but it was the search for, and subsequent discovery of, the enkephalins that gave credence to this idea.

Table 43.2 Functional effects associated with the main types of opioid receptor

Receptor	μ	δ	κ	NOP
Analgesia				
Supraspinal	+++	−?	−	Antiopioid[a]
Spinal	++	++	+	++
Peripheral	++	−	++	−
Respiratory depression	+++	−	−	−
Pupil constriction	++	−	+	−
Reduced gastrointestinal motility	++	++	+	−
Euphoria	+++	−	−	−
Dysphoria and hallucinations	−	−	+++	−
Sedation	++	−	++	−
Catatonia	−	−	−	++
Physical dependence	+++	−	−	−

[a]NOP receptor agonists were originally thought to produce nociception or hyperalgesia but it was later shown that they reverse the supraspinal analgesic effects of endogenous and exogenous μ receptor agonists.

Opioid receptors

- μ Receptors are responsible for most of the analgesic effects of opioids, and for some major unwanted effects (e.g. respiratory depression, constipation, euphoria, sedation and dependence).
- δ Receptor activation results in analgesia but also can be proconvulsant.
- κ Receptors contribute to analgesia at the spinal level and may elicit sedation, dysphoria and hallucinations. Some analgesics are mixed κ agonists/μ antagonists.
- NOP receptors are also members of the opioid-receptor family. Activation results in an antiopioid effect (supraspinal), analgesia (spinal), immobility and impairment of learning.
- σ Receptors are not true opioid receptors but are the site of action of certain psychotomimetic drugs, with which some opioids also interact.
- All opioid receptors are linked through G_i/G_o proteins and thus open potassium channels (causing hyperpolarisation) and inhibit the opening of calcium channels (inhibiting transmitter release). In addition, they inhibit adenylyl cyclase and activate the MAP kinase (ERK) pathway.
- Functional heteromers, formed by combination of different types of opioid receptor or with other types of G protein–coupled receptor, may occur and give rise to further pharmacological diversity.

ORL_1) are all G protein–coupled receptors (see Ch. 3).[7] The main behavioural effects resulting from their activation are summarised in Table 43.2.

The development of genetically modified mouse strains lacking each of the opioid receptor types has revealed that the major pharmacological effects of morphine, including analgesia, are mediated by the μ receptor.

All four opioid receptors appear to form homomeric as well as heteromeric receptor complexes (see Ch. 3). Opioid receptors are, in fact, quite promiscuous and can form heteromers with non-opioid receptors. Heteromerisation between opioid receptors has been shown to result in pharmacological characteristics distinct from those observed with the monomeric receptors and may explain some of the subtypes of each receptor that have been proposed (see Fujita et al., 2014). Another level of complexity may reflect 'bias' (see Ch. 3), whereby different ligands acting on the same opioid receptor can elicit different cellular responses and differential receptor trafficking (see Kelly, 2013).[8]

MECHANISM OF ACTION OF OPIOIDS

The opioids have probably been studied more intensively than any other group of drugs in the effort to understand their powerful effects in molecular, cellular and physiological terms, and to use this understanding to develop new drugs as analgesics with significant advantages over morphine. Even so, morphine – described by Osler as 'God's own medicine' – remains the standard against which any new analgesic is assessed.

Cellular actions

All four types of opioid receptor belong to the family of G_i/G_o protein–coupled receptors. Opioids thus exert powerful effects on ion channels on neuronal membranes through a direct G protein coupling to the channel. Opioids promote the opening of potassium channels (see Ch. 4) and inhibit the opening of voltage-gated calcium channels. These membrane effects decrease neuronal excitability (because the increased K^+ conductance causes hyperpolarisation of the membrane making the cell less likely to fire action potentials) and reduce transmitter release (due to inhibition of Ca^{2+} entry). The overall effect is therefore inhibitory at the cellular level. Nonetheless, opioids do increase activity in some neuronal pathways (Fig. 43.4). They cause excitation of projection neurons by suppressing the activity of inhibitory interneurons that tonically inhibit the projection neurons, a process referred to as 'disinhibition' (see Ch. 37).

At the biochemical level, all four receptor types inhibit adenylyl cyclase and cause MAP kinase (ERK) activation (see Ch. 3). These cellular responses are likely to be important in mediating the long-term adaptive changes

[7]The opioid receptors are unusual among G protein–coupled receptors. First, in that there are many (20 or more) opioid peptides but only four receptors. In contrast, 5-HT, for example, is a single mediator interacting with many (about 14) receptors, which is the more common pattern. Second, all four receptors couple to the same types of G protein (G_i/G_o) and therefore activate the same spectrum of cellular effector mechanisms. In contrast, other receptor families (e.g. muscarinic receptors) couple to different types of G proteins and therefore give rise to different cellular responses (see Ch. 14).

[8]Claims have been made that 'G protein biased' μ opioid receptor ligands will show a reduced side-effect profile in comparison to morphine which is 'unbiased', but recent research does not support this hypothesis (Gillis et al., 2020, Trends Pharmacol Sci 41, 947–959).

that occur in response to prolonged receptor activation and which, for μ receptor agonists, may underlie the phenomenon of physical dependence (see Ch. 50).

At the cellular level, therefore, all four types of opioid receptor mediate very similar effects. It is their heterogeneous anatomical distributions across the central nervous system (CNS) that give rise to the different behavioural responses seen with selective agonists for each type of receptor.

Sites of action of opioids to produce analgesia

Opioid receptors (μ, δ and κ) are widely distributed in the brain and spinal cord. Opioids are effective as analgesics when injected in minute doses into a number of specific brain nuclei (such as the insular cortex, amygdala, hypothalamus, PAG region and RVM) as well as into the dorsal horn of the spinal cord (see Fig. 43.4). Supraspinal analgesia results primarily from μ receptor activation but there is some evidence for the involvement of supraspinal δ receptors as well. Supraspinal opioid analgesia involves disinhibition resulting in endogenous opioid peptide release both at supraspinal and spinal sites and of serotonin (5-HT) from descending inhibitory fibres in the dorsal horn of the spinal cord. Surgical interruption of the descending pathway from the RVM to the spinal cord reduces analgesia induced by opioids that have been given systemically or microinjected into supraspinal sites, implying that a combination of effects at supraspinal and spinal sites contributes to the analgesic response.

At the spinal level, opioids inhibit transmission of nociceptive impulses through the dorsal horn and suppress nociceptive spinal reflexes, even in patients with spinal cord transection. They can act presynaptically to inhibit release of various neurotransmitters from primary afferent terminals in the dorsal horn as well as acting postsynaptically to reduce the excitability of dorsal horn neurons.

There is also evidence (see Sawynok, 2003) that opioids inhibit the discharge of nociceptive afferent terminals in the periphery, particularly under conditions of inflammation, in which the expression of opioid receptors by sensory neurons is increased. Injection of morphine into the knee joint following surgery to the joint provides effective analgesia, undermining the age-old belief that opioid analgesia is exclusively a central phenomenon.

PHARMACOLOGICAL ACTIONS

Morphine is typical of many opioid analgesics and will be taken as the reference compound. Its effects are mediated predominately through μ receptors.

The most important effects of morphine are on the CNS and the gastrointestinal tract, although numerous effects of lesser significance on many other systems have been described.

Effects on the central nervous system

Analgesia

Morphine and other opioids are highly effective in most kinds of acute pain as well as in 'end of life' pain resulting from cancer. They are much less effective in treating neuropathic and other chronic pain states (see later).

Hyperalgesia

In both animal studies and in patients receiving opioids for pain relief, prolonged exposure to opioids may paradoxically induce a state of hyperalgesia in which pain sensitisation or allodynia occurs (see Lee et al., 2011). This can appear as a reduced analgesic response to a given dose of opioid but should not be confused with tolerance, which is a reduced responsiveness due in large part to μ receptor desensitisation and occurs with other opioid-induced effects such as euphoria and to a lesser extent respiratory depression. Hyperalgesia appears to have peripheral, spinal and supraspinal components. At the neuronal level, an array of mediators and mechanisms have been proposed to contribute to this phenomenon (Roeckel et al., 2016). These include NO, PKC and NMDA receptor activation. In addition, $P2X_4$ receptor expression in microglia is up-regulated resulting in BDNF release, TrkB signalling and down-regulation of the K^+/Cl^- co-transporter KCC2. In mice in which BDNF has been deleted from microglia, hyperalgesia to morphine does not occur, whereas antinociception and tolerance are unaffected.

Opioid-induced hyperalgesia declines on cessation of opioid administration. Clinically, it can be reduced by opioid rotation – switching from one to another opioid drug (e.g. from morphine to fentanyl or methadone, the latter having weak NMDA-receptor antagonist action which may be helpful). Another approach is to co-administer an adjuvant such as ketamine (an NMDA antagonist), propofol (an intravenous anaesthetic), dexmedetomidine (an α_2-adrenoceptor agonist) or a cyclo-oxygenase (COX)-2 inhibitor.

Euphoria

Morphine causes a powerful sense of contentment and well-being (see also Ch. 50). This may contribute to its analgesic effect. If morphine or diamorphine (heroin) is given intravenously, the result is a sudden 'rush' likened to an 'abdominal orgasm'. The euphoria produced by morphine depends considerably on the circumstances. In patients who have become accustomed to pain, morphine causes analgesia with little or no euphoria. Some patients report restlessness rather than euphoria under these circumstances.

Euphoria is mediated through μ receptors, whereas κ receptor activation produces dysphoria and hallucinations (see Table 43.2). Thus, different opioid drugs vary greatly in the amount of euphoria that they produce. It does not occur with codeine to any marked extent. There is evidence that antagonists at the κ receptor have antidepressant properties which may indicate that release of endogenous κ agonists may occur in depression.

Respiratory depression

Respiratory depression occurs with a normal analgesic dose of morphine or related compounds, although in patients in severe pain the degree of respiratory depression produced may be less than anticipated. For drug users who inject illicit opioids (see Ch. 50), respiratory depression leading to overdose death is a constant danger.

Respiratory depression results from μ receptor activation in several regions of the brainstem including the pre-Bötzinger complex, which controls inspiratory drive, and the Kölliker-fuse and lateral parabrachial nuclei, which control upper airway coordination and termination of inspiration. The overall effect produced is a reduction in respiratory rate. The depressant effect is also associated with a decrease in the sensitivity of the respiratory centres to arterial P_{CO_2}. Changes in P_{CO_2} are detected by chemosensitive neurons in a number of brain stem and medullary nuclei. Increased arterial CO_2 (hypercapnia) thus normally results in a compensatory increase in minute ventilation rate (V_E).

Depression of cough reflex

Cough suppression (antitussive effect; see also Ch. 28), surprisingly, does not correlate closely with the analgesic and respiratory depressant actions of opioids, and its mechanism at the receptor level is unclear. In general, increasing substitution on the phenolic hydroxyl group of morphine increases antitussive relative to analgesic activity. **Codeine** and **pholcodine** suppress cough in subanalgesic doses but they cause constipation as an unwanted effect.

Dextromethorphan, the dextro-isomer of the opioid analgesic **levorphanol**, suppresses cough but has very low affinity for opioid receptors and its cough suppressing action, unlike that of opioids, is not antagonised by naloxone. It is an uncompetitive NMDA receptor antagonist – this might explain why at high doses it evokes CNS effects similar to ketamine and may be used for its psychoactive effects (see Ch. 49) – and has putative actions at σ receptors. It is believed to work at various sites in the brain stem and medulla to suppress cough. In addition to its antitussive action, dextromethorphan is neuroprotective (see Ch. 40) and has an analgesic action in neuropathic pain.

Nausea and vomiting

Nausea and vomiting occur in up to 40% of patients to whom morphine is given, and do not seem to be separable from the analgesic effect among a range of opioid analgesics. The site of action is the *area postrema* (chemoreceptor trigger zone), a region of the medulla where chemical stimuli of many kinds may initiate vomiting (see Ch. 30).[9] Nausea and vomiting following morphine injection are usually transient and disappear with repeated administration, although in some individuals they persist and can limit patient compliance.

Pupillary constriction

Pupillary constriction is caused by μ and κ receptor-mediated stimulation of the oculomotor nucleus. Pinpoint pupils are an important diagnostic feature in opioid poisoning[10] because most other causes of coma and respiratory depression produce pupillary dilatation. Tolerance does not develop to the pupillary constriction induced by opioids and therefore can be observed in opioid-dependent drug users who may have been taking opioids for a considerable time.

Effects on the gastrointestinal tract

Opioids increase tone and reduce motility in many parts of the gastrointestinal system, resulting in constipation, which may be severe and very troublesome to the patient.[11] The resulting delay in gastric emptying can considerably retard the absorption of other drugs. Pressure in the biliary tract increases because of contraction of the gall bladder and constriction of the biliary sphincter. Opioids should be avoided in patients suffering from biliary colic due to gallstones, in whom pain may be increased rather than relieved. The rise in intrabiliary pressure can cause a transient increase in the concentration of amylase and lipase in the plasma.

The action of morphine on visceral smooth muscle is probably mediated mainly through the intramural nerve plexuses, because the increase in tone is reduced or abolished by atropine. It is also partly mediated by a central action, because intracerebroventricular injection of morphine inhibits propulsive gastrointestinal movements. **Methylnaltrexone bromide** (see also Ch. 9), **alvimopan**, **naloxegol** and **naldemedine** are opioid antagonists that do not cross the blood–brain barrier. They have been developed to reduce unwanted peripheral side effects of opioids, such as constipation, without significantly reducing analgesia or precipitating withdrawal in dependent individuals.

Other actions of opioids

Morphine releases histamine from mast cells by an action unrelated to opioid receptors. Pethidine and fentanyl do not produce this effect. The release of histamine can cause local effects, such as urticaria and itching at the site of the injection, or systemic effects, namely bronchoconstriction and hypotension.

Hypotension and bradycardia occur with large doses of most opioids, due to an action on the medulla. With morphine and similar drugs, histamine release may contribute to the hypotension.

Effects on smooth muscle other than that of the gastrointestinal tract and bronchi are slight, although spasms of the ureters, bladder and uterus sometimes occur. Opioids also exert complex immunosuppressant effects, which may be important as a link between the nervous system and immune function. The pharmacological significance of this is not yet clear, but there is evidence in humans that the immune system is depressed by long-term opioid use, and that in drug users suffering from AIDS the use of opioids may exacerbate the immune deficiency.

Actions of morphine

- The main pharmacological effects are:
  - analgesia
  - euphoria and sedation
  - respiratory depression
  - suppression of cough
  - nausea and vomiting
  - pupillary constriction
  - reduced gastrointestinal motility, causing constipation
  - histamine release, causing itch, bronchoconstriction and hypotension
- The most troublesome unwanted effects are nausea and vomiting, constipation and respiratory depression.
- Acute overdosage with **morphine** produces coma and respiratory depression.
- **Diamorphine** (heroin) is inactive at opioid receptors but is rapidly cleaved in the brain to 6-acetylmorphine and **morphine.**
- **Codeine** is also converted to **morphine** but more slowly by liver metabolism.

[9]The chemically related compound apomorphine is more strongly emetic than morphine, through its action as a dopamine agonist; despite its name, it is inactive on opioid receptors.

[10]The exception is pethidine, which causes pupillary dilatation because it also blocks muscarinic receptors.

[11]In treating pain, constipation is regarded as an undesirable side effect. However, opiates such as codeine and morphine can be used to treat diarrhoea.

TOLERANCE, PHYSICAL DEPENDENCE AND ADDICTION

Tolerance to many of the actions of opioids (i.e. an increase in the dose needed to produce a given pharmacological effect) develops within a few days during repeated administration. There is some controversy over whether significant tolerance develops to the analgesic effects of morphine, especially in palliative care patients with severe cancer pain (see McQuay, 1999; Ballantyne and Mao, 2003). Drug rotation (changing from one opioid to another) is frequently used clinically to overcome loss of effectiveness.

In animal experiments, tolerance can be detected even with a single dose of morphine. Tolerance extends to most of the pharmacological effects of morphine, including analgesia, emesis, euphoria and respiratory depression, but affects the constipating and pupil-constricting actions much less. As tolerance is likely to depend upon the level of receptor occupancy, the degree of tolerance observed may reflect the response being assessed, the intrinsic efficacy of the drug and the dose being administered (see Hayhurst and Durieux, 2016). The cellular mechanisms responsible for tolerance are discussed in Chapter 2. Tolerance results in part from desensitisation of the μ receptors (i.e. at the level of the drug target) as well as from long-term adaptive changes at the cellular, synaptic and network levels (see Williams et al., 2013). Cross-tolerance occurs between drugs acting at the same receptor, but not between opioids that act on different receptors.

Physical dependence refers to a state in which cessation of drug treatment causes adverse physiological effects, i.e. a withdrawal syndrome (see also Ch. 50). Although it can develop along with tolerance the two adaptive phenomena result from different adaptive cellular mechanisms (see Williams et al., 2013). In experimental animals (e.g. rats), abrupt withdrawal of morphine after repeated administration for a few days, or the administration of an antagonist such as naloxone, causes an increase in diarrhoea, loss of weight and a variety of abnormal behaviour patterns, such as body shakes, writhing, jumping and signs of aggression. These reactions decrease after a few days, but abnormal aggression persists for many weeks. The signs of physical dependence are much less intense if the opioid is withdrawn gradually. Patients on an opioid for pain relief often experience withdrawal symptoms such as restlessness, runny nose, diarrhoea, shivering and piloerection when drug administration is stopped.[12]

Addiction refers to the compulsive use of opioid drugs. Misuse of prescription and illicit opioids can result in the development of addiction. The processes involved in opioid addiction are described in Chapter 50.

PHARMACOKINETIC ASPECTS

Table 43.3 summarises the pharmacokinetic properties of the main opioid analgesics. The absorption of morphine congeners by mouth is variable. Morphine itself is slowly and erratically absorbed, and is commonly given by intravenous injection to treat acute severe pain; oral morphine is, however, often used in treating prolonged pain, and slow-release preparations are available to increase its duration of action. Oxycodone is also available as a slow-release oral preparation. Codeine is well absorbed

[12]Other symptoms include goose pimples and restless leg syndrome. These are the origin of the terms 'cold turkey' and 'kicking the habit' often used to describe the effect of opioid withdrawal.

Tolerance and physical dependence

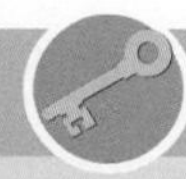

- Tolerance and physical dependence develop on repeated administration of μ receptor agonists.
- The mechanism of tolerance involves receptor desensitisation. It is not pharmacokinetic in origin.
- Physical dependence is evidenced by the appearance of withdrawal symptoms on cessation of drug administration and lasts for a few days. The withdrawal syndrome can also be precipitated by μ receptor antagonists such as naloxone.
- Certain opioid analgesics, such as **codeine**, **buprenorphine** and **tramadol**, are much less likely to cause physical dependence.

and normally given by mouth. Most morphine-like drugs undergo considerable first-pass metabolism, and are therefore markedly less potent when taken orally than when injected.

Opioids that have no free hydroxyl in the 3 position (i.e. diamorphine, codeine) are inactive at opioid receptors. The substitution at the 3 position must be cleaved and replaced with a hydroxyl for the molecule to become pharmacologically active. With diamorphine the conversion occurs rapidly in the plasma and brain but with codeine the effect is slower and occurs by metabolism in the liver.

The plasma half-life of most morphine analogues is 3–6 h. Hepatic metabolism is the main mode of inactivation, usually by conjugation with glucuronide. This occurs at the 3- and 6-OH groups (see Fig. 43.7), and these glucuronides constitute a considerable fraction of the drug in the bloodstream. Morphine-6-glucuronide is more active as an analgesic than morphine itself, and contributes to the pharmacological effect. Morphine-3-glucuronide has been claimed to antagonise the analgesic effect of morphine, but the significance of this experimental finding is uncertain, as this metabolite has little or no affinity for opioid receptors. Morphine glucuronides are excreted in the urine, so the dose needs to be reduced in cases of renal failure. Glucuronides also reach the gut via biliary excretion, where they are hydrolysed, most of the morphine being reabsorbed (enterohepatic circulation). Because of low conjugating capacity in neonates, morphine-like drugs have a much longer duration of action; because even a small degree of respiratory depression can be hazardous, morphine congeners should not be used in the neonatal period, nor used as analgesics during childbirth. Pethidine is a safer alternative for this purpose.

Morphine produces very effective analgesia when administered intrathecally, and is used in this way by anaesthetists, the advantage being that the sedative and respiratory depressant effects are reduced, although not completely avoided. **Remifentanil** is rapidly hydrolysed and eliminated with a half-life of 3–4 min. The advantage of this is that when given by intravenous infusion during general anaesthesia, the level of the drug can be manipulated rapidly when required (see Ch. 11 for a description of how, for intravenous infusion, both the rate of rise and the rate of decay of the plasma concentration are determined by the half-time of elimination).

Table 43.3 Characteristics of the main opioid analgesic drugs

Drug	Use(s)	Route(s) of administration	Pharmacokinetic aspects	Main adverse effects	Notes
Morphine	Widely used for acute and cancer pain	Oral, including sustained-release form Injection[a] Intrathecal	Half-life 3–4 h Converted to active metabolite (morphine-6-glucuronide)	Sedation Respiratory depression Constipation Nausea and vomiting Itching (histamine release) Tolerance and dependence Euphoria	Tolerance and withdrawal effects not common when used for analgesia
Diamorphine (heroin)	Acute and cancer pain	Oral Injection	Acts more rapidly than morphine because of rapid brain penetration.	As morphine	Not available in all countries Metabolised to morphine and other active metabolites
Tramadol	Acute (mainly postoperative), cancer and chronic pain	Oral Intravenous	Well absorbed Half-life 4–6 h	Dizziness May cause convulsions No respiratory depression	Has to be metabolised to active moiety Weak agonist at opioid receptors Also inhibits monoamine uptake. **Tapentadol** is similar
Oxycodone	Acute and cancer pain	Oral, including sustained-release form Injection	Half-life 3–4.5 h	As morphine	Has become a major drug of abuse in North America Hydrocodone is similar
Hydromorphone	Acute and cancer pain	Oral Injection	Half-life 2–4 h No active metabolites	As morphine but allegedly less sedative	**Levorphanol** is similar, with longer duration of action
Fentanyl	Acute pain Anaesthesia	Intravenous Sublingual Transdermal patch	Half-life 1–2 h	As morphine	High potency allows transdermal administration **Sufentanil** is similar
Remifentanil	Anaesthesia	Intravenous infusion	Half-life 5 min	Respiratory depression	Very rapid onset and recovery
Pethidine	Acute pain	Oral Intramuscular injection	Half-life 2–4 h Active metabolite (norpethidine) may account for stimulant effects	As morphine Anticholinergic effects Risk of excitement and convulsions	Known as **meperidine** in United States Interacts with monoamine oxidase inhibitors (see Ch. 48)
Methadone	Cancer pain Maintenance of opioid users	Oral Injection	Long half-life (>24 h) Slow onset	As morphine but less euphoric effect Accumulation may occur	Slow recovery results in attenuated withdrawal syndrome because of long half-life
Buprenorphine	Acute and cancer pain Maintenance of opioid users	Sublingual Injection Transdermal patch Intrathecal	Half-life about 12 h Slow onset Inactive orally because of first-pass metabolism	As morphine but less pronounced Respiratory depression not reversed by naloxone (therefore not suitable for obstetric use) May precipitate opioid withdrawal (partial agonist)	A sustained release preparation for subcutaneous administration has recently been developed for substitution therapy in opioid users
Codeine	Mild pain	Oral	Acts as prodrug Metabolised to morphine and other active metabolites	Mainly constipation Low dependence liability	Effective only in mild pain. Often referred to as a 'weak' opioid Also used to suppress cough **Dihydrocodeine** is similar

Continued

Table 43.3 Characteristics of the main opioid analgesic drugs—cont'd

Drug	Use(s)	Route(s) of administration	Pharmacokinetic aspects	Main adverse effects	Notes
Dextropro-poxyphene	Mild pain	Mainly oral	Half-life ~4 h Active metabolite (norpropoxyphene) with half-life ~24 h	Respiratory depression May cause convulsions (possibly by action of norpropoxyphene)	Similar to codeine No longer recommended
Dipipanone	Moderate to severe pain	Oral	Half-life 3.5 h (although there are longer values quoted)	In addition to effects similar to morphine it produces psychosis	Marketed in combination with **cyclizine** (Diconal) and became a popular intravenous drug of abuse

[a]Injections may be given intravenously, intramuscularly or subcutaneously for most drugs.

In postoperative and cancer pain, opioids are often given 'on demand' (patient-controlled analgesia). The patients are provided with an infusion pump that they control, the maximum possible rate of administration being limited to avoid acute toxicity. Patients show little tendency to use excessively large doses and so do not become dependent; instead, the dose is adjusted to achieve analgesia without excessive sedation, and is reduced as the pain subsides. Being in control of their own analgesia, the patients' anxiety and distress are reduced, and analgesic consumption actually tends to decrease. In cancer pain, patients often experience sudden, sharp increases in the level of pain they are experiencing. This is referred to as breakthrough pain. To combat this, there is a therapeutic need to be able to increase rapidly the amount of opioid being administered. This has led to the development of touch-sensitive transdermal patches containing potent opioids such as fentanyl that rapidly release drug into the bloodstream. Fentanyl lozenges and lollipops, producing rapid absorption through the buccal mucosa, are also used.

The opioid antagonist, naloxone, has a shorter biological half-life than most opioid agonists. In the treatment of opioid overdose, it must be given repeatedly to avoid the respiratory depressant effect of the agonist reoccurring once the naloxone has been eliminated. Naltrexone has a longer biological half-life.

UNWANTED EFFECTS

The main unwanted effects of morphine and related drugs are listed in Table 43.3.

Acute overdosage with morphine results in coma and respiratory depression, with characteristically constricted pupils. It is treated by giving naloxone. This also serves as a diagnostic test, for failure to respond to naloxone suggests a cause other than opioid poisoning for the comatose state. There is a danger of precipitating a severe withdrawal response with naloxone, because opioid poisoning occurs mainly in illicit opioid users (see Ch. 50).

Individual variability

Individuals vary by as much as 10-fold in their sensitivity to opioid analgesics. This can be due to altered metabolism or altered sensitivity of the receptors (for extensive review, see Rollason et al., 2008). For morphine, reduced responsiveness may result from mutations in a number of genes including that for the drug transporter, P-glycoprotein (see Chs 9 and 12), for glucuronyltransferase that metabolises morphine and for the μ receptor itself. Mutations of various cytochrome P450 (CYP) enzymes influence the metabolism of codeine, oxycodone, methadone, tramadol and dextromethorphan. Genotyping could in principle be used to identify opioid-resistant individuals, but first the contribution of genotype to clinical outcome must be confirmed in the population at large.

OTHER OPIOID ANALGESICS

Diamorphine (heroin) is 3,6-diacetylmorphine; it can be considered as a prodrug because its high analgesic potency is attributable to rapid conversion first to 6-monoacetylmorphine (6-MAM) and then to morphine. Its effects are indistinguishable from those of morphine following oral administration. It is said to be less emetic than morphine, but the evidence for this is limited. It is still available in Britain for use as an analgesic, although it is banned in many countries. Its only advantage over morphine is its greater solubility, which allows smaller volumes to be given orally, subcutaneously or intrathecally. It exerts the same respiratory depressant effect as morphine and, if given intravenously, is more likely to cause dependence.

Codeine (3-methoxymorphine) is also a prodrug but, unlike heroin, undergoes demethylation by CYP2D6 in the liver to produce morphine. It has 20% or less of the analgesic potency of morphine, as a large proportion of the absorbed drug is not converted to morphine but instead undergoes hepatic glucuronidation and is then excreted. Its analgesic effect does not increase appreciably at higher dose levels, presumably because of limited conversion to morphine, and so it is sometimes referred to as a weak opioid. It is more reliably absorbed by mouth than morphine and is therefore used mainly as an oral analgesic for mild types of pain (headache, acute backache, etc.). About 10% of the population is resistant to the analgesic effect of codeine, because they lack the demethylating enzyme that converts it to morphine. Unlike morphine, it causes little or no euphoria and is rarely addictive. It is often combined with **paracetamol** in proprietary analgesic preparations (see later section on combined use of opioids and NSAIDs). In relation to its analgesic effect, codeine produces the same degree of respiratory depression as morphine, but the limited response, even at high doses, means that it is seldom a problem in practice. It does, however, cause constipation. Codeine has marked antitussive activity and is often used in cough mixtures (see Ch. 28). **Dihydrocodeine** is pharmacologically very similar, having no substantial advantages or disadvantages over codeine.

Oxycodone is used in the treatment of acute pain, for example after an operation or a serious injury, and cancer pain. The suggestion that it acts on a subtype of κ opioid receptor is not generally accepted. Claims that it has less euphoric effect and less abuse potential are unfounded. It is available as a slow-release oral preparation, as is **hydrocodone** which is similar in action. Overprescribing of these drugs led to them becoming a major drug problem especially in North America (see Ch. 50).

Tramadol and **tapentadol** are widely used as analgesics for postoperative pain. Tramadol comprises two structural enantiomers – (+)-tramadol inhibits 5-HT reuptake and (−)-tramadol inhibits noradrenaline (NA) reuptake – and the major metabolite of (+)-tramadol, O-desmethyltramadol, activates the μ receptor. Tapentadol inhibits NA reuptake and activates the μ receptor. They are effective analgesics and appear to have a better side-effect profile than most opioids, although psychiatric reactions have been reported. They are given by mouth or by intramuscular or intravenous injection for acute and chronic pain, including musculoskeletal pain and the pain associated with diabetic neuropathy.

Fentanyl, **alfentanil**, **sufentanil** and **remifentanil** are highly potent phenylpiperidine derivatives, with actions similar to those of morphine but with a more rapid onset and shorter duration of action, particularly remifentanil. They are used extensively in anaesthesia, and they may be given intrathecally. Fentanyl, alfentanil and sufentanil are also used in patient-controlled infusion systems or administered via patches applied to the skin. The rapid onset is advantageous in breakthrough pain. Fentanyl has minimal cardiovascular effects and does not release histamine. **Carfentanil** is a highly potent fentanyl analogue used to sedate large animals for veterinary procedures. In recent years, illicitly produced fentanyl, carfentanil and a range of other analogues have become a major drug problem, especially in North America (see Ch. 50). Unlike other opioids, they are easily synthesised, without the need to harvest poppies.

Methadone is orally active and pharmacologically similar to morphine, the main difference being that its duration of action is considerably longer (plasma half-life >24 hours). The increased duration seems to occur because the drug is bound in the extravascular compartment and slowly released. On withdrawal, the physical abstinence syndrome is less acute than with morphine. Methadone is widely used as a heroin substitution treatment (see Ch. 50).[13] Methadone also has actions at other sites in the CNS, including block of potassium channels, NMDA receptors and 5-HT receptors, that may explain its CNS side-effect profile. There is interindividual variation in the response to methadone, probably due to genetic variability between individuals in its metabolism.

Pethidine (meperidine) is very similar to morphine in its pharmacological effects, except that it tends to cause restlessness rather than sedation. It was originally investigated as a new antimuscarinic agent but was found to have opioid analgesic activity, its residual antimuscarinic action being responsible for its side effects of dry mouth and blurring of vision. It produces a very similar euphoric effect. Its duration of action is the same or slightly shorter than that of morphine, but the route of metabolic degradation is different. Pethidine is partly *N*-demethylated in the liver to norpethidine, which has hallucinogenic and convulsant effects. These become significant with large oral doses of pethidine, producing an overdose syndrome rather different from that of morphine. Pethidine is preferred to morphine for analgesia during labour, because it does not reduce the force of uterine contraction. Pethidine is only slowly eliminated in the neonate, and naloxone may be needed to reverse respiratory depression in the newborn (morphine is even more problematic in this regard, because the conjugation reactions on which the excretion of morphine, but not of pethidine, depends are deficient in the newborn). Severe reactions, consisting of excitement, hyperthermia and convulsions, have been reported when pethidine is given to patients receiving monoamine oxidase inhibitors. This seems to be due to inhibition of an alternative metabolic pathway, leading to increased norpethidine formation, but the details are unclear.

Buprenorphine is a partial agonist on μ receptors that produces strong analgesia but there is a ceiling to its respiratory depressant effect. Due to extensive first-pass elimination it is administered sublingually or by injection. Because of its antagonist actions, it can produce mild withdrawal symptoms in patients dependent on other opioids. It dissociates slowly from the receptors and so has a long duration of action. Like methadone, it is also used in substitution treatment for people dependent on opioids (see Ch. 50).

Meptazinol is an opioid of unusual chemical structure. It can be given orally or by injection and has a duration of action shorter than that of morphine. It is a μ receptor partial agonist and seems to be relatively free of morphine-like side effects, causing neither euphoria nor dysphoria, nor severe respiratory depression. It does, however, produce nausea, sedation and dizziness, and has atropine-like actions. Because of its short duration of action and lack of respiratory depression, it may have advantages for obstetric analgesia.

Etorphine is a morphine analogue with a potency more than 1000 times that of morphine, but otherwise very similar in its actions. Its high potency confers no particular human clinical advantage, but it is used in veterinary practice, especially in large animals. It can be used in conjunction with sedative agents (neuroleptanalgesia) to immobilise wild animals.[14]

Nalbuphine is an analgesic that has activity at κ, μ and, to a lesser extent, δ receptors. It acts as an agonist at κ receptors and as a partial agonist at μ receptors. **Pentazocine**, rarely used clinically nowadays, also combines a degree of κ agonist and μ antagonist (or weak partial agonist) activity. These agents are thought to produce less euphoria than μ receptor agonists. **Cebranopadol**, currently awaiting

[13]The benefits come mainly from removing the risks of self-injection and the need to finance the drug habit through crime.

[14]The required dose of etorphine, even for an elephant, is small enough to be incorporated into a dart or pellet.

regulatory approval, is an agonist at all four opioid receptors.

Loperamide is a μ receptor agonist that is effectively extruded from the brain by P-glycoprotein and therefore lacks analgesic activity. It inhibits peristalsis, and is used to control diarrhoea (see Ch. 30).

OPIOID ANTAGONISTS

Naloxone was the first pure opioid antagonist, with affinity for all three classic opioid receptors (μ > κ ≥ δ). It blocks the actions of endogenous opioid peptides as well as those of morphine-like drugs and has been extensively used as an experimental tool to determine the physiological role of these peptides, particularly in pain transmission.

Given on its own, naloxone produces very little effect in normal subjects but produces a rapid reversal of the effects of morphine and other opioids. It has little effect on pain threshold under normal conditions but causes hyperalgesia under conditions of stress or inflammation, when endogenous opioids are produced. This occurs, for example, in patients undergoing dental surgery, or in animals subjected to physical stress. Naloxone also inhibits acupuncture analgesia, which is known to be associated with the release of endogenous opioid peptides, but does not reduce meditation-induced analgesia. Analgesia produced by PAG stimulation is also prevented by naloxone.

The main clinical uses of naloxone are to treat respiratory depression caused by opioid overdosage (see Ch. 50), and occasionally to reverse the effect of opioid analgesics, used during labour, on the respiration of the newborn baby. It can be administered nasally, intramuscularly or intravenously, and its effects are rapid in onset. It is rapidly metabolised by the liver, and its effect lasts only 2–4 h, which is considerably shorter than that of most morphine-like drugs and therefore it may have to be given repeatedly.

Naloxone has no important unwanted effects of its own but precipitates withdrawal symptoms in opioid users. It can be used to detect opioid dependence.

Naltrexone is very similar to naloxone but with the advantage of a much longer duration of action (half-life about 10 h). It may be of value in opioid users who have been 'detoxified', because it nullifies the effect of a subsequent dose of an opioid should the patient's resolve fail. For this purpose, it is available in a slow-release subcutaneous implant formulation. It is also effective in reducing alcohol consumption in heavy drinkers (see Ch. 50), the rationale being that part of the high from alcohol comes from the release of endogenous opioid peptides. **Nalmefene**, another non-selective opioid antagonist, is also used to treat patients with alcohol use disorder. Naltrexone may also have beneficial effects in septic shock. It is effective in treating chronic itching (pruritus), as occurs in chronic liver disease. Again, this may indicate the involvement of endogenous opioid peptides in the pathophysiology of such itch conditions.

Methylnaltrexone bromide, **alvimopan**, **naloxegol** and **naldemedine** are μ receptor antagonists that do not cross the blood–brain barrier. They can be used in combination with opioid agonists to block unwanted effects, most notably reduced gastrointestinal motility, nausea and vomiting.

Opioid antagonists

- Pure antagonists include **naloxone** (short acting) and **naltrexone** (longer acting). They block μ, δ and κ receptors. Selective antagonists are available as experimental tools.
- **Alvimopan**, **naloxegol** and **naldemedine** are μ receptor antagonists that do not cross the blood–brain barrier. They block opioid-induced constipation, nausea and vomiting.
- **Naloxone** does not affect pain threshold normally but blocks stress-induced analgesia and can exacerbate clinical pain.
- **Naloxone** rapidly reverses opioid-induced analgesia and respiratory depression, and is used mainly to treat opioid overdose or to improve breathing in newborn babies affected by opioids given to the mother.
- **Naloxone** precipitates withdrawal symptoms in opioid-dependent patients or animals. **Buprenorphine** (a partial agonist) can also precipitate withdrawal due to its antagonist action against higher efficacy opioid agonists.

PARACETAMOL

NSAIDs (covered in detail in Ch. 25) are widely used to treat painful inflammatory conditions and to reduce fever. **Paracetamol** (known as **acetaminophen** in the United States) deserves special mention here. It was first synthesised more than a century ago, and since the 1950s has (alongside aspirin and ibuprofen) been the most widely used over-the-counter remedy for minor aches and pains. Paracetamol differs from other NSAIDs in producing analgesic and antipyretic effects while lacking anti-inflammatory effects. It also lacks the tendency of other NSAIDs to cause gastric ulceration and bleeding. The reason for the difference between paracetamol and other NSAIDs is unclear. Biochemical tests showed it to be only a weak COX inhibitor, with some selectivity for brain COX, possibly because of the unique reducing environment in neurons (see Ch. 25). Interestingly, the antinociceptive and antipyretic effects of paracetamol are absent in mice lacking the TRPA1 receptor. These effects appear to be mediated by a metabolite (*N*-acetyl-*p*-benzoquinoneimine), not by paracetamol itself. This activates TRPA1 and thus reduces voltage-gated calcium and sodium currents in primary sensory neurons.

Paracetamol is well absorbed following oral administration, and its plasma half-life is about 3 h. It is metabolised by hydroxylation, conjugated mainly as glucuronide, and excreted in the urine. In therapeutic doses, it has few adverse effects. However, in overdose, paracetamol causes severe liver damage, which is commonly fatal (see Chs 25 and 58), and the drug is often used in attempted suicide.

USE OF OPIOIDS AND NSAIDs IN COMBINATION

The rationale behind co-administration of two drugs that produce analgesia by different mechanisms is that, if the effects are additive, less of each drug can therefore be given but the same degree of analgesia produced. This has the effect of reducing the intensity of the unwanted side effects produced by each drug. In the case of opioids (e.g. codeine) in combination with paracetamol or aspirin, the combination appears to produce synergy rather than simple additivity. The combination of dextropropoxyphene and paracetamol was withdrawn in the United Kingdom due to concerns about overdosing.

CHRONIC PAIN

The International Association for the Study of Pain (IASP) has classified chronic pain (pain that persists for more than three months) into two types (Treede et al., 2019):

- chronic secondary pain in which the underlying or initiating cause is known. Common conditions of this type are neuropathic pains (e.g. those that are a consequence of diabetes, shingles or herpes zoster infection, as well as sciatica and trigeminal neuralgia), posttraumatic and postsurgical pain (e.g. following a stroke, spinal cord injury or phantom limb pain) and musculoskeletal pain.
- chronic primary pain in which there is no obvious cause. Common conditions of this type are nonspecific low back pain and fibromyalgia.[15]

Chronic pain involves not only the processing of nociceptive information but also comprises emotional and psychosocial components (e.g. mood, circumstance, stress, duration, meaning, acceptance, expectation and fear), more so than acute or cancer-related pain (see Stannard, 2016). These other components may render most opioid drugs less effective in the long-term treatment of chronic pain.[16] The British Medical Association concluded that 'There is a lack of good-quality evidence to support a strong clinical recommendation for the long-term use of opioids for patients with chronic pain' (see BMA, 2017). Psychological treatments such as acceptance and commitment therapy (ACT) and cognitive behavioural therapy (CBT) are useful in reducing the impacts of chronic pain. A number of non-opioid drugs are used to treat chronic pains but for many of them sound evidence for their efficacy or an understanding of the mechanisms underlying their effects in chronic pain is somewhat lacking (see Dworkin et al., 2010; BMA, 2017). Their use to treat chronic pain results largely from serendipitous observations rather than a rational programme of drug discovery. An important component of pain is its emotional and cognitive effects (Fig. 43.8). In acute pain these serve important roles including focusing attention on the cause of the pain and facilitating learning so that future behaviours are adapted to avoid pain. However, in chronic pain, these effects can be detrimental and are thought to contribute to the high prevalence of depression in patients with chronic pain. It may be that drugs used to treat chronic pain primarily work through targeting these cognitive and emotional symptoms.

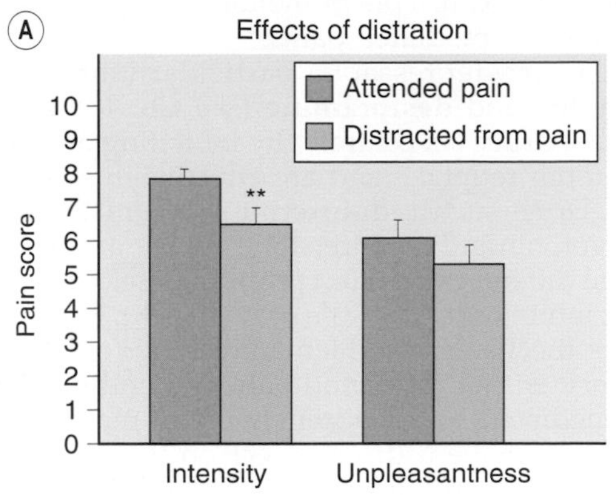

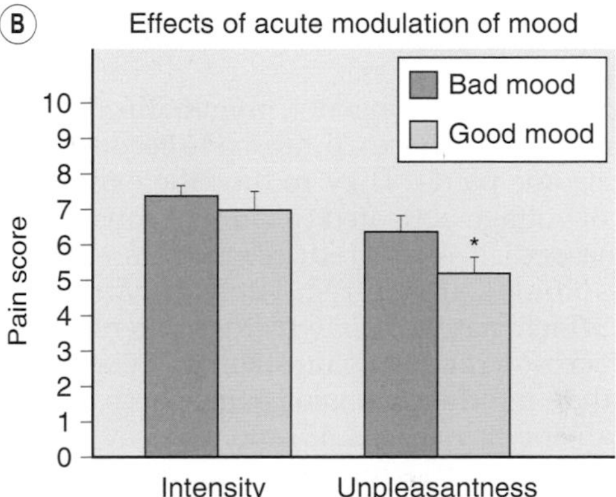

Fig. 43.8 Experimental manipulations to take attention away from the painful sensation or to change mood can change a patient's perception of pain. (A) Manipulating attention away from the pain primarily alters the perceived intensity of the pain sensation without significantly altering the perceived unpleasantness of the pain. (B) By contrast, altering the mood state using acute manipulations, e.g. using emotive music or recalling emotional memories, alters the perceived unpleasantness of the pain without altering the intensity of the sensation. These data suggest that the effects of these higher level cognitive and emotional mechanisms alter pain via distinct descending modulatory systems. Although the effects may seem modest, these are likely to be associated with improvements in patient well-being.

TREATMENT OF CHRONIC SECONDARY PAIN

Musculoskeletal pain affects bones, joints, ligaments, tendons or muscles. Arthritic conditions can be especially painful. Treatment can be targeted at disease modification or at reducing inflammation and pain (described in detail in Ch. 25). Inflammation and pain in these conditions respond to NSAIDs.

The pathophysiological mechanisms underlying neuropathic pain are poorly understood, although spontaneous activity in damaged sensory neurons, due to overexpression or redistribution of voltage-gated sodium channels, is thought to be a factor. In addition, central sensitisation occurs. The sympathetic nervous system also plays a part, because damaged sensory neurons can express α_1 adrenoceptors and develop a sensitivity to noradrenaline that they do not possess under normal conditions. Thus, physiological stimuli that evoke sympathetic responses can

[15]Sciatica, characterized by pain, numbness and tingling in the thigh and leg, is often discussed along with chronic low back pain but its cause can in fact often be defined (e.g. nerve compression by a herniated lumbar disc) and is therefore better described as a chronic secondary pain.
[16]Over the past 30 years, there has been widespread long-term prescribing of opioids for chronic pain in the developed world leading to an alarming increase in addiction to prescription opioids and to overdose deaths (see Ch. 50).

produce severe pain, a phenomenon described clinically as sympathetically mediated pain.

Tricyclic antidepressants, particularly **amitriptyline**, **nortriptyline** and **desipramine** (see Ch. 48), are widely used. These drugs act centrally by inhibiting noradrenaline and serotonin reuptake and are effective in some, but not all, cases. Drugs such as **duloxetine** and **venlafaxine**, which inhibit serotonin and noradrenaline uptake, are also effective and have a different side-effect profile, but selective serotonin reuptake inhibitors show little or no benefit. Little is known about the mechanisms which contribute to these effects. One theory is that they modulate descending inhibitory control mediated by noradrenaline and maybe serotonin and therefore have a direct effect on the pain pathway. However, they may also work centrally by affecting the emotional effects of chronic pain via mechanisms similar to those associated with their antidepressant and anxiolytic effects. Depression and anxiety are also highly comorbid in patients with chronic pain.

Gabapentin and its congener, **pregabalin**, first introduced as antiepileptic drugs (see Ch. 46), have become widely used to treat chronic pains. They reduce the expression of $\alpha_2\delta$ subunits of voltage-activated calcium channels on the nerve membrane (see Ch. 4) and reduce neurotransmitter release. The $\alpha_2\delta$ subunits are up-regulated in damaged sensory neurons, which may explain why these agents may be more effective across a range of pain states associated with nerve damage than in other forms of pain. These drugs are also effective anxiolytics (see Ch. 45) and this may also contribute to their overall benefits for these patients.

Carbamazepine, another type of antiepileptic drug, is effective in trigeminal neuralgia but evidence for effectiveness against other neuropathic pains is lacking. Carbamazepine blocks voltage-gated sodium channels (see Ch. 4) being slightly more potent in blocking $Na_v1.8$ than $Na_v1.7$ and $Na_v1.3$ channels; all of these channel subtypes are thought to be up-regulated by nerve damage and contribute to the sensation of pain. At higher concentrations, it inhibits voltage-activated calcium channels. **Phenytoin** administered intravenously is sometimes used in cases of severe trigeminal neuralgia. Other antiepileptic agents such as **valproic acid**, **lamotrigine**, **oxcarbazepine**, **topiramate** and **levetiracetam** may have some efficacy in some neuropathic pain states.

Tramadol and **tapentadol** have been reported to have efficacy in treating diabetic peripheral neuropathy, chronic low back pain and sciatica. In addition to their agonist action at μ opioid receptors, their ability to reduce monoamine reuptake (discussed earlier in this chapter) may be important.

Lidocaine (lignocaine), a local anaesthetic drug (see Ch. 44), can be used topically to relieve neuropathic pain. It probably acts by blocking spontaneous discharges from damaged sensory nerve terminals. Some antidysrhythmic drugs (e.g. **mexiletine**, **tocainide**, **flecainide**; see Ch. 20) are effective orally.

Capsaicin can be applied topically to areas of localised neuropathic and osteoarthritic pain. It activates nociceptors before subsequently desensitising them and so it initially produces short-lived, localised sensations of burning, or pain. A single application can produce relief of pain for up to 3 months.

Although some drug treatments may only partially alleviate chronic secondary pain for sufferers any decrease in pain intensity can be a welcome improvement to their condition. The abundance of drugs and mechanisms deployed to alleviate chronic secondary pain reflects the current lack of drugs that work effectively and reliably in these common and serious conditions.

Drugs used to treat neuropathic pain

- Certain antidepressants (e.g. **amitriptyline**, **duloxetine**) provide therapeutic benefit.
- **Gabapentin** and **pregabalin** are now used more to treat neuropathic pain than as antiepileptic agents.
- **Carbamazepine**, as well as some other antiepileptic agents that block sodium channels, can be effective in treating trigeminal neuralgia.
- **Capsaicin and lidocaine** may provide relief when applied topically.

TREATMENT OF CHRONIC PRIMARY PAIN

The National Institute for Clinical Care (UK) recently concluded that in people suffering from chronic primary pains, pharmacological treatment with some antidepressants (**amitriptyline, citalopram, duloxetine, fluoxetine, paroxetine** and **sertraline**) can be beneficial (NICE Guideline, 2021) but they considered the evidence of efficacy for most other drugs currently used to treat chronic primary pain states to be insufficient.

Fibromyalgia is characterised by widespread musculoskeletal pain, fatigue and insomnia. Its cause is unknown, with no obvious characteristic pathology being apparent. It is associated with allodynia. Classical analgesics (i.e. NSAIDs and opioids) are not very effective in treating this disorder. As with chronic secondary pain, some antidepressant drugs can bring relief. However, while **gabapentin and pregabalin** and benzodiazepines (e.g. **clonazepam**, **zopiclone**; see Ch. 45) are currently used to treat fibromyalgia, convincing evidence of their efficacy is still lacking.

OTHER DRUGS USED TO TREAT PAIN

Nefopam, an inhibitor of amine uptake with some sodium channel-blocking properties, is sometimes used in the treatment of persistent pain unresponsive to opioid drugs. It does not depress respiration but does produce sympathomimetic and antimuscarinic side effects.

Ketamine, a dissociative anaesthetic (see Ch. 41), **memantine** and **dextromethorphan** work by blocking NMDA receptor channels, and probably reduce the wind-up phenomenon in the dorsal horn (see Fig. 43.2). Given intrathecally, ketamine's effects on memory and cognitive function are largely avoided. It is used for acute relief rather than long-term treatment.

Ziconotide, a synthetic analogue of the N-type calcium-channel blocking peptide ω-conotoxin MVIIA, is effective when administered by the intrathecal route. It is used in patients whose pain does not respond to other analgesic agents. Blockers of low voltage-activated T-type calcium channels may also be effective analgesics in some pain states.

Cannabinoids (see Ch. 18) acting at CB_1 receptors are effective pain-relieving agents in animal models of pain, including models of acute, antinociceptive, inflammatory and neuropathic pain. There is also mounting evidence that these agents are effective in reducing pain in humans (see Barnes and Barnes, 2016). However, good quality, large, long-term randomised controlled trials are required to define their effectiveness in different pain states. The strongest evidence of therapeutic benefit is for central neuropathic pain in multiple sclerosis. Effective cannabinoids include **nabilone** and **dronabinol** (synthetic (−)-trans-Δ^9-tetrahydrocannabinol) as well as natural cannabinoids such as **nabiximols** (formerly known by its trade name **Sativex**). **Nabiximols** is an extract of the cannabis plant containing Δ^9-tetrahydrocannabinol (THC) and cannabidiol that has been suggested to have improved therapeutic efficacy. CB_2 receptor agonists may also be potential analgesic agents.

In addition, cannabinoids and related drugs that lack agonist action at CB_1 receptors have been observed to induce analgesia by potentiating the actions of the inhibitory amino acid glycine at the ionotropic glycine receptor (see Ch. 38) in the spinal cord. This may lead to the development of new therapeutic agents lacking the unwanted effects of CB_1 agonism.

Botulinum toxin injections are effective in relieving back pain and the pain associated with spasticity. This effect is due mainly to a relief of muscle spasm (see Ch. 14).

Ropinirole, **pramipexole** and **rotigotine**, dopamine-receptor agonists (see Ch. 39), are used to treat restless leg syndrome, which can be painful in some individuals.

Clinical uses of analgesic drugs (1)

- Analgesics are used to treat and prevent pain, for example:
  - pre- and postoperatively
  - common painful conditions including headache, dysmenorrhoea, labour, trauma and burns
  - many medical and surgical emergencies (e.g. myocardial infarction and renal colic)
  - terminal disease (especially metastatic cancer)
- Opioid analgesics are used in some non-painful conditions, for example acute heart failure (because of their haemodynamic effects) and terminal chronic heart failure (to relieve distress).
- The choice and route of administration of analgesic drugs depend on the nature and duration of the pain.
- A progressive approach is often used, starting with NSAIDs, supplemented first by weak opioid analgesics and then by strong opioids.
- In general, severe acute pain is treated with strong opioids (e.g. **morphine**, **fentanyl**) given by injection. Mild inflammatory pain (e.g. sprains, mild arthralgia) is treated with NSAIDs (e.g. **ibuprofen**) or by **paracetamol** supplemented by weak opioids (e.g. **codeine**). Severe pain (e.g. cancer pain) is treated with strong opioids given orally, intrathecally, epidurally or by subcutaneous injection. Patient-controlled infusion systems are useful postoperatively.
- Chronic neuropathic pain is less responsive to NSAIDS or opioids and can be treated with tricyclic antidepressants (e.g. **amitriptyline**) or anticonvulsants (e.g. **carbamazepine**, **gabapentin**).

Clinical uses of analgesic drugs (2)

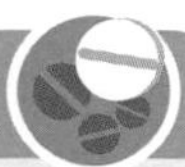

- NSAIDs (see first clinical box), including **paracetamol**, are useful for musculoskeletal and dental pain and for dysmenorrhoea. They reduce opioid requirements in acute (e.g. postoperative) and chronic (e.g. bone metastasis) pain.
- Weak opioids (e.g. **codeine**) combined with **paracetamol** are useful in moderately severe pain if non-opioids are not sufficient. **Tramadol** and **tapentadol** (a weak opioid with additional action on 5-HT and noradrenaline uptake) are alternatives.
- Strong opioids (e.g. **morphine**) are used for severe pain, particularly of visceral origin.
- Note that:
  - the intravenous route provides rapid relief from pain and distress;
  - the intravenous dose is much lower than the oral dose because of presystemic metabolism;
  - **morphine** is given orally as a solution or as 'immediate-release' tablets every 4 h;
  - dose is titrated; when the daily requirement is apparent, the preparation is changed to a modified-release formulation to allow once- or twice-daily dosing;
  - **morphine** and **oxycodone** can be given orally in slow-release tablet form;
  - transdermal administration (e.g. patches of **fentanyl**) is an alternative, rapid means of pain relief;
  - adverse effects (nausea, constipation) are anticipated and treated pre-emptively;
  - addiction is not an issue in the setting of terminal care.
- Subanaesthetic doses of **nitrous oxide** (see Ch. 41) are analgesic, and self-administration of a mixture of **nitrous oxide** with oxygen is widely used during labour, following acute injury or for painful dressing changes.

REFERENCES AND FURTHER READING

General

Apkarian, A.V., Bushnell, M.C., Schweinhardt, P., 2013. Representation of pain in the brain. In: McMahon, S.B., Koltzenburg, M., Tracey, I., Turk, D.C. (Eds.), Wall & Melzack's Textbook of Pain, sixth ed. Elsevier, Philadelphia, pp. 111–128.

McMahon, S.B., Koltzenburg, M., Tracey, I., Turk, D.C. (Eds.), 2013. Wall & Melzack's Textbook of Pain, sixth ed. Elsevier, Philadelphia.

Todd, A.J., Koerber, H.R., 2013. Neuroanatomical substrates of spinal nociception. In: McMahon, S.B., Koltzenburg, M., Tracey, I., Turk, D.C. (Eds.), Wall & Melzack's Textbook of Pain, sixth ed. Elsevier, Philadelphia, pp. 77–93.

Yaksh, T.L., 1999. Spinal systems and pain processing: development of novel analgesic drugs with mechanistically defined models. Trends Pharmacol. Sci. 20, 329–337.

TRP channels and ASICs

Dibas, J., Al-Saad, H., Dibas, A., 2019. Basics on the use of acid-sensing ion channel inhibitors as therapeutics. Neural Regen. Res. 14 (3), 395–398.

Jardin, I., Lopez, J.J., Diez, R., et al., 2017. TRPs in pain sensation. Front. Physiol. 8, 392.

Nilius, B., Szallasi, A., 2014. Transient receptor potential channels as drug targets: from the science of basic research to the art of medicine. Pharmacol. Rev. 66, 676–814.

BDNF and TrkA

Mantyh, P.W., Koltzenburg, M., Mendell, L.M., Tive, L., Shelton, D.L., 2011. Antagonism of nerve growth factor-TrkA signaling and the relief of pain. Anesthesiology 115, 189–204.

Opioids

Bagley, E.E., Ingram, S.L., 2020. Endogenous opioid peptides in the descending pain modulatory circuit. Neuropharmacology 173, 108131.

Ballantyne, J.C., Mao, J., 2003. Opioid therapy for chronic pain. N. Engl. J. Med. 349, 1943–1953.

Bingel, U., Tracey, I., Wiech, K., 2012. Neuroimaging as a tool to investigate how cognitive factors influence analgesic drug outcomes. Neurosci. Lett. 520, 149–155.

BMA, 2017. Chronic Pain: Supporting Safer Prescribing of Analgesics. Available at: https://www.bma.org.uk/media/2100/analgesics-chronic-pain.pdf.

Corbett, A.D., Henderson, G., McKnight, A.T., et al., 2006. 75 years of opioid research: the exciting but vain search for the holy grail. Br. J. Pharmacol. 147, S153–S162.

Fujita, W., Gomes, I., Devi, L.A., 2014. Revolution in GPCR signaling: opioid receptor heteromers as novel therapeutic targets: IUPHAR review 10. Br. J. Pharmacol. 171, 4155–4176.

Gillis, A., Kliewer, A., Kelly, E., et al., 2020. Critical assessment of G protein-biased agonism at the μ-opioid receptor. Trends Pharmacol. Sci. 41, 947–959.

Hayhurst, C.J., Durieux, M.E., 2016. Differential opioid tolerance and opioid-induced hyperalgesia: a clinical reality. Anesthesiology 124, 483–488.

Kelly, E., 2013. Efficacy and ligand bias at the μ-opioid receptor. Br. J. Pharmacol. 169, 1430–1446.

Lee, M., Silverman, S.M., Hansen, H., Patel, V.B., Manchikanti, L., 2011. A comprehensive review of opioid-induced hyperalgesia. Pain Physician 14, 145–161.

McQuay, H., 1999. Opioids in pain management. Lancet 353, 2229–2232.

Roeckel, L.A., Le Coz, G.M., Gavériaux-Ruff, C., Simonin, F., 2016. Opioid-induced hyperalgesia: cellular and molecular mechanisms. Neuroscience 338, 160–182.

Rollason, V., Samer, C., Piquet, V., et al., 2008. Pharmacogenetics of analgesics: towards the personalization of prescription. Pharmacogenomics 9, 905–933.

Sawynok, J., 2003. Topical and peripherally acting analgesics. Pharmacol. Rev. 55, 1–20.

Stannard, C., 2016. Opioids and chronic pain: using what we know to change what we do. Curr. Opin. Support. Palliat. Care 10, 129–136.

Williams, J.T., Ingram, S.L., Henderson, G., et al., 2013. Regulation of μ-opioid receptors: desensitization, phosphorylation, internalization, and tolerance. Pharmacol. Rev. 65, 223–254.

Chronic pain

Barnes, M.P., Barnes, J.C., 2016. Cannabis: The Evidence for Medical Use. All Party Parliamentary Group on Drug Policy Reform Report. Available at: https://www.drugsandalcohol.ie/26086/1/Cannabis_medical_use_evidence.pdf.

Dworkin, R.H., O'Connor, A.B., Audette, J., et al., 2010. Recommendations for the pharmacological management of neuropathic pain: an overview and literature update. Mayo Clin. Proc. 85 (Suppl. 3), S3–S14.

NICE Guideline, 2021. Chronic Pain (Primary and Secondary) in over 16s: Assessment of All Chronic Pain and Management of Chronic Primary Pain. Available at: https://www.nice.org.uk/guidance/ng193/chapter/Recommendations#managing-chronic-primary-pain.

Treede, R.D., Rief, W., Barke, A., et al., 2019. Chronic pain as a symptom or a disease: the IASP classification of chronic pain for the international classification of diseases (ICD-11). Pain 160, 19–27.

Local anaesthetics and other drugs affecting sodium channels

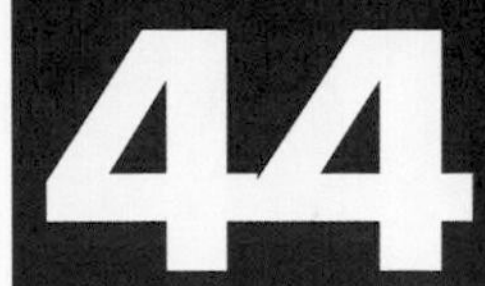

OVERVIEW

As described in Chapter 4, the property of electrical excitability is what enables the membranes of nerve and muscle cells to generate propagated action potentials, which are essential for communication in the nervous system and for the initiation of mechanical activity in striated muscle. Initiation of the action potential depends on voltage-gated sodium channels, which open transiently when the membrane is depolarised. Here we discuss local anaesthetics, which act mainly by blocking sodium channels, and mention briefly other drugs that affect sodium-channel function.

There are, broadly speaking, two ways in which channel function may be modified, namely block of the channels and modification of gating behaviour. Blocking sodium channels reduces excitability. On the other hand, different types of drugs can either facilitate channel opening, and thus increase excitability, or inhibit channel opening and reduce excitability.

LOCAL ANAESTHETICS

Although many drugs can, at high concentrations, block voltage-sensitive sodium channels and inhibit the generation of the action potential, the only drugs used clinically for this effect are the local anaesthetics, various antiepileptic and analgesic drugs (see Chs 42, 43 and 46) and class I antidysrhythmic drugs (see Ch. 20).

HISTORY

Coca leaves have been chewed for their psychotropic effects for thousands of years (see Ch. 49) by Native South American tribes, who knew about the numbing effect they produced on the mouth and tongue. **Cocaine** was isolated in 1860 and proposed as a local anaesthetic for surgical procedures. Sigmund Freud, who tried unsuccessfully to make use of its 'psychic energising' power, gave some cocaine to his ophthalmologist friend in Vienna, Carl Köller, who reported in 1884 that reversible corneal anaesthesia could be produced by dropping cocaine on to the eye. The idea was rapidly taken up, and within a few years cocaine anaesthesia was introduced into dentistry and general surgery. A synthetic substitute, **procaine**, was discovered in 1905, and many other useful compounds were later developed.

CHEMICAL ASPECTS

Local anaesthetic molecules consist of an aromatic part linked by an ester or amide bond to a basic side chain (Fig. 44.1). They are weak bases, with pK_a values mainly in the range 8–9, so that they are mainly, but not completely, ionised at physiological pH (see Ch. 9 for an explanation of how pH influences the ionisation of weak bases). This is important in relation to their ability to penetrate the nerve sheath and axon membrane; quaternary derivatives such as QX-314, which are fully ionised irrespective of pH, are ineffective as local anaesthetics but have important experimental uses. **Benzocaine**, an atypical local anaesthetic, has no basic group.

The presence of the ester or amide bond in local anaesthetic molecules is important because of its susceptibility to metabolic hydrolysis. The ester-containing compounds are fairly rapidly inactivated in the plasma and tissues (mainly liver) by non-specific esterases. Amides are more stable, and these anaesthetics generally have longer plasma half-lives.

MECHANISM OF ACTION

Local anaesthetics block the initiation and propagation of action potentials by preventing the voltage-dependent increase in Na^+ conductance (see Ch. 4 and Hille, 2001; Strichartz and Ritchie, 1987). At low concentrations they decrease the rate of rise of the action potential, increasing its duration, and increase the refractory period thus reducing the firing rate. At higher concentrations they prevent action potential firing. Currently available local anaesthetic agents do not, by and large, distinguish between different sodium-channel subtypes, although their potencies vary (see Ch. 4). They block sodium channels by physically plugging the transmembrane pore (Fig 44.2), interacting with various amino acid residues of the S6 transmembrane helical domains of the channel protein (see Catterall et al., 2020).

Local anaesthetic activity is strongly pH dependent, being increased at alkaline extracellular pH (i.e. when the proportion of ionised molecules is low) and reduced at acid pH. This is because the compound first needs to penetrate the nerve sheath and the axon membrane to gain access to the pore of the sodium channel (where the local anaesthetic-binding site resides). Because the ionised form is not membrane-permeant, penetration is very poor at acid pH. Once inside the pore, it is primarily the ionised form of the local anaesthetic molecule that binds to the channel and blocks it (Fig. 44.2), the unionised form having only weak channel-blocking activity. This pH dependence can be clinically important, because the extracellular fluid of inflamed tissues is often relatively acidic and such tissues are thus somewhat resistant to local anaesthetic agents.

Many drugs that block sodium channels do so in a state-dependent manner, depending on the resting membrane potential and the frequency of action potential firing. They exhibit the property of *'use-dependent' block* of sodium channels, as well as affecting, to some extent, the gating of the channels. Use-dependence means that the more the channels are opened, the greater the block becomes. It is a prominent feature of the action of many class I antidysrhythmic drugs (see Ch. 20) and antiepileptic drugs (see Ch. 46), and occurs because the blocking molecule enters the channel much more readily when the channel is open than when it is closed. Furthermore, for local anaesthetics that rapidly dissociate

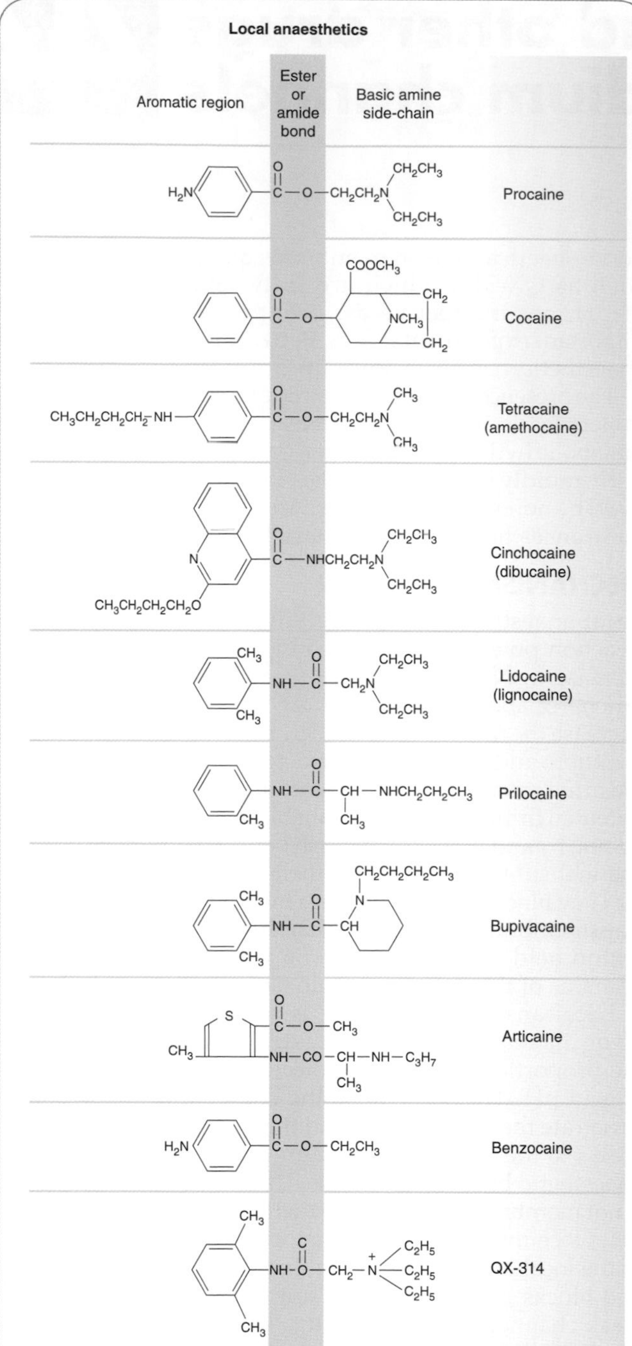

Fig. 44.1 Structures of some local anaesthetics. The general structure of local anaesthetic molecules consists of an aromatic group *(left)*, ester or amide group *(shaded blue)* and amine group *(right)*.

from the channel, block only occurs at high frequencies of action potential firing when the time between action potentials is too short for drug dissociation from the channel to occur. The channel can exist in three functional states: resting, open and inactivated (see Ch. 4). Many local anaesthetics bind most strongly to the inactivated state of the channel. Therefore, at any given membrane potential, the equilibrium between resting and inactivated channels will, in the presence of a local anaesthetic, be shifted in favour of the inactivated state, and this factor contributes to the overall blocking effect by reducing the number of channels available for opening, and by prolonging the refractory period following an action potential. The passage of a train of action potentials, for example, in response to a painful stimulus, causes the channels to cycle through the open and inactivated states, both of which are more likely to bind local anaesthetic molecules than the resting state; thus both mechanisms contribute to use-dependence, which explains in part why pain transmission may be blocked more effectively than other sensory modalities.

Quaternary amine local anaesthetics only work when applied to the inside of the membrane and the channels must be cycled through their open state a few times before the blocking effect appears. With tertiary amine local anaesthetics, block can develop even if the channels are not open, and it is likely that the blocking molecule (uncharged) can reach the channel either directly from the membrane phase through fenestrations in the channel protein that allow uncharged molecules to access the pore of the channel in the resting (closed) state or from the intracellular side via the open gate (see Fig. 44.2). The fenestrations can change size and shape in the inactivated state and this might explain the preferential binding of local anaesthetics and related drugs to inactivated sodium channels. The relative importance of the two blocking pathways – the hydrophobic pathway via the fenestrations and the hydrophilic pathway via the inner mouth of the channel – varies according to the chemical properties of the drug.

In general, local anaesthetics block conduction in small-diameter nerve fibres more readily than in large fibres. Because nociceptive impulses are carried by Aδ and C fibres (see Ch. 43), pain sensation is blocked more readily than other sensory modalities (touch, proprioception, etc.). Motor axons, being large in diameter, are also relatively resistant. The differences in sensitivity among different nerve fibres, although easily measured experimentally, are not of much practical importance, and it is not possible to block pain sensation without affecting other sensory modalities.

Local anaesthetics, as their name implies, are mainly used to produce local nerve block. At low concentrations, they are also able to suppress the spontaneous action potential discharge in sensory neurons that occurs in neuropathic pain (see Ch. 43). The properties of individual local anaesthetic drugs are summarised in Table 44.1.

UNWANTED EFFECTS

When used clinically as local anaesthetics, the main unwanted effects involve the central nervous system (CNS) and the cardiovascular system (see Table 44.1). Their action on the heart can also be of use in treating cardiac arrhythmias (see Ch. 20). Although local anaesthetics are usually administered in such a way as to minimise their spread to other parts of the body, they are ultimately absorbed into the systemic circulation.

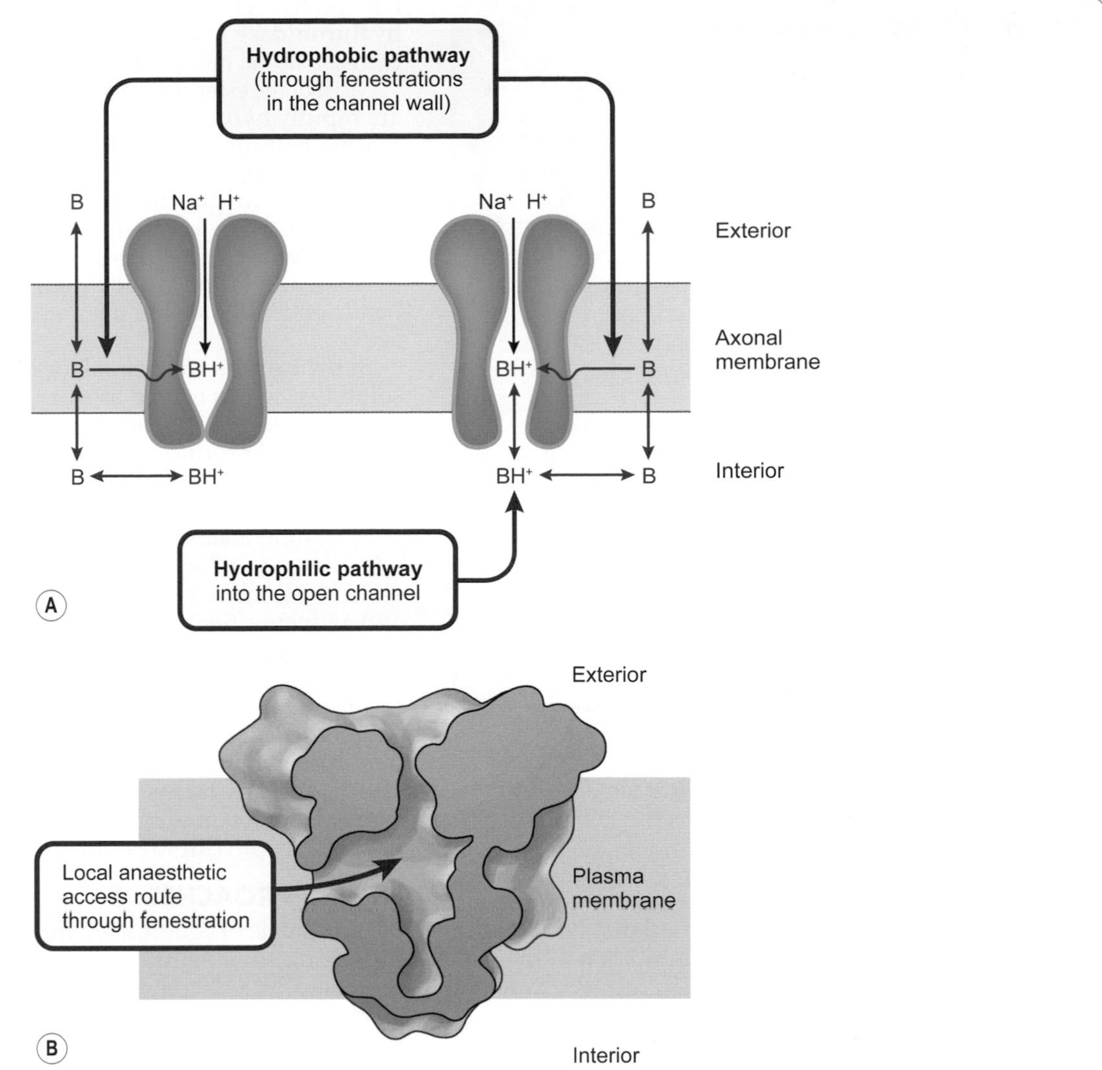

Fig. 44.2 (A) Interaction of local anaesthetics with sodium channels. The blocking site within the channel can be reached via the open channel gate on the inner surface of the membrane by the charged species BH^+ *(hydrophilic pathway)*, or directly from the membrane through fenestrations in the channel wall by the uncharged species B *(hydrophilic pathway)*. (B) Side view section through the sodium channel crystal structure showing a fenestration in the channel wall through which a local anaesthetic can enter and block the pore. (Adapted from Catterall, W.A., Swanson, T.M., 2015. Structural basis for pharmacology of voltage-gated sodium and calcium channels. Mol. Pharmacol. 88, 141–150.)

They may also be injected into veins or arterioles in error.

Most local anaesthetics produce a mixture of depressant and stimulant effects on the CNS. Depressant effects predominate at low plasma concentrations, giving way to stimulation at higher concentrations, resulting in restlessness, tremor and sometimes convulsions, accompanied by subjective effects ranging from confusion to extreme agitation. Further increasing the dose produces profound CNS depression and death due to respiratory depression. The only local anaesthetic with markedly different CNS effects is **cocaine** (see Ch. 49), which produces euphoria at doses well below those that cause other CNS effects. This relates to its specific effect to inhibit monoamine uptake, an effect not shared by other local anaesthetics. **Procaine** is particularly liable to produce unwanted central effects, and has been superseded in clinical use by agents such as **lidocaine** and **prilocaine**. Studies with **bupivacaine**, a widely used long-acting local anaesthetic prepared as a racemic mixture of two optical isomers, suggested that its CNS and cardiac effects were mainly due to the *S*(+) isomer. The *R*(−) isomer (**levobupivacaine**) has a better margin of safety.

Actions of local anaesthetics

- Local anaesthetics block action potential generation by blocking sodium channels.
- Local anaesthetics are amphiphilic molecules with a hydrophobic aromatic group and a basic amine group.
- Local anaesthetics are weak bases that act in their cationic form but must reach their site of action by penetrating the nerve sheath and axonal membrane as un-ionised species.
- Many local anaesthetics show use-dependence (depth of block increases with action potential frequency). This arises:
  - because anaesthetic molecules gain access to the channel more readily when the channel is open;
  - because anaesthetic molecules gain access to the channel more readily when the channel is open;
  - because anaesthetic molecules have higher affinity for inactivated than for resting channels.
- Use-dependence is mainly of importance in relation to antidysrhythmic and antiepileptic effects of sodium-channel blockers.
- Local anaesthetics block conduction in peripheral nerves in the following order: small myelinated axons, non-myelinated axons, large myelinated axons. Nociceptive and sympathetic transmission is thus blocked first.
- Sodium-channel block in cardiac muscle and in CNS neurons is exploited in the therapy of cardiac dysrhythmias (see Ch. 20) and epilepsy (see Ch. 46).

The adverse cardiovascular effects of local anaesthetics are due mainly to myocardial depression, conduction block and vasodilatation. Reduction of myocardial contractility probably results indirectly from an inhibition of the Na^+ current in cardiac muscle (see Ch. 20). The resulting decrease of $[Na^+]_i$ in turn reduces intracellular Ca^{2+} stores (see Ch. 4), and this reduces the force of contraction. Interference with atrioventricular conduction can result in partial or complete heart block, as well as other types of dysrhythmia. **Ropivacaine** has less cardiotoxicity than bupivacaine.

Vasodilatation, mainly affecting arterioles, is due partly to a direct effect on vascular smooth muscle, and partly to inhibition of the sympathetic nervous system. This leads to a fall in blood pressure, which may be sudden and life-threatening. Cocaine is an exception in respect of its cardiovascular effects, because of its ability to inhibit noradrenaline reuptake (see Ch. 15). This enhances sympathetic activity, leading to tachycardia, increased cardiac output, vasoconstriction and increased arterial pressure.

Hypersensitivity reactions sometimes occur with local anaesthetics, usually in the form of allergic dermatitis but rarely as an acute anaphylactic reaction. Other unwanted effects that are specific to particular drugs include mucosal irritation (cocaine) and methaemoglobinaemia (which occurs after large doses of prilocaine, because of the production of a toxic metabolite).

PHARMACOKINETIC ASPECTS

Local anaesthetics vary a good deal in the rapidity with which they penetrate tissues, and this affects the rate at which they cause nerve block when injected into tissues, and the rate of onset of, and recovery from, anaesthesia (see Table 44.1; see Becker and Reed, 2012). It also affects their usefulness as surface anaesthetics for application to mucous membranes. They are sometimes administered along with **hyaluronidase** to break down the intercellular matrix and increase tissue permeation of the local anaesthetic.

Most of the ester-linked local anaesthetics (e.g. **tetracaine**) are rapidly hydrolysed by plasma cholinesterase, so their plasma half-life is short. Procaine – now rarely used – is hydrolysed to *p*-aminobenzoic acid, a folate precursor that interferes with the antibacterial effect of sulfonamides (see Ch. 52). The amide-linked drugs (e.g. lidocaine and prilocaine) are metabolised mainly in the liver, usually by *N*-dealkylation rather than cleavage of the amide bond, and the metabolites are often pharmacologically active.

Benzocaine is an unusual local anaesthetic of very low solubility, which is used as a dry powder to dress painful skin ulcers, or as throat lozenges. The drug is slowly released and produces long-lasting surface anaesthesia.[1]

The routes of administration, uses and main adverse effects of local anaesthetics are summarised in Table 44.2.

Most local anaesthetics have a direct vasodilator action, which increases the rate at which they are absorbed into the systemic circulation, thus increasing their potential toxicity and reducing their local anaesthetic action. **Adrenaline (epinephrine)**, **phenylephrine** or **felypressin**, a short-acting vasopressin analogue (see Ch. 33), may be added to local anaesthetic solutions injected locally to cause vasoconstriction. Adrenaline and phenylephrine absorbed into the circulation may induce unwanted cardiovascular effects such as tachycardia and vasoconstriction, and felypressin may cause coronary artery constriction. Their use in patients with cardiovascular disease is contraindicated.

NEW APPROACHES

Blocking specific sodium-channel subtypes is seen as a promising therapeutic strategy for a variety of clinical conditions, including epilepsy (see Ch. 46), neurodegenerative diseases and stroke (see Ch. 40), neuropathic pain (see Ch.

Unwanted effects and pharmacokinetics of local anaesthetics

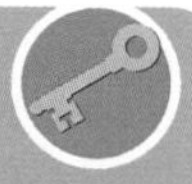

- Local anaesthetics are either esters or amides. Esters are rapidly hydrolysed by plasma and tissue esterases, and amides are metabolised in the liver. Plasma half-lives are generally short, about 1–2 h.
- Unwanted effects are due mainly to escape of local anaesthetics into the systemic circulation.
- Main unwanted effects are:
  - CNS effects, namely agitation, confusion, tremors progressing to convulsions and respiratory depression;
  - cardiovascular effects, namely myocardial depression and vasodilatation, leading to a fall in blood pressure;
  - occasional hypersensitivity reactions.
- Local anaesthetics vary in the rapidity with which they penetrate tissues, and in their duration of action. **Lidocaine** (lignocaine) penetrates tissues readily and is suitable for surface application; **bupivacaine** has a particularly long duration of action.

[1]Benzocaine is also used in 'endurance' condoms to delay ejaculation.

Table 44.1 Properties of local anaesthetics

Drug	Onset	Duration	Tissue penetration	Plasma half-life (h)	Main unwanted effects	Notes
Cocaine	Medium	Medium	Good	~1	Cardiovascular and CNS effects owing to block of amine uptake	Rarely used, only as a nasal spray for upper respiratory tract analgesia
Procaine	Medium	Short	Poor	<1	CNS: restlessness, shivering, anxiety, occasionally convulsions followed by respiratory depression Cardiovascular system: bradycardia and decreased cardiac output; vasodilatation, which can cause cardiovascular collapse	The first synthetic agent No longer used **Chloroprocaine** is also short acting and is used to produce intrathecal anaesthesia
Lidocaine (lignocaine)	Rapid	Medium	Good	~2	As procaine but less tendency to cause CNS effects	Widely used for local anaesthesia Also used intravenously for treating ventricular dysrhythmias, although no longer as first choice (Ch. 20)
Mepivacaine	Rapid	Medium	Good	~2	As procaine	Less vasodilatation (may be administered without a vasoconstrictor)
Tetracaine (amethocaine)	Very slow	Long	Moderate	~1	As lidocaine	Applied topically to the eye for ocular anaesthesia, **Proxymetacaine** and **oxybuprocaine** also used in this way May be applied to skin before venepuncture or venous cannulation
Bupivacaine	Slow	Long	Moderate	~2	As lidocaine but greater cardiotoxicity due to slow dissociation from sodium channels	Widely used because of long duration of action that can be further extended when formulated as a slow-release liposomal preparation (see Ch. 9) **Ropivacaine** is similar, with less cardiotoxicity **Levobupivacaine** causes less cardiotoxicity and CNS depression than the racemate, bupivacaine
Prilocaine	Medium	Medium	Moderate	~2	No vasodilator activity Can cause methaemoglobinaemia	Widely used; not for obstetric analgesia because of risk of neonatal methaemoglobinaemia
Articaine	Rapid	Short	Good	~0.5	As lidocaine	Used in dentistry While its chemical structure contains an amide linkage it also has an ester group on a side chain (see Fig. 44.1). Hydrolysis of the side chain inactivates the drug
Benzocaine	Rapid	Short	Good	<1	As procaine May cause methemoglobinemia	Used for surface anaesthesia. Not for use in children

CNS, Central nervous system.

Table 44.2 Methods of administration, uses and adverse effects of local anaesthetics

Method	Uses	Drug(s)	Notes and adverse effects
Surface anaesthesia	Nose, mouth, trachea and bronchi (usually in spray form), cornea, urinary tract, uterus (for hysteroscopy), rectum and anus (to treat painful haemorrhoids) Not very effective for skin[a]	**Lidocaine, tetracaine (amethocaine), cinchocaine (dibucaine), benzocaine**	Risk of systemic toxicity when high concentrations and large areas are involved **Chloroethane** (ethyl chloride) applied to the skin produces a mild chilling and local numbing. It can be used for minor surgical procedures
Infiltration anaesthesia	Direct injection into tissues to reach nerve branches and terminals Used in minor surgery	Most	**Adrenaline** (epinephrine) or **felypressin** often added as vasoconstrictors (not with fingers or toes, for fear of causing ischaemic tissue damage) Suitable for only small areas, otherwise serious risk of systemic toxicity
Intravenous regional anaesthesia	LA injected intravenously distal to a pressure cuff to arrest blood flow; remains effective until the circulation is restored Used for limb surgery	Mainly **lidocaine, prilocaine**	Risk of systemic toxicity when cuff is released prematurely; risk is small if cuff remains inflated for at least 20 min
Nerve block anaesthesia	LA is injected close to nerve trunks (e.g. brachial plexus, intercostal or dental nerves) to produce a loss of sensation peripherally Used for surgery, dentistry, analgesia	Most	Less LA needed than for infiltration anaesthesia Accurate placement of the needle is important Onset of anaesthesia may be slow Duration of anaesthesia may be increased by addition of vasoconstrictor
Spinal anaesthesia[b]	LA injected into the subarachnoid or intrathecal space (containing cerebrospinal fluid) to act on spinal roots and spinal cord Sometimes formulated with glucose ('hyperbaricity') so that spread of LA can be controlled by tilting the patient Used for surgery to the abdomen, pelvis or leg LA can be used alone or in conjunction with a general anaesthetic to reduce stress Provides good postoperative pain relief	Mainly **lidocaine**	Main risks are bradycardia and hypotension (owing to sympathetic block), respiratory depression (owing to effects on phrenic nerve or respiratory centre); avoided by minimising cranial spread Postoperative urinary retention (block of pelvic autonomic outflow) is common
Epidural anaesthesia[c]	LA injected into epidural space, blocking spinal roots Uses as for spinal anaesthesia; also for painless childbirth	Mainly **lidocaine, bupivacaine, ropivacaine**	Unwanted effects similar to those of spinal anaesthesia but less probable, because longitudinal spread of LA is reduced Postoperative urinary retention common

[a]Surface anaesthesia does not work well on the skin, although a non-crystalline mixture of lidocaine and prilocaine (eutectic mixture of local anaesthetics, or EMLA) has been developed for application to the skin, producing complete anaesthesia in about 1 h. Lidocaine is available in a patch preparation that can be applied to the skin to reduce pain in conditions such as post-herpetic neuralgia (shingles).
[b]Use of spinal anaesthesia is declining in favour of epidural administration.
[c]Intrathecal or epidural administration of LA in combination with an opioid (see Ch. 43) produces more effective analgesia than can be achieved with the opioid alone. Only a small concentration of LA is needed, insufficient to produce appreciable loss of sensation or other side effects. The mechanism of this synergism is unknown, but the procedure has proved useful in pain treatment.
LA, Local anaesthetic.

43) and myopathies (see Ch. 20). As our understanding of the role of specific sodium-channel subtypes in different pathophysiological situations increases, so too will be the likelihood that selective blocking agents can be developed for use in different clinical situations.

OTHER DRUGS THAT AFFECT SODIUM CHANNELS

TETRODOTOXIN AND SAXITOXIN

Tetrodotoxin (TTX) is produced by a marine bacterium and accumulates in the tissues of a poisonous Pacific fish, the puffer fish. The puffer fish is regarded in Japan as a special delicacy, partly because of the mild tingling sensation that follows eating its flesh. To serve it in public restaurants, however, the chef must be registered as sufficiently skilled in removing the toxic organs (especially liver and ovaries) to make the flesh safe to eat. Accidental TTX poisoning is quite common, nonetheless. Historical records of long sea voyages often contained reference to attacks of severe weakness, progressing to complete paralysis and death, caused by eating puffer fish. It was suggested that the powders used by voodoo practitioners to induce zombification may contain TTX but this is disputed.

Saxitoxin (STX) is produced by a marine microorganism that sometimes proliferates in very large numbers and even colours the sea, giving the *red tide* phenomenon. At such times, marine shellfish can accumulate the toxin and become poisonous to humans.

These toxins, unlike conventional local anaesthetics, act exclusively from the outside of the membrane. Both are complex molecules, bearing a positively charged guanidinium moiety. The guanidinium ion is able to permeate voltage-sensitive sodium channels, and this part of the TTX or STX molecule lodges in the channel, while the rest of the molecule blocks its outer mouth. In the manner of its blockade of sodium channels, TTX can be likened to a champagne cork. In contrast to local anaesthetics, there is no interaction between the gating and blocking reactions with TTX or STX – their association and dissociation are independent of whether the channel is open or closed. Some voltage-sensitive sodium channels expressed in cardiac muscle or up-regulated in sensory neurons in neuropathic pain (i.e. $Na_V1.5$, $Na_V1.8$ and $Na_V1.9$) are relatively insensitive to TTX (see Ch. 43).

Both TTX and STX are unsuitable for clinical use as local anaesthetics, being expensive to obtain from their exotic sources and poor at penetrating tissues because of their very low lipid solubility. They have, however, been important as experimental tools for the study of sodium channels (see Ch. 4).

AGENTS THAT AFFECT SODIUM-CHANNEL GATING

Various substances modify sodium-channel gating in such a way as to *increase* the probability of opening of the channels (see Hille, 2001). They include various toxins, mainly from frog skin (e.g. batrachotoxin), scorpion or sea anemone venoms; plant alkaloids such as **veratridine**; and insecticides such as dichlorodiphenyltrichloroethane (DDT) and the pyrethrins. They facilitate sodium-channel activation so that sodium channels open at more negative potentials close to the normal resting potential; they also inhibit inactivation, so that the channels fail to close if the membrane remains depolarised. The membrane thus becomes hyperexcitable, and the action potential is prolonged. Spontaneous discharges occur at first, but the cells eventually become permanently depolarised and inexcitable. All these substances affect the heart, producing extrasystoles and other dysrhythmias, culminating in fibrillation; they also cause spontaneous discharges in nerve and muscle, leading to twitching and convulsions. The very high lipid solubility of substances like DDT makes them effective as insecticides, for they are readily absorbed through the integument. Drugs in this class are useful as experimental tools for studying sodium channels but have no clinical uses.

Clinical uses of local anaesthetics

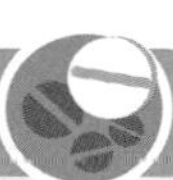

- Local anaesthetics may be injected into soft tissue (e.g. of gums) or to block a nerve or nerve plexus.
- Co-administration of a vasoconstrictor (e.g. **adrenaline**) prolongs the local effect.
- Lipid-soluble drugs (e.g. **lidocaine**) are absorbed from mucous membranes and are used as surface anaesthetics.
- **Bupivacaine** has a slow onset but long duration. It is often used for epidural blockade (e.g. to provide continuous epidural blockade during labour) and spinal anaesthesia. Its isomer **levobupivacaine** is less cardiotoxic if it is inadvertently administered into a blood vessel.

REFERENCES AND FURTHER READING

Becker, D.E., Reed, K.L., 2012. Local anesthetics: review of pharmacological considerations. Anesth. Progr. 59, 90–102.

Catterall, W.A., Lenaeus, M.J., Gamal El-Din, T.M., 2020. Structure and pharmacology of voltage-gated sodium and calcium channels. Annu. Rev. Pharmacol. Toxicol. 60, 133–154.

Hille, B., 2001. Ionic Channels of Excitable Membranes. Sinauer, Sunderland.

Strichartz, G.R., Ritchie, J.M., 1987. The action of local anaesthetics on ion channels of excitable tissues. Handb. Exp. Pharmacol. 81, 21–52.

45 Anxiolytic and hypnotic drugs

OVERVIEW

In this chapter we discuss the nature of anxiety and the drugs used to treat it (anxiolytic drugs), as well as drugs used to treat insomnia (hypnotic drugs). Historically there was overlap between these two groups, reflecting the fact that older anxiolytic drugs commonly caused a degree of sedation and drowsiness. Newer anxiolytic drugs show much less sedative effect and other hypnotic drugs have been introduced that lack specific anxiolytic effects. Many of the drugs now used to treat anxiety were first developed, and are still used, to treat other disorders such as depression (see Ch. 48), epilepsy (see Ch. 46) and schizophrenia (see Ch. 47). Here we will focus on their use as anxiolytics.

THE NATURE OF ANXIETY AND ITS TREATMENT

The normal fear response to threatening stimuli comprises several components, including defensive behaviours, autonomic reflexes, arousal and alertness, corticosteroid secretion and negative emotions. It is also normal to experience these reactions in anticipation of activities which are associated with a fearful or stressful situations, but these should be transient and not adversely affect normal activities. The distinction between a 'pathological' and a 'normal' state of anxiety is not clear-cut but to meet the diagnosis of an anxiety disorder the symptoms need to cause significant personal distress and be associated with impairments to everyday function. The term *anxiety* is applied to several distinct disorders. A useful division of anxiety disorders that may help to explain why different types of anxiety respond differently to different drugs is (i) disorders that involve *fear* (panic attacks and phobias) and (ii) those that involve a more general feeling of *anxiety* (often categorised as general anxiety disorder).

Anxiety disorders recognised clinically include the following:

- *generalised anxiety disorder* (an ongoing state of excessive anxiety lacking any clear reason or focus)
- *social anxiety disorder or social phobia* (fear of being with and interacting with other people)
- *phobias* (strong fears of specific objects or situations, e.g. snakes, open spaces, flying)
- *panic disorder* (sudden attacks of overwhelming fear that occur in association with marked somatic symptoms, such as sweating, tachycardia, chest pains, trembling and choking). Such attacks can be induced experimentally in normal individuals by infusion of sodium lactate or exposure to inhalation of 35% CO_2.
- *post-traumatic stress disorder* (PTSD; distress triggered by recall of past stressful experiences)
- *obsessive–compulsive disorder* (recurrent obsessive ruminations, images or impulses, and/or recurrent physical or mental rituals driven by unfounded and specific anxieties, e.g. fear of contamination).
- *illness anxiety disorder* (a somatic symptom related disorder characterised by excessive or disproportionate preoccupations with having or acquiring a serious illness).

Extensive descriptions of anxiety disorders can be found in *DSM-5*.[1]

Treatment of anxiety disorders requires careful consideration of the individual patient, probable cause and severity of the symptoms (Fig. 45.1). Psychological therapies are important as well as drug treatments and, for most patients, drug treatments alone are unlikely to achieve long-term recovery. The traditional approach to treating anxiety was the use of anxiolytic/hypnotic agents (i.e. benzodiazepines and barbiturates). These drugs are referred to as sedative anxiolytics as they produce both anxiolytic effects at low doses and sedation at higher doses. However, the sedative side effects even at low doses, amnesic effects and propensity to induce tolerance and physical dependence limit their value for the long-term treatment of anxiety disorders. Anxiolytic effects have been observed with drugs also used to treat other brain disorders (e.g. some antidepressants, antiepileptic and antipsychotic drugs) or 5-hydroxytryptamine (5-HT)$_{1A}$-receptor agonists (e.g. **buspirone**) that have no hypnotic effects and this has led to a new class of non-sedating anxiolytics which are now first-line treatments for most anxiety disorders. Another important distinction between classes of anxiolytics is their rate of onset of clinical benefit, with benzodiazepines acting within 30 min while the antidepressants and buspirone require several weeks of treatment before a benefit becomes apparent. Clinically, the choice of drug needs to consider whether acute management of anxiety is required, e.g. for a patient undergoing a stressful procedure or where they are required in acute situations, versus long-term management where the side effects and abuse liability of the benzodiazepines outweigh their short-term benefits. However, there remain situations where, contrary to the widely used <3-week recommendation, poor response to other treatments leads to their longer-term use despite these risks. Anxiety symptoms are also highly comorbid with depression, and for these patients antidepressants are more likely to provide benefits in the long term even though there is an initial delay in the onset of therapeutic effects.

[1]DSM-5: Diagnostic and Statistical Manual of Mental Disorders. fifth ed. American Psychiatric Association, Washington, DC, 2013.

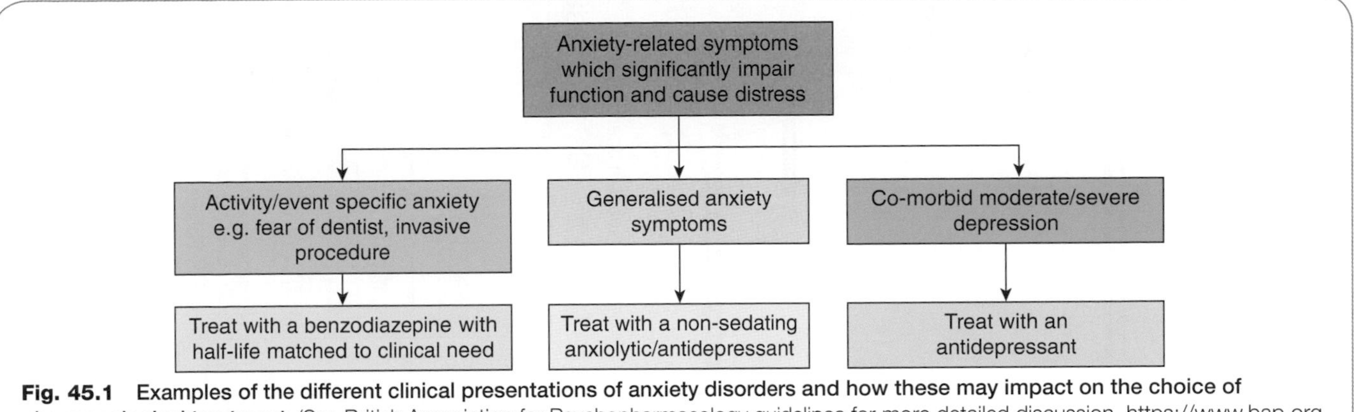

Fig. 45.1 Examples of the different clinical presentations of anxiety disorders and how these may impact on the choice of pharmacological treatment. (See British Association for Psychopharmacology guidelines for more detailed discussion, https://www.bap.org.uk/pdfs/BAP_Guidelines-Anxiety.pdf)

In recent years a number of over-the-counter 'relaxation' drinks containing CNS neurotransmitters, their precursors or other hormones and amino acids have been marketed, without any evidence of efficacy.[2]

MEASUREMENT OF ANXIOLYTIC ACTIVITY

ANIMAL MODELS OF ANXIETY

Anxiety is a state defined by the subjective, self-reported experience of humans and cannot be directly measured in animals; however, many of the behavioural and physiological effects associated with fear or anticipation/expectation of aversive events can be measured in experimental animals. The development of some of the first animal models of anxiety was based on natural behavioural responses which could be modulated by traditional anxiolytic drugs such as benzodiazepines. Methods which capitalised on natural fear behaviours in animals were used to establish pharmacological assays that could be used to predict anxiolytic effects in patients. The 'elevated plus maze' and 'open field test' were developed to capitalise on this behaviour (Fig. 45.2). Rodents spend most of their time in the closed arms or close to the perimeter but administration of benzodiazepine-type anxiolytics reduces time to start exploring and increases the time spent in the open areas but without an increase in motor activity.

An alternative approach is to use learnt behaviours including fear conditioning and conflict tests. Normally, the rat ceases responding or freezes (behavioural inhibition) and an anxiolytic drug reduces this suppressive effect. Other types of psychotropic drug are not effective, nor are analgesic drugs, thus providing some indication of selective anxiolytic effects. However, these fear-related tests and conflict models are less effective for studying non-sedating anxiolytics. The novelty suppressed feeding test is another conflict-type model and depends on a natural response in rodents to a novel environment, hyponeophagia (suppression of food intake). However it still remains a challenge to the development of new anxiolytic drugs to have animal tests that give a good guide to efficacy in humans, and much ingenuity has gone into developing and validating such tests (for more discussion on animal models for anxiety research see Campos et al., 2013, Ennaceur and Chazot, 2016).

[2]Because 'relaxation' drinks are classified as dietary supplements they are not subject to the same efficacy and safety tests as drugs (see Editorial in Nature Neuroscience, 2012, vol. 15, p. 497).

QUANTIFYING ANXIETY IN HUMANS

Diagnosis of anxiety disorders and response to treatment largely depend on subjective self-report questionnaires. Objective methods that directly quantify the physiological and psychological effects of anxiety disorders provide an alternative, and potential more reliable and translational approach. For example, galvanic skin reactions – a measure of sweat secretion – provide a direct measure of autonomic activation in anxiety. Neuropsychological tests, based on computer tasks, have been developed and have revealed that anxiety disorders change a person's responses to certain emotional expressions and words, referred to as affective biases. For example, an anxious patient shows a shift in their attention towards fearful faces referred to as an *attentional bias*. Experimental medicine has also sought to develop human models of anxiety disorders where healthy volunteers are subjected to acute manipulations which generate a transient state of anxiety. An experience akin to a panic attack can be induced in many subjects by breathing a single inhalation of 35% CO_2 whilst a state more akin to generalised anxiety disorder is triggered by a more prolonged period of inhalation of 7.5% CO_2 (see Fig. 45.2).

The challenge remains to develop better human and animal models to study anxiety as well as objective and translational methods to quantify the impacts of anxiety. One example of a translational model is the conflict test described earlier where in humans, substitution of money for food pellets and the use of graded electric shocks as punishment generate similar suppression of responding which is attenuated by administration of the benzodiazepine diazepam although the subjects reported no change in the painfulness of the electric shock.

DRUGS USED TO TREAT ANXIETY

The main groups of drugs are as follows:

- Antidepressants (see Ch. 48 for details). Selective serotonin (5-HT) reuptake inhibitors (SSRIs; e.g. **escitalopram**, **sertraline** and **paroxetine**) and serotonin/noradrenaline reuptake inhibitors (SNRIs; e.g. **venlafaxine and duloxetine**) are effective in the

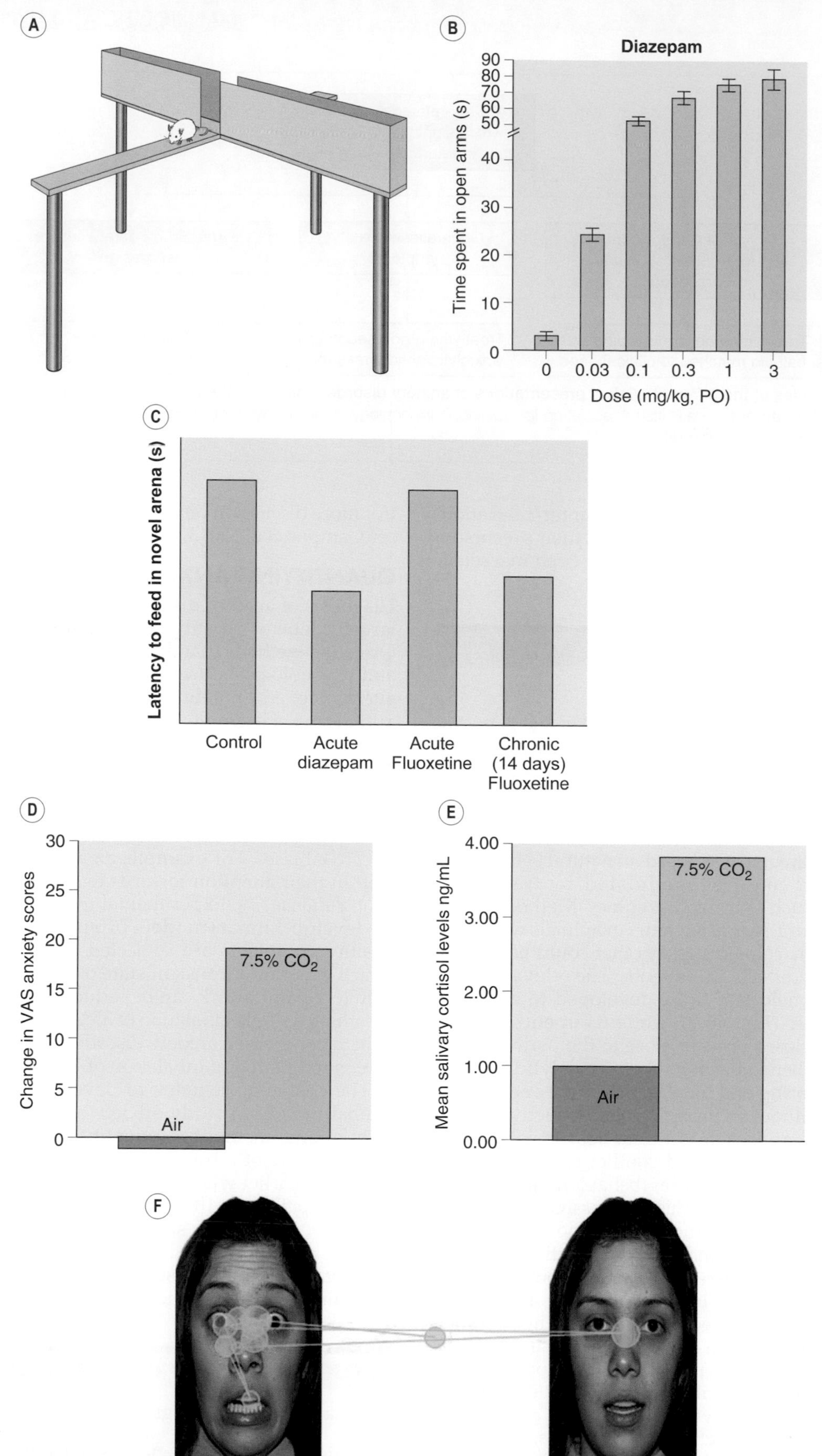

Fig. 45.2 Anxiety testing. (A) Illustration of the elevated plus maze with open and closed arms. (B) Effects of a single dose of diazepam on time spent by rats in the open arms. Each bar represents time spent with movement in the open arms during a 5-min test period. (C) Effects of a single dose of diazepam (benzodiazepine) versus a single or chronic treatment with fluoxetine on novelty suppressed feeding in mice. (D) and (E) Effects of a 7.5% CO_2 challenge for 20 min on anxiety, measured on a visual analogue scale (VAS) and salivary cortisol levels in human subjects. (F) Example of eye tracking and an attentional bias towards a fearful facial image in an anxious individual. *PO,* Oral administration.

treatment of generalised anxiety disorder, phobias, social anxiety disorder, PTSD and obsessive–compulsive disorder. Older antidepressants (tricyclic antidepressants (TCAs) and monoamine oxidase inhibitors (MAOIs)) are also effective, but a lower side-effect profile favours the use of SSRIs. Some of the newer receptor blocking antidepressants (mirtazapine and agomelatine) have effects on 5-HT receptors which may contribute to their anxiolytic effects particularly antagonism at 5-HT_2 receptors. These agents have the additional advantage of reducing depression, which is not uncommonly associated with anxiety. The 5-HT_{1A} partial agonist **buspirone**, whilst not an antidepressant, has been used as an anxiolytic and acts via the serotonin system.
- **Benzodiazepines.** Used to treat acute anxiety. Those used to treat anxiety have a long biological half-life (Table 45.1). They may be co-administered during stabilisation of a patient on an SSRI and may also be useful in patients who have failed to respond to other treatments.
- **Gabapentin** and **pregabalin (gabapentinoids)** are used to treat general anxiety disorder (Wensel et al., 2012), although trial data on gabapentin are limited. Other antiepileptic drugs such as **tiagabine, valproate** and **levetiracetam** (see Ch. 46) may also be effective in treating generalised anxiety disorder.
- Some atypical antipsychotic agents (see Ch. 47) such as **olanzapine**, **risperidone**, **quetiapine** and **ziprasidone** may be effective in generalised anxiety disorder and PTSD.
- β-Adrenoceptor antagonists (e.g. **propranolol**; see Ch. 15). These are used to treat some forms of anxiety, particularly where physical symptoms such as sweating, tremor and tachycardia are troublesome.[3] Their effectiveness depends on block of peripheral sympathetic responses rather than on any central effects.

Antidepressants (see Ch. 48), antiepileptics (see Ch. 46), antipsychotics (see Ch. 47) and β-adrenoceptor antagonists (see Ch. 15) are described in detail elsewhere in this book. Here we will first focus on how drugs affecting the serotonin system are thought to exert their anxiolytic activity and then discuss in detail the benzodiazepines, the primary use of which is to treat anxiety.

Classes of anxiolytic drugs

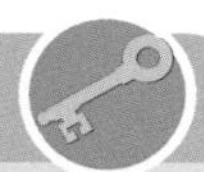

- Antidepressant drugs (SSRIs, SNRIs, TCAs and MAOIs, receptor-blocking antidepressants – see Ch. 48) are effective anxiolytic agents.
- Benzodiazepines are used for treating acute anxiety and insomnia.
- **Gabapentin** and **pregabalin** drugs have anxiolytic properties.
- **Buspirone** is a 5-hydroxytryptamine (5-HT)$_{1A}$-receptor agonist with anxiolytic activity but little sedative effect.
- Some atypical antipsychotic agents (e.g. **quetiapine**) can be useful to treat some forms of anxiety, but have significant unwanted effects.
- β-Adrenoceptor antagonists (e.g. **propranolol**) are used mainly to reduce physical symptoms of anxiety (tremor, palpitations, etc.); no effect on affective component.

Table 45.1 Characteristics of benzodiazepines in humans

Drug(s)	Half-life of parent compound (h)	Active metabolite	Half-life of metabolite (h)	Overall duration of action	Main use(s)
Midazolam[a]	2–4	Hydroxylated derivative	2	Ultrashort (<6 h)	Hypnotic Midazolam used as intravenous anaesthetic and anticonvulsant
Zolpidem[b]	2	No	—	Ultrashort (~4 h)	Hypnotic
Lorazepam, oxazepam, temazepam, lormetazepam	8–12	No	—	Short (12–18 h)	Anxiolytic, hypnotic. Lorazepam used as anticonvulsant
Alprazolam	6–12	Hydroxylated derivative	6	Medium (24 h)	Anxiolytic, antidepressant
Nitrazepam	16–40	No	—	Medium	Anxiolytic, hypnotic[c]
Diazepam, chlordiazepoxide	20–40	Nordazepam	60	Long (24–48 h)	Anxiolytic, muscle relaxant Diazepam used as anticonvulsant
Flurazepam	1	Desmethyl-flurazepam	60	Long	Anxiolytic, hypnotic[c]
Clonazepam	50	No	—	Long	Anticonvulsant, anxiolytic (especially mania)

[a]Another short-acting benzodiazepine, triazolam, has been withdrawn from use in the United Kingdom on account of side effects.
[b]Zolpidem is not a benzodiazepine but acts in a similar manner. Zopiclone and zaleplon are similar.
[c]Due to their long half-life, drowsiness is common on waking.

DELAYED ANXIOLYTIC EFFECT OF DRUGS ACTING VIA SEROTONERGIC MECHANISMS

The time course of clinical improvements in anxiety varies for the different classes and this has important implications for their use (see Fig. 45.1). The anxiolytic effects of SSRIs (e.g. **escitalopram** and **sertraline**) and, where used, **buspirone** are not immediate but take up to 4 weeks to develop after commencing drug therapy. Recent clinical findings suggest that the main effect of these drugs is to generate an emotional blunting which reduces the subjective experience of anxiety and this may be linked to their ability to induce an adaptive change in serotonin receptor expression, particularly 5-HT_{1A} receptors.

5-HT_{1A} receptors are expressed on the soma and dendrites of 5-HT-containing neurons, where they function as inhibitory autoreceptors, as well as being expressed on other types of neuron (e.g. noradrenergic locus coeruleus neurons) where, along with other types of 5-HT receptor (see Ch. 39), they mediate the postsynaptic actions of 5-HT. Postsynaptic 5-HT_{1A} receptors are highly expressed within the cortico-limbic circuits implicated in emotional behaviour. One theory of how SSRIs and buspirone produce their anxiolytic effect is that over time they induce desensitisation of somatodendritic 5-HT_{1A} autoreceptors, resulting in heightened excitation of serotonergic neurons and enhanced 5-HT release (see Ch. 48, Fig. 48.3). This might also explain why early in treatment, anxiety can be worsened by these drugs due to the initial activation of 5-HT_{1A} autoreceptors and inhibition of 5-HT release. Drugs with combined 5-HT_{1A} antagonism and SSRI properties have been developed but have not been found to be effective in man, perhaps because they block both 5-HT_{1A} autoreceptors and postsynaptic receptors, the latter effect occluding the beneficial effect of the former. Elevated 5-HT levels may also induce other postsynaptic adaptations. 5-HT_2 receptors have also been implicated, down-regulation of which may be important for anxiolytic action. Drugs with 5-HT_2 and 5-HT_3 receptor antagonist activity are in clinical trials for treating anxiety and the receptor blocking antidepressants mirtazapine and agomelatine (Ch. 48) block 5-HT_2 receptors. **Vortioxetine** and **vilazodone** exhibit dual action inhibiting the serotonin reuptake transporters and acting as agonists at 5-HT_{1A} receptors and therefore may work like an SSRI and buspirone combined.

Antidepressants as anxiolytic drugs

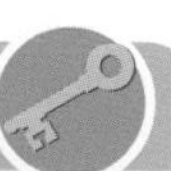

- Anxiolytic effects take days or weeks to develop.
- Antidepressants (selective serotonin reuptake inhibitors (SSRIs), serotonin/noradrenaline reuptake inhibitors SNRIs, tricyclic antidepressants and monoamine oxidase inhibitors (MAOIs) – see Ch. 48):
  - effective treatments for generalised anxiety disorder, phobias, social anxiety disorder and post-traumatic stress disorder;
  - may also reduce depression associated with anxiety.

BENZODIAZEPINES AND RELATED DRUGS

The first benzodiazepine, **chlordiazepoxide**, was synthesised by accident in 1961, the unusual seven-membered ring having been produced as a result of a reaction that went wrong in the laboratories of Hoffman–La Roche. Its unexpected pharmacological activity was recognised in a routine screening procedure, and benzodiazepines quite soon became the most widely prescribed drugs in the pharmacopoeia.

The basic chemical structure of benzodiazepines consists of a seven-membered ring fused to an aromatic ring, with four main substituent groups that can be modified without loss of activity. Thousands of compounds have been made and tested, and about 20 are available for clinical use, the most important ones being listed in Table 45.1. They are basically similar in their pharmacological actions, although some degree of selectivity has been reported. For example, some, such as **clonazepam**, show anticonvulsant activity with less marked sedative effects. From a clinical point of view, differences in pharmacokinetic behaviour among different benzodiazepines (see Table 45.1) are more important than differences in profile of activity. Drugs with a similar structure have been discovered that reverse the effects of the benzodiazepines, for example, **flumazenil** (see later).

The term *benzodiazepine* refers to a distinct chemical structure. Also discussed here are 'Z-drugs' such as **zaleplon**, **zolpidem** and **zopiclone**[4] as well as **abecarnil** – a β-carboline (not licensed for clinical use) – which have different chemical structures but bind to the same sites as the benzodiazepines.

MECHANISM OF ACTION

Benzodiazepines act selectively on $GABA_A$ receptors (see Ch. 38), which mediate inhibitory synaptic transmission throughout the CNS. They act as positive allosteric modulators (see Ch. 2) to facilitate the opening of γ-aminobutyric acid (GABA)–activated chloride channels thus enhancing the response to GABA (see Ch. 38, Fig. 38.5). They bind specifically to a modulatory site on the receptor, distinct from the GABA-binding sites, and act allosterically to increase the affinity of GABA for the receptor. Single-channel recordings show an increase in the frequency of channel opening by a given concentration of GABA, but no change in the conductance or mean open time, consistent with an effect on GABA binding rather than the channel-gating mechanism. Benzodiazepines do not affect receptors for other amino acids, such as glycine or glutamate (see Fig. 45.3).

The $GABA_A$ receptor is a ligand-gated ion channel (see Ch. 3) consisting of a pentameric assembly of different subunits, the main ones being α, β and γ (see Ch. 38). The $GABA_A$ receptor should actually be thought of as a family of receptors as there are six different subtypes of α subunit, three subtypes of β and three subtypes of γ. Although the potential number of combinations is therefore large, certain combinations predominate in the adult brain (see Ch. 38). The various combinations occur in different parts of the brain, have different physiological functions and have subtle differences in their pharmacological properties.

[4]Z-drugs are used primarily to induce sleep and so should perhaps be called 'Zzzzzz drugs'.

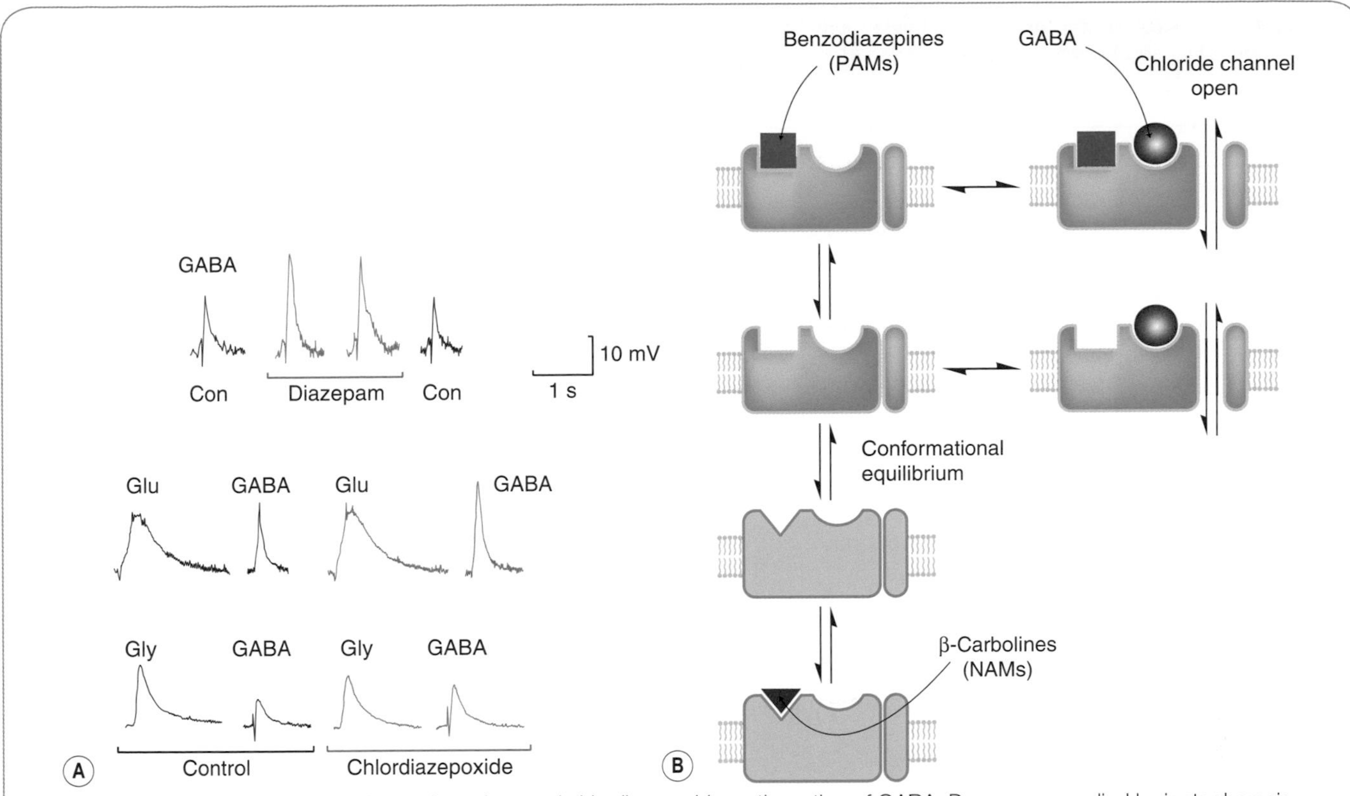

Fig. 45.3 (A) Potentiating effect of benzodiazepines and chlordiazepoxide on the action of GABA. Drugs were applied by iontophoresis to mouse spinal cord neurons grown in tissue culture, from micropipettes placed close to the cells. The membrane was hyperpolarised to −90 mV, and the cells were loaded with Cl^- from the recording microelectrode, so inhibitory amino acids (GABA and glycine (Gly)), as well as excitatory ones (glutamate (Glu)), caused depolarising responses. The potentiating effect of diazepam is restricted to GABA responses, glutamate and glycine responses being unaffected. (B) Model of benzodiazepine/$GABA_A$-receptor interactions. Benzodiazepines and related drugs bind to a modulatory site on the $GABA_A$ receptor distinct from the GABA-binding site. This mode envisages a conformational equilibrium between states in which the benzodiazepine site binds positive allosteric modulators (PAMs) (i) and negative allosteric modulators (NAMs) (ii). In the latter state, the $GABA_A$ receptor has a much reduced affinity for GABA; consequently the chloride channel remains closed. *Con*, Control; *GABA*, γ-aminobutyric acid.

Benzodiazepines bind across the interface between the α and γ subunits but only to receptors that contain γ2 and α1, α2, α3 or α5 subunits. Genetic approaches have been used to study the roles of different subunits in the different behavioural effects of benzodiazepines. Behavioural analysis of mice with various mutations of the $GABA_A$ receptor subunit indicates that α1-containing receptors mediate the anticonvulsant, sedative/hypnotic and addictive effects but not the anxiolytic effect of benzodiazepines, whereas α2-containing receptors mediate the anxiolytic effect, α2-, α3- and α5-containing receptors mediate muscle relaxation and α1- and α5-containing receptors mediate the amnesic effects (Tan et al., 2011).

The obvious next step was to try to develop subunit-selective drugs. Unfortunately, this has proved difficult, due to the structural similarity between the benzodiazepine binding site on different α subunits. The α-subunit selectivity of some benzodiazepines is given in Table 45.2. It was hoped that selective efficacy at α2-containing receptors would produce anxiolytic drugs lacking the unwanted effects of sedation and amnesia. However, such compounds have not translated into human therapeutic agents (Skolnick, 2012). **Pagoclone**, reported to be a full agonist at α3 with less efficacy at α1, α2 and α5, has little or no sedative/hypnotic or amnesic actions. Clinical trials of this drug as a treatment for stammering proved unsuccessful; however, it has been suggested that this could form the basis for a new class of social drugs which could deliver the effects of alcohol with less side effects.

ANTAGONISM AND NEGATIVE ALLOSTERIC MODULATION

Flumazenil is a benzodiazepine-like compound that competes with benzodiazepines at their binding site on $GABA_A$ receptors but has zero efficacy and so acts as an antagonist. Originally reported to lack effects on behaviour or on drug-induced convulsions when given on its own, subsequent studies found it to possess some 'anxiogenic' and proconvulsant activity which may indicate weak negative allosteric modulatory activity. Flumazenil can be used to reverse the effect of benzodiazepine overdosage (normally used only if respiration is severely depressed), or to reverse the effect of benzodiazepines such as midazolam used for minor surgical procedures. Flumazenil acts quickly and effectively when given by injection, but its action lasts for only about 2 h, so drowsiness tends to return. Convulsions may occur in patients treated with flumazenil, and this is more common in patients receiving TCAs (see Ch. 48). Reports that flumazenil improves the mental state of patients with severe liver disease (hepatic

Table 45.2 GABA$_A$-receptor α-subunit selectivity of some therapeutically used benzodiazepines

Drug	Subunit selectivity
Diazepam	α1, α2, α3, α4, α5, α6
Flunitrazepam	α1, α2, α5
Midazolam	α1, α2, α3, α4, α5, α6
Zolpidem	α1
Flumazenil	Antagonist at α1, α2, α3, α4, α5, α6

GABA, γ-aminobutyric acid.
Adapted from Tan, K.R., Rudolph, U., Lüscher, C., 2011. Hooked on benzodiazepines: GABA$_A$-receptor subtypes and addiction. Trends Neurosci. 34, 188–197.

encephalopathy) and alcohol intoxication have not been confirmed in controlled trials.

Drugs that bind to the benzodiazepine site and exert the opposite effect to that of conventional benzodiazepines (negative allosteric modulators, see Ch. 2) produce signs of increased anxiety, panic and convulsions. These include ethyl-β-carboline-3-carboxylate (βCCE) and some benzodiazepine analogues.

PHARMACOLOGICAL EFFECTS AND USES

The main effects of benzodiazepines are:

- reduction of anxiety and aggression;
- induction of sleep (see section on hypnotic drugs);
- reduction of muscle tone;
- anticonvulsant effect;
- anterograde amnesia.

Reduction of anxiety and aggression

Benzodiazepines have rapid anxiolytic effects, reducing anxiety in both humans and animal models following a single dose. With the possible exception of alprazolam (see Table 45.1), benzodiazepines do not have antidepressant effects. Benzodiazepines may paradoxically produce an increase in irritability and aggression in some individuals. This appears to be particularly pronounced with the ultrashort-acting drug triazolam (and led to its withdrawal in the United Kingdom and some other countries), and is generally more common with short-acting compounds. It is probably a manifestation of the benzodiazepine withdrawal syndrome, which occurs with all these drugs but is more acute with drugs whose action wears off rapidly.

Benzodiazepines are recommended for treating acute anxiety states, behavioural emergencies and during procedures such as endoscopy. They are also used as premedication before surgery (both medical and dental). Under these circumstances their anxiolytic, sedative and amnesic properties may be beneficial. Intravenous midazolam can be used to induce anaesthesia (see Ch. 41).

Reduction of muscle tone

Benzodiazepines reduce muscle tone by a central action on GABA$_A$ receptors, primarily in the spinal cord.

Increased muscle tone is a common feature of anxiety states in humans and may contribute to the aches and pains, including headache, that often trouble anxious patients. The relaxant effect of benzodiazepines may therefore be clinically useful. A reduction of muscle tone appears to be possible without appreciable loss of coordination. However, with intravenous administration in anaesthesia and in overdose when these drugs are being used non-medicinally, airway obstruction may occur. Other clinical uses of muscle relaxants are discussed in Chapter 14.

Anticonvulsant effects

All the benzodiazepines have anticonvulsant activity in experimental animal tests. They are highly effective against chemically induced convulsions caused by **pentylenetetrazol, bicuculline** and similar drugs that act by blocking GABA$_A$ receptors (see Chs 38 and 46) but less so against electrically induced convulsions.

Clonazepam (see Table 45.1), **diazepam, midazolam** and **lorazepam** are used to treat epilepsy (see Ch. 46). They can be given intravenously to control life-threatening seizures in status epilepticus. Diazepam can be administered rectally to children to control acute seizures. Tolerance develops to the anticonvulsant actions of benzodiazepines.

Anterograde amnesia

Benzodiazepines prevent memory of events experienced while under their influence, an effect not seen with other CNS depressants. Minor surgical or invasive procedures can thus be performed without leaving unpleasant memories. **Flunitrazepam** (better known to the general public by one of its trade names, Rohypnol) is infamous as a date rape drug and victims frequently have difficulty in recalling exactly what took place during the attack.

Amnesia is thought to be due to benzodiazepines binding to GABA$_A$ receptors containing the α5 subunit. α5-Knock-out mice show an enhanced learning and memory phenotype. This raises the possibility that an α5 subunit-selective negative allosteric modulator could be memory enhancing.

Pharmacokinetic aspects

Benzodiazepines are well absorbed when given orally, usually giving a peak plasma concentration in about 1 h. Some (e.g. oxazepam, lorazepam) are absorbed more slowly. They bind strongly to plasma protein, and their high lipid solubility causes many of them to accumulate gradually in body fat. They are normally given by mouth but can be given intravenously (e.g. diazepam in status epilepticus, midazolam in anaesthesia), buccally or rectally. Intramuscular injection often results in slow absorption.

Benzodiazepines are all metabolised and eventually excreted as glucuronide conjugates in the urine. They vary greatly in duration of action and can be roughly divided into short-, medium- and long-acting compounds (see Table 45.1). Duration of action influences their use, short-acting compounds being useful hypnotics with reduced hangover effect on wakening, long-acting compounds being more useful for use as anxiolytic and anticonvulsant drugs. Several are converted to active metabolites such as *N*-desmethyldiazepam (**nordazepam**), which has a half-life of about 60 h, and which accounts for the tendency of many benzodiazepines to produce cumulative effects and long hangovers when they are given repeatedly. The short-acting compounds are those that are metabolised directly by conjugation with glucuronide.

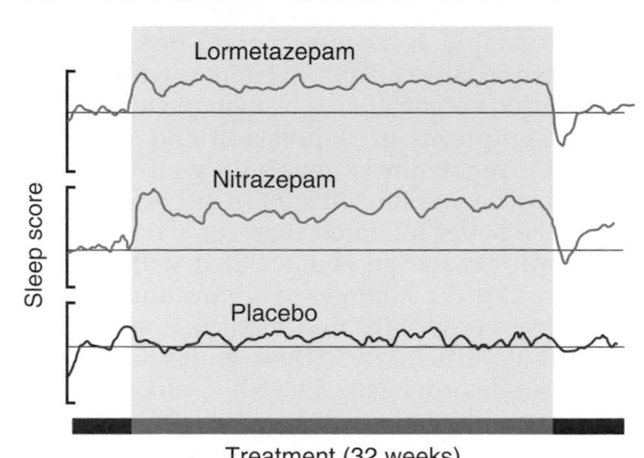

Fig. 45.4 Effects of long-term benzodiazepine treatment on sleep quality. A group of 100 poor sleepers were given, under double-blind conditions, lormetazepam 5 mg, nitrazepam 2 mg or placebo nightly for 24 weeks, the test period being preceded and followed by 4 weeks of placebo treatment. They were asked to assess, on a subjective rating scale, the quality of sleep during each night, and the results are expressed as a 5-day rolling average of these scores. The improvement in sleep quality was maintained during the 24-week test period, and was followed by a 'rebound' worsening of sleep when the test period ended. (From Oswald, I., et al., 1982. Br. Med. J. 284, 860–864.)

Advancing age affects the rate of oxidative reactions more than that of conjugation reactions. Thus the effect of the long-acting benzodiazepines tends to increase with age, and it is common for drowsiness and confusion to develop insidiously for this reason.[5]

UNWANTED EFFECTS

These may be divided into:

- toxic effects resulting from acute overdosage;
- unwanted effects occurring during normal therapeutic use;
- tolerance and dependence.

Acute toxicity

Benzodiazepines in acute overdose are considerably less dangerous than other anxiolytic/hypnotic drugs. Because such agents are often used in attempted suicide, this is an important advantage. In overdose, benzodiazepines cause prolonged sleep, without serious depression of respiration or cardiovascular function. However, in the presence of other CNS depressants, particularly alcohol and opioids, benzodiazepines can cause severe, even life-threatening, respiratory depression. This is a frequent problem when benzodiazepines are used non medicinally (see Chs 50 and 59). The availability of an effective antagonist, flumazenil, means that the effects of an acute overdose can be counteracted,[6] which is not possible for most CNS depressants.

Side effects during therapeutic use

The main side effects of benzodiazepines are drowsiness, confusion, amnesia and impaired coordination, which considerably impairs manual skills such as driving performance. Benzodiazepines enhance the depressant effect of other drugs, including alcohol, in a more than additive way. The long and unpredictable duration of action of many benzodiazepines is important in relation to side effects. Long-acting drugs such as nitrazepam are rarely used as hypnotics, and even shorter-acting compounds such as lorazepam can produce a substantial day-after impairment of job performance and driving skill.

Tolerance and dependence

Tolerance (i.e. a gradual escalation of dose needed to produce the required effect) occurs with all benzodiazepines, as does dependence, which is their main drawback. Tolerance appears to represent a change at the receptor level, but the mechanism is not well understood.

At the receptor level, the degree of tolerance will be governed both by the number of sites occupied (i.e. the dose) and the duration of site occupancy (which may vary according to the therapeutic use). Therefore marked tolerance develops when benzodiazepines are used continuously to treat epilepsy, whereas less tolerance occurs to the sleep-inducing effect of short-acting agents when the subject is relatively drug free during the day. It is not clear to what degree tolerance develops to the anxiolytic effect.

Benzodiazepines produce dependence, and this is a major problem and the main reason they are not recommended as a first-line treatment for anxiety disorders. In human subjects and patients, abrupt cessation of benzodiazepine treatment after weeks or months causes a rebound heightened anxiety, together with tremor, dizziness, tinnitus, weight loss and disturbed sleep due to enhanced rapid eye movement (REM) sleep. It is recommended that benzodiazepines be withdrawn gradually by stepwise lowering of the dose. Withdrawal after chronic administration causes physical symptoms, namely nervousness, tremor, loss of appetite and sometimes convulsions.[7] The withdrawal syndrome is slower in onset than with opioids, probably because of the long plasma half-life of most benzodiazepines. With diazepam, the withdrawal symptoms may take up to 3 weeks to become apparent. Short-acting benzodiazepines cause more abrupt withdrawal effects.

The physical and psychological withdrawal symptoms make it difficult for patients to give up taking benzodiazepines, but craving (i.e. severe psychological dependence that outlasts the physical withdrawal syndrome), which occurs with many drugs of abuse (see Ch. 50), is less of an issue.

[5]At the age of 91 years, the grandmother of one of the authors was growing increasingly forgetful and mildly dotty, having been taking nitrazepam for insomnia regularly for years. To the author's lasting shame, it took a canny general practitioner to diagnose the problem. Cancellation of the nitrazepam prescription produced a dramatic improvement.

[6]In practice, patients are usually left to sleep it off, because there is a risk of seizures with flumazenil; however, flumazenil may be useful diagnostically to rule out coma of other causes.

[7]Withdrawal symptoms can be more severe. A relative of one of the authors, advised to stop taking benzodiazepines after 20 years, suffered hallucinations and one day tore down all the curtains, convinced that they were on fire.

NON-MEDICINAL USE

Benzodiazepines are frequently used for non-medicinal purposes, often taken in combination with other drugs such as opioids or alcohol (see Ch. 50). Most illicit use comes from diversion of prescribed benzodiazepines although illicitly synthesised etizolam has recently become widely available, especially in Scotland. They induce a feeling of calm and reduced anxiety, with users describing a dream state where they are cushioned from reality. The risk of overdose is greatly increased when used in combination with alcohol. Tolerance and physical dependence occur as described earlier.

Benzodiazepines

- Act by binding to a specific allosteric modulatory site on the $GABA_A$ receptor, thus enhancing the inhibitory effect of GABA. Subtypes of the $GABA_A$ receptor exist in different regions of the brain and differ in their functional effects.
- Anxiolytic benzodiazepines are agonists at this modulatory site. Other benzodiazepines (e.g. **flumazenil**) are antagonists or weak negative allosteric modulators and prevent the actions of the anxiolytic benzodiazepines. Strong negative allosteric modulators (not used clinically) are anxiogenic and proconvulsant.
- Anxiolytic effects are mediated by $GABA_A$ receptors containing the $\alpha 2$ subunit, while sedation occurs through those with the $\alpha 1$ subunit.
- Benzodiazepines cause:
  - reduction of anxiety and aggression
  - sedation, leading to improvement of insomnia
  - muscle relaxation and loss of motor coordination
  - suppression of convulsions (antiepileptic effect)
  - anterograde amnesia
- Differences in the pharmacological profile of different benzodiazepines are minor; **clonazepam** appears to have more anticonvulsant action in relation to its other effects.
- Benzodiazepines are active orally and differ mainly in respect of their duration of action. Short-acting agents (e.g. **lorazepam** and **temazepam**, half-lives 8–12 h) are metabolised to inactive compounds and are used mainly as sleeping pills. Some long-acting agents (e.g. **diazepam** and **chlordiazepoxide**) are converted to a long-lasting active metabolite (**nordazepam**).
- Some are used intravenously, for example, **diazepam and lorazepam** in status epilepticus, **midazolam** in anaesthesia.
- Benzodiazepines are relatively safe in overdose. Their main disadvantages are interaction with alcohol, long-lasting 'hangover' effects and the development of tolerance and physical dependence – characteristic withdrawal syndrome on cessation of use.

GABAPENTINOIDS

Originally developed as drugs to treat epilepsy the gabapentinoid, **pregabalin** is now a second-line anxiolytic drug used in patients who do not respond to a serotonergic drug or patients who cannot tolerate the side effects of SSRI/SNRIs (Baldwin et al., 2011). Their clinical effects develop more quickly than those of the SSRIs and are usually apparent within a week of starting treatment but they are not as rapid as the effects of the benzodiazepines. They also have sedative effects. In patients with generalised anxiety disorder, pregabalin has been found to also improve associated symptoms of depression and reduce sleep disturbance. Pregabalin is generally well tolerated but can cause drowsiness and dizziness although these side effects may be better tolerated than some other treatment options. Abrupt cessation is associated with withdrawal suggesting adaptive changes develop and there is an increasing awareness of the non-medicinal potential of the gabapentinoids particularly in those with a history of other substance use disorder (see Ch. 50). Unlike many other anxiolytics, pregabalin is excreted unchanged which may be advantageous in patients with hepatic impairments but not those with renal disease.

OTHER POTENTIAL ANXIOLYTIC DRUGS

PTSD is caused by experiencing stressful, frightening or distressing events. Sufferers often relive the traumatic events through nightmares and flashbacks, and may experience feelings of isolation, irritability and guilt. Symptoms include anxiety, depression and insomnia. If treatment with psychological therapies is unsuccessful then drug therapy with anxiolytic/antidepressant drugs (see Ch. 48) (e.g. **paroxetine**, **sertraline** and **mirtazapine)** may be tried. In addition, hypnotic agents (see later) may aid sleeping.

A recent development has been the recognition that the unpleasant, negative memories that underlie fear are not necessarily permanent. When such memories are reactivated (recalled) they return transiently to a labile state that can be disrupted. In humans, propranolol administered before memory reactivation may erase the negative emotions associated with traumatic memories (see AlOkda et al., 2019). Ketamine, psilocybin, lysergic acid diethylamide (LSD), dimethyltryptamine (found in ayahuasca) and 3,4-methylenedioxymethamphetamine (MDMA or ecstasy) may have a similar effect (Glavonic et al., 2022). Disrupting unpleasant memories in this way may provide a new treatment for PTSD.

Besides the GABA and 5-HT mechanisms discussed before, many other transmitters and hormones have been implicated in anxiety and panic disorders, particularly noradrenaline, glutamate, melatonin, corticotrophin-releasing factor, cholecystokinin (CCK), substance P, neuropeptide Y, galanin, orexins and neurosteroids. The melatonin agonist agomelatine has been licensed to treat depression (Ch. 48), and noradrenaline and serotonin reuptake inhibitors are used as an alternative to SSRIs but other potential targets have yet to yield new treatments

Clinical use of drugs as anxiolytics

- Antidepressants (selective serotonin reuptake inhibitors (SSRIs) or serotonin/noradrenaline reuptake inhibitors (SNRIs)) are now the main drugs used to treat anxiety, especially when this is associated with depression. Their effects are slow in onset (>2 weeks).
- Benzodiazepines are now recommended only as a short-term measure, usually limited to acute relief of severe and disabling anxiety.

DRUGS USED TO TREAT INSOMNIA (HYPNOTIC DRUGS)

Insomnia can be *transient*, in people who normally sleep well but have to do shift work or have jet lag; *short-term*, usually due to illness or emotional upset; or *chronic*, where there is an underlying cause such as anxiety, depression, drug use disorder, pain, pruritus or dyspnoea. While in anxiety and depression the underlying psychiatric condition should be treated, improvement of sleep patterns can improve the underlying condition. The drugs used to treat insomnia are:

- Benzodiazepines. Short-acting benzodiazepines (e.g. lorazepam and temazepam) are used for treating insomnia as they have little hangover effect. The short half-life gives more time drug free so reducing the development of tolerance. Diazepam, which is longer-acting, can be used to treat insomnia associated with daytime anxiety.
- Z-drugs (e.g. **zaleplon**, **zolpidem** and **zopiclone**). Although chemically distinct, these short-acting hypnotics act at the benzodiazepine site on $GABA_A$ receptors containing the α1 subunit. They lack appreciable anxiolytic activity. **Eszopiclone** is the active stereoisomer of zopiclone.
- **Clomethiazole.** It acts as a positive allosteric modulator of $GABA_A$ receptors acting at a site distinct from the benzodiazepines.
- Melatonin receptor agonists. **Melatonin**, **ramelteon** and **tasimelteon** are agonists at MT_1 and MT_2 receptors (see Ch. 39). They are effective in treating insomnia in the elderly and autistic children as well as in totally blind individuals.
- Orexin receptor antagonist. **Suvorexant** is an antagonist of OX_1 and OX_2 receptors which mediate the actions of the orexins, peptide transmitters in the CNS that are important in setting diurnal rhythm. Orexin levels are normally high in daylight and low at night, so the drug reduces wakefulness.
- Antihistamines[8] (see Ch. 25; e.g. **diphenhydramine** and **promethazine**) can be used to induce sleep. They are included in various over-the-counter preparations. **Mirtazapine** is a receptor blocking antidepressant (see Ch. 48) with histamine H_1- and H_2-receptor antagonist properties and many of the older antidepressants (TCAs and MAOIs) as well as some antipsychotic drug (see Table 47.1) include H_1 antagonism and can benefit insomnia.
- Miscellaneous other drugs (e.g. **chloral hydrate** and **meprobamate**). They are no longer recommended, but therapeutic habits die hard and they are occasionally used.

[8]This is an interesting example of an initial unwanted side effect – sedation is undesired when treating hay fever – subsequently becoming a therapeutic use.

INDUCTION OF SLEEP BY BENZODIAZEPINES

Benzodiazepines decrease the time taken to get to sleep, and increase the total duration of sleep, although the latter effect occurs only in subjects who normally sleep for less than about 6 h each night. With agents that have a short duration of action (e.g. zolpidem or temazepam), a pronounced hangover effect on wakening can be avoided.

On the basis of electroencephalography measurements, several levels of sleep can be recognised. Of particular psychological importance are REM sleep, which is associated with dreaming, and slow-wave sleep, which corresponds to the deepest level of sleep when the metabolic rate and adrenal steroid secretion are at their lowest and the secretion of growth hormone is at its highest (see Ch. 33). Most hypnotic drugs reduce the proportion of REM sleep, although benzodiazepines affect it less than other hypnotics, and zolpidem least of all. Artificial interruption of REM sleep causes irritability and anxiety, even if the total amount of sleep is not reduced, and the lost REM sleep is made up for at the end of such an experiment by a rebound increase. The same rebound in REM sleep is seen at the end of a period of administration of benzodiazepines or other hypnotics. The proportion of slow-wave sleep is significantly reduced by benzodiazepines, although growth hormone secretion is unaffected.

Fig. 45.4 shows the improvement of subjective ratings of sleep quality produced by a benzodiazepine, and the rebound decrease at the end of a 32-week period of drug treatment. It is notable that, although tolerance to objective effects such as reduced sleep latency occurs within a few days, this is not obvious in the subjective ratings.

Benzodiazepines are now, however, only recommended for short courses of treatment of insomnia. Tolerance develops over 1–2 weeks with continuous use, and on cessation rebound insomnia and withdrawal occur.

Hypnotic drugs

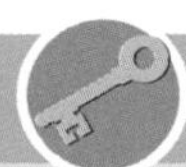

- Drugs that potentiate the action of GABA at $GABA_A$ receptors (e.g. benzodiazepines, **zolpidem**, **zopiclone**, **zaleplon** and **clomethiazole**) are used to induce sleep.
- Drugs with shorter half-lives in the body reduce the incidence of hangover the next morning.
- Drugs with H_1-receptor antagonist properties induce sedation and sleep.
- Drugs with novel mechanisms of action have been developed, e.g. melatonin receptor agonists and orexin receptor antagonists.

Clinical use of hypnotics ('sleeping tablets')

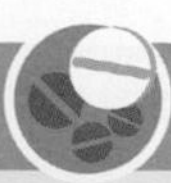

- The cause of insomnia should be established before administering hypnotic drugs. Common causes include alcohol or drug use disorder (see Ch. 50) and physical or psychiatric disorders (especially depression).
- Tricyclic antidepressants (see Ch. 48) cause drowsiness, so can kill two birds with one stone if taken at night by depressed patients with sleep disturbance.
- Optimal treatment of chronic insomnia is often by changing behaviour (e.g. increasing exercise, staying awake during the day) rather than with drugs.
- Benzodiazepines should be used only for short periods (<4 weeks) and for severe insomnia. They can be useful for a few nights when transient factors such as admission to hospital, jet lag or an impending procedure cause insomnia.
- Drugs used to treat insomnia include:
  - benzodiazepines (e.g. **temazepam**) and related drugs (e.g. **zolpidem**, **zopiclone**, which also act at the benzodiazepine binding site);
  - **chloral hydrate** and **triclofos**, which were used formerly in children, but this is seldom justified;
  - sedating antihistamines (e.g. **promethazine**), which cause drowsiness (see Ch. 25) are less suitable for treating insomnia. They can impair performance the next day.

REFERENCES AND FURTHER READING

AlOkda, A.M., Nasr, M.M., Amin, S.N., 2019. Between an ugly truth and a perfect lie: wiping off fearful memories using beta-adrenergic receptors antagonists. J. Cell. Physiol. 234, 5722–5727.

Baldwin, D., Woods, R., Lawson, R., Taylor, D., 2011. Efficacy of drug treatments for generalised anxiety disorder: systematic review and meta-analysis. BMJ 342, d1199.

Bandelow, B., Michaelis, S., Wedekind, 2017. Treatment of anxiety disorders. Dialogues Clin. Neurosci. 19, 93–107.

British Association for Psychopharmacology guidelines for treatment of anxiety disorders. Available at: https://www.bap.org.uk/pdfs/BAP_Guidelines-Anxiety.pdf.

Campos, A.C., V Fogaça, M., Aguiar, D.C., Guimarães, F.S., 2013. Animal models of anxiety disorders and stress. Braz. J. Psychiatry 35 (Suppl. 2), S101–S111.

Ennaceur, A., Chazot, P.L., 2016. Preclinical animal anxiety research – flaws and prejudices. Pharmacol. Res. Perspect. 4, e00223.

Garakani, A., Murrough, J.W., Freire, R.C., et al., 2020. Pharmacotherapy of anxiety disorders: current and emerging treatment options. Front. Psychiatry. 11, 595584.

Glavonic, E., Mitic, M., Adzic, M., 2022. Hallucinogenic drugs and their potential for treating fear-related disorders: through the lens of fear extinction. J. Neurosci. Res. 100, 947–969.

Jacob, T.C., Michels, G., Silayeva, L., Haydonm, J., Succol, F., Moss, S.J., 2012. Benzodiazepine treatment induces subtype-specific changes in $GABA_A$ receptor trafficking and decreases synaptic inhibition. Proc. Natl. Acad. Sci. U. S. A. 109, 18595–18600.

Murrough, J.W., Yaqubi, S., Sayed, S., Charney, D.S., 2015. Emerging drugs for the treatment of anxiety. Expert Opin. Emerg. Drugs 20, 393–406.

Skolnick, P., 2012. Anxioselective anxiolytics: on a quest for the holy grail. Trends Pharmacol. Sci. 33, 611–620.

Tan, K.R., Rudolph, U., Lüscher, C., 2011. Hooked on benzodiazepines: $GABA_A$ receptor subtypes and addiction. Trends Neurosci. 34, 188–197.

Wensel, T.M., Powe, K.W., Cates, M.E., 2012. Pregabalin for the treatment of generalized anxiety disorder. Ann. Pharmacother. 46, 424–429.

46 Antiepileptic drugs

OVERVIEW

In this chapter we describe the nature of epilepsy, the neurobiological mechanisms underlying it and the animal models that can be used to study it. We then proceed to describe the various classes of drugs that are used to treat it, the mechanisms by which they work and their pharmacological characteristics.

Centrally acting muscle relaxants are discussed briefly at the end of the chapter.

INTRODUCTION

Epilepsy is a very common disorder, characterised by *seizures*, which take various forms and result from episodic neuronal discharges, with the form of the seizure depending on the part of the brain affected. Epilepsy affects 0.5%–1% of the population, i.e. ~50 million people worldwide. It may be genetic in origin (often referred to as idiopathic) or develop after brain damage, such as trauma, stroke, infection or tumour growth, or other kinds of neurological disease. In many instances the cause is unknown. Epilepsy is treated mainly with drugs, although brain surgery may be used for suitable severe cases. Current antiepileptic drugs are effective in controlling seizures in about 70% of cases, but their use is often limited by side effects. In addition to their use in patients with epilepsy, antiepileptic drugs are used to treat or prevent convulsions caused by other brain disorders, for example trauma (including following neurosurgery), infection (as an adjunct to antibiotics), brain tumours and stroke. For this reason, they are sometimes termed *anticonvulsants* rather than *antiepileptics*. Increasingly, some antiepileptic drugs have been found to have beneficial effects in non-convulsive disorders such as neuropathic pain (see Ch. 43), bipolar depression (see Ch. 48) and anxiety (see Ch. 45). Many new antiepileptic drugs have been developed over the past 30 years in attempts to improve efficacy and side-effect profiles. Improvements have been steady rather than spectacular, and epilepsy remains a difficult problem.

THE NATURE OF EPILEPSY

The term *epilepsy* is used to define a group of neurological disorders, all of which exhibit periodic seizures. Epilepsy may be genetic in origin or result from structural, infectious, metabolic and immune insults. For information on the underlying causes of epilepsy see Shorvon et al. (2019). As explained later, not all seizures involve convulsions. Seizures are associated with episodic high-frequency discharge of impulses by a group of neurons (sometimes referred to as the *focus*) in the brain. What starts as a local abnormal discharge may then spread to other areas of the brain. The site of the primary discharge and the extent of its spread determine the symptoms that are produced, which range from a brief lapse of attention to a full convulsive seizure lasting for several minutes, as well as odd sensations or behaviours. The particular symptoms produced depend on the function of the region of the brain that is affected. Thus, involvement of the motor cortex causes convulsions, involvement of the hypothalamus causes peripheral autonomic discharge, and involvement of the reticular formation in the upper brain stem leads to loss of consciousness.

Abnormal electrical activity during and following a seizure can be detected by electroencephalography (EEG) recording from electrodes distributed over the surface of the scalp. Various types of seizure can be recognised on the basis of the nature and distribution of the abnormal discharge (Fig. 46.1). Modern brain imaging techniques, such as magnetic resonance imaging and positron emission tomography, are now routinely used in the evaluation of patients with seizures (Fig. 46.2) (Bernasconi et al., 2019).

TYPES OF EPILEPSY

The clinical classification of epilepsy is done on the basis of the characteristics of the seizure rather than on the cause or underlying pathology. There are two major seizure categories, namely *partial* (localised to part of the brain) and *generalised* (involving the whole brain).

PARTIAL SEIZURES

Partial (focal) seizures are those in which the discharge begins locally and often remains localised. The symptoms depend on the brain region or regions involved, and include involuntary muscle contractions, abnormal sensory experiences or autonomic discharge, or the effects on mood and behaviour – often termed *psychomotor epilepsy* – which may arise from a focus within a temporal lobe. The EEG discharge in this type of epilepsy is normally confined to one hemisphere (see Fig. 46.1D). Partial seizures can often be attributed to local cerebral lesions, and their incidence increases with age. In complex partial seizures, loss of consciousness may occur at the outset of the attack, or somewhat later, when the discharge has spread from its site of origin to regions of the brain stem reticular formation. In some individuals, a partial seizure can, during the seizure, become generalised when the abnormal neuronal activity spreads across the whole brain.

An epileptic focus in the motor cortex results in attacks, sometimes called *Jacksonian epilepsy*,[1] consisting of repetitive jerking of a particular muscle group, beginning on one side of the body, often in the thumb, big toe or angle of

[1]After Hughlings Jackson, a distinguished 19th-century Yorkshire neurologist who published his outstanding work in the *Annals of the West Riding Lunatic Asylum*.

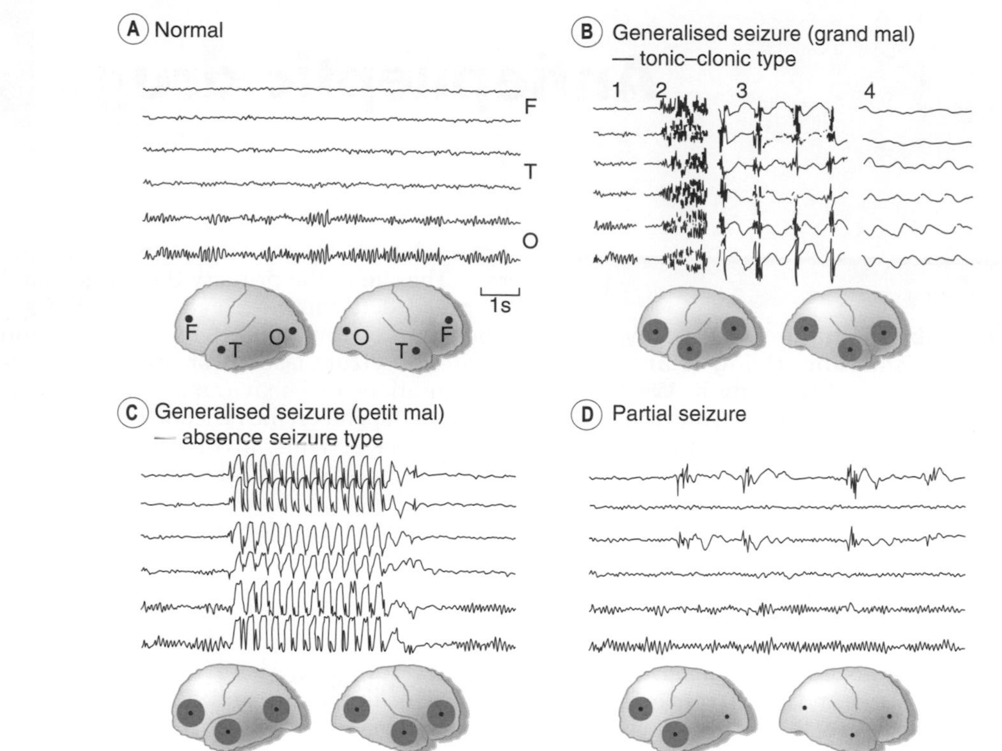

Fig. 46.1 Electroencephalography (EEG) records in epilepsy. (A) Normal EEG recorded from frontal *(F)*, temporal *(T)* and occipital *(O)* sites on both sides, as shown in the inset diagram. The α rhythm (10/s) can be seen in the occipital region. (B) Sections of EEG recorded during a generalised tonic–clonic (grand mal) seizure: *1*, normal record; *2*, onset of tonic phase; *3*, clonic phase; *4*, postconvulsive coma. (C) Generalised absence seizure (petit mal) showing sudden brief episode of 3/s 'spike-and-wave' discharge. (D) Partial seizure with synchronous abnormal discharges in left frontal and temporal regions. (From Eliasson, S.G., et al., 1978. Neurological Pathophysiology, second ed. Oxford University Press, New York.)

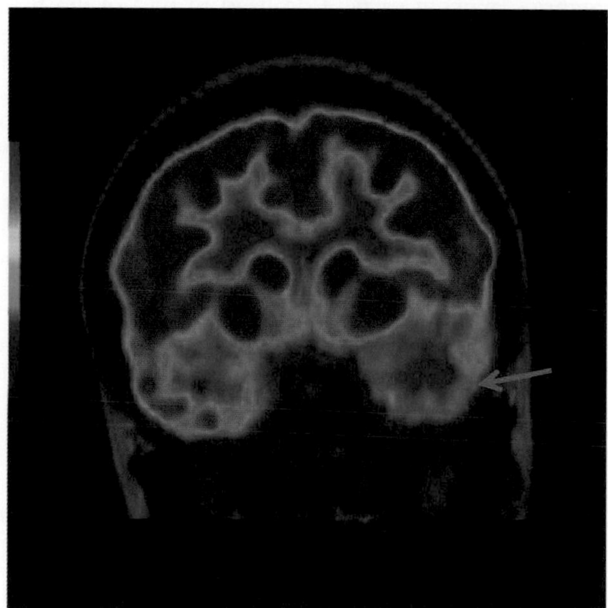

Fig. 46.2 Positron emission tomography (PET) image using [^{18}F]-fluoro-2-deoxyglucose (FDG) of the brain of a female patient suffering from temporal lobe epilepsy. The interictal area of hypometabolism in the left temporal lobe *(arrow)* is suggestive of the site of the epileptic focus. (Image kindly provided by Prof. John Duncan and Prof. Peter Ell, UCL Institute of Neurology, London.)

the mouth, which spreads and may involve much of the body within about 2 min before dying out. The patient loses voluntary control of the affected parts of the body but does not necessarily lose consciousness. In *psychomotor epilepsy* the attack may consist of stereotyped purposive movements such as rubbing or patting movements, or much more complex behaviour such as dressing, walking or hair combing. The seizure usually lasts for a few minutes, after which the patient recovers with no recollection of the event. The behaviour during the seizure can be bizarre and accompanied by a strong emotional response.

GENERALISED SEIZURES

Generalised seizures involve the whole brain, including the reticular system, thus producing abnormal electrical activity throughout both hemispheres. Immediate loss of consciousness is characteristic of generalised seizures. There are a number of types of generalised seizure – two important categories are *tonic–clonic* seizures (formerly referred to as grand mal, see Fig. 46.1B) and *absence seizures* (petit mal, see Fig. 46.1C); others include myoclonic, tonic, atonic and clonic seizures.

A *tonic–clonic seizure* consists of an initial strong contraction of the whole musculature, causing a rigid extensor spasm and an involuntary cry. Respiration stops, and defecation, micturition and salivation often occur. This tonic phase lasts for about 1 min, during which the face is suffused and becomes blue (an important clinical distinction from syncope, the main disorder from which epileptic seizures must be distinguished, where the face is ashen pale), and is followed by a series of violent, synchronous jerks that gradually die out in 2–4 min. The patient stays unconscious for a few more minutes and then gradually recovers, feeling ill and confused. Injury may occur during the convulsive episode. The EEG shows generalised continuous high-frequency activity in the tonic phase and an intermittent discharge in the clonic phase (see Fig. 46.1B).

Absence seizures occur in children; they are much less dramatic but may occur more frequently (many seizures each day) than tonic–clonic seizures. The patient abruptly ceases whatever he or she was doing, sometimes stopping speaking in mid-sentence, and stares vacantly for a few seconds, with little or no motor disturbance. Patients are unaware of their surroundings and recover abruptly with no after-effects. The EEG pattern shows a characteristic rhythmic discharge during the period of the seizure (see Fig. 46.1C). The rhythmicity appears to be due to oscillatory feedback between the cortex and the thalamus, the special properties of the thalamic neurons being dependent on the T-type calcium channels that they express. The pattern differs from that of partial seizures, where a high-frequency asynchronous discharge spreads out from a local focus. Accordingly, the drugs used specifically to treat absence seizures act mainly by blocking T-type calcium channels, whereas drugs effective against other types of epilepsy act mainly by blocking sodium channels or enhancing GABA-mediated inhibition.

A particularly severe kind of epilepsy, *Lennox–Gastaut syndrome*, occurs in children and is associated with progressive intellectual disability, possibly a reflection of excitotoxic neurodegeneration (see Ch. 40).

As detection techniques have advanced it has become increasingly evident that many forms of epilepsy result from genetic abnormalities (Perucca et al., 2020). While some are due to a single genetic mutation, most result from polygenetic mutations. A number of genes associated with familial epilepsies encode neuronal ion channels closely involved in controlling action potential generation (see Ch. 4), such as voltage-gated sodium and potassium channels, GABA receptors and nicotinic acetylcholine receptors (see Weber and Lerche, 2008). Some other genes encode proteins that interact with ion channels.

Status epilepticus refers to a seizure that lasts longer than 5 min, or having more than one seizure within a 5-min period, without returning to a normal level of consciousness between episodes. This is a medical emergency that may lead to permanent brain damage or death.

NEURAL MECHANISMS AND ANIMAL MODELS OF EPILEPSY

The underlying neuronal abnormality in epilepsy is poorly understood. In general, excitation will naturally tend to spread throughout a network of interconnected neurons but is normally prevented from doing so by inhibitory mechanisms. Thus *epileptogenesis* can arise if excitatory transmission is facilitated or inhibitory transmission is reduced (exemplified by $GABA_A$ receptor antagonists causing convulsions; see Ch. 38). In certain respects, epileptogenesis resembles long-term potentiation (see Ch. 38), and similar types of use-dependent synaptic plasticity may be involved. Neurons from which the epileptic discharge originates display an unusual type of electrical behaviour, termed the paroxysmal depolarising shift (PDS), during which the membrane potential suddenly decreases by about 30 mV and remains depolarised for up to a few seconds before returning to normal. A burst of action potentials often accompanies this depolarisation (Fig. 46.3). This event probably results from the abnormally exaggerated and prolonged action of an excitatory transmitter. Activation of *N*-methyl-D-aspartate (NMDA) receptors (see Ch. 38) produces 'plateau-shaped' depolarising responses very similar to the PDS.

Because detailed studies are difficult to carry out on epileptic patients, many different animal models of epilepsy have been investigated (see Bialer and White, 2010; Grone and Baraban, 2015). Genetically altered mouse strains have been reported that show spontaneous seizures. They include knock-out mutations of various ion channels, receptors and other synaptic proteins. Local application of penicillin crystals to the cerebral cortex results in focal seizures, probably by interfering with inhibitory synaptic transmission. Convulsant drugs (e.g. **pentylenetetrazol** [PTZ]) are often used, as are seizures caused by electrical stimulation of the whole brain. In the *kainate model* a single injection of the glutamate receptor agonist kainic acid into the amygdaloid nucleus of a rat can produce spontaneous seizures 2–4 weeks later that continue indefinitely. This is believed to result from excitotoxic damage to inhibitory neurons.

In the *kindling model*, brief low-intensity electrical stimulation of certain regions of the limbic system, such as the amygdala, normally produces no seizure response but if repeated daily for several days, the response gradually increases until very low levels of stimulation will evoke a full seizure, and eventually seizures occur spontaneously. This kindled state can persist indefinitely but is prevented by NMDA receptor antagonists or deletion of the neurotrophin receptor, TrkB, consistent with a mechanism involving synaptic plasticity.

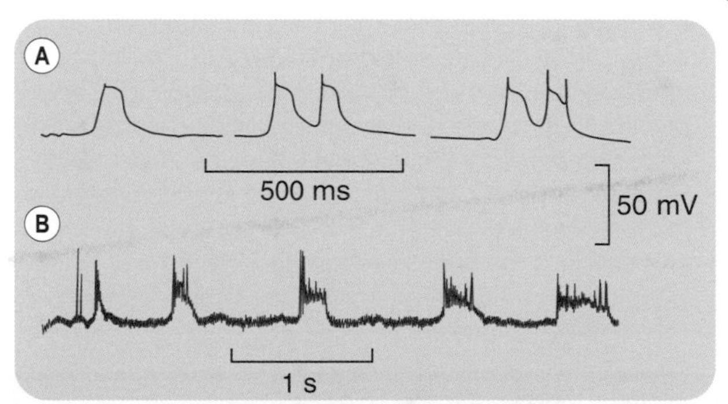

Fig. 46.3 'Paroxysmal depolarising shift' (PDS) compared with experimental activation of glutamate receptors of the *N*-methyl-D-aspartate (NMDA) type. (A) PDS recorded with an intracellular microelectrode from cortical neurons of anaesthetised cats. Seizure activity was induced by topical application of penicillin. (B) Intracellular recording from the caudate nucleus of an anaesthetised cat. The glutamate analogue NMDA was applied by ionophoresis from a nearby micropipette. (A from Matsumoto, H., Marsan, C.A., 1964. Exp. Neurol. 9, 286; panel B from Herrling, P.L. et al., 1983. J. Physiol. 339, 207.)

In human focal epilepsies, surgical removal of a damaged region of cortex may fail to cure the condition, as though the abnormal discharge from the region of primary damage had somehow produced a secondary hyperexcitability elsewhere in the brain. Furthermore, following severe head injury, prophylactic treatment with antiepileptic drugs reduces the incidence of post-traumatic epilepsy, which suggests that a phenomenon similar to kindling may underlie this form of epilepsy.

Most recently, zebrafish have been used to study epileptic phenotypes resulting from genetic manipulation, both gene knock-out and knock-in of specific mutations. There is promise for this approach in the screening of drugs with activity against specific forms of genetic epilepsies (Grone and Baraban, 2015; Gawel et al., 2020).

Nature of epilepsy

- Epilepsy affects about 0.5% of the population.
- The characteristic event is the seizure, which may be associated with convulsions but may take other forms.
- The seizure is caused by an asynchronous high-frequency discharge of a group of neurons, starting locally and spreading to a varying extent to affect other parts of the brain. In absence seizures, the discharge is regular and oscillatory.
- Partial seizures affect localised brain regions, and the attack may involve mainly motor, sensory or behavioural phenomena. Unconsciousness occurs when the reticular formation is involved.
- Generalised seizures affect the whole brain. Two common forms of generalised seizure are the tonic–clonic and the absence seizures. Status epilepticus is a life-threatening condition in which seizure activity is uninterrupted.
- Partial seizures can become secondarily generalised if the localised abnormal neuronal activity subsequently spreads across the whole brain.
- The neurochemical basis of the abnormal discharge is not well understood. It may be associated with enhanced excitatory amino acid transmission, impaired inhibitory transmission or abnormal electrical properties of the affected cells. Several susceptibility genes, mainly encoding neuronal ion channels, have been identified.
- Repeated epileptic discharge can cause neuronal death (excitotoxicity).
- Current drug therapy is effective in 70%–80% of patients.

ANTIEPILEPTIC DRUGS

Antiepileptic (sometimes known as *anticonvulsant*) drugs are used to treat epilepsy as well as non-epileptic convulsive disorders.

When patients fail to respond to single drugs (monotherapy) then combination therapy with two or even three antiepileptic drugs may bring benefit. With optimal drug therapy, epilepsy is controlled completely in about 75% of patients, but about 10% (50,000 in Britain) continue to have seizures at intervals of 1 month or less, which severely disrupts their life and work. There is therefore a need to improve the efficacy of therapy.

Patients with epilepsy usually need to take drugs continuously for many years, so avoidance of side effects and drug interactions (see Ch. 58) is particularly important. Nevertheless, some drugs that have considerable adverse effects are still quite widely used even though they are not drugs of choice for newly diagnosed patients.[2] There is still a need for more effective drugs, and a number of new drugs have been introduced for clinical use. Long-established antiepileptic drugs are listed in Table 46.1. Newer drugs (see Table 46.2) with similar mechanisms of action to older drugs or novel mechanisms of action may offer advantages in terms of efficacy in drug-resistant epilepsies, better pharmacokinetic profile, improved tolerability, lower potential for interaction with other drugs (see Ch. 58) and fewer adverse effects. The appropriate use of drugs from this large available menu depends on many clinical factors (see Shih et al., 2017).

MECHANISM OF ACTION

Antiepileptic drugs aim to inhibit the abnormal neuronal discharge rather than to correct the underlying cause. Three main mechanisms of action appear to be important:

1. Enhancement of GABA action.
2. Inhibition of sodium channel function.
3. Inhibition of calcium channel function.

More recently, newer drugs with other, novel mechanisms of action have been developed.

Antiepileptic drugs may exert more than one beneficial action, prime examples being **valproate** and **topiramate** (see Tables 46.1 and 46.2). The relative importance and contribution of each of these actions to the therapeutic effect are somewhat uncertain.

As with drugs used to treat cardiac dysrhythmias (see Ch. 20), the aim is to prevent the paroxysmal discharge without affecting normal transmission. It is clear that properties such as use dependence and voltage dependence of channel-blocking drugs (see Ch. 4) are important in achieving this selectivity, but our understanding remains fragmentary.

Enhancement of GABA action

Several antiepileptic drugs (e.g. **phenobarbital, stiripentol** and **benzodiazepines**) enhance the activation of $GABA_A$ receptors, thus facilitating the GABA-mediated opening of chloride channels (see Chs 3 and 45).[3] **Vigabatrin** acts by irreversibly inhibiting the enzyme GABA transaminase that is responsible for inactivating GABA (see Ch. 38) in astrocytes and GABAergic nerve terminals. **Tiagabine** is an inhibitor of the 'neuronal' GABA transporter GAT1 that is expressed on GABAergic nerve terminals, and, to a lesser extent, on neighbouring astrocytes, thus inhibiting the removal of GABA from the synapse. It elevates

[2]Bromide was the first antiepileptic agent. Its propensity to induce sedation and other unwanted side effects has resulted in it being largely withdrawn from human medicine, although it is still approved for human use in some countries and may have uses in drug-resistant childhood epilepsies. It is still widely used in veterinary practice to treat epilepsy in dogs and cats.

[3]Absence seizures, paradoxically, are often exacerbated by drugs that enhance GABA activity and better treated by drugs acting by different mechanisms such as T-type calcium-channel inhibition.

Table 46.1 Properties of long-established antiepileptic drugs

Drug	Site of action				Main uses	Main unwanted effect(s)	Pharmacokinetics
	Sodium channel	$GABA_A$ receptor	Calcium channel	Other			
Carbamazepine[a]	+	–	–	–	All types except absence seizures Especially focal seizures such as temporal lobe epilepsy Also trigeminal neuralgia	Sedation, ataxia, blurred vision, water retention, hypersensitivity reactions, leukopenia, liver failure (rare)	Half-life 12–18 h (longer initially) Strong induction of liver enzymes, so risk of drug interactions
Phenytoin[b]	+	–	–	–	All types except absence seizures	Ataxia, vertigo, gum hypertrophy, hirsutism, megaloblastic anaemia, fetal malformation, hypersensitivity reactions	Half-life ~24 h Saturation kinetics, therefore unpredictable plasma levels Plasma monitoring often required
Valproate	+	?+	+	GABA transaminase inhibition	Most types, including absence seizures	Generally less than with other drugs Nausea, hair loss, weight gain, fetal malformations	Half-life 12–15 h
Ethosuximide[c]	–	–	+	–	Absence seizures May exacerbate tonic–clonic seizures	Nausea, anorexia, mood changes, headache	Long plasma half-life (~60 h)
Phenobarbital[d]	?+	+	–	–	All types except absence seizures	Sedation, depression	Long plasma half-life (>60 h) Strong induction of liver enzymes, so risk of drug interactions (e.g. with phenytoin)
Benzodiazepines (e.g. clonazepam, clobazam, lorazepam, midazolam, diazepam)	–	+	–	–	Lorazepam used intravenously to control status epilepticus	Sedation Withdrawal syndrome (see Ch. 45)	See Ch. 45

[a]Oxcarbazepine and eslicarbazepine, recently introduced, are similar; claimed to have fewer side effects.
[b]Fosphenytoin is a water-soluble phenytoin prodrug that is safer than phenytoin when given by injection.
[c]Trimethadione is similar to ethosuximide in that it acts selectively against absence seizures but has greater toxicity (especially the risk of severe hypersensitivity reactions and teratogenicity).
[d]Primidone is pharmacologically similar to phenobarbital and is converted to phenobarbital in the body. It has no clear advantages and is more liable to produce hypersensitivity reactions, so is now rarely used.

Table 46.2 Properties of newer antiepileptic drugs

Drug	Site of action: Sodium channel	Site of action: GABA$_A$ receptor	Site of action: Calcium channel	Site of action: Other	Main uses	Main unwanted effect(s)	Pharmacokinetics
Vigabatrin	–	–	–	GABA transaminase inhibition	All types Appears to be effective in patients resistant to other drugs	Sedation, behavioural and mood changes (occasionally psychosis) Visual field defects	Short plasma half-life, but enzyme inhibition is long-lasting
Lamotrigine	+	–	?+	Inhibits glutamate release	All types	Dizziness, sedation, rashes	Plasma half-life 24–36 h
Gabapentin Pregabalin	–	–	+	–	Partial seizures	Few side effects, mainly sedation	Plasma half-life 6–9 h Excreted unchanged
Tiagabine	–	–	–	Inhibits GABA uptake	Partial seizures	Sedation Dizziness, light-headedness	Plasma half-life ~7 h Liver metabolism
Topiramate	+	?+	?+	AMPA-receptor block	Partial and generalised tonic–clonic seizures Lennox–Gastaut syndrome	Sedation Fewer pharmacokinetic interactions than phenytoin Fetal malformation	Plasma half-life ~20 h Excreted unchanged
Levetiracetam[a]	–	–	–	Binds to SV2A protein	Partial and generalised tonic–clonic seizures	Sedation (slight)	Plasma half-life ~7 h Excreted unchanged
Zonisamide	+	?+	+	–	Partial seizures	Sedation (slight) Appetite suppression, weight loss	Plasma half-life ~70 h
Rufinamide	+	–	–	–	Partial seizures	Headache, dizziness, fatigue	Plasma half-life 6–10 h
Perampanel	–	–	–	Non-competitive AMPA antagonist	Partial seizures	Dizziness, weight gain, sedation impaired coordination changes in mood and behaviour	Plasma half-life 70–100 h
Lacosamide	+	–	–	–	Partial seizures	Nausea and vomiting dizziness, visual disturbances impaired coordination mood changes	Plasma half-life 13 h
Stiripentol	–	+	–	Enhances GABA release	Dravet syndrome	Drowsiness, decreased appetite, agitation, ataxia, weight decreased, hypotonia, nausea, tremor, dysarthria and insomnia	Plasma half-life increases with dose, ranging from 4.5 to 13 h
Cenobamate	+	–	–	Enhances GABA release	Partial seizures	Drowsiness (in up to 40% of people taking the drug), dizziness and fatigue	Plasma half-life increases with dose, and ranges from 30 to 76 h

Table 46.2 Properties of newer antiepileptic drugs—cont'd

Drug	Site of action				Main uses	Main unwanted effect(s)	Pharmacokinetics
	Sodium channel	$GABA_A$ receptor	Calcium channel	Other			
Cannabidiol (CBD)	–	–	–	?	Adjunct treatment of Lennox–Gastaut and Dravet syndromes	Relatively minor – dry mouth, reduced appetite, drowsiness and fatigue, diarrhoea	Plasma half-life 18–32 h
Felbamate	+	+	?+	? NMDA receptor block	Used mainly for severe epilepsy (Lennox–Gastaut syndrome) because of risk of adverse reaction	Few acute side effects but can cause aplastic anaemia and liver damage (rare but serious)	Plasma half-life ~20 h Excreted unchanged
Ganaxolone	–	+	–	–	Seizures associated with CDKL5 deficiency disorder	Drowsiness, dizziness, and fatigue	Biphasic decay with terminal plasma half-life of 37–70 h

[a]Brivaracetam is a structural analogue.
AMPA, α-amino-3-hydroxy-5-methyl-4-isoxazolepropionic acid; *NMDA*, *N*-methyl-D-aspartate; *SV2A*, synaptic vesicle protein 2A.

the extracellular GABA concentration, as measured in microdialysis experiments, and also potentiates and prolongs GABA-mediated synaptic responses in the brain.

Inhibition of sodium channel function

Many antiepileptic drugs (e.g. **carbamazepine, phenytoin, lamotrigine** and **cenobamate**; see Tables 46.1 and 46.2) affect membrane excitability by an action on voltage-dependent sodium channels (see Chs 4 and 44), which carry the inward membrane current necessary for the generation of an action potential. Their blocking action shows the property of use-dependence; in other words, they block preferentially the excitation of cells that are firing repetitively, and the higher the frequency of firing, the greater the block produced. This characteristic, which is relevant to the ability of drugs to block the high-frequency discharge that occurs in an epileptic seizure without unduly interfering with the low-frequency firing of neurons in the normal state, arises from the ability of blocking drugs to discriminate between sodium channels in their resting, open and inactivated states (see Chs 4 and 44). Depolarisation of a neuron (such as occurs in the PDS described previously) increases the proportion of the sodium channels in the inactivated state. Some antiepileptic drugs bind preferentially to channels in this state, preventing them from returning to the resting state, and thus reducing the number of functional channels available to generate subsequent action potentials. **Lacosamide** enhances sodium channel inactivation, but unlike other antiepileptic drugs it appears to affect slow rather than rapid inactivation processes.

Inhibition of calcium channels

Drugs that are used to treat absence seizures (e.g. **ethosuximide** and **valproate**) share the ability to block T-type low-voltage-activated calcium channels (see Ch. 4). T-type channel activity is important in determining the rhythmic discharge of thalamic neurons associated with absence seizures (Khosravani et al., 2004).

Gabapentin, although designed as a simple analogue of GABA that would be sufficiently lipid soluble to penetrate the blood–brain barrier, owes its antiepileptic effect mainly to an action on P/Q-type calcium channels. By binding to a particular channel subunit (α2δ1), both gabapentin and **pregabalin** (a related analogue) reduce the trafficking to the plasma membrane of calcium channels containing this subunit, thereby reducing calcium entry into the nerve terminals and reducing the release of various neurotransmitters and modulators.

Other mechanisms

Many of the newer antiepileptic drugs were developed empirically on the basis of activity in animal models. Their mechanism of action at the cellular level is not fully understood.

Levetiracetam is believed to interfere with neurotransmitter release by binding to synaptic vesicle protein 2A (SV2A), which is involved in synaptic vesicle docking and fusion. **Brivaracetam**, a related antiepileptic agent, also binds to SV2A with 10-fold higher affinity.

While a drug may appear to work by one of the major mechanisms described, close scrutiny often reveals other actions that may also be therapeutically relevant. For example, **phenytoin** not only causes use-dependent block of sodium channels but also affects other aspects of membrane function, including calcium channels and post-tetanic potentiation, as well as intracellular protein phosphorylation by calmodulin-activated kinases, which could also interfere with membrane excitability and synaptic function.

Antagonism at ionotropic excitatory amino acid receptors has been a major focus in the search for new antiepileptic drugs. Despite showing efficacy in animal models, by and large they did not prove useful in the clinic, because the margin between the desired anticonvulsant effect and unacceptable side effects, such as loss of motor coordination, was too narrow. However, **perampanel**, a non-competitive α-amino-3-hydroxy-5-methyl-4-isoxazolepropionic acid (AMPA)-receptor antagonist, has been approved as an add-on treatment for partial seizures.

Mechanism of action of antiepileptic drugs

- The major antiepileptic drugs are thought to act by three main mechanisms:
  - reducing electrical excitability of cell membranes, mainly through use-dependent block of sodium channels;
  - enhancing GABA-mediated synaptic inhibition; this may be achieved by an enhanced postsynaptic action of GABA, by inhibiting GABA transaminase or by inhibiting GABA uptake into neurons and glial cells;
  - inhibiting T-type calcium channels (important in controlling absence seizures).
- Newer drugs act by other mechanisms, some yet to be elucidated.

CARBAMAZEPINE

Carbamazepine is chemically related to the tricyclic antidepressant drugs (see Ch. 48) and was found in a routine screening test to inhibit electrically evoked seizures in mice. Pharmacologically and clinically, its actions resemble those of phenytoin, although it appears to be particularly effective in treating certain partial seizures (e.g. psychomotor epilepsy). It is also used to treat other conditions, such as neuropathic pain (see Ch. 43) and bipolar disorder (see Ch. 48).

Pharmacokinetic aspects

Carbamazepine is slowly but well absorbed after oral administration. Its plasma half-life is about 30 h when it is given as a single dose, but it is a strong inducer of hepatic enzymes, and the plasma half-life shortens to about 15 h when it is given repeatedly. Some of its metabolites have antiepileptic properties. A slow-release preparation is used for patients who experience transient side effects coinciding with plasma concentration peaks following oral dosing.

Unwanted effects

Carbamazepine produces a variety of unwanted effects ranging from drowsiness, dizziness and ataxia to more severe mental and motor disturbances.[4] It can also cause water retention (and hence hyponatraemia; see Ch. 29) and a variety of gastrointestinal and cardiovascular side effects. The incidence and severity of these effects are relatively low, however, compared with other drugs. Treatment is usually started with a low dose, which is built up gradually to avoid dose-related toxicity. Severe bone marrow depression, causing neutropenia, and other severe forms of hypersensitivity reaction can occur, especially in people of Asian origin (see Ch. 12).

Carbamazepine is a powerful inducer of hepatic microsomal enzymes, and thus accelerates the metabolism of many other drugs, such as phenytoin, oral contraceptives, warfarin and corticosteroids, as well as of itself. When starting treatment, the opposite of a 'loading dose' strategy is employed: small initial doses are gradually increased, as when dosing is initiated, metabolising enzymes are not induced and so even low doses may give rise to adverse effects (notably ataxia); as enzyme induction occurs, increasing doses are needed to maintain therapeutic plasma concentrations. In general, it is inadvisable to combine it with other antiepileptic drugs, and interactions with other drugs (e.g. warfarin) metabolised by cytochrome P450 (CYP) enzymes are common and clinically important. **Oxcarbazepine** is a prodrug that is metabolised to a compound closely resembling carbamazepine, with similar actions but less tendency to induce drug-metabolising enzymes. Another structurally related drug, **eslicarbazepine**, may have less effect on metabolising enzymes.

PHENYTOIN

Phenytoin is the most important member of the hydantoin group of compounds, which are structurally related to the barbiturates. It is highly effective in reducing the intensity and duration of electrically induced convulsions in mice, although ineffective against PTZ-induced convulsions. Owing to its many side effects and unpredictable pharmacokinetic behaviour, phenytoin usage is declining. Phenytoin is effective against various forms of partial and generalised seizures, although not against absence seizures, which it may even worsen. **Fosphenytoin** is a phosphorylated, prodrug form of phenytoin that is water soluble and can be administered by intravenous infusion or intramuscular injection in situations where oral phenytoin administration would be inappropriate, e.g. during status epilepticus or vomiting.

Pharmacokinetic aspects

Phenytoin has certain pharmacokinetic peculiarities that need to be taken into account when it is used clinically. It is well absorbed when given orally, and about 80%–90% of the plasma content is bound to albumin. Other drugs, such as salicylates, phenylbutazone and valproate, inhibit this binding competitively (see Ch. 58). This increases the free phenytoin concentration but also increases hepatic clearance of phenytoin, so may enhance or reduce the effect of the phenytoin in an unpredictable way. Phenytoin is metabolised by the hepatic mixed function oxidase system and excreted mainly as glucuronide. It causes enzyme induction, and thus increases the rate of metabolism of other drugs (e.g. oral anticoagulants). The metabolism of phenytoin itself can be either enhanced or competitively inhibited by various other drugs that share the same hepatic enzymes. **Phenobarbital** produces both effects, and because competitive inhibition is immediate whereas induction takes time, it initially enhances and later reduces the pharmacological activity of phenytoin. **Ethanol** has a similar dual effect.

The metabolism of phenytoin shows the characteristic of saturation (see Ch. 10), which means that over the therapeutic plasma concentration range the rate of inactivation does not increase in proportion to the plasma concentration. The consequences of this are that:

[4]One of the authors who was a keen hockey player played in a team with a goalkeeper who sometimes made silly errors early in the match. It turned out that he suffered from epilepsy and had taken his dose of carbamazepine too close to the start of the match.

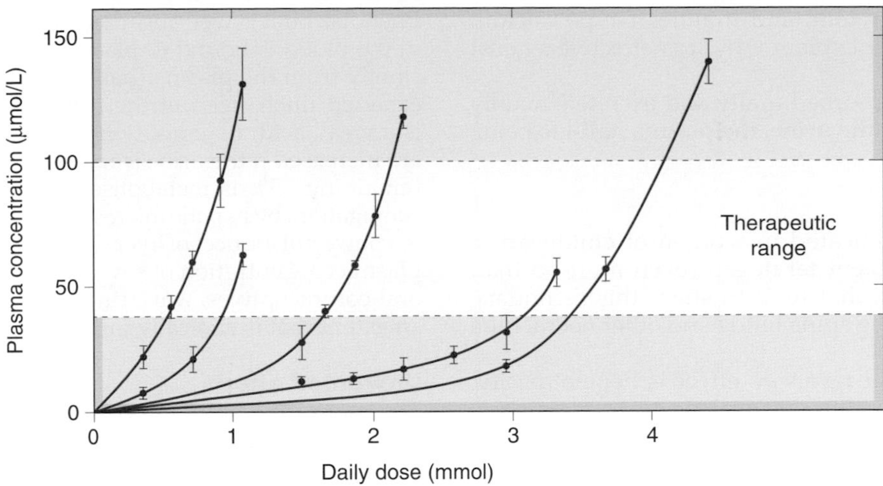

Fig. 46.4 Non-linear relationship between daily dose of phenytoin and steady-state plasma concentration in five individual human subjects. The daily dose required to achieve the therapeutic range of plasma concentrations (40–100 μmol/L) varies greatly between individuals, and for any one individual the dose has to be adjusted rather precisely to keep within the acceptable plasma concentration range. (Redrawn from Richens, A., Dunlop, A., 1975. Lancet 2, 247.)

- the plasma half-life (approximately 20 h) increases as the dose is increased
- the steady-state mean plasma concentration, achieved when a patient is given a constant daily dose, varies disproportionately with the dose. Fig. 46.4 shows that, in one patient, increasing the dose by 50% caused the steady-state plasma concentration to increase more than four-fold.

The range of plasma concentration over which phenytoin is effective without causing excessive unwanted effects is quite narrow (approximately 40–100 μmol/L). The very steep relationship between dose and plasma concentration and the many interacting factors mean that there is considerable individual variation in the plasma concentration achieved with a given dose. Regular monitoring of plasma concentration has helped considerably in achieving an optimal therapeutic effect. The past tendency was to add further drugs in cases where phenytoin alone failed to give adequate control. It is now recognised that much of the unpredictability can be ascribed to pharmacokinetic variability, and regular monitoring of plasma concentration has reduced the use of polypharmacy.

Unwanted effects

Side effects of phenytoin begin to appear at plasma concentrations exceeding 100 μmol/L and may be severe above about 150 μmol/L. The milder side effects include vertigo, ataxia, headache and nystagmus, but not sedation. At higher plasma concentrations, marked confusion with intellectual deterioration occurs; a paradoxical increase in seizure frequency is a particular trap for the unwary prescriber. These effects occur acutely and are quickly reversible. Hyperplasia of the gums often develops gradually, as does hirsutism and coarsening of the features, which probably result from increased androgen secretion. Megaloblastic anaemia, associated with a disorder of folate metabolism, sometimes occurs, and can be corrected by giving folic acid (see Ch. 24). Hypersensitivity reactions, mainly rashes, are quite common. Phenytoin has also been implicated as a cause of the increased incidence of fetal malformations in children born to epileptic mothers, particularly the occurrence of cleft palate, associated with the formation of an epoxide metabolite. Severe idiosyncratic reactions, including hepatitis, skin reactions and neoplastic lymphocyte disorders, occur in a small proportion of patients.

VALPROATE

Valproate is a simple monocarboxylic acid usually administered as the sodium salt (**sodium valproate**). **Valproic acid** acts similarly to sodium valproate **and semisodium valproate** is equimolar amounts of sodium valproate and valproic acid. Valproate is chemically unrelated to any other class of antiepileptic drug, and in 1963 it was discovered quite accidently to have anticonvulsant properties in mice. It inhibits most kinds of experimentally induced convulsions and is effective in many kinds of epilepsy, being particularly useful in certain types of infantile epilepsy, where its low toxicity and lack of sedative action are important, and in adolescents who exhibit both tonic–clonic or myoclonic seizures in addition to absence seizures, because valproate (unlike most antiepileptic drugs) is effective against each. Like carbamazepine, valproate is also used in psychiatric conditions such as bipolar disorder (see Ch. 48).

Valproate works by several mechanisms (see Table 46.1), the relative importance of which remains to be clarified. It causes a significant increase in the GABA content of the brain and is a weak inhibitor of the enzyme system that inactivates GABA, namely GABA transaminase and succinic semialdehyde dehydrogenase (see Ch. 38), but in vitro studies suggest that these effects would be very slight at clinical dosage. Other more potent inhibitors of these enzymes (e.g. **vigabatrin**) also increase GABA content and have an anticonvulsant effect in experimental animals. There is some evidence that it enhances the action of GABA by a postsynaptic action, but no clear evidence that it affects inhibitory synaptic responses. It inhibits sodium channels, but less so than phenytoin, and inhibits T-type calcium channels, which might explain why it is effective against absence seizures.

Valproate is well absorbed orally and excreted, mainly as the glucuronide, in the urine, the plasma half-life being about 15 h.

Unwanted effects

Valproate is contraindicated in women of childbearing age because it is a potent teratogen (even more so than other anticonvulsants that tend to share this secondary pharmacology), causing spina bifida and other neural tube defects.

Another serious but rare side effect is hepatotoxicity. An increase in plasma glutamic oxaloacetic transaminase, which signals liver damage of some degree, commonly occurs, but proven cases of valproate-induced hepatitis are rare. The few cases of fatal hepatitis in valproate-treated patients may well have been caused by other factors. More commonly, valproate causes thinning and curling of the hair, in about 10% of patients.

ETHOSUXIMIDE

Ethosuximide is another drug developed empirically by modifying the barbituric acid ring structure. Pharmacologically and clinically, however, it is different from the drugs so far discussed, in that it is active against PTZ-induced convulsions in animals and against absence seizures in humans, with little or no effect on other types of epilepsy. It supplanted **trimethadione**, the first drug found to be effective in absence seizures, which had major side effects. Ethosuximide is used clinically for its selective effect on absence seizures.

Ethosuximide and trimethadione, unlike other antiepileptic drugs, act mainly by inhibition of T-type calcium channels, which play a role in generating the firing rhythm in thalamic relay neurons that generates the 3/s spike-and-wave EEG pattern characteristic of absence seizures.

Ethosuximide is well absorbed and metabolised and excreted much like phenobarbital, with a plasma half-life of about 60 h. Its main side effects are nausea and anorexia, sometimes lethargy and dizziness, and it is said to precipitate tonic–clonic seizures in susceptible patients. Very rarely, it can cause severe hypersensitivity reactions.

PHENOBARBITAL

Phenobarbital was one of the first barbiturates to be developed but is rarely used nowadays. Its clinical effectiveness closely resembles that of phenytoin; it affects the duration and intensity of artificially induced seizures, rather than the seizure threshold, and is (like phenytoin) ineffective in treating absence seizures. **Primidone** acts by being metabolised to phenobarbital. It may cause hypersensitivity reactions and is rarely used nowadays to treat epilepsy but is used for the treatment of essential tremor (see Ch. 40). The clinical uses of phenobarbital are virtually the same as those of phenytoin, but it is seldom used now because it causes sedation. For some years, phenobarbital was widely used in children, including as prophylaxis following febrile convulsions in infancy, but it can cause behavioural disturbances and hyperkinesias. It is, however, widely used in veterinary practice.

Pharmacokinetic aspects

Phenobarbital is well absorbed, and about 50% of the drug in the blood is bound to plasma albumin. It is eliminated slowly from the plasma (half-life 50–140 h). About 25% is excreted unchanged in the urine. Because phenobarbital is a weak acid, its ionisation and hence renal elimination are increased if the urine is made alkaline (see Ch. 10). The remaining 75% is metabolised, mainly by oxidation and conjugation, by hepatic microsomal enzymes. Phenobarbital is a powerful inducer of liver CYP enzymes, and it lowers the plasma concentration of several other drugs (e.g. steroids, oral contraceptives, warfarin, tricyclic antidepressants) to an extent that is clinically important.

Unwanted effects

The main unwanted effect of phenobarbital is sedation, which often occurs at plasma concentrations within the therapeutic range for seizure control. This is a serious drawback, because the drug may have to be used for years on end. Some degree of tolerance to the sedative effect seems to occur, but objective tests of cognition and motor performance show impairment even during long-term treatment. Other unwanted effects that may occur with clinical dosage include megaloblastic anaemia (similar to that caused by phenytoin), mild hypersensitivity reactions and osteomalacia. Like other barbiturates, it must not be given to patients with porphyria (see Ch. 12). In overdose, phenobarbital depresses brain stem function, producing coma and respiratory and circulatory failure, as do all barbiturates.

BENZODIAZEPINES

Benzodiazepines can be used to treat both acute seizures, especially in children – **midazolam** given buccally or **diazepam** being administered rectally – and status epilepticus (a life-threatening condition in which epileptic seizures occur almost without a break) for which agents such as **lorazepam**, diazepam or **clonazepam** are administered intravenously. The advantage in status epilepticus is that they act very rapidly compared with other antiepileptic drugs. With most benzodiazepines (see Ch. 45), the sedative effect is too pronounced for them to be used for maintenance therapy and tolerance develops over 1–6 months. **Clonazepam** is unique among the benzodiazepines in that in addition to acting at the $GABA_A$ receptor, it also inhibits T-type calcium channels. Both this and the related compound **clobazam** are claimed to be relatively selective as antiepileptic drugs. Sedation is the main side effect of these compounds, and an added problem is the withdrawal syndrome, which results in an exacerbation of seizures if the drug is stopped abruptly.

NEWER ANTIEPILEPTIC DRUGS

VIGABATRIN

Vigabatrin, the first 'designer drug' in the epilepsy field, is a vinyl-substituted analogue of GABA that was designed as an irreversible inhibitor of the GABA-metabolising enzyme GABA transaminase. In animal studies, vigabatrin increases the GABA content of the brain and also increases the stimulation-evoked release of GABA, implying that GABA transaminase inhibition can increase the releasable pool of GABA and effectively enhance inhibitory transmission. In humans, vigabatrin increases the content of GABA in the cerebrospinal fluid. Although its plasma half-life is short, it produces a long-lasting effect because the enzyme is blocked irreversibly, and the drug can be given by mouth once daily.

Vigabatrin's licence is restricted to patients with resistant epilepsy who have not responded or tolerated other appropriate drug combinations. A major drawback of vigabatrin is the development of irreversible peripheral visual field defects in a proportion of patients on long-term therapy, thus necessitating systematic screening examinations of the visual fields at regular intervals. Vigabatrin may cause depression, and occasionally psychotic disturbances and hallucinations, in a minority of patients.

LAMOTRIGINE

Lamotrigine, although chemically unrelated, resembles phenytoin and carbamazepine in its pharmacological effects but it appears that, despite its similar mechanism of action, lamotrigine has a broader therapeutic profile than the earlier drugs, with significant efficacy against absence seizures (it is also used to treat unrelated psychiatric disorders). Its main side effects are nausea, dizziness and ataxia, and hypersensitivity reactions (mainly mild rashes, but occasionally more severe). Its plasma half-life is about 24 h, with no particular pharmacokinetic anomalies, and it is taken orally.

GABAPENTIN AND PREGABALIN

Gabapentin and pregabalin are effective against partial seizures. Side effects (drowsiness, headache, fatigue, dizziness and weight gain) are less severe than with many antiepileptic drugs. The absorption of gabapentin from the intestine depends on the L-amino acid carrier system and shows the property of saturability, which means that increasing the dose does not proportionately increase the amount absorbed. Pregabalin is more readily absorbed from the gut. Gabapentin and pregabalin have a plasma half-life of about 6 h, requiring dosing two to three times daily. As these drugs are excreted unchanged in the urine they must be used with care in patients whose renal function is impaired. Both drugs are also used as analgesics to treat neuropathic pain (see Ch. 43) and as anxiolytics in the treatment of general anxiety disorders (see Ch. 45). Recently gabapentin and pregabalin misuse has become popular, especially amongst heroin users, and may contribute to opioid overdose deaths (see Ch. 50).

TIAGABINE

Tiagabine is an analogue of GABA that is able to penetrate the blood–brain barrier. It has a short plasma half-life and is mainly used as an add-on therapy for partial seizures. Its main side effects are drowsiness and confusion, dizziness, fatigue, agitation and tremor.

TOPIRAMATE

Topiramate is a drug that appears to do a little of everything, blocking sodium and calcium channels, enhancing the action of GABA, blocking AMPA receptors and, for good measure, weakly inhibiting carbonic anhydrase. Its clinical effectiveness resembles that of phenytoin, and it is claimed to produce less severe side effects, as well as being devoid of the pharmacokinetic properties that cause trouble with phenytoin. Currently, it is mainly used as add-on therapy in refractory cases of partial and generalised seizures.

LEVETIRACETAM

Levetiracetam was developed as an analogue of **piracetam**, a drug developed to improve cognitive function, and discovered by accident to have antiepileptic activity in animal models. Unusually, it lacks activity in conventional models such as electroshock and PTZ tests, but is effective in the audiogenic and kindling models. Levetiracetam is excreted unchanged in the urine. Common side effects include headaches, inflammation of the nose and throat, sleepiness, vomiting and irritability. **Brivaracetam** is similar to levetiracetam.

ZONISAMIDE

Zonisamide is a sulfonamide compound originally intended as an antibacterial drug and found accidently to have antiepileptic properties. It is mainly free of major unwanted effects, although it causes drowsiness, and of serious interaction with other drugs. It tends to suppress appetite and cause weight loss and is sometimes used for this purpose. Zonisamide has a long plasma half-life of 60–80 h, and is partly excreted unchanged and partly converted to a glucuronide metabolite. It is licensed for use as an adjunct treatment of partial and generalised seizures but may be effective as a monotherapy.

RUFINAMIDE

Rufinamide is a triazole derivative structurally unrelated to other antiepileptic drugs. It is licensed for treating Lennox–Gastaut syndrome and may also be effective in partial seizures. It has low plasma protein binding and is not metabolised by CYP enzymes.

PERAMPANEL

Perampanel is effective in refractory partial seizures. Side effects include dizziness, sedation, fatigue, irritability, weight gain and loss of motor coordination. There is a risk of serious psychiatric problems (violent, even homicidal, thoughts and threatening behaviour) in some individuals.

LACOSAMIDE

Lacosamide is a functionalised amino acid used alone or in combination with other drugs to treat partial seizures. Side effects include nausea, dizziness, sedation and fatigue. It produces relief of pain caused by diabetic neuropathy.

STIRIPENTOL

Stiripentol is used as an adjunctive therapy for Dravet's syndrome in children. It enhances GABA release and prolongs GABA-mediated synaptic events in a manner similar to phenobarbital. It also inhibits lactate dehydrogenase (LDH) which may reduce the metabolic energy production required to maintain seizures. It inhibits cytochrome P450 isoenzymes and so interacts with several antiepileptic drugs as well as other drugs (see Ch. 58).

CENOBAMATE

Cenobamate is used as an adjunct therapy for partial onset seizures. It is well absorbed from the gut and reaches peak plasma concentrations after 1 to 4 h.

CANNABIDIOL

Cannabidiol, a major phytocannabinoid devoid of the psychoactive properties of **Δ^9-tetrahydrocannabinol** (Δ^9-

THC; see Ch. 18), has been approved for the treatment of Dravet syndrome and Lennox–Gastaut syndrome as well as for seizures associated with tuberous sclerosis complex, a rare genetic condition that causes mainly non-cancerous tumours to develop. The mechanisms underlying its antiepileptic efficacy are unclear as it has low affinity for CB_1 and CB_2 cannabinoid receptors. Other phytocannabinoids may also have anticonvulsant properties.

FELBAMATE

Felbamate is an analogue of an obsolete anxiolytic drug, **meprobamate**. It is active in many animal seizure models and has a broader clinical spectrum than earlier antiepileptic drugs, but its mechanism of action at the cellular level is uncertain. Its acute side effects are mild, mainly nausea, irritability and insomnia, but it occasionally causes severe reactions resulting in aplastic anaemia or hepatitis. For this reason, its recommended use is limited to intractable epilepsy (e.g. in children with Lennox–Gastaut syndrome) that is unresponsive to other drugs. Its plasma half-life is about 24 h, and it can enhance the plasma concentration of other antiepileptic drugs given concomitantly.

NEW DRUGS

There are a number of new antiepileptic agents with novel mechanism of action approved or in late stages of clinical trials.[5] **Ganaxolone**, structurally resembling endogenous neurosteroids (see Ch. 38), is a positive allosteric modulator of $GABA_A$ receptors containing δ subunits that has recently been approved for the treatment of CDLK5 disorder, a rare form of genetic epilepsy predominantly affecting young girls. It may be effective against other forms of epilepsy especially in children. Side effects include drowsiness, dizziness and fatigue. **Everolimus**, an inhibitor of mammalian target of rapamycin (mTOR, see Ch. 25), is in a phase III clinical trial for partial seizures. **Tonabersat** is a novel neuronal gap junction inhibitor that shows early promise.

OTHER USES OF ANTIEPILEPTIC DRUGS

Antiepileptic drugs have proved to have much wider clinical applications than was originally envisaged, and clinical trials have shown many of them to be effective in the following conditions:

- bipolar disorder (**valproate**, **carbamazepine**, **oxcarbazepine**, **lamotrigine**, **topiramate**; see Ch. 48)
- migraine prophylaxis (**valproate**, **gabapentin**, **topiramate**; see Ch. 42)
- anxiety disorders (**gabapentin, pregabalin**; see Ch. 45)
- neuropathic pain (**gabapentin**, **pregabalin**, **carbamazepine**, **lamotrigine, lacosamide**; see Ch. 43)

This surprising multiplicity of clinical indications may reflect the fact that similar neurobiological mechanisms, involving synaptic plasticity and increased excitability of interconnected populations of neurons, underlie each of these disorders.

[5]The Epilepsy Foundation website (http://www.epilepsy.com/accelerating-new-therapies/new-therapies-pipeline#drugs) gives details on the large number of drugs currently in development for the treatment of epilepsies.

ANTIEPILEPTIC DRUGS AND PREGNANCY

There are several important implications for women taking antiepileptic drugs. By inducing hepatic CYP3A4 enzymes, some antiepileptic drugs may increase oral contraceptive metabolism, thus reducing their effectiveness (see Ch. 35). Taken during pregnancy, drugs such as phenytoin, carbamazepine, lamotrigine, topiramate and valproate are thought to have some risk of teratogenic effects, although the magnitude of risk appears greatest with valproate. It remains to be clarified if newer agents also have this problem. Induction of CYP enzymes may result in vitamin K deficiency in the newborn (see Ch. 24).

Clinical uses of antiepileptic drugs

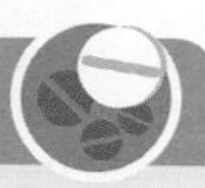

- Generalised tonic–clonic seizures:
  - **valproate**, **lamotrigine** or **carbamazepine**;
  - use of a single drug is preferred, when possible, to avoid pharmacokinetic interactions;
  - newer agents include **topiramate**, **levetiracetam.**
- Partial (focal) seizures: **carbamazepine**, or **lamotrigine**; alternatives include **valproate**, **levetiracetam**, **clobazam**, **gabapentin**, **topiramate**, **levetiracetam.**
- Absence seizures: **ethosuximide**, **valproate**
  - **valproate** is the first-choice drug when absence seizures coexist with tonic–clonic seizures, because most other drugs used for tonic–clonic seizures can worsen absence seizures.
- Myoclonic seizures: **valproate**, **topiramate**, **levetiracetam.**
- Status epilepticus: **lorazepam** intravenously (or in the absence of accessible veins, intramuscular or oromucosal **midazolam** or **diazepam** rectally).
- Neuropathic pain: for example **carbamazepine**, **gabapentin** (see Ch. 43).
- To stabilise mood in mono- or bipolar affective disorder (as an alternative to **lithium**): for example, **carbamazepine**, **valproate** (see Ch. 48).

MUSCLE SPASM AND MUSCLE RELAXANTS

Many diseases of the brain and spinal cord produce an increase in muscle tone, which can be painful and disabling. Spasticity resulting from birth injury or cerebral vascular disease and the paralysis produced by spinal cord lesions are examples. Multiple sclerosis is a neurodegenerative disease that is triggered by inflammatory attack on the central nervous system (see Ch. 40). When the disease has progressed for some years it can cause muscle stiffness and spasms, as well as other symptoms such as pain, fatigue, difficulty passing urine and tremors. Local injury or inflammation, as in arthritis, can also cause muscle spasm, and chronic back pain is also often associated with local muscle spasm.

Certain centrally acting drugs are available that have the effect of reducing the background tone of the muscle without seriously affecting its ability to contract transiently under voluntary control. The distinction between voluntary movements and 'background tone' is not clear-cut, and the selectivity of those drugs is not complete. Postural control, for example, is usually jeopardised by centrally acting muscle relaxants. Furthermore, drugs that affect motor control generally produce rather widespread effects on the central nervous system, and drowsiness and confusion turn out to be very common side effects of these agents.

Baclofen (see Ch. 38) is a chlorophenyl derivative of GABA originally prepared as a lipophilic GABA-like agent in order to assist penetration of the blood–brain barrier, which is impermeable to GABA itself. Baclofen is a selective agonist at $GABA_B$ receptors (see Ch. 38). The antispastic action of baclofen is exerted mainly on the spinal cord, where it inhibits both monosynaptic and polysynaptic activation of motor neurons. It is effective when given by mouth and is used in the treatment of spasticity associated with multiple sclerosis or spinal injury. However, it is ineffective in cerebral spasticity caused by birth injury.

Baclofen produces various unwanted effects, particularly drowsiness, motor incoordination and nausea, and it may also have behavioural effects. It is not useful in epilepsy.

Benzodiazepines are discussed in detail in Chapter 45. They produce muscle relaxation by an effect in the spinal cord. They are also anxiolytic.

Tizanidine is an α_2-adrenoceptor agonist that relieves spasticity associated with multiple sclerosis and spinal cord injury.

For many years anecdotal evidence suggested that smoking **cannabis** (see Ch. 18) relieves the painful muscle spasms associated with multiple sclerosis. **Sativex**, a cannabis extract containing Δ^9-THC (also known as **dronabinol**; see Ch. 18) and cannabidiol, is licensed in some countries as a treatment for spasticity in multiple sclerosis. It also has pain-relieving properties (see Chs 18 and 43).

Methocarbamol is used to treat muscle pain and stiffness. Its mechanism of action is unclear.

Dantrolene acts peripherally rather than centrally to produce muscle relaxation (see Ch. 4).

Botulinum toxin (see Ch. 14) injected into a muscle inhibits acetylcholine release, causing long-lasting paralysis confined to the site of injection; its use to treat local muscle spasm is increasing. Its non-medicinal use as a 'beauty' treatment has become widespread.

REFERENCES AND FURTHER READING

General

Shorvon, S., Guerrini, R., Schachter, S., Trinka, E., 2019. The Causes of Epilepsy: Common and Uncommon Causes in Adults and Children. Cambridge University Press, Cambridge.

Pathogenesis and types of epilepsy

Bernasconi, A., Cendes, F., Theodore, W.H., et al., 2019. Recommendations for the use of structural magnetic resonance imaging in the care of patients with epilepsy: a consensus report from the international league against epilepsy neuroimaging task force. Epilepsia 60, 1054–1068.

Gawel, K., Langlois, M., Martins, T., et al., 2020. Seizing the moment: zebrafish epilepsy models. Neurosci. Biobehav. Rev. 116, 1–20.

Grone, B.P., Baraban, S.C., 2015. Animal models in epilepsy research: legacies and new directions. Nat. Neurosci. 18, 339–343.

Khosravani, H., Altier, C., Simms, B., et al., 2004. Gating effects of mutations in the $Ca_v3.2$ T-type calcium channel associated with childhood absence epilepsy. J. Biol. Chem. 279, 9681–9684.

Perucca, P., Bahlo, M., Berkovic, S.F., 2020. The genetics of epilepsy. Annu. Rev. Genom. Hum. Genet. 21, 205–230.

Weber, Y.G., Lerche, H., 2008. Genetic mechanisms in idiopathic epilepsies. Dev. Med. Child Neurol. 50, 648–654.

Antiepileptic drugs

Bialer, M., White, H.S., 2010. Key factors in the discovery and development of new antiepileptic drugs. Nat. Rev. Drug Discov. 9, 68–82.

Shih, J.J., Whitlock, J.B., Chimato, N., Vargas, E., Karceski, S.C., Frank, R.D., 2017. Epilepsy treatment in adults and adolescents. Epilepsy Behav. 69, 186–222.

47 Antipsychotic drugs

OVERVIEW

Antipsychotic drugs are used to treat disorders associated with psychosis, particularly schizophrenia, which affects about 1% of the population. As with other treatments for psychiatric disorders, the relationship between the mechanisms of action of antipsychotic drugs and the underlying pathology of the disorders is poorly understood. There has also been a similar tendency to relate the pharmacology of the treatments to the cause of the disorder but with relatively limited empirical evidence. We include here discussion of these various neurochemical hypotheses and their relationship to the actions of the main types of antipsychotic drug.

INTRODUCTION

Psychotic illnesses include various disorders, but the term *antipsychotic drugs* – previously known as *neuroleptic drugs, antischizophrenic drugs* or *major tranquillisers* – conventionally refers to those used to treat schizophrenia. These same drugs are also used to treat mania (see Ch. 48) and other acute behavioural disturbances including drug-induced psychosis, e.g. resulting from non-medical use of stimulants or *N*-methyl-D-aspartate (NMDA) receptor antagonists such as phencyclidine (PCP or 'Angel Dust') (see Ch. 49). Pharmacologically, most are dopamine receptor antagonists, although many of them also act on other targets, particularly 5-hydroxytryptamine$_2$ (5-HT$_2$) receptors, which may contribute to their clinical efficacy as well as affecting their side effect profile. Existing drugs still have many drawbacks in terms of their efficacy and side effects. Gradual improvements have been achieved with newer drugs, but radical new approaches will require a better understanding of the causes and underlying pathology of the disease, which are still poorly understood.[1]

THE NATURE OF SCHIZOPHRENIA

Schizophrenia[2] (see Stahl, 2021) affects about 1% of the population. It is one of the most important forms of psychiatric illness, because it affects young people, is often chronic and is usually highly disabling.[3] There is a strong hereditary factor in its aetiology, and evidence suggestive of a fundamental biological disorder. The main clinical features of the disease are as follows.

Positive symptoms

- Delusions (often paranoid in nature).
- Hallucinations (often in the form of voices, which may be exhortatory in their message).
- Thought disorder (comprising wild trains of thought, delusions of grandeur, garbled sentences and irrational conclusions).
- Abnormal, disorganised behaviour (such as stereotyped movements, disorientation and occasionally aggressive behaviours).
- Catatonia (can be apparent as immobility or purposeless motor activity).

Negative symptoms

- Withdrawal from social contacts.
- Flattening of emotional responses.
- Anhedonia (an inability to experience pleasure).
- Reluctance to perform everyday tasks.

Cognition

- Deficits in cognitive function (e.g. cognitive flexibility, attention, memory).

In addition to the more recognised psychotic symptoms, anxiety, guilt, depression and self-punishment are often present, leading to suicide attempts in up to 50% of cases, about 10% of which are successful. The clinical phenotype varies greatly, particularly with respect to the balance between positive and negative symptoms, and this may have a bearing on the efficacy of antipsychotic drugs in individual cases. Schizophrenia can present dramatically, usually in young people, with predominantly positive features such as hallucinations, delusions and uncontrollable behaviour, or more insidiously in older patients with negative features such as flat mood and social withdrawal. The latter may be more debilitated than those with a florid presentation, and the prognosis is generally worse. Cognitive impairment may be evident even before the onset of other symptoms. Schizophrenia can follow a relapsing and remitting course, or be chronic and progressive, particularly in cases with a later onset. Chronic schizophrenia used to account for most of the patients in long-stay psychiatric hospitals; following the closure of many of these in the United Kingdom, it now accounts for many of society's outcasts.

A characteristic feature of schizophrenia is a defect in 'selective attention'. Whereas most people quickly accommodate to stimuli of a familiar or inconsequential

[1]In this respect, the study of schizophrenia lags some years behind that of Alzheimer's disease (Ch. 40), where understanding of the pathogenesis has progressed rapidly to the point where promising drug targets have been identified. On the other hand, pragmatists can argue that drugs against Alzheimer's disease are so far only marginally effective, whereas current antipsychotic drugs deliver great benefits even though we do not quite know how they work.

[2]Schizophrenia is a condition where the patient exhibits symptoms of psychosis (e.g. delusions, hallucinations and disorganised behaviour). Psychotic episodes may also occur as a result of taking certain drugs for non-medicinal reasons (see Ch. 49); as an adverse effect of drug treatment, for example steroid-induced psychoses; or in disorders such as mania, bipolar disorder, depression (see Ch. 48) and dementias (see Ch. 40).

[3]A compelling account of what it is like to suffer from schizophrenia is contained in Kean (2009), *Schizophrenia Bulletin* 35, 1034–1036. The author is a pharmacology graduate and now a lecturer in mental health.

nature, and respond only to stimuli that are unexpected or significant, the ability to discriminate between significant and insignificant stimuli seems to be impaired in people with schizophrenia. Thus the ticking of a clock may command as much attention as the words of a companion; a chance thought, which a normal person would dismiss as inconsequential, may become an irresistible imperative.

AETIOLOGY AND PATHOGENESIS OF SCHIZOPHRENIA

GENETIC AND ENVIRONMENTAL FACTORS

The causes of schizophrenia remain unclear but involve a combination of genetic and environmental factors. Thus a person may have a genetic predisposition to schizophrenia, but exposure to environmental factors is required for schizophrenia to develop. As with other mental health conditions, stress is a major risk factor for the development of schizophrenia. The different forms that gene–environment interaction can take are discussed in detail in Ayhan et al. (2016).

The disease shows a strong, but incomplete, hereditary tendency. In first-degree relatives, the risk is about 10%, but even in monozygotic (identical) twins, one of whom has schizophrenia, the probability of the other being affected is only about 50%, pointing towards the importance of environmental factors. Genetic linkage studies have identified more than 100 genetic regions (loci) associated with a risk of schizophrenia (McCutcheon et al., 2020). There are significant associations between polymorphisms in individual genes and the likelihood of an individual developing schizophrenia but there appears to be no single gene that has an overriding influence. Some of the genes implicated in schizophrenia are also associated with bipolar disorder (see Ch. 48).

The most robust associations are with genes that control neuronal development, synaptic connectivity and glutamatergic neurotransmission. These include *complement component 4A (C4A), neuregulin, dysbindin, DISC-1, TCF4* and *NOTCH4*. Increases in C4A expression result in increased synaptic pruning (the process of synapse elimination that occurs between early childhood and the onset of puberty) and may help explain the reduced numbers of synapses in the brains of patients with schizophrenia. Genetically altered mice that underexpress neuregulin-1, a protein involved in synaptic development and plasticity and which controls NMDA receptor expression, show a phenotype resembling human schizophrenia in certain respects. Dysfunction of NMDA receptors is further implicated by genetic association with the genes for D-amino acid oxidase (DAAO), the enzyme responsible for metabolising D-serine, an allosteric modulator of NMDA receptors (see Ch. 39), and for DAAO activator (G72). Dysbindin is located in postsynaptic density domains and may be involved in tethering receptors including NMDA receptors. DISC-1 – which stands for **d**isrupted **in** **sc**hizophrenia-**1** – is a protein that associates with cytoskeletal proteins and is involved with cell migration, neurite outgrowth and receptor trafficking. Population genetic studies have suggested that *NOTCH4*, a developmentally expressed gene, and TCF-4, a gene also associated with intellectual disability, are strongly associated with susceptibility for schizophrenia-like symptoms but their precise roles in its aetiology remain to be elucidated. Among other suggested susceptibility genes, some (such as the genes for monoamine oxidase A (MAO-A), tyrosine hydroxylase and the D_2 dopamine receptor) are involved in monoamine transmission in the central nervous system. However, the weight of current evidence seems to suggest that schizophrenia results from neurodevelopmental consequences of both genetic and environmental factors. These affect the way the neuronal circuits develop and the connections between different regions of the brain and it is these abnormal brain networks that cause the disorder rather than a deficit in any one transmitter system.

Some environmental influences early in development have been identified as possible predisposing factors, particularly maternal virus infections, leading to changes in the cerebral cortex which occur in the first few months of prenatal development. These developmental changes seem to then manifest in adolescence as the brain undergoes synaptic pruning during this important stage in brain development. It is also when key regions such as the prefrontal cortex undergo maturation. This view is supported by brain imaging studies showing neuroanatomical changes in the early course of the disease which may increase with time and correlate with the progression of the disorder (Fusar-Poli et al., 2012). Functional whole-brain network architecture is also altered (Kambeitz et al., 2016).

THE NEUROANATOMICAL AND NEUROCHEMICAL BASIS OF THE SYMPTOMS OF SCHIZOPHRENIA

The symptoms of schizophrenia appear to result from dysfunction in neuronal circuits which regulate behaviour; however, there is a lack of reliable evidence of gross anatomical or neurochemical changes in any one brain region or neurotransmitter system. Instead, neurodevelopmental changes in the cerebral cortex are thought to lead to altered regulation of subcortical regions leading to positive symptoms whilst also contributing to emotional and cognitive impairments and hence the negative and cognitive symptoms in schizophrenia. The behavioural manifestation of the positive symptoms of schizophrenia is similar to that seen in healthy subjects following ingestion of drugs which induce neurochemical changes in either subcortical dopamine (e.g. amphetamine, cocaine) or cortical glutamatergic pathways (e.g. NMDA receptor antagonists, 5-HT_{2A} agonists). These observations, alongside identification of the main drug targets for antipsychotic drugs, have led to different neurochemical hypotheses of schizophrenia although with inconclusive clinical evidence. More recent studies have shifted the focus to theories based on changes in neural connectivity including synaptic pruning, excitatory-inhibitory balance in regions such as the prefrontal cortex and also immune-mediated mechanisms but no specific pathology has yet been established.

Dopamine

The original dopamine theory of schizophrenia was proposed by Carlson[4] on the basis of indirect pharmacological evidence in humans and experimental animals. **Amphetamine** releases dopamine in the brain and can produce in humans a behavioural syndrome reminiscent of an acute schizophrenic episode. Also, hallucinations are a side effect of **levodopa** and dopamine agonists used for

[4]Carlson was awarded a Nobel Prize in 2000 for this work.

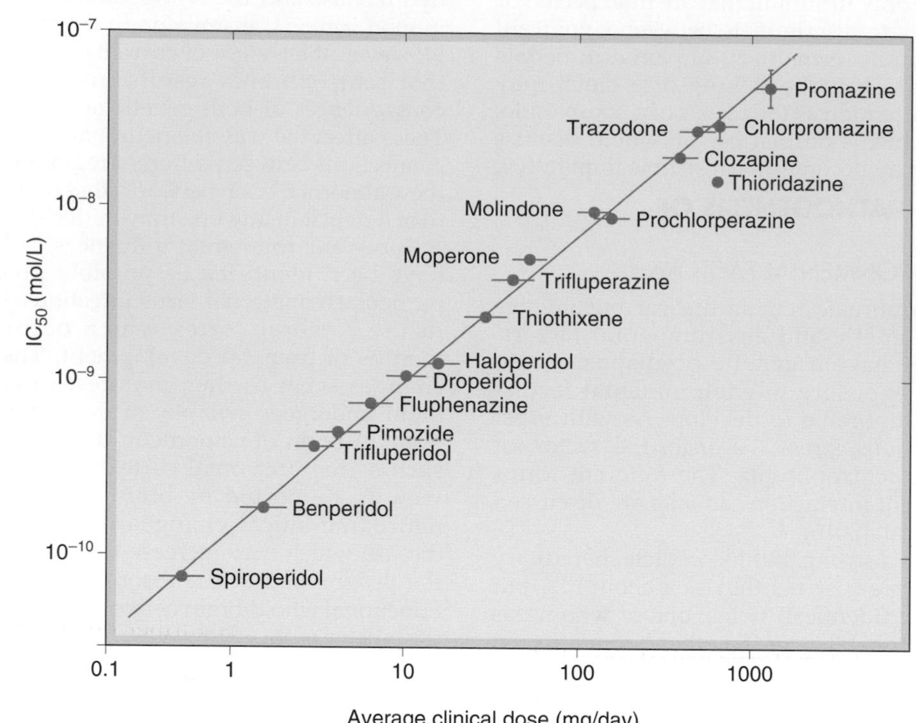

Fig. 47.1 Correlation between the clinical potency and affinity for dopamine D_2 receptors among antipsychotic drugs. Clinical potency is expressed as the daily dose used in treating schizophrenia, and binding activity is expressed as the concentration needed to produce 50% inhibition of haloperidol binding. (From Seeman, P., et al., 1976. Nature 361, 717.)

Parkinson's disease (see Ch. 40). In animals, dopamine release causes a specific pattern of stereotyped behaviour that resembles the repetitive behaviours sometimes seen in patients with schizophrenia. Potent D_2 receptor agonists, such as **bromocriptine**, produce similar effects in animals, and these drugs, like amphetamine, exacerbate the symptoms of patients with schizophrenia. Furthermore, dopamine antagonists and drugs that block neuronal dopamine storage (e.g. **reserpine**) are effective in controlling the positive symptoms of schizophrenia, and in preventing amphetamine-induced behavioural changes.

There is a strong correlation between antipsychotic potency in reducing positive symptoms and activity in blocking D_2 receptors (Fig. 47.1) and receptor imaging studies have shown that clinical efficacy of antipsychotic drugs is achieved when D_2 receptor occupancy reaches 65%–80% with first-generation antipsychotics but can be lower with second-generation antipsychotics (Fig. 47.2).[5]

An increase in dopamine receptor density in schizophrenia has been reported in some studies, but not consistently. There have also been mixed findings in terms of evidence of increased mesolimbic dopamine levels or altered regulation of dopamine release, and the interpretation is complicated by the fact that chronic antipsychotic drug treatment is known to increase dopamine receptor expression. In fact,

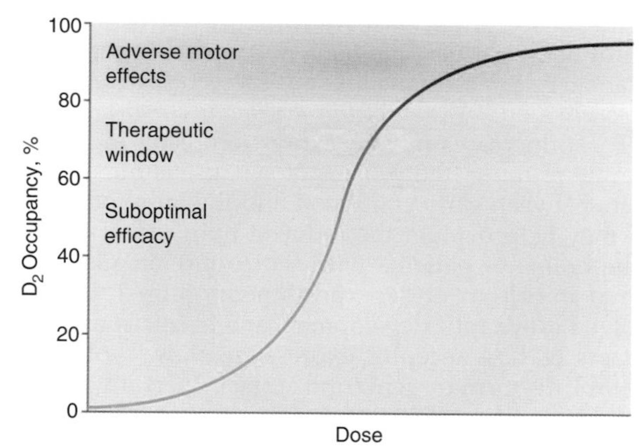

Fig. 47.2 Striatal D2 receptor occupancy greater than 60% is needed for the therapeutic effects of antipsychotics but more than 80% occupancy results in motor side effects. Studies using positron emission tomography of D2-antagonist antipsychotic drugs suggest that there is a therapeutic window between 60% and 80% D2-receptor occupancy. This is associated with beneficial effects in terms of the positive symptoms but with reduced risk of extrapyramidal side effects. This is true for most D2 antagonists but there are exceptions with clozapine achieving therapeutic effects at lower levels of D2 occupancy and partial agonists require higher occupancy.

[5]There are, however, exceptions to this simple rule. Up to one-third of patients with schizophrenia fail to respond even when D_2 receptor blockade exceeds 90%, and clozapine (see Table 47.1) can be effective at much lower levels of block.

a side effect of antipsychotic treatment is the increased risk of rebound psychosis if patients are taken off medication.

Glutamate

In humans, NMDA receptor antagonists such as **PCP**, **ketamine** and **dizocilpine** (see Ch. 39) can reproduce symptoms characteristic of the positive, negative and cognitive deficit symptoms - in contrast to amphetamine, which produces only positive symptoms. Many of the genes linked to schizophrenia are involved in synapse formation which play a critical role in the development of neuronal networks particularly during adolescent brain development and it has been postulated that these manifest in altered glutamatergic neurotransmission. An interesting insight into the possible role of altered glutamate signalling in schizophrenia comes from a rare autoimmune disorder, anti-NMDA receptor encephalitis, where patients often present with symptoms very similar to schizophrenia but which result from impaired NMDA receptor function.

Another class of drugs which induce altered glutamatergic signalling and can also affect subcortical dopamine are the 5-HT_{2A} receptor antagonists. Highly enriched in cortical regions and particularly associated with effects in the prefrontal cortex, 5-HT_{2A} receptors modulate intracortical and cortical-subcortical glutamatergic neurotransmission, and agonists and partial agonists induce potent psychedelic effects which include altered perception, hallucinations and changes in cognitive and emotional processing.

Glutamatergic neurons and GABAergic neurons play complex roles in controlling the level of activity in neuronal pathways involved in schizophrenia. NMDA receptor hypofunction is thought to *reduce* the level of activity in mesocortical dopaminergic neurons. This would result in a decrease in dopamine release in the prefrontal cortex and could thus give rise to negative symptoms of schizophrenia. NMDA receptor hypofunction in the cortex may affect GABAergic interneurons and alter cortical processing, giving rise to cognitive impairment. In addition, NMDA receptor hypofunction on GABAergic neurons would reduce inhibition of the excitatory cortical input to the ventral tegmental area (VTA) and thus *enhance* activity in the mesolimbic dopaminergic pathway. Thus NMDA receptor hypofunction could give rise to enhanced dopamine release in limbic areas such as the nucleus accumbens, resulting in the production of positive symptoms.

Given the evidence that schizophrenic symptoms may be due to a reduction in NMDA receptor function, efforts have been made to develop new drugs to enhance NMDA-mediated signalling but not to a level where it becomes neurotoxic (see Ch. 40), e.g. by activating the facilitatory glycine site on the NMDA receptor (see Ch. 38) with an agonist or by raising extracellular glycine levels by inhibiting the GlyT1 transporter. However, **bitopertin**, a GlyT1 inhibitor, failed as an antipsychotic drug in clinical trials. An alternative approach to modulating glutamate signalling is to target autoreceptors, however clinical trials of mGlu2/3 (Ch. 38) agonists failed in clinical trials despite showing promising effects in animal models.

Other glutamate pathways thought to be involved in schizophrenia are the corticostriatal, thalamocortical, corticothalamic and cortico-brain stem pathways. The thalamus normally functions as a sensory filter to limit unnecessary sensory input to the cortex. Disruption of the normal inputs to the thalamus, for example from a reduction in glutamatergic or GABAergic transmission, disables this 'sensory gate' function, allowing uninhibited input to reach the cortex. The role of the thalamus in schizophrenia is reviewed by Pergola et al. (2015).

Animal models

Traditional pharmacological models of schizophrenia by and large reflect behaviours resulting from heightened dopaminergic transmission in the brain and provide a useful screen for drugs which have dopamine receptor-antagonist activity. Models based on inhibition of NMDA function by PCP or 5-HT_{2A} agonist–induced behaviours such as the head twitch response also provide a useful screen but do not reflect the underlying aetiology of schizophrenia. With increasing understanding of genetic and environmental risk factors, various genetic and developmental models have been evaluated to try to provide a more relevant phenotype. However, it is difficult to fully recapitulate the multifactorial genetic and environmental factors which contribute to the human disorder, many of which are not yet fully understood, in an animal model and laboratory setting. Models of cognitive deficits and negative symptoms are also lacking. For further details of behavioural tasks used for evaluating schizophrenia-like symptoms and an overview of animal models of schizophrenia see Ang et al. (2021) and Winship et al. (2019).

The nature of schizophrenia

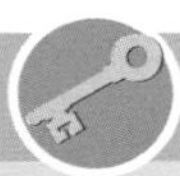

- Psychotic illness characterised by delusions, hallucinations and thought disorder (positive symptoms), together with social withdrawal and flattening of emotional responses (negative symptoms), and cognitive impairment.
- Acute episodes (mainly positive symptoms) frequently recur and may develop into chronic schizophrenia, with predominantly negative symptoms.
- Incidence is about 1% of the population, with a significant hereditary component. Genetic linkage studies suggest involvement of multiple genes, but no single 'schizophrenia gene'.
- Neurodevelopmental changes linked to both genetic risk and environmental factors resulting in increased grey matter loss and aberrant network organisation seem the most likely cause of schizophrenia, but no single gene, brain region or neurotransmitter system has consistently been found to underlie the disorder.

ANTIPSYCHOTIC DRUGS

CLASSIFICATION OF ANTIPSYCHOTIC DRUGS

More than 80 different antipsychotic drugs are available for clinical use. These have been divided into two groups – those drugs that were originally developed (e.g. **chlorpromazine**, **haloperidol** and many similar compounds), often referred to as *first-generation, typical* or *conventional antipsychotic drugs*, and more recently developed agents (e.g. **clozapine**, **risperidone**), which are termed *second-generation* or *atypical* *antipsychotic drugs*. Table 47.1 summarises the main drugs that are in clinical use.[6]

The term *atypical* refers to the diminished tendency to cause unwanted motor side effects, but it is also used to describe compounds with a different pharmacological profile from first-generation compounds. In practice, however, it often serves - not very usefully - to distinguish the large group of similar first-generation dopamine antagonists from the more diverse group of later compounds.

The therapeutic activity of the prototype drug, chlorpromazine, in patients with schizophrenia was discovered through the acute observations of a French surgeon, Laborit, in 1947. He tested various substances, including **promethazine**, for their ability to alleviate signs of stress in patients undergoing surgery, and concluded that promethazine had a calming effect that was different from mere sedation. Elaboration of the phenothiazine structure led to chlorpromazine, the antipsychotic effect of which was demonstrated in man, at Laborit's instigation, by Delay and Deniker in 1953. This drug was unique in controlling the symptoms of patients with psychotic disorders. The clinical efficacy of phenothiazines was discovered long before their mechanism was guessed at, let alone understood.

Pharmacological investigation showed that phenothiazines, the first-generation antipsychotic agents, block many different mediators, including dopamine, histamine, catecholamines, acetylcholine and 5-HT, and this multiplicity of actions led to the trade name Largactil for chlorpromazine.

Classification of antipsychotic drugs

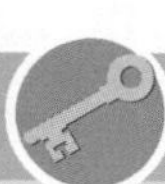

- Main categories are:
  - first-generation ('typical', 'classical' or 'conventional') antipsychotics (e.g. **chlorpromazine**, **haloperidol**, **fluphenazine**, **flupentixol**, **zuclopenthixol**);
  - second-generation ('atypical') antipsychotics (e.g. **clozapine**, **risperidone**, **quetiapine**, **amisulpride**, **aripiprazole**, **ziprasidone**).
- The distinction between first- and second-generation drugs is not clearly defined but rests on:
  - receptor profile;
  - incidence of extrapyramidal side effects (EPSs) (less in second-generation group);
  - efficacy (specifically of **clozapine**) in 'treatment-resistant' patients;
  - efficacy against negative and cognitive symptoms although whether this is due to specific beneficial effects or rather reduced side effects compared with first-generation drugs is still debated.

CLINICAL EFFICACY IN TREATMENT OF SCHIZOPHRENIA

The clinical efficacy of antipsychotic drugs in enabling patients with schizophrenia to lead more normal lives has been demonstrated in many controlled trials (see Leucht et al., 2013). The inpatient population (mainly patients with chronic schizophrenia) of psychiatric hospitals declined sharply in the 1950s and 1960s. The introduction of antipsychotic drugs was a significant enabling factor, as well as the changing public and professional attitudes towards hospitalisation of people with psychiatric disorders.

Antipsychotic drugs have severe drawbacks that include:

- Not all patients with schizophrenia respond to drug therapy. It is recommended to try clozapine in patients who are resistant to other antipsychotic drugs. The 30% of patients who do not respond are classed as 'treatment resistant' and present a major therapeutic problem. The reason for the difference between responsive and unresponsive patients is unknown at present.
- While they control the positive symptoms (thought disorder, hallucinations, delusions, etc.) effectively, most are ineffective in relieving the negative symptoms (emotional flattening, social isolation) and cognitive impairment and some antipsychotics may worsen these symptoms.
- They induce a range of side effects that include extrapyramidal motor, endocrine and sedative effects (see Table 47.1) that can be severe and limit patient compliance.
- They may produce unwanted cardiac (proarrhythmic) effects (see Ch. 21).

Second-generation antipsychotic drugs were believed to overcome these shortcomings to some degree. However, a meta-analysis (Leucht et al., 2013) concluded that only some of the second-generation antipsychotic drugs examined showed better overall efficacy. An important consideration in this discussion is the extent to which a reduced side effect burden, particularly in relation to cognitive and emotional side effects, may improve overall outcomes but this is not directly linked to drug-induced efficacy.

Abrupt cessation of antipsychotic drug administration may lead to a rapid-onset psychotic episode linked to the adaptive changes induced by the antipsychotic drug treatment and is distinct from the underlying illness.

OTHER USES OF ANTIPSYCHOTIC DRUGS

A common emerging theme with centrally acting drugs is that while they were initially developed to treat one brain disorder they have been subsequently found to be effective in treating other disorders. This is also the case with antipsychotic drugs, which are now used to manage behavioural symptoms associated with a range of disorders, including:

- bipolar disorder, mania and depression (see Ch. 48)
- psychomotor agitation and severe anxiety (**chlorpromazine** and **haloperidol**)
- agitation and restlessness in the elderly including patients with dementia (**risperidone**), although this is discouraged due to the potential for adverse long term outcomes
- psychosis associated with Parkinson's disease (**pimavanserin**) (see Ch. 41)
- restlessness and pain in palliative care (**levomepromazine**)
- nausea and vomiting (e.g. **chlorpromazine** and **haloperidol**) reflecting antagonism at dopamine, muscarinic, histamine and possibly 5-HT receptors

[6]Wikipedia (https://en.wikipedia.org/wiki/List_of_antipsychotics) lists no fewer than 49 first-generation and 33 second-generation agents approved for clinical use. Despite this huge investment by the pharmaceutical industry and plethora of me-too compounds, clinical benefits remain modest.

- motor tics and intractable hiccup (**chlorpromazine** and **haloperidol**)
- antisocial sexual behaviour (**benperidol**)
- involuntary movements caused by Huntington's disease (mainly **haloperidol**; see Ch. 40)

PHARMACOLOGICAL PROPERTIES

DOPAMINE RECEPTORS

The classification of dopamine receptors in the central nervous system is discussed in Chapter 39 (see Table 39.1). There are five subtypes, which fall into two functional classes: the D_1 type, comprising D_1 and D_5, and the D_2 type, comprising D_2, D_3 and D_4. Antipsychotic drugs owe their therapeutic effects mainly to blockade of D_2 receptors.[7] As stated previously, antipsychotic effects develop when occupancy reaches between 65% and 80% whilst occupancy

[7]The D_4 receptor attracted attention on account of the high degree of genetic polymorphism that it shows in human subjects, and because some of the newer antipsychotic drugs (e.g. clozapine) have a high affinity for this receptor subtype. However, a specific D_4 receptor antagonist proved ineffective in clinical trials.

Table 47.1 Characteristics of some major antipsychotic drugs

	Receptor affinity						Main side effects				
Drug	D_1	D_2	α_1	H_1	mACh	$5\text{-}HT_{2A}$	EPS	Sed	Hypo	Other	Notes
Chlorpromazine	++	++	+++	+++	++	+++	++	+++	++	Increased prolactin (gynaecomastia)	Phenothiazine class
										Hypothermia	Perphenazine and prochlorperazine are similar.
										Anticholinergic effects	
										Hypersensitivity reactions	Fluphenazine and trifluoperazine are similar but: • do not cause jaundice • cause less hypotension • cause more EPS.
										Obstructive jaundice	
											Fluphenazine available as depot preparation
											Pericyazine causes less EPS probably due to its greater muscarinic antagonist actions.
											Pipotiazine has been withdrawn.
Haloperidol	++	+++	++	+	–	++	+++	–	+	As chlorpromazine but does not cause jaundice	Butyrophenone class
										Fewer anticholinergic side effects	Widely used antipsychotic drug
											Strong EPS tendency
											Available as depot preparation
Flupentixol	+++	+++		+++	–	+	++	+	+	Increased prolactin (gynaecomastia)	Thioxanthene class
										Restlessness	Zuclopenthixol is similar.
											Available as depot preparation

Table 47.1 Characteristics of some major antipsychotic drugs—cont'd

	Receptor affinity						Main side effects				
Drug	**D_1**	**D_2**	**α_1**	**H_1**	**mACh**	**$5\text{-}HT_{2A}$**	**EPS**	**Sed**	**Hypo**	**Other**	**Notes**
Amisulpride	–	++	–	–	–	–	+	+	–	Increased prolactin (gynaecomastia)	Benzamide class (includes sulpiride)
											Selective D_2/D_3 antagonist
											Less EPS than haloperidol (reason for this unclear, but could result from action at D_3 or very weak partial agonism at D_2)
											Increases alertness in apathetic patients
											Poorly absorbed
											Amisulpride and pimozide (long-acting) are similar.
Clozapine	+	+	+++	++++	++	+++	–	++	++	Risk of agranulocytosis (~1%): regular blood counts required	Dibenzodiazepine class
										Seizures	No EPS (first second-generation antipsychotic)
Clozapine, cont'd										Salivation	Shows efficacy in 'treatment-resistant' patients and reduces incidence of suicide
										Anticholinergic side effects	Effective against negative and positive symptoms
										Weight gain	Olanzapine is somewhat less sedative, without risk of agranulocytosis, but questionable efficacy in treatment-resistant patients
Risperidone	+	+++	+++	++	–	++++ (IA?)	+	++	++	Weight gain	Significant risk of EPS
										EPS at high doses	? Effective against negative symptoms
										Hypotension	Potent on D_4 receptors
											Available as depot preparation
											Paliperidone is a metabolite of risperidone.

Continued

Table 47.1 Characteristics of some major antipsychotic drugs—cont'd

	Receptor affinity						Main side effects				
Drug	**D_1**	**D_2**	**α_1**	**H_1**	**mACh**	**$5\text{-}HT_{2A}$**	**EPS**	**Sed**	**Hypo**	**Other**	**Notes**
											Iloperidone reported to have low incidence of EPS and weight gain
Quetiapine	+	+	+++	+++	+	+	–	++	++	Tachycardia	Low incidence of EPS
										Drowsiness	No increase in prolactin secretion
										Dry mouth	$5\text{-}HT_{1A}$ partial agonist
										Constipation	Short-acting (plasma half-life ~6 h)
										Weight gain	
Aripiprazole	+	++++ (PA)	++	++	–	+++	–	+	–	–	Long-acting (plasma half-life ~3 days)
											Unusual D_2 partial agonist profile may account for paucity of side effects.
											Also a $5\text{-}HT_{1A}$ partial agonist
											No effect on prolactin secretion
											No weight gain
											Available as a depot preparation
											Brexpiprazole may also be useful in the treatment of depression.
Ziprasidone	++	+++	+++	++	–	++++	+	–	+	Tiredness	Low incidence of EPS
										Nausea	No weight gain
											Lurasidone is similar.
											? Effective against negative symptoms
											Short-acting (plasma half-life ~8 h) but a depot preparation is available
Lumateperone	++	++	+	–	–	++++	–	+	–	Sleepiness	High affinity for serotonin transporter
											Indirectly modulates glutamate transmission

+, pKi 5–7; ++, pKi 7–8; +++, pKi 8–9; +++, pKi >9.
$5\text{-}HT_{1A}$, $5\text{-}HT_{2A}$, 5-Hydroxytryptamine types 1A and 2A receptors; α_1, α_1 adrenoceptor; *D_1, D_2, D_3, D_4*, dopamine types 1, 2, 3 and 4 receptor, respectively; *EPS*, extrapyramidal side effects; *H_1*, histamine type 1 receptor; *Hypo*, hypotension; *IA*, inverse agonist; *mACh*, muscarinic acetylcholine receptor; *PA*, partial agonist; *Sed*, sedation.
Table based on data contained in Guide to Pharmacology (http://www.guidetopharmacology.org/) and NIMH Psychoactive Drug Screening Program database (http://pdsp.med.unc.edu/). Where available, data obtained on human receptors are given.

over 80% has been linked to motor side effects (see Fig. 47.2). The first-generation compounds show some preference for D_2 over D_1 receptors, whereas some of the later agents (e.g. **sulpiride, amisulpride**) are highly selective for D_2 receptors. D_2 antagonists that dissociate rapidly from the receptor (e.g. **quetiapine**) and D_2 partial agonists (e.g. **aripiprazole**) were introduced in an attempt to reduce extrapyramidal motor side effects. **Cariprazine**, a new antipsychotic drug, is a D_2 and D_3 partial agonist with higher affinity for D_3 than D_2 receptors.

It is the antagonism of D_2 receptors in the mesolimbic pathway that is believed to reduce the positive symptoms of schizophrenia (Fig. 47.3). Unfortunately, systemically administered antipsychotic drugs do not discriminate between D_2 receptors in distinct brain regions and D_2 receptors in other brain pathways will also be blocked. Thus antipsychotic drugs produce unwanted motor effects (block of D_2 receptors in the nigrostriatal pathway), enhance prolactin secretion (block of D_2 receptors in the tuberoinfundibular pathway), produce emotional blunting and anhedonia (block of D_2 receptors in the reward component of the mesolimbic pathway) and perhaps even worsen the cognitive and negative symptoms of schizophrenia (Fig. 47.3). Expression of D_2 receptors in the prefrontal cortex is low but D_1 receptors are in greater abundance. This is particularly relevant for the first-generation antipsychotics which are also potent D_1- antagonists. While all first-generation antipsychotic drugs block D_2 receptors and should therefore in theory induce all of these unwanted effects, some have additional pharmacological activity (e.g. mACh receptor antagonism and 5-HT_{2A} receptor antagonism) that, to varying degrees, ameliorate some of the unwanted effects.

Antipsychotic drugs have classically been thought to have a delayed onset to their therapeutic actions, even though their dopamine receptor-blocking action is immediate. This view has, however, been called into question (Kapur et al., 2005; Leucht et al., 2005). In animal studies, chronic antipsychotic drug administration does produce compensatory changes in the brain, for example, a reduction in the activity of dopaminergic neurons and proliferation of dopamine receptors, detectable as an increase in haloperidol binding, with a pharmacological supersensitivity to dopamine reminiscent of the phenomenon of denervation supersensitivity (see Ch. 13). The mechanism(s) of these delayed effects are poorly understood. They are likely to contribute to the development of unwanted *tardive dyskinesias* and also contribute to acute rebound psychosis

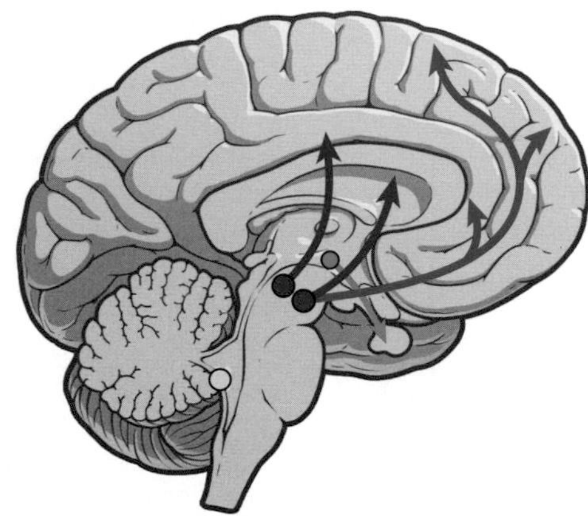

Dopamine$_2$-receptor antagonism and dopamine pathways

- Mesolimbic – antipsychotic
- Mesocortical – cognitive, emotional impairment
- Nigrostriatal – extrapyramidal side effects
- Tuberohypophyseal – hyperprolactinaemia
- Chemoreceptor trigger zone – antiemetic

Key receptors linked to efficacy and side effects of typical and atypical antipsychotics

RECEPTOR TARGET	ROLE IN EFFICACY	ROLE IN SIDE EFFECTS
D_2-receptor antagonism	Antipsychotic	EPS, hyperprolactinaemia, emotional blunting, cognitive impairment
5-HT_{2A} receptor antagonism	Antipsychotic	Reduced EPS, reduces akathisia induced by D2 antagonism
5-HT_{2C} receptor antagonism	?	Increased appetite, metabolic effects
Muscarinic$_1$ receptor antagonism	?	Constipation, dry mouth, blurred vision Reduced EPS
Histamine$_1$ receptor antagonism	Sedation*	Sedation*
α-adrenoceptor antagonism	?	Postural hypotension
SERT/NAT	Antidepressant	?

*Depending on the circumstances sedation may contribute to efficacy or side effects i.e. in acute psychosis, sedation may be beneficial

Fig. 47.3 Receptors affected by antipsychotic drugs and their relationship to efficacy and side effects. The figure illustrates the effects of D2 antagonism in the different dopamine pathways in the brain whilst the table details some of the receptors commonly affected at therapeutic doses. The beneficial effects and side effects associated with individual antipsychotics depend on their specific receptor profile. *EPS,* Extrapyramidal side effects; *5-HT,* 5-hydroxytryptamine; *NAT,* noradrenaline transporter; *SERT,* serotonin transporter.

if the antipsychotic is stopped abruptly. The sedating effect of some antipsychotic drugs is immediate, making them useful in acute behavioural emergencies.

Mechanism of action of antipsychotic drugs

- Most antipsychotic drugs are antagonists or partial agonists at D_2 dopamine receptors, but they vary in their potency and also block a variety of other receptors.
- Efficacy in treating positive symptoms generally runs parallel to activity on D_2 receptors, but activities at 5-HT_{2A} receptors are thought to contribute to efficacy whilst interactions with other receptors (e.g. 5-HT_{2A} and muscarinic) may reduce extrapyramidal side effects (EPS).
- Activity at muscarinic, H_1 and α receptors may determine unwanted side effect profile.
- Imaging studies suggest that therapeutic effects typically require 65%–80% occupancy of D_2 receptors with occupancy >80% linked to EPSs.

5-HYDROXYTRYPTAMINE RECEPTORS

The idea that 5-HT dysfunction could be involved in schizophrenia has drifted in and out of favour many times. It was originally based on the fact that LSD, a partial agonist at 5-I IT_{2A} receptors (see Chs 16 and 49), can induce psychosis with some similarities to the symptoms of schizophrenia. Most of the newer atypical antipsychotics have affinity for 5-HT receptors and antagonism at the 5-HT_{2A} receptor, and to a lesser extent the 5-HT_{1A} receptor, is linked to both therapeutic effects and reduced EPSs. Pharmacological manipulation of 5-HT receptor activity, combined with D_2 receptor antagonism, has resulted in drugs with improved therapeutic profiles (see Table 47.1).[8] There is a plethora of 5-HT receptors (see Chs 16 and 39), with disparate functions in the body. Interestingly, antagonism at the 5-HT_{2A} receptor is not only a feature of some antipsychotics but also some antidepressants (see Ch. 48) and has been associated with anxiolytic, antidepressant and antipsychotic effects. It remains unknown exactly why the 5-HT_{2A} receptor is a common target for many of these drugs but this receptor is an important therapeutic target in psychiatry. 5-HT_{2A} receptors can induce pleiotropic effects dependent on their associated intracellular signalling. The most common intracellular mechanism is to increase calcium signalling via Gq-mediated stimulation of phospholipase C and inositol triphosphate production but other mechanisms have also been reported depending on the brain region and cell type being studied. Drugs with 5-HT_{2A} antagonist properties (e.g. olanzapine and risperidone) are able to enhance dopamine release in the striatum by reducing the inhibitory effect of 5-HT. This may reduce EPSs (see later). In contrast, in the mesolimbic pathway, the combined effects of D_2 and 5-HT_{2A} antagonism are thought to have beneficial effects on the positive symptoms of schizophrenia. Further, enhancing both dopamine and glutamate release in the mesocortical circuit, 5-HT_{2A} receptor antagonism may improve the negative symptoms of schizophrenia (Stahl, 2021). Pimavanserin, a drug recently introduced for the treatment of psychosis associated with Parkinson's disease (see Ch. 40) and which may be beneficial as an adjunct to other antipsychotic drugs in the treatment of schizophrenia, is an inverse agonist at the 5-HT_{2A} receptor and has no activity at dopaminergic receptors.

5-HT_{1A} receptors are found post-synaptically as well as functioning as somatodendritic autoreceptors that inhibit 5-HT release (see Ch. 39). Antipsychotic drugs that are agonists or partial agonists at 5-HT_{1A} receptors (e.g. quetiapine; see Table 47.1) may work by decreasing 5-HT release, thus enhancing dopamine release in the striatum and prefrontal cortex.

MUSCARINIC ACETYLCHOLINE RECEPTORS

Some phenothiazine antipsychotic drugs (e.g. **pericyazine**) have been reported to produce fewer EPSs than others, and this was thought to correlate with their muscarinic antagonist actions. Also, some second-generation drugs possess muscarinic antagonist properties (e.g. olanzapine). In the striatum, dopaminergic nerve terminals are thought to innervate cholinergic interneurons that express inhibitory D_2 receptors (Pisani et al., 2007). It is suggested that there is normally a balance between D_2 receptor activation and muscarinic receptor activation. Blocking D_2 receptors in the striatum with an antipsychotic agent will result in enhanced acetylcholine release on to muscarinic receptors, thus producing EPSs, which are counteracted if the antipsychotic also has muscarinic antagonist activity. Maintaining the dopamine/acetylcholine balance was also the rationale for the use of the muscarinic antagonist **benztropine** to reduce extrapyramidal effects of antipsychotic drugs. Muscarinic antagonist activity does, however, induce side effects such as constipation, dry mouth and blurred vision.

UNWANTED EFFECTS

EXTRAPYRAMIDAL MOTOR DISTURBANCES

Antipsychotic drugs produce two main kinds of motor disturbance in humans: *acute dystonias* and *akathisia,* and *tardive dyskinesias*, collectively termed *extrapyramidal side effects (EPSs)*. These all result directly or indirectly from D_2 receptor blockade in the nigrostriatal pathway. EPSs constitute one of the main disadvantages of first-generation antipsychotic drugs. Second-generation drugs were defined based on their ability to induce lower incidence of EPSs at doses which were effective against positive symptoms of schizophrenia. Whilst there may be a reduction in EPS, second-generation antipsychotics are not devoid of these motor side effects and a long-term study of olanzapine, risperidone, quetiapine and **ziprasidone** concluded that they too can induce EPSs (see Lieberman and Stroup, 2011). Even aripiprazole, which is a D_2 partial agonist, has been reported to produce this unwanted effect.

[8]Early antipsychotic drugs (e.g. chlorpromazine) had actions at various receptors but also had unwanted side effects that resulted from activity at other receptors. Towards the end of the 20th century, drug development, not just of antipsychotic drugs, was focused largely on developing agents with a single action with the intention of reducing unwanted side effects. This philosophy drove the search for selective D_4 receptor antagonists, which proved ineffective. What is now apparent is that drugs with selected multiple actions (e.g. a combination of D_2 antagonism and 5-HT_{2A} antagonism) may have a better therapeutic profile.

Acute dystonias are involuntary movements (restlessness, muscle spasms, protruding tongue, fixed upward gaze, neck muscle spasm), and ***akathisia,*** an urge to move that you can't control, are symptoms of Parkinson's disease (see Ch. 40). They occur commonly in the first few weeks, often declining with time, and are reversible on stopping drug treatment. The timing is consistent with block of the dopaminergic nigrostriatal pathway. Concomitant block of muscarinic receptors and 5-HT_{2A} receptors may mitigate the motor effects of dopamine receptor antagonists (see earlier).

Tardive dyskinesia (see Klawans et al., 1988) develops after months or years (hence 'tardive') in 20%–40% of patients treated with first-generation antipsychotic drugs and is one of the main problems of antipsychotic therapy. Its seriousness lies in the fact that it is a disabling and often irreversible condition, which often gets worse when antipsychotic therapy is stopped and is resistant to treatment. The syndrome consists of involuntary movements, often of the face and tongue, but also of the trunk and limbs, which can be severely disabling. It resembles that seen after prolonged treatment of Parkinson's disease with levodopa (see Ch. 40). The incidence depends greatly on drug, dose and age (being commonest in patients who are over 50 years of age).

There are several theories about the mechanism of tardive dyskinesia (see Casey, 1995). One is that it is associated with a gradual increase in the number of D_2 receptors in the striatum, which is less marked during treatment with second-generation than with first-generation antipsychotic drugs. Another possibility is that chronic block of inhibitory dopamine receptors enhances catecholamine and/or glutamate release in the striatum, leading to excitotoxic neurodegeneration (see Ch. 41).

Drugs that rapidly dissociate from D_2 receptors (e.g. clozapine, olanzapine) induce less severe EPSs. A possible explanation for this (see Kapur and Seeman, 2001) is that with a rapidly dissociating compound, a brief surge of dopamine can effectively overcome the block by competition (see Ch. 2), whereas with a slowly dissociating compound, the level of block takes a long time to respond to the presence of endogenous dopamine, and is in practice non-competitive. Adverse motor effects may be avoided if fractional receptor occupation by the antagonist falls during physiological surges of dopamine. An extension of this idea is that perhaps a little D_2 receptor activation may be beneficial. This could be produced, for example, by drugs that are D_2 partial agonists (e.g. aripiprazole) in contrast to simple antagonists. It is thought that partial agonists reduce D_2 hyperactivation in the mesolimbic pathway, thus alleviating positive symptoms of schizophrenia, but provide enough D_2 receptor stimulation in the mesocortical pathway to prevent negative symptoms, and in the nigrostriatal pathway to lower the incidence of EPSs.

Theories for reduced EPS with second-generation antipsychotics include antagonism at 5-HT_{2A} receptors as well as rapid dissociation from the D_2 receptor and improved pharmacokinetic profile that enable D_2 receptor occupancy to be more easily maintained between levels which are antipsychotic but do not cause EPS.

ENDOCRINE EFFECTS

Dopamine, released in the median eminence by neurons of the tuberohypophyseal pathway (see Chs 33 and 39), acts physiologically via D_2 receptors to inhibit prolactin secretion. Blocking D_2 receptors by antipsychotic drugs can therefore increase the plasma prolactin concentration (Fig. 47.4), resulting in breast swelling, pain and lactation (known as 'galactorrhoea'), which can occur in men as well as in women. As can be seen from Fig. 47.4, the effect is maintained during chronic antipsychotic administration, without any habituation. Other less pronounced endocrine changes have also been reported, including a decrease of growth hormone secretion, but these, unlike the prolactin response, are believed to be relatively unimportant clinically. Because of its D_2 receptor partial agonist action aripiprazole, unlike other antipsychotic drugs, reduces prolactin secretion.

Antipsychotic-induced motor disturbances

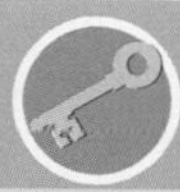

- Major problem of antipsychotic drug treatment.
- Two main types of disturbance occur:
  - acute, reversible dystonias, akathesis and Parkinson-like symptoms (indeed, antipsychotic drugs generally worsen Parkinson's disease and block the actions of drugs used to treat the disorder);
  - slowly developing tardive dyskinesia, often irreversible.
- Acute symptoms comprise involuntary movements, tremor and rigidity, and are probably the direct consequence of block of nigrostriatal dopamine receptors.
- Tardive dyskinesia comprises mainly involuntary movements of the face and limbs, appearing after months or years of antipsychotic treatment. It may be associated with proliferation of dopamine receptors in the corpus striatum. Treatment is generally unsuccessful.
- The incidence of acute dystonias and tardive dyskinesia is less with newer, second-generation antipsychotics, and particularly low with **clozapine**, **aripiprazole** and **zotepine.**

OTHER UNWANTED EFFECTS

Most antipsychotic drugs block a variety of receptors, particularly acetylcholine (muscarinic), histamine (H_1), noradrenaline (α) and 5-HT receptors (see Table 47.1). This gives rise to a wide range of side effects (Fig. 47.3).

They can produce sexual dysfunction – decreased libido and decreased arousal as well as erection and ejaculation difficulties in men – through block of dopamine, muscarinic and α_1 receptors.

Drowsiness and sedation, which tend to decrease with continued use, occur with many antipsychotic drugs. Antihistamine (H_1) activity is a property of some phenothiazine antipsychotics (e.g. chlorpromazine and **methotrimeprazine**) and contributes to their sedative and antiemetic properties (see Ch. 30), but not to their antipsychotic action.

While block of muscarinic receptors produces a variety of peripheral effects, including blurring of vision and increased intraocular pressure, dry mouth and eyes, constipation and urinary retention (see Ch. 14), it may, however, also be beneficial in relation to EPSs.

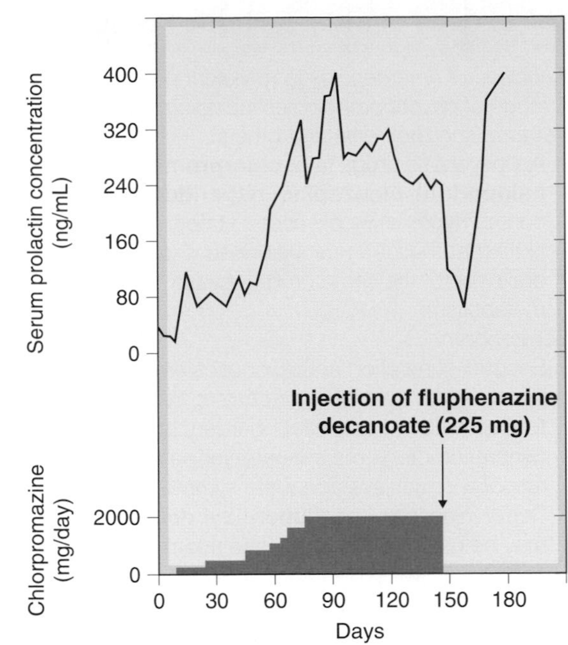

Fig. 47.4 Effects of antipsychotic drugs on prolactin secretion in a patient with schizophrenia. When daily dosage with chlorpromazine was replaced with a depot injection of fluphenazine, the plasma prolactin initially dropped, because of the delay in absorption, and then returned to a high level. (From Meltzer, H.Y., et al., 1978. In: Lipton et al. (Eds). Psychopharmacology: A Generation in Progress. Raven Press, New York.)

Blocking α adrenoceptors causes *orthostatic hypotension* (see Ch. 15) but does not seem to be important for their antipsychotic action.

Weight gain is a common and serious side effect particularly associated with second-generation antipsychotics and is linked to antagonism at the 5-HT_{2C} receptor leading to effects on both appetite and metabolism. Increased risk of diabetes and cardiovascular disease occurs with several second-generation antipsychotic drugs. Antagonist actions at H_1 and muscarinic receptors may also contribute to these effects.

Antipsychotic drugs can prolong the QT interval in the heart (see Ch. 20) giving rise to arrhythmia and risk of sudden death (Jolly et al., 2009). As such, a range of baseline measurements are usually recommended prior to starting antipsychotic drugs; these include weight, blood pressure, blood glucose, and electrocardiogram.

Various idiosyncratic and hypersensitivity reactions can occur, the most important being the following:

- *Jaundice*, which occurs with older phenothiazines such as chlorpromazine. The jaundice is usually mild, associated with elevated serum alkaline phosphatase activity (an 'obstructive' pattern), and disappears quickly when the drug is stopped or substituted by a chemically unrelated antipsychotic.
- *Leukopenia* and *agranulocytosis* are rare but potentially fatal, and occur in the first few weeks of treatment. The incidence of leukopenia (usually reversible) is less than 1 in 10,000 for most antipsychotic drugs, but much higher (1%–2%) with clozapine, whose use therefore requires regular monitoring of blood cell counts. Provided the drug is stopped at the first sign of leukopenia or anaemia, the effect is reversible. Olanzapine appears to be free of this disadvantage.
- *Urticarial skin reactions* are common but usually mild. Excessive sensitivity to ultraviolet light may also occur.
- *Antipsychotic malignant syndrome* is a rare but serious complication similar to the malignant hyperthermia syndrome seen with certain anaesthetics (see Ch. 41). Muscle rigidity is accompanied by a rapid rise in body temperature and mental confusion. It is usually reversible, but death from renal or cardiovascular failure occurs in 10%–20% of cases.

Unwanted effects of antipsychotic drugs

- Important side effects common to many drugs are:
  - motor disturbances (see Antipsychotic-induced motor disturbances box);
  - endocrine disturbances (increased prolactin release);
  - these are secondary to dopamine receptor block.
- Sedation, hypotension and weight gain are common.
- Obstructive jaundice sometimes occurs with phenothiazines.
- Other side effects (dry mouth, blurred vision, hypotension, etc.) are due to block of other receptors, particularly muscarinic receptors and α adrenoceptors.
- Some antipsychotic drugs cause agranulocytosis as a rare and serious idiosyncratic reaction. With **clozapine**, leukopenia is common and requires routine monitoring.
- Antipsychotic malignant syndrome is a rare but potentially dangerous idiosyncratic reaction.

PHARMACOKINETIC ASPECTS

Chlorpromazine, in common with other phenothiazines, is erratically absorbed after oral administration. Fig. 47.5 shows the wide range of variation of the peak plasma concentration as a function of dosage in 14 patients. Among four patients treated at the high dosage level of 6–8 mg/kg, the variation in peak plasma concentration was nearly 90-fold; two showed marked side effects, one was well controlled and one showed no clinical response.

The relationship between the plasma concentration and the clinical effect of antipsychotic drugs is highly variable, and the dosage has to be adjusted on a trial-and-error basis. This is made even more difficult by the fact that at least 40% of patients with schizophrenia fail to take drugs as prescribed. It is remarkably fortunate that the acute toxicity of antipsychotic drugs is slight, given the unpredictability of the clinical response.

The plasma half-life of most antipsychotic drugs is 15–30 h, clearance depending entirely on hepatic transformation by a combination of oxidative and conjugative reactions.

Most antipsychotic drugs can be given orally or in urgent situations by intramuscular injection. Slow-release (depot) preparations of many are available, in which the active drug is esterified with heptanoic or decanoic acid and dissolved

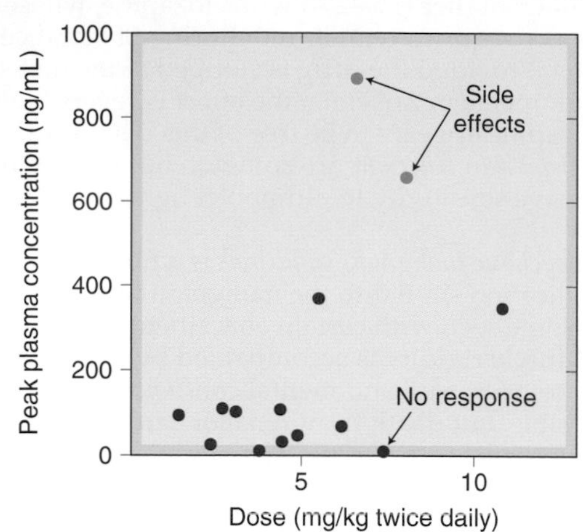

Fig. 47.5 Individual variation in the relation between dose and plasma concentration of chlorpromazine in a group of patients with schizophrenia. (Data from Curry, S.H., et al., 1970. Arch. Gen. Psychiatry 22, 289.)

in oil. Given as an intramuscular injection, the drug acts for 2–4 weeks, but initially may produce acute side effects. These preparations are widely used to minimise compliance problems.

The more predictable pharmacokinetic profile of the second-generation antipsychotics as well as their more dynamic interactions with the D_2 receptor may be a factor in their improved EPS profile. Imaging studies suggest that >80% occupancy of D_2 receptors in the nigrostriatal pathway leads to EPS. The pharmacology of first-generation antipsychotics can make it difficult to achieve the optimal dose but it is easier with many of the second-generation drugs because of their more predictable pharmacokinetics and more rapid association and dissociation from the D2 receptor.

Clinical uses of antipsychotic drugs

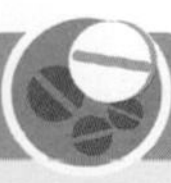

- *Behavioural emergencies* (e.g. violent patients with a range of psychopathologies including *mania*, *toxic delirium*, *schizophrenia* and others):
  - Antipsychotic drugs (e.g. **chlorpromazine**, **haloperidol**, **olanzapine**, **risperidone**) can rapidly control hyperactive psychotic states.
  - Note that the intramuscular dose is lower than the oral dose of the same drug because of presystemic metabolism.
- Schizophrenia:
  - Second-generation antipsychotics are recommended as a first-line treatment for chronic treatment due to their reduced side effect burden; however, first-generation drugs are still used for patients who fail to respond or achieve adequate symptomatic control. Depot injections (e.g. **flupentixol decanoate**) may be useful for maintenance treatment when compliance with oral treatment is a problem.
  - **Flupentixol** has antidepressant properties distinct from its antipsychotic action.
  - **Clozapine** can cause *agranulocytosis* and is reserved for patients whose condition remains inadequately controlled despite previous use of two or more antipsychotic drugs, of which at least one is a second-generation drug. Blood count is monitored weekly for the first 18 weeks, and less frequently thereafter.

FUTURE DEVELOPMENTS

Progress in the development of new antipsychotics has been disappointing with much of the enthusiasm around glutamate-based treatments being crushed when drugs designed to modify glutamatergic transmission failed in clinical trials despite showing promise in both animal models and early trials in humans. This includes the orthosteric and allosteric agonists of $mGluR_2$ and $mGluR_3$ metabotropic glutamate receptors and $mGluR_5$ receptor agonists (see Ch. 38). An alternative approach to modulating glutamatergic function is positive allosteric modulation at the AMPA receptor, one such drug, BIIB-104, is currently under development for the treatment of cognitive symptoms in schizophrenia.

Roluperidone is a 5-HT_{2A} and σ_2 receptor antagonist and has an active metabolite with some affinity at H_1 receptors. However, after initial promise, the most recent phase III data are disappointing. Other drugs currently undergoing clinical trial include those with more novel mechanisms of action including, muscarinic M_1 and M_4 agonists such as **xanomeline** which have been shown to have potential as antipsychotic and pro-cognitive drugs but their peripheral side effects (see Ch. 14) have limited progress. A combination of xanomeline and the peripherally restricted muscarinic antagonist **trospium** is currently undergoing clinical trials in schizophrenia. It may also be useful to treat cognitive impairments in other disorders such as Alzheimer's disease. A novel phosphodiesterase10A inhibitor, TAK-063, is also in stage II clinical trial.

Using a different approach to classical drug development methods (see Ch. 60), a non-D_2 psychotropic drug was identified based on a novel high-throughput, high-content, mouse-behaviour phenotyping platform, in combination with in vitro screening. The mechanism(s) of action of the arising lead molecule, ulotaront (SEP-363856), has yet to be fully elucidated but includes trace amine-associated receptor-1 and 5-HT_{1A} receptor agonism. Its path through clinical trials will be interesting to follow and, if successful, could provide an example of a different approach to identify new molecules and targets for complex psychiatric disorders – a sort of 'targeted serendipity'.

REFERENCES AND FURTHER READING

General reading

Gross, G., Geyer, M.A., 2012. Current Antipsychotics. Handbook of Experimental Pharmacology. Springer Verlag.

Kean, C., 2009. Silencing the self: schizophrenia as a self-disturbance. Schizophr. Bull. 35 (6), 1034–1036.

McCutcheon, R.A., Reis Marques, T., Howes, O.D., 2020. Schizophrenia—an overview. JAMA Psychiatr. 77 (2), 201–210.

Stahl, S.M., 2021. Stahl's Essential Psychopharmacology Neuroscientific Basis and Practical Applications, fifth ed. Cambridge University Press, Cambridge.

Pathogenesis of schizophrenia

Ayhan, Y., McFarland, R., Pletnikov, M.V., 2016. Animal models of gene-environment interaction in schizophrenia: a dimensional perspective. Prog. Neurobiol. 136, 1–27.

Fusar-Poli, P., Radua, J., McGuire, P., Borgwardt, S., 2012. Neuroanatomical maps of psychosis onset: voxel-wise meta-analysis of antipsychotic-naive VBM studies. Schizophr. Bull. 38 (6), 1297–1307.

Kambeitz, J., Kambeitz-Ilankovic, L., Cabral, C., et al., 2016. Aberrant functional whole-brain network architecture in patients with schizophrenia: a meta-analysis. Schizophr. Bull. 42 (Suppl. 1): S13–S21.

Pergola, G., Selvaggi, P., Trizio, S., et al., 2015. The role of the thalamus in schizophrenia from a neuroimaging perspective. Neurosci. Biobehav. Rev. 54, 57–75.

Animal models

Ang, M.J., Lee, S., Kim, J.-C., Kim, S.-H., Moon, C., 2021. Behavioral tasks evaluating schizophrenia-like symptoms in animal models: a recent update. Curr. Neuropharmacol. 19 (5), 641–664.

Winship, I.R., Dursun, S.N., Baker, G.B., et al., 2019. An overview of animal models related to schizophrenia. Can. J. Psychiatry 64 (1), 5–17.

Antipsychotic drugs

Jolly, K., Gammage, M.D., Cheng, K.K., Bradburn, P., Banting, M.V., Langman, M.J., 2009. Sudden death in patients receiving drugs tending to prolong the QT interval. Br. J. Clin. Pharmacol. 68, 743–751.

Kapur, S., Arenovich, T., Agid, O., et al., 2005. Evidence for onset of antipsychotic effects within the first 24 hours of treatment. Am. J. Psychiatry 162, 939–946.

Kapur, S., Seeman, P., 2001. Does fast dissociation from the dopamine D_2 receptor explain the action of atypical antipsychotics? A new hypothesis. Am. J. Psychiatry 158, 360–369.

Leucht, S., Busch, R., Hamann, J., Kissling, W., Kane, J.M., 2005. Early-onset hypothesis of antipsychotic drug action: a hypothesis tested, confirmed and extended. Biol. Psychiatry 57, 1543–1549.

Leucht, S., Cipriani, A., Spineli, L., et al., 2013. Comparative efficacy and tolerability of 15 antipsychotic drugs in schizophrenia: a multiple-treatments meta-analysis. Lancet 382, 951–962.

Extrapyramidal side effects

Casey, D.E., 1995. Tardive dyskinesia: pathophysiology. In: Bloom, F.E., Kupfer, D.J. (Eds.), Psychopharmacology: A Fourth Generation of Progress. Raven Press, New York.

Klawans, H.L., Tanner, C.M., Goetz, C.G., 1988. Epidemiology and pathophysiology of tardive dyskinesias. Adv. Neurol. 49, 185–197.

Lieberman, J.A., Stroup, T.S., 2011. The NIMH-CATIE Schizophrenia Study: what did we learn? Am. J. Psychiatry 68, 770–775.

Pisani, A., Bernardi, G., Ding, J., Surmeier, D.J., 2007. Re-emergence of striatal cholinergic interneurons in movement disorders. Trends Neurosci. 30, 545–553.

48 Antidepressant drugs

OVERVIEW

Depression is an extremely common psychiatric condition but with limited understanding of the underlying neurobiology or how antidepressants reduce symptoms. Bipolar disorder is less common but equally poorly understood. It is a field in which therapeutic empiricism has led the way, with mechanistic understanding tending to lag behind, part of the problem being that it has been difficult to develop animal models that replicate the characteristics that define the human condition. In this chapter, we discuss the current understanding of the nature of the disorder, and describe the major drugs that are used to treat it.

THE NATURE OF DEPRESSION

Depression and anxiety are the most common psychiatric disorders and are highly comorbid. Symptoms of depression may range from a very mild condition, bordering on normality, to severe (psychotic) depression accompanied by hallucinations and delusions. Worldwide, depression is a major cause of disability and premature death. In addition to the significant suicide risk, individuals with depression are more likely to die from other causes, such as heart disease or cancer. Depression is a heterogeneous disorder, with patients presenting with one or more core symptoms, and depression is often associated with other psychiatric conditions, including anxiety, eating disorders, schizophrenia, Parkinson's disease and drug use disorder.

The symptoms of depression include emotional and biological components. Emotional symptoms include:

- low mood, excessive rumination of negative thought, misery, apathy and pessimism
- low self-esteem: feelings of guilt, inadequacy and ugliness
- indecisiveness, loss of motivation
- anhedonia, loss of interest in previously rewarding activities

Biological symptoms include:

- retardation of thought and action
- loss of libido
- sleep disturbance and loss of appetite

There are two distinct types of depressive syndrome, namely *unipolar depression*, in which the mood changes are always in the same direction, and *bipolar disorder*, in which depression alternates with mania. Mania is in most respects exactly the opposite, with excessive exuberance, enthusiasm and self-confidence, accompanied by impulsive actions, these signs often being combined with irritability, impatience and aggression, and sometimes with grandiose delusions. As with depression, the mood and actions are inappropriate to the circumstances.

Unipolar depression is commonly (about 75% of cases) non-familial, clearly associated with stressful life events, and usually accompanied by symptoms of anxiety and agitation; this type is sometimes termed *reactive depression*. Other cases (about 25%, sometimes termed *endogenous depression*) show a familial pattern, less obviously related to external stresses and with a somewhat different symptomatology. This distinction is made clinically, but there is little evidence that antidepressant drugs show significant selectivity between these conditions. After an inauspicious start, population genetic studies have begun to identify novel genetic variations associated with depression, but depression is probably a polygenic disorder where a number of individual genetic variations as well as environmental factors contribute to the disorder. As illustrated in Fig 48.1, depression is linked to both genetic and environmental risk factors which increase vulnerability with precipitating factors related to adolescent and adult stress. These stressors can be psychological and/or physiological with depression a common feature of patients with other chronic illnesses. Some interesting theories have also emerged relating to the role of inflammation and the role of the gut microbiome and the benefit of these microflora on mental health (for those interested in exploring these further see Bastiaanssen et al., 2020; Duman et al., 2021; Gonda et al., 2019; Pariante, 2017; Saavedra and Salazar, 2021).

Depression cannot be attributed to altered neuronal activity within a single brain region; rather, the circuitry linking different parts of the brain is likely to be more important. Brain imaging studies have indicated that the prefrontal cortex, amygdala and hippocampus may all be involved in components of these disorders. These regions play a critical role in cognitive and emotional behaviour and it is likely that psychological factors are also important but understanding how these biological and experience-dependent factors interact is not straightforward.

Bipolar disorder, which usually appears in early adult life, is less common and results in oscillating depression and mania over a period of weeks/months. It can be difficult to differentiate between mild bipolar disorder and unipolar depression. Also, bipolar manic episodes can be confused with episodes of schizophrenic psychosis (see Ch. 47). There is a stronger hereditary tendency for bipolar disorder, and gene-wide association studies (GWASs) have identified a number of new susceptibility genes that may have an effect on the brain functions affected in bipolar disorder but to date these have not impacted on drug therapy of the disorder.

THEORIES OF DEPRESSION

Several theories have been proposed to explain the causes of depression although with limited clinical evidence and mainly inferred from the pharmacological effects of antidepressant treatments, e.g. the monoamine hypothesis which arose from the observation that monoamine transmitters were the primary target for antidepressant

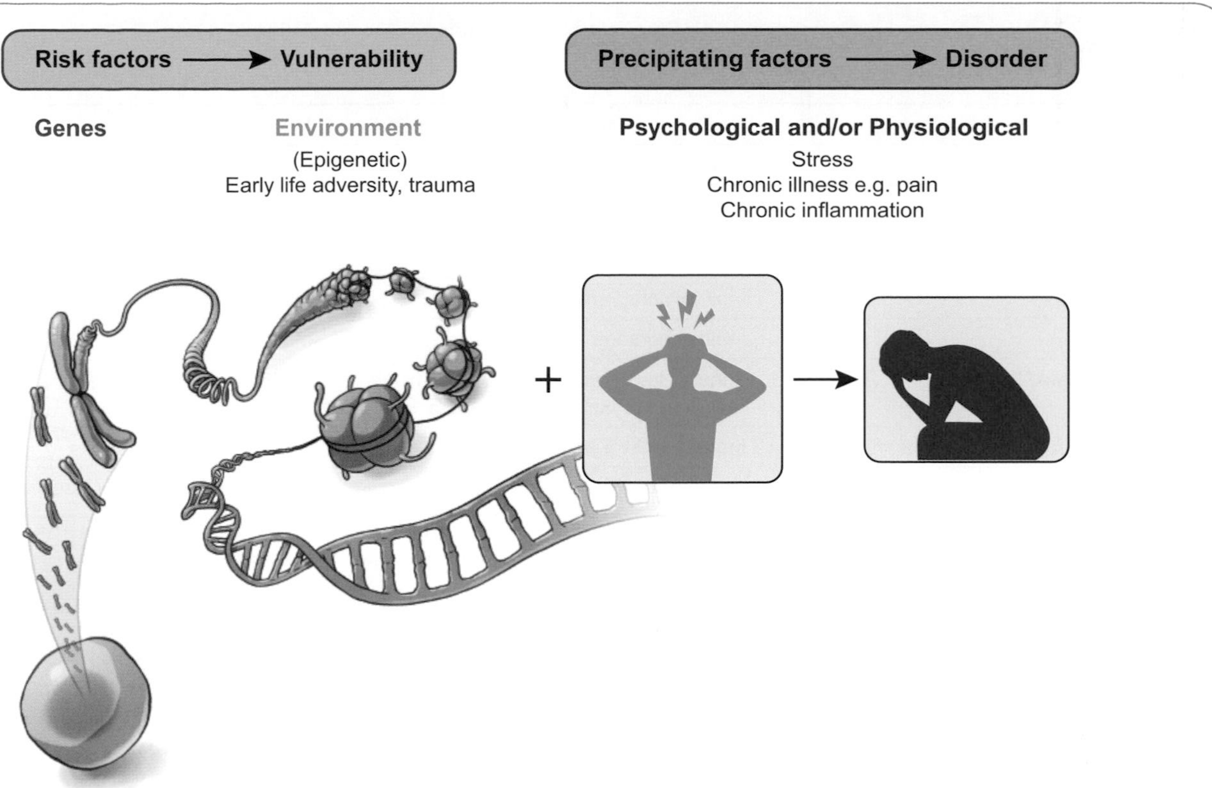

Fig. 48.1 Genetic and environmental factors which contribute to the risks of developing depression. The causes of depression are complex and poorly understood but this diagram illustrates the different risk factors which have been linked to the development of mood disorders. Genetic factors and early life events, e.g. childhood abuse, neglect or trauma, lead to increased vulnerability possibly due to a sensitisation of the stress system. Precipitating factors in adolescence and adulthood then lead to the development of depression. Stress, particularly uncontrollable stress and social stress, as well as other chronic illnesses and chronic inflammatory disorders have all been linked to precipitating an episode of depression. More vulnerable individuals may develop depression more readily when exposed to chronic stress but even those who have low vulnerability may experience events in adulthood which can lead to the development of depression. Decades of research have failed to find a specific biological impairment or biomarker which can be attributed to causing depression.

drugs, and studies in animal models. None fully explain all of the observations and no biological marker has been identified to date. Much of what has been established in the last 70 years has recently had to be re-evaluated in light of the discovery that some drugs, e.g. **ketamine**, have both rapid and sustained antidepressant effects. This is contrary to what had been seen previously with classical antidepressant drugs, now referred to as conventional antidepressants or delayed-onset antidepressants reflecting the widely observed 4–6-week delay from onset of drug treatment before clinical improvement in symptoms is observed. Any theory of depression must now take account of the fact that the direct neurochemical effects of most antidepressant drugs appear very rapidly (minutes to hours), whereas the therapeutic benefits of conventional antidepressant take weeks to fully develop. They also need to incorporate the developments of the last 20 years following the discovery that low doses of the *N*-methyl-D-aspartate (NMDA) receptor antagonist ketamine has rapid and sustained antidepressant effects. The discovery of ketamine's antidepressant effects has also led to a new class of antidepressants referred to as rapid-acting antidepressants (RAADs).

To explain the delayed-onset phenomenon, proponents of the monoamine theory have suggested that secondary, slow adaptive changes in monoamine receptors, rather than the primary drug effect, are responsible for the clinical improvement. Others have favoured a neurotrophic hypothesis where the effects on brain monoamine systems result in longer-term trophic effects including neurogenesis, increases in dendritic arborisation and synapses, the time course of which is paralleled by mood changes. More recently, a neuropsychological model of antidepressant efficacy has been proposed which links the biological effects of the antidepressant with psychological effects. Here we summarise the main theories as they relate to the mechanisms of action of current drug therapies. A more comprehensive review and analysis of these theories are provided by Harmer et al. (2017) and Duman et al. (2021).

THE MONOAMINE THEORY

The monoamine theory of depression, first proposed by Schildkraut in 1965, states that depression is caused by a functional deficit of the monoamine transmitters, noradrenaline and 5-hydroxytryptamine (5-HT) at certain sites in the brain, while mania results from a functional excess.

The monoamine hypothesis grew originally out of associations between the clinical effects of various drugs

Table 48.1 Pharmacological evidence supporting the role of monoamines in the regulation of mood

Drug(s)	Principal action	Effect in patients with depression
Tricyclic antidepressants	Block noradrenaline and 5-HT reuptake	Mood ↑
MAO inhibitors	Increase stores of noradrenaline and 5-HT	Mood ↑
Tetrabenazine	Reversibly inhibits vesicular monoamine transporter 2 leading to depletion of monoamine storage	Mood ↓
α-Methyltyrosine	Inhibits noradrenaline synthesis	Mood ↓ (calming of manic patients)
Methyldopa	Inhibits noradrenaline synthesis	Mood ↓
Electroconvulsive therapy	? Increases central nervous system responses to noradrenaline and 5-HT	Mood ↑
Tryptophan (5-hydroxytryptophan)	Increases 5-HT synthesis	Mood ? ↑ in some studies
Tryptophan depletion	Decreases brain 5-HT synthesis	Induces relapse in SSRI-treated patients[a]

[a]Although initially seen as evidence supporting a monoamine hypothesis of depression, these effects may be more related to the adaptive changes induced by SSRIs which are also linked to emotional blunting and symptoms of withdrawal (see Fig 48.3).
5-HT, 5-Hydroxytryptamine; *MAO,* monoamine oxidase; *SSRI,* selective serotonin reuptake inhibitor.

that cause or alleviate symptoms of depression and their known neurochemical effects on monoaminergic transmission in the brain. This pharmacological evidence, which is summarised in Table 48.1, gives general support to the role of monoamine in the modulation of mood. It provides a potential explanation for how drugs which alter monoamine levels in the brain can alter mood but evidence of a deficit in patients has not been established. Studies into monoamine metabolism in patients with depression or by measuring changes in the number of monoamine receptors in postmortem brain tissue have been inconsistent and the interpretation is often problematic, because the changes described are not specific to depression.

Clinically, it seems that inhibitors of noradrenaline reuptake and of 5-HT reuptake are similarly effective as antidepressants, although individual patients may respond better to one or the other. Given the close interactions between these two transmitter systems, this may not be that surprising.

NEUROENDOCRINE MECHANISMS

Various attempts have been made to test for a functional deficit of monoamine pathways in depression linked to neuroendocrine responses, particularly relating to stress hormones. Hypothalamic neurons controlling pituitary function receive noradrenergic and 5-HT inputs, which control the discharge of these cells. Hypothalamic cells release corticotrophin-releasing factor (CRF; also known as *corticotrophin-releasing hormone*), which stimulates pituitary cells to secrete adrenocorticotrophic hormone (ACTH), leading in turn to release of the stress hormone, cortisol (see Ch. 33). The plasma cortisol concentration is sometimes higher in patients with depression. Other hormones in plasma are also sometimes affected; for example, growth hormone concentration is reduced and prolactin is increased in some studies. While these changes are consistent with deficiencies in monoamine transmission, they are not specific to depressive syndromes or found reliably across patients.

NEUROTROPHIC EFFECTS AND NEUROPLASTICITY

It has been suggested that lowered levels of brain-derived neurotrophic factor (BDNF) or dysfunction of its receptor, TrkB, plays a significant role in the pathology of depression. There has been some evidence of a reduction in BDNF expression in patients, and treatment with antidepressants elevates BDNF levels as well as potentiating downstream signalling via mammalian target of rapamycin (mTOR) or glycogen synthase kinase 3 beta (GSK3β). Changes in glutamatergic neurotransmission have been linked to this loss of neurons and atrophy in the hippocampus and prefrontal cortex. As with other theories of depression, most studies have focused on the actions of antidepressants and animal studies and then generated hypotheses from this about a possible pathological process which the drugs are able to reverse. This is likely to be too simplistic given the complex biological, psychological and environmental factors which contribute to depression. However, preclinical studies have shown that both conventional and RAADs induce positive effects on both neuroplasticity and neurogenesis.[1] The RAAD ketamine has been found to increase synaptogenesis, the development of new synapses, whilst conventional antidepressants increase BDNF and associated downstream effects including neurogenesis, possibly via effects on monoamine transmitters. The mood stabiliser, lithium, has also been shown to interact with GSK3β and has been linked to neuroprotective and neurotrophic effects (Won and Kim, 2017). Key evidence supporting a role for neuroplastic and neurotrophic mechanism in depression and antidepressant efficacy include:

[1]Neurogenesis (see Ch. 40) – the formation of new neurons from stem cell precursors – occurs to a significant degree in the adult hippocampus, and possibly elsewhere in the brain, contradicting the old dogma that it occurs only during brain development.

- Brain imaging and postmortem studies show reductions in volume of the hippocampus and prefrontal cortex of patients with depression, with loss of neurons and glia. Functional imaging reveals altered brain activity in emotional circuits possibly linked to this neuronal loss.
- In animals, the same effect is produced by chronic stress of various kinds, or by administration of glucocorticoids, mimicking the increased cortisol secretion in human depression. Excessive glucocorticoid secretion in humans (Cushing's syndrome; see Ch. 33) often causes depression.
- In experimental animals, antidepressant drugs, or other treatments such as electroconvulsions (see later section on *Brain Stimulation Therapies*), promote neurogenesis in the hippocampus, and (as in humans) restore functional activity. Preventing hippocampal neurogenesis prevents the behavioural effects of antidepressants in rats.
- 5-HT and noradrenaline, whose actions are enhanced by many antidepressants, promote neurogenesis, probably through activation of 5-HT_{1A} receptors and α_2 adrenoceptors, respectively. This effect may be mediated by BDNF.
- Exercise has been shown to promote neurogenesis in animals and to be effective in some patients with mild to moderate depression.
- Ketamine and other putative RAAD increase the development of new synapses on glutamatergic neurons in the prefrontal cortex (Krystal et al., 2019; Vargas et al., 2021).

NEUROPSYCHOLOGICAL HYPOTHESIS

People suffering from depression tend to perceive events in a negative way, focus on negative information and recall information in a negative rather than positive manner - a behaviour pattern that psychologists term *negative affective biases*. Studies in healthy volunteers and patients with depression suggest that antidepressant drugs may indeed exert acute effects on the way information is processed (cognitive processing), leading to a positive effect on emotional behaviour. For example, when presented with a series of pictures showing facial expressions of different levels of happiness or sadness, patients with depression consider fewer of the faces to be happy than do healthy volunteers presented with the same faces. But after a single dose of an antidepressant both healthy volunteers and patients now consider more of the same faces to be happy (i.e. their perception of what is happy (positive) has changed) (Fig 48.2). It is suggested that patients with depression may not initially be consciously aware of the effect the antidepressant drug has produced, but with prolonged drug administration, these neuropsychological effects positively bias new learning which, over time, leads to a subjective improvement in mood. Using translational animal models of affective biases, similar acute neuropsychological effects have been observed in animals and humans performing memory tasks (Fig 48.2).

Theories of depression

- The *monoamine theory*, first proposed in 1965, suggests that depression results from functionally deficient monoaminergic (noradrenaline and/or 5-hydroxytryptamine) transmission in the central nervous system (CNS).
- The theory is based on the ability of most antidepressant drugs (tricyclic antidepressants (TCAs) and monoamine oxidase inhibitors (MAOIs)) to facilitate monoaminergic transmission, and of drugs which deplete monoamines such as **tetrabenazine and reserpine** to cause depression.
- Although the *monoamine hypothesis* in its simple form is insufficient as an explanation of depression, pharmacological manipulation of monoamine transmission remains the most successful therapeutic approach.
- The *neuropsychological hypothesis* of antidepressant efficacy suggests that drugs may produce immediate psychological effects but patients receiving the drugs need time for these to bias new learning before they become aware of the improvements in their mood.
- Depression may be associated with neurodegeneration in brain regions regulating emotional behaviour and reduced neurogenesis in the hippocampus, effects which can be reversed by both conventional delayed onset and rapid acting antidepressants (RAADs).

  Biochemical studies in patients with depression do not clearly support any single hypothesis with no biological marker identified which shows reliable changes in all patients.
- The discovery of RAADs such as ketamine requires us to re-evaluate many of these hypotheses but research to date has provided evidence of both neurotrophic and neuropsychological effects associated with RAADs.

ANTIDEPRESSANT DRUGS

TYPES OF ANTIDEPRESSANT DRUG

With the emergence of a new class of RAADs, types of antidepressants can be divided into two main types based on the rate of onset of therapeutic effects. *Conventional antidepressants* is a term often now used to describe drugs which have a delayed onset and target monoamine systems whilst those which have immediate and sustained antidepressant effects are referred to as RAADs. Antidepressant drugs fall into the following pharmacological categories:

Inhibitors of monoamine reuptake

- Selective serotonin (5-HT) reuptake inhibitors (SSRIs) (e.g. fluoxetine, fluvoxamine, paroxetine, sertraline, citalopram, escitalopram, vilazodone).
- Classic TCAs (e.g. imipramine, desipramine, amitriptyline, nortriptyline, clomipramine). These

vary in their activity and selectivity with respect to inhibition of noradrenaline and 5-HT reuptake.

- Mixed 5-HT and noradrenaline reuptake inhibitors (e.g. venlafaxine (somewhat selective for 5-HT, although less so than SSRIs), desvenlafaxine, duloxetine).
- Noradrenaline reuptake inhibitors (e.g. **reboxetine, atomoxetine, bupropion** (also a dopamine reuptake inhibitor)).

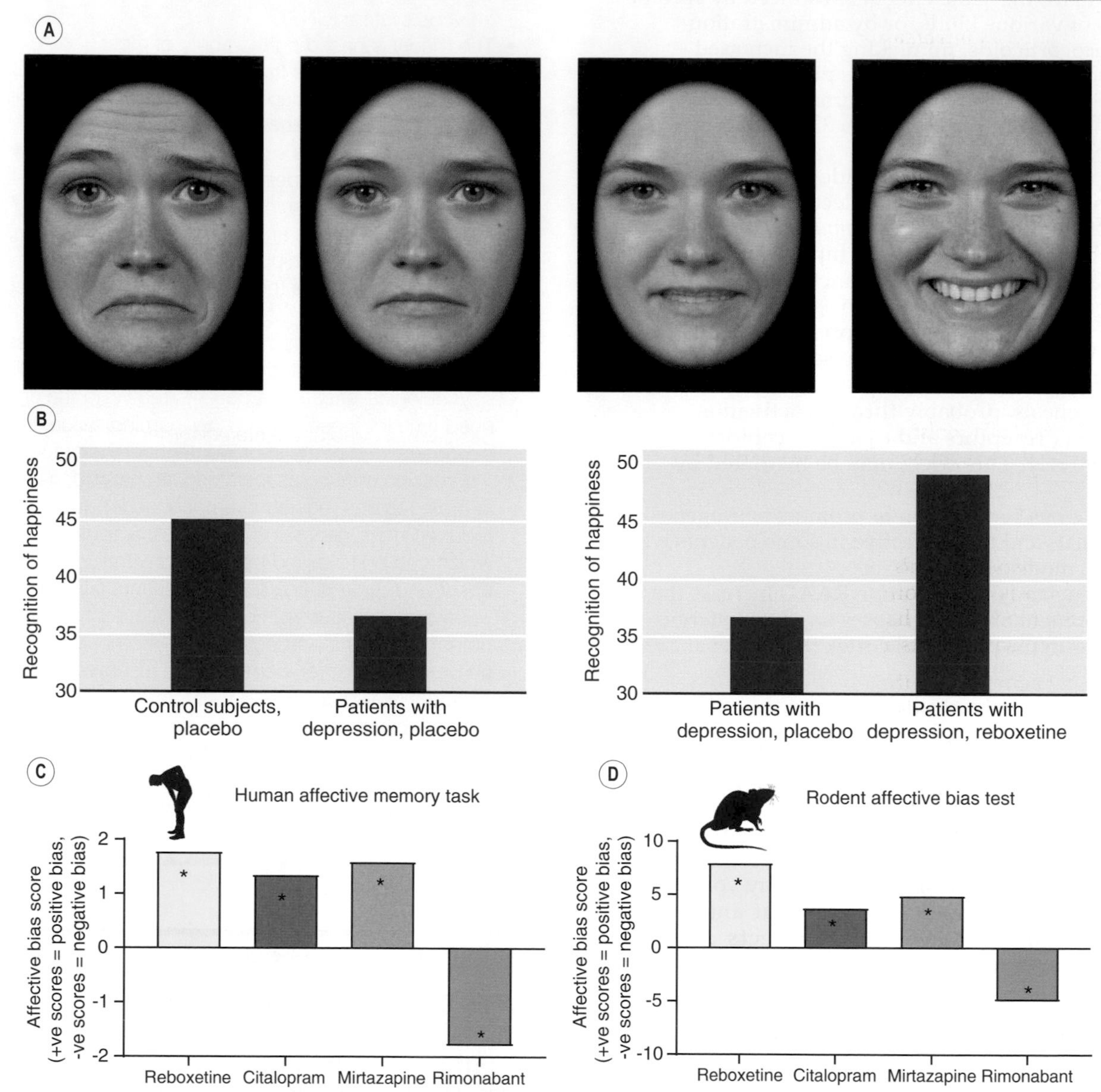

Fig. 48.2 Acute neuropsychological effects of different pharmacological treatments on affective biases in humans and rodents. Affective biases describe how information processing can be altered by the emotional state of the subject and can be measured in humans or animals. (A) illustrates the happy and sad facial expressions used to assess how well patients with depression recognise happy faces. When presented with an array of faces, such as those in (A), patients with depression considered fewer faces to be happy than did control subjects. After an acute dose of reetine, patients with depression considered more of the facial expressions to be happy. (B) Using tasks which measure affective biases associated with learning and memory has also revealed that acute treatment with antidepressant drugs induces positive memory bias while the pro-depressant cannabinoid$_1$-receptor antagonist, rimonabant, induces a negative memory bias with similar effects seen in humans (C) and rats (D). (Faces in (A) are reprinted from the P1vital Oxford Emotional Test Battery, P1vital Products Ltd. Data in (B) are adapted from Harmer, et al., 2009. Am. J. Psychiatry 166, 1178–1184.) (C and D) created using data from Harmer, C.J., Shelley, N.C., Cowen, P.J., et al., 2004. Am. J. Psychiatry 161, 1586–1592; Harmer et al., 2013; Harmer, C.J., Shelley, N.C., Cowen, P.J., et al., 2004. Am. J. Psychiatry 161, 1256–1263; Pringle, A., Browning, M., Cowen, P.J., et al., 2011. Prog. Neuropsychopharmacol. Biol. Psychiatry 35, 1586–1592; Horder, J., Browning, M., Di Simplicio, M., et al., 2012. J. Psychopharmacol. 26, 125–32; Arnone, D., Horder, J., Cwen, P.J. et al., 2009. Psychopharmacology (Berl) 203, 685–691; and Stuart, S.A., Butler, P., Munafo, M.R., et al., 2013. Neuropsychopharmacology 38, 1625–1635.)

- The herbal preparation St John's wort, the main active ingredient of which is hyperforin: it has similar clinical efficacy to most of the prescribed antidepressants. It is a weak monoamine uptake inhibitor but also has other actions.[2]

Receptor blocking antidepressants

- Drugs such as **mirtazapine** and **mianserin** inhibit a range of amine receptors including α_2 adrenoceptors and 5-HT_2 receptors. **Trazodone** has a mixture of agonist and antagonist effects at a range of monoamine receptors and weak effects on monoamine uptake.

Monoamine oxidase inhibitors (MAOIs)

- Irreversible, non-competitive inhibitors (e.g. **phenelzine**, **tranylcypromine**), which are non-selective with respect to the monoamine oxidase (MAO)-A and -B subtypes.
- Reversible, MAO-A-selective inhibitors (e.g. **moclobemide**).

Melatonin receptor agonist

- **Agomelatine** is an agonist at MT_1 and MT_2 melatonin receptors, and a weak 5-HT_{2C} antagonist.

Rapid-acting antidepressants

- **Ketamine** is a non-competitive NMDA receptor channel blocker and has rapid and sustained antidepressant effects at low doses.

Table 48.2 summarises the main features of these types of drug. Mention should also be made of electroconvulsive therapy (ECT), electromagnetic therapy, deep brain stimulation and vagus stimulation, which can be effective in patients who have failed to respond to drug therapy and usually act more rapidly than conventional antidepressant drugs.

To some extent, the term *antidepressant drug* is misleading, as many of these drugs are now also used to treat disorders other than depression. These include:

- neuropathic pain (e.g. amitriptyline, nortriptyline, duloxetine; see Ch. 43)
- anxiety disorders (e.g. SSRIs, venlafaxine, duloxetine; see Ch. 45)
- fibromyalgia (e.g. duloxetine, venlafaxine, SSRIs, TCAs; see Ch. 43)
- bipolar disorder (e.g. fluoxetine in conjunction with **olanzapine**; see later)
- smoking cessation (e.g. bupropion; see Ch. 50)
- attention deficit/hyperactivity disorder (e.g. atomoxetine; see Ch. 49)

[2]Although relatively free of acute side effects, hyperforin activates cytochrome P450, resulting in loss of efficacy (see Ch. 10), with serious consequences, of several important drugs, including ciclosporine, oral contraceptives, some anti-HIV and anticancer drugs and oral anticoagulants – underlining the principle that herbal remedies are not inherently safe, and must be used with the same degree of informed caution as any other drug.

Types of antidepressant drugs

- Main types are:
  - monoamine uptake inhibitors (tricyclic antidepressants, selective serotonin reuptake inhibitors, newer inhibitors of noradrenaline and 5-HT reuptake);
  - monoamine receptor antagonists;
  - monoamine oxidase (MAO) inhibitors.
- Monoamine uptake inhibitors act by inhibiting uptake of noradrenaline and/or 5-HT by monoaminergic nerve terminals.
- α_2-Adrenoceptor antagonists can indirectly elevate 5-HT release (Fig 48.3).
- MAOIs inhibit one or both forms of brain MAO, thus increasing the cytosolic stores of noradrenaline and 5-HT in nerve terminals. Inhibition of type A MAO correlates with antidepressant activity. Most are non-selective; **moclobemide** is specific for MAO-A.
- Most antidepressant drugs appear to take at least 2 weeks to produce any perceived beneficial effects.
- Esketamine, one of the stereoisomers of ketamine, is delivered as a nasal spray whilst ketamine is also used as an intravenous infusion (off license) and produces a rapid response lasting for up to 2 weeks.

TESTING OF ANTIDEPRESSANT DRUGS

ANIMAL MODELS

Progress in unravelling the neurochemical mechanisms is, as in so many areas of psychopharmacology, limited by the lack of good animal models of the clinical condition. Investigating complex psychiatric disorders in animals poses at least two significant challenges. A model of the disorder is needed to understand the underlying pathophysiology and readouts which are relevant to human symptoms of depression to test the effects of novel treatments. Methods which expose animals to stress can generate behavioural despair (e.g. forced swim test, learned helplessness) and these behaviours are sensitive to the original monoaminergic antidepressants but interpretation of these models in the context of underlying disease processes or non-monoaminergic drugs is limited. Somewhat more success has been achieved using different types of stress to induce a depression-like phenotype including early life adversity and experience of chronic social and/environmental stressors. Detecting changes in the animal's emotional behaviour mostly focuses on changes in reward-related behaviours akin to the anhedonia seen in many patients. More recently, attempts to improve the translation between human and animal studies have led to novel neuropsychological models based on negative affective biases. For a more detailed discussion around the limitations of current animal models of depression and future prospects see Gururajan et al. (2019).

TESTS ON HUMANS

Clinically, the effect of antidepressant drugs is usually measured by a subjective rating scale such as the Hamilton

Table 48.2 Types of antidepressant drugs and their characteristics

Type and examples	Action(s)	Unwanted effects	Risk of overdose	Pharmacokinetics	Notes
Monoamine uptake inhibitors					
(1) SSRIs	Selective for 5-HT	Nausea, diarrhoea, agitation, insomnia, anorgasmia Inhibit metabolism of other drugs, so risk of interactions Withdrawal effects	Low risk in overdose but must not be used in combination with MAO inhibitors	—	—
Fluoxetine	As above	As above	As above	Long $t_{1/2}$ (24–96 h)	—
Fluvoxamine	As above	As above	As above	$t_{1/2}$ 18–24 h	Less nausea than with other SSRIs
Paroxetine	As above	As above	As above	$t_{1/2}$18–24 h	Withdrawal reaction
Citalopram	As above	As above	As above	$t_{1/2}$ 24–36 h	—
Escitalopram	As above	As above	As above	$t_{1/2}$ 24–36 h	Active *S* isomer of citalopram Fewer side effects
Sertraline	As above	As above	As above	$t_{1/2}$ 24–36 h	—
Vilazodone	As above. Also has 5-HT_{1A} receptor partial agonist activity	As above	As above	$t_{1/2}$ 25 h	—
Vortioxetine	As above. Also has partial agonist activity at 5-HT_{1A} and 5-HT_{1B} receptors and antagonist activity at 5-HT_{3A} receptors	As above	As above	$t_{1/2}$ >60 h	—
(2) Classical TCA group[a]	Inhibition of NA and 5-HT reuptake	Sedation Anticholinergic effects (dry mouth, constipation, blurred vision, urinary retention, etc.) Postural hypotension Seizures Impotence Interaction with CNS depressants (especially alcohol, MAO inhibitors) Withdrawal effects	Ventricular dysrhythmias High risk in combination with CNS depressants	—	'First-generation' antidepressants, still very widely used, although newer compounds generally have fewer side effects and lower risk with overdose
Imipramine	Non-selective Converted to desipramine	As above	As above	$t_{1/2}$ 4–18 h	—
Desipramine	NA selective	As above	As above	$t_{1/2}$ 12–24 h	—
Amitriptyline	Non-selective	As above	As above	$t_{1/2}$ 12–24 h; converted to nortriptyline	Widely used, also for neuropathic pain (see Ch. 43)

Continued

Table 48.2 Types of antidepressant drugs and their characteristics—cont'd

Type and examples	Action(s)	Unwanted effects	Risk of overdose	Pharmacokinetics	Notes
Nortriptyline	NA selective (slight)	As above	As above	Long $t_{1/2}$ (24–96 h)	Long duration, less sedative
Clomipramine	Non-selective	As above	As above	$t_{1/2}$ 18–24 h	Also used for anxiety disorders
(3) Other 5-HT/NA uptake inhibitors[b]					
Venlafaxine	Weak non-selective NA/5-HT uptake inhibitor Also, non-selective receptor-blocking effects	As SSRIs Withdrawal effects common and troublesome if doses are missed or reduced too quickly	Safe in overdose	Short $t_{1/2}$ (~5 h) Converted to desvenlafaxine which inhibits NA uptake	Claimed to act more rapidly than other antidepressants, and to work better in 'treatment-resistant' patients Usually classed as non-selective NA/5-HT uptake blocker, although in vitro data show selectivity for 5-HT
Duloxetine	Potent non-selective NA/5-HT uptake inhibitor No action on monoamine receptors	Fewer side effects than venlafaxine Sedation, dizziness, nausea Sexual dysfunction	See SSRIs above	$t_{1/2}$ ~14 h	Also used to treat urinary incontinence (see Ch. 30) and for anxiety disorders
St John's wort (active principle: hyperforin)	Weak non-selective NA/5-HT uptake inhibitor Also, non-selective receptor-blocking effects	Few side effects reported Risk of drug interactions due to enhanced drug metabolism (e.g. loss of efficacy of ciclosporin, antidiabetic drugs, etc.)	—	$t_{1/2}$ ~12 h	Freely available as crude herbal preparation Similar efficacy to other antidepressants, with fewer acute side effects but risk of serious drug interactions
(4) NA-selective inhibitors					
Bupropion	Selective inhibitor of NA over 5-HT uptake but also inhibits dopamine uptake Converted to active metabolites (e.g. radafaxine)	Headache, dry mouth, agitation, insomnia	Seizures at high doses	$t_{1/2}$ ~12 h Plasma half-life ~20 h	Used in depression associated with anxiety Slow-release formulation used to treat nicotine dependence (see Ch. 50)
Reboxetine	Selective NA uptake inhibitor	Dizziness Insomnia Anticholinergic effects	Safe in overdose (low risk of cardiac dysrhythmia)	$t_{1/2}$ ~12 h	Less effective than TCAs The related drug atomoxetine now used mainly to treat ADHD (see Ch. 49)
Maprotiline	Selective NA uptake inhibitor	As TCAs; no significant advantages	As TCAs	Long $t_{1/2}$ ~40 h	No significant advantages over TCAs

Table 48.2 Types of antidepressant drugs and their characteristics—cont'd

Type and examples	Action(s)	Unwanted effects	Risk of overdose	Pharmacokinetics	Notes
Monoamine receptor antagonists					
Mirtazapine	Blocks α_2, 5-HT_{2C} and 5-HT_3 receptors	Dry mouth Sedation Weight gain	No serious drug interactions	$t_{1/2}$ 20–40 h	Claimed to have faster onset of action than other antidepressants
Trazodone	Blocks 5-HT_{2A} and 5-HT_{2C} receptors as well as H_1 receptors Weak 5-HT uptake inhibitor (enhances NA/5-HT release)	Sedation Hypotension Cardiac dysrhythmias	Safe in overdose	$t_{1/2}$ 6–12 h	Nefazodone is similar
Mianserin	Blocks α_1, α_2, 5-HT_{2A} and H_1 receptors	Milder antimuscarinic and cardiovascular effects than TCAs Agranulocytosis, aplastic anaemia	—	$t_{1/2}$ 10–35 h	Blood count advised in early stages of use
MAO inhibitors	Inhibit MAO-A and/or MAO-B Earlier compounds have long duration of action due to covalent binding to enzyme				
Phenelzine	Non-selective	'Cheese reaction' to tyramine-containing foods (see text) Anticholinergic side effects Hypotension Insomnia Weight gain Liver damage (rare)	Many interactions (TCAs, opioids, sympathomimetic drugs) – risk of severe hypertension due to 'cheese reaction'	$t_{1/2}$ 1–2 h Long duration of action due to irreversible binding	—
Tranylcypromine	Non-selective	As phenelzine	As phenelzine	$t_{1/2}$ 1–2 h Long duration of action due to irreversible binding	—
Isocarboxazid	Non-selective	As phenelzine	As phenelzine	Long $t_{1/2}$ ~36 h	—
Moclobemide	MAO-A selective Short acting	Nausea, insomnia, agitation	Interactions less severe than with other MAO inhibitors; no 'cheese reactions' reported	$t_{1/2}$ 1–2 h	Safer alternative to earlier MAO inhibitors
Melatonin agonist					
Agomelatine	MT_1 and MT_2 receptor agonist. Weak 5-HT_{2C} antagonist	Headache, dizziness, drowsiness, fatigue, sleep disturbance, anxiety, nausea, GI disturbances, sweating	Limited data available at present	$t_{1/2}$ 1–2 h	Should not be combined with ethanol Usually taken once daily before bed

Continued

Table 48.2 Types of antidepressant drugs and their characteristics—cont'd

Type and examples	Action(s)	Unwanted effects	Risk of overdose	Pharmacokinetics	Notes
NMDA antagonist					
Ketamine	NMDA-channel blocker	Psychotomimetic effects (see Ch. 49) Prolonged use of high doses can cause cystitis Abuse liability	Deaths from overdose are rare	$t_{1/2}$ 2–4 h Given intravenously	Rapid onset antidepressant action lasting for a few days after single IV dose Effective in patients resistant to other antidepressants Potentially metabolites of ketamine are responsible for the antidepressant effects

[a]Other TCAs include dosulepin, doxepin, lofepramine, trimipramine.
[b]Other 5-HT/NA uptake inhibitors include milnacipran and levomilnacipran.
5-HT, 5-Hydroxytryptamine; *ADHD,* attention deficit/hyperactivity disorder; *CNS,* central nervous system; *GI,* gastrointestinal; *IV,* intravenous; *MAO,* monoamine oxidase; *NA,* noradrenaline; *NMDA, N*-methyl-D-aspartate; *SSRI,* selective serotonin reuptake inhibitor; *TCA,* tricyclic antidepressant.

Rating Scale or the Beck Depression Inventory. Clinical depression takes many forms, and the symptoms vary between patients and over time. Quantitation is therefore difficult, and the many clinical trials of antidepressants have generally shown rather weak effects, after allowance for quite large placebo responses. There is also a high degree of individual variation, with 30%–40% of patients failing to show any improvement, possibly due to genetic factors (see later section on Clinical Effectiveness). Objective methods based on computerised tasks have been developed for experimental medicine research and are now starting to be used alongside traditional rating scales in early clinical studies.

MECHANISM OF ACTION OF CONVENTIONAL ANTIDEPRESSANT DRUGS

CHRONIC ADAPTIVE CHANGES

There is a discrepancy between the immediate neurochemical effects of conventional antidepressants and the patient's subjective experience of their mood with therapeutic benefits not usually seen for several weeks after the start of treatment. There has been little evidence that different types of conventional antidepressant are effective over different timescales although early studies with imipramine did report more rapid onset of effects than seen in studies with the second-generation antidepressants.

The initial focus of research into the delayed onset was the adaptive changes which arise in certain monoamine receptors e.g. 5-HT_{1A}, α_2 adrenoceptors, α_1 adrenoceptors, following chronic treatment. Similar effects have also been seen following ECT.

Receptor down-regulation has been shown to occur experimentally in human and animals and can involve both pre- and post-synaptic receptors. Changes in autoreceptor density, which provide negative feedback and regulate further neurotransmitter release, have been of particular interest.

On acute administration, one would expect inhibition of 5-HT uptake (e.g. by SSRIs) to increase the level of 5-HT at the synapse by inhibiting reuptake into the nerve terminals. However, the increase in synaptic 5-HT levels has been observed to be less than expected. This is because the increased activation of 5-HT_{1A} receptors on the soma and dendrites of 5-HT-containing raphe neurons (Fig. 48.3A) inhibits these neurons and thus reduces 5-HT release, thus cancelling out to some extent the effect of inhibiting reuptake into the terminals. On prolonged drug treatment, the elevated level of 5-HT in the somatodendritic region desensitises the 5-HT_{1A} receptors, reducing their inhibitory effect on 5-HT release from the nerve terminals. Similar effects may also explain the down-regulation of α_2 adrenoceptors observed when chronic noradrenaline re-uptake inhibitors or mixed re-uptake inhibitors are given chronically.

If autoreceptor activation is the major cause of the delayed onset then co-administration of a 5-HT_{1A} or α_2 adrenoceptor antagonist might lead to a more rapid onset of clinical effects. Attempts with 5-HT_{1A} antagonists have largely failed to find beneficial effects but α_2 adrenoceptor antagonists such as mirtazapine and mianserin have proved to be effective antidepressants although not with more rapid clinical benefits.

Block of presynaptic α_2 autoreceptors on noradrenergic nerve terminals throughout the CNS will reduce the negative feedback from released noradrenaline and thus enhance further noradrenaline release (see Chs 15 and 37). In addition, α_2 adrenoceptor antagonists can indirectly enhance 5-HT release through enhanced activation of α_1 adrenoceptors which are found on the raphe nuclei cell bodies and increase firing rate.

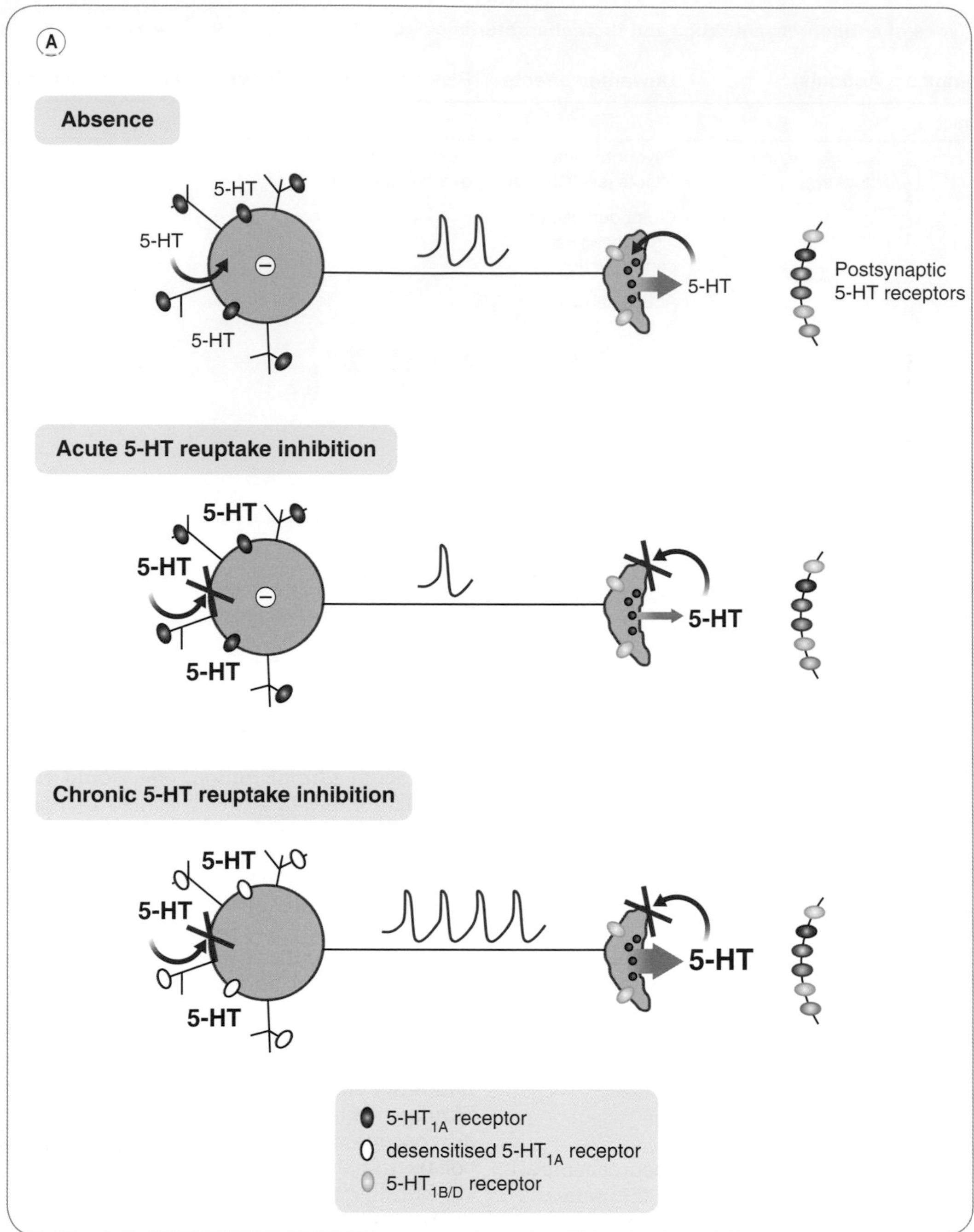

Fig. 48.3 Control of 5-hydroxytryptamine (5-HT) release and the impact of chronic treatment with selective serotonin reuptake inhibitors (SSRIs). (A) 5-HT release is controlled by the inhibitory action of 5-HT on somatodendritic 5-HT_{1A} receptors. Acute inhibition of 5-HT reuptake results in increased extracellular levels of 5-HT but this increases somatodendritic 5-HT_{1A} receptor–mediated inhibition, hence synaptic 5-HT levels do not rise as much as expected. 5-HT_{1A} receptors eventually desensitise, resulting in reduced inhibition and thus greater 5-HT release. These adaptive changes may contribute to the effects of SSRIs on mood and are also likely to contribute to the withdrawal effects experienced by patients when they stop taking their medication.

GENE EXPRESSION AND NEUROGENESIS

An alternative perspective is that the adaptive changes are not directly related to efficacy and the delayed onset is linked to downstream activation of neurotrophic factors which mediate a slow reversal of the stress-induced neuronal loss. As described earlier, several antidepressant drugs appear to promote neurogenesis in the hippocampus, a mechanism that could account for the slow development of the therapeutic effect. This offers the potential to target directly these mechanisms but if neurogenesis is the primary mediator of the antidepressant effects, then rapid changes in depression would not be expected even with more direct modulation of these pathways.

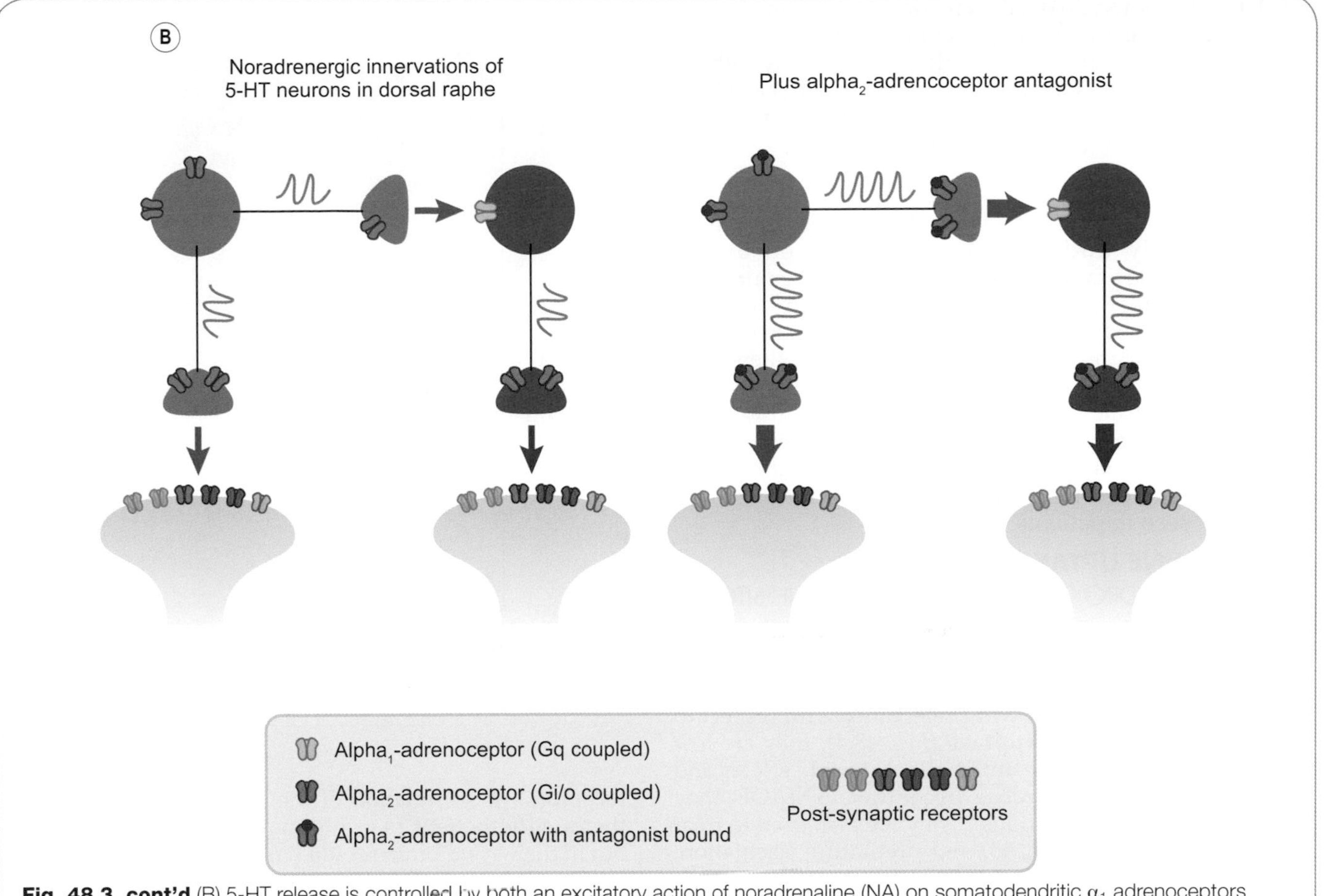

Fig. 48.3, cont'd (B) 5-HT release is controlled by both an excitatory action of noradrenaline (NA) on somatodendritic α_1 adrenoceptors and an inhibitory action on α_2 adrenoceptors on serotonergic nerve terminals. Block of α_2 adrenoceptors located on noradrenergic neurons enhances noradrenaline release resulting in further excitation of serotonergic neurons, while block of α_2 adrenoceptors on serotonergic neurons removes presynaptic inhibition and thus 5-HT release is enhanced. NA can therefore function as both an accelerator and brake on the 5-HT neurons.

Impact of the discovery of rapid-acting antidepressants

A major challenge to receptor adaptation and neurotrophic theories about delayed onset came with the publication of a landmark paper in 2000 which showed that a single, low-dose intravenous infusion of the NMDA receptor antagonist, ketamine, induced a rapid (<24 h) and sustained (~7 days) antidepressant effect. Subsequent studies also found ketamine induced an immediate and sustained attenuation of suicidal ideation in bipolar disorder. Receptor adaptation was very unlikely to account for these effects but studies in animals revealed that low-dose ketamine induced rapid changes in synapse formation in the prefrontal cortex. These synaptogenic effects have yet to be studied in humans but there is a growing literature from animal studies, including imaging studies, showing how synapses which are lost due to chronic stress can be reinstated following acute ketamine or esketamine treatment.

Based on a series of clinical trials, it has emerged that not only ketamine has rapid and sustained antidepressant effects, but also similar effects are seen with the muscarinic antagonist scopolamine and the psychedelic 5-HT agonist, psilocybin (see Ch. 49). These drugs all act on different primary targets but have all been shown to result in enhancement of glutamate transmission in prefrontal cortex which has been suggested to lead to enhanced BDNF signalling which acts via downstream mediators such as mTOR to induce rapid changes in synaptic plasticity and synaptogenesis. There is now growing interest in these drugs as a possible new class of 'psychoplastogens' which can promote synaptic plasticity and rapidly reverse maladaptive changes which have led to depression (Vargas et al., 2021).

Neuropsychological effects of conventional and rapid-acting antidepressants

An important but often overlooked factor contributing to depression is the psychological experience of the patient. Mood arises from a complex integration of past experiences (memories), current circumstances and future expectations, and a purely biochemical explanation of depression does not consider these psychological factors. The neuropsychological hypothesis of antidepressant efficacy posits that conventional antidepressants generate a neurochemical state which facilitates more positive emotional learning and memory, but the patient needs to form new memories to outweigh the accumulated negatively biased memories. Preclinical studies also suggest that RAAD antidepressants contrast with conventional antidepressants and do not depend on new learning but can modify biases associated with previously learnt memories. For more detailed discussion of this emerging hypothesis see Godlewska and Harmer (2021) and Harmer et al. (2017) for a discussion of an integration of both the neurotrophic and neuropsychological hypotheses.

SUMMARY

The mechanisms which underlie antidepressant effects remain poorly understood and hampered by the challenges of the limitations of animal models, complexity of psychological and biological factors and disease heterogeneity. The emergence of the RAAD is an exciting development for the field but presents new challenges to established theories and is leading to a rapid reappraisal. It is also feasible that the complexity of emotional regulation and mood disorders means that more than one mechanism may be involved and aspects of all these different hypotheses may yet emerge as contributing to the symptoms seen in patients.

MONOAMINE UPTAKE INHIBITORS

SELECTIVE 5-HYDROXYTRYPTAMINE UPTAKE INHIBITORS

These are the most commonly prescribed group of antidepressants. Examples include **fluoxetine**, **fluvoxamine**, **paroxetine**, **citalopram**, **escitalopram** and **sertraline** (see Table 48.2). As well as showing selectivity with respect to 5-HT over noradrenaline uptake (Fig. 48.4), they are less likely than TCAs to cause anticholinergic side effects and are less dangerous in overdose. In contrast to MAOIs, they do not cause 'cheese reactions'. They are also used to treat anxiety disorders (see Ch. 45) and premature ejaculation. **Vortioxetine** is a novel SSRI that is an agonist at 5-HT_{1A}, a partial agonist at 5-HT_{1B} receptors and an antagonist at other 5-HT receptors including 5-HT_{3A} receptors.

Individual patients may respond more favourably to one SSRI than another. This may reflect other pharmacological properties of each individual drug as none is devoid of other actions. Fluoxetine has 5-HT_{2C} antagonist activity, a property it shares with other non-SSRI antidepressants such as **mirtazapine**. Sertraline is a weak inhibitor of dopamine uptake. Escitalopram is the *S* isomer of racemic citalopram. It lacks the antihistamine and CYP2D6 inhibitory properties of the *R* isomer.

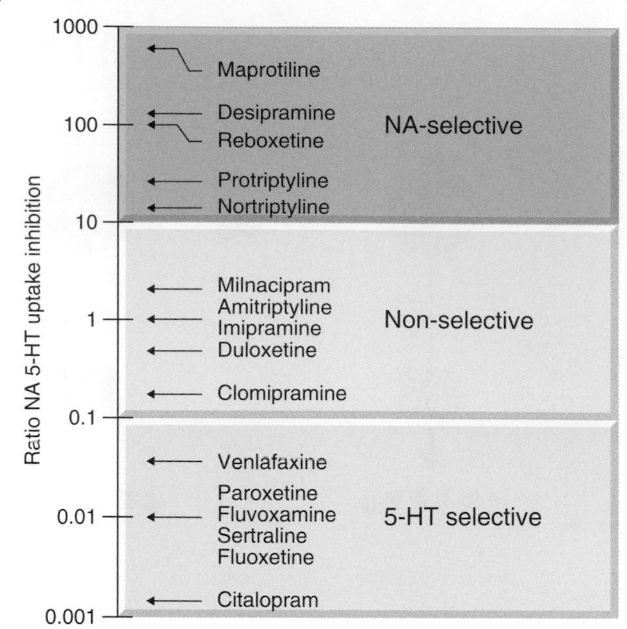

Fig. 48.4 Selectivity of inhibition of noradrenaline (NA) and 5-hydroxytryptamine (5-HT) uptake by various antidepressants.

Pharmacokinetic aspects

The SSRIs are well absorbed when given orally, and most have plasma half-lives of 18–24 h (fluoxetine is longer acting: 24–96 h). Paroxetine and fluoxetine are not used in combination with TCAs, whose hepatic metabolism they inhibit through an interaction with CYP2D6, for fear of increasing TCA toxicity.

Unwanted effects

Common side effects include nausea, anorexia, insomnia, loss of libido and failure of orgasm.[3] Some of these unwanted effects result from the enhanced stimulation of postsynaptic 5-HT receptors as a result of the drugs increasing the levels of extracellular 5-HT. This can be either stimulation of the wrong type of 5-HT receptor (e.g. 5-HT_2, 5-HT_3 and 5-HT_4 receptors) or stimulation of the same receptor that gives therapeutic benefit (e.g. postsynaptic 5-HT_{1A} receptors) but in the wrong brain region (i.e. enhanced stimulation of 5-HT receptors can result in both therapeutic and adverse responses).

A common problem for patients taking reuptake inhibitors is the withdrawal effects they can experience if they stop taking their medication abruptly or try to reduce their dose too quickly. Possibly linked to the adaptive changes induced by chronic treatment, the symptoms include increased anxiety and agitation and a careful programme of dose reduction is needed to manage these.

In combination with MAOIs, SSRIs can cause a 'serotonin syndrome' characterised by tremor, agitation, increased reflexes, hyperthermia and cardiovascular collapse, from which deaths have occurred.

There have been reports of increased aggression, and occasionally violence, in patients treated with fluoxetine, but these have not been confirmed by controlled studies. The use of SSRIs is not recommended for treating depression in children under 18, in whom efficacy is doubtful and adverse effects, including excitement, insomnia and aggression in the first few weeks of treatment, may occur. The possibility of increased suicidal ideation is a concern in this age group. Despite this, SSRIs, particularly fluoxetine, are increasingly being prescribed to patients under 18 years of age.

Despite the apparent advantages of 5-HT uptake inhibitors over TCAs in terms of side effects, the combined results of many trials show little overall difference in terms of efficacy (Cipriani et al., 2018).

They are relatively safe in overdose, compared with TCAs (see later section, *Suicide and antidepressants*), but can prolong the cardiac QT interval, giving rise to ventricular arrhythmias (see Ch. 22) and risk of sudden death.

[3]Thus conversely, SSRIs can be used to treat premature ejaculation. Dapoxetine has a short half-life and is taken 1–3 h before sex.

5-HT uptake inhibitors are used in a variety of other psychiatric disorders including anxiety disorders, obsessive–compulsive disorder and eating disorders (see Ch. 45).

Selective serotonin reuptake inhibitors (SSRIs)

- Examples include fluoxetine, fluvoxamine, paroxetine, sertraline, citalopram, escitalopram.
- Antidepressant actions are similar in efficacy and time course to tricyclic antidepressants (TCAs).
- Acute toxicity (especially cardiotoxicity) is less than that of monoamine oxidase inhibitors (MAOIs) or TCAs, so overdose risk is reduced.
- Side effects include nausea, insomnia and sexual dysfunction. SSRIs are less sedating and have fewer antimuscarinic side effects than the older TCAs.
- No food reactions, but dangerous 'serotonin reaction' (hyperthermia, muscle rigidity, cardiovascular collapse) can occur if given with MAOIs.
- There is concern about the use of SSRIs in children and adolescents, due to reports of an increase in suicidal thoughts on starting treatment.
- Also used for some other psychiatric indications (e.g. anxiety and obsessive–compulsive disorder).

TRICYCLIC ANTIDEPRESSANT DRUGS

TCAs (**imipramine**, **desipramine**, **amitriptyline**, **nortriptyline**, **clomipramine**) are still widely used. They are, however, far from ideal in practice, and it was the need for drugs that produce fewer side effects and are less hazardous in overdose that led to the introduction of newer 5-HT reuptake inhibitors and other antidepressants.

TCAs are closely related in structure to the phenothiazines (see Ch. 47) and were initially synthesised (in 1949) as potential antipsychotic drugs. Several are tertiary amines and are quite rapidly demethylated in vivo (Fig. 48.5) to the corresponding secondary amines (e.g. imipramine to desipramine, amitriptyline to nortriptyline), which are themselves active and may be administered as drugs in their own right. Other tricyclic derivatives with slightly modified bridge structures include **doxepin**. The pharmacological differences between these drugs are not very great and relate mainly to their side effects, which are discussed later.

Some TCAs are also used to treat neuropathic pain (see Ch. 43).

Mechanism of action

As discussed previously, the main immediate effect of TCAs is to block the uptake of amines by nerve terminals, by competition for the binding site of the amine transporter (see Ch. 15). Most TCAs inhibit noradrenaline and 5-HT uptake (see Fig. 48.4) but have much less effect on dopamine uptake. It has been suggested that improvement of emotional symptoms reflects mainly an enhancement of 5-HT-mediated transmission, whereas relief of biological symptoms results from facilitation of noradrenergic transmission. Interpretation is made difficult by the fact that the major metabolites of TCAs have considerable pharmacological activity (in some cases greater than that of the parent drug) and often differ from the parent drug in respect of their noradrenaline/5-HT selectivity (Table 48.3).

In addition to their effects on amine uptake, most TCAs affect other receptors, including muscarinic acetylcholine receptors, histamine receptors, α adrenoceptors and 5-HT receptors.

Unwanted effects

In human subjects without depression, TCAs cause sedation, confusion and motor incoordination. These effects occur also in patients with depression in the first few days of treatment, but tend to wear off over 1–2 weeks as tolerance develops.

TCAs produce a number of troublesome side effects, mainly due to interference with autonomic control.

Anti-muscarinic effects include dry mouth, blurred vision, constipation and urinary retention. These effects are strong with amitriptyline and much weaker with desipramine. Postural hypotension, mainly due to α_1 adrenoceptor antagonism, occurs with TCAs. The other common side effect is sedation due to histamine$_1$ receptor antagonism, and the long duration of action means that daytime performance is often affected by drowsiness and difficulty in concentrating.

TCAs, particularly in overdose, may cause ventricular dysrhythmias associated with prolongation of the QT interval (see Ch. 60). Usual therapeutic doses of TCAs increase, slightly, but significantly, the risk of sudden cardiac death.

Withdrawal effects similar to those seen with the specific re-uptake inhibitors are also seen with TCAs and gradual dose reduction should be used.

Interactions with other drugs

TCAs are particularly likely to cause adverse effects when given in conjunction with other drugs (see Ch. 58). They rely on hepatic metabolism by microsomal cytochrome P450 (CYP) enzymes for elimination, and this may be inhibited by competing drugs (e.g. antipsychotic drugs and some steroids).

TCAs potentiate the effects of alcohol and anaesthetic agents, for reasons that are not well understood, and deaths have occurred as a result of this, when severe respiratory depression has followed a bout of drinking. TCAs also interfere with the action of various antihypertensive drugs (see Ch. 21), with potentially dangerous consequences, so their use in hypertensive patients requires close monitoring.

Acute toxicity

TCAs are dangerous in overdose and were at one time commonly used for suicide attempts, which was an important factor prompting the introduction of safer antidepressants. The main effects are on the CNS and the heart. The initial effect of TCA overdosage is to cause excitement and delirium, which may be accompanied by convulsions. This is followed by coma and respiratory depression lasting for some days. Atropine-like effects are pronounced, including dry mouth and skin, mydriasis and inhibition of gut and bladder. Anticholinesterase drugs have been used to counter atropine-like effects but are no

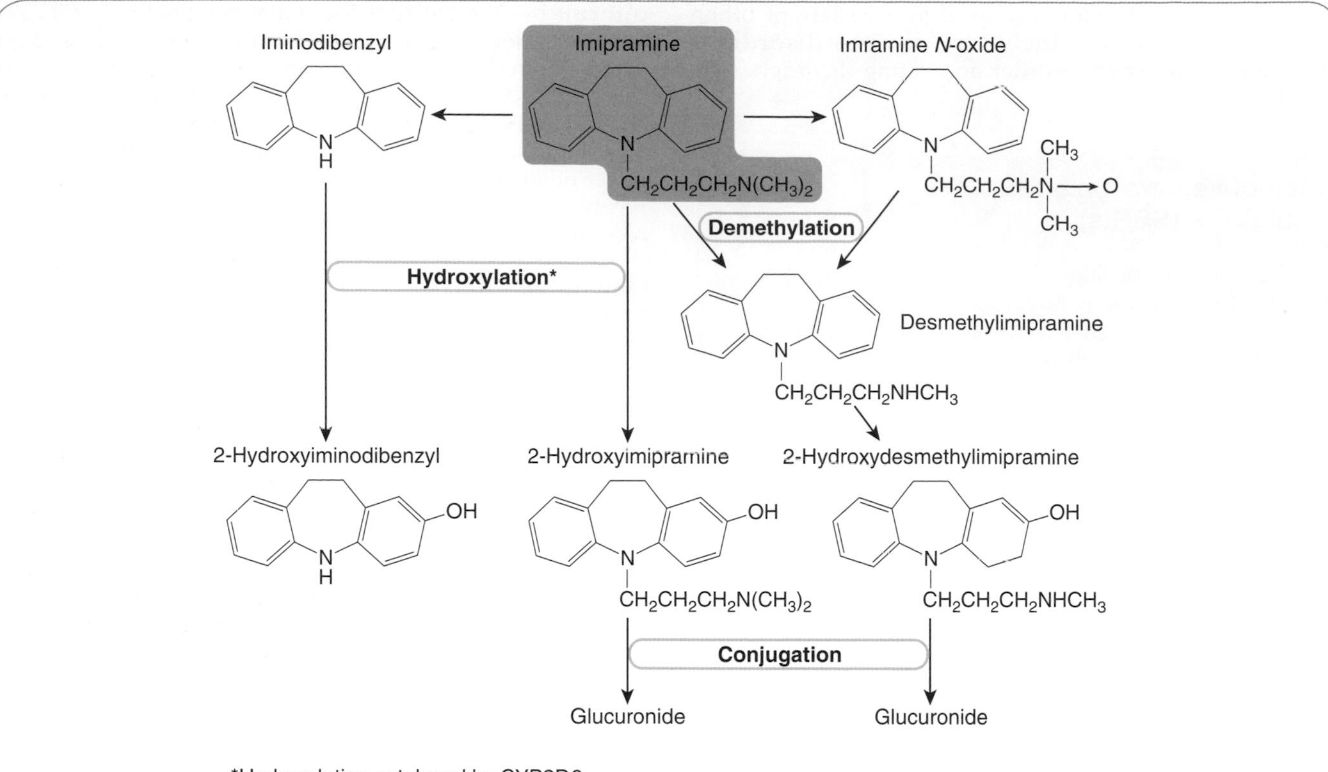

Fig. 48.5 Metabolism of imipramine, which is typical of that of other tricyclic antidepressants. *The hydroxylating enzyme CYP2D6 is subject to genetic polymorphism, which may account for individual variation in response to tricyclic antidepressants (see Ch. 12).

longer recommended. Cardiac dysrhythmias are common, and sudden death may occur from ventricular fibrillation.

Pharmacokinetic aspects

TCAs are all rapidly absorbed when given orally and bind strongly to plasma albumin, most being 90%–95% bound at therapeutic plasma concentrations. They also bind to extravascular tissues, which accounts for their generally very large distribution volumes (usually 10–50 L/kg; see Ch. 9) and low rates of elimination. Extravascular sequestration, together with strong binding to plasma albumin, means that haemodialysis is ineffective as a means of increasing drug elimination.

TCAs are metabolised in the liver by two main routes, *N*-demethylation and ring hydroxylation (see Fig. 48.5). Both the desmethyl and the hydroxylated metabolites commonly retain biological activity (Table 48.4). During prolonged treatment with TCAs, the plasma concentration of these metabolites is usually comparable to that of the parent drug, although there is wide variation between individuals. Inactivation of the drugs occurs by glucuronide conjugation of the hydroxylated metabolites, the glucuronides being excreted in the urine.

The overall half-times for elimination of TCAs are generally long, ranging from 10 to 20 h for imipramine and desipramine to about 80 h for **protriptyline**. They are even longer in elderly patients. Therefore gradual accumulation is possible, leading to slowly developing side effects.

Tricyclic antidepressants

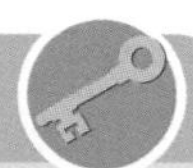

- Tricyclic antidepressants are chemically related to phenothiazine antipsychotic drugs (see Ch. 47), and some have similar non-selective receptor-blocking actions.
- Important examples are **imipramine**, **amitriptyline** and **clomipramine.**
- Most are long acting, and they are often converted to active metabolites.
- Important side effects: sedation (H_1 block); postural hypotension (α-adrenoceptor block); dry mouth, blurred vision, constipation (muscarinic block); occasionally mania and convulsions. Risk of ventricular dysrhythmias.
- Dangerous in acute overdose: confusion and mania, cardiac dysrhythmias.
- Liable to interact with other drugs (e.g. alcohol, anaesthetics, hypotensive drugs and non-steroidal anti-inflammatory drugs; should not be given with monoamine oxidase inhibitors).
- Also used to treat neuropathic pain.

SEROTONIN AND NORADRENALINE UPTAKE INHIBITORS

These drugs are relatively non-selective for 5-HT and noradrenaline uptake. They include **venlafaxine**, **desvenlafaxine** and **duloxetine** (see Table 48.2).

Table 48.3 Inhibition of neuronal noradrenaline (NA) and 5-hydroxytryptamine (5-HT) uptake by tricyclic antidepressants and their metabolites

Drug/metabolite	NA uptake	5-HT uptake
Imipramine	+++	++
Desmethylimipramine (DMI) (also known as desipramine)	++++	+
Hydroxy-DMI	+++	–
Clomipramine (CMI)	++	+++
Desmethyl-CMI	+++	+
Amitriptyline (AMI)	++	++
Nortriptyline (desmethyl-AMI)	+++	++
Hydroxynortriptyline	++	++

Table 48.4 Substrates and inhibitors for type A and type B monoamine oxidase

	Type A	Type B
Preferred substrates	Noradrenaline 5-Hydroxytryptamine	Phenylethylamine Benzylamine
Non-specific substrates	Dopamine Tyramine	Dopamine Tyramine
Specific inhibitors	Clorgyline Moclobemide	Selegiline
Non-specific inhibitors	Pargyline Tranylcypromine Isocarboxazid	Pargyline Tranylcypromine Isocarboxazid

As the dose of venlafaxine is increased, its efficacy also increases, which has been interpreted as demonstrating that its weak action to inhibit noradrenaline reuptake may add to its 5-HT uptake inhibition that occurs at lower doses, the combination providing additional therapeutic benefit. They are all active orally; slow-release formulations are available that reduce the incidence of nausea. Venlafaxine, desvenlafaxine and duloxetine are effective in some anxiety disorders (see Ch. 45). Desvenlafaxine may be useful in treating some perimenopausal symptoms such as hot flushes and insomnia. Duloxetine is also used in the treatment of neuropathic pain and fibromyalgia (see Ch. 43) and urinary incontinence.

Venlafaxine and duloxetine are metabolised by CYP2D6. Venlafaxine is converted to desvenlafaxine, which shows greater inhibition of noradrenaline reuptake. The unwanted effects of these drugs – largely due to enhanced activation of adrenoceptors – include headache, insomnia, sexual dysfunction, dry mouth, dizziness, sweating and decreased appetite. The most common symptoms in overdose are CNS depression, serotonin toxicity, seizure and cardiac conduction abnormalities. Duloxetine has been reported to cause hepatotoxicity and is contraindicated for patients with hepatic impairment.

OTHER NORADRENALINE UPTAKE INHIBITORS

Bupropion inhibits both noradrenaline and dopamine (but not 5-HT) uptake but, unlike cocaine and amphetamine (see Ch. 49), does not induce euphoria and has so far not been observed to have abuse potential. It is metabolised to active metabolites. It is also used to treat nicotine dependence (see Ch. 50). At high doses it may induce seizures. Reboxetine and atomoxetine are highly selective inhibitors of noradrenaline uptake but their efficacy in depression is less than SSRIs and TCAs, possibly related to poor tolerability (Cipriani et al., 2018). Atomoxetine is approved for the treatment of attention deficit/hyperactivity disorder (see Ch. 49).

Other monoamine uptake inhibitors

- **Venlafaxine** is a 5-HT uptake inhibitor, but less selective for 5-HT versus noradrenaline than SSRIs. It is metabolised to **desvenlafaxine**, which is also an antidepressant.
- **Duloxetine** inhibits noradrenaline and 5-HT uptake.
- **Bupropion** is a noradrenaline and dopamine uptake inhibitor.
- Generally similar to tricyclic antidepressants but lack major receptor-blocking actions, so fewer side effects.
- Less risk of cardiac effects, so safer in overdose than tricyclic antidepressants.
- Can be used to treat other disorders:
  - **venlafaxine, desvenlafaxine** and **duloxetine** – anxiety disorders
  - **duloxetine** – neuropathic pain and fibromyalgia
  - **duloxetine** – urinary incontinence
  - **bupropion** – nicotine dependence.

RECEPTOR BLOCKING ANTIDEPRESSANTS

Mirtazapine blocks not only α_2 adrenoreceptors but also other receptors, including 5-HT_2 and 5-HT_3 receptors, which may contribute to its antidepressant actions and reduce some of the side effects arising from increased 5-HT release. Block of α_2 adrenoceptors will not only increase noradrenaline release but will also enhance 5-HT release (see Fig. 48.3B); however, by simultaneously blocking 5-HT_{2A} and 5-HT_3 receptors, it will reduce the unwanted effects mediated through these receptors (e.g. sexual dysfunction and nausea) but leave intact stimulation of postsynaptic 5-HT_{1A} receptors. It also blocks histamine H_1 receptors, which causes sedation sedation particularly at low doses. **Trazodone** is a mixed agonist and antagonist of various 5-HT receptors, antagonist of adrenoceptors, weak histamine H_1 receptor antagonist and weak serotonin reuptake inhibitor. The combined 5-HT_{2A} and 5-HT_{2C} receptor antagonism with weak 5-HT reuptake inhibition may lead to antidepressant effects with reduced 5-HT_2-related side effects, e.g. sleep disturbance, sexual dysfunction and anxiety.

Mianserin, another α_2 adrenoceptor antagonist that also blocks H_1, 5-HT_{2A} and α_1 adrenoceptors (reducing effects of 5-HT relative to mirtazapine), can cause bone marrow depression, requiring regular blood counts, so its use has declined in recent years.

Monoamine receptor antagonist antidepressant drugs

- **Mirtazapine** blocks α_2 adrenoceptors, 5-HT_2 and 5-HT_3 receptors, enhancing noradrenaline and 5-HT release and reducing 5-HT-related side effects.
- **Mirtazapine** causes less nausea and sexual dysfunction than SSRIs but can lead to weight gain due to 5-HT_{2C} effects.
- **Trazodone** blocks 5-HT_{2A} and 5-HT_{2C} receptors and blocks 5-HT reuptake.
- **Mianserin** is an antagonist at multiple 5-HT receptors (including 5-HT_{2A}) as well as at H_1, α_1 and α_2 receptors. It is also an inverse agonist at H_1 receptors. Use is declining because of risk of bone marrow depression. Regular blood counts are advisable.
- Cardiovascular side effects of these drugs are fewer than those of tricyclic antidepressants.
- **Vortioxetine** has both 5-HT uptake inhibition and multiple 5-HT receptor partial agonist, full agonist or antagonist actions.

MONOAMINE OXIDASE INHIBITORS

MAOIs were among the first drugs to be introduced clinically as antidepressants but were largely superseded by other types of antidepressants, whose clinical efficacies were considered better and whose side effects are generally less than those of MAOIs. The main examples are **phenelzine**, **tranylcypromine** and **iproniazid**. These drugs cause irreversible inhibition of the enzyme and do not distinguish between the two main isozymes (see later). The discovery of reversible inhibitors that show isozyme selectivity has rekindled interest in this class of drug. Although several studies have shown a reduction in platelet MAO activity in certain groups of patients with depression, there is no clear evidence that abnormal MAO activity is involved in the pathogenesis of depression.

MAO (see Ch. 15) is found in nearly all tissues, and exists in two similar molecular forms coded by separate genes (see Table 48.4). MAO-A has a substrate preference for 5-HT and noradrenaline, and is the main target for the antidepressant MAOIs. MAO-B has a substrate preference for phenylethylamine and dopamine. Type B is selectively inhibited by **selegiline**, which is used in the treatment of Parkinson's disease (see Ch. 40). Most antidepressant MAOIs act on both forms of MAO, but clinical studies with subtype-specific inhibitors have shown clearly that antidepressant activity, as well as the main side effects of MAOIs, is associated with MAO-A inhibition. MAO is located intracellularly, mostly associated with mitochondria, and has two main functions:

1. Within nerve terminals, MAO regulates the free intraneuronal concentration of noradrenaline or 5-HT. It is not involved in the inactivation of released transmitter.
2. MAO in the gut wall is important in the inactivation of endogenous and ingested amines such as tyramine that would otherwise produce unwanted effects.

Chemical aspects

MAOIs are substrate analogues with a phenylethylamine-like structure, and most contain a reactive group (e.g. hydrazine, propargylamine, cyclopropylamine) that enables the inhibitor to bind covalently to the enzyme, resulting in a non-competitive and long-lasting inhibition. Recovery of MAO activity after inhibition takes several weeks with most drugs, but is quicker after **tranylcypromine**, which forms a less stable bond with the enzyme. **Moclobemide** acts as a reversible competitive inhibitor.

MAOIs are not specific in their actions, and inhibit a variety of other enzymes as well as MAO, including many enzymes involved in the metabolism of other drugs. This is responsible for some of the many clinically important drug interactions associated with MAOIs.

Pharmacological effects

MAOIs cause a rapid and sustained increase in the 5-HT, noradrenaline and dopamine content of the brain, 5-HT being affected most and dopamine least. Similar changes occur in peripheral tissues such as heart, liver and intestine, and increases in the plasma concentrations of these amines are also detectable. Although these increases in tissue amine content are largely due to accumulation within neurons, transmitter release in response to nerve activity is not increased. In contrast to the effect of TCAs, MAOIs do not increase the response of peripheral organs, such as the heart and blood vessels, to sympathetic nerve stimulation. The main effect of MAOIs is to increase the cytoplasmic concentration of monoamines in nerve terminals, without greatly affecting the vesicular stores that are releasable by nerve stimulation. The increased cytoplasmic pool results in an increased rate of spontaneous leakage of monoamines, and also an increased release by indirectly acting sympathomimetic amines such as amphetamine and tyramine (see Ch. 15 and Fig. 15.7). Tyramine thus causes a much greater rise in blood pressure in MAOI-treated animals than in controls. This mechanism is important in relation to the 'cheese reaction' produced by MAOIs in humans (see later).

In normal human subjects, MAOIs cause an immediate increase in motor activity; euphoria and excitement develop over the course of a few days. This is in contrast to TCAs, which cause only sedation and confusion when given to subjects without depression. The effects of MAOIs on amine metabolism develop rapidly, and the effect of a single dose lasts for several days. There is a clear discrepancy, as with SSRIs and TCAs, between the rapid biochemical response and the delayed antidepressant effect.

Unwanted effects and toxicity

Many of the unwanted effects of MAOIs result directly from MAO inhibition, but some are produced by other mechanisms.

Hypotension is a common side effect; indeed, **pargyline** was at one time used as an antihypertensive drug. One possible explanation for this effect – the opposite of what might have been expected – is that amines such as dopamine or octopamine accumulate within peripheral sympathetic nerve terminals and displace noradrenaline from the storage vesicles, thus reducing noradrenaline release associated with sympathetic activity.

Excessive central stimulation may cause tremors, excitement, insomnia and, in overdose, convulsions.

Increased appetite, leading to weight gain, can be so extreme as to require the drug to be discontinued.

Atropine-like side effects (dry mouth, blurred vision, urinary retention, etc.) are common with MAOIs, although they are less of a problem than with TCAs.

MAOIs of the hydrazine type (e.g. phenelzine and iproniazid) produce, very rarely (less than 1 in 10,000), severe hepatotoxicity, which seems to be due to the hydrazine moiety of the molecule. Their use in patients with liver disease is therefore unwise.

Interaction with other drugs and foods

Interaction with other drugs and foods is the most serious problem with MAOIs and is the main factor that caused their clinical use to decline. The special advantage claimed for the new reversible MAOIs, such as moclobemide, is that these interactions are reduced.

The 'cheese reaction' is a direct consequence of MAO inhibition and occurs when normally innocuous amines (mainly tyramine) produced during fermentation are ingested. Tyramine is normally metabolised by MAO in the gut wall and liver, and little dietary tyramine reaches the systemic circulation. MAO inhibition allows tyramine to be absorbed, and also enhances its sympathomimetic effect, as discussed earlier. The result is acute hypertension, giving rise to a severe throbbing headache and occasionally even to intracranial haemorrhage. Although many foods contain some tyramine, it appears that at least 10 mg of tyramine needs to be ingested to produce such a response, and the main danger is from ripe cheeses and from concentrated yeast products such as Marmite. Administration of indirectly acting sympathomimetic amines (e.g. **ephedrine** – a nasal decongestant – or **amphetamine**) also causes severe hypertension in patients receiving MAOIs; directly acting agents such as noradrenaline (used, for example, in conjunction with local anaesthetics; see Ch. 44) are not hazardous. Moclobemide, a specific MAO-A inhibitor, does not cause the 'cheese reaction', probably because tyramine can still be metabolised by MAO-B and through competition with moclobemide at MAO-A.

Hypertensive episodes have been reported in patients given TCAs and MAOIs simultaneously. The probable explanation is that inhibition of noradrenaline reuptake further enhances the cardiovascular response to dietary tyramine, thus accentuating the 'cheese reaction'. This combination of drugs can also produce excitement and hyperactivity.

MAOIs can interact with **pethidine** (see Ch. 43) to cause severe hyperpyrexia, with restlessness, coma and hypotension. The mechanism is uncertain, but it is likely that an abnormal pethidine metabolite is produced because of inhibition of demethylation.

MELATONIN AGONIST

Agomelatine is a potent agonist at MT_1 and MT_2 receptors (see Ch. 39) with weak antagonist activity at $5\text{-}HT_{2A,2B,2C}$ receptors (almost 1000-fold lower potency). It has a short biological half-life and does not give rise to the side effects associated with other antidepressant drugs. Used to treat severe depression, it is usually taken once daily before bed and may work by correcting disturbances in circadian rhythms often associated with depression. There are reports of hepatotoxicity in a few patients, and it should not be used in patients with liver disease.

RAPID-ACTING ANTIDEPRESSANTS

Esketamine is the S(+) enantiomer of ketamine and has been licensed as a nasal spray for once or twice weekly administration for treatment-resistant depression. The S(+) enantiomer of ketamine is about four-fold more potent at the NMDA receptor. It is currently licensed in the United States. In the UK there is a growing number of clinics offering intravenous infusions of low doses of the racemic mixture of ketamine for patients who have failed to respond to conventional antidepressants. A single, sub-anaesthetic dose of ketamine or intranasal esketamine induces an initial dissociative effect accompanied by increased blood pressure and can cause a variety to unpleasant side effects (see Ch. 41). These only last for a brief period of time (<1 h) however and the antidepressant effects emerge within a few hours and are sustained for up to 14 days. Ketamine is a non-competitive NMDA channel blocker (see Ch. 41); however, it also has effects at a number of other receptors at clinical doses including actions at μ-opioid receptors. To date, clinical trials with other NMDA receptor antagonists, e.g. memantine, have failed to find similar antidepressant effects. There is controversy surrounding whether the putative antidepressant effect is produced by ketamine itself, and which receptor is the primary mediator, or by its metabolite, R,R-hydroxynorketamine. Hydroxynorketamine would have the added advantage that, unlike ketamine, it may not produce psychotomimetic effects as it has low affinity for the NMDA receptor, and thus would be unlikely to be abused (see Ch. 50).

Several other classes of hallucinogenic drugs have been investigated as RAADs. The muscarinic antagonist, **scopolamine** (see Ch. 14), which is also referred to as a 'deliriant' reflecting is potent induction of a state of delirium, was found to have rapid and sustained antidepressant effects. Psychedelic serotonin agonists are potent $5\text{-}HT_{2A}$ agonists (as well as acting at other 5-HT receptors) and include drugs such as psilocybin, dimethyltryptamine and lysergic acid diethylamide (LSD). Several clinical trials have now been undertaken and suggest that these drugs may also induce rapid and sustained antidepressant effects including some evidence for effects lasting several months after a single treatment. Although previously used in drug-assisted psychotherapy, until they were banned in the 1970s, research is only just starting to unlock the clinical efficacy of these drugs and how they interact with psychological treatments to generate their effects. A challenge with all these RAADs is their history as drugs which have been used non-medically and their powerful dissociative, deliriant or psychedelic effects requiring intensive patient care. Although still in the early days, the discovery of RAADs has provided a new avenue for research which will hopefully generate new insights into the mechanisms which underlie the antidepressant efficacy of these drugs and may even help us learn more about conventional antidepressants.

Monoamine oxidase inhibitors (MAOIs)

- Main examples are **phenelzine**, **tranylcypromine**, **isocarboxazid** (irreversible, long-acting, non-selective between MAO-A and -B) and **moclobemide** (reversible, short-acting, MAO-A selective).
- Long-acting MAOIs:
  - main side effects: postural hypotension (sympathetic block); atropine-like effects (as with tricyclic antidepressants (TCAs)); weight gain; CNS stimulation, causing restlessness, insomnia; hepatotoxicity and neurotoxicity (rare);
  - acute overdose causes CNS stimulation, sometimes convulsions;
  - 'cheese reaction', i.e. severe hypertensive response to tyramine-containing foods (e.g. cheese, beer, wine, well-hung game, yeast or soy extracts); such reactions can occur up to 2 weeks after treatment is discontinued.
- Interaction with other amines (e.g. **ephedrine** in over-the-counter decongestants, **clomipramine** and other TCAs) and some other drugs (e.g. **pethidine**) are also potentially lethal.
- **Moclobemide** is used for major depression and social phobia. 'Cheese reaction' and other drug interactions are less severe and shorter lasting than with irreversible MAOIs.
- MAOIs are used much less than other antidepressants because of their adverse effects and serious interactions. They are indicated for major depression in patients who have not responded to other drugs.

OTHER ANTIDEPRESSANT APPROACHES

Brexanolone is an allopregnanolone-based treatment recently licensed in the United States for postpartum depression. The drug acts as a neuroactive steroid and is a positive allosteric modulator at the $GABA_A$ receptor (see Ch. 38) which is thought to be the primary mechanism mediating its therapeutic effects.

Oestrogen, which is known to elevate mood in perimenopausal women, may also be of value for the treatment of postnatal depression. Its effectiveness in treating other forms of depression is unclear. In addition to its well-documented hormonal actions in the body (see Ch. 35), it also has actions on monoaminergic, GABAergic and glutamatergic systems in the brain (see Chs 38 and 39).

CLINICAL EFFECTIVENESS OF ANTIDEPRESSANT TREATMENTS

The overall clinical efficacy of antidepressants is generally accepted for severe depression, although there is concern that the published clinical trials evidence may be misleading, because many negative trials have gone unreported. However, 30%–40% of patients with depression fail to show improvement, and those who do may only show partial improvement, reinforcing the need for new drugs with novel mechanisms of action. Clear evidence of benefit from current antidepressant drugs in mild to moderate depression is lacking. Interpretation of trials data is complicated by a high placebo response, and spontaneous recovery independent of any treatment. Clinical trial data do not suggest that drugs currently in use differ in terms of efficacy. Nevertheless, clinical experience suggests that individual patients may, for unknown reasons, respond better to one drug than another. Current treatment guidelines recommend evidence-based psychological procedures as first-line treatments in most cases, before antidepressant drugs.

Pharmacogenetic factors

The individual variation in response to antidepressants and the incidence of adverse effects may be partly due to genetic factors (Crisafulli et al., 2014). Two genetic factors have received particular attention, namely:

- polymorphism of cytochrome P450 genes, especially *CYP2D6 and CYP2C19, which are responsible for hydroxylation and demethylation of TCAs and SSRIs;*
- polymorphism of serotonin and noradrenaline transporter genes.

Up to 10% of Caucasians possess a dysfunctional *CYP2D6* gene, and consequently may be susceptible to the side effects of antidepressants and various other drugs (see Ch. 12) that are metabolised by this route. The opposite effect, caused by duplication of the gene, is common in Eastern European and East African populations, and may account for a lack of clinical efficacy in some individuals. There is some evidence to suggest that responsiveness to SSRIs and serotonin and noradrenaline uptake inhibitors (SNRIs) is related to polymorphism of the serotonin and noradrenaline transporter genes.

Although genotyping may prove to be a useful approach in the future to individualising antidepressant therapy, its practical realisation is still some way off.

Suicide and antidepressants

SSRI and SNRI antidepressants can increase the risk of 'suicidality' and increase aggression in children, adolescents and young adults (see Sharma et al., 2016). The term *suicidality* encompasses suicidal thoughts and planning as well as unsuccessful attempts; actual suicide, although one of the major causes of death in young people, is much rarer than suicidality. The risk is less in older age groups. However, the risk has to be balanced against the beneficial effects of these drugs, not only on depression but also on anxiety, panic and obsessive–compulsive disorders (see Ch. 45).

Clinical uses of drugs in depression

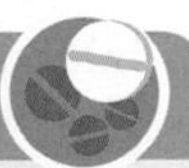

- Mild depression is often best treated initially with non-drug measures (such as cognitive behavioural therapy), with antidepressant drugs being used in addition if the response is poor.
- The use of antidepressant drugs is advisable in the treatment of moderate to severe depression.
- The clinical efficacy of antidepressant drugs is limited, and varies between individuals. Clinical trials have produced inconsistent results, because of placebo responses and spontaneous fluctuations in the level of depression.
- Different classes of antidepressant drugs have similar efficacy but different side effects.
- Choice of drug is based on individual aspects including concomitant disease treatment, suicide risk and previous response to treatment. Other things being equal, a SSRI is preferred as these are usually better tolerated and are less dangerous in overdose.
- Conventional antidepressant drugs take several weeks before taking effect, so decisions on dose increment or switching to another class should not be made precipitately. Use of MAOIs is managed by specialists.
- An effective regimen should be continued for at least 2 years.
- Treatment-resistant patients may benefit from treatment with the rapid-acting antidepressant, ketamine.
- Anxiolytic (e.g. benzodiazepine, see Ch. 45) or antipsychotic (see Ch. 47) drugs are useful adjuncts in some patients.

FUTURE ANTIDEPRESSANT DRUGS

The successive failures of adjunct therapies targeting autoreceptors has limited further progress in this area and most new clinical trials in depression focus on the RAADs. This includes ongoing clinical trials with different NMDA receptor antagonists, particularly those targeting the NR2B subunit which have been hypothesised to achieve similar RAAD effects as ketamine but with reduced dissociation and abuse liability. There is also interest in methods which could prolong the effects of ketamine (and possibly other RAAD) through targeting of downstream effects thought to mediate the neurotrophic effects. Clinical trials with the psychedelics are ongoing and preclinical projects are seeking to identify novel targets which could achieve these RAAD effects but with reduced dissociative and hallucinogenic effects and abuse liability.

BRAIN STIMULATION THERAPIES

A number of brain stimulation techniques are now being used or developed to treat depression. Bright light stimulation has been proposed as a treatment for seasonal affective disorder. The most established brain stimulation techniques are ECT and repetitive transcranial magnetic stimulation (TMS). Brain stimulation treatments are often used as the therapeutic approach of last resort for patients who have not responded to antidepressant drugs.

ECT involves stimulation through electrodes placed on either side of the head, with the patient lightly anaesthetised, paralysed with a short-acting neuromuscular-blocking drug (e.g. **suxamethonium**; see Ch. 14) to avoid physical injury, and artificially ventilated. Controlled trials have shown ECT to be at least as effective as antidepressant drugs, with response rates ranging between 60% and 80%; it appears to be an effective treatment for severe suicidal depression and has the advantage of producing a fast-onset response. The main disadvantage of ECT is that it often causes confusion and memory loss lasting for days or weeks. TMS gives electrical stimulation without anaesthesia or convulsion and does not produce cognitive impairment, but comparative studies suggest that its antidepressant efficacy is less than that of conventional ECT.

The effect of ECT on experimental animals has been carefully analysed to see if it provides clues as to the mode of action of antidepressant drugs, but the clues it gives are enigmatic. 5-HT synthesis and uptake are unaltered, and noradrenaline uptake is somewhat increased (in contrast to the effect of TCAs). Decreased β adrenoceptor responsiveness, both biochemical and behavioural, occurs with both ECT and long-term administration of antidepressant drugs, but changes in 5-HT-mediated responses tend to go in opposite directions.

There have been reports that deep brain stimulation, which has also been used in the treatment of Parkinson's disease (see Ch. 40), in which stimulation is delivered in a specific brain region through surgically implanted electrodes, is effective in patients not responding to other treatments (see Sullivan et al., 2021). The effectiveness of another technique, vagal stimulation, in producing long-term benefit in depression is still unclear.

Novel-acting antidepressants

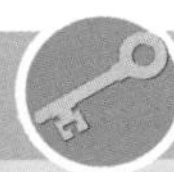

- **Agomelatine** is an agonist at MT_1 and MT_2 melatonin receptors that improves mood, probably by improving sleep patterns.
- **Ketamine**, an NMDA receptor channel blocker, produces rapid and sustained antidepressant effects in patients resistant to other therapies.

DRUG TREATMENT OF BIPOLAR DISORDER

The main class of drugs used to manage the symptoms of bipolar disorder are the mood stabilisers. The major drugs are:

- **lithium**;
- certain antiepileptic drugs, e.g. **carbamazepine, valproate, lamotrigine**; and
- some antipsychotic drugs, e.g. **olanzapine, risperidone, quetiapine, aripiprazole, brexpiprazole, cariprazine.**

Other agents that may have some beneficial effects in the treatment of bipolar disorder are benzodiazepines (to calm, induce sleep and reduce anxiety), **memantine**, **amantadine** (to improve depression and cognitive impairments) and **ketamine** (to treat suicidal ideation).

The use of antidepressant drugs in bipolar disorder is somewhat controversial. It is recommended that they are given in combination with an antimanic agent because, in some patients, they may induce or enhance mania.

Used prophylactically in bipolar disorder, these drugs prevent the swings of mood and thus can reduce both the depressive and the manic phases of the illness. They are given over long periods, and their beneficial effects take 3–4 weeks to develop. Given in an acute attack, they are effective only in reducing mania, but not the depressive phase (although lithium is sometimes used as an adjunct to antidepressants in severe cases of unipolar depression). Very little is known about the pathophysiology of bipolar disorder although it has a much higher genetic risk than unipolar depression and some aspects of the disorder reflect symptoms seen in schizophrenia. The mechanisms of action of mood stabilisers are also poorly understood and even though the molecular targets have been investigated, how actions at these receptors or downstream signalling pathways translate to effects on mood remains unknown.

LITHIUM

The psychotropic effect of lithium was discovered in 1949 by Cade, who had predicted that urate salts should prevent the induction by uraemia of a hyperexcitability state in guinea pigs. He found lithium urate to produce an effect, quickly discovered that it was due to lithium rather than urate and went on to show that lithium produced a rapid improvement in a group of manic patients.

Antiepileptic and atypical antipsychotic drugs (see later) are equally effective in treating acute mania; they act more quickly and are considerably safer, so the clinical use of lithium is mainly confined to prophylactic control of bipolar disorder. The use of lithium is declining.[4] It is relatively difficult to use, as plasma concentration monitoring is required, and there is the potential for problems in patients with renal impairment and for drug interactions, for example with diuretics (see Ch. 58).

Pharmacological effects and mechanism of action

Lithium is clinically effective at a plasma concentration of 0.5–1 mmol/L, and above 1.5 mmol/L it produces a variety of toxic effects, so the therapeutic window is narrow. In normal subjects, 1 mmol/L lithium in plasma has no appreciable psychotropic effects. It does, however, produce many detectable biochemical changes, and it is still unclear how these may be related to its therapeutic effect.

Lithium is a monovalent cation that can mimic the role of Na^+ in excitable tissues, being able to permeate the voltage-gated Na^+ channels that are responsible for action potential generation (see Ch. 4). It is, however, not pumped out by the Na^+-K^+-ATPase, and therefore tends to accumulate inside excitable cells, leading to a partial loss of intracellular K^+ and depolarisation of the cell.

The biochemical effects of lithium are complex, and it inhibits many enzymes that participate in signal transduction pathways. Those that are thought to be relevant to its therapeutic actions are as follows:

- Inhibition of inositol monophosphatase, which blocks the phosphatidylinositol (PI) pathway (see Ch. 3) at the point where inositol phosphate is hydrolysed to free inositol, resulting in depletion of PI. This prevents agonist-stimulated inositol trisphosphate formation through various PI-linked receptors, and therefore blocks many receptor-mediated effects.
- Inhibition of GSK3 isoforms, possibly by competing with magnesium for its association with these kinases. GSK3 isoforms phosphorylate a number of key enzymes involved in pathways leading to apoptosis and amyloid formation. Lithium can also affect GSK3 isoforms indirectly by interfering with their regulation by Akt, a closely related serine/threonine kinase regulated through PI-mediated signalling and by arrestins (see Ch. 3).

Neuroprotective and neurotrophic effects may account for its delayed onset and prophylactic efficacy and lithium's beneficial effects in neurodegenerative diseases such as Alzheimer's disease (see Ch. 40).

Lithium inhibits G protein function, thus reducing K^+ channel activation and hormone-induced cAMP production. It also blocks other cellular responses (e.g. the response of renal tubular cells to antidiuretic hormone, and of the thyroid to thyroid-stimulating hormone; see Chs 29 and 34, respectively). This is not, however, a pronounced effect in the brain.

The cellular selectivity of lithium appears to depend on its selective uptake, reflecting the activity of sodium channels in different cells. This could explain its relatively selective action in the brain and kidney, even though many other tissues use the same second messengers. Notwithstanding such insights, our ignorance of the nature of the disturbance underlying the mood swings in bipolar disorder leaves us groping for links between the biochemical and prophylactic effects of lithium.

Pharmacokinetic aspects and toxicity

Lithium is given by mouth as carbonate salt and is excreted by the kidney. About half of an oral dose is excreted within about 12 h – the remainder, which presumably represents lithium taken up by cells, is excreted over the next 1–2 weeks. This very slow phase means that, with regular dosage, lithium accumulates slowly over 2 weeks or more before a steady state is reached. The narrow therapeutic window means that monitoring of the plasma concentration is essential. Na^+ depletion reduces the rate of excretion by increasing the reabsorption of lithium by the proximal tubule, and thus increases the likelihood of toxicity. Diuretics that act distal to the proximal tubule (see Ch. 29) also have this effect, and renal disease also predisposes to lithium toxicity.

The main toxic effects that may occur during treatment are as follows:

- nausea, vomiting and diarrhoea;
- tremor;
- renal effects: polyuria (with resulting thirst) resulting from inhibition of the action of antidiuretic hormone. At the same time, there is some Na^+ retention associated with increased aldosterone secretion. With prolonged treatment, serious renal

[4] The decline in lithium use may have been influenced by the imbalance in the marketing of this simple inorganic ion versus more profitable pharmacological agents.

tubular damage may occur, making it essential to monitor renal function regularly in lithium-treated patients;
- thyroid enlargement, sometimes associated with hypothyroidism;
- weight gain;
- hair loss.

Acute lithium toxicity results in various neurological effects, progressing from confusion and motor impairment to coma, convulsions and death if the plasma concentration reaches 3–5 mmol/L.

ANTIEPILEPTIC DRUGS

Carbamazepine, **valproate** and **lamotrigine** (see Ch. 46) have fewer side effects than lithium and have proved efficacious in the treatment of bipolar disorder.

It is assumed that the mechanisms of action of anticonvulsant drugs in reducing bipolar disorder are related to their anticonvulsant activity although they can also interact with intracellular signalling molecules linked to the effects of lithium. While each drug has multiple actions (see Table 46.1), the antiepileptic drugs effective in bipolar disorder share the property of sodium-channel blockade, although there are subtle differences in their effectiveness against the different phases of bipolar disorder. Valproate and carbamazepine are effective in treating acute attacks of mania and in the long-term treatment of the disorder, although carbamazepine may not be as effective in treating the depression phase. Valproate is sometimes given along with other drugs such as lithium. Lamotrigine is effective in preventing the recurrence of both mania and depression.

SECOND-GENERATION ANTIPSYCHOTIC DRUGS

An ever-increasing number of second-generation antipsychotic drugs (e.g. **olanzapine**, **risperidone**, **quetiapine**, **aripiprazole**, **cariprazine**, **brexpiprazole**, **asenapine**) (see Ch. 47) are proving effective in the treatment of bipolar disorder. These agents have D_2 dopamine and $5\text{-}HT_{2A}$ receptor antagonist properties as well as actions on other receptors and amine transporters that may contribute to their effectiveness. All appear to be effective against mania while some may also be effective against bipolar depression. In bipolar depression, they are often used in combination with lithium or valproate. Olanzapine is given in combination with the antidepressant fluoxetine. Haloperidol, a first-generation antipsychotic drug, is also sometimes used to treat bipolar disorder.

Treatment of bipolar disorder

- **Lithium**, an inorganic ion, taken orally as lithium carbonate.
- Mechanism of action is not understood. The main biochemical possibilities are:
  - interference with inositol trisphosphate formation
  - inhibition of kinases
  - effects on neurotrophic mechanisms leading to neuroprotective effects
- Antiepileptic drugs (e.g. carbamazepine, valproate, lamotrigine):
  - better side effect and safety profile.
- Atypical antipsychotic drugs (e.g. olanzapine, risperidone, quetiapine, aripiprazole) and also haloperidol.

Clinical uses of mood-stabilising drugs

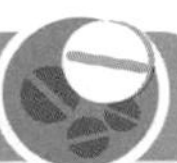

- **Lithium** (as the carbonate) is the classical drug. It is used:
  - in prophylaxis and treatment of *mania*, and in the prophylaxis of *bipolar* or *unipolar disorder* (bipolar disorder or recurrent depression).
- Points to note include the following:
  - there is a narrow therapeutic window and long duration of action;
  - acute toxic effects include cerebellar effects, nephrogenic *diabetes insipidus* (see Ch. 29) and renal failure;
  - dose must be adjusted according to the plasma concentration;
  - elimination is via the kidney and is reduced by proximal tubular reabsorption. Diuretics increase the activity of the reabsorptive mechanism and hence can precipitate lithium toxicity;
  - thyroid disorders and mild cognitive impairment occur during chronic use.
- **Carbamazepine valproate** and **lamotrigine** (sodium-channel blockers with antiepileptic actions; see Ch. 46) are used for:
  - the prophylaxis and treatment of manic episodes in patients with *bipolar disorder*;
  - the treatment of *bipolar disorder* (**valproate**, **lamotrigine**).
- **Olanzapine**, **risperidone**, **quetiapine**, **aripiprazole** (atypical antipsychotic drugs) are primarily used to treat *mania.*

REFERENCES AND FURTHER READING

Pathogenesis of depressive illness

Bastiaanssen, T.F.S., Cussotto, S., Claesson, M.J., Clarke, G., Dinan, T.G., Cryan, J.F., 2020. Gutted! unraveling the role of the microbiome in major depressive disorder. Harv. Rev. Psychiatry. 28, 26–39.

Duman, R.S., Deyama, S., Fogaça, M.V., 2021. Role of BDNF in the pathophysiology and treatment of depression: activity-dependent effects distinguish rapid-acting antidepressants. Eur. J. Neurosci. 53, 126–139.

Gonda, X., Petschner, P., Eszlari, N., et al., 2019. Genetic variants in major depressive disorder: from pathophysiology to therapy. Pharmacol. Ther. 194, 22–43.

Pariante, C.M., 2017. Why are depressed patients inflamed? A reflection on 20 years of research on depression, glucocorticoid resistance and inflammation. Eur. Neuropsychopharmacol. 27, 554–559.

Saavedra, K., Salazar, L.A., 2021. Epigenetics: a missing link between early life stress and depression. Adv. Exp. Med. Biol. 1305, 117–128.

Animal models

Gururajan, A., Reif, A., Cryan, J.F., Slattery, D.A., 2019. The future of rodent models in depression research. Nat. Rev. Neurosci. 20, 686–701.

Conventional antidepressant treatments

Cipriani, A., Furukawa, T.A., Salanti, G., 2018. Comparative efficacy and acceptability of 21 antidepressant drugs for the acute treatment of adults with major depressive disorder: a systematic review and network meta-analysis. Lancet 391, 1357–1366.

Cleare, A., Pariante, C.M., Young, A.H., 2015. Evidence-based Guidelines for Treating Depressive Disorders with Antidepressants: A Revision of the 2008 British Association for Psychopharmacology Guidelines. Available at: https://www.bap.org.uk/pdfs/BAP_Guidelines-Antidepressants.pdf.

Godlewska, B.R., Harmer, C.J., 2021. Cognitive neuropsychological theory of antidepressant action: a modern-day approach to depression and its treatment. Psychopharmacology 238, 1265–1278.

Harmer, C.J., Duman, R.S., Cowen, P.J., 2017. How do antidepressants work? new perspectives for refining future treatment approaches. Lancet Psychiatr. 4, 409–418.

Jolly, K., Gammage, M.D., Cheng, K.K., Bradburn, P., Banting, M.V., Langman, M.J., 2009. Sudden death in patients receiving drugs tending to prolong the QT interval. Br. J. Clin. Pharmacol. 68, 743–751.

Sharma, T., Guski, L.S., Freund, N., Gøtzsche, P.C., 2016. Suicidality and aggression during antidepressant treatment: systematic review and meta-analyses based on clinical study reports. Brit. Med. J. 352, i65.

Sullivan, C.R.P., Olsen, S., Widge, A.S., 2021. Deep brain stimulation for psychiatric disorders: from focal brain targets to cognitive networks. Neuroimage 225, 117515.

Rapid acting antidepressants

Krystal, J.H., Abdallah, C.G., Sanacora, G., Charney, D.S., Duman, R.S., 2019. Ketamine: a paradigm shift for depression research and treatment. Neuron 101, 774–778.

Malhi, G.S., Byrow, Y., Cassidy, F., et al., 2016. Ketamine: stimulating antidepressant treatment? Brit. J. Psychiatry Open 2, e5–e9.

Vargas, M.V., Meyer, R., Avanes, A.A., Rus, M., Olson, D.E., 2021. Psychedelics and other psychoplastogens for treating mental illness. Front. Psychiatry 12, 727117.

Pharmacogenetic factors

Crisafulli, C., Drago, A., Calabro, M., et al., 2014. Pharmacogenetics of antidepressant drugs; an update. Hosp. Pharmacol. 1, 33–51.

Lithium

Malhi, G.S., Tanious, M., Das, P., et al., 2013. Potential mechanisms of action of lithium in bipolar disorder. CNS Drugs 27, 135–153.

Won, E., Kim, Y., 2017. An oldie but goodie: lithium in the treatment of bipolar disorder through neuroprotective and neurotrophic mechanisms. Int. J. Mol. Sci. 2017 18 (12), 2679.

49 Psychoactive drugs

OVERVIEW

In its broadest sense, the term *psychoactive drug* would cover all drugs that act on the brain to produce changes in perception, mood, consciousness and behaviour, and would thus include anaesthetic, anxiolytic, antipsychotic and antidepressant drugs, which are described elsewhere in this book. Here we describe psychoactive drugs that are not covered in detail elsewhere. Some of these drugs have proven therapeutic usefulness in the treatment of behavioural disorders such as attention deficit/hyperactive disorder and narcolepsy. Others may prove to have clinical potential as antidepressants, anxiolytics and cognition enhancers. Drugs such as nicotine and ethanol have little or no medicinal value but their use is legal in many countries whereas most others are illegal.

Further information on psychoactive drugs is contained in Miller (2015).

INTRODUCTION

Attempting to classify psychoactive drugs according to their pharmacological mechanisms of action and their behavioural effects is a challenging task. Several of the drugs exert more than one important pharmacological action, drugs with apparently similar pharmacological activity can induce different subjective experiences (e.g. amphetamine and 3,4-methylenedioxymethamphetamine [MDMA]) and for a single drug the behavioural response may change with dose (e.g. ethanol induces excitement at low doses but is depressant at higher doses). Here, for convenience, we have grouped psychoactive drugs as

- Psychomotor stimulants
- Psychedelics
- Dissociatives
- Depressants
- Synthetic cannabinoid receptor agonists (SCRAs)

The 21st century has seen an explosion in the availability of novel psychoactive substances (NPS). By and large, these have been developed to circumvent legal restrictions on more established drugs (e.g. amphetamines, cocaine, MDMA and cannabinoids) and were for a time referred to as 'legal highs'. This has led to changes in the law in many countries to make them illegal. The array of psychoactive substances is vast;[1] in this chapter we concentrate on psychoactive drugs for which good evidence of their behavioural effects and mechanisms of action are available.

[1]The Drugs Wheel (http://www.thedrugswheel.com/) provides an up-to-date, easily understood classification of the more prevalent psychoactive drugs.

PSYCHOMOTOR STIMULANTS

Table 49.1 lists the major psychomotor stimulants, their mechanisms of action and clinical uses.

AMPHETAMINES[2]

DL-amphetamine (*speed* or *billy whizz*), its active dextroisomer **dextroamphetamine** (*dexies*) and **methamphetamine** (*crystal meth* or *ice*) have very similar chemical structures (Fig. 49.1) and pharmacological properties.

Pharmacological effects

The amphetamines act by releasing monoamines, primarily dopamine (DA) and noradrenaline (NA), from nerve terminals in the brain. They do this in a number of ways. They are substrates for the neuronal plasma membrane transporters for dopamine (DAT) and noradrenaline (NET) but not the transporter for 5-hydroxytryptamine (SERT) (see Chs 15, 16 and 39), and thus act as competitive inhibitors, reducing the reuptake of DA and NA. In addition, they enter nerve terminals via the uptake processes or by diffusion and interact with the vesicular monoamine pump VMAT-2 to inhibit the uptake into synaptic vesicles of cytoplasmic DA and NA. The amphetamines are taken up into the storage vesicles by VMAT-2 and displace the endogenous monoamines from the vesicles into the cytoplasm. At high concentrations, amphetamines can inhibit monoamine oxidase, which otherwise would break down cytoplasmic monoamines, and monoamine oxidase inhibitors (see Ch. 48) potentiate the effects of amphetamine. The cytoplasmic monoamines can then be transported out of the nerve endings via the plasma membrane DAT and NET transporters working in reverse, a process that is thought to be facilitated by amphetamine binding to these transporters. All of these will combine to increase the concentration of extracellular DA and NA in the vicinity of the synapse (see Chs 15 and 39).

In animals, prolonged administration results in degeneration of monoamine-containing nerve terminals and eventually cell death. This effect is observed with toxic doses and is probably due to the accumulation of reactive metabolites of the parent compounds within the nerve terminals. In human brain-imaging studies a reduction in the levels of DAT and D_2 receptors has been observed in the brains of amphetamine users. It is unclear, however, whether this is due to long-term exposure to the drug-inducing nerve damage or is an underlying vulnerability that was responsible for drug seeking in the first instance.

[2]As discussed in the Preface to this book, in Chapters 49 and 50, where mainly illicit drug use is being described, we use common drug names and spellings (e.g. amphetamine and heroin) rather than their recommended international non-proprietary names (amfetamine and 3,6-diacetyl morphine).

Table 49.1 Major central nervous system psychomotor stimulants

Drugs	Mode(s) of action	Clinical significance	Notes
Amphetamine and related compounds (e.g. dexamphetamine, methamphetamine)	Release of DA and NA Inhibition of DA and NA uptake	Dexamphetamine used to treat ADHD in children; Some use to treat narcolepsy	Risk of dependence, sympathomimetic side effects and pulmonary hypertension **Fenethylline** is a prodrug that is broken down to release both amphetamine and theophylline. It is a popular drug in Arab countries
Methylphenidate	Inhibition of DA and NA uptake	Used to treat ADHD in children	Structurally related to amphetamines (see Fig. 49.1) **Ethylphenidate** has similar actions
Modafinil	Inhibition of DA reuptake	May have use to reduce fatigue and enhance cognition	–
Cocaine	Inhibition of DA, 5-HT and NA uptake Local anaesthetic	Risk of fetal damage Occasionally used for nasopharyngeal and ophthalmic anaesthesia (see Ch. 44)	Widespread non medicinal use
MDMA (ecstasy)	Releases 5-HT and inhibits uptake	May have potential in the treatment of post-traumatic stress disorder	Other related drugs are **3,4-methylenedioxyamphetamine** (MDA), **4-bromo-2,5-dimethoxyphenethylamine** (2CB) and **4-methylthioamphetamine** (4-MTA)
Paramethoxyam phetamine (PMA)	Releases 5-HT and blocks uptake	–	Often added to, or sold as, MDMA; **paramethoxymethamphetamine** (PMMA) is similar but less potent
Benzofuran derivatives	Releases 5-HT and NA and inhibit uptake	–	Have both MDMA and amphetamine-like properties Examples include **1-(benzofuran-5-yl)-propan-2-amine** (5APB) and **1-(benzofuran-6-yl)-propan-2-amine** (6APB)
Cathinone	Releases DA and inhibits DA, NA and 5-HT uptake	–	Chemically related to amphetamines but with a ketone functional group. Present in khat
Mephedrone	Inhibition of DA and 5-HT uptake	–	Derived from cathinone **Methedrone** and **mexedrone** are similar
Methylone	Inhibition of NA, DA and 5-HT uptake	–	Cathinone derivative containing the dioxy ring of MDMA **Ethylone** and **butylone** are similar
Benzylpiperazine (BZP)	Inhibition of DA, NA and 5-HT uptake α_2-adrenoceptor agonist, 5-HT_{2A} agonist	–	Effects are comparable to amphetamine but less potent
Methylxanthines (e.g. caffeine, theophylline)	Inhibition of phosphodiesterase Antagonism of adenosine A_2 receptors	Theophylline used for action on cardiac and bronchial muscle (see Chs 20 and 28)	Caffeine is a constituent of beverages and tonics. It is also available in tablet form
Nicotine	Stimulates and desensitises nicotinic receptors (see Chs 14 and 39)	–	Consumed as tobacco or by vaping
Arecoline	Muscarinic agonist	–	Mild stimulant contained in betel nut. Use is widespread in India, Thailand, Indonesia and other Asian countries

ADHD, Attention deficit/hyperactivity disorder; *DA,* dopamine; *5-HT,* 5-hydroxytryptamine; *NA,* noradrenaline.

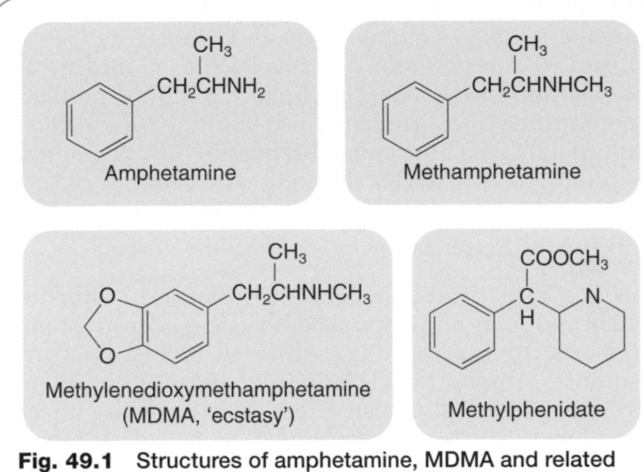

Fig. 49.1 Structures of amphetamine, MDMA and related drugs.

The main central effects of amphetamine-like drugs are:

- locomotor stimulation
- euphoria and excitement
- insomnia
- increased stamina
- anorexia
- long-term psychological effects: psychotic symptoms, anxiety, depression and cognitive impairment

In addition, amphetamines have peripheral sympathomimetic actions (see Ch. 15), producing a rise in blood pressure and inhibition of gastrointestinal motility.

In humans, amphetamines cause euphoria; with intravenous injection, this can be so intense as to be described as 'orgasmic'. Rats quickly learn to press a lever in order to obtain a dose of amphetamine – an indication that the drug is acutely reinforcing. Humans become confident, hyperactive and talkative, and sex drive is said to be enhanced. Fatigue, both physical and mental, is reduced. Amphetamines (and similar drugs such as **dexfenfluramine** and **sibutramine**) cause marked anorexia, but with continued administration this effect wears off and food intake returns to normal. They are no longer used clinically for weight reduction (see Ch. 32).

Adverse effects of amphetamines include feelings of anxiety, irritability and restlessness. High doses may induce panic and paranoia.

The locomotor and rewarding effects of amphetamine are due mainly to release of DA rather than NA, since in animal models destruction of the DA-containing nucleus accumbens (see Ch. 39) or administration of D_2 receptor antagonists (see Ch. 47) inhibits these responses and the effects were absent in mice genetically engineered to lack DAT.

Chronic use, tolerance and dependence

If amphetamines are taken repeatedly over a few days, a state of 'amphetamine psychosis' can develop, resembling an acute schizophrenic attack (see Ch. 47), with hallucinations, paranoia and aggressive behaviour. At the same time, repetitive stereotyped behaviour may develop. The close similarity of this condition to schizophrenia, and the effectiveness of antipsychotic drugs in controlling it, is consistent with a DA-mediated effect (see Ch. 47).

Tolerance develops rapidly to euphoric and anorexic effects of amphetamines, but more slowly to the other effects. Presumably tolerance is due to depletion of DA in nerve terminals or DA receptor desensitisation.

Addiction to amphetamines, a consequence of the insistent memory of euphoria, is very strong (see Ch. 50). When drug taking is stopped there is usually a period of deep sleep, and on awakening the subject feels lethargic, depressed, anxious, irritable (sometimes even suicidal) and hungry. These after-effects may be the result of depletion of the normal stores of DA and NA. It is estimated that about 10%–15% of users progress to full dependence, the usual pattern being that the dose is increased as tolerance develops, and then uncontrolled 'binges' occur in which the user takes the drug repeatedly over a period of a day or more, remaining continuously intoxicated. Large doses may be consumed in such binges, with a high risk of acute toxicity, and the demand for the drug displaces all other considerations.

Experimental animals, given unlimited access to amphetamine, take it in such large amounts that they die from the cardiovascular effects within a few days. Given limited amounts, they too develop a binge pattern of dependence.

Pharmacokinetic aspects

Amphetamines are readily absorbed from the gastrointestinal tract, but to increase the intensity of the hit the drugs can be snorted or injected. In crystal form, the free base of methamphetamine can be ignited and smoked in a manner similar to crack cocaine. Amphetamines freely penetrate the blood–brain barrier; methamphetamine is reported to cross the blood–brain barrier fastest which may in part explain its more potent and addictive nature. They are more readily brain penetrant than other indirectly acting sympathomimetic amines such as **ephedrine** or **tyramine** (see Ch. 15), which probably explains why they produce more marked central effects than those drugs. Amphetamines are mainly excreted unchanged in the urine, and the rate of excretion is increased when the urine is made more acidic (see Fig. 10.6).

Amphetamines

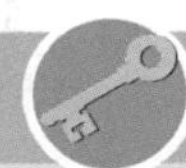

- The main effects are:
  - increased motor activity
  - euphoria and excitement
  - insomnia
  - anorexia
  - with prolonged administration, stereotyped and psychotic behaviour
- Effects are due mainly to release of catecholamines, especially DA and NA.
- Stimulant effect lasts for a few hours and is followed by depression and anxiety.
- Tolerance to the stimulant effects develops rapidly, although peripheral sympathomimetic effects may persist.
- Amphetamines are highly addictive.
- Amphetamine psychosis, which closely resembles schizophrenia, can develop after prolonged use.
- Amphetamines may be useful in treating narcolepsy, and also (paradoxically) to control hyperkinetic children. They are no longer prescribed as appetite suppressants.
- Their main importance is as non-medicinally used drugs.

METHYLPHENIDATE

Methylphenidate (*Ritalin*) inhibits the NET and DAT transporters on the neuronal plasma membrane. Unlike the amphetamines, methylphenidate is not a substrate for these transporters and thus does not enter the nerve terminals to facilitate NA and DA release (Heal et al., 2009). It nevertheless produces a profound and sustained elevation of extracellular NA and DA.

Methylphenidate is orally active, being absorbed from the intestine, but it undergoes presystemic metabolism such that only ~20% enters the systemic circulation. Absorption is slow following oral administration – T_{max} ~2 h – which may limit the intensity of any euphoric response to the drug. It is metabolised by carboxylesterase and has a half-life of ~2–4 h. It is used therapeutically to treat attention deficit/hyperactivity disorder (ADHD) and may also have cognition-enhancing effects.

MODAFINIL

Modafinil is the primary metabolite of **adrafinil**, a drug that was introduced as a treatment for narcolepsy in the 1980s. Since 1994, modafinil has been available as a drug in its own right. It inhibits DA reuptake by binding to DAT but with low potency. In the human brain, modafinil blocks DAT and increases extracellular DA levels in the caudate, putamen and nucleus accumbens. It also produces a number of other effects including α_1-adrenoceptor activation; enhanced release of 5-hydroxytryptamine (5-HT), glutamate and histamine; and inhibition of GABA release, as well as enhanced electrotonic coupling between neurons. The contribution of each action to the behavioural effects of modafinil remains to be clarified. Modafinil enhances some aspects of cognitive performance and has gained popularity as a 'lifestyle drug' (see Ch. 59) for this reason.

Modafinil is well absorbed from the gut, is metabolised in the liver and has a half-life of 10–14 h. While reported to 'brighten mood' there is little evidence that modafinil produces significant levels of euphoria when administered by mouth, but tablets can be crushed and snorted to obtain a quicker onset of effect. Modafinil is too insoluble for intravenous injection to be practical.

CLINICAL USE OF STIMULANTS

Attention deficit/hyperactivity disorder (ADHD)

The main use of amphetamines and methylphenidate is in the treatment of ADHD, a common and increasingly diagnosed condition, estimated as occurring in up to 9% of children whose overactivity and limited attention span disrupt their education and social development. The efficacy of drug treatment (e.g. with methylphenidate) has been confirmed in controlled trials, but there is concern as to the possible long-term adverse effects since treatment is sometimes continued into adolescence and beyond. Drug treatment should be part of a programme that includes psychological and behavioural interventions, and is started after the diagnosis has been confirmed by an expert.

Slow-release formulations of amphetamine and methylphenidate have been developed to deliver more stable concentrations of the drug, lower than that required to produce euphoria. D-amphetamine conjugated to lysine (**lisdexamphetamine**) is an inactive prodrug that, following oral administration, is cleaved enzymatically to release D-amphetamine, resulting in a slower onset of action.

Other drug treatments for ADHD include the NA reuptake inhibitors **atomoxetine** and **viloxazine** (see Ch. 48), and α_2-adrenoceptor agonists such as **clonidine** and **guanfacine**. The monoamine uptake inhibitor modafinil is not approved for paediatric use but may be effective in adult ADHD, as is **bupropion**. **Melatonin** (Ch. 39) improves sleep patterns in ADHD sufferers. The pharmacology of drugs used to treat ADHD is reviewed by Heal et al. (2009).

Narcolepsy

This is a rare, disabling sleep disturbance in which the patient suddenly and unpredictably falls asleep at frequent intervals during the day, while suffering nocturnal insomnia. Amphetamine is helpful but not completely effective. Modafinil is also effective in reducing attacks. Narcolepsy is often accompanied by *cataplexy* (abrupt onset of paralysis of variable extent often triggered by emotion, sometimes with 'frozen' posture). Treatment is usually with **fluoxetine**, a selective 5-HT reuptake inhibitor, or **venlafaxine**, a 5-HT and norepinephrine reuptake inhibitor (see Ch. 48). **Sodium oxybate**, the sodium salt of γ-hydroxybutyrate (also known as GHB; see Chs 38 and 59), is a CNS depressant that paradoxically is used to prevent cataplexy.

Clinical uses of CNS stimulants

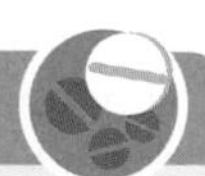

- CNS stimulants have few legitimate therapeutic indications. Where appropriate they are usually initiated by experts.
- ADHD: **methylphenidate**, **atomoxetine** (see Ch. 48). **Dexamphetamine** is an alternative in children who do not respond.
- Narcolepsy: **modafinil** for the excessive sleepiness; **oxybate** to reduce cataplexy (which can be associated with narcolepsy).
- Apnoea of prematurity: *xanthine alkaloids* (under expert supervision in hospital) are effective; **caffeine** is preferred to **theophylline.**

COCAINE

Cocaine is found in the leaves of the South American shrub coca. These leaves are used for their stimulant properties by natives of South America, particularly those in mountainous areas, who use it to reduce fatigue during work at high altitude.

Considerable mystical significance was attached to the powers of cocaine to boost the flagging human spirit, and Freud tested it extensively on his patients and his family, publishing an influential monograph in 1884 advocating its use as a psychostimulant.[3] Freud's ophthalmologist colleague, Köller, obtained supplies of the drug and discovered its local anaesthetic action (see Ch. 44), but the psychostimulant effects of cocaine have not proved to be clinically useful although they have led to its widespread non-medicinal use in Western countries. The mechanisms and treatment of cocaine addiction are discussed in Chapter 50.

[3]In the 1860s a Corsican pharmacist, Mariani, devised cocaine-containing beverages, Vin Mariani and Thé Mariani, which were sold very successfully as tonics. Imitators soon moved in, and Thé Mariani became the forerunner of Coca-Cola. In 1903, cocaine was removed from Coca-Cola because of its growing association with addiction and criminality.

Pharmacological effects

Cocaine binds to and inhibits the transporters NET, DAT and SERT (see Chs 15, 16 and 39), thereby producing a marked psychomotor stimulant effect, and enhancing the peripheral effects of sympathetic nerve activity.

In humans, cocaine produces euphoria, garrulousness, increased motor activity and a magnification of pleasure. Users feel alert, energetic and physically strong and believe they have enhanced mental capabilities. Its effects resemble those of amphetamines, although it has less tendency to produce stereotyped behaviour, delusions, hallucinations and paranoia. Evidence from transgenic knock-out mice indicates that the euphoric effects of cocaine involve inhibition of both DA and 5-HT reuptake. The peripheral sympathomimetic actions lead to tachycardia, vasoconstriction and an increase in blood pressure. Body temperature may increase, owing to the increased motor activity coupled with reduced heat loss. With excessive dosage, tremors and convulsions, followed by respiratory and vasomotor depression, may occur.

Experimental animals rapidly learn to press a lever to self-administer cocaine and will consume toxic amounts of the drug if access is not limited. In transgenic mice lacking the D_2 receptor, the enhanced locomotor effects of cocaine are reduced, but surprisingly self-administration of cocaine is increased, in contrast to what is found with other self-administered drugs such as ethanol and morphine.

Chronic use, addiction and tolerance

Cocaine is highly addictive (see Ch. 50), but there is some debate about whether or not its continued use induces tolerance and physical dependence. Users may increase their intake of the drug but this may reflect a desire for an increased effect rather than the development of tolerance. In experimental animals, sensitisation (the opposite of tolerance) can be observed but the relevance of this to the situation in humans is unclear. Cocaine does not produce a clear-cut withdrawal syndrome but depression, dysphoria and fatigue may be experienced following the initial stimulant effect. Cocaine induces addiction where users crave the drug's euphoric and stimulatory effects. The cellular mechanisms underlying craving, and pharmacological approaches to reduce craving, are discussed in Chapter 50. The pattern of drug use, evolving from occasional use through escalating dosage to compulsive binges, is similar to that seen with amphetamines.

Pharmacokinetic aspects

Cocaine is readily absorbed by many routes. For many years illicit supplies have consisted of the hydrochloride salt, which could be taken by nasal inhalation or intravenously. The latter route produces an intense and immediate euphoria, whereas nasal inhalation produces a less dramatic sensation and also tends to cause atrophy and necrosis of the nasal mucosa and septum.

Cocaine use changed dramatically when the free-base form ('crack') became available as a street drug. When an aqueous solution of cocaine hydrochloride is heated with sodium bicarbonate, free-base cocaine, water, CO_2 and NaCl are produced. The free-base cocaine is insoluble in water, precipitates out and can then be rolled into 'rocks' of crack. Free-base cocaine vaporises at around 90°C, much lower than the melting point of cocaine hydrochloride (190°C), which burns rather than vaporises. Thus crack can be smoked, with the uncharged free base being rapidly absorbed across the large surface area of the alveolae, giving rise to a greater CNS effect than that obtained by snorting cocaine. Indeed, the effect is nearly as rapid as that of intravenous administration. The social and economic consequences of this small change in formulation have been far-reaching.

The duration of its stimulant effect, about 30 min, is much shorter than that of amphetamine. It is rapidly metabolised in the liver. Heroin users may inject cocaine and heroin together intravenously (known as *speedballing*) to obtain the rapid effect of cocaine before the prolonged effect of heroin kicks in.

A cocaine metabolite is deposited in hair, and analysis of its content along the hair shaft allows the pattern of cocaine consumption to be monitored, a technique that has revealed a much higher incidence of cocaine use than was voluntarily reported. Cocaine exposure in utero can be estimated from analysis of the hair of neonates.

Cocaine is still occasionally used topically as a local anaesthetic, mainly in ophthalmology and minor nose and throat surgery, where its local vasoconstrictor action is an advantage, but has no other clinical uses.

Adverse effects

Toxic effects occur commonly in cocaine users. The main acute dangers are serious cardiovascular events (cardiac dysrhythmias, aortic dissection, and myocardial or cerebral infarction or haemorrhage). Progressive myocardial damage can lead to heart failure, even in the absence of a history of acute cardiac effects.

Cocaine can severely impair brain development in utero. The brain size is significantly reduced in babies exposed to cocaine in pregnancy, and neurological and limb malformations are increased. The incidence of ischaemic and haemorrhagic brain lesions, and of sudden infant death, is also higher in cocaine-exposed babies. Interpretation of the data is difficult because many cocaine users also take other illicit drugs that may affect fetal development, but the probability is that cocaine is highly detrimental.

Cocaine addiction has potentially severe effects on quality of life (see Ch. 50).

Cocaine

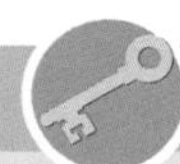

- **Cocaine** acts by inhibiting catecholamine uptake (especially DA) by nerve terminals.
- The behavioural effects of cocaine are very similar to those of amphetamines, although psychotomimetic effects are rarer. Duration of action is shorter.
- **Cocaine** used in pregnancy impairs fetal development and may produce fetal malformations.
- **Cocaine** regular use can lead to addiction.

MDMA

MDMA (*ecstasy* or *molly*) and related drugs are widely used as 'party drugs' because of the feelings of empathy and euphoria, and the loss of inhibitions, heightened sensations and energy surge, that they produce. They are sometimes referred to as 'empathogens' or 'enactogens'. They also have mild hallucinogenic effects. Common examples are listed in Table 49.1. In conjunction with psychotherapy, MDMA is in phase III clinical trials for the treatment of post-traumatic stress disorder (PTSD).

Pharmacological effects

Although an amphetamine derivative (see Fig. 49.1), MDMA affects monoamine function in a different manner from the amphetamines. It inhibits monoamine transporters, principally the 5-HT transporter, and also releases 5-HT, the net effect being a large increase in free 5-HT in certain brain regions, followed by depletion. Similar but smaller changes occur in relation to DA and NA release. Simplistically, the effects on 5-HT function determine the psychotomimetic effects, while DA and NA changes may account for the initial euphoria and later rebound dysphoria. MDMA does not induce physical dependence or addiction but its use carries several serious risks. Unintentional consumption of high doses may occur if pills have a higher than expected MDMA content or when MDMA is taken in powdered form. Also, illicit MDMA tablets or powders may be contaminated with or entirely substituted with ***para*-methoxyamphetamine** (PMA), a more dangerous psychoactive agent.

Common adverse effects of MDMA ingestion are:

- Feeling nauseous is common but vomiting is much less likely to occur.
- Acute hyperthermia (Fig. 49.2), resulting in damage to skeletal muscle and consequent renal failure. It is still unclear how hyperthermia is produced in humans. It may be mediated centrally through release of 5-HT, DA and NA acting on various receptors for these monoamines (Docherty and Green, 2010). It could also reflect an action of MDMA on mitochondrial function. It is exacerbated by energetic dancing and high ambient temperature and certain individuals may be particularly susceptible to this danger.
- Excess water intake and water retention. Users may consume large amounts of water as a result of increased physical activity and feeling hot. In addition, MDMA causes inappropriate secretion of antidiuretic hormone (see Ch. 33). This can lead to overhydration and hyponatraemia ('water intoxication'). Symptoms include dizziness and disorientation, leading to collapse into coma.
- Heart failure in individuals with an undiagnosed heart condition.

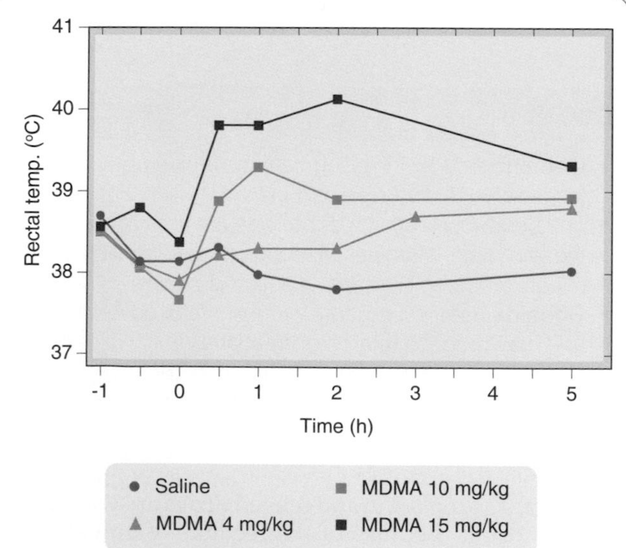

Fig. 49.2 A single injection of 3,4-methylenedioxymethamphetamine (MDMA) causes a dose-related increase in body temperature in rats. Drug administered at time zero. (Reproduced with permission from Green et al., 2004. Eur. J. Pharmacol. 500, 3–13.)

The after-effects of MDMA persist for a few days and comprise symptoms of depression, anxiety, irritability and increased aggression – the 'mid-week blues'. There is also evidence of long-term deleterious effects on memory and cognitive function in heavy MDMA users. In animal studies, MDMA can cause degeneration of 5-HT and DA neurons, but whether this occurs in humans is uncertain (see Green et al., 2012).

Potential therapeutic use

PTSD is a common and debilitating condition. Current treatments include selective serotonin reuptake inhibitor (SSRI) drugs (see Ch. 48) and psychotherapies such as cognitive behavioural therapy. The effectiveness of these, however, is limited and many sufferers fail to respond or continue to have significant symptoms. Recent clinical trials have demonstrated marked improvements in sufferers receiving MDMA along with psychotherapy (see Ch. 45 and Mitchell et al., 2021). The potential for MDMA in the treatment of alcohol use disorder is currently being evaluated.

MDMA (ecstasy)

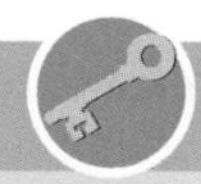

- **MDMA** is an amphetamine analogue that has powerful psychostimulant as well as mild psychotomimetic effects.
- **MDMA** inhibits monoamine transporters, principally the 5-HT transporter, and releases 5-HT.
- **MDMA** can cause an acute hyperthermic reaction as well as overhydration and hyponatraemia, sometimes fatal.
- **MDMA** does not cause physical dependence.
- **MDMA** has shown benefit in the treatment of PTSD.

CATHINONES

Cathinone and **cathine** are the active ingredients in the khat shrub. Chewing the leaves is popular in parts of Africa, such as Ethiopia and Somalia, and its use is spreading through immigrant populations in Western countries. They are chemically related to amphetamines but with a ketone functional group rather than a methyl group on the side chain.

Synthetic cathinone derivatives have become popular street drugs as they produce feelings of elevated mood and improved mental function. **Mephedrone** elevates extracellular levels of both DA and 5-HT, possibly by inhibiting reuptake and enhancing release.

METHYLXANTHINES

Various beverages, particularly tea, coffee and cocoa, contain methylxanthines, to which they owe their mild central stimulant effects. The main compounds responsible are **caffeine** and **theophylline**. The nuts of the cola plant also contain caffeine, which is present in cola-flavoured soft drinks. However, the most important sources, by far, are coffee and tea, which account for more than 90% of caffeine consumption. Further information on the pharmacology and toxicology of caffeine is presented by Fredholm et al. (1999).

Pharmacological effects

Methylxanthines have the following major pharmacological actions:

- CNS stimulation
- mild diuresis, not clinically significant
- stimulation of cardiac muscle (see Ch. 20)
- relaxation of smooth muscle, especially bronchial muscle (see Ch. 28)

The latter two effects resemble those of β-adrenoceptor stimulation (see Chs 15, 20 and 28). This is thought to be because methylxanthines (especially **theophylline**) inhibit phosphodiesterase, which is responsible for the intracellular metabolism of cAMP (see Ch. 3). They thus increase intracellular cAMP and produce effects that mimic those of mediators that stimulate adenylyl cyclase. Methylxanthines also antagonise many of the effects of adenosine, acting on both A_1 and A_2 receptors (see Ch. 16). Transgenic mice lacking functional A_2 receptors are abnormally active and aggressive, and fail to show increased motor activity in response to caffeine, suggesting that antagonism at A_2 receptors accounts for part, at least, of its CNS stimulant action. Caffeine also sensitises ryanodine receptors (see Ch. 4) but this effect occurs at higher concentrations (>10 mmol/L) than those achieved by recreational intake of caffeine. The concentration of caffeine reached in plasma and brain after two or three cups of strong coffee – about 100 μmol/L – is sufficient to produce appreciable adenosine receptor block and a small degree of phosphodiesterase inhibition. Adenosine receptor block probably causes the diuretic effect by reducing proximal tubular reabsorption of sodium.

Caffeine and theophylline have very similar stimulant effects on the CNS. Human subjects experience a reduction of fatigue, with improved concentration and a clearer flow of thought. This is confirmed by objective studies, which have shown that caffeine reduces reaction time and produces an increase in the speed at which simple calculations can be performed (although without much improvement in accuracy). Performance at motor tasks, such as typing and simulated driving, is also improved, particularly in fatigued subjects. Mental tasks, such as syllable learning, association tests and so on, are also facilitated by moderate doses (up to about 200 mg of caffeine, or about two cups of coffee) but impaired by larger doses. Insomnia is common. By comparison with amphetamines, methylxanthines produce less locomotor stimulation and do not induce euphoria, stereotyped behaviour patterns or a psychotic state, but their effects on fatigue and mental function are similar.

Tolerance and habituation develop to a small extent, but much less than with amphetamines; withdrawal effects are modest but can be troublesome.[4] Caffeine is not classified as a dependence-producing drug.

Clinical use and unwanted effects

There are few clinical uses for caffeine. It is included with aspirin in some preparations for treating headaches and other aches and pains, and with ergotamine in some antimigraine preparations, the objective being to produce a mildly agreeable sense of alertness. Methylxanthines are effective respiratory stimulants in the treatment of apnoea of prematurity (a developmental disorder caused by immaturity of central respiratory control), for which indication caffeine is preferred to theophylline because of its long half-life and safety. Theophylline (formulated as **aminophylline**) is used mainly as a bronchodilator in treating severe asthmatic attacks (see Ch. 28). In vitro tests show that it has mutagenic activity, and large doses are teratogenic in animals. However, epidemiological studies have shown no evidence of carcinogenic or teratogenic effects of tea or coffee drinking in humans. Some people have heightened sensitivity to caffeine and in these individuals it can trigger cardiac tachycardia and arrhythmias.

Methylxanthines

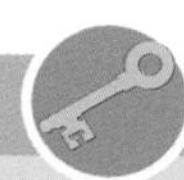

- **Caffeine** and **theophylline** produce psychomotor stimulant effects.
- Average **caffeine** consumption from beverages is about 200 mg/day.
- Main psychological effects are reduced fatigue and improved mental performance, without euphoria. Even large doses do not cause stereotyped behaviour or psychotomimetic effects.
- Methylxanthines act mainly by antagonism at A_2 purine receptors, and partly by inhibiting phosphodiesterase.
- Peripheral actions are exerted mainly on heart, smooth muscle and kidney.
- **Theophylline** is used clinically as a bronchodilator; **caffeine** is used as a respiratory stimulant for apnoea of prematurity and as an additive in many beverages and over-the-counter analgesics.

NICOTINE

Nicotine[5] is the psychoactive ingredient in tobacco.

Tobacco growing, chewing and smoking were indigenous throughout the American subcontinent and Australia at the time that European explorers first visited these places. Smoking spread through Europe during the 16th century, coming to England mainly as a result of its enthusiastic espousal by Walter Raleigh at the court of Elizabeth I. James I strongly disapproved of both Raleigh and tobacco, and in the early 17th century initiated the first antismoking campaign, with the support of the Royal College of Physicians. Parliament responded by imposing a substantial duty on tobacco, thereby giving the state an economic interest in the continuation of smoking at the same time that its official expert advisers were issuing emphatic warnings about its dangers.

[4]Caffeine withdrawal symptoms are a well-recognised cause of adverse events (headache, irritability) in residential phase I clinical trial units where caffeine-containing beverages are routinely prohibited.

[5]From the plant *Nicotiana*, named after Jean Nicot, French ambassador to Portugal, who presented seeds to the French king in 1560, having been persuaded by natives of South America of the medical value of smoking tobacco leaves. Smoking was believed to protect against illness, particularly the plague.

Until the latter half of the 19th century, tobacco was smoked in pipes, and primarily by men. Cigarette manufacture began at the end of the 19th century. Filter cigarettes (which give a lower delivery of carcinogenic tars and nicotine than standard cigarettes) and 'low-tar' cigarettes (which are also low in nicotine) became available in the 1950s and were thought to be less harmful.[6] More recently, the use of electronic cigarettes (e-cigarettes) to deliver nicotine, without the carcinogenic tars of cigarette smoke, has become popular. Laws banning smoking in public places and the increased use of e-cigarettes have led to a reduction in cigarette consumption in some countries. The World Health Organization (WHO) estimate, however, that over 80% of the world's 1.3 billion tobacco users live in low- and middle-income countries where there are fewer controls.

PHARMACOLOGICAL EFFECTS OF NICOTINE

EFFECTS ON THE CNS

At the neuronal level, nicotine acts on nicotinic acetylcholine receptors (nAChRs) (see Ch. 39), which are widely expressed in the brain, particularly in the cortex and hippocampus, and are believed to play a role in cognitive function, as well as in the ventral tegmental area (VTA), from which dopaminergic neurons project to the nucleus accumbens (the reward pathway, Fig. 39.3). nAChRs are ligand-gated cation channels located both pre- and postsynaptically, causing, respectively, enhanced transmitter release and neuronal excitation (see Wonnacott et al., 2005). Nicotine increases the firing rate and phasic activity of VTA dopaminergic neurons (see Fig. 49.3). Of the various subtypes of nAChR (see Table 39.2), the α4β2, α6β2 and α7 subtypes have received most attention, but other subtypes may also be involved in the rewarding effects of nicotine. As well as activating the receptors, nicotine also causes desensitisation, so the effects of a dose of nicotine are diminished after sustained exposure to the drug. Chronic nicotine administration leads to a substantial increase in the number of nAChRs (an effect opposite to that produced by sustained administration of most receptor agonists), which may represent an adaptive response to prolonged receptor desensitisation. It is likely that the overall effect of nicotine reflects a balance between activation of nAChRs, causing neuronal excitation, and desensitisation, causing synaptic block.

The higher-level functioning of the brain, as reflected in the subjective sense of alertness or by the electroencephalography (EEG) pattern, can be affected in either direction by nicotine, according to dose and circumstances. Nicotine wakes people up when they are drowsy and calms them down when they are tense, and EEG recordings broadly bear this out. It also seems that small doses of nicotine tend to cause arousal, whereas large doses do the reverse. Tests of motor and sensory performance (e.g. reaction time measurements or vigilance tests) in humans generally show improvement with nicotine, and nicotine enhances learning in rats. Nicotine and other nicotinic agonists such as **epibatidine** has analgesic activity in animal models, but, taken in the form of tobacco smoke or administered by other delivery systems such as patch or nasal spray, has only a weak analgesic effect in humans.

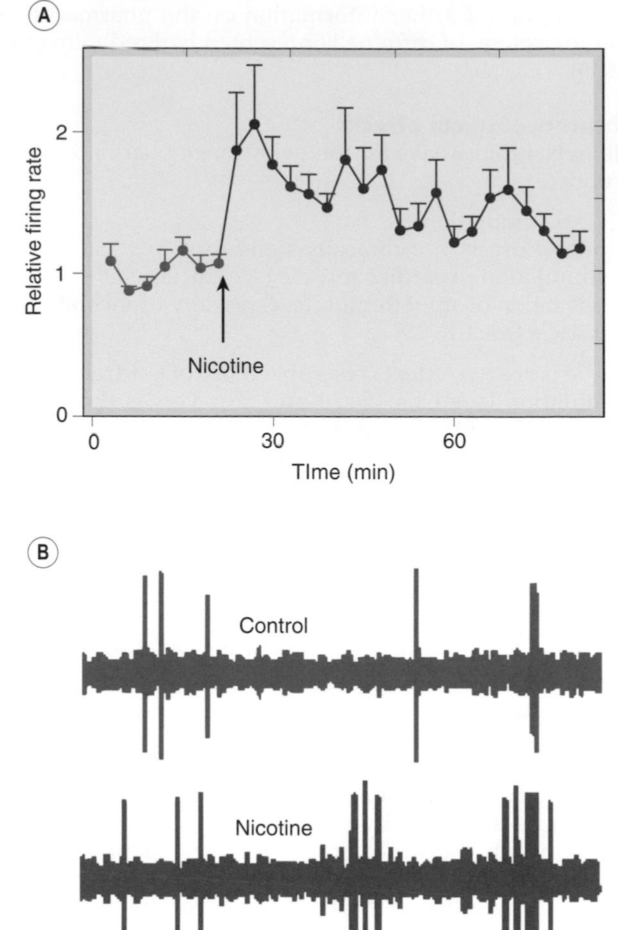

Fig. 49.3 Nicotine alters action potential firing characteristics of ventral tegmental area (VTA) dopaminergic neurons in freely moving rats. (A) Neuronal firing rate increases after nicotine injection i.p. (B) Action potential firing is phasic after nicotine injection. (Adapted from De Biasi, M., Dani, J.A., 2011. Reward, addiction, withdrawal to nicotine. Annu. Rev. Neurosci. 34, 105–130.)

PERIPHERAL EFFECTS

The peripheral effects of small doses of nicotine result from stimulation of autonomic ganglia (see Ch. 14) and of peripheral sensory receptors, mainly in the heart and lungs. Stimulation of these receptors produces tachycardia, increased cardiac output and arterial pressure, sweating, and a reduction of gastrointestinal motility. When people take nicotine for the first time, they usually experience nausea and sometimes vomit, probably because of stimulation of sensory receptors in the stomach. All these effects decline with repeated dosage, although the central effects remain. Secretion of adrenaline and NA from the adrenal medulla contributes to the cardiovascular effects, and release of antidiuretic hormone from the posterior pituitary causes a

[6]Smokers, however, adapted by smoking more low-tar cigarettes and inhaling more deeply to maintain their nicotine consumption.

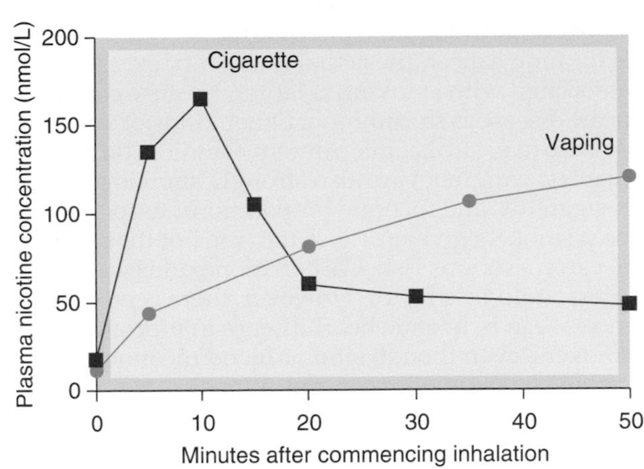

Fig. 49.4 Nicotine concentration in plasma during smoking or vaping. The subjects were habitual users who inhaled from a traditional cigarette or an e-cigarette according to their usual habit. (Data from Bowman, W.C., Rand, M., 1980. Chapter 4. In: Textbook of Pharmacology. Blackwell, Oxford; and Farsalinos et al., 2015. Sci. Rep. 5, 11269.)

decrease in urine flow.[7] The plasma concentration of free fatty acids is increased, probably owing to sympathetic stimulation and adrenaline secretion.

Smokers weigh, on average, about 4 kg less than non-smokers, mainly because of reduced food intake; giving up smoking usually causes weight gain associated with increased food intake.

PHARMACOKINETIC ASPECTS

Nicotine is rapidly absorbed from the lungs but less readily from the mouth and nasopharynx.[8] Therefore inhalation is required to give appreciable absorption of nicotine, each puff delivering a distinct bolus of drug to the CNS. The amount of nicotine absorbed varies greatly with the habits of the user and the way in which nicotine is self-administered.

An average cigarette, smoked over 10 min, causes the plasma nicotine concentration to rise to 15–30 ng/mL (100–200 nmol/L), falling to about half within 10 min and then more slowly over the next 1–2 h (Fig. 49.4). The rapid decline results mainly from redistribution between the blood and other tissues; the slower decline is due to hepatic metabolism, mainly by oxidation to an inactive ketone metabolite, *cotinine*. This has a long plasma half-life, and measurement of urinary cotinine provides a useful indication of nicotine consumption.

E-cigarettes work by heating a liquid (usually propylene glycol and glycerine) to generate a vapour containing nicotine which is then inhaled (a process commonly referred to as vaping). Vaping avoids inhalation of the toxic chemicals present in tobacco smoke. Early e-cigarette devices were found to deliver only minimal amounts of nicotine to the user. However, the technology has advanced rapidly and new-generation devices have been developed that deliver more nicotine more rapidly, but as yet, not quite as fast as a traditional cigarette (see Fig. 49.4).

Other routes of nicotine administration that provide a more sustained delivery are used by smokers trying to quit. A transdermal nicotine patch applied for 24 h causes the plasma concentration of nicotine to rise to 75–150 nmol/L over 6 h and to remain fairly constant for about 20 h. Administration by nasal spray or chewing gum results in a time course intermediate between that of smoking and the nicotine patch.

ADDICTION AND TOLERANCE

Nicotine is a highly addictive drug. Regular use also results in the development of tolerance. For reviews on nicotine and addiction see De Biasi and Dani (2011) and Leslie et al. (2013).

The effects of nicotine associated with peripheral ganglionic stimulation show rapid tolerance, perhaps as a result of desensitisation of nAChRs. With large doses of nicotine, this desensitisation produces a block of ganglionic transmission (see Ch. 14). Tolerance to the central effects of nicotine (e.g. in the arousal response) is much less than in the periphery. The increase in the number of nAChRs in the brain produced by chronic nicotine administration in animals also occurs in heavy smokers. Because the cellular effects of nicotine are diminished, it is possible that the additional binding sites represent desensitised rather than functional receptors.

The addictiveness of nicotine is due to the effects of the drug combined with the ritual of taking it (see Le Foll and Goldberg, 2005). Rats choose to drink dilute nicotine solution in preference to water if given a choice, and in a situation in which lever pressing causes an injection of nicotine to be delivered – admittedly at high doses – they quickly learn to self-administer it. Similarly, monkeys who have been trained to smoke, by providing a reward in response to smoking behaviour, will continue to do so spontaneously (i.e. unrewarded) if the smoking medium contains nicotine, but not if nicotine-free tobacco is offered instead. Humans, however, are unlikely to become addicted to nicotine delivered from patches, suggesting that other factors are also involved, such as the controlled pulsatile delivery associated with smoking and vaping.

Like other addictive drugs, nicotine causes excitation of the mesolimbic reward pathway and increased DA release in the nucleus accumbens. Transgenic mice lacking the β2 subunit of the nAChR lose the rewarding effect of nicotine and its DA-releasing effect, confirming the importance of the β2-containing nAChR subtypes and mesolimbic DA release in the response to nicotine. In contrast to normal mice, the mutant mice could not be induced to self-administer nicotine, even though they did so with cocaine.

In contrast to euphoria, induction of physical dependence involves nicotinic receptors containing α5 and β4 subunits in the medial habenula–interpeduncular nucleus pathway. A physical withdrawal syndrome occurs in humans on cessation of smoking. Its main features are increased irritability, impaired performance of psychomotor tasks, aggressiveness and sleep disturbance. The withdrawal syndrome is much less severe than that produced by opioids, and can be alleviated by replacement nicotine. It lasts for 2–3 weeks, although the craving for cigarettes persists for much longer than this; relapses during attempts to quit occur most commonly at a time when the physical withdrawal syndrome has long since subsided.

[7]This may explain why, in years gone by, men smoked cigars while chatting over drinks after dinner.

[8]Nicotine absorbed from cigar smoke is via the buccal mucosa but cigars deliver a much higher dose per puff than cigarettes, so a substantial amount gets in despite a low fraction absorbed.

Pharmacology of nicotine

- At the cellular level, **nicotine** acts on nicotinic acetylcholine receptors (nAChRs) to enhance neurotransmitter release and increase neuronal excitation. Its central effects are blocked by receptor antagonists such as **mecamylamine.**
- At the behavioural level, nicotine produces a mixture of inhibitory and excitatory effects.
- **Nicotine** shows reinforcing properties, associated with increased activity in the mesolimbic dopaminergic pathway, and self-administration can be elicited in animal studies.
- Electroencephalography changes show an arousal response, and subjects report increased alertness accompanied by a reduction of anxiety and tension.
- Learning, particularly under stress, is facilitated by **nicotine.**
- The peripheral effects of **nicotine** are due mainly to ganglionic stimulation: tachycardia, increased blood pressure and reduced gastrointestinal motility. Tolerance develops rapidly to these effects.
- **Nicotine** is metabolised to cotinine, mainly in the liver, within 1–2 h.
- **Nicotine** gives rise to tolerance, physical dependence and addiction. Attempts at long-term cessation succeed in only about 20% of cases.
- **Nicotine** replacement therapy (e-cigarettes, chewing gum or skin patch preparations) improves the chances of giving up smoking when combined with active counselling.

HARMFUL EFFECTS OF TOBACCO SMOKING

The life expectancy of smokers is shorter than that of non-smokers. Smoking causes almost 90% of deaths from lung cancer, about 80% of deaths from bronchitis and emphysema and 17% of deaths from heart disease. The increased use of e-cigarettes should reduce the number of such deaths. About one-third of all cancer deaths can be attributed to smoking. Smoking is, by a large margin, the biggest preventable cause of death, responsible for about 1 in 10 adult deaths worldwide. Despite the introduction of e-cigarettes, deaths from smoking worldwide are continuing to rise. It is estimated that in 2021 smoking was responsible for some 7 million deaths (and 1.2 million additional deaths of non-smokers from involuntary secondary inhalation).

The main health risks are as follows:

- *Cancer, particularly of the lung and upper respiratory tract but also of the oesophagus, pancreas and bladder.* Smoking 20 cigarettes per day is estimated to increase the risk of lung cancer about 10-fold. Tar, rather than nicotine, is responsible for the cancer risk. Genetic variants of nicotinic-receptor subunits have been associated with lung cancer although the mechanisms behind this association are unclear (see Hung et al., 2008).
- *Coronary heart disease and other forms of peripheral vascular disease.* The mortality among men aged 55–64 from coronary thrombosis is about 60% greater in men who smoke 20 cigarettes per day than in non-smokers. Although the increase in risk is less than it is for lung cancer, the actual number of excess deaths associated with smoking is larger, because coronary heart disease is so common. Other kinds of vascular disease (e.g. stroke, intermittent claudication and diabetic gangrene) are also strongly smoking related. E-cigarettes and nicotine preparations, used to help smokers give up cigarettes, are not thought to carry a serious risk. Carbon monoxide (see later) could be a factor. However, there is no clear increase in ischaemic heart disease in pipe and cigar smokers, even though similar blood nicotine and carboxyhaemoglobin concentrations are reached, suggesting that other factors may be responsible for the risk associated with cigarettes.
- *Chronic obstructive pulmonary disease* (COPD; see Ch. 28) is a major global health problem. Cigarette smoking is the main cause. Stopping smoking slows the progression of the disease. Bronchitis, inflammation of the mucous membranes of the bronchi, is much more common in smokers than in non-smokers. These effects are probably due to tar and other irritants rather than nicotine.
- *Harmful effects in pregnancy.* Smoking, particularly during the latter half of pregnancy, significantly reduces birth weight (by about 8% in women who smoke 25 or more cigarettes per day during pregnancy) and increases perinatal mortality (by an estimated 28% in babies born to mothers who smoke in the last half of pregnancy). There is evidence that children born to smoking mothers remain behind, in both physical and mental development, for at least 7 years. By 11 years of age, the difference is no longer significant. These effects of smoking, although measurable, are much smaller than the effects of other factors, such as social class and birth order. Various other complications of pregnancy are also more common in women who smoke, including spontaneous abortion (increased 30%–70% by smoking), premature delivery (increased about 40%) and placenta praevia (where the placenta obstructs normal vaginal delivery, increased 25%–90%). Nicotine is excreted in breast milk in sufficient amounts to cause tachycardia in the infant.

The agents probably responsible for the harmful effects are as follows:

- Tar and irritants, such as nitrogen dioxide and formaldehyde. Cigarette smoke tar contains many known carcinogenic hydrocarbons, as well as tumour promoters, which together account for the high cancer risk. It is likely that the various irritant substances are also responsible for the increase in bronchitis and emphysema.
- Nicotine probably accounts for retarded fetal development because of its vasoconstrictor properties.
- Carbon monoxide. Cigarette smoke contains about 3% carbon monoxide. Carbon monoxide has a high affinity for haemoglobin, and the average carboxyhaemoglobin content in the blood of

cigarette smokers is about 2.5% (compared with 0.4% for non-smoking urban dwellers). In very heavy smokers, up to 15% of haemoglobin may be carboxylated, a level that affects fetal development in rats. Fetal haemoglobin has a higher affinity for carbon monoxide than adult haemoglobin, and the proportion of carboxyhaemoglobin is higher in fetal than in maternal blood.
- Increased oxidative stress may contribute to atherogenesis (see Ch. 22) and COPD (see Ch. 28).

OTHER EFFECTS OF TOBACCO SMOKING

Parkinson's disease is approximately twice as common in non-smokers as in smokers. It is possible that this reflects a protective effect of nicotine. Ulcerative colitis appears to be a disease of non-smokers. Former smokers are at high risk for developing ulcerative colitis, while current smokers have the least risk. This tendency indicates that smoking cigarettes may prevent the onset of ulcerative colitis. In contrast, smoking tends to worsen the effects of Crohn's disease (another type of inflammatory bowel disease). Earlier reports that Alzheimer's disease is less common in smokers have not been confirmed; indeed there is evidence that smoking may increase the occurrence of Alzheimer's disease in some genetic groups.

Effects of tobacco smoking

- Smoking accounts for more than 10% of deaths worldwide, mainly due to:
  - cancer, especially lung cancer, of which about 90% of cases are smoking related; carcinogenic tars are responsible;
  - chronic bronchitis; tars are mainly responsible.
- Smoking in pregnancy reduces birth weight and retards childhood development. It also increases abortion rate and perinatal mortality. **Nicotine** and possibly carbon monoxide are responsible.
- Use of e-cigarettes (vaping) avoids the inhalation of tar and carbon monoxide that occurs with smoking.
- The incidence of Parkinson's disease is lower in smokers than in non-smokers.

COGNITION-ENHANCING DRUGS

'Cognition' embraces many aspects of mental function, including memory, reasoning and problem-solving skills, situational judgements, decision-making and executive function. A variety of different test batteries have been designed to measure these functions in humans (e.g. Cambridge Neuropsychological Test Automated Battery [CANTAB]) and test the effects of drugs. Many clinical disorders, such as dementia (see Ch. 40), schizophrenia (see Ch. 47), depression (see Ch. 48) and drug addiction (see Ch. 50), impair these functions, and the hope is to develop cognition-enhancing drugs to restore them. Progress has been limited, although much hyped, as much with the questionable aim of 'improving' mental function in healthy humans, as in alleviating deficits in the sick.

Drugs currently available have been shown to:

- alter memory processing (i.e. enhance memory);
- reduce fatigue (stimulants), thus permitting the user to function for longer (i.e. perform complex tasks, study for examinations, overcome jet lag);
- increase motivation, energy, confidence and concentration.

They are also referred to as 'smart drugs' or 'nootropics'.

Drugs for which there is some evidence of an ability to enhance cognitive performance are **caffeine, amphetamines, methylphenidate, modafinil, arecoline, donepezil, vortioxetine** and **piracetam** but the clinical efficacy of these drugs is limited, and development of more effective cognition enhancers could have significant benefits for many patient groups.

Cognition-enhancing drugs are also used by healthy individuals aiming to enhance their performance, e.g. in revising for and taking examinations (D'Angelo et al., 2017) or in demanding professional roles. The use of drugs by healthy individuals to enhance academic performance does raise ethical issues in relation to fairness, academic pressure and fears of coercion by 'pushy' parents. There are also safety issues. Although many of the drugs taken are available as medicines (i.e. have gone through standard drug safety testing) there is still a lack of information on their acute and long-term effects in children and adolescents, whose brains are still in development. In healthy individuals, cognitive performance can be enhanced by improved sleep and mood as well as reduced anxiety. It would seem more appropriate to achieve this by lifestyle changes and behavioural therapy rather than resorting to the use of drugs.[9]

Effectiveness

While the effectiveness of cognition enhancers on healthy individuals is often trumpeted by individuals who use them and in the media, their actual effectiveness as assessed in scientific studies is somewhat inconclusive and ambiguous.[10] Also, drugs may affect different forms of memory differently (D'Angelo et al., 2017). It is important to distinguish between drugs that only improve a subject's abilities when they are fatigued and those that might improve cognitive ability in non-fatigued individuals.

Many studies have shown that amphetamines improve mental performance in fatigued subjects. Mental performance is improved for simple tedious tasks much more than for difficult tasks. Amphetamines are thought to increase ability to focus and maintain self-control. In addition to reducing fatigue, methylphenidate has a positive effect on long-term memory consolidation. Amphetamines and modafinil have

[9]A popular phenomenon is 'microdosing' with very small quantities of psychedelic drugs such as LSD, psilocybin or mescaline every few days with the aim of improving concentration, creativity and problem solving. At such low doses users do not experience psychedelic effects. Properly controlled scientific studies have revealed that while psychological outcomes do improve over time, the placebo group also improved and there were no significant differences between microdosing with a psychedelic drug and placebo.

[10]A survey of information available on the www came up with 142 substances (plants, herbs and drugs) for which claims of cognition enhancing ability have been made (Napoletano et al., 2020). However, for most of the agents little or no good scientific evidence was available to support claims of efficacy.

been used to improve the performance of soldiers, military pilots and others who need to remain alert under extremely fatiguing conditions. Modafinil appears to enhance cognition in non-fatigued individuals (Battleday and Brem, 2015) while also improving wakefulness, memory and executive functions in sleep-deprived individuals. Evidence for efficacy in patients with chronic cognitive impairment is controversial.

NON-STIMULANT DRUGS

The novel antidepressant **vortioxetine** (see Ch. 48) improves cognitive dysfunction in patients suffering from major depression.

Piracetam, which is a positive allosteric modulator at AMPA receptors (see Ch. 38), enhances memory in non-fatigued adults, and there is limited clinical evidence of reading improvement in dyslexic children. **Phenylpiracetam** is said to be more potent and may also have nicotinic antagonist properties. As with many CNS disorders, the possible importance of glutamate and its receptors was widely speculated on, but new, effective drugs acting on the glutamatergic system are still awaited (see, for example, Collingridge et al., 2013; Harms et al., 2013).

PSYCHEDELIC DRUGS

Psychedelic drugs (also sometimes referred to as *hallucinogenic* or *psychotomimetic* drugs) affect thought, perception and mood, without causing marked psychomotor stimulation or depression (see Nichols, 2004). Thoughts and perceptions tend to become distorted and dream-like, rather than being merely sharpened or dulled, and the change in mood is likewise more complex than a simple shift in the direction of euphoria or depression. Importantly, psychedelic drugs do not cause dependence. Common psychedelic drugs are listed in Table 49.2.

LYSERGIC ACID DIETHYLAMIDE, PSILOCYBIN AND MESCALINE

Lysergic acid diethylamide (LSD) is an exceptionally potent psychotomimetic drug capable of producing strong effects in humans in doses less than 1 µg/kg. It is a chemical derivative of lysergic acid, which occurs in the cereal fungus ergot (see Ch. 16).

LSD was first synthesised by Hoffman in 1943. Hoffman deliberately swallowed about 250 µg of LSD (the threshold dose is now known to be around 20 µg) and wrote 30 years later of the experience: 'the faces of those around me appeared as grotesque coloured masks … marked motoric unrest, alternating with paralysis … heavy feeling in the head, limbs and entire body, as if they were filled with lead … clear recognition of my condition, in which state I sometimes observed, in the manner of an independent observer, that I shouted half insanely.' These effects lasted for a few hours, after which Hoffman fell asleep, 'and awoke next morning feeling perfectly well.' Apart from these dramatic psychological effects, LSD has few physiological effects in humans at doses that cause hallucinations.

Mescaline, which is derived from the Mexican peyote cactus and has been known as a hallucinogenic agent for many centuries, was made famous by Aldous Huxley in *The Doors of Perception*.

Psilocybin is obtained from fungi ('magic mushrooms'). It is rapidly dephosphorylated to psilocin, the active moiety. Its effects are similar to those experienced with LSD.

The potential of LSD and psilocybin as treatments for depression and some forms of anxiety is discussed in Chapters 45 and 48.

Pharmacological effects

The main effects of these drugs are on mental function, most notably an alteration of perception in such a way that sights and sounds appear distorted and fantastic. Hallucinations – visual, auditory, tactile or olfactory – also occur, and sensory modalities may become confused, so that sounds are perceived as visions. Thought processes tend to become illogical and disconnected, but subjects retain insight into the fact that their disturbance is drug induced, and generally find the experience exhilarating. Occasionally, especially if the user is already anxious, LSD produces a syndrome that is extremely disturbing (the 'bad trip'), in which the hallucinatory experience takes on a menacing quality and may be accompanied by paranoid delusions. 'Flashbacks' of the hallucinatory experience may occur subsequent to drug use.

LSD acts on various 5-HT receptor subtypes (see Chs 16 and 39); its psychotomimetic effects are thought to be

Table 49.2 Major psychedelic drugs

Drugs	Mode(s) of action	Notes
LSD	Interacts with 5-HT and DA receptors Psychedelic effects are thought to be mainly through 5-HT_{2A} receptor activation	Potential as an antidepressant is currently being evaluated (see Ch. 48)
Mescaline	Lower potency partial agonist at 5-HT_{2A} and other 5-HT receptors Chemically related to amphetamine	No current clinical use Found in Peyote cactus plant
Psilocybin	Rapidly metabolised to psilocin, a partial agonist at 5-HT receptors including 5-HT_{1A} and 5-HT_{2A} receptors Chemically related to 5-HT	May have potential for the treatment of depression and some forms of anxiety (see Chs 45 and 48)
DMT	Interacts with a wide range of amine receptors, including 5-HT_{2A} receptors	Major component of Ayahuasca, a psychoactive 'tea' that originates from the Amazon region
Salvinorin A	κ Opioid receptor agonist (see Ch. 43)	No clinical use Found in *Salvia divinorum* (plant)

DA, Dopamine; *DMT*, dimethyltryptamine; *5-HT*, 5-hydroxytryptamine; *LSD*, lysergic acid diethylamide.

mediated mainly by its 5-HT_{2A} receptor agonist actions (see Nichols, 2004). It inhibits the firing of 5-HT-containing neurons in the raphe nuclei (see Ch. 39), apparently by acting as an agonist on the inhibitory somatodendritic 5-HT_{1A} receptors on these cells. The significance of this response to its psychotomimetic effects is unclear. Psilocybin is dephosphorylated to psilocin, which is a weak agonist at several 5-HT receptors including the 5-HT_{2A} receptor. The mechanism of action of mescaline is less well defined. It has lower affinity and efficacy at 5-HT_{2A} receptors than LSD and psylocybin. The binding affinity and agonist efficacies of LSD, psilocybin, mescaline and other psychedelic drugs at monoamine receptors and transporters are described in detail by Rickli et al. (2016).

Addictive liability

LSD, psilocybin and mescaline are seldom self-administered by experimental animals. Indeed, in contrast to most of the psychoactive drugs that are widely used by humans, they have aversive rather than reinforcing properties in behavioural tests. Tolerance to their effects develops quite quickly, but there is no physical withdrawal syndrome in animals or humans.

Psychedelic drugs induce head twitching in rodents through activation of 5-HT_{2A} receptors. However, the main effects of these psychedelic drugs in humans are subjective, so it is not surprising that animal tests that model psychedelic activity in humans have not been devised.[11]

OTHER PSYCHEDELIC DRUGS

Salvinorin A is a hallucinogenic agent contained in the American sage plant *Salvia divinorum*, a member of the mint family. It was originally used by the Mazatecs in Mexico; in recent years its use has spread and it has become known as *herbal ecstasy*. It is a κ opioid receptor agonist (see Ch. 43).[12] It also produces dissociative effects (see later) and, at high doses, delirium.

Other hallucinogens include **α-MT** (methyltryptamine) and **DMT** (dimethyltryptamine), which are naturally occurring, and **DPT** (dipropyltryptamine) and **DOM** (2,5-dimethoxy-4-methylamphetamine).

Muscarinic receptor antagonists (see Chs 14 and 39), **hyoscine**, **hyoscyamine** and **atropine**, are contained in various plants, including henbane and mandrake. Consumption can cause hallucinations, drowsiness, disorientation, amnesia and delirium

Ibogaine is contained in the root bark of iboga shrubs in Africa, South America and Australia. At high doses, it is hallucinogenic. Users have reported experiencing a reduced desire to take other drugs such as cocaine and heroin, leading to ibogaine being used as treatment for drug craving (see Ch. 50).

[11]One of the more bizarre attempts involves spiders, whose normal elegantly symmetrical webs become jumbled and erratic if the animals are treated with LSD. Search the web (worldwide rather than arachnid) for 'spiders LSD' to see images.

[12]In phase I clinical trials of synthetic κ-opioid receptor agonists as potential analgesic agents, the drugs were reported to induce a feeling of dysphoria. Perhaps the 'normal' volunteers in those trials were disturbed by the hallucinations they probably experienced. Interesting then that a naturally occurring κ agonist has now become popular amongst some people who use drugs.

Psychedelic drugs

- The main types are lysergic acid diethylamide (LSD), psilocybin and mescaline.
- LSD and psilocybin are 5-HT_{2A} receptor agonists.
- They cause sensory distortion and hallucinatory experiences.
- **LSD** is exceptionally potent, producing a long-lasting sense of dissociation and disordered thought. Hallucinatory episodes can recur after a long interval.
- In animal behavioural tests, they exhibit aversive rather than rewarding properties.
- **Salvinorin A** is a κ opioid receptor agonist that causes hallucinatory and dissociative effects.

DISSOCIATIVE DRUGS

Ketamine (*Special K*), a dissociative anaesthetic (see Ch. 41) with antidepressant properties (see Ch. 48), is also used for its psychoactive properties (see Morgan and Curran, 2012). Its fore-runner, **phencyclidine** (PCP, *angel dust*), was a popular hallucinogen in the 1970s but its use has declined. These drugs produce a feeling of euphoria. At higher doses they cause hallucinations and feelings of detachment, disorientation and numbness. PCP was reported to cause psychotic episodes and is used in experimental animals to produce a model of schizophrenia (see Ch. 47 and Morris et al., 2005).

Pharmacological effects

Their main pharmacological effect is non-competitive block of the *N*-methyl-D-aspartate (NMDA) receptor channel (see Ch. 38). **Methoxetamine**, a chemical derivative of ketamine, is an NMDA antagonist as well as an inhibitor of 5-HT reuptake, which may contribute to its CNS effects.

Adverse effects

Tolerance develops with repeated use of ketamine, resulting in higher doses being taken to achieve the same effect. Repeated use is associated with serious and persistent toxic effects, including abdominal pain, ulcerative cystitis (with associated severe bladder pain), liver damage and cognitive impairment (Morgan and Curran, 2012). Combination of ketamine with depressant drugs such as **alcohol**, **barbiturates** and **heroin** can result in dangerous overdose.

Nitrous oxide is a weak general anaesthetic with analgesic properties that acts as an antagonist at NMDA receptors (see Ch. 41). It is a colourless, slightly sweet-smelling gas that is also used in catering to whip cream. Recreational users normally purchase nitrous oxide in the form of small whipped-cream chargers from which they fill a balloon and then inhale the gas.[13] Users experience a brief rush of dizziness, euphoria – it is often referred to as 'laughing gas' – relaxation and dissociation that lasts only for a few minutes and so they may take a number of 'hits' over the space of a few hours. Regular and prolonged use

[13]Taking the gas directly into the mouth from the pressurised container can result in severe freezing of the lips and mouth as the temperature may be as low as -40°C. Breathing only nitrous oxide (e.g. by filling a large bag and placing it over the head) is extremely dangerous as there will be no oxygen in the inhaled gas (see Ch. 41).

Table 49.3 Depressant drugs

Drugs	Described further in Chapter	Notes
Benzodiazepines (diazepam, temazepam, alprazolam, etizolam)	45	Etizolam and pyrazolam are derived from benzodiazepines and act similarly
Zopiclone and other Z drugs	45	Short acting but similar effects to benzodiazepines
Gabapentin and pregabalin	46	Often taken in high doses to induce a feeling of drunkenness and stupor May enhance likelihood of overdose in opioid users
γ-Hydroxybutyric acid (GHB)	39, 59	γ-Butyrolactone (GBL) and 1,4-butanediol (BD) are broken down to GHB in the body
Ethanol	This chapter	
Propofol	42	Sub-anaesthetic doses induce a general feeling of well-being, euphoria and sexual disinhibition

can result in vitamin B_{12} deficiency which causes peripheral neuropathy (see Ch. 41).

DEPRESSANTS

Many CNS depressant drugs (Table 49.3) that are used for their psychoactive effects also have important therapeutic uses that are described in detail elsewhere in this book. Here we will concentrate on ethanol, which has little or no therapeutic value but is widely used in many countries for its psychoactive properties.

ETHANOL

It may at first seem strange to categorise ethanol as a depressant drug[14] given that its consumption in alcoholic beverages can make people excited, garrulous and violent. However, as with general anaesthetics (see Ch. 41), at low concentrations ethanol depresses inhibitions, resulting in apparent behavioural stimulation, whereas at higher concentrations all brain functions are depressed.

Judged on a molar basis, the consumption of ethanol far exceeds that of any other drug. The ethanol content of various drinks ranges from about 2.5% (weak beer) to about 55% (strong spirits), and the size of the normal measure is such that a single drink usually contains about 8–12 g (0.17–0.26 mol) of ethanol. Its low pharmacological potency is reflected in the range of plasma concentrations needed to produce pharmacological effects: minimal effects occur at about 10 mmol/L (46 mg/100 mL), and 10 times this concentration may be lethal. The average per capita consumption of ethanol in the United Kingdom doubled between 1970 and 2007, but has fallen slightly since then. There has been an increase in non-drinkers, mainly amongst young people. Amongst those who do drink, the main changes have been a growing consumption of wine in preference to beer among adults, greater consumption in the home and an increasing tendency for binge drinking, especially among young people.

For practical purposes, ethanol intake is often expressed in terms of units. One unit is equal to 8 g (10 mL) of ethanol, and is the amount contained in half a pint of normal-strength beer, one measure of spirits or one small glass of wine. The current UK government's guidelines state that for both men and women it is safest not to drink regularly more than 14 units per week, and that if as much as 14 units per week are drunk, it is best to spread this evenly over 3 days or more. It is estimated that in the United Kingdom, about 31% of men and 16% of women exceed these levels. Governments in most developed countries are attempting to curb alcohol consumption.

An excellent detailed review of all aspects of alcohol and alcoholism is provided by Spanagel (2009).

PHARMACOLOGICAL EFFECTS OF ETHANOL

Effects on CNS neurons

The main effects of ethanol are on the CNS, where its depressant actions resemble those of volatile anaesthetics (see Ch. 41). At a neuronal level, the effect of ethanol is depressant, although it increases neuronal activity – presumably by disinhibition – in some parts of the CNS, notably in the mesolimbic dopaminergic pathway that is involved in reward. The main acute cellular effects of ethanol that occur at concentrations (5–100 mmol/L) relevant to alcohol consumption by humans are:

- enhancement of both GABA- and glycine-mediated inhibition
- inhibition of Ca^{2+} entry through voltage-gated calcium channels
- activation of certain types of K^+ channel
- inhibition of ionotropic glutamate receptor function
- inhibition of adenosine transport

For review, see Harris et al. (2008).

Ethanol enhances the action of GABA on $GABA_A$ receptors in a similar way to benzodiazepines (see Ch. 45). Its effect is, however, smaller and less consistent than that of benzodiazepines, and no clear effect on inhibitory synaptic transmission in the CNS has been demonstrated

[14]In some countries ethanol is classed as a food, not a drug! This reflects the lobbying power of the alcohol industry. Ethanol meets the criteria for 'What is a drug?' given in Chapter 1.

for ethanol. This may be because the effect of ethanol is seen only on some subtypes of $GABA_A$ receptor (see Ch. 38), e.g. the extrasynaptic $\alpha6\beta3\delta$ $GABA_A$ receptor subtype has been reported to be sensitive to ethanol. Ethanol may also act presynaptically to enhance GABA release.

Ethanol enhances glycine receptor function, due both to a direct interaction with the $\alpha1$ subunit of the glycine receptor and to indirect effects mediated through protein kinase C (PKC) activation. Ethanol can also enhance glycine release from nerve terminals.

Ethanol reduces transmitter release in response to nerve terminal depolarisation by inhibiting the opening of voltage-gated calcium channels in neurons. It also reduces neuronal excitability by activating G protein–activated inwardly rectifying K^+ (GIRK) channels as well as potentiating calcium-activated potassium (BK) channel activity.

The excitatory effects of glutamate are inhibited by ethanol at concentrations that produce CNS depressant effects in vivo. NMDA receptor activation is inhibited at lower ethanol concentrations than are required to affect AMPA receptors (see Ch. 38). Other effects produced by ethanol include an enhancement of the excitatory effects produced by activation of nAChRs and $5\text{-}HT_3$ receptors. The relative importance of these various effects in the overall effects of ethanol on CNS function is not clear.

The depressant effects of ethanol on neuronal function resemble those of adenosine acting on A_1 receptors (see Ch. 16). Ethanol in cell culture systems increases extracellular adenosine by inhibiting adenosine uptake, and there is some evidence that inhibition of the adenosine transporter may account for some of its CNS effects.

Endogenous opioids also play a role in the CNS effects of ethanol, because both human and animal studies show that the opioid receptor antagonist **naltrexone** reduces the reward associated with ethanol.

Behavioural effects

The effects of acute ethanol intoxication in humans are well known and include slurred speech, motor incoordination, increased self-confidence and euphoria. The effect on mood varies among individuals, most becoming louder and more outgoing, but some becoming morose and withdrawn. At higher levels of intoxication, the mood tends to become highly labile, with euphoria and melancholy, aggression and submission, often occurring successively. The association between alcohol consumption and violence is well documented.

Intellectual and motor performance and sensory discrimination are impaired by ethanol, but subjects are generally unable to judge this for themselves.[15] Much effort has gone into measuring the effect of ethanol on driving performance in real life, as opposed to artificial tests under experimental conditions. In a US study of city drivers, it was found that the probability of being involved in an accident was unaffected at blood ethanol concentrations up to 50 mg/100 mL (10.9 mmol/L); by 80 mg/100 mL (17.4 mmol/L) the probability was increased about four-fold, and by 150 mg/100 mL (32.6 mmol/L), about 25-fold. In Scotland, driving with a blood ethanol concentration greater than 50 mg/100 mL is illegal whereas in the rest of the United Kingdom the legal limit is 80 mg/100 mL.

The relationship between plasma ethanol concentration and effect is highly variable. A given concentration produces a larger effect when the concentration is rising than when it is steady or falling. A substantial degree of cellular tolerance develops in habitual drinkers, with the result that a higher plasma ethanol concentration is needed to produce a given effect. In one study, 'gross intoxication' (assessed by a battery of tests that measured speech, gait and so on) occurred in 30% of subjects between 50 and 100 mg/100 mL and in 90% of subjects with more than 150 mg/100 mL. Coma generally occurs at about 400 mg/100 mL, and death from respiratory failure is likely at levels exceeding 500 mg/100 mL.

Ethanol significantly enhances – sometimes to a dangerous extent – the CNS depressant effects of many other drugs, including benzodiazepines, antidepressants, antipsychotic drugs and opioids.

Neurotoxicity

In addition to the acute effects of ethanol on the nervous system, chronic administration also causes irreversible neurological damage (see Harper and Matsumoto, 2005). This may be due to ethanol itself, or to metabolites such as acetaldehyde or fatty acid esters, or to dietary deficiencies (e.g. of thiamine) that are common in alcoholics. Binge drinking is thought to produce greater damage, probably due to the high brain concentrations of ethanol achieved and to repeated phases of withdrawal between binges. Heavy drinkers often exhibit convulsions and may develop irreversible dementia and motor impairment associated with thinning of the cerebral cortex (apparent as ventricular enlargement) detectable by brain-imaging techniques. Degeneration of the cerebellar vermis, the mammillary bodies and other specific brain regions can also occur, as well as peripheral neuropathy.

Effects on other systems

The main acute cardiovascular effect of ethanol is to produce cutaneous vasodilatation, central in origin, which causes a warm feeling but actually increases heat loss.[16] It has been proposed that mild consumption of ethanol reduces the incidence of coronary heart disease, by increasing circulating levels of high-density lipoprotein (HDL), thus reducing the incidence of atherosclerosis (see Ch. 22). The much hyped notion that a glass of red wine each day (red wine contains the antioxidant, resveratrol) reduces coronary artery disease has come in for criticism in recent years. Moderate ethanol consumption may protect against ischaemic heart disease, especially in older people, perhaps partly by inhibiting platelet aggregation. This effect occurs at ethanol concentrations in the range achieved by moderate drinking (10–20 mmol/L) and probably results from inhibition of arachidonic acid formation from phospholipid. However, chronic or intermittent drinking of excessive

[15]Bus drivers were asked to drive through a gap that they selected as the minimum for their bus to pass through; ethanol caused them not only to hit the barriers more often at any given gap setting, but also to set the gap to a narrower dimension, often narrower than the bus.

[16]The image of a large St Bernard dog carrying a small keg of brandy around its neck to revive avalanche victims is an apocryphal one created by the English painter Edwin Landseer, who in 1820 produced a painting called 'Alpine Mastiffs Reanimating a Distressed Traveller'. With their keen sense of smell, such dogs were useful in searching for people buried in the snow, but taking a tot of brandy would only have enhanced the victim's heat loss.

amounts of ethanol causes raised blood pressure, which is one of the most important risk factors for having a heart attack or a stroke.

Diuresis is a familiar effect of ethanol. It is caused by inhibition of antidiuretic hormone secretion, and tolerance develops rapidly, so that the diuresis is not sustained. There is a similar inhibition of oxytocin secretion, which can delay parturition.

Ethanol increases salivary and gastric secretion, perhaps a reason in some cultures for the popularity of a glass of sherry before dinner. However, heavy consumption of spirits causes damage directly to the gastric mucosa, causing chronic gastritis. Both this and the increased acid secretion are factors in the high incidence of gastric bleeding in alcoholics. CNS depression predisposes to aspiration pneumonia and lung abscess formation. Acute pancreatitis may become chronic with pseudocyst formation (collections of fluid in the peritoneal sac), fat malabsorption and ultimately loss of B-cell function, and insulin-dependent diabetes mellitus.

Ethanol produces a variety of endocrine effects. In particular, it increases the output of adrenal steroid hormones by stimulating the anterior pituitary gland to secrete adrenocorticotrophic hormone. However, the increase in plasma hydrocortisone usually seen in alcoholics (producing a 'pseudo-Cushing's syndrome' [see Ch. 33]) is due partly to inhibition by ethanol of hydrocortisone metabolism in the liver.

Acute toxic effects on muscle are exacerbated by seizures and prolonged immobility; severe myositis ('rhabdomyolysis') with myoglobinuria can cause acute renal failure. Chronic toxicity affects particularly cardiac muscle, giving rise to alcoholic cardiomyopathy and chronic heart failure.

Chronic ethanol consumption may also result in immunosuppression, leading to increased incidence of infections such as pneumonia (immunisation with pneumococcal vaccine is important in chronic alcoholics) and increased cancer risk, particularly of the mouth, larynx and oesophagus.

Male alcoholics are often impotent and show signs of feminisation. This is associated with impaired testicular steroid synthesis, but induction of hepatic microsomal enzymes by ethanol, and hence an increased rate of testosterone inactivation, also contributes.

Effects of ethanol on the liver

Together with brain damage, liver damage is the most common serious long-term consequence of excessive ethanol consumption (see Lieber, 1995). Ethanol increases fat accumulation in the liver even after a single dose. Increased fat accumulation (fatty liver) progresses to hepatitis (i.e. inflammation of the liver) and eventually to irreversible hepatic necrosis and fibrosis. Cirrhosis is an end stage, with extensive fibrosis and foci of regenerating hepatocytes that are not correctly 'plumbed in' to the blood and biliary systems. Diversion of portal blood flow around the cirrhotic liver often causes portal hypertension and the development of oesophageal varices, which can bleed suddenly and catastrophically.

With chronic ethanol consumption, many other factors contribute to the liver damage. One is malnutrition, for alcoholic individuals may satisfy much of their calorie requirement from ethanol itself. Three hundred grams of ethanol (equivalent to one bottle of whisky) provides about 2000 kcal but, unlike a normal diet, it provides no vitamins, amino acids or fatty acids. Thiamine deficiency is an important factor in causing chronic neurological damage. Folate deficiency (see Ch. 24) is also common in alcoholics, often associated with macrocytosis of red blood cells.

The overall incidence of chronic liver disease is a function of cumulative ethanol consumption over many years. An increase in the plasma concentration of the liver enzyme γ-glutamyl transpeptidase (a marker of cytochrome P450 induction; see Ch. 10) often raises the suspicion of ethanol-related liver damage, although not specific to ethanol.

The effect of ethanol on fetal development

Drinking alcohol, especially in the first 3 months of pregnancy, increases the risk of miscarriage, premature birth and low birth weight. The adverse effect of heavier ethanol consumption during pregnancy on fetal development was demonstrated in the early 1970s, when the term *fetal alcohol syndrome* (FAS) was coined.

The features of full FAS include:

- abnormal facial development, with wide-set eyes, short palpebral fissures and small cheekbones;
- reduced cranial circumference;
- growth restriction;
- intellectual disability and behavioural abnormalities, often taking the form of hyperactivity and difficulty with social integration;
- other anatomical abnormalities, which may be major or minor (e.g. congenital cardiac abnormalities, malformation of the eyes and ears).

A lesser degree of impairment, termed *alcohol-related neurodevelopmental disorder* (ARND), results in behavioural problems, and cognitive and motor deficits, often associated with reduced brain size. Full FAS occurs in about 3 per 1000 live births and affects about 30% of children born to alcoholic mothers. It is rare with mothers who drink less than about 5 units/day, and most common in binge drinkers who sporadically consume much larger amounts, resulting in high peak levels of ethanol. ARND is about three times as common. Although there is no clearly defined safe threshold, there is no evidence that amounts less than about 2 units/day are harmful. There is no critical period during pregnancy when ethanol consumption is likely to lead to FAS, although one study suggests that FAS incidence correlates most strongly with ethanol consumption very early in pregnancy, even before pregnancy is recognised, implying that not only pregnant women but also women who are likely to become pregnant should be advised not to drink heavily. Experiments on rats and mice suggest that the effect on facial development may be produced very early in pregnancy (up to 4 weeks in humans), while the effect on brain development is produced rather later (up to 10 weeks).

Effects of ethanol

- **Ethanol** acts as a general CNS depressant, similar to volatile anaesthetic agents, producing the familiar effects of acute intoxication.
- Several cellular mechanisms are postulated: enhancement of GABA and glycine action, inhibition of calcium channel opening, activation of potassium channels and inhibition at NMDA receptors.
- Effective plasma concentrations:
  - threshold effects: about 20 mg/100 mL (5 mmol/L)
  - severe intoxication: about 150 mg/100 mL
  - death from respiratory failure: about 500 mg/100 mL
- Main peripheral effects are self-limiting diuresis (reduced antidiuretic hormone secretion), and cutaneous vasodilatation.
- Neurological degeneration occurs with heavy and binge drinking, causing dementia and peripheral neuropathies.
- Long-term ethanol consumption causes liver disease, progressing to cirrhosis and liver failure.
- Excessive consumption in pregnancy causes impaired fetal development, associated with small size, abnormal facial development and other physical abnormalities, and intellectual disability.
- Addiction, physical dependence and tolerance all occur with **ethanol.**

PHARMACOKINETIC ASPECTS

Metabolism of ethanol

Ethanol is rapidly absorbed, an appreciable amount being absorbed from the stomach. A substantial fraction is cleared by first-pass hepatic metabolism. Hepatic metabolism of ethanol shows saturation kinetics (see Chs 10 and 11) at quite low ethanol concentrations, so the fraction of ethanol removed decreases as the concentration reaching the liver increases. Thus if ethanol absorption is rapid and portal vein concentration is high, most of the ethanol escapes into the systemic circulation, whereas with slow absorption more is removed by first-pass metabolism. This is one reason why drinking ethanol on an empty stomach produces a much greater pharmacological effect. Ethanol is quickly distributed throughout the body water, the rate of its redistribution depending mainly on the blood flow to individual tissues, as with volatile anaesthetics (see Ch. 41).

Ethanol is about 90% metabolised, 5%–10% being excreted unchanged in expired air and in urine. This fraction is not pharmacokinetically significant but provides the basis for estimating blood ethanol concentration from measurements on breath or urine. The ratio of ethanol concentrations in blood and alveolar air, measured at the end of deep expiration, is relatively constant, 80 mg/100 mL of ethanol in blood producing 35 μg/100 mL in expired air; this being the basis of the breathalyser test. The concentration in urine is more variable and provides a less accurate measure of blood concentration.

Ethanol metabolism occurs almost entirely in the liver, and mainly by a pathway involving successive oxidations, first to acetaldehyde and then to acetic acid (Fig. 49.5). Since ethanol is often consumed in large quantities (compared with most drugs), 1–2 mol daily being by no means unusual, it constitutes a substantial load on the hepatic oxidative systems. The oxidation of 2 mol of ethanol consumes about 1.5 kg of the co-factor nicotinamide adenine dinucleotide (NAD^+). Availability of NAD^+ limits the rate of ethanol oxidation to about 8 g/h in a normal adult, independently of ethanol concentration (Fig. 49.6), causing the process to show saturating kinetics (see Ch. 10). It also leads to competition between the ethanol and other metabolic substrates for the available NAD^+ supplies, which may be a factor in ethanol-induced liver damage (see Ch. 58).

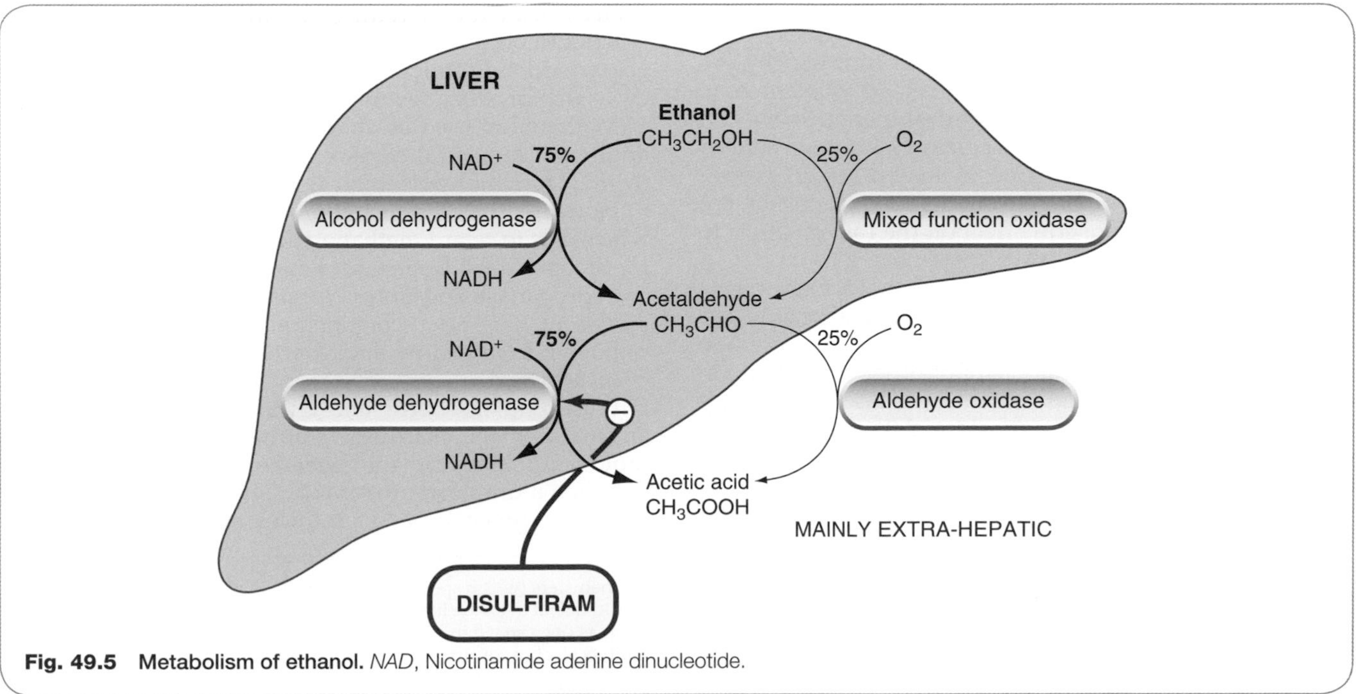

Fig. 49.5 Metabolism of ethanol. *NAD*, Nicotinamide adenine dinucleotide.

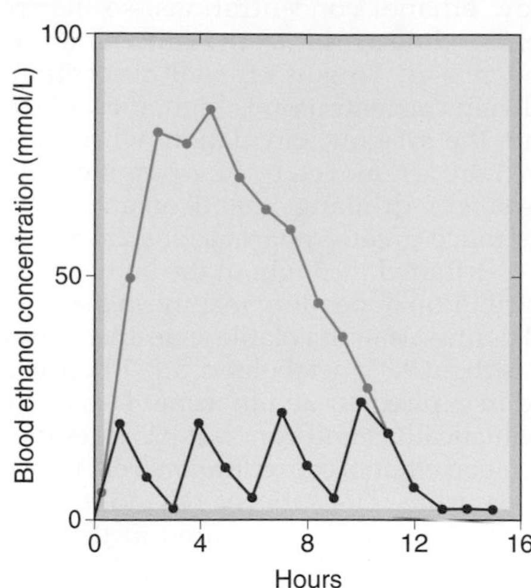

Fig. 49.6 Zero-order kinetics of ethanol elimination in rats. Rats were given ethanol orally (104 mmol/kg) either as a single dose or as four divided doses. The single dose results in a much higher and more sustained blood ethanol concentration than the same quantity given as divided doses. Note that, after the single dose, ethanol concentration declines linearly, the rate of decline being similar after a small or large dose, because of the saturation phenomenon. (From Kalant, H., et al., 1975. Biochem. Pharmacol. 24, 431.)

The intermediate metabolite, acetaldehyde, is a reactive and toxic compound, and this may also contribute to the hepatotoxicity. A small degree of esterification of ethanol with various fatty acids also occurs in the tissues, and these esters may also contribute to long-term toxicity.

Alcohol dehydrogenase is a soluble cytoplasmic enzyme, confined mainly to liver cells, which oxidises ethanol at the same time as reducing NAD^+ to NADH (see Fig. 49.5). Ethanol metabolism causes the ratio of NAD^+ to NADH to fall, and this has other metabolic consequences (e.g. increased lactate and slowing down of the Krebs cycle). The limitation on ethanol metabolism imposed by the limited rate of NAD^+ regeneration has led to attempts to find a 'sobering up' agent that works by regenerating NAD^+ from NADH. One such agent is fructose, which is reduced by an NADH-requiring enzyme. In large doses, it causes a measurable increase in the rate of ethanol metabolism, but not enough to have a useful effect on the rate of return to sobriety.

Normally, only a small amount of ethanol is metabolised by the microsomal mixed function oxidase system (see Ch. 10), but induction of this system occurs in alcoholics. Ethanol can affect the metabolism of other drugs that are metabolised by the mixed function oxidase system (e.g. **phenobarbital**, **warfarin** and **steroids**), with an initial inhibitory effect produced by competition, followed by enhancement due to enzyme induction.

Nearly all the acetaldehyde produced is converted to acetate in the liver by *aldehyde dehydrogenase* (see Fig. 49.5). Normally, only a little acetaldehyde escapes from the liver, giving a blood acetaldehyde concentration of 20–50 μmol/L after an intoxicating dose of ethanol in humans. The circulating acetaldehyde usually has little or no effect, but the concentration may become much larger under certain circumstances and produce toxic effects. This occurs if aldehyde dehydrogenase is inhibited by drugs such as **disulfiram**. In the presence of disulfiram, which produces no marked effect when given alone, ethanol consumption is followed by a severe reaction comprising flushing, tachycardia, hyperventilation and considerable panic and distress, which is due to excessive acetaldehyde accumulation in the bloodstream. This reaction is extremely unpleasant but not usually harmful, at least in otherwise relatively healthy drinkers, and disulfiram can be used as aversion therapy to discourage people from taking ethanol. Some other drugs (e.g. **metronidazole**; see Ch. 52) produce similar reactions to ethanol. Interestingly, a Chinese herbal medicine used traditionally to cure alcoholics contains **daidzin**, a specific inhibitor of aldehyde dehydrogenase.[17]

Genetic factors

In 50% of Asian people, an inactive genetic variant of one of the aldehyde dehydrogenase isoforms (ALDH-2) is expressed; these individuals experience a disulfiram-like reaction after alcohol, and the incidence of alcoholism in this group is extremely low (see Tyndale, 2003).

Metabolism and toxicity of methanol and ethylene glycol

Methanol is metabolised in the same way as ethanol but produces formaldehyde instead of acetaldehyde from the first oxidation step. Formaldehyde is more reactive than acetaldehyde and reacts rapidly with proteins, causing the inactivation of enzymes involved in the tricarboxylic acid cycle. It is converted to another toxic metabolite, formic acid. This, unlike acetic acid, cannot be utilised in the tricarboxylic acid cycle and is liable to cause tissue damage. Conversion of alcohols to aldehydes occurs not only in the liver but also in the retina, catalysed by the dehydrogenase responsible for retinol–retinal conversion. Formation of formaldehyde in the retina accounts for one of the main toxic effects of methanol, namely blindness, which can occur after ingestion of as little as 10 g. Formic acid production and derangement of the tricarboxylic acid cycle also produce severe acidosis.

Methanol is used as an industrial solvent and also to adulterate industrial ethanol in order to make it unfit to drink. Methanol poisoning is quite common, and used to be treated by administration of large doses of ethanol, which acts to retard methanol metabolism by competition for alcohol dehydrogenase. **Fomepizole** inhibits alcohol dehydrogenase and is now preferred, if available. Such treatment may be in conjunction with haemodialysis to remove unchanged methanol, which has a small volume of distribution.

Poisoning with ethylene glycol, used in automobile antifreeze and brake fluid, is a medical emergency. It is rapidly absorbed from the gut and metabolised to glycolate and then more slowly to oxalate. Glycolate interferes with metabolic processes and produces metabolic acidosis. It

[17]In hamsters (which spontaneously consume alcohol in amounts that would defeat even the hardest two-legged drinker, while remaining, as far as one can tell in a hamster, completely sober), daidzin markedly inhibits alcohol consumption.

affects the brain, heart and kidneys. Treatment is with fomepizole or, with caution, ethanol,[18] and haemodialysis.

TOLERANCE AND PHYSICAL DEPENDENCE

Tolerance to the effects of ethanol can be demonstrated in both humans and experimental animals, to the extent of a two- to three-fold reduction in potency occurring over 1–3 weeks of continuing ethanol administration. A small component of this is due to the more rapid elimination of ethanol. The major component is cellular tolerance, which accounts for a roughly two-fold decrease in potency and which can be observed in vitro (e.g. by measuring the inhibitory effect of ethanol on transmitter release from synaptosomes) as well as in vivo. The mechanism of this tolerance is not known for certain. Ethanol tolerance is associated with tolerance to many anaesthetic agents, and alcoholics are often difficult to anaesthetise.

Chronic ethanol administration produces various changes in CNS neurons, which tend to oppose the acute cellular effects that it produces. There is a small reduction in the density of $GABA_A$ receptors, and a proliferation of voltage-gated calcium channels and NMDA receptors.

A well-defined physical abstinence syndrome develops in response to ethanol withdrawal. As with most other dependence-producing drugs, this is probably important as a short-term factor in sustaining the drug habit, but other (mainly psychological) factors are more important in the longer term (see Ch. 50). The physical abstinence syndrome usually subsides in a few days, but the craving for ethanol and the tendency to relapse last for very much longer. Treatment of alcohol dependence is described in Chapter 50.

The physical abstinence syndrome in humans, in severe form, develops after about 8 h. In the first stage, the main symptoms are tremor, nausea, sweating, fever and sometimes hallucinations. These last for about 24 h. This phase may be followed by seizures ('rum fits'). Over the next few days, the condition of 'delirium tremens' develops, in which the patient becomes confused, agitated and often aggressive, and may suffer much more severe hallucinations. Treatment of this medical emergency is by sedation with large doses of a benzodiazepine such as **chlordiazepoxide** (see Ch. 45) together with large doses of thiamine.

SYNTHETIC CANNABINOID RECEPTOR AGONISTS

The endogenous cannabinoid system and cannabinoids contained in the *Cannabis sativa* plant (phytocannabinoids) are described in detail in Chapter 18. Here we will focus on SCRAs, which are sometimes referred to colloquially as *Spice*, *K2* or *Black Mamba*. The chemical structures of SCRAs are diverse, with over 10 chemical families having been described (see Davidson et al., 2017; Advisory Council on the Misuse of Drugs, 2020). Some originated from legitimate attempts by pharmaceutical companies to develop new therapeutic compounds but more recently others have been developed purely for non-medicinal purposes. SCRA solutions are often sprayed on herbal material or paper and subsequently smoked, but SCRAs are also available in crystal and powder form. Smoking, vaping, insufflation and ingestion are the main ways in which SCRAs are used. They are full agonists at the CB_1 cannabinoid receptor, the target through which **Δ^9-tetrahydrocannabinol** (THC), the major psychoactive ingredient in cannabis, has its effects. THC is a partial agonist at CB_1 receptors. SCRAs are said to exert a 'more forceful' activation of the CB_1 receptor, in that users often become 'zombie-like' or cataleptic. This may explain their popularity amongst the homeless and prisoners in jail, allowing them a period of escape from their daily lives.

Unlike cannabis itself, SCRAs are quite harmful and can induce hallucinations, psychotic episodes, panic attacks, seizures, respiratory depression and death. The precise reasons for these toxic effects are not known. They may have 'off-target' effects unrelated to their actions on CB_1 receptors. Furthermore, when smoked, the parent compounds are subject to pyrolysis giving rise to unexpected derivatives, which may be responsible for some of the damaging effects. Quality control is not a priority for the producers of these agents and so there may be toxic contaminants in occasional batches of chemicals. Cessation of use can result in withdrawal symptoms in heavy users.

Metabolism of ethanol

- **Ethanol** is metabolised mainly by the liver, first by alcohol dehydrogenase to acetaldehyde, then by aldehyde dehydrogenase to acetate. About 25% of the acetaldehyde is metabolised extrahepatically.
- Small amounts of **ethanol** are excreted in urine and expired air.
- Hepatic metabolism shows saturation kinetics, mainly because of limited availability of nicotinamide adenine dinucleotide (NAD^+). The maximal rate of **ethanol** metabolism is about 10 mL/h. Thus plasma concentration falls linearly rather than exponentially.
- Acetaldehyde may produce toxic effects. Inhibition of aldehyde dehydrogenase by **disulfiram** accentuates nausea, etc., caused by acetaldehyde, and can be used in aversion therapy.
- **Methanol** is similarly metabolised to formic acid, which is toxic, especially to the retina.
- Asian people show a high rate of genetic polymorphism of alcohol and aldehyde dehydrogenase, associated with alcoholism and alcohol intolerance, respectively.

[18]When presented with a late evening emergency poisoning of a dog with ethylene glycol, a veterinarian colleague of one of the authors ran to the local supermarket and purchased a bottle of vodka – the dog survived!

REFERENCES AND FURTHER READING

General reference

Miller, R.J., 2015. Drugged: The Science and Culture behind Psychotropic Drugs. Oxford University Press, Oxford.

Stimulants

Docherty, J.R., Green, A.R., 2010. The role of monoamines in the changes in body temperature induced by 3,4-methylenedioxymethamphetamine (MDMA, ecstasy) and its derivatives. Br. J. Pharmacol. 160, 1029–1044.

Fredholm, B.B., Battig, K., Holmes, J., et al., 1999. Actions of caffeine in the brain with special reference to factors that contribute to its widespread use. Pharmacol. Rev. 51, 83–133.

Green, A.R., King, M.V., Shortall, S.E., Fone, K.C., 2012. Lost in translation: preclinical studies on 3,4-methylenedioxymethamphetamine provide information on mechanisms of action, but do not allow accurate prediction of adverse events in humans. Br. J. Pharmacol. 166, 1523–1536.

Heal, D.J., Cheetham, S.C., Smith, S.L., 2009. The neuropharmacology of ADHD drugs in vivo: insights on efficacy and safety. Neuropharmacology 57, 608–618.

Mitchell, J.M., Bogenschutz, M., Lilienstein, A., et al., 2021. MDMA-assisted therapy for severe PTSD: a randomized, double-blind, placebo-controlled phase 3 study. Nat. Med. 27, 1025–1033.

Nicotine

De Biasi, M., Dani, J.A., 2011. Reward, addiction, withdrawal to nicotine. Annu. Rev. Neurosci. 34, 105–130.

Hung, R.J., McKay, J.D., Gaborieau, V., et al., 2008. A susceptibility locus for lung cancer maps to nicotinic acetylcholine receptor subunit genes on 15q25. Nature 452, 633–637.

Le Foll, B., Goldberg, S.R., 2005. Control of the reinforcing effects of nicotine by associated environmental stimuli in animals and humans. Trends Pharmacol. Sci. 26, 287–293.

Leslie, F.M., Mojica, C.Y., Reynaga, D.D., 2013. Nicotinic receptors in addiction pathways. Mol. Pharmacol. 83, 753–758.

Wonnacott, S., Sidhpura, N., Balfour, D.J.K., 2005. Nicotine: from molecular mechanisms to behaviour. Curr. Opin. Pharmacol. 5, 53–59.

Cognition enhancers

Battleday, R.M., Brem, A.K., 2015. Modafinil for cognitive neuroenhancement in healthy non-sleep-deprived subjects: a systematic review. Eur. Neuropsychopharmacol. 25, 1865–1881.

Collingridge, G.L., Volianskis, A., Bannister, N., et al., 2013. The NMDA receptor as a target for cognitive enhancement. Neuropharmacology 64, 13–26.

D'Angelo, L.S.C., Savulich, D., Sahakian, B.J., 2017. Lifestyle use of drugs by healthy people for enhancing cognition, creativity, motivation and pleasure. Br. J. Pharmacol. 174, 3257–3267.

Harms, J.E., Benveniste, M., Maclean, J.K., Partin, K.M., Jamieson, C., 2013. Functional analysis of a novel positive allosteric modulator of AMPA receptors derived from a structure-based drug design strategy. Neuropharmacology 64, 45–52.

Napoletano, F., Schifano, F., Corkery, J.M., et al., 2020. The psychonauts' world of cognitive enhancers. Front. Psychiatr. 11, 546796.

Psychedelics

Nichols, D.E., 2004. Hallucinogens. Pharmacol. Ther. 101, 131–181.

Rickli, A., Moning, O.D., Hoener, M.C., Liechti, M.E., 2016. Receptor interaction profiles of novel psychoactive tryptamines compared with classic hallucinogens. Eur. Neuropsychopharmacol. 26 (8), 1327–1337.

Ethanol

Garbutt, J.C., 2009. The state of pharmacotherapy for the treatment of alcohol dependence. J. Subst. Abuse Treat. 36, S15–S21.

Harper, C., Matsumoto, I., 2005. Ethanol and brain damage. Curr. Opin. Pharmacol. 5, 73–78.

Harris, R.A., Trudell, J.R., Mihic, S.J., 2008. Ethanol's molecular targets. Sci. Signal. 1, re7.

Lieber, C.S., 1995. Medical disorders of alcoholism. N. Engl. J. Med. 333, 1058–1065.

Spanagel, R., 2009. Alcoholism: a systems approach from molecular physiology to addictive behaviour. Physiol. Rev. 89, 649–705.

Tyndale, R.F., 2003. Genetics of alcohol and tobacco use in humans. Ann. Med. 35, 94–121.

Dissociative drugs

Morgan, C.J., Curran, H.V., 2012. Ketamine use: a review. Addiction 107, 27–38.

Morris, B.J., Cochran, S.M., Pratt, J.A., 2005. PCP: from pharmacology to modelling schizophrenia. Curr. Opin. Pharmacol. 5, 101–106.

Synthetic cannabinoid receptor agonists

Advisory Council on the Misuse of Drugs, 2020. Synthetic cannabinoid receptor agonists (SCRA). Available at: https://assets.publishing.service.gov.uk/government/uploads/system/uploads/attachment_data/file/929909/FOR_PUBLICATION_-_ACMD_SCRA_report_final.pdf.

Davidson, C., Opacka-Juffry, J., Arevalo-Martin, A., Garcia-Ovejero, D., Molina-Holgado, E., Molina-Holgado, F., 2017. Spicing up pharmacology: a review of synthetic cannabinoids from structure to adverse events. Adv. Pharmacol. 80, 135–168.

50 Drug use and addiction

OVERVIEW

In other chapters, we have considered how drugs that are taken because some people find their effects pleasurable (hedonic) exert their profound effects in the brain. In this chapter, we now focus on factors that relate specifically to their use – routes of administration, harms involved in drug taking, compulsive drug use (addiction). Finally, pharmacological treatments for compulsive drug use are described. The reasons why the use of a particular drug may be viewed as a problem by some societies, but not others, are complex and largely outside the scope of this book. The use of drugs to enhance sexual arousal is discussed separately in Chapter 59.

DRUG USE

A number of terms are used, sometimes interchangeably and sometimes incorrectly, to describe drug use and the consequences of taking drugs which have not been prescribed for that person or for that purpose. Terms that are best avoided are listed in Table 50.1. Other, more useful, terms are defined in the text.

A vast and ever-increasing array of drugs is used to alter mood and perception.[1] These include drugs that are also used as medicines – anxiolytics (see Ch. 45), opioids (see Ch. 43), general anaesthetics (see Ch. 41), cannabinoids (see Ch. 18) and some stimulants (see Ch. 49) – as well as non-medicinal psychoactive drugs (see Ch. 49) and volatile organic solvents (present in glues and aerosols). The popularity of each varies between different societies across the world, and within societies popularity differs among different groups of individuals.[2] Frequently, users will take more than one drug concomitantly (e.g. heroin users will inject cocaine and heroin together, an activity known as *speedballing*) or sequentially. Sequential use is often intended to reduce adverse effects that occur when coming down off the first drug (e.g. use of benzodiazepines when coming down from stimulants). Polydrug use is an under-researched area in regard to why it is done, how different drugs may interact and the potential harm that may arise from such practices. For example, ethanol alters cocaine metabolism, resulting in the production of *cocaethylene*, which is more potent than cocaine and has potentially greater cardiovascular toxicity.

The drugs taken are an extremely heterogeneous pharmacological group; we can find little in common in the behavioural effects produced by say, **heroin**, **cocaine** and **LSD** (lysergic acid diethylamide). What links them is that some people find their effects pleasurable (hedonic) and tend to want to repeat the experience. The drug experience may take the form of intense euphoria, mood elevation, hallucinations, stimulation, calming or sedation, depending upon the specific drug taken. Many drug users have existing mental health problems and for them drug taking is a means of self-medicating to alleviate symptoms they are experiencing.

The popularity and availability of drugs change with time. For example, over the last 20 years the opioid epidemic in the United States has been fuelled first by the ease of obtaining prescription opioids such as **oxycodone**, and more recently by the widespread availability of illicitly produced **fentanyl** and related drugs (**fentanyls**), such that in 2019 in the United States, of over 70,000 drug overdose deaths, some 52% involved **fentanyls**, 20% involved prescription opioids (e.g. **oxycodone**) and only 20% involved **heroin** (official name **diamorphine**). The situation is different in other countries such as the United Kingdom, where heroin remains the predominant opioid that is available.

Drug use involves effects on the brain that can be both acute and chronic (Fig. 50.1). The immediate, acute effect on mood is the reason the drug is taken. For some drugs (e.g. **amphetamines** and **3,4-methylenedioxymethamphetamine (MDMA)**, see Ch. 49), this may be followed by a rebound negative or depressed phase. Persistent use of a drug may lead to compulsive drug use and to the development of tolerance.

DRUG ADMINISTRATION

For drugs that induce strong feelings of euphoria, there are two components to the experience: an initial rapid effect (the *rush* or *buzz*) and a more prolonged pleasurable effect (the *high*) that may for some drugs (e.g. gabapentinoids or opioids) be accompanied by a period of sedation (*gouching*). The intensity of the initial effect is determined by how fast the drug enters the brain and activates its effector mechanism. For many casual drug users, ease of administration defines how the drug is taken (e.g. smoking, swallowing or snorting a drug is relatively easy). However, for other drug users chasing a more intense experience, the route of administration and the choice of individual drug become important. Intravenous injection or smoking results in faster absorption of a drug than when it is taken orally. Heroin, cocaine, amphetamines, tobacco and cannabis are all taken by one or other of these routes. Heroin is more popular as a street drug than morphine despite its lack of activity at μ-opioid receptor (see Ch. 43). This is because heroin is rapidly deacetylated to an active

[1]The Drugs Wheel (http://www.thedrugswheel.com/) provides an up-to-date, easily understood classification of the ever-expanding array of drugs. Most are illegal, although there are strong lobbies to legalise those that are considered less harmful, a process that is well underway for cannabis in several countries.

[2]A survey in one UK city showed that among Friday-night clubbers, the choice of drug was associated with the type of music the clubs played (Measham and Moore, 2009).

Table 50.1 Glossary of frequently used and 'abused' terms

Addict	Person for whom the desire to experience a drug's effects overrides any consideration for the serious physical, social or psychological problems that the drug may cause to the individual or others. Often used in non-scientific circles to convey criminal intent and so has fallen out of favour with those involved in treating people with drug use disorders
Junkie	Pejorative term for someone who has a drug use disorder usually involving opioids
Drug abuse and drug misuse	Non-medicinal drug use (it is debatable whether taking drugs to alter mood/induce hallucinations should be described as 'misuse' or 'abuse')
Recreational drug use	Originally used to describe all drug use, it is now sometimes used to describe drug use in the bar/club/dance scene.
Narcotics	Originally used as a term to describe opioids as they induce sleep (narcosis). Subsequently this term has been used by non-scientists to describe a wide range of drugs (including cocaine, which is a stimulant!).

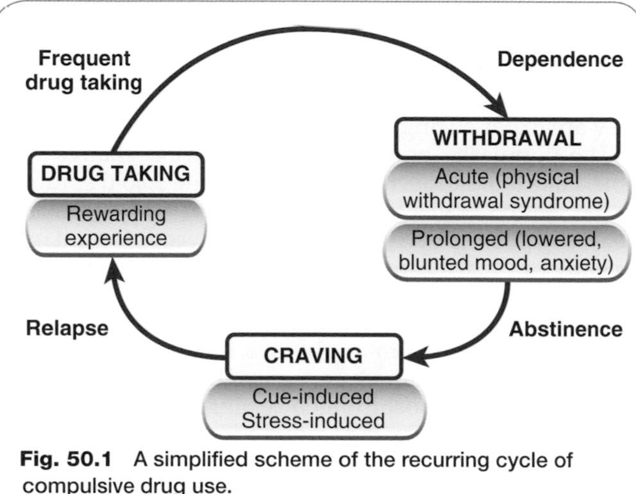

Fig. 50.1 A simplified scheme of the recurring cycle of compulsive drug use.

metabolite, 6-acetylmorphine, which rapidly enters the brain and stimulates the receptors (Gottås et al., 2013). The subsequent conversion of 6-acetylmorphine to morphine occurs relatively slowly.

DRUG HARM

All drugs are harmful but to varying degrees. Adverse effects can be the result of drug overdose (e.g. respiratory depression produced by opioids), of effects on tissues other than the brain (e.g. necrosis of the nasal septum resulting from chronic cocaine use), of the route of administration (e.g. HIV, hepatitis C and other infections in drug users who share needles), of effects unrelated to the specific actions of the drug (e.g. carcinogenicity of tobacco smoke, severe bladder pain in regular **ketamine** users) or of use for nefarious purposes (e.g. **flunitrazepam** or **γ-hydroxybutyrate** (**GHB**) as date-rape drugs). Many major harms relate to the addictive nature of some drugs (e.g. psychostimulants, opioids, ethanol and tobacco) or to their ability to reveal a susceptibility to psychotic illness in some individuals (e.g. amphetamines and cannabis).

There have been attempts by expert panels in the UK, European Union and Australia to produce a rational scale of drug harm, based on assessment of harms to users and harms to others, that results from their physical, psychological and social effects (see Bonomo et al., 2019). Ethanol was ranked the most harmful substance overall in each study. While there were differences between the panels on the relative harms of other drugs, there was general agreement that tobacco (nicotine), methamphetamine, heroin, fentanyls, crack cocaine and cocaine are the most harmful after ethanol, with **LSD** and **MDMA** much less so.[3]

DRUG ADDICTION

Drug addiction, also referred to as *substance use disorder*,[4] describes the human condition in which:

- drug taking becomes compulsive, taking precedence over other needs;
- there is a loss of control of the amount of drug taken;
- physical and psychological changes occur when access to drug is denied.

Addiction thus involves both psychological and physiological components and can be considered as a three-stage process around which drug using individuals recycle (see Fig. 50.1). As addiction progresses, taking the drug may only reverse the lowered mood that develops between doses rather than produce the high that was initially experienced at earlier stages of using the drug. The neurobiology of drug addiction is described in detail by Koob and Volkow (2016).

Drug addiction becomes a problem when the need becomes so insistent that it dominates the lifestyle of the individual and damages their quality of life, and the drug use itself causes actual harm to the individual or the community. Examples of the latter are the mental incapacity and liver damage caused by ethanol, the many diseases associated with smoking tobacco, the high risk of infection when injecting intravenously (especially HIV and hepatitis C), the serious risk of overdose with most opioids and the criminal behaviour resorted to when drug users need to finance their drug taking.

Not all psychoactive drugs induce severe addiction. Highly addictive drugs are nicotine, ethanol, opioids, crack

[3]This order of harm is not reflected in the classification of drugs under UK law where LSD and MDMA are Class A whereas ethanol and tobacco are legal.

[4]Pharmacologists are more likely to favour the term *drug use disorder* over *substance use disorder* as to them alcohol and solvents are drugs (see Ch. 1 for a pharmacological definition of what is a drug) but other interested parties have decided upon the term *substance use disorder*.

and powdered cocaine, methamphetamine, amphetamine and benzodiazepines. On the other hand, cannabis, MDMA and psychedelic drugs are less addictive.

Not everyone who takes a drug progresses to become addicted to it. Family studies show clearly that susceptibility to addiction is an inherited characteristic. Around 50% of the risk of becoming addicted is genetic. Variants of many different genes may each make a small contribution to the overall susceptibility of an individual to addiction – a familiar scenario that provides few pointers for therapeutic intervention. Polymorphisms in ethanol-metabolising genes (see Ch. 49) are the best example of genes that directly affect the tendency to use a drug.

Other factors that contribute to drug addiction are developmental (adolescents are more at risk than adults) and environmental, e.g. stress, social pressures and drug availability. Many individuals who become addicted will also suffer from mental illness – *severe anxiety, depression, attention-deficit hyperactivity disorder (ADHD), bipolar disorder personality disorders or schizophrenia* – or have been physically or mentally abused. These underlying issues may contribute to their wish to take drugs as well as to their inability to stop taking drugs.

DRUG-INDUCED REWARD

The common feature of the various types of psychoactive drugs that are addictive is that all produce a *rewarding* experience (e.g. an elevation of mood or a feeling of euphoria or calmness).

In animal studies, where the state of mood cannot be inferred directly, reward is manifest as *positive reinforcement*, i.e. an increase in the probability of occurrence of any behaviour that is associated with the drug experience. In *conditioned place preference* studies, animals receive a drug or placebo and are then placed in different environments. Subsequently, when tested in a drug-free state, they will spend more time in the environment associated with a previous rewarding drug experience. Another way of determining if a drug is rewarding is to test whether or not animals will self-administer the drug by pressing a lever to obtain it. Stimulants and opioids are self-administered by experimental animals whereas psychedelic drugs are less likely to be self-administered, which may indicate that, unlike humans, they find the experience non-rewarding.

Humans have a choice as to whether or not they wish to experiment with and continue taking drugs – there may therefore be an element of risk-taking when experimenting with drugs. In behavioural tests, some rats have been observed to be much more impulsive than others (Jupp et al., 2013). The impulsive rats showed a higher rate of cocaine, nicotine, alcohol and methylphenidate self-administration and had a lower level of expression of D_2 and D_3 dopamine receptors in the nucleus accumbens (see later for the importance of this brain region in drug use). Impulsive rats were not, however, more prone to self-administering opioids.

REWARD PATHWAYS

Virtually all of the major addictive drugs so far tested, including opioids, nicotine, amphetamines, ethanol and cocaine, activate the *reward pathway* – the mesolimbic dopaminergic pathway (see Ch. 39), that runs, via the medial forebrain bundle, from the ventral tegmental area (VTA) of the midbrain to the nucleus accumbens and limbic region. Even though for some of these drugs their primary sites of action may be elsewhere in the brain, they all increase the extracellular level of dopamine in the nucleus accumbens, as shown by microdialysis in animals and in vivo brain-imaging techniques in humans. Opioids enhance the firing of VTA dopaminergic neurons by reducing the level of GABAergic inhibition (disinhibition) within the VTA, whereas amphetamine and cocaine act on dopaminergic nerve terminals in the nucleus accumbens to release dopamine or prevent its reuptake (see Ch. 15). Given that dopamine release in the nucleus accumbens is also enhanced by naturally rewarding stimuli, such as food, water, sex and nurturing, it would appear that drugs are simply activating, or overactivating, the body's own pleasure system. In experienced drug users the anticipation of the effect may become sufficient to elicit the release of dopamine. Paradoxically, brain-imaging studies have revealed that in chronic users the increase in dopamine may be less than expected when compared with what is seen in naïve individuals, even though the subjective high is still intense. This may reflect some degree of sensitisation, but the mechanism is not well understood.

Chemical or surgical interruption of the VTA–accumbens dopaminergic pathway impairs drug-seeking behaviours in many experimental situations. Deletion of D_2 receptors in a transgenic mouse strain was shown to eliminate the rewarding properties of morphine administration without reducing other opioid effects, and it did not prevent the occurrence of physical withdrawal symptoms in morphine-dependent animals (Maldonado et al., 1997), suggesting that the dopaminergic pathway is responsible for the positive reward but not for the negative withdrawal effects. However, D_2-receptor antagonists (antipsychotic drugs; see Ch. 47) have not been successful in treating addiction, and more recent evidence suggests that D_1 receptors activated by steep increases in dopamine release and possibly also D_3 receptors play important roles. The translation of preclinical studies into the development of D_3-receptor antagonists or partial agonists as treatments for drug addiction has been extremely slow (see Galaj et al., 2020).

PHYSICAL DEPENDENCE

This is characterised by a *withdrawal* or *abstinence syndrome* whereby on cessation of drug administration or on administering an antagonist, adverse physiological effects are experienced. On prolonged cessation of drug administration the withdrawal effects can persist for a period of days or weeks, the precise withdrawal responses being characteristic of the type of drug taken. The intensity of the withdrawal syndrome also varies between drugs of the same type according to their pharmacokinetic characteristics. The desire to avoid or suppress the withdrawal syndrome increases the drive to retake the drug. In individuals undergoing drug detoxification treatment (detox) pharmacological intervention can be used to reduce the intensity of drug withdrawal (Table 50.2).

The mechanisms responsible for the withdrawal syndrome have been most fully characterised for opioid dependence but similar mechanisms may apply to cocaine and ethanol withdrawal. At the cellular level, opioids inhibit cAMP formation, and withdrawal results in a rebound increase as a result of 'superactivation' of adenylyl cyclase, as well as up-regulation of the amount of this enzyme. This results in activation of

Table 50.2 Pharmacological approaches to treating drug addiction

Mechanism	Example(s)
Agonist therapies	• Methadone (orally active opioid agonist with long biological half-life) and buprenorphine (oromucosal absorbed opioid partial agonist now also available as a subcutaneous prolonged release preparation) or legal heroin (administered IM or IV) to maintain opioid-dependent patients • Nicotine patches or chewing gum to alleviate nicotine withdrawal symptoms and reduce craving
Blocking pleasurable response	• Naltrexone (non-selective opioid antagonist) to block opioid effects in drug-withdrawn patients • Naltrexone and nalmefene (non-selective opioid agonist/weak partial agonist) to reduce ethanol use (presumably by blocking the effects of endogenous opioids released by ethanol in the brain) • Mecamylamine (nicotinic antagonist) to block nicotine effects • Immunisation against nicotine, cocaine and opioids to produce circulating antibodies (still being developed)
Aversive therapies	• Disulfiram (aldehyde dehydrogenase inhibitor) to induce unpleasant response to ethanol
To alleviate withdrawal symptoms	• Methadone or buprenorphine used short term to blunt opioid withdrawal • Ibogaine (a naturally occurring psychoactive agent) used by some to reduce opioid withdrawal symptoms • Lofexidine (α_2-adrenoceptor agonist to diminish opioid, alcohol and nicotine withdrawal symptoms • Propranolol (β-adrenoceptor antagonist) to diminish excessive peripheral sympathetic activity • Varenicline ($\alpha 4\beta 2$ nicotinic receptor partial agonist) to alleviate nicotine withdrawal symptoms. Treatment can be continued in abstinent individuals to reduce risk of relapse • Benzodiazepines (e.g. chlordiazepoxide), clomethiazole, topiramate and GHB to blunt alcohol withdrawal symptoms
Reducing continued drug use (may act by reducing craving)	• Bupropion (antidepressant with some nicotinic receptor antagonist activity) and nortriptyline (noradrenaline reuptake inhibiting antidepressant) to reduce tobacco use • Clonidine (α_2-adrenoceptor agonist) to reduce craving for nicotine[a] • Acamprosate (NMDA receptor antagonist) to treat alcoholism[a] • Topiramate and lamotrigine (antiepileptic agents) to treat alcoholism and cocaine use[a] • GHB reported to reduce craving for alcohol and cocaine[a] • Baclofen ($GABA_B$ receptor agonist) reported to reduce opioid, alcohol and stimulant use[a] • Modafinil (dopamine reuptake inhibitor) to reduce cocaine use[a] • Ibogaine (natural product hallucinogen) reported to reduce craving for stimulants and opioids[a] • MDMA, psilocybin and LSD may have beneficial effects in the treatment of alcoholism[a]

[a]The effectiveness of these agents at reducing the continued use of other drugs over and above the ones listed remains to be determined. Antidepressant, mood stabilising, anxiolytic and antipsychotic medications are useful when treating patients who, in addition to their drug use, also suffer from other mental disorders. The cannabinoid CB_1-receptor antagonist rimonabant, in addition to its antiobesity effects, also reduces nicotine, ethanol, stimulant and opioid consumption. However, it also induces depression and its use has been discontinued.
GHB, γ-Hydroxybutyric acid; *LSD*, lysergic acid diethylamide; *MDMA*, 3,4-methylenedioxymethamphetamine; *NMDA*, *N*-methyl-D-aspartate.

protein kinase A (PKA), in an increase in adenosine as a consequence of the conversion of cAMP to adenosine and in activation of a transcription factor – cAMP response element binding protein (CREB). The rise in PKA activity increases the excitability of nerve terminals by phosphorylating neurotransmitter transporters to increase their ionic conductance (see Bagley et al., 2005), as well as increasing neurotransmitter release by a direct action on the secretory process (Williams et al., 2001). Withdrawal results in enhanced GABA release in various parts of the brain, probably through the mechanisms described earlier (see Bagley et al., 2011). The release of other neurotransmitters is also likely to be enhanced. On the other hand, the enhanced extracellular levels of adenosine, acting on presynaptic A_1 receptors (see Ch. 16), inhibit glutamate release at excitatory synapses, and thus counteract the neuronal hyperexcitability that occurs during drug withdrawal, suggesting the possibility – not yet clinically proven – that adenosine agonists might prove useful in reducing the withdrawal syndrome. CREB, which is up-regulated in the nucleus accumbens by prolonged administration of opioids or cocaine, plays a key role in regulating various components of cAMP signalling pathways, and transgenic animals lacking CREB show reduced withdrawal symptoms (see Chao and Nestler, 2004).

Several types of therapeutic drug, including antidepressant and antipsychotic agents, also produce withdrawal symptoms on cessation of administration, but it is important to distinguish this type of commonly observed 'rebound' phenomenon from the physical dependence associated with drug use. A degree of physical dependence is common when patients receive opioid analgesics in hospital for several days, but this rarely leads to addiction.

PSYCHOLOGICAL CHANGES

During periods of drug abstinence, individuals experience irritability, stress, anxiety, low mood and blunted responses to experiences that would normally be pleasurable. These aversive behavioural changes can be long lasting and contribute to the drive to retake the drug to escape from what is a negative emotional state (*negative affect*). Furthermore, the memory of previous drug-induced experiences can be very intense and long lasting, giving rise to *craving*; it may drive an individual to take the drug again – referred to as *relapse* – even after a prolonged period of abstinence (see Weiss, 2005). The relative effort required to transition through detoxification into abstinence and recovery is illustrated in Fig. 50.2.

Craving may be triggered by stress or by cues, such as experiencing the environment that a person associates with previously taking the drug or the sight of drug administration paraphernalia, e.g. a crack pipe or syringe. This suggests that associative learning may be important (Robbins et al., 2008). It has been suggested that drugs alter memory formation to enhance the recollection of previous drug experience. In this regard, it is of interest that several drugs such as cocaine, morphine, nicotine and ethanol can produce changes in synaptic plasticity, a cellular correlate of memory formation (see Ch. 38), in both the VTA and the nucleus accumbens (Hyman et al., 2006; Nestler and Lüscher, 2019).

Drug addiction

- Addiction occurs when, as a result of repeated administration of the drug, the desire to experience the effects of a drug again becomes compulsive.
- Addiction occurs with a wide range of psychotropic drugs, acting by many different mechanisms.
- The common feature of the major addictive drugs is that they have a positive reinforcing action ('reward') associated with activation of the mesolimbic dopaminergic pathway.
- Physical dependence is characterised by a withdrawal syndrome on cessation of drug use, and varies in type and intensity for different classes of drug.
- Drug withdrawal also results in prolonged mood changes – irritability, stress, anxiety, depression and blunted responses to normally rewarding experiences – and craving.
- Craving can be triggered by stress or cues relating to previous drug experience and may occur in individuals who have been drug-free for some considerable time.
- On repeated drug administration, tolerance may occur to the effects of the drug.
- Although genetic factors contribute to drug-seeking behaviour, no specific genes have yet been identified.

The psychological factors in drug addiction are discussed in detail by Koob and Volkow (2016) and summarised in Fig. 50.3.

TOLERANCE

Tolerance (see Ch. 2) describes the decrease in pharmacological effect on repeated administration of a drug – it develops over time, as does physical dependence. It does not occur with all drugs. Contrary to earlier thinking, physical dependence and tolerance are now thought to involve different cellular mechanisms (see Bailey and Connor, 2005).

For drugs such as opioids that are agonists at specific receptors (see Ch. 43), cellular tolerance results in part from desensitisation of the receptors. On prolonged activation by an agonist, the μ receptor is phosphorylated by various intracellular kinases (Williams et al., 2013) – which either directly desensitises the receptor or causes the binding to the

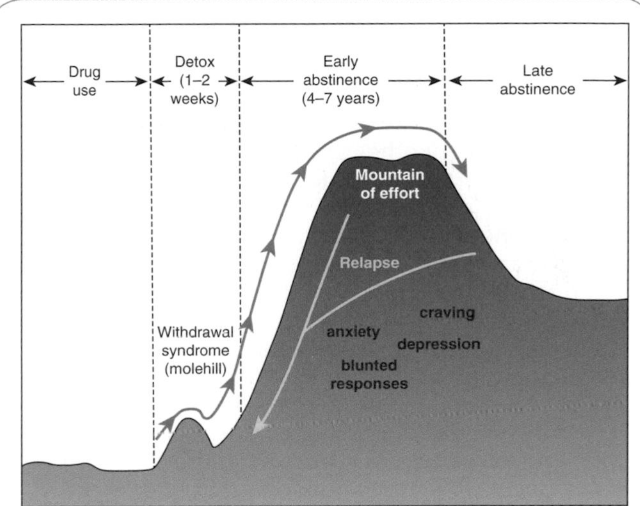

Fig. 50.2 The molehill of detox versus the mountain of abstinence. The graph illustrates the effort required to go through detoxification and maintain abstinence. Adapted from Diaper, A.M., Law, F.M., Melichar, J.K., 2014. Pharmacological strategies for detoxification. Brit. J. Clin. Pharmacol. 77, 302-314.

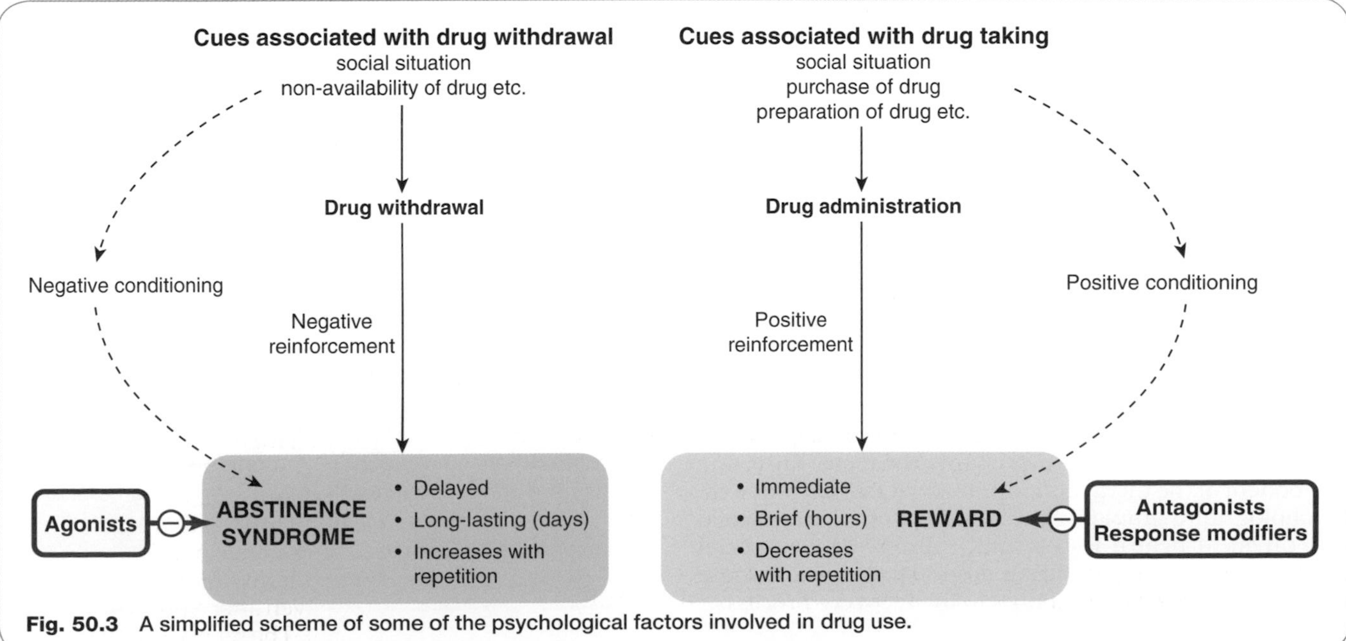

Fig. 50.3 A simplified scheme of some of the psychological factors involved in drug use.

receptor of other proteins, such as arrestins, that uncouple the receptor from its G protein (see Ch. 3). In the intact animal, inhibition or knock-out of these kinases reduces the level of tolerance.

PHARMACOLOGICAL APPROACHES TO TREATING DRUG ADDICTION

There are a number of different approaches taken to treat drug addiction. Specific examples of the drugs used in each are given in Table 50.2.

- Agonist therapy, in which a medicinal grade drug is provided long term to *'maintain'* the individual, preventing them from going into withdrawal and reducing the craving to take drugs. For heroin users this form of treatment has been shown to also reduce criminal activities to fund illicit drug purchase, to reduce associated health hazards such as HIV and hepatitis C infection and to decrease overdose deaths.
- Facilitating drug withdrawal (detox) by either substituting a drug in the same class from which subsequent withdrawal is less intense or by administration of other drugs during the withdrawal process that reduce the intensity of the withdrawal symptoms.
- Blocking the effects of a drug by prior administration of an antagonist so that if the individual has detoxed but relapses and retakes the drug again they will not experience the pleasurable effects of the drug. For this to be successful, the antagonist has to be long lasting or administered in the form of a prolonged release preparation that releases the antagonist over a prolonged period.
- Blocking the effects of a drug by immunisation to produce circulating antibodies that sequester the drug and prevent it crossing the blood–brain barrier. Vaccines against nicotine, heroin, fentanyls or cocaine have shown efficacy in animal tests but to date have proved less effective in human trials. Lack of efficacy in humans may be due to low antibody titres or to subjects just taking greater amounts of drug to overcome the sequestering effects of the antibodies generated (Truong and Kosten, 2022)
- Making the drug experience unpleasant. The best example of this approach is for ethanol which is rapidly metabolised to acetic acid by a two-step process (see Ch. 49, Fig. 49.5). Disulfiram, an aldehyde dehydrogenase inhibitor, inhibits the second step, resulting in the build-up of acetaldehyde which elicits an unpleasant response when ethanol is consumed.
- Reducing craving for a drug. A range of drugs have been suggested to reduce craving for various drugs. Their effectiveness is an ongoing area of debate and research.

Drug addiction involves many psychosocial and some genetic factors, as well as neuropharmacological mechanisms, and so while pharmacological approaches to drug treatment are important, they are only one component of the therapeutic approaches that are required. Psychological therapies, treatment for underlying mental and physical health issues and improvement in social circumstances (e.g. providing accommodation for those who are homeless) are essential to the recovery process.

HARM REDUCTION

For intravenous drug users, the provision of sterile injection equipment (needles, syringes, spoons and water) reduces equipment sharing and the spread of blood-borne diseases such as HIV and hepatitis C. Opioid overdose results in severe respiratory depression that can lead to death. Opioid-induced respiratory depression is rapidly reversed by administration of the opioid antagonist, **naloxone**. Supervised injection rooms and the distribution of naloxone (either as an intramuscular injection kit or in the form of a nasal spray) within the drug-using community are ways to reduce opioid overdose deaths.

Clinical use of drugs in substance use disorders

Tobacco

- Short-term **nicotine** is an adjunct to behavioural therapy in smokers committed to giving up; **varenicline** is also used as an adjunct but has been linked to suicidal ideation.
- **Bupropion** is also effective but lowers seizure threshold, so is contraindicated in people with risk factors for seizures (and also if there is a history of eating disorder).

Alcohol

- Long-acting benzodiazepines (e.g. **chlordiazepoxide**) can be used to reduce withdrawal symptoms and the risk of seizures; they should be tapered over 1–2 weeks and then discontinued.
- **Disulfiram** is used as an adjunct to behavioural therapy in suitably motivated patients with alcohol use disorder after detoxification; it is contraindicated for patients in whom hypotension would be dangerous (e.g. those with coronary or cerebral vascular disease).
- **Acamprosate** can help to maintain abstinence; it is started as soon as abstinence has been achieved and maintained if relapse occurs, and it is continued for 1 year.

Opioids

- **Naloxone**, a competitive opioid antagonist, has become available for use in community settings to reverse respiratory depression from opioid overdose. It can be administered as a nasal spray or by intramuscular injection.
- Opioid agonists or partial agonists (e.g. respectively, **methadone** or **buprenorphine**) administered orally or sublingually may be substituted for injectable narcotics, many of whose harmful effects are attributable to the route of administration.
- **Naltrexone**, a long-acting opioid antagonist, is used as an adjunct to help prevent relapse in opioid users who have been detoxified (opioid free for at least 1 week).
- **Lofexidine**, an α_2 agonist (cf. **clonidine**; see Ch. 15), is used short term (usually up to 10 days) to ameliorate symptoms of opioid withdrawal, and is then tapered over a further 2–4 days.

REFERENCES AND FURTHER READING

General

Chao, J., Nestler, E.J., 2004. Molecular neurobiology of addiction. Annu. Rev. Med. 55, 113–132.

Gottås, A., Øiestad, E.L., Boix, F., et al., 2013. Levels of heroin and its metabolites in blood and brain extracellular fluid after i.v. heroin administration to freely moving rats. Br. J. Pharmacol. 170, 546–556.

Koob, G.F., Volkow, N.D., 2016. Neurobiology of addiction: a neurocircuitry analysis. Lancet Psychiatr. 3, 760–773.

Measham, F., Moore, K., 2009. Repertoires of distinction. exploring patterns of weekend polydrug use within local leisure scenes across the English night time economy. Criminol. Crim. Justice 9, 437–464.

Drug harm

Bonomo, Y., Norman, A., Biondo, S., et al., 2019. The Australian drug harms ranking study. J. Psychopharmacol. 33, 759–768.

Nutt, D., King, L.A., Phillips, L.D., 2010. Drug harms in the UK: a multicriteria decision analysis. Lancet 376, 558–565.

van Amsterdam, J., Nutt, D., Phillips, L., van den Brink, W., 2015. European rating of drug harms. J. Psychopharmacol. 29, 655–660.

Reward

Galaj, E., Newman, A.H., Xi, Z.X., 2020. Dopamine D3 receptor-based medication development for the treatment of opioid use disorder: rationale, progress, and challenges. Neurosci. Biobehav. Rev. 114, 38–52.

Hyman, S.E., Malenka, R.C., Nestler, E.J., 2006. Neural mechanisms of addiction: the role of reward-related learning and memory. Annu. Rev. Neurosci. 29, 565–598.

Jupp, B., Caprioli, D., Dalley, J.W., 2013. Highly impulsive rats: modelling an endophenotype to determine the neurobiological, genetic and environmental mechanisms of addiction. Dis. Model. Mech. 6, 302–311.

Maldonado, R., Saiardi, A., Valverde, O., et al., 1997. Absence of opiate rewarding effects in mice lacking dopamine D_2 receptors. Nature 388, 586–589.

Nestler, E.J., Lüscher, C., 2019. The molecular basis of drug addiction: linking epigenetic to synaptic and circuit mechanisms. Neuron 102, 48–59.

Physical dependence and tolerance

Bagley, E.E., Gerke, M.B., Vaughan, C.W., et al., 2005. GABA transporter currents activated by protein kinase A excite midbrain neurons during opioid withdrawal. Neuron 45, 433–445.

Bagley, E.E., Hacker, J., Chefer, V.I., et al., 2011. Drug-induced GABA transporter currents enhance GABA release to induce opioid withdrawal behaviors. Nat. Neurosci. 14, 1548–1554.

Bailey, C.P., Connor, M., 2005. Opioids: cellular mechanisms of tolerance and physical dependence. Curr. Opin. Pharmacol. 5, 60–68.

Robbins, T.W., Ersche, K.D., Everitt, B.J., 2008. Drug addiction and the memory systems of the brain. Ann. N. Y. Acad. Sci. 1141, 1–21.

Weiss, F., 2005. Neurobiology of craving, conditioned reward and relapse. Curr. Opin. Pharmacol. 5, 9–19.

Williams, J.T., Christie, M.J., Manzoni, O., 2001. Cellular and synaptic adaptations mediating opioid dependence. Physiol. Rev. 81, 299–343.

Williams, J.T., Ingram, S.L., Henderson, G., et al., 2013. Regulation of μ-opioid receptors: desensitization, phosphorylation, internalization, and tolerance. Pharmacol. Rev. 65, 223–254.

Treatment

Truong, T.T., Kosten, T.R., 2022. Current status of vaccines for substance use disorders: a brief review of human studies. J. Neurol. Sci. 434, 120098.

51 Basic principles of antimicrobial chemotherapy

OVERVIEW

The term *chemotherapy* was originally used to describe the use of drugs that were 'selectively toxic' to microbial pathogens (e.g. bacteria, viruses, protozoa, fungi and helminths) while having minimal effects on the host. It also refers to the use of drugs to treat tumours and, in the public mind at least, is usually associated with those cytotoxic anticancer drugs that cause distressing and unwanted effects such as loss of hair, nausea and vomiting. In this chapter, we focus on antimicrobial chemotherapy; anticancer drugs are covered in Chapter 57. The feasibility of the selective toxicity strategy depends on the ability to exploit such biochemical differences as may exist between the infecting organism and the host. While the bulk of this section of the book describes the drugs used to combat such infections, in this introductory chapter we consider the nature of these biochemical differences, outline the molecular targets of drug action and discuss the grave problem of antibiotic resistance and its possible solutions.

BACKGROUND

All living organisms are vulnerable to infection. Humans, being no exception, are susceptible to diseases caused by microorganisms including viruses, bacteria, protozoa and fungi (collectively referred to as *microbial pathogens*) as well as by some larger parasites such as helminths. The concept of 'chemotherapeutic agents' dates back to the work of Ehrlich and others and to the development of selectively toxic arsenical drugs such as **salvarsan** for the treatment of syphilis.[1] Indeed, it was Ehrlich himself who coined the term *chemotherapy* to describe the use of synthetic chemicals to destroy such pathogens, and over time, the definition of the term has been broadened to include *antibiotics* – strictly speaking, substances produced by microorganisms (although latterly by pharmaceutical chemists as well) – that kill or inhibit the growth of other microorganisms. The successful development of these drugs during the 'golden age' of antibiotic research (1940s–1970s) constitutes one of the most important therapeutic advances in the history of medicine.

Unhappily, our success in developing drugs to neutralise these invaders has been paralleled by their own success in counteracting their effects, resulting in the emergence of *drug resistance*. And at present, the invaders – particularly some bacteria – seem close to gaining the upper hand. This is a very important clinical problem, and so we will devote some space to the mechanisms of resistance and the means by which it is spread.

THE MOLECULAR BASIS OF CHEMOTHERAPY

Chemotherapeutic agents, then, are chemicals intended to be toxic to a pathogenic organism but innocuous to the host. It is important to remember that many microorganisms share our body spaces (e.g. the gut[2]) without causing disease (these are called *commensals*), although they may become pathogenic under adverse circumstances (i.e. if the host is immunocompromised or if barrier breakdown results in them setting up shop in an inappropriate location elsewhere in our bodies).

Cells without nuclei (e.g. bacteria) are termed *prokaryotes*, while cells that contain nuclei (e.g. protozoa, fungi, helminths and most of the cells in our own bodies) are *eukaryotes*. In a separate category are the viruses, which need to utilise the metabolic machinery of the host cell to replicate, and thus present a particular kind of problem for chemotherapeutic attack. Lurking in the taxonomic shadows, there remain those mysterious infectious proteins, the *prions* (see Ch. 40), which cause disease but resist all attempts at classification and treatment.

Virtually all creatures, host and parasite alike, utilise the same genetic code and while there are differences in genetic make-up, many biochemical processes are common to most, if not all, organisms. It follows that finding drugs that affect only pathogens but not other host cells necessitates finding either qualitative or quantitative biochemical or genetic differences between them which can be exploited therapeutically.

BACTERIA

Bacteria are a common cause both of mild and severe infectious disease. Fig. 51.1 shows, in simplified diagrammatic form, the main components of a notional bacterial cell and their functions. Surrounding the bacterium is the *cell wall*, which characteristically contains *peptidoglycan* (*Mycoplasma pneumoniae*, a very small bacterium that causes an atypical lung infection – 'pneumonia' – resistant to several antibiotics, is an exception). Peptidoglycan is unique to prokaryotic cells and has no counterpart in eukaryotes. Within the cell wall is the *plasma membrane*, which, like that of eukaryotic cells, consists of a phospholipid bilayer and associated proteins. It functions as a selectively permeable membrane with specific transport mechanisms for various

[1]Toxic mercury-containing compounds were also once commonly used for treating syphilis. 'One night with Venus, a lifetime with Mercury' was a common saying prior to the advent of the antibiotic era.

[2]Humans harbour about 2 kg of bacteria in the gut, comprising a large 'forgotten organ' in the body which has important metabolic functions. Together with the commensals living on our skin and other organs, these are collectively known as the *microbiome*.

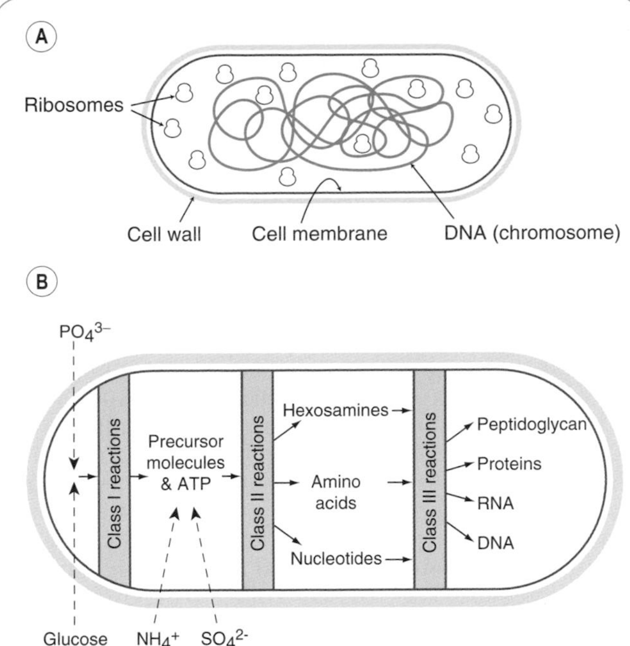

Fig. 51.1 Diagram of the structure and metabolism of a 'typical' bacterial cell. (A) Schematic representation of a bacterial cell. (B) Flow diagram showing the synthesis of the main types of macromolecule of a bacterial cell. *Class I reactions* result in the synthesis of the precursor molecules necessary for *class II reactions*, which result in the synthesis of the constituent molecules; these are then assembled into macromolecules by *class III reactions*. (Modified from Mandelstam, J., McQuillen, K., Dawes, I. (Eds), 1982. Biochemistry of Bacterial Growth. Blackwell Scientific, Oxford.)

ions and nutrients. However, the plasma membrane in bacteria, unlike that of mammals, does not contain *sterols* (e.g. cholesterol), and this may alter the penetration of some drugs.

The cell wall supports the underlying plasma membrane, which is subject to an internal osmotic pressure of about 5 atmospheres in *gram-negative* organisms, and about 20 atmospheres in *gram-positive* organisms (see Ch. 52 for an explanation of Gram staining). The plasma membrane and cell wall together comprise the *bacterial envelope*.

As in eukaryotic cells, the plasma membrane surrounds the *cytoplasm* and cellular organelles. Bacterial cells have no nucleus or mitochondria. Instead, the genetic material takes the form of a single *chromosome* which lies within the cytoplasm with no surrounding nuclear membrane and cellular energy is generated by enzyme systems located in the plasma membrane rather than dedicated organelles such as mitochondria.

Biochemical reactions that are potential targets for antibacterial drugs are shown in Fig. 51.1. These can be broadly classified into three overlapping groups: a drug may affect more than one class of reactions or more than one subgroup of reactions within a class.

- *Class I*: catabolic reactions involved in the utilisation of glucose, or some alternative carbon source, for the generation of energy (ATP) and synthesis of simple carbon compounds used as precursors in the next class of reactions.
- *Class II*: synthetic pathways which utilise these precursors in an energy-dependent synthesis of all the amino acids, nucleotides, phospholipids, amino sugars, carbohydrates and growth factors required by the cell for survival and growth.
- *Class III*: anabolic reactions which assemble these small molecules into macromolecules - proteins, RNA, DNA, polysaccharides and peptidoglycan.

Other potential drug targets include *formed structures*, for example, the cell membrane, the *microtubules* in fungi or the neuromuscular junction in helminths. Also, in an era in which biopharmaceuticals are impacting upon the treatment of disease (see Ch. 5), we must mention the pathogen genome as a potential target.

In our discussion, emphasis will be placed on bacteria because we have a reasonable understanding of bacterial chemotherapy, but reference will also be made to protozoa, helminths, fungi and viruses.

The molecular basis of antibacterial chemotherapy

- Chemotherapeutic drugs should be toxic to invading organisms and innocuous to the host. Such selective toxicity depends on the identification of biochemical differences between the pathogen and the host that can be appropriately exploited.
- Three general classes of biochemical reaction are potential targets for chemotherapy of bacteria:
  - *class I*: biochemical reactions that utilise glucose and other carbon sources to produce ATP and simple carbon compounds
  - *class II*: metabolic pathways utilising energy and class I compounds to make small molecules (e.g. amino acids and nucleotides)
  - *class III*: anabolic pathways that convert small molecules into macromolecules such as proteins, nucleic acids and peptidoglycan

BIOCHEMICAL REACTIONS AS POTENTIAL TARGETS

CLASS I REACTIONS

Class I reactions are generally not promising targets for two reasons. First, bacterial and human cells use similar mechanisms to obtain energy from glucose (the *Embden–Meyerhof pathway* and the *tricarboxylic acid cycle*). Second, even if glucose oxidation is blocked, many other compounds (amino acids, lactate, etc.) can be utilised by bacteria as an alternative energy source.

CLASS II REACTIONS

Class II reactions are better targets because some pathways exist in pathogens, but not in human cells. There are several examples, with one of the most significant being the folate biosynthesis pathway.

Folate biosynthesis and utilisation

Folate is required for DNA synthesis in both bacteria and in humans (see Chs 24 and 52) but in humans, which have no biosynthetic pathway, it must be obtained from the diet and concentrated in cells by specific uptake mechanisms. Fortunately for pharmacologists, most species of bacteria, as well as the asexual forms of malarial protozoa, lack these transport mechanisms and therefore must synthesise folate de novo. **Sulfonamides** contain a moiety that is a structural analogue of *p*-aminobenzoic acid (PABA). PABA is essential in bacterial synthesis of folate (see Ch. 52) and sulfonamides compete with it, inhibiting bacterial growth without impairing mammalian cell function.

The intracellular utilisation of folate, in the form of *tetrahydrofolate*, as a co-factor in thymidylate synthesis is a good example of a pathway where human and bacterial enzymes exhibit a differential sensitivity to chemicals (Table 51.1; see Volpato and Pelletier, 2009). Although the pathway is virtually identical in microorganisms and humans, one of the key enzymes, *dihydrofolate reductase*, which reduces dihydrofolate to tetrahydrofolate (see Ch. 52), is many times more sensitive to the drug **trimethoprim** in bacteria than in humans. In some malarial protozoa, this enzyme is somewhat less sensitive than the bacterial enzyme to **trimethoprim** but more sensitive to **pyrimethamine** and **proguanil**, which are used as antimalarial agents (see Ch. 55). The relative IC_{50} values (the concentration causing 50% inhibition) for bacterial, malarial, protozoal and mammalian enzymes are given in Table 51.1. The human enzyme, by comparison, is very sensitive to the effect of the folate analogue **methotrexate**, which is used to treat severe psoriasis (see Ch. 26), cancer (see Ch. 57) and inflammatory arthritis (see Ch. 25), although in the latter case, inhibition of folate metabolism is not its main mode of action.

Treatment with a combination of two drugs that affect the same pathway at different points, for example sulfonamides and the folate antagonists, may be more successful than the use of either alone. Thus pyrimethamine and a sulfonamide (**sulfadoxine**) are used to treat *falciparum* malaria (see Ch. 55). **Co-trimoxazole** is an antibacterial formulation that contains both a sulfonamide and **trimethoprim.** Once widely used, this combination has become less popular for treating bacterial infections because **trimethoprim** alone is similarly effective and does not cause sulfonamide-specific adverse effects; its use is now mainly restricted to treatment of *Pneumocystis jirovecii*, an opportunistic infection of immunosuppressed patients such as those with acquired immunodeficiency disease (AIDS) and for which high doses are required (see Chs 52 and 53).

Table 51.1 Specificity of inhibitors of dihydrofolate reductase

	IC_{50} (µmol/L) for dihydrofolate reductase		
Inhibitor	**Human**	**Protozoal**	**Bacterial**
Trimethoprim	260	0.07	0.005
Pyrimethamine	0.7	0.0005	2.5
Methotrexate	0.001	~0.1[a]	Inactive

[a]Tested on *Plasmodium berghei*, a rodent malaria.
IC_{50}, Concentration causing 50% inhibition.

CLASS III REACTIONS

As pathogens cannot take up their own unique macromolecules, class III reactions are particularly good targets for selective toxicity, and there are sometimes distinct differences between mammalian and parasitic cells in this respect. Once again, there are several examples.

The synthesis of peptidoglycan

The cell wall of bacteria contains *peptidoglycan*, a substance that does not occur in eukaryotes and which contains D-amino acids and unusual sugars. It is the equivalent of a non-stretchable string bag enclosing the whole bacterium. In gram-negative bacteria, this bag consists of a single thickness, but in gram-positive bacteria there may be as many as 40 layers of peptidoglycan. Each layer consists of multiple backbones of amino sugars – alternating *N*-acetylglucosamine and *N*-acetylmuramic acid residues (Fig. 51.2) – the latter having short peptide side-chains that are cross-linked to form a polymeric lattice. These may constitute up to 10%–15% of the dry weight of the cell and the lattice is strong enough to resist the high internal osmotic pressure. The cross-links differ in different species. In *staphylococci*, for example, they consist of five glycine residues.

To build up this very large insoluble peptidoglycan layer on the outside of the cell membrane, the bacterial cell has the problem of how to transport the hydrophilic cytoplasmic 'building blocks' through the hydrophobic cell membrane structure. This is accomplished by linking them to a very large lipid carrier, containing 55 carbon atoms, which 'tows' them across the membrane. The process of peptidoglycan synthesis is outlined in Fig. 51.3. First, *N*-acetylmuramic acid, attached to uridine diphosphate (UDP) and a pentapeptide,

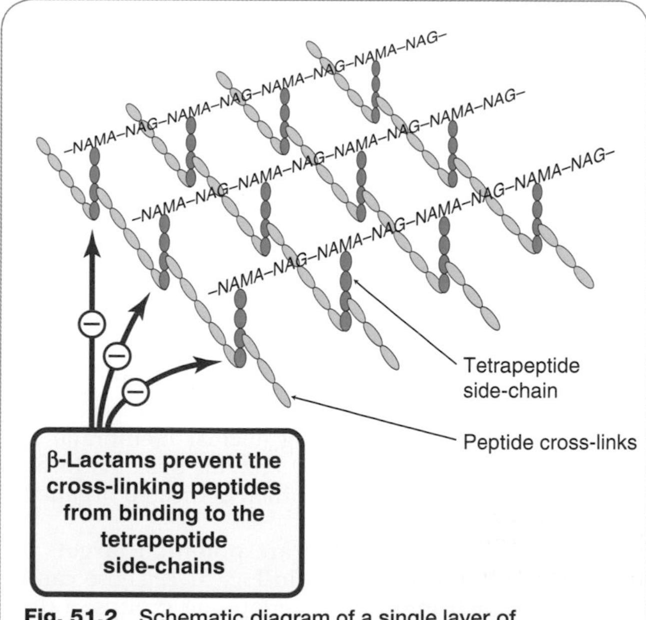

Fig. 51.2 Schematic diagram of a single layer of peptidoglycan from a bacterial cell (e.g. *Staphylococcus aureus*), showing the site of action of the β-lactam antibiotics. In *S. aureus* the peptide cross-links consist of five glycine residues. Gram-positive bacteria have several layers of peptidoglycan. More detail in Fig. 51.3. *NAG*, *N*-Acetylglucosamine; *NAMA*, *N*-acetylmuramic acid.

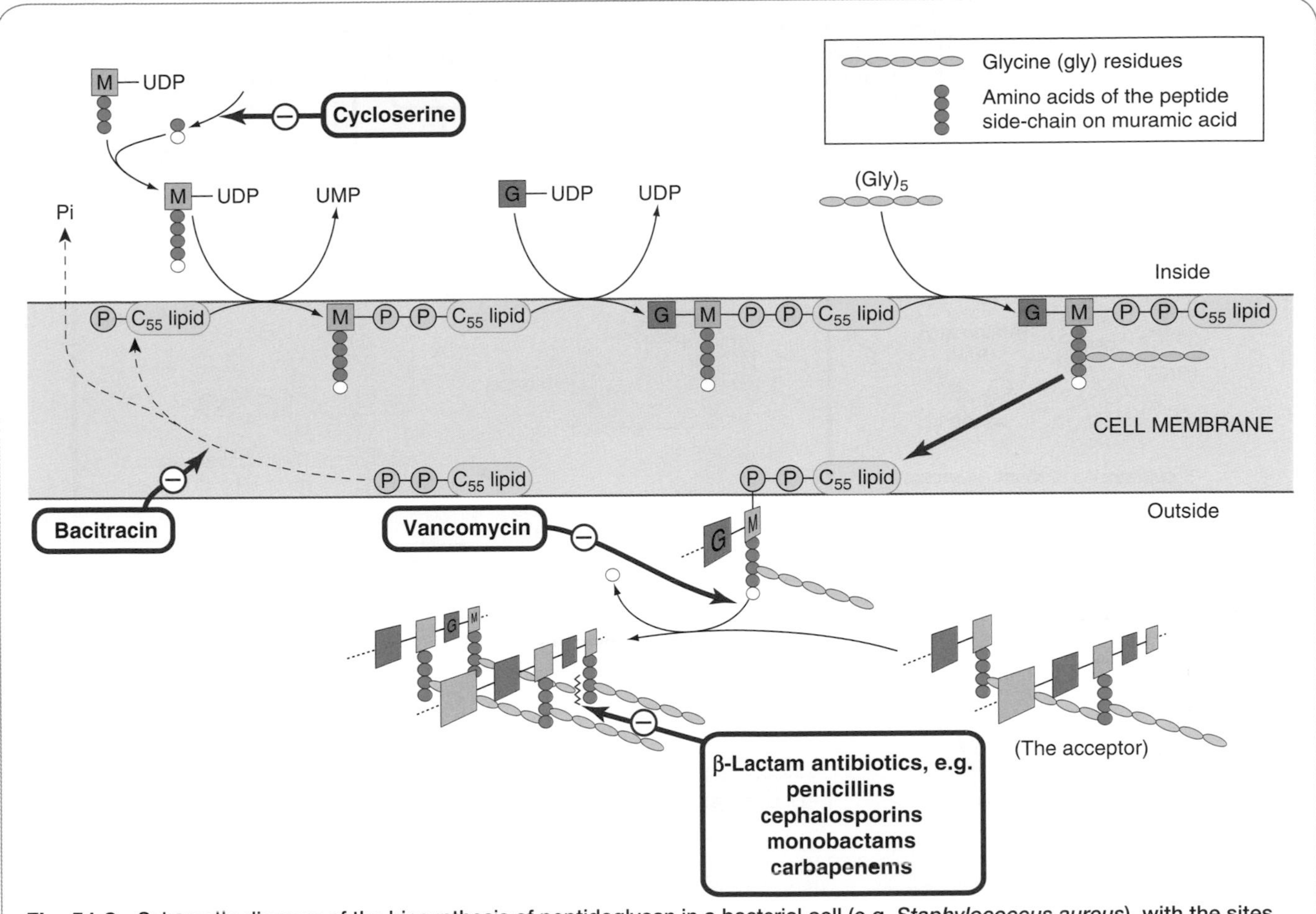

Fig. 51.3 Schematic diagram of the biosynthesis of peptidoglycan in a bacterial cell (e.g. *Staphylococcus aureus*), with the sites of action of various antibiotics. The hydrophilic disaccharide–pentapeptide is transferred across the lipid cell membrane attached to a large lipid (C_{55} lipid) by a pyrophosphate bridge (–P–P–). On the outside, it is enzymically attached to the 'acceptor' (the growing peptidoglycan layer). The final reaction is a transpeptidation, in which the loose end of the (Gly) 5 chain is attached to a peptide side-chain of an M in the acceptor and during which the terminal amino acid (alanine) is lost. The lipid is regenerated by loss of a phosphate group (Pi) before functioning again as a carrier. *G*, *N*-Acetylglucosamine; *M*, *N*-acetylmuramic acid; *UDP*, uridine diphosphate; *UMP*, uridine monophosphate.

is transferred to the C55 lipid carrier in the membrane, with the release of uridine monophosphate. This is followed by a reaction with UDP-*N*-acetylglucosamine, resulting in the formation of a disaccharide–pentapeptide complex attached to the carrier. This complex is the basic building block of the peptidoglycan. In *Staphylococcus aureus*, the five glycine residues are attached to the peptide chain at this stage. The building block is now transported out of the cell and added to the growing end of the peptidoglycan, the 'acceptor', with the release of the C55 lipid, which still has two phosphates attached. The lipid carrier then loses one phosphate group and thus becomes available for another cycle. Cross-linking between the peptide side-chains of the sugar residues in the peptidoglycan layer then occurs, the hydrolytic removal of the terminal alanine supplying the requisite energy.

This synthesis of peptidoglycan is a vulnerable step and can be blocked at several points by antibiotics (see Fig. 51.3 and Ch. 52). Cycloserine, which is a structural analogue of D-alanine, prevents the addition of the two terminal alanine residues to the initial tripeptide side-chain on *N*-acetylmuramic acid by competitive inhibition. **Vancomycin** inhibits the release of the building block unit from the carrier, thus preventing its addition to the growing end of the peptidoglycan. **Bacitracin** interferes with the regeneration of the lipid carrier by blocking its dephosphorylation. Penicillins, cephalosporins and other β-lactams inhibit the final transpeptidation by forming covalent bonds with *penicillin-binding proteins* that have transpeptidase and carboxypeptidase activities, thus preventing formation of the cross-links.

Protein synthesis

Another very important class III target is protein synthesis. This takes place at the ribosomes, but eukaryotic and prokaryotic ribosomes are different, and this provides the basis for the selective action of some antibiotics. The bacterial ribosome consists of a 50S subunit and a 30S subunit (Fig. 51.4), whereas in the mammalian ribosome the subunits are 60S and 40S. The other elements involved in peptide synthesis are messenger RNA (mRNA), which forms the template for protein synthesis, and transfer RNA (tRNA), which specifically transfers the individual amino acids to the ribosome. The ribosome has three binding sites for tRNA, termed the *A, P* and *E sites*. Notably, the final peptidyl transferase reaction by which the growing peptide chain is extended is catalysed not by a protein, but a *ribozyme*. This means that, unlike the vast majority of other

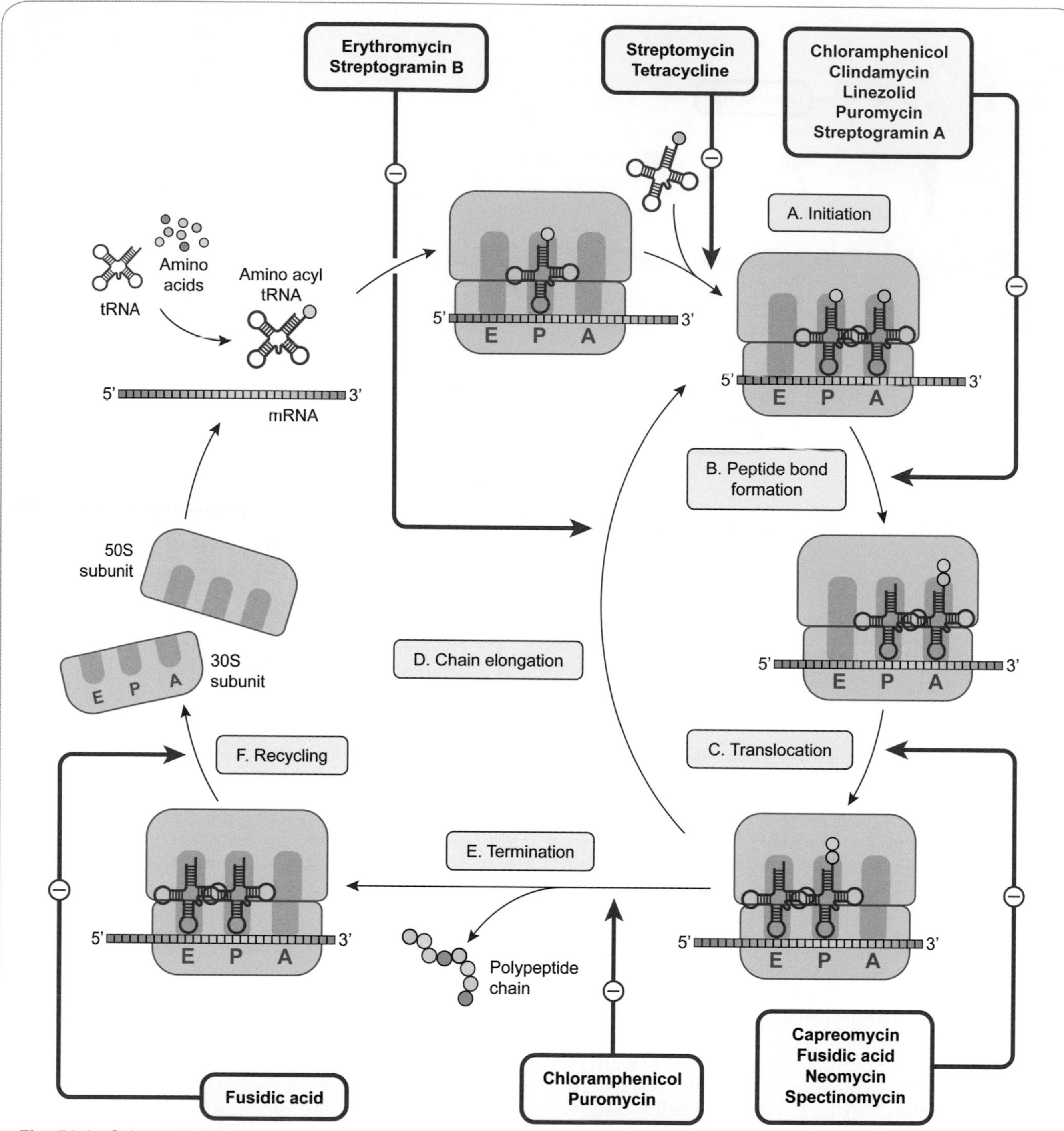

Fig. 51.4 Schematic diagram of bacterial protein synthesis, indicating the points at which some common antibiotics inhibit the process. mRNA is attached to the assembled ribosomes; amino acids, bound to their corresponding aminoacyl tRNA carriers, are attached to the *P* site of the 30S subunit and at (A) the dipeptide is linked together by the aminoacyl tRNA synthase ribozyme at the *A* site on the ribosome (B). The mRNA molecule then translocates, moving the dipeptide to the *P* site. The 'empty' tRNA is then released. This process of chain elongation (D) continues until a stop codon is reached. At this point (E) the nascent polypeptide is released, the ribosomal apparatus dissociates, and the components are recycled (F) to begin again. Note that some antibiotics can act at several points in the process. For the sake of simplicity, cofactors in this process have been omitted. (Adapted and modified from Wilson, D.N., 2014. Ribosome-targeting antibiotics and mechanisms of bacterial resistance. Nat. Rev. Microbiol. 12, 35–48.)

drugs, the antibiotics in question act upon a polynucleotide, rather than a protein target.

In a technical tour de force in 2000, the complete fine structure of the bacterial 30S subunit was elucidated (Carter et al., 2000, and others), earning a Nobel Prize for Venki Ramakrishnan, Thomas Steitz and Ada Yonath in 2009. This, together with other work (reviewed in Wilson, 2014), provided fresh information about the detailed site of action of antibiotics and providing new leads for antibiotic research and discovery.

A highly simplified version of the ribosomal protein synthesis system in bacteria and the sites of action of some antibiotics are shown in Fig. 51.4. To initiate translation, mRNA, transcribed from the DNA template, is attached to the 30S subunit of the ribosome. The 50S subunit then binds to the 30S subunit to form a 70S subunit,[3] which moves along the mRNA such that successive codons of the messenger pass along the ribosome from the A position to the P position.

Nucleic acid synthesis

Gene expression and cell division also require nucleic acid synthesis, and this class III reaction is an important site of action of many chemotherapeutic drugs as well as some biopharmaceuticals. It is possible to interfere with nucleic acid synthesis in several different ways:

- by inhibiting the synthesis of nucleotides;
- by altering the base-pairing properties of the DNA template;
- by inhibiting either DNA or RNA polymerase;
- by inhibiting DNA gyrase, which uncoils supercoiled DNA to allow transcription;
- by interfering with the transcription of microbial genes;
- by a direct effect on DNA itself. Some anticancer (but no antimicrobial) drugs work in this way.

[3]You query whether 30S + 50S = 70S? Yes, it does, because we are talking about *Svedberg units*, which measure sedimentation *rate*, which is only partly dependent on *mass*.

Inhibition of the synthesis of nucleotides

This can be accomplished by an effect on the metabolic pathways that generate nucleotide precursors. Examples of agents that have such an effect have been described under class II reactions.

Alteration of the base-pairing properties of the template

Agents that intercalate in the DNA have this effect. Examples include acridines (**proflavine** and **acriflavine**), which are used topically as antiseptics. The acridines double the distance between adjacent base pairs and cause a *frameshift mutation*, whereas some purine and pyrimidine analogues cause base *mispairing*.

Inhibition of either DNA or RNA polymerase

Specific inhibitors of bacterial RNA polymerase that act by binding to this enzyme in prokaryotic, but not in eukaryotic, cells include **rifamycin** and **rifampicin**, which are particularly useful for treating tuberculosis (see Ch. 52). **Aciclovir** (an analogue of guanine) is phosphorylated in cells infected with herpes virus, the initial phosphorylation being by a virus-specific kinase to give the active metabolite **aciclovir trisphosphate**, which inhibits the DNA polymerase of the herpes virus (see Ch. 53).

RNA retroviruses have a *reverse transcriptase* (viral RNA-dependent DNA polymerase) that copies the viral RNA into DNA that then integrates into the host cell genome as a *provirus*. Antiviral drugs such as **zidovudine** and **didanosine** are phosphorylated by cellular enzymes to

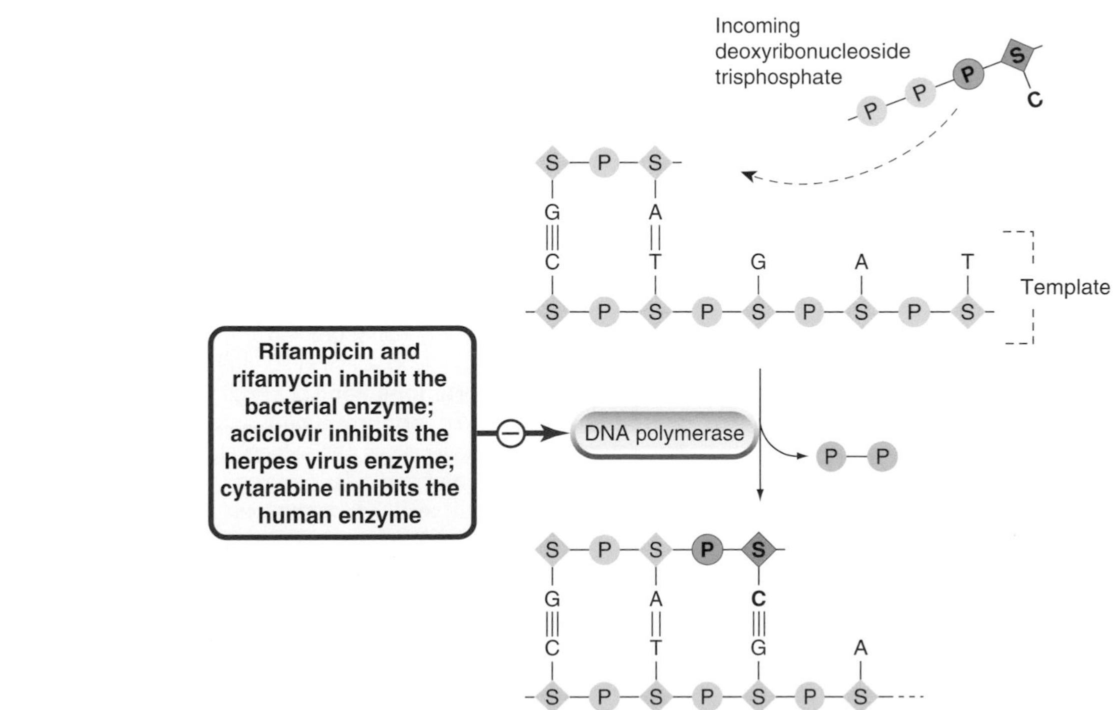

Fig. 51.5 Schematic diagram of DNA replication, showing some antibiotics that inhibit it by acting on DNA polymerase. Nucleotides are added, one at a time, by base pairing to an exposed template strand, and are then covalently joined together in a reaction catalysed by DNA polymerase. The units that pair with the complementary residues in the template consist of a base linked to a sugar and three phosphate groups. Condensation occurs with the elimination of two phosphates. The elements added to the template are shown in darker colours and bold type. *A*, Adenine; *C*, cytosine; *G*, guanine; *P*, phosphate; *S*, sugar; *T*, thymine.

the trisphosphate forms, which compete with the host cell precursors essential for the formation by the viral reverse transcriptase of proviral DNA.

Interfering with the transcription of microbial genes
RNA-based biopharmaceuticals (see Ch. 5) such as antisense agents have been used to prevent viral replication. For example, the anti-cytomegalovirus drug **fomivirsen** blocks transcription of a key gene for the viral protein IE2. This halts the progress of cytomegalovirus retinitis, although it was subsequently withdrawn for commercial reasons.

Inhibition of DNA gyrase
Fig. 51.6 is a simplified scheme showing the functional action of DNA gyrase. The *fluoroquinolones* (**cinoxacin**, **ciprofloxacin**, **nalidixic acid** and **norfloxacin**) act by inhibiting DNA gyrase and are selective for the bacterial enzyme. These chemotherapeutic agents are particularly useful for treating infections with gram-negative organisms (see Ch. 52).

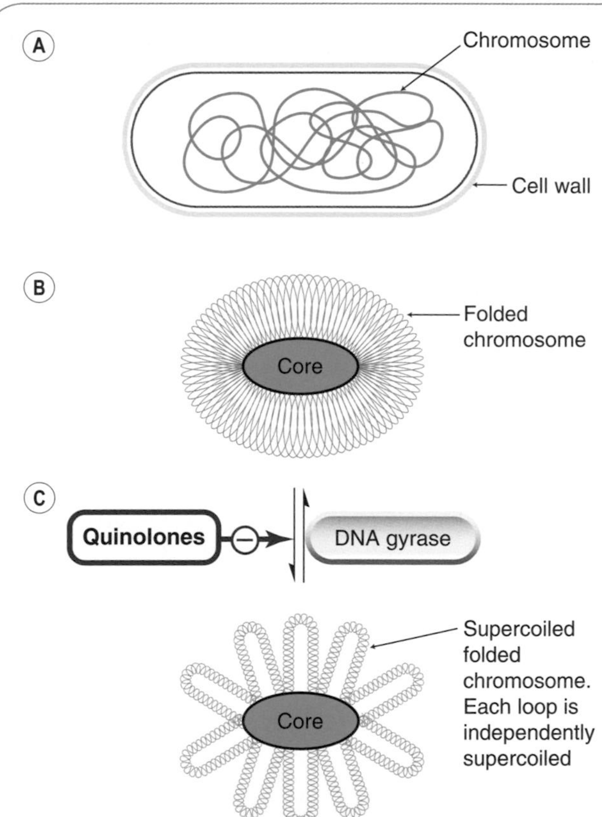

Fig. 51.6 Schematic diagram of the action of DNA gyrase: the site of action for quinolone antibacterials. (A) Conventional diagram used to depict a bacterial cell and chromosome (e.g. *Escherichia coli*). Note that the *E. coli* chromosome is 1300 mm long and is contained in a cell envelope of 2 μm × 1 μm; this is approximately equivalent to a 50 m length of cotton folded into a matchbox. (B) Chromosome folded around RNA core, and then (C) supercoiled by DNA gyrase (topoisomerase II). Quinolone antibacterials interfere with the action of this enzyme. (Modified from Smith, J.T., 1985. In: Greenwood, D., O'Grady, F. (Eds). Scientific Basis of Antimicrobial Therapy. Cambridge University Press, Cambridge, p. 69.)

THE FORMED STRUCTURES OF THE CELL AS POTENTIAL TARGETS

THE MEMBRANE

Several important antimicrobials act on cell membranes. The plasma membrane of bacterial cells is similar to that in mammalian cells in that it consists of a phospholipid bilayer in which proteins are embedded, but it can be more easily disrupted in certain bacteria and fungi.

Polymyxins are cationic peptide antibiotics, containing both hydrophilic and lipophilic residues, which have a selective effect on bacterial cell membranes. They act as detergents, disrupting the phospholipid components of the membrane structure, thus killing the cell.

Unlike mammalian and bacterial cells, fungal cell membranes contain large amounts of *ergosterol*. This facilitates the attachment of *polyene antibiotics* (e.g. **nystatin** and **amphotericin**; see Ch. 54), which act as ionophores and cause leakage of cations from the cytoplasm.

Azoles such as **itraconazole** kill fungal cells by inhibiting ergosterol synthesis, thereby disrupting the function of membrane-associated enzymes. The azoles also affect gram-positive bacteria, their selectivity being associated with the presence of high levels of free fatty acids in the membrane of susceptible organisms (see Ch. 54).

Biochemical reactions as potential targets for chemotherapy

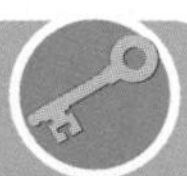

- Class I reactions are poor targets.
- Class II reactions are better targets:
  - *folate synthesis* in bacteria is inhibited by sulfonamides;
  - *folate utilisation* is inhibited by folate antagonists, for example **trimethoprim** (bacteria), **pyrimethamine** (malarial parasite).
- Class III reactions are important targets:
  - *peptidoglycan synthesis* in bacteria can be selectively inhibited by β-lactam antibiotics (e.g. **penicillin**);
  - *bacterial protein synthesis* can be selectively inhibited by antibiotics that prevent binding of tRNA (e.g. tetracyclines), promote misreading of mRNA (e.g., aminoglycosides), inhibit transpeptidation (e.g. **chloramphenicol**) or inhibit translocation of tRNA (e.g. **erythromycin**); antisense RNA biopharmaceuticals can selectively prevent the expression of particular proteins;
  - *nucleic acid synthesis* can be inhibited by altering base pairing of DNA template (e.g. the antiviral **vidarabine**), by inhibiting DNA polymerase (e.g. the antivirals **aciclovir** and **foscarnet**) or by inhibiting DNA gyrase (e.g. the antibacterial **ciprofloxacin**).

INTRACELLULAR ORGANELLES

Mitochondria

Mitochondria probably originated as a result of a symbiotic relationship between a prokaryotic and a eukaryotic cell during evolution. Since prokaryotes do not contain mitochondria, drugs such as **atovaquone** (see Ch. 55) that target these organelles in parasites are ineffective in bacteria. However, they can damage the host mitochondria, and this can contribute to the host toxicity encountered during their use.

Microtubules and/or microfilaments

The benzimidazoles (e.g. **albendazole**) exert their antihelminthic action by binding selectively to parasite tubulin and preventing microtubule formation (see Ch. 56).

Food vacuoles

The erythrocytic form of the malaria plasmodium feeds on host haemoglobin, which is digested by proteases in the parasite food vacuole, the final product, haem, being detoxified by polymerisation. **Chloroquine** and several other antimalarials exert their antimalarial actions by inhibiting plasmodial haem polymerase (see Ch. 55).

Ion channels and receptors

Some antihelminthic drugs have a selective action on helminth muscle cells (see Ch. 56). **Piperazine** acts as an agonist on parasite-specific chloride channels gated by GABA in nematode muscle, hyperpolarising the muscle fibre membrane and paralysing the worm; avermectins increase Cl^- permeability in helminth muscle - possibly by a similar mechanism. **Pyrantel** and **levamisole** are agonists at nematode acetylcholine nicotinic receptors on muscle, causing contraction followed by paralysis (see Ch. 56).

Formed structures of the cell that are targets for chemotherapy

- The bacterial cell wall may be affected by several classes of antibiotics, including the β-lactams.
- The plasma membrane is affected by:
  - **amphotericin**, which acts as an ionophore in fungal cells
  - azoles, which inhibit fungal membrane ergosterol synthesis
- Microtubule function is disrupted by:
  - benzimidazoles (antihelminthics)
- Muscle fibres are affected by:
  - avermectins (antihelminthics), which increase Cl^- permeability
  - **pyrantel** (antihelminthic), which stimulates nematode nicotinic receptors, eventually causing muscle paralysis by depolarising neuromuscular block

RESISTANCE TO ANTIBACTERIAL DRUGS

The development and use of sulfonamides in the 1930s, and of antibiotics proper in the 1940s, to treat bacterial and other infections have revolutionised medical treatment, and the morbidity and mortality associated with these diseases have been dramatically reduced. Unfortunately, this welcome development has been accompanied by the spread of drug-resistant organisms and, with it, the fear that we are moving towards a 'post antibiotic' era. It is worth noting here that 'resistance' to therapeutic intervention is a general problem which is not restricted to antibiotics: vaccines too can lose efficacy either because of mutation and natural selection within the target organisms or random 'antigenic drift'.

The WHO has termed antimicrobial (especially antibiotic) resistance '...one of the biggest threats to global health, food security, and development today' and the growing concern has prompted several supra-national and domestic political responses. The WHO has formulated a *Global Action Plan on Antibiotic Resistance* and regularly issues updated fact sheets on the problem. Other organisations supported by the WHO include the *Global Antibiotic Resistance Development Partnership* (GARDP), the *Global Antimicrobial Resistance Surveillance System* (GLASS) and the *Interagency Coordination Group on Antimicrobial Resistance* (IACG). These bodies have been monitoring the emergence of resistant strains around the world since 2009 and advising on local treatment strategies. There have been domestic initiatives too: in the United States, a national action plan was announced in 2015 and many other countries have introduced similar, if less formal, strategies to implement the advice arising from the WHO, GARDP and other organisations. Developing countries often struggle to introduce such measures and, because they are often burdened with large numbers of immunocompromised patients, lack of access to clean water, drugs and healthcare systems, lack of enforceable policies, poor hygiene and infection control, poverty and overcrowding, are (as always) faring less well.

So, what is the cause of this problem? The prevailing view used to be that antibiotic resistance was a phenomenon unique to our age and which arose largely through human mismanagement of antibiotic resources. This 'anthropogenic' view seemed to be supported by the relative absence of resistance elements in samples of bacteria taken from remote locations (such as the Galapagos islands) or from ancient samples that predated the antibiotic era. On the other hand, sequencing of recovered DNA from Pleistocene fossils (around 30,000 years old) suggested that at least some of the antibiotic resistance elements had a very ancient origin (see Bhullar et al., 2012). This presumption was dramatically confirmed by (among others) the discovery, in New Mexico, of multidrug-resistant bacteria in a deep cave system, which had been isolated from human and animal contact for 4–7 million years (Bhullar et al., 2012). A detailed analysis of one of the species recovered, *Paenibacillus*, which is resistant to most clinically used antibiotics, found that resistance genes in this bacterium had evidently been conserved for millions of years. Not only that, but this study also uncovered several hitherto-unknown resistance mechanisms (Pawlowski et al., 2016).

Interestingly, while resistance to naturally occurring antibiotics (e.g. penicillin) was extensive among these organisms, little resistance to synthetic drugs such as **linezolid** was observed. Furthermore, none of these genes were expressed in samples of this bacterium collected from the nearby cave surface, suggesting that the organisms in the cave expressed these under some selection pressure. Findings such as these have led to a reappraisal of the origin and role of the bacterial 'resistome' (the pool of genes involved in antibiotic resistance) and the issue of antibiotic resistance in general and it is now clear that we have to take a more nuanced view of the problem.

Many clinically used antibiotics are complex, naturally occurring chemicals derived from bacteria or fungi. These are released as part of a defensive strategy by these organisms. Obviously, organisms which release antibiotics must also protect themselves against the effects of these substances, perhaps explaining, at least in part, why the resistome is so significant in soil-dwelling organisms. In addition, it is now thought that these endogenous antibiotics together with their resistance mechanisms may also have a 'physiological' role: perhaps regulating metabolic pathways, acting as communication molecules or as part of bacterial 'quorum sensing' mechanisms.[4] Many of the resistance genes are located on mobile elements of DNA, and transfer between organisms in the soil by *horizontal gene transfer* (as opposed to the *vertical gene transfer* that occurs during reproduction) is common. This in part explains why the incidence of resistance is high in sites where bacteria proliferate and antibiotic usage is high, such as in agriculture or in hospitals.

Under the 'selection pressure' of intense clinical usage (and especially *mis*-usage) of antibiotics, multiple resistance elements have accumulated in pathogens. This obviously imposes serious constraints on the options available for the medical treatment of many bacterial infections. While resistance to chemotherapeutic agents can also develop in protozoa and multicellular parasites (and in populations of malignant cells; see Ch. 57), we will confine our discussion here mainly to the mechanisms of resistance in bacteria as this is the most studied.

THE SPREAD OF ANTIBIOTIC RESISTANCE

Antibiotic resistance may be *innate* – pre-existing in a particular strain – or *acquired* in some way from other bacterial cells. In either case, *natural selection* works to favour resistant strains when the antibiotic is prevalent in the environment. Fundamental to the whole issue is how bacterial resistance genes are moved around between chromosomal DNA and mobile elements both *within* and *between* bacteria.

Several basic mechanisms have been identified:

- By transfer of resistance genes between genetic elements *within* bacteria, on transposons.
- By transfer of resistance genes *between* bacteria by mobile elements (such as plasmids).
- By transfer of resistant bacteria between people or animals.

An understanding of these mechanisms is crucial for the sensible clinical use of existing medicines ('antibiotic stewardship') as well as in the design of new antibacterial drugs. We look first at the mechanisms whereby genetic information can be exchanged and then at how these transferred genes undermine the activity of antibiotics.

MOVEMENT OF GENETIC INFORMATION

Plasmids and mobile elements

In addition to chromosomal DNA, many species of bacteria contain *extrachromosomal* genetic elements called plasmids that exist free in the cytoplasm. These genetic elements can replicate independently. Structurally, they are closed loops of DNA that may comprise a single gene, as many as 500, or in some cases even more. Only a few plasmid copies may exist in the cell, but often multiple copies are present, and there may also be more than one type of plasmid in each bacterial cell. Plasmids that carry genes for resistance to antibiotics (*r genes*) are referred to as *R plasmids*. Much of the drug resistance encountered in clinical medicine is plasmid-determined.

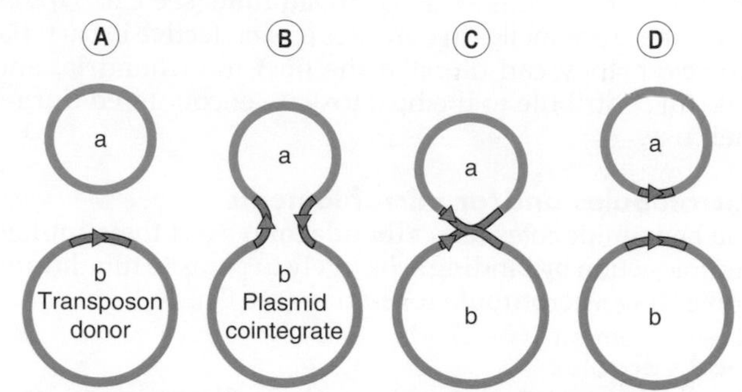

Fig. 51.7 An example of the transfer and replication of a transposon (which may carry genes coding for resistance to antibiotics). (A) Two plasmids, *a* and *b*, with plasmid *b* containing a transposon (shown in brown). (B) An enzyme encoded by the transposon cuts DNA of both donor plasmid and target plasmid a to form a cointegrate. During this process, the transposon replicates. (C) An enzyme encoded by the transposon resolves the cointegrate. (D) Both plasmids now contain the transposon DNA.

The whole process can occur with frightening speed. *S. aureus*, for example, is a past master of the art of antibiotic resistance. Having become completely resistant to **penicillin** through plasmid-mediated mechanisms, this organism, within only 1–2 years, was able to acquire resistance to its β-lactamase-resistant (see later) descendant, **meticillin** (de Lencastre et al., 2007).

Transposons

Some stretches of DNA are readily transferred (transposed) from one plasmid to another and also from plasmid to chromosome or vice versa.[5] This is because integration of these segments of DNA, which are called *transposons*, into the acceptor DNA can occur independently of the normal mechanism of homologous genetic recombination. Unlike plasmids, transposons are not able to replicate independently, although some may replicate during the process of integration (Fig. 51.7), resulting in a copy in both the donor and the acceptor DNA. Transposons may carry one or more resistance genes and can 'hitch-hike' on a plasmid to a new species of bacterium. Even if the plasmid is unable to replicate in the new host, the transposon may integrate into its chromosome or into its indigenous plasmids. This probably accounts for the widespread distribution of certain resistance genes on different R plasmids and among unrelated bacteria.

Gene cassettes and integrons

Plasmids and transposons do not complete the tally of mechanisms that natural selection has provided to confound the hopes of the microbiologist/chemotherapist. Resistance – in fact, multidrug resistance – can also be spread by

[4]Quorum sensing is a mechanism by which bacterial colonies can regulate their gene expression (and other metabolic activity) according to their population density.

[5]According to one school of thought, viruses may have arisen as transposons that escaped from cells and now continued to ply their trade independently.

another mobile element, the *gene cassette*, which consists of a resistance gene attached to a small recognition site. Several cassettes may be packaged together in a *multi-cassette array*, which can, in turn, be integrated into a larger mobile DNA unit termed an *integron*. The integron (which may be located on a transposon) contains a gene for an enzyme, *integrase* (recombinase), which inserts the cassette(s) at unique sites into the host DNA. This system – transposon/integron/multi-resistance cassette array – allows particularly rapid and efficient transfer of multidrug resistance between genetic elements both within and between bacteria.

THE TRANSFER OF RESISTANCE GENES BETWEEN BACTERIA

Horizontal gene transfer between bacteria of the same, or indeed of different, species is considered the most significant mechanism whereby antibiotic resistance is spread. There are several important mechanisms including conjugation, transduction, transformation and vesiduction, with the former being the most important. These mechanisms have assumed new significance in the light of the discovery that antibiotic resistance genes are abundant in the environment especially in the soil, in wastewater and in agricultural waste.

Conjugation

Conjugation is the main mechanism for the spread of resistance genes. It involves cell-to-cell contact during which chromosomal or extrachromosomal DNA is transferred from one bacterium to another. The ability to conjugate is encoded in *conjugative plasmids*: these are plasmids that contain transfer genes that, in (for example) coliform bacteria, code for the production by the host bacterium of proteinaceous surface tubules termed *sex pili*, which connect the two cells. The conjugative plasmid then passes across from one bacterial cell to another (generally of the same species).

Many gram-negative and some gram-positive bacteria can conjugate. Some promiscuous plasmids can even cross the species barrier, adopting one host as readily as another. Many R plasmids are conjugative. Non-conjugative plasmids, if they co-exist in a 'donor' cell with conjugative plasmids, can hitchhike from one bacterium to the other with the conjugative plasmids. The transfer of resistance by conjugation is particularly significant in populations of bacteria that are normally found at high densities, as in the gut.

Transduction

Transduction is a process by which plasmid DNA is enclosed in a virus that infects bacteria (termed a *phage*) and transferred to another bacterium of the same species. It is a relatively ineffective means of transfer of genetic material but is clinically important in the transmission of resistance genes between strains of *staphylococci* and of *streptococci*.

Transformation

Under natural conditions a few species of bacteria can undergo transformation by taking up DNA from the environment and incorporating it into their genome by normal homologous recombination. Astonishingly, bacteria able to do this can import just a single strand of the DNA through special pili on their surface, subsequently degrading the unwanted strand (Ellison et al., 2018).

Vesiduction

Another, recently proposed mechanism for DNA transfer is termed *vesiduction* (Soler and Forterre, 2020). This refers to a well-studied process whereby vesicles containing various cargoes are released from (e.g.) bacterial cells and fuse with the membranes of nearby cells releasing their contents intracellularly. Notably, this can occur between cells of different species, including from prokaryote to eukaryote. These vesicles can include DNA and thus can spread their genetic payload.

Resistance to antibiotics

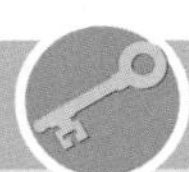

- Antibiotic resistance is a naturally occurring phenomenon which plays a role in the normal bacterial ecology.
- In many bacterial species, resistance genes (*r* genes) are of ancient origin and are normally expressed in the presence of the antibiotic.
- R genes may be moved around between genetic elements within individual bacteria. There are several mechanisms:
  - Plasmids are extrachromosomal genetic elements that can replicate independently and can carry genes coding for resistance to antibiotics.
  - Transposons are stretches of DNA that can be transposed from one plasmid to another, from a plasmid to a chromosome or vice versa. A plasmid containing an r gene–bearing transposon may code for enzymes that cause the plasmid to be integrated with another. Following their separation, this transposon replicates so that both plasmids then contain the r gene.
- R genes, including *multi-cassette arrays* of drug resistance genes, can also be transferred to other bacteria of the same, or different, species. There are several mechanisms:
  - The main method of transfer of r genes from one bacterium to another is by conjugative plasmids. The bacterium forms a connecting tube with other bacteria through which the plasmids pass.
  - A less common method of transfer is by transduction, i.e. the transmission by a bacterial virus (phage) of a plasmid bearing an r gene into another bacterium.

CHROMOSOMAL MUTATIONS

The spontaneous mutation rate in bacterial populations for any particular gene is very low: only approximately one cell in 10 million will bear a mutation and pass it on. However, as there are likely to be very many more cells than this over the course of an infection, the probability of a mutation causing a change from drug sensitivity to drug resistance can be quite high. Fortunately, the presence of a few mutants is not generally sufficient to produce resistance: despite the selective advantage that the resistant mutants possess, the drastic reduction of the population by the antibiotic usually enables the host's natural defences (see

Ch. 7) to prevail at least in acute, if not chronic, infections. However, the outcome may not be quite so desirable if the primary infection is caused by a drug-resistant strain.

GENE AMPLIFICATION

Gene duplication and *amplification* are important mechanisms for resistance in some organisms (Sandegren and Andersson, 2009). According to this idea, treatment with antibiotics can induce an increased number of copies for pre-existing resistance genes such as antibiotic-destroying enzymes and efflux pumps.

BIOCHEMICAL MECHANISMS OF RESISTANCE TO ANTIBIOTICS

Resistance genes are translated into proteins that subvert the action of antibiotics in several ways. Here we discuss several of these, but new mechanisms are constantly being uncovered (Pawlowski et al., 2016). Fig. 51.8 illustrates the main mechanisms by which resistance can occur.

THE PRODUCTION OF ENZYMES THAT INACTIVATE DRUGS

Inactivation of β-lactam antibiotics

Perhaps the most important example of resistance caused by inactivation is that of the β-lactam antibiotics. The enzymes concerned are *β-lactamases*, which cleave the β-lactam ring of penicillins and cephalosporins (see Ch. 52). Cross-resistance between the two classes of antibiotic is not complete, because some β-lactamases have a preference for penicillins and some for cephalosporins.

Staphylococci are the principal bacterial species producing β-lactamase, and the genes coding for the enzymes are on plasmids that can be transferred by transduction. In this species, the enzyme is inducible and is barely expressed in the absence of the drug. Minute, sub-inhibitory, concentrations of antibiotics de-repress the gene and result in a 50- to 80-fold increase in expression. The enzyme passes through the bacterial envelope and inactivates antibiotic molecules in the surrounding medium. The grave clinical problem posed by resistant staphylococci secreting β-lactamase was tackled by developing semisynthetic penicillins (such as **meticillin**) and new β-lactam antibiotics (the monobactams and carbapenems), and cephalosporins (such as **cefamandole**), that are less susceptible to inactivation. In addition to acquiring resistance to β-lactams, some strains of *S. aureus* have even become resistant to some antibiotics that are not significantly inactivated by β-lactamase (e.g. **meticillin**), because they express an additional β-lactam-binding protein coded for by a mutated chromosomal gene. See Lambert (2005) for other examples of this type of action.

Gram-negative organisms can also produce β-lactamases, and this is a significant factor in their resistance to the semisynthetic broad-spectrum β-lactam antibiotics. In these organisms, the enzymes may be coded by either chromosomal or plasmid genes. In the former case, the enzymes may be inducible, but in the latter, they are produced constitutively. When this occurs, the enzyme does not inactivate the drug in the surrounding medium but instead remains attached to the cell wall, preventing access of the drug to membrane-associated target sites. Many of these β-lactamases are encoded by transposons, some of which may also carry resistance determinants to several other antibiotic classes.

Inactivation of chloramphenicol

Chloramphenicol is inactivated by *chloramphenicol acetyltransferase*, an enzyme produced by resistant strains of both gram-positive and gram-negative organisms, the resistance gene being plasmid borne. In gram-negative bacteria, the enzyme is produced constitutively, resulting in levels of resistance five-fold higher than in gram-positive bacteria, in which the enzyme is inducible.

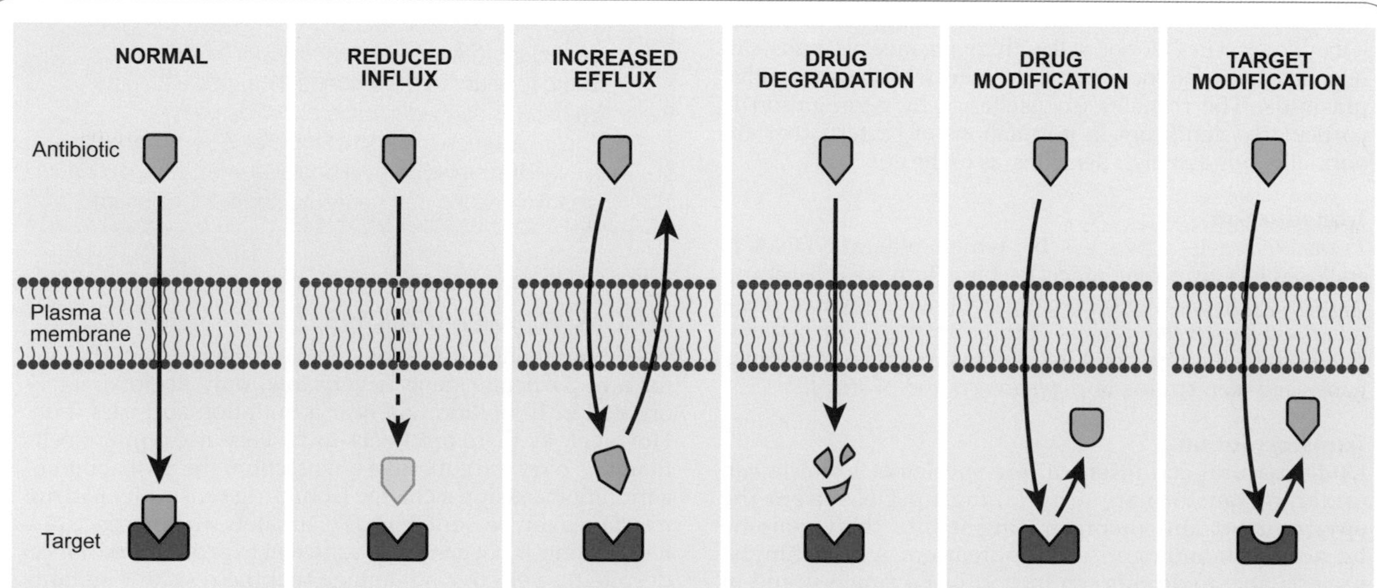

Fig. 51.8 The principal mechanisms of biochemical resistance to antibiotics. (Adapted and modified from Wilson, D.N., 2014. Ribosome-targeting antibiotics and mechanisms of bacterial resistance. Nat. Rev. Microbiol. 12, 35–48.)

Inactivation of aminoglycosides

Aminoglycosides are inactivated by phosphorylation, adenylation or acetylation, and the requisite enzymes are found in both gram-negative and gram-positive organisms. The resistance genes are carried on plasmids, and several are found on transposons. Many other examples of this kind are given by Wright (2005) and Giedraitiene et al. (2011).

ALTERATION OF DRUG-BINDING SITE

The aminoglycoside-binding site on the 30S subunit of the ribosome may be altered by chromosomal mutation. A plasmid-mediated alteration of the binding site protein on the 50S subunit also underlies resistance to **erythromycin**, and decreased binding of fluoroquinolones because of a point mutation in DNA gyrase A has also been described. An altered DNA-dependent RNA polymerase determined by a chromosomal mutation is reported to be the basis for **rifampicin** resistance.

DECREASED ACCUMULATION OF DRUGS BY BACTERIA

An important example of decreased drug accumulation is the plasmid-mediated resistance to tetracyclines encountered in both gram-positive and gram-negative bacteria. In this case, resistance genes in the plasmid code for inducible protein pumps in the bacterial membrane, which promote energy-dependent efflux of the tetracyclines, and hence resistance. This type of resistance is common and has greatly reduced the therapeutic value of the tetracyclines in human and veterinary medicine. Resistance of *S. aureus* to **erythromycin** and other macrolides, and to fluoroquinolones, is also brought about by energy-dependent efflux. Notably, these pumps may be selective for one antibiotic class or may be more promiscuous in their action – an important problem in multidrug resistance of cancer cells (see Ch. 57). Inhibitors of such pumps may be useful adjuncts to antibiotics (Thakur et al., 2021) .

There is also recent evidence of plasmid-determined inhibition of porin synthesis, which could affect those hydrophilic antibiotics that enter the bacterium through these water-filled channels in the outer membrane. Altered permeability as a result of chromosomal mutations involving the polysaccharide components of the outer membrane of gram-negative organisms may also confer enhanced resistance to ampicillin. Mutations affecting envelope components have been reported to affect the accumulation of aminoglycosides, β-lactams, **chloramphenicol**, peptide antibiotics and **tetracycline**.

ALTERATION OF ENZYME SELECTIVITY

Resistance to **trimethoprim** is the result of plasmid-directed synthesis of a *dihydrofolate reductase* with low or zero affinity for trimethoprim. It is transferred by transduction and may be spread by transposons.

Sulfonamide resistance in many bacteria is plasmid mediated and results from the production of a form of *dihydropteroate synthetase* with a low affinity for sulfonamides but no change in affinity for PABA. Bacteria causing serious infections and carrying plasmids with resistance genes to both sulfonamides and **trimethoprim** have been reported.

Biochemical mechanisms of resistance to antibiotics

The principal mechanisms are as follows:

- *Production of enzymes that inactivate the drug*: for example, β-lactamases, which inactivate **penicillin**; acetyltransferases, which inactivate **chloramphenicol**; kinases and other enzymes, which inactivate aminoglycosides.
- *Alteration of the drug-binding sites*: this occurs with aminoglycosides, **erythromycin**, **penicillin.**
- *Reduction of drug uptake by the bacterium or enhanced efflux*: for example, tetracyclines.
- *Alteration of enzyme sensitivity*: for example, dihydrofolate reductase becomes insensitive to **trimethoprim.**

CURRENT STATUS OF ANTIBIOTIC RESISTANCE IN BACTERIA

The latest WHO assessment (2020) stresses that antibiotic resistance is now found in every country. Estimates of the global burden of this problem vary but one (Antibiotic Research UK) cites a figure of 700,000 deaths per annum rising to 10 million by 2050. Without effective antibiotics, many routine surgical procedures and other medical interventions are impossible. The WHO also highlights the following cases as being of special significance:

- *Klebsiella pneumoniae.* Resistance of this intestinal organism to 'last-resort' antibiotics such as carbapenem drugs has spread around the world and in many countries, treatment fails in about half of all cases.
- *Escherichia coli.* In many countries this organism has become resistant to fluoroquinolone antibiotics and again, treatment fails in about half of the patients in some parts of the world. Resistance to the last-resort treatment, **colistin**, is also spreading.
- *Neisseria gonorrhoea.* In many countries this organism has acquired resistance to almost all common antibiotics, with the last-resort drug, **ceftriaxone**, being the final remaining hope for treating resistant strains.
- *S. aureus.* Resistance of this skin organism to first-line drugs is now widespread and patients with **meticillin**-resistant *S. aureus* (MRSA) are more than twice as likely to die following infection. While mortality is declining in the North America and Europe, it is increasing in developing countries.
- *Enterobacteriaceae.* These organisms can cause life-threatening infections and recently resistance to the 'last-resort' drug **colistin** has been reported.
- *Mycobacterium tuberculosis.* This hitherto treatable disease has now become a major global health emergency. In 2018 WHO estimated that half a million new cases of **rifampicin-**resistant TB were seen annually and that the majority of these cases harboured multidrug-resistant strains of the disease. Cure rates are less than 60% in such cases.

Multidrug resistance

Some pathogenic bacteria have developed resistance to many or most commonly used antibiotics. Examples include the following:

- Some strains of staphylococci and enterococci that are resistant to virtually all current antibiotics, the resistance being transferred by transposons and/or plasmids; such organisms can cause serious and virtually untreatable hospital-acquired (so-called nosocomial) infections.
- Some strains of *Mycobacterium tuberculosis* that have become resistant to most antituberculosis agents.

RESISTANCE TO OTHER ANTIMICROBIALS

While we have stressed bacterial resistance to antibiotics in this chapter, it is important to realise that this problem extends to all antimicrobial agents. The WHO has warned that resistance to most antiviral agents has developed. A particularly stark example is the emergence of a strain of HIV which is fully resistant to the current portfolio of antiretroviral drugs (see Ch. 53). More than half of all infants with HIV in sub-Saharan Africa are already infected with this resistant strain. Patients infected with HIV are immunocompromised and thus fungal infections are easily able to gain a foothold in their weakened immune systems. It is depressing to note that some *Candida* strains also have developed resistance to a battery of antifungal drugs including those in the azole group and **amphotericin** (see Ch. 56). The situation with antimalarial drugs is equally serious, with some parasite strains in Africa and Asia developing resistance to a key drug, **artemisinin**, as well as other conventional antimalarial agents.

So what is the way forward? Regardless of the ancient origin of bacterial resistance mechanisms, all parties agree that indiscriminate use of antibiotics in agriculture, human and veterinary medicine, and their use in animal foodstuffs, has undoubtedly encouraged the spread of resistant strains. The situation is particularly acute in the developing world where poverty, overcrowding, lack of clean water and minimal sanitation exacerbate the problem.

The current trend is to tackle clinical drug resistance as part of a more holistic 'One Health' approach which embraces not only human health, but also that of plants and that of all animals, both land dwelling and aquatic, as well as agricultural, environmental and ecological practices (e.g. Ben et al., 2019). To support this the WHO has published numerous reports, updates, guidelines, policies and lists of 'priority pathogens' and launched several initiatives, most recently the annual *World Antimicrobial Awareness Week* in 2020 with its slogan 'Antimicrobials: Handle with Care'.

Prescribers and consumers alike must bear a measure of responsibility for the burgeoning problem of resistance. Most members of the general public have only a vague notion of the causes of the problem, its likely ultimate implications and their role in its development (McCullough et al., 2016). More worryingly, even many clinicians, while realising the scope of the problem, also seem unaware of their crucial role in its spread (McCullough et al., 2015).

Some authors (e.g.Chaudhary, 2016) have advocated tackling the problem at the point of diagnosis and prescription suggesting that bacterial susceptibility testing should be mandatory before the drug is dispensed. Unnecessary prescribing (e.g. for viral infections), inadequate dosing or inappropriate duration of treatment (which often leads to resistance) should all be scrupulously avoided and more rigorous adherence by patients to antibiotic regimes would help. Therapy using multiple antibiotics acting through different mechanisms can be a useful strategy in some cases and a number of other unconventional therapies have been proposed (Kumar et al., 2021). Public health measures such as infection control procedures also play a key role. The removal of antibiotic resistance genes from the soil and wastewater is of particular importance and several innovative solutions have been proposed, including the construction of artificial wetlands and other measures (Herraiz-Carbone et al., 2021; Liu et al., 2019).

Another problem (which not only applies to antimicrobials but to other fields of medicine as well) is the funding model for such research. The antimicrobial drug 'pipeline' is depressingly slim, but the pharmaceutical industry is wary of investment in the field since the potential profits are unlikely to cover the huge development costs and most governments have no stomach for the eye-watering risks associated with investing in drug discovery either. Various techniques to counteract resistance have been proposed, including the repurposing of other drugs, combination therapies as well as the use of artificial Intelligence (AI) and associated techniques (Alvarez-Martinez et al., 2020) to predict likely candidate drugs. A number of public/private partnerships such as the *Antimicrobial Resistance Multi Partner Trust Fund* and the *Global Antibiotic Research & Development Partnership* have stepped in to fill the funding vacuum. Let's all hope that this action is not too late.

REFERENCES AND FURTHER READING

Books

Davies, S., 2013. The Drugs Don't Work: A Global Threat. Penguin, London, p. 272.

Ramakrishnan, V., 2018. Gene Machine. Oneworld Publications Ltd, London, p. 112.

Original papers and reviews

Alvarez-Martinez, F.J., Barrajon-Catalan, E., Micol, V., 2020. Tackling antibiotic resistance with compounds of natural origin: a comprehensive review. Biomedicines 8, 405.

Arias, C.A., Murray, B.E., 2012. The rise of the *Enterococcus*: beyond vancomycin resistance. Nat. Rev. Microbiol. 10, 266–278.

Barrett, C.T., Barrett, J.F., 2003. Antibacterials: are the new entries enough to deal with the emerging resistance problem? Curr. Opin. Biotechnol. 14, 621–626.

Bax, R., Mullan, N., Verhoef, J., 2000. The millennium bugs – the need for and development of new antibacterials. Int. J. Antimicrob. Agents 16, 51–59.

Ben, Y., Fu, C., Hu, M., Liu, L., Wong, M.H., Zheng, C., 2019. Human health risk assessment of antibiotic resistance associated with antibiotic residues in the environment: a review. Environ Res. 169, 483–493.

Bhullar, K., Waglechner, N., Pawlowski, A., et al., 2012. Antibiotic resistance is prevalent in an isolated cave microbiome. PLoS One 7, e34953.

Carter, A.P., Clemons, W.M., Brodersen, D.E., Morgan-Warren, R.J., Wimberly, B.T., Ramakrishnan, V., 2000. Functional insights from the structure of the 30S ribosomal subunit and its interactions with antibiotics. Nature 407, 340–348.
Chaudhary, A.S., 2016. A review of global initiatives to fight antibiotic resistance and recent antibiotics discovery. Acta. Pharm. Sin. B. 6, 552–556.
Cox, G., Wright, G.D., 2013. Intrinsic antibiotic resistance: mechanisms, origins, challenges and solutions. Int. J. Med. Microbiol. 303, 287–292.
de Lencastre, H., Oliveira, D., Tomasz, A., 2007. Antibiotic resistant *Staphylococcus aureus*: a paradigm of adaptive power. Curr. Opin. Microbiol. 10, 428–435.
Ellison, C.K., Dalia, T.N., Vidal Ceballos, A., et al., 2018. Retraction of DNA-bound type IV competence pili initiates DNA uptake during natural transformation in Vibrio cholerae. Nat. Microbiol. 3, 773–780.
Giedraitiene, A., Vitkauskiene, A., Naginiene, R., Pavilonis, A., 2011. Antibiotic resistance mechanisms of clinically important bacteria. Medicina 47, 137–146.
Herraiz-Carbone, M., Cotillas, S., Lacasa, E., et al., 2021. A review on disinfection technologies for controlling the antibiotic resistance spread. Sci. Total Environ. 797, 149150.
Knodler, L.A., Celli, J., Finlay, B.B., 2001. Pathogenic trickery: deception of host cell processes. Mol. Cell. Biol. 2, 578–588.
Kumar, M., Sarma, D.K., Shubham, S., et al., 2021. Futuristic non-antibiotic therapies to combat antibiotic resistance: a review. Front. Microbiol. 12, 609459.
Lambert, P.A., 2005. Bacterial resistance to antibiotics: modified target sites. Adv. Drug Deliv. Rev. 57, 1471–1485.
Levy, S.B., 1998. The challenge of antibiotic resistance. Sci. Am. 278, 32–39.
Liu, X., Guo, X., Liu, Y., et al., 2019. A review on removing antibiotics and antibiotic resistance genes from wastewater by constructed wetlands: performance and microbial response. Environ. Pollut. 254, 112996.
McCullough, A.R., Parekh, S., Rathbone, J., Del Mar, C.B., Hoffmann, T.C., 2016. A systematic review of the public's knowledge and beliefs about antibiotic resistance. J. Antimicrob. Chemother. 71, 27–33.
McCullough, A.R., Rathbone, J., Parekh, S., Hoffmann, T.C., Del Mar, C.B., 2015. Not in my backyard: a systematic review of clinicians' knowledge and beliefs about antibiotic resistance. J. Antimicrob. Chemother. 70, 2465–2473.
Nesme, J., Simonet, P., 2015. The soil resistome: a critical review on antibiotic resistance origins, ecology and dissemination potential in telluric bacteria. Environ. Microbiol. 17, 913–930.
Pawlowski, A.C., Wang, W., Koteva, K., Barton, H.A., McArthur, A.G., Wright, G.D., 2016. A diverse intrinsic antibiotic resistome from a cave bacterium. Nat. Commun. 7, 13803.
Sandegren, L., Andersson, D.I., 2009. Bacterial gene amplification: implications for the evolution of antibiotic resistance. Nat. Rev. Microbiol. 7, 578–588.
Shlaes, D.M., 2003. The abandonment of antibacterials: why and wherefore? Curr. Opin. Pharmacol. 3, 470–473.
Soler, N., Forterre, P., 2020. Vesiduction: the fourth way of HGT. Environ. Microbiol. 22, 2457–2460.
St Georgiev, V., 2000. Membrane transporters and antifungal drug resistance. Curr. Drug Targets 1, 184–261.
Thakur, V., Uniyal, A., Tiwari, V., 2021. A comprehensive review on pharmacology of efflux pumps and their inhibitors in antibiotic resistance. Eur. J. Pharmacol. 903, 174151.
Van Bambeke, F., Pages, J.M., Lee, V.J., 2006. Inhibitors of bacterial efflux pumps as adjuvants in antibiotic treatments and diagnostic tools for detection of resistance by efflux. Recent. Pat. Antiinfect. Drug Discov. 1, 157–175.
Volpato, J.P., Pelletier, J.N., 2009. Mutational 'hot-spots' in mammalian, bacterial and protozoal dihydrofolate reductases associated with antifolate resistance: sequence and structural comparison. Drug Resist. Updat. 12, 28–41.
Walsh, C., 2000. Molecular mechanisms that confer antibacterial drug resistance. Nature 406, 775–781.
Wilson, D.N., 2014. Ribosome-targeting antibiotics and mechanisms of bacterial resistance. Nat. Rev. Microbiol. 12, 35–48.
Woodford, N., 2005. Biological counterstrike: antibiotic resistance mechanisms of gram-positive cocci. Clin. Microbiol. Infect. 3, 2–21.
Wright, G.D., 2005. Bacterial resistance to antibiotics: enzymatic degradation and modification. Adv. Drug Deliv. Rev. 57, 1451–1470.
Zasloff, M., 2002. Antimicrobial peptides of multicellular organisms. Nature 415, 389–395.

Useful web resources

The World Health Organisation (WHO) hosts web pages that deal with the global problem of microbial resistance, and the regularly updated *Antibiotic Resistance* Fact Sheet (see https://www.who.int/news-room/fact-sheets/detail/antibiotic-resistance) contains definitive information on the current situation around the world.

The AntiBiotic Research UK website also contains some interesting data relevant to this problem and also offers support for patients (see https://www.antibioticresearch.org.uk).

52 Antibacterial drugs

OVERVIEW

In this chapter we discuss antibacterial drugs. Bacteriology is a vast subject and a detailed discussion is beyond the scope of this book, but information about some clinically significant pathogens is included to provide necessary context. The pharmacological properties and therapeutic effects of the major classes of antibacterial drugs are described. We conclude with an assessment of the prospects for new antibacterials and the attendant risks if we fail to do so.

INTRODUCTION

Working at St Mary's Hospital in London in 1928, Alexander Fleming discovered that a culture plate on which staphylococci were being grown had become contaminated with a mould of the genus *Penicillium*. He made the crucial observation that bacterial growth in the vicinity of the mould had been inhibited. He subsequently isolated the mould in pure culture and demonstrated that it produced an antibacterial substance, which he named **penicillin**. This substance was subsequently prepared in bulk, extracted and its antibacterial effects analysed by Florey, Chain, Heatley and their colleagues at Oxford in 1940. They demonstrated that **penicillin** was non-toxic to the host but killed the pathogens in infected mice and in doing so they ushered in the 'antibiotic era'. Since then, many new types of antibiotics have been discovered and the practice of medicine today would be unthinkable without them.

GRAM STAINING AND ITS SIGNIFICANCE FOR DRUG ACTION

Most bacteria can be classified as being either *gram-positive* or *gram-negative*, depending on whether they stain with *Gram stain*.[1] This reflects fundamental differences in the structure of their cell walls and has important implications for the action of antibiotics (Table 52.1).

The cell wall of gram-positive organisms is a relatively simple structure. It is some 15–50 nm thick and comprises about 50% peptidoglycan (see Ch. 51), 40%–45% acidic polymer together with 5%–10% proteins and polysaccharides. The cell surface is highly polar and negatively charged and this influences the penetration of some drugs.

The cell wall of gram-negative organisms is much more complex. From the plasma membrane outwards, it consists of the following:

- A *periplasmic space* containing enzymes and other components.
- A *peptidoglycan layer* 2 nm in thickness, forming 5% of the cell wall mass. This is often linked to outwardly projecting lipoprotein molecules.
- An *outer membrane* consisting of a lipid bilayer, similar in some respects to the plasma membrane, that contains protein molecules and (on its inner aspect) lipoproteins linked to the peptidoglycan. Other proteins form transmembrane water-filled channels, termed *porins*, through which some hydrophilic antibiotics can move freely (see also Ch. 9).
- *An outer surface rich in complex polysaccharides.* These differ between strains of bacteria and are the main determinants of their antigenicity. They are also the source of *endotoxin*, a lipopolysaccharide which, when shed in vivo, triggers various aspects of the inflammatory reaction by activating complement and releasing cytokines, causing fever, etc. (see Ch. 7).

The cell wall lipopolysaccharide is a major barrier to penetration of some antibiotics, including **benzylpenicillin**, **meticillin**, the macrolides, **rifampicin**, **fusidic acid** and **vancomycin** and difficulty in penetrating this complex outer layer explains why some antibiotics are less active against gram-negative than gram-positive bacteria. It is also one reason for the extraordinary antibiotic resistance exhibited by *Pseudomonas aeruginosa*, a pathogen that can cause life-threatening infections in neutropenic patients and those with burns and wounds, as well as a chronic bronchial infection in patients with cystic fibrosis.

BACTERIOSTATIC AND BACTERICIDAL DRUGS

Antibiotics that interfere with bacterial cell wall synthesis (e.g. penicillins) or inhibit crucial enzymes (such as the quinolones) generally kill bacteria (i.e. they are *bactericidal*), while those that inhibit protein synthesis, such as the tetracyclines, are generally *bacteriostatic*, that is they do not kill cells but rather prevent growth and replication. This distinction is not especially clinically significant, as the therapeutic outcome of antibiotic therapy depends critically on the host response in dealing with compromised bacterial load.

In discussing the pharmacology of antibacterial drugs, it is convenient to divide them into different groups based upon their mechanism of action.

ANTIBACTERIAL AGENTS THAT INTERFERE WITH FOLATE SYNTHESIS OR ACTION

(See Figs 52.1 and 52.2.)

SULFONAMIDES

In a landmark discovery in the 1930s, prior to the advent of penicillin into the clinic, Domagk demonstrated that it

[1]Named after its inventor, Hans Christian Gram, a 19th century Danish bacteriologist.

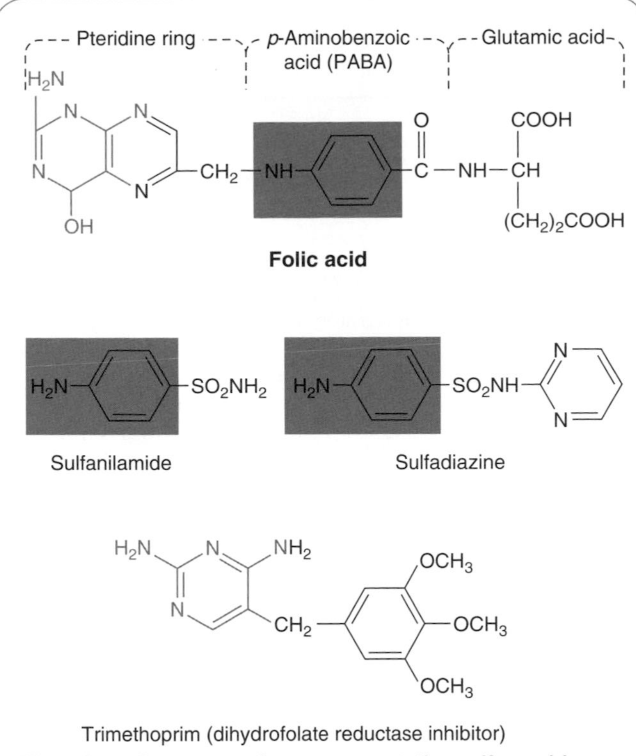

Fig. 52.1 Structures of two representative sulfonamides and trimethoprim. The structures illustrate the relationship between the sulfonamides and the *p*-aminobenzoic acid moiety in folic acid *(orange box)*, as well as between the antifolate drugs and the pteridine moiety *(orange)*. Co-trimoxazole is a mixture of sulfamethoxazole and trimethoprim.

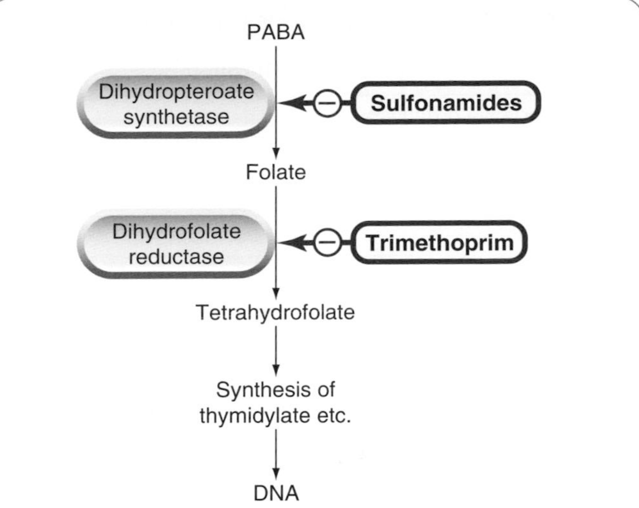

Fig. 52.2 The action of sulfonamides and trimethoprim on bacterial folate synthesis. See Chapter 24 for more detail of tetrahydrofolate synthesis, and Chapter 51 for comparisons of antifolate drugs. *PABA*, *p*-aminobenzoic acid.

was possible for a drug to suppress a bacterial infection. The drug was a dye called **prontosil rubrum**,[2] which proved to be an inactive prodrug that was metabolised in vivo to an active product, **sulfanilamide** (see Fig. 52.1). Many sulfonamides have been developed since, but their importance has declined in the face of increasing resistance. The only sulfonamide drugs still commonly used as *systemic* antibacterials are **sulfamethoxazole** (usually in combination with **trimethoprim** as **co-trimoxazole**) and **sulfasalazine**, which is poorly absorbed by the gastrointestinal (GI) tract but is widely used to treat ulcerative colitis and Crohn's disease (see Chs 25 and 30). **Silver sulfadiazine** is another sulfonamide; it is used topically to treat infected burns. Some drugs with quite different clinical uses (e.g. the antiplatelet drug **prasugrel**, see Ch. 23, and the carbonic anhydrase inhibitor **acetazolamide**, see Ch. 30) are also sulfonamides and share some of the off-target adverse effects of this class (see later).

[2]Domagk believed, wrongly as it happens, that the staining property of azo dyes, such as prontosil, was responsible for their antibacterial selectivity. He used **prontosil** – a red dye – to treat his young daughter for a life-threatening streptococcal infection. She survived but was left with permanently red-stained skin – a testament to its lack of selectivity for the invading bacteria.

Clinical uses of sulfonamides

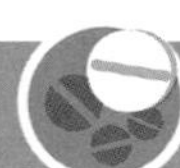

- Combined with **trimethoprim** (**co-trimoxazole**) for *Pneumocystis carinii* (now known as *P. jirovecii*), for toxoplasmosis and nocardiasis.
- Combined with **pyrimethamine** for drug-resistant malaria (see Ch. 55) and for toxoplasmosis.
- In inflammatory bowel disease: **sulfasalazine** (sulfapyridine–aminosalicylate combination) is used (see Ch. 30).
- For infected burns (silver **sulfadiazine)** given topically

Mechanism of action

Sulfanilamide, the active metabolite of **prontosil**, is a structural analogue of *p*-aminobenzoic acid (PABA; see Fig. 52.1), which is an essential precursor in the biosynthesis of folic acid and is required for the synthesis of DNA and RNA in bacteria (see Ch. 51). Sulfonamides compete with PABA for the enzyme *dihydropteroate synthetase*, and the effect of the sulfonamide may be overcome by adding excess PABA. This is why local anaesthetics which are PABA esters (such as **procaine**; see Ch. 44) antagonise the antibacterial effect of these agents.

Sulfonamide action is vitiated in the presence of pus or products of tissue breakdown, because these contain thymidine and purines which bacteria utilise directly, bypassing the requirement for folic acid. Resistance to sulfonamides, which is common, is plasmid mediated (see Ch. 51) and results from the synthesis of a bacterial enzyme insensitive to the drugs.

Pharmacokinetic aspects. Most sulfonamides can be given orally and, apart from **sulfasalazine** and **silver sulfadiazine** (see earlier), are well absorbed and widely distributed in the body. The drugs pass into inflammatory exudates and cross both placental and blood–brain barriers.

Table 52.1 Some clinically significant pathogenic bacteria

Genus	Morphology	Species	Disease
Gram-negative organisms			
Bordetella	Cocci	*B. pertussis*	Whooping cough
Brucella	Curved rods	*B. abortus*	Brucellosis (cattle and humans)
Campylobacter	Spiral rods	*C. jejuni*	Food poisoning
Escherichia	Rods	*E. coli*	Septicaemia, wound infections, UTIs
Haemophilus	Rods	*H. influenzae*	Acute respiratory tract infection, meningitis
Helicobacter	Motile rods	*H. pylori*	Peptic ulcers, gastric cancer
Klebsiella	Capsulated rods	*K. pneumonia*	Pneumonia, septicaemia
Legionella	Flagellated rods	*L. pneumophila*	Legionnaires' disease
Neisseria	Cocci, paired	*N. gonorrhoeae*	Gonorrhoea
Pseudomonas	Flagellated rods	*P. aeruginosa*	Septicaemia, respiratory infections, UTIs
Rickettsiae	Cocci or threads	*Several spp.*	Tick- and insect-borne infections
Salmonella	Motile rods	*S. typhimurium*	Food poisoning
Shigella	Rods	*S. dysenteriae*	Bacillary dysentery
Yersinia	Rods	*Y. pestis*	Bubonic plague
Vibrio	Flagellated rods	*V. cholera*	Cholera
Gram-positive organisms			
Bacillus	Rods, chains	*B. anthrax*	Anthrax
Clostridium	Rods	*C. tetani*	Tetanus
Corynebacterium	Rod	*C. diphtheria*	Diphtheria
Mycobacterium	Rods	*M. tuberculosis*	Tuberculosis
		M. leprae	Leprosy
Staphylococcus	Cocci, clusters	*S. aureus*	Wound infections, boils, septicaemia
Streptococcus	Cocci, pairs	*S. pneumoniae*	Pneumonia, meningitis
	Cocci, chains	*S. pyogenes*	Scarlet fever, rheumatic fever, cellulitis
Other			
Chlamydia	Gram 'uncertain'	*C. trachomatis*	Eye disease, infertility
Treponema	Flagellated spiral rods	*T. pallidum*	Syphilis

UTI, Urinary tract infection.

They are metabolised mainly in the liver, the major product being an acetylated derivative that lacks antibacterial action. There is a risk of sensitisation or allergic reactions when these drugs are given topically.

Unwanted effects. Serious adverse effects necessitating cessation of therapy include hepatitis, hypersensitivity reactions (rashes including severe forms of erythema multiforme, fever, anaphylactoid reactions – see Ch. 58), bone marrow depression and acute renal failure due to interstitial nephritis or crystalluria. This last effect results from the precipitation of acetylated metabolites in the urine (see Ch. 29). Cyanosis caused by methaemoglobinaemia may occur but is a lot less alarming than it looks. Mild to moderate side effects include nausea and vomiting, headache and mental depression.

TRIMETHOPRIM

Mechanism of action

Trimethoprim is chemically related to the antimalarial drug **pyrimethamine** (see Ch. 55), both being folate antagonists. Structurally it resembles the pteridine moiety of folate and the similarity is close enough to fool the bacterial *dihydrofolate reductase*, which is many times more sensitive to **trimethoprim** than is the equivalent enzyme in humans.

Trimethoprim is active against most common bacterial pathogens as well as protozoa, and is used to treat various urinary, pulmonary and other infections. It is sometimes given in combination with **sulfamethoxazole** as **co-trimoxazole**. Because sulfonamides inhibit a different stage on the same bacterial metabolic pathway, they can potentiate the action of **trimethoprim,** but to be effective, they must have a similar *pK* to the drug. **Sulfamethoxazole** has this property. In the United Kingdom, the use of **co-trimoxazole** is generally restricted to the treatment of Pneumocystis pneumonia, an opportunistic infection with which AIDS may present (see Ch. 53), caused by the fungus *Pneumocystis carinii* (now known as *Pneumocystis jirovecii*), toxoplasmosis (a protozoan infection) or nocardiasis (a bacterial infection).

Pharmacokinetic aspects. **Trimethoprim** is well absorbed orally, and widely distributed throughout the tissues and body fluids. It reaches high concentrations in the lungs and kidneys, and fairly high concentrations in the cerebrospinal fluid (CSF). When given with **sulfamethoxazole,** the only sulfonamide with similar *p*K to trimethoprim, about half the dose of each is excreted within 24 h. Because **trimethoprim** is a weak base, its elimination by the kidney increases with decreasing urinary pH.

Unwanted effects. Folate deficiency can result from long-term administration of **trimethoprim** resulting in megaloblastic anaemia (see Ch. 24). Other unwanted effects include nausea, vomiting, blood disorders and rashes.

Antimicrobial agents that interfere with the synthesis or action of folate

- Sulfonamides are bacteriostatic; they act by interfering with folate synthesis and thus with nucleotide synthesis. Unwanted effects include crystalluria and hypersensitivities.
- **Trimethoprim** is bacteriostatic. It acts by antagonising folate.
- **Co-trimoxazole** is a mixture of **trimethoprim** with **sulfamethoxazole**, which affects bacterial nucleotide synthesis at two points in the pathway.
- **Pyrimethamine** and **proguanil** are also antimalarial agents (see Ch. 55).

β-LACTAM ANTIBIOTICS AND OTHER AGENTS THAT INTERFERE WITH BACTERIAL WALL OR MEMBRANE SYNTHESIS

(See Ch. 51 and Fig. 52.3 and Table 52.2.)

PENICILLINS

The remarkable antibacterial effects of systemic penicillin in humans were clearly demonstrated in 1941. A small amount of **penicillin**, extracted laboriously from crude cultures in the laboratories of the Dunn School of Pathology in Oxford, was given to a desperately ill policeman with septicaemia and multiple abscesses. Although sulfonamides were available, they would have had no effect in the presence of pus. Intravenous injections of **penicillin** were given every 3 h. All of the patient's urine was collected, and each day the bulk of the excreted **penicillin** was extracted and reused. After 5 days, the patient's condition was vastly improved, and there was obvious resolution of the abscesses. Furthermore, there seemed to be no toxic effects of the drug. Unfortunately, when the supply of **penicillin** was finally exhausted his condition gradually deteriorated and he died a month later.

Penicillins, often combined with other antibiotics, remain crucially important in antibacterial chemotherapy, but regrettably they are destroyed by bacterial *amidases* and *β-lactamases* (*penicillinases*) which limits their effectiveness. This is one of the principal types of antibiotic resistance.

Clinical uses of the penicillins

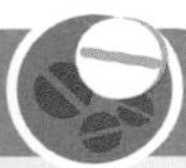

- Penicillins are given by mouth or, in more severe infections, intravenously, and often in combination with other antibiotics.
- Uses are for sensitive organisms and may (but may not: individual sensitivity testing is often appropriate depending on local conditions) include:
  - *bacterial meningitis* (e.g. caused by *Neisseria meningitidis*, *Streptococcus pneumoniae*): **benzylpenicillin**, high doses intravenously;
  - *bone* and *joint infections* (e.g. with *Staphylococcus aureus*): **flucloxacillin**;
  - *skin* and *soft tissue infections* (e.g. with *Streptococcus pyogenes* or *S. aureus*): **benzylpenicillin**, **flucloxacillin**; animal bites: **co-amoxiclav**;
  - *pharyngitis* (from *S. pyogenes*): **phenoxymethylpenicillin**;
  - *otitis media* (organisms commonly include *S. pyogenes*, *Haemophilus influenzae*): **amoxicillin**;
  - *bronchitis* (mixed infections common): **amoxicillin**;
  - *pneumonia*: **amoxicillin**;
  - *urinary tract infections* (e.g. with *Escherichia coli*): **amoxicillin**;
  - *gonorrhoea*: **amoxicillin** (plus **probenecid**);
  - *syphilis*: **procaine benzylpenicillin**;
  - *endocarditis* (e.g. with *Streptococcus viridans* or *Enterococcus faecalis*): high-dose intravenous **benzylpenicillin** sometimes with an aminoglycoside;
  - serious infections with *P. aeruginosa*: **ticarcillin**, **piperacillin.**

This list is not exhaustive. In severe infection, especially sepsis, treatment with penicillins, often in combination with an aminoglycoside, is often started empirically while awaiting the results of laboratory tests to identify the organism and determine its antibiotic susceptibility.

Mechanisms of action

All β-lactam antibiotics interfere with the synthesis of the bacterial cell wall peptidoglycan. After attachment to **penicillin**-binding proteins on bacteria (there may be seven or more types in different organisms), they inhibit the transpeptidation enzyme that cross-links the peptide chains attached to the backbone of the peptidoglycan.

The final bactericidal event is the inactivation of an inhibitor of autolytic enzymes in the cell wall, leading to lysis of the bacterium. Some organisms, referred to as 'tolerant', have defective autolytic enzymes in which case lysis does not occur in response to the drug. Resistance to **penicillin** may result from a number of different causes and is discussed in detail in Chapter 51.

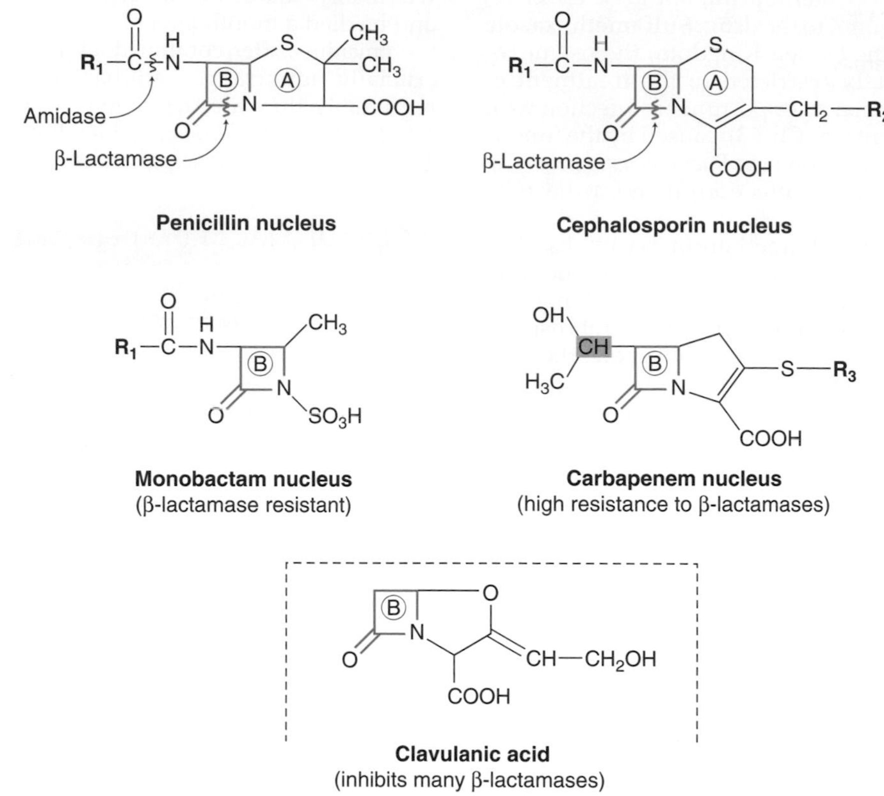

Penicillin nucleus

Cephalosporin nucleus

Monobactam nucleus
(β-lactamase resistant)

Carbapenem nucleus
(high resistance to β-lactamases)

Clavulanic acid
(inhibits many β-lactamases)

Fig. 52.3 Basic structures of four groups of β-lactam antibiotics and clavulanic acid. The structures illustrate the β-lactam ring (marked B; outlined in orange) and the sites of action of bacterial enzymes that inactivate these antibiotics (*A*, thiazolidine ring). Various substituents are added at R1, R2 and R3 to produce agents with different properties. In carbapenems, the stereochemical configuration of the part of the β-lactam ring shown shaded in *orange* here is different from the corresponding part of the penicillin and cephalosporin molecules; this is probably the basis of the β-lactamase resistance of the carbapenems. The β-lactam ring of clavulanic acid is thought to bind strongly to β-lactamase, meanwhile protecting other β-lactams from the enzyme.

Types of penicillin and their antimicrobial activity

The first penicillins were the naturally occurring **benzylpenicillin (penicillin G)** and its congeners, including **phenoxymethylpenicillin (penicillin V)**. **Benzylpenicillin** is active against a wide range of organisms and is still the drug of first choice for many infections (see clinical box). Its main drawbacks are inactivation by gastric acid and hence generally poor absorption in the GI tract (which means it must be given by injection).

Semisynthetic penicillins, incorporating different side-chains attached to the penicillin nucleus (at R1 in Fig. 52.3), include β-lactamase-resistant penicillins (e.g. **meticillin**,[3] **flucloxacillin, temocillin**) and broad-spectrum penicillins (e.g. **ampicillin, amoxicillin**). Extended-spectrum penicillins (e.g. **ticarcillin, piperacillin**) with activity against *Pseudomonas* have gone some way to overcoming the problem of serious infections caused by *P. aeruginosa*. **Amoxicillin** and **ticarcillin** are sometimes given in combination with the β-lactamase inhibitor **clavulanic** acid (e.g. **co-amoxiclav**). **Pivmecillinam** is a prodrug of **mecillinam**, which also has a wide spectrum of action.

Pharmacokinetic aspects. Oral absorption of penicillins varies, depending on their stability in acid and their adsorption to foodstuffs in the gut. Penicillins can also be given by intravenous injection. Preparations for intramuscular injection are also available, including slow-release preparations such as **benzathine benzylpenicillin** which is useful for treating syphilis since *Treponema pallidum* is a very slowly dividing organism. Intrathecal administration of **benzylpenicillin** (used historically to treat meningitis) is no longer used as penicillin is not excluded by the inflamed blood–brain barrier (see Ch. 9), and overdosage via the intrathecal route causes convulsions.[4]

The penicillins are widely distributed in other body fluids, passing into joints; into pleural and pericardial cavities; into bile, saliva and milk and across the placenta. Being lipid-insoluble, they do not enter mammalian cells.

[3]**Meticillin** (previous name: **methicillin**) was the first β-lactamase-resistant **penicillin**. It is not now used clinically because it was associated with interstitial nephritis, but is remembered in the acronym 'MRSA' – **meticillin**-resistant *S. aureus*, which are resistant to other β-lactamase-resistant penicillins as well as **meticillin**.

[4]Indeed, penicillins applied topically to the cortex are used to induce convulsions in an animal model of epilepsy (see Ch. 46).

Table 52.2 Antibiotics which inhibit bacterial wall or membrane synthesis

Site of action	Family	Type	Examples	Typical target organism
Bacterial membrane or cell wall/ peptidoglycan synthesis (Generally bactericidal)	β-Lactams	Penicillins	Benzylpenicillin, phenoxymethylpenicillin	Overall, mainly gram-positive spp.; some gram-negative spp.
			Penicillinase-resistant penicillins Flucloxacillin, temocillin	Used for staphylococcal infections
			Broad-spectrum penicillins Amoxicillin, ampicillin	A wide range of gram-positive and gram-negative spp.
			Antipseudomonal penicillins Piperacillin, ticarcillin (used with β-lactamase inhibitors)	Selected gram-negative spp., especially *P. aeruginosa*
		Mecillinams	Pivmecillinam	Mainly gram-negative spp.
		Cephalosporins	Cefaclor, cefadroxil, cefalexin, cefixime, cefotaxime, cefradine, ceftaroline, ceftazidime, ceftriaxone, cefuroxime	Broad spectrum of activity against gram-negative and positive spp.
		Carbapenems	Ertapenem, imipenem, meropenem	Many gram-negative and positive spp. Some anaerobes
		Monobactams	Aztreonam	Gram-negative aerobes
	Glyco-/ Lipopeptides	–	Vancomycin, teicoplanin, telavancin, dalbavancin, and daptomycin (actually a lipopeptide)	Many gram-positive spp. Including MRSA
	Phosphonic acids	–	Fosfomycin	Many gram-positive and gram-negative spp. Treatment of UTI
Bacterial outer cell membrane structure (Generally bactericidal)	**Polymyxins**	–	Colistitin (polymyxins B and E)	Gram-negative spp.

Drug mixtures (e.g. co-fluampicil – flucloxacillin with ampicillin) are not shown.
MRSA, Methicillin-resistant staphylococcus aureus; *UTI*, urinary tract infection.
Sources: BNF (2021) and others.

Elimination of most penicillins occurs rapidly and is mainly renal, 90% being through tubular secretion. The relatively short plasma half-life is a potential problem in the clinical use of **benzylpenicillin**, although because **penicillin** works by preventing cell wall synthesis in dividing organisms, intermittent rather than continuous exposure to the drug can be an advantage.

Unwanted effects. Penicillins are relatively free from direct toxic effects (other than their proconvulsant effect when given intrathecally). The main unwanted effects are hypersensitivity reactions caused by the degradation products of penicillin, which combine with host protein and become antigenic. Rashes and fever are common; a delayed type of serum sickness occurs infrequently. Much more serious is *acute anaphylactic shock* which, although rare, may be fatal. When given orally, penicillins, particularly the broad-spectrum type, also alter the bacterial flora in the gut. This very commonly causes diarrhoea, and predisposes to suprainfection by other, ***penicillin****-insensitive*, microorganisms leading less commonly to serious problems such as *pseudomembranous colitis* (caused by *Clostridium difficile*; see later).

CEPHALOSPORINS AND CEPHAMYCINS

First isolated from fungi in seawater near a sewage outlet in Sardinia, cephalosporins and cephamycins are also β-lactam antibiotics and have the same mechanism of action as penicillins. Semisynthetic broad-spectrum cephalosporins have been produced by addition, to the cephalosporin C nucleus, of different side-chains at R_1 and/or R_2 (see Fig. 52.3). This group of agents is water soluble and relatively acid stable. They vary in susceptibility to β-lactamases.

Many cephalosporins and cephamycins are now available for clinical use. Resistance to this group of drugs has increased because of plasmid-encoded or chromosomal β-lactamase. The latter is present in nearly all gram-negative bacteria, and it is more active in hydrolysing cephalosporins than penicillins. In several organisms a single mutation can result in high-level constitutive production of this enzyme. Resistance also occurs when there is decreased penetration of the drug as a result of alterations to outer membrane proteins, or mutations of the binding-site proteins.

Pharmacokinetic aspects. Some cephalosporins are given orally, but most are given parenterally, intramuscularly (which may be painful) or intravenously. After absorption, they are widely distributed in the body and some, such as **cefotaxime**, **cefuroxime** and **ceftriaxone**, cross the blood–brain barrier. Excretion is mostly via the kidney, largely by tubular secretion, but 40% of **ceftriaxone** is eliminated in the bile.

Unwanted effects. Hypersensitivity reactions, very similar to those seen with penicillin, may occur, and there may be some cross-sensitivity; about 10% of penicillin-sensitive individuals will also have allergic reactions to cephalosporins. Nephrotoxicity has been reported (especially with **cefradine**), as has drug-induced alcohol intolerance – a ***disulfiram***-like effect (see Ch. 50) because the methylthiotetrazole moiety inhibits aldehyde dehydrogenase. Diarrhoea is common and can be due to *C. difficile*.

Clinical uses of the cephalosporins

Cephalosporins are used to treat infections caused by sensitive organisms. As with other antibiotics, patterns of sensitivity vary geographically, and treatment is often started empirically. Many different kinds of infection may be treated, including:

- *septicaemia* (e.g. **cefuroxime**, **cefotaxime**)
- *pneumonia* caused by susceptible organisms
- *meningitis* (e.g. **ceftriaxone**, **cefotaxime**)
- *biliary tract infection*
- *urinary tract infection* (especially in pregnancy or in patients unresponsive to other drugs)
- *sinusitis* (e.g. **cefadroxil**)

OTHER β-LACTAM ANTIBIOTICS

Carbapenems and monobactams (see Fig. 52.3) were developed to deal with β-lactamase-producing gram-negative organisms resistant to penicillins. Most carbapenems are not orally active and are used only in special situations.

CARBAPENEMS

Imipenem, an example of a carbapenem, acts in the same way as the other β-lactams. It has a very broad spectrum of antimicrobial activity, being active against many aerobic and anaerobic gram-positive and gram-negative organisms. However, many of the '**meticillin**-resistant' staphylococci are less susceptible, and resistant strains of *P. aeruginosa* have emerged during therapy. Resistance to **imipenem** was initially low but is increasing as some organisms now have chromosomal genes that code for **imipenem**-hydrolysing β-lactamases.

Imipenem is sometimes given together with **cilastatin**, which inhibits its inactivation by renal enzymes. **Meropenem** is similar but is not metabolised by the kidney. **Ertapenem** has a broad spectrum of antibacterial actions but is licensed only for a limited range of indications.

Unwanted effects are generally similar to those seen with other β-lactams, nausea and vomiting being the most frequently seen. Neurotoxicity can occur with high plasma concentrations.

MONOBACTAMS

The main monobactam is **aztreonam**, which is resistant to most β-lactamases. It is given by injection and has a plasma half-life of 2 h. **Aztreonam** has an unusual spectrum of activity and is effective only against gram-negative aerobic bacilli such as *Pseudomonas* species, *Neisseria meningitidis* and *Haemophilus influenzae*. It has no action against gram-positive organisms or anaerobes.

Unwanted effects are, in general, similar to those of other β-lactam antibiotics, but this agent does not necessarily cross-react immunologically with **penicillin** and its products and does not usually cause allergic reactions in **penicillin**-sensitive individuals.

β-Lactam antibiotics

Bactericidal because they inhibit peptidoglycan synthesis.

Penicillins

- The first choice for many infections.
- **Benzylpenicillin**:
  - given by injection, has a short half-life and is destroyed by β-lactamases;
  - spectrum: gram-positive and gram-negative cocci and some gram-negative bacteria;
  - many staphylococci are now resistant.
- β-Lactamase-resistant penicillins (e.g. **flucloxacillin**):
  - given orally;
  - spectrum: as for **benzylpenicillin**;
  - many staphylococci are now resistant.
- Broad-spectrum penicillins (e.g. **amoxicillin**):
  - given orally; they are destroyed by β-lactamases;
  - spectrum: as for **benzylpenicillin** (although less potent); they are also active against gram-negative bacteria.
- Extended-spectrum penicillins (e.g. **ticarcillin**):
  - given orally; they are susceptible to β-lactamases;
  - spectrum: as for broad-spectrum penicillins; they are also active against pseudomonads.
- Unwanted effects of penicillins: mainly hypersensitivities.
- A combination of **clavulanic acid** plus **amoxicillin** or **ticarcillin** is effective against many β-lactamase-producing organisms.

Cephalosporins and cephamycins

- Second choice for many infections.
- Oral drugs (e.g. **cefaclor**) are used in urinary infections.
- Parenteral drugs (e.g. **cefuroxime**, which is active against *S. aureus*, *H. influenzae*, Enterobacteriaceae).
- Unwanted effects: mainly hypersensitivities.

Carbapenems

- **Imipenem** is a broad-spectrum antibiotic.
- **Imipenem** is used with **cilastatin**, which prevents its breakdown in the kidney.

Monobactams

- **Aztreonam**: active only against gram-negative aerobic bacteria and resistant to most β-lactamases.

(See Table 52.2 for further examples.)

OTHER ANTIBIOTICS THAT INHIBIT BACTERIAL CELL WALL PEPTIDOGLYCAN SYNTHESIS

GLYCOPEPTIDES

Vancomycin is a glycopeptide antibiotic, and **teicoplanin** is similar but longer lasting. **Vancomycin** inhibits cell wall synthesis. It is effective mainly against gram-positive bacteria. **Vancomycin** is not absorbed from the gut and is only given by the oral route for treatment of GI infection with *C. difficile*.

The main clinical use of **vancomycin** is the treatment of **meticillin**-resistant *Staphylococcus aureus* (MRSA). It is often the drug of last resort for this condition, an alarming consideration since **vancomycin**-resistant *S. aureus* (VRSA) has now emerged. **Vancomycin** is also valuable in some other serious infections including severe staphylococcal infections in patients allergic to both penicillins and cephalosporins.

Pharmacokinetic aspects. For systemic use, it is given intravenously and has a plasma half-life of about 8 h.

Unwanted effects include fever, rashes and phlebitis at the infusion site. Ototoxicity and nephrotoxicity can occur, and hypersensitivity reactions are occasionally seen.

Daptomycin is a lipopeptide antibacterial with a similar spectrum of actions to **vancomycin**. It is used, in combination with other drugs, for the treatment of MRSA. **Telavancin** (another lipopeptide) is also active against MRSA and has a longer duration of action than **vancomycin**.

POLYMYXINS

The polymyxin antibiotics include **polymyxins B** and **E**, **colistitin** and **colistimethate** (its sulphomethate salt). They have cationic detergent properties and disrupt the bacterial outer cell membrane. They have a selective, rapidly bactericidal action on gram-negative bacilli, especially pseudomonads and coliform organisms, and can bind to, and neutralise, some bacterial endotoxins. They are increasingly used to treat multidrug-resistant (MDR) organisms.

Pharmacokinetic aspects. They are not absorbed from the GI tract and must therefore be given systemically. Clinical use of these drugs is limited by their toxicity and is generally confined to intestinal infections and topical treatment of ear, eye or skin infections caused by susceptible organisms.

Unwanted effects include neurotoxicity and nephrotoxicity which may be serious.

Also related to this group is **fosfomycin,** a small organic molecule originally found in *Streptomyces*, which blocks peptidoglycan synthesis by inactivating a key enzyme *Mur A*. It has a good spectrum of activity but, currently, fairly limited use in the treatment of urinary tract infections.

Miscellaneous antibacterial agents that prevent cell wall or membrane synthesis

- *Glycopeptide antibiotics.* **Vancomycin** is bactericidal, acting by inhibiting cell wall synthesis. It is used intravenously for multiresistant staphylococcal infections and orally for pseudomembranous colitis. Unwanted effects include ototoxicity and nephrotoxicity.
- *Polymyxins* (e.g. **colistimethate**). By disrupting bacterial cell membranes these are bactericidal. They are highly neurotoxic and nephrotoxic and are only used topically. (See Table 52.2 for further examples.)

ANTIMICROBIAL AGENTS AFFECTING BACTERIAL PROTEIN SYNTHESIS

(See Table 52.3.)

TETRACYCLINES

The tetracyclines are broad-spectrum antibiotics. The group includes **tetracycline**, **oxytetracycline**, **demeclocycline**, **lymecycline**, **doxycycline**, **minocycline** and **tigecycline**.

Clinical uses of tetracyclines

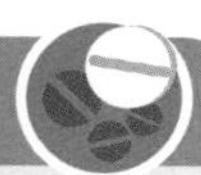

- The use of tetracyclines declined because of widespread drug resistance, but has staged a comeback, e.g. for respiratory infections, as resistance has receded with reduced use. Most members of the group are microbiologically similar; **doxycycline** is given once daily and may be used in patients with renal impairment. Uses (sometimes in combination with other antibiotics) include:
  - rickettsial and chlamydial infections, brucellosis, anthrax and Lyme disease;
  - as useful second choice, for example in patients with allergies, for several infections (see Table 52.3), including mycoplasma and leptospira;
  - respiratory tract infections (e.g. exacerbations of chronic bronchitis, community-acquired pneumonia);
  - acne;
  - inappropriate secretion of antidiuretic hormone (e.g. by some malignant lung tumours), causing hyponatraemia: **demeclocycline** inhibits the action of this hormone by an entirely distinct action from its antibacterial effect (see Ch. 33).

Mechanism of action

Following uptake into susceptible organisms by active transport, tetracyclines exert a bacteriostatic effect by inhibiting protein synthesis as explained in Chapter 51.

Antibacterial spectrum

The spectrum of antimicrobial activity of the tetracyclines is very wide and includes gram-positive and gram-negative bacteria, *Mycoplasma, Rickettsia, Chlamydia* spp., spirochaetes and some protozoa (e.g. amoebae). **Minocycline** is also effective against *N. meningitidis* and has been used to eradicate this organism from the nasopharynx of carriers. However, widespread resistance to these agents has decreased their usefulness. This is transmitted mainly by plasmids and, because the genes controlling resistance to tetracyclines are closely associated with genes for resistance to other antibiotics, organisms may develop resistance to many drugs simultaneously.

Pharmacokinetic aspects. The tetracyclines are generally given orally but can also be administered parenterally. **Minocycline** and **doxycycline** are well absorbed orally. The absorption of most other tetracyclines is irregular and incomplete but is improved in the absence of food. Because tetracyclines chelate metal ions (calcium, magnesium, iron, aluminium), forming non-absorbable complexes, absorption is decreased in the presence of milk, certain antacids and iron preparations.

Table 52.3 Antibiotics which inhibit bacterial protein or DNA synthesis

Site of action	Family	Examples	Typical target organism
Bacterial protein synthesis (multiple mechanisms inhibited including initiation, transpeptidation and translocation; see Ch. 51) (Generally bacteriostatic)	**Tetracyclines**	Demeclocycline, doxycycline, lymecycline, minocycline, oxytetracycline, tetracycline tigecycline	Broad-spectrum activity against many gram-negative and gram-positive spp.
	Aminoglycosides	Amikacin, gentamicin, neomycin, streptomycin, tobramycin	Many gram-negative, some gram-positive spp.
	Macrolides	Azithromycin, clarithromycin, erythromycin	Similar to penicillin
	Oxazolidinones	Linezolid, tedizolid	Gram-positive spp. including MRSA
	Lincosamides	Clindamycin	Gram-positive spp. Many anaerobes
	Amphenicols	Chloramphenicol	Broad-spectrum activity against gram-negative and gram-positive spp.
	Streptogramins	Quinupristin – dalfopristin	Gram-positive spp. Especially *Enterococcus faecium*
	Steroidals	Fusidic acid	Narrow spectrum Gram-positive spp.
Bacterial DNA synthesis, structure or replication (Generally bacteriostatic)	**Quinolones**	Ciprofloxacin, levofloxacin, moxifloxacin, nalidixic acid, norfloxacin, ofloxacin	Gram-negative and gram-positive spp.

MRSA, Methicillin-resistant staphylococcus aureus.
Sources: BNF (2021) and others.

Unwanted effects. The commonest unwanted effects are GI disturbances caused initially by direct irritation and later by modification of the gut flora. Vitamin B complex deficiency can occur, as can suprainfection. Because they chelate Ca^{2+}, tetracyclines are deposited in growing bones and teeth, causing staining and sometimes dental hypoplasia and bone deformities. They should therefore not be given to children, pregnant women or nursing mothers. Another hazard to pregnant women is hepatotoxicity. Phototoxicity (sensitisation to sunlight) has also been seen, particularly with **demeclocycline**. **Minocycline** can produce vestibular disturbances (dizziness and nausea). High doses of tetracyclines can decrease protein synthesis in host cells, an anti-anabolic effect that may result in renal damage. Long-term therapy can cause disturbances of the bone marrow.

CHLORAMPHENICOL

Chloramphenicol was originally isolated from cultures of *Streptomyces*. It inhibits bacterial protein synthesis by inhibiting peptide bond formation and chain termination (Ch. 51).

Antibacterial spectrum

Chloramphenicol has a wide spectrum of antimicrobial activity, including gram-negative and gram-positive organisms and rickettsiae. It is bacteriostatic for most organisms but kills *H. influenzae*. Resistance, caused by the production of *chloramphenicol acetyltransferase*, is plasmid-mediated.

Pharmacokinetic aspects. Given orally, chloramphenicol is rapidly and completely absorbed and reaches its maximum concentration in the plasma within 2 h. It can also be given parenterally. The drug is widely distributed throughout the tissues and body fluids including the CSF. Its half-life is approximately 2 h. About 10% is excreted unchanged in the urine, and the remainder is inactivated in the liver.

Unwanted effects. The most important unwanted effect of **chloramphenicol** is severe, idiosyncratic depression of the bone marrow, resulting in *pancytopenia* (a decrease in all blood cell elements) – an effect that, although rare, can occur even with low doses in susceptible individuals. **Chloramphenicol** must be used with great care in newborns, with monitoring of plasma concentrations, because inadequate inactivation and excretion of the drug can result in the 'grey baby syndrome' – vomiting, diarrhoea, flaccidity, low temperature and an ashen-grey colour – which carries 40% mortality. Hypersensitivity reactions can occur, as can GI disturbances secondary to alteration of the intestinal microbial flora.

Clinical uses of chloramphenicol

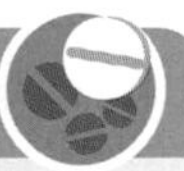

- Systemic use should be reserved for serious infections in which the benefit of the drug outweighs its uncommon but serious haematological toxicity. Such uses may include:
  - infections caused by *H. influenzae* resistant to other drugs;
  - *meningitis* in patients in whom penicillin cannot be used;
  - *typhoid fever*, but **ciprofloxacin** or **amoxicillin** and **co-trimoxazole** are similarly effective and less toxic.
- Topical use: safe and effective in bacterial conjunctivitis.

AMINOGLYCOSIDES

The aminoglycosides are a group of antibiotics of complex chemical structure, resembling each other in antimicrobial activity, pharmacokinetic characteristics and toxicity. The main agents are **gentamicin**, **streptomycin**, **amikacin**, **tobramycin** and **neomycin**.

Mechanism of action

There are several possible sites of action by which aminoglycosides inhibit bacterial protein synthesis. Their penetration through the cell membrane of the bacterium depends partly on oxygen-dependent active transport by a polyamine carrier system (which, incidentally, is blocked by **chloramphenicol**) and they have minimal action against anaerobic organisms. The effect of the aminoglycosides is bactericidal and is enhanced by agents that interfere with cell wall synthesis (e.g. penicillins).

Resistance

Resistance to aminoglycosides is becoming a problem. It occurs through several different mechanisms, the most important being inactivation by microbial enzymes, of which nine or more are known. **Amikacin** was designed to be a poor substrate for these enzymes, but some organisms can inactivate this agent as well. Resistance as a result of failure of penetration can be largely overcome by the concomitant use of **penicillin** and/or **vancomycin**, at the cost of an increased risk of severe adverse effects.

Antibacterial spectrum

The aminoglycosides are effective against many aerobic gram-negative and some gram-positive organisms. They are most widely used against gram-negative enteric organisms and in sepsis. They may be given together with a penicillin in streptococcal infections and those caused by *Listeria* spp. and *P. aeruginosa*. **Gentamicin** is the aminoglycoside most commonly used, although **tobramycin** is slightly more active against *P. aeruginosa* infections. **Amikacin** has the widest antimicrobial spectrum and can be effective in infections with organisms resistant to **gentamicin** and **tobramycin**. **Streptomycin**, the first aminoglycoside to be discovered, is active against *Mycobacterium tuberculosis*, and is seldom used for other indications.

Pharmacokinetic aspects. The aminoglycosides are polycations and therefore polar at neutral pH. They are not absorbed from the gastrointestinal tract and are usually given intramuscularly or intravenously. They cross the placenta but do not cross the blood–brain barrier, although high concentrations can be attained in joint and pleural fluids. The plasma half-life is 2–3 h. Elimination is by glomerular filtration in the kidney, 50%–60% of a dose being excreted unchanged within 24 h. If renal function is impaired, accumulation occurs rapidly, with a resultant increase in those toxic effects (such as ototoxicity and nephrotoxicity) that are dose related.

Unwanted effects. Serious, dose-related toxic effects, which may increase as treatment proceeds, can occur with the aminoglycosides, the main hazards being ototoxicity and nephrotoxicity. The former involves progressive damage to, and eventually destruction of, the sensory cells in the cochlea and vestibular organ of the ear. The result, usually irreversible, may manifest as vertigo, ataxia and loss of balance in the case of vestibular damage, and auditory disturbances or deafness in the case of cochlear damage. Any aminoglycoside may produce both types of effect, but **streptomycin** and **gentamicin** are more likely to interfere with vestibular function, whereas **neomycin** and **amikacin** mostly affect hearing. Ototoxicity is potentiated by the concomitant use of other ototoxic drugs (e.g. loop diuretics, see Ch. 29, and **vancomycin,** see earlier) and susceptibility is genetically determined via mitochondrial DNA (see Ch. 12). Unlike nephrotoxicity, regular monitoring of plasma aminoglycoside concentration does not mitigate the risk of ototoxicity reliably.

The nephrotoxicity consists of damage to the kidney tubules and may necessitate dialysis, although function usually recovers if administration ceases as soon as renal toxicity is detected. Nephrotoxicity is more likely to occur in patients with pre-existing renal disease or in conditions in which urine volume is reduced, and concomitant use of other nephrotoxic agents (e.g. first-generation cephalosporins, **vancomycin**) increases the risk. As the elimination of these drugs is almost entirely renal, this nephrotoxic action can impair their own excretion and a vicious cycle may develop. Plasma concentrations should be monitored repeatedly, and the dose or dose interval adjusted accordingly.

A rare but serious toxic reaction is paralysis caused by long-lasting neuromuscular blockade. This is usually seen only if the agents are given concurrently with neuromuscular-blocking agents. It results from inhibition of the Ca^{2+} uptake necessary for the exocytotic release of acetylcholine (see Ch. 14).

MACROLIDES

The term *macrolide* relates to a structural feature of this group, a many-membered lactone ring to which one or more deoxy sugars are attached. The main macrolide and related antibiotics are **erythromycin**, **clarithromycin** and **azithromycin**. **Telithromycin** is of minor utility.

Mechanism of action

The macrolides inhibit bacterial protein synthesis by acting at different sites in the synthesis of new bacterial proteins (see Ch. 51).

Antimicrobial spectrum

The antimicrobial spectrum of **erythromycin** is very similar to that of **penicillin**, and it is a safe and effective alternative for **penicillin**-sensitive patients. **Erythromycin** is effective against gram-positive bacteria and spirochaetes but not against most gram-negative organisms, exceptions being *Neisseria gonorrhoeae* and, to a lesser extent, *H. influenzae*. *M. pneumoniae*, *Legionella* spp. and some chlamydial organisms are also susceptible (see Table 52.3). Resistance can occur and results from a plasmid-controlled alteration of the binding site for **erythromycin** on the bacterial ribosome.

Azithromycin is less active than **erythromycin** against gram-positive bacteria but is considerably more effective against *H. influenzae* and may be more active against *Legionella*. It can be used to treat *Toxoplasma gondii*, as it kills the cysts. **Clarithromycin** is as active, and its metabolite is twice as active, against *H. influenzae* as **erythromycin**. It is also effective against *Mycobacterium avium-intracellulare* (which can infect immunologically compromised individuals and elderly patients with chronic lung disease), and it may also be useful in leprosy and against *Helicobacter pylori* (see Ch. 30). Both these macrolides are also effective in *Lyme disease*.

Pharmacokinetic aspects. The macrolides are administered orally or parenterally, although intravenous injections can cause local thrombophlebitis. They diffuse readily into most tissues but do not cross the blood–brain barrier, and there is poor penetration into synovial fluid. The plasma half-life of **erythromycin** is about 90 min; that of **clarithromycin** is three times longer, and that of **azithromycin** is 8–16 times longer. Macrolides enter and indeed are concentrated within phagocytes – **azithromycin** concentrations in phagocyte lysosomes can be 40 times higher than in the blood – and they can enhance intracellular killing of bacteria by phagocytes.

Erythromycin is partly inactivated in the liver; **azithromycin** is more resistant to inactivation, and **clarithromycin** is converted to an active metabolite. Inhibition of the P450 cytochrome system by these agents can affect the bioavailability of other drugs leading to clinically important interactions, for example, with **theophylline** (see Ch. 12). The major route of elimination is in the bile.

Unwanted effects. GI disturbances are common and unpleasant but not serious. With **erythromycin**, the following have also been reported: hypersensitivity reactions such as rashes and fever, transient hearing disturbances and rarely, following treatment for longer than 2 weeks, cholestatic jaundice. Opportunistic infections of the GI tract or vagina can occur.

OXAZOLIDINONES

Following their discovery in the mid-1990s, the oxazolidinones were originally hailed as the 'first truly new class of antibacterial agents to reach the marketplace in several decades' (Zurenko et al., 2001). The group inhibits bacterial protein synthesis by a novel mechanism: inhibition of *N*-formylmethionyl-tRNA binding to the 70S ribosome. **Linezolid** was the first member of this new antibiotic family to be introduced. It is active against a wide variety of gram-positive bacteria and is particularly useful for the treatment of drug-resistant bacteria such as MRSA, **penicillin**-resistant *Streptococcus pneumoniae* and **vancomycin**-resistant enterococci. The drug is also effective against some anaerobes, such as *C. difficile*. Most common gram-negative organisms are not susceptible to the drug. **Linezolid** can be used to treat pneumonia, septicaemia and skin and soft tissue infections. Its use is restricted to serious bacterial infections where other antibiotics have failed, and there have so far been few reports of resistance.

Unwanted effects include thrombocytopenia, diarrhoea, nausea and, rarely, rash and dizziness. **Linezolid** is a non-selective inhibitor of monoamine oxidase, and appropriate precautions need to be observed (see Ch. 48).

FUSIDIC ACID

Fusidic acid is a narrow-spectrum steroidal antibiotic active mainly against gram-positive bacteria. It acts by inhibiting bacterial protein synthesis, but resistance commonly emerges if it is used as a single agent. It is used in combination with other anti-staphylococcal agents in staphylococcal sepsis, and also used topically for staphylococcal infections (e.g. as eye drops or cream).

Pharmacokinetic aspects. As the sodium salt, the drug is well absorbed from the gut and is distributed widely in the tissues. Some is excreted in the bile and some metabolised.

Unwanted effects such as GI disturbances are fairly common. Skin eruptions and jaundice can occur. Resistance occurs if it is used systemically as a single agent, so it is always combined with other antibacterial drugs when used systemically.

STREPTOGRAMINS

Dalfopristin and **quinupristin** are cyclic peptides used in combination. They inhibit bacterial protein synthesis by binding to the 50S subunit of the bacterial ribosome. Other members of the family include **pristinamycin** and **virginiamycin**. **Dalfopristin** changes the structure of the ribosome so as to promote the binding of **quinupristin**. Individually, they exhibit only very modest bacteriostatic activity, but combined together as an intravenous injection they have good activity against many gram-positive bacteria. The combination is used to treat serious infections, usually where no other antibacterial is suitable being effective, for example, against MRSA and **vancomycin**-resistant *Enterococcus faecium*.

Pharmacokinetic aspects. Both drugs undergo extensive first-pass hepatic metabolism and must therefore be given by intravenous infusion. The half-life of each compound is 1–2 h.

Unwanted effects include inflammation and pain at the infusion site, arthralgia, myalgia and nausea, vomiting and diarrhoea. To date, resistance to **quinupristin** and **dalfopristin** does not seem to be a major problem.

CLINDAMYCIN

The lincosamide **clindamycin** is active against gram-positive cocci, including many penicillin-resistant staphylococci and many anaerobic bacteria such as *Bacteroides* spp. It acts in the same way as macrolides and **chloramphenicol**. In addition to its use in infections caused by *Bacteroides* organisms, it is used to treat staphylococcal infections of bones and joints. It is also given topically, as eye drops, for staphylococcal conjunctivitis and used as an anti-protozoal drug (see Ch. 55).

Unwanted effects consist mainly of GI disturbances, ranging from uncomfortable diarrhoea to potentially lethal pseudomembranous colitis, caused by a toxin-forming *C. difficile*.[5]

---

[5]This may also occur with broad-spectrum penicillins and cephalosporins as a result of cross-infection (usually within hospital) by *C. difficile* in patients susceptible because of the disturbance caused to their gut microbiome by the broad-spectrum antibiotic. Hand washing by staff with soap and water can prevent this (alcohol rub is less effective as it does not kill bacterial spores).

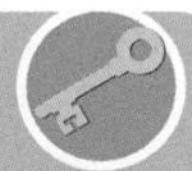

Antimicrobial agents affecting bacterial protein synthesis

- *Tetracyclines* (e.g. **minocycline**). These are orally active, bacteriostatic, broad-spectrum antibiotics. Resistance is increasing. GI disorders are common. They also chelate calcium and are deposited in growing bone. They are contraindicated in children and pregnant women.
- ***Chloramphenicol.*** This is an orally active, bacteriostatic, broad-spectrum antibiotic. Serious toxic effects are possible, including bone marrow depression and 'grey baby syndrome'. Systemic use should be reserved for life-threatening infections.
- *Aminoglycosides* (e.g. **gentamicin**). These are given by injection. They are bactericidal, broad-spectrum antibiotics (but with low activity against anaerobes, streptococci and pneumococci). Resistance is increasing. The main unwanted effects are dose-related nephrotoxicity and ototoxicity. Serum levels should be monitored. (**Streptomycin** is an aminoglycoside used to treat tuberculosis.)
- *Macrolides* (e.g. **erythromycin**). Can be given orally and parenterally. They are bactericidal/bacteriostatic. The antibacterial spectrum is the same as for **penicillin**. **Erythromycin** can cause jaundice. Newer agents are **clarithromycin** and **azithromycin.**
- *Lincosamides* (e.g. **clindamycin**). Can be given orally and parenterally. It can cause pseudomembranous colitis.
- *Streptogramins* (e.g. **quinupristin/dalfopristin**). Given by intravenous infusion as a combination. Considerably less effective when administered separately. Active against several strains of drug-resistant bacteria.
- ***Fusidic acid.*** This is an anti-staphylococcal antibiotic that acts by inhibiting protein synthesis. It penetrates bone. Unwanted effects include GI disorders. It is used systemically in combination with other anti-staphylococcal drugs (e.g. **flucloxacillin**), and topically for staphylococcal conjunctivitis.
- ***Linezolid.*** Given orally or by intravenous injection. Active against several strains of drug-resistant bacteria. (See Table 52.3 for further examples.)

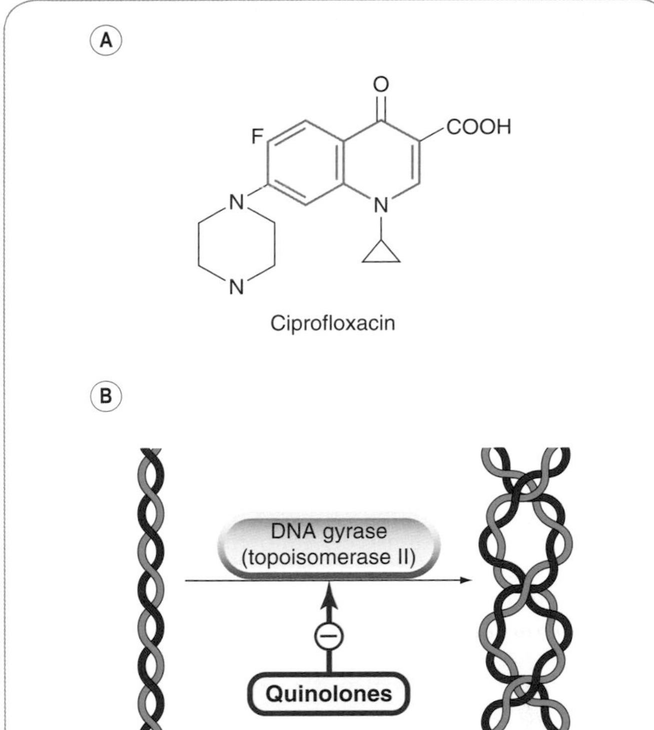

Fig. 52.4 A simplified diagram of the mechanism of action of the fluoroquinolones. (A) An example of a quinolone (the quinolone moiety is shown in *orange*). (B) Schematic diagram of *(left)* the double helix and *(right)* the double helix in supercoiled form (see also Ch. 51). In essence, the DNA gyrase unwinds the RNA-induced positive supercoil (not shown) and introduces a negative supercoil.

ANTIMICROBIAL AGENTS AFFECTING TOPOISOMERASE

QUINOLONES

The quinolones include the broad-spectrum agents **ciprofloxacin**, **levofloxacin**, **ofloxacin**, **norfloxacin** and **moxifloxacin** as well as **nalidixic acid**, a narrow-spectrum drug used in urinary tract infections. Most are fluorinated (fluoroquinolones). These agents inhibit *topoisomerase II*, a bacterial DNA gyrase that produces a negative supercoil in DNA and thus permits transcription or replication (see Fig. 52.4 and Table 52.3).

Antibacterial spectrum and clinical use

Ciprofloxacin is widely used and is typical of the group. It is a broad-spectrum antibiotic effective against both gram-positive and gram-negative organisms, including the Enterobacteriaceae (enteric gram-negative bacilli), many organisms resistant to penicillins, cephalosporins and aminoglycosides, and against *H. influenzae*, penicillinase-producing *N. gonorrhoeae*, *Campylobacter* spp. and pseudomonads. Of the gram-positive organisms, streptococci and pneumococci are only weakly inhibited, and there is a high incidence of staphylococcal resistance. **Ciprofloxacin** should be avoided in MRSA infections. Clinically, the fluoroquinolones are best reserved for infections with facultative and aerobic gram-negative bacilli and cocci.[6] Resistant strains of *S. aureus* and *P. aeruginosa* have emerged.

Pharmacokinetic aspects. Fluoroquinolones are well absorbed following oral administration. The drugs accumulate in several tissues, particularly in the kidney, prostate and lung. All quinolones are concentrated in phagocytes. Most fail to cross the blood–brain barrier, but **ofloxacin** does so. Aluminium and magnesium antacids interfere with the absorption of the quinolones. Elimination of **ciprofloxacin** and **norfloxacin** is partly by hepatic metabolism by P450 enzymes (which they can inhibit, giving rise to interactions

[6]When **ciprofloxacin** was introduced, clinical pharmacologists and microbiologists sensibly suggested that, to prevent emergence of resistance, it should be reserved for organisms already refractory to the effects of other drugs. However, by 1989 it was already estimated that it was prescribed for 1 in 44 of Americans, so it would seem that the horse had not only left the stable but had bolted into the therapeutic blue!

with other drugs) and partly by renal excretion. **Ofloxacin** is excreted in the urine.

Unwanted effects. In hospitals, infection with *C. difficile* may prove hazardous. *Tendonitis* is commoner in children and adults over 60 years old and can lead to tendon rupture so treatment must be discontinued immediately if tendonitis is suspected; co-treatment with corticosteroids is a risk factor. There is also a risk of aortic dissection and aortic aneurysm. GI disorders are common and rashes can occur. Central nervous system (CNS) symptoms – headache and dizziness – have occurred, as have, less frequently, convulsions associated with CNS pathology or concurrent use of a non-steroidal anti-inflammatory drug (NSAID; see Ch. 25).

There is a clinically important interaction between **ciprofloxacin** and **theophylline** (through inhibition of P450 enzymes), which can lead to **theophylline** toxicity (including convulsions) in asthmatics treated with the fluoroquinolones. The topic is discussed further in Chapter 28. **Moxifloxacin** prolongs the electrocardiographic QT interval and is used extensively, following FDA guidance, as a positive control in studies in healthy volunteers examining possible effects of new drugs on cardiac repolarisation.

Antimicrobial agents affecting DNA topoisomerase II

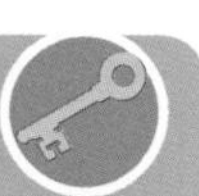

- The quinolones interfere with the supercoiling of DNA.
- **Ciprofloxacin** has a wide antibacterial spectrum, being especially active against gram-negative enteric coliform organisms, including many organisms resistant to penicillins, cephalosporins and aminoglycosides; it is also effective against *H. influenzae*, penicillinase-producing *N. gonorrhoeae*, *Campylobacter* spp. and pseudomonads. There is a high incidence of staphylococcal resistance.
- Unwanted effects include tendonitis, tendon rupture, rarely aortic dissection and aortic aneurysm; GI tract upsets are common, hypersensitivity reactions and, rarely, CNS disturbances can occur.
(See Table 52.3 for further examples.)

MISCELLANEOUS ANTIBACTERIAL AGENTS

Fidaxomicin was originally discovered in actinomycetes. It inhibits bacterial RNA polymerase. It is not used to treat systemic infections as it is poorly absorbed from the gut but has a role in treating *C. difficile* infections.

METRONIDAZOLE

Metronidazole was introduced as an antiprotozoal agent (see Ch. 55), but it is also active against anaerobic bacteria such as *Bacteroides*, *Clostridia* spp. and some streptococci. It is effective in the therapy of pseudomembranous colitis and is important in the treatment of serious anaerobic infections (e.g. sepsis secondary to bowel disease). It has a disulfiram-like action (see Ch. 50), so patients must avoid alcohol during treatment.

NITROFURANTOIN

Nitrofurantoin is a synthetic compound active against a range of gram-positive and gram-negative organisms. The development of resistance in susceptible organisms is rare, and there is no cross-resistance. Its mechanism of action is probably related to its ability to damage bacterial DNA.

Pharmacokinetic aspects. **Nitrofurantoin** is given orally and is rapidly and totally absorbed from the GI tract and just as rapidly excreted by the kidney. Its use is confined to the treatment of bladder infections ('cystitis') and prophylactically in the prevention of such infections in patients with recurrent cystitis.

Unwanted effects. GI disturbances are relatively common, and hypersensitivity reactions involving the skin and the bone marrow (e.g. leukopenia) can occur. Hepatotoxicity and peripheral neuropathy have been reported.

ANTIMYCOBACTERIAL AGENTS

(See Table 52.4.)

The main mycobacterial infections in humans are tuberculosis (TB) and leprosy, which are chronic infections caused by *M. tuberculosis* and *Mycobacterium leprae*, respectively. Another mycobacterial infection is *M. avium-intracellulare* (actually two organisms), which can infect some AIDS patients. A particular problem with mycobacteria is that they can survive inside macrophages after phagocytosis, unless these cells are 'activated' by cytokines produced by T-helper (Th) 1 lymphocytes (see Ch. 7). Drugs in this section are usually considered separately since some of them are specific for mycobacteria or used only to treat these infections for other reasons.

DRUGS USED TO TREAT TUBERCULOSIS

For centuries, TB was a major killer disease, but the introduction of **streptomycin** in the late 1940s followed by **isoniazid** and, in the 1960s, of **rifampicin** and **ethambutol** revolutionised therapy and TB came to be regarded as an easily treatable condition. Regrettably, this is no longer true. Strains with increased virulence or exhibiting multidrug resistance are now common (Bloom and Small, 1998), and at the time of writing, TB now causes more deaths than any other single infectious agent apart from COVID-19. Even though infection rates are falling at a rate of about 2% annually, some 10 million people fell ill with the disease in 2020 (including 1.1 million children) and there were 1.5 million deaths from the disease according to the latest WHO figures. While TB is a global disease, about 86% of new infections can be accounted for by 30 countries with India and China being the worst affected. MDR TB is common and because of an ominous synergy between mycobacteria (e.g. *M. tuberculosis*, *M. avium-intracellulare*) and HIV, infections with the latter increase the risk of catching the disease some 20-fold and about a quarter of HIV-associated deaths are caused by TB.

Treatment is usually initiated with **isoniazid**, **rifampicin**, **rifabutin**, **ethambutol** and **pyrazinamide**. Second-line drugs include **capreomycin**, **cycloserine**, **streptomycin** (rarely used for this purpose now in the United Kingdom), **clarithromycin** and **ciprofloxacin**. These are used to treat infections likely to be resistant to first-line drugs, or when the first-line agents have to be abandoned because of adverse effects. Two newer drugs, **bedaquiline** and **delamanid**, have been introduced for use in MDR cases of TB, usually in conjunction with other agents.

Table 52.4 Antibiotics with miscellaneous mechanisms of action

Site of action	Family	Examples	Typical target organism
Various unrelated mechanisms (including inhibition of membrane components and protein synthesis; see text)	**Anti-mycobacterials**	Bedaquiline, capreomycin, clofazimine, cycloserine, delamanid, dapsone, ethambutol, isoniazid, pyrazinamide, rifabutin, rifampicin[a]	Mostly used for mycobacterial infections only; e.g. *Mycobacterium tuberculosis* and *Mycobacterium leprae*
Prodrug of formaldehyde (Bacteriostatic)	**Miscellaneous**	Methenamine	Gram-negative UTIs

[a]These drugs are often used in combination.
UTI, Urinary tract infection.
Sources: BNF (2021) and others.

To decrease the probability of the emergence of resistant organisms, combination drug therapy is usually mandatory.[7] This commonly involves:

- an initial phase of treatment (about 2 months) with a combination of **isoniazid**, **rifampicin** and **pyrazinamide** (plus **ethambutol** if the organism is suspected to be resistant);
- a second, continuation phase (about 4 months) of therapy, with **isoniazid** and **rifampicin.** Longer-term treatment is needed for patients with meningitis, bone/joint involvement or drug-resistant infection.

ISONIAZID

The antibacterial activity of **isoniazid** is limited to mycobacteria. It halts the growth of resting organisms (i.e. is bacteriostatic) but can also kill dividing bacteria. It passes freely into mammalian cells and is thus effective against intracellular organisms. **Isoniazid** is a prodrug that must be activated by bacterial enzymes before it can exert its inhibitory activity on the synthesis of *mycolic acids*, important constituents of the cell wall peculiar to mycobacteria. Resistance to the drug, secondary to reduced penetration into the bacterium, may be present, but cross-resistance with other tuberculostatic drugs does not occur.

Pharmacokinetic aspects. **Isoniazid** is readily absorbed from the gastrointestinal tract and is widely distributed throughout the tissues and body fluids, including the CSF. An important point is that it penetrates well into 'caseous' tuberculous lesions (i.e. necrotic lesions with a cheese-like consistency). Metabolism, which involves acetylation, depends on genetic factors that determine whether a person is a slow or rapid acetylator of the drug (see Ch. 12), with slow inactivators enjoying a better therapeutic response. The half-life in slow inactivators is 3 h and in rapid inactivators, 1 h. **Isoniazid** is excreted in the urine partly as unchanged drug and partly in the acetylated or otherwise inactivated form.

Unwanted effects depend on the dosage and occur in about 5% of individuals, the commonest being allergic skin eruptions. A variety of other adverse reactions have been reported, including fever, hepatotoxicity, haematological changes, arthritic symptoms and vasculitis. Adverse effects involving the central or peripheral nervous systems are largely consequences of pyridoxine deficiency and were common in malnourished patients before supplementation of this vitamin during isoniazid treatment became routine. **Isoniazid** may cause haemolytic anaemia in individuals with glucose 6-phosphate dehydrogenase deficiency, and it decreases the metabolism of the antiepileptics **phenytoin**, **ethosuximide** and **carbamazepine**, resulting in an increase in the plasma concentration and toxicity of these drugs.

[7]An exception is the use of **isoniazid** monotherapy in selected healthy people with latent tuberculosis. This is diagnosed by a positive whole blood test based on interferon gamma release in response to mycobacterial antigens ('IGRA' test).

RIFAMPICIN

Rifampicin (also called **rifampin**) acts by binding to, and inhibiting, *DNA-dependent RNA polymerase* in prokaryotic but not in eukaryotic cells (see Ch. 51). It is one of the most active antituberculosis agents known and is also effective against leprosy and most gram-positive bacteria as well as many gram-negative species, but it is usually reserved for the treatment of TB and leprosy. It enters phagocytic cells and kills intracellular tubercle bacilli. Resistance can develop rapidly in a one-step process in which a chromosomal mutation changes its target site on microbial DNA-dependent RNA polymerase, so it is used in combination with other antituberculous antibiotics.

Pharmacokinetic aspects. **Rifampicin** is given orally and is widely distributed in the tissues and body fluids (including CSF), giving an orange tinge to saliva, sputum, tears and sweat. It is excreted partly in the urine and partly in the bile, some of it undergoing enterohepatic cycling. The metabolite retains antibacterial activity but is less well absorbed from the GI tract. The half-life is 1–5 h, becoming shorter during treatment because of induction of hepatic microsomal enzymes.

Unwanted effects are relatively infrequent. The commonest are skin eruptions, fever and GI disturbances. Liver damage with jaundice has been reported and has proved fatal in a very small proportion of patients, so liver function should be assessed before treatment is started. **Rifampicin** induces hepatic metabolising enzymes (see Ch. 11), increasing the degradation of **warfarin**, glucocorticoids, narcotic analgesics, oral antidiabetic drugs, **dapsone** and oestrogens, the last effect leading to failure of oral contraception.

ETHAMBUTOL

Ethambutol has no effect on organisms other than mycobacteria. It is taken up by the bacterial cells and exerts a bacteriostatic effect after a period of 24 h, probably by inhibiting mycobacterial cell wall synthesis. Resistance emerges rapidly if the drug is used alone.

Pharmacokinetic aspects. **Ethambutol** is given orally and is well absorbed. It can reach therapeutic concentrations in the CSF in tuberculous meningitis. In the blood, it is taken up by erythrocytes and slowly released. **Ethambutol** is partly metabolised and is excreted in the urine.

Unwanted effects. These are uncommon, the most significant being optic neuritis, which is dose related and is more likely to occur if renal function is decreased. This results in visual disturbances manifesting initially as red–green colour blindness progressing to a decreased visual acuity. Colour vision should be monitored before and during prolonged treatment.

Antituberculosis drugs

To avoid the emergence of resistant organisms, combination therapy is used (e.g. three drugs initially, followed by a two-drug regimen later).

First-line drugs

- **Isoniazid** kills actively growing mycobacteria within host cells. Given orally, it penetrates necrotic lesions, also the CSF. 'Slow acetylators' (genetically determined) respond well. It has low toxicity. Pyridoxine deficiency increases risk of neurotoxicity. No cross-resistance with other agents.
- **Rifampicin** is a potent, orally active drug that inhibits mycobacterial RNA polymerase. It penetrates CSF. Unwanted effects are infrequent (but serious liver damage has occurred). It induces hepatic drug-metabolising enzymes. Resistance can develop rapidly.
- **Ethambutol** inhibits growth of mycobacteria. It is given orally and can penetrate CSF. Unwanted effects are uncommon, but optic neuritis can occur. Resistance can emerge rapidly.
- **Pyrazinamide** is tuberculostatic against intracellular mycobacteria. Given orally, it penetrates CSF. Resistance can develop rapidly. Unwanted effects include increased plasma urate and liver toxicity with high doses.

Second-line drugs

- **Capreomycin** is given intramuscularly. Unwanted effects include damage to the kidney and to the auditory nerve.
- **Cycloserine** is a broad-spectrum agent. It inhibits an early stage of peptidoglycan synthesis. Given orally, it penetrates the CSF. Unwanted effects affect mostly the CNS.
- **Streptomycin**, an aminoglycoside antibiotic, acts by inhibiting bacterial protein synthesis. It is given intramuscularly. Unwanted effects are ototoxicity (mainly vestibular) and nephrotoxicity.

(See Table 52.4 for further examples.)

PYRAZINAMIDE

Pyrazinamide is inactive at neutral pH but tuberculostatic at acid pH. It is effective against the intracellular organisms in macrophages because, after phagocytosis, the organisms are contained in phagolysosomes where the pH is low. The drug probably inhibits bacterial fatty acid synthesis. Resistance develops rather readily, but cross-resistance with **isoniazid** does not occur.

Pharmacokinetic aspects. The drug is well absorbed after oral administration and is widely distributed, penetrating the meninges. It is excreted through the kidney, mainly by glomerular filtration.

Unwanted effects include gout, which is associated with high concentrations of plasma uric acid with which pyrazinamide competes for the renal tubular OAT (see Chs 9 and 10). GI upsets, malaise and fever have also been reported. Serious hepatic damage due to high doses was once a problem but is less likely with lower dose/shorter course regimens now used; nevertheless, liver function should be assessed before treatment.

CAPREOMYCIN

Capreomycin is a peptide antibiotic given by intramuscular injection. Its principal mechanism of action is thought to be through inhibition of translocation thereby inhibiting protein synthesis, but it may also have other effects on the bacterial cell membrane.

Unwanted effects are many and the drug should be used with great caution. They include kidney damage and injury to the auditory nerve, with consequent deafness and ataxia. The drug should not be given at the same time as **streptomycin** or other drugs that may cause deafness. It is usually reserved for patients with disease due to drug-resistant organisms.

CYCLOSERINE

Cycloserine is a broad-spectrum antibiotic that inhibits the growth of many bacteria, including coliforms and mycobacteria. It is water soluble and destroyed at acid pH. It acts by competitively inhibiting bacterial cell wall synthesis. It is an analogue of D-alanine and inhibits the formation of the D-Ala-D-Ala dipeptide that is added to the initial tripeptide side-chain on *N*-acetylmuramic acid; i.e. it prevents completion of the major building block of peptidoglycan. It is administered orally and distributed throughout the tissues and body fluids, including CSF. Its use is limited to the treatment of TB that is resistant to other drugs.

Pharmacokinetic aspects. Most of the drug is eliminated in active form in the urine, but approximately 35% is metabolised.

Unwanted effects are mainly on the CNS possibly through an inhibitory effect on GABA-transaminase. A wide variety of disturbances may occur, ranging from headache and irritability to depression, convulsions and psychotic states.

DRUGS USED TO TREAT LEPROSY

Leprosy is one of the most ancient diseases known to mankind and has been mentioned in texts dating back to 600 BC. The causative organism is *M. leprae*. It is a chronic disfiguring illness with a long latency and, historically, sufferers have been ostracised and forced to live apart from their communities, even though the disease is not particularly contagious. Once viewed as incurable, the introduction in the 1940s of **dapsone**, and subsequently, in the 1960s, of **rifampicin** and **clofazimine**, completely changed our perspective on leprosy. It is now generally curable, and the global figures show that the prevalence rates for the disease have now fallen by about 99% as a result of public health measures and the **M**ulti**d**rug **T**reatment (MDT; essential to avoid drug resistance) regimens implemented by WHO since

1981 with support from some pharmaceutical companies. The disease has been now eliminated from all but a few small countries; nevertheless, the WHO reported some 127,000 new cases in 2020, mainly in Asia and Africa.

There are two forms:

- *Paucibacillary leprosy*, leprosy characterised by one to five numb patches, is mainly *tuberculoid*[8] in type and is generally treated for 6 months with **dapsone** and **rifampicin.**
- *Multibacillary leprosy*, characterised by more than five numb skin patches, is mainly *lepromatous* in type and is treated for at least 2 years with **rifampicin**, **dapsone** and **clofazimine.**

DAPSONE

Dapsone is chemically related to the sulfonamides. Its action is antagonised by PABA and so the drug probably acts through inhibition of bacterial folate synthesis. Resistance to **dapsone** has steadily increased since its introduction and treatment in combination with other drugs is now recommended.

Pharmacokinetic aspects. **Dapsone** is given orally; it is well absorbed and widely distributed through the body water and in all tissues. The plasma half-life is 24–48 h, but some drug persists in liver, kidney and, to some extent, skin and muscle for much longer periods. There is enterohepatic recycling of the drug, but some is acetylated and excreted in the urine. **Dapsone** is also used to treat *dermatitis herpetiformis*, a chronic blistering skin condition associated with coeliac disease.

Unwanted effects occur fairly frequently and include haemolysis of red cells (although usually not severe enough to lead to frank anaemia), methaemoglobinaemia, anorexia, nausea and vomiting, fever, allergic dermatitis and neuropathy. *Lepra reactions* (an exacerbation of lepromatous lesions) can occur, and a potentially fatal syndrome resembling infectious mononucleosis has occasionally been seen.

CLOFAZIMINE

Clofazimine is a dye of complex structure. Its mechanism of action against leprosy bacilli may involve an action on DNA. It also has anti-inflammatory activity and is useful in patients in whom **dapsone** causes inflammatory side effects.

Pharmacokinetic aspects. **Clofazimine** is given orally and accumulates in the body, being sequestered in the mononuclear phagocyte system. The plasma half-life may be as long as 8 weeks. The anti-leprotic effect is delayed and is usually not evident for 6–7 weeks.

Unwanted effects may be related to the fact that **clofazimine** is a dye. The skin and urine can develop a reddish colour and the lesions a blue-black discoloration. Dose-related nausea, giddiness, headache and GI disturbances can also occur.

[8]The difference between *tuberculoid* and *lepromatous* disease appears to be that the T cells from patients with the former vigorously produce interferon-γ, which enables macrophages to kill intracellular microbes, whereas in the latter case the immune response is dominated by interleukin-4, which blocks the action of interferon-γ (see Ch. 17).

Antileprosy drugs

- For *tuberculoid leprosy*: **dapsone** and **rifampicin** (**rifampin**).
  - **Dapsone** is sulfonamide-like and inhibits folate synthesis. It is given orally. Unwanted effects are fairly frequent; a few are serious. Resistance is increasing.
  - **Rifampicin** (see *Antituberculosis drugs* box).
- For *lepromatous leprosy*: dapsone, **rifampicin** and **clofazimine.**
  - **Clofazimine** is a dye that is given orally and can accumulate by sequestering in macrophages. Action is delayed for 6–7 weeks, and its half-life is 8 weeks. Unwanted effects include red skin and urine, sometimes GI disturbances.

(See Table 52.4 for further examples.)

PROSPECTS FOR NEW ANTIBACTERIAL DRUGS

During the 5 years ending in 2020, only 12 'new' antibiotics were approved by the FDA and, as a recent review has made plain, virtually all of these were essentially variations upon existing antibiotic structures with only one **cephalosporin** derivative acting through a novel mechanism (Provenzani et al., 2020).

Historically, antibiotics were one of the mainstays of the pharmaceutical industry. The rapid discoveries and developments that characterised the 'heroic' years of antibiotic research, which spanned approximately 1930–1960, led to the discovery of some 20 novel classes of antibiotics which even today constitute the core of our arsenal of antibacterial drugs. The depressing message is that to compensate for the loss of drug efficacy to resistance mechanisms, we would need another 20 new classes of antibiotics within the next 50 years. Despite the emergence of isolated reports of new antibiotic mechanisms in the scientific literature, there is, at present, little prospect of achieving this goal.

Hubris is partly to blame. The antibiotics originally discovered were so successful that by 1970, it was thought that infectious diseases had been effectively vanquished.[9] Many pharmaceutical companies scaled down their efforts in the area, despite the continuing need for compounds acting by novel mechanisms to keep pace with the adaptive potential of pathogens.

One might legitimately ask how this has been allowed to happen given the cardinal importance of this group of drugs. The reasons are multifactorial. Innovation by the pharmaceutical industry has been beset by regulatory problems and ethical issues with the clinical trials of new antibiotics. Perhaps most important though is the financial backing for new drug discovery. The private sector is the major initiator of drug discovery but with an eye-watering outlay currently estimated at about US$2.9 billion

[9]In 1967 the US Surgeon General announced (in effect) that infectious diseases had been vanquished, and that the researchers should turn their attention to chronic diseases instead.

(Provenzani et al., 2020) required to develop such drugs, the payback to the pharmaceutical industry is seldom sufficient to recoup such a massive investment. Evidence of antibiotic efficacy is difficult to generate and 'success' is rewarded by a product that will used for the shortest duration possible to minimise the emergence of resistance, and which probably cannot be afforded by the peoples in poor countries who often have the greatest need for such drugs. These and other complex reasons for the failure to develop new antibiotics have been analysed in detail by Coates et al. (2011).

Legislation and government initiatives have been introduced in some countries (e.g. United States) which promise fast-track regulatory approval and extended patent life for those wishing to take the huge financial risks. These, and other potentially useful strategies, have been reviewed by Renwick et al. (2016) but have seemingly made little impact thus far.

At the same time, drug resistance has been increasing and can develop with shocking rapidity. Bax et al. (2000) noted the appearance of resistant strains within 2 years or so of the introduction of a new agent and Costelloe et al. (2010) concluded that most patients prescribed antibiotics for a respiratory or urinary tract infection develop individual resistance to the drug within a few weeks and that this may persist for up to a year after treatment. In fact, deaths from drug-resistant bacteria now exceed those caused by HIV/AIDS or malaria with *Escherichia coli*, *S. aureus* and *Klebsiella pneumoniae* topping the list of frequent killers (Murray, 2022).[10] Since about half the antibiotic use is for veterinary purposes, it is not just human medicine that is compromised by this phenomenon.

The stark reality is that unless substantial progress is made, we will soon be entering the 'post-antibiotic' era and medicine, as we know it today, will not be possible. But perhaps we should not underestimate the collective ingenuity of biomedical scientists. Many labs, both academic and commercial, are utilising the power of high-throughput screens to search for, and assess, new naturally occurring antibiotic candidates. Others are exploring different types of antibacterials such as biopharmaceuticals (see Ch. 5) or devising increasingly sophisticated ways of defeating bacterial resistance mechanisms. In all cases their endeavours are informed by the latest conceptual tools such as bioinformatic analysis of pathogen genomes. In the meantime, the world awaits further therapeutic developments with bated breath.

[10]The worst offenders are sometimes collectively referred to, rather fittingly, as 'ESKAPE pathogens'. The acronym is formed of the initial letters of *E. faecium*, *S. aureus*, *K. pneumonia*, *A. baumanii*, *P. aeruginosa* and *Enterobacter* spp.

REFERENCES AND FURTHER READING

Allington, D.R., Rivey, M.P., 2001. Quinupristin/dalfopristin: a therapeutic review. Clin. Ther. 23, 24–44.

Ball, P., 2001. Future of the quinolones. Semin. Resp. Infect. 16, 215–224.

Bax, R., Mullan, N., Verhoef, J., 2000. The millennium bugs – the need for and development of new antibacterials. Int. J. Antimicrob. Agents 16, 51–59.

Bloom, B.R., Small, P.M., 1998. The evolving relation between humans and *Mycobacterium tuberculosis*. Lancet 338, 677–678.

Blondeau, J.M., 1999. Expanded activity and utility of the new fluoroquinolones: a review. Clin. Ther. 21, 3–15.

Coates, A.R., Halls, G., Hu, Y., 2011. Novel classes of antibiotics or more of the same? Br. J. Pharmacol. 163, 184–194.

Costelloe, C., Metcalfe, C., Lovering, A., Mant, D., Hay, A.D., 2010. Effect of antibiotic prescribing in primary care on antimicrobial resistance in individual patients: systematic review and meta-analysis. BMJ 340, c2096.

Draenert, R., Seybold, U., Grutzner, E., Bogner, J.R., 2015. Novel antibiotics: are we still in the pre-post-antibiotic era? Infection 43, 145–151.

Duran, J.M., Amsden, G.W., 2000. Azithromycin: indications for the future? Expert Opin. Pharmacother. 1, 489–505.

Escaich, S., 2008. Antivirulence as a new antibacterial approach for chemotherapy. Curr. Opin. Chem. Biol. 12, 400–408.

Falconer, S.B., Brown, E.D., 2009. New screens and targets in antibacterial drug discovery. Curr. Opin. Microbiol. 12, 497–504.

Jagusztyn-Krynicka, E.K., Wyszynska, A., 2008. The decline of antibiotic era – new approaches for antibacterial drug discovery. Pol. J. Microbiol. 57, 91–98.

Ji, Y., Lei, T., 2013. Antisense RNA regulation and application in the development of novel antibiotics to combat multidrug resistant bacteria. Sci. Prog. 96, 43–60.

Livermore, D.M., 2000. Antibiotic resistance in staphylococci. J. Antimicrob. Agents 16, S3–S10.

Loferer, H., 2000. Mining bacterial genomes for antimicrobial targets. Mol. Med. Today 6, 470–474.

Lowy, F.D., 1998. *Staphylococcus aureus* infections. N. Engl. J. Med. 339, 520–541.

Michel, M., Gutman, L., 1997. Methicillin-resistant *Staphylococcus aureus* and vancomycin-resistant enterococci: therapeutic realities and possibilities. Lancet 349, 1901–1906.

Murray, C.J.L., 2022. BSAC vanguard series: tracking the global rise of antimicrobial resistance. J. Antimicrob. Chemother. 77, 2586–2587.

O'Neill, A.J., 2008. New antibacterial agents for treating infections caused by multi-drug resistant gram-negative bacteria. Expert Opin. Invest. Drugs 17, 297–302.

Perry, C.M., Jarvis, B., 2001. Linezolid: a review of its use in the management of serious gram-positive infections. Drugs 61, 525–551.

Provenzani, A., Hospodar, A.R., Meyer, A.L., et al., 2020. Multidrug-resistant gram-negative organisms: a review of recently approved antibiotics and novel pipeline agents. Int. J. Clin. Pharm. 42, 1016–1025.

Renwick, M.J., Brogan, D.M., Mossialos, E., 2016. A systematic review and critical assessment of incentive strategies for discovery and development of novel antibiotics. J. Antibiot. (Tokyo) 69, 73–88.

Shimada, J., Hori, S., 1992. Adverse effects of fluoroquinolones. Prog. Drug Res. 38, 133–143.

Zurenko, G.E., Gibson, J.K., Shinabarger, D.L., et al., 2001. Oxazolidinones: a new class of antibacterials. Curr. Opin. Pharmacol. 1, 470–476.

Books

Davies, S., Grant, J., Catchpole, M., 2013. The Drugs Don't Work: A Global Threat. Penguin Books, London. pp 112.

Useful website

http://www.who.int

Antiviral drugs 53

OVERVIEW

This chapter deals with drugs used to treat infections caused by viruses. We first provide some basic information about viruses, including a simple outline of their structure and classification as well as a brief summary of their life cycle. We continue with a consideration of the host–virus interaction: the defences deployed by the human host against viruses and the strategies employed by viruses to evade these measures. We next discuss the various types of antiviral drugs and their mechanisms of action. We illustrate this discussion with particular reference to severe acute respiratory syndrome coronavirus 2 (SARS-CoV-2) infection, which causes COVID-19, and the human immunodeficiency virus (HIV), which is responsible for a dangerous acquired immunodeficiency syndrome (AIDS).

BACKGROUND INFORMATION ABOUT VIRUSES

AN OUTLINE OF VIRUS STRUCTURE

Viruses are small infective agents which range in size between the tiny parvovirus (~20 nm) and the (relatively) giant Ebola virus (>900 nm). Their distinguishing feature is that they lack any metabolic machinery or capacity and which must therefore infect other cells in order to replicate. The 'free-living' virus particle is termed a *virion* and consists of segments of nucleic acid enclosed in a protein coat comprised of symmetrical repeating structural units and called a *capsid* (Fig. 53.1). The viral coat, together with the nucleic acid core, is termed the *nucleocapsid*. Some viruses have a further external lipoprotein envelope, which may be decorated with antigenic viral glycoproteins or phospholipids acquired from its host when the nucleocapsid buds through the membranes of the infected cell.[1] Nobody knows how many individual species of viruses exist, but they probably number in the millions (at least).[2] It is now thought that they play a crucial role in the planetary ecosystem and that they have been instrumental in the evolution of living beings – so not all the news is bad.[1]

[1]In 1960, the British immunologist Peter Medawar opined that: 'It has been well said that a virus is a piece of bad news wrapped up in protein.'
[2]The number of copies of viral genes on earth is "…beyond astronomical. There are hundreds of billions of stars in the Milky way and a couple of trillion galaxies in the observable universe. The virions in the surface waters of any smallish sea handily outnumber all the stars in all the skies that science could ever speak of." – *'The viral universe'*, Economist, 22 August 2020.

Viruses can infect virtually all living organisms. Whilst by no means all are pathogenic – the human genome itself is estimated to contain 8%–10% viral material – they are nevertheless a common and important cause of disease in humans. Some important examples are as follows:

- *DNA viruses*: poxviruses (smallpox), herpesviruses (chickenpox, shingles, cold sores, glandular fever), adenoviruses (sore throat, conjunctivitis) and papillomaviruses (warts, cervical carcinoma).
- *RNA viruses*: orthomyxoviruses (influenza), paramyxoviruses (measles, mumps), coronaviruses (respiratory tract infections including COVID-19), rubella virus (German measles), rhabdoviruses (rabies), picornaviruses (colds, meningitis, poliomyelitis), retroviruses (AIDS, T-cell leukaemia), arenaviruses (meningitis, Lassa fever), hepadnaviruses (serum hepatitis) and arboviruses (various **ar**thropod-**bo**rne illnesses, e.g. encephalitis, yellow fever).

Despite being so numerous, only some 9000 viruses have been characterised and classified. Unlike animals or plants, viruses have not descended from a common ancestry and so classification is therefore a problem. Two systems are in use: one is based upon their morphology (e.g. rotaviruses, coronaviruses etc.), the other on their mode of replication. From the pharmacologist's viewpoint, the latter is the more useful scheme because it suggests useful drug targets.

THE LIFECYCLE OF VIRUSES

To replicate, viruses must first attach to and penetrate a living host cell – be it an animal, plant or bacterial cell – and hijack its metabolic capability. The first step in this process is facilitated by polypeptide binding sites on the envelope or capsid which interact with corresponding attachment points on the host cell. These viral 'receptors' are actually normal membrane constituents, receptors for cytokines, neurotransmitters or hormones, ion channels or other integral membrane glycoproteins. COVID-19, for example, uses *angiotensin converting enzyme 2* (ACE2) for this purpose while the virus that produces AIDS utilises the CD4 protein. Sometimes other accessory proteins are co-opted to aid viral entry. In the former case, the transmembrane protease, serine 2 (TMPRSS2) is used while in the latter case, chemokine receptors are involved. Some other examples of cellular viral receptors are listed in Table 53.1.

Following attachment, the receptor–virus complex enters the cell, often utilising receptor-mediated endocytosis (though some viruses bypass this route). The virus coat is removed by host cell enzymes (often lysosomal in nature) and the virion is dismantled, thereby liberating the genetic material together with any other viral enzymes or other factors important for replication. What follows is known as the *eclipse phase* of viral infection because individual virus particles can no longer be observed within the host cell.

The viral nucleic acid then utilises the host cellular machinery to synthesise viral proteins and further copies of the viral genetic material. Following processing, these components are then assembled into new virus particles in specialised complexes in the Golgi membranes and released from the cell during the final *shedding* (or *budding*) phase. The new viral particles are then free to infect further cells.

MECHANISMS OF VIRAL REPLICATION

When they infect cells, viruses have to solve two problems: they must produce more viral proteins, but they must also regenerate and synthesise further copies of their genetic material.

Since viruses lack ribosomes, the host cell cannot directly translate their genetic information to make further viral proteins and several enzymatic steps may be required to transform the viral genetic material into a form that can be 'read' by the host. How this is achieved depends upon whether their genetic material comprises either *DNA* or *RNA*, whether this is in a single- or double-stranded configuration and whether these are in a (+) sense or (-) sense form (in other words whether they are the same as (+), or complementary to (-), the final mRNA molecule). The actual enzymology is complex, sometimes involving viral and sometimes host enzymes, but the manner in which viruses produce a readable mRNA is the basis for commonly used classification system known as the *Baltimore system*.[3] Fig. 53.2 and the text later provide a simplified summary of this system

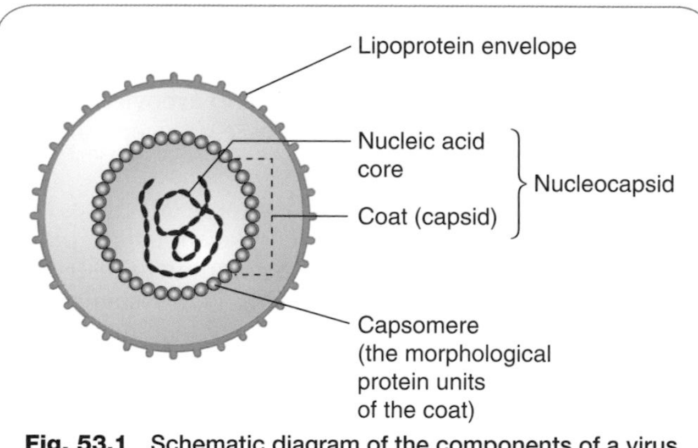

Fig. 53.1 Schematic diagram of the components of a virus particle or virion.

REPLICATION OF DNA VIRUSES

The mechanisms by which viral DNA replication occurs depends upon its configuration. In some cases, a conventional DNA–mRNA–protein pathway can be utilised. The double-stranded DNA of poxviruses or herpesviruses for example is transcribed directly by a host or viral *DNA-dependent RNA polymerase* into mRNA which can then be translated by the host cell to make viral proteins in the usual way. Some of these proteins are enzymes while others are structural proteins which comprise the viral coat and envelope. To synthesise further copies of viral DNA a separate *DNA-dependent DNA polymerase* must be used, and again, this may originate from the virus or the host.

The final assembly of coat proteins around the new viral DNA takes place in specialised structures in the Golgi and the mature virions are released by shedding or following host cell lysis.

In the case of viruses such as those of the parvovirus family, the DNA is in a single stranded (+) form, so a complementary (-) species must first be produced to form a replicative form of dsDNA which can then be transcribed into viral mRNA and thence translated into viral proteins by the host ribosomes. This dsRNA species is also used to regenerate the viral genomic material.

The dsDNA hepadnaviruses, such as the hepatitis virus utilise yet another method. Because their dsDNA genome contains stretches of single-stranded DNA, leaving 'gaps'

[3]Named after David Baltimore, the American biologist and Nobel Laureate (1975) who devised this system.

Table 53.1 Some host cell surface structures that can function as receptors for virus entry

Host cell structure[a]	Virus(es)
Acetylcholine receptor on skeletal muscle	Rabies virus
Angiotensin converting enzyme 2 (ACE2)	Coronaviruses including SARS-CoV and SARS-CoV-2 (COVID-19[b])
β-Adrenoceptors	Infantile diarrhoea virus
B lymphocyte complement C3d receptor	Glandular fever virus
CCR5 receptor for chemokines MCP-1 and RANTES	HIV (causing AIDS)
CXCR4 chemokine receptor for cytokine SDF-1	HIV (causing AIDS)
Helper T lymphocytes CD4 glycoprotein	HIV (causing AIDS)
MHC molecules	Adenoviruses (causing sore throat and conjunctivitis) T-cell leukaemia viruses
T lymphocyte interleukin-2 receptor	T-cell leukaemia viruses

[a]For more detail on complement, interleukin-2, the CD4 glycoprotein on helper T lymphocytes, MHC molecules, etc., see Chapter 7.
[b]COVID-19 also utilises TMPRSS2 (transmembrane serine protease 2).
MCP-1, Monocyte chemoattractant protein-1; *MHC,* major histocompatibility complex; *RANTES,* regulated on activation normal T cell expressed and secreted; *SDF-1,* stromal cell-derived factor-1.

Group	Examples	Viral genome	In the host
I	**Herpes viruses, pox viruses, adenoviruses, papilloma viruses.**	dsDNA	→ mRNA → VP
II	**Parvoviruses** (many animal diseases)	+ssDNA	→ –ssDNA → dsDNA → mRNA → VP
III	**Reoviruses** (e.g., Diarrheal rotavirus diseases)	dsRNA	→ mRNA → VP
IV	**Coronaviruses, picornaviruses, togaviruses** (e.g., Polio, respiratory diseases, hepatitis A and C)	+ssRNA	→ (–) ssRNA → mRNA → VP
V	**Orthomyxoviruses, rhabdoviruses.** (e.g., Ebola, measles, influenza, rabies)	–ssRNA	→ mRNA → VP
VI	**Retroviruses** (e.g., HIV)	+ssRNA (+RT)	→ dsRNA → dsDNA → mRNA → VP
VII	**Hepadnaviruses** (e.g., Hepatitis B)	dsDNA (+ RT)	→ +ssRNA → dsRNA → dsDNA → mRNA → VP

Fig. 53.2 A simplified schematic diagram of the Baltimore system of virus classification. This system categorises viruses depending on how they produce a readable mRNA from their genomes. Note that the regeneration of viral genomic material, which is obviously essential for viral reproduction, is not shown here. *VP*, Viral protein.

in the coding sequence, enzymes in the host nucleus must first add additional bases to produce a replication-capable dsRNA copy. From this, a (+) ssRNA is synthesised so that a dsRNA species can be produced. A *reverse transcriptase* enzyme (an *RNA-dependent DNA polymerase* enzyme) uses this template to synthesise dsDNA which can then be utilised by the host to produce mRNA for subsequent translation.

REPLICATION OF RNA VIRUSES

The replication of RNA viruses again reflects the complexity of the different configurations adopted by the viral genome. Reoviruses, such as the rotaviruses for example, contain dsRNA which can be transcribed into a useable mRNA for the host cell to translate and also copied by an *RNA-dependent RNA polymerase* to replicate the viral genome. This must occur within the viral capsid itself because cells can detect and destroy dsRNA species.

(+) ssRNA viruses such as coronaviruses or rabies virus can be modified by the attachment of a poly A tail and a 5′ cap to furnish a source of useable mRNA but this (+) ssRNA is amplified by a viral *RNA-dependent RNA polymerase*, producing a (-) ssRNA copy as a template for producing more (+) ssRNA which can then be used to synthesise further proteins as well as to replenish the viral genome. In the case of (-) ssRNA viruses, such as the influenza virus, this can be transcribed directly into mRNA and copied to produce a (+) ssRNA strand using the viral *RNA-dependent RNA polymerase*. This is used as a template for producing further (-) ssRNA species for the nascent viruses.

The human immunodeficiency virus (HIV) bears a (+) ssRNA genome. In this case, however, a viral *reverse transcriptase* uses this to synthesise a dsDNA species via a dsRNA intermediate. In addition to using this source for mRNA, the dsDNA can be inserted into the host genome forming a stable *provirus*; it can remain in the host indefinitely, becoming activated under certain circumstances. RNA viruses such as HIV which utilise reverse transcriptase in this fashion are known as *retroviruses*.

Like some DNA viruses, retroviruses may remain associated with the host genome and in some cases (e.g. HIV) replicated together with host genetic material when the cell divides. This accounts for the periodic nature of some viral diseases, such as those caused by *herpes labialis* (cold sores) or *varicella zoster* – another type of herpes virus (which causes chickenpox and shingles), which can recur when viral replication is reactivated by some factor (or when the immune system is compromised in some way). Other RNA retroviruses (e.g. the *Rous sarcoma* virus) can transform normal cells into malignant cells (a serious concern with use of retroviral vectors for gene therapy, see Ch. 5).

THE HOST–VIRUS INTERACTION

HOST DEFENCES AGAINST VIRUSES

The host's first line of defence is the simple barrier function of intact skin, which most viruses are unable to penetrate. Mucous membranes and broken skin (e.g. at sites of wounds or insect bites) are another matter and are more vulnerable to viral attack. Should the virus gain entry to the body, then the host will deploy both an innate and, subsequently, an adaptive immune response (see Ch. 7) to limit the incursion. An infected cell presents viral peptides, complexed with major histocompatibility complex (MHC) class I molecules on its surface. This is recognised by T lymphocytes, which then kill the infected cell (Fig. 53.3). Killing may be accomplished by the release of lytic proteins (such as perforins, granzymes) or by triggering the apoptotic pathway of the infected cell by activation of its Fas receptor ('death receptor', see Ch. 6). The latter may also be triggered indirectly through the release of a cytokine such as tumour necrosis factor (TNF)-α. Natural killer (NK) cells will also react to the absence of normal MHC molecules by killing the cell. This is called the 'mother turkey' strategy (kill everything that does not sound exactly like a baby turkey; see Ch. 7). The virus may escape immune detection by cytotoxic lymphocytes by modifying the expression of the peptide–MHC complex, but still fall victim to NK cells, although some viruses have also developed ways of evading NK cells (see later).

Within the cell itself, *gene silencing* provides a further level of protection (see Schutze, 2004). Short double-stranded fragments of RNA, such as those that could arise as a result of the virus's attempts to recruit the host's transcription/translational machinery, actually cause the gene coding for the RNA to be 'silenced' – to be switched off. The gene is then no longer able to direct further viral protein synthesis and replication is halted. This mechanism can be exploited for experimental purposes in many areas of biology, and tailored siRNA (*small- or short-interfering RNA*) is a cheap[4] and useful technique to suppress the expression of a particular gene of interest. Attempts to harness the technique for viricidal and more general therapeutic purposes have met with some success (see Barik, 2004; Bo et al., 2020), and are beginning to find their way into clinical use (see Ch. 5).

VIRAL PLOYS TO CIRCUMVENT HOST DEFENCES

Viruses have evolved a variety of strategies to ensure successful infection, some entailing redirection of the host's response to the advantage of the virus (see Xu et al., 2021; Konig and Munk, 2021, for recent reviews).

Subversion of the immune response

Viruses can inhibit the synthesis or action of cytokines, such as interleukin-1, TNF-α and antiviral interferons (IFNs), the chemical signals that normally coordinate innate and adaptive immune responses. For example, following infection, some poxviruses express proteins that mimic the extracellular ligand-binding domains of cytokine receptors. These pseudoreceptors bind cytokines, preventing them from reaching their natural targets on cells of the immune system and thus inhibiting the normal immune response to virus-infected cells. Other viruses that can interfere with cytokine signalling include human cytomegalovirus, Epstein–Barr virus, herpesvirus and adenovirus.

[4]The technique is indeed cheap in the laboratory, but siRNA drugs certainly are not. Treatment with **givosiran**, the siRNA drug pictured on the front cover of this book, costs some $US0.5 million per annum.

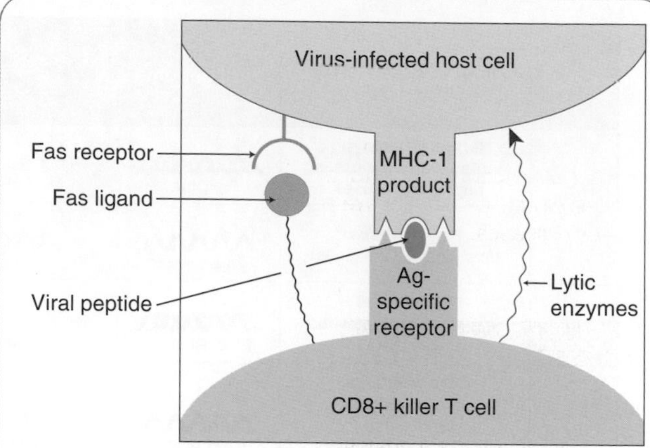

Fig. 53.3 How a CD8+ T cell kills a virus-infected host cell. The virus-infected host cell expresses a complex of virus peptides plus major histocompatibility complex class I product (MHC-I) on its surface. This is recognised by the CD8+ T cell, which then releases lytic enzymes into the virus-infected cell. The killer T cell also expresses a Fas ligand which triggers apoptosis in the infected cell by stimulating its Fas 'death receptor'.

Evasion of immune detection and attack by killer cells

Once within host cells, viruses may also escape immune detection and evade lethal attack by cytotoxic lymphocytes and NK cells in various ways, these include:

- *Interference with the surface protein markers on the infected cells essential for killer cell recognition and attack.* Some viruses inhibit generation of the antigenic peptide and/or the presentation of MHC–peptide molecules that signals that the cells are infected. In this way, they can remain undetected. Examples include adenovirus, herpes simplex virus, human cytomegalovirus, Epstein–Barr virus and influenza virus.
- *Interference with the apoptotic pathway.* Adenovirus, human cytomegalovirus and Epstein–Barr virus can also subvert this pathway to ensure their own survival.
- *Fooling the 'baby turkey' ploy.* Other viruses (e.g. cytomegalovirus) get round the 'mother turkey strategy' of NK cells by expressing a homologue of MHC class I (the equivalent of a turkey chick's chirping) that is close enough to the real thing to hoodwink NK cells.

It is evident that natural selection has equipped pathogenic viruses with many efficacious tactics for circumventing host defences, and understanding these in more detail is likely to suggest new types of antiviral therapy. Fortunately, the biological arms race is not one sided, and evolution has also equipped the host with sophisticated countermeasures. In the majority of cases these prevail, and most viral infections eventually resolve spontaneously, except in immunocompromised hosts. The situation does not always end happily though; some viral infections, such as Lassa fever and Ebola virus infection, have a high mortality or can lead to chronic ill health and we now discuss a two further examples of hazardous viruses: HIV and the COVID-19 coronavirus. Whilst different in many ways, these examples exhibit many of the features common to other viral infections. The scale of the global AIDS problem pushed HIV up the priority list of antiviral targets and at the time or writing, the world is in the grip of a COVID-19 pandemic which, as well as inflicting illness on a huge number of people, has had a profound effect on the global economy and has halted research into, and diverted precious healthcare resources from, the treatment of other diseases.

Viruses

- Viruses are small infective agents consisting of nucleic acid (RNA or DNA) enclosed in a protein coat.
- They are not cells and, having no metabolic machinery of their own, are obligate intracellular parasites, utilising the metabolic processes of the host cell to replicate.
- *DNA viruses* (e.g. herpes virus) usually enter the host cell nucleus and direct the generation of new viruses.
- *RNA viruses* (e.g. COVID-19 virus) usually direct the generation of new viruses without involving the host cell nucleus (the influenza virus is an exception).
- *RNA retroviruses* (e.g. HIV, T-cell leukaemia virus) contain an enzyme, reverse transcriptase, which makes a DNA copy of the viral RNA. This DNA copy is integrated into the host cell genome and directs the generation of new virus particles. The infection may remain latent in the host genome becoming reactivated during periods of stress or immunosuppression.

HIV AND AIDS

HIV is an RNA retrovirus. Two forms are known: *HIV-1* is the principal organism responsible for human AIDS. The *HIV-2* organism is similar to the HIV-1 virus in that it also causes immune suppression, but it is less virulent. HIV-1 is distributed around the world, whereas HIV-2 is confined to parts of Africa. While it was first identified in the West in the 1960s, it is thought that the virus actually passed from chimpanzees to humans sometime in the late 19th or early 20th century. Since then almost 80 million people have become infected with the virus and over 36 million have died. Recent assessments by the The Joint United Nations Programme on HIV/AIDS (UNAIDS, 2021) suggest that over 37 million people are presently living with HIV, including over 1.7 million children (a particularly horrid thought), and that new infections are appearing at the rate of about 1.5 million per year.

The search for effective drugs to treat patients with HIV was responsible for dramatic advances in antiviral pharmacotherapy and thanks to the current availability of antiviral medicines, the global situation is improving, and the number of AIDS-related deaths is declining. HIV/AIDS is currently overwhelmingly centred on sub-Saharan Africa, which accounts for two-thirds of the total global number of infected persons, and where the adult prevalence is over 10 times greater than in Europe. It is estimated that there are currently some 28 million people receiving these drugs – approximately three quarters of all those suffering from the disease. Overall, mortality has fallen by over half since the peak of the pandemic and by a third in the last decade. For a review of the pathogenesis (and many other aspects) of AIDS, see Moss (2013).

INDUCTION OF THE DISEASE

The interaction of HIV with the host's immune system is complex; cytotoxic T lymphocytes (CTLs; $CD8^+$ T cells) and $CD4^+$ helper T lymphocytes ($CD4^+$ cells) are the main targets although other cells may be involved. The HIV virion cannily attaches to CD4 (the glycoprotein marker of a particular group of helper T lymphocytes) and CCR5 (a co-receptor for certain chemokines, including monocyte chemoattractant protein-1 and RANTES; see Ch. 7 and Fig. 53.4A). Antibodies are produced by the host to various HIV components, but it is the action of the CTLs and $CD4^+$ cells that initially prevents the spread of HIV within the host. CTLs directly kill virally infected cells and produce and release antiviral cytokines. The lethal event is lysis of the target cell, but induction of apoptosis by interaction of Fas ligand (see Ch. 6) on the CTL with Fas receptors on the virally infected cell also plays a part. $CD4^+$ cells have an important role as helper cells and may have a direct role in the control of HIV replication (e.g. lysis of target cells: Norris et al., 2004). It is the progressive loss of these cells that is the defining characteristic of HIV infection.

The CTLs are effective during the initial stages of the infection but are not able to stop the progression of the disease. It is believed that this is because they become 'exhausted' and unable to maintain their protective function. Different mechanisms may be involved (see Jansen et al., 2004, and Barber et al., 2006, for further details).

CD4+ cells normally orchestrate the immune response to viruses, but HIV virtually cripples this aspect of the immune response. Evidence from exposed individuals who somehow evade infection indicates that CCR5 also has a central role in HIV pathogenesis. Drugs that inhibit the entry of HIV into cells by blocking CCR5 are now used clinically.

When immune surveillance finally breaks down, other mutated strains of HIV arise within an individual patient which recognise other host cell surface molecules. For example, gp120, a surface glycoprotein on the HIV envelope binds to CD4 and also to the T-cell chemokine co-receptor CXCR4. Another viral glycoprotein, gp41, then causes fusion of the viral envelope with the plasma membrane of the cell.

PROGRESS OF INFECTION

New HIV virions produced following infection (usually within 48 h) can lead to the release of a staggering 10^{10} new virus particles each day.

Viral replication is highly error prone. Many mutations occur daily at each site in the HIV genome, so HIV soon escapes recognition by the original cytotoxic lymphocytes (a particularly virulent new strain is currently circulating in Europe at the time of writing). Although other cytotoxic lymphocytes arise that recognise the altered virus protein(s), further mutations eventually allow escape from surveillance by these cells too. It is suggested that wave after wave of cytotoxic lymphocytes act against new mutants as they arise, gradually depleting a T-cell repertoire already seriously compromised by the loss of $CD4^+$ helper T cells, until eventually the immune response falters or completely fails.

Intracellular HIV may remain 'silent' (latent) for a long time before clinical signs emerge and there is considerable variability in the progress of the disease, but the usual

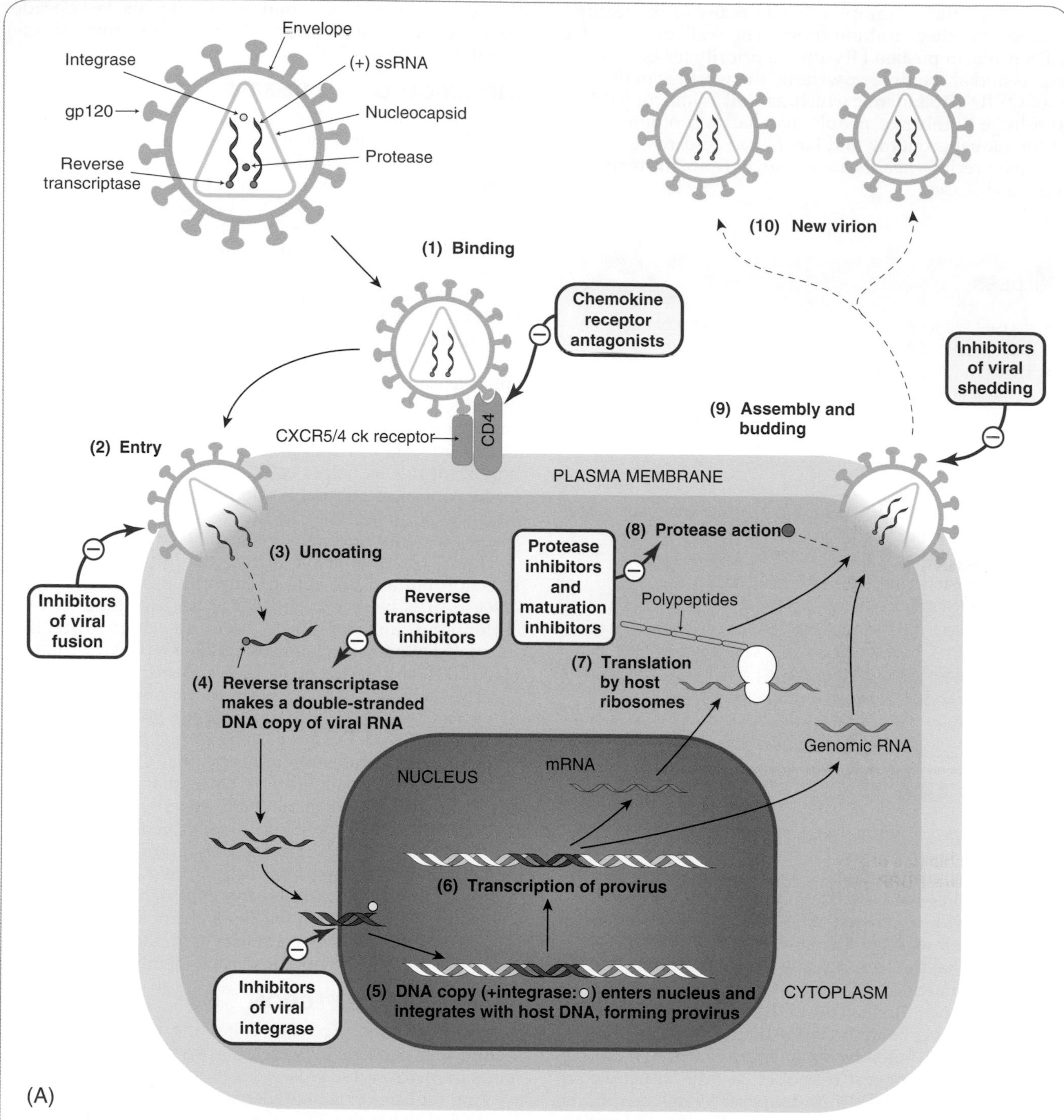

Fig. 53.4 Schematic diagrams of infection by (A) the HIV virion and (B) the COVID-19 coronavirus, with the sites of action of the main classes of antiviral drugs. (A) The HIV virus uses the CD4 co-receptor and the chemokine (ck) receptors CCR5/CXCR4 as binding sites to facilitate entry into the cell, where it becomes incorporated into host DNA (steps *1–5*). When transcription occurs (step *6*), the T cell itself is activated and the transcription factor nuclear factor κB initiates transcription of both host cell and provirus DNA. A viral protease cleaves the nascent viral polypeptides (steps *7* and *8*) into enzymes (integrase, reverse transcriptase, protease) and structural proteins for new virions. These are assembled and released from the cells, initiating a fresh round of infection (steps *9* and *10*). The sites of action of anti-HIV drugs are shown.

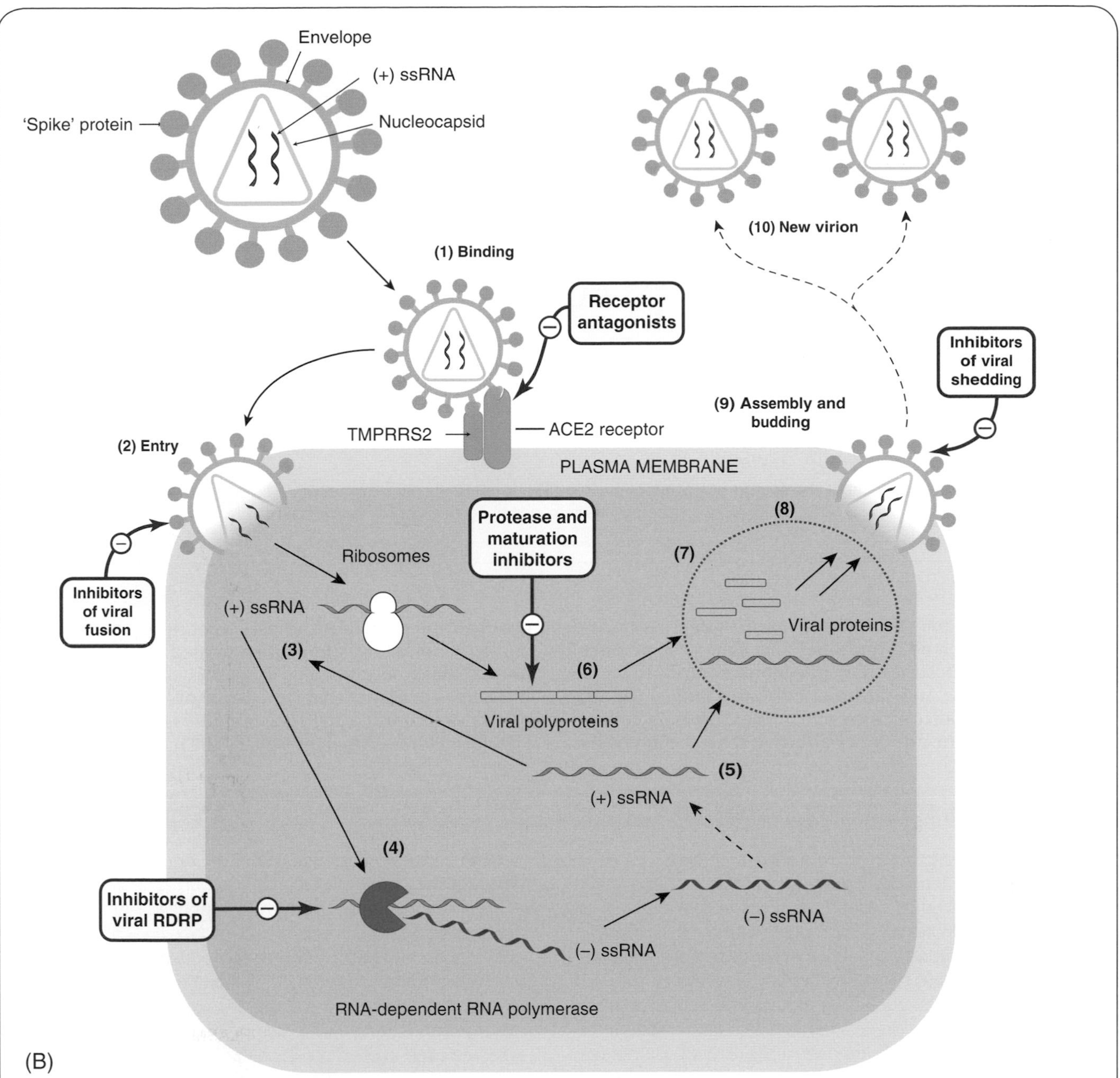

Fig. 53.4—cont'd (B) Infection of respiratory epithelial cell by the COVID-19 coronavirus virion. The virus attaches to the ACE2 receptor using its 'spike' protein *(1)*. This may be modified by the transmembrane protease TMPRSS2 which facilitates fusion and entry of the virion into the cell *(2)*. The (+) ssRNA viral genome may be used as mRNA *(3)* but it also is used as a template for synthesis (by RNA-dependent RNA polymerase) of (-) ssRNA *(4)* which can be used as a template to produce further (+) ssRNA for protein synthesis or for packaging into new virions *(5)*. Host ribosomes produce viral polyproteins *(6)* which are cleaved *(7)* into viral proteins. These are packaged *(8)* together with copies of (+) ssRNA into new virions *(9)* and released *(10)*. Note that some organelles and other cellular components have been omitted to improve clarity.

clinical course of an untreated HIV infection is shown in Fig. 53.5. An initial acute influenza-like illness is associated with an increase in the number of virus particles in the blood, their widespread dissemination through the tissues and the seeding of lymphoid tissue with the virion particles. Within a few weeks, this viraemia is reduced by the action of cytotoxic lymphocytes as explained earlier.

The acute initial illness is followed by a symptom-free period during which there is reduction in the viraemia accompanied by silent virus replication in the lymph nodes, associated with damage to lymph node architecture and the loss of $CD4^+$ lymphocytes and dendritic cells. Clinical latency (median duration 10 years) comes to an end when the immune response finally fails and the signs and symptoms of AIDS appear – opportunistic infections (e.g. *Pneumocystis* pneumonia or tuberculosis), neurological symptoms (e.g. confusion, paralysis, dementia) caused by direct infection of neuronal tissue by HIV or

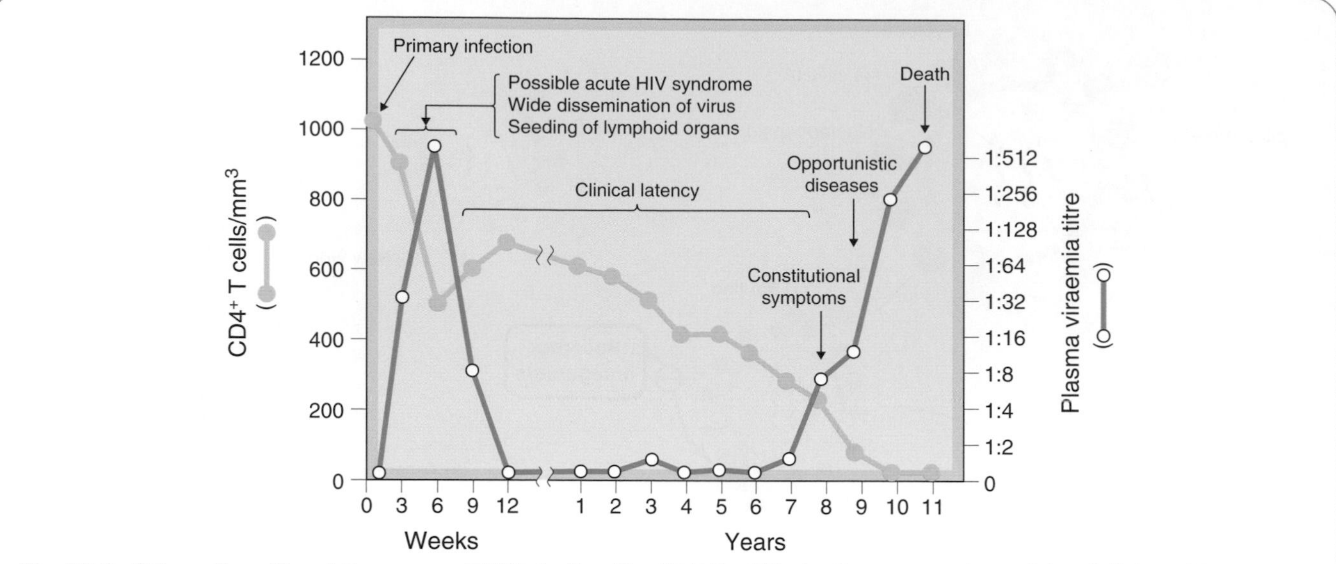

Fig. 53.5 Schematic outline of the course of HIV infection. The CD4+ T-cell titre is often expressed as cells/mm^3. (Adapted from Pantaleo, G., Graziosi, C., Fauci, A.S., 1993. New concepts in the immunopathogenesis of human immunodeficiency virus infection. N. Engl. J. Med. 328, 327–335.)

by opportunistic infections, bone marrow depression and malignancies such as lymphoma and Kaposi's sarcoma.[5] Chronic gastrointestinal (GI) infections contribute to the severe weight loss, and cardiovascular and kidney damage can also occur. In an untreated patient, death usually follows within 2 years. The advent of effective drug regimens has greatly improved the prognosis in countries that are able to deploy them, and patients thus treated may enjoy a near-normal life expectancy.

There is evidence that genetic factors play an important role in determining the susceptibility – or resistance – to HIV (see Flores-Villanueva et al., 2003).

Drug mechanisms in HIV infections

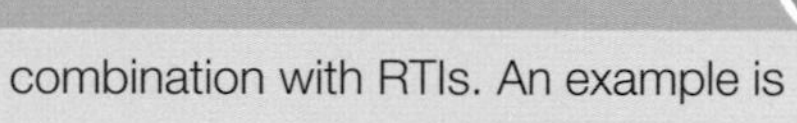

- Reverse transcriptase inhibitors (RTIs):
  - *nucleoside (or nucleotide) analogue RTIs* are phosphorylated by host cell enzymes to give the 5′-trisphosphate, which competes with the equivalent host cellular trisphosphates that are essential substrates for the formation of proviral DNA by viral reverse transcriptase (examples are **zidovudine** and **abacavir**); they are used in combination with protease inhibitors.
  - *non-nucleoside RTIs* are chemically diverse compounds that bind to the reverse transcriptase near the catalytic site and denature it; an example is **nevirapine.**
- Protease inhibitors inhibit cleavage of the nascent viral protein into functional and structural proteins. They are often used in combination with RTIs. An example is **saquinavir.**
- Combination therapy is essential in treating HIV; this characteristically comprises two nucleoside RTIs with either a non-nucleoside RTI or one or two protease inhibitors. Other drugs, such as the HIV integrase inhibitor **raltegravir**, the chemokine receptor antagonist **maraviroc** and the HIV fusion inhibitor **enfuvirtide**, may also be used in such combination therapy regimens. 'Once-daily' combination therapies greatly improve patient compliance and longer-lasting (e.g. once monthly, or longer) formulations are in prospect.

COVID-19

The first reports of this viral disease surfaced in December 2019 from the city of Wuhan in China prompted by cases of an unfamiliar type of pneumonia which progressed to serious respiratory disease. Whilst the origin of the initial infection is still uncertain – and indeed the continuing subject of speculation and conspiracy theories – it may be significant that all of the original 10 victims were connected in some way with the Wuhan Seafood Wholesale Market which, in addition to fish, also sells live animals including bats, poultry and snakes.

The causative agent was soon identified as a novel coronavirus genomically similar (>95%) to a bat coronavirus, RaTG13 (Wacharapluesadee et al., 2021) suggesting that it was a zoonotic infection acquired through an intermediate

[5]A tumor caused by infection with human herpesvirus 8 (HHV8), also known as Kaposi's sarcoma-associated herpesvirus (KSHV) or KS agent, was originally described by Moritz Kaposi, a Hungarian dermatologist practicing at the University of Vienna in 1872. It became more widely known as one of the AIDS-defining illnesses in the 1980s.

animal host. At least seven other coronaviruses were known to be pathogenic in humans and two previous global epidemics of coronavirus-mediated respiratory disease were already well documented: SARS-CoV which was again first reported in China and MERS (Middle Eastern respiratory syndrome) which appeared in Saudi Arabia in 2012. The new agent was named SARS-CoV-2, and the disease it causes was termed COVID-19.

No doubt facilitated by the ease of international travel, the virus quickly spread around the world: according to the latest (2022) global data from the WHO, there have been an astonishing total of almost 316 million *confirmed* infections with the virus since it was first reported. There have also been some 5.5 million confirmed COVID-19-related deaths, but the true death toll is estimated to be 3–5 times higher. Europe and the Americas have seen the highest numbers of infections, followed by SE Asia, which experienced about a third as many.

The virus is spread from person to person primarily in exhaled respiratory droplets and any illness usually develops within a few days following infection. Although the symptomatology is varied, those who do become ill usually present with a dry cough, fever, myalgia and fatigue and a change in the sensations of smell and taste, although many other effects of the virus have been described. In some people, these initial symptoms can progress to a severe respiratory illness characterised by widespread alveolar damage, and ARDS (acute respiratory distress syndrome) requiring intensive medical care including supplemental oxygen usually administered non-invasively but in the most severe cases, by mechanical ventilation. Most hospitalised patients are over 50 years old, and men are slightly more susceptible than women. Generally, children under the age of 15 years are unaffected. Between 10% and 20% of those who become ill may experience *long COVID* – which is usually taken to mean that their disease symptoms last more than 3 months. Many of those infected with the COVID-19 virus are asymptomatic and this cohort is probably mainly responsible for spreading the infection.

Since the initial detection of the disease, several variant forms, generally with mutations in the characteristic coronavirus 'spike' protein, have been identified around the world. The WHO has given these variants Greek names, with the *alpha* variant being the original virus identified, soon followed by a further *beta, gamma* and (until recently the dominant) *delta* strain. More recently (late 2021), a further rapidly spreading *omicron* variant was detected. Evolution of variants with even higher transmissibility is inevitable while global cases remain so high; virulence of such future variants is unpredictable.

The virus gains access to cells by binding to the cell surface receptor *angiotensin converting enzyme 2* (ACE-2), a protein which is known to be used by other coronaviruses such as SARS-CoV as an entry point. This enzyme is expressed in many tissues around the body including the gut epithelium and ciliated cells of the lower and, particularly, the upper respiratory tract. A co-receptor, TMPRSS2 (a transmembrane serine protease mentioned previously), aids this binding by proteolytically modifying the spike protein such that the virus is more capable of fusing with the cell membrane. However, this latter enzyme is much less abundant in the lower respiratory tract perhaps explaining why the omicron variant, which is unable to enter cells without this cofactor, is less damaging to alveolar cells.

Fig. 53.4B shows how the COVID-19 virus infects cells. Like HIV, its genome is comprised of (+) single-strand RNA but, unlike HIV, it does not utilise a reverse transcriptase, its viral RNA itself acting as mRNA.

ANTIVIRAL DRUGS

Because viruses hijack many of the metabolic processes of the host cell itself, it is difficult to find drugs that are selective for the pathogen. Happily, there are some enzymes that are (relatively or wholly) virus specific, and these have proved to be useful drug targets. Most currently available antiviral agents (excluding vaccines) are effective only while the virus is replicating. Because the initial phases of viral infection are often asymptomatic, treatment is characteristically not initiated until the infection is well established. This is unfortunate because, as is often the case with infectious diseases, an ounce of pharmacological prevention is worth a pound of cure, hence the importance of pre-exposure prophylaxis wherever possible.

Antiviral drugs, of which many are now available, may be conveniently grouped according to their mechanisms of action. Table 53.2 shows the commonest agents, together with some of the diseases they are used to treat. Since the antiviral pharmacology of HIV has been so well explored, Table 53.3 separately lists the principal agents specifically used in this disease.

DNA POLYMERASE INHIBITORS

Aciclovir

The development of the landmark drug **aciclovir** launched the era of effective selective antiviral therapy. Typical of drugs of this type, it is a guanosine derivative that is converted to the monophosphate by viral thymidine kinase. This viral enzyme is much more effective in carrying out the phosphorylation than the enzyme of the host cell, so **aciclovir** is predominantly activated in infected cells. Kinases in the host cell then convert the monophosphate to the trisphosphate, the active form that inhibits viral DNA polymerase, terminating the nucleotide chain. It is 30 times more potent against the herpes virus enzyme than the host enzyme. **Aciclovir trisphosphate** is inactivated within the host cells, presumably by cellular phosphatases. Resistance caused by changes in the viral genes coding for thymidine kinase or DNA polymerase has been reported, and **aciclovir**-resistant herpes simplex virus can cause pneumonia, encephalitis and mucocutaneous infections in immunocompromised patients.

Aciclovir can be given orally, intravenously or topically. When it is given orally, only 20% of the dose is absorbed. The drug is widely distributed and reaches effective concentrations in the cerebrospinal fluid (CSF). It is excreted by the kidneys, partly by glomerular filtration and partly by tubular secretion.

Unwanted effects are minimal. Local inflammation can occur during intravenous injection if there is extravasation of the solution. Renal dysfunction has been reported when **aciclovir** is given intravenously but slow infusion reduces the risk. Nausea and headache can occur and, rarely, encephalopathy.

There are now other drugs with a similar action to **aciclovir** such as **famciclovir** and **valaciclovir** (see list in Table 53.2). **Foscarnet** achieves the same effect through a slightly different mechanism.

Table 53.2 Some drugs used to treat viral infections (excluding HIV)

Therapeutic use	Drug	Mechanism of action
Cytomegalovirus	Cidofovir, foscarnet, ganciclovir, valganciclovir	Ns or Nc analogues and other drugs which inhibit viral DNA polymerase
Hepatitis B	Adefovir, entecavir, lamivudine, telbivudine, tenofovir	Ns or Nc analogues which inhibit reverse transcriptase
Hepatitis C	Elbasvir, ledipasvir, ombitasvir, pibrentasvir, ritonavir	NS 5A protease inhibitors
	Glecaprevir, grazoprevir, paritaprevir, velpatasvir, voxilaprevir	NS 3/4 protease inhibitors
	Dasabuvir, sofosbuvir	NS 5B RNA polymerase inhibitor
Hepatitis B and C	Interferon-a, pegylated interferon-a	Immunostimulant
Herpes	Aciclovir, famciclovir[a] (penciclovir), valaciclovir	Ns and other viral DNA polymerase inhibitors
	Inosine pranobex	Immunomodulator
Influenza	Oseltamivir, zanamivir	Neuraminidase inhibitors
Respiratory syncytial virus	Palivizumab	Targets viral protein crucial for cellular internalisation

NB some drugs are only used as components of combination therapies.
[a]Prodrug of penciclovir.
Nc, Nucleotide; *Ns,* nucleoside.
Data from various sources including BNF (2021).

Clinical uses of drugs for herpes viruses

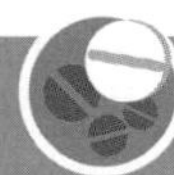

- *Varicella zoster* infections (chickenpox, shingles):
  - orally (e.g. **famciclovir**) including in immunocompetent patients;
  - intravenously (e.g. in encephalitis, **aciclovir**) including in immunocompromised patients.
- *Herpes simplex* infections: *genital* herpes (systemic and/or topical treatment depending on severity, whether immunocompromised and whether or not a first attack), *mucocutaneous* herpes (e.g. **aciclovir** or, if unresponsive, **foscarnet**) and herpes *encephalitis* (e.g. intravenous aciclovir).
- Prophylactically:
  - patients who are to be treated with immunosuppressant drugs or radiotherapy and who are at risk of herpesvirus infection owing to reactivation of a latent virus;
  - in individuals who suffer from frequent recurrences of genital infection with herpes simplex virus.
- Cytomegalovirus (CMV)
  - CMV, while a herpes virus, is less sensitive to **aciclovir** than is *herpes simplex* or *herpes zoster.* **Valaciclovir** is licensed for prevention of CMV during immunosuppression following organ transplantation. **Ganciclovir** and **valganciclovir** are more active against CMV than **aciclovir**, but are more toxic; they are used by specialists for serious problems such as CMV retinitis in patients with AIDS.

REVERSE TRANSCRIPTASE INHIBITORS

These include *nucleoside or nucleotide analogues*, exemplified by **zidovudine** and **tenofovir**, respectively. Nucleosides are first phosphorylated to the corresponding nucleotides and can then act as false substrates, being further phosphorylated by host cell enzymes and incorporated into the growing DNA chain but causing chain termination. While mammalian α-DNA polymerase is relatively resistant, the mitochondrial γ-DNA polymerase is susceptible to inhibition by these drugs, and unwanted effects may result at high doses. The main use of these drugs is the treatment of HIV, but several have useful activity against other viruses also (e.g. hepatitis B, which, though not a retrovirus, also uses reverse transcriptase for replication).

Zidovudine

Zidovudine (or **azidothymidine**, AZT) was the first drug to be introduced for the treatment of HIV and retains an important place in therapy. It can prolong life in HIV-infected individuals and diminish HIV-associated dementia. Given during pregnancy and then to the newborn infant, it can reduce mother-to-baby transmission by more than 20%. It is generally administered orally two to three times each day but can also be given by intravenous infusion. Its plasma half-life is 1 h, but the intracellular half-life of the active trisphosphate is 3 h. The concentration in CSF is 65% of the plasma level. Most of the drug is metabolised to the inactive glucuronide in the liver, only 20% of the active form being excreted in the urine.

Table 53.3 Some drugs used to treat HIV infection

Drug	Mechanism of action
Abacavir, bictegravir, didanosine, emtricitabine, lamivudine, stavudine, tenofovir, zidovudine	Ns or Nc reverse transcriptase inhibitors
Doravirine, efavirenz, etravirine, nevirapine, rilpivirine	Non-Ns reverse transcriptase inhibitors
Atazanavir, darunavir, fosamprenavir (PD), indinavir, lopinavir, ritonavir, saquinavir, tipranavir	Protease inhibitors
Enfuvirtide	Inhibitor of HIV fusion with host cells
Cabotegravir, dolutegravir, elvitegravir, raltegravir	HIV integrase inhibitor
Maraviroc	Chemokine receptor antagonist (CCR5)
Cobicistat[a]	Pharmacokinetic enhancer

[a]No intrinsic antiviral activity but prolongs the action of atazanavir and darunavir.
NB some drugs are only used as components of combination therapies.
Nc, Nucleotide; *Ns*, nucleoside; *PD*, prodrug.
Data from various sources including BNF (2021).

Because of rapid mutation, the virus is a constantly moving target, and resistance develops with long-term use of **zidovudine**, particularly in late-stage HIV infection. Furthermore, resistant strains can be transferred between individuals. Other factors that underlie loss of efficacy include decreased activation of **zidovudine** to the trisphosphate and increased virus load as the host immune response fails.

Unwanted effects include GI disturbances (e.g. nausea, vomiting, abdominal pain), blood disorders (sometimes anaemia or neutropenia) and central nervous system (CNS) effects (e.g. insomnia, dizziness, headache), as well as the risk of lactic acidosis (possibly secondary to mitochondrial toxicity) in some patients; all these effects are shared by this entire group of drugs to a greater or lesser extent.

Other, currently approved, antiviral drugs in this group include **abacavir**, **adefovir**, **emtricitabine**, **entecavir**, **lamivudine**, **stavudine**, **telbivudine** and **tenofovir** which are used for hepatitis B as well as treatment of HIV infection.

NON-NUCLEOSIDE REVERSE TRANSCRIPTASE INHIBITORS

Non-nucleoside reverse transcriptase inhibitors are chemically diverse compounds that bind to the reverse transcriptase enzyme near the catalytic site and inactivate it. Most are also, to varying degrees, inducers, substrates or inhibitors of the liver cytochrome P450 enzyme system (see Ch. 10). Currently available drugs include **efavirenz** and **nevirapine**, and the related compounds **etravirine** and **rilpivirine**.

Efavirenz (plasma half-life ~50 h) is given orally, once daily. It is 99% bound to plasma albumin, and its CSF concentration is ~1% of that in the plasma. Its major adverse effects are insomnia, bad dreams and sometimes psychotic symptoms. It is teratogenic.

Nevirapine has good oral bioavailability and penetrates into the CSF. It is metabolised in the liver, and the metabolite is excreted in the urine. **Nevirapine** can prevent mother-to-baby transmission of HIV.

Unwanted effects include rash (common) as well as a cluster of other effects.

PROTEASE INHIBITORS

In many cases, the viral mRNA is initially translated into biochemically inert *polyproteins*. A virus-specific protease then converts the polyproteins into various structural and functional proteins by cleavage at the appropriate positions. Because this functionally critical protease does not occur in the host, it is a useful target for chemotherapeutic intervention. HIV infection generates two such polyproteins named *Gag* and *Gag-Pol*. Specific protease inhibitors bind to the site where cleavage occurs, and their use, in combination with reverse transcriptase inhibitors, has transformed the therapy of AIDS. In the case of the hepatitis C virus, two protease targets have also been identified, *non-structural protein (NS) 3*, a serine protease, and *NS 5A*, which appears to act as an accessory protein for NS3. Examples of currently available protease inhibitors are shown in Tables 53.2 and 53.3.

Darunavir, a typical example, binds tightly to the specific retropepsin proteases from HIV-1 or HIV-2, inactivating the catalytic site. **Ritonavir** acts in a similar way but also inhibits the P450 enzymes that metabolise these drugs potentiating their activity and for this reason is often given in combination with other protease inhibitors (e.g. **lopinavir**).

Unwanted effects that are shared among this group include GI disturbances (e.g. nausea, vomiting, abdominal pain), blood disorders (sometimes anaemia or neutropenia) and CNS effects (e.g. insomnia, dizziness, headache) as well as the risk of hyperglycaemia.

Drug interactions are numerous, clinically important and unpredictable. As with other antiretroviral drugs, it is essential to check possible interactions before prescribing any other drugs in patients receiving antiretroviral treatment.

NEURAMINIDASE INHIBITORS AND INHIBITORS OF VIRAL COAT DISASSEMBLY

Viral neuraminidase is one of three transmembrane proteins coded by the influenza genome. Infection with these RNA viruses begins with the attachment of the viral haemagglutinin to neuraminic (sialic) acid residues on host cells. The viral particle then enters the cell by endocytosis. The endosome is acidified following influx of H^+ through another viral protein, the *M2 ion channel*. This facilitates the disassembly of the viral structure, allowing the RNA to enter the host nucleus, thus initiating a round of viral replication. Newly replicated virions escape from the host cell by budding from the cell membrane. Viral neuraminidase promotes this by severing the bonds linking the particle coat and host sialic acid.

The neuraminidase inhibitors **oseltamivir** and **zanamivir** are active against both influenza A and B viruses and are licensed for use at early stages in the infection or when use of the vaccine is impossible. **Zanamivir** is available as a powder for inhalation, and **oseltamivir** as an oral preparation. Although **oseltamivir** has in the past been 'stockpiled' by governments when flu pandemics (e.g. 'swine' flu – H1N1) are forecast, clinical trials suggest that its efficacy in reducing disease severity is very limited.

Unwanted effects of **oseltamivir** include GI symptoms (nausea, vomiting, dyspepsia and diarrhoea), but these are less frequent and severe in the inhaled preparation. **Zanamivir** commonly causes a rash.

DRUGS ACTING THROUGH OTHER MECHANISMS

Enfuvirtide inhibits the fusion of HIV with host cells. It is generally given by subcutaneous injection in combination with other drugs to treat HIV when resistance becomes a problem or when the patient is intolerant of other antiretroviral drugs.

Unwanted effects include flu-like symptoms, central effects such as headache, dizziness, alterations in mood, GI effects and, sometimes, hypersensitivity reactions.

Raltegravir and related agents (see Table 53.3) act by inhibiting HIV DNA integrase, the enzyme that splices viral DNA into the host genome when forming the provirus. It is used for the treatment of HIV as part of combination therapy and is generally reserved for cases that are resistant to other antiretroviral agents.

Maraviroc. CCR5, together with CXCR4, are cell surface chemokine receptors that have been exploited by some strains of HIV to gain entry to the cell (see earlier). In patients who harbour 'R5' strains, the chemokine receptor antagonist **maraviroc** may be used, in combination with more conventional antiretroviral drugs (see Dhami et al., 2009). Its use, in combination with other antiretroviral drugs, is currently restricted to CCR5-tropic HIV infection in patients previously treated with other antiretrovirals.

Cobicistat is classed as a *pharmacokinetic enhancer*. It has no intrinsic activity but potentiates the actions of **atazanavir** and **darunavir** by inhibiting CYP3A enzymes and hence inhibiting drug metabolism.

Antiviral drugs

Most antiviral drugs generally fall into the following groups:

- *Nucleoside (or nucleotide) analogues* that inhibit the viral reverse transcriptase enzyme, preventing replication (e.g. **lamivudine**, **zidovudine**).
- *Non-nucleoside analogues* that have the same effect (e.g. **efavirenz**).
- *Inhibitors of proteases* that prevent viral protein processing (e.g. **saquinavir**, **indinavir**).
- *Inhibitors of viral DNA polymerase* that prevent replication (e.g. **aciclovir**, **famciclovir**).
- *Inhibitors of HIV integrase* that prevent the incorporation of viral DNA into the host genome (**raltegravir**).
- *Inhibitors of viral fusion with cells* (e.g. **enfuvirtide**).
- *Inhibitors of viral entry* that block the use of host cell surface receptors, which are used as entry points by viruses (**maraviroc**).
- *Inhibitors of neuraminidase* that prevent viral escape from infected cells (e.g. **oseltamivir**).
- *Immunomodulators* that generally enhance host defences (e.g. interferons and **inosine pranobex**).
- *Immunoglobulin and related preparations* that contain neutralising antibodies to various viruses.

BIOPHARMACEUTICAL ANTIVIRAL DRUGS

Biopharmaceuticals (see Ch. 5) that have been recruited in the fight against virus infections include immunoglobulin preparations, IFNs and monoclonal antibodies.

Immunoglobulins

Pooled immunoglobulin contains antibodies against various viruses present in the population. The antibodies are directed against the viral envelopes and can 'neutralise' some viruses and prevent their attachment to host cells. If used before the onset of signs and symptoms, it may attenuate or prevent measles, German measles, infectious hepatitis, rabies or poliomyelitis. *Hyperimmune* globulin, specific against particular viruses, is used against hepatitis B, varicella zoster and rabies and, more recently, COVID-19.

Palivizumab

Related in terms of its mechanism of action to immunoglobulins is **palivizumab**, a monoclonal antibody (see Ch. 5) directed against a glycoprotein on the surface of respiratory syncytial virus. Given by intramuscular injection under specialist supervision, it has proved useful in children at high risk to prevent infection by this organism.

Interferons

IFNs are a family of inducible proteins synthesised by mammalian cells and now generally produced commercially by recombinant DNA technology. There are at least three types, α, β and γ, constituting a family of hormones involved in cell growth and regulation and the modulation of immune reactions. IFN-γ, termed *immune interferon*, is produced mainly by T lymphocytes as part of an immunological response to both viral and non-viral antigens, the latter including bacteria and their products, rickettsiae, protozoa, fungal polysaccharides and a range of polymeric chemicals and other cytokines. IFN-α and IFN-β are produced by B and T lymphocytes, macrophages and fibroblasts in response to the presence of viruses and cytokines. The general actions of the IFNs are described briefly in Chapter 7.

The IFNs bind to specific ganglioside receptors on host cell membranes. They induce, in host cell ribosomes, the production of enzymes that inhibit the translation of viral mRNA into viral proteins, thus halting viral replication. They have a broad spectrum of action and inhibit the replication of most viruses in vitro. Given intravenously, IFNs have a half-life of 2–4 h. They do not cross the blood–brain barrier.

IFN-α-2a is used for treatment of hepatitis B infections and AIDS-related Kaposi's sarcomas; **IFN-α-2b** is used for hepatitis C (a chronic viral infection which can progress insidiously in apparently healthy people, leading to end-stage liver disease or liver cancer). There are reports that IFNs can prevent reactivation of herpes simplex after trigeminal root section in animals and can prevent spread of herpes zoster in cancer patients. Preparations of IFNs conjugated with polyethylene glycol (pegylated IFNs) have a longer lifetime in the circulation.

Unwanted effects are common and resemble the symptoms of influenza (which are mediated by cytokine release) including fever, lassitude, headache and myalgia. Repeated injections cause chronic malaise. Bone marrow depression, rashes, alopecia and disturbances in cardiovascular, thyroid and hepatic function can also occur.

OTHER AGENTS

Immunomodulators are drugs that act by modulating the immune response to viruses or use an immune mechanism to target a virus or other organism. **Inosine pranobex** may interfere with viral nucleic acid synthesis but also has immune-potentiating actions on the host. It is sometimes used to treat herpes infections of mucosal tissues or skin.

Tribavirin (**ribavirin**) is a synthetic nucleoside, similar in structure to guanosine. It interferes with the synthesis of viral mRNA although the exact mechanism of action is unclear. While it inhibits a wide range of DNA and RNA viruses, including many that affect the lower airways, it is used mainly to treat infections with *respiratory syncytial virus* (an RNA paramyxovirus) using an aerosol or tablet form. It has also been shown to be effective in hepatitis C as well as Lassa fever, an extremely serious *arenavirus* infection. When given promptly to victims of the latter disease, it has been shown to reduce to fatality rates (usually about 76%) by approximately eight-fold.

COMBINATION THERAPY FOR HIV

Because the two main classes of antiviral drugs used to treat HIV (reverse transcriptase inhibitors and protease inhibitors) have different mechanisms of action (see Fig 53.4A), they can usefully be deployed in synergistic combinations, and this has dramatically improved the prognosis of the disease. Such combination treatment was originally known as **h**ighly **a**ctive **a**nti**r**etroviral **t**herapy (HAART; sometimes simply abbreviated to ART). A typical HAART three- or four-drug combination would involve two nucleoside reverse transcriptase inhibitors with either a non-nucleoside reverse transcriptase inhibitor or one or two protease inhibitors.

Using a HAART protocol, HIV replication is inhibited, the presence in the plasma of HIV RNA is reduced to undetectable levels and patient survival is greatly prolonged – so much so that near-normal life spans can now be achieved, given prompt diagnosis and treatment and good patient adherence. The latter is a key point – an adherence rate of 95% or higher is required to achieve this result and prevent treatment failure. This is difficult to achieve because the daily multiple dosing regimens are complex, and these drugs have many unwanted effects. Since lifelong treatment is necessary, 'treatment fatigue' is a real issue.

To circumvent at least some of these problems, several 'once-a-day' formulations have been devised. The first one to be approved, **Atripla**, comprised a fixed-dose mixture of nucleoside and non-nucleoside reverse transcriptase inhibitors (**tenofovir**, **emtricitabine** and **efavirenz**). Several other proprietary combinations have also been approved with different constituent drugs. It is estimated that switching to a 'once-daily' administration doubles the likelihood of maintaining the 95% adherence rate that is crucial to treatment success (see Truong et al., 2015). More recently, such three-drug combinations have been successfully replaced with two-drug combinations comprising a DNA integrase inhibitor such as **dolutegravir** together with the reverse transcriptase inhibitor **rilpivirine** for example. Perhaps the most important step forward for patients, however, is the use of long-lasting injectable drug combinations. At the time of writing (January 2022), the UK National Institute for Health and Care Excellence has just approved the use of **cabotegravir** and **rilpivirine** for injectable use every 2 months in selected patients with a pre-existing good level of control. The use of combination therapy of this type has been successfully applied to other viral infections in addition to HIV.

Unwelcome interactions can occur between the component drugs of HAART combinations, and there may be inter-individual variations in absorption. Metabolic and cardiovascular complications attend the usage of these drugs and pose a problem to patients requiring lifelong therapy (see Hester, 2012). Some drugs penetrate poorly into the brain, and this could lead to local proliferation of the virus. So far there is little cross-resistance among the three groups of drugs, but the virus has a high mutation rate – so this could be a problem in the future.

The choice of drugs to treat pregnant or breastfeeding women with HIV is difficult and depends upon whether the patient is already well controlled with HAART or not. The main aims are to avoid damage to the fetus and to prevent transmission of the disease to the neonate. Specialist advice is essential and while combination therapy is highly effective, it increases the chances of fetal toxicity.

Other applications that require special consideration are prophylaxis for individuals who may have been exposed to the virus accidently or who are likely to become infected.

The former case is *post-exposure prophylaxis* and, the latter, *pre-exposure prophylaxis*. **Emtricitabine** with **tenofovir disoproxil** is often used in these cases but, once again, specialist advice is essential.

Treatment of HIV/AIDS

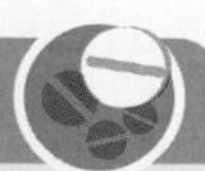

- Current treatment (supervised by experienced physicians) is not curative, but aims to optimise quantity and quality of life using HAART. This consists of combinations of drugs (e.g. of two nucleoside reverse transcriptase inhibitors with either a non-nucleoside reverse transcriptase inhibitor or with a boosted protease inhibitor or with an integrase inhibitor). Drugs with additive or synergistic therapeutic effects are selected to minimise the emergence of resistance, minimise toxicity and optimise adherence to lifelong therapy.
- Plasma viral load and CD4$^+$ cell count are monitored; viral sensitivity is determined before starting treatment and before changing drugs if the viral load increases.
- Treatment is started based on CD4$^+$ cell count and aims to reduce viral load as much as possible for as long as possible.
- Special situations (e.g. prophylaxis following accidental exposure via needle-stick injury, treatment of children and during pregnancy) are best managed by specialists.

COVID-19 PHARMACOTHERAPY

The progress of the AIDS virus may have been arrested by modern medicines but has certainly not yet been vanquished and neither has the COVID-19 virus. The former is not eradicated by drug treatment but lies latent in the host genome of memory T cells, ready to reactivate if therapy is stopped. The COVID-19 virus still ravages healthcare systems and economies around the world, with only a few countries now untouched. Vaccination has been shown to be a safe and effective strategy in controlling infection (but see Ch. 58). At the time of writing, there are some 120 vaccine candidates undergoing trial with 17 already approved in multiple countries (Mohammed et al., 2022), but until global coverage is achieved, new mutations with increased transmissibility will emerge. COVID-19 is likely to become endemic with different variants becoming dominant each winter (in the Northern hemisphere), and a need for repeat vaccination.

In contrast to HIV, the pharmacotherapy of COVID-19 is, as yet, relatively undeveloped. There have been several attempts to identify useful drugs to treat the acute infection and these fall into two main classes: 'repurposed' drugs – medicines originally designed to treat other disorders but for which presumptive evidence suggests some antiviral or other potentially beneficial action – and secondly, drugs with established antiviral properties which are usually already used to treat other types of viral infections.

The first group included as candidates the quinolone antimalarials, **chloroquine** and **hydroxychloroquine** (see Ch. 55), the antiparasitic drug **ivermectin** (see Ch. 56), the antibiotic **azithromycin** (see Ch. 52) and the glucocorticoid **dexamethasone** (see Chs 3 and 25).[6] While some of these drugs exhibited some antiviral activity in vitro, subsequent clinical trials have ruled them out as ineffective and harmful. The exception is **dexamethasone** which has proved effective and safe in seriously ill patients potentially requiring ventilation. In this group, the administration of the drug reduces mortality by approximately a third. However, this is not due to any antiviral action but likely because it prevents local pulmonary inflammation which exacerbates the severity of the viral pneumonia.

The second group of drugs trialled as anti-COVID therapies are existing antiviral drugs. This group includes **tribavirin** (**ribavirin**, an inhibitor of viral RNA synthesis), **remdesivir** and **favipiravir** (inhibitors of RNA-dependent RNA polymerase) and **umifenovir** (an inhibitor of viral entry). Newer orally active agents such as **molnupiravir**, which provides a modest protection (see Fig. 53.6), and **paxlovid** (a combination of **ritonavir** and **nirmatrelvir**) have been authorised in some countries including the UK.

This hugely important area has been reviewed by Ahsan et al. (2020), Ghasemiyeh and Mohammadi-Samani (2020) and Siddiqui et al. (2021).

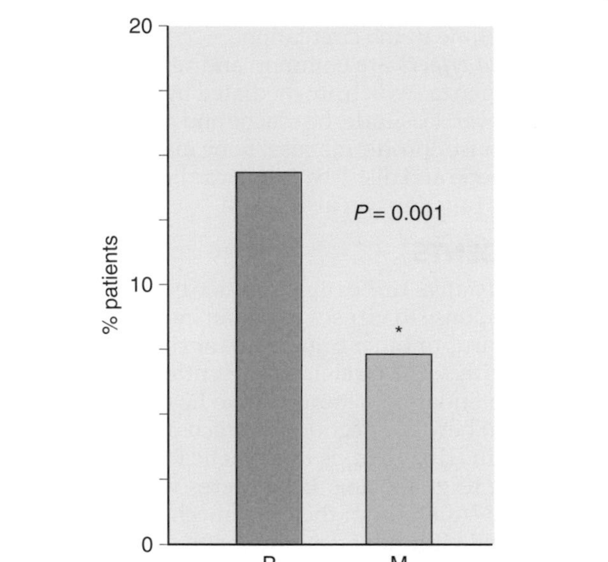

Fig. 53.6 The nucleoside analogue molnupiravir, which inhibits viral RNA synthesis, reduces the rate of hospitalisation or death in unvaccinated patients with COVID-19. The bar graph summarises the data at 29 days: compared to placebo (P) treatment, **molnupiravir** (M) reduced the percentage of patients who were hospitalised or who died following COVID-19 infection from 14.1% to 7.3% in a randomised double-blind trial. (Data from Jayk Bernal, A., Gomes da Silva, M.M., Musungaie, D.B., et al., 2022. Molnupiravir for oral treatment of Covid-19 in nonhospitalized patients. N. Engl. J. Med. 386, 509-520.)

[6]At a press conference in April 2021, President Trump horrified his medical advisors by suggesting that bleach and disinfectants should be trialled used as intravenous anti-COVID treatments. Although he later dismissed this as a prank, the US Centre for Disease Control and Prevention noted a surge in calls to poison centres the following month and several suppliers of 'cleaning products' which claimed efficacy were subsequently prosecuted.

PROSPECTS FOR NEW ANTIVIRAL DRUGS

At the beginning of the 1990s, there were only five drugs available to treat viral infections, but this number has increased some 10-fold during the intervening years. Our understanding of the biology of pathogenic viruses and their actions in the host has grown enormously. This has led to the discovery and development of antiviral drugs and the formulation and implementation of HAART which has been a triumph in the fight against HIV, transforming the lives of millions of people in a dramatic manner. However, the ultimate weapon in the fight against HIV would be vaccination. This has proved to be highly effective in the past against diseases such as polio and smallpox, measles, mumps, rubella and more recently against influenza (both types), hepatitis B, COVID-19 and other pathogens. Such a development would have several advantages including the fact that it would be of great benefit to many people in developing countries who are unable to afford expensive retroviral drugs and also, that while the latter are extremely effective when the dosing regime is strictly adhered to, their protection can falter when doses are missed.

Since the late 1980s, hundreds of vaccine candidates have been tested but unfortunately, and despite some encouraging results in animal models, clinical trials have proved disappointing There are various reasons for this relative lack of success: as well as the fact that patients may be infected with one or the other, or a mixture of, different viral subtypes, *antigenic drift* is a major problem. The HIV reverse transcriptase is highly prone to errors, resulting in changes to the viral coating hence different antigenic properties.

Despite these problems, there have recently been some partially successful attempts. A vaccine trial (RV144) which tested a combination of two vaccines that had proved ineffective when given separately had an efficacy of 60% a year after vaccination, declining to about 30% at 3.5 years. However, this trial was chiefly important because it confirmed that a vaccine-based approach to HIV was at least feasible, if difficult to achieve. Today, attempts to produce a long-lasting immunity to the disease with a vaccine are concentrating upon mRNA-based vaccines and improving understanding of mucosal immunity mechanisms in the female genital tract and the human rectal mucosa as these are the most common sites of infection. The whole area has been comprehensively reviewed (see Hargrave et al., 2021; Sobia and Archary, 2021, for recent assessments of the field).

Antigenic drift is also an issue with COVID-19 vaccines. Variant strains may arise following evolutionary pressure caused by treatment with a vaccine minimising the chance of an effective and long-lasting immune response. Five variant COVID-19 strains have arisen at the time of writing all of which have different infective characteristics. A vaccine which induces *broad neutralising antibody* production by the host is today considered to be a key objective.

REFERENCES AND FURTHER READING

Ahsan, W., Alhazmi, H.A., Patel, K.S., et al., 2020. Recent advancements in the diagnosis, prevention, and prospective drug therapy of COVID-19. Front. Public Health 8, 384.

Barber, D.L., Wherry, E.J., Masopust, D., et al., 2006. Restoring function in exhausted CD8 T cells during chronic viral infection. Nature 439, 682–687.

Barik, S., 2004. Control of nonsegmented negative-strand RNA virus replication by siRNA. Virus Res. 102, 27–35.

Bo, H., Liping, Z., Yuhua, W., et al., 2020. Therapeutic siRNA: state of the art. signal transduct. Targeted Ther. 5, 101.

Dhami, H., Fritz, C.E., Gankin, B., et al., 2009. The chemokine system and CCR5 antagonists: potential in HIV treatment and other novel therapies. J. Clin. Pharm. Ther. 34, 147–160.

Flores-Villanueva, P.O., Hendel, H., Caillat-Zucman, S., et al., 2003. Associations of MHC ancestral haplotypes with resistance/susceptibility to AIDS disease development. J. Immunol. 170, 1925–1929.

Ghasemiyeh, P., Mohammadi-Samani, S., 2020. COVID-19 outbreak: challenges in pharmacotherapy based on pharmacokinetic and pharmacodynamic aspects of drug therapy in patients with moderate to severe infection. Heart Lung 49, 763–773.

Hargrave, A., Mustafa, A.S., Hanif, A., Tunio, J.H., Hanif, S.N.M., 2021. Current status of HIV-1 vaccines. Vaccines (Basel) 9, 1026.

Hester, E.K., 2012. HIV medications: an update and review of metabolic complications. Nutr. Clin. Pract. 27, 51–64.

Jansen, C.A., Piriou, E., Bronke, C., et al., 2004. Characterisation of virus-specific CD8(+) effector T cells in the course of HIV-1 infection: longitudinal analyses in slow and rapid progressors. Clin. Immunol. 11, 299–309.

Konig, R., Munk, C., 2021. Special Issue: "Innate Immune Sensing of Viruses and Viral Evasion". Viruses 13, 567–569.

Mohammed, I., Nauman, A., Paul, P., et al., 2022. The efficacy and effectiveness of the COVID-19 vaccines in reducing infection, severity, hospitalization, and mortality: a systematic review. Hum. Vaccin. Immunother. 18, 2027160.

Moss, J.A., 2013. HIV/AIDS review. Radiol. Technol. 84, 247–267.

Murphy, P.M., 2001. Viral exploitation and subversion of the immune system through chemokine mimicry. Nat. Immunol. 2, 116–122.

Norris, P.J., Moffett, H.F., Brander, C., et al., 2004. Fine specificity and cross-clade reactivity of HIV type 1 Gag-specific CD4+ T cells. AIDS Res. Hum. Retroviruses 20, 315–325.

Pantaleo, G., Graziosi, C., Fauci, A.S., 1993. New concepts in the immunopathogenesis of human immunodeficiency virus infection. N. Engl. J. Med. 328, 327–335.

Schutze, N., 2004. siRNA technology. Mol. Cell. Endocrinol. 213, 115–119.

Siddiqui, A.J., Jahan, S., Ashraf, S.A., et al., 2021. Current status and strategic possibilities on potential use of combinational drug therapy against COVID-19 caused by SARS-CoV-2. J. Biomol. Struct. Dyn. 39, 6828–6841.

Sobia, P., Archary, D., 2021. Preventive HIV Vaccines-leveraging on lessons from the past to pave the way forward. Vaccines (Basel) 9, 1011–1032.

Truong, W.R., Schafer, J.J., Short, W.R., 2015. Once-daily, single-tablet regimens for the treatment of HIV-1 Infection. P. T. 40, 44–55.

Wacharapluesadee, S., Tan, C.W., Maneeorn, P., et al., 2021. Evidence for SARS-CoV-2 related coronaviruses circulating in bats and pangolins in Southeast Asia. Nat. Commun. 12, 972.

Xu, C., Chen, J., Chen, X., 2021. Host innate immunity against hepatitis viruses and viral immune evasion. Front. Microbiol. 12, 740464.

Useful Web resources

https://www.aidsinfo.nih.gov/ (also deals with COVID-19 infections).

https://www.unaids.org/en (The Joint United Nations Programme on HIV/AIDS (UNAIDS))

54 Antifungal drugs

OVERVIEW

Fungal infections (*mycoses*) are widespread in the population. In temperate climates, such as the United Kingdom, they are generally associated with the skin (e.g. 'athlete's foot') or mucous membranes (e.g. 'thrush').[1] In otherwise healthy people, these infections are mainly minor, being more of a nuisance than a threat. However, they can pose a more serious (sometimes fatal) problem when the immune system is compromised or when the fungal organism gains access to the systemic circulation. In this chapter, we will briefly review the main types of fungal infections and discuss the drugs that can be used to treat them.

FUNGI AND FUNGAL INFECTIONS

Fungi are non-motile eukaryotic cells and thousands of species have been characterised. Unlike green plants, they cannot photosynthesise, and many are parasitic or saprophytic in nature. Many are of economic importance, either because they are edible (e.g. mushrooms), useful in manufacturing other products (e.g. yeast in brewing and in the production of antibiotics), or because of the damage they cause to other animals, crops or foodstuffs. Along with bacteria, fungi are the major *decomposers* in most terrestrial ecosystems.

Approximately 50 species are potentially pathogenic in humans. These organisms are present in the environment or may co-exist with humans as *commensals* (i.e. not pathogenic) without causing any overt risks to health. However, since the 1970s there has been a steady increase in the incidence of serious secondary systemic fungal infections, causing some 2 million deaths per year, usually in immunologically vulnerable individuals. One of the contributory factors has been the widespread use of broad-spectrum antibiotics,[2] which eradicate the non-pathogenic bacterial populations that normally compete with fungi for nutritional resources. Other causes include diseases in which the immune system is compromised, such as AIDS as well as the widespread use of immunosuppressant, and cancer chemotherapy agents. The result has been an increased prevalence of *opportunistic infections*, that is, infections that exploit vulnerabilities in host immune systems. Older people, people with diabetes, pregnant women and burn wound victims are particularly at risk of fungal infections such as *candidiasis*. Primary systemic fungal infections, once rare in the temperate world, are also now encountered more often because of increased international travel.

Clinically important fungi may be classified into four main types on the basis of morphological and other characteristics. Of particular taxonomic significance is the presence of *hyphae* – filamentous projections that can knit the fungal cells together to form a complex *mycelium*, a mat-like structure that is responsible for the characteristic appearance of moulds.

Fungi are remarkably specific in their choice of preferred location. The main groups are:

- yeasts (e.g. *Cryptococcus neoformans*)
- yeast-like fungi that produce a structure resembling a mycelium (e.g. *Candida albicans*)
- filamentous fungi with a true mycelium (e.g. *Aspergillus fumigatus*)
- 'dimorphic' fungi which, depending on nutritional constraints, may grow as either yeasts or filamentous fungi (e.g. *Histoplasma capsulatu*[3])

Most fungi only cause systemic infections in immunocompromised individuals, but the dimorphic fungi can infect healthy individuals. Another organism, *Pneumocystis jirovecii* (formerly known as *P. carinii*), described in Chapter 55, shares characteristics of both protozoa and fungi; it is an important opportunistic pathogen in patients with compromised immune systems, but is not susceptible to antifungal drugs.

Superficial fungal infections can be classified into the *dermatomycoses* and *candidiasis*. Dermatomycoses include infections of the skin, hair and nails (*onychomycosis*). They are most commonly caused by *Trichophyton*, *Microsporum* or *Epidermophyton*, giving rise to circular rashes known as 'ringworm' or, generically, *tinea* (not to be confused with genuine helminth infections; see Ch. 56). *Tinea capitis* affects the scalp; *Tinea cruris*, the groin ('dhobie itch', 'Jock itch'); *Tinea pedis*, the feet ('athlete's foot'); and *Tinea corporis*, the body. Superficial candidiasis, caused by the yeast-like organism *Candida*, may infect the mucous membranes of the mouth or vagina (thrush), or the skin in an area where two skin surfaces are in contact and can rub together ('intertriginous' areas), such as under the breast, in the groin or between the toes. Secondary bacterial infections may complicate the course and treatment of these conditions.

Systemic (or 'disseminated') fungal diseases are much more serious than superficial infections. The commonest

[1]However, they may also 'infect' buildings and contribute to 'sick building syndrome'.

[2]In the days when tetracycline use was widespread, a common physical sign in chronic users was a black tongue – caused by overgrowth of commensal *Aspergillus niger*: dramatic and potentially alarming but harmless in that situation.

[3]Histoplasma is endemic in the mid-West United States. The organism is taken up intracellularly by histiocytes where they can survive and provoke a granulomatous reaction like tuberculosis (TB). Individuals are often asymptomatic, and past infection is picked up on X-rays as calcifications in various organs such as lung, spleen, etc., due to calcified granulomata like old TB but more densely calcified. As with TB the adrenal glands can be infected and, like TB, it is a cause of Addison's disease.

Table 54.1 Some clinically significant fungal infections (mycoses) and a typical first choice of antifungal drug therapy

Organism(s) responsible		Principal disease(s)	Common drug treatments
Yeasts	*Cryptococcus neoformans*	Meningitis	Amphotericin, flucytosine, fluconazole
Yeast-like fungi	*Candida albicans*	Thrush (and other superficial infection)	Fluconazole, itraconazole, miconozole
		Systemic candidiasis	Echinocandins, amphotericin, fluconazole, other azoles
Filamentous fungi	*Trichophyton* spp. *Epidermophyton floccosum* *Microsporum* spp.	All these organisms cause skin and nail infections and are referred to as tinea or 'ringworm'	Itraconazole, terbinafine, griseofulvin
	Aspergillus fumigatus	Pulmonary aspergillosis	Amphotericin, capsofungin, voriconazole, other azoles
Dimorphic fungi	*Histoplasma capsulatum*	Histoplasmosis	Itraconazole, amphotericin
	Coccidioides immitis	Coccidiomycosis	
	Blastomyces dermatitidis	Blastomycosis	

in the United Kingdom is *Candidiasis*. Other serious conditions include *cryptococcal meningitis*, endocarditis (particularly of artificial valves), *pulmonary aspergillosis* and *rhinocerebral mucormycosis*. Invasive *pulmonary aspergillosis* is now a leading cause of death in recipients of bone marrow transplants or those with neutropenia. Colonisation by *Aspergillus* of the lungs of patients with asthma or cystic fibrosis can lead to a condition termed allergic *bronchopulmonary aspergillosis* and growth of *Aspergillus* within a pathological cavity in lung tissue (usually caused by prior tuberculosis) can result in a fungus ball known as an *aspergilloma*. Aspergillomas may be asymptomatic but if they invade pulmonary vessels can cause death by massive haemoptysis.

In other parts of the world, systemic fungal infections include *blastomycosis*, *histoplasmosis* (which produces characteristic calcifications on chest X-rays), *coccidiomycosis* and *paracoccidiomycosis*; these are often *primary* infections; that is, they are not secondary to reduced immunological function or altered commensal microorganisms.

In addition to a free-floating lifestyle, some fungi can develop and grow in *biofilms*, that is, fungal communities attached to the surface of inert (e.g. catheters) or living (e.g. implants) surfaces. Such colonies are highly resistant to stress and to antifungal drugs, making them very difficult to treat.

DRUGS USED TO TREAT FUNGAL INFECTIONS

Drugs vary in their efficacy between the different fungal groups. Table 54.1 gives examples of each type of organism and lists some of the diseases they cause and the most common choice of drug used to treat them. Serious infections are often treated with combinations of these drugs.

The current therapeutic agents can be broadly classified into two groups: first, the naturally occurring antifungal antibiotics such as the *polyenes* and *echinocandins*, and second, synthetic drugs including *azoles* and *fluorinated pyrimidines*. Because many fungal infections are superficial, there are many topical preparations. Many antifungal agents are quite toxic, and when systemic therapy is required, this is generally undertaken under expert medical supervision.

Fig. 54.1 shows sites of action of common antifungal drugs.

ANTIFUNGAL ANTIBIOTICS

AMPHOTERICIN

Amphotericin (also called **amphotericin B**) was originally a mixture of antifungal substances derived from cultures of *Streptomyces*. Structurally, the pure compound is a large ('macrolide') molecule belonging to the polyene group of antifungal agents.

Like other polyene antibiotics (see Ch. 52), the site of **amphotericin** action is the fungal cell membrane. The hydrophilic core of the doughnut-shaped amphotericin molecule creates a transmembrane ion channel, causing gross disturbances in ion balance with the loss of intracellular K+, altering cellular permeability and disrupting transport systems. **Amphotericin** has a selective action, binding avidly to the membranes of fungi and some protozoa, less avidly to mammalian cells and not at all to bacteria. The basis of this relative specificity is the drug's greater avidity for ergosterol, a fungal membrane sterol that is not found in animal cells (where cholesterol is the principal sterol). **Amphotericin** is active against most fungi and yeasts and is the gold standard for treating disseminated infections caused by organisms including *Aspergillus* and *Candida*. **Amphotericin** also enhances the antifungal effect of **flucytosine**, providing a useful synergistic combination.

Pharmacokinetic aspects

Amphotericin is very poorly absorbed when given orally, and this route is used only for treating fungal infections of the upper gastrointestinal (GI) tract. It can be used topically,

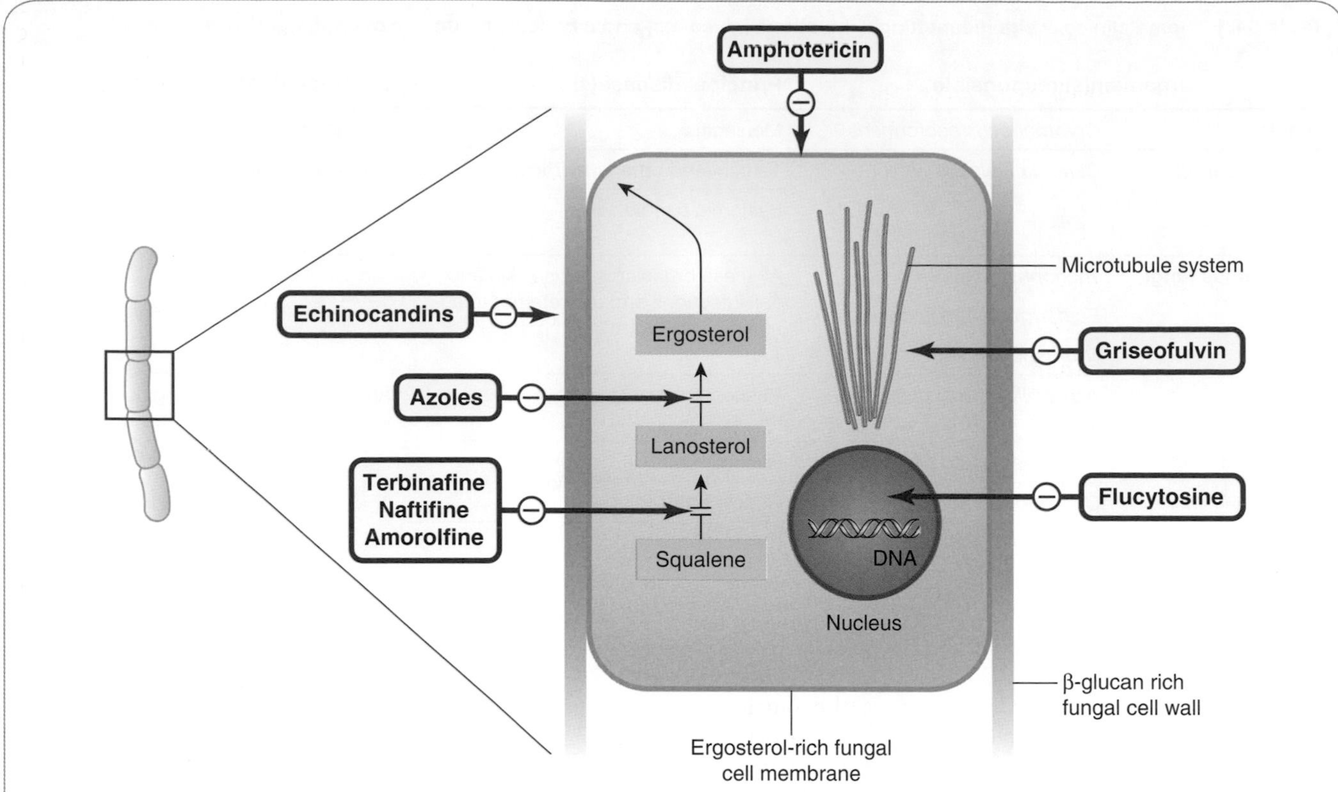

Fig. 54.1 Sites of action of common antifungal drugs. Fungi are morphologically very diverse organisms, and this schematic diagram of a 'typical' fungal cell is not intended to be structurally accurate. The principal sites of action of the main antifungal agents mentioned in this chapter are indicated as shown in *red-bordered boxes*.

but for systemic infections it is generally formulated in liposomes or other lipid-containing preparations and given by slow intravenous infusion. This improves the pharmacokinetics and reduces the (considerable) burden of harmful effects.

Amphotericin is highly protein bound. It penetrates tissues and membranes poorly although it is found in fairly high concentrations in inflammatory exudates and may cross the blood–brain barrier quite readily when the meninges are inflamed. Intravenous **amphotericin** is essential in the treatment of cryptococcal meningitis, often with **flucytosine**. It is excreted very slowly via the kidney; traces being found in the urine for 2 months or more after administration has ceased.

Unwanted effects

The commonest (indeed almost invariable) adverse effects of **amphotericin** include rigors, fever, chills and headache during drug infusion; hypotension and anaphylactoid reactions occur in more severely affected individuals. The (considerably more expensive) liposome-encapsulated and lipid-complexed preparations have no greater efficacy than the native drug but cause much less frequent and less severe infusion reactions.

The most serious unwanted effect of **amphotericin** is renal toxicity. Some reduction of renal function occurs in more than 80% of patients receiving the drug; although this generally improves after treatment is stopped, some impairment of glomerular filtration may remain. Hypokalaemia occurs in 25% of patients, because of the action of the drug on renal tubular cells, and often requires potassium chloride supplementation. Hypomagnesaemia also occurs for the same reason. Acid–base disturbance and anaemia can be further problems. Other unwanted effects include impaired hepatic function and thrombocytopenia. The drug is irritant to the endothelium of the veins and can cause local thrombophlebitis. Intrathecal injections can cause neurotoxicity, and topical applications cause a rash.

GRISEOFULVIN

Griseofulvin is a narrow-spectrum antifungal agent isolated from cultures of *Penicillium griseofulvum*. It interferes with mitosis by binding to fungal microtubules. It can be used to treat dermatophyte infections of skin or nails when local administration is ineffective, but treatment needs to be prolonged. It potently induces cytochrome P450 enzymes and causes several clinically important drug interactions, and because of this is now seldom used.

ECHINOCANDINS

Echinocandins comprise a ring of six amino acids linked to a lipophilic sidechain. All drugs in this group are synthetic modifications of **echinocandin B**, which is found naturally in *Aspergillus nidulans*. As a group, the echinocandins are fungicidal for *Candida* and fungistatic for *Aspergillus*. The drugs inhibit the synthesis of 1,3-β-glucan, a glucose polymer that is necessary for maintaining the structure of fungal cell walls. In the absence of this polymer, fungal cells lose integrity and lyse. Resistance genes have been identified in *Candida* (Chen et al., 2011).

Caspofungin is active in vitro against a wide variety of fungi, and it has proved effective in the treatment of candidiasis and forms of invasive aspergillosis that are refractory to **amphotericin**. Oral absorption is poor, and it is given intravenously, once daily. **Anidulafungin** is used mainly for invasive candidiasis; again, it is given intravenously. The principal side effects of both drugs include nausea, vomiting and diarrhoea, and rash. The relatively new **micafungin** is also mainly used for treating invasive candidiasis. It shares many of the side effects of the group but may also cause serious hepatotoxicity.

NYSTATIN

Nystatin (also called **fungicidin**) is a polyene macrolide antibiotic similar in structure to **amphotericin** and with the same mechanism of action. Its use is mainly limited to *Candida* infections of the oral mucosa; it is not absorbed through mucous membranes or skin and is administered as an oral suspension. ***Unwanted effects*** may include nausea, vomiting and diarrhoea.

SYNTHETIC ANTIFUNGAL DRUGS

AZOLES

The azoles are a group of synthetic fungistatic agents with a broad spectrum of antifungal activity. **Clotrimazole**, **econazole**, **fenticonazole**, **ketoconazole**, **miconazole**, **tioconazole** and **sulconazole** (not available in United Kingdom) are based on the imidazole nucleus and **isavuconazole**, **itraconazole**, **posaconazole**, **voriconazole** and **fluconazole** are triazole derivatives.

The azoles inhibit the fungal cytochrome P450 3A enzyme, *lanosine 14α-demethylase*, which converts lanosterol to ergosterol, the main sterol in fungal cell membranes. The resulting depletion of ergosterol alters the fluidity of the membrane, and this interferes with the action of membrane-associated enzymes. The net effect is an inhibition of replication. Azoles also inhibit the transformation of candidal yeast cells into hyphae – the invasive and pathogenic form of the organism. Depletion of membrane ergosterol reduces the binding of **amphotericin** but it is not known if this leads to a clinically important interaction.

Ketoconazole

Ketoconazole was the first azole that could be given orally to treat systemic fungal infections. It is effective against several different types of organism. It is, however, toxic, and relapse is common after apparently successful treatment. It is well absorbed from the GI tract and is distributed widely throughout the tissues and tissue fluids although it does not reach therapeutic concentrations in the central nervous system unless high doses are given. It is inactivated in the liver and excreted in bile and in urine. Its half-life in the plasma is 8 h.

Unwanted effects

The main hazard of **ketoconazole** is liver toxicity, which is rare but can prove fatal. Liver function is therefore monitored before and during treatment. Other adverse effects include GI disturbances and pruritus. Inhibition of adrenocortical steroid and testosterone synthesis has been recorded with high doses, the latter resulting in gynaecomastia in some male patients. There may be adverse interactions with other drugs. **Ciclosporin** and **astemizole** compete with **ketoconazole** for cytochrome P450 mixed function oxidase enzymes, causing increased plasma concentrations of both parties. Drugs that reduce gastric acidity decrease the absorption of **ketoconazole**, and **rifampicin** reduces the plasma concentration by induction of metabolising enzymes.

Fluconazole

Fluconazole is well absorbed and can be given orally or intravenously. It reaches high concentrations in the cerebrospinal fluid and ocular fluids and is used as a second-line agent to treat most types of fungal meningitis. Fungicidal concentrations are also achieved in vaginal tissue, saliva, skin and nails. It has a half-life of ~25 h and is mainly excreted unchanged in the urine.

Unwanted effects

Unwanted effects, which are generally mild, include nausea, headache and abdominal pain. However, exfoliative skin lesions (including, on occasion, Stevens–Johnson syndrome[4]) have been seen in some individuals – primarily in AIDS patients who are being treated with multiple drugs. Hepatitis has been reported, although this is rare, and **fluconazole**, in usual doses, does not inhibit steroidogenesis and hepatic drug metabolism to the same extent as occurs with **ketoconazole**.

Itraconazole

Itraconazole is active against a range of dermatophytes. It may be given orally but, after absorption (which is variable), undergoes extensive hepatic metabolism. It is highly lipid-soluble (and water-insoluble), and a formulation in which the drug is retained within pockets of β-cyclodextrin is available. In this form, **itraconazole** can be administered intravenously, thereby overcoming the problem of variable absorption from the GI tract. It does not penetrate the cerebrospinal fluid. When administered orally, its half-life is about 36 h, and it is excreted in the urine.

Unwanted effects

The most serious are hepatoxicity and Stevens–Johnson syndrome. GI disturbances, headache and allergic skin reactions can occur. Inhibition of steroidogenesis has not been reported. Drug interactions as a result of inhibition of cytochrome P450 enzymes occur (similar to **ketoconazole**).

Miconazole

Miconazole is generally used topically (often as a gel) for oral and other infections of the GI tract or for skin or mucosal fungal infection. If significant systemic absorption occurs, drug interactions can present a problem.

Other azoles

Clotrimazole, **econazole**, **tioconazole** and **sulconazole** are used only for topical application. **Clotrimazole** interferes with amino acid transport into the fungus by an action on the cell membrane. It is active against a wide range of fungi, including *Candida*. These drugs are sometimes combined with anti-inflammatory glucocorticoids (see Ch. 25). **Isavuconazole, posacanazole** and **voriconazole** are

---

[4]This is a severe and sometimes fatal condition involving blistering of the skin, mouth, GI tract, eyes and genitalia, often accompanied by fever, polyarthritis and kidney failure.

used mainly for the treatment of invasive life-threatening infections such as aspergillosis.

OTHER ANTIFUNGAL DRUGS

Flucytosine is a synthetic, orally active antifungal agent that is effective against a limited range (mainly yeasts) of systemic fungal infections. In fungal, but not human, cells it is converted to the antimetabolite 5-fluorouracil which inhibits thymidylate synthetase and thus DNA synthesis (see Chs 6 and 57). If given alone, drug resistance commonly arises during treatment, so it is usually combined with **amphotericin** for severe systemic infections such as systemic candidiasis and cryptococcal meningitis.

Flucytosine is usually given by intravenous infusion (because such patients are often too ill to take medicine by mouth) but can also be given orally. It is widely distributed throughout the body fluids, including the cerebrospinal fluid. About 90% is excreted unchanged via the kidneys, and the plasma half-life is 3–5 h. The dosage should be reduced if renal function is impaired.

Unwanted effects include GI disturbances, anaemia, neutropenia, thrombocytopenia and alopecia (possibly due to formation of fluorouracil [see Ch. 57] from **flucytosine** by gut bacteria), but these are usually manageable. Uracil is reported to decrease the toxic effects on the bone marrow without impairing the antimycotic action. Hepatitis has been reported but is rare.

Terbinafine is a highly lipophilic, keratinophilic fungicidal compound active against a wide range of skin pathogens. It is particularly useful against nail infections. It acts by selectively inhibiting the enzyme *squalene epoxidase*, which catalyses a key step in the synthesis of ergosterol from squalene in the fungal cell wall. The accumulation of squalene within the cell is toxic to the organism.

When used to treat ringworm or fungal infections of the nails, it is given orally. The drug is rapidly absorbed and is taken up by skin, nails and adipose tissue. Given topically, it penetrates skin and mucous membranes. It is metabolised in the liver by the cytochrome P450 system, and the metabolites are excreted in the urine.

Unwanted effects occur in about 10% of individuals and are usually mild and self-limiting. They include GI disturbances, rashes, pruritus, headache and dizziness. Joint and muscle pains have been reported and, more rarely, hepatitis.

Naftifine is similar in action to **terbinafine**. Among other developments, a morpholine derivative, **amorolfine**, which interferes with fungal sterol synthesis, is available as a nail lacquer, being effective against onychomycoses.

FUTURE DEVELOPMENTS

Fungal infections are on the rise no doubt encouraged by the prevalence of cancer chemotherapy, the increase in type 2 diabetes and transplant-associated immunosuppression. Many existing drugs have low efficacy, and problems with toxicity and new strains of commensal-turned-pathogenic fungi are emerging. Furthermore, increasing numbers of fungal strains are becoming resistant to the current antifungal drugs (see Ch. 51) as they develop resistance genes or acquire naturally occurring protective mutations. The capacity of some species to develop biofilms exacerbates this problem (although also offering other opportunities for drug design; see de Mello et al., 2017). It is fortunate that drug resistance is not transferable between fungi as it is in bacteria.

There is therefore a pressing need for more antifungals. Encouragingly, several new synthetic compounds are in development (see Gintjee et al, 2020), including novel azole drugs and new **amphotericin** derivatives as well as some with novel mechanisms of action such as **ibrexafungerp** (approved in the United States for vulvo-vaginal candidiasis), an oral inhibitor of glucan synthase, and **olorofim** (the first of a new class of antifungals), which is highly active against *Aspergillus* species. **Rezafungin** is a novel echinocandin antifungal derived by chemical modification of **anidulafungin** which has been approved in the United States and EU (but not yet in the UK). It is characterised by high potency against a range of fungal pathogens and a long-lasting effect requiring only a once weekly administration.

New therapeutic strategies are being developed too, including novel drug formulations (Asadi et al., 2021; Nagaraj et al., 2021) and the deployment of naturally occurring substances including microbial peptides (Li et al., 2021) and herbal extracts (Hsu et al., 2021). An ideal solution would be an antifungal vaccine(s). The idea was first mooted in the 1960s but so far success has proved elusive and there is no clinically approved antifungal vaccine available at the time of writing. Several approaches are being trialled (see Taborda and Nosanchuk, 2017). One promising development has been the use of 'hybrid' molecules bearing peptide and carbohydrate antigens. This strategy has already been shown to provoke robust immune responses in animals (Liao et al., 2019) but one fundamental problem with any vaccine-based solution is that it is dependent upon an appropriate function of the patient's immune system and it is precisely immunocompromised patients who often require treatment.

REFERENCES AND FURTHER READING

Asadi, P., Mehravaran, A., Soltanloo, N., Abastabar, M., Akhtari, J., 2021. Nanoliposome-loaded antifungal drugs for dermal administration: a review. Curr. Med. Mycol. 7, 71–78.

Chen, S.C., Slavin, M.A., Sorrell, T.C., 2011. Echinocandin antifungal drugs in fungal infections: a comparison. Drugs 71, 11–41.

Datta, K., Hamad, M., 2015. Immunotherapy of fungal infections. Immunol. Invest. 44, 738–776.

de Mello, T.P., de Souza Ramos, L., Braga-Silva, L.A., et al., 2017. Fungal biofilm – a real obstacle against an efficient therapy: lessons from Candida. Curr. Top. Med. Chem.

Denning, D.W., 2003. Echinocandin antifungal drugs. Lancet 362, 1142–1151.

Gintjee, T.J., Donnelley, M.A., Thompson 3rd, G.R., 2020. Aspiring antifungals: review of current antifungal pipeline developments. J. Fungi. (Basel) 6, 28.

Hadrich, I., Makni, F., Neji, S., et al., 2012. Invasive aspergillosis: resistance to antifungal drugs. Mycopathologia 174, 131–141.

Hsu, H., Sheth, C.C., Veses, V., 2021. Herbal extracts with antifungal activity against *Candida albicans*: a systematic review. Mini Rev. Med. Chem. 21, 90–117.

Li, T., Li, L., Du, F., et al., 2021. Activity and mechanism of action of antifungal peptides from microorganisms: a review. Molecules 26, 3438.

Liao, J., Pan, B., Liao, G., et al., 2019. Synthesis and immunological studies of beta-1,2-mannan-peptide conjugates as antifungal vaccines. Eur. J. Med. Chem. 173, 250–260.
Lupetti, A., Nibbering, P.H., Campa, M., et al., 2003. Molecular targeted treatments for fungal infections: the role of drug combinations. Trends Mol. Med. 9, 269–276.
Nagaraj, S., Manivannan, S., Narayan, S., 2021. Potent antifungal agents and use of nanocarriers to improve delivery to the infected site: a systematic review. J. Basic Microbiol. 61, 849–873.
Nanjappa, S.G., Klein, B.S., 2014. Vaccine immunity against fungal infections. Curr. Opin. Immunol. 28, 27–33.
Noel, T., 2012. The cellular and molecular defense mechanisms of the Candida yeasts against azole antifungal drugs. J. Mycol. Med. 22, 173–178.
Sant, D.G., Tupe, S.G., Ramana, C.V., et al., 2016. Fungal cell membrane-promising drug target for antifungal therapy. J. Appl. Microbiol. 121 (6), 1498–1510.
Taborda, C.P., Nosanchuk, J.D., 2017. Editorial: vaccines, immunotherapy and new antifungal therapy against fungi: updates in the new frontier. Front. Microbiol. 8, 1743.
Thursky, K.A., Playford, E.G., Seymour, J.F., et al., 2008. Recommendations for the treatment of established fungal infections. Intern. Med. J. 38, 496–520.

55 Antiprotozoal drugs

OVERVIEW

Protozoa are motile, unicellular eukaryotic organisms that have colonised virtually every habitat and ecological niche are collectively responsible for an enormous burden of illness in humans as well as domestic and wild animal populations. Historically, malaria has been one of mankind's greatest afflictions. Even today there are over 200 million cases of malaria each year and some half a million deaths, with pregnant women and children constituting the bulk of the victims. In this chapter, we will first review some general features of protozoa, discuss the interactions of these parasites with their hosts and then consider the therapy of each group of diseases in turn. In view of its continuing global importance, malaria is the main topic.

BACKGROUND

Protozoa may be conveniently classified into four main groups on the basis of their mode of locomotion: *amoebas*, *flagellates* and *sporozoa* are easily characterised, but the final group which includes *ciliates* also contain other organisms of uncertain affiliation, such as the *Pneumocystis jirovecii* mentioned in the last chapter. Protozoa have diverse feeding behaviour, with some being parasitic. Many have extremely complex life cycles, sometimes involving several hosts, reminiscent of the helminths discussed in Chapter 56. Table 55.1 lists some of the clinically important organisms, together with the diseases that they cause and an overview of current anti-infective drugs.

HOST–PARASITE INTERACTIONS

While mammals have developed very efficient mechanisms for defending themselves against invading parasites, many species have, in turn, evolved sophisticated evasion tactics. One common parasite ploy is to take refuge within the cells of the host, where antibodies cannot reach them. Most protozoa do this; for example, *Plasmodium* species take up residence in red cells, *Leishmania* species infect macrophages exclusively, while *Trypanosoma* species invade many other cell types. The host deals with these intracellular fugitives by deploying cytotoxic $CD8^+$ T cells and T helper (Th) 1 pathway cytokines, such as interleukin (IL)-2, tumour necrosis factor (TNF)-α and interferon-γ. These cytokines (see Ch. 17) activate macrophages, which can then kill the infected cells along with the intracellular parasites.

As we explained in Chapter 7, the Th1 pathway responses can be down-regulated by Th2 pathway cytokines (e.g. transforming growth factor-β, IL-4 and IL-10) and some intracellular parasites have exploited this by stimulating the production of Th2 cytokines thus reducing their vulnerability to Th1-driven activated macrophages. For example, the invasion of macrophages by *Leishmania* species induces transforming growth factor-β and IL-10, inactivates complement pathways and down-regulates many other intracellular defence mechanisms (Singh et al., 2012). Similar parasite countermeasures operate during worm (helminth) infestations (see Ch. 56).

Toxoplasma gondii has evolved a different, counterintuitive, gambit – *up-regulation* of host defence responses. The definitive host (i.e. in which sexual recombination occurs) of this protozoon is the cat, but humans can inadvertently become intermediate hosts, harbouring the asexual form of the parasite. In humans, *T. gondii* infects numerous cell types and has a highly virulent replicative stage. To ensure that its host survives, it stimulates production of interferon-γ, modulating the host's cell-mediated responses to promote encystment (and thus persistence) of the parasite in the tissues.

MALARIA AND ANTIMALARIAL DRUGS

Malaria[1] is caused by parasites belonging to the genus *Plasmodium*. Four main species infect humans: *Plasmodium falciparum*, *Plasmodium vivax*, *Plasmodium ovale* and *Plasmodium malariae*. A related parasite that infects monkeys, *Plasmodium knowlesi*, can also infect humans and is causing increasing concern in some regions, such as South-East Asia. The insect vector in all cases is the female *Anopheles* mosquito. This breeds in stagnant water and the disease it spreads is estimated to have killed half the human beings who have ever existed. Despite substantial therapeutic advances, it shows little sign of abandoning its murderous rampage.

Malaria was eradicated from most temperate countries in the 20th century, and the WHO attempted to eradicate malaria elsewhere using the powerful 'residual' insecticides and highly effective antimalarial drugs, such as **chloroquine**, which had, by then, become available. By the end of the 1950s, the incidence of malaria had dropped dramatically. However, it was clear by the 1970s that this attempt at eradication had failed, mainly because of the increasing resistance of the mosquito to the insecticides, and of the parasite to antimalarial drugs.

Massive increases in spending on public health campaigns, sponsored by a partnership of private, national governments and transnational organisations such as the WHO and the World Bank, have yielded significant successes and the global death toll has fallen by 60% over the last 20 years. In the latest World Malaria Report, the WHO has estimated that 1.5 million infections had been

[1]The disease was once considered to arise from marshy land and be somehow airborne, hence the Latin name '*mal aria*', meaning bad or poisonous air.

Table 55.1 Principal protozoal infections and common drug treatments

Type	Species	Disease	Common drug treatment
Amoeba	*Entamoeba histolytica*	Amoebic dysentery	Metronidazole, tinidazole, diloxanide
Flagellates	*Trypanosoma brucei rhodesiense* *Trypanosoma brucei gambiense*	Sleeping sickness	Suramin, pentamidine, melarsoprol, eflornithine, nifurtimox
	Trypanosoma. cruzi	Chagas disease	Nifurtimox, benznidazole
	Leishmania tropica *Leishmania donovani* *Leishmania mexicana* *Leishmania braziliensis*	Kala-azar Chiclero's ulcer Espundia Oriental sore	Sodium stibogluconate, amphotericin, pentamidine isethionate
	Trichomonas vaginalis	Vaginitis	Metronidazole, tinidazole
	Giardia lamblia	Diarrhoea, steatorrhoea	Metronidazole, tinidazole, mepacrine
Sporozoa	*Plasmodium falciparum*[a] *Plasmodium vivax* *Plasmodium ovale* *Plasmodium malariae*	Malignant tertian malaria Benign tertian malaria Benign tertian malaria Quartan malaria	Artemether, atovaquone, chloroquine, clindamycin, dapsone, doxycycline, lumefantrine, mefloquine, primaquine, proguanil, pyrimethamine, quinine, sulfadoxine, tafenoquine and tetracycline
	Toxoplasma gondii	Encephalitis, congenital malformations, eye disease	Pyrimethamine–sulfadiazine
Ciliates and others	*Pneumocystis carinii*[b]	Pneumonia	Co-trimoxazole, atovaquone, pentamidine isethionate

[a]See also Table 55.2.
[b]This organism is of uncertain classification. See text for details and Chapter 54 for further comments.

averted and 7.6 million lives saved. Progress in Sub-Saharan Africa which bears the greatest burden of disease has been particularly impressive, with the mortality rate falling by over 40% in the last decade. In Southeast Asia, the fall in infections was 75% and in the Indian subcontinent, 70%.

Despite these successes, the overall global statistics are still deeply concerning. According to the latest reported (2019) figures there were almost 230 million cases and 409,000 deaths, not much different from the previous year. Half the world's population is still at risk from the disease with Sub-Saharan Africa reporting some 94% of all cases. Even those who survive may suffer lasting impairment, with pregnant women, refugees and labourers entering endemic regions being at particularly high risk. Malaria also imposes a huge economic burden on countries where the disease is rife.

Also of concern is the fact that malaria has gained a foothold in other countries where it is not normally endemic. In Europe (declared 'Malaria free' in 2015), for example, virtually all reported cases (>8641 in 2019) of the disease are imported malaria[2] and this figure has remained fairly constant, unlike the global fall in cases. This phenomenon is partly due to increasing international travel, partly due to immigration from countries where the disease is endemic and (possibly) partly caused by global warming.

[2]More terminology: 'Airport malaria' is caused by infected mosquitoes in aircraft arriving from areas where the disease is endemic; 'baggage malaria' is caused by their presence in luggage arriving from such areas; and 'runway malaria' has been contracted by some rather unlucky passengers who have stopped in endemic areas even though they have not actually left the aircraft.

Malaria

Malaria is caused by various species of plasmodia, which are carried by the infected female *Anopheles* mosquito. Sporozoites (the asexual form of the parasite) are introduced into the host following insect bite and these develop in the liver into:

- schizonts (the pre-erythrocytic stage), which liberate merozoites – these infect red blood cells, forming motile trophozoites, which, after development, release another batch of erythrocyte-infecting merozoites, causing fever; this constitutes the *erythrocytic cycle*;
- dormant hypnozoites, which may liberate merozoites later (the exoerythrocytic stage).

The main malarial parasites causing tertian ('every third day') malaria are:

Malaria—cont'd

- *P. vivax*, which causes benign tertian malaria;
- *P. falciparum*, which causes malignant tertian malaria; unlike *P. vivax*, this plasmodium has no exoerythrocytic stage.

Some merozoites develop into gametocytes, the sexual forms of the parasite. When ingested by the mosquito, these give rise to further stages of the parasite's life cycle within the insect.

THE LIFE CYCLE OF THE MALARIA PARASITE

The symptoms of malaria include fever, shivering, pain in the joints, headache, repeated vomiting, generalised convulsions and coma. Symptoms, which appear during the erythrocytic phase of infection, only become apparent 7–9 days after being bitten by an infected mosquito. By far the most dangerous parasite is *P. falciparum* (predominant in Africa) followed by *P. vivax* (the dominant form of the parasite in other countries).

The life cycle of the parasite consists of a *sexual cycle*, which takes place in the female *Anopheles* mosquito, and an *asexual cycle*, which occurs in humans (Fig. 55.1 and the 'Malaria' box). Therefore, it is the mosquito, not the human, that is the *definitive* host for plasmodia. Indeed, it has been said that the only function of humans is to enable the parasite to infect more mosquitoes so that further sexual recombination can occur.

The sexual cycle in the mosquito involves fertilisation of the female *gametocyte* by the male gametocyte, with the formation of a *zygote*, which develops into an *oocyst (sporocyst)*. A further stage of division and multiplication takes place, leading to rupture of the sporocyst with release of *sporozoites*, which then migrate to the mosquito's salivary glands and thus enter the human host following mosquito bites.

When sporozoites enter the human host, they disappear from the bloodstream within 30 min and enter the parenchymal cells of the liver where, during the next 10–14 days, they undergo a *pre-erythrocytic* stage of development and multiplication. The parasitised liver cells then rupture, and a host of fresh *merozoites* are released. These bind to and enter erythrocytes and develop into motile intracellular parasites termed *trophozoites*. During the *erythrocytic stage*, the parasite remodels the host cell, inserting parasite proteins and phospholipids into the red cell membrane. The host's haemoglobin is transported to the parasite's food vacuole, where it is digested, providing a source of amino acids. Free haem, which would be toxic to the plasmodium, is rendered harmless by polymerisation to *haemozoin*. Some antimalarial drugs act by inhibiting the haem polymerase enzyme responsible for this step.

Following mitotic replication, the parasite in the red cell is termed a *schizont*, and its rapid growth and division, *schizogony*. Another phase of multiplication results in the production of further *merozoites*, which are released when the red cell ruptures. These merozoites then bind to and enter fresh red cells, and the erythrocytic cycle begins again. In certain forms of malaria, some sporozoites entering the liver cells form *hypnozoites*, or 'sleeping' forms of the parasite, which can be reactivated months or years later to continue an *exoerythrocytic* cycle of multiplication.

Malaria parasites can multiply in the body at a phenomenal rate – a single parasite of *P. vivax* can give rise to 250 million merozoites in 14 days. To appreciate the therapeutic challenges this entails, note that destruction of 94% of the parasites every 48 h will serve only to maintain equilibrium and will not further reduce their number or their propensity for proliferation. Some merozoites, on entering red cells, differentiate into male and female gametocytes. These can complete their life cycle only when taken up again by the mosquito, when it sucks the blood from the infected host.

The periodic episodes of fever that characterise malaria result from the synchronised rupture of red cells with release of merozoites and cell debris. The rise in temperature is associated with a rise in the concentration of TNF-α in the plasma. Relapses of malaria are likely to occur with those forms of malaria that have an exoerythrocytic cycle, because the dormant hypnozoite form in the liver may emerge after an interval of weeks or months to start the infection again.

The characteristic clinical presentations of the different forms of human malaria are as follows:

- *P. falciparum*, which has an erythrocytic cycle of 48 h in humans, produces *malignant tertian malaria* – 'tertian' because the fever was believed to recur every third day (actually it varies) and 'malignant' because it is the most severe form of malaria and is responsible for most malaria deaths. The plasmodium induces adhesion molecules on the infected cells, which then stick to uninfected red cells forming clusters (rosettes). These adhere to, and obstruct the vessels of the microcirculation, interfering with tissue blood flow and causing organ dysfunction including renal failure and encephalopathy (cerebral malaria). *P. falciparum* does not have an exoerythrocytic stage, so if the erythrocytic stage is eradicated, relapses do not occur.
- *P. vivax* produces *benign tertian malaria*, less severe than falciparum malaria and rarely fatal. However, exoerythrocytic forms may persist for years and cause relapses.
- *P. ovale*, which has a 48-h cycle and an exoerythrocytic stage, is the cause of a rare form of malaria.
- *P. malariae*, which is said to cause *quartan malaria*, has a 72-h cycle. It has no exoerythrocytic cycle.

Individuals living in areas where malaria is endemic may acquire a natural immunity, but this may be lost if the individual is absent from the area for more than 6 months. *Sickle cell disease*, which is also common in Africa, may have persisted in the population because those carrying the single copy of the mutated haemoglobin gene (and who do not therefore develop the disease) have about 30% less incidence of malaria. The best way to prevent malaria is to prevent mosquito bites by suitable clothing, insect repellents and bed nets. Bed nets sprayed with insecticides such as permethrin are very effective and form the cornerstone of many public health campaigns.

Sometimes mistaken for malaria is *babesiosis* which is caused by tickborne parasites of the *Babesia* sp. (five examples known). The main vector seems to be the arthropod, *Ixodes ricinus*. The disease is endemic in many

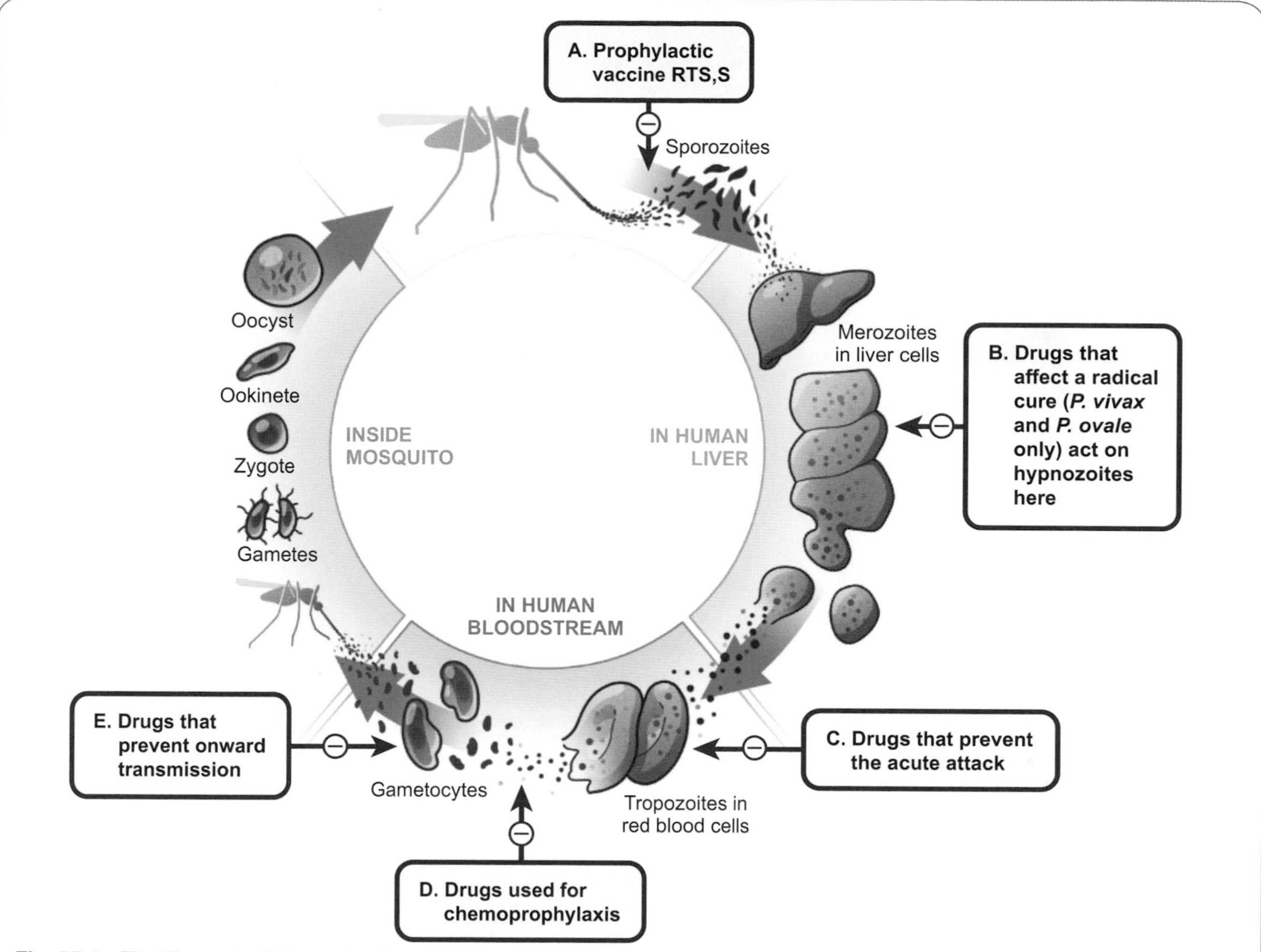

Fig. 55.1 The life cycle of the malarial parasite and the site of action of some current antimalarial drugs. Infection is initiated by the bite of a parasite-bearing female *Anopheles* mosquito, which introduces the asexual sporozoite form of the parasite into the victim's blood. These are susceptible to immune-mediated clearance by the RTS,S vaccine *(yellow box A)*. The sporozoites then enter a *pre-* or *exoerythrocytic cycle* in the liver infecting the liver cells entering the merozoite stage. Here, the merozoites multiply, eventually rupturing the liver cells and releasing vesicles containing large numbers of the parasite. Some may re-enter other liver cells to become hypnozoites, dormant forms of the parasite. In the case of *Plasmodium vivax* and *Plasmodium ovale* these may reactivate years later causing relapses in the disease. Drugs that affect a radical cure act here *(yellow box B)*. Once released into the blood the merozoites begin the erythrocytic phase of their life cycle, entering red blood cells, dividing and multiplying (schizogony). Drugs which prevent acute attacks of malaria can act at this point *(yellow box C)*. Eventually the infected erythrocytes rupture, releasing large numbers of motile trophozoites into the blood; it is at this point that the characteristic clinical symptoms of the disease appear. Drugs which block the link between the exoerythrocytic stage and the erythrocytic stage that are used for chemoprophylaxis act here *(yellow box D)*. Some merozoites develop into male and female gametocytes in red cells. If consumed by another mosquito, these gametocytes can mature in the insect's gut to form oocysts. These pass into the mosquito salivary glands where they give rise to further sporozoites which may enter the next victim to begin the cycle again. Drugs which block onward transmission of the infection act at this step *(yellow box E)*. (Adapted and modified from http://www.malariavaccine.org/malaria-and-vaccines/vaccin-development/life-cycle-malaria-parasite)

countries including Europe but cases are rare and may be asymptomatic. Like malaria, the life cycle of the parasite also includes an erythrocytic stage. Treatment, if required, is usually with **clindamycin**, **quinine** or **atovaquone**.

ANTIMALARIAL DRUGS

In general, antimalarial drugs are classified in terms of their action against the different stages of the life cycle of the parasite (see Fig. 55.1). Fig. 55.2 shows chemical structures of some significant agents and Fig. 55.3 summarises what is known about their molecular targets. Most current drugs are only effective against the erythrocytic phase of the parasitic life cycle (**primaquine** is an exception). Some are used prophylactically to prevent malaria (Table 55.2), while others are used to treat acute attacks.

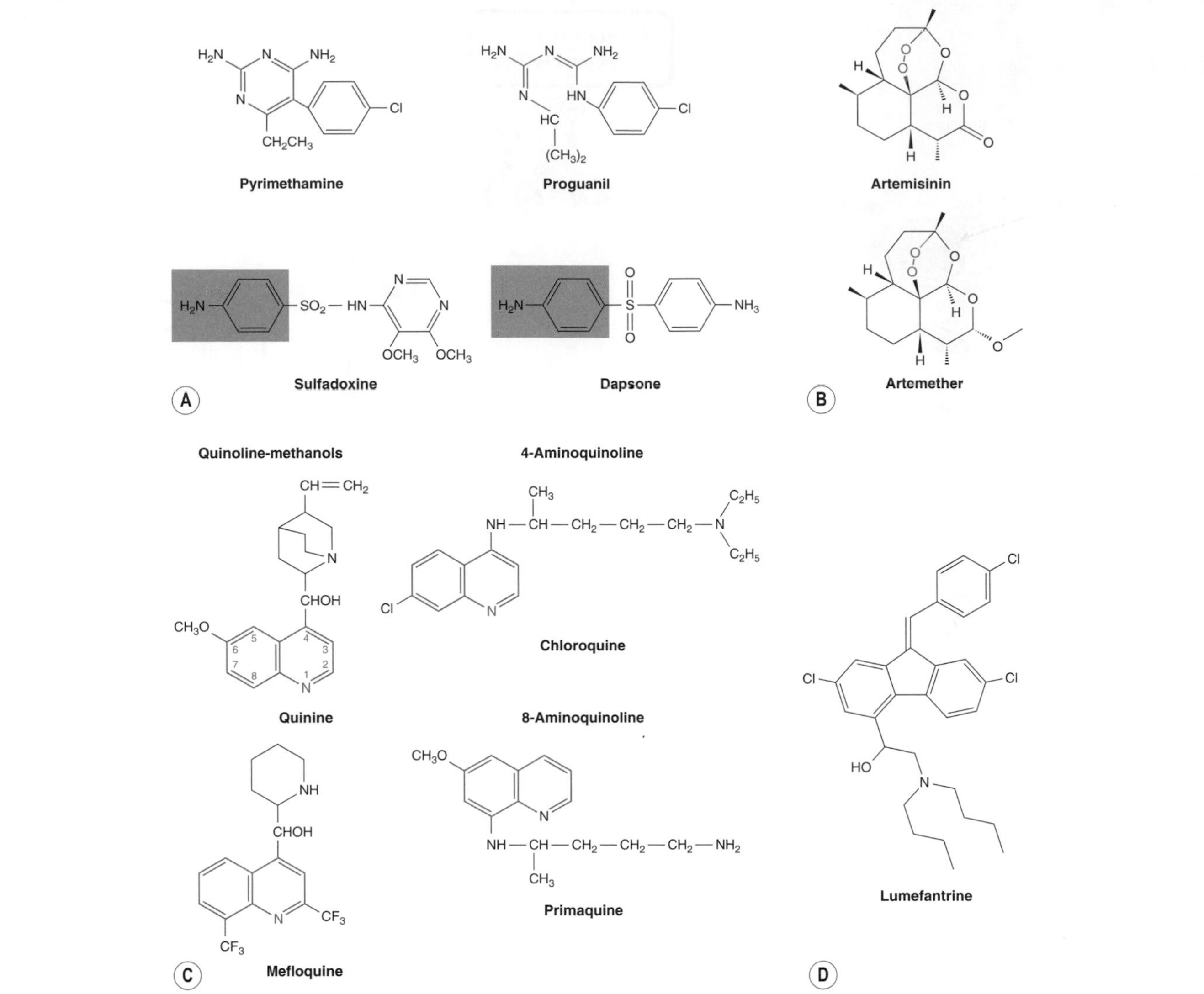

(A) Pyrimethamine, Proguanil, Sulfadoxine, Dapsone

(B) Artemisinin, Artemether

(C) Quinoline-methanols: Quinine, Mefloquine; 4-Aminoquinoline: Chloroquine; 8-Aminoquinoline: Primaquine

(D) Lumefantrine

Fig. 55.2 Structures of some significant antimalarial drugs. (A) Drugs that act on the folic acid pathway of the plasmodia. Folate antagonists (**pyrimethamine**, **proguanil**) inhibit dihydrofolate reductase; the relationship between these drugs and the pteridine moiety is shown in *orange*. Sulfones (e.g. **dapsone**) and sulfonamides (e.g. **sulfadoxine**) compete with p-aminobenzoic acid for dihydropteroate synthetase (relationship shown in *orange box*; see also Chs 51 and 52). (B) **Artemisinin** and a derivative artemether. Note the endoperoxide bridge structure *(in orange)* that is crucial to their action. (C) Some quinolone antimalarials. The quinoline moiety is shown in *orange*. (D) The aryl amino alcohol **lumefantrine**.

The use of antimalarials has changed considerably during the last half-century, mainly because resistance developed to **chloroquine** and other successful early drug combinations (see Butler et al., 2010). Where this has occurred, monotherapy has largely been abandoned in favour of **artemisinin**-based combination therapy (ACT) regimes. The WHO 'malaria' page (see Further Reading list) provides links to their latest recommendations covering all areas in the world and the 'Antimalarial drugs' box and Table 55.2 provide a brief summary of currently recommended treatment regimens. Only antimalarial drugs in common use are described in this chapter.

Drugs used to treat acute malaria

Blood schizonticidal agents which act on the erythrocytic forms of the plasmodium (see Fig. 55.1, site A) can suppress the acute manifestations of the disease. In the case of *P.*

Antimalarial therapy and the parasite life cycle

Drugs used in the treatment of malaria are directed at several sites of action and no single agent is able to target all phases of the parasite life cycle.

The main agents used are:

- Drugs which treat the acute attack of malaria by acting on the parasites in the blood; these can cure infections with parasites (e.g. *P. falciparum*) that have no exoerythrocytic stage.
- Drugs which provide prophylactic protection act on merozoites emerging from liver cells.
- Drugs which effect a 'radical cure' are active against parasites in the liver.
- Some drugs act on gametocytes and prevent transmission by the mosquito.

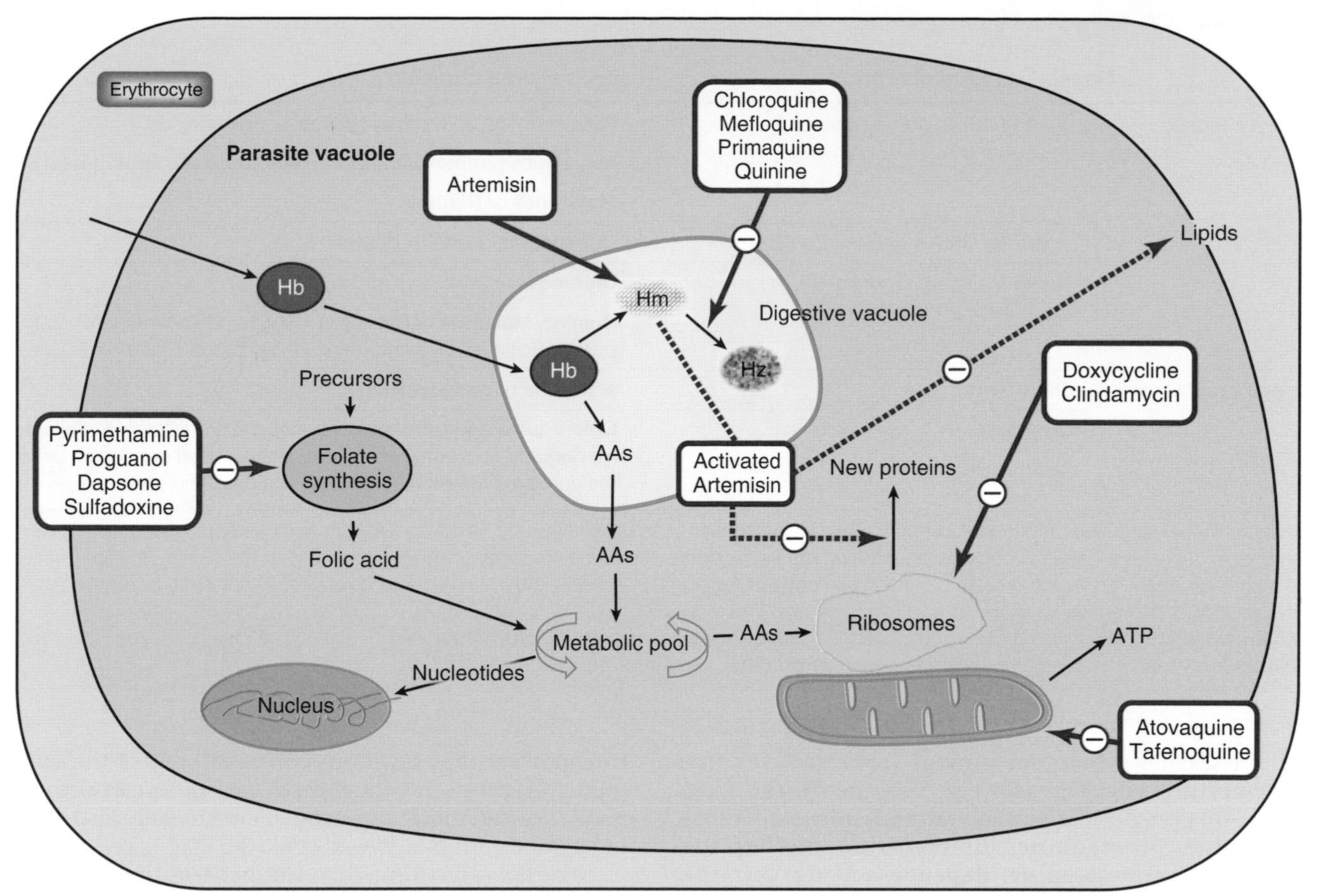

Fig. 55.3 Schematic diagram showing the sites of action of antimalarial drug targets in plasmodia. During the *erythrocytic stage* of infection the parasite lives within erythrocytes in a *parasitophorus vacuole* and feeds on haemoglobin (Hb) which is imported into the *digestive vacuole* where it is metabolised to amino acids (AAs) for use by the parasite. The haem (Hm) residue remaining is toxic to the parasite, so this is metabolised to haemozoin (Hz). Some quinolone antimalarials (e.g. **chloroquine**) prevent the detoxification of haem, thus poisoning the parasite. Other drugs (e.g. **pyrimethamine**) prevent the synthesis of folic acid, which is essential for nucleotide synthesis, target the synthesis of nascent proteins by ribosomes (e.g. antibiotics such as **clindamycin**) or inhibit mitochondrial function (e.g. **atovaquone**). **Artemisinin** and its derivatives enter the digestive vacuole where they are 'activated' by haem to form compounds that react with, and thus damage, proteins and lipids. (After Blasco, B., Leroy, D., Fidock, D.A., 2017. Antimalarial drug resistance: linking *Plasmodium falciparum* parasite biology to the clinic. Nat. Med. 23, 917–928.)

falciparum or *P. malariae*, which have no exoerythrocytic stage, these drugs effect a 'suppressive' or 'clinical' cure; however, in the case of *P. vivax* or *P. ovale*, which have exoerythrocytic forms, the parasite can re-emerge later to cause relapses.

This group of drugs includes:

- **artemisinin** and related compounds derived from the Chinese herb *qinghao*, which are usually used in combination with other drugs;
- the quinoline-methanols (e.g. **quinine** and **mefloquine**) and various 4-aminoquinolines (e.g. **chloroquine**);
- agents that interfere either with the synthesis of folate (e.g. **dapsone**) or with its action (e.g. **pyrimethamine** and **proguanil**);
- **atovaquone**, which affects mitochondrial function.

Combinations of these agents are frequently used. Some antibiotics, such as the tetracycline **doxycycline** (see Ch. 52), have proved useful when combined with the above agents. They have an antiparasitic effect in their own right, but also control other concomitant infections.

Drugs that effect a radical cure

Tissue schizonticidal agents effect a 'radical' cure by eradicating *P. vivax* and *P. ovale* parasites in the liver (see Fig. 55.1, site B). Only the 8-aminoquinolines (e.g. **primaquine** and **tafenoquine**) have this action. These drugs also destroy gametocytes and thus reduce the spread of infection.

Drugs used for chemoprophylaxis

Drugs used for chemoprophylaxis (also known as *causal prophylactic drugs*) block the link between the exoerythrocytic stage and the erythrocytic stage, and thus prevent the development of malarial attacks. True causal prophylaxis – the prevention of infection by the killing of the sporozoites on entry into the host – is not feasible with present drugs, although it may be possible with vaccines (see later). Clinical attacks can be prevented by chemoprophylactic drugs that

Table 55.2 Examples of drug treatment and chemoprophylaxis of malaria[a]

Reason for administration		Typical drug choices
Active infection	...with *Plasmodium falciparum*	**Quinine** followed by **doxycycline** or **clindamycin** Sometimes **pyrimethamine** with **sulfadoxine** if appropriate, **or** **Malarone**[b] or **Riamet**[c]
	....with unknown or mixed organisms	**Quinine**, **Malarone** or **Riamet**
	...with *Plasmodium malariae*, *Plasmodium vivax* or *Plasmodium ovale*	**Chloroquine** (if not in a resistant area) **or** **Quinine**, **Malarone** or **Riamet** (if in a chloroquine-resistant area) possibly followed by **primaquine** in the case of *P. vivax* or *P. ovale*
Chemoprophylaxis	Short-term	**Malarone** or **doxycycline**
	Long-term	**Chloroquine** and **proguanil** are often the first choice. **Malarone**, **mefloquine** and **doxycycline** can also be used depending upon the duration of treatment required and drug tolerance.

[a]This information is based on current UK recommendations including the *British National Formulary* 2022. It must be appreciated that this is only a summary, not a definitive guide to prescription, as the recommended drug combinations vary depending on the patient, the area visited, the overall risk of infection, the presence of resistant forms of the disease and specialised help should be sought. Also, these regimes must be used with other preventive measures.
[b]**Malarone** is a proprietary fixed-dose combination of **atovaquone** and **proguanil hydrochloride**.
[c]**Riamet** is a proprietary fixed-dose combination of **artemether** and **lumefantrine**

kill the parasites when they emerge from the liver after the pre-erythrocytic stage (see Fig. 55.1, site C). The drugs used for this purpose are mainly **artemisinin** derivatives, **chloroquine**, **piperaquine**, **lumefantrine**, **mefloquine**, **proguanil**, **pyrimethamine**, **dapsone** and **doxycycline**. They are often used in combinations with other drugs.

Chemoprophylactic agents are given to individuals who intend travelling to an area where malaria is endemic. Administration should start at least 1 week before entering the area and should be continued throughout the stay and for at least a month afterwards. No chemoprophylactic regimen is 100% effective, and unwanted effects may occur. A further problem is the complexity of some regimens, which require different drugs to be taken at different times, and the fact that different agents may be required for different travel destinations. For a brief summary of currently commonly recommended regimens of chemoprophylaxis, see Table 55.2.

Drugs used to prevent transmission

Some drugs (e.g. **primaquine**, **proguanil** and **pyrimethamine**) can also destroy gametocytes (see Fig. 55.1, site D), preventing transmission by the mosquito and thus diminishing the human reservoir of the disease, although they are rarely used for this action alone.

Drug resistance

Parasite resistance is a serious and ongoing problem with almost all antimalarial drugs, with the possible exception of **lumefantrine**. In many cases, resistant strains of the parasite appear within a decade, or even less, of the introduction of a novel drug. Most of the resistance is due to the appearance of spontaneously arising point mutations in (for example) target proteins such as dihydrofolate reductase (which confers resistance to antifolate drugs such as **proguanil**) or in the mitochondrial cytochrome B subunit (which confers resistance to **atovaquone**). Mutations in parasite transporters that facilitate entry, or control the exit of, quinolone drugs into the digestive vacuoles can also confer resistance and mutations in other enzymes are also thought to be important (see Blasco et al., 2017).

A rather alarming development is the increase in *multidrug resistance* in certain parts of the world. This may be linked to poor compliance, poor therapy or local variations in host immune responses to infection

CHLOROQUINE

The 4-aminoquinoline **chloroquine** dates from the 1940s but is still widely used as a blood schizonticidal agent (see Fig. 55.1, site A), effective against the erythrocytic forms of all four plasmodial species (in areas where resistance is not an issue), but it does not have any effect on sporozoites, hypnozoites or gametocytes. It is uncharged at neutral pH and can therefore diffuse freely into the parasite lysosome. At the acid pH of the lysosome, it is converted to a protonated, membrane-impermeable form and is 'trapped' inside the parasite. Its chief antimalarial action derives from an inhibition of *haem polymerase*, the enzyme that polymerises toxic free haem to harmless *haemozoin*. This poisons the parasite and prevents it from utilising the amino acids from haemoglobin proteolysis. **Chloroquine** has also been used as a disease-modifying antirheumatoid drug (see Ch. 25) and also has some **quinidine**-like actions on the heart (see Ch. 20).

Resistance

P. falciparum is now resistant to **chloroquine** in most parts of the world. Resistance appears to result from enhanced efflux of the drug from parasitic vesicles as a result of mutations in plasmodia transporter genes (Baird, 2005). Resistance of *P. vivax* to **chloroquine** is also a growing problem.

Administration and pharmacokinetic aspects

Chloroquine is generally administered orally, but severe falciparum malaria may be treated by frequent intramuscular or subcutaneous injection of small doses, or by slow continuous intravenous infusion. Following oral dosing, it is completely absorbed, extensively distributed throughout the tissues and concentrated in parasitised red cells. Release from tissues and infected erythrocytes is slow. The drug is metabolised in the liver and excreted in the urine, 70% as unchanged drug and 30% as metabolites. Elimination is slow, the major phase having a half-life of 50 h, and a residue persists for weeks or months.

Unwanted effects

Chloroquine has few adverse effects when given for chemoprophylaxis. However, unwanted effects, including nausea and vomiting, dizziness and blurring of vision, headache and urticarial symptoms, can occur when larger doses are administered to treat acute attacks of malaria. Large doses have also sometimes resulted in retinopathies and hearing loss. Bolus intravenous injections of **chloroquine** may cause hypotension and, if high doses are used, fatal dysrhythmias. **Chloroquine** is considered to be safe for use by pregnant women.

Amodiaquine has very similar action to chloroquine. It was withdrawn several years ago because of the risk of agranulocytosis but has now been reintroduced in several areas of the world where **chloroquine** resistance is endemic. **Piperaquine** is also structurally related to **chloroquine** and shares a similar pharmacology. It is often used in combination with **artenimol**.

QUININE

Quinine, derived from cinchona bark, has been used for the treatment of 'fevers' since the 16th century, when Jesuit missionaries brought the bark, and the knowledge of its action, to Europe from Peru. It is a blood schizonticidal drug effective against the erythrocytic forms of all four species of *Plasmodium* (see Fig. 55.1, site A), but it has no effect on exoerythrocytic forms or on the gametocytes of *P. falciparum*. Its mechanism of action is the same as that of **chloroquine**, but **quinine** is not so extensively concentrated in the plasmodium as **chloroquine**, so other mechanisms could also be involved. With the emergence and spread of **chloroquine** resistance, **quinine** is now the main chemotherapeutic agent for *P. falciparum* in certain parts of the world. Pharmacological actions on host tissue include a depressant action on the heart, a mild oxytocic effect on the uterus in pregnancy, a marginal blocking action on the neuromuscular junction and a weak antipyretic effect.

Resistance

Some degree of resistance to **quinine** has developed because of increased expression of plasmodial drug efflux transporters.

Pharmacokinetic aspects

Quinine is well absorbed and is usually administered orally as a 7-day course, but it can also be given by slow intravenous infusion for severe *P. falciparum* infections and in patients who are vomiting. A loading dose may be required, but bolus intravenous administration is contraindicated because of the risk of cardiac dysrhythmias. The half-life of the drug is 10 h; it is metabolised in the liver and the metabolites are excreted in the urine within about 24 h.

Unwanted effects

Quinine has a bitter taste, and oral compliance is often poor.[3] It is irritant to the gastric mucosa and can cause nausea and vomiting. 'Cinchonism' – characterised by nausea, dizziness, tinnitus, headache and blurring of vision – is likely to occur if the plasma concentration exceeds 30–60 μmol/L. Excessive plasma levels may also cause hypotension, cardiac dysrhythmias and severe central nervous system (CNS) disturbances such as delirium and coma.

Other, infrequent, unwanted reactions that have been reported are bone marrow depression (mainly thrombocytopenia) and hypersensitivity reactions. **Quinine** can stimulate insulin release. Patients with marked falciparum parasitaemia may develop hypoglycaemia for this reason and also because of glucose consumption by the parasite. This can make a differential diagnosis between a coma caused by cerebral malaria and low blood sugar difficult. A rare result of treating malaria with **quinine**, or of erratic and inappropriate use of the drug, is *Blackwater fever*, a severe and often fatal condition in which acute haemolytic anaemia is associated with renal failure.

MEFLOQUINE

Mefloquine (see Fig. 55.2) is a blood schizonticidal compound active against *P. falciparum* and *P. vivax* (see Fig. 55.1, site A); however, it has no effect on hepatic forms of the parasites, so treatment of *P. vivax* infections is usually followed by a course of **primaquine** to eradicate the hypnozoites. **Mefloquine** acts in the same way as quinine and is frequently combined with **pyrimethamine**.

Resistance

P. falciparum is resistant to **mefloquine** in some areas – particularly in South-East Asia – and is thought to be caused, as with **quinine**, by increased expression in the parasite of drug efflux transporters.

Pharmacokinetic aspects and unwanted effects

Mefloquine is given orally and is rapidly absorbed. It has a slow onset of action and a very long plasma half-life (up to 30 days), which may be the result of enterohepatic cycling or tissue storage.

When **mefloquine** is used for treatment of the acute attack, about 50% of subjects complain of GI disturbances. Transient CNS side effects – giddiness, confusion, dysphoria and insomnia – can occur, and there have been a few reports of aberrant atrioventricular conduction and, rarely, serious skin diseases or severe neuropsychiatric reactions. It is contraindicated in pregnant women or in those liable to become pregnant within 3 months of stopping the drug, because of its long half-life and uncertainty about its teratogenic potential. When used for chemoprophylaxis, the unwanted actions are usually milder, but the drug should not be used in this way unless

[3]Quinine may be the first documented anti-infective agent. The Scottish doctor George Leghorn is credited with re-introducing it as a remedy for 'fevers' (often malarial in origin) in the 18th century. British soldiers stationed in India in the 1870s were encouraged to take the drug to counteract the risk of this disease. The bitter taste of the quinine was masked by incorporating it into palatable drinks, which included fruit, gin, vodka and other beverages. Originally named 'Indian Tonic Water' it is still popular today, although less quinine is used in its preparation.

there is a high risk of acquiring **chloroquine**-resistant malaria.

LUMEFANTRINE

This aryl amino alcohol drug is related to an older compound, **halofantrine**, which is now seldom used. **Lumefantrine** is never used alone but is combined with **artemether**. Its mode of action is probably to prevent parasite detoxification of haem. The pharmacokinetics of the combination are complex (see Ezzet et al., 1998). Unwanted effects of the combination may include GI and CNS symptoms.

DRUGS AFFECTING FOLATE METABOLISM

Whilst known as antibacterial drugs, agents which affect folate metabolism also have antiprotozoal activity. **Pyrimethamine** and **proguanil** inhibit dihydrofolate reductase, which prevents the utilisation of folate in DNA synthesis. Used together, they block the folate pathway at different points, thus acting synergistically.

Pyrimethamine is similar in structure to the antibacterial drug **trimethoprim** (see Ch. 52). **Proguanil** has a slightly different structure but its (active) metabolite can assume a similar configuration. Both drugs have a greater affinity for the plasmodium enzyme than for the human enzyme. They have a slow action against the erythrocytic forms of the parasite (see Fig. 55.1, site A), and **proguanil** is believed to have an additional effect on the initial hepatic stage (see Fig. 55.1) but not on the hypnozoites of *P. vivax* (see Fig. 55.1, site B). **Pyrimethamine** is used only in combination with either a sulfone or a sulfonamide.

Sulfonamides and sulfones inhibit the synthesis of folate in plasmodia by competing with p-aminobenzoic acid (see Ch. 52). The main sulfonamide used in malaria treatment is **sulfadoxine**, and the only sulfone used is **dapsone**. Details of these drugs are given in Chapter 52. The sulfonamides and sulfones are active against the erythrocytic forms of *P. falciparum* but are less active against those of *P. vivax*; they have no activity against the sporozoite or hypnozoite forms of the plasmodia. **Pyrimethamine–sulfadoxine** has been extensively used for chloroquine-resistant malaria, but unfortunately resistance to this combination has developed in many areas.

Resistance

Point mutations in the enzymes of the folate synthesis pathway can confer resistance to these drugs.

Pharmacokinetic aspects

Both **pyrimethamine** and **proguanil** are given orally and are well, although slowly, absorbed. **Pyrimethamine** has a plasma half-life of 4 days, and effective 'suppressive' plasma concentrations may last for 14 days; it is taken once a week. The half-life of **proguanil** is 16 h. It is a prodrug and is metabolised in the liver to its active form, *cycloguanil*, which is excreted mainly in the urine. It must be taken daily.

Unwanted effects

These drugs have few untoward effects in therapeutic doses. Larger doses of the **pyrimethamine–dapsone** combination can however cause serious reactions such as haemolytic anaemia, agranulocytosis and lung inflammation. The **pyrimethamine–sulfadoxine** combination can cause serious skin reactions, blood dyscrasias and allergic alveolitis and it is no longer recommended for chemoprophylaxis. In high doses, **pyrimethamine** may inhibit mammalian dihydrofolate reductase and cause a *megaloblastic anaemia* (see Ch. 24) and folic acid supplements should be given if this drug is used during pregnancy. Resistance to antifolate drugs may arise from single-point mutations in the genes encoding parasite dihydrofolate reductase.

PRIMAQUINE

Primaquine is an 8-aminoquinoline drug, which is (almost uniquely among clinically available antimalarial drugs) active against liver hypnozoites (see Fig. 55.2). **Etaquine** and **tafenoquine** are more active and slowly metabolised analogues of **primaquine**. These drugs can effect a radical cure of *P. vivax* and *P. ovale* malaria in which the parasites have a dormant stage in the liver. **Primaquine** does not affect sporozoites and has little if any action against the erythrocytic stage of the parasite. However, it has a gametocidal action and is the most effective antimalarial drug for preventing transmission of all four species of plasmodia. It is almost invariably used in combination with another drug, usually **chloroquine**. The pharmacology of **primaquine** and similar drugs has been reviewed by Shanks et al. (2001).

Resistance

Resistance to primaquine is (happily) scarce, although evidence of a decreased sensitivity of some *P. vivax* strains has been reported.

Pharmacokinetic aspects

Primaquine is given orally and is well absorbed. Its metabolism is rapid, and very little drug is present in the body after 10–12 h. The half-life is 3–6 h. **Tafenoquine** is metabolised much more slowly and therefore has the advantage that it can be given on a weekly basis.

Unwanted effects

Primaquine has few unwanted effects in most patients when used in normal therapeutic dosage. Dose-related GI symptoms may occur however, and large doses may cause methaemoglobinaemia with cyanosis.

Primaquine can also cause haemolysis in individuals with the X chromosome-linked genetic metabolic condition, *glucose 6-phosphate dehydrogenase deficiency*, in red cells (see Ch. 12). When this deficiency is present, the red cells are not able to regenerate nicotinamide adenine dinucleotide phosphate (NADPH), which is depleted by the oxidant metabolic derivatives of **primaquine**. As a consequence, the metabolic functions of the red cells are impaired, and haemolysis occurs. The deficiency of the enzyme occurs in up to 15% of black males and is also fairly common in some other ethnic groups. Glucose 6-phosphate dehydrogenase activity should be estimated before giving **primaquine**.

ARTEMISININ AND RELATED COMPOUNDS

The importance of this group cannot be overstated as they are often the only effective treatment for drug-resistant *P. falciparum*. These sesquiterpene lactones are derived from *sweet wormwood*, *qinghao*, a traditional Chinese remedy for fevers. The scientific name, conferred on the herb by

Linnaeus, is *Artemisia*.[4] **Artemisinin**, a poorly soluble chemical extract from *Artemisia*, is a fast-acting blood schizonticide effective in treating acute attacks of malaria (including **chloroquine**-resistant and cerebral malaria). In randomised trials, artemisinins have cured attacks of malaria, including cerebral malaria, more rapidly and with fewer unwanted effects than any other antimalarial agents. **Artemisinin** and derivatives are effective against multidrug-resistant *P. falciparum* in sub-Saharan Africa and, combined with **mefloquine**, against multidrug-resistant *P. falciparum* in South-East Asia.

Pharmacokinetic aspects

Derivatives of artemisinin, which include **artenimol** (dihydroartemisinin, the active metabolite of **artemisinin**), **artesunate** (a water-soluble derivative available in some countries) and **artemether,** are more potent and better absorbed than the parent compound. All artemisinins are concentrated in parasitised red cells. Upon entering the digestive vacuoles, haem iron activates their unusual 'endoperoxide bridge' giving rise to highly reactive oxygen-containing compounds. These cause irreversible damage to parasite proteins, lipid membranes and other targets. These drugs are without effect on liver hypnozoites.

Artemisinin can be given orally, intramuscularly or by suppository; **artemether** orally or intramuscularly; and artesunate intramuscularly or intravenously. They are rapidly absorbed and widely distributed and are converted in the liver to the active metabolite *dihydroartemisinin*. The half-life of **artemisinin** is about 4 h, of **artesunate** is 45 min and of **artemether** is 4–11 h.

Unwanted effects. are few. Transient heart block, decrease in blood neutrophil count and brief episodes of fever have been reported. In animal studies, **artemisinin** causes an unusual injury to some brain stem nuclei, particularly those involved in auditory function; however, there have been no reported incidences of neurotoxicity in humans.

In rodent studies, **artemisinin** potentiated the effects of **mefloquine**, **primaquine** and **tetracycline**, was additive with **chloroquine** and antagonised the sulfonamides and the folate antagonists. For this reason, **artemisinin** derivatives are frequently used in combination with other antimalarial drugs as part of ACT regimes; for example, **artemether** is often given in combination with **lumefantrine**.

Resistance

Initially resistance was not a major problem but, alarmingly, reports that the parasite in some areas of the world (e.g. South-East Asia) was becoming less sensitive to these drugs - either alone or in ACT combinations - began to appear about a decade ago (Blasco et al., 2017). The situation is being monitored very carefully.

[4]*Artemisia* extracts have been used for thousands of years in China for treating 'fevers'. *Artemisia* was the wife and sister of the 4th-century king of Halicarnassus. Upon his death, she was so distraught that she mixed his ashes with whatever she drank to make it bitter. Since 'sweet' wormwood is noted for its extreme bitterness, it was named in her honour. The biologically active compound artemisinin was isolated by Chinese chemists in 1972. This was ignored in the West for more than 10 years, until the WHO recognised its importance and, in 2002, placed it on their list of 'essential drugs' for malaria treatment. In 2015, the Chinese pharmacologist Youyou Tu was awarded the Nobel Prize for her role in developing this drug.

ATOVAQUONE

Atovaquone is a hydroxynaphthoquinone drug used prophylactically to prevent malaria, and to treat cases resistant to other drugs. It acts primarily to inhibit the parasite's mitochondrial electron transport chain, possibly by mimicking the natural substrate ubiquinone. **Atovaquone** is usually used in combination with the antifolate drug **proguanil**, because they act synergistically. The mechanism underlying this synergism is not known, but it is specific for this particular pair of drugs, because other antifolate drugs or electron transport inhibitors have no such synergistic effect. When combined with **proguanil**, **atovaquone** is highly effective and well tolerated. Few unwanted effects of such combination treatment have been reported, but abdominal pain, nausea and vomiting can occur. Pregnant or breastfeeding women should not take **atovaquone**.

Resistance

Resistance to **atovaquone** alone is rapid and results from a single-point mutation in the gene for cytochrome B. Resistance to combined treatment with **atovaquone** and **proguanil** is less common.

POTENTIAL NEW ANTIMALARIAL DRUGS

Malaria has been dubbed a 're-emerging disease', largely because of the increasing appearance of drug-resistant strains of the parasite. No new *synthetic* drug has been discovered for over 40 years and so progress has become a matter of some urgency.

In this context, Ceravolo et al. (2021) have reviewed the quest for naturally occurring substances with antimalarial actions (recall that the first antimalarial was **quinine**) and reported some success, while Nweze et al. (2021) have focused on products derived from marine organisms with antiprotozoal properties. Miller et al. (2019) discuss progress in the quest for novel drugs that inhibit of parasite digestive vacuole proteases. Coupled with a better understanding of the pharmacokinetic aspects of current drugs (Elewa and Wilby, 2017), these advances may enable novel, more selective treatment regimes in the future.

A significant development in existing antimalarial drugs has arisen through the application of synthetic biology to solve the problem of **artemisinin** production. **Artemisinin** is notoriously difficult to synthesise by conventional chemical techniques and awkward to harvest in large amounts. Using genetically modified yeast transfected with genes from *Artemisia* it has been possible to produce substantial amounts of the precursor *artemisinic acid*, which can be easily converted into **artemisinin** (Paddon et al., 2013), thus relieving the desperate shortage of the drug.

Historically, the creation of an antimalarial vaccine has proved technically problematic because of the different forms the parasite assumes during its life cycle, but after decades of frustration, 2021 finally saw a major breakthrough (see Laurens, 2020). The launch of the *RTS,S* vaccine (**Mosquirix**), the first antimalarial vaccine (and the first antiprotozoal vaccine ever) to be approved for clinical use, was the result of over 30 years of development funded by a private–public initiative which included substantial funding arising from the philanthropic Bill and Melinda Gates Foundation.

The vaccine was launched in 2020 and endorsed by the WHO as a treatment for vulnerable children (who constitute the majority of the victims) in Sub-Saharan Africa, a continent where the deadliest form of the parasite, *P. falciparum*, predominates. Its target is the *circumsporozoite antigen* which, as the name implies, is present in the earliest forms of the parasite introduced into the bloodstream by the infecting mosquito. It therefore prevents the spread of the parasite into the liver and therefore subsequent stages of its development. Studies have shown that the vaccine provides a 30% protection against *P. falciparum* infection. This may not sound much but is highly significant especially when considered together with other concomitant preventive measures such as insecticide impregnated mosquito nets, treatment of stagnant water, etc.

But perhaps the main lesson from the development of this vaccine is that it is technically feasible. Indeed, several other vaccines are in preparation (Almeida et al., 2021; Bonam et al., 2021) but whilst vaccine prophylaxis is indeed a breakthrough in public health treatment, it still important to remember that it cannot treat the acute disease and that antimalarial drugs will still be important even following the widespread adoption of the vaccine.

Antimalarial drugs

- **Chloroquine** is a blood schizonticide that is concentrated in the parasite and inhibits the haem polymerase. Resistance is now common. **Piperaquine** is a long-lasting derivative of **chloroquine.**
- **Quinine** is a blood schizonticide. It is usually given in combination therapy with:
  - **pyrimethamine**, a folate antagonist that acts as a slow blood schizonticide, and either
  - **dapsone**, a sulfone, or
  - **sulfadoxine**, a long-acting sulfonamide (orally active; half-life 7–9 days).
- **Proguanil**, a folate antagonist, is a slow blood schizonticide with some action on the primary liver forms of *P. vivax.*
- **Mefloquine** is a blood schizonticidal agent active against *P. falciparum* and *P. vivax* and which acts by inhibiting the parasite haem polymerase.
- **Primaquine** is effective against the liver hypnozoites and also gametocytes.
- **Artemisinin** derivatives are now widely used particularly in combination with other drugs such as **lumefantrine** and **artenimol.** They are fast-acting blood schizonticidal agents that are effective against both *P. falciparum* and *P. vivax.*
- **Artenimol** (dihydroxyartemisinin) is the active metabolite of **artemisinin.**
- **Artesunate** is water-soluble and can be given orally or by intravenous, intramuscular or rectal administration. Resistance is so far uncommon.
- **Atovaquone** (in combination with **proguanil**) is used for prevention, and for the treatment of, acute uncomplicated *P. falciparum* malaria. Resistance to **atovaquone** develops rapidly if it is given alone.

AMOEBIASIS AND AMOEBICIDAL DRUGS

Amoebiasis is caused by infection with one or more strains of *Entamoeba* organisms. Infection may be asymptomatic or provoke a range of GI symptoms, some of which may be serious. The main organism of concern is *Entamoeba histolytica*, the causative agent of amoebiasic dysentery, which can produce a severe colitis (dysentery) and, sometimes, liver abscesses.

The infection is encountered around the world, but more often in warmer climates, and is associated with poor sanitation. Approximately 50 million people are currently (2020) thought to harbour the disease, with some 100,000 deaths occurring each year as a result. It is considered to be the second-leading cause of death from parasitic diseases worldwide.

The organism has a simple life cycle, and humans are the chief hosts. Infection, generally spread by poor hygiene, follows the ingestion of the mature cysts in water or food that is contaminated with human faeces. The infectious cysts pass into the colon, where they develop into *trophozoites*. These motile organisms adhere to colonic epithelial cells, utilising a galactose-containing lectin on the host cell membrane. Here, the trophozoites feed, multiply, encyst and eventually pass out in the faeces, thus completing their life cycle. Some individuals are symptomless 'carriers' and harbour the parasite without developing overt disease, but cysts are present in their faeces, and they can infect other individuals. The cysts can survive outside the body for at least a week in a moist and cool environment.

Drugs used in amoebiasis

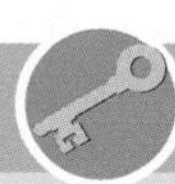

Amoebiasis is caused by infection with *E. histolytica*, which causes dysentery and liver abscesses. The organism may be present in motile invasive form or as a cyst. The main drugs are:

- **Metronidazole** given orally (half-life 7 h). Active against the invasive form in gut and liver but not the cysts. Unwanted effects (rare): gastrointestinal (GI) disturbances and CNS symptoms. **Tinidazole** is similar. Follow-on treatment directed at the GI lumen is needed to ensure eradication.
- **Diloxanide** is a luminal agent given orally with no serious unwanted effects. It is active, while unabsorbed, against the non-invasive form in the GI tract.

The trophozoite lyses the colonic mucosal cells (hence 'histolytica') using proteases, *amoebapores* (peptides that form pores in cell membranes) or by inducing host cell apoptosis. The organism then invades the submucosa, where it secretes factors to modify the host response which would otherwise prove lethal to the parasite. It is this process that produces the characteristic bloody diarrhoea and abdominal pain, although a chronic intestinal infection may be present in the absence of dysentery. In some patients, an *amoebic granuloma (amoeboma)* may be present in the intestinal wall. The trophozoites may also migrate through the damaged intestinal tissue into the portal blood and hence the liver, giving rise to the most common extra-intestinal symptom of the disease – amoebic liver abscesses.

The use of drugs to treat this condition depends largely on the site and type of infection. The drugs of choice, which are often used in combination for the various forms of amoebiasis, are:

- **metronidazole** (or **tinidazole**) followed by **diloxanide** for acute invasive intestinal amoebiasis resulting in acute severe amoebic dysentery;
- **diloxanide** for chronic intestinal amoebiasis;

- **metronidazole** followed by **diloxanide** for hepatic amoebiasis;
- **diloxanide** for the asymptomatic 'carrier' state.

METRONIDAZOLE

Metronidazole kills the trophozoites of *E. histolytica* but has no effect on the cysts. It is the drug of choice for invasive amoebiasis of the intestine or the liver, but it is less effective against organisms in the lumen of the gut. The drug is activated by anaerobic organisms to a compound that damages DNA, leading to parasite apoptosis.

Metronidazole is usually given orally and is rapidly and completely absorbed. Rectal and intravenous preparations are also available. It is distributed rapidly throughout the tissues, reaching high concentrations in the body fluids, including the cerebrospinal fluid. Some is metabolised, but most is excreted in urine.

Unwanted effects are mild. The drug produces a metallic, bitter taste in the mouth but causes few unwanted effects in therapeutic doses. Minor GI disturbances have been reported, as have CNS symptoms (dizziness, headache, sensory neuropathies). **Metronidazole** causes a **disulfiram**-like reaction to alcohol (see Ch. 50), which should be strictly avoided. It should not be used in pregnancy.

Tinidazole is similar to **metronidazole** in its mechanism of action and unwanted effects, but is eliminated more slowly, having a half-life of 12–14 h.

DILOXANIDE

Diloxanide and, more commonly, an insoluble ester, **diloxanide furoate**, are the drugs of choice for the asymptomatic infected patient and are often given as a follow-up after the disease has been reversed with metronidazole. Both drugs have a direct amoebicidal action, affecting the parasites before encystment. **Diloxanide furoate** is given orally and acts without being absorbed. Unwanted GI or other effects may be seen but it has an excellent safety profile.

Other drugs that are sometimes used include the antibiotic **paromomycin** (see Further Reading list for information). Some promising new candidate drugs have been identified by Shrivastav et al. (2020).

TRYPANOSOMIASIS AND TRYPANOCIDAL DRUGS

Trypanosomes belong to the group of pathogenic flagellate protozoa. Two subtypes of *Trypanosoma brucei* (*rhodesiense* and *gambiense*) cause sleeping sickness in Africa (also known as *HAT* – human African trypanosomiasis). In South America, another species, *Trypanosoma cruzi*, causes *Chagas disease* (also known as American trypanosomiasis).

Almost eliminated by 1960, HAT re-emerged but, because of concerted public health campaigns, the number of cases is now falling again. Thanks to improved awareness, treatment and preventive measures, WHO reported in 2019 less than 1000 cases detected (25,000 in 1995) out of some 60 million people at risk of contracting sleeping sickness. The disease is caused by *T. brucei gambiense* (TbG) and *T. brucei rhodesiense* (TbR) with TbR being the more aggressive form albeit less widespread. Civil unrest, famine, AIDS and pandemic diseases such as COVID-19 encourage the spread of the disease by reducing the chances of distributing medication or because patients are immunocompromised. Related trypanosome infections also pose a major risk to livestock and thus have a secondary impact on human health and well-being. In the case of Chagas disease, some 6–7 million people are believed to harbour the infection according to the latest WHO survey.

The vector of HAT is the tsetse fly. In both types of the disease, there is an initial local lesion at the site of entry, which may (in the case of TbR) develop into a painful *chancre* (ulcer or sore). This is followed by bouts of parasitaemia and fever as the parasite enters the haemolymphatic system. The parasites, and the toxins they release during the second phase of the disease, cause organ damage. This manifests as 'sleeping sickness' when parasites reach the CNS causing somnolence and progressive neurological breakdown. Left untreated, such infections are fatal.

T. cruzi is spread through other blood-sucking insects, including the 'kissing bugs'. The initial phases of the infection are similar, but the parasites damage the heart, muscles and sometimes liver, spleen, bone and intestine. Many people harbour chronic infections. The cure rate is good if treatment begins immediately after infection but is less successful if delayed. An accessible account of trypanosomiasis is given by Buscher et al. (2017).

The main drugs used for HAT are **suramin**, with **pentamidine** as an alternative, in the haemolymphatic stage of the disease, and the arsenical **melarsoprol** for the late stage with CNS involvement and/or **eflornithine** (see Burchmore et al., 2002; Burri and Brun, 2003). All have toxic side effects. **Nifurtimox**, **eflornithine** and **benznidazole** are used in Chagas disease: however, there is no totally effective treatment for this form of trypanosomiasis.

SURAMIN

Suramin was introduced into the therapy of trypanosomiasis in 1920. The drug binds firmly to host plasma proteins, and the complex enters the trypanosome by endocytosis, and is then liberated by lysosomal proteases. It inhibits key parasite enzymes inducing gradual destruction of organelles, such that the organisms are cleared from the circulation after a short interval.

Administration is by slow intravenous injection. The blood concentration drops rapidly during the first few hours and then more slowly over the succeeding days. A residual concentration remains for 3–4 months. **Suramin** tends to accumulate in mononuclear phagocytes, and in the cells of the proximal tubule in the kidney.

Unwanted effects are common. **Suramin** is relatively toxic, particularly in malnourished patients, the main organ affected being the kidney. Many other slowly developing adverse effects have been reported, including optic atrophy, adrenal insufficiency, skin rashes, haemolytic anaemia and agranulocytosis. A small proportion of individuals have an immediate idiosyncratic reaction to **suramin** injections, which may include nausea, vomiting, shock, seizures and loss of consciousness.

PENTAMIDINE

Pentamidine has a direct trypanocidal action in vitro. It is rapidly taken up into parasites by a high-affinity energy-dependent carrier and is thought to interact with their DNA. The drug is administered intravenously or by deep intramuscular injection, usually daily for 10–15 days. After absorption from the injection site, it binds strongly to tissues (especially in the kidney) and is eliminated slowly, only 50% of a dose being excreted over 5 days. Fairly high concentrations of the drug persist in the kidney, the liver and the spleen for several months, but it does not penetrate the blood–brain barrier. It is also active in *Pneumocystis* pneumonia (see Ch. 52). Its usefulness is limited by its unwanted effects – an immediate decrease in blood pressure, with tachycardia, breathlessness and vomiting, and later serious toxicity, such as kidney damage, hepatic impairment, blood dyscrasias and hypoglycaemia.

MELARSOPROL

This is an organic arsenical compound that is used mainly when the CNS is involved. It is given intravenously and enters the CNS in high concentrations, where it kills the parasite. It is a highly toxic drug that produces many unwanted effects including encephalopathy and, sometimes, immediate fatality. As such, it is only administered under strict supervision.

EFLORNITHINE

Eflornithine inhibits the parasite *ornithine decarboxylase* enzyme. It shows good activity against *TbG* and is used as a back-up for **melarsoprol**, although unfortunately it has limited activity against *TbR*. Side effects are common and may be severe but are readily reversed when treatment is discontinued. Combined therapy with **nifurtimox** and **eflornithine** has yielded promising results in patients with late-stage disease.

Until the recent introduction of **fexinidazole** (only approved in 2021 and not covered here), **eflornithine** was the only novel drug adopted in the last 30 years. There is therefore an urgent need for new agents to treat trypanosome infections, partly because of the toxicity of existing drugs and partly because of developing drug resistance. Several reviews detail recent progress in the area both in natural (Simoben et al., 2018) and other synthetic therapeutic agents (Altamura et al., 2022; Kourbeli et al., 2021).

OTHER PROTOZOAL INFECTIONS AND DRUGS USED TO TREAT THEM

LEISHMANIASIS

Leishmania organisms are flagellate protozoa, and the infection that they cause is spread by the female sandfly. According to the latest (2020) WHO figures, more than 1 billion people are at risk from the disease and some 30,000 cases of visceral *leishmaniasis* and 1 million cases of the cutaneous disease are currently seen worldwide. Many cases are asymptomatic so the disease is not found in all those infected. With increasing international travel, leishmaniasis is being imported into new areas and opportunistic infections are now being reported (particularly in AIDS patients).

The parasite exists in a flagellated form (*promastigote*) in the gut of the infected insect and a nonflagellated intracellular form (*amastigote*) in the mononuclear phagocytes of the infected mammalian host. Within these cells, the parasites thrive in modified phagolysosomes. By deploying an array of countermeasures (Singh et al., 2012), they promote the generation of Th2 cytokines and subvert the macrophage's microbiocidal systems to ensure their survival. The amastigotes multiply, and eventually the infected cell releases a new crop of parasites into the haemolymphatic system, where they can infect further macrophages and possibly other cells.

Different species of *Leishmania* exist in different geographical areas and cause distinctive clinical manifestations (see Table 55.1). Typical presentations include:

- a *cutaneous form*, which presents as an unpleasant chancre ('oriental sore', 'Chiclero's ulcer' and other names), which may heal spontaneously, but can leave scarring. This is the most common form and is found in the Americas, some Mediterranean countries and parts of central Asia;
- a *mucocutaneous form* ('espundia' and other names), which presents as large ulcers of the mucous membranes of the mouth, nose and throat; most cases are seen in South America;
- a serious *visceral form* ('kala-azar' and other names), where the parasite spreads through the bloodstream causing hepatomegaly, splenomegaly, anaemia and intermittent fever. This manifestation is encountered mainly in the Indian subcontinent and West Africa.

The main drugs used in visceral leishmaniasis are pentavalent antimony compounds such as **sodium stibogluconate** and **pentamidine** as well as **amphotericin** (see Ch. 54), which is sometimes used as a follow-up treatment. **Miltefosine**, an antitumour drug, is also used in some countries (not United Kingdom), as is **meglumine antimoniate**.

Sodium stibogluconate is given intramuscularly or by slow intravenous injection in a 10-day course. It is rapidly eliminated in the urine, 70% being excreted within 6 h. More than one course of treatment may be required. The mechanism of its action is not clear, but the drug may increase production of toxic oxygen free radicals in the parasite.

Unwanted effects include anorexia, vomiting, bradycardia and hypotension. Coughing and substernal pain may occur during intravenous infusion. Reversible hepatitis and pancreatitis are common.

Miltefosine (hexadecylphosphocholine) is also effective in the treatment of both cutaneous and visceral leishmaniasis. The drug may be given orally and is well tolerated. Side effects are mild and include nausea and vomiting. In vitro, the drug induces DNA fragmentation and apoptosis in the parasites.

Other drugs, such as antibiotics and antifungals, may be given concomitantly with the earlier agents. They may have some action on the parasite in their own right, but their main utility is to control the spread of secondary infections.

Resistance to current drugs, particularly the pentavalent antimonials (possibly caused by increased expression of an antimonial efflux pump), is a serious problem and there is no immediate prospect of a vaccine. The pharmacology of current drugs and prospects for new agents have been reviewed by Singh et al. (2012), Altamura et al. (2022) and Santana et al. (2020).

TRICHOMONIASIS

The principal *Trichomonas* organism that produces disease in humans is *Trichomonas vaginalis*. Virulent strains cause inflammation of the vagina and sometimes of the urethra in males. The main drug used in therapy is **metronidazole** (see Ch. 52), although resistance to this drug is on the increase. High doses of **tinidazole** are also effective, with few side effects.

GIARDIASIS

Giardia lamblia colonises the upper GI tract in its trophozoite form, and the cysts pass out in the faeces. Infection is then spread by ingestion of food or water contaminated with faecal matter containing the cysts. It is encountered worldwide, and epidemics caused by bad sanitation are not uncommon. **Metronidazole** is the drug of choice, and treatment is usually very effective. **Tinidazole** or **mepacrine** may be used as an alternative.

TOXOPLASMOSIS

The cat is the definitive host of *T. gondii*, a pathogenic member of this group of organisms (i.e. it is the only host in which the sexual cycle can occur). It expels the infectious cysts in its faeces; humans can inadvertently become intermediate hosts, harbouring the asexual form of the parasite. Ingested oocysts develop into sporozoites, then to trophozoites, and finally encyst in the tissues. In most individuals, the disease is asymptomatic or self-limiting, although intrauterine infections can severely damage the developing foetus and it may cause fatal generalised infection in immunosuppressed patients or those with AIDS, in whom *toxoplasmic encephalitis* may occur. In humans, *T. gondii* infects numerous cell types and has a highly virulent replicative stage.

The treatment of choice is **pyrimethamine–sulfadiazine** (to be avoided in pregnant patients); trimethoprim-**sulfamethoxazole** (**co-trimoxazole**, see Ch. 52); or combinations of **pyrimethamine** with **clindamycin**, **clarithromycin** or **azithromycin** (see Ch. 52).

PNEUMOCYSTIS

First recognised in 1909, *Pneumocystis carinii* (now known as *P. jirovecii*; see also Ch. 54) shares structural features with both protozoa and fungi, leaving its precise taxonomy uncertain. Previously considered to be a widely distributed but largely innocuous microorganism, it is now recognised as an important cause of opportunistic infections in immunocompromised patients. It is common in AIDS, where *P. carinii* pneumonia is often the presenting symptom as well as a leading cause of death.

High-dose **co-trimoxazole** (see Chs 51 and 52) is the drug of choice in serious cases, with parenteral **pentamidine** as an alternative. Treatment of milder forms of the disease (or prophylaxis) can be effected with **atovaquone**, **trimethoprim–dapsone** or **clindamycin–primaquine** combinations.

FUTURE DEVELOPMENTS

Antiprotozoal pharmacology is a huge global challenge, with each species posing its own distinct problems to the would-be designer of new antiprotozoal drugs. But it is not simply a lack of new drugs that is the problem: for political and economic reasons, the countries and populations most affected often lack an efficient infrastructure for the distribution and safe administration of the drugs that we already possess. Cultural attitudes, civil wars, famine, pandemics, the circulation of counterfeit or defective drugs, drought and natural disasters also exacerbate this problem.

REFERENCES AND FURTHER READING

Host–parasite interactions

Brenier-Pinchart, M.P., Pelloux, H., Derouich-Guergour, D., et al., 2001. Chemokines in host–parasite interactions. Trends Parasitol. 17, 292–296.

Langhorne, J., Duffy, P.E., 2016. Expanding the antimalarial toolkit: targeting host-parasite interactions. J. Exp. Med. 213, 143–153.

Malaria

Achieng, A.O., Rawat, M., Ogutu, B., et al., 2017. Antimalarials: molecular drug targets and mechanism of action. Curr. Top. Med. Chem. 17, 2114–2128.

Almeida, M.E.M., Vasconcelos, M.G.S., Tarrago, A.M., Mariuba, L.A.M., 2021. Circumsporozoite surface protein-based malaria vaccines: a review. Rev. Inst. Med. Trop. Sao Paulo 63, e11.

Baird, J.K., 2005. Effectiveness of antimalarial drugs. N. Engl. J. Med. 352, 1565–1577.

Basore, K., Cheng, Y., Kushwaha, A.K., Nguyen, S.T., Desai, S.A., 2015. How do antimalarial drugs reach their intracellular targets? Front. Pharmacol. 6, 91.

Blasco, B., Leroy, D., Fidock, D.A., 2017. Antimalarial drug resistance: linking *Plasmodium falciparum* parasite biology to the clinic. Nat. Med. 23, 917–928.

Bonam, S.R., Renia, L., Tadepalli, G., Bayry, J., Kumar, H.M.S., 2021. Plasmodium *falciparum* malaria vaccines and vaccine adjuvants. Vaccines (Basel) 9, 1–35.

Butler, A.R., Khan, S., Ferguson, E., 2010. A brief history of malaria chemotherapy. J. R. Coll. Physicians Edinb. 40, 172–177.

Ceravolo, I.P., Aguiar, A.C., Adebayo, J.O., Krettli, A.U., 2021. Studies on activities and chemical characterization of medicinal plants in search for new antimalarials: a ten year review on ethnopharmacology. Front. Pharmacol. 12, 734263.

Deu, E., 2017. Proteases as antimalarial targets: strategies for genetic, chemical, and therapeutic validation. FEBS J. 284 (16), 2604–2628.

Elewa, H., Wilby, K.J., 2017. A Review of Pharmacogenetics of Antimalarials and associated clinical implications. Eur. J. Drug Metab. Pharmacokinet. 42, 745–756.

Ezzet, F., Mull, R., Karbwang, J., 1998. Population pharmacokinetics and therapeutic response of CGP 56697 (artemether + benflumetol) in malaria patients. Br. J. Clin. Pharmacol. 46, 553–561.

Fidock, D.A., Rosenthal, P.J., Croft, S.L., et al., 2004. Antimalarial drug discovery: efficacy models for compound screening. Nat. Rev. Drug Discov. 3, 509–520.

Foley, M., Tilley, L., 1997. Quinoline antimalarials: mechanisms of action and resistance. Int. J. Parasitol. 27, 231–240.

Gorobets, N.Y., Sedash, Y.V., Singh, B.K., et al., 2017. An overview of currently available antimalarials. Curr. Top. Med. Chem. 17, 2143–2157.

Greenwood, B.M., Fidock, D.A., Kyle, D.E., et al., 2008. Malaria: progress, perils, and prospects for eradication. J. Clin. Invest. 118, 1266–1276.

Hoffman, S.L., Vekemans, J., Richie, T.L., Duffy, P.E., 2015. The march toward malaria vaccines. Am. J. Prev. Med. 49, S319–S333.

Laurens, M.B., 2020. RTS,S/AS01 vaccine (Mosquirix): an overview. Hum. Vaccin. Immunother. 16, 480–489.

Miller Iii, W.A., Teye, J., Achieng, A.O., et al., 2019. Antimalarials: review of plasmepsins as drug targets and HIV protease inhibitors interactions. Curr. Top. Med. Chem. 18, 2022–2028.

Mishra, M., Mishra, V.K., Kashaw, V., et al., 2017. Comprehensive review on various strategies for antimalarial drug discovery. Eur. J. Med. Chem. 125, 1300–1320.

Muregi, F.W., Wamakima, H.N., Kimani, F.T., 2012. Novel drug targets in malaria parasite with potential to yield antimalarial drugs with long useful therapeutic lives. Curr. Pharm. Des. 18, 3505–3521.

Nweze, J.A., Mbaoji, F.N., Li, Y.M., et al., 2021. Potentials of marine natural products against malaria, leishmaniasis, and trypanosomiasis parasites: a review of recent articles. Infect. Dis. Poverty 10, 9.

Paddon, C.J., Westfall, P.J., Pitera, D.J., et al., 2013. High-level semi-synthetic production of the potent antimalarial artemisinin. Nature 25, 528–532.

Shanks, G.D., Kain, K.C., Keystone, J.S., 2001. Malaria chemoprophylaxis in the age of drug resistance. II. Drugs that may be available in the future. Clin. Infect. Dis. 33, 381–385.

Thota, S., Yerra, R., 2016. Drug discovery and development of antimalarial agents: recent advances. Curr. Protein Pept. Sci. 17, 275–279.

Amoebiasis

Haque, R., Huston, C.D., Hughes, M., et al., 2003. Amebiasis. N. Engl. J. Med. 348, 1565–1573.

Shrivastav, M.T., Malik, Z., Somlata, 2020. Revisiting drug development against the neglected tropical disease, amebiasis. Front. Cell. Infect. Microbiol. 10, 628257.

Stanley, S.L., 2001. Pathophysiology of amoebiasis. Trends Parasitol. 17, 280–285.

Stanley, S.L., 2003. Amoebiasis. Lancet 361, 1025–1034.

Trypanosomiasis

Aksoy, S., Gibson, W.C., Lehane, M.J., 2003. Interactions between tsetse and trypanosomes with implications for the control of trypanosomiasis. Adv. Parasitol. 53, 1–83.

Altamura, F., Rajesh, R., Catta-Preta, C.M.C., Moretti, N.S., Cestari, I., 2022. The current drug discovery landscape for trypanosomiasis and leishmaniasis: challenges and strategies to identify drug targets. Drug Dev. Res. 83, 225–252.

Barrett, M.P., 2010. Potential new drugs for human African trypanosomiasis: some progress at last. Curr. Opin. Infect. Dis. 23, 603–608.

Brun, R., Don, R., Jacobs, R.T., Wang, M.Z., Barrett, M.P., 2011. Development of novel drugs for human African trypanosomiasis. Future Microbiol. 6, 677–691.

Burchmore, R.J., Ogbunude, P.O., Enanga, B., Barrett, M.P., 2002. Chemotherapy of human African trypanosomiasis. Curr. Pharm. Des. 8, 256–267.

Burri, C., Brun, R., 2003. Eflornithine for the treatment of human African trypanosomiasis. Parasitol. Res. 90 (Suppl. 1), S49–S52.

Buscher, P., Cecchi, G., Jamonneau, V., Priotto, G., 2017. Human African trypanosomiasis. Lancet 390, 2397–2409.

Denise, H., Barrett, M.P., 2001. Uptake and mode of action of drugs used against sleeping sickness. Biochem. Pharmacol. 61, 1–5.

Gehrig, S., Efferth, T., 2008. Development of drug resistance in *trypanosoma brucei rhodesiense* and *trypanosoma brucei gambiense*. treatment of human African trypanosomiasis with natural products (review). Int. J. Mol. Med. 22, 411–419.

Keiser, J., Stich, A., Burri, C., 2001. New drugs for the treatment of human African trypanosomiasis: research and development. Trends Parasitol. 17, 42–49.

Kourbeli, V., Chontzopoulou, E., Moschovou, K., Pavlos, D., Mavromoustakos, T., Papanastasiou, I.P., 2021. An overview on target-based drug design against kinetoplastid protozoan infections: human African trypanosomiasis, chagas disease and leishmaniases. Molecules 26, 1–41.

Simoben, C.V., Ntie-Kang, F., Akone, S.H., Sippl, W., 2018. Compounds from African medicinal plants with activities against selected parasitic diseases: schistosomiasis, trypanosomiasis and leishmaniasis. Nat. Prod. Bioprospect. 8, 151–169.

Leishmaniasis

Handman, E., Bullen, D.V.R., 2002. Interaction of *leishmania* with the host macrophage. Trends Parasitol. 18, 332–334.

Mishra, J., Saxena, A., Singh, S., 2007. Chemotherapy of leishmaniasis: past, present and future. Curr. Med. Chem. 14, 1153–1169.

Santana, W., de Oliveira, S.S.C., Ramos, M.H., et al, 2021. Exploring innovative leishmaniasis treatment: drug targets from pre-clinical to clinical findings. Chem. Biodivers. 18, e2100336.

Singh, N., Kumar, M., Singh, R.K., 2012. Leishmaniasis: current status of available drugs and new potential drug targets. Asian Pac. J. Trop. Med. 5, 485–497.

Useful Web resources

https://www.who.int.

56 Antihelminthic drugs

OVERVIEW

Some 1.5 billion people around the world suffer from *helminthiasis* – infection with various species of parasitic *helminths* (worms). Inhabitants of tropical or subtropical low-income countries are most at risk; children often become infected at birth (polyparasitaemia is common) and may remain so throughout their lives. The clinical consequences of helminthiasis vary: for example, threadworm infections mainly cause discomfort but infection with *schistosomiasis* (*bilharzia*) or hookworm is associated with serious morbidity. Anaemia, nutritional problems and cognitive impairment are common in helminth-infected children. Helminthiasis is often co-endemic with malaria, tuberculosis and HIV/AIDS, adding to the disease burden as well as interfering with vaccination campaigns. Helminth infections are an even greater concern in veterinary medicine, affecting both domestic pets and farm animals leading to significant welfare and economic challenges. Because of its prevalence and economic significance, the pharmacological treatment of helminthiasis with antihelminthics (or anthelmintics) is therefore of great practical therapeutic importance.

HELMINTH INFECTIONS

The helminths comprise two major groups: the *nemathelminths* (nematodes, roundworms) and the *platyhelminths* (flatworms). The latter group is subdivided into the *trematodes* (flukes) and the *cestodes* (tapeworms). Almost 350 species of helminths have been found in humans, and most colonise the gastrointestinal (GI) tract. The global range and occurrence of helminthiasis have been reviewed by Lustigman et al. (2012).

Helminths have a complex life cycle, often involving several host species. Infection may occur in many ways, with poor hygiene a major contributory factor. Humans are generally the *primary* (or *definitive*) host for relevant helminth infections, in the sense that they harbour the sexually mature reproductive form. Direct ingestion is common: eggs or larvae in the faeces of infected humans enter the soil then drinking water and subsequently are ingested and infect the *secondary* (*intermediate*) host. In some cases, the eggs or larvae may persist in the human host and become *encysted*, covered with granulation tissue, giving rise to *cysticercosis*. Encysted larvae may lodge in the muscles and viscera or, more seriously, in the eye or the brain.

Approximately 20 helminth species are considered to be clinically significant (see Figs 56.1 and 56.2) and these fall into two main categories – those in which the worm lives in the host's alimentary canal and those in which the worm lives in other tissues of the host's body.

The main examples of intestinal worms are:

- *Tapeworms*: *Taenia saginata*, *Taenia solium*, *Hymenolepis nana* and *Diphyllobothrium latum*. Some 85 million people in Asia, Africa and parts of America commonly harbour one or other of these tapeworm species. Only the first two are likely to be seen in the United Kingdom. Cattle and pigs are the usual intermediate hosts of the most common tapeworms (*T. saginata* and *T. solium*). Humans become infected by eating raw or undercooked meat containing the larvae, which have encysted in the animals' muscle tissue. *H. nana* may exist as both the adult (the intestinal worm) and the larval stage in the same host, which may be human or rodent, although some insects (fleas, grain beetles) can also serve as intermediate hosts. The infection is usually asymptomatic.[1] *D. latum* has two sequential intermediate hosts: a freshwater crustacean and a freshwater fish. Humans become infected by eating raw or incompletely cooked fish containing the larvae.
- *Intestinal roundworms*: *Ascaris lumbricoides* (common roundworm), *Enterobius vermicularis* (threadworm, called pinworm in the United States), *Trichuris trichiura* (whipworm), *Strongyloides stercoralis* (threadworm in the United States), *Necator americanus* and *Ancylostoma duodenale* (hookworms). Again, undercooked meat or contaminated food is an important cause of infection by roundworm, threadworm and whipworm, whereas hookworm is generally acquired when their larvae penetrate the skin. Intestinal blood loss is a common cause of anaemia in regions where hookworm is endemic.

The main examples of worms that live elsewhere in host tissues are:

- *Flukes*: *Schistosoma haematobium*, *Schistosoma mansoni* and *Schistosoma japonicum*. These cause schistosomiasis (bilharzia). The adult worms of both sexes live and mate in the veins or venules of the bladder or the gut wall. The female lays eggs that pass into the bladder or gut, triggering inflammation in these organs. This results in haematuria in the former case and, occasionally, loss of blood in the faeces in the latter. The eggs hatch in water after discharge from the body and thus enter the secondary host – in this case a particular species of snail. After a period of development in this host, free-swimming *cercariae* emerge. These are capable of infecting humans by penetration of the skin. About 200 million people are infected with schistosomes in this manner.

[1]A general principle is that the infecting vector (in this case helminths) spreads more efficiently if they are less detrimental to the hosts. The least effective vector would kill its secondary host quickly and thus not be very good at spreading among its population. Survival of the sneakiest.

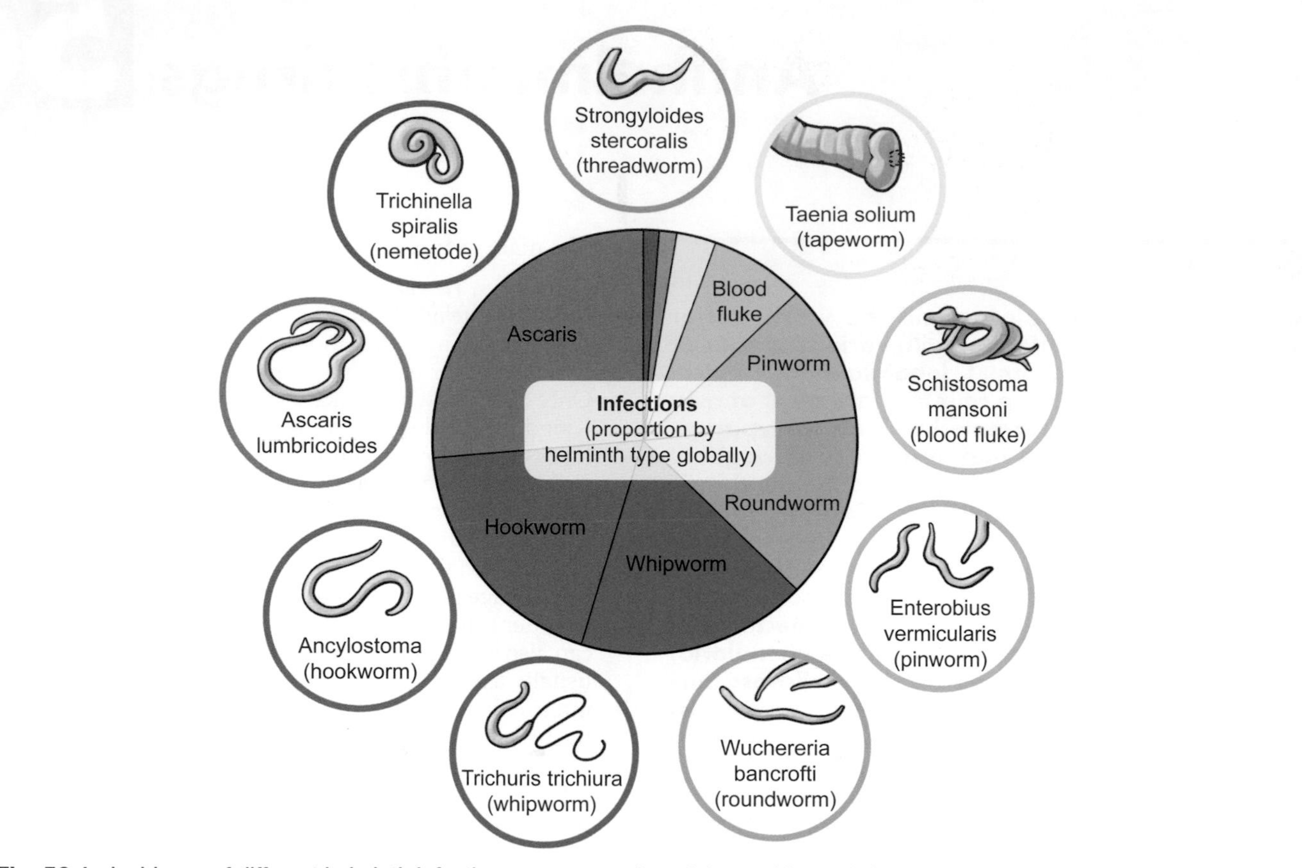

Fig. 56.1 Incidence of different helminth infections as a proportion of the world population and by type of infection. Surrounding illustrations show examples of species associated with each of the main genus.

- *Tissue roundworms: Trichinella spiralis, Dracunculus medinensis* (*guinea worm*) and the *filariae*, which include *Wuchereria bancrofti, Loa loa, Onchocerca volvulus* and *Brugia malayi*. The adult filariae live in the lymphatics, connective tissues or mesentery of the host and produce live embryos or *microfilariae*, which find their way into the bloodstream and may be ingested by mosquitoes or other biting insects. After a period of development within this secondary host, the larvae pass into the mouth parts of the insect and thus infect the next victim. Major filarial diseases are caused by *Wuchereria* or *Brugia*, which cause obstruction of lymphatic vessels, producing *elephantiasis* – hugely swollen legs. Other related diseases are *onchocerciasis* (in which the presence of microfilariae in the eye causes 'river blindness' – a leading preventable cause of blindness in Africa and Latin America) and *loiasis* (in which the microfilariae cause inflammation in the skin and other tissues). *T. spiralis* causes trichinosis; the larvae from the viviparous female worms in the intestine migrate to skeletal muscle, where they become encysted. In *guinea worm disease*,[2] larvae of *D. medinensis* released from crustaceans in wells and waterholes are ingested and migrate from the intestinal tract to mature and mate in the tissues; the gravid female then migrates to the subcutaneous tissues of the leg or the foot, and may protrude through an ulcer in the skin. The worm may be up to a metre in length and must be removed surgically or by slow mechanical winding of the worm on to a stick over a period of days, to ensure that the worm does not break, because the remains would putrefy.
- *Hydatid tapeworm*. These are cestodes of the *Echinococcus* species for which dogs are the primary hosts, and sheep the intermediate hosts. The primary, intestinal stage does not occur in humans, but under certain circumstances humans can function as the intermediate host, in which case the larvae develop into *hydatid cysts* within the tissues, sometimes with fatal consequences.

Some nematodes that generally live in the GI tract of animals may infect humans and penetrate tissues. A skin infestation, termed *creeping eruption* or *cutaneous larva migrans*, is caused by the larvae of dog and cat hookworms which often enter through the foot. Visceral larva migrans is caused by larvae of cat and dog roundworms of the *Toxocara* genus.

[2]Now, happily, eliminated from many parts of the world. There are no effective drug treatments for *guinea worm disease*, but clean drinking water and filtering larval-contaminated water through nylon mesh tights have helped reduce global infection from 3.5 million to 5 in only 30 years – the first globally eradicated parasitic disease.

ANTIHELMINTHIC DRUGS

The aim of treatment is to eliminate the parasite but without adversely affecting the biology of the host. Helminths being distinct species has the advantage of different biology,

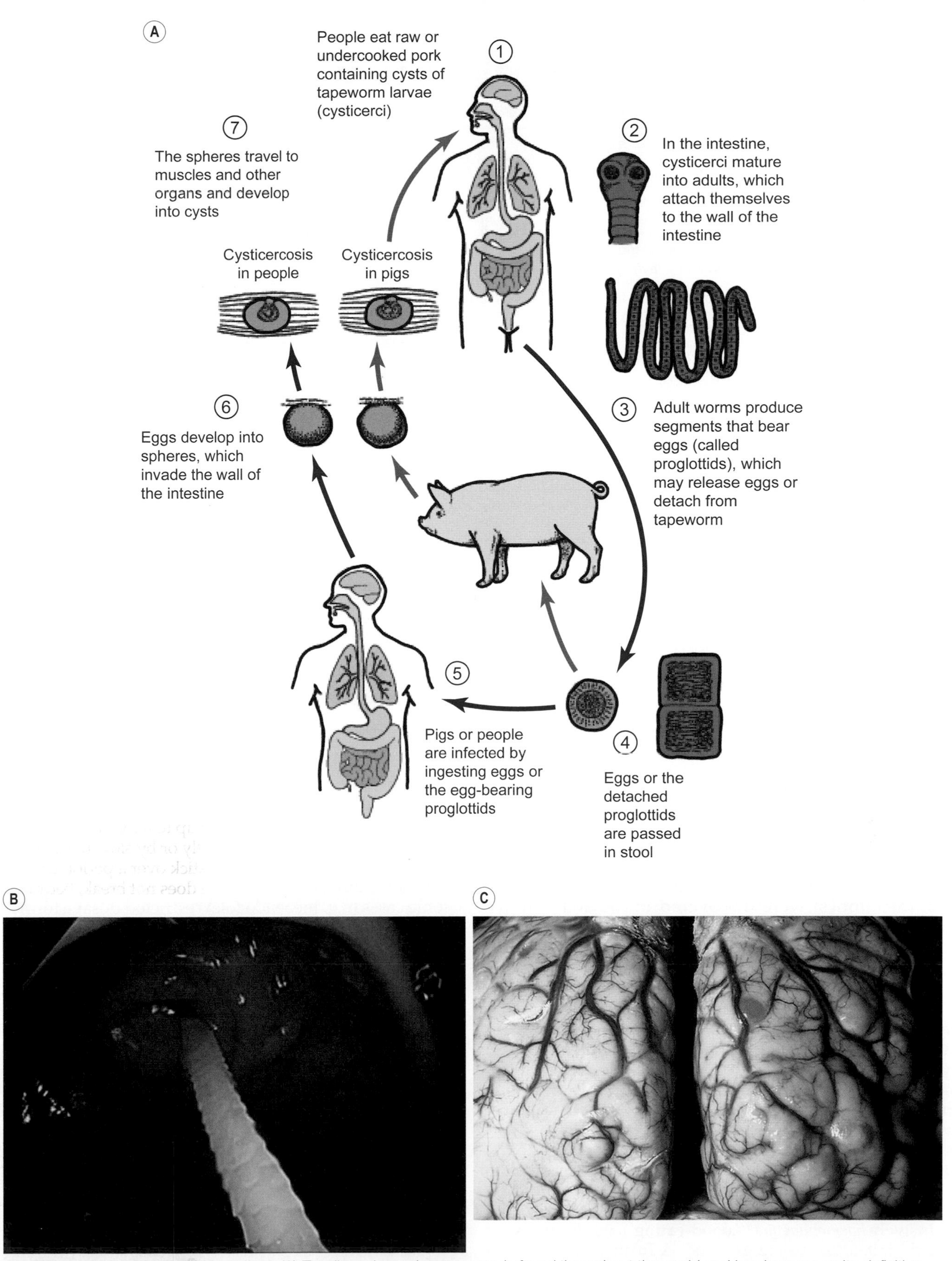

Fig. 56.2 **Life cycle of *Taenia solium.*** (A) *T. solium*, the pork tapeworm, is found throughout the world and has humans as its definitive host and pigs as the intermediate or secondary hosts. Humans can be infected by either eating undercooked pork meat that contains the intermediate cysts or eating food or drinking water contaminated with faeces which contain tapeworm eggs. (B) The former, known as taeniasis, results in adult tapeworm in the intestines which usually has no symptoms and is easily treated with anthelmintic medications. The later, known as cysticercosis, results in cysts forming in different organs of the body. This is usually muscle and has minimal symptoms but (C) the cysts can form in the brain with more serious symptoms.

Table 56.1 Principal drugs used in helminth infections and some common indications

	Helminth	Principal drug(s) used
Threadworm (pinworm)	*Enterobius vermicularis*	Mebendazole, piperazine (not United Kingdom)
	Strongyloides stercoralis (threadworm in the United States)	Ivermectin, albendazole, mebendazole
Common roundworm	*Ascaris lumbricoides*	Levamisole, mebendazole, piperazine (not United Kingdom)
Other roundworm (filariae)	Lymphatic filariasis 'elephantiasis' (*Wuchereria bancrofti*, *Brugia malayi*)	Diethylcarbamazine, ivermectin
	Subcutaneous filariasis 'eyeworm' (*Loa loa*)	Diethylcarbamazine
	Onchocerciasis 'river blindness' (*Onchocerca volvulus*)	Ivermectin
	Guinea worm (*Dracunculus medinensis*)	Praziquantel, mebendazole
	Trichiniasis (*Trichinella spiralis*)	Tiabendazole, mebendazole
	Cysticercosis (infection with larval *Taenia solium*)	Praziquantel, albendazole
	Tapeworm (*Taenia saginata*, *T. solium*)	Praziquantel, niclosamide
	Hydatid disease (*Echinococcus granulosus*)	Albendazole
	Hookworm (*Ancylostoma duodenale*, *Necator americanus*)	Mebendazole, albendazole, Levamisole
	Whipworm (*Trichuris trichiura*)	Mebendazole, albendazole, diethylcarbamazine
Blood flukes (*Schistosoma* spp.)	Bilharziasis: *Schistosoma haematobium*, *Schistosoma mansoni*, *Schistosoma japonicum*	Praziquantel
Cutaneous larva migrans	*Ancylostoma caninum*	Albendazole, tiabendazole, ivermectin
Visceral larva migrans	*Toxocara canis*	Albendazole, tiabendazole, diethylcarbamazine

e.g. motor function, metabolism offer a route to achieving selective toxicity, a similar concept to antibiotics for example (Ch. 51). These same principles rely on the selective toxicity of a drug, whereby the drug is more toxic to a parasite or cancer cell, than the host itself.

The first effective antihelminthic drugs (also known as anthelmintics) were discovered in the 20th century and incorporated toxic metals such as arsenic (*atoxyl*) or antimony (*tartar emetic*). They were used to treat trypanosome and schistosome infestations.

Current antihelminthic drugs generally act by paralysing the parasite (e.g. by preventing muscular contraction), by damaging the worm such that the host immune system can eliminate it or by altering parasite metabolism (e.g. by affecting microtubule function). Because the metabolic requirements of these parasites vary greatly from one species to another, drugs that are highly effective against one type of worm may be ineffective against others.

To bring about its action, the drug must penetrate the tough exterior cuticle of the worm or gain access to its alimentary tract. This may present difficulties, because helminths have different lifestyles with some worms being exclusively *haemophagous* ('blood-eating'), while others are best described as 'tissue grazers'. A further complication is that many helminths possess active drug efflux pumps that reduce the concentration of the drug in the parasite. The route of administration and dose of antihelminthic drugs are therefore important. In a reversal of the normal order of things, several antihelminthic drugs used in human medicine were originally developed for veterinary use.

Some individual antihelminthic drugs are described briefly here and indications for their use are given in Table 56.1. Many of these drugs are unlicensed in the United Kingdom but are used on a 'named patient' basis[3]: in some cases (e.g. mebendazole) restricted dosage forms are available from pharmacies.

BENZIMIDAZOLES

This group includes **mebendazole**, **tiabendazole** and **albendazole,** which are widely used broad-spectrum antihelminthics. They are thought to act by inhibiting the polymerisation of helminth β-tubulin, thus interfering with microtubule-dependent functions such as glucose uptake. They have a selective inhibitory action, being 250–400 times more effective in producing this effect in helminth, than in mammalian, tissue. However, the effect takes time to develop and the worms may not be expelled for several days. Cure rates are generally between 60% and 100% with most parasites.

[3]A situation in which the physician seeks access to an unlicensed drug from a pharmaceutical company to use in a named individual. The drug is either a 'newcomer' that has shown promise in clinical trials but has not yet been licensed or, as in these instances, an established drug that has not been licensed because the company has not applied for a product license for this indication (possibly for commercial reasons).

Only 10% of mebendazole is absorbed after oral administration, but a fatty meal increases absorption. It is rapidly metabolised; the products being excreted in the urine and the bile within 24–48 h. It is generally given as a single dose for threadworm, and twice daily for 3 days for hookworm and roundworm infestations. Tiabendazole is rapidly absorbed from the GI tract, and very rapidly metabolised and excreted in the urine in conjugated form. It may be given twice daily for 3 days for guinea worm and *Strongyloides* infestations, and for up to 5 days for hookworm and roundworm infestations. Albendazole is also poorly absorbed but, as with mebendazole, absorption is increased by food, especially fats. It is metabolised extensively by presystemic metabolism to sulfoxide and sulfone metabolites. The former is likely to be the pharmacologically active species.

Unwanted effects are few with albendazole or mebendazole, although GI disturbances can occasionally occur. Unwanted effects with tiabendazole are more frequent but usually transient, the commonest being GI disturbances, although headache, dizziness and drowsiness have been reported and allergic reactions (fever, rashes) may also occur. Mebendazole is considered unsuitable for pregnant women or children less than 2 years old, although more recent WHO guidance suggests albendazole or mebendazole could be suitable in pregnant women after their first trimester.

PRAZIQUANTEL

Praziquantel is a highly effective broad-spectrum antihelminthic drug that was introduced over 20 years ago. It is the drug of choice for all forms of schistosomiasis and is the agent generally used in large-scale schistosome eradication programmes. It is also effective in cysticercosis. The drug affects not only the adult schistosomes but also the immature forms and the cercariae – the form of the parasite that infects humans by penetrating the skin.

Praziquantel disrupts Ca^{2+} homeostasis in the parasite by binding to consensus protein kinase C-binding sites in a β subunit of schistosome voltage-gated calcium channels (Greenberg, 2005). This induces an influx of Ca^{2+}, a rapid and prolonged contraction of the musculature and eventual paralysis and death of the worm. Praziquantel also disrupts the tegument of the parasite, unmasking novel antigens, and may thus make the worm more susceptible to the host's normal immune responses.

Given orally, praziquantel is well absorbed; much of the drug is rapidly metabolised to inactive metabolites on first passage through the liver, and the metabolites are excreted in the urine. The plasma half-life of the parent compound is 60–90 min.

Praziquantel has minimal side effects in therapeutic dosage. Such unwanted effects as do occur are usually transitory and rarely of clinical importance. Effects may be more marked in patients with a heavy worm load because of products released from the dead worms. Praziquantel is considered safe for pregnant and lactating women, an important property for a drug that is commonly used in national disease control programmes. Some resistance has developed to the drug.

PIPERAZINE

Piperazine (discontinued in United Kingdom due to issues sourcing the raw ingredients) can be used to treat infections with the common roundworm (*A. lumbricoides*) and the threadworm (*E. vermicularis*). It reversibly inhibits neuromuscular transmission in the worm, probably by mimicking GABA (see Ch. 38), at GABA-gated chloride channels in nematode muscle. The paralysed worms are expelled alive by normal intestinal peristaltic movements. It is administered with a stimulant laxative such as **senna** (see Ch. 30) to facilitate expulsion of the worms.

Piperazine is given orally and some, but not all, is absorbed. It is partly metabolised, and the remainder is eliminated, unchanged, via the kidney. The drug has little pharmacological action in the host. When used to treat roundworm, piperazine is effective in a single dose. For threadworm, a longer course (7 days) at lower dosage is necessary.

Unwanted effects may include GI disturbances, urticaria and bronchospasm. Some patients experience dizziness, paraesthesia, vertigo and incoordination. The drug should not be given to pregnant patients or to those with compromised renal or hepatic function.

DIETHYLCARBAMAZINE

Diethylcarbamazine is a piperazine derivative that is active in filarial infections caused by *B. malayi*, *W. bancrofti* and *L. loa*. Diethylcarbamazine rapidly removes the microfilariae from the blood circulation and has a limited effect on the adult worms in the lymphatics, but it has little action on microfilariae in vitro. It may act by changing the parasite such that it becomes susceptible to the host's normal immune responses or by interfering with helminth arachidonate metabolism.

The drug is absorbed following oral administration and is distributed throughout the cells and tissues of the body, excepting adipose tissue. It is partly metabolised, and both the parent drug and its metabolites are excreted in the urine, being cleared from the body within about 48 h.

Unwanted effects are common but transient, subsiding within a day or so even if the drug is continued. Side effects from the drug itself include GI disturbances, joint pain, headache and a general feeling of weakness. Allergic side effects referable to the products of the dying filariae are common and vary with the species of worm. In general, these start during the first day's treatment and last 3–7 days; they include skin reactions, enlargement of lymph glands, dizziness, tachycardia and GI and respiratory disturbances. When these symptoms disappear, larger doses of the drug can be given without further problem. The drug is not used in patients with onchocerciasis, in whom it can have serious unwanted effects.

NICLOSAMIDE

Niclosamide is widely used for the treatment of tapeworm infections together with praziquantel. The *scolex* (the head of the worm that attaches to the host intestine) and a proximal segment are irreversibly damaged by the drug, such that the worm separates from the intestinal wall and is expelled. For *T. solium*, the drug is given in a single dose after a light meal, usually followed by a purgative 2 h later in case the damaged tapeworm segments release ova, which are not affected by the drug. For other tapeworm infections, this precaution is not necessary. There is negligible absorption of the drug from the GI tract.

Unwanted effects nausea, vomiting, pruritus and light-headedness may occur but generally such effects are few, infrequent and transient.

LEVAMISOLE

Levamisole is effective in infections with the common roundworm (*A. lumbricoides*). It has a nicotine-like action (see Ch. 14), stimulating and subsequently blocking the neuromuscular junctions. The paralysed worms are then expelled in the faeces. Ova are not killed. Given orally the drug is rapidly absorbed and is widely distributed crossing the blood–brain barrier. It is metabolised in the liver to inactive metabolites, which are excreted via the kidney. Its plasma half-life is 4 h. It has immunomodulatory effects and has in the past been used to treat various solid tumours.

It can cause central nervous system (CNS) and GI disturbances as well as several other unwanted effects, including agranulocytosis. The drug has been withdrawn from North American markets.

IVERMECTIN

First introduced in 1981 as a veterinary drug, **ivermectin** is a safe and highly effective broad-spectrum antiparasitic in humans.[4] It is frequently used in global public health campaigns,[5] and is the first choice of drug for the treatment of many filarial infections. It yields good results against *W. bancrofti*, which causes elephantiasis. A single dose kills the immature microfilariae of *O. volvulus* but not the adult worms. Ivermectin is also the drug of choice for onchocerciasis, which causes river blindness and reduces the incidence of this disease by up to 80%. It is also active against some roundworms: common roundworms, whipworms and threadworms of both the UK (*E. vermicularis*) and US (*S. stercoralis*) variety, but not hookworms.

Chemically, ivermectin is a semisynthetic agent derived from a group of natural substances, the *avermectins*, obtained from an actinomycete organism. The drug is given orally and has a half-life of 11 h. It is thought to kill the worm either by opening glutamate-gated chloride channels (found only in invertebrates) and increasing Cl^- conductance; by binding to GABA receptors; or by binding to a novel allosteric site on the acetylcholine nicotinic receptor to cause an increase in transmission, leading to motor paralysis.

Unwanted effects include skin rashes and itching but in general the drug is very well tolerated. One interesting exception in veterinary medicine is the CNS toxicity seen in Collie dogs.[6]

RESISTANCE TO ANTIHELMINTHIC DRUGS

Resistance to antihelminthic drugs is a widespread and growing problem affecting not only humans but also the animal health market. Understanding of the mechanisms of helminth mutations in drug-resistant forms is not as well understood or researched, as with other microbes. During the 1990s, helminth infections in sheep (and, to a lesser extent, cattle) developed varying degrees of resistance to a number of different drugs. Parasites that develop such resistance pass this ability on to their offspring, leading to treatment failure. The widespread use of antihelminthic agents in farming has been blamed for the spread of resistant species.

There are probably several molecular mechanisms that contribute to drug resistance. The presence of the P-glycoprotein transporter (see Ch. 10) in some species of nematode has already been mentioned, and agents such as **verapamil** that block the transporter in trypanosomes can partially reverse resistance to the benzimidazoles. However, some aspects of benzimidazole resistance may be attributed to alterations in their high-affinity binding to parasite β-tubulin. Likewise, resistance to levamisole is associated with changes in the structure of the target acetylcholine nicotinic receptor.

Of great significance is the way in which helminths evade the host's immune system. Even though they may reside in immunologically exposed sites such as the lymphatics or the bloodstream, many are long-lived and may co-exist with their hosts for many years without seriously affecting their health, or in some cases without even being noticed. It is striking that the two major families of helminths, while evolving separately, deploy similar strategies to evade destruction by the immune system. Clearly, this must be of major survival value for the species.

In addition to rapidly changing external antigens, which hamper immune recognition, it appears that many helminths secrete immunomodulatory products that steer the host's immune system away from a local Th1 response (see Ch. 7), which would damage the parasite, and instead promote a modified systemic Th2 type of response. This is associated with the production by the host of 'anti-inflammatory' cytokines such as interleukin-10 and is favourable to, or at least better tolerated by, the parasites. The immunology underlying this is fascinating but complex (see e.g. Harris, 2011; Harnett, 2014; McNeilly and Nisbet, 2014).

Ironically, the ability of helminths to modify the host immune response in this way may confer some survival value on the hosts themselves. For example, in addition to the local anti-inflammatory effect exerted by helminth infections, rapid wound healing is also seen. Clearly, this is of advantage to parasites that must penetrate tissues without killing the host, but may also be beneficial to the host as well. It has been proposed that helminth infections may mitigate some forms of malaria and other diseases, possibly conferring survival advantages in populations where these diseases are endemic. The deliberate, 'therapeutic' ingestion of helminths by patients has been evaluated as an (admittedly unappealing) strategy to induce remission of inflammatory diseases such as Crohn's disease, ulcerative colitis and even multiple sclerosis (see Ch. 30; Benzel et al., 2012; Heylen et al., 2014; Peon and Terrazas, 2016; Summers et al., 2005a, 2005b), although their effectiveness in clinical trials is mixed.

On the basis that Th2 responses reciprocally inhibit the development of Th1 diseases, it has also been hypothesised that the comparative absence of Crohn's disease, as well as some other autoimmune diseases, in the developing world may be associated with the high incidence of parasite infection, and that the rise of these disorders in the West is associated with superior sanitation and reduced helminth

[4]The Western World has collectively lost its mind over the potential use and repurposing of ivermectin as a possible treatment for COVID-19, surprising for a drug which won its inventors the Nobel Prize in 2015.
[5]Ivermectin is supplied by the manufacturers free of charge in countries where river blindness is endemic. Because the worms develop slowly, a single annual dose of ivermectin is sufficient to prevent the disease.
[6]A multidrug-resistance (MDR) gene (see Ch. 3) coding for a transporter that expels ivermectins from the CNS is mutated to an inactive form in Collie dogs.

infection! This type of argument is generally known as the 'hygiene hypothesis'.

On the negative side however, helminth infections may undermine the efficacy of tuberculosis and other vaccination programmes that depend upon a vigorous Th1 response (see, for example, Elias et al., 2006, and Apiwattanakul et al., 2014).

VACCINES AND OTHER NOVEL APPROACHES

Despite the enormity of the clinical (and economic) problems associated with helminth infection, there are few novel antihelminthic drugs in development, possibly because the similarity between helminth and mammalian targets makes achieving selective toxicity difficult. New candidates such as **tribendimidine** are being assessed in a range of human infections and have shown promise in liver fluke infection (Duthaler et al., 2016) and some new veterinary drugs (e.g. **derquantel**) also tested in humans (see Prichard et al., 2012). The identification of new parasite metabolic enzymes as targets may help with future drug design (Timson, 2016).

Public health measures to eliminate helminth infections depend upon promoting better sanitation and mass drug administration programmes (e.g. McCarty et al., 2014). The development of effective anti-helminth vaccines would be a major step forward in this endeavour. Using surface protein and glycoprotein antigens as immunogens, some success has been achieved with veterinary vaccines (e.g. Sciutto et al., 2013; Bassetto and Amarante, 2015). The use of sophisticated tools such as genomics, transcriptomics, proteomics, metabolomics, lipidomics (collectively known as 'OMICS') to identify novel antigens may facilitate progress (Loukas et al., 2011).

REFERENCES AND FURTHER READING

General papers on helminths and their diseases

Boatin, B.A., Basanez, M.G., Prichard, R.K., et al., 2012. A research agenda for helminth diseases of humans: towards control and elimination. PLoS Negl. Trop. Dis. 6, e1547.

Horton, J., 2003. Human gastrointestinal helminth infections: are they now neglected diseases? Trends Parasitol. 19, 527–531.

Lustigman, S., Prichard, R.K., Gazzinelli, A., et al., 2012. A research agenda for helminth diseases of humans: the problem of helminthiases. PLoS Negl. Trop. Dis. 6, e1582.

McCarty, T.R., Turkeltaub, J.A., Hotez, P.J., 2014. Global progress towards eliminating gastrointestinal helminth infections. Curr. Opin. Gastroenterol. 30, 18–24

Antihelminthic drugs

Burkhart, C.N., 2000. Ivermectin: an assessment of its pharmacology, microbiology and safety. Vet. Hum. Toxicol. 42, 30–35.

Croft, S.L., 1997. The current status of antiparasite chemotherapy. Parasitology 114, S3–S15.

Geary, T.G., Sangster, N.C., Thompson, D.P., 1999. Frontiers in anthelmintic pharmacology. Vet. Parasitol. 84, 275–295.

Greenberg, R.M., 2005. Are Ca^{2+} channels targets of praziquantel action? Int. J. Parasitol. 35, 1–9.

Prichard, R., Tait, A., 2001. The role of molecular biology in veterinary parasitology. Vet. Parasitol. 98, 169–194.

Prichard, R.K., Basanez, M.G., Boatin, B.A., et al., 2012. A research agenda for helminth diseases of humans: intervention for control and elimination. PLoS Negl. Trop. Dis. 6, e1549.

Robertson, A.P., Bjorn, H.E., Martin, R.J., 2000. Pyrantel resistance alters nematode nicotinic acetylcholine receptor single channel properties. Eur. J. Pharmacol. 394, 1–8.

Timson, D.J., 2016. Metabolic enzymes of helminth parasites: potential as drug targets. Curr. Protein Pept. Sci. 17, 280–295.

Antihelminthic vaccines

Bassetto, C.C., Amarante, A.F., 2015. Vaccination of sheep and cattle against haemonchosis. J. Helminthol. 89, 517–525.

Harris, N.L., 2011. Advances in helminth immunology: optimism for future vaccine design? Trends Parasitol. 27, 288–293.

Loukas, A., Gaze, S., Mulvenna, J.P., et al., 2011. Vaccinomics for the major blood feeding helminths of humans. OMICS 15, 567–577.

Sciutto, E., Fragoso, G., Hernandez, M., et al., 2013. Development of the S3Pvac vaccine against porcine *Taenia solium* cysticercosis: a historical review. J. Parasitol. 99, 686–692.

Immune evasion by helminths and therapeutic exploitation

Apiwattanakul, N., Thomas, P.G., Iverson, A.R., McCullers, J.A., 2014. Chronic helminth infections impair pneumococcal vaccine responses. Vaccine 32, 5405–5410.

Benzel, F., Erdur, H., Kohler, S., et al., 2012. Immune monitoring of *Trichuris suis* egg therapy in multiple sclerosis patients. J. Helminthol. 86, 339–347.

Duthaler, U., Sayasone, S., Vanobbergen, F., et al., 2016. Single-ascending-dose pharmacokinetic study of tribendimidine in *Opisthorchis viverrini*-infected patients. Antimicrob. Agents Chemother. 60, 5705–5715.

Elias, D., Akuffo, H., Britton, S., 2006. Helminths could influence the outcome of vaccines against TB in the tropics. Parasite Immunol. 28, 507–513.

Harnett, W., 2014. Secretory products of helminth parasites as immunomodulators. Mol. Biochem. Parasitol. 195, 130–136.

Heylen, M., Ruyssers, N.E., Gielis, E.M., et al., 2014. Of worms, mice and man: an overview of experimental and clinical helminth-based therapy for inflammatory bowel disease. Pharmacol. Ther. 143, 153–167.

McNeilly, T.N., Nisbet, A.J., 2014. Immune modulation by helminth parasites of ruminants: implications for vaccine development and host immune competence. Parasite 21, 51.

Peon, A.N., Terrazas, L.I., 2016. Immune-regulatory mechanisms of classical and experimental multiple sclerosis drugs: a special focus on helminth-derived treatments. Curr. Med. Chem. 23, 1152–1170.

Summers, R.W., Elliott, D.E., Urban Jr., J.F., Thompson, R., Weinstock, J.V., 2005a. *Trichuris suis* therapy in Crohn's disease. Gut 54, 87–90.

Summers, R.W., Elliott, D.E., Urban Jr., J.F., Thompson, R.A., Weinstock, J.V., 2005b. *Trichuris suis* therapy for active ulcerative colitis: a randomized controlled trial. Gastroenterology 128, 825–832.

57 Anticancer drugs

OVERVIEW

Cancer is one of the great challenges for pharmacology. There have been great strides in the overall treatment of cancer, with some cancer types seeing marked improvement in survival thanks to drug advances – many cancer types remaining stubbornly intractable, for now. A wealth of new drugs have been brought onto the market, due in part to the often terminal nature of the disease and the willingness of a sufferer to try a novel treatment in the hope of extending their life. Many of the toxicities associated with cancer treatments are tolerated in the hope of a cure. Companies continually strive to improve cancer drug effectiveness without increasing toxicity, resulting in a range of new anticancer therapies that have evolved and improved over recent decades. In this chapter, we consider cancer in general and anticancer drug therapy. We discuss first the pathogenesis of cancer and then describe the drugs that can be used to treat malignant disease. Finally, we consider the extent to which our new knowledge of cancer biology is leading to new therapies.

INTRODUCTION

'Cancer' is characterised by uncontrolled multiplication and spread of abnormal forms of the body's own cells. It is second only to cardiovascular disease as cause of death in developed nations, and one in every two people born in the United Kingdom after 1960 will be diagnosed with some form of cancer during their lifetime. According to Cancer Research UK (2018), over 375,000 new cases were reported per annum in the United Kingdom and mortality was in excess of 166,000 (global figures respectively are 17 and 9.6 million). Cancer is responsible for approximately 30% of all deaths in the United Kingdom. Lung and bowel cancers are the commonest malignancies, closely followed by breast and prostate cancer. Statistics from most other countries in the developed world tell much the same story.

A comparison of the incidence of cancer over the past 100 years or so gives the impression that the disease is increasing in developed countries, but this is not so. Cancer occurs mainly in later life and, with advances in public health and medical science, many more people now live to an age where malignancy is common.[1]

The terms *cancer*, *malignancy* and *malignant tumour* are often used synonymously.[2] Both benign and malignant tumours manifest uncontrolled proliferation, but the latter are distinguished by their capacity for *de-differentiation*, their *invasiveness* and their ability to *metastasise* (spread to other parts of the body). The appearance of these abnormal characteristics reflects altered patterns of gene expression in the cancer cells, resulting from inherited or acquired mutations.

There are three main approaches to treating established cancer – *surgical excision*, *irradiation* and *drug therapy* (previously often called *chemotherapy*, but now often including hormonal and biological agents as described later and in Chs 5 and 35) – and the relative value of each of these approaches depends on the disease and the stage of its development. Drug therapy may be used on its own or as an adjunct to other forms of therapy.

Compared with that of bacterial diseases, cancer chemotherapy presents a difficult conceptual problem. Microorganisms differ qualitatively from human cells (see Ch. 51), but cancer cells and normal cells are so similar in most respects that it is more difficult to find general, exploitable, biochemical differences between these differing cell types. Conventional *cytotoxic drugs* act on all cells and rely on a small margin of selectivity to be useful as anticancer agents, but the scope of cancer therapy has now broadened to include drugs that affect either the hormonal regulation of tumour growth or the defective cell cycle controls that underlie malignancy (see Ch. 6 and Croce, 2008; Weinberg, 1996). Numerous biopharmaceuticals including monoclonal antibodies (see Ch. 5), as well as other novel immunomodulators, have transformed the chemotherapeutic landscape.

THE PATHOGENESIS OF CANCER

It is important to consider the pathobiology in more detail to understand how anticancer drugs work and may be improved on in future.

Cancer cells manifest, to varying degrees, four characteristics that distinguish them from normal cells. These are

- *Uncontrolled proliferation*
- *De-differentiation and loss of function*
- *Invasiveness*
- *Metastasis*

[1]Cancer in general is a disease of older age – you have to be around long enough for all the mutations to accumulate in a cell and create a cancer phenotype that escapes the body's immune surveillance system. Clinical oncologists are gradually improving their treatment. Their goal is to keep you alive long enough so that you die of something other than cancer: a measure of their success.

[2]Blood cell malignancies – lymphomas and leukaemias – are non-tumour forming, and at times not referred to as cancers. Along with myelomas, they are generally classed as 'blood cancers'. In this account, 'cancer' is used to cover all malignancy types.

THE GENESIS OF A CANCER CELL

A normal cell turns into a cancer cell because of one or, more often, several mutations in its DNA. These can be inherited or acquired, usually through exposure to viruses or *carcinogens* (e.g. tobacco products, ultraviolet radiation, asbestos). A good example is breast cancer; women who inherit a single defective copy of either of the tumour suppressor genes *BRCA1* and *BRCA2* have a significantly increased *risk* of developing breast cancer. However, carcinogenesis is a complex multistage process, usually involving more than one genetic change as well as other, *epigenetic* factors (hormonal, co-carcinogen and tumour promoter effects – see later) that do not themselves produce cancer but which increase the *likelihood* that the genetic mutation(s) will eventually result in cancer. These mutations accumulate and lead to '*genomic instability*', which is a hallmark of carcinogenesis.

There are two main categories of relevant genetic change:

- The activation of *proto-oncogenes* to *oncogenes.* Proto-oncogenes are genes that normally control cell division, apoptosis and differentiation (see Ch. 6), but which can be converted by viruses or carcinogens to oncogenes that induce malignant change.
- The inactivation of *tumour suppressor genes.* Normal cells contain genes that suppress malignant change – termed *tumour suppressor genes* (*anti-oncogenes*) – and mutations of these genes are commonly involved in many different cancers. The loss of function of tumour suppressor genes can be the critical event in carcinogenesis.

The Cancer Gene Census has catalogued more than 500 genes with mutations that have a causal role in cancer (https://cancer.sanger.ac.uk/cosmic/census). Among the changes that lead to malignancy are mutations (e.g. inactivating mutations in tumour suppressor genes and missense mutations for dominant oncogenes), gene amplification or chromosomal translocation (see Hanahan and Weinberg, 2011).

THE SPECIAL CHARACTERISTICS OF CANCER CELLS

UNCONTROLLED PROLIFERATION

It is not generally true that cancer cells proliferate faster than normal cells. Many healthy cells, in the bone marrow and the epithelium of the gastrointestinal (GI) tract (for example), undergo continuous rapid division. Some cancer cells multiply slowly (e.g. those in plasma cell tumours) and some much more rapidly (e.g. the cells of *Burkitt's lymphoma*). The significant issue is that cancer cells *have escaped from the mechanisms that normally regulate cell division and tissue growth; the normal brakes on cell division, present in a healthy cell, have been cut.* It is this, rather than their rate of proliferation, that distinguishes them from normal cells.

What are the changes that lead to the uncontrolled proliferation of tumour cells? Inactivation of tumour suppressor genes or transformation of proto-oncogenes into oncogenes can confer autonomy of growth on a cell and thus result in uncontrolled proliferation by producing changes in cellular systems (Fig. 57.1), including:

- *growth factors*, their receptors and signalling pathways;
- the *cell cycle transducers*, for example, cyclins, cyclin-dependent kinases (cdks) or the cdk inhibitors;
- the *apoptotic machinery* that normally disposes of abnormal cells;
- *telomerase expression;*
- *local blood supply*, resulting from tumour-directed angiogenesis.

Potentially all the genes coding for the earlier components could be regarded as oncogenes or tumour suppressor genes (Fig. 57.2), although not all are equally prone to malignant transformation and malignant transformation of several components is needed for the development of cancer.

Resistance to apoptosis

Apoptosis is programmed cell death (see Ch. 6), and mutations in antiapoptotic genes are usually a prerequisite for cancer; indeed, resistance to apoptosis is a hallmark of malignant disease. It can be brought about by inactivation of proapoptotic factors or by activation of antiapoptotic factors.

Telomerase expression

Telomeres are specialised structures that cap the ends of chromosomes – like the small metal tubes on the end of shoelaces – protecting them from degradation, rearrangement and fusion with other chromosomes. Furthermore, DNA polymerase cannot easily duplicate the last few nucleotides at the ends of DNA, and telomeres prevent loss of these 'end' genes. With each round of cell division, a portion of the telomere is eroded, so that eventually it becomes non-functional. At this point, DNA replication ceases and the cell becomes senescent.[3]

Healthy stem cells express *telomerase*, a *terminal transferase* enzyme that maintains and elongates telomere ends. While it is absent from most fully differentiated somatic cells, about 95% of late-stage malignant tumours express telomerase enzymes to continuously rebuild the telomere end and extend the cell's replicative ability, thus elongating the telomere ends and effectively conferring 'immortality' on cancer cells (see Buys, 2000; Keith et al., 2004).

The control of tumour-related blood vessels

The factors described earlier lead to the uncontrolled proliferation of individual cancer cells, but other factors, particularly blood supply, determine the actual growth of a solid tumour. Tumours 1–2 mm in diameter can obtain nutrients by diffusion through their exterior wall boundary, but their further expansion requires *angiogenesis* to feed this propagating tumour with nutrients, the development of new blood vessels in response to growth factors produced by the growing tumour itself (see Griffioen and Molema, 2000).

[3]Once eroded down, telomere ends signal cells to stop replicating forever, which is why we humans have a limited life-span. Cancer cells however express telomerases to constantly build upon the telomere-end, and as such have lost this 'end replication' signal to limit their lifetime – some cancer cell lines have been replicating in the laboratory for many decades. The entire weight of an individual tumour line grown in all laboratories worldwide means that the original single cancer cell has now amassed many, many tonnes of itself in total – much heavier than the individual tumour it was derived from. The patient may have mouldered in the grave, but their cancer cells go marching on – theoretically forever!

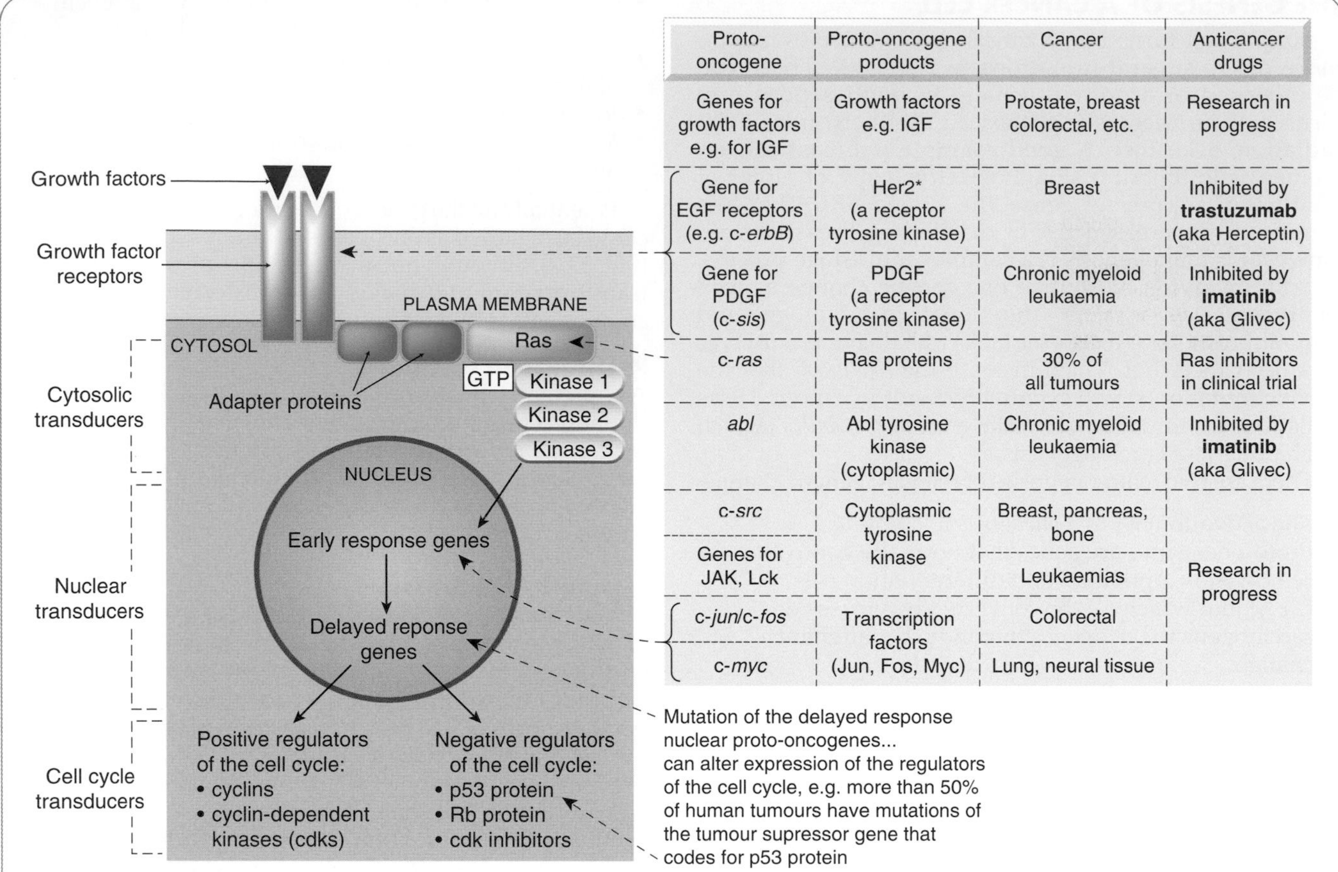

Proto-oncogene	Proto-oncogene products	Cancer	Anticancer drugs
Genes for growth factors e.g. for IGF	Growth factors e.g. IGF	Prostate, breast colorectal, etc.	Research in progress
Gene for EGF receptors (e.g. c-*erbB*)	Her2* (a receptor tyrosine kinase)	Breast	Inhibited by **trastuzumab** (aka Herceptin)
Gene for PDGF (c-*sis*)	PDGF (a receptor tyrosine kinase)	Chronic myeloid leukaemia	Inhibited by **imatinib** (aka Glivec)
c-*ras*	Ras proteins	30% of all tumours	Ras inhibitors in clinical trial
abl	Abl tyrosine kinase (cytoplasmic)	Chronic myeloid leukaemia	Inhibited by **imatinib** (aka Glivec)
c-*src*	Cytoplasmic tyrosine kinase	Breast, pancreas, bone	Research in progress
Genes for JAK, Lck		Leukaemias	
c-*jun*/c-*fos*	Transcription factors (Jun, Fos, Myc)	Colorectal	
c-*myc*		Lung, neural tissue	

Fig. 57.1 Signal transduction pathways initiated by growth factors and their relationship to cancer development. A few examples of proto-oncogenes and the products they code for are given in the table, with examples of the cancers that are associated with their conversion to oncogenes. Many growth factor receptors are receptor tyrosine kinases, the cytosolic transducers including adapter proteins that bind to phosphorylated tyrosine residues in the receptors. Ras proteins are guanine nucleotide-binding proteins and have GTPase action; decreased GTPase action means that Ras remains activated. **Her2* is also termed *her2/neu*. *EGF*, Epidermal growth factor; *IGF*, insulin-like growth factor; *PDGF*, platelet-derived growth factor.

DE-DIFFERENTIATION AND LOSS OF FUNCTION

The multiplication of normal cells in a tissue begins with division of the undifferentiated stem cells, giving rise to two *daughter cells*, one of which differentiates to become a mature non-dividing cell, ready to perform functions appropriate to that differentiated tissue. One of the main characteristics of cancer cells is that they de-differentiate to varying degrees. In general, poorly differentiated cancers carry a worse prognosis than well-differentiated cancers.

INVASIVENESS

Normal cells, other than those of the blood and lymphoid tissues, are not generally found outside their 'designated' tissue of origin. This is because, during differentiation and tissue or organ growth, they develop certain spatial relationships with respect to each other. These relationships are maintained by various tissue-specific survival factors that prevent apoptosis (see Ch. 6). In this way, any cells that escape accidently lose these survival signals and die.

For example, while the cells of the normal mucosal epithelium of the rectum proliferate continuously as the lining is shed, they remain as a lining epithelium. A cancer of the rectal mucosa, in contrast, invades other surrounding tissues. Cancer cells have not only lost, through mutation, the restraints that act on normal cells but also secrete enzymes (e.g. metalloproteinases; see Ch. 6) that break down the extracellular matrix, enabling them to move around.

METASTASIS

Metastases are *secondary tumours* ('secondaries') formed by cells that have been released from the initial or *primary tumour* and which have reached other sites through blood vessels or lymphatics, by transportation on other cells or as a result of being shed into body cavities. Often, the primary tumour is asymptomatic and it is not until the cancer spreads that the secondary tumours cause symptoms leading to diagnosis of illness. As such, metastases are the principal cause of mortality and morbidity in most solid tumours and constitute a major problem for cancer therapy[4] (see Chambers et al., 2002).

[4]Although not widely accepted, there is a school of thought that maintaining the primary tumour's integrity and stopping it spreading would prolong life in the cancer sufferer. It may seem anathema to nurture a tumour to keep it happy and avoid stressing it, to prevent any metastatic behaviour.

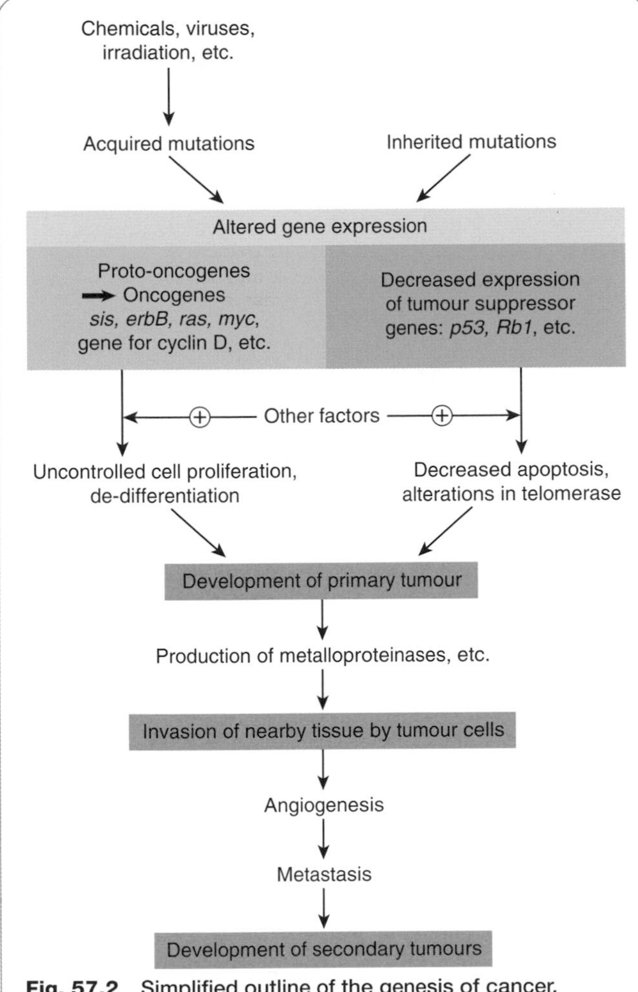

Fig. 57.2 Simplified outline of the genesis of cancer. The diagram summarises the information given in the text. The genesis of cancer is usually multifactorial, involving more than one genetic change. 'Other factors', as specified above, may involve the actions of promoters, co-carcinogens, hormones, etc., which, while not themselves carcinogenic, increase the likelihood that genetic mutation(s) will result in cancer.

As discussed earlier, displacement or aberrant migration of normal cells would lead to programmed cell death as a result of withdrawal of the necessary antiapoptotic factors. Cancer cells that metastasise have undergone a series of genetic changes that alter their responses to the regulatory factors that control the cellular architecture of normal tissues, enabling them to establish themselves 'extraterritorially'. Tumour-induced angiogenic growth of new blood vessels locally favours metastasis.

Secondary tumours occur more frequently in some tissues than in others. For example, metastases of mammary cancers are often found in brain, lung, bone and liver. The reason for this is that breast cancer cells express chemokine receptors such as CXCR4 (see Ch. 7 and Hughes and Nibbs, 2018) on their surfaces, and chemokines that recognise these receptors are expressed at high level in these tissues but not in others (e.g. kidney), facilitating the selective accumulation of cells at these sites, providing a microenvironmental niche for them to reside and thrive. Similarly, lung cancer most commonly spreads to brain, bone and adrenal gland; malignant melanoma to brain; colorectal and ovarian tumours most commonly spread to liver and pancreatic cancer typically to liver and lung.

GENERAL PRINCIPLES OF CYTOTOXIC ANTICANCER DRUGS

In experiments with rapidly growing transplantable leukaemias in mice, it has been found that a given therapeutic dose of a cytotoxic drug[5] destroys a constant fraction of the malignant cells. If used to treat a tumour with 10^{11} cells, a dose of drug that kills 99.99% of cells will still leave 10 million (10^7) viable malignant cells. As the same principle holds for fast-growing tumours in humans, schedules for chemotherapy are aimed at producing as near a total cell kill as possible because, in contrast to the situation that occurs in microorganisms, little reliance can be placed on the host's immunological defence mechanisms against the remaining cancer cells. If a tumour is removed (or at least *de-bulked*) surgically, any remaining *micro-metastases* are now more accessible to chemotherapy, hence its use as adjuvant therapy in these circumstances.

One of the major difficulties in treating cancer is that tumour growth is usually far advanced before cancer is diagnosed. Let us suppose that a tumour arises from a single cell and that the growth is exponential, as it may well be during the initial stages. 'Doubling' times vary, being, for example, approximately 24 h with Burkitt's lymphoma, 2 weeks in the case of some leukaemias, and 3 months with mammary cancers. Approximately 30 doublings would be required to produce a cell mass with a diameter of 2 cm, containing 10^9 cells. Such a tumour is within the limits of diagnostic procedures, although it could easily go unnoticed. A further 10 doublings would produce 10^{12} cells, a tumour mass that is likely to be lethal, and which would measure about 20 cm in diameter if it were one solid mass.

However, continuous exponential growth of this sort does not usually occur. In the case of most solid tumours, as opposed to *leukaemias* (tumours of white blood cells), the growth rate falls as the neoplasm grows. This is partly because the tumour outgrows its blood supply, and partly because not all the cells proliferate continuously. The cells of a solid tumour can be considered as belonging to three compartments:

1. *Compartment A* consists of dividing cells, possibly being continuously in the cell cycle.
2. *Compartment B* consists of resting cells (G_0 phase) which, although not dividing, are potentially able to do so.
3. *Compartment C* consists of cells that are no longer able to divide but which contribute to the tumour volume.

Essentially, only cells in *compartment A*, which may form as little as 5% of some solid tumours, are susceptible to the main current cytotoxic drugs. The cells in *compartment C* do not constitute a problem, but the existence of *compartment B* makes cancer chemotherapy difficult, because these cells

[5]The term *cytotoxic drug* applies to any drug that can damage or kill cells. In practice, it is used more restrictively to refer to drugs that inhibit cell division and are therefore potentially useful in cancer chemotherapy.

are not very sensitive to cytotoxic drugs and are liable to re-enter *compartment A* following chemotherapy.

Benign tumours can still grow (often more slowly) but are characteristically unable to metastasise and spread, and are thus considered much less dangerous to the individual. One example of such is basal cell carcinoma (BCC) skin cancer which continues to expand but will not metastasise, unlike malignant melanoma skin cancer, which readily metastasises to threaten critical organs, such as the brain. BCC still has the potential to transform from its benign form into a malignant form, and kill. Some benign tumours such as colonic polyps have the potential to become malignant, and therefore need close monitoring and removal. Conversely, other benign tumours (such as uterine fibroids) have low risk of turning malignant, and do not need surgical removal unless there are symptoms of bleeding or local compression of other organs.

Most current anticancer drugs, particularly cytotoxic agents, affect only one characteristic aspect of cancer cell biology – cell division – but have no specific inhibitory effect on invasiveness, the loss of a differentiated phenotype or the tendency to metastasise. In many cases, the antiproliferative action results from an action during S phase of the cell cycle (see Ch. 6), and the resultant damage to DNA initiates apoptosis. Furthermore, because their main target is cell division, they will affect all rapidly dividing normal tissues, and therefore are likely to produce, to a greater or lesser extent, the following general toxic effects:

- *bone marrow toxicity* (myelosuppression) with decreased leukocyte production and thus decreased resistance to infection;
- *impaired wound healing*;
- *loss of hair* (alopecia);
- damage to GI *epithelium* (including oral mucous membranes);
- *depression of growth* in children;
- *sterility*;
- *teratogenicity*;
- *carcinogenicity* – because many cytotoxic drugs are mutagenic themselves.

Rapid cell destruction also entails extensive purine catabolism, and urates may precipitate in the renal tubules and cause kidney damage. Finally, in addition to specific toxic effects associated with individual drugs, virtually all cytotoxic drugs produce severe nausea and vomiting, an 'inbuilt deterrent' now thankfully largely overcome by modern antiemetic drug prophylaxis (see Ch. 30).

Cytotoxic drugs, along with surgery and radiotherapy, remain the mainstay of cancer treatment, but newer treatments based on targeting the specific malfunctions of cell cycle control that characterise cancer cells, and on increasing their susceptibility to immunological attack, are becoming increasingly important. These include hormone antagonists, kinase inhibitors and monoclonal antibodies – drugs that are not cytotoxic in the conventional sense, and have a different range of side effects. Described later, they herald a significant shift in pharmacological approaches to cancer treatment. Often these newer types of therapy are guided by the genomic profile of the cancer they target – a principle that is coming more and more into reality for most drugs aimed at treating cancer (see also Ch. 12).

Cancer pathogenesis and cancer chemotherapy: general principles

- Cancer arises as a result of a series of genetic and epigenetic changes, the main genetic lesions being:
  - inactivation of tumour suppressor genes;
  - the activation of oncogenes (mutation of the normal genes controlling cell division and other processes).
- Cancer cells have four characteristics that distinguish them from normal cells:
  - uncontrolled proliferation;
  - loss of function because of lack of capacity to differentiate;
  - local invasiveness;
  - the ability to metastasise.
- Cancer cells have uncontrolled proliferation often because of changes in:
  - growth factors and/or their receptors;
  - intracellular signalling pathways, particularly those controlling the cell cycle and apoptosis;
  - telomerase expression.
- Proliferation may be supported by tumour-related angiogenesis.
- Most anticancer drugs are antiproliferative – most damage DNA and thereby initiate apoptosis. They also affect rapidly dividing normal cells and are thus likely to depress bone marrow, impair healing and depress growth. Most cause nausea, vomiting, sterility, hair loss and teratogenicity.

ANTICANCER DRUGS

The main anticancer drugs can be divided into the following general categories:

- *Cytotoxic drugs.* These include:
  - *alkylating agents* and related compounds, which act by forming covalent bonds with DNA and thus impeding its replication;
  - *antimetabolites*, which block or subvert one or more of the catabolic pathways involved in DNA synthesis;
  - *cytotoxic antibiotics*, i.e. substances of microbial origin that prevent mammalian cell division;
  - *plant derivatives* (e.g. vinca alkaloids, taxanes, camptothecins): most of these specifically affect microtubule function and hence the formation of the mitotic spindle.
- *Hormones*, especially steroids and their antagonists (see Chs 33 and 35).
- *Protein kinase inhibitors* which inhibit growth factor receptor signal transduction (see Krause and Van Etten, 2005) and other non-proliferative effects of tyrosine kinases, such as cell adhesion.
- Monoclonal antibodies.
- Miscellaneous agents.

The clinical use of anticancer drugs is the province of the specialist, who selects treatment regimens appropriate to the patient with the objective of curing, prolonging life or providing palliative therapy.[6] There are hundreds of drugs

[6]You will have gathered that many anticancer drugs are toxic. 'To be an oncologist,' one practitioner commented, 'one has to hate cancer more than one loves life.'

available in the UK for this purpose and they are often used in combination. The principal clinically used treatments are listed in Table 57.1. For reasons of space, we restrict our discussion of mechanisms of action to the more common examples from each group. Anticancer pharmacology is a rapidly expanding and changing field of new chemical entities (NCEs), with new drugs continuously being brought onto the market, and other drugs falling out of favour in the clinic. Further reading (Goldberg and Airley, 2020; Sun et al., 2017) provides more detailed information.

Table 57.1 An overview of anticancer drugs

Group	Examples (specific target, year of approval)	Main mechanism
Drug type: alkylating, and related, agents		
Nitrogen mustards	Mustine (1949), chlorambucil (1957), cyclophosphamide (1959), estramustine (ER, 1981),[a] ifosfamide (1988), melphalan (1992), bendamustine (2008)	Intrastrand cross-linking of DNA
Nitrosoureas	Lomustine (1976), carmustine (1977)	
Platinum compounds	Cisplatin (1978), carboplatin (1989), oxaliplatin (2002)	
Other	Busulfan (1954), procarbazine (1969), dacarbazine (1975), streptozotocine (1982), mitobronitol (1985), thiotepa (1994), temozolomide (1999), hydroxycarbamide (2010), treosulfan (2019)	
Drug type: antimetabolites		
Folate antagonists	Methotrexate (1953), raltitrexed (1986), pemetrexed (2004), pralatrexate (2009), trifluridine/tipiracil (2015)	Blocking the synthesis of DNA and/or RNA
Pyrimidine pathway	Floxuridine (1970), fluorouracil (1970), tegafur (1972), altretamine (1990), gemcitabine (1996), capecitabine (1998), cytarabine (1999), azacytidine (2004), decitabine (2006)	
Purine pathway	Mercaptopurine (1953), thioguanine (1966), cladribine (1993), fludarabine (1990), pentostatin (1991), clofarabine (2004), nelarabine (2005)	
Drug type: cytotoxic antibiotics		
Anthracyclines	Doxorubicin (1974), amsacrine (1992), idarubicin (1997), daunorubicin (1998), valrubicin (1998), epirubicin (1999), mitoxantrone (2000)	Multiple effects on DNA/RNA synthesis and topoisomerase action
Other	Dactinomycin (1964), bleomycin (1973), trabectedin (1996), mitomycin (2002)	
Drug type: plant derivatives and similar compounds		
Taxanes	Paclitaxel (1992), docetaxel (1996), ixabepilone (2007), cabazitaxel (2010)	Microtubule assembly; prevents spindle formation
Vinca alkaloids	Vincristine (1963), vinblastine (1965), vinorelbine (1994), vindesine (2009), eribulin (2010), vinflunine (2012)	
Camptothecins	Irinotecan (1996), topotecan (1996)	Inhibition of topoisomerase
Other	Etoposide (1983), teniposide (1992)	
Drug type: hormones/antagonists		
Hormones/analogues	Ethinyloestradiol (ER, 1943), diethylstilboestrol (ER, 1947), norethisterone (PR, 1957), methyltestosterone (AR, 1973), buserelin (GR, 1985), octreotide (SSR, 1988), goserelin (GR, 1989), megestrol (PR, 1993), triptorelin (GR, 2000), leuprorelin (GR, 2002), abarelix (GR, 2003), medroxyprogesterone (PR, 2004), histrelin (GR, 2005), enzalutamide (AR, 2012), pasireotide (SSR, 2012), lanreotide (SSR, 2014)	Act as physiological agonists, antagonists or hormone synthesis inhibitors to disrupt hormone-dependent tumour growth
Antagonists	Fluoxymesterone (AR, 1956), mitotane (AR, 1960), cyproterone (AR, 1973), tamoxifen (ER, 1977), flutamide (AR, 1989), bicalutamide (AR, 1995), nilutamide (AR, 1996), toremifene (ER, 1997), raloxifene (ER, 1997), fulvestrant (ER, 2001), degarelix (GR, 2008), darolutamide (AR, 2019), relugolix (GR, 2020)	
Aromatase inhibitors	Anastrozole (1995), letrozole (1997), exemestane (1999), abiraterone (2011)	

Continued

Table 57.1 An overview of anticancer drugs—cont'd

Group	Examples (specific target, year of approval)	Main mechanism
Drug type: protein kinase inhibitors		
BCR-Abl tyrosine kinase inhibitors	Imatinib (2001), dasatinib (2006), nilotinib (2007), bosutinib (2012), ponatinib (2012), asciminib (2021)	Inhibition of the Philadelphia chromosome
Tyrosine, or other kinase, inhibitors	Gefitinib (EGFR, 2003), erlotinib (EGFR, 2004), lapatinib (EGFR, 2007), crizotinib (ALK, 2011), ruxolitinib (JAK, 2011), vemurafenib (BRAF, 2011), trametinib (MEK, 2013), afatinib (EGFR, 2013), ibrutinib (BTK, 2013), debrafenib (BRAF, 2013), idelalisib (PI3K, 2014), ceritinib (ALK, 2014), icotinib (EGFR, 2014), palbociclib (CDK, 2015), cobimetinib (MEK, 2015), osimertinib (EGFR, 2015), alectinib (ALK, 2015), lenvatinib (VEGFR, 2016), olmutinib (EGFR, 2016), abemaciclib (CDK, 2017), acalabrutinib (BTK, 2017), ribociclib (CDK, 2017), tivozanib (VEGFR, 2017), copanlisib (PI3K, 2017), midostaurin (FLT3, 2017), duvelisib (PI3K, 2018), encorafenib (BRAF, 2018), binimetinib (MEK, 2018), gilteritinib (FLT3, 2018), ivosidenib (IDH, 2018), larotrectinib (Trk, 2018), dacomitinib (EGFR, 2018), fruquintinib (VEGFR, 2018), erdafitinib (FGFR, 2019), alpelisib (PI3K, 2019), selumetinib (MEK, 2020), pralsetinib (RET, 2020), selpercatinib (RET, 2020), capmatinib (MET, 2020), pemigatinib (FGFR, 2021), mobocertinib (EGFR, 2021), infigratinib (FGFR, 2021), tepotinib (MET, 2021), almonertinib (EGFR, 2021), zanubrutinib (BTK, 2021), trilaciclib (CDK, 2021), olutasidenib (IDH, 2022)	Inhibition of kinases involved in growth factor receptor transduction
Pan-kinase inhibitors	Sorafenib (2005), sunitinib (2006), temsirolimus (2007), everolimus (2009), pazopanib (2009), vandetanib (2011), axitinib (2012), cabozantinib (2012), regorafenib (2012), aflibercept (2012), dabrafenib (2012), nintedanib (2014), brigatinib (2017), enasidenib (2017), neratinib (2017), lorlatinib (2018), anlotinib (2018), entrectinib (2019), fedratinib (2019), avapritinib (2020), ripretinib (2020), umbralisib (2021), pacritinib (2022)	
Drug type: monoclonal antibodies		
Anti-EGF, EGF-2/EGFR	Trastuzumab (EGF-2, 1998), cetiximab (EGFR, 2004), panitumumab (EGFR, 2006), cetuximab (EGFR, 2009), pertuzumab (EGFR, 2012), necitumumab EGFR, 2019), margetuximab (EGF-2, 2020), tucatinib (EGF-2, 2020), amivantamab (EGF, 2021)	Blocks cell proliferation or angiogenesis
Anti-CD20/CD30/CD52/CD19	Rituximab (CD20, 1997), alemtuzumab (CD52, 2001), tositumomab (CD20, 2003), ofatumumab (CD20, 2009), obinutuzumab (CD20, 2013), tafasitamab (CD19, 2020)	Inhibition of lymphocyte proliferation
Anti-CD3/EpCAM/MHC/Bi-specific T-cell engager (BiTE)	Catumaxomab (2009), blinatumomab (2014), tebentafusp (2022), solitomab (2022)	Binds adhesion molecules promoting cell killing
Anti-CD22/CD33/IgG1, etc.	Gemtuzumab ozogamacin (CD33, 2000), inotuzumab ozogamacin (CD22, 2017), ibritumomab tiuxetan (IgG1, 2001), trastuzumab emtansine (2013), enfortumab vedotin (Nectin, 2019), polatuzumab vedotin (CD20, 2019), trastuzumab deruxtecan (HER2, 2019), moxetumomab pasudotox (CD22, 2020), belantamab mafodotin (BCMA, 2020), loncastuximab tesirine (CD19, 2021) mirvetuximab soravtansine-gynx (FR, 2022), teclistamab-cqyv (BCMA, 2022), mosunetuzumab-axgb (CD20, 2023)	Antibody-cytotoxin conjugate
Anti-PD-1/PD-L1 or CTLA4	Ipilimumab CTLA4, 2011), pembrolizumab (PD-1, 2014), nivolumab (PD-1, 2014), elotuzumab (SLAMF7, 2015), atezolizumab (PD-L1, 2016) avelumab (PD-L1, 2017), cemiplimab (PD-1, 2018), durvalumab (PD-L1, 2020), dostarlimab (PD-1, 2021)	Immune checkpoint inhibitors that prevent immune cell suppression
Anti-VEGF/VEGFR	Bevacizumab (VEGF, 2004), ramucirumab (VEGFR, 2014)	Prevents angiogenesis
Miscellaneous	Tocilizumab (IL6R, 2006), denosumab (TNFSF11, 2010), brentuxumab (TNFRSF8, 2011), mogamulizumab (CCR4, 2012), siltuximab (IL6, 2014), daratumumab (CD38, 2015), dinutuximab (GD2, 2015), Emapalumab (IFNAR, 2018), naxitamab (GD2, 2020), isatuximab (CD38, 2020), sotorasib (RAS, 2021), sacituzumab govitecan (EGP, 2021), adagrasib (RAS, 2022)	Multiple myeloma, prostate cancer, bone cancer, etc.

Continued

Table 57.1 An overview of anticancer drugs—cont'd

Group	Examples (specific target, year of approval)	Main mechanism
Drug type: miscellaneous		
Retinoic acid and Retinoid X receptor modulators	Alitretinoin (1999), bexarotene (1999)	Inhibits cell proliferation and differentiation
Proteasomal inhibition	Thalidomide (CRBN, 1998), bortezomib (PSMB, 2003), lenalidomide (CRBN, 2005), carfilzomib CRBN, 2012), pomalidomide (CRBN, 2013), ixazomib (PSMB, 2015)	Activation of programmed cell death
Enzyme	Asparaginase (1978), cristantaspase (2011)	Depletes asparagine
Receptor ligands	Interferon-α (IFNAR, 1986); aldesleukin (IL2R, 1992), imiquimod (TLR7, 1997), denileukin (IL2R, 1999), peginterferon (IFNAR, 2001), palifermin (FGF, 2004), vismodegib (SMO, 2012), sonidegib (SMO, 2015), luspatercept (TGF, 2015), glasdegib (SHH, 2018), tagraxofusp (IL3R, 2018), pexidartinib (CSF1R, 2019)	Receptor modulation
Photoactivated cytotoxics	Porfimer (1995), temoporfin (2001)	Accumulate in cells and kills them when activated by light
Histone deacetylase (HDAC) inhibitors	Vorinostat (2006), romidepsin (2009), belinostat (2014), panobinostat (2015), tazemetostat (2020), tucidinostat (2021)	Broad-spectrum epigenetic activities
Cell-based immunotherapies	Sipuleucel-T (PSA, 2010), talimogene laherparepvec (HSV, 2015), tisagenlecleucel (CD19, 2017), axicabtagene ciloleucel (CD19, 2017), brexucabtagene autoleucel (CD19, 2020), lisocabtagene maraleucel (CD19, 2021), idecabtagene vicleucel (TNFRSF17, 2021), ciltacabtegene autoleucel (TNFRSF17, 2022)	Including directed CAR-T cells
	Omacetaxine (2012), lurbinectedin (2020)	RNA synthesis/mixed
PARP inhibitors	Olaparib (2014), rucaparib (2016), niraparib (2017), talazoparib (2018)	Blocks DNA repair
BH3-mimetic	Venetoclax (2016)	Mitochondrial death
HIF inhibitors	Belzutifan (2021)	
Export inhibitors	Selinexor (2020)	
	Arsenic trioxide (2000)	Unknown

[a]A combination of oestrogen and chlormethine. Drugs in parentheses have similar pharmacological actions but are not necessarily chemically related.

ALK, Anaplastic lymphoma kinase; *AR*, androgen receptor; *BCMA*, B-cell maturation antigen; *BCR-A*, breakpoint cluster region protein-Abelson chimeric tyrosine kinase (Philadelphia chromosome); *BRAF*, B-Raf kinase; *BTK*, Bruton's tyrosine kinase; *CAR-T*, chimeric antigen receptor T-cell therapy *CCR*, chemokine receptor; *CD*, cluster of differentiation; *CDK*, cyclin-dependent kinases; *CRBN*, cereblon; *EGF*, epidermal growth factor; *EGFR*, EGF receptor; *EGP*, epithelial glycoprotein-1; *EpCAM*, epithelial cell adhesion molecule; *ER*, estrogenic receptor; *FGF*, fibroblast growth factor; *FGFR*, FGF receptor; *FLT3*, fms like tyrosine kinase 3; *FR*, folate receptor; *GR*; gonadotrophin-releasing hormone receptor; *HIF*, Hypoxia-inducible factor; *HSV*, herpes simplex virus; *IDH*, isocitrate dehydrogenase-1; *IFNAR*, interferon-α receptor; *ILxR*, interleukin-x receptor; *JAK*, Janus tyrosine kinase; *MEK*, MAP-kinase kinase; *MET*, protein tyrosine kinase; *MHC*, or histocompatibility complex; *PD*, programmed cell death protein; *PI3K*, phosphoinositide 3-kinase; *PR*, progesterone receptor; *PSA*, prostate specific antigen; *PSMB*, proteasome *RET*, receptor tyrosine kinase; β; *SHH*, Sonic hedgehog ligand; *SLAMF7*, surface antigen CD319; *SMO*, smoothened receptor of SHH; *SSR*, somatostatin receptor; *TGF*, transforming growth factor; *TLR7*, toll-like receptor-7; *TNFRSF*, tumour necrosis factor receptor super family; *TNFSF*, tumour necrosis factor super family;*VEGF*, vascular endothelial growth factor; *VEGFR*, VEGF receptor.

ALKYLATING AGENTS AND RELATED COMPOUNDS

Alkylating agents and related compounds contain chemical groups that can form covalent bonds with particular nucleophilic substances in the cell (such as DNA). With alkylating agents themselves, the first step is the formation of a *carbonium ion* – a carbon atom with only six electrons in its outer shell. Such ions are highly reactive and react instantaneously with an electron donor such as an amine, hydroxyl or sulfhydryl group. Most of the cytotoxic anticancer alkylating agents are *bifunctional*, i.e. they have two alkylating groups (Fig. 57.3).

The nitrogen at position 7 (N7) of guanine, being strongly nucleophilic, is probably the main molecular target for alkylation in DNA (see Fig. 57.3), although N1 and N3 of adenine and N3 of cytosine may also be affected. A bifunctional agent, by reacting with two groups, can cause intra- or inter-chain cross-linking. This interferes and prevents not only with transcription, but also with DNA replication, which is probably the critical effect of anticancer alkylating agents.

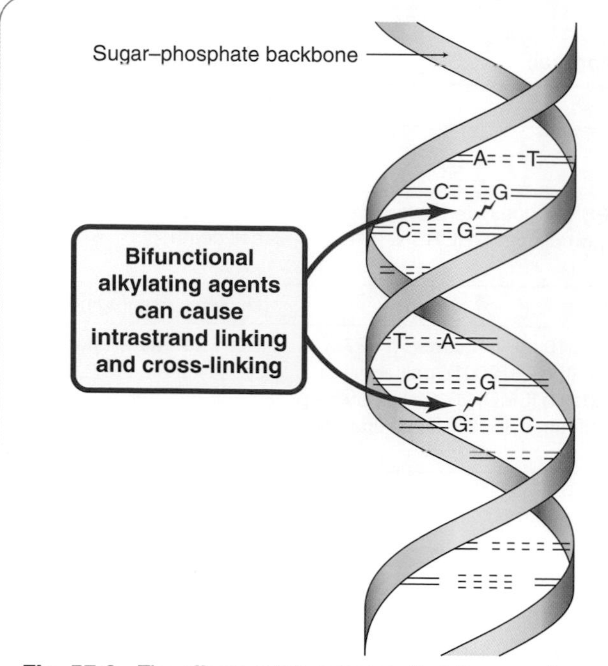

Fig. 57.3 The effects of bifunctional alkylating agents on DNA. Note the cross-linking of two guanines. *A*, Adenine; *C*, cytosine; *G*, guanine; *T*, thymine.

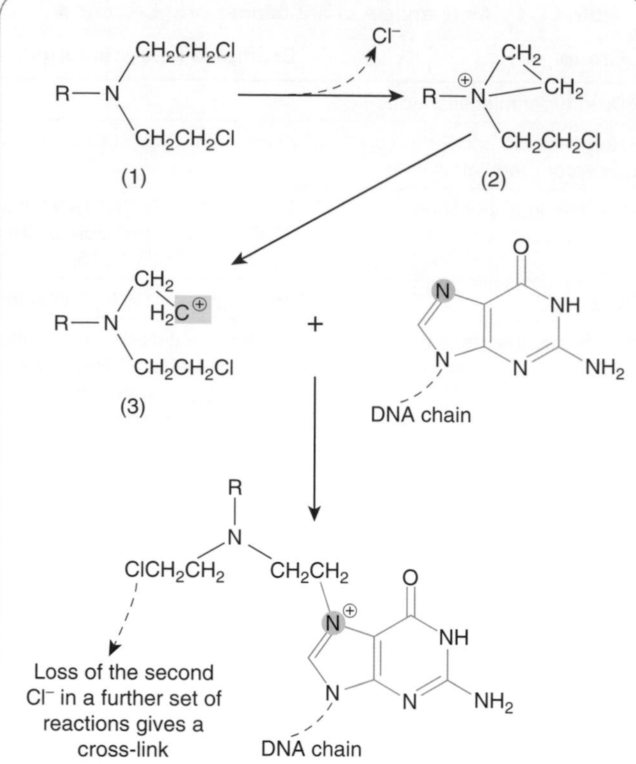

Fig. 57.4 An example of alkylation and cross-linking of DNA by a nitrogen mustard. A bis(chloroethyl)amine *(1)* undergoes intramolecular cyclisation, forming an unstable ethylene immonium cation *(2)* and releasing Cl^-, the tertiary amine being transformed to a quaternary ammonium compound. The strained ring of the ethylene immonium intermediate opens to form a reactive carbonium ion (in *yellow box*) *(3)*, which reacts immediately with N7 of guanine (in *green circle*) to give *7-alkylguanine* (bond shown in *blue*), the N7 being converted to a quaternary ammonium nitrogen. These reactions can then be repeated with the other $-CH_2CH_2Cl$ to give a cross-link.

All alkylating agents depress bone marrow function and cause hair loss and diarrhoea. Depression of gametogenesis, leading to sterility, and an increased risk of a second malignancy occur with prolonged use.

Alkylating agents are among the most commonly employed of all anticancer drugs. Only a few commonly used examples will be dealt with here.

Nitrogen mustards

Nitrogen mustards are related to the 'mustard gas' used during the First World War[7]; their basic formula (R-*N*-*bis*-[2-chloroethyl]) is shown in Fig. 57.4. In the body, each 2-chloroethyl side-chain undergoes an intramolecular cyclisation with the release of a Cl^-. The highly reactive *ethylene immonium* derivative so formed can interact with DNA (see Figs 57.3 and 57.4) and other molecules.

Cyclophosphamide is a commonly used alkylating agent. It is inactive until metabolised in the liver by the P450 mixed function oxidases (see Ch. 10). It has a pronounced effect on lymphocytes and can also be used as an immunosuppressant (see Ch. 25). It is given orally or by intravenous injection. Important toxic effects are nausea and vomiting, bone marrow depression and haemorrhagic cystitis. This last effect (which also occurs with the related drug **ifosfamide**) is caused by the metabolite acrolein and can be ameliorated by increasing fluid intake and administering compounds that are sulfhydryl donors, such as **N-acetylcysteine** or **mesna** (sodium-2-mercaptoethane sulfonate). These agents react with acrolein, to then form a non-toxic compound. (See also Chs 10 and 58.)

Other nitrogen mustards used include **bendamustine**, ifosfamide, **chlorambucil** and **melphalan**. **Estramustine** is a combination of **chlormethine** (mustine) with an oestrogen. It has both cytotoxic and hormonal action and is used for the treatment of prostate cancer.

Nitrosoureas

Examples include **lomustine** and **carmustine**. As they are lipid soluble and cross the blood–brain barrier, they are used to treat tumours of the brain and meninges. However, most nitrosoureas have a severe cumulative depressive effect on the bone marrow that starts 3–6 weeks after initiation of treatment.

Other alkylating agents

Busulfan has a selective effect on the bone marrow, depressing the formation of granulocytes and platelets in low dosage and of red cells in higher dosage. It has little or no effect on lymphoid tissue or the GI tract. It is used in chronic myeloid leukaemia (CML) and myelodysplastic syndromes, and also in patients with other haematological cancers before they undergo stem cell or bone marrow transplants

Dacarbazine, a prodrug, is activated in the liver, and the resulting compound is subsequently cleaved in the target cell to release an alkylating derivative. Unwanted effects include myelotoxicity and severe nausea and vomiting. **Temozolomide** is a related compound with a restricted usage (malignant glioma).

[7]It was the clinical insight of Alfred Goodman and Louis Gilman that led to the testing of (what became the first effective anticancer drug) mustine, a modified and stable version of 'mustard gas', to treat lymphomas. They also wrote what was to become a famous textbook of pharmacology.

Procarbazine inhibits DNA and RNA synthesis and interferes with mitosis at interphase. Its effects may be mediated by the production of active metabolites. It is given orally, and its main use is in Hodgkin's disease. It causes **disulfiram**-like actions with alcohol (see Ch. 50), exacerbates the effects of central nervous system depressants and, because it is a weak monoamine oxidase inhibitor, can produce hypertension if given with certain sympathomimetic agents (see Ch. 48). Other alkylating agents in clinical use include **hydroxycarbamide**, **mitobronitol**, **thiotepa** and **treosulfan**.

Platinum compounds

Cisplatin is a water-soluble planar coordination complex containing a central platinum atom surrounded by two chlorine atoms and two ammonia groups. Its action is analogous to that of the alkylating agents. When it enters the cell, Cl^- dissociates, leaving a reactive complex that reacts with water and then interacts with DNA. It causes intrastrand cross-linking, probably between N7 and O6 of adjacent guanine molecules, which results in local denaturation of DNA.

Cisplatin is clinically useful across a wide range of tumours, and is particularly important for solid tumours of the testes and ovary. Therapeutically, it is given by slow intravenous injection or infusion. It is seriously nephrotoxic, and strict regimens of hydration and diuresis must be instituted. It has low myelotoxicity but causes very severe nausea and vomiting which is best managed through prophylactic use of various combinations of antiemetic drugs (see below and Ch. 30). Tinnitus and hearing loss in the high-frequency range may occur, as may peripheral neuropathies, hyperuricaemia and anaphylactic reactions.

The newer cisplatin derivatives (**carboplatin** and **oxaliplatin**) are considered to have different patterns of toxicity and are potentially easier to administer because they are less likely to cause nephrotoxicity.

Anticancer drugs: alkylating agents and related compounds

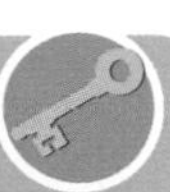

- Alkylating agents have groups that form covalent bonds with cell substituents; a carbonium ion is the reactive intermediate. Most have two alkylating groups and can cross-link DNA. This causes defective replication and chain breakage.
- Their principal effect occurs during DNA synthesis and the resulting damage triggers apoptosis.
- Unwanted effects include myelosuppression, sterility and risk of non-lymphocytic leukaemia.
- The main alkylating agents are:
  - nitrogen mustards, for example **cyclophosphamide**, which is converted to phosphoramide mustard (the cytotoxic molecule); **cyclophosphamide** myelosuppression affects particularly the lymphocytes.
  - nitrosoureas, for example **lomustine**, may act on non-dividing cells, can cross the blood–brain barrier and cause delayed, cumulative myelotoxicity.
- Platinum compounds (e.g. **cisplatin**) cause intrastrand linking in DNA. **Cisplatin** has low myelotoxicity but causes severe nausea and vomiting, and carries high risk of nephrotoxicity.

ANTIMETABOLITES

Folate antagonists

The main folate antagonist in cancer chemotherapy is **methotrexate** (see also Ch. 25 for its use as an immunosuppressant in rheumatology). Folates are essential for the synthesis of purine nucleotides and thymidylate, which in turn are essential for DNA synthesis and cell division. (This topic is also dealt with in Chs 24, 51 and 55.) The main action of the folate antagonists is to interfere with thymidylate synthesis. Folates consist of three elements: a pteridine ring, *p*-aminobenzoic acid and glutamic acid; methotrexate is structurally closely related (Fig. 57.5). Its effect on thymidylate synthesis is summarised in Fig. 57.6.

Methotrexate is usually given orally but can also be given intramuscularly, intravenously or intrathecally. It has low lipid solubility and thus does not readily cross the blood–brain barrier. It is, however, actively taken up into cells by the folate transport system and is metabolised to polyglutamate derivatives, which are retained in the cell for weeks or months even in the absence of continued extracellular drug. Resistance to methotrexate may develop in tumour cells by a variety of mechanisms.

Unwanted effects include depression of the bone marrow and damage to the epithelium of the GI tract. Pneumonitis can occur. In addition, high-dose regimens – doses 10 times greater than the standard doses, sometimes used in patients with methotrexate resistance – can lead to nephrotoxicity. This is caused by precipitation of the drug or a metabolite in the renal tubules. High-dose regimens must be followed by 'rescue' with folinic acid (a form of FH_4).

Also chemically related to folate are **raltitrexed**, which inhibits thymidylate synthetase, and **pemetrexed**, which inhibits thymidylate transferase.

Pyrimidine analogues

Fluorouracil, an analogue of uracil, also interferes with 2′-deoxythymidylate (dTMP) synthesis (see Fig. 57.6). It is converted into a 'fraudulent' nucleotide, *fluorodeoxyuridine monophosphate* (FdUMP). This interacts with thymidylate synthetase but cannot be converted into dTMP. The result is inhibition of DNA but not RNA or protein synthesis.

Fluorouracil is usually given parenterally, but it can be delivered in a more convenient oral formulation using its oralpro-drugs, **capecitabine** and **tegafur**. The main unwanted effects are GI epithelial damage and myelotoxicity. Cerebellar disturbances can also occur. Pharmacogenetic testing is recommended for patients receiving these agents so that treatment adjustments can be made based on metaboliser status and risk of toxicity (see Ch. 12).

Cytarabine (cytosine arabinoside (ara-C)) is an analogue of the naturally occurring nucleoside 2′-deoxycytidine. The drug enters the target cell and undergoes the same phosphorylation reactions as the endogenous nucleoside to give cytosine arabinoside trisphosphate, which inhibits DNA polymerase (Fig. 57.7). The main unwanted effects are on the bone marrow and the GI tract.

Gemcitabine, an analogue of cytarabine, has fewer unwanted actions, the main ones being an influenza-like syndrome and mild myelotoxicity. It is often given in combination with other drugs such as cisplatin. **Azacitidine** and **decitabine** inhibit DNA methylase.

Pteridine ring — *p*-Aminobenzoic acid (PABA) — Glutamyl residues

Folic acid

Methotrexate

Fig. 57.5 Structure of folic acid and methotrexate. Both compounds are shown as polyglutamates. In tetrahydrofolate, one-carbon groups (R, in *orange box*) are transported on N5 or N10 or both (shown *dotted*). The points at which methotrexate differs from endogenous folic acid are shown in the *blue boxes*.

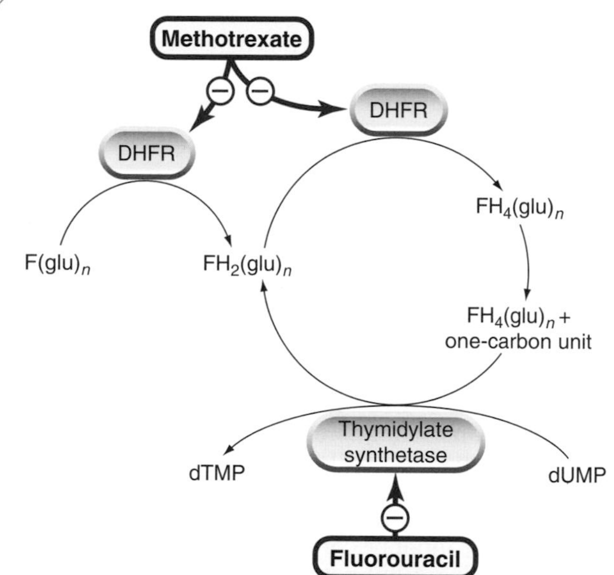

Fig. 57.6 Simplified diagram of action of methotrexate and fluorouracil on thymidylate synthesis. Tetrahydrofolate polyglutamate $FH_4(glu)_n$ functions as a carrier of a one-carbon unit, providing the methyl group necessary for the conversion of 2′-deoxyuridylate (dUMP) to 2′-deoxythymidylate (dTMP) by *thymidylate synthetase*. This one-carbon transfer results in the oxidation of $FH_4(glu)_n$ to $FH_2(glu)_n$. Fluorouracil is converted to FdUMP, which inhibits thymidylate synthetase. *DHFR*, Dihydrofolate reductase.

Purine analogues

The main anticancer purine analogues include cladribine, clofarabine, fludarabine, pentostatin, nelarabine, mercaptopurine and thioguanine.

Fludarabine is metabolised to the trisphosphate and inhibits DNA synthesis by actions similar to those of cytarabine. It is myelosuppressive. Pentostatin has a different mechanism of action. It inhibits adenosine deaminase, the enzyme that transforms adenosine to inosine. This action interferes with critical pathways in purine metabolism and can have significant effects on cell proliferation. Cladribine, mercaptopurine and thioguanine (tioguanine) are used mainly in the treatment of leukaemia.

Anticancer drugs: antimetabolites

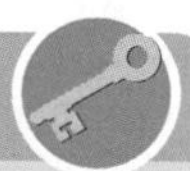

Antimetabolites block or subvert pathways of DNA synthesis.

- *Folate antagonists.* **Methotrexate** inhibits dihydrofolate reductase, preventing generation of tetrahydrofolate interfering with thymidylate synthesis.
- *Pyrimidine analogues.* **Fluorouracil** is converted to a 'fraudulent' nucleotide and inhibits thymidylate synthesis. **Cytarabine** in its trisphosphate form inhibits DNA polymerase. They are potent myelosuppressives.
- *Purine analogues.* **Mercaptopurine** is converted into fraudulent nucleotide. **Fludarabine** in its trisphosphate form inhibits DNA polymerase and is myelosuppressive. **Pentostatin** inhibits adenosine deaminase – a critical pathway in purine metabolism.

CYTOTOXIC ANTIBIOTICS

This is a widely used group of drugs that mainly produce their effects through direct action on DNA. As a rule, they should not be given together with radiotherapy, as the cumulative burden of toxicity is very high.

Doxorubicin and the anthracyclines

Doxorubicin, **idarubicin**, **daunorubicin** and **epirubicin** are widely used anthracycline antibiotics; **mitoxantrone** (**mitozantrone**) is a derivative.

Doxorubicin has several cytotoxic actions. It binds to DNA and inhibits both DNA and RNA synthesis, but its main cytotoxic action appears to be mediated through an effect on topoisomerase II (a DNA gyrase; see Ch. 51), the activity of which is markedly increased in proliferating cells. During replication of the DNA helix, reversible swivelling needs to take place around the replication fork in order to prevent the daughter DNA molecule becoming inextricably entangled during mitotic segregation. The 'swivel' is produced by

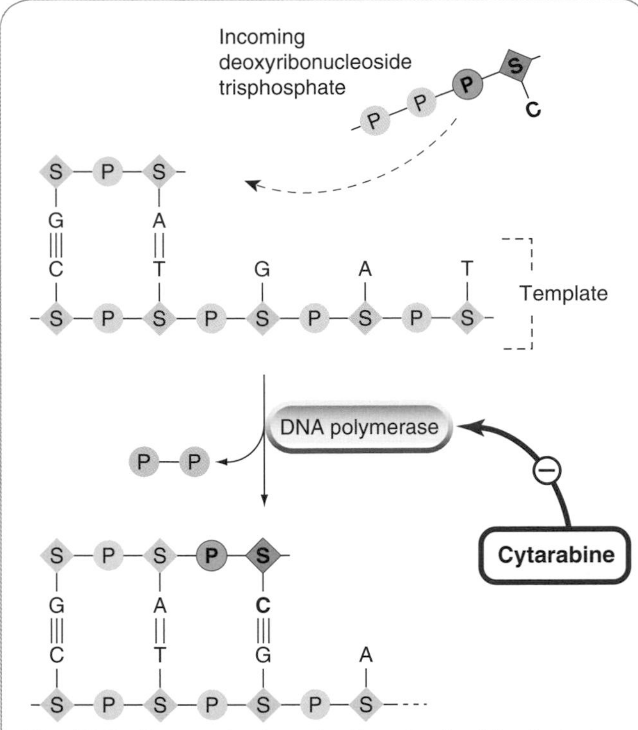

Fig. 57.7 The mechanism of action of cytarabine (cytosine arabinoside). For details of DNA polymerase action, see Fig. 51.5. *Cytarabine* is an analogue of cytosine.

topoisomerase II, which 'nicks' both DNA strands and subsequently reseals the breaks. Doxorubicin intercalates in the DNA, and its effect is, in essence, to stabilise the DNA–topoisomerase II complex after the strands have been nicked, thus halting the process at this point.

Doxorubicin is given by intravenous infusion. Extravasation at the injection site can cause local necrosis. The anthracyclines as a class a have very serious dose-related adverse effects on the heart, resulting in dysrhythmias and heart failure. This action may be the result of generation of iron-dependent free radical oxidative stress, as well as inhibition of topoisomerase 2β. Cardiac toxicity can be reduced through careful monitoring, limiting the maximal dose and prophylactic use of dexrazoxane (which binds metal ions) in high-risk patients.

Dactinomycin

Dactinomycin intercalates in the minor groove of DNA between adjacent guanosine–cytosine pairs, interfering with the movement of RNA polymerase along the gene and thus preventing transcription. There is also evidence that it has a similar action to that of the anthracyclines on topoisomerase II. It produces most of the toxic effects outlined previously, except cardiotoxicity. It is mainly used for treating paediatric cancers.

Bleomycins

The bleomycins are a group of metal-chelating glycopeptide antibiotics that degrade preformed DNA, causing chain fragmentation and release of free bases. This action is thought to involve chelation of ferrous iron and interaction with oxygen, resulting in the oxidation of the iron and generation of superoxide and/or hydroxyl radicals. **Bleomycin** is most effective in the G_2 phase of the cell cycle and mitosis, but it is also active against non-dividing cells (i.e. cells in the G_0 phase; Ch. 6, Fig. 6.4). It is often used to treat germline cancer. In contrast to most anticancer drugs, bleomycin causes little myelosuppression: its most serious toxic effect is pulmonary fibrosis, which occurs in 10% of patients treated and is reported to be fatal in 1%. Allergic reactions can also occur. About half the patients manifest mucocutaneous reactions (the palms are frequently affected), and many develop hyperpyrexia.

Mitomycin

Following enzymic activation, **mitomycin** functions as a bifunctional alkylating agent, binding preferentially at O6 of the guanine nucleus. It cross-links DNA and may also degrade DNA through the generation of free radicals. It causes marked delayed myelosuppression and can also cause kidney damage and fibrosis of lung tissue.

Anticancer drugs: cytotoxic antibiotics

- **Doxorubicin** inhibits DNA and RNA synthesis; the DNA effect is mainly through interference with topoisomerase II action. Unwanted effects include nausea, vomiting, myelosuppression and hair loss. The major problem is cardiotoxicity with high cumulative doses.
- **Bleomycin** causes fragmentation of DNA chains. It acts on non-dividing cells. Unwanted effects include fever, allergies, mucocutaneous reactions and pulmonary fibrosis. There is virtually no myelosuppression.
- **Dactinomycin** intercalates in DNA, interfering with RNA polymerase and inhibiting transcription. It also interferes with the action of topoisomerase II. Unwanted effects include nausea, vomiting and myelosuppression.
- **Mitomycin** is activated to give an alkylating metabolite.

PLANT DERIVATIVES

As with all branches of pharmacology, several naturally occurring plant products exert potent cytotoxic effects and have a use as anticancer drugs.

Vinca alkaloids

The vinca alkaloids are derived from the Madagascar periwinkle (*Catharanthus roseus*). The principal members of the group are **vincristine**, **vinblastine** and **vindesine**. **Vinflunine**, a fluorinated vinca alkaloid, and **vinorelbine** are semisynthetic vinca alkaloids with similar properties. The drugs bind to tubulin and inhibit its polymerisation into microtubules, preventing spindle formation in dividing cells and causing arrest at metaphase. Their effects become manifest only during mitosis. They also inhibit other cellular activities that require functioning microtubules, such as leukocyte phagocytosis and chemotaxis, as well as axonal transport in neurons.

As you would expect, the adverse effects of vinca alkaloids differ from other anticancer drugs. Vincristine has very mild myelosuppressive activity but is neurotoxic and commonly causes *paraesthesia* (sensory changes), abdominal pain and weakness. Vinblastine is less neurotoxic but causes leukopenia, while vindesine has both moderate myelotoxicity and neurotoxicity. All members of the group can cause reversible hair loss.

Paclitaxel and related compounds

These *taxanes* are derived from a naturally occurring compound found in the bark of the Pacific yew tree (*Taxus* spp.). The group includes **paclitaxel** and the semisynthetic derivatives **docetaxel** and **cabazitaxel**. These agents act on microtubules, stabilising them (in effect 'freezing' or 'trapping' them) in the polymerised state, achieving a similar effect to that of the vinca alkaloids. These drugs are usually given by intravenous infusion. They are generally used to treat breast and lung cancer, and paclitaxel, given with carboplatin, is the treatment of choice for ovarian cancer.

Unwanted effects, which can be serious, include bone marrow suppression and cumulative neurotoxicity. Resistant fluid retention (particularly oedema of the legs) can occur with docetaxel. Hypersensitivity to these compounds is common and requires pretreatment with corticosteroids and antihistamines.

Camptothecins

The camptothecins **irinotecan** and **topotecan**, isolated from the stem of the tree *Camptotheca acuminata*, bind to and inhibit topoisomerase I, high levels of which are present throughout the cell cycle. Diarrhoea and reversible bone marrow depression occur but, in general, these alkaloids have fewer unwanted effects than most other anticancer agents.

Etoposide

Etoposide is derived from mandrake root (*Podophyllum peltatum*). Its mode of action is not clearly known, but it may act by inhibiting mitochondrial function and nucleoside transport, as well as having an effect on topoisomerase II similar to doxorubicin. *Unwanted effects* include nausea and vomiting, myelosuppression and hair loss.

Compounds from marine sponges. Eribulin and trabectedin are naturally occurring compounds from marine sponges. Eribulin's main inhibitory action on cell division is through inhibition of microtubule function and it is used for the treatment of advanced breast cancer. **Trabectedin** also disrupts DNA but utilises a superoxide-related mechanism. It is used for treatment of soft-tissue sarcoma, as well as ovarian cancer.

Anticancer drugs: plant derivatives

- **Vincristine** (and related alkaloids) inhibits mitosis at metaphase by binding to tubulin. It is relatively non-toxic but can cause unwanted neuromuscular effects.
- **Etoposide** inhibits DNA synthesis by an action on topoisomerase II and also inhibits mitochondrial function. Common unwanted effects include vomiting, myelosuppression and alopecia.
- **Paclitaxel** (and other taxanes) stabilise microtubules, inhibiting mitosis; it is relatively toxic and hypersensitivity reactions occur.
- **Irinotecan** and **topotecan** inhibit topoisomerase I. Acute cholinergic syndrome can occur with irinotecan.

HORMONES

All tissues are sensitive to hormonal actions, but tumours arising in the more hormone-sensitive tissues (e.g. breast, uterus, prostate gland) may be fundamentally *hormone dependent*, an effect related to the enhanced presence of hormone receptors in those malignant cells, gauged by the receptors present in screened biopsy samples. Crucially, their growth can be inhibited by hormone agonists or antagonists, or by agents that inhibit the synthesis of the hormone.

Hormones or their analogues that have inhibitory actions on target tissues can be used in treatment of tumours of those tissues. Such procedures alone rarely effect a cure but do retard tumour growth and mitigate the symptoms of the cancer, and thus play an important part in the clinical management of sex hormone-dependent tumours.

Glucocorticoids

Glucocorticoids such as **prednisolone** have marked inhibitory effects on lymphocyte proliferation (see Chs 25 and 33) and are used in the treatment of leukaemias and lymphomas. The ability of **dexamethasone** to lower raised intracranial pressure is exploited in treating patients with brain tumours. Glucocorticoids mitigate some of the side effects of anticancer drugs, such as nausea and vomiting, making them useful as supportive co-therapies when treating other cancers, as well as in palliative care.

Oestrogens

Diethylstilboestrol and **ethinyloestradiol** are still occasionally used in the palliative treatment of androgen-dependent prostatic tumours. These tumours can also be treated with gonadotrophin-releasing hormone analogues (see Ch. 33).

Progestogens

Progestogens such as **megestrol**, **norethisterone** and **medroxyprogesterone** have a role in treatment of endometrial cancer.

Gonadotrophin-releasing hormone analogues

As explained in Chapter 35, analogues of the gonadotrophin-releasing hormones, such as **goserelin**, **buserelin**, **leuprorelin** and **triptorelin**, can, when administered chronically, inhibit gonadotrophin release. These agents are therefore used to treat advanced breast cancer in premenopausal women and prostate cancer. The effect of the transient surge of testosterone secretion that can occur in patients treated in this way for prostate cancer must be prevented by an antiandrogen such as **cyproterone**. **Degarelix** is a gonadotrophin-releasing hormone antagonist used for the treatment of prostate cancer.

Somatostatin analogues

Analogues of somatostatin such as **octreotide** and **lanreotide** (see Ch. 33) are used to relieve the symptoms of neuroendocrine tumours, including hormone-secreting tumours of the GI tract such as VIPomas, glucagonomas, carcinoid tumours and gastrinomas. These tumours express somatostatin receptors, activation of which inhibits cell proliferation as well as hormone secretion.

HORMONE ANTAGONISTS

In addition to the hormones themselves, hormone antagonists can also be effective in the treatment of several types of hormone-sensitive tumours.

Antioestrogens

An antioestrogen, **tamoxifen**, is effective in some cases of hormone-dependent breast cancer and may have a role in preventing these cancers. In breast tissue, tamoxifen competes with endogenous oestrogens for the oestrogen receptors (ERs) and therefore inhibits the transcription of oestrogen-responsive genes. Tamoxifen has less disruptive effects due to it being a partial agonist at the ER types found in endometrium, bone and the cardiovascular system. Other ER antagonists include **toremifene** and **fulvestrant**.

Unwanted effects are similar to those experienced by women following the menopause. Potentially more serious are hyperplastic events in the endometrium, which may progress to malignant changes, and the risk of thromboembolism. Drugs such as **raloxifene** are known as selective oestrogen receptor modulators (SERMs), meaning they have a mixture of both agonistic and antagonistic properties at the ER combinations in different tissues. For example it can be oestrogenic in bone (preventing osteoporosis) and simultaneously be anti-oestrogenic in breast and uterine tissue, if it is desirable to prevent oestrogen's positive effects in breast and uterine cancer treatment.

Aromatase inhibitors such as **anastrozole**, **letrozole** and **exemestane**, which suppress the synthesis of oestrogen from androgens in the adrenal cortex (but not in the ovary), are also effective in the treatment of breast cancer in postmenopausal (but not in premenopausal) women, in whom they are somewhat more effective than tamoxifen.

Antiandrogens

The androgen antagonists **flutamide**, **cyproterone** and **bicalutamide** may be used either alone or in combination with other agents to treat tumours of the prostate. They are also used to control the testosterone surge ('flare') that is seen when treating patients with gonadorelin analogues. Degarelix does not cause this flare. An interesting gene in prostate cancer is the transmembrane protease, serine 2 (TMPRSS2) gene that is up-regulated by androgenic hormones and down-regulated in androgen-independent prostate cancers. Some viruses such as SARS-CoV-2 use the TMPRSS2 protease activity to enter and infect their host cells.

Anticancer agents: hormones

Hormones or their antagonists are used in hormone-sensitive tumours:

- **Glucocorticoids** for leukaemias and lymphomas.
- **Tamoxifen** for breast tumours.
- **Gonadotrophin-releasing hormone analogues** for prostate and breast tumours.
- **Antiandrogens** for prostate cancer.
- **Aromatase inhibitors** for postmenopausal breast cancer.

MONOCLONAL ANTIBODIES

Monoclonal antibodies (see Ch. 5) are relatively recent additions to the anticancer armamentarium and are becoming a whole new class of go-to drugs in cancer treatment.[8] In some cases, binding of the antibody to its target activates the host's immune mechanisms and the cancer cell is killed by complement-mediated lysis or by killer T cells (see Ch. 7). Other monoclonal antibodies attach to and inactivate growth factors or their receptors on cancer cells, thus inhibiting the survival pathway and promoting apoptosis (see Ch. 6, Fig. 6.5). Unlike most of the cytotoxic drugs described earlier, they offer the prospect of a more highly targeted therapy without many of the side effects of conventional chemotherapy. This advantage is offset in most instances as they are often given in combination with more traditional drugs. More than 50 separate anticancer monoclonals are currently used clinically (see Table 57.1). Their high costs of development and manufacture are still significant problems. Here are some key examples of the monoclonals used to treat cancer.

Rituximab

Rituximab is a monoclonal antibody (mAb) that is used (in combination with other chemotherapeutic agents) for treatment of certain types of *lymphoma*, including non-Hodgkin's lymphoma. It lyses B lymphocytes by binding to the calcium-channel forming CD20 protein and activating complement. It also sensitises resistant cells to other chemotherapeutic drugs. It provides progression-free survival in 40%–50% of cases when combined with standard chemotherapy (in the clinic called **R-CHOP**; rituximab-cyclophosphamide, hydroxydaunorubicin (doxorubicin), oncovin (vincristine) plus prednisolone).

Rituximab is given by infusion, and its elimination half-life is approximately 3–4 weeks.

Unwanted effects include hypotension, chills and fever during the initial infusions and subsequent hypersensitivity reactions. A cytokine release reaction can occur and has been fatal. Rituximab (like several common anticancer drugs) may exacerbate cardiovascular disorders.

Alemtuzumab is another mAb that lyses B lymphocytes, and is used in the treatment of resistant chronic lymphocytic leukaemia. It may also cause a similar cytokine release reaction to that with rituximab. **Ofatumumab** is similar. **Brentuximab** additionally targets T cells but in a different manner. It is a conjugate of a cytotoxic drug attached to an antibody that binds to CD30 on malignant cells. It is used to treat *Hodgkin's lymphoma*.

HER2-receptor antibodies

Trastuzumab (Herceptin) is a humanised murine mAb that binds to an oncogenic protein termed *HER2* (the human epidermal growth factor receptor (EGFR) 2), a member of the wider family of receptors with integral tyrosine kinase activity (see Fig. 57.1). There is some evidence that, in addition to inducing host immune responses, trastuzumab induces cell cycle inhibitors p21 and p27 (see Ch. 6, Fig. 6.2). Immunological studies are conducted on breast tumour tissue to identify the roughly one in five breast cancers that overexpress this receptor and proliferate rapidly. Trastuzumab and related antibodies (e.g. pertuzumab, margetuximab) have demonstrable efficacy in various stages of HER2-positive breast cancer. However, heart failure is a recognised adverse effect that requires careful monitoring during chemotherapy with these agents.

[8]In 2022, 10 of the top 15 globally sold cancer drugs were monoclonal antibodies, and their proportion is only estimated to increase.

Two mechanistically related compounds are **cetuximab** and **panitumumab**, which bind to EGFRs (also overexpressed in a high proportion of tumours). They are used for the treatment of colorectal cancer usually in combination with other agents.

Bevacizumab

Bevacizumab is a humanised mAb that is used for the treatment of colorectal cancer and now used in a wide range of other cancers. It neutralises *VEGF* (vascular endothelial growth factor), thereby preventing the angiogenesis that is crucial to tumour survival. It is administered by intravenous infusion and is generally combined with other agents. Bevacizumab and other related VEGF inhibitors are also given by direct injection into the eye to retard the progression of wet-*acute macular degeneration* and other pathologies associated with ocular neovascularisation (see Ch. 27).

Catumaxomab

Catumaxomab attaches to an epithelial adhesion molecule, EpCAM, which is overexpressed in some malignant cells. It is given by intraperitoneal injection to treat malignant ascites, a collection of fluid and cancer cells in the peritoneal cavity. The antibody binds to this adhesion molecule and also to T lymphocytes and antigen-presenting cells, thus facilitating the action of the immune system in clearing the cancer.

Gemtuzumab

Gemtuzumab ozogamicin is a drug-conjugate linking a DNA-targeting calicheamicin cytotoxin (ozogamicin) to a mAb directed against the CD33 cell surface receptor. CD33 is found on the myeloid lineage of blood cells and gemtuzumab ozogamicin (aka Mylotarg) is used to treat acute myeloid leukaemias. Similarly, **inotuzumab ozogamicin** was approved in 2017, it being directed against CD22 instead, for the treatment of acute lymphocytic leukaemia. **Moxetumomab pasudotox** CD22 conjugate treats hairy cell leukaemia.

Nivolumab

Nivolumab is a fully humanised mAb against **p**rogrammed cell **d**eath protein-1 (PD-1) which is a cell surface receptor that dampens down the immune system to promote self-tolerance and suppress T-cell activation. Its ligand is PD-L1. Nivolumab has been used to re-prime the immune system so that it will re-recognise and destroy cancer cells that have previously evaded immunosurveillance. It has been approved for the treatment of metastatic melanoma, lymphoma, lung, kidney and head and neck cancers. **Pembrolizumab** is another approved variant of a PD-1 mAb. **Atezolizumab** is a mAb against PD-L1 approved in 2016 for the treatment of bladder cancer.

Ipilimumab

Approved in 2011 for the treatment of melanoma, **ipilimumab** targets the immune checkpoint system known as cytotoxic T-lymphocyte-associated protein 4 (CTLA-4) which functions similarly to the PD-1 system to 'stand down' the immune system. Cancers often employ both these mechanisms to evade immunodetection. Inhibitors of both systems are called 'immune *checkpoint inhibitors*'. Ipilimumab has been used in the treatment of melanoma, with efficacy shown in combating lung and pancreatic cancers. Trials combining both PD-1 and CTLA-4 inhibitors have proven that combined therapy of these checkpoint inhibitors is a useful strategy to reactivate our immune systems and target it against cancer cells in general.

These checkpoint inhibitor antibodies targeting PD-1/PD-L1 and CTLA-4 (see Table 57.1) represent a paradigm shift in cancer treatment, where drugs reactivate our immune system to render it once again capable of hunting out and destroying 'hidden' cancer cells (the immune system's day job).

PROTEIN KINASE INHIBITORS

Imatinib

Hailed as a conceptual breakthrough in targeted chemotherapy, **imatinib** (see Savage and Antman, 2002) is a small-molecule inhibitor of signalling pathway kinases. It inhibits an oncogenic cytoplasmic kinase (BCR-Abl (the Philadelphia chromosome), see Figs 57.1. and 57.8), considered to be a unique factor in the pathogenesis of CML. It has transformed the (hitherto poor) prognosis of patients with CML. It also inhibits two other tyrosine kinases, platelet-derived growth factor receptor (see Fig. 57.1) and the c-kit receptor (CD117), whose ligand is stem cell factor (SCF), and is licensed for the treatment of c-kit positive **GI s**tromal **t**umours (GISTs), not susceptible to surgery.

The drug is given orally. The half-life is about 18 h, and the main site of metabolism is in the liver, where approximately 75% of the drug is converted to a metabolite that is also biologically active. The bulk (81%) of the metabolised drug is excreted in the faeces.

Unwanted effects include GI symptoms (pain, diarrhoea, nausea), fatigue, headaches and sometimes rashes. Resistance to imatinib, resulting from mutation of the kinase gene, is a growing clinical problem. It results in little or no cross-resistance to other kinase inhibitors. Various second (**nilotinib**, **dasatinib**, **bosutinib**) and third (**ponatinib**) generation BCR-Abl tyrosine kinase inhibitors have been developed to combat, to varying degrees, a typical drug-resistant mutation in BCR-Abl (T315I) occurring in imatinib-treated CML patients.

Many similar tyrosine kinase inhibitors have recently been developed, including **axitinib**, **crizotinib**, **erlotinib**, **gefitinib**, **imatinib**, **lapatinib**, **pazopanib**, **sunitinib** and **vandetanib**. **Ruxolitinib** inhibits the JAK1 and JAK2 kinases and **vemurafenib** inhibits BRAF kinase. **Sorafenib**, **everolimus** and **temsirolimus** are pan-kinase inhibitors with a similar utility. **Ibrutinib, acalabrutinib** and **zanubrutinib** inhibit Bruton's tyrosine kinase (BTK) (see Ch. 7). They covalently modify residue C481 on BTK and irreversibly inhibit its cellular actions, which include chemotaxis and secretion of factors necessary for adhesion to the microenvironment. Interestingly their effectiveness in B lymphoid leukaemias and lymphomas derives from the ability to prevent migration and adhesion of these cancer cells to their resident tissues. Lymphocytosis (the extrusion of B cells from lymph nodes, spleen and bone marrow into the peripheral blood) is one of the first effects of these drugs, and is a marker of their chemotherapeutic effect. Thus, similar in nature to checkpoint inhibitors, such anticancer drugs with cellular responses other than simple direct cytotoxic actions represent a new approach to chemotherapeutics.

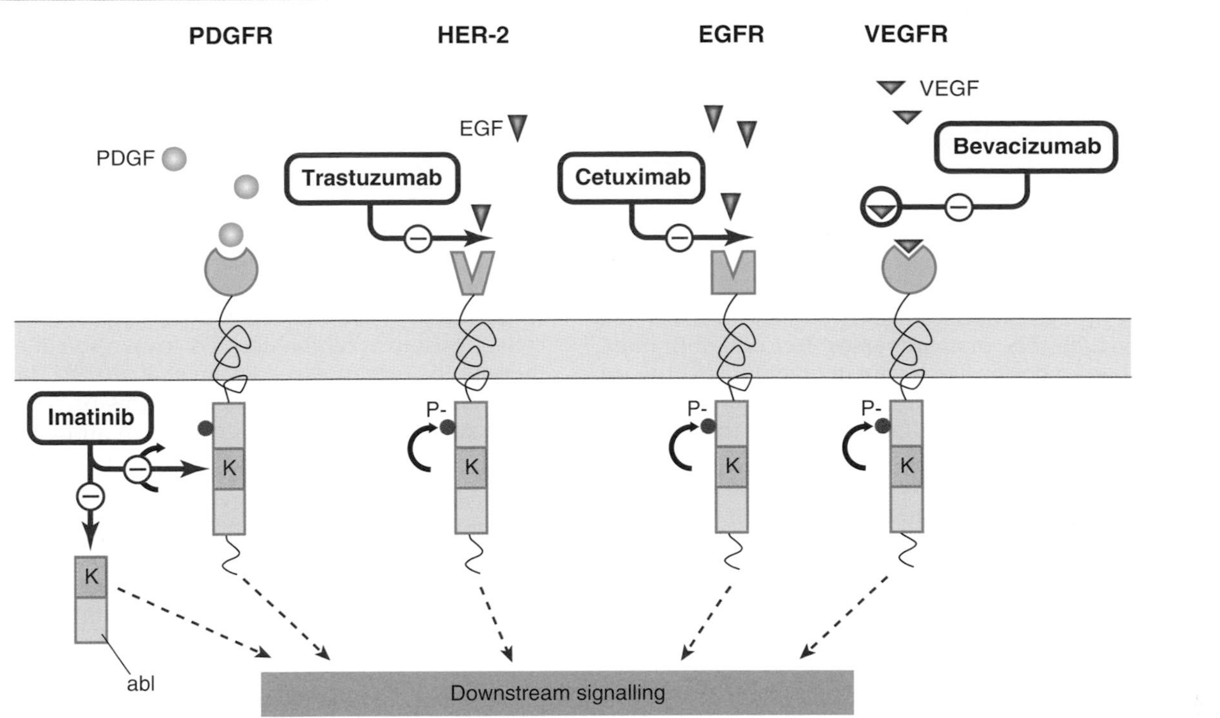

Fig. 57.8 The mechanism of action of anticancer monoclonal antibodies and protein kinase inhibitors. Many tumours overexpress growth factor receptors such as epidermal growth factor receptor *(EGFR)*, the proto-oncogene human epidermal growth factor 2 *(HER2)* or vascular endothelial growth factor receptor *(VEGFR)*. Therapeutic monoclonals can prevent this by interacting directly with the receptor itself (e.g. *trastuzumab, cetuximab*) or with the ligand (e.g. *bevacizumab*). An alternate way of reducing this drive on cell proliferation is by inhibiting the downstream signalling cascade. The receptor tyrosine kinases are good targets as are some oncogenic kinases such as BCR-Abl. *K*, Kinase domain in receptor; *P-*, phosphate group; *PDGFR*, platelet-derived growth factor receptor.

Anticancer drugs: monoclonal antibodies and protein kinase inhibitors

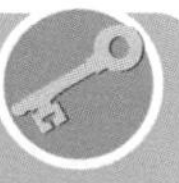

- Many tumours overexpress growth factor receptors that therefore stimulate cell proliferation and tumour growth. This can be inhibited by:
  - monoclonal antibodies, which bind to the extracellular domain of the epidermal growth factor (EGF) receptor (e.g. **panitumumab**), the oncogenic receptor HER2 receptor (e.g. **trastuzumab**), or which neutralise the growth factors themselves (e.g. VEGF; **bevacizumab**);
  - protein kinase inhibitors, which prevent downstream signalling triggered by growth factors by inhibiting specific oncogenic kinases (e.g. **imatinib**; BCR-Abl) or by inhibiting specific receptor tyrosine kinases (e.g. EGF receptor, **erlotinib;** BTK, **ibrutinib**) or several receptor-associated kinases as once (e.g. **sorafenib**).
  - checkpoint inhibitors (**nivolumab**, **ipilimumab**) act through PD-1/PD-L1 or CTLA-4 pathways to unblind cancer cells, allowing their targeting by a reawakened immune system
- Some monoclonals act directly on lymphocyte cell surface proteins to cause lysis (e.g. **rituximab**), thereby preventing proliferation.

MISCELLANEOUS AGENTS

Crisantaspase

Crisantaspase is a preparation of the enzyme *asparaginase*, given by injection. It converts asparagine to aspartic acid and ammonia, and is active against tumour cells, such as those of acute lymphoblastic leukaemia, which have lost the capacity to synthesise asparagine and therefore require an exogenous source. As most normal cells are able to synthesise asparagine, the drug has a fairly selective action and has very little suppressive effect on the bone marrow, the mucosa of the GI tract or hair follicles. The most clinically important adverse effects are hypersensitivity reactions and vascular thrombosis.

Hydroxycarbamide

Hydroxycarbamide (hydroxyurea) is a urea analogue that inhibits ribonucleotide reductase, thus interfering with the conversion of ribonucleotides to deoxyribonucleotides. It is mainly used to treat *polycythaemia rubra vera* (a myeloproliferative disorder of the red cell lineage) and (in the past) chronic myelogenous leukaemia. Its use (in somewhat lower dose) in sickle cell anaemia is described in Chapter 24. It has the familiar spectrum of unwanted effects, bone marrow depression being significant.

Bortezomib

Bortezomib is a boron-containing tripeptide that inhibits cellular proteasome function. For some reason, rapidly dividing cells are more sensitive than normal cells to this drug, making it a useful anticancer agent. Bortezomib inhibits components of the constitutive 26S proteasome β (PMSB) complex subunits (β5, β2 and β1). It is mainly used for the treatment of myeloma (a clonal malignancy of plasma cells).

Thalidomide

Investigations of the notorious teratogenic effect of **thalidomide** showed that it has multiple effects on gene transcription, angiogenesis and proteasome function, leading to trials of its efficacy as an anticancer drug.[9] In the event, it proved efficacious in myeloma, for which it is now widely used. The main adverse effect of thalidomide, apart from teratogenesis (irrelevant in myeloma treatment), is peripheral neuropathy, leading to irreversible weakness and sensory loss (see Ch. 58). It also increases the incidence of thrombosis and stroke.

A thalidomide derivative **lenalidomide** is thought to have fewer adverse effects, but unlike thalidomide, it can cause bone marrow depression and neutropenia. **Pomalidomide** is a newer derivative brought onto the market. These drugs act similarly to inhibit proteasomal degradation through modifying cereblon (CRBN), a receptor substrate of the E3 ubiquitin ligase complex.

PARP inhibitors

Poly ADP ribose polymerase (PARP) is an enzyme found in the nucleus that is involved in DNA repair to maintain genomic stability. Chemical or radiation-induced single-strand breaks are detected and repaired by PARP, to prevent DNA damage-induced apoptosis of our cells. Similar to proteasomal inhibition previously, cancer cells have evolved to ignore DNA damage-induced cell death mechanisms compared to normal non-cancerous cells, but are relatively susceptible to PARP inhibition. More recently developed anticancer agents, PARP inhibitors such as **olaparib**, **rucaparib**, **niraparib** and **talazoparib** are a newer branch of anticancer agents that are useful in the treatment of ovarian cancers and peritoneal cancer, particularly those cancers possessing mutations in their BRCA DNA repair enzymes. PARP inhibitors are often given alongside radiotherapy, which itself induces DNA damage of the tumourous tissues.

Biological response modifiers and others

Agents that enhance the host's response are referred to as *biological response modifiers*. Some, for example **interferon-α** (and its pegylated derivative), are used in treating some solid tumours and lymphomas, and **aldesleukin** (recombinant interleukin-2) is used in some cases of renal tumours. **Tretinoin** (a form of vitamin A/ATRA (all-trans retinoic acid); see Ch. 26) is a powerful inducer of differentiation in leukaemic cells and is used as an adjunct to chemotherapy to induce remission. A related compound is **bexarotene**, a retinoid X receptor antagonist (see Ch. 3) that inhibits cell proliferation and differentiation.

Porfimer and **temoporfin** are haematoporphyrin photosensitising agents. They accumulate in cells and kill them when excited by the appropriate wavelength light. They are administered intravenously as part of photodynamic therapy where the laser light source can be selectively aimed at the tumour (e.g. in the case of obstructing oesophageal tumours, or in head and neck squamous cancers).

RESISTANCE TO ANTICANCER DRUGS

The resistance that neoplastic cells manifest to cytotoxic drugs is said to be *primary* (present when the drug is first given) or *acquired* (developing during treatment with the drug). Acquired resistance may result from either *adaptation* of the tumour cells or *mutation*, with the emergence of cells that are less susceptible or resistant to the drug and consequently have a selective advantage over the sensitive cells. Resistance can be derived from a so-called selective therapeutic pressure (see Vasan et al., 2019). The following are examples of various mechanisms of resistance. See Mimeault et al. (2008) for a critical appraisal of this issue.

- *Decreased accumulation of cytotoxic drugs* in cells as a result of the increased expression of cell surface, energy-dependent drug transport proteins. These are responsible for multidrug resistance to many structurally dissimilar anticancer drugs (e.g. doxorubicin, vinblastine and dactinomycin; see Gottesman et al., 2002). An important member of this transporter group is *P-glycoprotein* (P-gp/MDR1; see Ch. 9). P-gp protects cells against environmental toxins. It functions as a hydrophobic 'vacuum cleaner', picking up foreign chemicals, such as drugs, as they enter the cell membrane and expelling them. Non-cytotoxic agents that reverse multidrug resistance are being investigated as potential adjuncts to treatment.
- *A decrease in the amount of drug taken up by the cell* (e.g. in the case of methotrexate).
- *Insufficient activation of the drug.* Some drugs require metabolic activation to manifest their antitumour activity. If this fails, they may no longer be effective. Examples include conversion of fluorouracil to FdUMP, phosphorylation of cytarabine and conversion of mercaptopurine to a fraudulent nucleotide.
- *Increase in inactivation* (e.g. cytarabine and mercaptopurine).
- *Increased concentration of target enzyme* (methotrexate).
- *Decreased requirement for substrate* (crisantaspase).
- *Increased utilisation of alternative metabolic pathways* (antimetabolites).
- *Rapid repair of drug-induced DNA damage* (alkylating agents).
- *Altered activity of target*, for example modified topoisomerase II (doxorubicin).
- *Mutations in various genes*, giving rise to resistant target molecules, for example, the *p53* gene, C481S mutation in BTK gene developing in ibrutinib resistance and overexpression of the *Bcl-2* gene family (several cytotoxic drugs).

COMBINATION THERAPIES

Treatment with combinations of anticancer agents increases the cytotoxicity against cancer cells without necessarily increasing the general toxicity. For example, methotrexate, which mainly has myelosuppressive toxicity, may be used in a regimen with vincristine, which has mainly neurotoxicity. The few drugs we possess with low

[9]Thalidomide had earlier been found, unexpectedly when used as a sedative, to cause shrinkage of the cutaneous swellings of leprosy (Ch. 52) and is approved for this indication as well as for myeloma.

myelotoxicity, such as cisplatin and bleomycin, are good candidates for combination regimens. Treatment with combinations of drugs also decreases the possibility of the development of resistance to individual agents. Drugs are often given in large doses intermittently in several courses, with intervals of 2–3 weeks between courses, rather than in small doses continuously, because this permits the bone marrow to regenerate during the intervals. Furthermore, it has been shown that the same total dose of an agent is more effective when given in one or two large doses than in multiple small doses.

Common combinations of drugs given together as standard therapy regimens include **ADE** (cytarabine, daunorubicin, etoposide), **FAC** (fluorouracil, doxorubicin, cyclophosphamide), **FEC** (fluorouracil, epirubicin, cyclophosphamide), **FOLFIRI** (leucovin, fluorouracil, irinotecan), **FOLFOX** (leucovin, fluorouracil, oxilaplatin), **XELIRI** (capecitabine, irinotecan), **PAD** (bortezomib, doxorubicin dexamethasone), **CHOP** (cyclophosphamide, doxorubicin, vincristine, prednisolone), **OFF** (gemcitabine, fluorouracil, leucovin), **BEP** (bleomycin, etoposide, cisplatin) and **VIP** (vinblastine, ifosfamide. cisplatin).

CONTROL OF EMESIS AND MYELOSUPPRESSION

EMESIS

The nausea and vomiting induced by many cancer chemotherapy agents are a serious deterrent to patient compliance. This problem can now be prevented by using combinations of different antiemetics which may include $5HT_3$ antagonists, corticosteroids, neurokinin antagonists or nabilone (see Ch. 30).

MYELOSUPPRESSION

Myelosuppression limits the use of many anticancer agents. Red cell and platelet transfusions can be used to support the patient, but febrile neutropaenia continues to pose a significant risk. Here, recombinant human granulocyte-colony stimulating factor (rhG-CSF) can be used after cytotoxic chemotherapy to stimulate neutrophil production and shorten the duration of the at-risk period for serious infections. Filgastrim (and its related compounds) can be given by daily injection at the end of each chemotherapy cycle to restore the white cell count.

FUTURE DEVELOPMENTS

As the reader will have judged by now, our current approach to cancer chemotherapy embraces an eclectic mixture of drugs – some very old and some very new – in an attempt to target cancer cells selectively. Real therapeutic progress has been achieved, although 'cancer' as a disease (actually many different diseases with a similar outcome) remains a massive challenge for future generations of researchers. In this therapeutic area, probably more than in any other, the debate about the risk–benefit of treatment and the patient quality of life issues has taken centre stage and remains a major area of concern (see Duric and Stockler, 2001; Klastersky and Paesmans, 2001).

Of the recent advances in drug therapy, the tyrosine kinase inhibitors and the biopharmaceuticals have arguably been the most innovative advances. Many drugs of the kinase inhibitor type have successfully entered the therapeutic arena and this area continues to be under active investigation (see Vargas et al., 2013; Cohen et al., 2021). Additionally, recent advances in BTK inhibitors primarily targeting non-cytotoxic signalling mechanisms, plus the use of immune checkpoint inhibitors to reset our immune systems so it can once more recognise and destroy cancer cells, are interesting paradigms for the future of intelligent cancer drug design. Moreover, the use of genetically modified cells as 'living drug' anticancer therapies is becoming a reality. For example, chimeric antigen receptor T cells (CAR-T cells) have been approved for the treatment of acute lymphoblastic leukaemia, with trials underway for other cancer types (see Table 57.1 for up-to-date examples). These cells express modified antigens that target and kill cancer cells. Advances in gene-editing technology (e.g. CRISPR-Cas9 (clustered regularly interspaced short palindromic repeats; CRISPR-associated protein 9) and TALENs (transcription activator-like effector nucleases)) have made it possible for patients to receive cancer-killing altered T cells generated from either their own T cells or from a donor (Delhove and Qasim, 2017). Impressive breakthroughs have been seen with these 'living drugs' in cancer patients whose previous treatment failed using standard chemotherapy.

Genotyping and immunological testing of tumour tissue are now widely used in clinical practice to guide selection of the optimal combination for personalising medicine, based on the particular characteristics of the tumour cells (see Ch. 12).

REFERENCES AND FURTHER READING

General textbook

Goldberg, G.S., Airley, R., 2020. Cancer Chemotherapy: Basic Science to the Clinic, second ed. Wiley-Blackwell, Chichester.

Mechanisms of carcinogenesis

Buys, C.H.C.M., 2000. Telomeres, telomerase and cancer. N. Engl. J. Med. 342, 1282–1283.

Chambers, A.F., Groom, A.C., MacDonald, I.C., 2002. Dissemination and growth of cancer cells in metastatic sites. Nat. Rev. Cancer 2, 563–567.

Croce, C.M., 2008. Oncogenes and cancer. N. Engl. J. Med. 358, 502–511.

Griffioen, A., Molema, G., 2000. Angiogenesis: potentials for pharmacologic intervention in the treatment of cancer, cardiovascular diseases and chronic inflammation. Pharmacol. Rev. 52, 237–268.

Hanahan, D., Weinberg, R.A., 2011. Hallmarks of cancer: the next generation. Cell 144, 646–674.

Hughes, C.E., Nibbs, R.J.B., 2018. A guide to chemokines and their receptors. FEBS J. 285, 2944–2971.

Mimeault, M., Hauke, R., Batra, S.K., 2008. Recent advances on the molecular mechanisms involved in the drug resistance of cancer cells and novel targeting therapies. Clin. Pharmacol. Ther. 83, 673–691.

Weinberg, R.A., 1996. How cancer arises. Sci. Am. 275 (3), 62–70.

Anticancer therapy

Gottesman, M.M., Fojo, T., Bates, S.E., 2002. Multidrug resistance in cancer: role of ATP-dependent transporters. Nat. Rev. Cancer 2, 48–56.

Krause, D.S., Van Etten, R., 2005. Tyrosine kinases as targets for cancer therapy. N. Engl. J. Med. 353, 172–187.

Savage, D.G., Antman, K.H., 2002. Imatinib mesylate – a new oral targeted therapy. N. Engl. J. Med. 346, 683–693.

Sun, J., Wei, Q., Zhou, Y., Wang, J., Liu, Q., Xu, H., 2017. A systematic analysis of FDA-approved anticancer drugs. BMC Syst. Biol. 11, 87.

New directions and miscellaneous

Cohen, P., Cross, D., Jänne, P.A., 2021. Kinase drug discovery 20 years after imatinib: progress and future directions. Nat. Rev. Drug Discov. 20, 551–569.

Dagogo-Jack, I., Shaw, A.T., 2018. Tumour heterogeneity and resistance to cancer therapies. Nat. Rev. Clin. Oncol. 15, 81–94.

Delhove, J.M.K.M., Qasim, W., 2017. Genome-edited T cell therapies. Curr. Stem Cell Rep. 3 (2), 124–136.

Duric, V., Stockler, M., 2001. Patients' preferences for adjuvant chemotherapy in early breast cancer. Lancet Oncol. 2, 691–697.

Ferrarotto, R., Hoff, P.M., 2013. Antiangiogenic drugs for colorectal cancer: exploring new possibilities. Clin. Colorectal Cancer 12, 1–7.

Keith, W.N., Bilsland, A., Hardie, M., Evans, T.R., 2004. Drug insight: cancer cell immortality – telomerase as a target for novel cancer gene therapies. Nat. Clin. Pract. Oncol. 1, 88–96.

Klastersky, J., Paesmans, M., 2001. Response to chemotherapy, quality of life benefits and survival in advanced non-small lung cancer: review of literature results. Lung Cancer 34, S95–S101.

Vargas, L., Hamasy, A., Nore, B.F., Smith, C.I., 2013. Inhibitors of BTK and ITK: state of the new drugs for cancer, autoimmunity and inflammatory diseases. Scand. J. Immunol. 78, 130–139.

Vasan, N., Baselga, J., Hyman, D.M., 2019. A view on drug resistance in cancer. Nature 575, 299–309.

Useful Web resources

http://www.cancer.org/.

http://www.cancerresearchuk.org/.

58 Harmful effects of drugs

OVERVIEW

This chapter addresses the harmful effects of drugs, both in the context of therapeutic use – so-called adverse drug reactions – and of deliberate or accidental overdose. We are concerned here with serious harm, sometimes life-threatening or irreversible, distinct from the minor side effects that virtually all drugs produce, as described throughout this book. The classification of adverse drug reactions is considered, followed by aspects of drug toxicity, namely toxicity testing in drug development, mechanisms of toxin-induced cell damage, mutagenesis and carcinogenicity, teratogenesis and allergic reactions.

INTRODUCTION

Paracelsus, a 16th-century alchemist, is credited with the aphorism that all drugs are poisons: '… the dosage makes it either a poison or a remedy'. Today, toxic effects of drugs remain clinically important in the context of overdose (self-poisoning accounts for approximately 10% of the workload of emergency medicine departments in the United Kingdom; by contrast, homicidal poisoning is extremely uncommon). Some susceptible individuals may experience dose-related toxicity even during therapeutic dosing and some of this susceptibility is genetically determined. There are now a wide range of genetic tests for identification and risk prediction of susceptible individuals, although relatively few of these tests are routinely used in current clinical practice (see Ch. 12).

Rigorous toxicity testing in animals (see later), including tests for carcinogenicity, teratogenicity and organ-specific toxicities, is carried out on potential new drugs during development (see Ch. 60), often leading to abandonment of the compound before it is tested in humans. These toxicity studies form part of the package of information routinely submitted to regulatory agencies by drug companies seeking approval to market a new drug. Nevertheless, harmful effects are often encountered after a drug is marketed for human use, due to the emergence of adverse effects not detected in animals. These harms are usually referred to as 'adverse drug reactions' (ADRs) and are of great concern to drug regulatory authorities, which are charged with establishing the safety, as well as the efficacy, of drugs. Unpredictable events are of particular concern. Some ADRs are predictable as a consequence of the main pharmacological effect of the drug and are relatively easily recognised, but some (e.g. immunological reactions) are unpredictable, sometimes serious, and likely to occur only in some patients.

Clinically important ADRs are common causes of hospital admission, costly and often avoidable (see Pirmohamed et al., 2004).[1] Any organ can be the principal target, and several organ systems can be involved simultaneously. The symptoms and signs sometimes closely shadow drug administration and discontinuation, but in other cases adverse effects only occur during prolonged use (*osteoporosis* during continued high-dose glucocorticoid therapy [see Ch. 33], or *tardive dyskinesia* during continuous use of antipsychotic drugs [see Ch. 47], for example). Some adverse effects occur on ending treatment, either within a few days (e.g. tachycardia on abrupt discontinuation of β-adrenoceptor blockade) or after a delay, first appearing months or years after treatment is discontinued, as in the case of some second malignancies following successful chemotherapy. Consequently, anticipating, avoiding, recognising and responding to ADRs are among the most challenging and important parts of clinical practice.

Evaluation of harm from unexpected or rare adverse reactions after long periods of therapy is especially problematic. Precise estimates of risk are seldom obtainable in such circumstances. Randomised trials may not have sufficiently large sample sizes or duration of follow-up for severe rare events, particularly if the trial excluded frail and multi-morbid patients who are most susceptible to adverse reactions. Although spontaneous reporting systems and healthcare database studies may lack the rigour of randomised trials, due especially to the difficulty in excluding various sources of bias between treated and untreated patient populations, these observational datasets are key contributors to our understanding of long-term or rare adverse reactions in large real-world populations. Here, it is worth noting that rare, serious harms such as vaccine-induced thrombotic-thrombocytopaenia or myocarditis were not picked up in thousands of randomised participants during clinical trials of COVID-19 vaccines, and these adverse events only became clear after millions of people had been vaccinated (see Ch. 53).

CLASSIFICATION OF ADVERSE DRUG REACTIONS

The harmful effects of drugs may or may not be related to the main known mechanism of action of the drug. In either case, individual variation (see Ch. 12) is a major factor in determining the response of a particular patient and their susceptibility to harm. Aronson and Ferner (2003) have suggested that ADRs are described according to the **do**se, **t**ime course and **s**usceptibility (DoTS). Potential susceptibility factors such as age and co-morbid conditions are thereby explicitly considered.

[1]Of hospital admissions in the United Kingdom, 6.5% were due to ADRs, at a projected annual cost of £466 million. Antiplatelet drugs, diuretics, non-steroidal anti-inflammatory drugs and anticoagulants between them accounted for 50% of the ADRs, and 2.3% of the patients died. Most events were avoidable.

ADVERSE EFFECTS RELATED TO THE KNOWN PHARMACOLOGICAL ACTION OF THE DRUG

Many adverse effects related to the known pharmacological actions of the drug are predictable, at least if these actions are well understood. They are sometimes referred to as type A ('augmented') adverse reactions in a classification proposed by Rawlins and Thompson (1977) and are related to dose and individual susceptibility. Many such reactions have been described in previous chapters. For example, postural hypotension occurs with α_1-adrenoceptor antagonists, bleeding with anticoagulants, sedation with anxiolytics and so on. In many instances, this type of unwanted effect is reversible, and the problem can often be dealt with by adjusting the dose to obtain a more favourable balance between efficacy and safety. Such effects are sometimes serious (e.g. intracerebral bleeding caused by anticoagulants, hypoglycaemic coma from insulin), and occasionally they are not easily reversible, for example, drug dependence produced by opioid analgesics (see Ch. 50).

Some adverse effects related to the main action of a drug result in discrete events rather than graded symptoms and can be difficult to detect. For example, drugs that block cyclo-oxygenase (COX)-2 (including 'coxibs', for example, **rofecoxib**, **celecoxib** and **valdecoxib**, as well as conventional non-steroidal anti-inflammatory drugs [NSAIDs]) increase the risk of myocardial infarction in a dose-dependent manner (see Ch. 25). This potential was predictable from the ability of these drugs to inhibit prostacyclin biosynthesis and increase arterial blood pressure, and early studies gave a hint of such problems. The effect was difficult to prove because of the background incidence of coronary thrombosis, and it was only when placebo-controlled trials were performed for another indication (in the hope that COX-2 inhibitors could prevent bowel cancer) that this effect was confirmed unequivocally.

ADVERSE EFFECTS UNRELATED TO THE KNOWN PHARMACOLOGICAL ACTION OF THE DRUG

Adverse effects unrelated to the main pharmacological effect may be predictable when a drug is taken in excessive dose, for example, **paracetamol** hepatotoxicity (see later) or **aspirin**-induced tinnitus, or when susceptibility is increased, for example, during pregnancy or by a predisposing disorder such as glucose 6-phosphate dehydrogenase deficiency (see Ch. 12).

Unpredictable reactions unrelated to the main effect of the drug (sometimes termed *idiosyncratic reactions*, or type B for Bizarre in the Rawlins and Thompson classification) are often initiated by a chemically reactive metabolite rather than the parent drug. Examples of such ADRs, which are often immunological in nature, include drug-induced hepatic or renal damage, bone marrow suppression, carcinogenesis and disordered fetal development. Uncommon but severe unpredictable adverse effects that have been mentioned in earlier chapters include aplastic anaemia from **chloramphenicol** and anaphylaxis in response to **penicillin**. They are usually severe – otherwise they would go unrecognised – and their existence is important in establishing the safety of medicines. The unpredictable nature of such reactions means that adjustment of the recommended therapeutic regimen (e.g. using a lower dose) may not prevent them.

Meyler's Side Effects of Drugs is an encyclopaedic source of regularly updated and detailed textbook coverage of ADRs and their clinical manifestations (Aronson, 2016).

DRUG TOXICITY

TOXICITY TESTING

Toxicity testing in animals is carried out on new drugs to identify potential hazards before they are administered to humans. It involves the use of a wide range of tests in different species, with long-term administration of the drug, regular monitoring for physiological or biochemical abnormalities and a detailed postmortem examination at the end of the trial to detect any gross or histological abnormalities. Toxicity testing is performed with doses well above the expected therapeutic range, and establishes which tissues or organs are likely 'targets' of toxic effects of the drug. Recovery studies are performed to assess whether toxic effects are reversible, and particular attention is paid to irreversible changes such as carcinogenesis or neurodegeneration. The basic premise is that the toxic effects caused by a drug are similar in humans and other animals. There are, however, wide interspecies variations, especially in drug-metabolising enzymes; consequently, a toxic metabolite formed in one species may not be formed in another, and so toxicity testing in animals is not always a reliable guide. **Pronethalol**, the first β-adrenoceptor antagonist synthesised, was not developed because it caused carcinogenicity in mice; it subsequently emerged that carcinogenicity occurred only in the one strain tested – but by then other β-blockers were already in development.

Toxic effects can range from negligible to so severe as to preclude further development of the compound. Intermediate levels of toxicity are more acceptable in drugs intended for severe illnesses (e.g. AIDS or cancers), and decisions on whether or not to continue development are often difficult. If development does proceed, safety monitoring can be concentrated on the system 'flagged' as a potential target of toxicity by the animal studies.[2] However, there may be a mismatch between the preclinical data and the subsequent clinical studies where low-risk but potentially effective new compounds are erroneously halted in the development pathway (see Vargas et al., 2021, for a thoughtful debate on QT prolongation and proarrhythmic risk). The *safety* of a drug (as distinct from toxicity) can be established only during use in humans.

[2]The value of toxicity testing is illustrated by experience with **triparanol**, a cholesterol-lowering drug marketed in the United States in 1959. Three years later, a team from the FDA, acting on a tip-off, paid the manufacturer a surprise visit that revealed falsification of toxicology data demonstrating cataracts in rats and dogs. The drug was withdrawn, but some patients who had been taking it for a year or more did develop cataracts. Regulatory authorities now require that toxicity testing is performed under a tightly defined code of practice (Good Laboratory Practice), which incorporates many safeguards to minimise the risk of error or fraud.

Types of drug toxicity

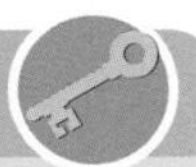

- Toxic effects of drugs can be:
  - related to the principal pharmacological action (e.g. bleeding with anticoagulants), and can usually be predicted from knowledge of the target sites;
  - unrelated to the principal pharmacological action (e.g. liver damage with **paracetamol**), This can be difficult to predict, and is sometimes referred to as 'off-target', collateral or bystander damage.
- Some adverse reactions that occur with ordinary therapeutic dosage are initially unpredictable, serious and uncommon (e.g. agranulocytosis with **carbimazole**). Such reactions (termed idiosyncratic) are almost inevitably detected only after widespread use of a new drug. It is sometimes possible to develop a test to exclude susceptible subjects from drug exposure (e.g. human leucocyte antigen status in patients who may need abacavir).
- Adverse effects unrelated to the main action of a drug are often caused by reactive metabolites and/or immunological reactions.

GENERAL MECHANISMS OF TOXIN-INDUCED CELL DAMAGE AND CELL DEATH

Toxic concentrations of drugs or drug metabolites can cause necrosis; however, programmed cell death (apoptosis; see Ch. 6) is increasingly recognised to be of equal or greater importance, especially in chronic toxicity.

Chemically reactive drug metabolites can form covalent bonds with target molecules or can damage tissue by non-covalent mechanisms. The liver is of great importance in drug metabolism (see Ch. 10), and hepatocytes are exposed to high concentrations of nascent metabolites. Drugs and their polar metabolites are concentrated in renal tubular fluid as water is reabsorbed, so renal tubules are exposed to higher concentrations than are other tissues. Several hepatotoxic drugs (e.g. paracetamol) are also nephrotoxic. Consequently, hepatic or renal damage are common reasons for abandoning development of drugs during toxicity testing and chemical pathology tests of hepatic damage (usually levels of transaminase enzymes measured in blood plasma or serum) and renal function (usually serum creatinine concentration) are routine.

NON-COVALENT INTERACTIONS

Reactive metabolites of drugs are implicated in several potentially cytotoxic, non-covalent processes, including:

- lipid peroxidation, which can initiate a chain reaction throughout the membrane lipids
- generation of toxic reactive oxygen species
- depletion of reduced glutathione (GSH)
- modification of sulfhydryl groups

COVALENT INTERACTIONS

Targets for covalent interactions include DNA, proteins/peptides, lipids and carbohydrates. Covalent bonding to DNA is a basic mechanism of mutagenic chemicals; this is dealt with later. Several non-mutagenic chemicals also form covalent bonds with macromolecules, but the relationship between this and cell damage is incompletely understood. For example, the cholinesterase inhibitor paraoxon (the active metabolite of the insecticide parathion) binds acetylcholinesterase at the neuromuscular junction (see Ch. 14) and causes necrosis of skeletal muscle. One toxin from an exceptionally poisonous toadstool, *Amanita phalloides*, binds actin, and another binds RNA polymerase, interfering with actin depolymerisation and protein synthesis, respectively.

General mechanisms of cell damage and cell death

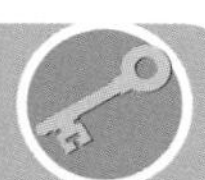

- Drug-induced cell damage/death is usually caused by reactive metabolites of the drug, involving non-covalent and/or covalent interactions with target molecules. Cell death often occurs by apoptosis.
- Non-covalent interactions include:
  - lipid peroxidation via a chain reaction;
  - generation of cytotoxic reactive oxygen species;
  - depletion of reduced glutathione;
  - modification of sulfhydryl groups on key enzymes (e.g. Ca^{2+}-ATPase) and structural proteins.
- Covalent interactions, for example adduct formation between a metabolite of **paracetamol** (*N*-acetyl-*p*-benzoquinone imine [NAPBQI]) and cellular macromolecules (see Fig. 58.1). Covalent binding to protein can produce an immunogen; binding to DNA can cause carcinogenesis and teratogenesis.

HEPATOTOXICITY

Many therapeutic drugs cause liver damage, manifested clinically as hepatitis or (in less severe cases) only by laboratory tests (e.g. increased activity of plasma aspartate transaminase, an enzyme released from damaged liver cells). **Paracetamol** and **halothane** cause hepatotoxicity by the mechanisms of cell damage outlined earlier. Genetic differences in drug metabolism (see Ch. 12) have been implicated in some instances (e.g. **isoniazid**, **phenytoin**). Mild drug-induced abnormalities of liver function are not uncommon, but the mechanism of liver injury is often uncertain (e.g. *statins*; see Ch. 22). It is not always necessary to discontinue a drug when such mild laboratory abnormalities occur, but the occurrence of cirrhosis as a result of long-term low-dose **methotrexate** treatment for arthritis or psoriasis (see Chs 25 and 26) argues for regular monitoring of liver function. Hepatotoxicity of a different kind, namely reversible obstructive jaundice, occurs with **chlorpromazine** (see Ch. 47) and androgens (see Ch. 35).

Hepatotoxicity caused by **paracetamol** overdose remains a common cause of death following self-poisoning. An outline is given in Chapter 25. Paracetamol poisoning exemplifies many of the general mechanisms of cell damage outlined previously. With toxic doses of paracetamol, the enzymes catalysing the normal conjugation reactions are saturated, and mixed-function oxidases instead convert the drug to the reactive metabolite NAPBQI. As explained in Chapter 10, paracetamol toxicity is increased in patients in whom P450 enzymes have been induced,

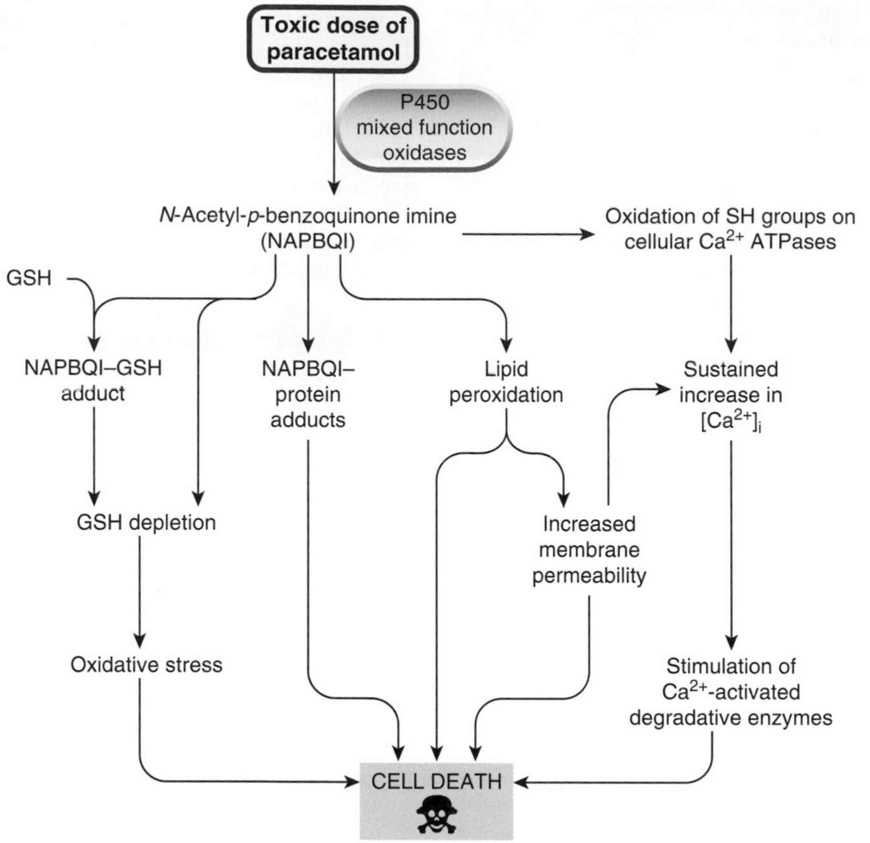

Toxic dose of paracetamol

P450 mixed function oxidases

N-Acetyl-*p*-benzoquinone imine (NAPBQI)

Oxidation of SH groups on cellular Ca^{2+} ATPases

GSH

NAPBQI–GSH adduct

NAPBQI–protein adducts

Lipid peroxidation

Sustained increase in $[Ca^{2+}]_i$

GSH depletion

Increased membrane permeability

Oxidative stress

Stimulation of Ca^{2+}-activated degradative enzymes

CELL DEATH

Fig. 58.1 Potential mechanisms of liver cell death resulting from the metabolism of paracetamol to *N*-acetyl-*p*-benzoquinone imine (NAPBQI). *GSH,* Glutathione. (Based on data from Boobis, A.R., et al., 1989. Trends Pharmacol. Sci. 10, 275–280; and Nelson, S.D., Pearson, P.G., 1990. Annu. Rev. Pharmacol. Toxicol. 30, 169.)

for instance by chronic excessive consumption of alcohol. NAPBQI initiates several of the covalent and non-covalent interactions described previously and illustrated in Fig. 58.1. Oxidative stress from GSH depletion is important in leading to cell death. Regeneration of GSH from glutathione disulfide (GSSG) depends on the availability of cysteine, the intracellular availability of which can be limiting. *Acetylcysteine* or *methionine* can substitute for cysteine, increasing GSH availability; intravenous N-acetylcysteine is the main treatment for paracetamol poisoning.

Liver damage can also be produced by immunological mechanisms (see later), which have been particularly implicated in halothane hepatitis (see Ch. 41).

Hepatotoxicity

- Hepatocytes are exposed to reactive metabolites of drugs as these are formed by P450 enzymes.
- Liver damage is produced by several mechanisms of cell injury; **paracetamol** exemplifies many of these (see Fig. 58.1).
- Some drugs (e.g. **chlorpromazine**, co-amoxiclav) can cause reversible cholestatic jaundice.
- Immunological mechanisms are sometimes implicated (e.g. **halothane**).

NEPHROTOXICITY

Drug-induced nephrotoxicity is a common clinical problem: NSAIDs (Table 58.1) and angiotensin-converting enzyme (ACE) inhibitors are among the commonest precipitants of acute renal failure, usually caused by the principal pharmacological actions of these drugs. Chronic kidney disease, associated with renal tubular or papillary damage, may be caused by a wide range of drugs, including aminoglycoside antibiotics, antiviral drugs and lithium. Nephrotoxic drugs are often well tolerated in healthy people but can cause renal failure in old people or children, or those with concurrent renal disease.

Nephrotoxicity

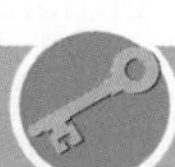

- Renal tubular cells are exposed to high concentrations of drugs and metabolites as urine is concentrated.
- Renal damage can cause papillary and/or tubular necrosis.
- Inhibition of prostaglandin synthesis by NSAIDs causes vasoconstriction and lowers glomerular filtration rate.

Table 58.1 Adverse effects of non-steroidal anti-inflammatory drugs on the kidney

Cause	Adverse effects
Principal pharmacological action (i.e. inhibition of prostaglandin biosynthesis)	Acute ischaemic renal failure Sodium retention (leading to or exacerbating hypertension and/or heart failure) Water retention Hyporeninaemic hypoaldosteronism (leading to hyperkalaemia)
Unrelated to principal pharmacological action (allergic-type interstitial nephritis)	Renal failure Proteinuria
Unknown whether or not related to principal pharmacological action (analgesic nephropathy)	Papillary necrosis Chronic renal failure

Adapted from Murray and Brater (1993).

MUTAGENESIS AND ASSESSMENT OF GENOTOXIC POTENTIAL

Drug-induced mutagenesis is one important cause of carcinogenesis and teratogenesis. Registration of pharmaceuticals requires a comprehensive assessment of their genotoxic potential. Because no single test is adequate, the usual approach is to carry out a battery of in vitro and in vivo tests for genotoxicity, usually comprising tests for gene mutation in bacteria, in vitro and in vivo tests for chromosome damage, and in vivo tests for reproductive toxicity and carcinogenicity (see later).

BIOCHEMICAL MECHANISMS OF MUTAGENESIS

Chemical agents cause mutation by covalent modification of DNA. Certain mutations result in carcinogenesis, because the affected DNA sequence codes for a protein that regulates cell growth. It usually requires more than one mutation in a cell to initiate the changes that result in malignancy, mutations in proto-oncogenes (which regulate cell growth) and tumour suppressor genes (which code for products that inhibit the transcription of oncogenes) being particularly implicated (see Chs 6, 12 and 57).

Mutagenesis and carcinogenicity

- Mutagenesis involves modification of DNA.
- Mutation of proto-oncogenes or tumour suppressor genes leads to carcinogenesis. More than one mutation is usually required.
- Drugs are relatively uncommon (but not unimportant) causes of birth defects and cancers.

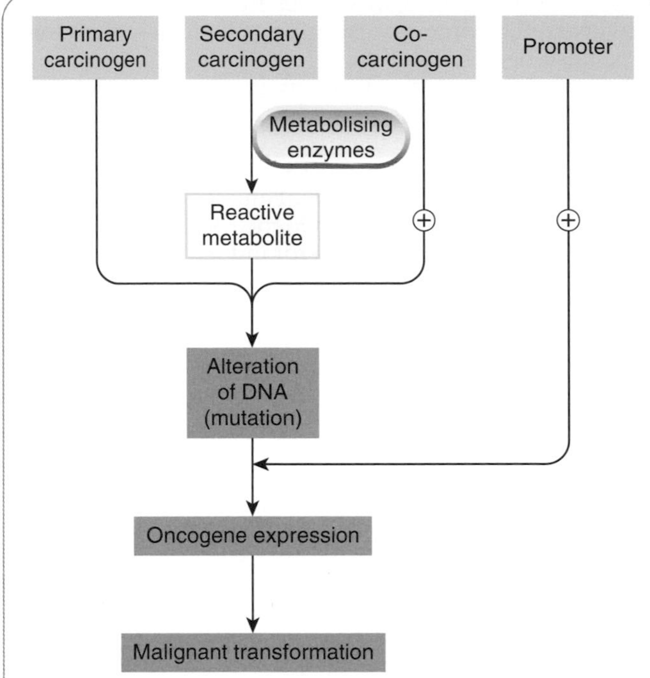

Fig. 58.2 Sequence of events in mutagenesis and carcinogenesis. Alterations to methylation and acetylation patterns of DNA and histones in an epigenetic manner can change gene expression during transcription, translation or even after translation, to increase the likelihood of carcinoma formation.

CARCINOGENESIS

Alteration of DNA is the first step in carcinogenesis (see Chs 6 and 57). Carcinogenic compounds can interact directly with DNA (genotoxic carcinogens) or act at a later stage to increase the likelihood that mutation will result in a tumour (epigenetic carcinogens; Fig. 58.2).

MEASUREMENT OF MUTAGENICITY AND CARCINOGENICITY

Much effort has gone into developing assays to detect mutagenicity and carcinogenicity. In vitro tests for *mutagenicity* are used to screen large numbers of compounds but are unreliable as predictors of carcinogenicity. Whole-animal tests for carcinogenicity are expensive and time-consuming but are usually required by regulatory authorities before a new drug is licensed for use in humans. The main limitation of this kind of study is that there are important species differences, mainly to do with the metabolism of the foreign compound and the formation of reactive products.

The widely used *Ames test* for mutagenicity measures the effect of substances on the rate of back-mutation (i.e. reversion from mutant to wild-type form) in *Salmonella typhimurium*. Additionally, the in vitro micronucleus test is used to detect formation of micronuclei that contain chromosomal fragments (breakage of DNA), or entire chromosomes from damage to the mitotic structure.

Other short-term in vitro tests for genotoxic chemicals include measurements of mutagenesis in mouse lymphoma cells, and assays for chromosome aberrations and sister chromatid exchanges in Chinese hamster ovary cells. However, all the in vitro tests give some false-positive and some false-negative results.

In vivo tests for carcinogenicity entail detection of tumours in groups of test animals. Carcinogenicity tests are inevitably slow, because there is usually a latency of months or years before tumours develop. Furthermore, tumours can develop spontaneously in control animals, and the results often provide only equivocal evidence of carcinogenicity of the test drug, making it difficult for industry and regulatory authorities to decide on further development and possible licensing of a product. None of the tests so far described can reliably detect epigenetic carcinogens. To do this, tests that measure the effect of the substance on tumour formation in the presence of a threshold dose of a separate genotoxic agent are being evaluated.

Few therapeutic drugs in clinical use are known to increase the risk of cancer, the most important groups being drugs that act on DNA, i.e. cytotoxic and immunosuppressant drugs (Chs 57 and 25, respectively), and sex hormones (e.g. *oestrogens*, see Ch. 35).

Carcinogens

- Carcinogens can be:
  - genotoxic, i.e. causing mutations directly (primary carcinogens) or after conversion to reactive metabolites (secondary carcinogens);
  - epigenetic, i.e. increasing the possibility that a mutagen will cause cancer, although not themselves mutagenic.
- New drugs are tested for mutagenicity and carcinogenicity.
- In vitro testing for mutagenicity includes the Ames test, as well as evaluation of micronuclei formation as evidence of chromosomal damage. Carcinogenicity testing:
  - involves chronic dosing of groups of animals;
  - is expensive and time-consuming;
  - does not readily detect epigenetic carcinogens.

TERATOGENESIS AND DRUG-INDUCED CONGENITAL ANOMALIES

Teratogenesis signifies the production of gross structural malformations during fetal development, in distinction from other kinds of drug-induced fetal damage such as growth impairment dysplasia (e.g. iodide-associated goitre) or the asymmetrical limb reduction resulting from vasoconstriction caused by **cocaine** (see Ch. 50) in an otherwise normally developing limb.

Other congenital anomalies may relate to neurobehavioural function. For instance, many psychoactive drugs (see Ch. 46) administered during pregnancy are known, or suspected, to increase the risk of cognitive and behavioural problems in offspring. Examples of drugs that affect fetal development adversely are given in Table 58.2.

The importance of X irradiation and rubella infection as causes of fetal malformation was recognised early in the 20th century, but it was not until 1960 that drugs were implicated as causative agents in teratogenesis: the shocking experience with **thalidomide** led to a widespread reappraisal of many other drugs in clinical use, and to the setting up of drug regulatory bodies in many countries. Most birth defects (about 70%) occur with no recognisable causative factor. Drug or chemical exposure during pregnancy is estimated to account for only approximately 1% of all fetal malformations. Fetal malformations are common, so the absolute numbers of children affected are substantial.

MECHANISM OF TERATOGENESIS

The timing of the teratogenic insult in relation to fetal development is critical in determining the type and extent of damage. Mammalian fetal development passes through three phases (Table 58.3):

1. Blastocyst formation
2. Organogenesis
3. Histogenesis and maturation of function

Cell division is the main process occurring during blastocyst formation. During this phase, drugs can kill the embryo by inhibiting cell division, but provided the embryo survives, its subsequent development does not generally seem to be compromised. Ethanol is an exception, affecting development even at this very early stage (see Ch. 50).

Drugs can cause gross malformations if administered during organogenesis (days 17–60 in humans). The structural organisation of the embryo occurs in a well-defined sequence: eye and brain, skeleton and limbs, heart and major vessels, palate, genitourinary system. The type of malformation produced thus depends on the time of exposure to the teratogen.

The cellular mechanisms by which teratogenic substances produce their effects are not at all well understood. There is a considerable overlap between mutagenicity and teratogenicity. In one large survey, among 78 compounds, 34 were both teratogenic and mutagenic, 19 were negative in both tests and 25 (among them thalidomide) were positive in one but not the other. Damage to DNA is important but not the only factor. The control of morphogenesis is poorly understood; vitamin A derivatives (retinoids) are involved and are potent teratogens (see later and Ch. 26). Known teratogens also include several drugs (e.g. **methotrexate** and **phenytoin**) that do not react directly with DNA but which inhibit its synthesis by their effects on folate metabolism (see Ch. 24). Administration of **folate** during pregnancy reduces the frequency of both spontaneous and drug-induced malformations, especially neural tube defects.

The fetus depends on an adequate supply of nutrients during the final stage of histogenesis and functional maturation, and development is regulated by a variety of hormones. Gross structural malformations do not arise from exposure to mutagens at this stage, but drugs that interfere with the supply of nutrients or with the hormonal milieu may have deleterious effects on growth and development. Exposure of a female fetus to androgens at this stage can cause masculinisation. **Stilbestrol** (a synthetic oestrogen, now seldom used, licensed to treat breast or prostate cancer) was commonly given to pregnant women with a history of recurrent miscarriage during the 1950s (for unsound reasons). Used in this way it caused dysplasia of the vagina of female infants and an increased incidence of carcinoma of the vagina, a rare malignancy with almost

Table 58.2 Some drugs reported to have adverse effects on human fetal development

Agent	Effect(s)	Risk of congenital anomaly[a]	See chapter
Thalidomide	Phocomelia, heart defects, gut atresia, etc.	K	This chapter
Warfarin	Saddle nose; impaired growth; defects of limbs, eyes, central nervous system	K	23
Corticosteroids	Cleft palate and congenital cataract – rare	–	33
Androgens	Masculinisation in female	–	35
Oestrogens	Testicular atrophy in male	–	35
Stilbestrol	Vaginal adenosis in female fetus, also vaginal or cervical cancer	20+ years later	35
Phenytoin	Cleft lip/palate, microcephaly, developmental delay	K	46
Valproate	Neural tube defects (e.g. spina bifida, facial anomalies)	K	46
Carbamazepine	Impaired fetal head growth	S	46
Cytotoxic drugs (especially folate antagonists)	Hydrocephalus, cleft palate, neural tube defects, etc.	K	57
Aminoglycosides	Deafness	–	52
Tetracycline	Staining of bones and teeth, thin tooth enamel, impaired bone growth	S	52
Ethanol	Fetal alcohol syndrome	K	50
Nicotine	Altered neurological function	K	49
Retinoids	Hydrocephalus, etc.	K	26
Angiotensin-converting enzyme inhibitors	Oligohydramnios, renal failure	K	21

[a]K, known to carry a high risk of congenital anomaly (in experimental animals and/or humans); S, suspected of causing or increasing risk of congenital anomaly (in experimental animals and/or humans).
Adapted from Juchau, M.R., 1989. Bioactivation in chemical teratogenesis. Ann. Rev. Pharmacol. Toxicol. 29, 165.

Table 58.3 The nature of drug effects on fetal development

Stage	Gestation period in humans	Main cellular process(es)	Affected by
Blastocyst formation	0–16 days	Division	Cytotoxic drugs, ?alcohol
Organogenesis	17–60 days approximately	Division	Teratogens
		Migration	Teratogens
		Differentiation	Teratogens
		Apoptosis	Teratogens
Histogenesis and functional maturation	60 days to term	As above	Miscellaneous drugs (e.g. alcohol, nicotine, antithyroid drugs, steroids)

no background incidence, in such offspring in their teens and twenties. Angiotensin II plays an important part in the later stages of fetal development and in renal function in the fetus, and ACE inhibitors and angiotensin receptor antagonists (see Ch. 21) cause oligohydramnios and renal failure if administered during later stages of pregnancy, and fetal malformations if given earlier.

TESTING FOR TERATOGENICITY

The thalidomide disaster dramatically brought home the need for teratogenicity and fetal developmental studies on new therapeutic drugs. Regulatory authorities typically require testing in a rodent as well as non-rodent species (e.g. rabbit), involving dosing both males and females. However, poor cross-species correlation means that tests of this kind are not reliably predictive in humans. Equally, the use of in vitro embryo testing has not yet reached the level where it can be fully relied upon as an accurate predictive tool for teratogenicity.

Detection of drug-induced teratogenesis in humans is a particularly difficult problem because the 'spontaneous' malformation rate is high (3%–10%, depending on the definition of a significant malformation) and highly variable between different regions, age groups and social classes. Nowadays, large-scale long-term studies are conducted on specific pregnancy or disease registries, but the results are often inconclusive because of difficulties controlling for the diversity of factors that pre-dispose to teratogenicity and developmental anomalies.

SOME DEFINITE AND PROBABLE HUMAN TERATOGENS

Although many drugs have been found to be teratogenic in varying degrees in experimental animals, relatively few are known to be teratogenic in humans (see Table 58.2). Some of the more important ones are discussed here.

Thalidomide

Thalidomide is almost unique in producing, at therapeutic dosage, virtually 100% malformed infants when taken in the first 3–6 weeks of gestation. It was introduced in 1957 as a hypnotic and sedative with the special feature that it was much less hazardous in overdosage than barbiturates, and it was even recommended specifically for use in pregnancy (with the advertising slogan 'the safe hypnotic'). It had been subjected to toxicity testing only in mice, which are resistant to thalidomide teratogenicity. Thalidomide was marketed energetically and successfully, and the first suspicion of its teratogenicity arose early in 1961 with reports of a sudden increase in the incidence of phocomelia ('seal limbs', an absence of development of the long bones of the arms and legs) that had hitherto been virtually unknown. At this time, a million tablets were being sold daily in West Germany. Reports of phocomelia came simultaneously from Hamburg and Sydney, and the connection with thalidomide was made.[3] The drug was withdrawn late in 1961, by which time an estimated 10,000 malformed babies had been born (Fig. 58.3 illustrates the use of data linkage in detecting delayed ADRs). Epidemiological investigation showed very clearly the correlation between the time of exposure and the type of malfunction produced (Table 58.4). Although the mechanism is not clearly understood, inhibition of blood vessel formation (angiogenesis) is thought to be involved.

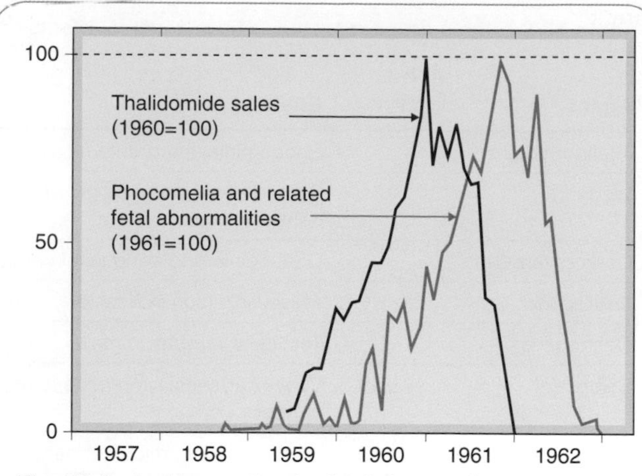

Fig. 58.3 Incidence of major fetal abnormalities in Western Europe following the introduction and withdrawal of thalidomide, linked to sales data for thalidomide.

Table 58.4 Thalidomide teratogenesis

Day of gestation	Type of deformity
21–22	Malformation of ears
	Cranial nerve defects
24–27	Phocomelia of arms
28–29	Phocomelia of arms and legs
30–36	Malformation of hands
	Anorectal stenosis

Cytotoxic drugs

Many alkylating agents (e.g. **chlorambucil** and **cyclophosphamide**) and antimetabolites (e.g. **azathioprine** and **mercaptopurine**) cause malformations when used in early pregnancy but more often lead to abortion (see Ch. 57). Folate antagonists (e.g. **methotrexate**) produce a much higher incidence of major malformations, especially neural tube defects evident in both liveborn and stillborn fetuses.

Retinoids

Etretinate, a retinoid (i.e. vitamin A derivative) with marked effects on epidermal differentiation, is a known teratogen and causes a high proportion of serious abnormalities (notably skeletal deformities) in exposed fetuses. Dermatologists use retinoids to treat skin diseases, including several, such as acne and psoriasis, that are common in young women. Etretinate accumulates in subcutaneous fat and is eliminated extremely slowly, detectable amounts persisting for many months after chronic dosing is discontinued. Because of this, women should avoid pregnancy for at least 2 years after treatment. **Acitretin** is an active metabolite of etretinate. It is equally teratogenic, but tissue accumulation is less pronounced and elimination may be more rapid.

Heavy metals

Lead, *cadmium* and *mercury* all cause fetal malformation in humans. The main evidence comes from *Minamata disease*, named after the locality in Japan where an epidemic occurred when the local population ate fish contaminated with methylmercury that had been used as an agricultural

[3]A severe peripheral neuropathy, leading to irreversible paralysis and sensory loss, was reported within a year of the drug's introduction and subsequently confirmed in many reports. The drug company responsible was less than punctilious in acting on these reports (see Sjöström and Nilsson, 1972), which were soon eclipsed by the discovery of teratogenic effects, but the neurotoxic effect was severe enough in its own right to have necessitated restriction of the drug from general use. Today, use of thalidomide has had a resurgence related to several highly specialised applications. It is prescribed by specialists (in dermatology, haematology, and oncology) under tightly controlled and restricted conditions. **Lenalidomide**, a teratogen and structural analogue of thalidomide, is used in treating myeloma (Ch. 57) and haematologic dysplastic syndromes with close supervision involving pregnancy testing every 4 weeks.

fungicide. This impaired brain development in exposed fetuses, resulting in cerebral palsy and developmental delay, often with microcephaly. Mercury, like other heavy metals, inactivates many enzymes by forming covalent bonds with sulfhydryl and other groups, and this is believed to be responsible for these developmental abnormalities.

Antiepileptic drugs (see Ch. 46)

Congenital malformations are increased two- to threefold in babies of epileptic mothers, especially of mothers treated with two or more antiepileptic drugs during the first trimester, and in association with above-therapeutic plasma concentrations. Many antiepileptic drugs have been implicated, including **phenytoin** (particularly cleft lip/palate), **valproate** (neural tube defects) and **carbamazepine** (spina bifida and hypospadias, a malformation of the male urethra) (see Ch. 46). The relative risks attributable to different antiepileptic drugs are not well defined, but valproate is considered to be particularly harmful (rate of congenital anomalies of about 10%, compared with 2%–3% in the general population), and is contraindicated in women of childbearing age.

Warfarin

Administration of **warfarin** (see Ch. 23) in the first trimester is associated with nasal hypoplasia and various central nervous system abnormalities, affecting roughly 25% of exposed babies. In the last trimester, it must not be used because of the risk of intracranial haemorrhage in the baby during delivery.

Teratogenesis and drug-induced fetal damage

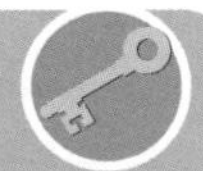

- Teratogenesis means production of gross structural malformations of the fetus (e.g. the absence of limbs after **thalidomide**). Less comprehensive damage can be produced by several drugs (see Table 58.2). Less than 1% of congenital fetal defects are attributed to drugs given to the mother.
- Gross malformations are produced only if teratogens act during organogenesis. This occurs during the first 3 months of pregnancy but after blastocyst formation. Drug-induced fetal damage is rare during blastocyst formation (exception: fetal alcohol syndrome) and after the first 3 months (exception: ACE inhibitors and sartans).
- The mechanisms of action of teratogens are not clearly understood, although DNA damage is a factor.

IMMUNOLOGICAL REACTIONS TO DRUGS

Biological agents (see Ch. 5) may provoke an immune response; antidrug antibodies to insulin are common in diabetic patients, although they seldom cause problems, but antidrug antibodies to erythropoietin and thrombopoietin can have serious consequences for patients treated with these agents (see Ch. 24). Measurement of antidrug antibodies is now routine during the development of biological products. Seemingly trivial differences in manufacturing process (e.g. between different batches, or when a new manufacturer makes a copy of a biological product after it is no longer protected by patent – so-called biosimilar products) can result in marked changes in immunogenicity.

Allergic reactions of various kinds are a common form of ADR. Low-molecular-weight drugs are not immunogenic in themselves. A drug or its metabolites can, however, act as a *hapten* by interacting with protein to form a stable immunogenic conjugate (see Ch. 7). The immunological basis of some allergic drug reactions has been well worked out, but often it is inferred from the clinical characteristics of the reaction, and direct evidence of an immunological mechanism is lacking. The existence of an allergic reaction is suggested by its delayed onset, or occurrence only after repeated exposure to the drug. Allergic reactions are generally unrelated to the main action of the drug, and conform to syndromes associated with types I, II, III and IV of the Gell and Coombs classification (see later and Ch. 7).

The overall incidence of allergic drug reactions is variously reported as being between 2% and 25%. Most are minor skin eruptions. Serious reactions (e.g. anaphylaxis, haemolysis and bone marrow depression) are rare. Penicillins, which are the commonest cause of drug-induced anaphylaxis, produce this response in an estimated 1 in 50,000 patients exposed. Rashes can be severe, and fatalities occur with the Stevens–Johnson syndrome/toxic epidermal necrolysis continuum (a group of life-threatening diseases affecting the skin, often provoked by drugs, for example, by sulfonamides, **allopurinol** or **carbamazepine**). The association between severe **carbamazepine**-induced skin disease and the gene for a particular human leukocyte antigen (HLA) allele *HLAB*1502* in people of Asian ancestry is mentioned in Chapter 12. Susceptibility to severe rashes in response to **abacavir** is closely linked to the variant *HLAB*5701* and this forms the basis of a clinically useful genomic test (see Ch. 12).

IMMUNOLOGICAL MECHANISMS

The formation of an immunogenic conjugate between a small molecule and an endogenous protein requires covalent bonding. In most cases, reactive metabolites, rather than the drug itself, are responsible. Such reactive metabolites can be produced during drug oxidation or by photoactivation in the skin. They may also be produced by the action of toxic oxygen metabolites generated by activated leukocytes. Rarely (e.g. in drug-induced lupus erythematosus), the reactive moiety interacts to form an immunogen with nuclear components (DNA, histone) rather than proteins. Conjugation with a macromolecule is usually essential, although penicillin is an exception because it can form sufficiently large polymers in solution to elicit an anaphylactic reaction in a sensitised individual even without conjugation to protein, although penicillin–protein conjugates can also act as the immunogen.

CLINICAL TYPES OF ALLERGIC RESPONSE TO DRUGS

Hypersensitivity reactions of types I, II and III (see Ch. 7) are antibody-mediated reactions, while type IV is cell mediated. Unwanted reactions to drugs involve both antibody- and cell-mediated reactions. The more important clinical manifestations of hypersensitivity include anaphylactic shock, haematological reactions, allergic liver damage and other hypersensitivity reactions.

ANAPHYLACTIC SHOCK

Anaphylactic shock – see also Chapters 7 and 28 – is a type I hypersensitivity response. It is a sudden and life-threatening reaction that results from the release of histamine, leukotrienes and other mediators. The main features include urticarial rash, swelling of soft tissues, bronchoconstriction and hypotension.

Penicillins account for about 75% of anaphylactic deaths, reflecting the frequency with which they are used in clinical practice. Other drugs that can cause anaphylaxis include enzymes, such as **asparaginase** (see Ch. 57); therapeutic monoclonal antibodies (see Ch. 5); hormones, for example, **corticotropin** (see Ch. 33); dextrans; radiological contrast agents; vaccines; and other serological products. Anaphylaxis can also be caused by local anaesthetics (see Ch. 44), the antiseptic chlorhexidine and many other medications (sometimes as a consequence of contaminants such as latex used to seal reusable vials or of excipients and colouring agents rather than the drug itself). Treatment of anaphylaxis is mentioned in Chapter 28.

It is sometimes feasible to carry out a skin test for the presence of hypersensitivity, which involves injecting a minute dose intradermally. A patient who reports that she or he is allergic to a drug such as penicillin may actually be allergic to fungal contaminants, which were common in early preparations, rather than to penicillin itself. The use of penicilloylpolylysine as a skin test reagent for penicillin allergy is an improvement over the use of penicillin itself, because it bypasses the need for conjugation of the test substance, thereby reducing the likelihood of a false-negative. Other specialised tests are available to detect the presence of specific immunoglobulin E in the plasma, or to measure histamine release from the patient's basophils, but these are not used routinely.

HAEMATOLOGICAL REACTIONS

Drug-induced haematological reactions can be produced by type II, III or IV hypersensitivity. Type II reactions can affect any or all of the formed elements of the blood, which may be destroyed by effects either on the circulating blood cells themselves or on their progenitors in the bone marrow. They involve antibody binding to a drug–macromolecule complex on the cell surface membrane. The antigen–antibody reaction activates complement, leading to lysis, or provokes attack by killer lymphocytes or phagocytic leukocytes (see Ch. 7). *Haemolytic anaemia* has been most commonly reported with sulfonamides and related drugs (see Ch. 52) and with an antihypertensive drug, **methyldopa** (see Ch. 15), which is still used to treat hypertension during pregnancy. With methyldopa, significant haemolysis occurs in less than 1% of patients, but the appearance of antibodies directed against the surface of red cells is detectable in 15% by the direct antiglobulin test. The antibodies are directed against Rh antigens, but it is not known how methyldopa produces this effect.

Drug-induced *agranulocytosis* (complete absence of circulating neutrophils) is usually delayed 2–12 weeks after beginning drug treatment but may then be sudden in onset. It often presents with mouth ulcers, a severe sore throat or other infection. Serum from the patient lyses leukocytes from other individuals, and circulating antileukocyte antibodies can usually be detected immunologically. Drugs associated with agranulocytosis include **carbimazole** (see Ch. 34), **clozapine** (see Ch. 47) and **sulfonamides** and related drugs (e.g. *thiazides* and *sulfonylureas*). Agranulocytosis is rare but life-threatening. Recovery when the offending drug is stopped is often slow or absent. Antibody-mediated leukocyte destruction must be distinguished from the direct effect of cytotoxic drugs (see Ch. 57), which cause granulocytopenia that is rapid in onset, predictably related to dose and reversible.

Thrombocytopenia (reduction in platelet numbers) can be caused by type II reactions to **quinine** (see Ch. 55), and **heparin** (see Ch. 23).

Some drugs (notably **chloramphenicol**) can suppress all three haemopoietic cell lineages, giving rise to *aplastic anaemia* (anaemia with associated agranulocytosis and thrombocytopenia).

The distinction between type III and type IV hypersensitivity reactions in the causation of haematological reactions is not clear cut, and either or both mechanisms can be involved.

ALLERGIC LIVER DAMAGE

Most drug-induced liver damage results from the direct toxic effects of drugs or their metabolites, as described earlier. However, hypersensitivity reactions are sometimes involved, a particular example being **halothane**-induced hepatic necrosis (see Ch. 41). *Trifluoracetylchloride*, a reactive metabolite of halothane, couples to a macromolecule to form an immunogen. Most patients with halothane-induced liver damage have antibodies that react with halothane–carrier conjugates. Halothane–protein antigens can be expressed on the surface of hepatocytes. Destruction of the cells occurs by type II hypersensitivity reactions involving killer T cells, and type III reactions can also contribute.

OTHER HYPERSENSITIVITY REACTIONS

The clinical manifestations of type IV hypersensitivity reactions are diverse, ranging from minor rashes to generalised autoimmune disease. Fever may accompany these reactions. Rashes can be antibody mediated but are usually cell mediated. They range from mild eruptions to fatal exfoliation. Stevens–Johnson syndrome/toxic epidermal necrolysis is now believed to be a continuum of very severe generalised rash extending into the alimentary tract and with blistering or exfoliation. In some cases, the lesions are photosensitive, probably because ultraviolet light converts the drug to reactive products.

Allergic reactions to drugs

- Drugs or their reactive metabolites can bind covalently to proteins to form immunogens. **Penicillin** (which can also form immunogenic polymers) is an important example.
- Drug-induced allergic (hypersensitivity) reactions may be antibody mediated (types I, II, III) or cell mediated (type IV). Important clinical manifestations include the following:
  - anaphylactic shock (type I): many drugs can cause this, and most deaths are caused by **penicillin**;
  - haematological reactions (type II, III or IV): including haemolytic anaemia (e.g. **methyldopa**), agranulocytosis (e.g. **carbimazole**), thrombocytopenia (e.g. **quinine**) and aplastic anaemia (e.g. **chloramphenicol**);
  - hepatitis (types II, III): for example, **halothane**, **phenytoin**;
  - rashes (type I, IV): are usually mild but can be life-threatening (e.g. Stevens–Johnson syndrome);
  - drug-induced systemic lupus erythematosus (mainly type II): antibodies to nuclear material are formed (e.g. **hydralazine**).

REFERENCES AND FURTHER READING

Adverse drug reactions

Aronson, J.K. (Ed.), 2016. Meyler's Side Effects of Drugs: The International Encyclopedia of Adverse Drug Reactions and Interactions, sixteenth ed. Elsevier Science, Amsterdam.

Aronson, J.K., Ferner, R.E., 2003. Joining the DoTS: a new approach to classifying adverse drug reactions. Br. Med. J. 327, 1222–1225

Pirmohamed, M., James, S., Meakin, S., et al., 2004. Adverse drug reactions as cause of admission to hospital: prospective analysis of 18820 patients. Br. Med. J. 329, 15–19.

Rawlins, M.D., Thompson, J.W., 1977. Pathogenesis of adverse drug reactions. In: Davies, D.M. (Ed.), Textbook of Adverse Drug Reactions. Oxford University Press, Oxford.

Talbot, J., Aronson, J.K. (Eds.), 2012. Stephens' Detection and Evaluation of Adverse Drug Reactions, sixth ed. Wiley-Blackwell, Oxford

Drug toxicity: general and mechanistic aspects

Andrade, E.L., Bento, A.F., Cavalli, J., et al., 2016. Non-clinical studies in the process of new drug development - part II: good laboratory practice, metabolism, pharmacokinetics, safety and dose translation to clinical studies. Braz. J. Med. Biol. Res. 49, e5646.

Drug toxicity: carcinogenesis, teratogenesis

Briggs, G.G., Freeman, R.K., Towers, C.V., Forinash, A.B., 2021. Briggs' Drugs in Pregnancy and Lactation, twelfth ed. Walters Kluwer, Philadelphia

Sjöström, H., Nilsson, R., 1972. Thalidomide and the Power of the Drug Companies. Penguin Books, London.

Drug toxicity: organ involvement

Hoetzenecker, W., Nägeli, M., Mehra, E.T., et al., 2016. Adverse cutaneous drug eruptions: current understanding. Semin. Immunopathol. 38, 75–86.

Gómez-Lechón, M.J., Tolosa, L., Donato, M.T., 2016. Metabolic activation and drug-induced liver injury: in vitro approaches for the safety risk assessment of new drugs. J. Appl. Toxicol. 36, 752–768

Ritter, J.M., Harding, I., Warren, J.B., 2009. Precaution, cyclooxygenase inhibition, and cardiovascular risk. Trends Pharmacol. Sci. 30, 503–514.

Vargas, H.M., Rolf, M.G., Wisialowski, T.A., et al., 2021. Time for a fully integrated nonclinical-clinical risk assessment to streamline QT prolongation liability determinations: a pharma industry perspective. Clin. Pharmacol. Ther. 109, 310–318

59 Lifestyle and drugs in sport

OVERVIEW

Drugs used for nontherapeutic reasons, but rather for cosmetic purposes, purely social reasons or to enhance athletic or other abilities are collectively referred to as *lifestyle drugs*. It is a diverse category of unrelated drugs and since many are also used for other conventional clinical purposes, their pharmacology is described elsewhere in this book. In this chapter we present an overview of lifestyle drugs illustrating the topic with three specific examples: cognitive enhancers, 'pharmacosex' and the use of drugs in sport. We also introduce some of the ethical, social and medico-legal problems associated with the 'lifestyle drug phenomenon' and also the related concept of 'human enhancement'.

WHAT ARE LIFESTYLE DRUGS?

Some commentators would describe lifestyle drugs as those which are used to treat 'lifestyle diseases' such as smoking or alcoholism but generally (and specifically in this chapter) the term refers to drugs or medicines that are taken by choice to satisfy an aspiration or a non-health-related goal rather than to treat an illness or disease. Since many are conventional therapeutics already used clinically for some purpose, a better term for this group might be *lifestyle uses* for drugs.

Some examples may make this clear. The vast majority of women who take the contraceptive pill are not 'ill'; they take these powerful drugs so they can plan their families, in other words, for lifestyle purposes. Likewise, while **sildenafil** is used clinically to treat male erectile dysfunction, this drug is mostly used by normal men who wish to improve their sexual prowess. Many people who use cognitive enhancers do so for lifestyle purposes, to improve concentration or exam performance for example, and not because they suffer from attention deficit hyperactivity disorder (ADHD). In the words of one commentator, lifestyle drugs are used to treat 'non-diseases' (Smith, 2002).

The lifestyle drug 'sector' is growing rapidly, with sales sometimes outstripping those of conventional medicines. Public demand is increased by the widespread availability of medical information on the internet and 'self-diagnosis'. Anyone with a computer can now look up their 'symptoms', their likely cause and the appropriate medical remedy. It is easy to locate advice on how drugs may ease your real or imagined problem or help with the realisation of some other physical or mental goal. Internet sites hosting 'patient support groups' provide a convenient forum where one can compare notes with others, learn which drugs are the best and even obtain advice on what to tell your doctor in order to ensure you receive your drug of choice. If this fails, online pharmacies are sure to oblige.

The lifestyle drug 'phenomenon' forms part of a larger debate which also embraces the concept of *human enhancement*, the use of pharmaceutical, genetic and other biotechnologies to augment human capabilities beyond those normally enjoyed by mankind. As you might imagine, these are controversial ideas, which will likely keep bioethicists and drug regulators busy for some time to come. The possibility, intensively pursued but so far regrettably unrealised, of finding drugs that prolong life by retarding the functional and degenerative changes characteristic of old age is another social and ethical minefield.

Whilst we touch upon some of these thorny issues later, we focus our attention mainly on the pharmacological aspects of lifestyle drugs, leaving other unresolved ethical issues to our more philosophically minded colleagues. For a more complete discussion of human enhancement by pharmacological means, see Buchanan (2011), Flower (2012) and Hofmann (2017).

CLASSIFICATION OF LIFESTYLE DRUGS

The 'lifestyle drug' category comprises a variety of chemically and pharmacologically unrelated groups of drugs and medicines. The classification scheme in Table 59.1 is based upon the work of several authors and since these drugs cut across the pharmacological classification used throughout this book, it includes the appropriate chapter cross-references.

The list embraces drugs that have been used for lifestyle choices based on historical precedent, such as oral contraceptives, agents used to manage potentially debilitating lifestyle illnesses such as addiction to smoking (e.g. **bupropion**), drugs such as **caffeine** and **alcohol** that are consumed on a massive scale around the world as components of drinks, nutritional supplements as well as drugs of abuse such as **cocaine** and 'NSPs' (novel psychoactive substances), increasing common street drugs.

Perhaps illustrating the potential pitfalls of any attempt to define lifestyle drugs, we may note how, over time, drugs can alternate between 'lifestyle' and 'clinical' categories, often depending upon the social mores of the day. For example, **cocaine** was used as a lifestyle drug by the indigenous peoples of South America. Early explorers commented that it 'satisfies the hungry, gives new strength to the weary and exhausted and makes the unhappy forget their sorrows'. Originally adopted into European medicine as a local anaesthetic, it is now largely returned to lifestyle drug status and, regrettably, is the basis of an illegal multimillion dollar international drugs industry. **Cannabis** is another good example of a drug that has been considered (in the West at least) as a purely recreational drug but which is now (as a plant extract containing **tetrahydrocannabinol** and **cannabidiol**) licensed for various clinical uses. There are many other examples (Flower, 2004).

Table 59.1 Some examples of lifestyle drugs and medicines (excluding drugs in sport)

Category	Example(s)	Clinical use (if any)	'Lifestyle' use	Chapter
Medicines approved for specific clinical indications and which have similar 'lifestyle' uses	Sildenafil[a]	Erectile dysfunction	Erectile enhancement	35
	Oral contraceptives	Preventing conception	Preventing conception	35
	Orlistat	Obesity	Weight loss	32
	Sibutramine	Anorectic agent (now withdrawn)	Weight loss	32
Medicines approved for specific clinical indications and which have different 'lifestyle' uses	Minoxidil	Hypertension	Regrowth of hair	21
	Methylphenidate	Treatment of ADHD	Cognitive enhancement	49
	Modafinil	Treatment of ADHD	Cognitive enhancement	49
	Opiates	Analgesia	'Recreational' usage	50
Drugs that have only minor, or no, current clinical use but which fall into the lifestyle category	Alcohol	None as such	Widespread component of drinks	50
	Botulinum toxin	Relief of muscle spasm	Cosmetic enhancement	14
	Caffeine	Former migraine treatment	Component of drinks	42, 49
	Cannabis (containing THC and CBD)	Managing chronic pain, nausea and possibly muscle spasm (THC) and some forms of epilepsy and seizures (CBD)	'Recreational' usage	18, 46, 50
Drugs (generally illegal) that have no clinical utility, but which are used to satisfy lifestyle requirements[b]	MDMA, 'ecstasy'	None (at present)	'Recreational' usage	49
	Tobacco (nicotine)	Nicotine preparations for tobacco addiction (e.g. patches etc.)	'Recreational' usage	50
	Cocaine (some formulations)	Local anaesthesia (now largely obsolete)	'Recreational' usage	44
	NSPs (novel psychoactive substances)	None	'Recreational' usage	50

[a]Obviously only in men.
[b]In addition, there are countless herbal preparations and other natural products, largely unregulated, which are marketed as health-promoting, life-enhancing and beneficial for many disorders, despite lack of rigorous evidence of therapeutic efficacy. Examples include numerous vitamin preparations, fish oils, melatonin, ginseng, *Echinacea*, *Ginkgo* and much besides.
ADHD, Attention deficit hyperactivity disorder; *MDMA*, methylenedioxy-methamphetamine ('ecstasy').
From Flower, 2004, after Gilbert et al., 2000, and Young, 2003.

Aside from those mentioned in Table 59.1, many widely used lifestyle 'drugs' or 'sports supplements' consist of natural products (e.g. *Ginkgo* extracts, melatonin, St John's wort, *Cinchona* extracts), the manufacture and sale of which have historically not been regulated.[1] Their composition is therefore highly variable, and their efficacy and safety generally untested. Many are 'spiked' with synthetic pharmacologically active drugs giving an illusion of efficacy (Rocha et al., 2016), or contain naturally occurring biologically active substances which, like synthetic drugs, can produce harmful as well as beneficial effects.

[1]Happily, this has now changed. Since 2014, the United Kingdom Medicines and Healthcare Products Regulatory Agency has a *Herbal Medicines Advisory Committee* designed to fulfil this demanding role. Many such compounds elude this regulation by implying some health benefit while avoiding any specific medical claims.

Because of the breadth of the lifestyle drug debate, we will consider only three particular topics in this chapter: cognitive enhancers, lifestyle drugs and sex and drugs in sport.

COGNITIVE ENHANCERS

At the time of writing, the lifestyle use of cognitive enhancers – *nootropic agents* – has become a topical (and divisive) issue much aired in the popular press.[2] Whilst the clinical use of drugs that improve cognitive defects in clinical conditions such as *attention deficit hyperactivity disorder* (ADHD), dementia, schizophrenia and depression is

[2]See 'Smart drugs "as common as coffee": media hype about neuroenhancement' (Partridge et al., 2011).

well established (see Chs 40 and 47–49), what has provoked controversy has been their use (mostly off-prescription) for improving intellectual performance or stamina in healthy people, particularly it appears, in academics and students (see d'Angelo et al., 2017).

The most common 'neuro-enhancers' (see also Ch. 49) used clinically include **modafinil**, **dextroamphetamine** (**Adderall**) and **methylphenidate**. Some anticholinergic agents such as **donepezil**, which are used to retard the mental decline associated with Alzheimer's disease, have also been also tested as cognitive enhancers. While their clinical actions are not disputed, evidence of their presumed activity on *healthy* people is often far from clear; as Sahakian's group put it '*...it may be that expectations of the effectiveness of these drugs exceed their actual effects*' (d'Angelo et al., 2017) although better and more effective drugs may well be forthcoming in the future. There are several reasons for this apparent disconnect, including the diversity of tests used to assess cognitive functioning by different groups, the ability of these drugs to produce effects on several neurotransmitter systems simultaneously as well as the fact that some of these drugs have bell-shaped dose–response curves, with larger doses producing reduced, rather than enhanced, scores. Another problem is the 'baseline effect'. While some cognitive enhancers such as **Adderall** and **methylphenidate** increase aspects of cognitive function when this is below par because of say, lack of sleep or jet lag, they have much less effect on 'normal' functioning. Of those drugs already mentioned, **modafinil** seems to produce consistent enhancement of cognitive indices effects in normal healthy, non-sleep-deprived, subjects. **Donepezil** has been reported in studies on pilots to improve training performance and ability to cope with emergencies but, in terms of other measures of effectiveness, seems once again to be more effective in sleep-deprived subjects than in rested subjects.

Notwithstanding some reservations about their real effects in normal people, the potential cognitive enhancers have been enthusiastically adopted by those faced with tasks requiring mental rather than physical application because of their potential benefits of. The scale of their use is striking. According to Sahakian's group (d'Angelo et al., 2017; Mohamed and Sahakian, 2012; Sahakian and Morein-Zamir, 2007), there has been a steep increase in this type of usage particularly among academic communities. In the United States, 16% of college students reported having illicitly obtained new prescription stimulants and, in the United Kingdom, a survey showed that 10% of students in 2009 were taking prescription drugs for cognitive enhancement, with 10%–20% of students at Oxford and Cambridge admitting to using them (cited in Teodorini et al., 2020). In 2008, the journal *Nature* conducted a poll (Maher, 2008) to gauge the usage of these drugs by healthy academics and some of the results were surprising. Responses from 1400 scientists from 60 countries revealed that about 20% used drugs for cognitive enhancement and approximately one-third of respondents had obtained these from internet sites where little, if any, medical assessment would have been made prior to supplying the drug.

The military too has long employed stimulants and cognitive enhancers to increase stamina, and to reduce the requirement for sleep among troops, and in military aviation, use of these substances to facilitate a pilot's concentration during long sorties is common (Tracey and Flower, 2014).

The apparent scale of student usage has led many to call for tighter rules to ensure that some students do not gain an unfair advantage in exams[3] although, as Sahakian has argued, it is difficult to know where to draw the line on such prohibitions. Presumably no one would complain if students took double espressos before an exam? And yet **caffeine** is a very effective stimulant in its own right being, perhaps equal too if not superior to many other 'enhancers' and only overlooked only because of its familiarity. So what is the difference?

DRUGS AND SEX

The use of lifestyle drugs to reduce inhibitions or increase the desire for, or the experience of, sex has become known as *pharmacosex*. The concept of 'aphrodisiac' drugs (usually in the form of plant extracts) is as old as history. A myriad of foods and natural products have been claimed to increase sexual desire (the original definition of an 'aphrodisiac') although there are actually very few agents with well-validated libidinous effects. In fact, drugs which actually enhance libido, as opposed to loosening inhibition (such as alcohol), are few, with **testosterone** being the obvious exception (in both sexes), although an aphrodisiac effect may be an incidental outcome of some drugs when used therapeutically: for example, **pramipexole**, a dopamine receptor agonist, is sometimes used to counteract the decrease in libido induced by serotonin-selective reuptake inhibitor (SSRI) antidepressant drugs. In a similar way, the antidepressant **fibanserin** (a 5-$HT_{1A/2A}$ agonist) has found a secondary utility in treating hypoactive sexual desire in premenopausal women.

The range of drugs which impact in some way or other upon the sexual experience is huge (see Table 59.2). A review of the experiences of people of many sexual orientations by Moyle et al. (2020) reports the use of many agents including **methylenedioxy-methamphetamine** (**MDMA)** ('ecstasy), **cocaine** and **GHB** (g-hydroxybutyrate) to intensify the experience of sex and in some cases produce an 'empathic effect' on their consumers, leading to feelings of greater intimacy and 'connectedness' (regrettably, usually only temporary). Often, such drugs are used in combinations ('polydrug' use) and there is some evidence that those who use such drugs in this way may be more likely to explore 'non-traditional' sexual behaviour (McCormack et al., 2021). However, it is sometimes difficult to disentangle the effects of agents which lower the inhibitory barriers to intimacy from those producing a genuine aphrodisiac effect.

Most other drugs in Table 59.2 would probably be more correctly termed 'sexual accessories' or 'enhancers', either promoting the ability to perform sex (e.g. **sildenafil** and other PDE5 inhibitors) or prolonging (e.g. **benzocaine**) or increasing (e.g. **MDMA**) the pleasure obtained from sexual activity.[4] The remainder are mainly drugs used to prevent negative consequences of sex such as unwanted pregnancies and HIV infection.

---

[3]'*"Exam boost" drugs that are said to improve cognitive ability are on sale to students for just £2, report shows.*' Mail Online, 8 April 2022.

[4]We have not included the numerous proprietary preparations such as 'vaginal-tightening creams' with names such as '*Forever Virgin*' and '*Virgin Again*', which promise rather alarming increases in vaginal grip strength.

Table 59.2 Drugs and sex

Type	Drug	Action	Notes
'Aphrodisiacs'	Testosterone (Ch. 35)	Stimulates desire, sexual development and function	Maintains and promotes sexual desire in both sexes
	Dopaminergic agents, e.g. pramipexole (Ch. 37)	Dopamine agonists	Dopamine is important in sexual desire and pleasure.
'Enhancers'	Amyl nitrite (Ch. 20)	Anal sphincter relaxation	'Poppers'; primarily used by gay men
	Benzocaine (Ch. 44)	Delays ejaculation	Contained in condoms for topical application to the penis
	Sildenafil and PDE5 inhibitors (Chs 19 and 35)	Maintain erection	To enhance male sexual function
	Flibanserin	Enhances female sexual pleasure	Used in premenopausal women to treat hypoactive sexual desire
Psychoactive drugs	Including methamphetamine (crystal meth), GHB, MDMA, cocaine and mephedrone (Ch. 50)	Said to intensify the sexual experience	Often taken in combination. May also relieve inhibitory restraints on intimacy and/or exert an empathogenic effect
Sexual medicine	Oestrogens and progestogens (Ch. 35)	Contraception	–
	Levonorgestrel (Ch. 35)	Postcoital contraception	The 'morning after' pill taken to avoid conception after unprotected sex
	Antiretroviral drugs (Ch. 53)	Pre- or post-exposure treatment for HIV infection	Used by gay men participating in unprotected sex

GHB, γ-Hydroxybutyrate; *MDMA*, methylenedioxy-methamphetamine ('ecstasy').

A subset of pharmacosexual practices is termed *chemsex*. This is usually applied to the use of drugs by gay men to increase the intensity and duration of sex, often with multiple partners, in sessions lasting several hours or days (see Moyle et al., 2020; McCall et al., 2015, for a fuller description). The drugs commonly taken include combinations of psychoactive drugs such as **mephedrone**, **γ-hydroxybutyrate** (GHB), and **methamphetamine** and **amyl nitrite**.

Lifestyle drugs

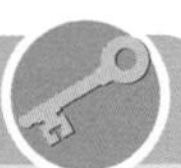

- More accurately called *lifestyle uses* for drugs, this is the term used to describe an unrelated group of drugs and medicines taken for non-medical reasons, including the illicit enhancement of athletic prowess in competitive sport.
- They include prescription drugs such as **sildenafil** and **methylphenidate**, substances such as **alcohol** and **caffeine**, drugs of abuse including other 'street' drugs and various nutritional preparations.
- Their use is linked to the concepts of 'self-diagnosis' and 'non-disease'.
- It is a growing sector of the pharmaceutical market.
- They are often brought to the consumer's attention through the internet or direct marketing.
- They form part of a larger debate on 'human enhancement'.

DRUGS IN SPORT

Although the use of drugs to enhance performance ('doping') in elite sporting competitions such as the Olympic Games is officially prohibited, it is evidently widespread. *The World Anti-Doping Agency* (WADA), which was established partly in response to some high-profile doping cases and drug-induced deaths among athletes, publishes an annually updated list of prohibited substances that may not be used by sportsmen or sportswomen either in or out of competition. This proscription is enforced by random and routine drug testing of an athlete's blood or urine using gas chromatography/mass spectrometry or immunoassay techniques. The testing protocols for such samples are strictly defined and must be performed by approved laboratories. Drug use by athletes for bona fide clinical reasons is allowed under the '*Therapeutic Use Exemptions*' scheme. According to this arrangement, which was introduced in the 1990s, an athlete may use a medicine (say, glucocorticoids for asthma) if it is determined clinically that this exemption is justified. Clearly, this system is open to abuse and has been so exploited on several occasions.

Infringements of the anti-doping regulations in professional sport are strictly punished but despite the threat of sanctions, there have been many instances where they have been flouted both by individual athletes and, in some cases, by entire teams. The American cyclist Lance Armstrong, for example, was a national hero. Having overcome testicular cancer, he went on to win the *Tour de France* on no less than seven occasions. For years, persistent accusations of drug abuse were strenuously denied but in January 2013, Armstrong finally admitted having used a cocktail of drugs to enhance his performance over the course of many years.[5] And it is not just individual athletes who have been caught out. An investigation into Russian athletics by WADA in 2016 concluded that a large-scale state-sponsored doping programme was routinely operating to conceal drug use by their athletes. This led to a ban on Russian participation in the subsequent Summer Olympics and other events although whether this had the desired salutary effect is debatable: at the 2022 Beijing Winter Olympics, the 15-year-old Russian skater, Kamila Valieva, already considered one of the top athletes in the sport, was found to have taken **trimetazidine,** a metabolic modulator used to improve coronary blood flow (and banned by WADA). According to a statement from the International Testing Agency she was provisionally suspended pending a further investigation. Shameful episodes such as these have prompted more than one commentator to despair of the 'charade of drug-free sport' (Sparling, 2013) with many believing that professional sport has been permanently damaged. Sadly, the practice is increasingly being extended to amateur and recreational sport also.

While athletes are easily persuaded of the potential of a wide variety of drugs to increase their chances of winning, controlled trials of such claims are difficult. In many cases these agents probably produce little or no effect, although of course, marginal improvements in performance (often 1% or less), which are difficult to measure experimentally, may make the difference between winning and losing, and the competitive instincts of athletes and their trainers generally carry more weight than scientific evidence.

Table 59.3 summarises the main classes of drugs used in sport, most of which are banned by WADA. A brief account of some of the more important drugs in common use follows. For a broader and more complete coverage, see La Gerche and Brosnan (2017), Reardon and Creado (2014) and Mottram (2005). Gould (2013) has reviewed the potential use of gene therapy in promoting athletic performance: another potential nightmare for the regulators!

ANABOLIC STEROIDS AND RELATED COMPOUNDS

Anabolic steroids (Ch. 35) include a large group of compounds with testosterone-like effects and include about 50 named compounds on the prohibited list. Together they constitute over half the number of 'doping' cases detected. They are often used in combination with **erythropoietin (EPO)** or other drugs to enhance performance in both endurance and strength events.

When given in combination with training and high protein intake, anabolic steroids undoubtedly reduce body fat, increase muscle mass and strength but probably not other parameters of sporting performance. They also have serious long-term effects, including male infertility, female masculinisation, liver and kidney tumours, hypertension, increased cardiovascular risk and (in adolescents) premature skeletal maturation causing irreversible cessation of growth. Anabolic steroids produce a feeling of physical well-being, increased competitiveness and aggressiveness, sometimes progressing to actual psychosis. Depression is common when the drugs are stopped and sometimes leads to long-term psychiatric problems. Mortality is increased among habitual users, with cardiac abnormalities being the principal cause of death. In attempt to circumvent the testing protocols, other drugs that release androgens (e.g. **human chorionic gonadotrophin; hCG**) or which modify their action, such as androgen receptor modulators, are increasingly used.

In addition to endogenous steroids, synthetic compounds such as **stanozolol** and **nandrolone** are also used and novel chemical derivatives ('designer steroids'), such as **tetrahydrogestrinone** (THG), are regularly developed and offered illicitly to athletes, posing a continuing problem to the authorities charged with detecting and identifying them. Since some are endogenous compounds (or their metabolites), their concentration can vary dramatically for physiological reasons, so results significantly above normal range are required to confirm illicit usage. Fortunately, isotope ratio techniques, based on the fact that endogenous and exogenous steroids have a slightly different ^{12}C:^{13}C composition, now enable the two to be distinguished analytically. Since anabolic steroids produce long-term effects and are normally used throughout training, rather than during the event itself, out-of-competition testing is essential.

Clenbuterol is a β-adrenoceptor agonist. Through an unknown mechanism of action, it produces anabolic effects similar to those of androgenic steroids, with apparently fewer adverse effects. It can be detected in urine and its use in sport is banned.

The use of **human growth hormone** (**hGH**) by athletes followed the availability of the recombinant form of the hormone, used clinically to treat endocrine disorders. It is given by injection and its effects appear to be similar to those of anabolic steroids. **hGH** is also reported to produce a similar feeling of well-being, although without the accompanying aggression and changes in sexual development and behaviour. It increases lean body mass, reduces fat and improves sprint capacity, but its effects on other aspects of athletic performance are unclear. It is claimed to increase the rate of recovery from tissue injury, allowing more intensive training routines. The main adverse effect of **hGH** is the development of acromegaly, causing overgrowth of the jaw and thickening of the fingers, but it may also lead to cardiac hypertrophy and cardiomyopathy, and possibly also an increased cancer risk.

Detection of **hGH** administration is difficult because physiological secretion is pulsatile, so normal plasma concentrations vary widely. The plasma half-life is short (20–30 min), and only trace amounts are excreted in urine. However, physiological **hGH** consists of three isoforms varying in molecular weight, whereas recombinant **hGH** contains only one, so measuring the relative amounts of the isoforms can be used to detect the exogenous material. Growth hormone acts partly by releasing insulin-like growth factor (**IGF-1**) from the liver, and this hormone itself is sometimes used by athletes. It also increases lean body mass, reduces fat and may accelerate recovery from tissue injury but also may cause cardiac hypertrophy, acromegaly, liver damage and increase cancer risk

[5]Among these were EPO, testosterone, diuretics, glucocorticoids and human growth hormone. He also used 'blood doping' techniques and presented fake documents to support his claims that he was 'drug free'.

Table 59.3 Some examples of drugs used in sport

Drug class	Example(s)	Effects	Chapter
Anabolic 'steroids'	Androgenic steroids (e.g. testosterone and nandrolone) and androgen receptor modulators	Increased muscle development, aggression and competitiveness; reduction in fat. Serious long-term side effects	35
	Clenbuterol	Combined anabolic and β_2 adrenoceptor agonist; may increase muscle strength	15
Hormones and related substances	Erythropoietin (also synthetic agonists)	Increased erythrocyte formation and oxygen transport. Increased blood viscosity causes hypertension and risk of strokes and coronary attacks. Often taken in combination with iron supplements. Used mainly in endurance sports[a]	24
	Human growth hormone, insulin-like growth factor-1	Increased lean body mass and reduced fat. May accelerate recovery from tissue injury. Causes cardiac hypertrophy, acromegaly, liver damage and increased cancer risk	33
	Insulin	Sometimes used (with glucose so as to avoid hypoglycaemia) to promote glucose uptake and energy production in muscle. Probably ineffective in improving performance	31
	Thyroxine	Increase in energy production	34
	Glucocorticoids	Multiple metabolic and anti-inflammatory effects which reduce physiological stress and injury	25, 33
Cardiovascular drugs	β_2-Adrenoceptor agonists (e.g. salbutamol)	Used by runners, cyclists, swimmers, etc. to increase oxygen uptake (by bronchodilatation) and increased cardiac function. Controlled studies show no improvement in performance.	15
	β-Adrenoceptor antagonists; (e.g. propranolol)	Used to reduce tremor and anxiety in 'precision' sports (e.g. shooting, archery, gymnastics, diving)	15
CNS 'stimulants'	Ephedrine and derivatives; amphetamines, cocaine, caffeine.	Trials have shown a slight increase in muscle strength and performance in non-endurance events (sprint, swimming, field events, etc.).	49
Narcotic analgesics and NSAIDs	Codeine, morphine, ibuprofen, etc.	Used to mask injury-associated pain	25, 42
Diuretics	Thiazides, furosemide	Used mainly to achieve rapid weight loss before 'weighing in'. Also used to 'mask' the presence of other agents in urine by dilution	29
'Masking agents'	Epitestosterone	Masks the administration of testosterone by altering the ratio between the hormone and its metabolite	35

[a]'Blood doping' (removal of 1–2 L of blood ahead of the competition, followed by re-transfusion immediately prior to the event) has a similar effect and is even more difficult to detect. Training at altitude or in a hypoxic environment achieves a similar effect and is not banned.
CNS, Central nervous system; *NSAIDs*, non-steroidal anti-inflammatory drugs.

DRUGS THAT INCREASE OXYGEN DELIVERY TO MUSCLES

EPO, which increases erythrocyte formation and oxygen transport, is given by injection for days or weeks prior to the competition to increase the erythrocyte count and hence boost the O_2-carrying capacity of blood. It is undoubtedly highly effective and is used extensively in endurance sports. The development of recombinant **EPO** has made it widely available and difficult to detect. Since **EPO** increases blood viscosity, it can cause hypertension and increase the risk of strokes and coronary attacks and neurologic disease. A doubling of the **EPO** plasma concentration is reported to increase heart failure by 25% over the following decade (cited in La Gerche and Brosnan, 2017). The administration of synthetic **EPO** agonists mimics the action of the native hormone itself and represents an alternate way to achieve the desired effect.

Another related way of increasing oxygen delivery to the muscle is by shifting the oxyhaemoglobin dissociation curve to the right which increases oxygen off-loading from blood to the tissues. The synthetic compound **efaproxiral** is said to improve tissue oxygenation in this way although there is little evidence that this happens in humans. Nevertheless, it is banned by WADA as a 'prohibited method' for enhancing performance. A further agent with similar effects is cobalt. Soluble cobalt salts such as cobalt chloride, probably acting through the hypoxia signalling mechanisms, stimulates erythropoiesis and angiogenesis producing a qualitatively similar effect to **EPO** and **efaproxiral**.

Insulin is sometimes used (with glucose so as to avoid hypoglycaemia) to promote glucose uptake and energy production in muscle but it is probably ineffective in improving athletic performance.

CARDIOVASCULAR DRUGS

β_2-Adrenoceptor agonists (e.g. **salbutamol**) have been used by runners, cyclists, swimmers, etc., to increase oxygen uptake (by bronchodilatation) and increase cardiac function, although controlled studies have shown little or no increase in performance. β-Adrenoceptor antagonists (e.g. **propranolol**) are taken by competitors to reduce tremor and anxiety in 'precision' sports (e.g. darts, snooker, shooting, gymnastics, diving) as does small amounts of alcohol. They are not explicitly banned in many sports because they may actually impair performance. **Sildenafil** is reportedly taken by athletes on the presumption that it will increase pulmonary blood flow yielding a concomitant increase in cardiac performance with less right ventricular load, although this has not been rigorously confirmed, at least in normoxic conditions.

COGNITIVE ENHANCERS AND STIMULANT DRUGS

Drugs of this type are used by athletes to improve focus and concentration (Smith et al., 2020) with some athletes apparently justifying their use on the basis of their alleged ADHD or other cognitive disorder. The apparent benefits include an increased ability to prepare mentally for forthcoming events, superior recall of important details of competitor strategies or of an opponent's team's strengths and weaknesses. Precision sports such as archery and shooting may particularly benefit from such drugs as well as those 'sports' which impose a substantial cognitive burden on the player (e.g. chess). The most commonly used are **methylephedrine**; various amphetamines and related compounds such as **modafinil** and **methylphenidate**; **cocaine**; and a variety of other central nervous system stimulants such as **nikethamide**, **amiphenazole** (no longer used clinically) and **strychnine**. **Caffeine** is also used: some commercially available 'energy drinks' contain **taurine** as well as **caffeine**. However, **taurine** is an agonist at glycine and extrasynaptic $GABA_A$ receptors. Its effects on the brain are therefore likely to be inhibitory rather than stimulatory. In this regard, **taurine** may be responsible for the post-energy-drink low that is experienced once the stimulatory effect of **caffeine** has worn off.

The psychological effect of stimulants is probably as important as their physiological effects. Rather surprisingly, and in contrast to anabolic steroids, some trials have shown stimulant drugs such as **ephedrine** improve performance in events such as sprinting, and under experimental conditions they increase muscle strength and reduce muscle fatigue significantly. Surprisingly, **caffeine** also appears to be more consistently effective in improving muscle performance than other more powerful stimulants and is among a few drugs (including **nicotine** and **alcohol**) that are not prohibited.

Regrettably, several deaths have occurred among athletes taking amphetamines and **ephedrine**-like drugs in endurance events. The main causes are coronary insufficiency, associated with hypertension; hyperthermia, associated with cutaneous vasoconstriction; and dehydration. The cyclist Tommy Simpson collapsed and died during the 1967 *Tour de France* as he attempted to ascend Mont Ventoux[6]. Amphetamines and alcohol were found in his blood stream.

Drugs in sport

- Drugs of many different types are used by athletes with to improve performance in competition.
- The main types used are:
  - anabolic agents, usually androgenic steroids and **clenbuterol**;
  - hormones, particularly **erythropoietin** and **human growth hormone**;
  - stimulants, mainly **amphetamine, ephedrine** derivatives and **caffeine**;
  - β-adrenoceptor antagonists, which reduce anxiety and tremor in 'precision' sports.
- The use of drugs in sport is officially prohibited – in most cases, in or out of competition.
- Detection depends mainly on analysis of the drug or its metabolites in urine or blood samples. Detection of abuse is difficult in the case of endogenous hormones such as **EPO**, **growth hormone** and **testosterone.**
- Controlled trials have shown that while some drugs (e.g. **EPO**) are extremely effective, many other drugs produce little improvement in sporting performance. Anabolic agents increase body weight and muscle volume but without clearly increasing strength. The effect of stimulants is often psychological rather than physiological.

REGULATORY, SOCIETAL AND ETHICAL ISSUES

Few aspects of the human enhancement/lifestyle drug debate have attracted more moral opprobrium than the use of drugs in sport. Doping is banned in professional sports because it is deemed to constitute an unfair advantage for the athletes who 'cheat' over those who don't. Many feel that it undermines the very purpose of sport which should surely be to encourage a sense of 'fair play', to inspire others to achieve physical excellence with (hopefully) a concomitant benefit to public health and wellbeing. Such critics feel that the very notion of professional sports has already been irrevocably tarnished and has become in reality, a competition not of athletic prowess, but rather the pharmaceutical ingenuity of their team physicians.

However, many factors are important in determining why one athlete may have an advantage over another – genetic makeup, for example – so one could argue that

[6]A memorial erected at the spot has become something of a site of pilgrimage for competitive cyclists.

there is no real 'level playing field' to begin with. Indeed, one school of thought argues that athletes should have unrestricted access to performance-enhancing drugs with the proviso that they do not impair the athlete's health (see Savulescu et al., 2004), although this view seems unlikely to gain public acceptance in the near future.

The financial and reputational inducements for athletes to take performance-enhancing drugs are great while the chance of getting caught is quite small, fuelling the search for better and less detectable agents. There are even reports that athletes have been used to test novel or experimental enhancers without the usual health and safety regulatory checks and balances. This in turn poses further analytical problems for the regulators who must devise screening tests to monitor an increasing range of agents, some of which are difficult to assay. The contest continues as new 'designer' drugs, *masking agents* (which make it more difficult to detect a particular substance in the blood or urine) or other procedures are devised by ingenious chemists and physicians to foil drug testing protocols.

While it easy to take sides in the polarised intellectual debate about lifestyle drugs and their use, some authors (see Chatterjee, 2004) have personalised the ethical quandaries by inviting us to answer some challenging questions about our own likely behaviour. Would you, for example, take cognitive enhancers yourself if it meant that you could accomplish a difficult task such as finishing your thesis on time, learn a language more rapidly or master a musical instrument? Would you give them to your child ahead of an exam if the other students in their class were known to be taking them? Since **donepezil** has been shown to speed reaction times of pilots in an aviation emergency, would you choose an airline which specified that its staff had received the drug?

Peer pressure and personal expediency, rather than bioethics, is likely to be a major determinant of your decision in many cases because ultimately one does not want to be disadvantaged when compared to one's colleagues.

CONCLUSION

The lifestyle drug phenomenon is one aspect of a broader debate about what actually constitutes 'disease', where the boundaries actually lie between therapy and enhancement and how far medical science and already overstretched healthcare systems should go to satisfy these aims.

Citizens of the affluent developed world are the principal consumers of lifestyle drugs, and the pharmaceutical industry is therefore incentivised to cater for this lucrative market, maybe even relying upon them to provide valuable income that can be diverted to other less profitable lines of research and development.

Despite the advantages that they can undoubtedly bring to their users, there are several reasons why lifestyle drugs – no matter how we choose to define them – are of concern to us as pharmacologists. Medicines have traditionally been developed to combat disease and the question of how one should search for, test or regulate, drugs designed to produce effects in healthy people suffering only 'non-diseases' has yet to be settled. The increasing availability of drugs (some counterfeit) from 'e-pharmacies', coupled with the lobbying power of patients, creates demands for these drugs, regardless of their potential costs or proven utility. This inevitably causes problems for physicians, drug regulators and ultimately those who set healthcare priorities for state-funded systems of social medicine.

Discussion of these complex issues is beyond the scope of this book but can be found in articles cited at the end of this chapter (e.g. Buchanan, 2011; Flower, 2004, 2012). The debate about the ethics and management of lifestyle drugs will undoubtedly run for a long time to come.

REFERENCES AND FURTHER READING

d'Angelo, L.C., Savulich, G., Sahakian, B.J., 2017. Lifestyle use of drugs by healthy people for enhancing cognition, creativity, motivation and pleasure. Br. J. Pharmacol. 174, 3257–3267.

Buchanan, A., 2011. Better than Human. The Promise and Perils of Enhancing Ourselves. Oxford University Press Inc., New York, p. 199.

Chatterjee, A., 2004. Cosmetic neurology: the controversy over enhancing movement, mentation, and mood. Neurology 63, 968–974.

Flower, R., 2012. The Osler Lecture 2012: pharmacology 2.0, medicines, drugs and human enhancement. QJM 105, 823–830.

Flower, R.J., 2004. Lifestyle drugs: pharmacology and the social agenda. Trends Pharmacol. Sci. 25, 182–185.

Gilbert, D., Walley, T., New, B., 2000. Lifestyle medicines. BMJ 321, 1341–1344.

Gould, D., 2013. Gene doping: gene delivery for olympic victory. Br. J. Clin. Pharmacol. 76, 292–298.

Hofmann, B., 2017. Limits to human enhancement: nature, disease, therapy or betterment? BMC Med. Ethics 18, 56.

La Gerche, A., Brosnan, M.J., 2017. Cardiovascular effects of performance-enhancing drugs. Circulation 135, 8999.

Maher, B., 2008. Poll results: look who's doping. Nature 452, 674–675.

McCall, H., Adams, N., Mason, D., Willis, J., 2015. What is chemsex and why does it matter? BMJ 351, h5790.

McCormack, M., Measham, F., Wignall, L., 2021. The normalization of leisure sex and reacreational drugs: exploring associations between polydrug use and sexual practices by English festival-goers. Contemp. Drug Probl. 48, 185–200.

Mohamed, A.D., Sahakian, B.J., 2012. The ethics of elective psychopharmacology. Int. J. Neuropsychopharmacol. 15, 559–571.

Mottram, D.R. (Ed.), 2005. Drugs in Sport, fourth ed. Routledge, London.

Moyle, L., Dymock, A., Aldridge, A., Mechen, B., 2020. Pharmacosex: reimagining sex, drugs and enhancement. Int. J. Drug Policy 86, 102943.

Partridge, B.J., Bell, S.K., Lucke, J.C., Yeates, S., Hall, W.D., 2011. Smart drugs "as common as coffee": media hype about neuroenhancement. PLoS One 6, e28416.

Reardon, C.L., Creado, S., 2014. Drug abuse in athletes. Subst. Abuse Rehabil. 5, 95–105.

Rocha, T., Amaral, J.S., Oliveira, M., 2016. Adulteration of dietary supplements by the illegal addition of synthetic drugs: a review. Compr. Rev. Food Sci. Food Saf. 15, 43–62.

Sahakian, B., Morein-Zamir, S., 2007. Professor's little helper. Nature 450, 1157–1159.

Savulescu, J., Foddy, B., Clayton, M., 2004. Why we should allow performance enhancing drugs in sport. Br. J. Sports Med. 38, 666–670.

Smith, A.C.T., Stavros, C., Westberg, K., 2020. Cognitive enhancing drugs in sport: current and future concerns. Subst. Use Misuse 55, 2064–2075.

Smith, R., 2002. In search of "non-disease". BMJ 324, 883–885.

Sparling, P.B., 2013. The Lance Armstrong saga: a wake-up call for drug reform in sports. Curr. Sports Med. Rep. 12, 53–54.

Teodorini, R.D., Rycroft, N., Smith-Spark, J.H., 2020. The off-prescription use of modafinil: an online survey of perceived risks and benefits. PLoS One 15, e0227818.

Tracey, I., Flower, R., 2014. The warrior in the machine: neuroscience goes to war. Nat. Rev. Neurosci. 15, 825–834.

Walley, T., 2002. Lifestyle medicines and the elderly. Drugs Aging 19, 163–168.

Young, S.N., 2003. Lifestyle drugs, mood, behaviour and cognition. J. Psychiatry Neurosci. 28, 87–89.

60 Drug discovery and development

OVERVIEW

With the emergence of the pharmaceutical industry towards the end of the 19th century, drug discovery became a highly focused and managed process and moved from the domain of inventive doctors to that of scientists hired for the purpose. The bulk of modern therapeutics, and of modern pharmacology, is based on drugs that originated from the laboratories of these pharmaceutical companies, without which neither the practice of therapeutics nor the science of pharmacology would be more than a pale fragment of what they have become.

In this chapter, we outline the main stages of the process, namely (1) the discovery phase, i.e. the identification of a new chemical entity as a potential therapeutic agent; and (2) the development phase, during which the compound is tested for safety and efficacy in one or more clinical indications, and suitable formulations and dosage forms devised. The aim is to achieve registration by one or more regulatory authorities, to allow the drug to be marketed legally as a medicine for human use. We also briefly mention some of the other routes to licensing which a new medicine can take, including repurposing, where a drug with an established preclinical and often a clinical development portfolio is trialled for a different indication. The rapidly initiated clinical trials and subsequent approval of new treatments for COVID-19 are excellent examples of this approach.

Our account is necessarily brief, and there are many detailed textbooks and review articles dedicated to this topic (for example Hill and Richards, 2021).

DRUG DISCOVERY: BACKGROUND

Diethyl ether ('sweet oil of vitriol') was synthesised in 1540 but not administered as an anaesthetic until 1846, while **morphine** was purified from poppy extract in 1806 and shown to be the active principle of opium. The impact of these seminal drug discoveries can be seen today, notably that chemistry is necessary but not sufficient – pharmacology is necessarily interdisciplinary – and that natural products remain potentially fertile starting points. Creating effective safe new drugs is difficult and expensive, and in this background section we briefly overview the relative importance of *serendipity* (exemplified by Fleming's culture plate on which the penicillium spores alighted) versus *rational drug design* – the design of new chemical entities predicted to have particular biological effects on the basis of the chemical structures of drugs and their targets. Currently both approaches remain highly productive.

Historically, chemists modified the structures of pharmacologically active drugs derived from plants or synthesised in the dye-stuffs industry and many 20th century drug discoveries stemmed from chemical modification of lead compounds. These approaches soon progressed to a more rational strategy based on the understanding of basic biochemical and physiological processes. Each of these discoveries required functional assays for their recognition driving the development of new technologies including, most recently, sophisticated in silico and even the introduction of methods incorporating artificial intelligence (AI).

George Hitchings and Gertrude Elion were among the first to design drugs directed at specific biochemical targets, which can be regarded as the forefather of structure-based drug discovery. They collaborated in the biochemistry laboratory of Burroughs Wellcome, and focused on the folic acid pathway which is key for the action of the sulfonamides and in particular on dihydrofolate reductase (see Ch. 52). They synthesised a series of purine and pyrimidine 'antimetabolites' with selectivity for different forms (mammalian, bacterial, protozoal) of the enzyme. Drugs that emerged from their program include the antibacterial **trimethoprim** (see Ch. 52), the antimalarial **pyrimethamine** (see Ch. 55), the antineoplasic **6-mercaptopurine** (see Ch. 57) and its prodrug the immunosuppressant **azathioprine** (see Ch. 25); spin-offs included **allopurinol** (xanthine oxidase inhibitor used to prevent gout – see Ch. 25 – and the urate-related complications of tumour lysis – see Ch. 57), **aciclovir** (one of the first antiviral drugs – see Ch. 53) and **zidovudine** (the first therapeutic reverse transcriptase inhibitor, still used in combination treatment for HIV – see Ch. 53). As with James Black's receptor-targeted drugs (β-adrenoceptor antagonists and H_2 antagonists among others) these outstanding discoveries were made using synthetic schemes where each step results in a single product, and capitalised on the interdisciplinary nature of pharmacology with collaborations between chemists, pharmacologists and physicians.

Meanwhile, *combinatorial chemistry* (see later) where large numbers (tens to millions) of compounds are prepared as product libraries was conceived and developed together with methods to deconvolute the compound libraries and extract those products with the desired properties from the complex mixtures of end-products. These methods were developed in parallel with sequencing of the human genome, which has enabled rapid cloning and synthesis of large quantities of purified proteins, and of determining the three-dimensional structures of many potential drug–target protein complexes. Much of modern drug discovery involves selection of a potential target protein such as a receptor for a neurotransmitter or an enzyme in a key pathophysiological pathway, followed by high-throughput screening to establish 'hit' molecules for testing on cells or tissues (see later). The evolution of in silico methods enabling detailed modelling of drug docking as well as cryogenic electron microscopy (cryo-EM) and crystal structures and the use of AI all support the identification of candidate molecules.

Despite the opportunities presented by advances in combinatorial chemistry, interest remains in drugs derived from natural products which have evolved over millennia. These exhibit much greater chemical diversity, particularly as regards numbers of chiral centres and drug structure rigidity, both of which are higher in natural products than in conventional combinatorial libraries. The discovery and development of organocatalysis, which has made it much easier to synthesise asymmetric molecules for use as starting blocks, may help to correct this (see, for example, the Nobel lectures from 2021 when the prize in chemistry was awarded for the discovery of organocatalysis – https://www.youtube.com/watch?v=IW4zgOHhefc). It has also led to resurgent interest in the search for natural products ('bioprospecting') and in semisynthetic derivatives of natural products.

Advances in the structural biology of different states of drug-bound receptor proteins, including proteins which reside naturally in a membrane environment (see later and Ch. 3), are such that it may be possible for mere mortals (lacking the chemical imaginations of Gertrude Elion or James Black) to predict with precision drug structures that will influence receptor structure in a desired manner. The number of potential organic molecules is astronomical and virtual libraries of billions of actual or make-on-demand compounds have been developed, together with 'less is more' strategies as explained later in more detail.

In the special case of RNA drugs, a 'precise prediction' structure-based drug discovery paradigm has already been achieved (see Ch. 5). This is thanks both to understanding how RNA codes protein synthesis (such as spike protein antigen for SARS-CoV-2 vaccines, see Ch. 53) and to the discovery of RNA silencing by short double-stranded sequences of interfering RNA (siRNA). If a particular protein is critical for the progression of a disease, suppressing its expression needs only a short and predictable sequence of double-stranded RNA to silence its expression. However, to work in vivo such RNA-silencing drugs must be delivered intracellularly to the cytoplasm of the cells where the specific protein target is translated. For example, this has been achieved for siRNA acting in liver hepatocytes by chemically modifying the ribose ring to increase stability and conjugating the modified RNA with tris-*N*-acetylgalactosamine (GalNAc). GalNAc is recognised by asialoglycoprotein (ASG) receptors in the sinusoidal membranes of hepatocytes, resulting in rapid binding to the ASG receptors and endocytosis of the drug complex into hepatocyte cytoplasm (see Springer and Dowdy, 2018, for a review). An example of such a drug in clinical use is **inclisiran** (see Ch. 22) which is given by subcutaneous injection twice a year, so is potentially suitable for administration in primary care. Other drugs utilising GalNAc delivery to the hepatocyte cytoplasm have been licensed, e.g. **givosiran** which, given subcutaneously once monthly, reduced the annual frequency of severe attacks of *acute hepatic porphyria* (see Ch. 12) by approximately 70%, and which is illustrated on our front cover.

Genomic epidemiology was the source of the idea that PSCK9 suppression would lower low-density lipoprotein (LDL) cholesterol safely, and other novel drugs for a multitude of unmet medical needs (both common and rare diseases) will be enabled if RNA drugs can be distributed into the relevant cell types (see Springer and Dowdy, 2018), potentially changing fundamentally the future practice of medicine.

THE STAGES OF A PROJECT

Fig. 60.1 shows in an idealised way the stages of a 'typical' project, aimed at producing a marketable drug that meets a particular medical need (e.g. to alleviate the symptoms of asthma, to retard the progression of cardiac failure or to treat an infection). It is important to note that the drug development process relies on a substantial body of fundamental research which occurs in both academia and industry and from which the new drug targets emerge and feed into the drug development process. A substantial amount of knowledge is now gained from the use of recombinant protein expression in cell lines. This has enabled high-throughput screens, mutagenesis studies and application of techniques such as cryo-EM to resolve receptor structures within their physiological membrane environment (see below), methods that are revolutionising drug discovery. Animal research plays an important role in both fundamental research and the drug development process but these technologies mean only the best candidates are progressed to in vivo studies. Fig 60.2 shows how animals are used in different areas of scientific research including the drug development process.

Broadly, the process can be divided into three main components designed to answer multiple specific questions:

1. *Drug discovery*, during which candidate molecules are chosen on the basis of their pharmacological properties.
2. *Preclinical development*, during which a wide range of non-human studies are carried out.
   a. Can pharmaceutical formulation be improved (optimisation may extend into clinical development)?
   b. What organs are most sensitive to its toxicity?
   c. Should specific safety tests (e.g. ophthalmic) be incorporated in future human studies?
   d. What is an appropriate first dose for human studies? Is the candidate effective in animal models of disease?
3. *Clinical development* (usually performed first in healthy – and then in patient – volunteers): Does the drug get to its site of action? Does it engage with its target? Does it cause the predicted desired biochemical and physiological effects? Is it tolerated (many plant-derived molecules are recognised as foreign and potentially poisonous in the chemoreceptor trigger zone in the brainstem and induce vomiting, see Ch. 30)? What dose regimens are appropriate for efficacy trials in patients? Does it work? Is it safe? These are deceptively simple questions that may have uncomfortable answers (e.g. positive inotrope drugs that improve symptoms of heart failure but reduce survival, see Ch. 20).

These phases do not necessarily follow in strict succession, as indicated in Fig. 60.1, but can overlap. The main factors influencing the timescales for drug development are financial (for a moderately successful

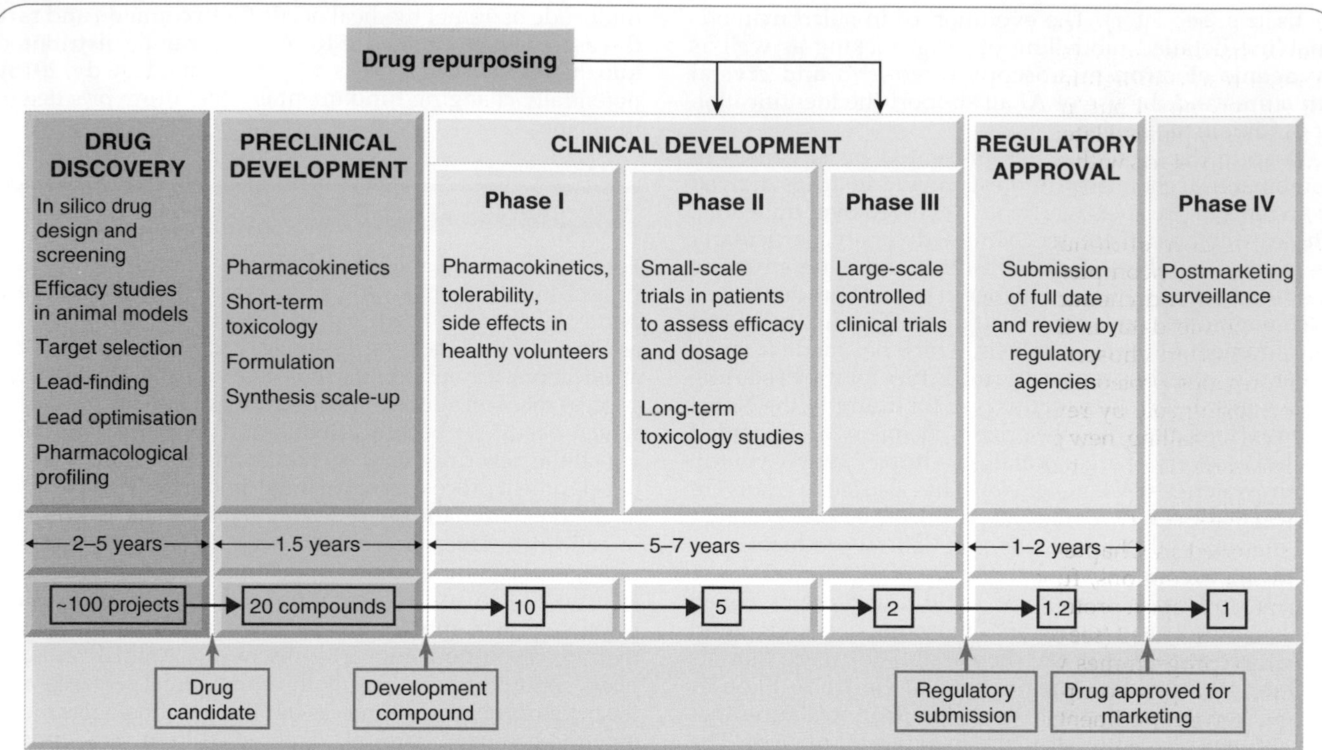

Fig. 60.1 The stages of development of a 'typical' new drug, i.e. a synthetic compound being developed for systemic use. Only the main activities undertaken at each stage are shown, and the details vary greatly according to the kind of drug being developed.

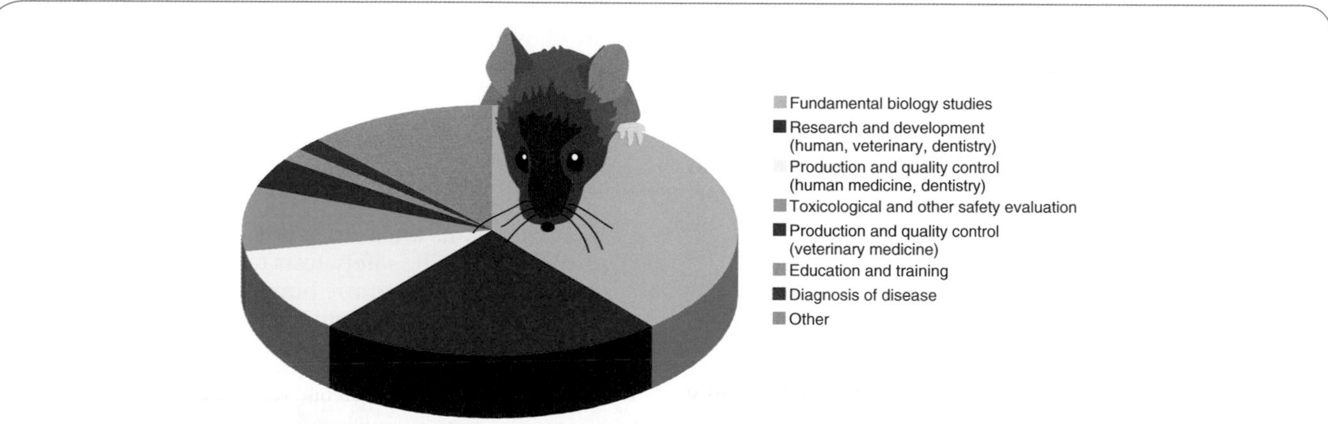

Fig. 60.2 Animal studies in the drug development process. The areas of the pie chart reflect the numbers of animals used annually in the UK in different components of the process from fundamental research supporting the identification of novel drug targets through to pharmacology and toxicology studies. Most of these studies involve rodent models. (Adapted from Dolgin, E., 2010. Nat. Med. 16, 1172.)

drug with sales of $40 million/year, each week's delay in development will cost the company roughly $8 million by reducing the competition-free sales window provided by patent protection) and balancing financial risks and so companies will often wait for each milestone and a risk re-evaluation before progressing to the next stage. As the drug development process progresses, costs increase disproportionately and so therefore does risk. As discussed later in this chapter, deviations from this 'standard' approach are not uncommon. For example, drug repurposing offers an alternative route to clinic. Costs, risk and the commercial interest associated with drug companies are usually necessary factors in the drug development process; however, alternative approaches such as the one set up by Cancer Research UK, the CRUK Centre for Drug Development, have enabled clinical evaluation of drugs and for indications which may not have progressed under a more typical commercial model.

THE DRUG DISCOVERY PHASE

Rational drug design (see earlier) is only feasible where there is strong fundamental biology and a clear hypothesis as seen for diseases such as diabetes mellitus (see Ch. 31). For many diseases, particularly those of the central nervous system, knowledge of the underlying pathology and pathophysiology (see Ch. 40) remains limited, and this can result in high failure rates. Many new drugs are not entirely novel but 'me-too' versions of drugs already in use.[1] As explained later, developing a new 'first-in-class' drug usually starts with identifying a new molecular target by following clues from a number of sources including serendipity, genomics and/or fundamental biology research. Conventional biological wisdom, drawing on a rich but incomplete fund of knowledge of disease mechanisms and chemical signalling pathways, coupled with genomic data, is the basis on which novel targets are most often chosen. Disciplines such as genomics, bioinformatics, proteomics and systems analysis are playing an increasing role by revealing new proteins involved in chemical signalling, new genes involved in disease and new models of disease progression.

TARGET SELECTION

As discussed in Chapter 2, drug targets are, with a few important exceptions, functional proteins (e.g. receptors, enzymes, transport proteins), but an increase in nucleic acid targets is anticipated (see earlier). Although, in the past, drug discovery programmes were often based – successfully – on measuring a complex response in vivo, such as prevention of experimentally induced seizures, lowering of blood sugar or suppression of an inflammatory response, without the need for prior identification of a molecular drug target, nowadays this is less common, and the first step is *target identification*. This most often comes from biological intelligence. It was known, for example, that inhibiting angiotensin-converting enzyme lowers blood pressure by suppressing angiotensin II formation, so it made sense to look for antagonists of the vascular angiotensin II receptor – hence the successful 'sartan' series of antihypertensive drugs (see Ch. 21). The success of biopharmaceuticals as treatments for a wide range of disorders from cancer to immune diseases builds from fundamental biology. However, for many disorders, particularly those involving the central nervous system, knowledge of the causal pathways remains poorly understood which, coupled with the complexity of the brain, has made rational drug design more challenging than in organs where the mechanism is better understood. Serendipity continues to play its part in the discovery of new treatments such as the example of severe infantile haemangioma (Ch. 15) which is now treated using propranolol after a baby with this tumour was treated with propranolol for coincident hypertrophic cardiomyopathy (HCM) leading to a large randomised controlled trial (RCT) which confirmed efficacy. A survey of 1194 FDA-approved human medicines (Santos et al., 2017) noted that they acted at a total of 893 targets, of which 667 were human proteins (comprising 549 small molecule and 146 biopharmaceutical drug targets) and a further 189 were pathogen protein targets. Based on knowledge derived from the human genome project, there are many thousands more potential drug targets for drug discovery awaiting therapeutic exploitation. Selecting *valid* and 'druggable' targets from this plethora is a major challenge.

LEAD FINDING

When the biochemical target has been decided and the feasibility of the project has been assessed, the next step is to find *lead compounds*. Here we focus on lead compounds derived from synthetic chemistry – see earlier in the chapter and Chapter 5 for biopharmaceutical leads from the biotech industry and academia. Commonly, lead finding involves cloning and expression of the human target protein. An assay system allowing the functional activity of the target protein to be measured is then used for high throughput screening. This could be a cell-free enzyme assay, a membrane-based binding assay or a cellular response assay and is engineered to run automatically, preferably with an optical read-out (e.g. fluorescence or optical absorbance), and in a miniaturised multiwell plate format (96-, 384-, 1536- or 3456-well versions are available) for reasons of speed and economy. Robotically controlled assay facilities capable of testing tens of thousands of compounds per day[2] in several parallel assays are now commonplace in the pharmaceutical industry and have become the standard starting point for most small molecule drug discovery projects. For details on high-throughput screening, see Ross and Bittker (2016).

To keep such hungry monsters running requires very large *compound libraries*. Large companies will typically maintain a growing collection of a million or more synthetic compounds, which will be routinely screened whenever a new assay is set up. Whereas, in the past, compounds were generally synthesised and purified one by one, often taking a week or more for each, the use of combinatorial chemistry allows large families of related compounds to be made simultaneously. By coupling such high-speed synthesis to high-throughput assay systems, the time taken over the initial lead-finding stage of projects has been reduced to a few months or less in most cases, having previously often taken several years.

In structure-based drug discovery use is made of X-ray crystallography and more recently of cryo-EM to provide knowledge of the three-dimensional structure of the target protein. This latter technique which evolved over decades was hailed in the press release for the 2017 Nobel Prize in chemistry, awarded to Jacques Dubochet, Joachim Frank and Richard Henderson, as having 'moved biochemistry into a new era'. It images vitrified biomolecules with associated water molecules, without the need for crystallisation so enabling study of transmembrane proteins and other difficult-to-crystallise complexes including intermediate and equilibrium states of ligand–protein complexes (Robertson et al., 2021). It has been embraced by big pharma and many academic laboratories and has already impacted structure-based drug design for G protein–coupled receptors (GPCRs), ion channels and solute carrier proteins (SLCs), as well as in vaccine development where it enables better antigen design. It is, however, still in its infancy compared with X-ray crystallography which currently

[1]Many commercially successful drugs have in the past emerged from exactly such 'me-too' projects; examples are the many β-adrenoceptor-blocking drugs developed in the wake of propranolol, the 'triptans' that followed the introduction of sumatriptan to treat migraine and selective serotonin reuptake inhibitors (SSRIs) for anxiety and depression. Quite small improvements (e.g. in pharmacokinetics or side effects), coupled with marketing, have often proved enough, but the barriers to registration are getting higher, so the emphasis has shifted towards developing innovative (first in class) drugs aimed at novel molecular targets.

[2]Testing up to 100,000 compounds per day is possible, and is known as ultra-high-throughput screening.

provides higher resolution where it is applicable (Lees at al., 2021). It thus seems likely that these two technologies will remain complementary for some time at least (Renaud et al., 2018).

Computer-based molecular modelling is used to identify possible lead structures within the compound library, in order to reduce the number of compounds to be screened. As mentioned earlier, molecular modelling can also be used to screen huge numbers of hypothetical – not yet synthesised – molecules to provide pointers for the synthesis and screening of new compound families. Refined in this way, screening can identify lead compounds that have the appropriate pharmacological activity and are amenable to further chemical modification. A recent method called V-SYNTH (virtual synthon hierarchical enumeration screening) has been described based on combining much smaller numbers (hundreds of thousands) of compound fragments ('synthons') with reliable known chemical reactions. This makes the synthesis of potential hits fast (4–6 weeks), reliable (>80% success) and affordable. The virtual library is screened by identifying the best scaffold–synthon combinations to initiate growth then iteratively elaborating such seeds. These can be used to build up molecules via progressive (cycle-by-cycle) additions of synthons to a growing scaffold with improved docking to the target at each cycle, cutting down very substantially on computing resource needed. This worked well in identifying hits for CB1 and CB2 receptors and for a kinase target (Sadybekov et al., 2022, and see Deane and Mokaya, 2022).

'Hits' detected in the initial screen often turn out to be molecules that have features undesirable in a drug, such as excessive molecular weight or polarity, or possession of groups known to be associated with toxicity. Computational 'prescreening' of compound libraries is often used to eliminate such compounds. Conversely some aspects of molecular structure, such as chirality and rigidity, have been associated with successful drugs, presenting the designer with choosing between screening out candidates that do not conform and potentially missing out on more novel possibilities.

The hits identified from the primary screen are used as the basis for preparing sets of homologues by combinatorial chemistry to establish the critical structural features necessary for binding selectively to the target. Several such iterative cycles of synthesis and screening are usually needed to identify one or more lead compounds for the next stage.

Natural products as lead compounds

Historically, natural products, derived mainly from fungal and plant sources, have proved to be a fruitful source of new therapeutic agents, particularly in the field of anti-infective, anticancer and immunosuppressant drugs. Familiar examples include **penicillin**, **streptomycin** and many other antibiotics; vinca alkaloids; **paclitaxel**; **ciclosporin** and **sirolimus** (**rapamycin**). NMR is often used to determine their complex structures. Recently, there has been renewed interest in psychedelic drugs, many of which are derived from plants and are being investigated as treatments for anxiety and depression and addiction (Chs 48 and 50). These substances presumably serve a specific protective function, having evolved to recognise, with great precision, vulnerable target molecules in an organism's enemies or competitors. The surface of this resource has barely been scratched, and many companies are actively engaged in generating and testing natural product libraries for lead-finding purposes. Fungi and other microorganisms are particularly suitable for this, because they are ubiquitous, highly diverse and easy to collect and grow in the laboratory. They have also had aeons of evolution to devise an armoury of effective substances fit for specific functions (e.g. antibacterial) which can sometimes be utilised as a starting compound in the search for our desired drug. However, compounds obtained from plants, animals or marine organisms are much more troublesome to produce commercially. Their main disadvantage as lead compounds is that they are often complex molecules that are difficult to synthesise or modify by conventional synthetic chemistry, so that *lead optimisation* may be difficult and commercial production very expensive.

LEAD OPTIMISATION

As mentioned earlier, the aim of lead optimisation is to increase the potency of the compound on its target and to optimise it with respect to other characteristics, such as selectivity and pharmacokinetic properties. Whilst this has been a widely adopted approach, in some areas such as psychiatric disorders, highly selective drugs acting at a single target have generally failed in clinical trials despite the predictions from animal models. It is often drugs with multiple sites of action, discovered through more traditional approaches, which have progressed, perhaps reflecting the complexity of brain disorders and our limited understanding of their pathophysiology.

The tests applied during lead optimisation include a broader range of assays than are used during initial screening, including studies to measure the activity and time course of the compounds in vivo (where possible in animal models mimicking aspects of the clinical condition; see Ch. 8), and checking for unwanted effects, evidence of genotoxicity and, where appropriate, oral availability. The objective of the lead optimisation phase is to identify one or more *drug candidates* suitable for further development.

As shown in Fig. 60.1, only about one project in five succeeds in generating a drug candidate, which can take up to 5 years. The most common problem is that lead optimisation proves to be impossible; despite much ingenious and back-breaking chemistry, the lead compounds, like antisocial teenagers, refuse to give up their bad habits. In other cases, the candidate leads, although they produce the desired effects on the target molecule and have no other obvious defects, fail to produce the expected effects in animal models of the disease, implying that the target may not be a useful one in humans either. The virtuous minority of drugs proceed to the next phase, preclinical development.

PRECLINICAL DEVELOPMENT

The aim of preclinical development is to satisfy all the requirements to enable approval for first-in-man studies. The work falls into four main categories:

1. *Safety pharmacology.* Pharmacological testing to check that the drug does not produce harmful effects, including studies to establish effects on the cardiovascular and respiratory systems and other major organs such as the liver and effects involving the central nervous system such as ataxia

(lacking coordinated muscle movement). Many drugs can fail at this early stage due to unwanted pharmacological effects such as QT prolongation (Ch. 20) which is an indicator that the drug can have serious cardiac side effects or effects on other major organs such as the liver. Drugs that inhibit hERG channel activity are routinely screened out, as this implies a QT prolongation effect with the potential to predispose to fatal ventricular dysrhythmia. Any drug which penetrates the brain or has targets within the central nervous system is required to undergo assessment for dependence liability. These studies are normally performed in rats and provide essential safety data.

2. *Toxicology*. Toxicological testing to eliminate genotoxicity and to determine the maximum non-toxic dose of the drug, usually when given daily for 28 days, and tested in two species of which one is a rodent. The more sensitive species is used to determine the 'no observed adverse effect level' (NOAEL), which is used in turn to estimate a 'human equivalent dose' (HED) based usually on scaling to estimated body surface area. The HED is combined with a safety factor determined by individual aspects of the preclinical pharmacology to select a suitable starting dose for the first-in-human study.[3] As well as being checked regularly for weight loss and other gross changes, the animals are examined *postmortem* at the end of the experiment to search for histological and biochemical evidence of tissue damage (see also Ch. 58). (Reproductive toxicity, relevant when a drug is likely to be used by women of child-bearing potential, is expensive and studies may overlap early clinical studies in men.)
3. *Pharmacokinetic and pharmacodynamic (PK/PD) testing*, including studies on the absorption, metabolism, distribution and elimination (*ADME studies*) in the species of laboratory animals used for toxicology testing, to link the pharmacological and toxicological effects to plasma concentration and drug exposure.
4. *Chemical and pharmaceutical development* to assess the feasibility of large-scale synthesis and purification, to assess the stability of the compound under various conditions and to develop a formulation suitable for clinical studies.

Much of the work of preclinical development, especially that relating to safety issues, is done under a formal operating code, known as *Good Laboratory Practice* (GLP), which covers such aspects as record-keeping procedures, data analysis, instrument calibration and staff training. The aim of GLP is to eliminate human error as far as possible and to ensure the reliability of the data submitted to the regulatory authority, and laboratories are regularly monitored for compliance to GLP standards. GLP standards are not usually adopted until projects get beyond the discovery phase.

Roughly half the compounds identified as drug candidates fail during the preclinical development phase; for the rest, a detailed dossier (the 'investigator brochure') is prepared for submission alongside specific study protocols to the responsible regulatory authority, such as the UK Medicines and Healthcare Products Regulatory Agency (MHRA), the European Medicines Agency or the US FDA. These organisations use the results from the preclinical studies to make a decision about whether to grant permission to proceed with studies in humans. This is not lightly given, and the regulatory authority may refuse permission or require further work to be done before giving approval.

Non-clinical development work continues throughout the clinical trials period, when much more data, particularly in relation to long-term and reproductive toxicity in animals, have to be generated. Failure of a compound at this stage is very costly, and considerable efforts are made to eliminate potentially toxic compounds much earlier in the drug discovery process using in vitro, or even in silico, methods.

CLINICAL DEVELOPMENT

Clinical development proceeds through four distinct but overlapping phases of clinical trials (see Ch. 8). Just as the regulatory authorities require GLP studies, clinical trials must be performed under equally strict *Good Clinical Practice* (GCP) conditions. Phase I–III trials are usually all placebo controlled, randomised and double blind – for detailed information, see Friedman et al. (2015).

- *Phase I studies* are performed on a small group (normally 20–80) of volunteers – often healthy young men but sometimes patients. Healthy volunteers are easier to recruit, better able to tolerate adverse effects if these occur and more homogeneous even in the absence of comedication that may be required by patients. Healthy volunteers are not appropriate when even low doses of test drug are expected to cause harm, as with cytotoxic drugs and some other anticancer agents, or when healthy men do not express the target on which the drug acts. Their aim is to check for signs of any potentially *harmful effects*, for example on cardiovascular,[4] respiratory, hepatic or renal function, and *tolerability* (does the drug produce any unpleasant symptoms, for example, headache, nausea, drowsiness?) and to explore its *pharmacokinetic properties* (Is the drug well absorbed? Is absorption affected by food? What is the time course of the plasma concentration in relation to dosing? Is there evidence of accumulation or non-linear kinetics?). These aspects are integrated to establish what dose regimen should be used for phase II studies and when PK sampling and drug effect recording should be undertaken during phase II. Phase I studies may also test for pharmacodynamic effects in volunteers, sometimes called 'proof-of-concept' experimental medicine

[3]A different approach is generally used for biopharmaceuticals, where a "minimum anticipated biologically effective level" (MABEL) is estimated from available relevant data such as effects on human (or humanized) cells or tissues. This was introduced after serious on-target toxicity from a monoclonal antibody biopharmaceutical TGN 1412 in healthy volunteers admitted to Northwick Park hospital in 2006 – see Ch. 5 and below.

[4]QT prolongation, a sign of potentially dangerous cardiac arrhythmias (see Ch. 22), is a common cause of failure in early development, and regulators demand extensive – and expensive – studies to test for this risk. Today, such studies are usually performed on cells expressing the hERG (human Ether-à-go-go-Related Gene – no, seriously!) that produces the $K_v11.1$ potassium channel. Drugs that inhibit hERG channel activity are routinely screened out, as this implies a QT prolongation effect with the potential to predispose to fatal ventricular dysrhythmia.

studies. These sometimes include challenge studies (e.g. does a novel analgesic compound block experimentally induced pain? Does a new anti-inflammatory drug block the effect of a small intravenous challenge dose of lipopolysaccharide endotoxin? How does the desired effect vary with dose?). Various trial designs are used, a common one being to start with single ascending doses in individual cohorts followed by multiple (repeated) ascending doses (so-called 'SAD/MAD' studies).

- *Phase II studies* are performed on groups of patients (typically 100–300) and are designed to determine clinically beneficial pharmacodynamic effects in patients, and to establish if the disease process alters the pharmacokinetics of the drug. If pharmacodynamic effect and acceptable pharmacokinetics are confirmed, the aim is to establish the dose regimen to be used in the definitive phase III study. Sometimes, such studies will cover several distinct clinical disorders, e.g. depression, anxiety states and phobias. When new drug targets are being studied, it is not until these phase II trials are completed that the team finds out whether or not its initial hypothesis was correct, and lack of the desired effect is a common reason for failure. Conversely, it is not uncommon for over-optimistic results to emerge from a phase II study that are not confirmed in phase III trials that use more rigorous clinical end-points (such as mortality) rather than just of drug effect on intermediate biochemical or physiological endpoints (see later).
- *Phase III studies* are the definitive studies almost always required for regulatory approval. They are commonly performed as multicentre trials on thousands of patients, aimed at comparing the new drug with commonly used alternatives or placebos as in studies of standard treatment + placebo versus standard therapy + experimental active. These are extremely costly and difficult to organise and often take years to complete, particularly if the treatment is designed to retard the progression of a chronic disease. It is not uncommon for a drug that seemed highly effective in the limited patient groups tested in phase II to look much less impressive under the more rigorous conditions of phase III trials. Increasingly, phase III trials now include a *pharmacoeconomic analysis* (see Ch. 1), such that not only the clinical but also economic impact of the new treatment is assessed.

  At the end of phase III, the drug will be submitted to the relevant regulatory authority for licensing. The dossier required for this is a massive and detailed compilation of preclinical and clinical data. Evaluation by the regulatory authority often takes a year or more. Eventually, about two-thirds of submissions gain marketing approval. Estimates vary but approximately 8% of compounds entering phase I are eventually approved. Increasing this proportion by better compound selection at the laboratory stage is one of the main challenges for the pharmaceutical industry.
- *Phase IV studies* comprise the obligatory postmarketing surveillance designed to detect any rare or long-term adverse effects resulting from the use of the drug in a clinical setting in many thousands of patients. Such events may necessitate limiting the use of the drug to particular patient groups, or even withdrawal of the drug.[5]

Disclosure and publication of trials data

Concern has been expressed that clinical trials showing negative or inconclusive results are less likely to be published than those giving positive results, so creating a more favourable impression of a new drug's clinical efficacy than would be the case if every trial was published. To ensure that all data, good and bad, are published and available to regulatory authorities and researchers, it is now mandatory to register the initiation of any trial in humans and to publish the results in full when the trial is completed. The difficult question of whether to require all past trials of currently registered drugs is under discussion. The accessibility of past data, much of it in the form of paper records in dusty repositories, and the cost of this exercise are serious problems.

BIOPHARMACEUTICALS

Biopharmaceuticals are discussed in Chapter 5. Such therapeutic agents now comprise about 30% of new products registered each year. The principles underlying the development and testing of biopharmaceuticals are basically the same as for synthetic drugs. In practice, biopharmaceuticals (often comprised of proteins or nucleic acids which are hydrolysed to their constituent amino acids or bases) generally run into fewer toxicological problems than synthetic drugs, but more problems relating to production, quality control, immunogenicity and drug delivery. Subtle but potentially harmful changes in the product when it is produced by another manufacturer are almost inevitable. This has regulatory consequences when products end their patent life and other companies wish to compete by producing and selling what is apparently the same product. Such competitor products are referred to as 'biosimilars' rather than 'bioequivalents' in acknowledgement of this, and a phase III efficacy trial is required for licensing approval. If this is successful, however, repeat phase III studies are not required for other indications for which the market leader is licensed. Walsh (2009) and Revers and Furczon (2010) cover this specialised field in more detail. In 2017 the first gene therapy products (for spinal muscular atrophy, see Ch. 40) and cell-based therapies for advanced cancer (see Ch. 57) were approved – significant milestones.

COMMERCIAL ASPECTS

Fig. 60.1 shows the approximate time taken for such a project and the attrition rate (at each stage and overall) based on recent data from several large pharmaceutical companies. The key messages are (1) that it is a high-risk business, with only about 1 drug discovery project in 50

[5]Recent high-profile cases include the withdrawal of rofecoxib (a cyclo-oxygenase-2 inhibitor; see Ch. 25) when it was found (in a phase III trial for a new indication) to increase the frequency of heart attacks, and of cerivastatin (Ch. 22), a cholesterol-lowering drug found to cause severe muscle damage in a few patients.

and 1 development compound in 10 reaching the goal of putting a new drug on the market, (2) that it takes a long time – about 12 years on average and (3) that it costs a lot of money to develop one drug – estimates vary hugely with the pharmaceutical industry claiming costs of up to $4 billion per drug whilst a more independent analysis in 2019 suggested costs closer to $1 billion (Wouters et al., 2020). For any one project, the costs escalate rapidly as development proceeds, phase III trials and long-term toxicology studies being particularly expensive. The time factor is crucial, because the new drug has to be patented, usually at the end of the discovery phase, and the period of exclusivity (20 years in most countries) during which the company is free from competition in the market starts on that date. After 20 years, the patent expires, and other companies, which have not supported the development costs, are free to make and sell the drug much more cheaply, so the revenues for the original company decrease rapidly thereafter. Reducing the development time after patenting is a major concern for all companies, but so far it has remained stubbornly fixed at around 10 years, partly because the regulatory authorities are demanding more clinical data before they will grant a license. In practice, only about one drug in three that goes on the market brings in enough revenue to cover its development costs. Success for the company relies on this one drug generating enough profit to pay for the rest.[6]

DRUG REPURPOSING

An alternative route to bringing forward a new treatment is to test drugs which have already gone through the initial stages of development for one indication but are then trialled for a different, often unrelated disease. Commonly referred to as repurposing or repositioning, this approach has been used for drugs which have failed due to a lack of efficacy in either phase II or III clinical trials and also drugs which have been licensed for a particular disease but are also found to be useful for a different condition (Pushpakom et al., 2019). Risks and costs are reduced because the drug has already passed most of the hurdles in the drug development process and has been found to be 'safe'. Several drugs for psychiatric disorders have been repurposed in this way; for example, certain drugs used to treat epilepsy (see Ch. 46) are also now prescribed for anxiety disorders (see Ch. 45) whilst others are used as mood stabilisers (see Ch. 48); antidepressants are now first-line treatments for generalised anxiety disorder (Chs 45 and 48) and some antipsychotics are also used for depression and bipolar disorder (Chs 47 and 48). Repurposing has been critical for the rapid testing and approval of treatments for COVID-19 infections (Chakraborty et al., 2021).

GENERIC DRUGS

New drugs brought to the market are protected initially by a patent (see earlier). A generic drug is the same chemical entity as the original, formulated to achieve bioequivalence, which is defined by the regulators such that the generic may safely be substituted for the original licensed product without loss of efficacy (see Ch. 9 on bioavailability and bioequivalence).

[6]But note that companies spend at least as much on marketing and administration as on research and development.

FUTURE PROSPECTS

Since about 1990, the drug discovery process has been in the throes of a substantial and ongoing methodological revolution, following the rapid ascendancy of molecular biology, genomics and informatics, amid high expectations that this would bring remarkable dividends in terms of speed, cost and success rate. High-throughput screening has emerged as a powerful lead-finding technology, but overall the benefits have not been realised: costs have risen steadily, the success rate has not improved and development times have not decreased.

Fig. 60.3 illustrates the trend in the number of new drugs launched in the major markets worldwide, which had until recently declined steadily despite escalating costs and improved technology, causing serious worries to the industry. There was much speculation as to the causes of the decline, the optimistic view being that fewer but better drugs were being introduced, and that the genomics revolution had yet to make its impact. This optimism may be well founded, for as Fig. 60.3 shows, the number of approvals has shown an encouraging upturn in recent years.

If the new drugs that are being developed improve the quality of medical care, there is room for optimism. In the latter half of the 20th century, synthetic drugs aimed at new targets (e.g. SSRIs, statins, kinase inhibitors and several monoclonal antibodies) have made major contributions to patient care. The ability of new technologies to make new targets available to the drug discovery machine is beginning to have a real effect on patient care. Creativity remains high, despite the rising costs and declining profits that remain a challenge to the pharmaceutical industry.

The drug development process continues to evolve, with biopharmaceuticals remaining an area of growth for many disorders particularly those involving the immune system and inflammatory disorders and the recent licensing of the first few of an anticipated wave of RNA drugs. Technologies that enable the drug development process continue to develop with more sophisticated methods for both in silico and high throughput in vitro drug screening. Novel tools include 'organs on a chip' and organoids which can recapitulate aspects of biology more complex than cultures of single cell lines. High-throughput methods combined with huge libraries of compounds should have improved the drug development process, but even when a novel drug target is identified, translating this into a new treatment is not as straightforward as it may at first appear. Antibody-based treatments against intra-neuronal amyloid plaques in Alzheimer's disease are a good example. Despite genetic and pathological evidence suggesting a key role for amyloid in the development of Alzheimer's disease, the phase III clinical trials produced disappointing clinical results. The idea of using patient genotype to 'individualise' treatments remains an important area in pharmacology (see Ch. 12) and the recommendations of a recent report by the Royal College of Physicians and British Pharmacological Society is aimed towards this becoming fully integrated into the NHS (Royal College of Physicians and British Pharmacological Society, 2022). This approach can improve patient outcomes by avoiding giving drugs to nonresponders or reducing the risk of adverse events through identifying those with genetic risk factors (Klein et al., 2017).

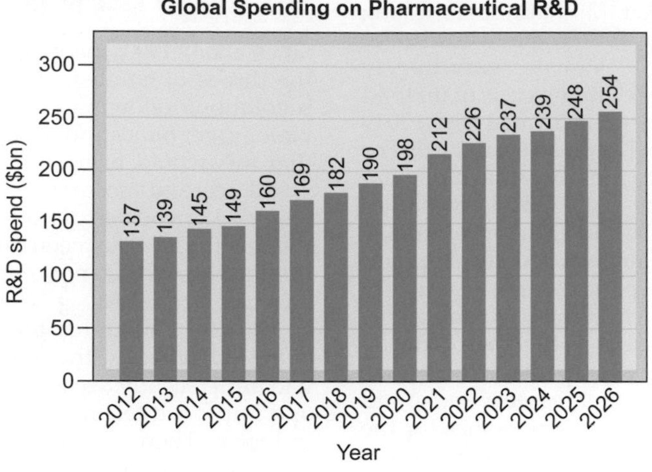

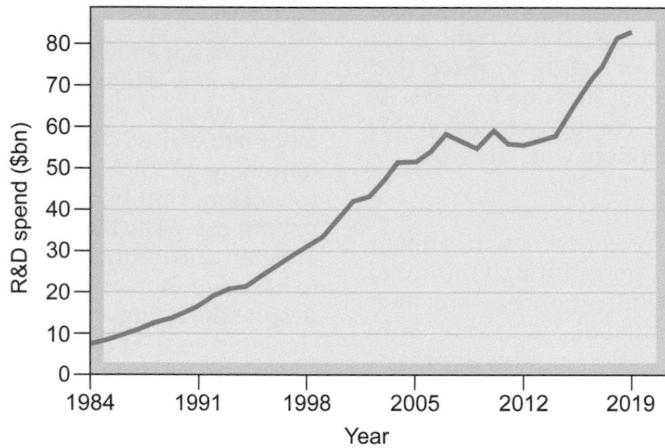

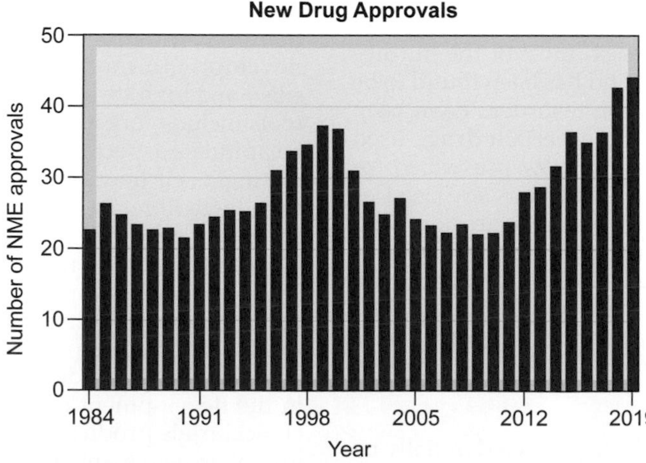

Fig. 60.3 Research and development (R&D) spend, sales and new drug registrations, 1980–2017. Registrations refer to new chemical entities (including biopharmaceuticals, excluding new formulations and combinations of existing registered compounds). The decline in registrations up to 2010 has since seen some reversal in more recent years. (Data from various sources, including the Centre for Medicines Research, Pharmaceutical Research and Manufacturers Association of America.)

A FINAL WORD

The pharmaceutical industry in recent years has attracted much adverse publicity, some of it well deserved, concerning drug pricing and profits, non-disclosure of adverse clinical trials data, reluctance to address major global health problems such as tuberculosis and malaria, aggressive marketing practices[7] and much else (see Angell, 2004; Goldacre, 2012). These perhaps more commercial aspects of the industry should not detract from the huge advances in fundamental biology and the development of important technologies which have been led by scientist working in the pharmaceutical industry. The pharmaceutical industry has been directly responsible for most of the therapeutic advances of the past half-century and has played a key role in the development of new technologies which underpin scientific advances. Without these new drugs, medical care would effectively have stood still. Innovation has by no means dried up. In the last decade, drug development has expanded beyond traditional small molecules, and biopharmaceuticals and RNA-based medicines are still in their infancy with many opportunities likely to emerge as we learn more. There has also been a shift in the structure of the industry with the preclinical development and even early clinical trials of new treatments being undertaken by small and medium-sized companies. Even psychiatry research has seen a renewed enthusiasm particularly in relation to the potential for psychedelic-based drugs to treat emotional disorders and addiction (Chs 48 and 50). Pharmacology remains a fast-moving field. In 2021 the European Medicines Agency approved 54 new active substances, many of which are first-in-class. Of these active substances, 7 related to COVID-19 but other indications were also widely represented: other infections (2), cardiovascular (3), metabolic (2), reproduction (3), gastro-intestinal (1), neurological (5), endocrine (4), skin (3), eyes (2), rheumatology (3), haematology (5), cancer (12) and vaccines other than those directed against SARS-CoV2 (2).

[7]The aggressive marketing of the opioid drug OxyContin (oxycodone) in the United States has been a major factor in the current opioid crisis. For those interested see Patrick Radden Keefe's 'Empire of Pain: The Secret History of the Sackler Dynasty'.

REFERENCES AND FURTHER READING

Angell, M., 2004. The Truth about the Drug Companies. Random House, New York.

Chakraborty, C., Sharma, A.R., Bhattacharya, M., 2021. The drug repurposing for COVID-19 clinical trials provide very effective therapeutic combinations: lessons learned from major clinical studies. Front. Pharmacol. 12, 704205.

Deane, C., Mokaya, M., 2022. A virtual drug-screening approach to conquer huge chemical libraries. Nature 601, 322–323.

Friedman, L.M., Furberg, C.D., DeMets, D.L., 2015. Fundamentals of Clinical Trials, fifth ed. Mosby, St Louis.

Goldacre, B., 2012. Bad Pharma. Fourth Estate, London.

Hill, R.G., Richards, D. (Eds.), 2021. Drug Discovery and Development, third ed. Elsevier, Amsterdam.

Klein, M.E., Parvez, M.M., Shin, J.G., 2017. Clinical implementation of pharmacogenomics for personalized precision medicine: barriers and solutions. J. Pharm. Sci. 106, 2368–2379.

Lees, J.A., Dias, J.M., Han, S., 2021. Applications of cryo-EM in small molecule and biologics drug design. Biochem. Soc. Trans. 49, 2627–2638.

Munos, B., 2009. Lessons from 60 years of pharmaceutical innovation. Nat. Rev. Drug Discov. 8, 959–968.

Pushpakom, S., Iorio, F., Eyers, P.A., et al., 2019. Drug repurposing: progress, challenges and recommendations. Nat. Rev. Drug Discov. 18, 41–58.

Renaud, J.-P., Chari, A., Ciferri, C., et al., 2018. Cryo-EM in drug discovery: achievements, limitations and prospects. Nat. Rev. Drug Discov. 17, 471–492.

Revers, L., Furczon, E., 2010. An introduction to biologics and biosimilars. Part II: subsequent entry biologics: biosame or biodifferent? Can. Pharm. J. 143, 184–191.

Robertson, M.J., Meyerowitz, J.G., Skiniotis, G., 2021. Drug discovery in the era of cryo-electron microscopy. Trends Biochem. Sci. 47, 124–135.

Ross, N.T., Bittker, J.A. (Eds.), 2016. High Throughput Screening Methods. Royal Society of Chemistry, Cambridge.

Royal College of Physicians and British Pharmacological Society, 2022. Personalised Prescribing: Using Pharmacogenomics to Improve Patient Outcomes. Report of a Working Party. RCP and BPS, London.

Sadybekov, A.A., Sadybekov, A.V., Liu, Y., et al., 2022. Synthon-based ligand discovery in virtual libraries of over 11 billion compounds. Nature 601, 452–459.

Santos, R., Ursu, O., Gaulton, A., et al., 2017. A comprehensive map of molecular drug targets. Nat. Rev. Drug Discov. 16, 19–34.

Springer, A.D., Dowdy, S.F., 2018. GalNAc-siRNA conjugates: leading the way for delivery of RNAi therapeutics. Nucleic Acid Therapeut. 28, 109–118.

Walsh, G., 2009. Biopharmaceuticals: Biochemistry and Biotechnology, second ed. Wiley, Chichester.

Wouters, O.J., McKee, M., Luyten, J., 2020. Estimated research and development investment needed to bring a new medicine to market, 2009–2018. JAMA 323 (9), 844–853.

Index

Note: Page numbers followed by "*f*," "*t*," and "*b*" refer to figures, tables, and boxes, respectively.

B

C

D

F

G

H

J

K

M

N

O

P

Q

R

S

U

V

W

X

Y

Z